Spinal Cord Medicine

Principles
and Practice

Spinal Cord Medicine

Principles and Practice

Second Edition

EDITOR

VERNON W. LIN, MD, PhD
Chairman
Department of Physical Medicine and Rehabilitation
Cleveland Clinic Lerner College of Medicine
Case Western Reserve University
Louis Stokes Cleveland VA Medical Center
Cleveland, Ohio

ASSOCIATE EDITORS

CHRISTOPHER M. BONO, MD

DIANA D. CARDENAS, MD, MHA

FREDERICK S. FROST, MD

MARGARET C. HAMMOND, MD

LAURIE B. LINDBLOM, MD

INDER PERKASH, MD, FACS, FRCS

STEVEN A. STIENS, MD, DO

ROBERT M. WOOLSEY, MD

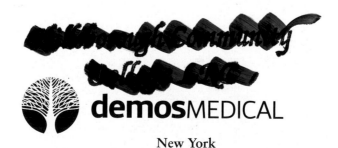

demosMEDICAL

New York

Acquisitions Editor: Beth Barry
Cover Design: Joe Tenerelli
Compositor: Publication Services, Inc.
Printer: Sheridan Press

Visit our website at www.demosmedpub.com

Medicine is an ever-changing science. Research and clinical experience are continually expanding our knowledge, in particular our understanding of proper treatment and drug therapy. The authors, editors, and publisher have made every effort to ensure that all information in this book is in accordance with the state of knowledge at the time of production of the book. Nevertheless, the authors, editors, and publisher are not responsible for errors or omissions or for any consequences from application of the information in this book and make no warranty, express or implied, with respect to the contents of the publication. Every reader should examine carefully the package inserts accompanying each drug and should carefully check whether the dosage schedules mentioned therein or the contraindications stated by the manufacturer differ from the statements made in this book. Such examination is particularly important with drugs that are either rarely used or have been newly released on the market.

Library of Congress Cataloging-in-Publication Data

Spinal cord medicine : principles and practice / editor, Vernon W. Lin ;
associate editors, Christopher M. Bono ... [et al.]. — 2nd ed.
    p. ; cm.
  Includes bibliographical references and index.
  ISBN 978-1-933864-19-8 (hardcover)
  1. Spinal cord—Wounds and injuries. I. Lin, Vernon W., 1959- II. Bono, Christopher M.
  [DNLM: 1. Spinal Cord Injuries. 2. Spinal Cord Diseases. WL 400 S757768
2010]
  RD594.3.S6696 2010
  617.4'82044—dc22   2009051599

Special discounts on bulk quantities of Demos Medical Publishing books are available to corporations, professional associations, pharmaceutical companies, health care organizations, and other qualifying groups. For details, please contact:

Special Sales Department
Demos Medical Publishing
11 W. 42nd Street, 15th Floor
New York, NY 10036
Phone: 800–532–8663 or 212–683–0072
Fax: 212–941–7842
E-mail: rsantana@demosmedpub.com

Made in the United States of America
10 11 12 13 14   5 4 3 2 1

Dedication

This book is dedicated to our teachers and mentors who have gone before us and paved the path for us to walk on; to our interdisciplinary colleagues, who work tirelessly with us and motivate us to provide the best care possible; to our family members and loved ones who love, support, and encourage us; to our patients who stimulate and challenge us to advance the field of spinal cord medicine and to provide the world class care that they deserve.

Special Dedication to Ms. Grace Pei-Lan Lin (1928–2009), a beloved public health nurse, mother, and grandmother.

Vernon W. Lin, MD, PhD

Contents

Foreword

It is a great pleasure to introduce the second edition of *Spinal Cord Medicine: Principles and Practice*. This successor to the highly successful first edition is another tribute to Dr. Lin's exceptional devotion to the field of spinal cord medicine and his seemingly inexhaustible motivation and energy.

The first modern comprehensive book on spinal cord medicine was Sir Ludwig Guttmann's seminal monograph, *Spinal Cord Injuries*, published in 1973. This book was based on Sir Ludwig's more than 35 years of research and experience treating spinal cord injured patients.

Though the field of spinal cord medicine rapidly expanded, no books summarizing this information appeared over the next 20 years. In 1995 Dr. Robert Young and I published the *Diagnosis and Management of Disorders of the Spinal Cord*, in which we attempted to produce a state-of-the-art review and, importantly, to include nontraumatic as well as traumatic myelopathies in our survey.

Another 5-year void ensued. In 2002 Dr. Lin and his associate editors produced the first edition of *Spinal Cord Medicine: Principles and Practice*, which was a truly encyclopedic treatment of the subject of spinal cord medicine. At about the same time, another excellent book appeared: *Spinal Cord Medicine*, edited by our friends and colleagues Drs. Kirshblum, Campagnolo, and DeLisa. Poverty had turned into riches.

The first edition of *Spinal Cord Medicine: Principles and Practice* was enthusiastically received by the spinal cord medicine community.

Subsequent scientific progress as well as the addition of new treatments and technologies to the field called for this new edition of Dr. Lin's book. All chapters from the first edition have been revised and updated by their authors. New chapters and new contributors have been added. I have had the opportunity to review much of the book and I am convinced it will be an information source of immense value. I again congratulate Dr. Lin and his collaborators.

Robert M. Woolsey, MD
Professor Emeritus of Neurology
Saint Louis University
Saint Louis, Missouri

Preface to the Second Edition

The goal for the first edition of *Spinal Cord Medicine: Principles and Practice* was to provide an up-to-date, interdisciplinary, comprehensive, yet user-friendly practical guide for practitioners, researchers, and learners in the field of spinal cord medicine. From the favorable reviews and commendations that we have received from our colleagues and trainees, I believe we have achieved our initial goal. To a certain extent, the first edition also defined the field of spinal cord medicine, which encompasses all the diseases and disorders that may affect the proper functioning of the spinal cord or spinal nerves, including but not limited to acute and chronic spinal cord injury (SCI), acute and chronic nontraumatic myelopathies, and other spine or spinal cord–related conditions. The second edition has been developed with a similar vision and goal, and many of the comments and constructive criticisms that we received from the first edition were incorporated into this new edition.

The second edition consists of nine sections, with 88 chapters (updated chapters from the first edition as well as 18 completely new chapters), and hundreds of new figures and tables. Some of the new topics to be found in this edition include: spinal cord pathology, functional assessment in spinal cord injury rehabilitation, neuro-critical care management of the patient with an acute spinal cord injury, nutrition in spinal cord injury, sexual dysfunction in women with spinal cord injury, new advances in the surgical treatment of nontraumatic myelopathies, surgical treatment of posttraumatic tethered and cystic spinal cords, scoliosis and spinal deformities: avoiding and managing neurologic deficits, the spondyloarthropathies, surgical management of spondyloarthropathies in the spinal cord injury patient, considerations for the translation of preclinical discoveries and valid spinal cord injury clinical trials, restoration of ventilation and cough with functional electrical stimulation: patient evaluation and comparison of currently available systems, and caring for spinal cord injury with complementary and alternative medicine.

Although it is not possible to include everything due to limitation of space, we have selected what we believe to be the most significant advances and innovations to bring this book into the next decade. This has been an immense effort, involving 150 authors and representing academic and clinical leaders in more than twenty medical disciplines. We truly appreciate and welcome feedback and constructive criticism from our colleagues in spinal cord medicine and from all readers in the medical and scientific community.

Vernon W. Lin, MD, PhD

Preface to the First Edition

Spinal cord medicine (SCM) is best described as the art and science underlying the diagnosis and treatment of patients with spinal cord injury (SCI) and spinal cord related disorders (SCD). The twentieth century was a landmark era in SCM, highlighted by the development of emergency medical services, the establishment of the specialized spinal cord centers, and advances in antibiotic use, modern therapies, and technology breakthroughs. Many patients with SCI and SCD are now living healthy lives, with life expectancies approaching that of the general population. Despite recent advances in SCM, considerable challenges remain and our patients suffer from multiorgan failures that require long-term and multidisciplinary care; and few residency training programs offer exposure or training in comprehensive SCI care.

This book had its origins in the first review course, *Spinal Cord Medicine—An Intensive Review* given at the annual meetings of the American Paraplegia Society, to prepare physicians to take the subspecialty board in spinal cord medicine. Our goal was to develop a comprehensive text that would cover the breadth and depth of the field of SCM, covering topics from acute medical and surgical management to cutting-edge research, rehabilitation, and psychosocial care.

Spinal Cord Medicine consists of 74 chapters in 10 sections. It begins with a review of anatomy and physiology, spinal cord imaging, and epidemiology, and is followed by a comprehensive discussion of acute spinal cord injury management that covers prehospital management, emergency room evaluation and intensive care, and con-

siderations relating to spine surgery. This is followed by sections that cover various aspects of medical management, and the management of bladder, bowel, and sexual dysfunctions. A section on the neurologic aspects of spinal cord care considers topics that include the neurologic assessment of SCI, electrophysiologic evaluation of the spinal tracts, myelopathies, multiple sclerosis, spasticity and pain management, autonomic dysfunction, and concomitant SCI and traumatic brain injury. The musculoskeletal care section addresses overuse injuries, osteoporosis and long bone fractures, and interdisciplinary approaches to upper extremity and pressure ulcer management. The rehabilitation section covers wheelchair and seating assessment, orthotics, activity of daily living training, vocational and driving training, and functional electrical stimulation. This is followed by discussions of recent advances in spinal cord research, including functional magnetic stimulation, spinal cord regeneration and repair strategies, and body weight supported ambulation. Special topics on aging, women's issues, pediatric care, and SCI prevention are also reviewed. The final section considers psychosocial issues, cost of care, SCI systems of care, and various supportive environments for SCI and SCD care.

This book was developed for all physicians, research scientists, and other health care professionals involved in the management of individuals with SCI, multiple sclerosis, and other spinal cord disorders. It is a practical guide, and has been developed to be the ultimate single source of information on SCM. It will be especially useful for physicians who are preparing for the subspecialty certification examination on Spinal Cord Injury Medicine. We are honored to have chapter contributions from over 130 authors, selected based upon their training, experience, and clinical leadership, and representing over 20 medical specialties and subspecialties. We welcome comments, suggestions, and constructive criticism from our colleagues in SCM and from all readers in the medical and scientific community.

Vernon W. Lin, MD, PhD

Acknowledgments

I must express my appreciation to two individuals, Mr. Vinoth Ranganathan and Dr. Ian Hsiao, for coordinating the various stages and assisting with the editing work for this second edition. I am grateful to the staff of Demos Medical Publishing for their assistance and guidance in publishing this book. I thank my secretary, Ms. Rebecca Randall, and Dr. Xiaoming Zhang for their assistance with editing this book. Finally, I would like to express my gratitude and appreciation to my wife, Grace Lin, and my children, Sarah, Daniel, and Rebecca, for their endless patience and support during the time spent on preparing this second edition.

In Memoriam

Asa J. Wilbourn died in 2007, at the age of 68. He left behind a wealth of publications on the subject of electrodiagnosis that has never been surpassed in clarity and comprehensiveness. Chapter 6 of this volume, largely unchanged from his chapter in the first edition, is an example of his best work. He was above all a clinical electromyographer. Entering the field of electromyography as it began to attain widespread use, Dr. Wilbourn recognized opportunities to define the usefulness of nerve conduction studies and electromyography in a number of conditions, including radiculopathy, plexopathy, and various mononeuropathies. In particular, he was fascinated by neurogenic thoracic outlet syndrome, both in regard to its proper diagnosis and how often the condition was inaccurately diagnosed, often to the patient's detriment. For those of us who care for patients with disorders of the peripheral nervous system, we can thank Dr. Wilbourn for making it easier to practice high-quality medical care.

Kerry Levin, MD
Chairman, Department of Neurology
Cleveland Clinic
Cleveland, Ohio

Contributors

Melanie Adams, PhD
Department of Kinesiology
McMaster University
Hamilton, Ontario

Dixie Lynne Reiko Aragaki, MD
Assistant Professor
Department of Medicine
David Geffen School of Medicine at University of
  California at Los Angeles
Assistant Program Director
VA Greater Los Angeles Health Care System
Los Angeles, California

Michal S. Atkins, MA, OTR/L
Occupational Therapy Clinical Instructor
Department of Occupational and Recreational
  Therapy
Rancho Los Amigos National Rehabilitation Center
Downey, California

Edmond Ayyappa, CPO, FAAOP
Clinical Director
Prosthetics
VA Desert Pacific Health Care Network
Long Beach, California

Ziyad Ayyoub, MD
Chief
Adult Brain Injury Rehabilitation Program
Ranchos Los Amigos National Rehabilitation
  Center
Assistant Clinical Professor
Department of Medicine
David Geffen School of Medicine at University of
  California at Los Angeles
Los Angeles, California

Cyril H. Barton, MD
Associate Professor of Medicine
Department of Medicine
Division of Nephrology
University of California Irvine
Orange, California

Ahmet Baydur, MD, FACL, FCCP
Professor of Clinical Medicine
Division of Pulmonary and Critical Care Medicine
Keck School of Medicine
University of Southern California
Los Angeles, California

Randal R. Betz, MD
Professor of Orthopaedic Surgery
Temple University
Chief of Staff
Shriners Hospital for Children
Philadelphia, Pennsylvania

Fin Biering-Sørensen, MD, DMSC
Professor and Head of Department
Clinic for Spinal Cord Injuries
Rigshospitalet and University of Copenhagen
Copenhagen, Denmark

George Kim Bigley, MD
Associate Clinical Professor of Medicine
Department of Neurology
University of Nevada School of Medicine
Reno, Nevada

Donald R. Bodner, MD
Professor of Urology
Department of Urology
UH Case Medical Center
Cleveland VA Medical Center
Cleveland, Ohio

Michael L. Boninger, MD
Professor and Chair
Department of Physical Medicine and
    Rehabilitation
University of Pittsburgh
Department of Veterans Affairs
Human Engineering Research Laboratories
Pittsburgh, Pennsylvania

Christopher M. Bono, MD
Chief
Department of Orthopedic Spine Service
Orthopedic Surgery
Brigham & Women's Hospital
Boston, Massachusetts

Helen Bosshart, MSW
Social Worker
Private Practice
Seabrook Island, South Carolina

Frank M. Brasile, BS, MS, PhD
Professor
Department of Health, Physical Education, and
    Recreation
University of Nebraska Omaha
Omaha, Nebraska

Robert Brown, BSC, MD
Director
Respiratory Acute Care Unit
Pulmonary Function Laboratory
Pulmonary and Critical Care Medicine Unit
Massachusetts General Hospital
Associate Professor of Medicine
Harvard Medical School
Boston, Massachusetts

Thomas N. Bryce, MD
Associate Professor
Department of Rehabilitation Medicine
Mount Sinai School of Medicine
New York, New York

Jack Burks, MD
President
Burks & Associates, Inc.
Chief Medical Officer
Multiple Sclerosis Association of America
Reno, Nevada

Diana D. Cardenas, MD, MHA
Professor and Chair
Department of Rehabilitation Medicine
University of Miami Miller School of Medicine
Medical Director
Jackson Memorial Rehabilitation Hospital
Miami, Florida

Susan B. Charlifue, PhD
Research Principal Investigator
Craig Hospital
Englewood, Colorado

David Chen, MD
Associate Professor
Department of Physical Medicine and
    Rehabilitation
Northwestern University Feinberg School of
    Medicine
Medical Director
Spinal Cord Injury Rehabilitation Program
Rehabilitation Institute of Chicago
Chicago, Illinois

Henrich Cheng, MD, PhD
Professor
Department of Neurosurgery
Taipei Veterans General Hospital
Taipei City, Taiwan

Sophia Chun, MD
Chief
Spinal Cord Injury Healthcare Group
VA Long Beach Healthcare System
Long Beach, California

Darrell Clark, BS
Director
Department of Orthotics
Rancho Los Amigos National Rehabilitation Center
Downey, California

Jerry Clayton, PhD
Director
Translational Medicine
Department of Physical Medicine and
    Rehabilitation
The Children's Hospital
Aurora, Colorado

Caryn J. Cohen, MS
Associate Director
Practice Guidelines
Paralyzed Veterans of America
Washington, District of Columbia

Jennifer L. Collinger, PhD
Research Biomedical Engineer
Human Engineering Research Laboratories
Department of Physical Medicine and
    Rehabilitation
Department of Veterans Affairs
University of Pittsburgh
Pittsburgh, Pennsylvania

Patrick J. Connolly, MD
Professor
Department of Orthopedic Surgery
University of Massachusetts Medical School
Worcester, Massachusetts

Rory A. Cooper, PhD
FISA/PVA Chair and Distinguished Professor
Department of Rehabilitation Science and
    Technology
University of Pittsburgh
Director and Senior Career Scientist
Department of Rehabilitation Science and
    Technology
Department of Verterans Affairs
Pittsburgh, Pennsylvania

Rosemarie Cooper, MPT, ATP
Director
Assistant Professor
Center for Assistive Technology
Department of Rehabilitation Science and
    Technology
University of Pittsburgh Medical Center
Pittsburgh, Pennsylvania

Daniel J. Culkin, MD, MBS/HCM
Professor and Chairman
Department of Urology
University of Oklahoma College of Medicine
Oklahoma City, Oklahoma

Catherine M. Curtin, MD
Assistant Professor
Department of Surgery
Stanford University
Palo Alto, California

Rabih O. Darouiche, MD
VA Distinguished Service Professor
Baylor College of Medicine and Michael E.
    Debakey VAMC
Houston, Texas

Michael J. DeVivo, DrPH
Professor
Department of Physical Medicine and
    Rehabilitation
University of Alabama at Birmingham
Birmingham, Alabama

Marcel P.J.M. Dijkers, PhD, FACRM
Research Professor
Department of Rehabilitation Medicine
Mount Sinai School of Medicine
New York, New York

Anthony F. DiMarco, MD
Professor of Medicine
Department of Physiology and Biophysics
Case Western Reserve University
Cleveland, Ohio

Angela E. Downes, MD
House Officer
Department of Neurosurgery
University of Mississippi Medical Center
Jackson, Mississippi

V. Reggie Edgerton, PhD
Professor
Department of Physiological Science,
    Brain Research Institute, Neurobiology
University of California, Los Angeles
Los Angeles, California

Stacy Elliott, BA, MD
Clinical Professor
Departments of Psychiatry and Urological Sciences
University of British Columbia
Director
BC Center for Sexual Medicine
Vancouver, BC, Canada

Ibrahim M. Eltorai, MD
Spinal Cord Injury
VA Long Beach Healthcare System
Long Beach, California

Mazen Elyan, MD, MS
Rheumatologist
Monroe Arthritis Clinic
Monroe, Michigan

Lawrence J. Epstein, MD
Instructor in Medicine
Division of Sleep Medicine
Harvard Medical School
Chief Medical Officer
Sleep HealthCenters
Boston, Massachusetts

Scott P. Falci, MD
Chief Neurosurgical Consultant
Neurosurgery
Craig Hospital
Englewood, Colorado

Rosemarie Filart, MD, MPH, MBA
Medical Officer
Department of Health and Human Services
National Institutes of Health
Rockville, Maryland

Philip R. Fine, PhD, MSPH
Director and Principal Investigator
Injury Control Research Center
The University of Alabama at Birmingham
Director and Principal Investigator
The Southern Consortium for Injury Biomechanics
Birmingham, Alabama

Cynthia S. Fok, MD
Chief Resident
Department of Urology
Loyola University Medical Center
Maywood, Illinois

Phillip Jeffrey Foster, Jr., MPH
Program Manager
Department of Rheumatory
Injury Control Research Center
Associate Director
The Southern Consortium for Injury Biomechanics
The University of Alabama at Birmingham
Birmingham, Alabama

Frederick S. Frost, MD
Staff Physician
Department of Physical Medicine and
    Rehabilitation
Cleveland Clinic Lerner College of Medicine
Cleveland, Ohio

Dudley Fukunaga, BS
Physician Assistant
Department of Orthopaedic Surgery
Rancho Los Amigos National Rehabilitation Center
Downey, California

Douglas E. Garland, MD
Clinical Professor
Department of Orthopedic Surgery
University of Southern California
Los Angeles, California

Susan V. Garstang, MD
Assistant Professor
New Jersey Medical School
Staff Physician
Veterans Affairs New Jersey Heatlthcare System
East Orange, New Jersey

Maria E. Gomez, OTR/L
Senior Occupational Therapist
Spinal Cord Unit
Department of Occupational Therapy
Jackson Memorial Hospital Rehabilitation Center
Miami, Florida

Peter H. Gorman, MD, MS
Chief
Division of Rehabilitation Medicine
Kernan Orthopaedics and Rehabilitation Hospital
Associate Professor
Department of Neurology
University of Maryland School of Medicine
Baltimore, Maryland

Harry G. Goshgarian, PhD
Professor of Anatomy/Cell Biology
Wayne State University
Detroit, Michigan

Barth A. Green, MD
Department of Neurological Surgery
Miller School of Medicine
University of Miami
Miami, Florida

Edward D. Hall, PhD
Director
Spinal Cord and Brain Injury Research Center
SCOBIRC Endowed Professor of Anatomy and
    Neurobiology, Neurosurgery, Neurology and
    Physical Medicine and Rehabilitation
University of Kentucky College of Medicine
Lexington, Kentucky

Margaret C. Hammond, MD
Chief Consultant
Spinal Cord Injury/Disorders Services
Veterans Health Administration
Professor
Department of Rehabilitation Medicine
University of Washington
Seattle, Washington

Susan J. Harkema, PhD
Associate Professor
Department of Neurological Surgery
Frazier Rehabilitation Institute
University of Louisville
Louisville, Kentucky

H. Louis Harkey, III, MD, FACS
Chairman and Professor of Neurosurgery
Department of Neurosurgery
University of Mississippi Medical Center
Jackson, Mississippi

Mitchel B. Harris, MD
Chief
Orthopedic Trauma Service
Orthopedic Surgery
Brigham & Women's Hospital
Boston, Massachusetts

Blaine L. Hart, MD
Professor of Radiology
University of New Mexico Health Sciences Center
Albuquerque, New Mexico

Jiping He, PhD
Professor of Bioengineering
Center for Neural Interface Design
School of Biological and Health Systems
    Engineering
Ira A. Fulton School of Engineering
Arizona State University
Tempe, Arizona

Vincent R. Hentz, MD
Professor of Surgery
Department of Surgery
Stanford University
Stanford, California

Richard Herman, MD
Research Professor
School of Biological and Health Systems
    Engineering
Arizona State University
Tempe, Arizona

Audrey L. Hicks, PhD
Professor and Associate Chair
Department of Kinesiology
McMaster University
Hamilton, Ontario

Haydon Harry Hill, MD
Associate Clinical Professor of Medicine
Department of Neurology
University of Nevada School of Medicine
Reno, Nevada

Chester H. Ho, MD
Chief
Spinal Cord Injury
Louis Stokes Cleveland VA Medical Center
Assistant Professor
Department of Physical Medicine and
  Rehabilitation
Case Western Reserve University
Cleveland, Ohio

Thomas Hodne, FAIA
Thomas Hodne Architects Inc.
Minneapolis, Minnesota

Dale Hoekema, MD, FCCP
Critical Care Unit
Kadlec Regional Medical Center
Richland, Washington

Joseph Hong, DO
Research Fellow
Spine/Orthopaedic Surgery
Rothman Institute
Philadelphia, Pennsylvania

An-Fu Hsiao, MD, PhD
Assistant Professor
University of California Irvine
Irvine, California
Department of Medicine
VA Long Beach Healthcare System
Long Beach, California

Ian Hsiao, PhD
Spinal Cord Injury/Disorders
VA Long Beach Healthcare System
Long Beach, California

Charlotte Indeck, MSN
Neurosurgical Clinical Assistant
Department of Neurosurgery
Craig Hospital
Englewood, Colorado

Amie Brown Jackson, MD
Professor and Chair
Department of Physical Medicine and
  Rehabilitation
Spain Rehabilitation Center
The University of Alabama at Birmingham
Birmingham, Alabama

Amitabh Jha, MD, MPH
Research Physician
Craig Hospital
Englewood, Colorado

Kurt L. Johnson, PhD
Professor
Department of Rehabilitation Medicine
University of Washington
Seattle, Washington

Anil K. Kesani, MD
Chief Resident
Orthopaedic Surgery
New Jersey Medical School
University of Medicine and Dentistry of New
  Jersey
Newark, New Jersey

Muhammad Asim Khan, MD, FRCP, MACP
Professor of Medicine
Department of Medicine
MetroHealth Medical Center
  Case Western Reserve University
Cleveland, Ohio

Ronald C. Kim, MD
Staff Neuropathologist
VA Long Beach Healthcare System
Long Beach, California
Clinical Professor
Department of Pathology and Neurology
University of California Irvine
Irvine, California

Alicia M. Koontz, PhD
Associate Director of Education and Outreach and
    Rehabilitation Scientist
Human Engineering Research Laboratories
Department of Veterans Affairs
Pittsburgh, Pennsylvania

Mark Allen Korsten, MD
Professor of Medicine
Department of Internal Medicine and
    Gastroenterology
JJP VA Medical Center
Mount Sinai School of Medicine
Bronx, New York

Sandra K. Kostyk, MD, PhD
Assistant Professor
Department of Neurology and Neuroscience
The Ohio State University
Columbus, Ohio

Andy Krieger, BS
Director
Paralyzed Veterans of America Sports and
    Recreation
Washington, District of Columbia

Timothy R. Kuklo, MD, JD
SpineAustin
Austin, Texas

Daniel P. Lammertse, MD
Medical Director of Research
Craig Hospital
Englewood, Colorado

Caroline Leclercq, MD
Attendino Hand Surgeon
Institut de la Main
Consultant
Centre de Reeducation
Neurologique of Fonetionnelle
Clinique Jouvenet
Paris, France

Roland R. Lee, MD, FACR
Professor of Radiology
University of California San Diego
VA San Diego Healthcare System
San Diego, California

Yu-Shang Lee, PhD
Assistant Professor
Department of Neurosciences
Lerner Research Institute
Cleveland Clinic
Cleveland, Ohio

Ching-Yi Lin, PhD
Assistant Professor
Department of Neurosciences
Lerner Research Institute
Cleveland Clinic
Cleveland, Ohio

Vernon W. Lin, MD, PhD
Chairman
Department of Physical Medicine and
    Rehabilitation
Cleveland Clinic Lerner College of Medicine
Case Western Reserve University
Louis Stokes Cleveland VA Medical Center
Cleveland, Ohio

Laurie B. Lindblom, MD
Service Line Chief
Spinal Cord Injury/Disorders
Hampton VA Medical Center
Hampton, Virginia

Frank Anthony Liporace, MD
Assistant Professor
Trauma Fellowship Director
Orthopaedics-Trauma Division
New Jersey Medical School
University of Medicine and Dentistry of New
    Jersey
Newark, New Jersey

Mark A. Lissens, MD, PhD
Professor, Physical Medicine and Rehabilitation
Department of Health Care and Chemistry
University College KHK
Geel, Belgium

James W. Little, MD, PhD
Professor
Department of Rehabilitation Medicine
University of Washington
Spinal Cord Injury Service
VA Puget Sound Health Care System
Seattle, Washington

Brenda Mallory, MD
Associate Clinical Professor of Rehabilitation
  Medicine
Department of Rehabilitation and Regenerative
  Medicine
Columbia University College of Physicians and
  Surgeons
New York, New York

Glen Manzano, MD
Department of Neurological Surgery
Miller School of Medicine
University of Miami
Miami, Florida

Ralph J. Marino, MD, MS
Associate Professor
Department of Rehabilitation Medicine
Thomas Jefferson University
Philadelphia, Pennsylvania

E. Jason Mask, MSW
Social Work Clinical Manager
Edward Hines, Jr., VA Hospital
Hines, Illinois

B. Cairbre McCann, MD
Director (Emeritus)
Department of Rehabilitation Medicine
Main Medical Center
Portland, Maine

Heather E. McCormack, PT
Instructor, Physical Therapy
Department of Physical Medicine and
  Rehabilitation
Mayo Clinic
Rochester, Minnesota

John David McGurl, MD
Staff Physician
Department of Medicine
VA Medical Center
Richmond, Virginia

Meena Midha, MD
Former Chief
Spinal Cord Injury Services
Hunter Holmes McGuire VA Medical Center
Consultant for Paralyzed Veterans of America
Richmond, Virginia

Robert E. Montroy, MD, FACS, FICS
Chief of Plastic Surgery
VA Medical Center Long Beach
Long Beach, California
Associate Clinical Professor of Surgery
Division of Plastic Surgery
University of California Irvine
Orange, California

Robert A. Moverman, PhD
Director
Psychology Services
Northeast Rehabilitation Health Network
Salem, New Hampshire
New England Neurological Associates, P.C.
Lawrence, Massachusetts

Mary Jane Mulcahey, PhD, OTR/L, LCP
Director
Rehabilitation and Clinical Research
Shriners Hospital for Children
Philadelphia, Pennyslvania

Kim S. Nalle
Manager
Clinical Practice Guidelines
Paralyzed Veterans of America
Washington, District of Columbia

Robert J. Nascimento, MD
Chief Resident
UMass Memorial Medical Center
Worchester, Massachusetts

Mark S. Nash, PhD, FACSM
Professor of Neurology Surgery and Rehabilitation
  Medicine
Director of Research in Rehabilitation Medicine
Department of Neurological Surgery and
  Rehabilitation Medicine
Miller School of Medicine
University of Miami
Miami, Florida

Ikechukwu Oguejiofor, MD
Fellow
Department of Urology
Loyola University Medical Center
Maywood, Illinois

Christina V. Oleson, MD
Assistant Professor
Department of Orthopaedics
Department of Physical Medicine and
    Rehabilitation
Dartmouth-Hitchcock Medical Center
Hanover, New Hampshire

Greg Paquin, BSc
Rehabilitation Engineer
California Department of Rehabilitation
Santa Fe Springs, California

Tamra Pelleschi, OTR/L, ATP
Program Manager
Instructor
Center for Assistive and Rehabilitative Technology
Department of Rehabilitation Science and
    Technology
Hiram G. Andrews Center
University of Pittsburgh
Pittsburgh, Pennsylvania

Inder Perkash, MD, MS, FRCS, FACS
Professor of Urology
Physical Medicine and Rehabilitation
PVA Professor Spinal Cord Injury Medicine
    (Emeritus)
Stanford School of Medicine
Stanford, California
Spinal Cord Injury Center
VA Palo Alto Health Care System
Palo Alto, California

Lily C. Pien, MD
Staff Physician
Pulmonary, Allergy, and Critical Care Medicine
Lerner College of Medicine
Cleveland Clinic
Cleveland, Ohio

Avraam Ploumis, MD, PhD
Assistant Professor
Orthopaedic Spine Surgeon
Department of Surgery
Division of Orthopaedics and Rehabilitation
University of Ioannina Medical School
Ioannia, Greece

Kornelis A. Poelstra, MD, PhD
Spine Surgeon
The Spine Institute at Orthopaedic Associates
Fort Walton Beach, Florida

Philip G. Popovich, PhD
Professor
Department of Molecular Viorology, Immunology,
    and Medical Genetics
Ohio State University
Columbus, Ohio

Heather Lynn Powell, MD
Assistant Professor of Neurology
Department of Physical Medicine and
    Rehabilitation Services
Integrated Department of Orthopaedics and
    Rehabilitation
Walter Reed Army Medical Center
Washington, District of Columbia

Michael Priebe, MD
Associate Professor
Department of Physical Medicine and
    Rehabilitation
Mayo Clinic
Rochester, Minnesota

Alexandre Rasouli, MD
Department of Neurological Surgery
Miller School of Medicine
University of Miami
Miami, Florida

J. Steven Richardson, PhD
Professor
Departments of Pharmacology and Psychiatry
University of Saskatchewan College of Medicine
Saskatoon, Canada

Roland R. Roy, PhD
Researcher
Brain Research Institute
University of California Los Angeles
Los Angeles, California

Sunil Sabharwal, MD
Chief of Spinal Cord Injury
West Roxbury VA Medical Center
Assistant Professor
Department of Physical Medicine and
    Rehabilitation
Harvard Medical School
Boston, Massachusetts

Catherine S.H. Sassoon, MD
Professor of Medicine
University of California Irvine
Irvine, California
Division of Pulmonary and Critical Care
VA Long Beach Healthcare System
Long Beach, California

James K. Schmitt, BA, MD
Chief General Internal Medicine
Hunter Holmes McGuire VA Medical Center
Professor of Medicine
Virginia Commonwealth University
Richmond, Virginia

Diane L. Schroeder, AB, MD
Chief Primary Care Service
Hunter Holmes McGuire VA Medical Center
Richmond, Virginia

Jack L. Segal, MD, FACP, FCP
Professor
University of California Los Angeles School of
    Medicine
Los Angeles, California
Director
Spinal Cord Injury Clinical Pharmacology
Los Amigos Research and Education Institute
Rancho Los Amigos National Rehabilitation Center
Downey, California

Andrew L. Sherman, MD
Associate Professor
Department of Rehabilitation Medicine
Miller School of Medicine
University of Miami
Miami, Florida

Robert W. Shields, Jr., MD
Co-Director
Center for Syncope and Automomic Disorders
Neurological Institute
Cleveland Clinic
Cleveland, Ohio

Ien Sie, MS, PT
University of Southern California
Downey, California

Norman F. Simoes, BS, MS
Senior Rehabilitation Engineer
Department of Rehabilitation
Mobility Evaluation Program, State of California
Santa Fe Springs, California

Andrew K. Simpson, MD, MHS
House Officer
Harvard Combined Orthopaedic Surgery
Massachusetts General Hospital
Boston, Massachusetts

Ashwani K. Singal, MD
GI Fellow
Division of Gastroenterology
Department of Internal Medicine
University of Texas Medical Branch
Galveston, Texas

Mandeep Singh, MD
French Creek Urology
Meadville, Pennsylvania

John D. Steeves, PhD
John and Penny Ryan BC Leadership Chair
Professor and Director of International
    Collaboration On Repair Discoveries
University of British Columbia
Vancouver Coastal Health
Vancouver, Canada

Steven A. Stiens, MD, MS
Associate Professor
Department of Rehabilitation Medicine
University of Washington
Director
Spinal Cord Medicine Fellowship
VA Puget Sound Health Care System
Seattle, Washington

Thomas Stripling
Director
Research and Education
Paralyzed Veterans of America
Washington, District of Columbia

Jelena N. Svircev, MD
Clinical Assistant Professor
Department of Rehabilitation Medicine
University of Washington
Spinal Cord Injury Service
VA Puget Sound Health Care System
Seattle, Washington

Emily Teodorski, MSW
Clinical Coordinator
Human Engineering Research Laboratories
Department of Veterans Affairs
University of Pittsburgh
Pittsburgh, Pennsylvania

Florian P. Thomas, MD, MA, PhD
Professor of Neurology
Saint Louis University
Director
Spinal Cord Injury/Dysfunction Service
Saint Louis VA Medical Center
Saint Louis, Missouri

Tricia Thorman, OTR/L
Occupational Therapist
Department of Occupational Therapy
The Children's Institute
Pittsburgh, Pennsylvania

Jared Toman, MD
Resident
Orthopedic Surgery
Boston University School of Medicine
Boston, Massachusetts

Andrea Underhill, MS, MPH, PhD
Associate Director
University of Alabama at Birmingham
University Transportation Center
Birmingham, Alabama

Alexander R. Vaccaro, MD, PhD
Professor
Department of Orthopaedics
The Rothman Institute
Philadelphia, Pennsylvania

Lawrence Cabell Vogel, MD
Assistant Chief of Staff, Medical
Chief of Pediatrics
Shriners Hospitals for Children
Professor of Pediatrics
Rush Medical College
Chicago, Illinois

Michael Y. Wang, MD
Department of Neurological Surgery
Miller School of Medicine
University of Miami
Miami, Florida

Robert L. Waters, MD
Orthopedic Surgeon/Research Scientist
Los Amigos Research and Education Institute, Inc.
Downey, California

Peter G. Whang, MD
Assistant Professor, Spine Services
Department of Orthopaedics and Rehabilitation
Yale University School of Medicine
New Haven, Connecticut

John S. Wheeler, Jr., MD
Professor
Department of Urology
Loyola University Medical Center
Maywood, Illinois

William D. Whetstone, MD
Associate Professor
Department of Emergency Medicine
University of California San Francisco
San Francisco, California

Asa J. Wilbourn, MD (Deceased)
Director, EMG Laboratory
Cleveland Clinic
Clinical Professor of Neurology
Case Western Reserve University
Cleveland, Ohio

Pamela E. Wilson, MD
Associate Professor
University of Colorado PM&R
The Children's Hospital
Aurora, Colorado

Stacey Quintero-Wolfe, MD
Department of Neurological Surgery
Miller School of Medicine
University of Miami
Miami, Florida

Robert M. Woolsey, MD
Professor of Neurology (Emeritus)
Saint Louis University
Director (Emeritus)
Spinal Cord Injury/Dysfunction Service
Saint Louis VA Medical Center
Saint Louis, Missouri

Lisa-Ann Wuermser, MD
Assistant Professor
Department of Physical Medicine and
   Rehabilitation
Mayo Clinic
Rochester, Minnesota

Ann Yamane, CO, MEd
Senior Lecturer
Department of Rehabilitation Medicine
University of Washington
Seattle, Washington

Omid Yousefian, BS
Psychobiology Student
Department of Psychology
University of California at Los Angeles School of
   Medicine
Los Angeles, California

Jeanne M. Zanca, PhD, MPT
Assistant Professor
Department of Rehabilitation Medicine
Mount Sinai School of Medicine
New York, New York

I

INTRODUCTION AND EVALUATION

1 Development, Anatomy, and Function of the Spinal Cord

Harry G. Goshgarian

This chapter is written for physicians and other practitioners who care for patients with spinal cord injury (SCI), and thus does not include all of the macroscopic and microscopic details of human spinal cord anatomy that may be included in standard medical texts. Only major topics are discussed and, whenever possible, the issues are covered from a perspective that is relevant to spinal cord medicine. For instance, in the discussion of the development of the spinal cord, a brief description of defects in neural tube closure (spinal bifida) is included. Moreover, although the function of several ascending and descending spinal pathways is discussed, emphasis is placed only on those that are most relevant to spinal cord injury. Finally, although the standard medical text description of the arterial blood supply to the spinal cord is included, there is also a discussion of how an understanding of the distribution pattern of these arteries may lead to a diagnosis of anterior cord syndrome. Details regarding the intrinsic neuroanatomic organization of the gray and white matter have been omitted, but references are included at the end of the chapter so that a reader may pursue this information if it should become necessary. This chapter is organized into four major sections, which cover the embryonic development, gross anatomy, neuroanatomic organization, and blood supply of the spinal cord.

EMBRYONIC DEVELOPMENT

The formation of the human spinal cord begins during the third week of gestation. Soon after gastrulation, the process that establishes all three germ layers (ectoderm, mesoderm, and endoderm), the axial portion of the neuroectoderm (neuroepithelium) thickens to form the neural plate dorsal to the mesodermal notochordal plate (Figure 1.1A, top). The neural plate thickens and eventually forms the neural groove (Figure 1.1A, middle). The lateral margins (folds) of the neural groove continue to thicken, approaching each other at the midline. As the neural plate thickens laterally, a group of cells appears along each edge (crest) of the neural folds (Figure 1.1A, middle). These ectoderm neural crest cells extend along the length of the neural groove.

Eventually, the neural groove closes and forms the neural tube. The neural crest cells then migrate laterally to ultimately give rise to the dorsal root ganglia of the spinal nerves and other cell types (Figure 1.1A, bottom). At about the same time as neural tube closure, the mesoderm of the notochordal plate is transformed into the notochord (Figure 1.1A, bottom). Both events occur at the 7–10 somite stage of development. The closure of the neural tube occurs at the cervical level of the future spinal cord and progresses both rostrally and caudally (Figure 1.1B). The junctional zones (at which neuroepithelial closure takes place) are known rostrally as the anterior neuropore and caudally as the posterior neuropore (Figure 1.1C). Final closure of the anterior neuropore occurs at the 18–20 somite stage of development (25th day), while the posterior neuropore of the lumbosacral spinal cord closes two days later, at the 25 somite stage. The closure of the neuroepithelium results in the spinal canal and cephalic brain vesicles. The ensuing mitosis of the surrounding neuroepithelial cells occurs in the fluid-filled humoral environment of the cerebrospinal ventricular system.

Mitosis of the neuroepithelial cells around the spinal canal gives rise to the primitive nerve cells, or neuroblasts, in the embryonic spinal cord. Collectively, these cells form the mantle layer around the neuroepithelial layer (Figure 1.2A). The mantle layer will develop into the future gray matter of the spinal cord. The peripheral marginal layer contains nerve fibers that grow out from the neuroblasts and will form the future white matter of the spinal cord (Figure 1.2B). During gestational weeks (GW) 3.5 and 4.5, the continuing mitosis of neuroepithelial cells results in a dorsal and ventral thickening on each side of the neural tube. There is a longitudinal groove in the central canal, the sulcus limitans, which marks the boundary between the dorsal and ventral thickenings (Figure 1.2A). The ventral thickenings are known as the basal plates, and these form the future ventral horns, or motor area of the spinal cord. The dorsal thickenings are the alar plates, and these form the future dorsal horns (sensory area) of the spinal cord (Figures 1.2A, B). The dorsal and ventral midline portions of the neural tube form the roof and floor plates, respectively (Figure 1.2A). These areas do not contain neuroblasts, but

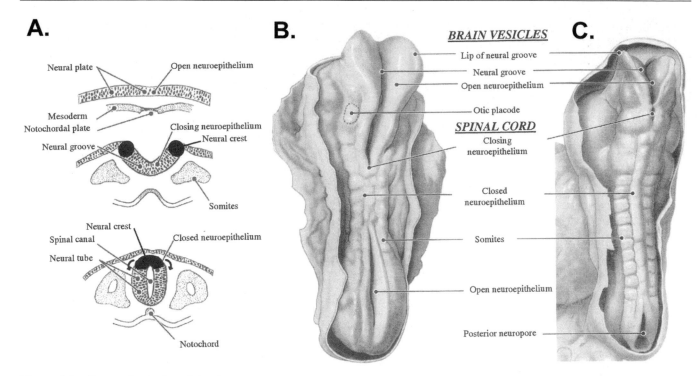

Figure 1.1   Stages of spinal cord development.

rather serve as substrates for axons crossing the midline of the spinal cord. The roof plate region will form the future dorsal gray commissure, while the floor plate will form the future ventral gray commissure of the spinal cord.

At GW 5.5 an intermediate thickening of the mantle layer is visible. This will ultimately form the intermediate horn of the spinal cord (Figure 1.2B) and will be the site of preganglionic sympathetic neurons found at all thoracic levels (T1–T12) and the first two lumbar levels (L1–L2).

By the end of the first trimester of development, the neuroepithelial cells that surround the central canal are replaced by ependymal cells, signaling the cessation of further neurogenesis. Motoneuron clusters in the ventral horn segregate into medial and lateral groups, and there is an expansion of the intermediate interneuronal field, a deepening of the dorsal funiculus, and a further growth and differentiation of the dorsal horn. The ventral median sulcus deepens considerably and is surrounded by the ventromedial funiculus.

Following the cessation of neuroblast production, gliablasts are formed from the neuroepithelium. These cells migrate from the neuroepithelial layer to the mantle and marginal layers, where they form both fibrous and protoplasmic astrocytes. Another glial cell type, most likely formed from gliablasts, is the oligodendroglial cell. This cell, which is found primarily in the marginal layer, is responsible for myelinating axons that remain within the central nervous system (CNS). The oligodendrocyte should be distinguished from the Schwann cell, which is derived from the neural crest. The Schwann cell myelinates axons in the PNS. Finally, during the second half of development, a third type of glial cell, the microglial cell, is derived from the mesenchyme. Microglia are the main phagocytic cells in the CNS. During the last 2–3 weeks of the first trimester, the gray matter of the spinal cord approximates its characteristic adult configuration.

The spinal cord lengthens more than threefold during the second half of the first trimester (Figures 1.3A–C). In fact, by the eleventh gestational week (GW11) the length of the spinal cord matches that of the vertebral column. By this time, the spinal nerves have passed through the intervertebral foramina at almost right angles and have established connections with the developing dermatomes and myotomes of the body somites. Starting at the beginning of the second (e.g., GW 14, Figure 1.3C) and progressing through the third trimester of development, there is a disparate growth of the vertebral column and spinal cord, with the vertebral column growing faster in length. The greater rate of growth of the vertebral column relative to that of the spinal cord continues beyond birth until the elongation of the body stops during adolescence.

The end result of the disparate growth of the spinal cord and vertebral column is that the end of the spinal cord is found at approximately the level of the first lumbar vertebra in the young adult. Thus, the spinal cord occupies the vertebral canal in the rostral 2/3 of the vertebral column in the adult. The neural connections between the spinal cord and body somites established during the first trimester are maintained during the second and

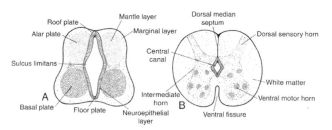

Figure 1.2   Embryonic formation of the dorsal, ventral, and intermediate horns.

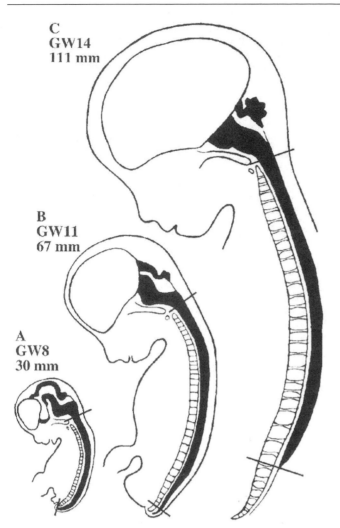

C
GW14
111 mm

B
GW11
67 mm

A
GW8
30 mm

Figure 1.3 The length of the spinal cord in relation to the vertebral column at three developmental periods. (GW, gestational week.)

ating tracts are found in the fasciculus gra of fasciculus cuneatus, the ventromedial a the marginal fasciculus. The tracts in th ascending exteroceptive and proprioce descending axons from the tectum responsible for the supraspinal control of the spinal cord.

Two conspicuous areas are not myelinated at the time of birth. These are Lissauer's tract (the posterolateral fasciculus), which remains unmyelinated postnatally, and the late-myelinating anterior and lateral corticospinal tracts. These last two pathways are part of the pyramidal motor system and do not become completely myelinated until the end of the first year after birth. There is a progressive rostral to caudal gradient in the growth and myelination of the corticospinal tracts in the newborn. At 3 days postnatally, the fasciculus gracilis, cuneatus, and ventral funiculus in the upper cervical spinal cord are well myelinated, but the lateral and anterior corticospinal tracts are not. By 4 months after birth, myelination of the lateral corticospinal tract is well under way at upper and lower cervical levels of the spinal cord, but the tract is not myelinated further caudally. This may be related to a 4-month infant being able to raise its head and reach for nearby objects, but not being able to voluntarily move its lower limbs. By the end of the first year of life, myelination of the lateral corticospinal tract is nearly complete and voluntary control of the lower limbs is possible. Walking behavior begins at this time. For a detailed description of the morphological maturation of the spinal cord and how it relates to behavioral development in the newborn, the reader should consult *Development of the Human Spinal Cord* by J. Altman and S. A. Bayer (2).

Neural Tube Defects

Most congenital defects of the spinal cord result from abnormal closure of the neural folds during GW 3 and 4. The defects that result may involve the meninges, vertebrae, muscles, and skin. Severe neural tube defects occur in approximately 1/1000 births, but the incidence varies depending upon the geographical area and may be as high as 1/100 births in some areas, such as northern China (3).

When the spinal region is involved, the general term used to describe neural tube defects is *spina bifida*. In spina bifida, the roof of the vertebral canal (vertebral arch) over one or more vertebrae fails to fuse dorsal to the spinal cord (Figure 1.4). This type of defect may or may not involve the underlying spinal cord. There are two types of spina bifida: *spina bifida occulta* and *spina bifida cystica*.

In spina bifida occulta, the vertebral arch is defective, but this is covered by skin and the defect usually does not involve the spinal cord (Figure 1.4A). It most often occurs in the lumbosacral region and is often accompanied by a patch of hair overlying the affected region.

In spinal bifida cystica, the meninges and, at times, the spinal cord protrude through the defect in the vertebral arch, forming a cystlike sac (Figures 1.4B, C). Spina bifida with *meningocele* is the term applied when only the meninges protrude through the defect (Figure 1.4B), but when the spinal cord also protrudes through the defect, the term used is spina bifida with *meningomyelocele* (Figure 1.4C). Hydrocephaly very often accompanies spina bifida cystica because the spinal cord is tethered to the vertebral column. Thus, as the vertebral column lengthens during development, tethering pulls the cerebellar tonsils down

third trimester (as well as postnatally) by the elongation of the central processes of the dorsal roots and ventral roots within the vertebral canal as well as the elongation of the peripheral nerves in the body. The resultant anatomy of the spinal cord and the clinical significance of this anatomy will be described later in this chapter.

Further development of the spinal cord during the second and third trimesters involves the establishment and growth of fibers systems that interconnect the spinal cord with supraspinal centers, the proliferation of glia throughout the spinal cord, and the myelination of developing ascending and descending tracts. The expansion of the white matter relative to the gray matter is a slow process that progresses over the entire second and third trimesters. The white matter enlarges in specific regions of the spinal cord, and myelination follows shortly thereafter in these regions. Myelination does not occur uniformly in the white matter. It is first seen in the lateral aspect of the fasciculus cuneatus (i.e., the "collateralization zone of the dorsal root" [1]) and in the white matter adjacent to the ventral horn (i.e., the "inferior circumferential fasciculus" [1]). The latter area contains the propriospinal and intraspinal tracts whose fibers "close" the intersegmental reflex circuits of the spinal cord. The next myelin-

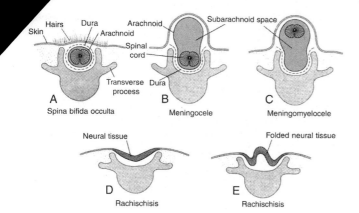

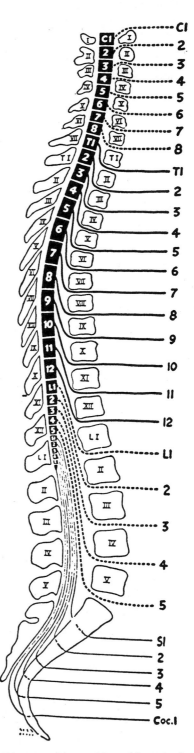

Figure 1.4 Types of neural tube defects involving the spinal cord.

extension found at lower cervical levels and the longest found at sacral levels. Thus, in adults, upper and mid-cervical spinal nerves have the shortest roots. From low cervical to sacral levels, the distance is progressively increased between the intervertebral foramen transmitting a nerve and the spinal cord segmental level giving rise to the roots of that nerve, and any particular spinal

into the foramen magnum and prevents the flow of cerebrospinal fluid out of the ventricles into the subarachnoid space. Spina bifida cystica can be treated by repairing the defect during in utero surgery at about 28 weeks of gestation. Preliminary results indicate that this approach reduces the incidence of hydrocephalus, improves bladder and bowel control, and increases motor development to the lower limbs (4).

There are instances in which the neural folds do not elevate during development, but remain flattened. In these cases, the neural tube does not close. In other instances the neural tissue folds, but there is still no closure of the neural tube. This is referred to as *spina bifida with rachischisis* (or sometimes *myeloschisis*, Figures 1.4D, E). In both types of rachischisis, the neural tissue is exposed and becomes necrotic.

The etiology of neural tube defects is multifactorial, and it is known that the likelihood of having a child with such a defect increases significantly after a first child is born with a defect. It is now established that folic acid (folate) reduces the incidence of neural tube defects by as much as 70% if 400 μg is taken daily 2 months before conception and throughout pregnancy (4).

GROSS ANATOMY

Extent and Appearance

The spinal cord in man is roughly cylindrical in shape and is slightly flattened anteriorly and posteriorly. It begins at the caudal end of the medulla oblongata and leaves the cranial vault by extending through the foramen magnum into the vertebral canal. At birth, the spinal cord terminates at the lower border of the third lumbar vertebra. In adults, the spinal cord is between 42 and 45 cm in length, weighs about 35 grams, and usually terminates at the level of the intervertebral disk between L1 and L2. However, the most inferior extent of the spinal cord, the conus medullaris, may be found as high as T12 or as low as L3. Thus, as pointed out earlier, the spinal cord does not extend the entire length of the vertebral canal, but rather occupies only its superior two-thirds in adults (Figure 1.5). The basis for the discrepancy in length between the vertebral column and spinal cord is embryologic, as explained in the first section of this chapter.

The result of this disparate growth between the spinal cord and vertebral column is a progressive increase in the length of spinal nerve roots within the vertebral canal, with the shortest

Figure 1.5 Diagram of the position of the spinal cord segments with reference to the bodies and spinous processes of the vertebrae.

cord segment lies somewhat higher than its corresponding numbered vertebra (Figure 1.5). It is important to appreciate that during development spinal nerves do not grow caudally in the vertebral canal to ultimately find their way to the appropriate intervertebral foramen and body segment. Rather, the connections are made early in development, and then the nerve roots elongate as the caudal half of the fetus grows in the later stages of development. The clinical significance of the anatomy of the "terminal end of the spinal cord" is explained below.

Relation of Spinal Nerves and Segments to the Vertebral Column

The thirty-one pairs of spinal nerves include eight cervical, twelve thoracic, five lumbar, five sacral, and one coccygeal pair. Spinal nerves emerge from the vertebral canal via the *intervertebral foramina*. The first seven cervical nerves pass out of intervertebral foramina *above* the vertebra having the corresponding number. For example, the sixth cervical nerve passes out of the foramen above the sixth cervical vertebra (Figure 1.5). Because there are eight pairs of cervical nerves, but only seven cervical vertebrae, it is best to remember that the eighth cervical nerve passes out *below* the seventh cervical vertebra. This establishes a pattern in which all remaining spinal nerves (thoracic, lumbar, sacral, and coccygeal) pass out *below* the vertebra with the corresponding number (Figure 1.5).

A knowledge of the anatomic relationship between spinal cord segments and the vertebral column is important for the diagnosis and treatment of certain spinal cord disorders, such as compression injury caused by a tumor. An appreciation of the relation of the spinal segment to overlying vertebra and spinous process is necessary when laminectomy is contemplated to relieve the spinal cord compression. As a general rule, at the upper cervical levels of the vertebral column (i.e., C2–C5) add 1 to the number of the spinous process to indicate the number of the underlying spinal segment at the tip of the process. Thus, the tip of the fourth cervical spinous process overlies the fifth cervical segment of the spinal cord. From mid-cervical to mid-thoracic levels (i.e., C6–T6), the underlying spinal cord segment at the process tip is identified by adding 2 to the number of the spinous process; and at mid-thoracic to low-thoracic levels (i.e., T7–T10), by adding 3 to this number. The eleventh and twelfth thoracic spinous processes overlie the five lumbar spinal cord segments, and the first lumbar spinous process overlies the five sacral segments. The part of the vertebral canal formed by the last four lumbar vertebrae and the sacrum contains a collection of long lumbar and sacral anterior and posterior roots known as the *cauda equina* (horse's tail) in addition to a specialization of the pia mater known as the *filum terminale.*

Surface Anatomy and Enlargements

The surface of the spinal cord displays a number of longitudinally oriented grooves (Figure 1.6). On the posterior (dorsal) surface in the midline is the shallow *posterior median sulcus.* This sulcus is continuous with the *posterior median septum,* a glial partition extending deeply to the gray matter. The *posterolateral sulcus* is a shallow groove that demarcates the entrance of the dorsal roots into the spinal cord bilaterally. In the cervical and

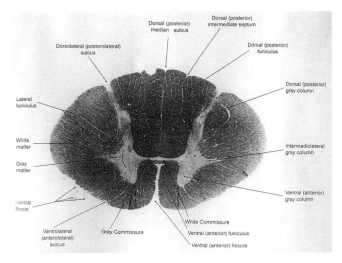

Figure 1.6 Photomicrograph of spinal cord showing division into gray and white matter.

upper six thoracic spinal cord segments, the *posterior intermediate sulcus* and underlying *posterior intermediate septum* is found between the posterior median and posterolateral sulci on each side of the spinal cord. On the anterior (ventral) surface, the prominent *anterior median fissure* penetrates the cord for a depth of approximately 3 mm and contains the sulcal branches of the anterior spinal artery and vein (Figure 1.6). The *anterolateral sulcus* marks the site at which the ventral root fibers exit the cord. However, because the ventral roots exit at less regular intervals and are not as numerous as dorsal roots, the anterolateral sulcus is not as easily seen as the posterolateral sulcus.

The spinal cord is not uniform in diameter; it contains two enlargements associated with the innervation of the upper and lower limbs. The *cervical enlargement* is the more prominent of the two and is found at the C5–T1 levels. These segmental levels are the same levels that give rise to the nerve roots that form the brachial plexus and thus provide innervation for the upper limbs. The *lumbar enlargement* gives rise to neurons and fibers that form the lumbar plexus (L1–L4) and the sacral plexus (L4–S2), both of which are involved in the innervation of the lower limbs. These enlargements are the natural result of the necessary increase in neurons and their processes at these levels for the innervation of limb musculature and skin.

Terminal End of the Spinal Cord

As mentioned earlier, the tapered end of the spinal cord is usually found at the level of the intervertebral disk between L1 and L2 and is called the *conus medullaris* (Figures 1.5 and 1.7). The conus medullaris consists of sacral spinal cord segments. It provides sensory innervation to the saddle area, motor innervation for the sphincters, and parasympathetic innervation for the bladder and lower bowel (i.e., from the left splenic flexure to the rectum). Here again an appreciation of the anatomic relationships between the spinal cord and vertebral column is useful in the diagnosis of some spinal cord disorders resulting from injury. Trauma in the lower back at the level of the L1 vertebra may result in *conus medullaris syndrome,* caused by a direct injury of the conus medullaris at this level (Figures 1.5 and 1.7). The signs and symptoms of this syndrome are permanent flaccid paralysis of the external anal sphincter and fecal incontinence, bladder distension and incontinence, impotence, and perianal or saddle anesthesia.

The flaccid paralysis of the external anal sphincter is caused by the destruction of the somatic lower motoneurons that innervate this voluntary muscle at the S2–S4 levels. These neurons normally project axons to the muscle via the inferior rectal branch of the pudendal nerve. Bladder distension and incontinence are caused by paralysis of the *detrusor muscle,* the smooth muscle wall of the bladder innervated by the pelvic splanchnic nerves arising from preganglionic parasympathetic neurons at S2–S4, and also by paralysis of the *urethral sphincter,* the striated (voluntary) muscle innervated by the perineal branch of the pudendal nerve (S2–S4). As in the bowel, the bladder dysfunction of conus medullaris syndrome is caused by the destruction of neurons at the S2–S4 levels of the spinal cord. Generally, the bladder is permanently areflexic in conus medullaris syndrome because of the loss of the sacral spinal neurons that give rise to the bladder reflexes. Thus, a "spastic" or "automatic" bladder does not develop as it would when the cord is injured at more rostral levels; the sacral bladder reflex circuitry is spared, and these neurons become hyperactive after recovery from spinal shock.

In conus medullaris syndrome, impotence is primarily caused by a loss of parasympathetic neurons at S2–S4. Erection is achieved normally when parasympathetic stimulation causes the smooth muscle of the arteries associated with the erectile tissue of the penis to relax. As a result, the arterial lumina enlarge and blood is allowed to flow into and dilate the cavernous spaces in the corpora of the penis. The bulbospongiosus and ischiocavernosus muscles are innervated by the deep branch of the perineal nerve, a branch of the pudendal nerve (S2–S4). Normally, during erection, these muscles contract and thus compress the venous plexuses at the periphery of the corpora cavernosa, preventing the return of venous blood. As a result, the penis becomes erect. Because it is likely that neurons innervating the bulbospongiosus and ischiocavernosus muscles will also be lost in conus medullaris syndrome, paralysis or paresis of these muscles contributes to impotence.

Loss of sensory neurons in the dorsal horn at S4 and S5 causes *perianal anesthesia* and *saddle anesthesia* (i.e., anesthesia of the posterior thigh). In conus medullaris syndrome, this anesthesia is caused predominantly by a loss of sensory neurons at the S2 level. In a pure conus lesion, normal sensory and motor function is retained in the lower limb (i.e., assuming only the conus medullaris is injured and lumbar roots of the cauda equina are spared). If the S1 level is spared, the ankle jerk is retained. Finally, if the conus medullaris lesion is incomplete, some of the signs and symptoms noted above may not occur.

Lesions of the cauda equina (Figure 1.7) below the L1 vertebral level result in *cauda equina syndrome.* The signs and symptoms of this syndrome are similar to those following conus lesions. However, cauda equina lesions usually affect not only peripheral nerve fibers from the sacral segments of the cord, but also a varying number of the lumbar dorsal and ventral nerve roots. The sensory and motor losses are, as a rule, more extensive and reach higher spinal levels (i.e., the lower limbs) following cauda equina lesions when compared to lesions of the conus medullaris. Furthermore, the distribution of motor and sensory

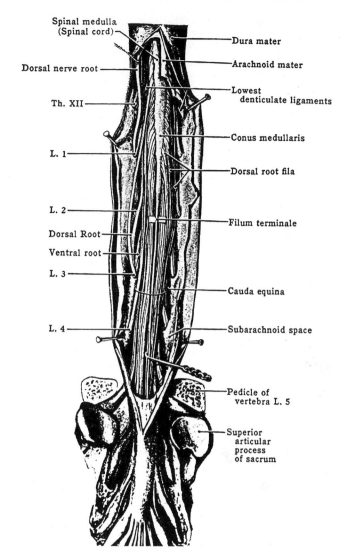

Figure 1.7   Posterior view of lower end of the dural sac.

loss is usually more irregular because some of the nerve roots will be damaged and others will be spared.

It is important to note that because of the anatomical proximity of the conus medullaris and cauda equina, a single lesion is likely to affect both structures, thus making the determination of the injury level and the specific syndrome difficult on the basis of a neurologic examination alone. In fact, the International Standards for Neurological and Functional Classification of Spinal Cord Injury (5) define conus medullaris syndrome as an injury of the sacral cord (conus) *and* lumbar nerve roots within the spinal canal that usually results in areflexic bladder, bowel, *and* lower limbs. Interestingly, cauda equina syndrome is defined as an injury to the lumbosacral nerve roots within the neural canal resulting in the same deficits noted under conus medullaris syndrome (5). In this chapter we define the syndromes differently and present a summary of the signs and symptoms that would occur following injury to either structure, but not both, to emphasize the anatomic and functional organization of the spinal cord. It is noteworthy that conus medullaris syndrome and cauda equina syndrome have been defined in this same manner in other textbooks (6).

Meninges of the Spinal Cord

The three membranous investments of the spinal cord—the dura mater, arachnoid, and pia mater—are continuous with the meningeal investments of the brain. The outermost covering, the *dura mater,* forms a long tubular sheath of dense, fibroelastic tissue around the spinal cord and cauda equina that extends from the foramen magnum to the level of the second sacral vertebra (Figure 1.7). In the cranial vault, the dura mater consists of two layers: an outer *periosteal* layer adherent to the inner surface of the cranium, and an inner *meningeal* layer. At various sites, the two layers of the cranial dura are separated by venous sinuses. In contrast, the spinal dura mater is single layered, devoid of venous sinuses, and continuous only with the meningeal layer of the cranial dura. There is a separate periosteal lining against the bone of the vertebral canal. The small space between this lining and the spinal dura mater is called the *epidural space.* This space contains epidural fat, areolar tissue, and the internal vertebral venous plexus. The spinal dura forms *dural root sleeves* that follow the dorsal and ventral roots into each intervertebral foramen (Figure 1.7, lower). At these sites, the sleeves end by blending with the epineurium of each spinal nerve. The dura is adherent to the periosteum lining the foramina at these sites. At the level of the second sacral vertebra, the tubular dural sac tapers down to a slender covering for the *filum terminale* (a specialization of the pia mater, described later). This covering, referred to as the *coccygeal ligament,* anchors the spinal cord with the vertebral canal where it descends and attaches to the periosteum of the coccyx (Figure 1.8). Cerebrospinal fluid (CSF) pushes the arachnoid directly up against the dura mater. Thus, there actually is no space between the dura and arachnoid under normal conditions. Several authors of anatomy have referred to a "potential" *subdural space,* which may be increased under pathologic conditions. For instance, rupture of bridging veins between the dura and arachnoid may result in the accumulation of blood and the expansion of this space, a condition known as *subdural hematoma.*

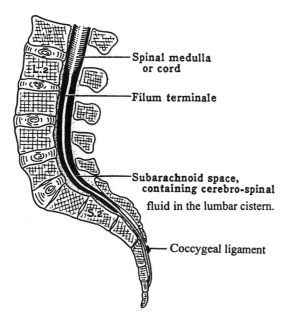

Figure 1.8 Spinal cord in situ.

- Spinal medulla or cord
- Filum terminale
- Subarachnoid space, containing cerebro-spinal fluid in the lumbar cistern.
- Coccygeal ligament

The arachnoid is continuous with the same layer surrounding the brain. This delicate avascular membrane completely lines the dural sac and its dural root sleeves and thus covers the nerve roots and dorsal root ganglia. Like the dura, the arachnoid blends with the epineurium of the spinal nerves. The arachnoid follows the dura inferiorly, where it ends as a sac at the level of the second sacral vertebra enclosing the cauda equina (Figure 1.7). The subarachnoid space, filled with CSF, surrounds the spinal cord and pia mater including its specializations (the denticulate ligaments and filum terminale described later). The space is largest inferiorly between the level of the second lumbar vertebra and the second sacral vertebra in a region known as the *lumbar cistern* (Figure 1.8). The lumbar cistern contains the cauda equina and filum terminale, which are free-floating within the CSF. Needles may be inserted into the lumbar cistern at the intervertebral space between L3 and L4 or L4 and L5 to draw off CSF for sampling (a "spinal tap") or to inject anesthetics (a "spinal block") without the risk of injuring the spinal cord, which ends as the conus medullaris at the first lumbar vertebral level. The nerve roots of the cauda equina are generally not injured by the procedure because, being suspended in fluid, they roll away from the needle point.

The *pia mater* is the innermost of the three meningeal investments and the only one that directly contacts the surface of the spinal cord (Figure 1.9). The pia also directly covers the roots of the spinal nerves and the spinal blood vessels. At the conus medullaris, the pia mater continues inferiorly into the lumbar cistern as a slender filament called the *filum terminale* (Figures 1.7, 1.8). Surrounded by the nerve roots of the cauda equina, the filum terminale pierces the arachnoid at the level of the second sacral vertebra and then becomes invested by dura mater to become the coccygeal ligament (Figure 1.8). By attaching to the periosteum of the coccyx, the coccygeal ligament centers the spinal cord within the lumbar cistern and serves as an anchor to maintain that position to prevent cord injury, especially under conditions of sudden jarring that could force delicate spinal tissue up against the bony walls of the vertebral canal.

Bilaterally thickened lateral extensions of the pia mater give rise to the *denticulate ligaments* (Figure 1.9). The two denticulate ligaments—one on the right and one on the left—are located between the dorsal and ventral roots on each side of the spinal cord. From each ligament twenty to twenty-two toothlike triangular processes extend further laterally, pierce the arachnoid, and fuse with the dura. The attachment of the processes of the ligament alternates with the passage of the nerve roots through the dura mater (Figure 1.9). The first attachment is at the level of the foramen magnum, whereas the most caudal attachment is between the T12 and L1 nerve roots (Figure 1.7). As in the filum terminale and coccygeal ligaments, the attachments of the denticulate ligaments to the dura mater provide an important fixation of the spinal cord, protecting it from sudden displacements.

Organization of a Spinal Nerve

Sensory information (i.e., pain, temperature, touch, etc.) is conveyed from the body into the spinal cord via the *dorsal roots,* which enter the spinal cord posteriorly along the *posterolateral sulcus* (Figure 1.9). The neuron cell bodies responsible for conveying the sensory (afferent) information are located in a distal

Posterior view

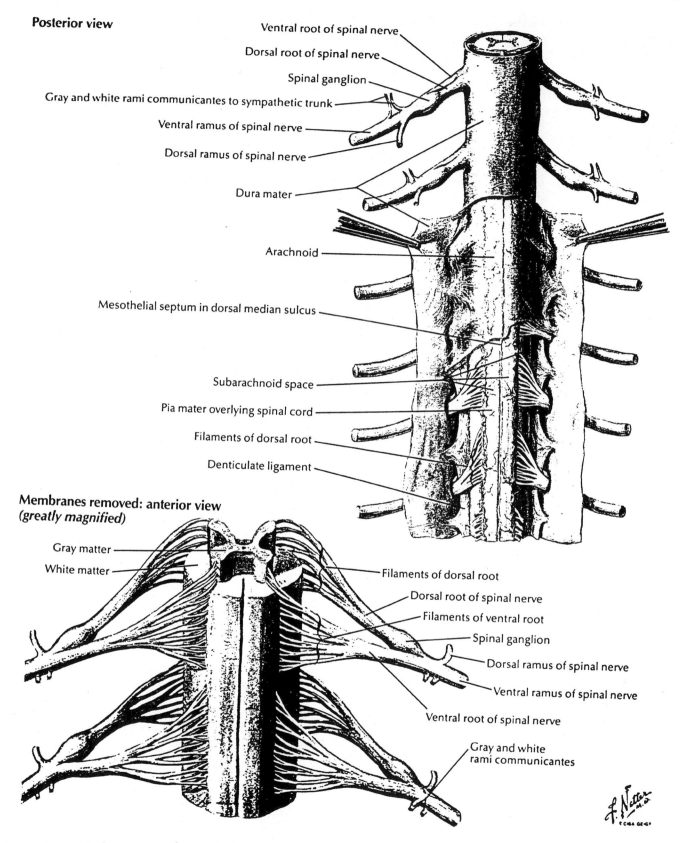

Ventral root of spinal nerve

Dorsal root of spinal nerve

Spinal ganglion

Gray and white rami communicantes to sympathetic trunk

Ventral ramus of spinal nerve

Dorsal ramus of spinal nerve

Dura mater

Arachnoid

Mesothelial septum in dorsal median sulcus

Subarachnoid space

Pia mater overlying spinal cord

Filaments of dorsal root

Denticulate ligament

**Membranes removed: anterior view
(*greatly magnified*)**

Gray matter

White matter

Filaments of dorsal root

Dorsal root of spinal nerve

Filaments of ventral root

Spinal ganglion

Dorsal ramus of spinal nerve

Ventral ramus of spinal nerve

Ventral root of spinal nerve

Gray and white
rami communicantes

Figure 1.9 Spinal meninges and nerve roots.

swelling of the dorsal root known as the *spinal ganglion.* The spinal ganglion is generally surrounded by bone and is found at the level of the intervertebral foramen. The *ventral roots* of the spinal cord convey motor (efferent) information from the spinal cord to skeletal muscle. Ventral root fibers exit the spinal cord at the *anterolateral sulcus* and also contain axons from preganglionic autonomic neurons (Figure 1.9). The dorsal and ventral roots that delineate a spinal cord segmental level fuse at the level of the intervertebral foramen just distal to the spinal ganglion to form the *spinal nerve* associated with that spinal cord segment. The spinal nerve is a *mixed nerve,* in that it contains both sensory and motor fibers from the dorsal and ventral roots, respectively. The first cervical nerve lacks dorsal roots in 50% of people, and the coccygeal nerves may be absent entirely (7). It should be noted that the spinal nerves are relatively short. Almost immediately after exiting the intervertebral foramen, each nerve bifurcates into a dorsal and ventral ramus (Figure 1.9). The *dorsal ramus* provides the cutaneous innervation of the back and the motor innervation of the intrinsic or deep back muscles. All the appendicular and remaining trunk muscle innervation and sensory innervation of the body (excluding the motor and sensory innervation provided by cranial nerves) is provided by the *ventral ramus* of each spinal nerve. It is important to appreciate that, whereas the dorsal and ventral *roots* convey pure sensory and motor fibers respectively, the dorsal and ventral *rami* are mixed nerves, each containing both sensory and motor fibers.

NEUROANATOMIC ORGANIZATION OF THE SPINAL GRAY AND WHITE MATTER

In cross section, the spinal cord is composed of a central portion of butterfly-shaped gray matter and peripherally oriented white matter (Figure 1.9). The gray matter is composed predominantly of neurons, their processes, and glial cells, and it has an enriched blood supply. The white matter contains ascending and descending fiber tracts and glial cells, and it appears white in unfixed tissue because of a predominance of myelin. The two halves of the gray matter are connected across the midline by a *dorsal* and *ventral gray commissure,* which are located above and below the central canal respectively (Figure 1.6). The gray matter is further subdivided into a *posterior* (dorsal) horn (column) and an *anterior* (ventral) *horn* (column). The thoracic and upper two lumbar spinal cord segments also display a wedge-shaped, intermediate *lateral horn* (intermediolateral gray column) (Figure 1.6).

The white matter on each side of the spinal cord is organized into three large areas, or *funiculi* (Figure 1.6). The *posterior funiculus* is the area of white matter between the posterior median sulcus and the posterolateral sulcus. The *lateral funiculus* is defined as the white matter between the *posterolateral sulcus* and an imaginary line from the medial border of the anterior horn to the anterior surface of the spinal cord. The *anterior funiculus* is the remaining white matter medial to the imaginary line noted above and lateral to the anterior median fissure (Figure 1.6). Each funiculus of the spinal cord is composed of bundles of fibers that run together and subserve the same function. Each bundle is referred to as a *tract,* or *fasciculus.* For instance, at cervical levels and the upper six thoracic levels of the spinal cord, the posterior funiculus is subdivided into two major fasciculi (gracilis

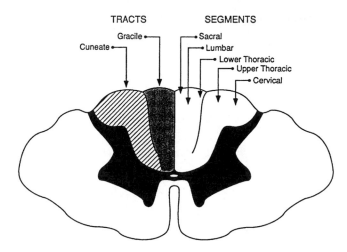

Figure 1.10   Diagram of the spinal cord showing the somatotopic organization of fibers in the posterior funiculus.

and cuneatus) by the posterior intermediate sulcus and septum (Figure 1.10). (The functional significance of these fiber tracts is discussed in the section "White Matter.")

Gray Matter

The posterior (dorsal) horn contains clusters of neurons concerned with sensory function. The central processes of spinal ganglion cells generally synapse on neurons in the dorsal horn, where sensory information is relayed either to higher centers in the brain or segmentally within the spinal cord.

The lateral (intermediate) horn is limited to the thoracic and upper two lumbar spinal cord segments. It contains *preganglionic sympathetic neurons* whose axons exit the spinal cord via the ventral roots. *Preganglionic parasympathetic neurons* are located in a comparable region of the gray matter at the S2–S4 levels of the spinal cord. However, a well-defined lateral horn is not found at these sacral levels. Axons of the preganglionic parasympathetic neurons distribute to the descending colon, sigmoid colon, rectum, and all pelvic viscera via the *pelvic splanchnic nerves.*

The anterior (ventral) horn contains both interneurons and motoneurons. Motoneuron axons innervating skeletal muscle comprise the major component of the ventral root. Alpha motoneurons of the anterior horn are somatotopically organized such that neurons supplying flexor muscles are located dorsally in the anterior horn and neurons supplying extensor muscles are located ventrally. In addition, neurons supplying the trunk musculature are located medially, whereas neurons innervating the limbs are located laterally within the anterior horn (Figure 1.11).

White Matter

Heavily myelinated nerve fibers in the posterior funiculus are concerned primarily with two general modalities related to conscious proprioception. These are *kinesthesia* (sense of position and movement) and *discriminative touch* (discriminating two points and localizing touch sensation). Injury to the spinal cord in the region of the posterior funiculus may result clinically in a loss or diminution of vibratory sense, position sense, two-point tactile

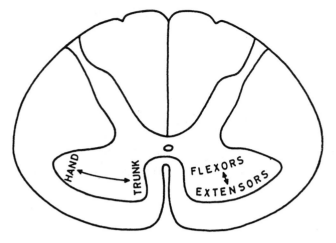

Figure 1.11 Diagram of the spinal cord showing the somatotopic organization of ventral horn motor neurons.

discrimination, and touch and weight perception in the body ipsilateral and caudal to the spinal cord lesion. The central processes of neurons whose cell bodies are located in spinal ganglia form the fibers of the posterior funiculus. The fibers that enter the spinal cord below the sixth thoracic segment form the *fasciculus gracilis* (gracile tract), whereas fibers that enter the cord above the sixth thoracic segment are located laterally and form the *fasciculus cuneatus* (cuneate tract). These two tracts are separated by the posterior intermediate sulcus and septum, which is found at all cervical levels of the spinal cord and the upper six thoracic levels. Thus, the nerve fibers in the posterior funiculus are somatotopically arranged, with the greatest number of medial fibers arising from the sacral levels and the greatest number of lateral fibers coming from the cervical levels (Figure 1.10). Fibers in the gracile and cuneate tract ascend ipsilaterally to the caudal medulla, where they synapse on neurons in the gracile and cuneate nuclei, respectively. Axons of these medullary neurons cross the midline and ascend as the medial lemniscus, which terminates on neurons in the thalamus (ventral posterolateral nucleus). Thalamic neurons, in turn, project to the cerebral cortex.

A functional relationship exists between the posterior funiculus and the tracts in the lateral funiculus of the spinal cord. For example, injury to the posterior funiculus augments all forms of sensation conveyed by the spinothalamic pathways in the lateral funiculus. Thus, painful stimuli are triggered by lower stimulation thresholds and nonpainful stimuli are interpreted as being painful. In both man and animals, there have been reports of lesions in the posterior funiculus that result in no loss of the sensory modalities presumably carried by this white matter region; the presence of the spinocervical thalamic tract in the lateral funiculus may compensate for some posterior funiculus deficits.

Sensory stimuli transmitted via the posterior funiculi are of three types: those impressed passively on the organism, those which have temporal or sequential components added to a spatial cue, and those which are not perceived without manipulation and active exploration by the digits. The first type of stimulus is exemplified by a vibrating tuning fork, two-point discrimination, or a touch by a piece of cotton. These passive stimuli are transmitted not only by the posterior funiculi, but also by a number of parallel pathways, such as the spinocervical thalamic tract. Thus, such passive sensations are often preserved following

lesions of the posterior funiculi. The second type of stimulus is exemplified by a determination of the direction of lines that are drawn on the skin or the direction of movement of a digit or toe. This type of stimulus, which contains temporal or sequential factors added to a spatial cue, is transmitted exclusively by the posterior funiculi. Thus, the information that concerns the relative changes in a stimulus over a period of time or the direction of a stimulus is transmitted to higher CNS centers only by the posterior funiculi. This is also the case with the third type of stimulus. Recognizing shapes and patterns by active exploration with the digits (i.e., stereognosis) is mediated only by the posterior funiculi, and the ability to recognize these shapes is often lost with lesions to this part of the spinal cord.

Position and movement sense is severely affected following injury to the posterior funiculi, especially in the distal part of the extremities. Small passive movements are not recognized as movements, but as touch or pressure. The direction of movement is seldom perceived. This loss of position sense greatly impairs motor function. The sensory loss causes movements to be clumsy, uncertain, and poorly coordinated, a condition referred to as *posterior column* or *sensory ataxia*.

Ascending Tracts in the Lateral and Anterior Funiculi

Posterior Spinocerebellar Tract

This ascending tract is located in the dorsal aspect of the lateral funiculus (Figure 1.12). The tract conveys to the cerebellum proprioceptive information from receptors located in muscles, tendons, and joints. The central processes of spinal ganglion cells enter the spinal cord via the dorsal root and then ascend or descend in the fasciculus gracilis for one or two segments before synapsing on neurons in the nucleus dorsalis of Clarke (Clarke's nucleus), located within the intermediate gray matter predominantly at thoracic spinal cord levels. Axons of neurons in the nucleus dorsalis form the posterior spinocerebellar tract. Because Clarke's nucleus is found only between C8 and L2, the posterior spinocerebellar tract is not found caudal to L2 in the spinal cord. The central processes of those spinal ganglion cells conveying proprioceptive information into the spinal cord below L2 ascend to the L2 level in the fasciculus gracilis before synapsing on cells

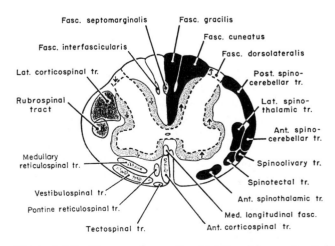

Figure 1.12 Diagram of ascending (right) and descending (left) pathways of the spinal cord.

in Clarke's nucleus. Similarly, incoming proprioceptive information entering the spinal cord rostral to C8 are carried by nerve fibers ascending in the fasciculus cuneatus. The cuneate tract nerve fibers synapse on neurons of the accessory cuneate nucleus in the medulla; this is homologous to the nucleus dorsalis. Both pathways are uncrossed.

The posterior spinocerebellar tract conveys to the cerebellum information pertaining to muscle contraction, including phase, rate, and strength of contraction. Clinical effects of posterior spinocerebellar tract destruction in spinal cord injury (SCI) are masked by the effects of destruction of the adjacent lateral corticospinal tract.

Spinocervical Thalamic Tract

Although the spinocervical thalamic tract has not been demonstrated in man, a description of this tract is included here because of its possible relevance to an explanation of some clinical cases involving preserved sensory function following SCI. In cats, the central processes of spinal ganglion cells conveying stimuli into the spinal cord from low-threshold cutaneous receptors, pressure receptors, and impulses following pinching of the skin synapse on neurons in the ipsilateral dorsal horn. These neurons send their axons into the dorsal aspect of the lateral funiculus, where they ascend to the upper two or three cervical segments and synapse on neurons of the *lateral cervical nucleus*. The lateral cervical nucleus is located lateral to the dorsal horn in the lateral funiculus of the upper three cervical segments of the cat spinal cord (8). The lateral cervical nucleus gives rise to axons that cross the midline in the *anterior white commissure* (Figure 1.6) at spinal levels C1 and C2 and ascend with the medial lemniscus to terminate in the contralateral ventral posterolateral (VPL) nucleus of the thalamus. This spinocervical thalamic tract has a somatotopic organization similar to that of the posterior funiculus pathways (i.e., sacral fibers are medially located and cervical fibers are the most laterally located [9]). It is important to appreciate that there is evidence that the pathways in the posterior funiculus (dorsal column–medial lemniscal system) are functionally linked with the spinocervical thalamic tract, because some spinocervical collaterals terminate in the dorsal column nuclei and some cells in the dorsal column nuclei project to the lateral cervical nucleus (10).

The putative clinical relevance of this information is that the spinocervical thalamic tract accounts for the persistence of kinesthesia and discriminative touch sensation following total interruption of the posterior funiculus in experimental animals. According to Afifi and Bergman (11), the presence of the spinocervical thalamic tract has been assumed in man because of the similar persistence of posterior funiculus sensations after total posterior funiculus lesions in patients. Thus, the old concept of the absolute necessity of the posterior funiculus for all discriminatory sensation is evolving into a newer concept that attributes to the posterior funiculus a role in the discrimination of those sensations that an animal must explore *actively* and to the spinocervical thalamic pathway a role in the perception of sensations that are impressed passively on the organism (12).

Lateral Spinothalamic Tract

One of the most clinically important pathways in the spinal cord is the *lateral spinothalamic tract,* which is concerned with the transmission of pain and temperature sensations (Figure 1.12). This tract is closely related to the *anterior spinothalamic tract,* and authors often combine the two pathways and refer to them together as the *anterolateral system* (ALS). In this chapter the pathways are discussed separately because of their clinical relevance.

Unmyelinated and thinly myelinated dorsal root fibers contributing to the lateral spinothalamic tract have their cell bodies in spinal ganglia. Incoming root fibers synapse on neurons of the dorsal horn. The dorsal horn neurons project axons across the midline in the anterior white commissure to the contralateral lateral funiculus and thus form the lateral spinothalamic tract. The crossing fibers of the lateral spinothalamic pathway ascend from one to two spinal segments above their entry level before entering the tract in the contralateral lateral funiculus. The fibers of the tract are somatotopically arranged with sacral fibers located laterally and cervical fibers located medially within the tract. Note that this arrangement is the reverse of the posterior funiculus pathways, in which sacral fibers are located medially and cervical fibers are laterally located. Once formed, the lateral spinothalamic tract ascends throughout the length of the spinal cord and brainstem to ultimately terminate on neurons of the VPL nucleus of the thalamus.

Lesions of the lateral spinothalamic tract in the lateral funiculus result in a loss of pain and temperature sensation in the contralateral half of the body, beginning one or two segments below the level of the lesion. This pattern of sensory loss is in marked contrast to the loss that occurs following injury to the dorsal roots, in which there is segmental or dermatomal loss of sensation ipsilateral to the lesion. Moreover, if pain and temperature fibers are injured as they cross the midline of the spinal cord in the anterior white commissure, there is a *bilateral* segmental loss of pain and temperature sensation in the dermatomes corresponding to the affected spinal cord segments. This last pattern of sensory loss is characteristic of *syringomyelia,* a condition caused by a centrally located cavitation of the spinal cord that destroys the anterior white commissure. Finally, in a *Brown-Séquard* lesion (hemisection of the spinal cord), the patient experiences *both* a contralateral loss of pain and temperature in the body (caused by the destruction of the lateral spinothalamic pathway in the lateral funiculus) *and* a bilateral segmental loss of pain and temperature (caused by a destruction of the anterior white commissure) that will be slightly higher than the contralateral loss of pain and temperature sensation, but still below the level of the lesion.

In the past, the lateral spinothalamic tract was sectioned surgically to relieve intractable pain. The procedure is referred to as *cordotomy* and may be carried out unilaterally or bilaterally. If bilateral cordotomy is performed, the lesions are made at slightly different levels in the spinal cord. During surgery, the denticulate ligament is used as a landmark; lesions are made just anterior to the denticulate ligament to locate and transect the lateral spinothalamic tract. A unilateral lesion of the tract results in anesthesia of the body wall and limbs, but not the viscera, which are bilaterally represented (12). Furthermore, the anogenital region is not markedly affected with unilateral lesions (13). Clinical results have indicated that after variable periods of time following bilateral cordotomies, there is often a return of pain and temperature sensation, thus suggesting that there may be other pathways in the spinal cord to convey this modality. These pathways may be multisynaptic and pass through the reticular formation (i.e., spinoreticular [14]) or involve shorter relays (i.e., spinospinal [13]). In addition, Afifi and Bergman (13) have suggested that pain sensation may be mediated through a spinotectal pathway, and Carpenter and Sutin (12) have suggested that uncrossed spinothalamic fibers may be responsible for the return of pain and temperature sensation following unilateral lesion of the lateral spinothalamic pathway.

Anterior Spinothalamic Tract

The dorsal root fibers conveying light touch sensation and certain types of pain impulses synapse on dorsal horn neurons. The axons of these dorsal horn neurons cross in the anterior white commissure over several segments and gather in the lateral and anterior funiculi to form the *anterior spinothalamic tract* (Figure 1.12). The course and termination of this tract in the spinal cord and brainstem are similar to those of the lateral spinothalamic tract.

Functionally, "light touch" is defined as the sensation provoked by stroking an area of skin devoid of hair (glabrous skin) with a feather or wisp of cotton (13). This type of sensation is conveyed to higher CNS centers in addition to the pressure sense and discriminatory tactile sensations conveyed by the posterior funiculus. Because tactile sensation is transmitted centrally by the posterior funiculi, the anterior spinothalamic tract, and the spinocervical thalamic tract, clinically this particular sensory modality is of little value in localizing injuries to the spinal cord (13). If the anterior spinothalamic tract is lesioned, there is little loss of tactile sensibility; however, the affective aspect of sensation may be lost. Bilateral destruction of the anterolateral funiculi may cause a complete loss of itching, tickling, and libidinous feeling (15); thus this region of the spinal cord has been associated with one's ability to judge the pleasant or unpleasant character of sensation. In addition to light touch stimuli, the anterior spinothalamic tract is thought to convey nondiscriminative pain sensations, in contrast to the lateral spinothalamic tract, which is thought to convey the well-localized discriminative pain sensations (15).

Other Ascending Tracts

There are several other ascending tracts in the spinal cord lateral and anterior funiculi that are of little clinical significance. These tracts include the spino-olivary, spinotectal, spinoreticular, spinocortical, spinovestibular, and anterior spinocerebellar. These multisynaptic pathways do not have a well-delineated functional significance, but may play a role in feedback control mechanisms or in the maintenance of the state of consciousness. For more detailed information on these pathways consult Carpenter and Sutin (15).

Descending Tracts of the Lateral and Anterior Funiculi

Corticospinal Tracts

As the name implies, neurons giving rise to the corticospinal tracts are found in the cerebral cortex. The axon of these neurons projects through the brainstem and terminates in the spinal cord. The corticospinal tracts comprise the largest, clinically important descending fiber system in the human neuraxis. The neurons that give rise to the tracts are located in the primary motor cortex (i.e., the precentral gyrus or Brodmann area 4), the premotor cortex (area 6), the primary sensory cortex (i.e., the postcentral gyrus or areas 3, 1, and 2), and adjacent parietal cortex (16, 17). Although both sensory and motor cortical areas contribute to the tracts, the primary motor cortex and the premotor cortex give rise to 80% of the tracts.

At the caudal level of the medulla oblongata, the majority of the corticospinal fibers cross the midline in the *pyramidal decussation* to form the *lateral corticospinal tract,* which is located in the dorsal aspect of the lateral funiculus (Figure 1.12). The lateral corticospinal tract extends the entire length of the spinal cord and is somatotopically organized. As in the lateral spinothalamic tract, cervical fibers are found medially. They are followed laterally by thoracic, lumbar, and then sacral fibers. Once again, it may be instructive to recall that the somatotopic organization of both the lateral corticospinal tract and the lateral spinothalamic pathway in the lateral funiculus is different from the somatotopic organization of the posterior funiculus in that, in the latter, sacral fibers are mostly medial and cervical fibers are located laterally.

The uncrossed corticospinal fibers descend from the medulla into the anterior funiculus of the spinal cord as the *anterior corticospinal tract* (bundle of Türck) (Figure 1.12). The anterior corticospinal tract extends only to the upper thoracic spinal cord and innervates neurons projecting to the muscles of the upper extremities and neck. The fibers of this tract generally cross the midline segmentally within the spinal cord before terminating on contralateral neurons. In rare cases, fibers do not cross the midline at all and form extremely large anterior corticospinal tracts (18).

Corticospinal fibers terminate mostly on interneurons in the spinal cord. Evidence also exists for a direct projection to alpha and gamma motoneurons. Because the corticospinal tracts innervate both alpha and gamma motoneurons, stimulation of corticospinal fibers leads to a co-contraction of both intrafusal and extrafusal muscle fibers. Because of the co-contraction of the two types of muscle fibers, there is increased sensitivity of the muscle spindle (intrafusal fiber) to changes in muscle length even when the muscle is shortening.

It has been estimated that 55% of all corticospinal fibers end in the cervical cord, 20% in the thoracic, and 25% in the lumbosacral segments (19). These data suggest that the corticospinal tracts have a greater control and influence over the upper extremities than over the lower. The corticospinal tracts are essential for skill and precision in movement and also for the execution of precise movements of the fingers. Interestingly, although the tracts are necessary for speed and agility during precise movements, they are not necessary for the initiation of voluntary movement. They also serve to regulate sensory relay processes and to determine which sensory modality reaches the cerebral cortex, as evidenced by terminations on sensory neurons in the spinal cord. The proper function of the corticospinal tracts is dependent on the extent of their myelination. Myelination of corticospinal fibers begins after birth and is not completed until the end of the first year of life.

Neurons in the cerebral cortex and their axons that form the corticospinal tracts have been referred to as *upper motor neurons.* The alpha motoneurons in the spinal cord ventral horns and their axons that directly innervate skeletal muscle are referred to as *lower motor neurons.* Lesion of the lateral corticospinal tract in the spinal cord lateral funiculus results in an upper motor neuron syndrome, which includes spasticity, hyperactive deep tendon reflexes, Babinski sign, clonus, and a loss or diminution of superficial reflexes, such as the abdominal or cremasteric reflex. In the acute phase of an SCI involving bilateral lesion of the lateral corticospinal tracts, a patient undergoes "spinal shock," in which there is a complete shutdown of neuronal activity in the spinal cord below the level of the injury. The signs of spinal shock include flaccid paralysis of muscles, hypotonia, and the absence of myotatic, bowel, and bladder reflexes. Depending on the level of injury, there may also be bradycardia and significant lowering of blood pressure. Following a variable period (days to weeks) the patient recovers from spinal shock and the upper motor neuron syndrome becomes apparent. The mechanisms underlying the induction and recovery from spinal shock are unknown. Lower motor neuron lesions result in signs similar to those of a patient in spinal shock. In lower motor neuron paralysis there is a loss of all movement, both reflex and voluntary, as well as a loss of muscle tone and subsequent atrophy of the affected muscles. Unlike the transient deficits associated with spinal shock, lower motor neuron deficits are permanent, assuming that there is no reinnervation of the denervated structures.

The signs associated with an upper motor neuron syndrome are not always indicative of injury or disease of the spinal cord. In older individuals, there is a tendency for the superficial abdominal reflexes to be absent; this occurs more often in females than in males (20). Although the Babinski sign is commonly associated with injury to the corticospinal system, it can also be elicited in the newborn infant, a sleeping or intoxicated adult, or following a generalized seizure. Interestingly, the Babinski sign may be absent in some patients with a known lesion of the corticospinal tract (21).

Rubrospinal Tract

The neurons that give rise to the axons of the rubrospinal tract are located in the posterior two-thirds of the red nucleus in the midbrain. The axons of the tract cross in the ventral tegmental decussation and descend to spinal levels, where the tract forms in the lateral funiculus mostly anterior to (partially overlapping) the lateral corticospinal tract (Figure 1.12). The fibers of the rubrospinal tract terminate in the same areas of the spinal gray matter as the lateral corticospinal tract and function to facilitate flexor motor neuron activity. Because the red nucleus receives an input from the cortex (corticorubral) and because of the similar terminations of both tracts in the spinal cord, the rubrospinal tract is thought to be functionally related to the lateral corticospinal tract.

Although the rubrospinal tract extends the length of the spinal cord in most mammals, it extends only to the thoracic segments in man (22), is thinly myelinated, and is thought to be rudimentary. Any effect of injury to the rubrospinal tract in patients will likely be masked by the severe motor deficits resulting from injury to the adjacent lateral corticospinal tract.

Lateral Vestibulospinal Tract

The neurons that give rise to this tract are found in the lateral vestibular nucleus located at the junction between the medulla and pons. The axons of the lateral vestibular nucleus descend uncrossed through the medulla and form the lateral vestibulospinal tract in the anterior aspect of the lateral funiculus along the entire length of the spinal cord (Figure 1.12). Fibers of the tract terminate mostly on interneurons in the spinal cord, but there are some direct terminations on alpha motor neuron dendrites.

The primary function of the lateral vestibulospinal tract is to facilitate extensor muscle tone to maintain an upright posture. With eyes closed and feet close together, a normal individual sways slightly from side to side. Balance is maintained because, for example, as the individual sways to the right, impulses from the right semicircular canals of the inner ear activate neurons in the ipsilateral lateral vestibular nucleus. These neurons, in turn, send impulses along the right vestibulospinal tract to extensor muscles, which correct for the sway and move the body back to the midline center of gravity. When the individual sways to the left, the left lateral vestibulospinal tract is activated. Similarly, if a walking individual stumbles, reflex extension of one of the lower extremities may prevent a fall, but if a fall is imminent, extension of the upper limbs often prevents severe injury to the face and head. Under these circumstances, the reflex extension of the limbs is also mediated by the lateral vestibulospinal tracts. If the eighth cranial nerve (vestibulocochlear), lateral vestibular nucleus, or the semicircular canals are injured on one side, a patient will often fall to that side or veer to the side of the injury while walking. The effects of injury to the lateral vestibulospinal tract in the spinal cord, however, are generally masked by the more severe deficits in motor capability that result from concomitant injury to the lateral corticospinal tract.

Medial Vestibulospinal Tract

The neurons that give rise to the medial vestibulospinal tract are located in the medial vestibular nucleus of the medulla. The fibers of these neurons descend through the medulla bilaterally in a composite bundle of several different fiber systems known as the *medial longitudinal fasciculus* (MLF). The MLF containing the medial vestibulospinal tract is located in the posterior aspect of the anterior funiculus of the cervical spinal cord (Figure 1.12). Fibers of the medial vestibulospinal tract terminate on interneurons in the spinal gray matter and play a role in the labyrinthine regulation of head positions.

Reticulospinal Tracts

The neurons that give rise to the reticulospinal tracts are located in the central core of the brainstem known as the *reticular formation,* at the level of the pons and medulla. Because of the different origins and locations of these tracts in the spinal cord, they are often referred to separately as the pontine and medullary reticulospinal tracts. The pontine reticulospinal tract is mostly ipsilateral and descends in the medial part of the anterior funiculus along the entire length of the spinal cord (Figure 1.12). The fibers terminate on interneurons. The medullary reticulospinal tract is also primarily ipsilateral and descends the length of the spinal cord in the anterior part of the lateral funiculus (Figure 1.12). The fibers of this pathway terminate on interneurons in close association with the termination of the fibers of the pontine reticulospinal tract, the rubrospinal tract, and the corticospinal tracts.

Animal studies have shown that stimulation of the brainstem reticular formation can facilitate or inhibit voluntary movement, cortically induced movement, and reflex activity; influence muscle tone; affect inspiratory phases of respiration; exert pressor or depressor effects on the circulatory system; and exert inhibitory effects on sensory transmission (23). Those areas of the medullary reticular formation giving rise to the medullary reticulospinal tract correspond closely with the regions from which inspiratory, inhibitory, and depressor effects are obtained (24–26). The areas of the reticular formation related to facilitatory effects, expiration, and pressor vasomotor responses are rostral to the medulla and extend beyond the regions that give rise to reticulospinal fibers (27). Thus, the reticulospinal tracts may not be the mediators of some facilitatory effects originating from neurons in the upper brainstem reticular formation.

Descending Autonomic Pathways

Fibers belonging to this important descending system originate primarily from the hypothalamus. Although there is evidence of direct projections from the hypothalamus to the spinal cord (28), polysynaptic routes also pass through various regions of the reticular formation before reaching the spinal cord. The descending autonomic pathways are located predominantly in the lateral funiculi and terminate on the preganglionic sympathetic and parasympathetic neurons located in the intermediate gray matter of T1–L2 and S2–S4, respectively.

Lesion of the descending autonomic pathways in spinal cord injury often leads to significant autonomic disturbances. If injury occurs at or above the T1 level, Horner syndrome results from injury to the sympathetic component of the descending autonomic pathways. The signs of this syndrome are seen predominantly in the eye ipsilateral to injury and consist of miosis caused by paralysis of the pupillary dilator muscle and slight ptosis caused by paralysis of the smooth muscle (tarsal plate) of the upper eyelid. In addition to the signs in the eye, the patient may have anhidrosis of the face because of the interruption of the sympathetic innervation of the sweat glands of the face ipsilateral to the spinal cord injury (29).

When the descending autonomic pathways innervating preganglionic parasympathetic neurons are lesioned bilaterally at any level of the spinal cord rostral to S2, the result is impotence and a loss of normal bowel and bladder function. However, after recovery from spinal shock, spontaneous or reflex erection of the penis (or clitoris) may occur and bowel and bladder reflexes may also return. This is in marked contrast to the deficits associated with the conus medullaris and cauda equina syndromes explained earlier in this chapter. In these latter cases, because the preganglionic parasympathetic neurons at S2–S4 are destroyed or their axons are severed, this usually results in a permanently areflexic bowel and bladder and the absence of spontaneous or reflex erections.

In contrast to erection, ejaculation is controlled by preganglionic sympathetic neurons located at the L1 and L2 levels of the spinal cord. During ejaculation, the seminal fluid from the seminal vesicles and prostate, as well as sperm from each epididymis, flows into the prostatic urethra and is ejected from the penis by rhythmic contractions of the smooth muscle associated with these structures. Thus, erection is controlled by parasympathetics and ejaculation is mediated by sympathetic neurons. During ejaculation, discharge of the semen into the bladder is prevented by the contraction of the sphincter vesicae, which is innervated by preganglionic sympathetics located at L1 and L2. When there is bilateral destruction of the descending autonomic pathways in SCI, there is not only a loss of erection, but also a loss of ejaculation. If the SCI is above lumbar levels, reflex ejaculation may be possible in some patients after recovery from spinal shock. Some patients may have a normal ejaculation, but without external emission because of the paralysis of the sphincter vesicae.

BLOOD SUPPLY OF THE SPINAL CORD

The spinal cord is supplied by three longitudinally oriented branches of the vertebral arteries and multiple *radicular arteries* that arise from various segmental vessels. The longitudinally oriented arteries are the *anterior spinal artery* and a pair of *posterior spinal arteries*.

Anterior Spinal Artery

On the anterior surface of the medulla, two branches from the vertebral arteries unite in the midline to form a single anterior spinal artery that descends the length of the spinal cord in the anterior median fissure (Figure 1.13). The *sulcal arteries* arising from the anterior spinal artery enter the spinal cord through the anterior median fissure. Successive sulcal arteries generally alternate in their distribution to the left and right side of the spinal cord, but occasionally a single sulcal artery will distribute to both sides (Figure 1.14). The sulcal arteries supply the anterior two-thirds of the spinal cord at any cross-sectional level. This is a clinically important feature of the anatomy of the spinal cord, because occlusion of the anterior spinal artery or its sulcal branches could result in *anterior cord (spinal artery) syndrome* (Figure 1.15). As in most vascular problems, the onset of signs and symptoms is rapid. Figure 1.15 shows the zone of distribution of the anterior spinal artery in the cross-hatched area. The posterior funiculus and horns are spared because these areas are supplied by the posterior spinal arteries. Initially, there is flaccid paralysis of the muscles in the body below the level of infarct because of spinal shock. In time, however, spastic paralysis and other upper motor neuron signs develop because of bilateral destruction of the corticospinal tracts. A variable degree of bowel and bladder dysfunction exists because of the interruption of the descending autonomic pathways. Initially, however, incontinence may be due to spinal shock. A cardinal sign of anterior cord syndrome is a dissociated sensory loss characterized by a loss of pain and temperature sensations (bilateral lateral spinothalamic tract lesion) with preservation of kinesthesia and discriminative touch sensations (sparing of posterior funiculi) in the body below the level of injury. Some patients develop painful dysesthesias about 6 to 8 months after the onset of neurologic symptoms. The source of this pain is unknown, but has been suggested to be attributed to the activation of previously latent pathways that mediate pain sensation. The anterior spinal artery is dependent on segmental contributions from anterior radicular arteries along the length of the spinal cord (Figure 1.13).

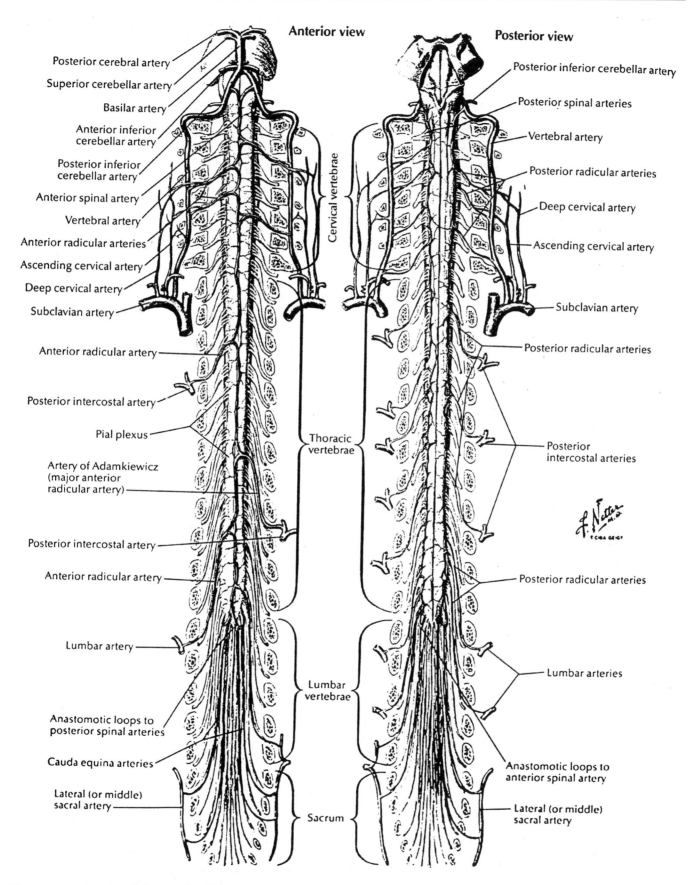

Figure 1.13 Arteries of the spinal cord.

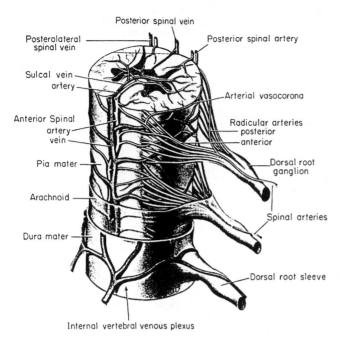

Figure 1.14 Arterial supply and venous drainage of the spinal cord.

Posterior Spinal Arteries

The paired posterior spinal arteries derived from the vertebral arteries descend on the posterior surface of the spinal cord just medial to the posterior roots (Figure 1.13). The arteries receive variable contributions from the posterior radicular arteries. At points along the cord, the posterior spinal arteries become so small that they appear to be discontinuous. The arteries supply blood to the posterior one-third of the spinal cord. The peripheral portions of the lateral funiculi are supplied by the *arterial vasocorona*, which is formed by an anastomosis between the anterior and posterior spinal arteries (Figure 1.14).

Radicular Arteries

The segmental vessels that pass through the intervertebral foramina divide into posterior and anterior radicular arteries, which follow the posterior and anterior roots respectively (Figure 1.14). At variable levels the radicular arteries continue coursing medially until they anastomose with either the anterior or posterior spinal arteries. The anterior radicular arteries contribute to the anterior spinal artery, and the posterior radicular arteries contribute to the posterior spinal arteries. In the lumbar region, one anterior radicular artery is quite large and is known as the *artery of Adamkiewicz* (Figure 1.13). This artery is usually found on the left, and it enters the vertebral canal by following an anterior root at either a low thoracic or upper lumbar level before anastomosing with the anterior spinal artery. The artery of Adamkiewicz reinforces the circulation to two-thirds of the spinal cord, including the lumbosacral enlargement. Occlusion of this artery may seriously compromise spinal cord circulation, which could lead to infarct and paraplegia.

The greatest distance between radicular arteries that contributes significantly to the anterior and posterior spinal arteries is found at the thoracic level of the spinal cord. At this level, occlusion of just one radicular artery could lead to significant infarct of spinal tissue. The T1–T4 levels of the thoracic cord are particularly vulnerable to infarct following occlusion of a radicular artery. Spinal cord segment L1 is another vulnerable region.

Collateral Circulation of the Spinal Cord

Severe trauma to the vertebral column on the left at the thoracic level can fracture the bodies of one or more vertebrae. A surgeon must often mobilize the descending aorta to the right to expose the fractured vertebral bodies, remove the bony fragments, and stabilize the spine. The aorta is mobilized by first tying off several posterior intercostal arteries close to their origin from the aorta, severing the arteries in this region, and then moving the aorta to the right (Figure 1.16). The upper thoracic spinal cord is particularly vulnerable to infarct if blood flow into the cord from an important segmental vessel is interrupted. The above surgical

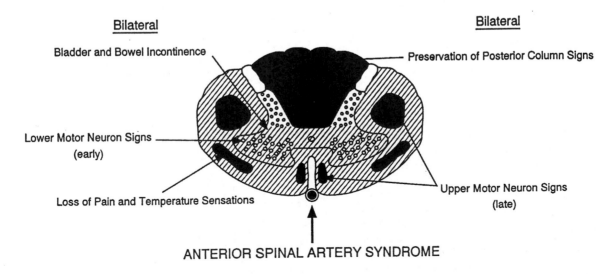

Figure 1.15 Diagram showing the extent of the lesion in anterior cord (spinal artery) syndrome and associated neurologic signs.

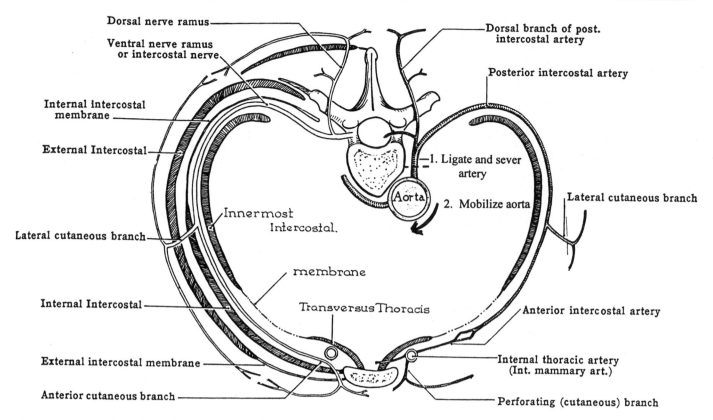

Figure 1.16 Collateral circulation of the spinal cord. When posterior intercostals are tied off surgically, blood flows to the spinal cord via internal thoracic and lateral thoracic (not shown) artery anastomoses with posterior intercostal arteries.

procedure, however, does not interrupt the flow of blood through the intervertebral foramen and thus to the spinal cord, because of collateral circulation. This collateral circulation results from the anastomosis of the internal thoracic artery (a branch of the subclavian artery) with the posterior intercostal artery. As soon as blood flow from the aorta is interrupted, blood begins retrograde flow from the internal thoracic artery through the posterior intercostal artery and into the spinal cord (Figure 1.16). Although this is not shown in the figure, Hollinshead and Rosse (30) have suggested that the lateral thoracic artery (a branch of the axillary artery) also has anastomoses with the posterior intercostals and thus provides a second source of blood flow to the spinal cord under these conditions.

Veins of the Spinal Cord

In general, the distribution pattern of the veins of the spinal cord is similar to that of the spinal arteries (Figure 1.17). Three longitudinally oriented posterior spinal veins and three anterior spinal veins communicate freely with each other and are drained by anterior and posterior radicular veins, which join the *internal vertebral (epidural) venous plexus* lying in the epidural space (Figure 1.17). This plexus of veins passes superiorly within the vertebral canal through the foramen magnum to communicate with the dural sinuses and veins within the skull (Figure 1.17). The internal vertebral venous plexus also communicates with the *external* vertebral venous plexus on the external surface of the vertebrae.

There are no valves in the spinous venous network. Thus, blood flowing in these vessels could pass directly into the systemic venous system. For instance, when intra-abdominal pressure is increased, blood from the pelvic venous plexus passes superiorly via the internal vertebral plexus. When the jugular veins are obstructed, blood leaves the skull by this same plexus. Because the prostatic plexus is continuous with the vertebral venous system, neoplasms originating in the prostate gland may metastasize and lodge in the vertebrae, spinal cord, brain, or skull (31).

References

1. Altman J, Bayer SA. Development of the human spinal cord. an interpretation based on experimental studies in animals. New York: Oxford University Press, 2001; 346.
2. Altman J, Bayer SA. Development of the human spinal cord. an interpretation based on experimental studies in animals. New York: Oxford University Press, 2001, Chapter 9, 458–503.
3. Sadler TW. Langman's medical embryology. 10th ed. Philadelphia: Lippincott Williams and Wilkins, 2006, 294.
4. Sadler TW. Langman's medical embryology. 10th ed. Philadelphia: Lippincott Williams and Wilkins, 2006, 295.
5. Maynard FM Jr (Chair). International standards for neurological and functional classification of spinal cord injury. Rev. 1996. Chicago: American Spinal Injury Association, 1996.
6. Brodal A. Neurological anatomy in relation to clinical medicine. 3rd ed. New York: Oxford University Press, 1981, 778–780.
7. Moore KL, Dalley AF. Clinically oriented anatomy. 4th ed. Philadelphia: Lippincott Williams and Wilkins, 1999, 477.
8. Rexed B, Brodal A. The nucleus cervicalis lateralis: a spinocerebellar relay nucleus. *J Neurophysiol* 1951; 14:399–407.

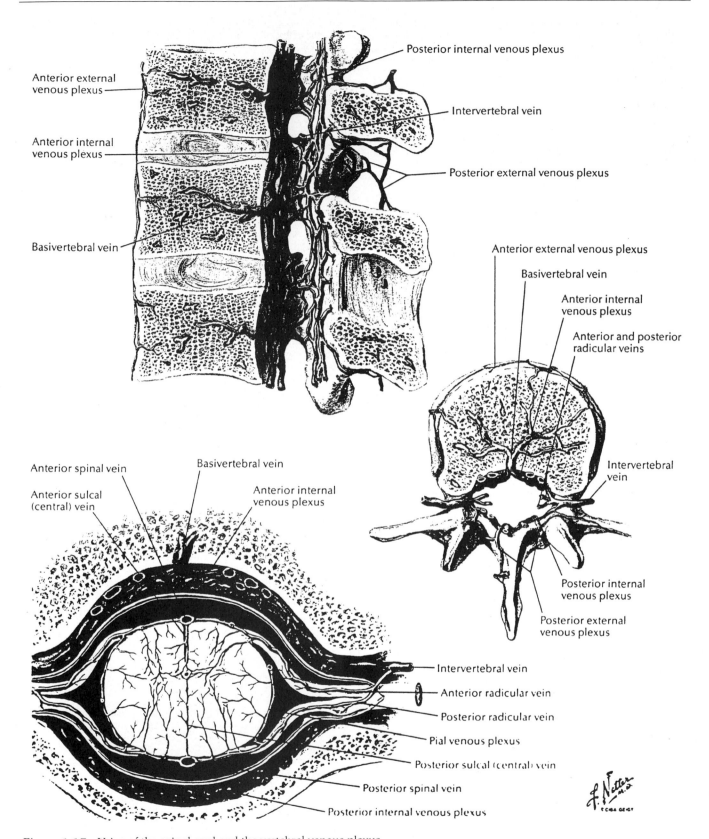

Anterior external venous plexus

Anterior internal venous plexus

Basivertebral vein

Posterior internal venous plexus

Intervertebral vein

Posterior external venous plexus

Anterior external venous plexus

Basivertebral vein

Anterior internal venous plexus

Anterior and posterior radicular veins

Intervertebral vein

Posterior internal venous plexus

Posterior external venous plexus

Anterior spinal vein

Anterior sulcal (central) vein

Basivertebral vein

Anterior internal venous plexus

Intervertebral vein

Anterior radicular vein

Posterior radicular vein

Pial venous plexus

Posterior sulcal (central) vein

Posterior spinal vein

Posterior internal venous plexus

Figure 1.17   Veins of the spinal cord and the vertebral venous plexus.

9. Craig AD Jr, Burton H. The lateral cervical nucleus in the cat: anatomical organization of cervicothalamic neurons. *J Comp Neurol* 1979; 185:329–346.

10. Craig AD Jr. Spinal and medullary input to the lateral cervical nucleus. *J Comp Neurol* 1978; 181:729–743.

11. Afifi AK, Bergman RA. *Functional Neuroanatomy. Text and Atlas.* New York: McGraw-Hill, Health Professions Division, 1998; 76–77.

12. Carpenter MB, Sutin J. *Human Neuroanatomy,* 8th Edition. Baltimore: Williams and Wilkins, 1983; 271–273.

13. Afifi AK, Bergman RA. *Functional Neuroanatomy. Text and Atlas.* New York: McGraw-Hill, Health Professions Divisions, 1998; 78.

14. Afifi AK, Bergman RA. *Functional Neuroanatomy. Text and Atlas.* New York: McGraw-Hill, Health Professions Divisions, 1998; 80–81.

15. Carpenter MB, Sutin J. *Human Neuroanatomy,* 8th Edition. Baltimore: Williams and Wilkins, 1983; 276–282.

16. Coulter JD, Ewing L, Carter C. Origin of primary sensorimotor cortical projections to lumbar spinal cord of cat and monkey. *Brain Res* 1976; 103:366–372.

17. Jones EG, Wise SP. Size, laminar and columnar distribution of efferent cells in the sensory-motor cortex of monkeys. *J Comp Neurol* 1977; 175:391–438.

18. Verhaart WJC, Kramer W. The uncrossed pyramidal tract. *Acta Psychiat Neurol Scand* 1952; 27:181–200.

19. Weil A, Lasser A. A quantitative distribution of the pyramidal tract in man. *Arch Neurol Psychiatry* 1929; 22:495–510.

20. Madonick MJ. Statistical control studies in neurology. VII: The cutaneous abdominal reflex. *Neurology (Minneap)* 1957; 7:459–465.

21. Nathan PW, Smith MC. Long descending tracts in man. I: Review of present knowledge. *Brain* 1955; 78:248–303.

22. Stern K. Note on the nucleus ruber magnocellularis and its efferent pathway in man. *Brain* 1938; 61:284–289.

23. Carpenter MB, Sutin J. *Human Neuroanatomy,* 8th Edition. Baltimore: Williams and Wilkins, 1983; 297.

24. Amoroso EC, Bell FR, Rosenberg H. The relationship of the vasomotor and respiratory regions of the medulla oblongata of the sheep. *J Physiol (Lond)* 1954; 126:86–95.

25. Pitts RF. The respiratory center and its descending pathways. *J Comp Neurol* 1940; 72:605–625.

26. Torvik A, Brodal A. The origin of reticulospinal fibers in the cat: an experimental study. *Anat Rec* 1957; 128:113–137.

27. Brodal A. *The Reticular Formation of the Brain Stem. Anatomical Aspects and Functional Correlations.* Springfield IL: Charles C. Thomas, 1957.

28. Saper CB, Loewry AD, Swanson LW, Cowan WM. Direct hypothalamo-autonomic connections. *Brain Res* 1976; 117:305–312.

29. Brodal A. *Neurological Anatomy in Relation to Clinical Medicine*, 3rd Edition. New York: Oxford University Press, 1981; 763.

30. Hollinshead WH, Rosse C. *Textbook of Anatomy,* 4th Edition. Philadelphia: Harper and Row, 1985; 182.

31. Batson OV. The function of the vertebral veins and their role in the spread of metastases. *Ann Surg* 1940; 112:138–149.

2 Spinal Cord Pathology

Ronald C. Kim

This chapter is structured to provide an overview of the morphologic findings in those disorders that physicians engaged in the practice of spinal cord medicine are most likely to encounter. It is written with an emphasis on clinicopathologic correlation and in such a manner as to provide the practitioner, where possible, with an insight into pathogenetic mechanisms.

SPINAL VASCULAR DISEASE

Spinal Arterial Infarction

Although all of the arterial blood supply to the spinal cord is ultimately derived from the aorta, it is provided by only seven to eight radiculomedullary branches (1). Because the cervical and upper two to three thoracic spinal segments are relatively richly supplied, arterial infarction in this region rarely occurs. The middle thoracic (T4–T8) region, however, is typically dependent on a single radicular artery that usually enters the spinal canal near the vertebral body of T7, and the thoracolumbar region is largely dependent on a single major artery, the artery of Adamkiewicz, which enters, usually on the left side, with the tenth, eleventh, or twelfth thoracic nerve root or, less often, the first or second lumbar nerve root. For this reason, the spinal cord from T5 downward is particularly susceptible to arterial insufficiency.

The radiculomedullary arteries, upon entry into the spinal canal, ramify over the surface of the spinal cord to form a perimedullary arterial network that coalesces into a single anterior and two posterior spinal arteries that send centripetally directed branches into the underlying white matter. The internal portion of the spinal cord is supplied by sulcal arteries coursing through the anterior median fissure and sending branches directed centrifugally, predominantly into gray matter. Because of the relatively rich anastomotic arterial network supplying the white matter, in contrast to the end-arterial supply of the gray matter, severe systemic circulatory impairment tends to produce damage mainly to the gray matter (2).

Arterial infarction of the spinal cord develops most commonly as a consequence of factors arising outside of the spinal canal (e.g., profound systemic circulatory impairment [shock or cardiac arrest] or surgical cross-clamping or disease of the aorta or its major branches). Under these circumstances the most common pattern of damage is one that is limited largely to the gray matter from upper to mid-thoracic levels downward (Figure 2.1), presumably because of the protective effect of the perimedullary anastomotic network exerted on the spinal white matter (3). Clinically, there will be persistent flaccid paraplegia (because of sparing of the corticospinal tracts) and loss of pain and temperature perception (because of interruption of the lateral spinothalamic pathways), with relative sparing of posterior column (proprioceptive) function.

Operative interruption of a major intercostal arterial feeder (such as ligation of the artery of Adamkiewicz during rib resection in preparation for thoracotomy for aortic surgery) will result in non-cavitary ischemic atrophy of the ventral portion

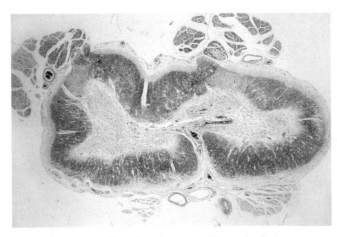

Figure 2.1 Spinal cord at S5 in a subject who became paraplegic after an episode of cardiac arrest and who died 9 weeks later. Tissue necrosis is limited almost exclusively to the gray matter.

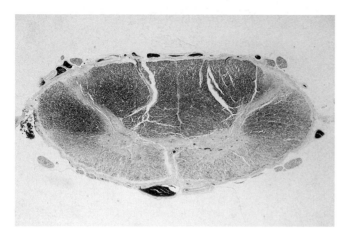

Figure 2.2 Ischemic atrophy of the ventral spinal cord at T12 in a man who had become paraplegic 4½ years earlier following resection of the left ninth and tenth ribs for repair of a thoracoabdominal aortic aneurysm.

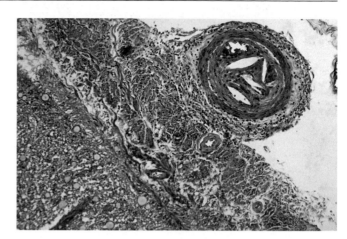

Figure 2.4 Atheromatous embolism to a dorsolateral spinal arterial branch, from the same patient described in Figure 2.3.

of the spinal cord (Figure 2.2) (4). In this situation lower extremity weakness is usually of upper motor neuron type (i.e., with spasticity) because of damage to the lateral corticospinal tracts.

Spinal Vascular Embolic Disease

Occlusion of the anterior spinal artery (ASA) with resultant cavitary infarction in its territory of supply is relatively uncommon but, when it occurs, is usually the result of atheromatous or fibrocartilaginous embolism (2). Atheromatous emboli (Figures 2.3 and 2.4) tend to appear in relatively elderly subjects with severe atherosclerotic vascular disease, and may affect smaller intramedullary arterial branches with resultant small infarcts, in which case the clinical manifestations may vary, depending upon their size and location. Fibrocartilaginous embolism (Figures 2.5 and 2.6), which may be observed on either the arterial or the

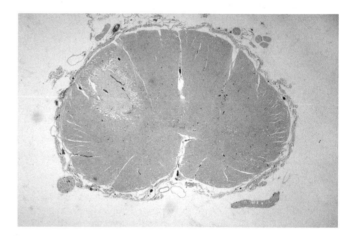

Figure 2.5 Coagulative necrosis within the lateral corticospinal tract following fibrocartilaginous embolism to the spinal circulation.

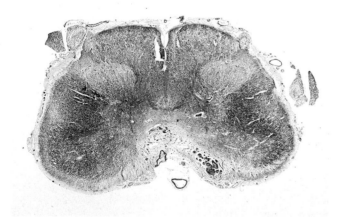

Figure 2.3 Cavitary necrosis of the tissue adjoining the anterior median fissure at spinal L4 in a man who developed sudden paraplegia following atheromatous embolism to the anterior spinal artery at spinal T10.

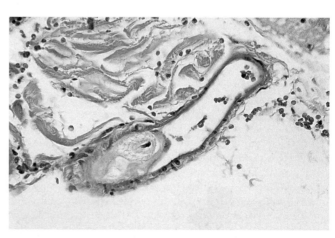

Figure 2.6 Same patient as in Figure 2.5, showing fibrocartilage embolus within a spinal vein.

venous side of the spinal circulation, tends to occur in either young adulthood or late middle life. A sizable proportion of affected subjects have a history of minor traumatic injury or of heavy lifting. It has been suggested that axial stress, such as that which is associated with heavy lifting, may result in herniation of fibrocartilaginous disc material into the bone marrow (Schmorl's nodes) and hence into the venous (and, if pressure is high enough, into the arterial) circulation (5). As is the case with atheromatous embolism, the neurologic manifestations will vary according to the size and location of the ischemic lesions produced.

Another form of spinal vascular embolism is that associated with decompression, either from ascending too quickly after a deep dive or from loss of aircraft cabin pressure. Approximately half of those afflicted have a patent foramen ovale (6). For reasons not well understood, when neurologic manifestations appear, spinal cord signs and symptoms tend to predominate, particularly those referable to the cervicothoracic region. In those subjects who have been examined postmortem, there are multiple small infarcts within the spinal gray and white matter. The pathogenesis of these lesions is poorly understood, but one group of observers noted, in an experimental model of decompression, the presence of gas bubbles within the spinal epidural veins (7).

Spinal Venous Infarction

Spinal venous thromboembolic occlusion is distinctly uncommon and tends to occur in hypercoagulable states. Epidural, leptomeningeal, or intraparenchymal veins may be affected. Venous infarction of the spinal cord may be either hemorrhagic or non-hemorrhagic. Hemorrhagic infarction is characterized by sudden onset with back pain, rapid progression, and short survival, whereas non-hemorrhagic infarction is more insidious and protracted, without back pain, and with relatively longer survival (8).

Spinal Vascular Malformations

Arteriovenous malformations, which presumably are of vascular embryological origin, may involve either a portion of or the entire cross-sectional extent of the spinal cord. They typically become manifest acutely (due to hemorrhage) in young adults. Pathologically, the parenchyma of the spinal cord is replaced by a network of abnormal, heavily collagenized vessels of greatly varying mural thickness that cannot be identified as either arterial or venous in nature.

Arteriovenous fistulas (AVFs) are acquired lesions that typically become manifest in middle life as slowly progressive lower extremity weakness. The fistulous communication is most frequently seen embedded within the dura ensheathing a nerve root in the thoracolumbar region, although myelopathy may occasionally be associated with fistulas at other sites, such as the pelvic or retroperitoneal region or within the cranial cavity. Pathologically, the walls of leptomeningal veins and of the spinal intraparenchymal venocapillary network are greatly thickened, an indication of venous hypertension and impairment of venous drainage of the spinal cord. This results in a venocongestive myelopathy, in which the cross-sectional area of the spinal cord may be reduced to one-half or less of its normal size (Figure 2.7).

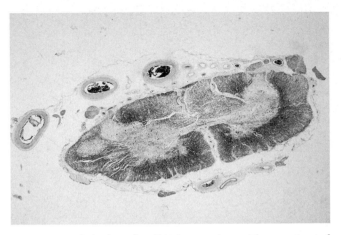

Figure 2.7 Spinal cord at T12 in a patient with an untreated dural AVF, showing ischemic atrophy and marked thickening of the walls of spinal leptomeningeal veins.

The pathological picture is identical to that described by Foix and Alajouanine under the heading of "subacute necrotic myelitis," and it is generally accepted that the so-called Foix-Alajouanine syndrome represents nothing more than the myelopathy associated with a spinal dural AVF (2).

TRAUMATIC INJURY TO THE SPINAL CORD

Patterns of Injury

The varied clinical expressions of traumatic spinal cord injury reflect the distribution and mechanism of damage (2). The anterior spinal cord syndrome (Figure 2.8) is typically the result of hyperflexion injury and is characterized by spastic weakness and loss of pain and temperature perception with relative preservation of posterior column (proprioceptive) sensation. The central spinal cord syndrome (Figure 2.9) is ordinarily a consequence of hyperextension injury (e.g., a diving accident) and is characterized by spastic weakness, loss of pain and temperature perception, and a variable loss of posterior column sensation. The

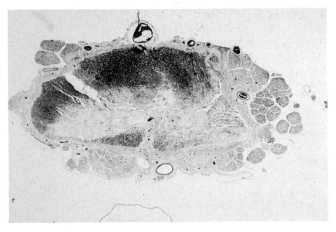

Figure 2.8 Ventrally predominant damage to the spinal cord at L2 in a subject who had become paraplegic following a hyperflexion injury in a motor vehicle accident 44 years earlier.

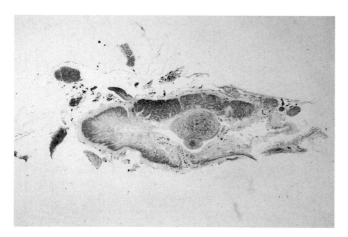

Figure 2.9 Centrally predominant damage to the spinal cord at C7 in a man who had become quadriplegic following a diving injury 27 years earlier. Note the large traumatic neuroma.

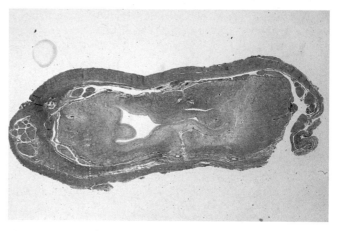

Figure 2.10 Delayed traumatic syringomyelia within the spinal cord at C8 in a man who developed C5 quadriplegia after chiropractic manipulation–associated vertebral osteomyelitis. Note the adhesive arachnoidopathy, characterized by proliferation of collagen within the subarachnoid compartment.

Brown-Séquard syndrome usually results from a stab wound and is characterized by ipsilateral motor weakness, contralateral loss of pain and temperature perception, and ipsilateral loss of posterior column sensation. The complete spinal cord syndrome results from crush injury or transection and is characterized by spastic weakness and by complete sensory loss below the level of the lesion.

Lesions developing directly as a result of the primary injury (e.g., laceration or crush) are typically segmental and hemorrhagic. Damage developing secondarily can be subdivided into early and delayed complications. Within 8 to 24 hours the white matter and the ascending and descending long spinal tracts contained therein show massive edema and diminished vascular perfusion. Other factors that contribute to the spread of tissue damage include the release of excitotoxic neurotransmitters, calcium and potassium ion shifts, generation of oxygen free radicals, and activation of the arachidonic acid cascade (2).

Weeks, months, or years after the injury, a number of additional morphologic alterations may appear. *Traumatic neuroma formation* (Figure 2.9) may be massive at the primary site of injury and is presumed to represent sprouting from dorsal spinal afferents. Visible evidence of *wallerian degeneration* of ascending tracts above and of descending tracts below the level of the lesion does not appear until approximately 6 to 8 weeks have elapsed. *Chronic adhesive arachnoidopathy* is an invariable consequence of traumatic spinal cord injury.

The most dramatic late consequence of traumatic injury with tethering of the spinal cord is *delayed traumatic syringomyelia,* in which, usually after several years have elapsed, one or more cavities appear within the spinal cord above or below (without necessarily being directly contiguous with) the injury site (9). Episodic elevation of venous back-pressure, such as that which may occur during Valsalva maneuvers or while coughing, sneezing, or straining at stool, may cause upward or downward extension of these cavities within an immobile spinal cord. This may in turn cause progression of the neurologic deficit; in extreme circumstances, for example, a paraplegic can, with upward extension of a syringomyelic cavity, become quadriplegic with a rising sensory level within a matter of hours, a situation

that calls for immediate surgical intervention. Pathologically, the cavity, which is typically asymmetrical and sometimes multiple, contains no epithelial lining and is bordered by a zone of gliosis (Figure 2.10).

MYELOPATHY DUE TO VERTEBRAL COLUMN DISEASE

Cervical Spondylosis

The most important vertebral column disease leading to structural damage to the spinal cord is cervical spondylosis. With advancing age the intervertebral discs lose water and elasticity, especially where spine mobility is greatest (i.e., at the C5-C6 and C6-C7 interspaces), and adjoining vertebral bodies may come into direct contact with each other, leading to the formation of bone spurs or osteophytes. When these bone spurs form along the posterior margins of the vertebral bodies, they may project into the spinal canal, thereby narrowing it. Narrowing of the spinal canal in this manner will not necessarily lead to symptomatic neurologic dysfunction in and of itself, but it may increase an individual's vulnerability to spinal cord damage when there is a superimposed stressful event, such as hyperextension of the neck after a rear-end motor vehicle collision.

The pattern of spinal cord damage that develops will vary according to the location of the bone spurs. For example, if they are laterally placed, they may encroach upon the neural foramina, resulting in a radiculopathy. A typical pattern of damage that is seen relatively commonly is associated with a posteriorly directed bone spur that is situated near the midline. In this situation, the spinal cord, as seen in transverse section, assumes an ovoid shape with a "butterfly" distribution of damage that affects both lateral corticospinal tracts (with resultant spastic lower extremity weakness and Babinski signs), the lateral spinal gray matter, and the ventral portions of the posterior columns (Figure 2.11) (2). The mechanism by which this pattern of damage develops is unclear, but there is imaging evidence to

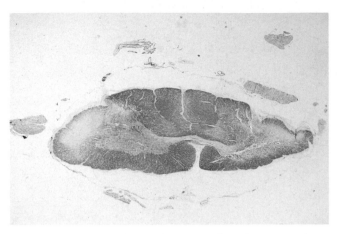

Figure 2.11 Cervical spondylotic myelopathy at spinal C5, showing pallor of myelin staining within the lateral and, to a lesser degree, the dorsal white matter. Note the ovoid contour of the spinal cord.

suggest that buckling of the ligamenta flava during hyperextension results in axonal disruption (10).

Rheumatoid Disease

Myelopathy may develop in subjects with rheumatoid disease, either as a result of direct involvement of the spinal cord or its coverings by the disease process (i.e., in the form of vasculitis or of rheumatoid nodule formation), or, more commonly, as a result of disease of the cervical spine (11). Vertebral column disease is typically the result of subluxation, most frequently atlantoaxial but sometimes subaxial. Atlantoaxial subluxation may occur either in a forward or in an upward direction; in the former circumstance the spinal cord may be pushed against the anterior wall of the spinal canal, resulting in a triangular spinal cord contour as seen in transverse sections, with a central pattern of damage (Figure 2.12).

DEGENERATIVE AND DEMYELINATIVE SPINAL CORD DISEASE

Friedreich's Ataxia

Friedreich's ataxia is the most common form of autosomal recessive ataxia. It is due to a mutation of a gene on chromosome 9q13 that leads to markedly reduced expression of a protein (frataxin) that appears to participate in the regulation of mitochondrial iron efflux (12, 13). In the vast majority of instances, there is a GAA trinucleotide repeat expansion.

The onset of illness usually occurs before the age of 20. The cardinal clinical manifestations are progressive ataxia of gait, pes cavus, kyphoscoliosis, hammer toes, areflexia, impaired proprioception, and hypertrophic or congestive cardiomyopathy with interstitial myocarditis and granular iron deposits.

The major neuropathologic findings are in the spinal cord (14). There is degeneration of the entire peripheral proprioceptive pathway, with loss of posterior column fibers, shrinkage of dorsal spinal nerve roots, loss of dorsal root ganglion cells, and loss of large myelinated fibers within peripheral nerves that is best seen in purely sensory nerves such as the sural nerve. Severe nerve cell loss is observed within the nucleus dorsalis of Clarke, with associated loss of nerve fibers from the dorsal spinocerebellar tract. Nerve fibers are also lost from the ventral spinocerebellar tracts and from the lateral and ventral corticospinal tracts (Figure 2.13). The cerebellum usually shows severe nerve cell loss within the dentate nuclei, with degeneration of their efferent fibers coursing through the superior cerebellar peduncles.

Hereditary Spastic Paraplegia

The hereditary spastic paraplegias (HSPs) are a clinically and genetically heterogeneous group of disorders characterized predominantly by progressive spastic weakness of the lower extremities. Several dozen different genetic loci have been identified. Most often the disorder is transmitted in autosomal dominant fashion, but autosomal or X-linked recessive forms have also

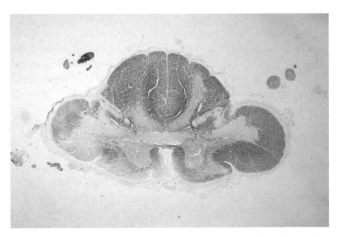

Figure 2.12 Spinal cord at C1 in a man with rheumatoid disease who became quadriplegic after C1/C2 vertebral subluxation, showing flattening of the ventral surface and damage within both gray and white matter.

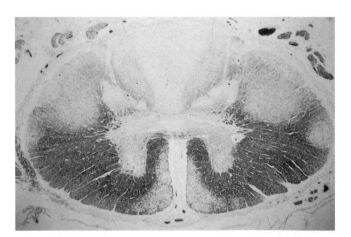

Figure 2.13 Upper thoracic spinal cord in a patient with Friedreich's ataxia, showing systematized loss of myelinated axons within the posterior columns, lateral and ventral corticospinal tracts, and dorsal and ventral spinocerebellar tracts.

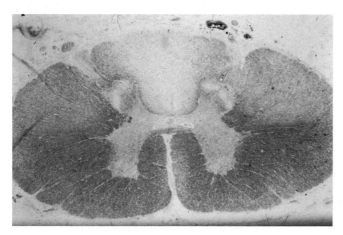

Figure 2.14 "Pure" hereditary spastic paraplegia, showing loss of myelinated axons within the posterior columns and lateral corticospinal tracts.

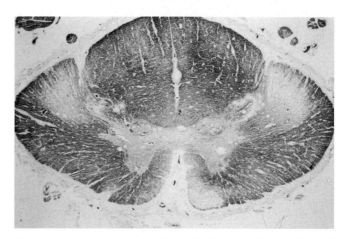

Figure 2.15 Amyotrophic lateral sclerosis, showing loss of myelinated axons within the lateral and (on one side) ventral corticospinal tracts. Loss of spinal anterior horn cells (not pictured) was also present.

been described. Mutations in the spastin gene (SPG4, encoded on chromosome 2p22) and in the atlastin gene (SPG3A, encoded on chromosome 14q12–q21) account for more than half of the autosomal dominant forms of HSP. The onset of illness may occur at any age, depending on the mutation. Pure phenotypes are characterized by spastic lower extremity weakness alone, whereas complex phenotypes are associated with other abnormalities, such as ataxia, dementia, seizures, visual dysfunction, or systemic manifestations (15, 16).

Pathologically, pure HSP is characterized by distally predominant loss of myelinated axons with the lateral corticospinal tracts and, sometimes, the posterior columns (Figure 2.14).

Amyotrophic Lateral Sclerosis

Amyotrophic lateral sclerosis (ALS) is often included, together with progressive muscular atrophy (PMA) and progressive bulbar palsy (PBP), under the broader heading of motor neuron disease (MND), and is characterized by degeneration of motor neurons within motor cortex, brain stem, and spinal cord. This is manifested clinically by the development, usually in older adult life, of progressive weakness that leads, within 2 to 5 years, to death from respiratory failure. Dementia of frontotemporal type is seen in about 5% of cases (17).

A small proportion (5%–10%) are familial (usually autosomal dominant), and of these, approximately 20% are associated with mutations of the gene encoding copper/zinc superoxide dismutase (SOD1) (17). Although classical sporadic ALS typically begins in the limbs and is characterized, at some time during the course of illness, by both upper motor neuron (UMN) and lower motor neuron (LMN) signs, PMA, which initially appears to be restricted to LMNs, and PBP, which seems at first to be limited to the brain stem, both usually progress to UMN involvement, a finding that is reflected in the distribution of CNS changes seen at autopsy.

Pathologically, LMN disease is characterized by nerve cell loss and astrocytosis within the spinal anterior horns and brain stem motor (especially the hypoglossal) nuclei, with striking atrophy of motor nerve roots, and UMN disease is characterized by dying-back degeneration of nerve fibers within the lateral and

ventral corticospinal tracts (Figure 2.15) (18, 19). With advanced disease the motor cortex may also be affected. Although sensory fibers are not ordinarily affected, in those subjects who have been maintained for long periods of time (5 years or more) on assisted ventilation, damage may be observed at sites that are typically spared, such as the lateral and ventral columns of the spinal cord and the third, fourth, and sixth cranial nerve nuclei and the nucleus of Onufrowicz in the sacral spinal cord (20). Cystatin C-immunoreactive Bunina bodies, small hyaline inclusions, and ubiquitin-immunoreactive skein-like inclusions may be observed within the cytoplasm of surviving spinal and brain stem motor neurons and are highly specific for ALS (17). Neurofilament-rich axonal spheroids may be seen within the most proximal axonal segments in the active stages of the disease. The familial forms of ALS show similar pathological features, although some may show either posterior column involvement or only minimal corticospinal tract involvement. Skeletal muscle that is deprived of its innervation will show denervation atrophy.

Primary Lateral Sclerosis

There is considerable debate as to whether or not primary lateral sclerosis is an entity that is separate and distinct from other forms of MND. Those who argue that it is describe a sporadic motor disorder that is dominated clinically by UMN dysfunction with little or no evidence of LMN involvement (i.e., spastic weakness with no fasciculations). Survival may be considerably longer than for classical ALS, often for 10 years or more. A few undergo progression into ALS. Pathologically, although damage to the corticospinal tracts is striking, the presence, on occasion, of some degree of loss of spinal anterior horn cells, together with the finding of ubiquitinated cytoplasmic inclusions, suggests that the disorder is a variant of ALS (21).

Spinal Muscular Atrophy

Spinal muscular atrophy (SMA) is a heterogeneous group of autosomal recessive disorders due to homozygous deletions in the survival motor neuron (SMN1) gene on chromosome 5q13

(21, 22). All are characterized clinically by LMN weakness, areflexia, fasciculations, absence of sensory signs, and EMG evidence of denervation. The classical infantile type (type I SMA or Werdnig-Hoffmann disease) is lethal and results in death at age 3 to 18 months. The chronic infantile type (type II SMA) is more slowly progressive and may be associated with survival into adulthood. Patients with the chronic childhood type (type III SMA or Kugelberg-Welander disease) progress very slowly and may have near-normal life expectancies.

Pathologically, in the severe infantile form, there is profound nerve cell loss and astrocytosis within the spinal anterior horns and brain stem motor nuclei, with atrophy of motor nerve roots. Skeletal muscle shows denervation atrophy.

Multiple Sclerosis

The vast majority of patients with multiple sclerosis will show clinical and pathological evidence of spinal cord involvement, usually in association with manifestations indicative of disease at other sites. In a sizable proportion, spinal cord dysfunction, in the form of spastic ataxia, spastic paraparesis, or impaired proprioception or vibratory sensation, may predominate.

As is the case elsewhere in the CNS, the characteristic pathologic finding is the presence of sharply circumscribed foci of demyelination with relative sparing of axons (23). These lesions may be visible on inspection of the surface of the spinal cord and may be associated with gross atrophy. As seen in transverse section, their boundaries bear no relation to gray–white matter interfaces or to fiber pathways (Figure 2.16). Active plaques are typically associated with perivascular "cuffs" of lymphocytes and plasma cells, axonal swellings, and lipid-laden macrophages. If several lesions are present, they may be in different histological stages of evolution. Within old plaques the concentration of oligodendrocytes is sharply reduced. "Shadow plaques" are those in which the staining density of the myelin is only partially reduced, and they represent remyelination with formation of short, thin myelin internodes. Foci of demyelination near nerve root entry zones may undergo remyelination by Schwann cells,

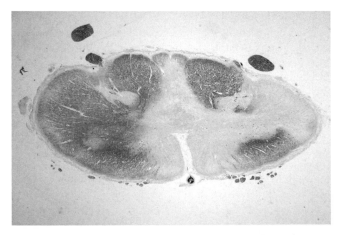

Figure 2.16 Sharply circumscribed plaques of demyelination within the spinal cord at C6 in a quadriplegic with long-standing multiple sclerosis. Note the presence of demyclination with both gray and white matter.

in which case the myelin that is formed is of peripheral rather than central type.

Neuromyelitis Optica

Neuromyelitis optica (NMO) is a relapsing, polyphasic inflammatory demyelinating disorder that appears to be separate and distinct from multiple sclerosis. The vast majority (90%) of affected subjects are women, and the median age of onset is toward the end of the fourth decade. The optic neuritis and myelitis may occur either sequentially or simultaneously, and over half of patients develop permanent visual or ambulatory impairment within 5 years of onset (24). A highly specific serum autoantibody (NMO-IgG) has been identified that binds to the water channel protein aquaporin 4, which appears to play a major role in water homeostasis within the CNS.

The histopathologic substrate of NMO is a necrotizing optic neuritis and longitudinally extensive myelitis in which an admixture of demyelination and cavitating necrosis, an inflammatory infiltrate containing many neutrophils and eosinophils, and vasocentrically distributed immune complex deposition are typically observed (25, 26). NMO also appears to occur in association with certain other autoimmune disorders, notably systemic lupus erythematosus and Sjögren's syndrome.

TOXIC/METABOLIC MYELOPATHIES

Postangiography Myelopathy

Postangiography myelopathy is an uncommon event and is typically encountered following aortography or, less frequently, vertebral angiography. It is a consequence of inadvertent administration of contrast material directly into the spinal circulation through radiculomedullary feeding arteries. Clinical manifestations (paraplegia or quadriplegia) appear within hours. Pathologically, there is centrally predominant necrosis that damages most of the gray matter (2). The arterial supply and venous drainage are intact. Margolis and his colleagues reproduced the myelopathy by injecting sodium acetrizoate (Urokon) into the aortas of dogs and concluded, on the basis of this work, that damage was the result of toxicity rather than ischemia (27).

Myelopathy after Intrathecal Injections

Myelopathy may follow the intrathecal administration of a wide variety of agents, including spinal anesthetics, alcohols, hypertonic saline, steroids, methylene blue, chemotherapeutic agents, ammonium sulfate, or magnesium sulfate. Pathologically, the pattern of damage is typically one of circumferentially distributed loss of myelinated axons (Figure 2.17) (2). Later there may be fibrous thickening of the leptomeninges. Bunge and his colleagues showed experimentally that simple CSF barbotage (i.e., slow, repeated withdrawal and reinjection of minute quantities of CSF without administering any exogenous material) could result in circumferential demyelination (28).

Chronic Adhesive Arachnoidopathy

Fibrous thickening of the leptomeninges may result from a wide variety of causes, including the intrathecal administration of any

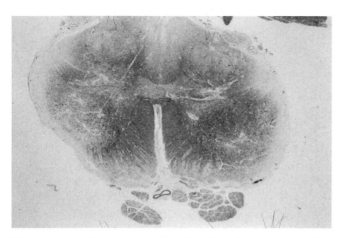

Figure 2.17 Circumferential pallor of myelin staining within the spinal cord at L4, following intrathecal administration of hypertonic saline for pain relief.

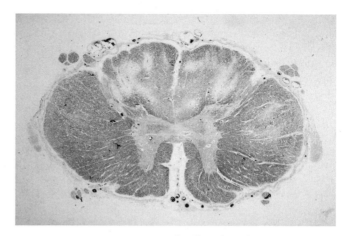

Figure 2.18 Non-systematized pallor of myelin staining within the dorsal and lateral white matter at spinal T8, in a patient with severe vitamin B12 deficiency.

one of a number of agents (particularly contrast media), tuberculous or pyogenic bacterial meningitis, traumatic injury or surgical intervention, and hemorrhage into the spinal subarachnoid compartment. In a sizable proportion of patients, the etiology is unclear. Depending on the mode of development, the pathologic findings may range from mild leptomeningeal opacification to dense collagenization within the subarachnoid compartment, with entrapment of nerve roots and blood vessels and adherence to the overlying dura (Figure 2.10) (2).

Vitamin B12 Deficiency Myeloneuropathy

The absorption within the distal ileum of vitamin B12 (cobalamin), which must be supplied by ingestion of meat and dairy products, requires binding to Castle's intrinsic factor, which is elaborated by gastric parietal cells. Vitamin B12 deficiency may therefore be induced in a variety of circumstances, including autoimmune gastritis, gastric or distal ileal surgery, Crohn's disease, tropical sprue, fish tapeworm infestation, dietary insufficiency (e.g., in vegeterians), or inborn errors of cobalamin metabolism. Neurologically symptomatic patients may not be anemic, although bone marrow examination will reveal the presence of megaloblasts. As the disease progresses over a period of weeks or months, gait ataxia, impaired proprioception and vibratory sensation, loss of deep tendon reflexes, and spasticity will develop, as will an unexplained psychosis.

Pathologically, the disease typically begins at mid-thoracic levels with small foci of ballooning degeneration of myelin sheaths within the central portions of the posterior columns and the peripheral portions of the lateral columns; these foci eventually coalesce to form large areas of myelin destruction (Figure 2.18) and secondary axonal damage, with permeation by macrophages and reactive astrocytosis (29). Although the terms "subacute combined degeneration" and "combined systems degeneration" are used to denote the pattern of damage, the destruction is *non-systematized* and does not affect entire tracts in the manner that Friedreich's ataxia or ALS do. Electron microscopy of experimentally induced vitamin B12 deficiency myelopathy in rhesus monkeys has shown that separation of myelin lamellae progresses sequentially to the formation of

intramyelinic vacuoles, degeneration of myelin sheaths, and degeneration of axons (30). Peripheral neuropathy appears in the majority of affected subjects, as evidenced by reduced nerve conduction velocity, and has been associated with both demyelination and axonal degeneration.

Chronic exposure to nitrous oxide (NO) may produce a similar clinical and pathologic picture. NO appears to inactivate methionine synthetase, a vitamin B12–dependent enzyme (31).

INFECTIONS WITHIN THE SPINAL CANAL

Spinal Epidural Abscess

Spinal epidural abscess formation typically develops in the presence of one or more predisposing factors, such as diabetes mellitus, chronic alcohol abuse, HIV infection, a prior operative procedure, placement of a stimulator or a catheter, or sepsis. It occurs more frequently posteriorly than anteriorly and in the thoracolumbar than in the cervical region. *Staphylococcus aureus* is the etiologic agent in at least two-thirds of cases (32). Clinically, the classical clinical triad consists of back pain, fever, and neurologic deficit (weakness), although not all components are always present. MRI is currently the most sensitive method of detection. Hematogenous dissemination, seen in approximately half of the affected subjects, typically results in an exudate in which neutrophils predominate, whereas contiguous spread from an adjoining focus of infection (such as vertebral osteomyelitis), which accounts for another third of those affected, often results in a mixed inflammatory response that contains an abundance of lymphocytes and plasma cells. The mechanism by which the spinal cord is damaged is unclear. Although Feldenzer and colleagues (1988), in their experimental animal model, found evidence of direct compression (33), studies at autopsy have shown the presence, on occasion, of thrombosis of small leptomeningeal arteries and veins (32).

Spinal Subdural Abscess

Spinal subdural abscess formation is considerably less common. Most of these lesions occur at cervical or thoracic levels and, as is the case with epidural infections, *Staphylococcus aureus* is the most commonly isolated agent (34). Although in most instances infection is believed to be the result of hematogenous dissemination, a primary focus at another site is often not found. Again, the mechanism of damage to the spinal cord is debated (i.e., compression vs. vasculitis).

Spinal Intramedullary Abscess

Intramedullary abscess formation is also distinctly uncommon. Such abscesses are usually solitary but may occur multiply. Most have been described at mid- to low thoracic levels. Over half appear to have resulted from hematogenous dissemination, and about 20% develop contiguously from an adjoining site of infection, such as vertebral osteomyelitis (35). *Staphylococcus aureus* is the most commonly isolated organism. The presence of a capsule and the predominating inflammatory cell type (lymphoplasmacytic or neutrophilic) will depend on whether the infection is chronic or acute.

Suppurative Spinal Leptomeningitis

Spinal subarachnoid suppuration accompanies that seen intracranially. Following upon large-scale immunization against type b *Hemophilus influenzae*, bacterial meningitis is now predominantly a disease of adults (36). In the post-neonatal period *Streptococcus pneumoniae* accounts for approximately one-half and *Neisseria meningitidis* for one-quarter to one-third of cases (37, 38).

Pathologically, the exudate tends to localize by gravity along the dorsal surface of the lower thoracic spinal cord (Figure 2.19). It consists mainly of neutrophils for the first few days, after which time lymphocytes and fibrin appear. After a week microglial cells within the underlying parenchyma begin to proliferate. If the exudate extends into the underlying neural parenchyma, the result is a meningomyelitis. Healing is characterized by fibroblastic organization of the exudates. Local complications may include occlusive vasculitis, abscess formation, or adhesive arachnoidopathy.

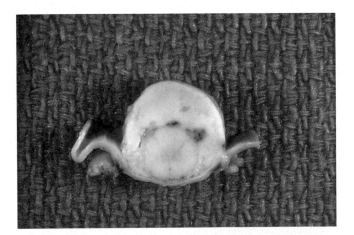

Figure 2.19 Acute suppurative leptomeningitis due to *Hemophilus influenzae* in a 14-month-old child. The exudate is confined within the subarachnoid compartment and is heavier along the dorsal surface.

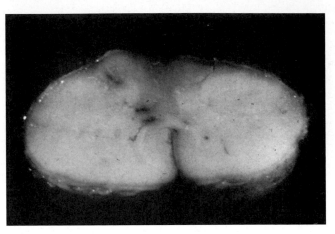

Figure 2.20 Tabes dorsalis within the cervical spinal cord, showing darkening within the posterior columns due to loss of myelinated axons.

Other Bacterial Infections

Tuberculosis of the spine may lead to vertebral body collapse, usually in the thoracic or lumbar region. Chronic epidural abscess formation may also occur. Tuberculous spinal meningitis is virtually always associated with concomitant intracranial infection.

Tabes dorsalis represents the classical spinal form of neurosyphilis and is rarely seen today. The lumbosacral region is most frequently affected. Pathologically, there is degeneration of the dorsal root ganglia, dorsal spinal roots, and posterior columns (Figure 2.20), without evidence of infiltration by inflammatory cells or stainable microorganisms. The pathogenesis of this condition is not understood.

Viral Infections of the Spinal Cord

Many viral agents are capable of producing myelitis. Only a few will be described here.

Poliovirus is a single-stranded RNA enterovirus that, on the rare occasion when symptomatic CNS involvement occurs, tends to damage spinal anterior horn cells and other motor neurons, presumably because they bear relatively large numbers of viral surface receptors. Histologically, in the active phase of the disease, the affected areas show the presence of many pleomorphic microglia with evidence of neuronophagia. At later stages there is striking focal tissue pallor (Figure 2.21) with nerve cell loss and astrocytosis and shrinkage of the ventral spinal roots.

West Nile virus, a culex mosquito-borne member of the flavivirus phylogenetic group, is harbored in birds but is capable of infecting many animals. Symptomatic CNS involvement is uncommon but, when it develops, is seen in widespread distribution. Pathologically, it is characterized by the presence of neuronal necrosis and neuronophagia, microglial nodule formation, and perivascular cuffing by mononuclear inflammatory cells. A small subset of patients will develop a poliomyelitis-like syndrome characterized by flaccid paralysis; in such cases, spinal anterior horn pathology is strikingly similar to that observed with poliovirus infection (39).

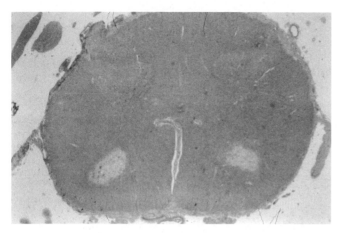

Figure 2.21 Focal tissue pallor within the spinal anterior horns of a patient who had suffered paralysis after having suffered acute anterior poliomyelitis 27 years earlier.

After *varicella-zoster virus* infection, the agent is typically stored within spinal dorsal root ganglia. In subjects who have been immunosuppressed (particularly those with AIDS), recrudescence of infection typically results in the appearance of a dermatomal eruption. Pathologically, the dorsal root ganglion at that level shows the presence of a ganglioradiculitis, sometimes with Cowdry type A intranuclear inclusion body formation. On rare occasion this may lead to the development of a granulomatous vasculitis or a focal necrotizing myelopathy.

HIV-infected individuals may develop a symptomatic myelopathy (*vacuolar myelopathy of AIDS*) that is characterized clinically by spastic paraparesis, impairment of proprioception, and posterior column ataxia, and pathologically by non-systematized vacuolar degeneration, particularly within the dorsal and lateral funiculi (Figure 2.22), that closely

resembles that associated with vitamin B12–deficiency myelopathy (40).

Other viral agents that may be associated with myelitis, such as herpes simplex virus types 1 and 2, cytomegalovirus, and human T-cell leukemia virus type I, typically produce necrotizing lesions.

NEOPLASMS WITHIN THE SPINAL CANAL

Although virtually any neoplasm that occurs within the cranial cavity can be seen within the spinal canal, the most common spinal neoplasms are nerve sheath tumors, meningiomas, ependymomas, astrocytomas, and secondary (metastatic) tumors (41, 42, 43).

Nerve sheath tumors are of two types, schwannomas and neurofibromas. Schwannomas, which account for roughly 30% of primary spinal neoplasms, are benign and tend to occur at and below lumbar regions. When multiple, they should raise the suspicion that NF-2 may be present. These sharply circumscribed extra-axial neoplasms, two-thirds of which are extradural, are usually situated within dorsal spinal nerve roots (Figure 2.23). They are composed of spindle-shaped cells

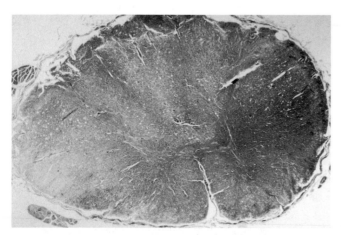

Figure 2.22 AIDS-associated vacuolar myelopathy, showing non-systematized microcystic rarefaction within the dorsal and lateral white matter. The pattern of damage closely resembles that of vitamin B12–deficiency myelopathy.

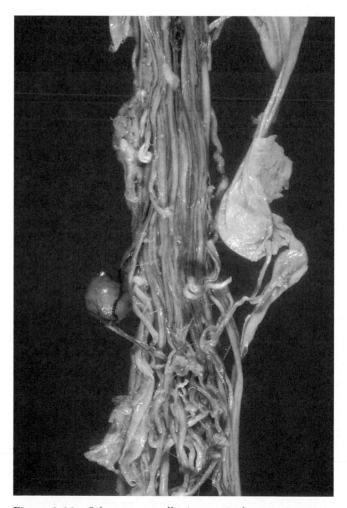

Figure 2.23 Schwannoma affecting a spinal nerve root.

arranged in interlacing fascicles, and typically show both compact (Antoni A) and loose-meshed (Antoni B) areas with nuclear palisading and Verocay body formation, nuclear atypia, vascular hyalinization, and immunoreactivity for S-100 protein.

Neurofibromas, which are also of Schwann cell origin, account for about 25% of primary spinal neoplasms. These benign tumors are typically encountered within the intradural portions of dorsal spinal nerve roots. They are usually solitary and, when seen multiply, should raise the suspicion that the patient may be suffering from NF-1. Pathologically, these fusiform lesions tend to separate rather than displace nerve fibers. Typically they are composed of spindle-shaped or stellate cells in a loose connective tissue matrix and, like schwannomas, show immunoreactivity for S-100 protein.

Meningiomas, which account for approximately 25% of primary spinal neoplasms, are benign intradural lesions that are most commonly observed at thoracic levels (Figure 2.24). Roughly 80% of affected subjects are women. When meningiomas occur multiply, the possibility of NF-2 should be considered. Pathologically, these tumors, which are of arachnoidal cell origin, are composed

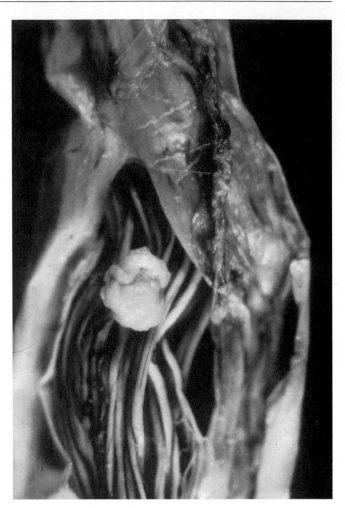

Figure 2.25   Filum terminale ependymoma.

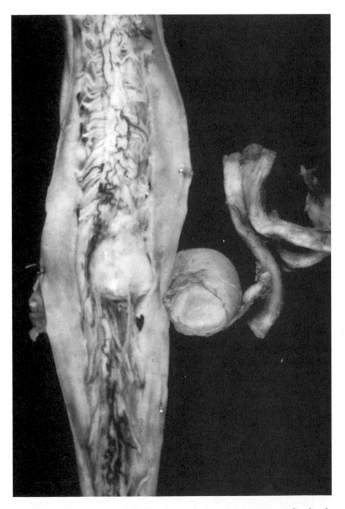

Figure 2.24 "Dumbbell" spinal meningioma with both extradural and intradural components.

of uniform, process-bearing cells with abundant cytoplasm and round to oval vesicular nuclei, with a tendency toward whorling and psammoma body formation.

Ependymomas are low-grade glial neoplasms that are observed most frequently within the cauda equina and the lumbosacral region. The most common site of origin is the filum terminale (Figure 2.25), presumably because of the presence there of residual nests of cells left by the embryonic ventriculus terminalis. Ependymomas are well-circumscribed lesions composed of process-bearing cells with uniform vesicular nuclei, a tendency toward perivascular pseudorosette formation, and, occasionally, the presence of ependymal rosettes. Most of the neoplasms arising in the cauda equina are of myxopapillary type and are characterized by the presence of tumor cells arranged around blood vessels that are separated by a mucopolysaccharide-rich stroma.

Some 80% to 85% of spinal *astrocytomas* arise in the cervical or thoracic regions. These infiltrative neoplasms are typically associated with fusiform enlargement of the spinal cord and are composed of stellate or spindle-shaped, process-bearing cells with rounded or oval vesicular nuclei that show immunoreactivity for glial fibrillary acidic protein. Higher-grade neoplasms

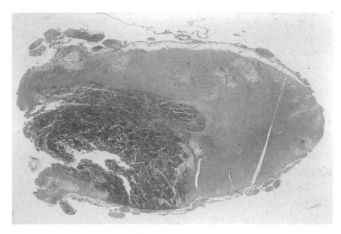

Figure 2.26 Spinal intramedullary metastasis of small cell carcinoma of the lung.

show a greater degree of nuclear pleomorphism, with a higher proliferation index, evidence of vascular hyperplasia, and tumor necrosis.

Metastases produce symptomatic spinal cord dysfunction usually following involvement of the vertebral column, especially in the thoracic region. Rarely, metastasis may develop within the spinal leptomeninges or within the spinal cord parenchyma (Figure 2.26). Lung and breast are the most common primary sites.

In most cases of spinal cord "compression" due to metastatic extradural disease, the spinal cord, when examined pathologically, typically does not show deformity of the type that might be expected on the basis of direct compression. Rather, there are wedge-shaped foci of perivenous microcystic rarefaction, often with hemorrhagic extravasation (Figure 2.27). This finding, coupled with experimental evidence, suggests that spinal cord damage associated with vertebral/epidural metastatic disease is attributable largely to epidural venous obstruction (44).

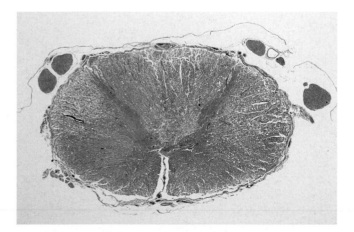

Figure 2.27 Ischemic perivenous microcystic rarefaction at spinal T7, particularly dorsally and laterally, owing to epidural venous obstruction by metastatic prostatic adenocarcinoma.

References

1. Lazorthes G. Pathology, classification and clinical aspects of vascular diseases of the spinal cord. In: Vinken PJ, Bruyn GW, eds. *Handbook of Clinical Neurology,* Vol. 12. Amsterdam: North Holland Publishing Company, 1972:492–506.
2. Kim RC. Pathology of non-neoplastic, regional disorders of the spinal cord. In Nelson JS, Mena H, Parisi JE, Schochet SS Jr, eds. *Principles and Practice of Neuropathology.* 2nd ed. New York: Oxford University Press, 2003:459–496.
3. Kim SW, Kim RC, Choi BH, Gordon SK. Non-traumatic ischaemic myelopathy: a review of 25 cases. *Paraplegia* 1988; 26:262–272.
4. Hughes JT, MacIntyre AG. Spinal cord infarction occurring during thoracolumbar sympathectomy. *J Neurol Neurosurg Psychiatry* 1963; 26:118–121.
5. Tosi L, Rigoli G, Beltramello A. Fibrocartilaginous embolism of the spinal cord: a clinical and pathogenetic reconsideration. *J Neurol Neurosurg Psychiatry* 1996; 60:55–60.
6. Wilmshurst PT, Byrne JC, Webb-Peploe MM. Relation between interatrial shunts and decompression sickness in divers. *Lancet* 1989; 2:1302–1306.
7. Hallenbeck JM, Bove AA, Elliott DH. Mechanisms underlying spinal cord damage in decompression sickness. *Neurology* 1975; 308–316.
8. Kim RC, Smith HR, Henbest ML, Choi BH. Non-hemorrhagic venous infarction of the spinal cord. *Ann Neurol* 1984; 156: 379–385.
9. Barnett HJM, Jousse AT, Ball MJ. Pathology and pathogenesis of progressive cystic myelopathy as a late sequel to spinal cord injury. In: Barnett HJM, Foster JB, Hudgson P, eds. *Syringomyelia*. Philadelphia: WB Saunders, 1973:179–219.
10. Quencer RM, Bunge RP, Egnor M, Green BA, et al. Acute traumatic central cord syndrome: MRI-pathological correlations. *Neuroradiology* 1992; 34:85–94.
11. Kim RC, Collins GH. The neuropathology of rheumatoid disease. *Hum Pathol* 1981; 12:5–15.
12. Koeppen AH. The hereditary ataxias. *J Neuropathol Exp Neurol* 1998; 57:531–543.
13. Albin RL. Dominant ataxias and Friedreich ataxia: an update. *Curr Opin Neurol* 2003; 16:507–514.
14. Lamarche JB, Lemieux, Lieu HB. The neuropathology of "typical" Friedreich's ataxia in Quebec. *Can J Neurol Sci* 1984; 11:592–600.
15. McDermott CJ, Shaw PJ. Hereditary spastic paraparesis. In: Eisen AA, Shaw PJ, eds. *Handbook of Clinical Neurology,* Vol. 12. Amsterdam: Elsevier, 2007:329–352.
16. Depienne C, Stevanin G, Brice A, Durr A. Hereditary spastic paraplegias: an update. *Curr Opin Neurol* 2007; 20:674–680.
17. Kato S, Shaw P, Wood-Allum C, Leigh PN, Shaw C. Amyotrophic lateral sclerosis. In: Dickson D, ed. *Neurodegeneration: The Molecular Pathology of Dementia and Movement Disorders.* Basel: ISN Neuropath Press, 2003:350–368.
18. Hays AP. The pathology of amyotrophic lateral sclerosis. In: Mitsumoto H, Przedborski S, Gordon PH, eds. *Amyotrophic Lateral Sclerosis.* New York: Taylor & Francis, 2006:43–80.
19. Kim RC, Sung JH. Motor system degenerations. In: Duckett S, ed. *Pathology of the Aging Human Nervous System.* Philadelphia: Lea & Febiger, 1991:159–171.
20. Bergmann M, Völpel M, Kuchelmeister K. Onuf's nucleus is frequently involved in motor neuron disease/amyotrophic lateral sclerosis. *J Neurol Sci* 1995; 129:141–146.
21. Swash M. Primary lateral sclerosis. In: Dickson D, ed. *Neurodegeneration: The Molecular Pathology of Dementia and Movement Disorders.* Basel: ISN Neuropath Press, 2003: 369–371.
22. Harding B. Spinal muscular atrophy. In: Dickson D, ed. *Neurodegeneration: The Molecular Pathology of Dementia and Movement Disorders.* Basel: ISN Neuropath Press, 2003:372–375.
23. Prineas JW, McDonald WI, Franklin RJM. Demyelinating diseases. In: Graham DI, Lantos PL, eds. *Greenfield's Neuropathology.* 7th ed. London: Arnold, 2002:471–550.
24. Wingerchuk DM, Lennon VA, Lucchinetti CF, Pittock SJ, Weinshenker BG. The spectrum of neuromyelitis optica. *Lancet Neurol* 2007; 6:805–815.
25. Mandler RN, Davis LE, Jeffery DR, Kornfeld M. Devic's neuromyelitis optica: a clinicopathological study of 8 patients. *Ann Neurol* 1993; 34:162–168.

26. Lucchinetti CF, Mandler RN, McGavern D, Bruck W, et al. A role for humoral mechanisms in the pathogenesis of Devic's neuromyelitis optica. *Brain* 2002; 125:1450–1461.

27. Margolis G, Tarazi AK, Grimson KS. Contrast medium injury to the spinal cord produced by aortography: pathologic anatomy of the experimental lesions. *J Neurosurg* 1956; 8:349–365.

28. Bunge RP, Bunge MB, Ris H. Electron microscopic study of demyelination in an experimentally induced lesion in adult cat spinal cord. *J Biophys Biochem Cytol* 1960; 7:685–696.

29. Pant SS, Asbury AK, Richardson EP Jr. The myelopathy of pernicious anemia: a neuropathological reappraisal. *Acta Neurol Scand* 1968; 44(Suppl 35):1–36.

30. Agamanolis DP, Victor V, Harris HW, Hines JD, et al. An ultrastructural study of subacute combined degeneration of the spinal cord in vitamin B12–deficient rhesus monkeys. *J Neuropathol Exp Neurol* 1978; 37:273–299.

31. Layzer RB. Myeloneuropathy after prolonged exposure to nitrous oxide. *Lancet* 1978; 2:1227–1230.

32. Darouiche RO. Spinal epidural abscess. *New Engl J Med* 2006; 355:2012–2020.

33. Feldenzer JA, McKeever PE, Schaberg DR, Campbell JA, Hoff JT. Experimental spinal epidural abscess: a pathophysiological model in the rabbit. *Neurosurgery* 1987; 20:859–867.

34. Levy ML, Wieder BH, Schneider J, Zee CS, Weiss MH. Subdural empyema of the cervical spine: clinicopathological correlates and magnetic resonance imaging; report of three cases. *J Neurosurg* 1993; 79:929–935.

35. Menezes AH, Graf CJ, Perret GE. Spinal cord abscess: a review. *Surg Neurol* 1977; 8:461–467.

36. Schuchat A, Robinson K, Wenger JD, Harrison LH, et al. Bacterial meningitis in the United States in 1995. *New Engl J Med* 1997; 337:970–976.

37. Swartz MN. Bacterial meningitis—a view of the past 90 years. *New Engl J Med* 2004; 351:1826–1828.

38. Van de Beek D, de Gans J, Spanjaard L, Weisfelt M, et al. Clinical features and prognostic factors in adults with bacterial meningitis. *New Engl J Med* 2004; 351:1849–1859.

39. Fratkin JD, Leis AA, Stokic DS, Slavinski SA, Geiss RW. Spinal cord neuropathology in human West Nile virus infection. *Arch Pathol Lab Med* 2004; 128:533–537.

40. Petito CK, Navia BA, Cho E-S, Jordan BD, et al. Vacuolar myelopathy pathologically resembling subacute combined degeneration in patients with the acquired immunodeficiency syndrome. *New Engl J Med* 1985; 312:874–879.

41. Slooff JL, Kernohan JW, MacCarty CS. *Primary Intramedullary Tumors of the Spinal Cord and Filum Terminale.* Philadelphia: WB Saunders, 1964.

42. Coons SW. Pathology of tumors of the spinal cord, spine, and paraspinous soft tissue. In: Dickman CA, Fehlings MG, Gokasian ZL, eds. *Spinal Cord and Spinal Column Tumors: Principles and Practice.* Stuttgart: Thieme, 2006:41–110.

43. Byrne TN, Waxman SG. *Spinal Cord Compression: Diagnosis and Principles of Management.* Philadelphia: FA Davis Company, 1990.

44. Arguello F, Baggs RB, Duerst RE, Johnstone L, et al. Pathogenesis of vertebral metastasis and epidural spinal cord compression. *Cancer* 1990; 65:98–106.

3 Imaging of the Spinal Cord

Roland R. Lee
Blaine L. Hart

Imaging—in vivo visualization—of the spine and spinal cord is extremely important in the evaluation of patients with spinal cord pathology. This chapter discusses the techniques used to image the spine and spinal cord, concentrating on magnetic resonance imaging (MRI). The contribution of imaging to the diagnosis of major categories of spinal cord pathology is then discussed and illustrated.

SPINAL IMAGING TECHNIQUES

For over a century, plain X-rays had been the imaging modality used to image the spine. The spinal vertebrae and their alignment are well evaluated, and the technique is simple and inexpensive, but the spinal cord proper cannot be visualized on X-rays.

Myelography, imaging of the spine by X-rays after introduction of contrast material into the thecal sac, for the first time enabled visualization of the silhouette of the spinal cord within contrast-enhanced cerebrospinal fluid (CSF), allowing diagnosis of epidural, intradural-extramedullary, and intramedullary lesions. The contrast between bone, spinal cord, and CSF is exquisite, but the procedure is invasive.

Computed tomography (CT) gives good cross-sectional depiction of primarily the bony anatomy and the paraspinal soft tissues. However, the spinal cord itself, and the spinal nerve roots, are not well distinguished from the surrounding intrathecal CSF. CT performed after myelography, however, does give excellent visualization of the spinal cord and nerve roots. However, it again relies on the instillation of nonionic contrast into the spinal canal. Also, images can only be obtained in the axial plane, although computer reconstructions in the sagittal and coronal planes may be obtained and may be of good quality if the axial slices are thin (3 mm or thinner). The wide availability of multislice, high-resolution CT scanning now makes possible high-quality reconstruction of images in sagittal, coronal, and oblique planes, and markedly decreases imaging time. This can be especially helpful in imaging traumatic injuries.

Spinal angiography is the best way to image the arteries and veins of the spine and spinal cord, with good depiction of vascular malformations and tumor vascularity. The diagnostic angiogram is a prerequisite en route to endovascular treatment of these lesions. However, spinal angiography is invasive and technically difficult; thus, its use is generally limited to diagnosis and treatment of spinal vascular malformations, and less commonly, vascular tumors.

Ultrasound is of limited utility in the diagnosis of spinal cord disease, because of the presence of the bony canal surrounding the theca and cord, which largely blocks transmission of sound waves. However, ultrasound is a portable, noninvasive, and relatively inexpensive modality that demonstrates good soft-tissue contrast. It is useful when the bony spinal elements are absent, such as during intraoperative visualization of the spinal cord after the bony laminae have been surgically removed, or in early infancy, when spinal ossification is limited.

Nuclear medicine studies, including planar bone scans, PET, and SPECT, enable functional detection of infection, cancer, or trauma. Indium-labeled CSF studies can be used to examine the distribution and flow of cerebrospinal fluid in the spine and head.

It has been little more than 20 years since the introduction of *MRI* to spinal imaging. Although it is more expensive than some of the techniques listed above, because of its noninvasive nature (no ionizing radiation), multiplanar imaging capabilities, superb soft tissue conspicuity, and ability to depict the spinal neural contents directly, MRI has established itself as the imaging modality of choice for the spine and spinal cord (1). In certain situations, however, one or more of the other modalities discussed above may be more useful than MRI.

Portions of this chapter were previously published in Lee RR: Recent advances in MRI of the spine, and Lee RR: Spinal tumors. In Lee RR (ed): *Spinal Imaging* (Spine: State of the Art Reviews, vol 9). Philadelphia: Hanley & Belfus, 1995, 45-60 and 261-286. Copyright Elsevier.

Basic Concepts of Imaging

Three major parameters that characterize an imaging modality are spatial resolution, signal-to-noise (S/N), and contrast resolution (1). Any improvement in image quality represents some combination of improved spatial resolution, increased S/N, and improved contrast resolution.

Spatial resolution, essentially the smallest size detectable by the technique, is determined by slice thickness, field of view (FOV), and the size of the acquisition and display matrices. In a digital system such as MRI, the unit of in-plane spatial resolution (defined as a pixel) is the FOV divided by the matrix size. Thus, using a field of view of 48 cm (which is roughly the length of the spinal cord) and a 512×512 matrix size yields a nominal in-plane spatial resolution of 0.94 mm, certainly adequate for imaging spinal structures. Ideally, to achieve good spatial resolution, thin sections (3 mm) with a large matrix (256×256, or up to 512×512) should be used, but unfortunately, as discussed in the following paragraph, there is a trade-off between improving spatial resolution and worsening signal-to-noise.

Signal-to-noise (S/N), as the name implies, is the ratio of the desired signal to be measured, divided by the inevitable noise that degrades and contaminates the signal. Because the MRI signal is proportional to the number of protons in the imaged volume element (voxel), increasing the volume sampled (i.e., increasing voxel and pixel size) increases the signal (more than the noise). However, increasing pixel size means decreasing spatial resolution.

However, an *intrinsic* increase in S/N, such as from increasing MRI magnet strength, or from improvements in coil technology, is extremely beneficial, not only because S/N is increased, but also because it allows for smaller pixel size, and hence improved spatial resolution.

Contrast resolution is the ability to discriminate between different tissues. MRI, which distinguishes matter not only by its density (as does X-ray and CT), but also by its different T1 and T2 relaxation parameters and diffusivity (i.e., diffusion-weighted imaging), is of unparalleled value in differentiating between soft tissues, such as gray and white matter, and normal vs. edematous tissue.

Imaging Speed

Imaging speed is another important parameter, in addition to the three listed above. Unlike the prior three parameters of image quality, which can be measured or calculated directly from the image itself, the time required to produce the image cannot (although it is measurable by other means). The imaging speed (i.e., the time required to obtain the image) is one of the most important benchmarks of an imaging system, and this is where many of the improvements in MRI and CT (and indeed all medical imaging) are being made.

Some portions of the human anatomy impose stringent requirements on imaging speed, most notably the beating heart or respiratory motion of the thorax, but the spine in a supine patient is relatively motion-free and considerably less demanding in this regard. However, both in the interests of patient comfort and to avoid degradation by patient motion (especially in those patients with severe back pain), it is desirable to minimize imaging time. Moreover, significant increases in imaging speed can yield major improvements in signal-to-noise, as discussed in the section on fast spin-echo (FSE), also known as the rapid acquisition relaxation enhanced (RARE) sequence.

As has historically occurred with all imaging modalities, including CT, improvements in image quality have been accompanied by increases in imaging speed. Faster and more powerful computers, better reconstruction algorithms, and hardware improvements have all resulted in these gains.

Phased-Array Surface Coils and Multichannel Parallel Imaging

Improved spatial resolution in spine imaging has long been achieved with the use of surface coils, with their higher signal-to-noise ratio, but with a penalty of a smaller field of view and a limited penetration into the body (2, 3). Fortunately, the spinal structures lie close to the posterior skin surface, so modern spine MRI uses posterior surface coils to receive the MR signals.

The development of the phased-array surface coil solved the problem of limited longitudinal field of view (FOV) by coupling many (four to six) such coils in a longitudinal array (4), mounted as a single long unit. This allows nearly the entire spine (48–50 cm) to be imaged in a single acquisition using a large FOV, with good resolution (using a 512×512 or 512×384 matrix), rather than requiring separate, time-consuming imaging of the cervical, thoracic, and lumbar regions individually (Figure 3.1). Various combinations of the phased coils may be electronically activated to view only the cervical, thoracic, or lumbar regions, or a combination thereof, without physically moving the coil or the patient.

This allows screening studies of the entire spine to be made in one acquisition, rather than treating the spine as three separate units (cervical, thoracic, and lumbar). It is particularly valuable in screening for metastatic disease; a screening 3-mm series of T1-weighted sagittal images of essentially the entire spine may be performed in a single 3- to 7-minute sequence, and selected axial images (T1 or fast spin-echo T2) should be obtained only through the levels of abnormality, rather than through the entire spine. A large FOV fast spin-echo (FSE) (discussed below) T2-weighted sagittal image may be obtained in about 3 to 6 minutes to clearly delineate regions of cord impingement (Figure 3.2). The total imaging time for this study is thus only about 20 minutes, which can generally be tolerated by almost any patient.

Also, screening for intrathecal disease throughout the spine can be performed with a single postgadolinium sagittal sequence in about 5 minutes, with a resolution of 0.9 mm (48 cm FOV/512 matrix), using selected axial images only through the regions of abnormal enhancement.

With recent advances in coil technology and reconstruction algorithms, multichannel phased-array radiofrequency coils can be used in parallel-imaging mode to markedly shorten scan times by factors of 2 or more. Parallel imaging is becoming widely used in brain MRI and is especially valuable at field strengths of 3 Tesla and higher (5). This technology will be employed to great advantage in spinal imaging as well (6).

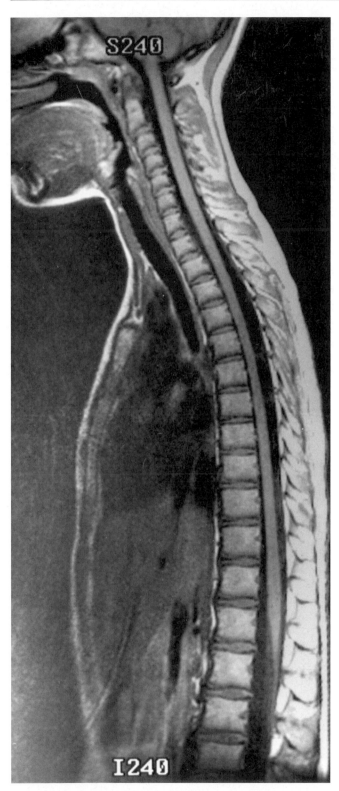

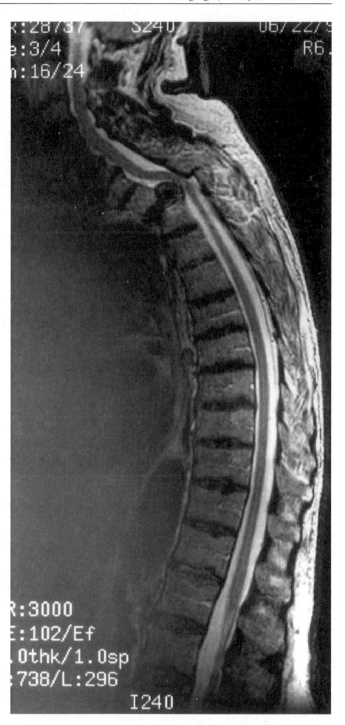

Figure 3.1 Sagittal T1 large field of view (48 cm, effective 512 × 512 matrix using rectangular field of view), using a phased-array coil, covers the entire spine of this normal 11-year-old girl from pons through L4, in only 4.5 minutes. Spatial resolution is 0.9 mm. Note the superb detail and uniform coverage of all anatomy (1).

Figure 3.2 Fast spin-echo T2 (FSE-T2) used with phased-array spinal coil. This screening FSE-T2 scan covered in only 6.5 minutes 48 cm (skull base through L3) in this kyphotic patient with metastatic thyroid carcinoma. Note the superb detail (0.9 mm resolution) and uniformity of signal throughout the length of the spine. T2-weighting yields an exquisite myelogram effect, clearly delineating the retropulsed tumor mass at T2 that is posteriorly displacing and compressing the spinal cord, as well as the spondylotic changes in the cervical region (1).

FAST-SCANNING TECHNIQUES: RATIONALE

To improve the signal-to-noise ratio (S/N), one may increase the signal by increasing the number of acquisitions (i.e., the number of times the image data is acquired—in effect, scanning the patient multiple times), but this obviously significantly lengthens the exam and increases the risk of image degradation from patient motion. However, if an imaging sequence is intrinsically very fast, doubling or tripling the (very short) imaging time is a feasible option, resulting in significant improvement in S/N and consequently allowing smaller pixels (i.e., better spatial resolution). Hence, recent developments have focused on decreasing scan time—techniques known as fast-scanning.

Gradient-Echo Imaging

Many fast-scanning methods have been developed, of which gradient-echo imaging (GRE) was one of the first. This technique relies on gradients to refocus the spins, rather than 180-degree pulses, as are used in conventional spin-echo imaging. Images are produced rapidly because of small flip angles and short repetition times (TRs) (7, 8). GRE's major advantage, besides speed, is the very thin slices obtainable (less than 1-mm thick), representing multiple thin partitions of a large three-dimensional (3D) imaging volume, in contrast to the usual 2-mm minimum slice thickness attainable with conventional 2D spin-echo slices. However, the signal characteristics of gradient-echo images do not correspond directly to conventional T1- or T2-weighted spin-echo imaging (9). In particular, GRE images of the spine are inferior to conventional T2-weighted or fast spin-echo images, because they consistently overestimate the hydration of the disks, overestimate the size of osteophytes because of susceptibility artifact, and provide poor visualization of the neural structures (9, 10). Also, because of the lack of the 180-degree refocusing pulse, gradient-echo scans are more prone to susceptibility artifacts from tissue and magnetic field inhomogeneity, and from motion (11).

In the spine, gradient-echo imaging currently has its most widespread application in 3D-volumetric thin-section axial images of the cervical spine, where the relatively small size of the anatomic structures necessitates contiguous thin-section images (12, 13).

Fast Spin-Echo (FSE or RARE) Imaging

Developed in 1990 by Melki and Mulkern et al. (14, 15) as a refinement of a technique first proposed by Hennig et al. (16), the RARE sequence and variations thereupon have been a major development in fast-scanning and have been particularly useful in spine MRI. This sequence, also known as fast spin-echo (FSE) or turbo spin-echo, gives good T2-weighted contrast in a fraction of the time required by true (conventional) spin-echo, thus resulting in better resolution and signal-to-noise than was previously practically attainable (Figure 3.2). (FSE generally requires only a few minutes per sequence, rather than about 20 minutes for an equivalent multiexcitation true T2-weighted acquisition.)

This sequence places several (from three to sixteen or more) different phase-encoding gradients followed by 180-degree radio frequency pulses after each 90-degree pulse, rather than just one phase-encode and one or two 180-degree pulses. This results in a much more efficient use of imaging time overall, cutting scanning time by a factor of 2 to 6 (or more).

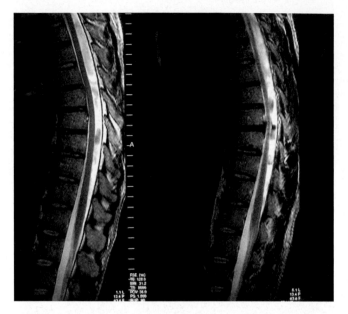

Figure 3.3 Consecutive sagittal FSE T2-weighted images of the thoracic spine show multiple focal signal voids in the CSF posterior to the spinal cord. These are common artifacts on this pulse sequence and must not be misinterpreted as a vascular malformation.

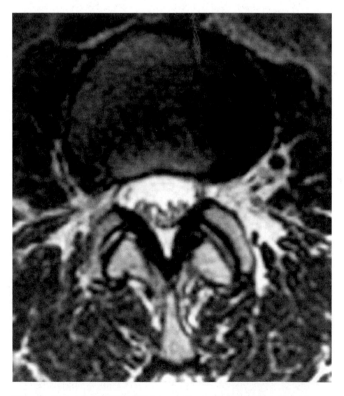

Figure 3.4 Axial FSE-T2 image through a lumbar disc shows a myelogram effect, with exquisite delineation of nerve roots in the thecal sac. The disc, bones, and facet joints, as well as the paravertebral soft tissues, are well visualized (1).

FSE images demonstrate less magnetic susceptibility artifact than true spin-echo images (17, 18), which minimizes artifacts from bone spurs and (to a certain degree) reduces artifact from surgical hardware (19) (see Figure 3.10). Possible disadvantages of FSE include bright signal from fat and decreased sensitivity to hemosiderin (old blood products), as well as some occasional blurring of images (16–18, 20). One major artifact on FSE imaging is caused by CSF pulsation in the rostral regions of the spine, which yields signal voids that could be misinterpreted as arteriovenous fistulas or AVMs in the CSF dorsal to the cord, especially on FSE images (17, 19) (Figure 3.3). Cardiac gating, flow compensation, and other special pulse sequences may decrease artifacts from pulsatile CSF (21, 22), but often some artifacts persist.

FSE sequences have dramatically improved spine imaging (19, 23). Good T2 weighting (extremely useful in the axial as well as the sagittal plane) (Figure 3.4) can be obtained in only a few (e.g., 3) minutes, as opposed to about 10 minutes for a true single-excitation T2-weighted sequence. As mentioned, this markedly faster sequence permits higher resolution and more excitations (better S/N) to be achieved. T1- and T2-weighted images may be obtained in both sagittal and axial planes, with good resolution and S/N, in very short imaging times (about 30 minutes total examination time, or less).

Recent development of three-dimensional volumetric FSE sequences (3D FSE-T2) provides thin-section, contiguous, high-resolution T2-weighted images that may be reconstructed in any plane, from a *single,* relatively rapid acquisition (24) (Figure 3.5).

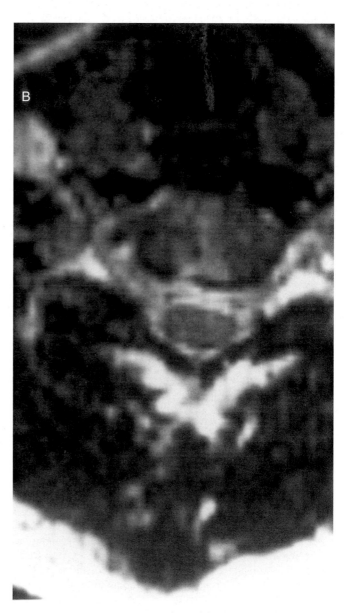

Figure 3.5 Three-dimensional fast spin-echo (3D FSE-T2) of cervical spine. **A**. 1.2-mm-thick sagittal fast spin-echo T2-weighted image was obtained as part of a 3D volume acquisition, with forty-eight slices in 7.5 minutes. Note the clear delineation between the vertebrae, CSF, and cord in this 36-year-old woman with prior C4–C5 fusion. **B**. 0.9-mm-thick axial T2-weighted image was reconstructed from the sagittal data acquired and shown in A. No axial images were directly acquired. Hence, both sagittal *and* axial views can be obtained in a single 7.5-minute acquisition, with a 1.2-mm resolution. Note the clear delineation of the spinal cord and neural foramina on this reconstructed image (1).

Other Fast-Imaging Techniques

Fast fluid-attenuated inversion recovery (FLAIR) is an effective technique in evaluating T2-bright signal in the brain, because confounding bright CSF signal is suppressed by the appropriate choice of inversion time (25). However, its use in evaluating the spinal cord is controversial, and some authors find that conspicuity of spinal cord lesions with FLAIR is inferior to that with conventional T2-weighted images (26).

Fast short inversion–time inversion–recovery (STIR) images have an appearance similar to that of standard T2-weighted images, with bright CSF and dark neural tissue. However, normal fatty bone marrow also appears dark on STIR images, compared with its relatively bright appearance on FSE-T2 (Figure 3.6). A comparative study concluded that fast STIR images more sensitively detected spinal cord lesions than FSE-T2 or fast FLAIR images (26).

All of these fast-imaging techniques continue to improve. There is a multitude of variables that may be optimized (27). For example, in FSE, variables include echo train length, partition of the various phase-encoding steps in k-space, number of echoes obtained, and interecho spacing, just to name a few.

Fast-Imaging Techniques in the Spine

The myelographic effect on T2-weighted images, whereby CSF is bright white, contrasting sharply with dark nerve roots and dark vertebrae and discs, is very valuable in the diagnosis of spinal pathology. Even more important, T2-weighted images directly demonstrate edema or gliosis within the spinal cord as bright T2-signal, contrasted with T2–dark normal tissue.

All the fast-imaging techniques discussed give a good myelographic effect, except for the fast FLAIR sequence. The best sequences for evaluating intrinsic spinal cord lesions are FSE-T2 and fast STIR, but the former also gives the best depiction of the intervertebral disc and other soft tissues. In our experience, FSE *proton-density* images are a useful adjunct to T2-weighted images in detecting spinal cord lesions; they corroborate lesions suspected on FSE-T2, often with increased conspicuity (Figure 3.6).

One use of GRE images is in detecting small amounts of hemosiderin (such as in spinal cord trauma) or calcium, which could be missed on FSE images and might be missed on SE T2-weighted images.

In summary, the screening MRI examination of the cervical spine should include a sagittal T1-weighted sequence; a sagittal flow-compensated, cardiac-gated conventional, or preferably FSE T2-weighted, sequence; and an axial 3D gradient-echo sequence. Alternatively, a sagittal 3D FSE sequence, with axial reformation, may replace the separate axial and sagittal T2-weighted sequences (Figure 3.5) (24).

Thoracic spine images should include sagittal T1-weighted and FSE T2-weighted sequences, with axial images obtained only through regions of abnormality.

In the lumbar spine, T1 and multiecho FSE T2-weighted images should be obtained in the sagittal plane, followed by axial T1 and FSE T2 images.

As discussed, the best technique for evaluating intrinsic spinal cord lesions includes sagittal FSE proton-density and T2-weighted images, supplemented with sagittal fast STIR

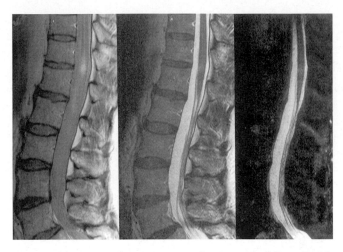

Figure 3.6 Sagittal MR images of a 58-year-old man with multiple sclerosis. **Left**. FSE proton-density image clearly demonstrates a small, ovoid, bright plaque in the distal conus. **Middle**. FSE T2-weighted image only subtly demonstrates the lesion. **Right**. Fast STIR image subtly demonstrates the plaque slightly better than FSE-T2, but not as well as FSE proton-density. Note the dark appearance of all the bony and soft tissue structures on the fast STIR image, with only CSF and lesion hyperintense.

images. T1-weighted images after intravenous administration of Gd-DTPA are necessary to evaluate intradural-extramedullary or intramedullary lesions.

Fat Saturation

Fat is bright on T1-weighted images and fairly bright on FSE-T2 images. This can be advantageous, providing natural contrast between the T1-dark CSF in the thecal sac, nerve roots in the neural foramina, and the surrounding epidural fat. However, there are two major circumstances in which the presence of bright fat can mask pathology: (1) enhancing structures on postgadolinium T1-weighted sequences may be masked by surrounding T1-bright fat, and (2) intrinsically T2-bright lesions in the vertebral marrow, such as metastases, may be masked by T2-bright fat on FSE images.

In both of these situations, suppression of the bright fat signal by special pulse sequences enables the enhancement or the T2-bright signal of lesions to be visualized; this may provide better conspicuity of inflammatory and neoplastic lesions in the spine (20, 28, 29). STIR is another method of fat suppression that may be especially useful in visualizing vertebral metastases (30). Fat suppression may be applied in combination with FSE sequences, as well as conventional spin-echo images, to improve lesion conspicuity in marrow (31), although T1-weighted images perhaps remain most sensitive (31).

Another valuable application of spectroscopic fat suppression is in the identification or diagnosis of fat-containing lesions. Because subacute blood, proteinaceous fluid, and occasionally calcium (32) can also be T1-bright, the selective saturation of T1-bright fat can be diagnostic in distinguishing among these possibilities (Figure 3.7). (The presence of chemical shift artifact is also a clue to the presence of fat, even without the use of fat saturation.)

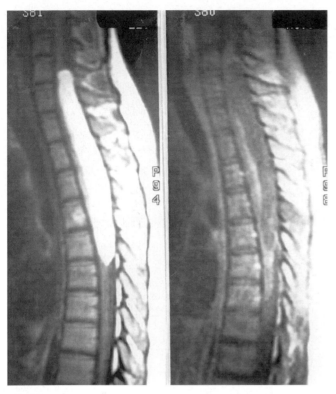

Figure 3.7 Use of fat saturation to diagnose intradural spinal lipoma. **Left**. Sagittal T1 shows a very large, well-circumscribed intradural-extramedullary T1-bright mass posterior to and compressing the upper thoracic cord. **Right**. Fat-saturated postgadolinium T1 image shows complete suppression of the T1-bright signal, proving the presence of fat rather than T1-bright blood. Hence, the diagnosis of lipoma rather than hematoma was made and confirmed at surgery. A subtle thin rim of enhancement is noted around the tumor capsule (1).

CSF Flow: MRI Measurements

MRI can qualitatively and quantitatively measure CSF flow because the phase of the precessing nuclei in the magnetic field gradients is very sensitive to motion within the field. In particular, the oscillatory motion of CSF in the brain and spinal canal (especially in the more rostral spine), driven by brain expansion and contraction during the cardiac cycle and by motion of the brain and cord itself, may be directly imaged by phase-contrast cine technique (20, 33–36). This technique can assess the degree of blockage of CSF flow within the spinal canal—for example, from congenital stenosis at the cervicomedullary junction, as seen in achondroplasia. Other possible uses include evaluating lack of normal cord motion in tethered cords and distinguishing between a intradural subarachnoid cyst versus a normally widened spinal canal, although the interpretation of such studies has yet to be perfected (20, 34).

Diffusion-Weighted Imaging and Diffusion-Tensor Imaging

Diffusion-weighted imaging (DWI) and diffusion-tensor imaging (DTI) are MRI techniques that measure the diffusivity of protons in tissue, providing another MRI parameter (besides T1, T2, proton density, and flow) to differentially characterize tissues and identify pathology. DWI can improve specificity of tissue characterization, for example in distinguishing between abscess and necrotic tumor, or between epidermoid tumor and arachnoid cyst (37). DWI is widely used in MRI of the brain to detect acute infarction and other pathologies with increased sensitivity and specificity; acutely infarcted tissue demonstrates restricted diffusion compared to normal tissue, as early as 30 minutes after arterial occlusion (38). DTI provides a three-dimensional map of the white matter fiber tracts (39).

DWI and DTI are now being applied to the spine and spinal cord, as well as the brain. It is technically more difficult to apply these techniques in the spine, due to the smaller axial dimensions of the spinal cord compared to the brain, artifacts from CSF pulsation in the spinal canal, and the presence of susceptibility differences between the spinal cord and bony canal (40). However, DWI has been successfully used to diagnose spinal cord ischemia (41); to evaluate cervical spondylotic myelopathy (42); and to distinguish between spinal epidermoid tumor and arachnoid cyst (43) (see Fig. 3.63), among other applications. Some applications of DTI include spinal cord trauma (40), spondylotic myelopathy (42), and multiple sclerosis (44). In the future, technical refinements will enable these techniques, as well as other techniques such as MR spectroscopy, to become more widely used in the spine (45).

Titanium Spinal Hardware

Imaging the postoperative spine by CT or MRI after implantation of fusion or stabilization metallic instrumentation is often frustrating and difficult because of excessive beam-hardening artifacts in CT or very extensive ferromagnetic susceptibility artifacts in MRI (Figure 3.8). Titanium is a strong metal that is less dense than stainless steel and is nonferromagnetic when

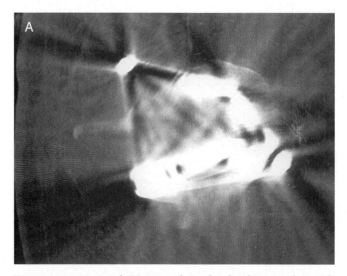

Figure 3.8 A. Axial CT image through a lumbar vertebra with stainless steel pedicle screws and vertebral body screw shows extensive beam-hardening artifact from the hardware, completely precluding evaluation of the spinal canal or the bony structures at this level.

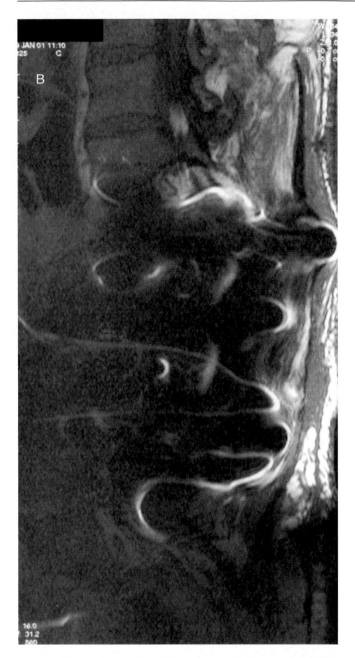

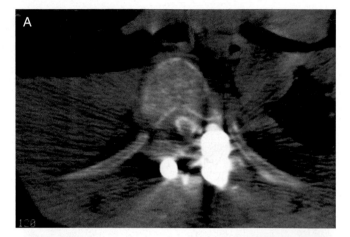

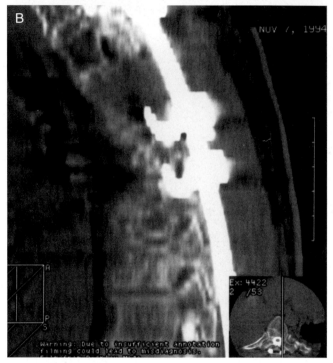

Figure 3.8 *(continued)* **B**. Sagittal T1-weighted MR image of the same patient with stainless steel pedicle screws shows severe metallic susceptibility artifact, rendering this lumbar MRI completely uninterpretable.

Figure 3.9 Titanium hardware minimizes artifact on CT. **A**. Axial CT-myelogram image at level of left-sided titanium laminar hook and right-sided rod shows only minimal artifact. Posterior elements and contents of the spinal canal, including cord and contrast-filled thecal sac, are clearly discernable. Steel hardware would have rendered this level uninterpretable. **B**. Sagittal reconstruction from the axial CT data again clearly demonstrates the titanium hardware and the spine, with only minimal beam-hardening artifact (1).

compared to steel. Consequently, the imaging of titanium implants both on CT and MRI, although far from perfect, is less fraught with artifacts than imaging steel hardware. Often the relevant structures can be adequately evaluated by a postoperative CT or MRI after titanium implants, whereas steel implants would have resulted in a nondiagnostic study secondary to extensive artifact (Figures 3.9 and 3.10) (46).

As discussed in the section on FSE, this fast spin-echo sequence should be used in concert with titanium instrumentation to minimize the metal susceptibility artifact.

Summary

There have been many recent developments in the fast-growing field of spinal imaging. Some (fast MR imaging, especially FSE; multichannel MRI coils employing parallel imaging techniques; and multislice CT) result in faster intrinsic imaging times, which can be exploited to yield improved signal-to-noise and spatial resolution. Other advances (variable bandwidth, phased-array coils, or increasing magnet field strength to 3 Tesla [47], for

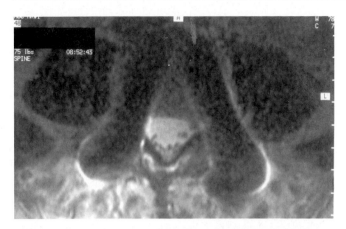

Figure 3.10 Titanium hardware minimizes artifact on MRI. Axial fast spin-echo (FSE) T2-weighted image of vertebra at level of bilateral titanium pedicle screws shows only minimal susceptibility artifact in the vicinity of the screws. The central canal is still clearly visualized, as are the individual nerve roots. Stainless steel hardware would have rendered this level uninterpretable. Use of fast spin-echo sequence also contributes to minimizing artifact (1).

example) yield improved signal-to-noise and secondarily result in faster imaging and improved patient comfort. Still others (fat saturation, diffusion-weighted imaging, and use of titanium instrumentation) improve contrast resolution or otherwise improve image quality.

All these developments are undergoing continual refinement, and advances in the future will continue to improve image quality, imaging speed, and ultimately, the quality of patient care.

CONGENITAL ABNORMALITIES

With the exception of early infancy, when ultrasound of the spine can be successfully performed because of the limited vertebral ossification at this age, MRI is the test of choice for imaging spinal malformations. In early infancy, sonography can visualize the spinal cord between the areas of early ossification. Tethering of the spinal cord can be demonstrated not only by a low position of the conus medullaris but by the failure of the spinal cord to move with positional changes and with cardiac and respiratory movement.

Plain radiographs are often very helpful to evaluate the bony structures of the spine. Spina bifida occulta is a common finding that may be seen with many different types of congenital malformations, but it is not specific in predicting congenital abnormalities. A rare but fairly specific plain-film finding is crossed laminar fusion, or diagonal fusion of laminae of adjacent vertebrae, which, when seen, is strongly associated with diastematomyelia, a malformation resulting from a split notochord. CT can be helpful to delineate bone abnormalities, identify bony or cartilaginous septa, and identify fat within the spinal canal. Myelography and postmyelography CT have a limited role in the evaluation of congenital abnormalities. For almost all congenital spine malformations, MRI is by far the best way to evaluate the spinal cord (48).

Myelomeningocele (Figure 3.11), which is an open neural tube defect, is obvious at birth, and the role of imaging is supplemental. Evaluation of the distal spinal cord for tethering is a common problem at later ages. Because a high percentage of patients with Chiari II malformation and myelomeningocele have hydrocephalus, CT or MRI of the head (or sonography in infancy) is commonly used to help evaluate the need for shunt catheter placement and to monitor function of a shunt catheter later. Syrinx can occur in Chiari II. Cervical spinal cord atrophy is occasionally seen, probably caused by compression from the downwardly displaced cerebellum in the upper cervical spinal canal (Figure 3.12).

Lipomyelomeningocele, despite its similar name, is a quite different entity than myelomeningocele. It results from the premature dysjunction of the skin from the neural tube before complete closure, thus exposing mesoderm to the developing CNS and inducing the formation of fat. Thus, the spinal cord

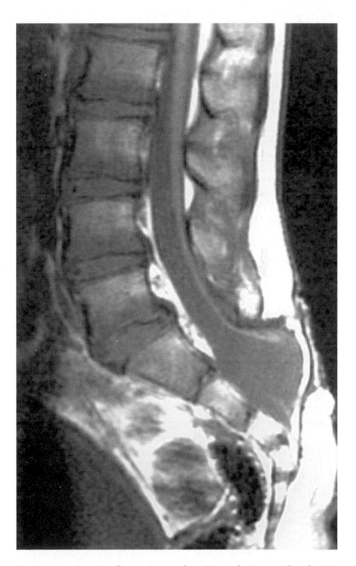

Figure 3.11 Myelomeningocele. Sagittal T1-weighted MR image of 6-year-old child with symptoms of tethered cord and previous surgery for myelomeningocele. The spinal cord extends inferiorly into the meningocele at the level of the sacrum.

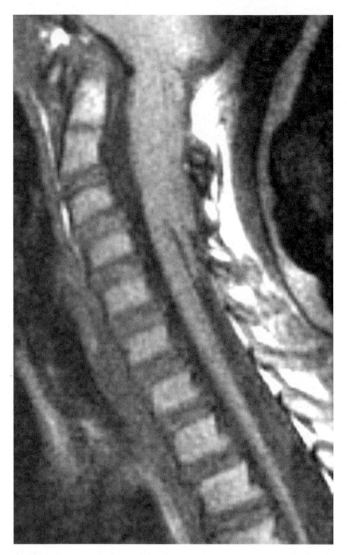

Figure 3.12 Chiari II and spinal cord atrophy. Sagittal T1-weighted MR image of a 6-year-old child with myelomeningocele shows downward displacement of the cerebellum far down into the cervical spinal canal. The cervical spinal cord is atrophied.

is intimately associated with fat that is continuous with subcutaneous fat and therefore tethered. Because the overlying skin is intact, the malformation may not present for years, or even for several decades. The lipoma can be demonstrated by CT but is especially well shown by MRI (Figure 3.13). Low attenuation on CT and similar signal intensity to fat elsewhere on MRI are specific for lipomas in the spinal canal. The position of the distal spinal cord is best demonstrated by MRI. Spina bifida occulta is seen at the site of communication with subcutaneous fat. Lipomyelomeningocele is not associated with the Chiari II malformation, and the incidence of hydrocephalus in these patients is similar to that of the general population.

A lipoma of the filum terminale may be associated with a tethered cord (Figure 3.14). Very small amounts of fat within the filum terminale are commonly seen and are of doubtful significance. The lipoma of the spinal cord is the least common

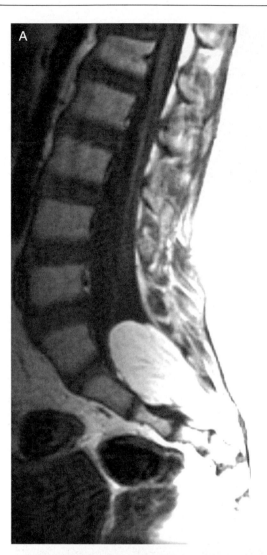

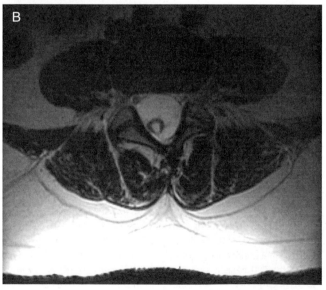

Figure 3.13 Lipomyelomeningocele. Twelve-year-old boy with lifelong urinary incontinence and no previous surgery. **A**. Sagittal T1-weighted MR image shows large lipoma within the distal spinal canal. **B**. Axial T2-weighted MR image discloses a syrinx (hydromyelia) of the distal spinal cord.

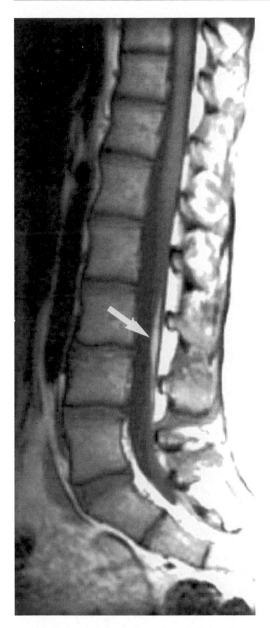

Figure 3.14 Tethered cord and filum lipoma. Sagittal T1-weighted MR image of a young adult with back pain shows high signal intensity (arrow) in a lipoma of the filum terminale.

of the spinal lipomas. It is actually a subpial collection of fat, nearly always along the dorsal surface of the spinal cord (Figure 3.15).

A focal failure of disjunction of the spinal cord from the overlying ectoderm leads to the formation of a dorsal dermal sinus tract, lined by epithelial tissue. When a dimple, patch of hair, or pigmented skin leads to suspicion of such a tract, MRI can demonstrate the tract. Such tracts often extend obliquely through the subcutaneous tissue. They may terminate anywhere from subcutaneous tissue to epidural space, to dura, to the spinal cord itself. In about half of dorsal dermal sinus tracts, a dermoid or epidermoid cyst is present. MRI shows such tumors or cysts as round or oval masses in the spinal canal and can show their relationship to the spinal cord.

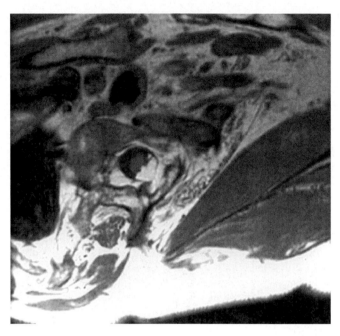

Figure 3.15 Intradural lipoma. Axial T1-weighted MR image of adult man with scoliosis shows high signal intensity fat dorsal to the spinal cord in the upper thoracic spine.

The spinal cord can be tethered from a variety of causes. Myelomeningocele and lipomyelomeningocele both imply that the spinal cord is tethered. However, errors in a later stage of development relating to the caudal cell mass can lead to a tethered cord without the more obvious abnormalities of the spinal cord and vertebra. The tip of the conus medullaris lies at the L2 level or above in 98% of people, and position of the conus medullaris at or below the L2–L3 level is generally considered abnormally low (49). Sagittal MR images alone can sometimes be confusing, because the nerve roots in the cauda equina may simulate the conus medullaris; additional coronal or axial images are often necessary to accurately image the distal spinal cord. T1-weighted images are often the most reliable way to identify the conus medullaris. As mentioned above, sonography is only possible early in life but has the advantage of providing dynamic information.

Diastematomyelia is a rare congenital malformation resulting from a split notochord. The spinal cord is segmentally divided in the sagittal plane, and the dural sac may be intact or may also be divided. In about half of these cases, there is a bony or cartilaginous septum through the spinal canal. Such septa are best demonstrated by CT but may be shown by MRI, especially with gradient-echo techniques. The split spinal cord and the length of the division are best shown by MRI.

TRAUMA

Imaging plays a key role in the evaluation of spine trauma, both in the acute situation and in the later imaging of complications. The complementary nature of various imaging modalities is especially important in imaging spine trauma.

Plain radiographs are part of the routine evaluation of patients in whom there is a strong suspicion of spine injury. Radiographic evaluation of the cervical spine is recommended for all patients with evidence of significant injury above the clavicles. There is no consensus on which views should be obtained, and numerous different opinions and protocols have been offered. A lateral view to include the cervicothoracic junction should always be obtained, and a typical radiographic series for cervical spine trauma includes AP and odontoid views as well. A "swimmer's" view is often helpful if the cervicothoracic junction is obscured by the shoulders. Additional projections such as oblique views or the "pillar" view may be obtained but are often reserved for special cases.

Radiographic evaluation of the thoracic and lumbar spine includes at least lateral, and often also AP, views. Oblique views of the thoracolumbar spine are rarely indicated in the evaluation of acute trauma.

In assessing spine radiographs, the interpreter should look at alignment, the bones themselves for presence of fractures, and adjacent soft tissue outlines (50). Focal kyphosis or subluxation should suggest the possibility of fracture or major ligamentous injury, although chronic degenerative change can cause minor abnormalities of alignment. In the cervical spine, anterior and posterior margins of the vertebral bodies, the spinolaminar line (along the posterior margin of the spinal canal and anterior margin of the spinous processes), and the posterior margin of the spinous processes should all demonstrate a regular, relatively smooth change. The prevertebral soft tissues in the cervical region can provide important clues to injury, especially in the upper half of the cervical spine. The presence of the esophagus adjacent to the lower cervical spine normally widens the soft tissues in this region and makes it more difficult to identify swelling. At the C3 vertebral body, the prevertebral tissues should normally not exceed 4 mm in thickness on a routine lateral view (183-cm [72-inch] distance); a portable technique using a shorter focal distance can cause magnification and slightly larger apparent thickness. In the thoracic spine, a paraspinous hematoma from a fracture is often visible on the AP view. Fractures may be visualized directly or inferred from the loss of vertebral body height or from increased density in the region of compressed bone. Fractures of the posterior elements are particularly difficult to identify with plain films, and as many as half of all posterior element fractures identified on CT are missed on plain film. The odontoid process should be inspected carefully for fractures.

CT is more sensitive than plain radiographs for the detection of fractures (51, 52). Fractures oriented in the axial plane may be difficult to identify on CT. Such injuries include fractures through the base of the odontoid process, some compression fractures, and Chance fractures (which are discussed later in this chapter, under thoracic and lumbar injury patterns). Sagittal and coronal reformatted views can be particularly helpful in such cases (Figure 3.16). Three-dimensional reconstructions are sometimes helpful in assessing alignment and displacement of fragments. Such reconstructions, as well as routine CT scanning of longer segments of the spine, are more readily performed with spiral or helical techniques. Modern multislice CT machines can quickly scan through the anatomy of interest within a few seconds, and they enable multiplanar and 3D reconstructions of excellent quality (Figure 3.17). CT of the spine should be performed with a slice thickness small enough to permit reformatted views and to identify fractures. In the authors' experience, slice thickness should not be more than 3 mm; in

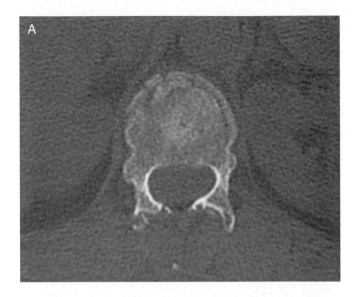

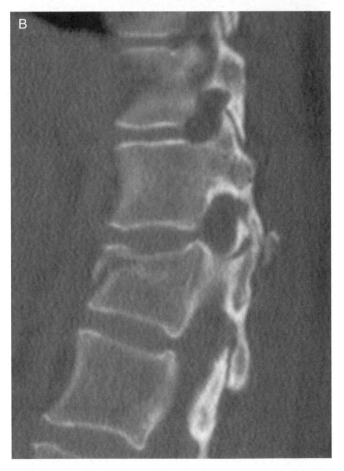

Figure 3.16 Chance injury. Young adult woman in a motor vehicle accident had anterior loss of height seen on plain X-rays at the T12 level. Axial CT scan (**A**) shows lucency and irregularity at the anterior margin of T12 and subtle lucency through the right lamina, representing fractures. Sagittal 2D reconstruction image (**B**) clarifies the anterior compression and posterior widening between the lamina in this Chance-type injury.

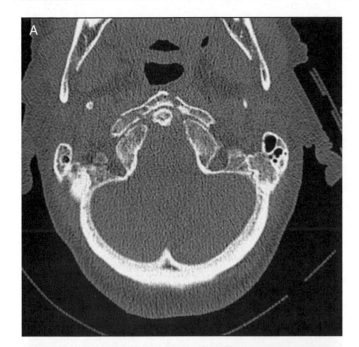

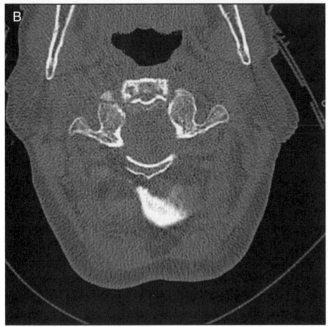

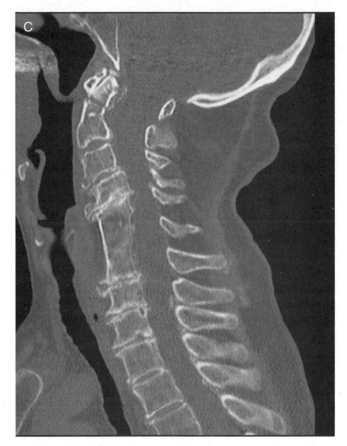

Figure 3.17 Multislice, high-resolution CT in trauma. CT of the cervical spine of an elderly woman in a motor vehicle accident. Axial images (**A**, **B**) show fractures of the C1 ring and of the base of the dens. Reconstructed sagittal image (**C**) demonstrates more clearly the horizontal fracture through the base of the dens, as well as old lower cervical spine fusion (C5 through C7), and extensive, multilevel degenerative changes. Scan was performed on a sixteen-slice helical scanner using 0.75-mm slice thickness.

areas such as the cervicocranial junction and odontoid process, thinner or overlapping slices may be necessary.

MRI is particularly helpful for visualization of the spinal cord and for identification of soft tissue injury. Hematomas, disk herniation, and spinal cord contusion, hemorrhage, or compression can be directly demonstrated by MRI, as is patency of the vertebral arteries (53). Indications for MRI in the setting of acute spine trauma include neurologic injury; evaluation of suspected complicating factors, such as disk herniation when surgery is being considered; and evaluation of soft tissue injury, especially in patients in whom clinical assessment is limited. Sagittal T1- and T2-weighted images can be used to screen the spinal cord, with axial images being used through areas of particular concern. Because normal paraspinal fat has high signal intensity on T2-weighted fast spin-echo (FSE), which could mask T2-bright edema from injury to the soft tissues, it is important to use a fat-suppression technique with FSE T2-weighted imaging. As discussed earlier in the section on fat saturation, inversion-recovery techniques (i.e., STIR) or chemical fat saturation can be used with fast spin-echo imaging.

Numerous types of cervical spine fractures can occur, and a comprehensive review is beyond the scope of this chapter. More extensive reviews are available, including entire books (54–56). However, it is useful to consider cervical spine fractures in terms of the major mechanisms of injury. Flexion injuries, resulting primarily from excessive force in flexion, include compression or wedge fracture, bilateral facet dislocation (Figure 3.18), spinous process fracture (clay-shoveler's), hyperflexion sprain, and flexion-teardrop fracture. Injuries resulting primarily from excessive force in extension include hyperextension dislocation, C1 anterior arch avulsion fracture, C1 posterior arch fracture,

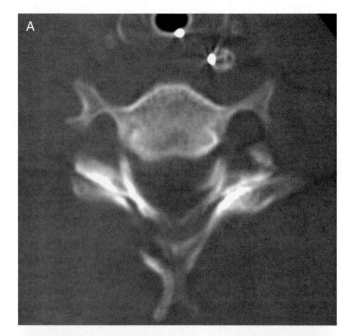

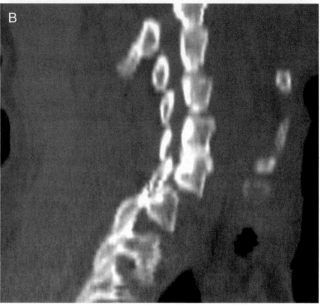

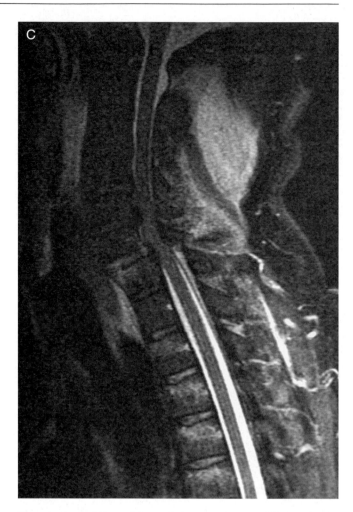

Figure 3.18 Bilateral facet dislocation in a middle-aged man with quadriplegia after motor vehicle accident. Axial CT (**A**) shows dislocation. Parasagittal 2D reconstruction view (**B**) demonstrates more directly the facet dislocation at C6–C7 on the right. Similar findings were present on the left side. Sagittal T2-weighted (inversion recovery) MR image (**C**) shows subluxation at C6–C7, spinal cord compression and edema, marrow edema in the upper thoracic spine, and extensive posterior paraspinal soft tissue edema.

laminar fracture, extension teardrop fracture, hangman's fracture (traumatic spondylolistheis) (Figure 3.19), and hyperextension fracture-dislocation. A combination of rotation and flexion causes unilateral facet dislocation (Figure 3.20). Rotation in combination with extension causes pillar or lateral mass fractures, which can be especially difficult to demonstrate on plain films. We have found that MRI can be helpful with these posterior-element fractures to demonstrate the extent of accompanying ligamentous injury, which may be an important factor in determining instability (57). More extensive ligamentous injury probably indicates a greater risk of instability in these lateral mass fractures. Combined fractures of the pedicle and lamina result in a separation of the lateral mass and risk of rotational instability (Figure 3.21).

Injuries resulting primarily from axial loading mechanisms include the Jefferson burst fracture of C1, burst fractures of C3 through C7, burst fractures involving the thoracic or lumbar spine, and oblique sagittal fractures (type 2) of the C2 body. The Jefferson fracture pattern includes two or more fractures through the ring of C1. CT is the best method for identifying this fracture (Figure 3.22). Plain film findings include lateral displacement of the lateral masses of C1 on the AP odontoid view, lucency through the posterior arch of C1 on the lateral view, and upper cervical prevertebral soft tissue swelling.

Burst fractures occur from C3 through the lower cervical and entire thoracic and lumbar spine. They result when axially directed force transmitted through a disk is transmitted to the centrum or body below, which then fractures. A prominent

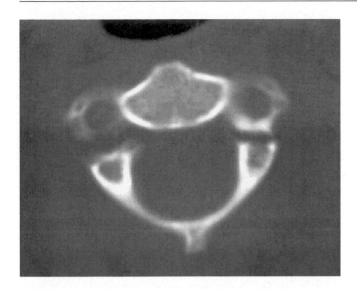

Figure 3.19 Hangman's fracture (traumatic spondylolisthesis). Axial CT at C2 shows bilateral fractures through the pars interarticularis.

sagittal component nearly always occurs; more extensive comminution of the vertebral body is variable. It is common for fragments to displace posteriorly into the spinal canal, possibly compromising the spinal cord.

The cervicocranial junction is complex, consisting of the articulations of C1 and C2 and the occiput, as well as multiple ligaments that contribute to stability and motion in multiple directions. In addition to the fractures of C1 and C2,

the occipital condyles can fracture. Such fractures are difficult to identify except with CT (58, 59) (Figure 3.23). Ligamentous injury can be inferred by soft tissue swelling and can be more directly demonstrated by MRI. The transverse ligament, responsible for maintaining the relationship between C1 and the odontoid process, is very strong and is damaged only by major injuries. The ligament can be visualized directly by MRI, but injury is often identified on the lateral X-ray by abnormal widening of the anterior atlantodental interval. This space should measure no more than 3 mm in adults. Widening of this space can occur from traumatic injury to the ligament, either rupture or avulsion from the tubercles on the lateral masses of C1, or from damage from rheumatoid arthritis or other inflammatory conditions, and some congenital conditions (Figure 3.24).

Atlanto-occipital dissociation (AOD) requires severe forces to tear the ligaments attaching the occiput to the atlas, especially the strong superior portion of the cruciate ligament. Such injuries are often fatal (60). Severe upper cervical prevertebral soft tissue swelling is present. Some patients with less severe displacement

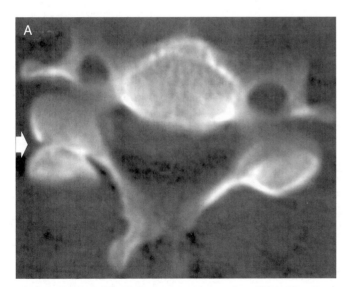

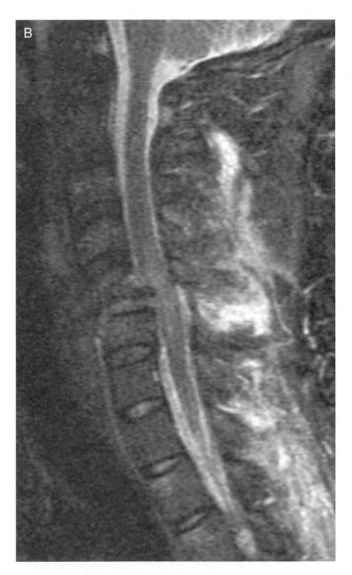

Figure 3.20 Unilateral facet dislocation. Axial CT (**A**) shows reversal of the usual relationship of the facets on the patient's right (arrow). Note that unlike Figure 3.17, bilateral facet dislocation, only one side is dislocated and there is less subluxation. Sagittal T2-weighted (inversion recovery) MR image (**B**) shows subluxation at C5–C6, spinal cord compression and edema, and dorsal soft tissue edema.

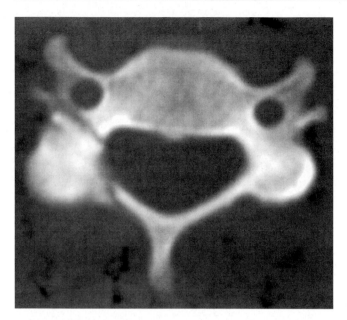

Figure 3.21 Pedicolaminar fracture pattern. CT shows fractures of the both the right pedicle and the right lamina.

can survive, and plain film findings of AOD can be subtle. A variety of measurements have been proposed to identify abnormalities of the relationship of C1, C2, and the occiput. The most reliable appear to be those described by Harris et al. (61). Two measurements are made from the basion, or inferior tip of the clivus. The distance from basion to the tip of the dens (basion–dental interval, or BDI) should not exceed 12 mm in adults as measured on a lateral radiograph obtained at 102-cm (40-inch) target-film distance. The distance from basion perpendicularly to a line extended rostrally from the posterior cortical margin of the body of C2 (basion–axial interval, or BAI) measured on a lateral radiograph should not exceed 12 mm in

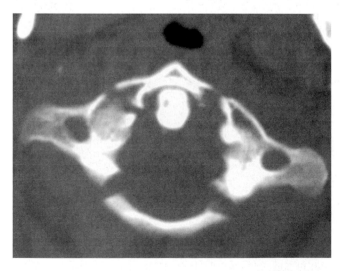

Figure 3.22 Jefferson burst fracture of C1. CT shows four fractures in the anterior and posterior arches of C1.

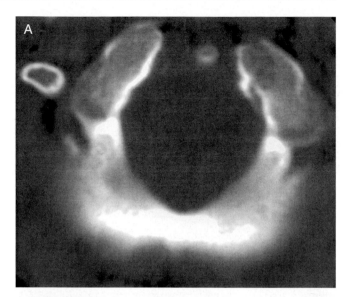

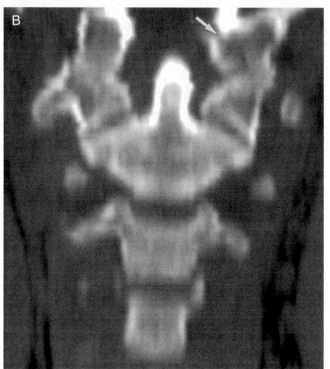

Figure 3.23 Occipital condyle fracture. Axial CT (**A**) shows subtle lucency through the left occipital condyle. Coronal 2D reconstruction (**B**) demonstrates the fracture more clearly (arrow).

children or adults. Normative values for the same measurements based on CT (62) are reported to be lower for BDI (95% of adults less than 9 mm) and difficult to measure for BAI (that is, poorly reproducible). MRI can more directly demonstrate ligamentous disruption (Figure 3.25).

Injury patterns in the thoracic and lumbar spine, in which motion is more restricted, are somewhat more limited than those in the cervical spine. Compression fractures are common injuries that result in loss of height of the vertebral body, anteriorly more

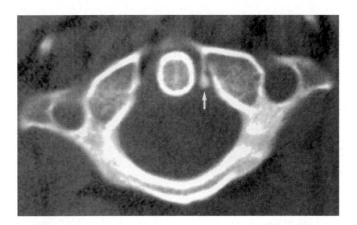

Figure 3.24 Avulsion of the transverse ligament attachment. Previous lateral cervical spine radiograph of a young woman in a motor vehicle accident showed widening of the anterior atlanto-dental interval to 5 mm. CT shows fracture through the tubercle where the transverse ligament attaches on the patient's left (arrow).

than posteriorly. In mild cases, radiographic findings include deformity of the cortical margins and end-plates. Axial loading can cause a burst fracture, in which the force transmitted through the intervertebral disk results in bursting of the centrum below. Posterior element fractures are usually present, there is nearly always a prominent sagittal component of the vertebral body fractures, and displacement into the spinal canal is variable. CT is usually helpful to define the extent of fractures and posterior element involvement (Figure 3.26). Fracture-dislocations involve complex, severe forces, variable amounts of dislocation of one vertebra on another, and usually multiple fractures. Neurologic deficits from spinal cord compression are common. Multiple imaging modalities are often helpful in management. The dislocation is usually initially demonstrated on plain radiographs, which are excellent for demonstrating alignment. CT of the affected vertebrae, especially high-resolution multidetector CT with multiplanar and 3D reconstructions, can be very helpful for planning surgical intervention. MRI is the best

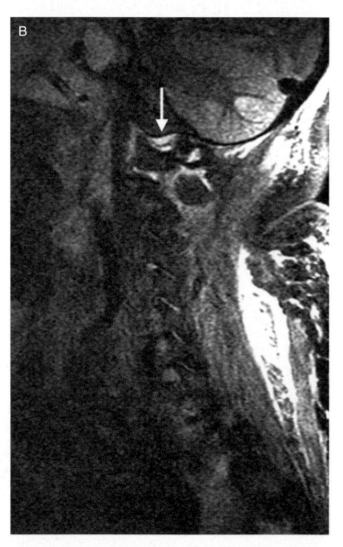

Figure 3.25 Atlanto-occipital dissociation. MRI was performed on a patient who was in a high-speed motor vehicle accident. Midline sagittal T2-weighted inversion recovery image (**A**) shows high signal intensity of severe anterior and posterior paraspinal soft tissue edema at the cervicocranial junction. Heterogeneous signal intensity within the spinal canal reflects some blood present. Parasagittal image (**B**) shows subluxation of the atlanto-occipital joint, with high signal intensity fluid between the occipital condyle and lateral mass of C1 (arrow).

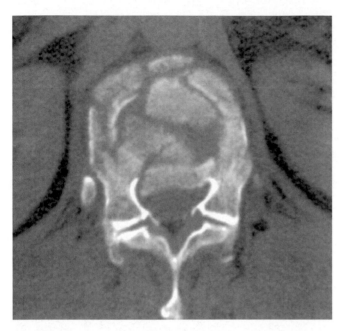

Figure 3.26 Burst fracture of T12 suffered in a parachuting accident. The patient had incomplete paraplegia. Axial CT shows numerous fractures in the body of T12, with posterior displacement of fragments into the spinal canal.

imaging method to evaluate the spinal cord (Figure 3.27). Finally, in any injury in which the surgical approach may be affected by the location of the artery of Adamkiewicz, spinal angiography may be indicated.

A combination of flexion and distraction results in a distinctive type of injury, usually in the upper lumbar or lower thoracic spine. The classic Chance fracture extends horizontally through the vertebral body and through both pedicles and may occur in automobile accidents when the patient is wearing a lap belt but not a shoulder harness. It is often best demonstrated on plain radiographs, because axial CT is less well suited to identifying axially oriented fractures (see Figure 3.16). However, other patterns of flexion-distraction injuries can also occur, still with an axial orientation and posterior distraction. In these injuries, shearing may occur through the disk space, with posterior subluxation or dislocation of the facet joints (63, 64).

In addition to mechanical narrowing of the spinal canal by displaced bone, the spinal cord can be compromised by traumatic disk protrusion, hematoma, transient hyperextension, hyperflexion, distraction, or ischemia. In all of these conditions, MRI is the best imaging test. Many cases of injury that would otherwise be considered *spinal cord injury without radiographic abnormality* (SCIWORA) have obvious abnormalities on MRI (65, 66) (Figure 3.28). Unexplained neurologic

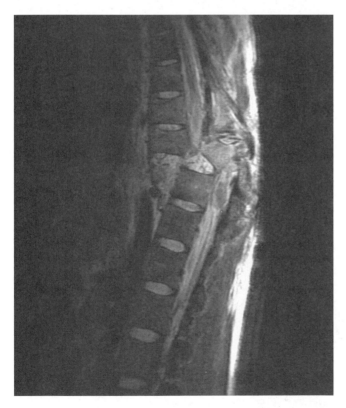

Figure 3.27 Thoracic fracture-dislocation. Sagittal T2-weighted inversion recovery image of a young adult who suffered severe T10–T11 fracture-dislocation in a logging accident shows dislocation and spinal cord transection.

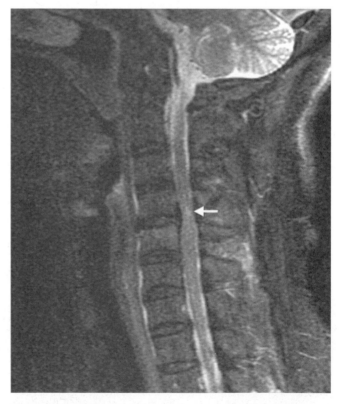

Figure 3.28 Spinal cord contusion without fracture. Sagittal T2-weighted inversion recovery MR image of a man who had upper extremity weakness after a motor vehicle accident shows stenosis of the cervical spinal canal, disc bulge or protrusion at C4–C5, and edema within the spinal cord at the same level (arrow).

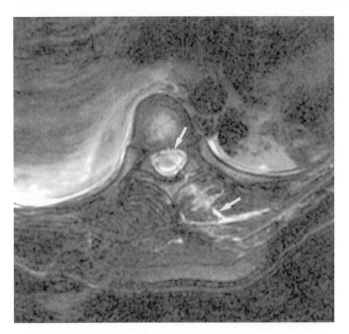

Figure 3.29 Stab injury of the spinal cord. Axial T2-weighted MR image shows linear high signal intensity along the knife track through the posterior soft tissues, left lamina of T10, and left side of the spinal cord (arrows). The patient had left lower extremity sensory loss, but intact strength.

deficits should be assessed with MRI when possible. In addition, MRI may aid in planning surgery by disclosing traumatic disc herniations that can compromise the spinal cord after reduction of fracture or dislocation (67). In the authors' experience, MRI within the first 2 to 3 days after injury can exclude any major ligamentous injury that may threaten the stability of the cervical spine (68).

Penetrating trauma of the spine can also damage the spinal cord and may be more difficult to image if bony injuries are minor. MRI can sometimes demonstrate spinal cord injury in these cases (Figure 3.29).

The late sequelae of traumatic spinal cord injury are best assessed by MRI. Syrinx appears as a region of fluid within the spinal cord, with CSF-signal intensity on both T1-weighted and T2-weighted images. MRI can demonstrate the size and extent of a posttraumatic syrinx and can be used to follow the results of intervention. Posttraumatic myelomalacia appears as a thinning of the spinal cord, often with the appearance of strandlike areas of soft tissue (Figure 3.30). Adhesions or cysts that may further limit spinal cord function can be visualized.

DEGENERATIVE DISEASE AND POSTOPERATIVE SPINAL IMAGING

Spinal degenerative disease is part of the normal aging process. Disc degeneration and associated end-plate osteophyte formation, as well as facet hypertrophy and the prominence of the ligamenta flava, may result in central or neural foraminal stenosis and spinal cord or nerve root compression. However, about 30% of all asymptomatic adults will have MRI findings of lumbar spinal degenerative disease, and 19% of asymptomatic people

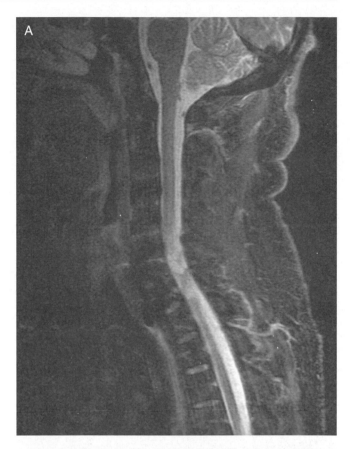

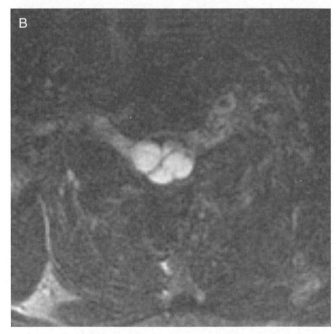

Figure 3.30 Posttraumatic changes. The patient who previously had a C5–C6 dislocation and subsequent anterior instrumentation returned after a new episode of more minor trauma. Sagittal T2-weighted inversion recovery image (**A**) shows loss of spinal cord contour at the level of the old injury. Myelomalacia is corroborated on axial T2-weighted image (**B**); there are multiple strandlike areas of soft tissue, with a suggestion of possible septations and cystic change.

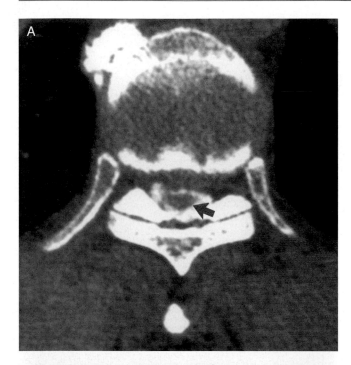

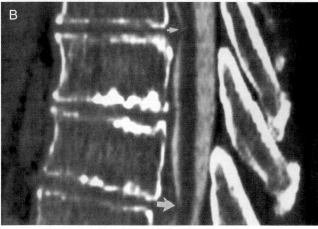

Figure 3.31 Sixty-seven-year-old man with multiple thoracic disc protrusions. **A.** Axial image from postmyelogram CT shows a broad-based central disc protrusion flattening the ventral thecal sac, compressing the spinal cord (black arrow), which is outlined by white contrast-laden CSF. **B.** Sagittal reconstruction from the axial CT data shows two thoracic disc protrusions (arrows) effacing the ventral CSF; the lower protrusion corresponds to A, slightly compressing the spinal cord.

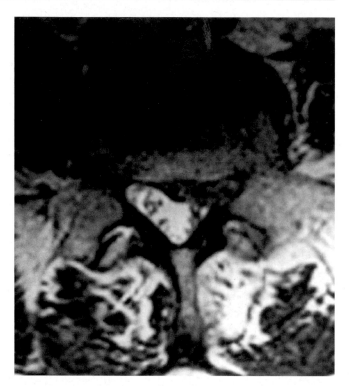

Figure 3.32 Axial FSE-T2 MR image shows a prominent disc protrusion posterior to the L5 vertebra in the left lateral recess, compressing and posteriorly displacing the traversing left L5 nerve root. There is superb delineation between the CSF, disc, and nerve roots (1).

were found to have significant abnormalities on cervical spine MRI (69, 70). Thus, it is essential for the physician to carefully interpret the imaging findings in light of the patient's symptoms (69). Moreover, the natural history of back pain is that about 80% of patients recover within 2 months without any treatment (71); therefore, spinal imaging for back pain should not be obtained emergently except in cases of known or suspected cancer, spinal infection, trauma, and the like.

Discogenic degeneration may be classified as disc bulge, protrusion, extrusion, and sequestered fragment, in order of increasing size and clinical symptomatology (72). Bulges are extremely common (one study [72] found disc bulges in 52% of asymptomatic normal adults) and are generally asymptomatic. These bulges are seen on MRI as a diffuse, nonfocal bulging of the disc beyond the normal contours of the disc and end-plate. Bulges may narrow the central spinal canal and inferior aspect of the neural foramina, but unless they are very large, they do not cause symptoms. Central canal stenosis and myelopathy may result from advanced disease; these disorders present with very large disc bulges and are commonly associated with marginal end-plate bony osteophytes (Figure 3.31).

Disc protrusions are defined as focal posterior deformities of the anulus fibrosus caused by posterior herniation of the nucleus pulposus, and generally have an intact posterior ligamentous complex (Figure 3.32). Disc protrusions have been incidentally found in 27% of asymptomatic volunteers (72); however, protrusions may also be symptomatic, causing spinal cord compression and resultant edema or gliosis within the spinal cord, which is manifested as T2-bright signal (Figure 3.33). Again, the physician must confirm the correlation between patient symptomatology and the MRI findings before intervening surgically.

Disc extrusions are generally larger than protrusions, and are generally associated with rupture of the posterior anuloligamentous complex. Extrusions are more likely to be symptomatic; only 1% of asymptomatic adults had disc extrusions (72).

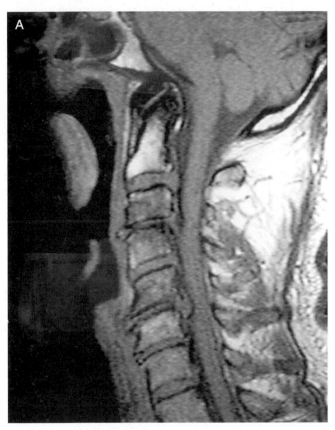
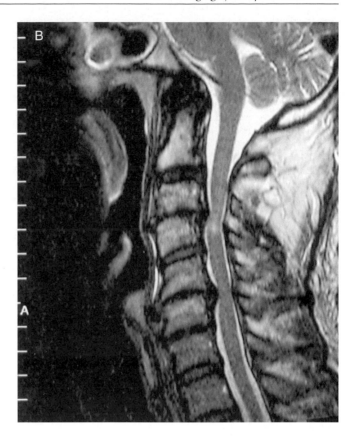

Figure 3.33 Cervical spinal cord compression and gliosis caused by large disc protrusions in a 62-year-old man. Sagittal (**A**) T1-weighted and (**B**) T2-weighted MR images show large disc protrusions at essentially all cervical levels, with spinal cord compression and flattening at C3–C4 and C5–C6. A small focus of T2-bright gliosis is present within the spinal cord (**B**) associated with the compression at C3–C4.

Sequestered fragments result when a disc extrusion becomes separated from the parent disc.

Ossification of the posterior longitudinal ligament (OPLL) is another less-common degenerative disorder, most common in Japanese but also seen in others, which can cause central stenosis and spinal cord compression (71) (Figure 3.34).

Postoperative Complications

Postoperative complications include postoperative hematomas, pseudomeningocele, infection, recurrent disc herniation, and arachnoiditis (73). Recurrent disc herniation can be distinguished from postoperative scar tissue in that, unlike normal scar tissue, recurrent disc herniations do not enhance with IV gadolinium-DTPA (74).

Arachnoiditis has many causes but may be associated with a history of pantopaque myelography or spinal surgery. On MRI, the nerve roots are thickened and clumped and exhibit variable enhancement. They may adhere to the periphery of the thecal sac. Intrathecal arachnoid bands or cysts may be present (Figure 3.35).

Another postoperative complication is improperly positioned spinal hardware. As discussed earlier, titanium hardware is better visualized on CT and MRI than stainless steel (Figures 3.8–3.10). Occasionally, CT demonstrates metal hardware directly impinging on spinal nerve roots (Figure 3.36).

INFLAMMATION AND DEMYELINATION

For purposes of evaluating demyelinating disease of the spinal cord and other inflammatory, intramedullary processes, MRI stands essentially alone as an imaging tool. Myelography and CT can show little more of the spinal cord than change in contour, whereas MRI reveals information about the contents of the spinal cord itself. However, the findings on MRI are often nonspecific, especially for a solitary lesion.

The plaques of multiple sclerosis (MS) appear as areas of high signal intensity within the spinal cord on T2-weighted images. They often occur at the dorsolateral margin of the spinal cord but can be seen elsewhere in the spinal cord. As in the brain, enhancement sometimes occurs in acute plaques, but lack of enhancement does not exclude a plaque (75). In the presence of acute plaques, the spinal cord can be enlarged, which can create concern for a possible neoplasm. For this reason, when a lesion is identified on MRI within the spinal cord, even if it enhances, it is appropriate to consider MS in the differential diagnosis and to obtain MRI of the brain to look for additional evidence of MS. Finding multiple spinal cord lesions increases the likelihood of MS and makes neoplasm much less likely (Figure 3.37).

Devic's disease, or neuromyelitis optica, usually lacks the typical brain findings seen in MS. Spinal cord lesions in Devic's disease are usually larger than MS plaques and have significant

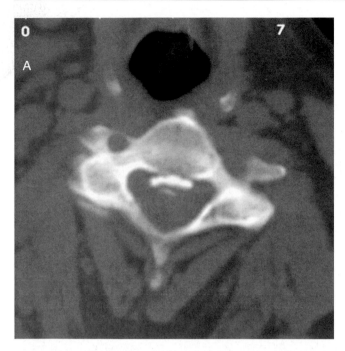

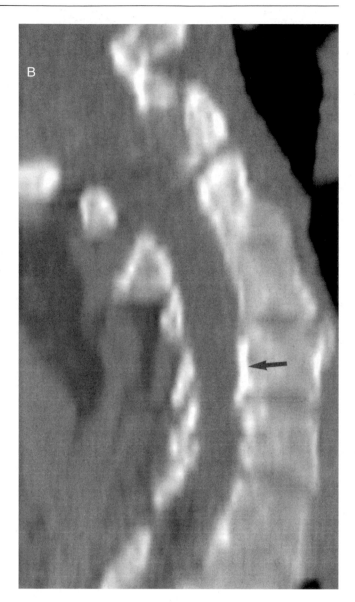

Figure 3.34 Ossification of posterior longitudinal ligament in a 60-year-old man. Axial CT image through C4 (**A**) and (**B**) sagittal CT reconstruction show a calcified, thickened posterior longitudinal ligament (black arrow) compromising the spinal canal.

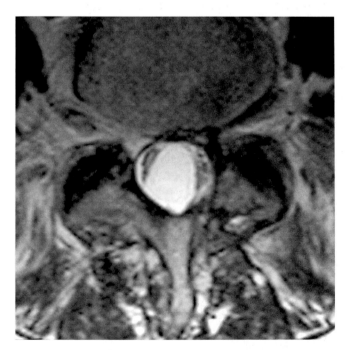

Figure 3.35 Pathologically proven arachnoiditis and central intradural arachnoid cyst in a 61-year-old man with prior lumbar surgery. Axial T2-weighted MR image at the L5-S1 level shows a central arachnoid cyst, with nerve roots clumped together and displaced lateral to the cyst. Old left hemilaminectomy defect noted.

longitudinal extent, often several spinal segments (Figure 3.38). Findings of optic neuritis help establish the diagnosis.

Transverse myelitis is usually readily apparent on MRI as a region of increased T2 signal intensity, often having an elongated or spindle shape on sagittal images (Figure 3.39). The term encompasses inflammation of the spinal cord from a variety of causes, but the imaging appearance is usually nonspecific (76).

Imaging plays an ancillary role in the evaluation of the patient with suspected Guillain-Barré syndrome. However, if MRI of the spine is performed, the nerve roots often appear thickened, and they enhance after intravenous contrast administration (Figure 3.40). Such enhancement is not specific and can also be seen with drop metastases or with infection. In Guillain-Barré syndrome, enhancement of both ventral and dorsal nerve roots or only ventral nerve roots can be seen; the latter is more specific (77, 78).

The spinal canal and cord can also be compromised by extradural inflammatory processes such as rheumatoid arthritis

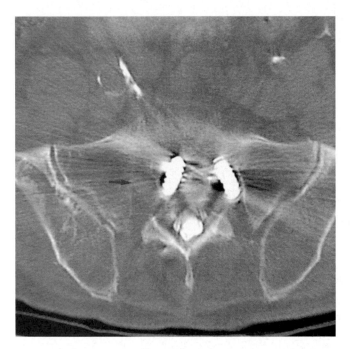

Figure 3.36 Sixty-four-year-old man with left S1 radiculopathy after spinal surgery. Axial image from postmyelogram CT shows the left pedicle screw incorrectly positioned, within the left S1 neural canal, obliterating the left S1 nerve root and correlating with the patient's symptoms. The right pedicle screw is malpositioned medial to the right S1 neural canal. The black arrow points to the right S1 nerve root in its neural canal.

(RA). A variety of conditions can affect the spinal cord, especially in the cervical spine. Erosions can lead to subluxation. Pannus in the region of the synovial space at the transverse ligament can lead to weakening or destruction of the ligament, with subsequent instability at C1–C2. The softening of bone and ligament destruction can result in basilar invagination, threatening the brainstem itself. Plain films and CT can demonstrate the erosive changes and subluxation, and MRI can show the pannus and the relationship of pannus and bone to the spinal cord (Figure 3.41).

Patients with longstanding ankylosing spondylitis may develop cauda equina syndrome. Their lumbar MRI may demonstrate a classic appearance of intrathecal arachnoiditis and a dilated thecal sac with erosion of the posterior elements (79), obviating the need for myelography (Figure 3.42).

SPINAL INFECTIONS

The incidence of central nervous system (CNS) infections, including spinal involvement, has increased in recent decades, largely because of AIDS (80). The most common site of spinal infection is the vertebral bodies and discs, which can then exert mass effect on the thecal sac, spinal cord, and nerve roots. Direct involvement of the epidural space is also common. Spinal infections can also involve the intradural space (Figure 3.43), being either extramedullary, involving the meninges, as in arachnoiditis, or intramedullary, involving the spinal cord and cauda equina directly (as in parenchymal myelitis, granuloma, or abscess).

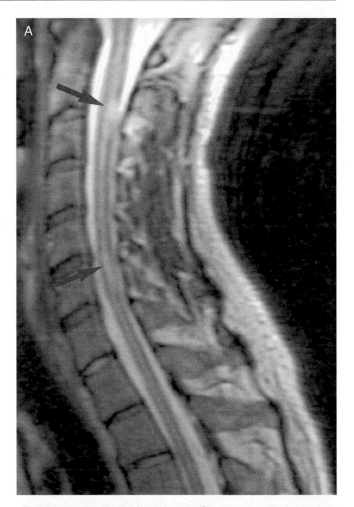

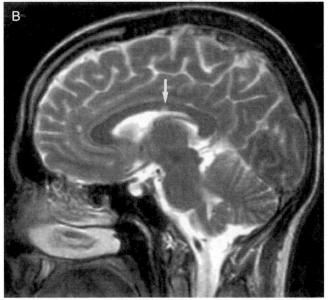

Figure 3.37 Multiple sclerosis. This young adult had lower and then upper extremity numbness. Sagittal T2-weighted image of the cervical spine cord (**A**) shows two separate areas of high signal intensity within the spinal cord (arrows). Sagittal T2-weighted image of the brain (**B**) shows a plaque in the inferior margin of the corpus callosum (arrow).

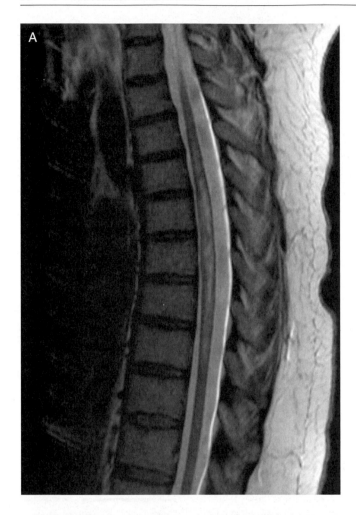

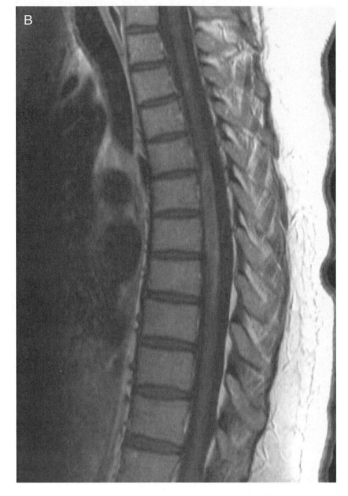

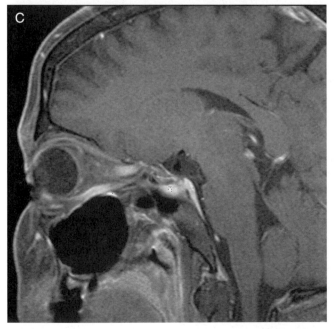

Figure 3.38 Devic's disease. Sagittal T2-weighted (**A**) and post-contrast T1-weighted (**B**) images of the lower thoracic spine show a long segment of T2-prolongation, mild expansion, and contrast enhancement within the lower thoracic spinal cord, extending over several spinal segments. Postcontrast fat-saturated sagittal T1 of the orbit and brain (**C**) shows marked enhancement of the optic nerve in the posterior orbit, representing optic neuritis.

Diagnostic imaging is essential in the diagnosis and treatment of patients with spinal infections. Conventional radiographs may be useful in initial evaluation of spinal infection involving the vertebrae and discs and can classically demonstrate the loss of height of the disc, erosion of the adjacent end-plates, and loss of vertebral body height. The most common bacterial organism is *Staphylococcus;* others are *Enterobacter, Salmonella, Pseudomonas,* and *Serratia* species (81). However, although associated soft-tissue masses may be demonstrated on plain films, only the bony cortical structures are well demonstrated.

CT demonstrates both the bony anatomy and soft tissue anatomy on cross-sectional images. However, the spinal cord is not delineated unless intrathecal contrast is introduced (myelography)—an invasive procedure. Computer-generated sagittal (and/or coronal) reconstructions are necessary to appreciate abnormalities of alignment and the three-dimensional anatomy of the infected spine.

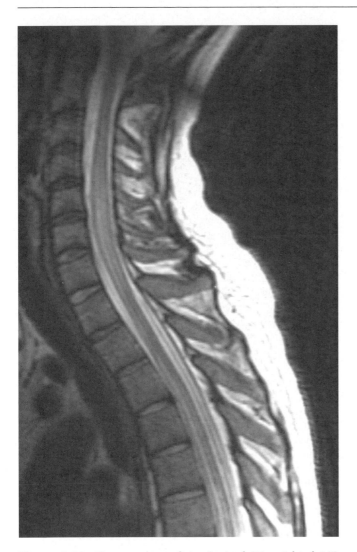

Figure 3.39 Transverse myelitis. Sagittal T2-weighted MR image of a patient who developed urinary retention and spinal cord level 3 weeks after a respiratory illness shows a region of high signal intensity in the cervical spinal cord. Abnormal signal continued into the thoracic spine.

MRI is the modality of choice in imaging spinal infections, because it noninvasively and clearly demonstrates soft tissue anatomy and pathology, including spinal cord or nerve root involvement, in addition to the bony anatomy demonstrated on plain X-rays. MRI can directly image in the sagittal (or any other) plane, in addition to in the axial plane.

Pyogenic infections generally involve the intervertebral disc and the adjacent portions of the vertebral bodies, with loss of demarcation of the end-plate cortex. The disc and vertebrae demonstrate decreased signal on T1-weighted images and increased signal on T2-weighted images (82) (Figure 3.44). A study by Modic et al. (82) reported that MRI has a sensitivity of 96%, a specificity of 93%, and an accuracy of 94% in the evaluation of osteomyelitis, equaling the results of combined bone and gallium scanning, but with the added benefits of superb anatomic resolution, as well as visualization of the soft tissues including the spinal cord, thecal sac, and paraspinal tissues.

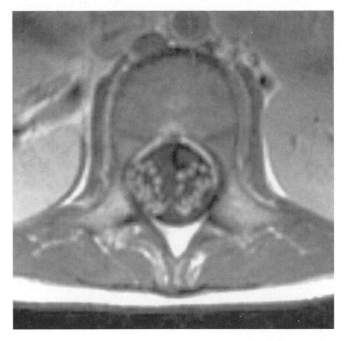

Figure 3.40 Guillain-Barré. Axial T1-weighted image through the lumbar spine after intravenous gadolinium-DTPA administration shows intense enhancement of the lumbar nerve roots.

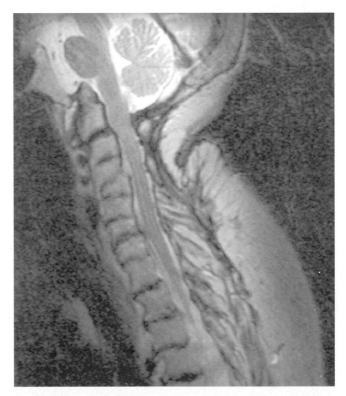

Figure 3.41 Rheumatoid arthritis (RA) and basilar invagination. Sagittal T2-weighted MR image of a woman with rheumatoid arthritis shows erosion of the dens and basilar invagination, with the dens nearly to the level of the pons. Subluxations at C2–C3 and C4–C5 typical of RA, are noted.

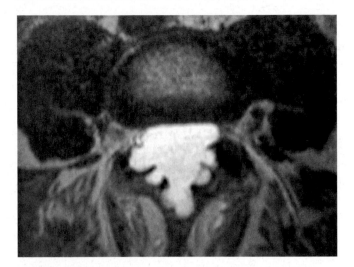

Figure 3.42 Cauda equina syndrome in 59-year-old man with longstanding ankylosing spondylitis. Axial T2-weighted image through the upper lumbar spine shows a patulous thecal sac with scalloped, eroded posterior elements. The inflamed, scarred nerve roots adhere to the walls of the thecal sac.

Epidural abscesses are often found in association with bony osteomyelitis and diskitis (Figure 3.44) but also may be an isolated finding (Figure 3.45). Again, MRI is the imaging modality of choice, especially with the use of intravenous gadolinium-DTPA. *Staphylococcus aureus* is the most common causative organism (occurring in about 60% of cases). Another 13% of cases are caused by other gram-positive cocci, and 15% are caused by gram-negative organisms (80, 83, 84). Most epidural abscesses enhance homogeneously with IV Gd-DTPA, suggesting that they are largely phlegmonous, but nonenhancing frank pus may also be recognized as a central collection of fluidlike T1-dark, T2-bright signal surrounded by an enhancing soft tissue rim (Figures 3.44 and 3.45).

Brucellosis presents with bony lytic lesions of the vertebral body, usually in the lower lumbar spine (85, 86).

Tuberculosis (87) differs from pyogenic bacterial infections in that the intervertebral disc is often relatively spared in early disease (possibly because mycobacteria lack proteolytic enzymes). It appears without abnormal T2-bright signal, more involvement of posterior aspects of the vertebrae, involvement of more than two vertebral bodies, and larger associated paraspinal masses. CT may show the small soft tissue calcifications suggestive of tuberculosis, which are not reliably shown on MRI (88). Chronic tuberculosis infection may result in a classic kyphotic deformity, known as Pott's disease, usually in the mid-thoracic region.

Patients with AIDS may often present with polyradiculopathy caused by viruses, most commonly cytomegalovirus (89). Gadolinium-enhanced MRI is by far the best modality to visualize the enhancing nerve roots of the cauda equina, which may appear normal on standard T1- and T2-weighted images; occasionally, enhancement extends diffusely throughout the spinal subarachnoid space (Figure 3.46). Infection of the spinal cord by the HIV virus has been found to cause vacuolar myelopathy

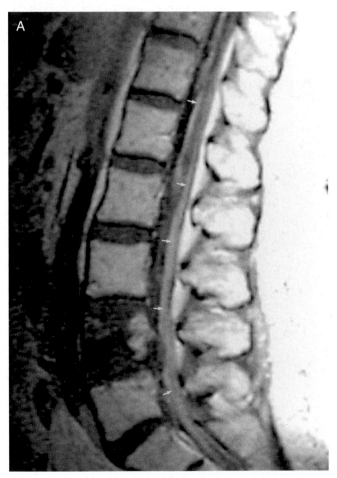

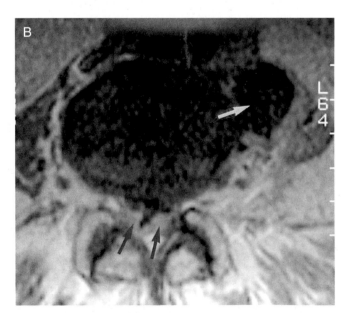

Figure 3.43 Fifty-seven-year-old woman with pyogenic spinal infection and left psoas abscess, with intradural extension. **A**. Sagittal postcontrast T1-weighted image shows diffuse thickening and abnormal enhancement of the cauda equina and enhancing intradural exudate around the distal spinal cord (small white arrows). The anterior portion of the L4 vertebra is infected. **B**. Axial postcontrast T1-weighted image again shows diffuse thickening and abnormal enhancement of the cauda equina (black arrows). White arrow points to pus in left psoas abscess.

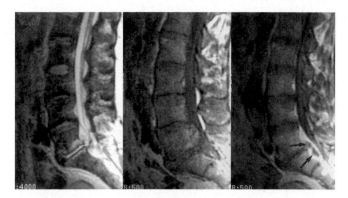

Figure 3.44 Pyogenic spinal infection in an adult male with L5–S1 diskitis, osteomyelitis, and epidural abscess. **Left**. Sagittal T2-weighted image shows T2-bright pus within the L5–S1 disc, extending posteriorly. T2-bright edema or infection is noted involving the adjacent end-plates. **Middle**. T1-weighted image better shows the associated epidural abscess compressing the distal thecal sac. **Right**. Postcontrast T1-weighted image again shows enhancing phlegmonous tissue compressing the anterior aspect of the thecal sac. T1-dark pus is noted centrally in the epidural abscess (arrows).

in AIDS patients. Spinal MRI may be normal but usually presents with spinal cord atrophy, or occasionally with T2-bright signal (90). Enhancement with IV contrast is not generally seen in AIDS-associated myelopathy (90).

VASCULAR LESIONS AND ISCHEMIA

Suspected vascular disease of the spine can be particularly challenging to verify with imaging. The spinal cord itself is best visualized with MRI, but angiography can have an important role in some cases.

Spinal cord infarction appears on MRI as a region of increased T2 signal intensity (Figure 3.47). This appearance is nonspecific, especially because the vascular territories are usually not as obvious in the spinal cord as in the brain. Distinction of spinal cord infarction from other entities, such as infectious or demyelinating processes, is therefore often more dependent on clinical information than on differences in imaging appearance.

Vascular malformations of the spine have been divided into four types: intramedullary glomus-type arteriovenous malformation (AVM), juvenile AVM, dural arteriovenous fistula, and perimedullary arteriovenous fistula (91). Patient age and the clinical presentations of these tend to differ. Symptoms can result from hemorrhage or from ischemia caused by venous hypertension or steal.

Hemorrhage within the spinal cord has an appearance similar to blood elsewhere in the CNS and depends on the age of the hemorrhage. The details of MRI appearance of hemorrhage are not reviewed here. It is important to consider the effect of the MRI technique on the appearance of hemorrhage. Fast spin-echo techniques, which are widely used for spine imaging because of the advantages in acquisition time and artifact reduction, also reduce the susceptibility changes of blood. This can make blood less conspicuous with fast spin-echo tech-

niques. Gradient-echo techniques, on the other hand, exaggerate magnetic susceptibility differences between blood and surrounding tissues. Although this can increase some artifacts, it has the potential advantage of making hemorrhage more conspicuous.

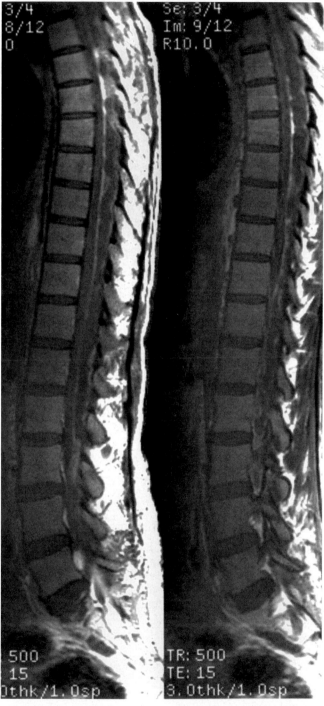

Figure 3.45 Twenty-one-year-old woman with autoimmune hepatitis, chronically on steroids, with diffuse posterior epidural cryptococcal abscess throughout her spine. Sequential postcontrast sagittal T1-weighted images of the thoracolumbar spine show an abscess with thin enhancing rind, located posterior to the thoracic spinal cord and cauda equina and compressing them. Note that the vertebrae and discs are normal.

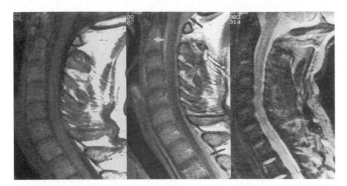

Figure 3.46 Thirty-one-year-old man with AIDS, who presented with bilateral leg pain and weakness and loss of bowel and bladder control. **Left**. Sagittal T1-weighted MR images of the cervical spine are normal, as are sagittal T2-weighted images, **Right**. (Patient is angulated on the T2-weighted images; the lower spinal cord is out of view so that CSF, rather than cord, is imaged; note that spinous processes are also out of field.) **Middle**. However, T1-weighted images after IV administration of gadolinium-DTPA show diffuse marked enhancement of inflammatory tissue throughout the spinal subarachnoid space (white and black arrows). Herpes simplex II virus was cultured from his CSF, and cytomegalovirus was cultured from his blood.

The differential diagnosis of hemorrhage within the spinal cord includes trauma (which would usually be obvious by history), vascular malformation, and neoplasm. The presence of multiple areas of flow void on MRI provides additional evidence of a high-flow vascular malformation. These may be present within the spinal cord in the case of intramedullary AVMs (Figure 3.48), or on the surface of the spinal cord or more peripherally in the case of AV fistulas (Figure 3.49). Tortuous draining veins are usually more conspicuous than the feeding arteries. Superficial vessels, especially enlarged draining veins, can be shown on myelography.

Angiography plays an important role in the diagnosis of spinal vascular malformations. It defines the location and number of feeding arteries, the size of the central nidus in the case of AVMs, and the location of the direct fistulous connection in fistulas (Figure 3.49B); it also shows the extent and direction of venous drainage. Depending on the nature and location of the malformation, endovascular therapy, such as embolization, can be used either alone or in combination with surgery to treat the condition. In some cases of suspected fistula, an exhaustive search of spinal arteries may be necessary, from the lowest lumbosacral branches up through the vertebral, cervical, and external carotid arteries.

Cavernous malformations can occur in the spinal cord as well in the brain, and the imaging characteristics are similar. Typically, blood products of varying age are present with a surrounding rim of dark T2-signal intensity from hemosiderin. Larger lesions often have a reticulated appearance because they contain pockets of methemoglobin, but small lesions may be seen only as hemosiderin scars. Acute hemorrhage within a cavernous malformation has a less-specific appearance unless the surrounding older blood products are visible.

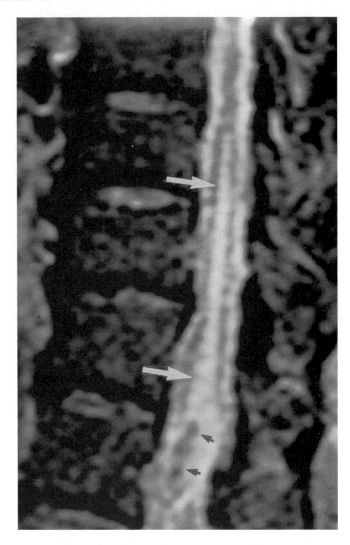

Figure 3.47 Spinal cord infarct in a 68-year-old man, sustained during surgical repair of abdominal aortic aneurysm. Sagittal T2-weighted image shows T2-bright edema (white arrows) within the distal thoracic spinal cord and conus, with small amount of dark intramedullary hemorrhage (black arrowheads) distally.

SPINAL TUMORS

An estimated one in four or five central nervous system tumors are located in the spine (92–94). A study by Kurland (95) estimated the incidence of primary spine tumors to be 2.5 per 100,000 people per year. MRI is the best single modality for imaging spine tumors (96). Its unsurpassed soft tissue differentiation (including the ability to differentiate between CSF and neural tissue without the use of intrathecal contrast), absence of beam-hardening artifact, and ability to image in multiple planes make it clearly superior to CT, myelography, plain films, and ultrasonography in evaluating epidural and intradural disease. For bony disease and primary bone tumors, plain X-rays and CT are still essential.

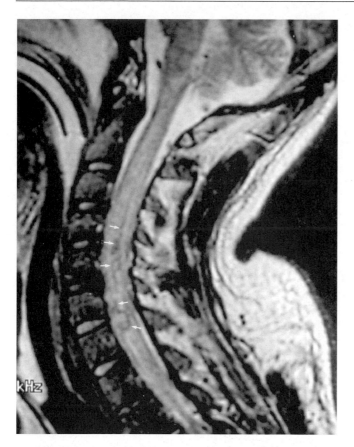

Figure 3.48 Intramedullary spinal arteriovenous malformation (AVM) in a 29-year-old man presenting with hemiparesis and difficulty breathing. Sagittal T2-weighted MRI image shows diffuse swelling and edema throughout the cervical spinal cord. Serpiginous linear flow voids of the intramedullary AVM and its draining vein extend from the C4 to C7 levels (small white arrows). The AVM was successfully endovascularly embolized via a right vertebral artery approach.

Technique

The screening MRI technique we use for the spine is sagittal TR 500–600, TE 11 and FSE sagittal TR 3000–4000, TE 102, which allow us to obtain a quick "myelogram" in about 4 minutes. Axial FSE T2-weighted images are obtained in a stacked fashion, rather than using oblique axials through the disc spaces only, which could result in missing portions of the tumor. Slice thickness should be preferably 3 mm on the sagittal images, and 4 mm axially, with a 1-mm gap to minimize partial-volume errors.

T1-weighted gadolinium-enhanced images (in sagittal and axial planes) are recommended to evaluate intradural tumors (97). Generally, intradural extramedullary tumors enhance significantly; enhancement of intramedullary tumors is more variable. However, in imaging vertebral metastases, gadolinium enhancement is not only not helpful, but may be detrimental, because T1-dark marrow metastases enhance and become isointense to normal T1-bright marrow, unless fat-saturation is employed.

To minimize CSF pulsation and other motion artifacts, flow compensation, cardiac gating, respiratory gating, and phase-frequency direction swapping are useful. However, in many systems, flow compensation is not yet available with fast spin-echo, and motion artifacts can be a problem for those inexperienced in reading FSE images.

The use of phased-array coils is extremely valuable in obtaining better signal-to-noise and obviating the need to move the coil or the patient when covering a large portion of the spine (as in screening for epidural cord compression).

In addition to T1-weighted images, inversion-recovery (IR) (or preferably, FSE IR) sequences also demonstrate vertebral marrow metastases by nulling the neighboring marrow fat (30, 31). Inversion-recovery images, like T2-weighted images, clearly demonstrate intramedullary edema or tumors as bright signal.

Coronal imaging may be useful, for example, in imaging cervicothoracic neurofibromas.

Gradient-echo T2* (GRE) images are generally not useful in the imaging of spinal tumors. The differentiation between soft tissue or tumor and CSF is poorer than on true-T2 or FSE-T2 images. GRE images are only useful for detecting small amounts of hemosiderin or calcium, which could be missed on FSE images and may be missed on SE T2-weighted images.

Spine tumors are generally classified according to anatomic location as extradural; intradural, extramedullary; or intramedullary.

Extradural Tumors

These account for about a third of all spine neoplasms and generally involve the vertebrae (92). The majority are metastases to bone. Metastases to the epidural space are less common, and even less common are tumors (benign or malignant) arising from the osseous or notochordal structures of the spine. A small fraction of neurofibromas and meningiomas are completely extradural.

Primary bone lesions may have a more characteristic appearance on plain X-rays than on MRI, because the cortical pattern and calcification are not well appreciated on MR. However, MRI detects changes in marrow, rather than in the bony matrix, and so is the most sensitive detector of vertebral body tumors (98).

Extradural Malignancy

Metastases to bone are by far the most common malignant tumors involving the spine encountered in everyday practice. Often the site of disease cannot be accurately localized clinically. Hence, it is important to be able to quickly and efficiently screen the entire spine in these patients. It is impractical and unnecessary to obtain sagittal and axial T1- and T2-weighted images, as well as pre- and postgadolinium images through all levels of the spine. These patients often suffer excruciating pain and are unable to lie motionless for even moderate lengths of time.

Instead, the screening examination should consist of first, a *single* T1-weighted sequence using a large field of view (48–50 cm) with a large matrix (512 × 512 or 512 × 384) in the sagittal plane. This will cover nearly the entire spine in a single acquisition of about 6 minutes or less (Figure 3.50). A fast spin-echo T2-weighted (FSE-T2) sagittal screening sequence can give a myelogram-effect scan in another few minutes, pointing out regions of CSF effacement by tumor. Then, 4-mm axial images (either T1 or fast spin-echo T2) may be obtained only

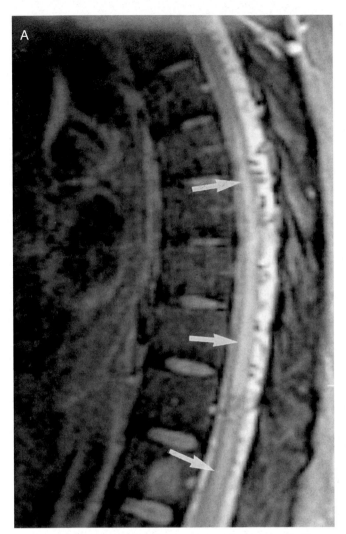

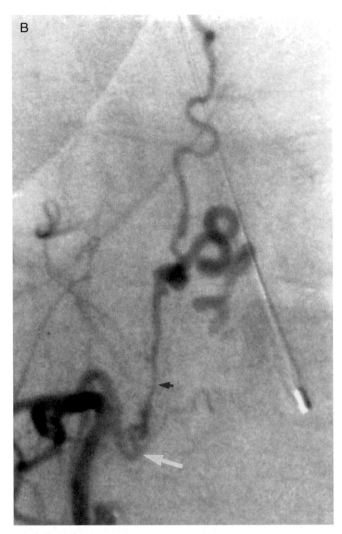

Figure 3.49 Spinal-dural arteriovenous fistula in a 42-year-old man presenting with paraplegia. **A.** Sagittal T2-weighted MRI image shows swelling and edema (white arrows) within the mid-lower thoracic spinal cord and multiple serpiginous flow-voids of an abnormal draining vein immediately dorsal to the spinal cord. **B.** Spinal angiogram with injection at the T7 level shows an abnormal fistulous connection (black arrowhead) between the radicular artery (white arrow) and the abnormal tortuous, dilated draining vein coursing superiorly. The patient's symptoms resolved within 2 minutes of endovascular embolization with glue.

at the levels of cord compression, to better delineate the degree of compression. Gadolinium is generally not needed to diagnose and evaluate cord compression from bony vertebral metastases. Hence, a complete examination can be obtained in about 20 minutes, which can be tolerated by almost all patients.

Good analgesia, such as morphine, is important to aid patient comfort and prevent image degradation by motion. Anxiolytics such as diazepam (Valium) or midazolam are less valuable; these patients move around in the scanner more from pain than from claustrophobia or anxiety.

Phased-array coils give superb signal-to-noise and enable complete spinal coverage without moving the patient or the coil. However, lacking a phased-array coil, the *body coil* should be used to screen the entire spine using the single large FOV T1-weighted sagittal sequence. Use of a conventional "license-plate" coil to initially separately screen the cervical spine, the thoracic spine, and the lumbar spine, using both T1- and T2-weighted

sequences in the axial and sagittal planes, followed by post-gadolinium sagittal and axial images of the cervical, thoracic, and lumbar regions will take hours, result in extreme patient discomfort, and generate reams of unnecessary and motion-degraded images.

As mentioned, T1-weighted SE images are sensitive to detecting these lesions, but their MRI appearance is not specific. They are dark on T1, are bright on T2, and enhance variably with contrast. Type I (fibrovascular) Modic degenerative changes and infection have similar signal characteristics. An important distinguishing characteristic between infection and tumor is that tumor generally spares the disc space, whereas infection (excepting tuberculosis) characteristically involves it. An infected disc appears as a very white T2-bright signal and often shows erosion of the adjacent end-plates. Conversely, Modic degenerative changes are associated with degenerated (i.e., T2-dark) discs, whereas tumor should not affect the disc signal.

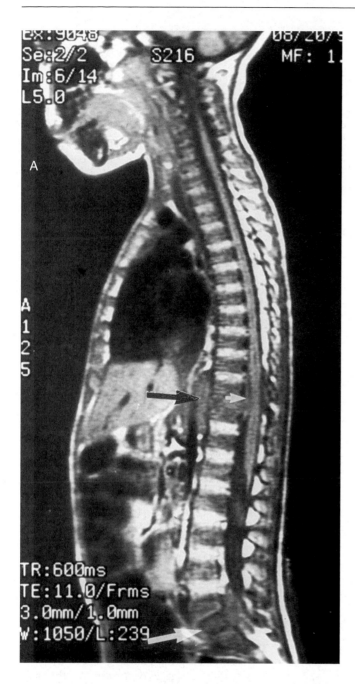

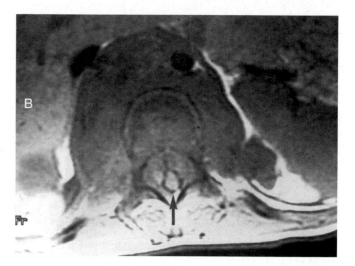

Figure 3.50 Metastatic bladder rhabdomyosarcoma in a 6-year-old girl. **A.** Sagittal T1-weighted large field-of-view image of the entire spine obtained in only 5 minutes shows the regions of vertebral tumor involvement (large arrows) and cord compression (arrowhead). **B.** Axial T1-image shows the large amount of vertebral and paraspinal tumor, which anteriorly displaces the aorta and vena cava and extends medially through the neural foramina into the spinal canal and compresses the cord (black arrow) from both sides (96).

Although some authors have tried to find radiographic signs distinguishing pathologic from osteoporotic fractures, such as complete replacement of marrow by T1-dark signal or posterior-convex vertebral body border indicating tumor, it is often not possible to make the distinction with certainty (99, 100).

Multiple Myeloma

Plasma cell neoplasms commonly involve the spine, usually in the thoracic region and generally in patients beyond middle age (101). The classic radiographic appearance of small "punched out" lytic lesions may also be seen as multiple small T1-dark foci in the vertebral body marrow on MRI. MRI is an efficient way to screen the entire spine for myeloma, and especially to evaluate for cord compression (Figure 3.51).

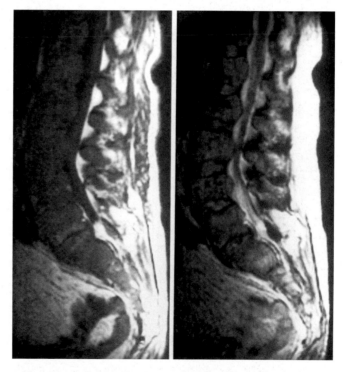

Figure 3.51 Multiple myeloma in a 61-year-old woman. **Left.** Sagittal T1-weighted image shows diffuse abnormal low intensity in all the marrow because of multiple myeloma infiltration. **Right.** Sagittal fast spin-echo T2-weighted image gives a myelogram effect and shows good conspicuity between the posteriorly bulging tumor-laden vertebrae and the CSF and neural structures (96).

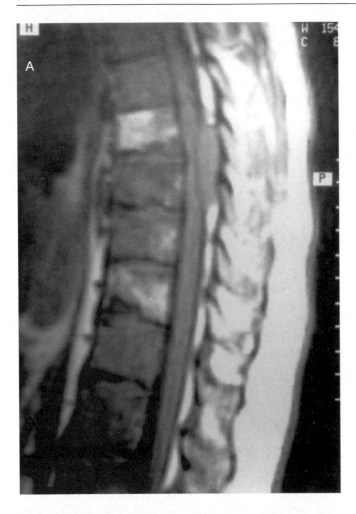

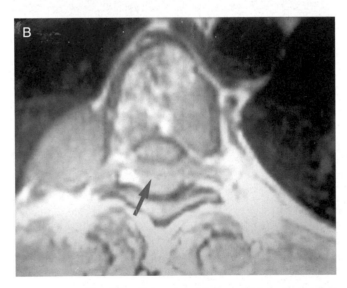

Leukemia and Lymphoma

The spinal marrow is often involved by these tumors of hematopoietic and lymphoid cells. Both may show variable radiographic appearance on MRI, including diffuse or patchy infiltration of marrow, sometimes causing cord impingement by compression fracture or by focal tumor deposits in bone. Extradural tumor may also present as separate epidural foci (102) (Figure 3.52).

Hemangioma

These tumors are very common incidental findings on MRI. They are found in 10% to 15% of patients at autopsy (101), increasing in incidence with age. In our experience, small bone hemangiomas are seen in almost every older patient. The most common location is the thoracic spine, followed by the lumbar spine (102). Mottled T1-bright signal caused by interspersed adipose tissue and a T2-bright signal of fluid and cells are characteristic (Figure 3.53). The hemangiomas are usually round and small when found incidentally but may occupy the entire vertebral body, expanding it and causing neurologic symptoms. The bony striations and spicules classically seen on plain films and CT may be seen on MRI.

Other Primary Bone Tumors

Giant Cell Tumor

Hemangiomas are the most common benign spinal bone tumor; giant cell tumors are the second most common (103). Their appearance on MRI is somewhat nonspecific, as is their appearance on plain films (Figure 3.54).

Aneurysmal Bone Cyst

These are expansile benign masses containing multiple blood-filled cysts, well seen on MRI. Signal intensity is somewhat variable depending on the state of the blood contents. Only 20% of aneurysmal bone cysts involve the spine (102).

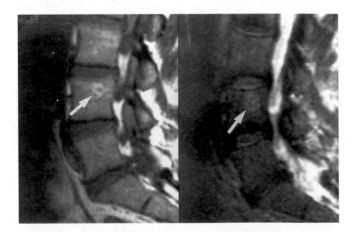

Figure 3.52 B-cell lymphoma in a 23-year-old man. **A.** Sagittal T1 MR-image shows patchy increased and decreased signal within the vertebral marrow, indicating tumor involvement. A large posterior epidural tumor mass compresses the cord from behind. **B.** Axial T1-image at this level shows vertebral marrow involvement, a large paravertebral tumor mass, and the posterior epidural mass (arrow) compressing the cord (96).

Figure 3.53 Small hemangioma (arrows) in a 38-year-old woman. **Left.** T1-weighted sagittal image. **Right.** T2-weighted sagittal image (96).

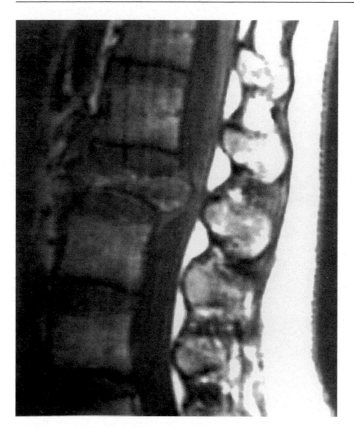

Figure 3.54 Giant cell tumor, with vertebral collapse and posterior retropulsion into the spinal canal in a 28-year-old man, shown on a sagittal T1-weighted MR image (96).

Other bone tumors include eosinophilic granuloma (histiocytosis X), osteoid osteoma, osteoblastoma, and the chondral tumors such as osteochondromas and chondrosarcomas.

Intradural-Extramedullary Tumors

Nerve Sheath Tumors

These comprise *schwannomas* (Figure 3.55) and *neurofibromas* (Figure 3.56) and occur most often in the thoracic spine. Most are intradural-extramedullary, although about 10% are both intradural and extradural; occasionally they are completely extradural (92). Schwannomas are usually solitary unless the patient has neurofibromatosis-2 (NF-2); these, along with meningiomas, are the usual intradural-extramedullary spinal neoplasm of NF-2 (Figure 3.57). (The typical intramedullary tumor of NF-2 is the ependymoma [104].) Most cases are seen in young to middle-aged adults (males slightly younger than females); males and females are equally affected, unlike the case with meningiomas, which have a strong female predominance (92). In a large series of intraspinal tumors cited in Slooff et al. (105), schwannomas (29%) had a slightly higher prevalence than meningiomas or gliomas.

Schwannomas and neurofibromas have a similar radiographic appearance. They are fairly isointense on T1 and bright on T2, and they enhance with contrast. Sometimes schwannomas have a cystic component (Figure 3.55), unlike neurofibromas (106). On postgadolinium and T2-weighted images, neurofibromas may have a central, nonenhancing, T2-dark focus (107) (Figures 3.56 and 3.58).

Meningioma

These occur in middle-aged and older adults, at a female-to-male ratio of greater than 4 to 1. Eighty percent are located in the

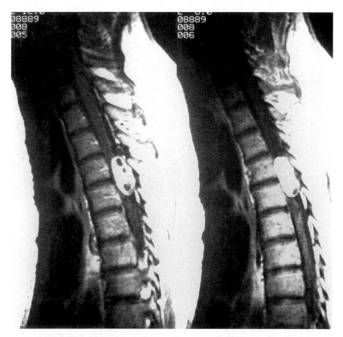

Figure 3.55 Schwannoma in a 52-year-old man. Consecutive sagittal postgadolinium T1 images show an oval, well-circumscribed intradural-extramedullary enhancing mass that contains darker cystic-appearing components and markedly compresses the mid thoracic spinal cord (96).

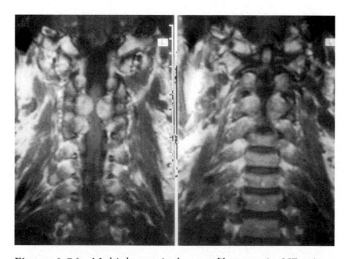

Figure 3.56 Multiple cervical neurofibromas in NF-1 in a 15-year-old boy. Consecutive postgadolinium coronal T1 MR images show multiple bilateral enhancing neurofibromas at nearly every level. The cord is markedly compressed by the bilateral tumors. Note the typical nonenhancing central core in these neurofibromas (96).

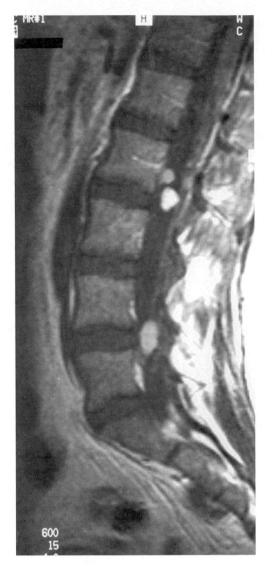

Figure 3.57 Multiple cauda equina schwannomas in NF-2 in an 18-year-old-woman. Sagittal postgadolinium T1-weighted MR image shows multiple nodular enhancing masses adherent to the cauda (96).

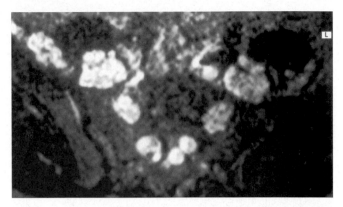

Figure 3.58 Multiple large sacral neurofibromas in NF-1, in an 8-year-old boy. Axial T2-weighted image shows multiple large bright neurofibromas involving all the sacral nerve roots within the nerve root canals, and extending out along the sacral ala into the pelvis. Note the typical central core of darker signal in the tumors (96).

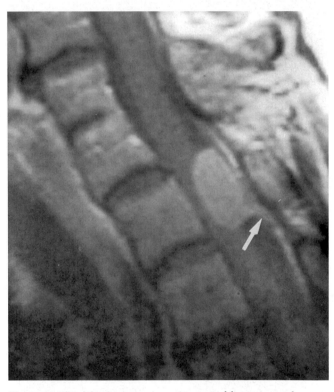

Figure 3.59 Meningioma in a 62-year-old woman, who presented with a several-month history of decreasing ability to walk. Postgadolinium sagittal T1 MR image shows uniform enhancement of the well-circumscribed intradural-extramedullary mass, which markedly compresses the thoracic spinal cord at the T2 level. Note the characteristic enhancing "dural tail" (arrow) (96).

thoracic region (Figure 3.59). About 6% are intradural-extradural, and an equivalent number are completely extradural (92). These have similar signal characteristics to schwannomas, enhance brightly and homogeneously (97), and characteristically are dural based. Rarely, a meningioma may have an intramedullary component.

Paraganglioma

Spinal paragangliomas have the same histology as their more familiar counterparts elsewhere in the body, such as the adrenal medulla and carotid body, and have similar imaging characteristics, including prominent contrast enhancement. They are found in adults and are generally attached to the filum terminale or cauda equina (106) (Figure 3.60).

Embryonal Tumors

Developmental tumors (e.g., epidermoids, lipomas, dermoids, teratomas) have a variable appearance on MRI, depending on the constituent components composing the tumor. Fat-saturation techniques in MRI are very helpful in making the diagnosis of fatty components (Figure 3.61). The presence of fat is also

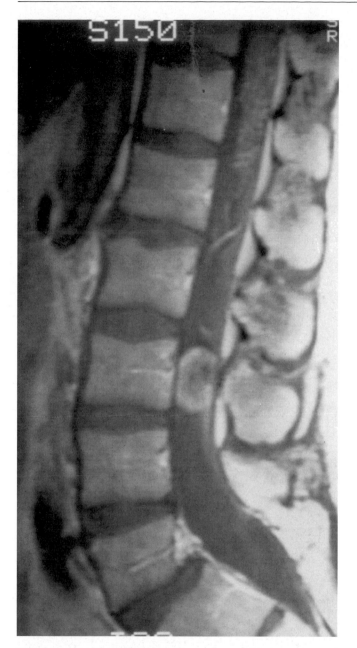

Figure 3.60 Paraganglioma in a 47-year-old man. Sagittal postgadolinium T1 MR image shows a well-circumscribed enhancing mass adherent to the filum terminale at the L3 level. Courtesy of Dr. P. Burger (96).

definitively diagnosed by CT (by fat's very low attenuation of approximately –100 Hounsfield units).

In the spine, as in the brain, epidermoids may be difficult to detect on MRI, because they may be isointense to CSF on all standard pulse sequences (108) (Figure 3.62). However, diffusion-weighted imaging (DWI) has proven very useful in distinguishing epidermoids (which usually demonstrate markedly restricted diffusion) from normal CSF or arachnoid cysts (which do not) (37, 43) (Figure 3.63).

Abnormalities of spinal development, such as meningomyeloceles or tethered cord, are commonly accompanied by developmental tumors, especially lipomas (Figure 3.64).

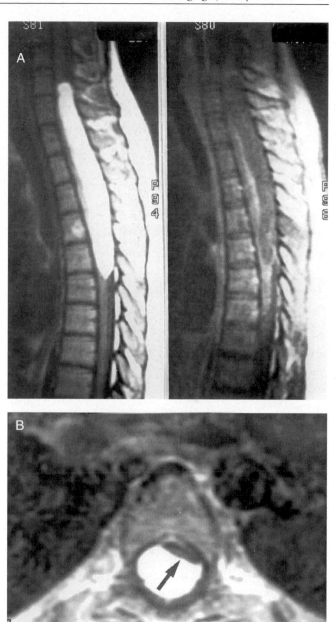

Figure 3.61 Intradural extramedullary lipoma in a 20-year-old woman. **A, Left**. Sagittal T1 MR image shows a very large, well-circumscribed intradural-extramedullary T1-bright mass posterior to and compressing the upper thoracic cord. **A, Right**. Fat-saturated postgadolinium T1 image shows complete suppression of the T1-bright signal, proving the presence of fat rather than T1-bright blood. A subtle thin rim of enhancement is noted around the tumor capsule. **B**. Axial T1 image shows the lipoma filling and expanding the thecal sac and spinal canal, markedly flattening the cord (arrow) (96).

Metastases

Spinal subarachnoid metastases result from CSF seeding from intracranial primary tumors such as medulloblastoma (Figure 3.65) or ependymoma, lung or breast cancer(Figure 3.66),

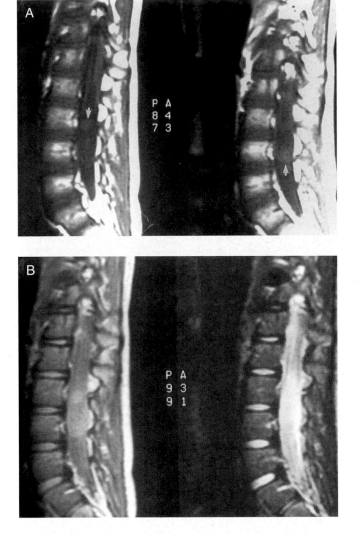

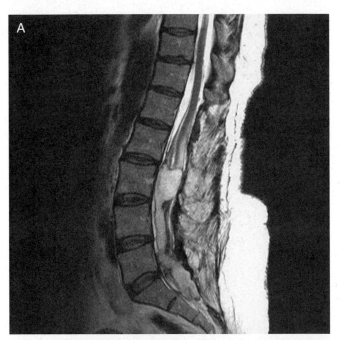

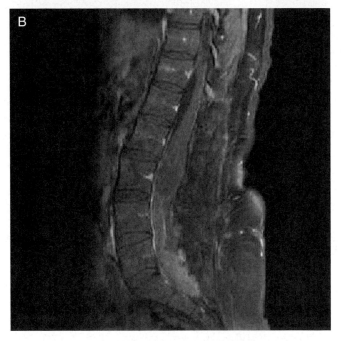

Figure 3.62 Epidermoid in a 5-year-old boy. **A.** Consecutive sagittal T1-images show a very subtle (almost undetectable) intradural bipartite mass (small arrows) below the conus, at the levels of L3 to L4. This lesion demonstrated no enhancement with gadolinium. **B. (Left)** Sagittal proton-density and **(right)** Sagittal T2-weighted images again show the very subtle mass which is almost isointense to CSF on all sequences, but is best seen on the proton-density images. At surgery, this mass was yellow-white in color. On being cut, it had the consistency and flake-like texture of a bar of soap (96).

or lymphoma. These metastases are often isointense or slightly hyperintense on T1, and somewhat hyperintense on T2, although this may be masked by T2-bright CSF. Gadolinium enhancement is extremely helpful in increasing the conspicuity of these intradural-extramedullary lesions, which enhance brightly (97).

Intramedullary Tumors

Glioma

These are the most common type of intramedullary tumor, particularly *ependymomas* (especially at the conus and filum terminale) in adults and *astrocytomas* in children. Sixty percent of

Figure 3.63 DWI distinguishes between postoperative arachnoid cyst and recurrent epidermoid neoplasm. Sagittal **(A)** fat-saturated postcontrast T1 and **(B)** FSE-T2 images show a rounded, large, nonenhancing intradural lesion at the L3 level, with signal characteristics similar to CSF, nearly filling the spinal canal. Extending anterior to the cauda equina from L4 to mid L5, and down to S2, is subtly enhancing intradural tissue, slightly hypointense to CSF on T2. Old L1 through S2 laminectomies are evident.

primary cord tumors are ependymomas (106). These expand the cord and are slightly dark on T1 and bright on T2. Associated cysts or syrinx may be seen either caudal or rostral to ependymomas, which generally enhance with contrast. Hemorrhage is not uncommonly associated with ependymomas, a fact stressed

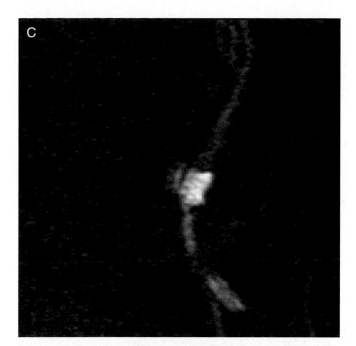

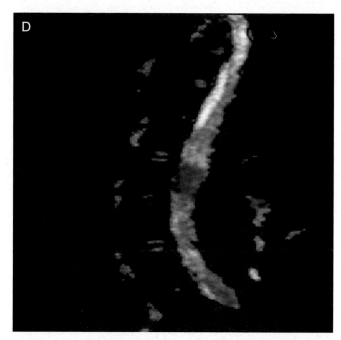

Figure 3.63 *(continued)* (**C**) Sagittal diffusion-weighted image (DWI) with corresponding (**D**) apparent diffusion coefficient (ADC) map shows marked restricted diffusion of the L3 intradural mass (bright on DWI, dark on ADC) and mild restricted diffusion of the lower intradural component from L4 through S2. DWI findings are consistent with recurrent epidermoid tumor rather than postoperative arachnoid cyst, and this was confirmed at surgery. Case courtesy of Dr. S. Imbesi (43).

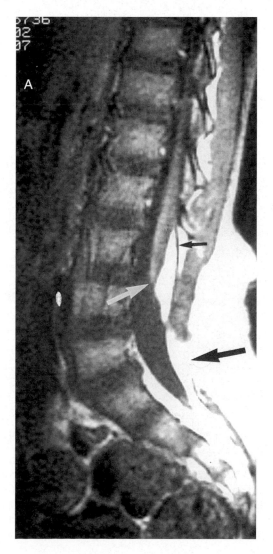

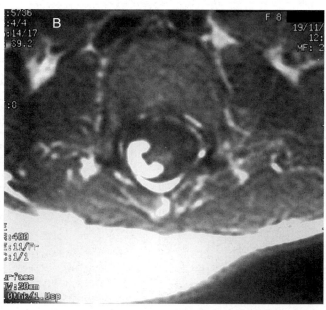

Figure 3.64 Tethered cord with conus lipomyelomeningocele in an 8-year-old girl. **A**. Sagittal T1 image shows a tethered cord with conus (white arrow) at the L3–L4 level, with posteriorly adherent T1-bright intradural lipoma. The posterior dura (small black arrow) is well visualized, outlined by fat. Note the absence of normal posterior elements at this level and the wide spina bifida defect (large black arrow). **B**. Axial T1-image shows the C-shaped T1-bright lipoma wrapped around the right side of the conus. Note also the epidural lipoma posterior to the thecal sac and the abnormal bony posterior elements (96).

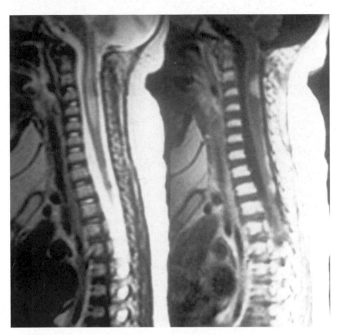

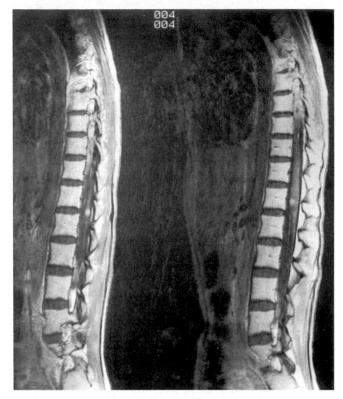

Figure 3.65 Intrathecal drop metastases from medulloblastoma in a 3-year-old boy. **Left**. T2-weighted image shows expansion and edema of the cervical cord, extending up to the medulla. Note that CSF occupies much of the midline posterior cranial fossa, because some cerebellum has been resected due to involvement by medulloblastoma. **Right**. Postgadolinium sagittal T1 image shows multiple enhancing subarachnoid metastases coating the posterior aspect of the cord, with some larger deposits appearing to extend into the cord, thus accounting for the edema (96).

Figure 3.66 Intrathecal metastases from lung cancer in a 25-year-old woman. Consecutive sagittal postgadolinium T1-weighted images show two small enhancing tumor nodules at the conus. There is also diffuse subtle enhancing tumor coating the posterior spinal cord and cauda equina. Precontrast images showed no involvement of the vertebral body marrow at any level (96).

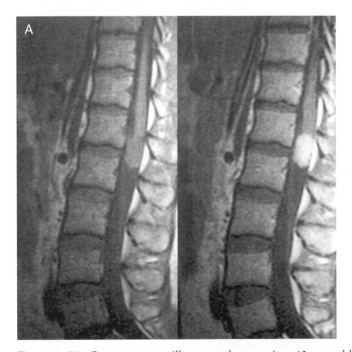

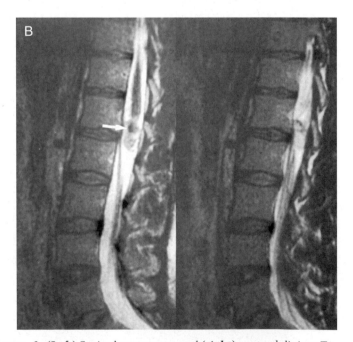

Figure 3.67 Conus myxopapillary ependymoma in a 43-year-old man. **A. (Left)** Sagittal precontrast and **(right)** postgadolinium T1-weighted images show a well-circumscribed enhancing mass at the conus. **B.** Consecutive sagittal T2-weighted images clearly demonstrate the mass. The small T2-dark focus (arrow) suggests the presence of hemosiderin (blood products), a useful clue favoring the diagnosis of ependymoma (96).

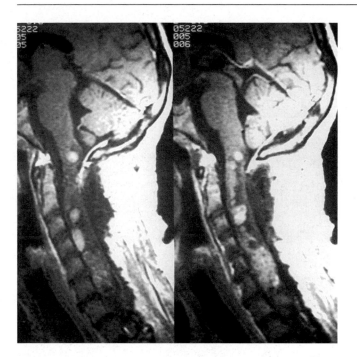

Figure 3.68 Recurrent cervical ependymoma in neurofibromatosis-2, in a 22-year-old woman. Consecutive postgadolinium sagittal images show an extensive enhancing mass expanding the cervical cord. Patient has had prior tumor resection, evidenced by postsurgical changes posteriorly (96).

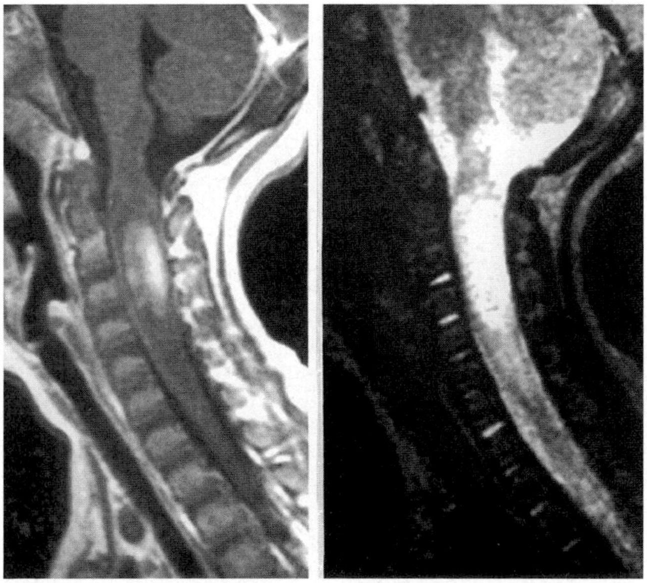

by Nemoto et al. in their study of cervical ependymomas (109). They may also contain calcification. (Gradient-echo T2* sequence may be helpful in demonstrating hemosiderin, which may be missed on FSE imaging.)

The myxopapillary subtype of ependymoma warrants special mention (106). These are well defined and almost exclusively found at the conus or filum terminale (Figure 3.67). They may become very large, filling and occasionally expanding the lower thecal sac with enhancing soft tissue. As mentioned, the intramedullary ependymoma tumor is classically associated with neurofibromatosis-2 (104) (Figure 3.68).

Astrocytomas usually show a fusiform expansion of the cord associated with T2 prolongation and (variable) enhancement (102) (Figures 3.69 and 3.70). Cysts may be present, either intrinsic to the tumor or at the edge of the tumor.

Spinal cord *oligodendrogliomas* are rare, comprising only 0.8% to 4.7% of intramedullary tumors of the spinal cord and filum (110). They are found in the cervicothoracic spine, usually in

Figure 3.69 Astrocytoma in a 4-year-old girl. **Left.** Sagittal postgadolinium T1 MR image shows fusiform expansion of the upper cervical cord, with mild partial enhancement, and extensive T1-dark edema extending up to the medulla and down to C6. **Right.** Sagittal T2 image again shows the fusiform cord expansion. The T2-bright edema is well demonstrated (96).

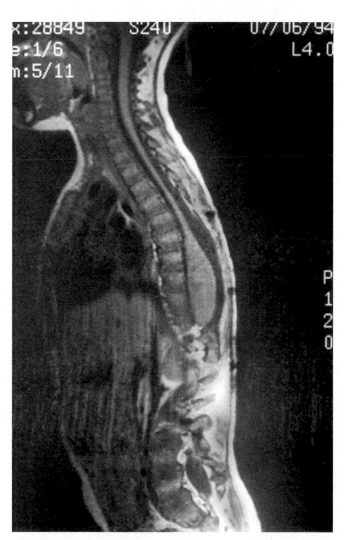

Figure 3.70 Astrocytoma in a 4-year-old boy. Sagittal T1-image shows marked fusiform expansion of the mid/lower thoracic cord (96).

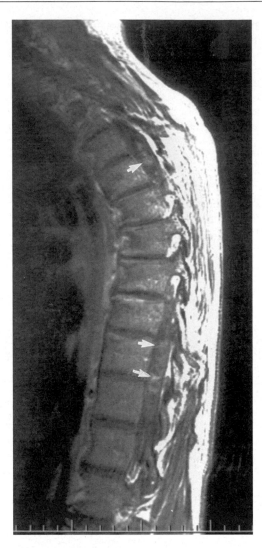

Figure 3.71 Oligodendroglioma: 64-year-old man presented with left leg atrophy and weakness. Postcontrast sagittal T1-weighted MR image shows an enhancing intramedullary mass (arrowheads), with some cystic components. (Because of patient's scoliosis, normal neural foramina are noted between the regions of tumor.)

patients in their fourth decade of life. One of the few published examples (110) has an appearance similar to our surgically proven case (Figure 3.71): an enhancing intramedullary expansile mass in the cervicothoracic cord, with adjacent cystic intramedullary component. Spinal oligodendrogliomas are often associated with meningeal or intracranial oligodendrogliomatosis (110, 111).

Hemangioblastoma

These tumors may occur sporadically but are often multiple and associated with the cerebellar hemangioblastomas of von Hippel–Lindau syndrome. They may exhibit the typical cyst with associated mural nodule, which enhances brightly with gadolinium (Figure 3.72). There may be associated edema and, as in the brain, they may have associated prominent vascularity (106).

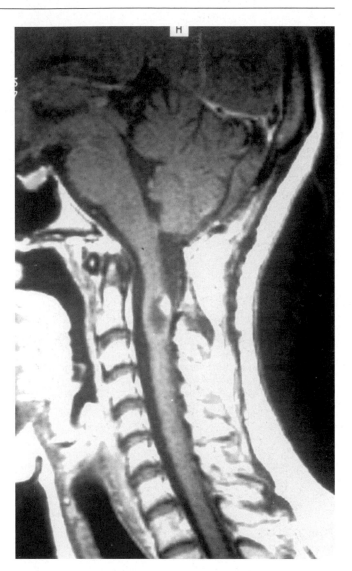

Figure 3.72 Hemangioblastoma in von Hippel–Lindau syndrome in a 28-year-old woman. Sagittal postgadolinium T1 image shows a small enhancing nodule in the posterior upper cervical cord, with an associated cyst that expands the cord slightly. Patient has had cerebellar hemangiomas resected previously (96).

Embryonal Tumor

These were previously discussed in the section on intradural-extramedullary tumors, but they may also occur in an intramedullary location. As mentioned, they may be associated with spinal dysraphism, especially lipomas. Dermoids and epidermoids have variable signal intensity, depending on their composition. Cystic teratomas may be found inside the cord substance (Figure 3.73).

Metastases

Rarely, these present as intramedullary lesions with a primary site in the brain or outside the CNS. Signal intensity is low on T1 and bright on T2; these usually enhance with intravenous contrast (Figure 3.74).

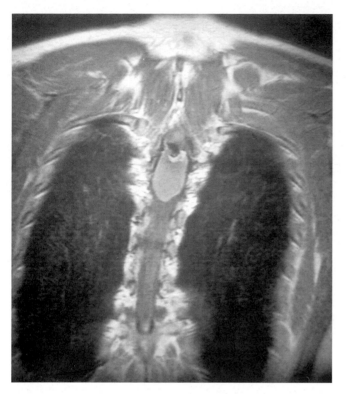

Figure 3.73 Recurrent intramedullary cystic teratoma in a 36-year-old woman. Coronal T1-weighted MR image shows cystic expansion of the cord by proteinaceous fluid. There was essentially no enhancement after IV contrast. At surgery this tumor contained keratin, hair, and mucus (96).

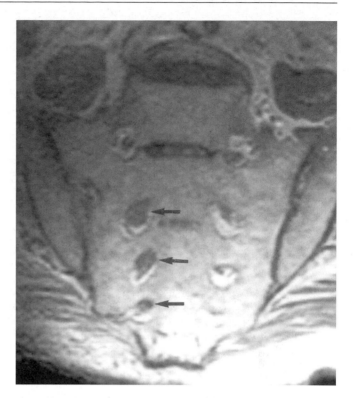

Figure 3.74 Metastatic prostate carcinoma invading sacral nerve roots in a 70-year-old man. Oblique-coronal postgadolinium T1-weighted MR image shows diffuse enlargement and subtle enhancement of the right-sided sacral nerve roots (arrows). At surgery, diffuse infiltration of the roots by prostate cancer was found. No involvement of the vertebral marrow was present (96).

*R*eferences

1. Lee RR. Recent advances in spinal MRI. In: Lee RR, ed. *Spinal Imaging* (Spine: State of the Art Reviews, Vol. 9). Philadelphia: Hanley & Belfus, 1995; 45–60.
2. Kneeland JB, Hyde JS. High-resolution MR imaging with local coils. *Radiology* 1989; 171:1–7.
3. Kulkarni MV, Patton JA, Price RR. Technical considerations for the use of surface coils in MRI. *AJR* 1986; 147:373–378.
4. Roemer PB, Edelstein WA, Hayes CE, Souza SP, Mueller OM. The NMR phased array. *Magn Reson Med* 1990; 16:192–223.
5. Jaermann T, Crelier G, Pruessmann KP, et al. SENSE-DTI at 3T. *Magn Reson Med* 2004; 51:230–236.
6. Noebauer-Huhmann IM, Glaser C, Dietrich O, et al. MRI of the cervical spine: assessment of image quality with parallel imaging compared to non-accelerated MR measurements. *Eur Radiol* 2007; 17:1147–1155.
7. Czervionke LF, Daniels DL, Ho PS, Yu S, et al. Cervical neural foramina: correlative anatomic and MR imaging study. *Radiology* 1988; 169:753–759.
8. Hedberg MC, Drayer BP, Flom RA, Hodak JA, Bird CR. Gradient echo (GRASS) MR imaging in cervical radiculopathy. *AJR* 1988; 150:683–689.
9. VanDyke C, Ross JS, Tkach J, Masaryk TJ, Modic MT. Gradient-echo MR imaging of the cervical spine: evaluation of extradural disease. *AJR* 1989; 153:393–398.
10. Enzmann DR, Rubin JB. Cervical spine: MR imaging with a partial flip angle, gradient-refocused pulse sequence: Part II. Spinal cord disease. *Radiology* 1988; 166:473–478.
11. Tsuruda JS, Remley K. Effects of magnetic susceptibility artifacts and motion in evaluating the cervical neural foramina on 3DFT gradient-echo MR imaging. *AJNR* 1991; 12:237–241.

12. Tsuruda JS, Norman D, Dillon W, Newton TH, Mills DG. Three-dimensional gradient-recalled MR imaging as a screening tool for the diagnosis of cervical radiculopathy. *AJNR* 1989; 10:1263–1271.
13. Yousem DM, Atlas SW, Goldberg HI, Grossman RI. Degenerative narrowing of the cervical spine neural foramina: evaluation with high-resolution 3DFT gradient-echo MR imaging. *AJNR* 1991; 12:229–236.
14. Melki PS, Mulkern RV, Panych LP, Jolesz FA. Comparing the FAISE method with conventional dual-echo sequences. *J Magn Reson Imaging* 1991:1:319–326.
15. Mulkern RV, Wong STS, Winalski C, Jolesz FA. Contrast manipulation and artifact assessment of 2D and 3D RARE sequences. *Magn Reson Imaging* 1990; 8:557–566.
16. Hennig J, Nauerth A, Friedburg H. RARE imaging: a fast imaging method for clinical MR. *Magn Reson Med* 1986; 3:823–833.
17. Jones KM, Mulkern RV, Schwartz RB, Oshio K, et al. Fast spin-echo MR imaging of the brain and spine: current concepts. *AJR* 1992; 158:1313–1320.
18. Mulkern RV, Wong STS, Winalski C, Jolesz FA. Contrast manipulation and artifact assessment of 2D and 3D RARE sequences. *Magn Reson Imaging* 1990; 8:557–566.
19. Sze G, Merriam M, Oshio K, Jolesz FA. Fast spin-echo imaging in the evaluation of intradural disease of the spine. *AJNR* 1992; 13:1383–1392.
20. Georgy BA, Hesselink JR. MR imaging of the spine: recent advances in pulse sequences and special techniques. *AJR* 1994; 162:923–934.
21. Rubin JB, Enzmann DR. Optimizing conventional MR imaging of the spine. *Radiology* 1987; 163:777–783.
22. Rubin JB, Enzmann DR, Wright A. CSF-gated MR imaging of the spine: theory and clinical implementation. *Radiology* 1987; 163:784–792.
23. Ross JS, Ruggieri P, Tkach J, Obuchowski N, et al. Lumbar degenerative disk disease: prospective comparison of conventional T2-weighted spin-echo imaging and T2-weighted rapid acquisition relaxation-enhanced imaging. *AJNR* 1993; 14:1215–1223.

24. Oshio K, Jolesz FA, Melki PS, Mulkern RV. T2 weighted thin slice imaging with multi-slab 3D RARE. *J Magn Reson Imaging* 1991; 1:695–700.

25. De Coene B, Hajnal JV, Gatehouse P, et al. MR of the brain using fluid-attenuated inversion recovery (FLAIR) sequences. *AJNR* 1992; 13:1555–1564.

26. Hittmair K, Mallek R, Prayer D, et al. Spinal cord lesions in patients with multiple sclerosis: comparison of MR pulse sequences. *AJNR* 1996; 17:1555–1565.

27. Sze G, Kawamura Y, Negishi C, Constable RT, et al. Fast spin-echo MR imaging of the cervical spine: influence of echo train length and echo spacing on image contrast and quality. *AJNR* 14:1203–1213, 1993.

28. Georgy BA, Hesselink JR. Evaluation of fat suppression in contrast-enhanced MR of neoplastic and inflammatory spine disease. *AJNR* 1994; 15:409–417.

29. Tien RD, Olson EM, Zee CS. Diseases of the lumbar spine: findings on fat-suppression MR imaging. *AJR* 1992; 159:95–99.

30. Dwyer AJ, Frank JA, Sank VJ, Reinig JW, et al. Short TI inversion-recovery sequence: analysis and initial experience in cancer imaging. *Radiology* 1988; 168:837–841.

31. Jones KM, Schwartz RB, Mantello MT, Ahn SS, et al. Fast spin-echo MR in the detection of vertebral metastases: comparison of three sequences. *AJNR* 1994; 15:401–407.

32. Henkelman RM, Watts J, Kucharczyk W. High signal intensity in MR images of calcified brain tissue. *Radiology* 1991; 179:199–206.

33. Enzmann DR, Pelc NJ. Normal flow patterns of intracranial and spinal cerebrospinal fluid defined with phase-contrast cine MR imaging. *Radiology* 1991; 178:467–474.

34. Levy LM, Di Chiro G. MR phase imaging and CSF flow in the head and spine. *Neuroradiology* 1990; 32:399–406.

35. Nitz WR, Bradley WG, Watanabe AS, Lee RR, et al. Flow dynamics of cerebrospinal fluid: assessment with phase-contrast velocity MR imaging performed with retrospective cardiac gating. *Radiology* 1992; 183:395–405.

36. Quencer RM, Donovan Post MJ, Hinks RS. Cine MR in the evaluation of normal and abnormal CSF flow: intracranial and intraspinal studies. *Neuroradiology* 1990; 32:371–391.

37. Tsuruda JS, Chew WM, Moseley ME, Norman D. Diffusion-weighted MR imaging of the brain: value of differentiating between extra-axial cysts and epidermoid tumors. *AJR* 1990; 155:1059–1065.

38. Gonzalez RG, Shaefer PW, Buonanno FS, et al. Diffusion-weighted MR imaging: diagnostic accuracy in patients imaged within 6 hours of stroke symptom onset. *Radiology* 1999; 210:155–162.

39. Mukherjee P, Berman JI, Chung SW, et al. Diffusion tensor MR imaging and fiber tractography: theoretic underpinnings. *AJNR* 2008; 29:632–641.

40. Shanmuganathan K, Gullapalli RP, Zhuo J, Mirvis SE. Diffusion tensor MR imaging in cervical spine trauma. *AJNR* 2008; 29:655–659.

41. Thurnher MM, Bammer R. Diffusion-weighted MR imaging (DWI) in spinal cord ischemia. *Neuroradiology* 2006; 48:795–801.

42. Demir A, Ries M, Moonen CTW, et al. DWI with apparent diffusion coefficient and apparent diffusion tensor maps in cervical spondylotic myelopathy. *Radiology* 2003; 229:37–43.

43. Tang L, Cianfoni A, Imbesi SG. Diffusion-weighted imaging distinguishes recurrent epidermoid neoplasm from postoperative arachnoid cyst in the lumbosacral spine. *J Comput Assist Tomogr* 2006; 30:507–509.

44. Agosta F, Benedetti B, Rocca MA, et al. Quantification of cervical cord pathology in primary progressive MS using DTI. *Neurology* 2005; 64:631–635.

45. Henning A, Schar M, Kollias SS, et al. Quantitative MR spectroscopy in the entire human cervical spinal cord and beyond at 3T. *Magn Reson Med* 2008; 59:1250–1258.

46. Rupp R, Ebraheim NA, Savolaine ER, Jackson WT. Magnetic resonance imaging evaluation of the spine with metal implants. *Spine* 1993; 18:379–385.

47. Shapiro MD. MR imaging of the spine at 3 Tesla. In: DeLano MC, ed. *3T MR Imaging* (MRI Clinics of North America, Vol. 14). Philadelphia: W.B. Saunders Co./Elsevier Inc., 2006; 97–108.

48. Barkovich AJ. *Pediatric Neuroimaging*. 3rd ed. Philadelphia: Lippincott Williams & Wilkins, 2000.

49. Wilson DA, Prince JR. MR imaging determination of the location of the normal conus medullaris throughout childhood. *AJR* 1989; 152:1029–1032.

50. Daffner RH, Deeb ZL, Rothfus WE. "Fingerprints" of vertebral trauma: a unifying concept based on mechanism. *Skeletal Radiol* 1986; 15:518–525.

51. Acheson MD, Livingston RR, Richardson ML, Stimac GK. High-resolution CT in the evaluation of cervical spine fractures: comparison with plain film examinations. *AJR* 187; 148:1179–1185.

52. Woodring JH, Lee C. The role and limitations of computed tomographic scanning in the evaluation of cervical trauma. *J Trauma* 1992; 33:698–708.

53. Lee RR. MR imaging and cervical spine injury. *Radiology* 1996; 201:617–618.

54. Hart BL, Butman JA, Benzel EC. Spine trauma. In: Orrison WW, ed. Philadelphia: W. B. Saunders, 2000; 1400–1439.

55. Harris JH Jr, Mirvis SE. *The Radiology of Acute Cervical Spine Trauma*. Baltimore: Williams & Wilkins, 1996.

56. Daffner RH. *Imaging of Vertebral Trauma*. Philadelphia: Lippincott-Raven, 1996.

57. Halliday AL, Henderson BR, Hart BL, Benzel EC. The management of unilateral lateral mass/facet fractures of the subaxial cervical spine. *Spine* 1997; 22:2614–2621.

58. Clayman DA, Sykes CH, Vines FS. Occipital condyle fractures: clinical presentation and radiologic adetection. *AJNR* 1994; 15:1309–1315.

59. Bettini N, Malagutti MC, Sintini M, et al. Fractures of the occipital condyles: report of four cases and review of the literature. *Skeletal Radiol* 1993; 22:187–190.

60. Bucholz RW, Burkhead WZ. The pathological anatomy of fatal atlanto-occipital dislocations. *J Bone Joint Surg Am* 1979; 61:248–250.

61. Harris JH Jr, Carson GC, Wagner LK, et al. Radiologic diagnosis of traumatic occipitovertebral dissociation: 2. Comparison of three methods of detecting occipitovertebral relationships on lateral radiographs of supine subjects. *AJR* 1994; 162:887–892.

62. Rojas CA, Bertozzi JC, Martinez CR, et al. Reassessment of the cranio-cervical junction: normal values on CT. *AJNR* 2007; 28:1819–1823.

63. Smith WS, Kaufer H. Patterns and mechanisms of lumbar injuries associated with lap seat belts. *J Bone Joint Surg Am* 1969; 51:239–254.

64. Gertzbein SD, Court-Brown CM. Flexion-distraction injuries of the lumbar spine: mechanisms of injury and classification. *Clin Orthop* 1988; 227:52–60.

65. Matsumura A, Meguro K, Tsurushima H, et al. Magnetic resonance imaging of SCI without radiologic abnormality. *Surg Neurol* 1990; 33:281–283.

66. Davis JW, Phreaner DL, Hoyt DB, Mackersie RC. The etiology of missed cervical spine injuries. *J Trauma* 1993; 34:342–346.

67. Robertson PA, Ryan MD. Neurological deterioration after reduction of cervical subluxation: mechanical compression by disk tissue. *J Bone Joint Surg Br* 1992; 74:224–227.

68. D'Alise MD, Benzel EC, Hart BL. Magnetic resonance imaging evaluation of the cervical spine in the comatose or obtunded trauma patient. *J Neurosurg* 1999; 91(1 Suppl):54–59.

69. Boden SD, Lee RR, Herzog RJ. MRI of the spine. In: Frymoyer J, ed. *The Adult Spine: Principles and Practice*. 2nd ed. New York: Raven Press, Ltd., 1996; 563–629.

70. Boden SD, McCowin PR, Davis DO, et al. Abnormal magnetic resonance scans of the cervical spine in asymptomatic subjects: a prospective investigation. *J Bone Joint Surg* 1990; 72A:1178–1184.

71. Modic MT. Degenerative disorders of the spine. In: Modic MT, Masaryk TJ, Ross JS, eds. *MRI of the Spine*. 2nd ed. St. Louis: Mosby, 1994; 80–150.

72. Jensen MC, Brant-Zawadzki MN, Obuchowski N, Modic MT, et al. MRI of the lumbar spine in people without back pain. *N Engl J Med* 1994; 331:69–73.

73. Gundry CR, Heithoff KB, Pollei SR. Imaging of the postoperative lumbar spine. In: Lee RR, ed. *Spinal Imaging* (Spine: State of the Art Reviews, Vol. 9). Philadelphia: Hanley & Belfus, 1995.

74. Bundschuh CV, Stein L, Slusser JH, et al. Distinguishing between scar and recurrent herniated disk in postoperative patients: value of contrast-enhanced CT and MR imaging. *AJNR* 1990; 11:949–958.

75. Larsson E-M, Holtas S, Nilsson O. GD-DTPA-enhancement of suspected spinal multiple sclerosis. *AJNR* 1989; 10:1071–1076.

76. Barakos JA, Mark AS, Dillon DW, Norman D. MR imaging of acute transverse myelitis and AIDS myelopathy. *J Comput Assist Tomogr* 1990; 14:45–50.

77. Bryn WM, Park WK, Park BH, Ahn SH, et al. Guillain-Barré syndrome: MR imaging findings of the spine in eight patients. *Radiology* 1998; 208:137–141.

78. Gorson KC, Ropper AH, Muriello MA, Blair R. Prospective evaluation of MRI lumbosacral nerve root enhancement in acute Guillain-Barré syndrome. *Neurology* 1996; 47:813–817.

79. Kerslake RW, Mitchell LA, Worthington BS. Case report: CT and MRI of the cauda equina syndrome in ankylosing spondylitis. *Clin Radiol* 1992; 45:134–136.

80. Reddy S, Leite CC, Jinkins JR. Imaging of infectious disease of the spine. In: Lee RR, ed. *Spinal Imaging* (Spine: State of the Art Reviews, Vol. 9). Philadelphia: Hanley & Belfus, 1995.

81. Sklar EM, Post MJD, Lebwohl NH. Imaging of infection of the lumbosacral spine. *Neuroimaging Clin N Am* 1993; 3:577–590.

82. Modic MT, Feiglin DH, Piraino DW, et al. Vertebral osteomyelitis: assessment using MR. *Radiology* 1985; 157:157–166.

83. Hlavin ML, Kaminski HJ, Ross JS, Ganz E. Spinal epidural abscess: a ten-year perspective. *Neurosurgery* 1990; 27:177–184.

84. Angtuaco EJC, McConnell JR, Chadduck WM, et al. MR imaging of spinal epidural sepsis. *AJNR* 1987; 8:879–883.

85. Sharif HS, Osarugue AA, Clark DC, et al. Brucellar and tuberculous spondylitis: comparative imaging features. *Radiology* 1989; 171:419–425.

86. Sharif HS, Clark DC, Aabed M, et al. Granulomatous spinal infections: MR imaging. *Radiology* 1990; 177:101–107.

87. Smith AS, Weinstein MA, Mizushima A, et al. MR imaging characteristics of tuberculous spondylitis vs. vertebral osteomyelitis. *AJR* 1989; 153:399–405.

88. Roos AD, van Meerten El, Bloem JL, et al. MRI of tuberculosis spondylitis. *AJR* 1987; 146:79–82.

89. Talpos D, Tien RD, Hesselink JR. MRI of AIDS-related polyradiculopathy. *Neurology* 1991; 41:1996–1997.

90. Chong J, Di Rocco A, Tagliati M, et al. MR findings in AIDS-associated myelopathy. *AJNR* 1999; 20:1412–1416.

91. Anson JA, Spetzler RF. Interventional neuroradiology for spinal pathology. *Clin Neurosurg* 1992; 39:388–417.

92. Nittner K. Spinal meningiomas, neurinomas and neurofibromas and hourglass tumors. In: Vinken PJ, Bruyn GW, eds. *Handbook of Clinical Neurology.* New York: Elsevier, 1976; 20:177–322.

93. Vinken PJ, Bruyn GW, eds. *Handbook of Clinical Neurology.* Vol. 19: Spinal cord tumors: Part I. New York: Elsevier, 1975.

94. Vinken PJ, Bruyn GW, eds. *Handbook of Clinical Neurology.* Vol. 20: Spinal cord tumors: Part II. New York: Elsevier, 1976.

95. Kurland LT. The frequency of intraspinal neoplasms in the resident population of Rochester, Minnesota. *J Neurosurg* 1958; 15:627–641.

96. Lee RR. Spinal tumors. In: Lee RR, ed. *Spinal Imaging* (Spine: State of the Art Reviews, Vol. 9). Philadelphia: Hanley & Belfus, 1995; 261–286.

97. Sze G, Abramson A, Krol G, et al. Gadolinium-DTPA in the evaluation of intradural extramedullary spinal disease. *AJR* 1988; 150:911–921.

98. Avrahami E, Tadmor R, Dally O, et al. Early MR demonstration of spinal metastases in patients with normal radiographs and CT and radionuclide bone scans. *J Comput Assist Tomogr* 1989; 13:598–602.

99. Baker LL, Goodman SB, Perkash I, Lane B, Enzmann DR. Benign versus pathologic compression fractures of vertebral bodies: assessment with conventional spin-echo, chemical-shift, and STIR MR imaging. *Radiology* 1990; 174:495–502.

100. Yuh WT, Zachar CK, Barloon TJ, Sato Y, et al. Vertebral compression fractures: distinction between benign and malignant causes with MR imaging. *Radiology* 1989; 172:215–218.

101. Burger PC, Scheithauer BW, Vogel FS. *Surgical Pathology of the Nervous System and Its Coverings.* 3rd ed. New York: Churchill Livingstone, 1991, Chapter 8: Spine and epidural space, 569–603.

102. Masaryk TJ. Spinal tumors. In: Modic MT, Masaryk TJ, Ross JS, eds. *MRI of the Spine.* St. Louis: Mosby, 1994; 249–314.

103. Dahlin DC, Unni KK. *Bone Tumors: General Aspects and Data on 8,542 Cases.* Springfield: Charles C. Thomas, 1986:62–69.

104. Egelhoff JC, Bates DJ, Ross JS, et al. Spinal MR findings in neurofibromatosis types 1 and 2. *AJNR* 1992; 13:1071–1077.

105. Slooff JL, Kernohan JW, MacCarty CS. *Primary Intramedullary Tumors of the Spinal Cord and Filum Terminale.* Philadelphia: Saunders, 1964.

106. Burger PC, Scheithauer BW, Vogel FS. *Surgical Pathology of the Nervous System and Its Coverings.* 3rd ed. New York: Churchill Livingstone, 1991, Chapter 9: Spinal meninges, spinal nerve roots, and spinal cord, 605–660.

107. Burk DL Jr., Brumberg JA, Kanal E, et al. Spinal and paraspinal neurofibromatosis: surface coil MR imaging at 1.5T. *Radiology* 1987; 162:797–801.

108. Barkovich AJ, Edwards MSB, Cogen PH. MR evaluation of spinal dermal sinus tracts in children. *AJNR* 1991; 12:123–129.

109. Nemoto Y, Inoue Y, Tashiro T, et al. Intramedullary spinal cord tumors: significance of associated hemorrhage at MR imaging. *Radiology* 1992; 82:793–796.

110. Fortuna A, Celli P, Palma L. Oligodendrogliomas of the spinal cord. *Acta Neurochir* 1980; 52:305–329.

111. Gilmer-Hall HS, Ellis WG, Imbesi SG, Boggan JE. Spinal oligodendroglioma with gliomatosis in a child: case report. *J Neurosurg Spine* 2000; 92:109–113.

4 Epidemiology of Spinal Cord Injury

Michael J. DeVivo

Spinal cord injury (SCI) epidemiology has been studied extensively over the past 40 years. Early population-based epidemiologic investigations of SCI in the United States (U.S.) include the studies of eighteen northern California counties conducted by Kraus et al., Olmsted County Minnesota conducted by Griffin et al., and national studies conducted by both Kalsbeek et al. and Bracken et al. (1–4) These investigations were limited to descriptive epidemiology, including the documentation of overall SCI incidence, age at time of injury, gender, racial or ethnic group, cause of injury, and mortality prior to either hospital admission or discharge.

In the early 1970s, the model SCI care system program was initiated with funding from what is now the National Institute on Disability and Rehabilitation Research in the U.S. Department of Education. All funded model systems of care were required to submit data on patients they treated to a national database. This database, the National Spinal Cord Injury Statistical Center (NSCISC) Database, began in Phoenix, Arizona, and was moved to the University of Alabama at Birmingham (UAB) in 1983, where it remains today (5, 6).

In 1987, three Shriners Hospital SCI units contracted with UAB to develop and maintain a longitudinal database in parallel with the model systems. Although the NSCISC and Shriners Hospital Databases have been used extensively to develop a descriptive profile of new SCIs that occur in the United States each year, they are not population based (7–12). Therefore, they cannot be used to calculate actual incidence rates or directly assess risk factors for obtaining SCI. However, the NSCISC and Shriners Hospital Databases have several advantages, including large sample size, geographic diversity, the range of information they contain, and excellent data quality.

Beginning in the 1980s, the Centers for Disease Control and Prevention began funding population-based SCI surveillance systems (registries) in many states (13–25). Data from these state registries have been used to demonstrate slight biases in the NSCISC Database toward overrepresentation of more severe injuries, non-whites, and injuries due to acts of violence (8). Given the complementary nature of the NSCISC Database, the Shriners Hospital Database, and the population-based state registries, a relatively complete description of the epidemiology of SCI in the United States during the 1980s and 1990s was obtained. Unfortunately, due to funding limitations, most of these state registries no longer exist, and there have been no recently published results to compare with those of the NSCISC or Shriners Hospital Database. Moreover, the number and locations of model systems changed in 2000 and again in 2006. Therefore, the direction and magnitude of current biases in the NSCISC and Shriners Hospital Databases are less clear.

OVERALL INCIDENCE

Published reports of the incidence of SCI in the United States vary from 25 new cases per million population per year in West Virginia to 59 new cases per million population per year in Mississippi (Table 4.1). Variation in SCI incidence rates among states is caused by differences in population demographic characteristics, the definition of SCI, and the data collection methodology that is used in each state. Overall, based on a combination of state registry information, the incidence rate of SCI in the United States is approximately 40 cases per million population, or approximately 12,000 new cases per year. Moreover, although there have been changes in the most common underlying causes of SCI during the past three decades, the overall incidence of new cases each year has remained relatively stable (26).

This annual incidence rate of 40 new cases per million population does not include persons who die at the scene of the accident. Most population-based state registries do not report deaths that occur prior to hospital admission. An exception is the state of Utah, where the incidence of prehospital SCI deaths from 1989–1991 was reported to be approximately four cases per million population per year, or 9.3% of the incidence rate for hospitalized cases (15). Nonetheless, incomplete reporting of these prehospital deaths is possible, and this estimate of fatal SCI incidence is probably conservative.

Table 4.1 Annual SCI Incidence Rates Derived from
Population-based State Registries

State	Dates	Annual Incidence Rate/10^6
Arkansas (13)	1980–89	27
New York (21)	1982–88	43
West Virginia (16)	1985–88	25
Oklahoma (14)	1988–90	40
Utah (15)	1989–91	43
Colorado (19)	1989–96	45
Virginia (23)	1990–92	30
Louisiana (22)	1991	46
Georgia (24)	1991–92	46
Mississippi (17)	1992–95	59
Kentucky/Indiana (25)	1993–98	27

Epidemiologic data from many other countries have also been reported. Table 4.2 contains a summary of 23 studies of the epidemiology of SCI by country of origin. It includes the time frame of each study, the incidence rate of SCI during that period of time, the mean age of persons at the time of injury, the proportion of SCIs that occurred among males, the proportion of injuries that involved the cervical spine, and the proportion of injuries that were neurologically complete. Blanks appearing in Table 4.2 reflect data that were not reported.

With the notable exception of Australia, where a national population-based registry has been established (27–29), the tail end of a 20-year German study (30), and a study conducted in Ireland (31), all of these international studies cited in Table 4.2 cover a period of time that is now more than 10 years old. Studies covering more recent time periods have not been done.

In Europe, the reported annual incidence rate of SCI varies from eight cases per million population in Spain (32) to 26 cases per million population in Greenland (33), with an average of about 16 cases per million population (34–41). Findings are similar in the Middle East, Australia, Fiji, Taipei, and South Africa (27–29, 42–51). These incidence rates are all considerably lower than those reported for any region of the United States (13–25). In fact, only two studies have produced incidence rates similar to those found in the United States. One study in Japan found an incidence rate of 39 cases per million population (47) while a study in a rural province of Taiwan found an incidence rate of 56 cases per million population (49).

Differences in reported annual incidence rates of SCI across countries are due to a number of factors. Many of these studies were not population-based, with a presumption being made that all cases of SCI would be treated at particular hospitals included in the studies. Therefore, case ascertainment in many of these studies is likely to be somewhat incomplete. Less severely injured persons who never got referred to specialized centers and those who died in outlying hospitals prior to referral to the specialized centers would be the most likely to be uncounted. The degree of under-ascertainment most likely varies with the

Table 4.2 Annual Incidence and Characteristics of SCI by Country

Location	Date	Incidence/10^6	Age(mean)	Male(%)	Complete(%)	Cervical(%)
Europe						
Italy (34, 35)	1989–94	20	39	80	51	40
Portugal (36)	1989–92	25	50	77	56	51
Germany (30)	1976–96	14		72		38
Norway (37)	1974–75	17	37	83	48	53
Switzerland (38)	1960–67	15	36	79	50	33
Spain (32)	1984–85	8	42	72	38	38
The Netherlands (39)	1994	10	44	77	49	58
The Netherlands (40)	1982–93	16	45	77	41	47
Denmark (33)	1975–84	9	33	77	36	51
Greenland (33)	1965–86	26				
France (41)	1970–75	13	39	79		
Ireland (31)	2000	13	37	87	39	50
Middle East						
Southeast Turkey (42)	1994	17	31	85		41
Istanbul Turkey (43)	1992	21	33	76		33
Turkey (44)	1992	13	36	71		32
Jordan (45)	1993	18	33	85	54	32
Israel (46)	1962–92		35	77	30	37
Pacific						
Japan (47)	1990	39	49	81	35	74
Taipei, Taiwan (48)	1978–81	15	36	83	58	47
Hualien, Taiwan (49)	1986–90	56	44	80	52	70
Fiji (50)	1985–94	10	38	87	61	53
Australia (27)	1996–97	13	39	80	44	45
Africa						
South Africa (51)	1988–93			80	66	25

exact study methodology that was employed. It is also important to note that these are crude incidence rates that have not been adjusted for differences in underlying study population characteristics such as age, gender, or race. Nonetheless, some variation is to be expected given differences in geography, climate, socio-economic characteristics, and other known risk factors for SCI that exist across countries. In fact, it is the relative consistency of all these reported incidence rates that is most striking.

One reason for the uniformly lower incidence rate of SCI in the rest of the world compared to the United States is the high rate of injuries caused by acts of violence in the United States (13–25). Violence (typically gunshot wounds inflicted by other people) caused 24.1% of SCIs treated at model systems in the United States between 1989 and 1993, when many of these international studies were conducted (52). In other countries, injuries caused by acts of violence are rare and typically involve failed suicide attempts. Nonetheless, differences in violence-induced SCIs alone are not sufficient to explain overall differences between the United States and other countries. In the case of less-developed countries, one possibility is that patients may die at the scene of the accident who would survive long enough to reach the hospital in the United States. The lower rates of tetraplegia and complete lesions reported in many countries relative to the United States may lend some support to that hypothesis. Other reasons for the relatively high incidence rate of SCIs in the United States undoubtedly exist and await further study.

RISK FACTORS

Age at Injury

Comparisons of age-specific SCI incidence rates are difficult among the state registries because of the lack of uniform categorization of reported age ranges. Nonetheless, several trends are apparent. SCI incidence rates are lowest for the pediatric age group, highest for persons in their late teens and early twenties, and decline consistently thereafter (13, 14, 16, 19, 22). The state of Oklahoma is typical, where age-specific SCI incidence rates per million population for 1988–1990 were 6 for age 0–14 (3% of cases), 94 for age 15–19 (18% of cases), 85 for age 20–24 (15% of cases), 71 for age 25–29 (14% of cases), 47 for age 30–44 (27% of cases), 32 for age 45–59 (12% of cases), and 26 for persons who were at least 60 years of age (11% of cases) (14).

A similar pattern emerges from the combined NSCISC and Shriners Hospital databases, where the mean age at time of injury is 32.4 years (+16.6 years), the median age at injury is 28 years, and the most common age at injury is 18 years (Table 4.3). Overall, 49.7% of persons enrolled in the combined NSCISC and Shriners Hospital databases since 1973 were between the ages of 16 and 30 at the time of their injury. However, these overall figures mask a rather substantial trend toward increasing age at injury in recent years. From 1973–1979, the mean age at injury for persons enrolled in the two databases was 28.9 years, whereas among persons injured since 2000, the mean age at injury was 35.6 years.

Table 4.3   Trends in Demographic and Injury Characteristics of Persons Enrolled in the NSCISC and Shriners Hospital SCI Databases by Year of Injury

CHARACTERISTIC	1973–79	1980–89	1990–99	2000+	TOTAL
Age at Injury (percent)					
1–15	7.0	6.0	7.1	6.8	6.8
16–30	60.1	56.0	44.3	40.2	49.7
31–45	18.4	21.9	25.8	24.7	23.2
46–60	9.9	9.7	12.8	17.8	12.3
61–75	4.0	5.0	7.4	7.8	6.2
76+	0.6	1.4	2.6	2.7	1.9
Age at injury (mean)	28.9	30.8	33.9	35.6	32.4
Male (percent)	80.9	81.2	78.9	77.1	79.6
Race/Ethnicity (percent)					
White	77.2	70.2	61.1	64.9	67.2
African American	14.6	19.4	23.2	18.6	19.8
Hispanic descent	5.4	7.7	12.3	13.6	10.0
Asian American	0.8	1.2	2.1	1.9	1.6
Native American	1.8	1.1	0.5	0.5	0.9
Other race	0.2	0.4	0.8	0.5	0.5
Etiology (percent)					
Motor vehicle	47.6	44.5	41.4	48.3	44.5
Violence	13.0	16.0	21.0	12.0	16.6
Sports	14.2	12.4	8.8	10.0	10.9
Falls	16.2	18.5	19.9	21.8	19.4
Other	9.0	8.5	8.9	7.9	8.6
Injury Severity					
C1–C8 Level (percent)	50.7	53.2	52.6	55.7	53.1
Complete (percent)	53.6	47.2	51.0	48.7	49.8

These figures mirror the increasing average age of the general United States population, which was 28 years in 1970 and 34.9 years in 1997, although changes in underlying age-specific incidence rates cannot be ruled out as also contributing to this trend in age at time of SCI (9).

The reported mean age at time of injury in Europe was approximately 40 years, varying from a low of 33 years in Denmark (33) to a high of 50 years in Portugal (36). In the Pacific region, reported average age at time of injury is comparable to that reported in Europe, but in the Middle East, the reported age at time of injury is somewhat lower (approximately 34 years). There are proportionately more violence-related spinal cord injuries in the Middle East than Europe, and most of these typically occur among younger persons. Given the time periods in which these studies were conducted and the overall aging of the general population, it is likely that the average age of someone injured today in Europe or the Middle East would be somewhat higher than reported in Table 4.2.

Gender

SCI occurs predominantly among men. Gender-specific SCI annual incidence rates have been reported by several state registries, with men ranging from a 4.6 times higher incidence rate in West Virginia (41 new cases per million men vs. 9 new cases per million women) to only a 2.3 times higher incidence rate in Louisiana (67 new cases per million men vs. 29 new cases per million women) (16, 22). The percentage of SCIs that occur among men is 79.6% for persons enrolled in the combined NSCISC and Shriners Hospital Databases (Table 4.3); 80% for Oklahoma and Arkansas; 78% for Virginia; 76% for Utah, Colorado, and Georgia; and 69% for Louisiana (9, 13–15,19, 22–24). This four-to-one ratio of male to female SCIs has remained very consistent over time despite significant trends in age at injury, ethnicity, and etiology of injury (Table 4.3).

The proportion of SCIs by gender is quite similar throughout the world, varying from a low of 72% in Spain (32) and Germany (30) to a high of 87% in Fiji (50). Unless meaningful changes in the typical causes of SCI in Europe were to occur, it is unlikely that the gender ratio of new injuries would vary much from figures reported in the past.

Race and Ethnicity

Fewer state registries have reported race and ethnicity data than information on age and gender. Nonetheless, some clear patterns have emerged. SCI incidence rates are substantially and consistently higher for African Americans than whites. In Oklahoma, the annual SCI incidence rate for African Americans was 57 new cases per million population compared to 40 new cases per million population for whites and 29 new cases per million population for Native Americans (14). In Louisiana, the difference is even more striking, with African Americans having an annual SCI incidence rate of 72 new cases per million population compared to 36 new cases per million population for whites (22). In fact, when race and gender were considered together, the SCI annual incidence rate per million population in Louisiana in 1991 was 127 for African American men, 41 for white men, 31 for white women, and 26 for African American women (22).

Unfortunately, state registries have not yet published SCI incidence rates for other racial and ethnic groups, such as Asian Americans and persons of Hispanic descent.

Since 2000, 64.9% of newly injured persons enrolled in the combined NSCISC and Shriners Hospital Databases were white; 18.6% were African American; 13.6% were Hispanic; 1.9% were Asian American; and 0.5% were Native American (Table 4.3). However, between 1973 and 1979, 77.2% of new persons enrolled in these two databases were white; 14.6% were African American; 5.4% were Hispanic; 0.8% were Asian American; and 1.8% were Native American. This trend toward an increasing percentage of new SCIs occurring among minority populations may be caused by periodic changes in the location of the model systems that participate in the NSCISC Database and changes in referral patterns to model systems and Shriners Hospitals. However, some changes in underlying race-specific SCI incidence rates may also have occurred.

Interestingly, the average age at injury varies by racial and ethnic group. Among persons enrolled in the combined NSCISC and Shriners Hospital Databases, persons of Hispanic descent have the youngest average age at injury (28.5 years), followed by Native Americans (28.6 years), whites (32.8 years), African Americans (33.5 years), and Asian Americans (35.9 years). Moreover, since 1973, the average age at time of injury for persons enrolled in these two databases has increased by about 9 years for whites while increasing only 6 years for Hispanics and only 4 years for African Americans and Asians.

ETIOLOGY OF INJURY

Cause-specific incidence rates have been reported by gender for Arkansas, by race for Oklahoma, and by both gender and race for Louisiana (13, 14, 22). Other states often report data on causes of SCI only in percentage terms that are heavily influenced by the racial and ethnic composition of the general population of each state (15, 16, 19). Overall, motor vehicle crashes are the leading cause of SCI in all states. In most states, such as Colorado, Oklahoma, Utah, West Virginia, and Arkansas, falls rank second, followed by sports and acts of violence (13–16, 19). However, in states like Louisiana and Mississippi, with greater proportions of African Americans and/or persons of Hispanic descent, acts of violence are the second leading cause of SCI (17, 22).

In fact, Oklahoma data reveal that the higher annual incidence of SCI among African Americans is caused entirely by acts of violence (14). Overall in Oklahoma, the annual incidence rate of SCI was 17 new cases per million population higher for African Americans than whites (57 vs. 40), whereas the cause-specific annual incidence rate of SCI caused by violence was 18 new cases per million population higher for African Americans than whites (21 vs. 3). There were no other meaningful differences in cause-specific annual SCI incidence rates among the races in Oklahoma (14).

Although motor vehicle crashes are the overall leading cause of SCI for the population as a whole, among African American men, violence ranks first. In Louisiana during 1991, the annual cause-specific SCI incidence rate per million population caused by acts of violence was 71 for African American men, but only 10 for African American women, 5 for white women, and 4 for white men (22). By comparison, annual cause-specific SCI incidence rates per million population caused by motor vehicle crashes in Louisiana during 1991 were 26 for African American men, 22 for white men, 17 for white women, and 13 for African American women (22).

SEVERITY OF INJURY

Most, but not all published studies provide at least some information on the severity of SCIs that occur each year. Table 4.2 reveals substantial international variability in the proportion of persons with tetraplegia and the proportion of neurologically complete injuries. In Europe, the proportion of new injuries resulting in either tetraplegia or tetraparesis ranges from a low of 33% in Switzerland (38) to a high of 58% in The Netherlands (39). However, the Swiss study is among the oldest to have been conducted, and given improved survival rates for tetraplegia today, it likely underestimates current proportions of tetraplegia and tetraparesis. The next lowest figures for tetraplegia and tetraparesis come from Spain (32) and Germany (30) at 38% each, but these results are also somewhat out of date. Under the circumstances, it is reasonable to presume that at least 40% and not more than 60% of new SCIs in Europe today would be cervical injuries. However, in the Middle East where a higher proportion of injuries were due to acts of violence that usually result in paraplegia, and acute survival rates for tetraplegics may not be as high as in Europe, the reported proportion of cervical injuries was lower (41–45). In the United States, about half of new injuries involve the cervical region of the spinal cord, and this has been increasing over time (52).

In Europe, about half of all new injuries were reported to be neurologically complete, ranging from a low of 36% in Denmark (33) to a high of 56% in Portugal (36). Unfortunately, competing trends over time make it difficult to assess the current applicability of these estimates of percentages of complete injuries. Improved methods of emergency management might minimize initial damage to the spinal cord and result in a higher percentage of neurologically incomplete injuries today. Conversely, improved survival of persons with more severe neurologically complete injuries could increase the proportion of those cases relative to persons with incomplete lesions. Any trends in etiology of injury over time could also impact the distribution of complete and incomplete paraplegia and tetraplegia. For example, acts of violence usually result in neurologically complete paraplegia, and sports injuries are typically in the cervical region of the spinal cord. Falls among the elderly usually result in incomplete cervical injuries. Therefore, new studies are needed to assess the distribution of SCI severities in Europe today. In the United States, approximately half of all new injuries continue to be neurologically complete (52).

PREVALENCE

Although incidence reflects the number of new cases that occur each year, prevalence is defined as the number of persons with an SCI who are currently alive. There are two ways to estimate prevalence. One approach is based on the epidemiologic relationship between prevalence, incidence, and the duration of the condition (as measured in the case of SCI by life expectancy). When a condition occurs relatively rarely, as is the case with SCI, then the prevalence rate can be estimated as the product of the incidence rate and average duration. Using this mathematical formula and the best available data at the time, the prevalence of SCI in the United States in 1980 was estimated to be 906 persons per million population, or just under 200,000 existing cases (53). However, an underlying assumption when making this calculation is that both incidence and life expectancy have remained constant over time. Because life expectancy at time of injury for persons with SCI has increased, and a current estimate of life expectancy was used, prevalence will be slightly overestimated by using this formula (54, 55).

Of course, the more straightforward way to estimate prevalence is simply to count people using standard sampling and survey techniques. For many years, this was not attempted because of the large sample size, time, and expense that would be required to produce an accurate estimate of prevalence for a condition as rare as SCI. Eventually, substantial funding was provided by the Paralyzed Veterans of America to use a sophisticated probability sampling plan of small geographic areas and institutions to estimate conservatively the prevalence of SCI in the United States at 721 persons per million population, or approximately 176,965 persons in 1988 (56).

More recently, current estimates of age–sex-specific incidence and mortality have been combined with the results of the 1988 survey to project the growth in prevalence of SCI in the United States over time (57). Using new mathematical models, the prevalence of SCI in the United States was projected to increase to 246,882 persons by 2004, and 276,281 persons by 2014 (57). This projected growth in prevalence is anticipated to occur exclusively from improved life expectancies rather than any change in SCI incidence rates. Conversely, prevalence of SCI among veterans in the United States was estimated to decline from 45,626 in 1994 to 40,950 by 2004 and 33,055 by 2014, in conjunction with similar decreases in the overall U.S. veteran population (57).

Because of the lifetime duration of SCI, as well as differences in life expectancy for persons with different demographic characteristics and degrees of SCI impairment, the profile of persons with SCI who are alive today is different from the typical characteristics of persons who incur these injuries each year. For example, the median current age of all persons with SCI who were alive in 1988 was estimated to be 41 years (15 years older than the median age of new cases occurring at that time) (56). Among U.S. veterans, mean age of persons with SCI who were alive in 1988 was estimated to be 47 years (57). Moreover, because that estimate of median age is now 19 years old, and because the median age of new cases that occur each year is increasing, the median age of all persons with SCI who are alive today would be somewhat higher than it was in 1988 (but less than 19 years higher because of higher mortality rates among older persons).

Similarly, it was estimated in 1988 that only 71% of persons with SCI who were alive at that time were men, compared to 82% of new cases enrolled in the NSCISC Database at that time (56). Again, the percentage of persons with SCI who are alive today and who are men will be slightly lower than 71%, because men have shorter life expectancies than women. However, there have been no new attempts to develop a profile of prevalence of persons with SCI since 1988, so one can only speculate about current SCI population characteristics such as age, gender, race, neurologic level of injury, and degree of injury completeness.

There have been only two published studies of the prevalence of SCI outside the United States. One study was conducted in Stockholm, Sweden, between 1991 and 1994, and identified 379 persons with SCI living in the surrounding geographic region with a total population of 1.67 million people, resulting in a prevalence rate of 227 cases per million population (58). This is considerably lower than prevalence estimates from the United States, but would be consistent with the much lower incidence rates reported by European countries relative to the United States. In the Stockholm study, the mean age of persons with SCI was 42 years, the average time post-injury was 11 years, 81% were men, 42% had cervical injuries, and 40% had neurologically complete injuries. Lower proportions of cervical and complete injuries would be expected in a prevalence population compared to an incidence series of cases due to the lower survival rates for more severe injuries over time. Therefore, the results of the Stockholm prevalence study seem consistent with the many European studies of SCI incidence.

Prevalence of SCI in Australia was estimated to be 681 cases per million population in 1997 based on current estimates of incidence and life expectancy (59). Again, because of increases in life expectancy over time, this is probably a slight overestimate of actual prevalence.

CONCLUSION

Thanks to the initiation of population-based SCI registries in several states, the continued existence of the NSCISC and Shriners Hospital Databases, and a recent comprehensive review of literature on SCI incidence, prevalence, and epidemiology (60), much is now known about the descriptive worldwide epidemiology of SCI. Future epidemiologic efforts should focus on developing a more accurate profile of persons with SCI who are alive today (SCI prevalence), as well as detailed investigations of the exact circumstances surrounding how these injuries occur. Such research might provide important clues to developing cost-effective primary prevention programs.

*R*eferences

1. Kraus JF, Franti CE, Riggins RS, Richards D, Borhani NO. Incidence of traumatic spinal cord lesions. *J Chron Dis* 1975; 28:471–492.
2. Griffin MR, Opitz JL, Kurland LT, Ebersold MJ, O'Fallon WM. Traumatic SCI in Olmsted County, Minnesota, 1935–1981. *Am J Epidemiol* 1985; 121:884–895.
3. Kalsbeek WD, McLaurin RL, Harris BSH, Miller JD. The national head and spinal cord injury survey: Major findings. *J Neurosurg* 1980; 53(Suppl):19–31.
4. Bracken MB, Freeman DH, Hellenbrand K. Incidence of acute traumatic hospitalized spinal cord injury in the United States, 1970–1977. *Am J Epidemiol* 1981; 113:615–622.
5. Stover SL, DeVivo MJ, Go BK. History, implementation, and current status of the national spinal cord injury database. *Arch Phys Med Rehabil* 1999; 80:1365–1371.
6. DeVivo MJ, Go BK, Jackson AB. Overview of the national spinal cord injury statistical center database. *J Spinal Cord Med* 2002; 25:335–338.
7. DeVivo MJ, Rutt RD, Black KJ, Go BK, Stover SL. Trends in spinal cord injury demographics and treatment outcomes between 1973 and 1986. *Arch Phys Med Rehabil* 1992; 73:424–430.
8. Go BK, DeVivo MJ, Richards JS. The epidemiology of spinal cord injury. In: Stover SL, DeLisa JA, Whiteneck GG, eds. *Spinal Cord Injury: Clinical Outcomes from the Model Systems.* Gaithersburg, MD: Aspen Publishers, 1995:21–55.
9. Nobunaga AI, Go BK, Karunas RB. Recent demographic and injury trends in people served by the model spinal care injury care systems. *Arch Phys Med Rehabil* 1999; 80:1372–1382.
10. Vogel LC, DeVivo MJ. Pediatric spinal cord injury issues: etiology, demographics, and pathophysiology. *Top Spinal Cord Inj Rehabil* 1997; 3(2):1–8.
11. DeVivo MJ, Vogel LC. Epidemiology of spinal cord injury in children and adolescents. *J Spinal Cord Med* 2004; 27(Suppl):S4–S10.
12. Jackson AB, Dijkers M, DeVivo MJ, Poczatek RB. A demographic profile of new traumatic spinal cord injuries: change and stability over 30 years. *Arch Phys Med Rehabil* 2004; 85:1740–1748.
13. Acton PA, Farley T, Freni LW, Ilegbodu VA, Sniezek JE, Wohlleb JC. Traumatic spinal cord injury in Arkansas, 1980–1989. *Arch Phys Med Rehabil* 1993; 74:1035–1040.
14. Price C, Makintubee S, Herndon W, Istre GR. Epidemiology of traumatic spinal cord injury and acute hospitalization and rehabilitation charges for spinal cord injuries in Oklahoma, 1988–1990. *Am J Epidemiol* 1994; 139:37–47.
15. Thurman DJ, Burnett CL, Jeppson L, Beaudoin DE, Sniezek JE. Surveillance of spinal cord injuries in Utah, USA. *Paraplegia* 1994; 32:665–669.
16. Woodruff BA, Baron RC. A description of nonfatal spinal cord injury using a hospital-based registry. *Am J Prev Med* 1994; 10:10–14.
17. Surkin J. *Spinal Cord Injury: Mississippi's Facts and Figures.* Jackson, MS: Mississippi State Department of Health, 1995.
18. Surkin J, Smith M, Penman A, Currier M, Harkey HL, Chang Y-F. Spinal cord injury incidence in Mississippi: a capture-recapture approach. *J Trauma* 1998; 45:502–504.
19. Colorado Department of Public Health and Environment, Disease Control and Environmental Epidemiology Division. 1996 *Annual Report of the Traumatic Spinal Cord Injury Early Notification System.* Denver, CO: Colorado Department of Transportation Printing Office, 1997.
20. Johnson RL, Gabella BA, Gerhart KA, McCray J, Menconi JC, Whiteneck GG. Evaluating sources of traumatic spinal cord injury surveillance data in Colorado. *Am J Epidemiol* 1997; 146:266–272.
21. Relethford JH, Standfast SJ, Morse DL. Trends in traumatic spinal cord injury—New York, 1982–1988. *MMWR* 1991; 40:535–537, 543.
22. Bayakly AR, Lawrence DW. *Spinal Cord Injury in Louisiana 1991 Annual Report.* New Orleans, LA: Louisiana Office of Public Health, 1992.
23. Virginia Department of Rehabilitation Services. *Spinal Cord Injury in Virginia: A Statistical Fact Sheet.* Fishersville, VA: Virginia Spinal Cord Injury System, 1993.
24. Johnson SC. Georgia Central Registry: *Spinal Cord Disabilities and Traumatic Brain Injury.* Warm Springs, GA: Roosevelt Warm Springs Institute for Rehabilitation, 1992.
25. Burke DA, Linden RD, Zhang YP, Maistre AC, Shields CB. Incidence rates and populations at risk for spinal cord injury: a regional study. *Spinal Cord* 2001; 39:274–278.
26. Glick T. SCI surveillance: Is there a decrease in incidence? [abstract] *J Spinal Cord Med* 2000; 23Suppl:61.
27. http://www.nisu.flinders.edu.au/pubs/bulletin18.
28. O'Connor PJ. Forecasting of spinal cord injury annual case numbers in Australia. *Arch Phys Med Rehabil* 2005; 86:48–51.
29. O'Connor PJ. Trends in spinal cord injury. *Accident Anal Prev* 2006; 38:71–77.
30. Exner G, Meinecke FW. Trends in the treatment of patients with spinal cord lesions seen within a period of 20 years in German centers. *Spinal Cord* 1997; 35:415–419.
31. O'Connor RJ, Murray PC. Review of spinal cord injuries in Ireland. *Spinal Cord* 2006; 44:445–448.
32. Garcia-Reneses J, Herruzo-Cabrera R, Martinez-Moreno M. Epidemiological study of SCI in Spain 1984–1985. *Paraplegia* 1991; 28:180–190.
33. Biering-Sorensen F, Pedersen V, Clausen S. Epidemiology of spinal cord lesions in Denmark. *Paraplegia* 1990; 28:105–118.
34. Pagliacci MC, Celani MG, Zampolini M, Spizzichino L, Franceschini M, Baratta S, Finali G, Gatta G, Perdon L. An Italian survey of traumatic spinal cord injury. The gruppo Italiano studio epidemiologico mielolesioni study. *Arch Phys Med Rehabil* 2003; 84:1266–1275.
35. Celani MG, Spizzichino L, Ricci S, Zampolini M, Franceschini M. Spinal cord injury in Italy: a multicenter retrospective study. *Arch Phys Med Rehabil* 2001; 82:589–596.
36. Martins F, Freitas F, Martins L, Dartigues JF, Barat M. Spinal cord injuries—epidemiology in Portugal's central region. *Spinal Cord* 1998; 36:574–578.
37. Gjone R, Nordlie L. Incidence of traumatic paraplegia and tetraplegia in Norway: a statistical survey of the years 1974 and 1975. *Paraplegia* 1978; 16:88–93.

38. Gehrig R, Michaelis LS. Statistics of acute paraplegia and tetraplegia on a national scale: Switzerland 1960–67. *Paraplegia* 1968; 6(2):93–95.

39. Van Asbeck FWA, Post MWM, Pangalila RF. An epidemiological description of spinal cord injuries in The Netherlands in 1994. *Spinal Cord* 2000; 38:420–424.

40. Schonherr MC, Groothoff JW, Mulder GA, Eisma WH. Rehabilitation of patients with spinal cord lesions in The Netherlands: an epidemiological study. *Spinal Cord* 1996; 34:679–683.

41. Minaire P, Castanier M, Girard R, Berard E, Deidier C, Bourret J. Epidemiology of spinal cord injury in the Rhone-Alpes region, France, 1970–75. *Paraplegia* 1978; 16:76–87.

42. Karamehmetoglu SS, Nas K, Karacan I, Sarac AJ, Koyuncu H, Ataoglu S, Erdogan F. Traumatic spinal cord injuries in Southeast Turkey: an epidemiological study. *Spinal Cord* 1997; 35:531–533.

43. Karamehmetoglu SS, Unal S, Karacan I, Yilmaz H, Togay HS, Ertekin M, Dosoglu M, Ziyal MI, Kasaroglu D, Hakan T. Traumatic spinal cord injuries in Istanbul, Turkey. An epidemiological study. *Paraplegia* 1995; 33:469–471.

44. Karacan I, Koyuncu H, Pekel O, Sumbuloglu G, Kirnap M, Dursun H, Kalkan A, Cengiz A, Yalinkilc A, Unalan HI, Nas K, Orkum S, Tekeoglu I. Traumatic spinal cord injuries in Turkey: a nation-wide epidemiological study. *Spinal Cord* 2000; 38:697–701.

45. Otom AS, Doughan AM, Kawar JS, Hattar EZ. Traumatic spinal cord injuries in Jordan—an epidemiological study. *Spinal Cord* 1997; 35:253–255.

46. Ronen J, Itzkovich M, Bluvshtein V, Thaleisnik M, Goldin D, Gelernter I, David R, Gepstein R, Catz A. Length of stay in hospital following spinal cord lesions in Israel. *Spinal Cord* 2004; 42:353–358.

47. Shingu H, Ikata T, Katoh S, Akatsu T. Spinal cord injuries in Japan: a nationwide epidemiological survey in 1990. *Paraplegia* 1994; 32:3–8.

48. Chen CF, Lien IN. Spinal cord injuries in Taipei, Taiwan, 1978–1981. *Paraplegia* 1985; 23:364–370.

49. Lan C, Lai JS, Chang KH, Jean YC, Lien IN. Traumatic spinal cord injuries in the rural region of Taiwan: an epidemiological study in Hualien county, 1986–1990. *Paraplegia* 1993; 31:398–403.

50. Maharaj JC. Epidemiology of spinal cord paralysis in Fiji: 1985–1994. *Spinal Cord* 1996; 34:549–559.

51. Hart C, Williams E. Epidemiology of spinal cord injuries: a reflection of changes in South African society. *Paraplegia* 1994; 32:709–714.

52. DeVivo MJ. Epidemiology of traumatic spinal cord injury. In: Kirshblum S, Campagnolo DI, DeLisa JA, eds. *Spinal Cord Medicine.* Philadelphia: Lippincott Williams & Wilkins, 2002:69–81.

53. DeVivo MJ, Fine PR, Maetz HM, Stover SL. Prevalence of spinal cord injury: A reestimation employing life table techniques. *Arch Neurol* 1980; 37:707–708.

54. DeVivo MJ, Krause JS, Lammertse DP. Recent trends in mortality and causes of death among persons with spinal cord injury. *Arch Phys Med Rehabil* 1999; 80:1411–1419.

55. Strauss DJ, DeVivo MJ, Paculdo DR, Shavelle RM. Trends in life expectancy after spinal cord injury. *Arch Phys Med Rehabil* 2006; 87:1079–1085.

56. Berkowitz M, Harvey C, Greene CG, Wilson SE. *The Economic Consequences of Traumatic Spinal Cord Injury.* New York: Demos Publishers, 1992.

57. Lasfargues JE, Custis D, Morrone F, Carswell J, Nguyen T. A model for estimating spinal cord injury prevalence in the United States. *Paraplegia* 1995; 33:62–68.

58. Levi R, Hulting C, Nash MS, Seiger A. The Stockholm spinal cord injury study: 1. Medical problems in a regional SCI population. *Paraplegia* 1995; 33:308–315.

59. O'Connor PJ. Prevalence of spinal cord injury in Australia. *Spinal Cord* 2005; 43:42–46.

60. Wyndaele M, Wyndaele J-J. Incidence, prevalence and epidemiology of spinal cord injury: what learns a worldwide literature survey? *Spinal Cord* 2006; 44:523–529.

5 Neurological Assessment of Spinal Cord Dysfunction

Ralph J. Marino

This chapter reviews the assessment of neurological function after traumatic spinal cord injury (SCI). The examination follows the *International Standards for Neurological Assessment of SCI*, hereafter referred to as the *Standards* (1). The classification system is often used in individuals with nontraumatic spinal cord dysfunction, but because different pathologic mechanisms are at work, the prognostic significance of findings is not the same as for traumatic injuries. However, the classification may succinctly convey current neurological status.

PURPOSE OF NEUROLOGICAL ASSESSMENT

The purpose of the neurological examination after a traumatic injury varies with circumstances, as does the detail required. The initial examination in the emergency department is done to diagnose SCI. It is important to determine if neurological deficits can be localized to the spinal cord as soon as possible after a traumatic injury so that appropriate interventions can be instituted. Methylprednisolone, for example, was shown in one study to improve neurological outcome after SCI if treatment was started within 8 hours of injury (2). A neurological level that differs significantly from the vertebral level of injury may point to a noncontiguous spinal fracture, which occurs in 10% to 15% of traumatic spinal injuries (3–4). This initial examination may not be as detailed as later examinations because of time constraints and the need to identify and treat injuries to other organ systems in the trauma patient. It should, however, be thorough enough to determine the sensory and motor levels, complete or incomplete status, and American Spinal Injury Association (ASIA) Impairment Scale (AIS) grade, all of which are described later in this chapter.

After the initial examination, a careful determination of the level and severity of injury is important to monitor progress. For this purpose it is useful to go beyond the *Standards* and examine several muscles innervated by root levels at and around the neurological level of injury. For example, in a C5 injury, monitoring of biceps, deltoid, and perhaps upper trapezius muscles is helpful. The reliability of manual muscle testing is such that, in order to detect a difference, an individual muscle score should change by more than one grade (5). A deterioration in strength of several muscles in the zone of injury would point to true deterioration rather than normal fluctuations in a muscle grade. The ascension of neurological level or other deterioration in neurological status should initiate reevaluation of spinal column stability and spinal cord compression, and may be an indication for surgical or medical intervention (6–7).

A third purpose of neurological assessment is to determine prognosis. For this purpose, it is best to delay the examination for a few days after injury. Complications and medical and surgical interventions over the first few days after injury may adversely or favorably influence spinal cord recovery. It is sometimes difficult to obtain a complete, reliable examination in the emergency room. Concomitant injuries, such as head injury, may make it difficult to be certain that an injury is truly complete (8). Other factors such as the need for intubation or sedation, or the presence of licit and illicit drugs may interfere with the accuracy of the early examination (9). For these reasons, the examination performed after 72 hours may more reliably predict recovery than the examination performed on the day of injury (10).

ELEMENTS OF NEUROLOGICAL ASSESSMENT

Neurological assessment is based on the *Standards* of ASIA and the International Spinal Cord Society (ISCoS). Elements of the examination include the determination of light touch and pinprick sensation, strength of key muscles, neurological rectal examination, and reflex testing. The 2002 *Standards* are described in this chapter. Further details can be found in the booklet describing the *Standards* (1) and the reference manual (11), updated in 2003 and available from ASIA at *http://www.asia-spinalinjury.org/publications/store.php*. In addition, ASIA has developed an online e-learning program for assessment and classification of SCI that became available in the spring of 2009. This interactive program consists of 6 modules with video clips and self-assessment tests to reinforce learning objectives.

Sensory Examination

The sensory examination consists of testing a key point in each of twenty-eight dermatomes on the right and left sides of the body (Figure 5.1). All dermatomes from C2 through S5 are tested, with S4–S5 tested as one level. The key points are tested for appreciation of light touch and pinprick sensation.

To test for light touch sensation, use a cotton swab or a cotton strand pulled out from a cotton applicator stick. Sometimes, for clinical purposes, you may pull the end of an examination glove away from a finger and use this to lightly tough the patient. Ask the patient to close his or her eyes. Move the cotton strand about 1 cm along the skin at the test point. Grade light touch as normal, impaired, or absent. Normal sensation is established by comparison with sensation on the face, or another area with normal sensation, if sensation of the face is affected. Impaired sensation is any sensation that differs from that on the normal area. Both hyperesthesia and diminished sensation are considered abnormal. If the patient does not feel the stimulus, light touch sensation in that dermatome is absent.

Testing for pinprick sensation is performed using a disposable safety pin. Establish normal pinprick sensation by lightly touching the sharp end of the safety pin to the face, or another area determined to be normal, if the face is affected. Normal pinprick sensation means that the sensation of sharpness in the area being tested is identical to that in the normal area. Abnormal sensation means that either the sensation is somewhat sharp, but not as sharp as the normal area, or that the sensation is more painful than normal. Absent means that there is no feeling of sharpness, or that the patient cannot distinguish the sharp from the blunt end of the safety pin. Note that the patient may feel a touch or a pressure sensation from the pin, but no sensation of sharpness. In this case pinprick sensation should be graded as absent. Also, in areas of hyperesthesia, all sensation may be perceived as sharp. In areas where the pin feels sharper than normal, the patient must be able to differentiate the sharp from the blunt end of the pin to receive a grade of impaired; otherwise grade pinprick sensation as absent.

Clinically, it is important to test for deep pressure sensation and position sense in the extremities. These modalities have functional significance, but are not used in the classification of spinal cord dysfunction. Deep pressure sensation may be present in individuals who have no light touch or pinprick sensation, but does not designate an incomplete injury unless it is present in the perianal area.

Pitfalls in Sensory Examination

The primary difficulties that occur in performing the sensory examination concern the pinprick sensation and evaluation of the T3 dermatome. As noted above, the assessment of pinprick sensation requires careful testing when there is hyperesthesia present. First, it must be determined that the patient can distinguish between the pointed and blunt end of the pin in a given testing point. If not, pinprick is graded as absent at that point. If able to distinguish sharp from dull, then the degree of sharpness is compared to that on the face to determine whether the pinprick sensation is impaired or normal.

The T3 dermatome is probably the most difficult to evaluate, because there is considerable variation in the distance that the C4 dermatome extends down the anterior chest wall. In cervical injuries, if testing for T3 sensation occurs too high on the chest, it may seem to be present because of C4 innervation. As described in the *Reference Manual for the International Standards*, if sensation is absent in T1 and T2, seems to be present in T3, and is absent in T4, it is recommended that the T3 dermatome be scored as absent (11, p.19).

Motor Examination

The motor examination consists of testing twenty muscles, five muscles in each extremity, representing ten spinal cord myotomes (see Figure 5.2). The muscles are graded by manual muscle testing (MMT) using a six-point scale (Table 5.1). It is important to score each muscle based on the identification of neurological weakness. Only muscles that are thought to be weak due to neurological injury should be scored less than Grade 5. If a muscle is felt to be slightly weak because of disuse rather than neurological weakness, then it should be graded as normal (Grade 5*). Similarly, if the patient is inhibited by pain or hypertonicity, but gives a forceful contraction (perhaps briefly), it may be graded normal (Grade 5*) if the examiner feels that the muscle would test normal were it not for these factors. The asterisk indicates that there was difficulty with MMT but that the examiner felt the muscle was not

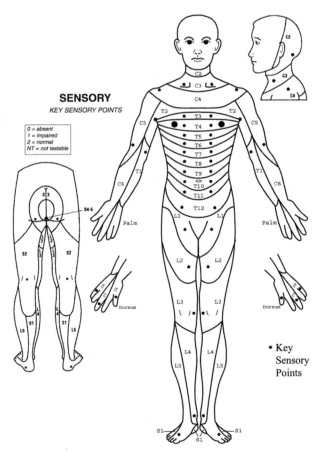

Figure 5.1 Sensory dermatomes and key sensory points. (With permission from the American Spinal Injury Association. Standards for Neurological Classification of SCI Worksheet 2006; http://www.asia-spinalinjury.org/publications/2006_Classif_worksheet.pdf.)

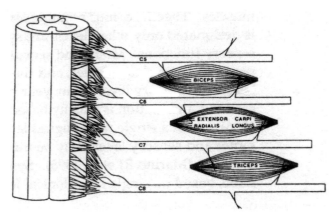

Figure 5.2 Schematic depiction of innervation of each of three key muscles by two nerve segments. (With permission from the American Spinal Injury Association. *International Standards for Neurological Classification of SCI,* revised 2002. Chicago, IL: American Spinal Injury Association, 2002; p.17.)

weak. The reason for using the asterisk should be noted in the comment box on the examination worksheet. If a muscle cannot be tested because of inhibiting factors, or if it is unable to be tested because of associated injuries or contracture, then it should be graded as not testable (NT). Note that according to the *Standards,* if range of motion of the joint on which the muscle acts is reduced by more than 50%, then the muscle should be graded NT.

Clinically it is important to examine other muscles in addition to the 10 key muscles needed for classification. Grading additional muscles at the level of injury is important in monitoring the progression of deficits and recovery. Other clinically significant muscles include the diaphragm, the deltoids, the abdominals (evaluation for Beevor's sign [12]), and the hip extensor muscles. It is not unusual during the early recovery period to find patients who can contract their hip adductor

muscles or toe flexors but who cannot activate any of the lower extremity key muscles.

Pitfalls in Motor Examination

Accurate MMT requires proper positioning of the extremity being tested and an awareness of substitution patterns. Perhaps the most difficult muscle to examine in the upper extremity is the triceps. When testing for grade 2 triceps, care must be taken to maintain the forearm in a horizontal position over the chest. Frequently the patient will externally rotate and abduct the shoulder, whereupon momentum and gravity will allow the elbow to extend. Careful positioning, as well as palpation and visual inspection of the triceps muscle, will minimize the chance of being fooled by this substitution pattern.

Testing the flexor digitorum profundus muscle requires stabilization of the wrist and proximal phalanx of the finger to isolate the muscle. Finger flexion can occur through tenodesis effect (passive pull of the flexor tendon) when the wrist is extended. Although this effect is often clinically useful, it can confound attempts to grade finger flexor strength. Finally, in the upper extremities, care must be taken when testing the finger abductors. In subjects with active finger extension, this motion (extension) results in some abduction of the fingers, usually with hyperextension at the metacarpophalangeal joints. The fingers should be positioned in extension on a flat surface and kept from hyperextending by applying gentle pressure on the dorsal proximal phalanges. The abductor digiti minimi should be observed and palpated when this muscle is being tested.

In the lower extremities, care should be taken when testing the ankle dorsiflexors and plantarflexors in patients with proximal leg movement. When the heel is in contact with the bed, hip movement may cause passive ankle movement that can be confused with active movement. When in doubt, the examiner should lift the leg and repeat the examination with the foot off the bed.

Reflex withdrawal and hypertonicity can also be confused with voluntary movement. The act of touching or grabbing the limb may set off a flexion withdrawal response. Some patients are able to trigger a lower extremity spasm when asked to move the limb. Careful testing is required to distinguish these involuntary movements from volitional muscle contractions.

Reflex Testing

The third component of the neurological examination is testing of reflexes. Deep tendon reflexes should be evaluated for biceps, wrist extensors, triceps, and finger flexors in the upper extremities. In the lower extremities, the patellar and Achilles reflexes should be assessed. In the days following an acute SCI, it is useful to test for the delayed plantar reflex. This test is conducted similarly to the Babinski test, stroking the plantar surface of the foot with a blunt object from the heel to lateral forefoot and medially across the metatarsal heads, using firm pressure. In a positive test, there is a slow flexion and relaxation of the toes lasting several seconds, and starting about 1/2 second or so after the stimulation starts. The delayed planter response is seen in most complete injuries and some incomplete injuries, and is replaced by the Babinski response over a period of 1–2 weeks. (13)

Table 5.1 Manual Muscle Test Grades

GRADE	DEFINITION
0	Total paralysis (no visible or palpable contraction)
1	Palpable or visible muscle contraction
2	Active movement, full range of motion (ROM) with gravity eliminated
3	Active movement, full ROM against gravity
4	Active movement, full ROM against moderate resistance
5	(Normal) active movement, full ROM against full resistance
5*	Sufficient resistance to be considered "normal" if identifiable inhibiting factors were not present (see text)
NT	Not testable

Adapted from ASIA 2002 (ref. 1), p.13, with permission.

Neurological Rectal Examination

The neurological rectal examination differs from the general medical rectal examination. In the neurological rectal examination, the purpose is to determine the function of the conus and S3–S5 nerve roots. It is critical for determining whether the injury is complete or incomplete in a severely injured individual. Any reliable sensory perception in the anal area or any voluntary sphincter contraction means that the injury is incomplete. Similar to the neurological assessment described thus far, the exam has three components: sensory testing, motor testing, and reflex testing.

Test the S3 and S4–S5 dermatomes for light touch and pinprick sensation using the methods described previously. In addition, perform a digital rectal exam and ask the patient if he or she feels any sensation to the gloved finger or any sensation of pressure as the finger is moved against the anal sphincter. Grade sensation as present or absent. Next examine the anal sphincter for any voluntary contraction. To do this, with a gloved finger in the rectum, ask the patient to squeeze (not bear down) as if he or she is holding in a bowel movement. Be careful not to move your finger or you may initiate a reflex contraction of the sphincter. Remember, resting tone is NOT voluntary. Grade voluntary anal sphincter contraction as present or absent. If voluntary contraction of the anal sphincter is present, then the injury is motor incomplete.

Finally, the anal wink and bulbocavernosus (BC) reflexes should be assessed. These reflexes have significance for bowel and bladder functioning, and their presence indicates the emergence from spinal shock. For anal wink, lightly poke the skin with a safety pin at the anocutaneous junction on the right and left sides, and look for a reflex contraction of the anal sphincter (the "wink"). For the BC reflex, insert a gloved finger into the patient's rectum. Then give a firm, quick squeeze to the head of the penis, and feel for a reflex contraction of the anal sphincter. In women, give a quick tug on the foley catheter if present, or poke the clitoris with a cotton applicator.

RELIABILITY OF NEUROLOGICAL EXAMINATION

Several studies have looked at reliability of the motor and sensory components of the examination, looking at total scores, individual dermatome/myotome scores, or both. Although findings on the digital rectal exam may determine whether an injury is complete or incomplete, reliability of this part of the exam has not been reported. Reliability of total scores is generally reported using the Pearson or intraclass correlation coefficient (ICC), with the ICC being preferred. For individual item scores, measures of agreement such as the kappa statistic or the weighted kappa are used; the latter giving partial credit for being close when there are more than two possible scores (14).

Cohen and Bartko (15) found high reliability of the summed LT, PP, and motor scores in trained examiners; inter-rater reliability values ranged from 0.96–0.98 and intra-rater reliability values were 0.98–0.99 for the three scales (Table 5.2). Savic et al. (16) had two experienced examiners test 45 patients with SCI and found ICC values above 0.98 for motor and sensory total scores. Marino et al. (17) looked at the reliability of 16 examiners who tested 3 of 16 patients. Results were similar to those of Cohen and Savic except for pinprick scores, where the ICC was only 0.89.

Table 5.2   Reliability Values for Total Scores[a] of Neurological Examination

	LIGHT TOUCH SCORE	PINPRICK SCORE	MOTOR SCORE
Inter-rater			
Cohen 1994	.96	.96	.98
Savic 2007	.99 (.99)	.99 (.97)	.99 (.99)
Marino 2008	.96 (.90)	.89 (.77)	.98 (.96)
Intra-rater			
Cohen 1994	.99	.98	.99
Mulcahey 2007	.97 (.95)	.97 (.96)	.89 (.82)
Marino 2008	.99 (.97)[b]	.99 (.94)[b]	.98 (.79)[b]

[a]Scores represent reliability coefficient (lower limit of 95% confidence interval).
[b]Complete injuries only.

Mulcahey et al. (18) evaluated the reliability of the motor and sensory data in children and youths. They found that the exam was not reliable or could not be done in children less than 4 years of age, and children under 10 were distressed by the pinprick exam, limiting the usefulness in these age groups. In children 4 years and older, ICC values were generally high, although results were inconclusive for total motor scores in children under 15 due to wide confidence intervals.

Jonsson et al. evaluated inter-rater agreement for individual sensory dermatome scores and muscle test scores, but did not look at reliability of the entire scales (19). They found weak inter-rater reliability, but used kappa values rather than the more appropriate weighted kappa. On the other hand, Savic et al. (16) found substantial agreement in scores for the 10 key muscles (weighted kappa > 0.93 for all except the biceps).

Perhaps more important than reliability for the sensory and motor scores is the repeatability—how close scores will be when repeated on stable patients. Using Bland and Altman's measure of repeatability (twice the SD of mean difference), Savic et al. found that 95% of repeat light touch and motor scores would differ by less than 4 points, and pinprick scores would differ by less than 8 points (16). Marino et al. (17) found good repeatability values when patients with complete injuries were tested—about 6 points for light touch and pinprick scores, and 2 points for motor scores. There were only a few patients with incomplete injuries tested, and repeatability values were higher at least partly due to the small sample.

CLASSIFICATION OF SPINAL CORD INJURY

The *Standards* were designed for describing the level and severity of injury in an acute traumatic SCI. The classification may not be as meaningful if used to describe nontraumatic spinal cord disorders. In addition, the *Standards* are difficult to apply when the spinal cord dysfunction is multifocal, as occurs in some traumatic injuries and with diseases such as multiple sclerosis. There are four components to classification: determination of levels of injury, completeness of injury, AIS grade, and for complete injuries, the zone of partial preservation (ZPP).

Table 5.3   Reliability of Classification of Spinal Cord Injury in Experienced Classifiers

YEAR OF STANDARDS (CITATION)	SENSORY LEVEL (AGREEMENT)	MOTOR LEVEL (AGREEMENT)	AIS GRADE (AGREEMENT)	AIS GRADE (KAPPA)
1987 (Donovan 1990)	81%	66%	73%	
1989 (Priebe 1991)	93%	85%	81%	.66
2002 (Marino 2004)	94%	93%	87%[a]	.81

[a]Agreement 95% for the 5 cases used by Donovan 1990.

Reliability of Classification

The *Standards* have been revised to clarify the definitions and criteria for determining motor level. Because there is a correct answer for classification, agreement statistics are not as relevant as accuracy or percent correct. Donovan et al. (20) reported accuracy for sensory levels, motor levels, and Frankel grade as 81%, 66% and 73%, respectively, using the 1987 *Standards* (Table 5.3). Because of the low accuracy for motor level designation, the operational definition of motor level was revised. Accuracy of classification improved with the 1989 *Standards* to 93% for sensory levels, 85% for motor levels, and 81% for Frankel grades (21). Using the 2002 *Standards,* experienced clinicians correctly determined motor levels 93% of the time, and AIS grade 87% of the time (22). To achieve this degree of accuracy, a systematic approach to classification is needed.

Steps in Classification of SCI

The worksheet provided in the ASIA/ISCoS booklet should be used to record the examination. Using the completed worksheet, the following steps should be performed in the order given to correctly classify patients with SCI. Most mistakes are made when rules and definitions are applied inappropriately or at the wrong time. It is assumed here that the patient has motor and sensory deficits due only to a single traumatic SCI, and that MMT grades less than 5 have been recorded only for muscles with neurological weakness and not for deconditioning or pain during testing. Basic terms used in the classification of SCI are defined in Table 5.4.

1. *Determine the sensory levels.* The sensory level for the right and left side is the most caudal segment of the spinal cord where both pinprick and light touch (and all rostral levels) are normal. Start from the top of the sensory columns on the worksheet and run down the right side scores until you come to a "1" or a "0" for either light touch or pinprick. The level immediately above (where both light touch and pinprick are "2") is the sensory level. Do the same thing for the left side.
2. *Determine the motor levels.* Although the motor level is the most caudal segment of the spinal cord with normal motor function, this does not mean that the key muscle must have normal strength. The key muscles have been selected in part because they are innervated predominantly by two myotomes (Figure 5.2). By convention, if the muscle has at least a grade of 3, it is considered to have intact innervation by the more rostral segment. If the upper myotome of a key muscle is

intact, for example the C7 myotome for the triceps, then the triceps strength should be at least grade 3. Also, the next rostral key muscle, in this example the radial wrist extensors, should be fully innervated and therefore have normal (grade 5) strength.

Operationally, then, the motor level is defined as the lowest key muscle that has a grade of at least 3, provided that the key muscles above that level are judged to be normal (grade 5). To assign a motor level of C5 or L2, where there is no key muscle immediately above to test, normal sensation in the C4 or L1 dermatome is considered equivalent to a normal (grade 5) muscle. If there is no muscle to test at a given segment, such as in the thoracic segments and the C2–C4 segments, then the motor level is determined by the sensory level.

Table 5.4   Definitions of Terms Used in the Classification of SCI

Neurological Level	The most caudal segment of the spinal cord with normal sensory and motor function.
Sensory Level	The most caudal segment of the spinal cord with normal sensory function (light touch and pinprick). Right and left levels are determined separately.
Motor Level	The most caudal segment of the spinal cord with normal motor function. Right and left levels are determined separately.
Complete Injury	An injury is considered complete if there is no sensory or motor function in the lowest sacral segments (S4–S5), including absent anal sensation and voluntary anal sphincter contraction.
Incomplete Injury	An injury is considered incomplete if any of the following are present: (1) sensation in the S4–S5 segments, (2) any anal sensation during a digital rectal examination, or (3) voluntary anal sphincter contraction.
Zone of Partial Preservation (ZPP)	Applicable only if the injury is complete, the ZPP is the caudal extent of any sensory or motor function beyond the level of injury.

Adapted from *ASIA* 2002 (Ref. 1), pp. 6–7, with permission.

3. *Determine the single neurological level.* The single neurological level is the most caudal segment of the spinal cord where sensory function and motor function on both sides are normal. When the lesion is asymmetric, a single neurological level should not be used to characterize the lesion. Instead, the individual sensory and motor levels should be used; for example, right C5 sensory-C6 motor, left C6 sensory-C7 motor level. However, the single neurological level is sometimes needed to determine the AIS grade. In the example above, the single neurological level would be C5.

4. *Determine if the injury is complete or incomplete.* The criterion for an incomplete injury is based on the detection of sacral sparing, after work by Waters et al. (23). Earlier versions of the *Standards* defined a lesion as incomplete if there was some preservation of motor or sensory function more than three levels below the neurological level (24). Waters et al. (23) compared this definition to a "sacral sparing" definition of incomplete; namely, the preservation of some sensory and/or motor function in the sacral segments. They found that the sacral sparing definition was more stable than the "more than 3 levels" definition. Subsequently, the sacral sparing definition was incorporated into the *Standards.* Thus, an injury is considered *complete* if neither motor nor sensory function is present in the lowest sacral segments. Conversely, an injury is considered *incomplete* if there is partial preservation of sensory or motor function below the neurological level that includes the lower sacral segments. This sacral sensation can be light touch or pinprick sensation at the anal mucocutaneous junction, or any anal sensation felt during a digital rectal examination. Motor function in the lowest sacral segment is determined by the presence of voluntary contraction of the external anal sphincter. Note that reflex contraction as obtained with the bulbocavernosus reflex or anal wink reflex is not voluntary.

A complete injury can be easily determined using the worksheet by looking for the "N-0-0-0-0-N" sign (Figure 5.3). If there is an "N" in the box for *voluntary anal contraction,* "0" in the S4–S5 sensory scores, and "N" in the box for *any anal sensation,* then the injury is complete. Otherwise the injury is incomplete.

5. *Determine the ASIA Impairment Scale grade.* The AIS is a modification of the Frankel scale (25), which describes the degree of incompleteness below the level of a spinal cord lesion. The degree of incompleteness is graded on a 5-point scale from A to E (Table 5.5). In determining the AIS grade, one first determines whether or not the injury is complete or incomplete, as described above. If complete, the grade is A. If incomplete, then determine whether or not the injury is motor complete or incomplete. To be motor incomplete

Table 5.5	ASIA Impairment Scale Grade Definitions
A = complete	No sensory or motor function is preserved in the sacral segments S4–S5.
B = incomplete	Sensory but not motor function is preserved below the neurological level and includes the sacral segments S4–S5.
C = incomplete	Motor function is preserved below the neurological level and *more than half* of key muscles below the neurological level have a muscle grade less than 3 (grades 0–2).
D = incomplete	Motor function is preserved below the neurological level, and *at least half* of key muscles below the neurological level have a muscle grade of 3 or more.
E = normal	Motor and sensory functions are normal.

From *ASIA* 2002 (Ref. 1), pp. 18–19, with permission.

there must be *either* (1) voluntary anal sphincter contraction *or* (2) some sparing of motor function more than three levels caudal to the motor level on a given side. If neither of these conditions is met, the patient is AIS grade B. For example, an individual with an L2 sensory and motor level, perianal sensation, no voluntary anal sphincter contraction, grade 2 ankle dorsiflexor strength (L4), and no movement in more distal muscles would be AIS grade B (L4 is only 2 levels below the L2 motor level). On the other hand, if the same individual had grade 1 plantarflexor strength (S1), he would receive an AIS grade of C (S1 is 4 levels below the L2 motor level). Note that motor sparing need not be in a key muscle. An individual with sensory sacral sparing and a C7 motor level with lower extremity voluntary movement only in the toe flexors would be motor incomplete.

If the injury is motor incomplete, the final distinction is between AIS grades C and D. In a motor incomplete lesion, count the number of key muscles on both sides of the body below the *single neurological level.* Determine the number of these key muscles with a MMT grade of at least 3. If *less than half* of the muscles are at least grade 3, then the AIS grade is C. If *at least half* of the muscles are grade 3 or better, then the AIS grade is D.

The AIS grade E is used to describe someone with a prior SCI who has recovered normal sensory and motor function. Deep tendon reflexes may still be abnormal. It should not be used for someone with a spine fracture but no neurological deficits. The use of AIS grade E implies that there were prior motor and sensory deficits that have since resolved.

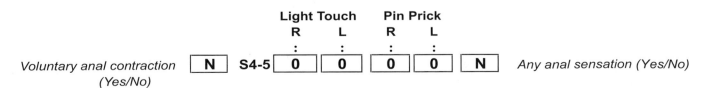

Figure 5.3 The N-0-0-0-0-N sign for classifying a spinal cord injury as complete. (Modified with permission from the American Spinal Injury Association. Standards for Neurological Classification of SCI Worksheet 2006; http://www.asia-spinalinjury.org/publications/2006_Classif_worksheet.pdf.)

Zone of Partial Preservation (ZPP)

The ZPP applies only when an injury is complete, and refers to the dermatomes and myotomes caudal to the neurological level that remain partially innervated. On the worksheet, record the lowest dermatome or myotome with some function on either side of the body. For the sensory ZPP, start at the bottom of the sensory columns and go up until you first encounter a "1" or a "2" for light touch or pinprick on a side. Record the corresponding dermatome for the ZPP. For motor ZPP, do the same with the motor scores. Note that unlike the motor level, the motor ZPP is not based on sensory function; there must be some motor function detected below the motor level to have a motor ZPP. There is prognostic significance to having an extended ZPP. Patients whose sensory ZPP extends for more than 3 levels have a greater chance of converting to motor incomplete than those with a shorter ZPP (26).

CONCLUSION

Accurate neurological classification after SCI requires careful neurological examination and a thorough understanding of the ASIA/ISCoS *Standards*. Testing sensation at the key dermatome points and muscle testing in the prescribed test positions will facilitate consistency across examinations. Although there will always be some patients with atypical injuries that are difficult to classify, use of the classification algorithm will help users avoid the most common errors in classification.

*R*eferences

1. American Spinal Injury Association. *International standards for neurological classification of spinal cord injury.* Revised 2000, reprinted 2002. Chicago, IL: American Spinal Injury Association; 2002.
2. Bracken MB, Holford TR. Effects of timing of methylprednisolone or naloxone administration on recovery of segmental and long-tract neurological function in NASCIS 2. *J Neurosurg* 1993; 79:500–507.
3. Henderson RL, Reid DC, Saboe LA. Multiple noncontiguous spine fractures. *Spine* 1991; 16:128–131.
4. Vaccaro AR, An HS, Lin S, Sun S, Balderston RA, Cotler JM. Noncontiguous injuries of the spine. *J Spinal Disord* 1992; 5:320–329.
5. Cohen ME, Sheehan TP, Herbison GJ. Content validity and reliability of the International Standards for Neurological Classification of Spinal Cord Injury. *Top Spinal Cord Inj Rehabil* 1996; 1(4):15–31.
6. Poonnoose PM, Ravichandran G, McClelland MR, Poonnoose PM, Ravichandran G, McClelland MR. Missed and mismanaged injuries of the spinal cord. *J Trauma* 2002; 53:314–320.
7. Harrop JS, Sharan AD, Vaccaro AR et al. The cause of neurologic deterioration after acute cervical spinal cord injury. *Spine* 2001; 26:340–346.
8. Maynard FM, Reynolds GG, Fountain S, Wilmot CB, Hamilton R. Neurologic prognosis after traumatic quadriplegia: three-year experience of California regional spinal cord injury care system. *J Neurosurg* 1979; 50:611–616.
9. Burns AS, Lee BS, Ditunno JFJ, Tessler A. Patient selection for clinical trials: the reliability of the early spinal cord injury examination. *J Neurotrauma* 2003; 20:477–482.
10. Brown PJ, Marino RJ, Herbison GJ, Ditunno JF, Jr. The 72-hour examination as a predictor of recovery in motor complete quadriplegia. *Arch Phys Med Rehabil* 1991; 72(8):546–548.
11. American Spinal Injury Association. *Reference Manual for the International Standards for Neurological Classification of Spinal Cord Injury.* Chicago, IL: American Spinal Injury Association; 2003.
12. Pearce JM, Pearce JMS. Beevor's sign. *Eur Neurol* 2005; 53:208–209.
13. Ko HY, Ditunno JFJ, Graziani V, Little JW. The pattern of reflex recovery during spinal shock. *Spinal Cord* 1999; 37:402–409.
14. Landis JR, Koch GG. The measurement of observer agreement for categorical data. *Biometrics* 1977; 33:159–174.
15. Cohen ME, Bartko JJ. Reliability of ISCSCI-92 for neurological classification of spinal cord injury. In: Ditunno JF, Donovan WH, Maynard FM, eds. *Reference Manual for the International Standards for Neurological and Functional Classification of Spinal Cord Injury.* Atlanta: American Spinal Injury Association, 1994:59–66.
16. Savic G, Bergstrom EMK, Frankel HL, Jamous MA, Jones PW. Inter-rater reliability of motor and sensory examinations performed according to American Spinal Injury Association standards. *Spinal Cord* 2007; 45:444–451.
17. Marino RJ, Jones L, Kirshblum S, Tal J, Dasgupta A. Reliability and repeatability of the motor and sensory examination of the International Standards for Neurological Classification of Spinal Cord Injury. *J Spinal Cord Med* 2008; 31:166–70.
18. Mulcahey MJ, Gaughan J, Betz RR, Johansen KJ. The International Standards for Neurological Classification of Spinal Cord Injury: reliability of data when applied to children and youths. *Spinal Cord* 2007; 45:452–459.
19. Jonsson M, Tollback A, Gonzales H, Borg J. Inter-rater reliability of the 1992 international standards for neurological and functional classification of incomplete spinal cord injury. *Spinal Cord* 2000; 38:675–679.
20. Donovan WH, Wilkerson MA, Rossi D, Mechoulam F, Frankowski RF. A test of ASIA guidelines for classification of spinal cord injuries. *J Neuro Rehabil* 1990; 4(1):39–53.
21. Priebe MM, Waring WP. The interobserver reliability of the revised American Spinal Injury Association standards for neurological classification of spinal injury patients. *Am J Phys Med Rehabil* 1991; 70:268–270.
22. Marino RJ, Kirshblum S, Jones L, Tal J. Agreement in neurological classification of spinal cord injury using the 2002 Standards. *J Spinal Cord Med* 2004; 27:415–416.
23. Waters RL, Adkins RH, Yakura JS. Definition of complete spinal cord injury. *Para* 1991; 29:573–581.
24. American Spinal Injury Association. *Standards for Neurological Classification of Spinal Injury Patients.* Chicago, IL: American Spinal Injury Association; 1989.
25. Frankel HL, Hancock DO, Hyslop G, et al. The value of postural reduction in the initial management of closed injuries of the spine with paraplegia and tetraplegia, part I. *Para* 1969; 7:179–192.
26. Marino RJ, Ditunno JFJ, Donovan WH, Maynard FJ. Neurologic recovery after traumatic spinal cord injury: data from the Model Spinal Cord Injury Systems. *Arch Phys Med Rehabil* 1999; 80:1391–1396.

6 The Electrodiagnostic Examination in Spinal Cord Disorders

Asa J. Wilbourn
Robert W. Shields, Jr.

The spinal cord is the long, cylindrical, caudal component of the central nervous system (CNS) that resides within the bony vertebral canal (1). The majority of the maladies that affect the brain portion of the CNS may also affect the spinal cord portion. Because the peripheral motor axons originate within the spinal cord, and the peripheral sensory fibers are linked to the spinal cord via their cell bodies in the dorsal root ganglia (DRGs) and the primary sensory roots, many of the disorders that affect the spinal cord have peripheral nervous system (PNS) manifestations, which can be detected by the electrodiagnostic (EDX) examination. This chapter focuses principally on these particular CNS disorders.

ANATOMY

The spinal cord extends from the upper border of the first cervical vertebrae—the *atlas* (where it is continuous with the medulla oblongata of the brainstem)—to the lower border of the first, or the upper border of the second lumbar vertebrae, where it tapers and ultimately is continuous with the filum terminale. The latter is composed mainly of fibrous tissue; it passes caudally in the vertebral canal to attach to the first segment of the coccyx. The spinal cord is approximately 45 cm in length in the average male, 2 to 3 cm shorter in the female. Similar to the brain, it is surrounded by the meninges: three protective membranes which, from peripheral to central, consist of the dura mater, the arachnoid, and the pia mater. In cross section, the spinal cord is essentially round but somewhat flattened anterioposteriorly. It is increased in diameter by enlargements in the cervical and lumbar regions. The cervical enlargement extends from approximately the fifth cervical to the second thoracic vertebra. It is from this region that the somatic nerve fibers arise that innervate the upper limbs, as well as the autonomic fibers that supply the head, neck, and upper limbs. The lumbar enlargement extends from approximately the ninth to the twelfth thoracic vertebrae. As it narrows caudally it is continuous with the conus medullaris, which is the most inferior portion of the spinal cord. It is from the latter and the lumbar enlargement that the somatic nerve fibers originate

to innervate the lower limbs, as well as the autonomic fibers that supply the lower limbs, genitourinary system, and much of the gastrointestinal system (Figure 6.1). Most of these axons, consisting of the primary motor and sensory (i.e., preganglionic) roots, must pass caudal to the conus medullaris to reach the intervertebral foramina, through which they exit the intraspinal canal. Those traveling several vertebral segments inferiorly do so almost vertically to reach beyond the conus medullaris. This collection of roots forms the cauda equina (1–3).

The spinal cord, on cross section, consists of grey matter surrounded by white matter. The grey matter is in the form of the letter "H," with the dorsal (or posterior) segments (or horns) containing sensory fibers, and the ventral (or anterior) segments containing the alpha motor neurons or anterior horn cells (AHCs), whose very long peripheral extensions, labeled *axons*, comprise the somatic motor portion of the PNS. Thus, the cell bodies of origin of the motor axons are within the spinal cord. In contrast, the cell bodies of origin of the sensory fibers are situated in ganglia, called dorsal root ganglia (DRG), which are located on the very distal portion of the primary sensory roots, at the entrance to or within the intervertebral foramina (1, 4).

The basic organization of the somatic portion of the PNS requires brief review. The motor portions of the PNS (i.e., the AHC and its axon) are two of the major components of the "motor unit": one AHC and all the muscle fibers that it innervates, via its axon, the latter's many terminal branches, and the interposed neuromuscular junctions. By this arrangement, whenever a single AHC fires, all the muscle fibers that it innervates are depolarized and fire almost simultaneously. (The exact number of muscle fibers that do so varies with the particular muscle, and whether it has ever been denervated and subsequently reinnervated in the past. In human limb muscles, the innervation ratio varies from approximately 200 to 250 to greater than 1,600) (5, 6). If a needle recording electrode is within the muscle when the latter is activated, the electrical activity generated by the muscle fibers composing one motor unit registers as a *motor unit action potential* (MUAP). On the sensory side, unipolar cell bodies located in the DRGs send one process

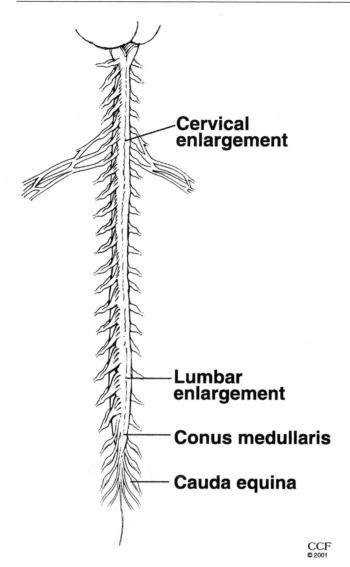

Figure 6.1 The spinal cord, frontal view. Of note is that the only motor nerve fibers arising from the spinal cord that can be optimally assessed in the electrodiagnostic laboratory are those that originate from the cervical and lumbar enlargements and the conus medullaris.

centrally into the spinal cord (pregangliotic component) and another peripherally (postganglionic component), the latter being the somatic sensory axon. From each spinal cord segment, both somatic motor and sensory axons originate. A *myotome* contains all the muscles innervated by a single spinal cord segment, whereas a *dermatome* is the cutaneous sensory area supplied by a single spinal cord segment (4).

SPINAL CORD DISORDERS

Spinal cord disorders (SCDs) may be focal, multifocal, or diffuse (7). They have numerous causes. Consequently, even a partial list of the many entities that can harm the spinal cord is formidable (Table 6.1). The frequency with which such injuries occur varies not only with different areas of the world, but also with the era.

Table 6.1   Some Spinal Cord Disorders
Anterior Horn Cell Disorders
Spinal muscle atrophies
Werdnig–Hoffmann
Wohlfort–Kugelberg–Welander
Adult onset progressive
Scapuloperoneal
Facioscapulohumeral
Monomelic/segmental amyotrophy
Amyotrophic lateral sclerosis
Syringomyelia (congenital; traumatic)
Epidural neoplasms
Metastatic
Myelitis
Viral (e.g., anterior poliomyelitis)
Bacterial (e.g., syphilis)
Post infectious
Multiple sclerosis
Myelopathy
Traumatic
Degenerative Spinal Disorders (e.g., spondylosis)
2° to bony/cartilaginous
Physical agents (e.g., radiation)
Toxins (e.g., tri-o-cresyl phosphate)
Metabolic/nutritional (e.g., pernicious anemia)
Vascular malformations (arterial, venous)
Neoplasms
Intramedullary ependymoma

Thus, acute poliomyelitis, which was a worldwide scourge before the 1950s (prior to the development of the Salk vaccine), is now very rarely encountered in the industrialized countries. Instead, the residual of that disease, post-polio atrophy, is its malevolent legacy (8, 9). In contrast, the incidence of certain age-related disorders, such as amyotrophic lateral sclerosis (ALS) and degenerative spinal disorders is increasing because of the greater longevity of the population. Meanwhile, traumatic myelopathies continue to contribute to the overall number of SCDs occurring yearly, as they have for centuries, fluctuating somewhat between periods of peace and war.

Because such a great number of causes exist for SCDs, no attempt will be made in this chapter to discuss the EDX findings with every entity. Rather, the typical EDX changes with SCDs in general will be described, and then the specific EDX findings with a few of these will be reviewed, at times with appropriate case reports.

THE ELECTRODIAGNOSTIC EXAMINATION

In most EDX laboratories, the basic EDX examination consists of three parts: nerve conduction studies (NCS)—motor, sensory, and mixed; needle electrode examination (NEE); and special studies—a variety of additional procedures, most of which are variations on NCS, such as F-wave and H-reflex testing (5, 6). Several other more specialized techniques are available, including motor-evoked potentials (10–12). These may be performed in EDX laboratories along with the basic studies, in EDX laboratories dedicated to them, and in some cases in electroencephalography (EEG) laboratories. None of these specialized techniques will be discussed in this chapter. Instead, the focus will be solely on the basic EDX examination, whose three components will now be reviewed.

Nerve Conduction Studies

During motor NCS, a mixed nerve or a "pure" motor nerve is stimulated at one or two points (the latter, if possible) along its course while the resulting response generated by a muscle it innervates is recorded, preferably with surface electrodes. This response, called a *compound muscle action potential* (CMAP), is a function not only of the motor nerve fibers stimulated, but also of the muscle fibers that produced it, and of the intervening neuromuscular junctions situated between the terminal motor nerve fibers and the muscle fibers. Thus, the motor NCS assesses motor nerve fibers only indirectly. This arrangement has one principal benefit and one major liability. The paramount benefit is that for every motor axon capable of conducting impulses, hundreds of muscle fibers are depolarized (the exact number depending on the innervation ratio of the particular muscle) on the stimulation of a single motor axon. In regard to the intrinsic hand muscles that serve as recording points, the innervation ratio generally is considered to be approximately 1/200 to 1/250. Thus, activation of a single ulnar motor axon that innervates muscle fibers in the hypothenar muscle causes near-simultaneous activation of 200 to 250 of those muscle fibers. This results in a striking "magnification" of the nerve action potentials. Consequently, CMAPs are large enough to be measured in millivolts (mV). The major liability is that a low amplitude or unelicitable CMAP is not necessarily evidence of a disorder of the motor component of the peripheral nervous system (PNS). Instead, the cause could reside in the neuromuscular junctions or the muscle fibers themselves (5, 6).

In contrast to the motor NCS, sensory NCS directly assess the sensory component of mixed nerves, or "pure" sensory (i.e., cutaneous) nerves. As a result, a low-amplitude or unelicitable sensory nerve action potential (SNAP) is indicative of an abnormality of the peripheral sensory fibers being assessed, or of the DRGs from which they derive, if various technical and physiologic factors can be excluded. The latter, unfortunately, often have significant adverse consequences on the sensory NCS, the main reason being that the SNAPs, lacking the magnification effect of the CMAPs, are tiny in comparison, being measured in microvolts (μV). As a result, physical factors (e.g., limb edema); physiologic factors (e.g., advanced patient age, in-phase cancellation of responses); and anatomic factors (e.g., the cutaneous nerves being quite superficial and thus vulnerable to minor trauma) can compromise recording SNAPs in otherwise normal persons. Whereas motor NCS assesses the peripheral neuromuscular system from the AHCs located in the spinal cord to the muscle fibers of the recorded muscle, the sensory NCS assesses sensory axons from their cell bodies in the DRGs to the most distal recording or stimulating electrode (specifically, the active recording electrode and the cathode), whichever is situated most distally along the nerve fibers. Thus, sensory NCS, unlike motor NCS, do not assess the most distal portions of the axons being studied (5, 6).

During mixed NCS, both the motor and sensory axons of a mixed nerve are assessed simultaneously by stimulating a nerve trunk distally (e.g., median nerve at wrist) while recording a nerve action potential from it more proximally (e.g., median nerve at elbow). In most instances, mixed NCS provide little information not already obtained from the motor and sensory NCS. The notable exceptions are those used to assess the palmar and plantar nerves (6). Because they play almost no role in the EDX evaluation of patients with suspected SCDs, mixed NCS are not mentioned further.

Every time an NCS is performed, the response that results contains several measurable components, each one of which provides information regarding the anatomic and physiologic status of the nerve fibers being assessed. For motor NCS, which usually involve stimulation of the nerve at two points along its course, these components are amplitude, duration, latency, and conduction velocity (CV). For each of these, measurements can be determined and reported separately for the proximal and the distal response; that is, the responses elicited on proximal and distal stimulations. Generally, the durations, although noted, are not formally reported, and the proximal latency is not reported directly, as is the distal latency. Instead, it is used to calculate a CV (see below). Thus, characteristically, the distal amplitude, distal latency, and the CV are reported for each motor NCS. During sensory NCS, typically the nerve is stimulated at only one point along its course, so that the measurable components include the amplitude, duration, and distal or peak latency. Only the amplitude and latency are reported (Figure 6.2). These components will now be discussed individually.

Amplitude

This is the height of the response, measured from baseline to peak, for CMAPs and for most SNAPs, and from negative to positive peak for the remaining SNAPs. Its primary importance is as an indicator of the number of axons capable of being stimulated and of conducting impulses between the stimulating and recording points. It is also (along with duration) a reflection of the relative rate of conduction along those axons. Moreover, it is also a function of a number of physical factors (e.g., the type and size of recording electrodes used, and the amount of intervening tissues between the nerve or muscle fibers generating the response and the surface recording electrode). Finally, in regard to motor NCS, it also conveys information regarding the status of neuromuscular transmission and of the muscle fibers of the recorded muscle. As already noted, the amplitude of the CMAP is reported in mV, whereas that of the SNAP is reported in μV (6).

Duration

This is the time period between the onset and termination of the response, measured in milliseconds (ms). It is an indicator primarily of the relative rates of conduction along those fibers transmitting impulses between the stimulation and recording points. Duration is obviously related to the amplitude: as the duration increases, the amplitude must decrease if the area under the curve is to remain constant. As the distance between the stimulating and recording electrodes increases, slight differences in the rate of conduction along each individual axon become accentuated. Consequently, the responses on proximal stimulation are somewhat increased in duration and lower in

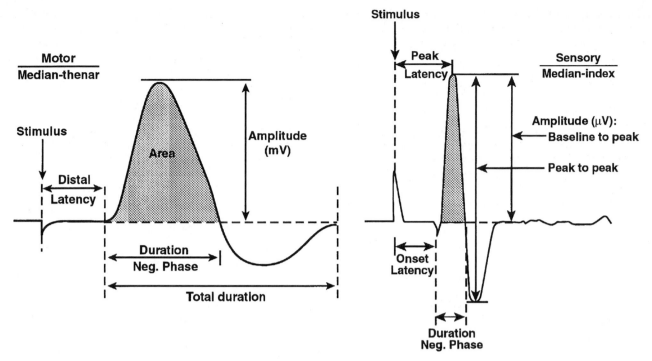

Figure 6.2   The various components of motor and sensory nerve conduction responses. (From Isley MR, Drass GL, Levin KH, Litt B, Shields RW, Wilbourn AJ. *Electromyography/Electroencephalography*. Redford, WA: Spacelabs Medical, 1993, with permission.)

amplitude when compared to those on distal stimulation. This phenomenon, termed *temporal dispersion,* has relatively little effect in motor fibers. Generally, the amplitude on proximal stimulation usually decreases less than 15% or so, compared to that obtained on distal stimulation. In contrast, whenever sensory fibers are stimulated at two points along their course, very often a substantial decrease in amplitude occurs, because of in-phase cancellation. This is because the duration of the SNAP is so much shorter than the CMAP's. Thus, stimulation of the sensory axons in the normal median nerve at the elbow and wrist while recording from the digital nerves of the index or ring finger can result in an amplitude drop of more than 50%. This is the principal reason why conduction blocks (discussed below) are difficult to detect using sensory NCS, compared to motor NCS (13).

Distal or Peak Latency

This is a rate measurement, determined from the moment of stimulation to either the onset of the response (distal latency) or to the peak of the response (peak latency). For motor NCS, distal latencies are always employed. For sensory NCS, some electrodiagnosticians use distal latencies, whereas others prefer peak latencies. Of particular note is that the distal latency provides almost no information regarding the number of axons that are conducting impulses, beyond the fact that at least a few must be doing so, or it could not be determined (6).

Conduction Velocity

Conduction velocity is also a rate measurement. Most often it is obtained by stimulating the nerve at two points along its course,

subtracting the latency elicited on distal stimulation (i.e., distal latency) from that obtained on proximal stimulation (i.e., proximal latency), and then dividing the difference (in ms) into the distance (in mm) between the two stimulation points, as determined with surface recording electrodes. The result is a CV measured in meters per second (m/s). Determining the rate of impulse transmission in this manner allows direct comparison to be made between assessments performed on identical nerves of different limbs, even in patients with different limb lengths; for example, the forearm for median and ulnar motor CVs, and the leg for the routine peroneal and tibial motor CVs. Although the proximal latency can serve the same purpose in a specific limb, comparisons would not be possible unless all limb segments were of the same length, or unless complicated normograms were constructed for different limb lengths. The use of CVs eliminates these problems (6).

Needle Electrode Examination

The second major component of the EDX examination, the NEE, is sometimes also called *needle* EMG. Similar to the motor NCS, it essentially assesses the entire motor unit from the AHCs to the muscle fibers peripherally. However, it does so in a different fashion. Consequently, the motor NCS and the NEE complement rather than duplicate each other (6).

The NEE customarily is described as having three phases: insertion, rest, and MUAP activation. (*abbreviation already cited)

Insertion Phase

The term "insertion" applies not only to the single instance in which the needle recording electrode is thrust through the skin into a particular muscle, but also to each of the several times it is advanced within that muscle while the latter is being assessed. Whenever a needle recording electrode is advanced in any normally innervated, healthy muscle, a brief burst of electrical activity is generated, which persists for approximately one-third of a second. This is labeled *normal insertional activity*. During the insertion phase, the electrical activity generated by needle advancement is assessed in regard to its presence or absence, and if present, whether it is accompanied or followed by abnormal discharges. Under various circumstances, different types of electrical activity triggered by the needle movement follow the normal insertional activity; these vary in their persistence and significance. *Snap, crackle, and pop* is one type of abnormal insertional activity. It most commonly is seen in young, mesomorphic males, and is considered a normal variant. *Insertional positive sharp waves* are another abnormal type. These unsustained potentials can be seen as a normal variant, but are also present when very recently denervated muscles are sampled at a time before spontaneous fibrillation potentials (see below) have had sufficient time to appear. Needle insertions also can initiate runs of *myotonic discharges,* a type of insertional and spontaneous activity most often seen with certain myopathies. (6, 13).

At-Rest Phase

During this segment of the NEE, the needle is held fixed in a muscle that is not being contracted (i.e., one in which muscle fibers are not firing). During this stage, various types of abnormal potentials can be observed, which collectively are known as *spontaneous activity*. The most important of these by far, and the most commonly seen, are *fibrillation potentials*. These are quite nonspecific in nature, in that they can occur with both lower motor neuron (LMN) and myopathic disorders, as well as with some abnormalities in neuromuscular transmission. (As will be noted subsequently, they also have been reported with upper motor neuron [UMN] lesions.) In regard to LMN disorders, these regularly firing potentials are generated by otherwise healthy single muscle fibers that lost their nerve supply at least 2 to 3 weeks previously. Initially, the denervated muscle fibers individually begin to produce fibrillation potentials only in an unsustained fashion, and after being injured by the needle recording electrode. These potentials (already described), are referred to as insertional positive sharp waves. Within several days, however, the denervated muscle fibers start to produce such potentials spontaneously, and in a sustained manner. Depending on whether the tip of the needle recording electrode has actually injured the muscle fibers that are responsible for these potentials, or is simply near them, this spontaneous activity has either a positive sharp wave or a biphasic spike appearance; both types are referred to as fibrillation potentials (5, 6, 13).

Fasciculation potentials are another type of spontaneous activity. In contrast to fibrillation potentials, which are produced by single denervated muscle fibers, fasciculation potentials are generated by motor units or portions of motor units. Thus, they are considerably larger than the typical fibrillation potential. Moreover, because the motor unit generating them must be intact to do so, they are evidence of motor unit irritation, rather than motor unit disintegration, as are fibrillation potentials. Finally, from the viewpoint of recognition, fasciculation potentials typically fire irregularly, whereas fibrillation potentials

characteristically fire with metronomic regularity. Although fasciculation potentials theoretically can be seen with any PNS disorder, in fact they are relatively uncommon and most often limited to those that are causing focal demyelination and are chronic in nature (e.g., ulnar neuropathy at the elbow, radiation plexopathy, multifocal motor neuropathy). In regard to intraspinal canal disorders, fasciculation potentials may occur with almost any one of them, including intramedullary neoplasms and radiculopathies, although they rarely have any diagnostic significance in these instances. The sole exception is one of the AHC disorders, ALS, in which their presence is nearly mandatory for diagnosis. The most common situation in which fasciculation potentials appear, however, is the *benign fasciculation syndrome.* As its name implies, this disorder (if it can be designated as such) consists solely of an otherwise healthy person's experiencing widespread, persistent fasciculations, and often cramps as well. (Because both fasciculations and cramps are caused by muscle membrane irritability, they are often seen together) (5, 9, 13).

Complex repetitive discharges are another type of spontaneous activity. They are caused by the repetitive firing of a group of muscle fibers, two of which serve as primary and secondary pacemakers, respectively. They are nonspecific in nature, in that they can be seen with both neurogenic and myopathic disorders. Nonetheless, their presence is not needed for diagnosis in any instance. However, they do demonstrate that the abnormal process is chronic because they rarely are seen with any disorder of less than 6 months duration (6).

Cramp potentials consist of involuntary sustained firing of MUAPs at high rates (200 to 300Hz). (As is mentioned below, normally MUAPs fire no faster than 30 to 40Hz.) Cramp potentials often are seen in patients who manifest fasciculations because, as noted, both are signs of abnormal motor unit irritability (i.e., a lowered threshold for activation) (6).

Although many other types of spontaneous activity can be observed during this phase of the NEE, they are of little importance in regard to SCDs and, therefore, are not discussed.

Motor Unit Action Potential Activation Phase

During this portion of the NEE, the patient voluntarily contracts the muscle in which the needle recording electrode has been inserted, and the MUAPs that are generated are assessed in regard to their firing frequency, stability on repeated firing, external configuration (e.g., amplitude, duration), and internal configuration (e.g., serrations, polyphasicity). Two MUAP firing patterns are of importance with spinal cord disorders.

With *reduced MUAP recruitment*, a significant number of motor units in the muscle being assessed by NEE do not fire on attempted AHC activation, either because the AHC or motor axon of the motor unit has degenerated, or the AHC is unable to initiate an impulse, or conduction is blocked along the axon. As a result, the MUAPs that can fire are observed to do so not only in decreased numbers, but also faster than their basal firing rate of approximately 10 Hz. There is nothing abnormal about MUAPs firing faster than 10 Hz; in fact, it is a normal component of the MUAP recruitment process. Thus, whenever progressively stronger muscle contractions are made, progressively more MUAP activation occurs, first by spatial recruitment, and then via temporal recruitment. During the latter, to increase the force of contraction, motor units that were firing at 5 Hz and 10 Hz shift their firing frequency to 30 Hz or greater. By this process, the same number of motor units can produce three times or more the amount of force generated by spatial recruitment alone. However, if there is a normal complement of motor units firing, then the fact that they begin to fire at faster rates on maximal activation goes undetected, because too many of them are firing simultaneously for the characteristics of individual ones to be discerned. Only if a substantial number of MUAPs are not being activated when they should—that is, they have "dropped-out"—can the firing rates of individual ones be recognized. Reduced MUAP recruitment is unequivocal evidence of an LMN lesion, and its severity has a high correlation with the clinical weakness of the recorded muscle. Thus, if the MUAPs are firing in substantially decreased numbers at 25 to 35 Hz, the muscle being assessed will appear weak on clinical examination; if only one or two MUAPs fire on maximal activation at faster than 10 Hz, the muscle will essentially be paralyzed. Although by far the most common cause for reduced MUAP recruitment seen in the EDX laboratory is axon loss (from the destruction of either the AHC or its axon), exactly the same MUAP firing abnormality is produced when demyelinating conduction block affects the axon.

Incomplete MUAP activation is seen whenever the patient is requested to vigorously contract the muscle and the MUAPs fire in reduced numbers, but at a slow-to-moderate rate (i.e., less than 10 Hz). Unlike reduced MUAP recruitment, incomplete MUAP activation is not a sign of an LMN lesion. Its cause varies: pain on muscle contraction, conversion reaction and malingering, and, in the context of this chapter, UMN lesions.

Another aspect of MUAP firing, besides recruitment or activation, is the constancy of the appearance of the MUAPs on consecutive firings. Under normal circumstances, this changes little from one firing to the next, thereby producing MUAP firing stability. However, in the presence of early reinnervation and of primary neuromuscular transmission disorders, a variable number of the endplates cannot conduct consecutive impulses, thus resulting in MUAP firing instability (6, 13).

The internal and external configurations of the MUAPs are altered by a great number of neurogenic and myopathic processes. With the former, if entire motor units had been lost and first a few and then progressively more of the denervated muscle fibers are reinnervated, then the MUAPs that initially fire are very low in amplitude, quite prolonged in duration, and highly polyphasic in internal configuration. As time passes, however, these *early reinnervational MUAPs* undergo remodeling, so that ultimately they may resume a normal appearance, or if much of the reinnervation was through the process of collateral sprouting, they may be permanently abnormal in appearance, have increased duration, and sometimes increased amplitude as well. Such *chronic neurogenic MUAP* changes generally indicate that the responsible nerve damage is of at least several months' duration. A great number of denervating processes (e.g., axon loss polyneuropathies and focal nerve trunk injuries) produce chronic neurogenic MUAP changes in which the MUAPs, although of increased duration, are of normal amplitude. However, in rather severe axon loss lesions that have affected the proximal portions of the motor system (i.e., the AHCs, roots, or very proximal portions of the plexuses), particularly those that are static and quite remote or very chronic in nature, the MUAPs frequently are not only of substantially increased duration, but

also of increased amplitude as well. Such prominent chronic neurogenic MUAP changes typically require years to develop (6).

In regard to the alterations of the internal configuration of MUAPs, these consist of their being either serrated or polyphasic. Serrated MUAPs are those that contain so-called "turns" (i.e., abrupt changes in direction or notches in the various peaks of the MUAP that do not cross the baseline). Conversely, when MUAPs are polyphasic, they contain more than four phases (changes in direction of the signal that cross the baseline). Many electrodiagnosticians consider serrated MUAPs to be simply the initial or early stages of a polyphasic MUAP. There are a number of situations in which polyphasic MUAPs customarily are found. These include disorders of the PNS, the neuromuscular junctions, and the muscle fibers themselves. Moreover, a certain proportion of the MUAPs (approximately 10%) in any muscle normally may be polyphasic. Thus, polyphasic MUAPs are nonspecific in nature and not necessarily abnormal. In regard to neurogenic lesions, they are an impressive component of early reinnervational MUAPs, and they almost always are a component of chronic neurogenic MUAPs (i.e., with chronic neurogenic MUAP changes, the MUAPs not only are of increased duration and sometimes amplitude, but are also polyphasic as well). The key point in these circumstances is that the MUAPs are of increased duration, not that they are polyphasic. Thus, the often-used term to describe these chronic neurogenic MUAP changes, *polyphasic MUAPs of long duration,* emphasizes the less important constituent of the MUAP alteration. Whether PNS lesions can solely cause polyphasia without alterations in the external configuration of the MUAP has been much debated by electrodiagnosticians, and there remains no general agreement on this point. Most often, this controversy arises in regard to chronic radiculopathies—can radiculopathies be reliably diagnosed by the detection of polyphasic MUAPs of normal duration in a myotome distribution (5, 13)?

What appear to be MUAPs of increased duration and polyphasic configuration are commonly seen whenever tremor is present, caused either by a UMN disorder or by conversion reaction or malingering. The *pseudopolyphasic* MUAPs in these instances are caused by the partial superimposition of two or more MUAPs, which are firing in poorly synchronized groups.

Special Studies

Although a number of specialized EDX tests are grouped under this title, only two are of concern in this chapter, the so-called late responses: F-waves and H-reflexes. The first of these, F-waves, are caused by stimulation-induced impulses traveling antidromically along motor axons, causing the AHCs to backfire, and thereby sending impulses back down the motor axons to the recorded muscle. Thus, F-waves assess solely motor axons and their parent AHC within the spinal cord; they do not evaluate any of the sensory portion of the PNS. In contrast to H-reflexes (discussed below), F-waves are elicited by supramaximal stimulation and can be recorded after stimulation of most of the major limb nerves. However, they are more easily detected when obtained from distal limb muscles because often they are obscured by the direct M-response when more proximal muscles are used for recording purposes. Only a fraction of the nerve impulses that travel antidromically up motor fibers each time the nerve is stimulated cause recurrent activation of the AHC and therefore produce F-waves. The percentage of supramaximal nerve stimulations to an individual axon that result in F-wave generation varies from one peripheral nerve to another, and is altered by several different physiologic variables (5, 13).

The second of these, the H-reflex, is a spinal monosynaptic reflex initiated by nerve stimulation, as opposed to tendon percussion, such as deep tendon reflex (DTR) assessment. H-reflexes are elicited by submaximal stimulation of a mixed nerve. As the stimulus strength is increased, a direct response (M-wave) also appears and increases in amplitude. As this occurs, there is a corresponding decrease in the H-wave amplitude. Eventually, when near-supramaximal stimulation is delivered to the nerve, the H-wave often becomes unelicitable. In adults with spasticity and in young children, H-waves can be elicited by stimulating many peripheral nerves. However, in healthy adults, usually the stimulation of only one upper and one lower limb nerve—the median at the elbow and particularly the posterior tibial at the popliteal fossa—results in H-waves being recorded from the pronator teres-flexor carpi radialis muscles and the gastrocnemius-soleus muscles, respectively. In most EDX laboratories, H-reflexes usually are elicited only in the lower limb. Thus, only the S1 root and the S1 segment of the spinal cord are assessed. H-reflexes are very sensitive (in that they are often abnormal) in two PNS disorders: S1 radiculopathies and generalized polyneuropathies. Often overlooked is the fact that whenever an H-reflex is being elicited by recording from the gastrocnemius-soleus muscles, a direct M-response (i.e., a tibial CMAP) can be recorded from those same muscles as well. The amplitude of this CMAP, recorded on supramaximal stimulation, can be very helpful in determining the amount of axon loss sustained by these muscles. The CMAP amplitude recorded from the anterior and lateral compartment muscles of the leg on supramaximal stimulation of the common peroneal nerve at the fibular head is also very useful (5, 6, 13). H-reflexes may also be abnormal in CNS disorders that involve the central pathways of the reflex at the S1 segment in the distal aspect of the spinal cord (11, 14).

PATHOPHYSIOLOGY

Virtually all the changes seen on the EDX examination are caused by alterations in physiology through the course of various pathologic processes. In regard to the PNS, although axons can be damaged by a great number of injurious processes—compression, traction, excess cold or heat, chemicals, radiation, etc.—their ability to respond to such injuries is extremely limited pathologically. Thus, the large myelinated axons, which are the only size of nerve fibers assessed by any component of the standard EDX examination, have only two reactions: *axon degeneration* (also known as axon loss), and *focal demyelination*. With the former, which is by far the most common of the two, the nerve fibers are interrupted at the lesion site and the entire distal portion of the nerve fibers undergoes Wallerian degeneration. This affects not only the axons but also the structures to which they are connected, directly or indirectly—sensory receptors, neuromuscular junctions, and muscle fibers. Thus, with axon loss, the ultimate effects are never limited to the site of injury. In contrast, with focal demyelination, the only alteration to the nerve fiber is that the myelin at the lesion site is damaged to varying degrees, which can result in several different types of abnormalities. Focal disturbances in conduction are critical for the electrodiagnostician. However, in contradistinction

to axon loss lesions, in focal demyelination the axons are not interrupted at the lesion site and the portions of nerves distal to that point are not disturbed in any manner: the axon and myelin are intact and conduction is normal in all respects distal to a focal demyelinating injury (6).

Although only two fundamental types of nerve pathology result from focal nerve damage, the pathophysiologic responses they cause, as detected on EDX studies, are more numerous. Two different pathophysiologic reactions can be seen following an axon loss lesion, whereas three may result from a focal demyelinating one. Moreover, various combinations are common. These five processes will now be reviewed, beginning with the two caused by axon loss.

Axon Loss

If an EDX examination is performed within the first several days after a mixed nerve has sustained a focal, substantial axon loss lesion, a characteristic combination of NCS and NEE changes is seen. On NCS, if the nerve is stimulated proximal and distal to the site of injury while recording further distally, a conduction block pattern is observed. The evoked response on stimulating distal to the lesion is normal, or low in amplitude, and the response on stimulating proximal to it is even lower in amplitude or unelicitable, depending on whether the lesion is partial or complete. This type of conduction block, termed an *axon-discontinuity conduction block,* is seen because those portions of the axons comprising the distal stump, although in the early stages of degeneration, are still capable of conducting impulses. This contrasts with the segments of the axons at the injury site, which have not been capable of impulse transmission since the instant of injury. Axon-discontinuity conduction blocks are short-lived phenomena because by 10 to 11 days after injury, all the distal stump fibers have degenerated sufficiently that they are incapable of transmitting impulses. Daily assessments of conduction along such injured fibers have revealed that the amplitudes of the CMAPs on distal stimulation remain normal for 2 to 3 days after injury, then drop steeply. By 7 days after injury, if the lesion is complete, CMAPs cannot be elicited on stimulation either proximal or distal to the lesion site. The time course of changes is somewhat different for sensory NCS. The SNAP amplitudes usually do not begin to drop until approximately 5 days after injury, and then reach their nadir at 10 to 11 days. Although it may superficially appear that the motor and sensory axons distal to a lesion are degenerating at different rates, in fact the differences in their conducting properties are caused by two other factors. These are a) dissimilarities in their recording methods and b) the degeneration of nerve fibers is always the most advanced along their most distal segments. With motor NCS, the impulses must traverse the most distal portion of the axons to reach the neuromuscular junctions. Hence, the CMAP amplitudes invariably are affected by the advanced degeneration along those distal portions. In contrast, during sensory NCS, the most distal portion of the sensory axons is not assessed. For these reasons, progressive changes seen with the SNAP amplitudes always lag a few days behind those of the CMAP amplitudes. On NEE, at these very early stages of axon loss, typically the only finding is that of reduced MUAP recruitment. The duration of the lesion is such that fibrillation potentials, or even insertional positive sharp waves, have not had time to develop (6, 13).

With substantial axon loss lesions, by 11 days after onset, the CMAPs and SNAPs elicited by stimulations applied at any point along the nerve—proximal, distal, or at the lesion site—are always equally affected. Thus, with incomplete axon loss injuries, the amplitudes of the CMAPs are uniformly low, whereas with complete lesions, they are uniformly unelicitable. This combination of NCS changes is designated the *conduction failure pattern*. It is by far the most common pattern of NCS change seen following focal nerve injuries, because the majority of the latter are axon loss in type, and nearly all are assessed 10 or more days after onset, at a time when the axon-discontinuity conduction block pattern has converted to the conduction failure pattern. In these lesions, reduced MUAP recruitment will be seen whenever the weak muscles are assessed with NEE. However, fibrillation potentials usually will not appear until some 2.5 to 5 weeks (average 3 weeks) after lesion onset. When the lesion is of several months' duration, depending on its severity and the relative efficiency of the reinnervating process, chronic neurogenic MUAP changes will be present. Once denervated muscle fibers are reinnervated, they cease to fibrillate. Consequently, fibrillation potentials usually are no longer present, or at least they are markedly reduced in numbers whenever static lesions of more than 1 to 1.5 years duration are assessed. By 2 years after injury, any muscles that were not reinnervated usually have degenerated, and once this occurs, they stop fibrillating. For this reason, fibrillation potentials tend to be seen in meager numbers if at all, with remote, static axon loss lesions (6).

In regard to the CMAP and SNAP amplitude changes seen with axon loss lesions, an important fact must be appreciated. For uncertain reasons, whenever focal incomplete axon loss involves mixed nerves, the SNAP amplitudes usually ultimately are more affected than the CMAP amplitudes, even though very early after injury the latter are the first to decrease in amplitude. Thus, when the focal nerve injury apparently has resulted in an approximate 30% loss of motor axons as manifested by a 30% fall in the CMAP on NCS performed 11 days or more after onset, the SNAP amplitudes will be substantially more decreased, by approximately 60%. With even more severe axon loss, whenever the CMAP amplitudes are only 40% to 50% of normal, the SNAP responses usually are unelicitable. Thus, the CMAP amplitudes customarily are more accurate indicators of the actual amount of axon loss that has been sustained, whereas the SNAP amplitudes are more reactive to axon loss. The reason for the SNAP amplitudes' being so "hypersensitive" to axon loss is unknown. Nonetheless, in very practical terms, this means that the SNAP amplitudes are the most sensitive NCS indicator of axon loss (6).

Focal Demyelination

Nerve lesions that cause focal demyelination manifest conduction abnormalities at the lesion site, consisting of either slowing or blocking. These can be detected by NCS if the nerve is stimulated proximal and distal to the point of injury. Two types of conduction slowing can be recognized: a) that in which the nerve impulses traversing all the large myelinated nerve fibers are slowed to the same degree, a process called focal or synchronized slowing; and b) that in which the fastest conducting fibers are not affected, but conduction along all the others is slowed to various degrees, resulting in desynchronized or differential slowing. With demyelinating conduction block, a process identical in its physiologic aspects to that of axon-discontinuity conduction block, nerve impulses are stopped at the lesion site and cannot progress beyond it, even though the conduction properties of the segments of nerve distal to that point are normal. In contradistinction to lesions causing axon loss, those causing focal demyelination produce very little change on NEE. With conduction slowing, the NEE of the recorded muscle is normal; it is inconsequential that all or some of the nerve impulses activating the MUAPs in the recorded muscle are slowed transiently as they traverse the lesion site. With demyelinating conduction block, no abnormalities are seen on NEE of the recorded muscle until the process is substantial. At that point, reduced MUAP recruitment is observed, identical to that resulting from axon loss, if the same number of motor axons are involved. Also, although theoretically fibrillation potentials are not seen with "pure" demyelinating conduction block injuries, because no motor axons have been killed, and therefore no muscle fibers denervated, in fact they are often observed in these circumstances. Presumably, this is because at least a minimal amount of motor axon loss customarily coexists with substantial demyelinating conduction block lesions (6).

Two facts should be appreciated regarding nerve pathophysiology, in regard to their EDX and clinical manifestations:

- Only those pathophysiologic processes that affect the amplitudes of the CMAPs and SNAPs have any relationship to clinical changes; more specifically, only those that affect the amplitudes without causing increased duration. Thus, axon-discontinuity conduction block, conduction failure, and demyelinating conduction block cause weakness or paralysis whenever they involve a substantial number or all of the motor axons, and they cause sensory deficits whenever they affect a substantial number of sensory axons. Concerning the latter, however, there is some discordance between those processes causing axon loss and those causing demyelination. Axon loss produces clinical deficits involving all sensory modalities, including pain and temperature. Focal demyelination, because it affects only large myelinated fibers, produces sensory changes limited to position, vibration, and light touch.

  In contrast to the above, demyelinating conduction slowing, either focal or differential in type, is responsible for essentially no clinical changes. The one exception is that differential slowing is manifest on those portions of the formal neurologic examination that require nerve impulses to pass along the sensory nerves in compact volleys. Thus, it alters the DTRs as well as vibration and two-point discrimination testing.

- Whereas the motor NCS, the NEE, or both, may be abnormal with PNS disorders causing both negative (e.g., weakness, sensory loss) and positive (e.g., cramps, fasciculations) phenomena, sensory NCS are abnormal only with those lesions that are producing negative manifestations (i.e., causing sensory deficits); those injuries of large myelinated sensory axons causing only positive phenomenon (e.g., paresthesias) do not register abnormalities on the sensory NCS (6).

Electrodiagnostic Changes with Spinal Cord Disorders

Much of the previous discussion regarding the various types of pathophysiology and their effects on different aspects of the EDX examination pertains to motor and sensory axons, not to their cell bodies within the intraspinal canal. This is pertinent because the literature suggests that certain rules concerning how the various EDX components are affected by lesions at various sites along the plexuses and peripheral nerves may not apply in regard to spinal cord involvement. Consequently, the EDX manifestation seen under three different circumstances will now be described; specifically, in regard to a focal SCD, when spinal cord segments are assessed that (a) are cephalad to it, (b) are affected by it, or (c) are caudal to it. The latter includes changes that are also seen with UMN lesions caused by spinal cord abnormalities.

Superior to the Level of the Lesion

As would be expected, generally all aspects of the EDX examination are normal when spinal cord segments cephalad to a focal SCD are assessed. Thus, the amplitudes and latencies of the CMAPs and SNAPs are normal whereas the NEE reveals no spontaneous activity and the MUAPs demonstrate a normal firing pattern and are of normal configuration. Consequently, in a patient having a focal lower thoracic myelopathy, EDX examination of the upper limbs typically reveals no abnormalities. One important note is that the actual rostral extent of a focal SCD may be higher than assumed, based on neuroimaging studies (14).

At the Level of the Lesion

The somatic motor axons that traverse the various plexuses and peripheral nerves to innervate the muscles of the limbs and trunks have their cell bodies of origin—the alpha motor neurons or AHCs—located in the ventral gray matter (the so-called anterior horn) of the spinal cord. Damage to the AHCs in the spinal cord or to the motor nerve fibers within the ventral portion of the spinal cord that link them to the primary motor roots alters the CMAP amplitudes recorded from muscles that they innervate. Specifically, as more AHCs are destroyed, more denervated muscle fibers in the recorded muscle cannot contribute to the CMAP, and therefore lower the CMAP amplitude. It must be remembered, however, that nearly all muscles receive innervation from more than one spinal cord segment (4). Consequently, unless all the spinal cord segments supplying the recorded muscle are involved, and all the AHCs within them are destroyed, the CMAPs are more likely to be of low amplitude than to be unelicitable. Also, the CMAP amplitudes in these instances are affected by the duration of the lesion, particularly if the latter is incomplete. This is because a variable number of the denervated muscle fibers in the recorded muscle will be reinnervated by sprouts arising from intramuscular axons whose cell bodies in the spinal cord were not injured. Under these circumstances, although the number of motor axons supplying the recording muscle remains severely reduced, the number of innervated muscle fibers in the recorded muscle that can respond to nerve stimuli increases. As a result, the CMAP responses, which for the first few months after onset of symptoms were quite low, will slowly begin to increase in amplitude. Ultimately, they often reach the normal range. Consequently, when motor NCS are performed many months following a focal SCD, the amount of denervation sustained by the recorded muscle may be seriously underestimated. This will be obvious when NEE is performed on the recorded muscle: reduced MUAP recruitment will be evident, and the MUAPs that can be activated will show prominent chronic neurogenic changes, indicating that the innervation ratio of the recorded muscle has been substantially altered (6, 13).

The cell bodies of origin of the peripheral sensory axons, assessed by sensory NCS, are not within the spinal cord; rather, as noted, they are located in the DRGs, which are situated along the very distal portion of the primary sensory roots. A sensory NCS that assesses axons derived from a DRG that resides in the intraspinal canal region that contains an SCD may be abnormal. Theoretically at least, this depends on whether the DRG or the proximal postganglionic sensory axons contiguous to it have been damaged, along with the spinal cord itself. Thus, it is certainly plausible that neoplastic invasion or a traumatic injury resulting from a vertebral fracture with displacement could destroy not only a localized portion of the spinal cord but also the intraspinal sensory structures linked to it. Under these circumstances, the SNAPs, as well as the CMAPs that assess axons derived from the involved level(s), should be of low amplitude or unelicitable. Conversely, there appears to be little justification for assuming that those situations in which SCDs occur in isolation, as when simultaneous involvement of the DRG or the post-ganglionic sensory axons does not happen, would alter the SNAPs in any manner. The most obvious examples in which the SNAPs should remain normal are those SCDs that purportedly involve solely the AHCs and not the sensory system at all.

However, rather surprisingly, there have been several reports describing reduction in the SNAP amplitudes occurring with at least one AHC disorder: ALS (11, 15, 16). Usually, however, demonstrating these SNAP abnormalities has required the use of specialized techniques such as near-nerve recording electrodes. Moreover, the findings typically have been labeled "subtle." Generally, this means that even though the SNAP amplitudes (and latencies) in patients with ALS may be altered statistically when compared to those obtained from a normal patient population, in the individual case they would be within normal limits. Nonetheless, to add to the debate, at least one report has described SNAP amplitudes as being abnormally increased in amplitude with certain myelopathies such as cervical spondylosis, cervical syrinxes, and arteriovenous malformations (17).

Despite the conflicting reports, in our experience the SNAP amplitudes characteristically are within the range of normal (i.e., neither too high nor abnormally low) in patients with AHC disorders and most other SCDs when sensory axons derived from the affected levels are assessed. There are two exceptions, however. First, coexisting or age-related problems often are present. Thus, many patients have abnormally low amplitude median sensory SNAPs because of superimposed carpal tunnel syndrome (CTS), whereas many patients over the age of 60 years have unelicitable lower extremity SNAPs (sural, superficial peroneal sensory) because of age factors. Second, one type of SCD, Kennedy's disease, although often considered to be principally an AHC disease, characteristically manifests abnormalities on the sensory NCS (e.g., low amplitude or unelicitable responses), as well as the NEE, and often the motor NCS as well (6, 9).

The late responses are affected, as in all other components of the EDX examination, when the involved spinal cord segments are assessed. F-waves, which are generated by AHCs, may not be elicitable. This typically is seen when the CMAPs recorded from the same muscles are low in amplitude because of severe denervation. With lesser involvement of the AHCs resulting in partial denervation of the recorded muscles, F-waves typically are more difficult to elicit and sometimes are prolonged in latency. The latter presumably is caused by loss of the largest motor neurons whose axons are the fastest conducting. The H-reflex not only assesses sensory axons, including their preganglionic components, but also certain portions of the spinal cord as well. Consequently, it characteristically is unelicitable when the S1 spinal cord segment is involved, even in those instances in which the direct M-response recorded from the gastrocnemius-soleus muscle is only modestly low in amplitude. Presumably, the H abnormalities in these instances are caused by involvement of the intramedullary pathways, specifically the sensory component (11, 14).

Inferior to the Level of the Lesion

It seems logical to contend, at least in regard to the NCS and NEE, that the EDX findings on assessing the portion of the spinal cord distal to a lesion should be predictable. Thus, the motor NCS should be normal, unless a superimposed lesion of plexuses or peripheral nerves coexists. Also, it is conceivable that, because of marked disuse atrophy of the recorded muscle, a CMAP amplitude could be low. In our experience, however, this situation is restricted to small muscles. We have never seen large muscles, such as the deltoid, quadriceps, or tibialis anterior generate low amplitude CMAPs for this reason, regardless of the degree of atrophy present. The sensory NCS, of course, should be normal as well, unless there is some superimposed PNS lesion. Finally, on NEE, the only abnormality present should be one of MUAP activation; either no MUAPs at all should be observed on voluntary effort, or a substantially decreased number, firing at a slow rate (i.e., showing incomplete MUAP activation.) Any MUAPs seen should be normal in appearance. A pertinent point is that fibrillation potentials should not be observed because the muscles being sampled are paretic or paralyzed because of a UMN rather than an LMN disorder.

Despite the seeming reasonableness of all these pronouncements, as Dumitru has observed regarding this topic, "This apparent logical conclusion, however, is not the case" (13). In fact, nearly all of the above statements have been challenged by various investigators. In regard to the motor NCS, several authors have reported finding CMAPs that are low in amplitude and often slow in CV when assessing nerves whose AHCs of origin were situated caudal to a focal SCD. Similarly, under the same circumstances, the SNAP responses have been reported to be prolonged in latency, and both low in amplitude and abnormally high in amplitude. Certainly the most intriguing finding has concerned one aspect of the NEE—specifically, the presence of fibrillation potentials in muscles affected by UMN lesions. In 1967, Goldkamp reported finding fibrillation potentials in paretic or paralyzed muscles in a large number of patients who had suffered cerebral strokes. Of the 116 patients evaluated, he detected fibrillation potentials in 66 (56.8%) in one or both hemiparetic limbs. He detected them in both limbs in 32% of patients, and in the upper limbs alone in 28% (18). Since that early report, many others (more than two dozen) have appeared, describing essentially the same findings, not only in limb muscles paretic

because of cerebral disorders, but also in those affected by focal SCDs situated cephalad to the spinal cord segments being assessed by the NEE. Some investigators have reported finding fibrillations in virtually all muscles sampled in these instances (19–25). Most, however, have found them in the majority—a sizable majority—of muscles sampled, ranging from 50% to more than 90% (26–34). Noteworthy is that the number of muscles assessed in each limb by the various investigators varied considerably, ranging from just one to many. Probably the most common scenario was for four muscles to be sampled in the affected limb, with each muscle receiving its innervation from a different segment (root) level. Several investigators also noted that in hemiplegic limbs fibrillation potentials were found more often or in greater density in upper limb muscles than in lower limb muscles, and that in a given limb, they were often of higher density in the more distal, compared to the more proximal muscles (20, 22, 35). Most reports did not concern NEE of the paraspinal muscles, and among the relatively few that did, the results reported were mixed. Thus, Nyboer detected fibrillation potentials in them as well as in the limb muscles, whereas Krueger et al. did not (30, 32).

Not all investigators agree that fibrillation potentials are present in muscles affected by UMN lesions. Thus, Alpert and co-workers, in two separate studies dealing with a total of 65 patients, reported that fibrillation potentials seldom occur under these circumstances, and when they do, they are not the result of UMN disorders (36, 37). Others share this view (38, 39). Moreover, even among the investigators who generally agree that fibrillation potentials are seen, there are significant differences on many specific points. Most of these relate to the cause for their presence, and to the timing of the NEE examination in regard to the duration of the disability. Thus, are these fibrillation potentials essentially found only relatively early after onset, during the period of spinal shock? Or are they found with equal incidence later, during the spasticity stage? When are they first likely to appear, when do they reach their maximum density, and when have they usually resolved? Concerning those found in the lower limbs with cervical spinal cord injuries, are they as prominent (i.e., have the same density) as those seen in muscles innervated by the spinal cord segments at the level of the lesion? Does their presence or density have any relationship to the results of NCS, particularly motor NCS, performed on the same limb? Moreover, the consensus regarding the presence of these fibrillation potentials does not at all extend to the cause for their presence. Instead, a number of different mechanisms have been proposed, including traction on the root and plexus fibers; traction or compression of various peripheral nerves; dysfunction of AHCs due to spinal shock; absence of a specific antifibrillation factor (AFF); transsynaptic degeneration of the alpha motor neuron; and AHC dysfunction because of transsynaptic influences, which cause alterations in axoplasmic flow, producing a "dying back" phenomenon in the peripheral nerves (7, 18, 19, 22–32, 38, 40, 41). Some version of the last two explanations appears to be the most popular.

The controversy regarding the presence of fibrillation potentials in muscles of hemiparetic, paraplegic, and quadriplegic limbs can be summarized as follows:

1. A few investigators contend that they are not seen under these circumstances, or their incidence is so low as to be insignificant.

2. A few investigators believe that they are observed, but are caused by superimposed LMN problems involving the plexuses or peripheral nerves (39).
3. The majority believe that they are seen, and in some manner the UMN lesion is responsible for their presence.

A resolution of this controversy is unlikely to occur in the foreseeable future, because the topic appears to be of little interest to any current investigators. Most of the articles on this subject were published in the 1960s, and particularly the 1970s. To the authors' knowledge, none have appeared over the past decade. An important point regarding this topic is that many electrodiagnosticians rarely, if ever, perform NEE on these types of patients because generally they are unnecessary for diagnostic purposes. Most who do so, as would be expected, specialize in rehabilitation medicine; that is, they are physiatrists and not neurologists. This is undoubtedly the reason why most of the articles on the topic can be found in the physical medicine literature. At an international EMG meeting held in the 1970s, one of the authors (Asa J. Wilbourn) attended a session at which two very eminent electrodiagnosticians were present: Edward Lambert and Fritz Buchthal. Although the author cannot recall the specific details of the subject under discussion, he vividly remembers both of them being directly asked if they had ever seen fibrillation potentials under these circumstances, and both replied, "No." Unfortunately, the obvious follow-up question was omitted: "How often do you perform NEEs on hemiparetic, paraplegic, or quadriplegic limbs?" If their experience is similar to that of most neurologists, the predicted answers to that would have been "Very infrequently." The author has encountered what may be examples of this phenomena in very few patients, but this is to be expected, considering that he rarely performs EDX examinations on limbs that could manifest these findings. However, one such patient merits describing:

CASE REPORT A young woman sustained multiple injuries, principally to the head and the right lower limb, when she was struck by an automobile while attempting to aid a stranded motorist on a snowy evening. She had a left hemiplegia and right lower limb paralysis, with the latter attributed not only to a femur fracture but also to a probable coexisting sciatic nerve lesion. On EDX examination performed 4.5 weeks after injury, there was evidence of a severe axon loss sciatic neuropathy on the right, located at or proximal to the mid-thigh (i.e., proximal to the motor branches supplying the hamstring muscles). However, an inexplicable aspect of the study was that when muscles in the hemiparetic left lower limb were assessed, solely for comparison purposes, they also showed fibrillation potentials. Ultimately, after an extensive EDX examination, it was evident that most of the muscles in both the left upper and lower hemiparetic limbs contained fibrillation potentials in the distribution of all segments, with a distal-proximal gradient. In contrast, no NEE abnormalities were present in the muscles of the normal right upper limb. Moreover, extensive motor and sensory NCS performed on the left lower limb were normal, in sharp contrast to those done on the right.

In regard to NCS changes in limbs affected by UMN disorders, the reported findings have been rather diverse. Concerning motor CVs, several authors have reported either normal results, or only slight slowing in a few of the subjects assessed (18, 20, 30, 42–44), and sometimes involving only the lower limb motor NCS. Conversely, a few investigators have described differences in side-to-side assessments of patients, with those performed on the hemiparetic limbs being slower. Nonetheless, in these reports the slowing has typically been so slight, averaging just a few m/s, or has involved other than the maximal CV, that it is of significance only when groups of patients rather than individuals are considered (39, 45–48). Proposed causes for this slowing have included reduced limb temperature and decreased diameter of nerve fibers (39, 48). A more significant point regarding motor NCS changes has been the fact that the CMAP amplitudes often decrease. Most of the reports have been concerned with the lower limb CMAPs, recording intrinsic foot muscles; that is, the tibial, and particularly the peroneal CMAPs have either been low in amplitude or unelicitable (24, 32, 33, 38, 41 49, 50). Brown and Snow, however, performed motor NCS while recording from distal, mid, and proximal muscles in both the upper and lower limbs, and demonstrated that all the motor NCS responses decreased somewhat in amplitude; these occurred earlier than the third to fourth weeks after onset and persisted through the seventh week (20). Spaans and coworkers observed that, in two patients, the peroneal CMAPs were unelicitable over several assessments, being first detected 7 to 9 months after onset (24). In contrast, Taylor and coworkers noted that the peroneal CMAP amplitudes gradually decreased over time, becoming unavailable 40 to 60 days after onset (42).

Concerning the sensory NCS, the results are equally varied. Some investigators have found the SNAPs (usually sural) to be normal (24, 27, 44, 50). Others reported them as being low in amplitude or unelicitable (29, 31, 46, 47, 51). Even when abnormalities were seen, they were noted to be quite variable from patient to patient and from one side to another in those with paraplegia and quadriplegia (51). They have also been linked to the tone of the limb—flaccid versus spastic—with the SNAP abnormalities being far more prominent in the former (32).

In regard to the late responses, far less has been published in the EDX literature about them and there is somewhat more agreement regarding the findings in limbs affected with UMN disorders. Concerning F-waves, initially (within the first 4 weeks of onset) they show decreased responsiveness: a decrease in the F-wave persistence, the average F-amplitude ratio, or both. Later they are more persistent, and more of them are of large amplitude. As a result, their averaged amplitudes are increased, as are their durations (52, 53). The latencies, according to Fisher, are slowed, whereas according to Liberson they may or may not be slowed (42, 54). Concerning the H-reflex, typically they are suppressed for 24 hours or so after an acute spinal cord lesion. Soon, however, they reappear, and they characteristically increase in amplitude (approximately 50%) by 3 months after injury. Because the amplitude of the M-component of the H-reflex test (i.e., the direct motor response recorded from the gastrocnemius and soleus muscles) does not change in the affected limb, this results in an increase in the H/M ratio. In contrast to the F-waves, the M and H latency are not altered in affected limbs (14, 54–57).

LIMITATIONS OF THE ELECTRODIAGNOSTIC EXAMINATION

Usually, it is customary in reviews such as this to discuss the benefits of a particular diagnostic procedure before cataloging its limitations. However, in this instance, the constraints on the EDX examination are considerable, and consequently play a major role in defining its utility; therefore, three of its major limitations will be reviewed first.

Location of Focal Spinal Cord Lesions

Unlike neuroimaging studies, the EDX examination does not assess all portions of the spinal cord with the same thoroughness. In practical terms, it provides comprehensive assessments only for two limited portions: (a) the C5 through T1 segments, and (b) the L3 through S1 segments. These, not coincidentally, are the portions of the spinal cord from which the motor and sensory nerves arise that supply the limbs. As a result, motor and sensory NCS can be performed on many of the axons arising from these segments, although "nonstandard" NCS are often required (Table 6.2), and most of the muscles innervated by these segments can be surveyed on NEE. For most of the remainder of the spinal cord—and this includes the majority overall—the EDX assessment is much less optimal. For practical purposes, the C1 through C4 spinal cord segments simply cannot be evaluated with any degree of accuracy. Similarly, the EDX assessment of the T2 through L2 segments consists solely of NEE of the paraspinal

muscles, the abdominal muscles, and the intercostal muscles. The problems with assessing each of these three groups of muscles have been reviewed in several publications concerned with radiculopathy assessment (4). In regard to the thoracic paraspinal muscles, these limitations include the fact that a) in many patients it is notoriously difficult to obtain adequate relaxation to enable a satisfactory search for fibrillation potentials to be made; b) at times, very small MUAPs are observed, which are readily mistaken for fibrillation potentials if their firing pattern (i.e., not metronomically regular) is not appreciated (4); and c) in obese patients, in whom the tips of the spinous processes cannot be palpated because of overlying tissue (and thus the exact location of the paraspinal muscles cannot be determined), the possibility exists of inducing a pneumothorax by inserting the needle electrode too far laterally from the midline. Such were the circumstances in our EDX laboratory when a pneumothorax was produced, the only known occurrence over a 28-year period, during which time more than 65,000 EDX examinations were performed. Concerning the NEE of the abdominal muscles, it is very important to advance the needle electrode only while the muscles are being actively contracted, and to stop advancing it when they are reached. Otherwise, the needle tip may enter the peritoneal cavity. In the case of SCDs, patients may not be able to voluntarily contract these muscles, so this safety factor is compromised. Even in those instances in which both the thoracic paraspinal and abdominal muscles contain fibrillation potentials because of a focal SCD, localization usually is quite inexact, both as to the level of the lesion and its longitudinal extent. This is primarily caused by the cascade effect of innervation of these muscles. Thus, often an SCD involving a single spinal cord segment causes fibrillation potentials to be found in the paraspinal muscles only several segments caudally, or spread over several segments from the level of injury (4). Concerning the abdominal muscles, generally the goal is simply to determine if fibrillation potentials involve the upper abdominal muscles or the lower; more precise localization is not attempted. In regard to the intercostal muscles, most electrodiagnosticians do not consider it worth the risk to assess them, because when doing so, the needle tip is so close to the pleural space. (Thus, most electrodiagnosticians, even those who are brave of heart, choose to follow the dictum of Campbell (58), stated in another context but quite appropriate in this instance: "Don't press your luck.")

The major effect the position of a focal SCD can have on the effectiveness of the EDX examination for localization was illustrated in a brief 1988 report concerned with the EDX assessment of primary intraspinal canal neoplasms. Of the 12 patients studied, the lesions were located in the higher cervical region (C1–C5) in four, and in only one (25%) of these was the EDX examination helpful. Conversely, in the remaining eight, the lesions were located in the lumbosacral region (at or below L5), and seven (87.5%) of these had definite EDX findings. Thus, for practical purposes, the EDX examination has little utility in patients with focal SCDs located above the C5 level or between the T2 and L2 segments (59).

Limited EDX Findings

With "pure" focal SCDs (i.e., those not also involving the DRGs), the EDX abnormalities often are quite restricted. Unless

---

Table 6.2   Standard and Nonstandard NCS

NCS	AHC	DRG
STANDARD NCS		
Median (S)—D2		(C6) C7
Ulnar (S)—D5		C8
Radial (S)—D1 base		(C6) (C7)
Median (M)—thenar	(C8), T1	
Ulnar (M)—hypothenar	C8, (T1)	
Sural (S)		S1
Peroneal (M)—EDB	L5 (S1)	
Tibial (M)—AH	S1 (S2)	
H response	S1	S1
NONSTANDARD NCS		
Median (S)—D1		C6
Median (S)—D3		C7
Lat antebrachial cutaneous (S)		C6
Med antebrachial cutaneous (S)		T1
Radial (M)—ext indicis prop	(C7) C8	
Radial (M)—brachioradialis	C6 (C7)	
Musculocutaneous (M)—biceps	(C5), C6	
Axillary (M)—deltoid	C5, (C6)	
Super peroneal sensory (S)		L5
Peroneal (M)—tibialis anterior	(L4), L5	
Tibial (M)—ADQP	S1, (S2)	
Femoral (M)—quadriceps	L2–L4	

Standard and nonstandard nerve conduction studies that are performed, and the anterior horn cells (motor) and dorsal root ganglia (sensory) they assess. (NCS = nerve conduction studies; AHC = anterior horn cells; DRG = dorsal root ganglia; S = sensory NCS; M = motor NCS; D = digit; EDB = extensor digitorum brevis; AH = abductor hallucis; ADQP = abductor digiti quinti pedis) For recorded muscles, lesser source of root innervation is in parenthesis.

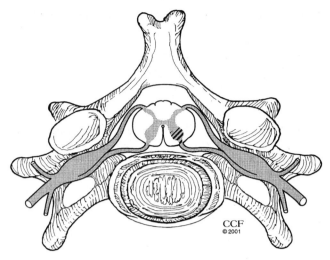

Figure 6.3 For the electrodiagnostic examination to show evidence of a lower motor neuron lesion, the small areas (shown with hatching) must be injured. A cross section of the cervical spinal cord is shown.

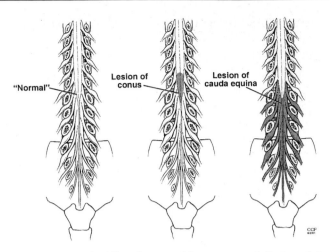

Figure 6.4 Only diffuse lesions of the conus medullaris and the cauda equina have identical electrodiagnostic manifestations: both affect intraspinal canal elements proximal to the dorsal root ganglia.

the AHCs or the fibers linking them to the primary motor roots are affected (Figure 6.3), the only detectable abnormality on the basic EDX examination may be the incomplete MUAP recruitment seen on NEE of the muscles innervated by spinal cord segments caudal to the lesion. Even when the AHCs are affected, the abnormalities may consist of nothing more than fibrillation potentials and the reduced MUAP recruitment found in muscles receiving their innervation from the damaged spinal cord segment. The motor NCS will be normal, unless one or more recorded muscles receive substantial innervation from the affected spinal cord segment. In these instances, the CMAP response may be low in amplitude, or even unelicitable (if contiguous spinal cord segments are involved, both of which supply innervation to the recorded muscle). Thus, the NCS are of rather limited utility in assessing SCDs, in contrast to their often impressive value in the assessment of the plexus and major peripheral nerve lesions. SCDs share this limitation with another, and far more common intraspinal canal lesion: radiculopathies (4).

Differentiating Spinal Cord Lesions

Electrodiagnosticians have a very limited ability to distinguish not only one SCD from another, but also one intraspinal canal lesion from another. Thus, both focal radiculopathies and focal SCDs may have identical EDX presentations. Moreover, because the incidences of root lesions and focal SCDs are so dissimilar, the EDX changes caused by a focal SCD frequently are attributed to one (or more) radiculopathies. This means that whenever clinical and EDX changes are present in L5 and S1 distributions bilaterally, typically the lesion is assumed to be affecting the cauda equina and not the conus medullaris (Figure 6.4). Nonetheless, because occasionally the EDX abnormalities in these circumstances are caused by an SCD and not a root problem, we always report such changes as being evidence of an "intraspinal canal lesion involving the (specific) segments or roots," rather than a radiculopathy (or cauda equina lesion). Ironically, at least

one of our former trainees, on entering private practice, was chided for following this advice; he was instructed by a senior colleague to simply call these "root lesions," so as not to "cause confusion."

A similar situation sometimes arises when the electrodiagnostician attempts to determine the specific etiology of an SCD, unless the latter has a characteristic presentation in regard to its distribution, its EDX manifestations, and the like. Thus, as will be noted later in more detail, it is a relatively easy task (if the EDX examination is of sufficient extent) to recognize ALS when fibrillation potentials, fasciculation potentials, and chronic neurogenic MUP changes are found in multiple segment distributions in the upper and the lower extremities, as well as in the mid-thoracic paraspinal muscles, and in at least one of the cranial nerve–innervated muscles. In contrast, it is extremely difficult to distinguish ALS from other intraspinal canal lesions in its very early stages, when it is manifested solely as fibrillation potentials and some MUAP loss in a single unilateral segment distribution. The problem is even more formidable when the referring physician requests that one SCD be identified in the presence of a preexisting one. This situation most often is encountered when middle-aged to elderly patients who had poliomyelitis in their youth develop new symptoms, particularly weakness. Almost all of them are referred with the same differential diagnosis: postpolio atrophy; developing ALS; a radiculopathy; or a generalized myopathy—disorders diagnosed in the EDX laboratory almost solely by NEE. The NCS typically are normal or, at most, one or more of the CMAPs are low in amplitude or unelicitable. Unfortunately, in the presence of markedly distorted MUAPs caused by remote poliomyelitis, none of these disorders can be diagnosed (or excluded) with any confidence. The only helpful finding would be the presence of fibrillation potentials in more than moderate numbers in the distribution of one or more segments. Because these would be unlikely to be the result of a long-standing static process, such as remote poliomyelitis, they would be consistent with a superimposed, more active process within the intraspinal canal.

ADVANTAGES OF THE ELECTRODIAGNOSTIC EXAMINATION

One of the major benefits of the EDX examination is that it can often unequivocally distinguish SCDs from other disorders with which they may be clinically confused. As noted, the EDX examination is very limited in its ability to differentiate an SCD from a radiculopathy because both are intraspinal canal lesions. Usually, however, disorders of the plexuses and peripheral nerves are readily distinguished from SCDs, for three reasons:

- The NCS, as well as the NEE, frequently are affected, particularly the SNAP amplitudes, which immediately excludes almost all SCDs (but not necessarily an intraspinal canal lesion involving the DRG as well as the spinal cord).

- In many instances, the pathophysiology is one of focal demyelination rather than axon loss, and the responsible lesion is located at some point along the peripheral neuraxis, where it can be detected during the NCS because it is causing conduction slowing or conduction block.

- The NEE of limb muscles having distal plexus and peripheral nerve lesions reveals abnormalities other than a segmental distribution. Conversely, with proximal plexus lesions (e.g., upper trunk) the distribution of the NEE abnormalities can be similar to that seen with SCDs (except for the presence of paraspinal fibrillation potentials in the rhomboids serratus anterior and paraspinal muscles), so that the value of the NEE with lesions at this proximal level is more limited.

In the authors' EDX laboratory, the EDX examination has been helpful on several occasions when SCDs were confused clinically with other disorders; a few of these will be briefly mentioned.

- Two patients with bilaterally symmetrical conus medullaris lesions were thought clinically to have a peripheral polyneuropathy as the cause of their bilateral foot numbness; the EDX examination revealed bilateral S1 intraspinal canal lesions and thereby excluded this possibility.

- A patient with a 2-month history of quadriparesis (moderately severe in the lower limbs and mild in the uppers), along with generalized hyperreflexia, bilateral sustained foot clonus, and a sensory loss for pain and vibration from the T6 level distally, was thought clinically to have multiple sclerosis. On EDX examination, however, there was evidence of widespread intraspinal canal lesions involving the C6 through T1 and the L5 through S2 segments bilaterally. A myelogram subsequently revealed multiple neoplasms within the intraspinal canal, which originated from an ependymoblastoma in the mid-thoracic region.

- An elderly patient rendered quadriplegic by an automobile accident 13 years previously, who had regained enough lower limb strength to ambulate with a walker, was referred with a 4-year history of constant burning sensation in the left lower limb; these symptoms were attributed to an ischemia-caused nerve problem—ischemic monomelic neuropathy. This disorder has characteristic EDX findings that were not seen when the EDX examination was performed on his left lower limb (and the right lower limb for control).

- Several months prior to his EDX examination, a middle-aged man was "scissored" between players while refereeing a professional football game. Since that time he had experienced paresthesias and sensory loss of the left lower limb and weakness of the right. On clinical examination, his quadriceps DTRs were brisk bilaterally, right greater than left, and the Achilles DTRs were normal bilaterally. Sensory loss was noted throughout most of his left lower limb, extending to the inferior portion of the left abdomen. Prior to his EDX examination, one of his physicians had attributed his hyperreflexia to a remote neck injury, and his sensory complaints to either a mid-lumbar radiculopathy or a femoral neuropathy, or possibly an ilioinguinal nerve entrapment. A CT scan of the lumbosacral spine was normal but did not visualize above the L3 level. On EDX examination requested to assess for a left lumbosacral radiculopathy, the only abnormality noted on bilateral lower limb evaluation was incomplete MUAP activation in the muscles of the right lower limb; the sural and superficial peroneal sensory SNAPs on the left were normal and equal to those on the right. Based on the rarely made EDX diagnosis of "suggestive Brown-Séquard syndrome," the patient underwent a myelogram, which revealed a T10 disc herniation with some spinal cord compression.

At times the EDX examination can definitely prove that new symptoms in a patient with a long-standing SCD are caused by a superimposed PNS lesion, as the following case report illustrates.

CASE REPORT. (FDI = first dorsal interosseous; D = digit) This middle-aged man had had bilateral upper limb motor and sensory changes for several years because of a cervical syrinx. Pain and temperature sensations were decreased from the C2 through C5 levels on the left, and the C3 through T1 levels on the right. A prior EDX examination had demonstrated prominent MUAP loss in the C7 through T1 distributions on the left and the C8, T1 distributions on the right. The extent of denervation in different intrinsic hand muscles was variable, as reflected by the median (recording thenar) and ulnar (recording hypothenar and FDI) CMAPs bilaterally. The right median CMAP and the left ulnar CMAP, recording hypothenar, were both less than one mV in amplitude. In contrast, the left median CMAP was only slightly low (4.8 mV), whereas the remaining ulnar motor CMAPs bilaterally (right hypothenar and bilateral FDI) were normal. The patient was being reassessed in the EDX laboratory because of the recent onset of new weakness in the distribution of his right ulnar nerve. This was accompanied by loss of light touch and position sense in the right fifth digit. (Pain and temperature sensation were abnormal throughout most of both upper limbs because of the cervical syrinx.) On EDX examination, in addition to the findings noted on the earlier assessment, the right ulnar SNAP (recording D5) was now unelicitable, and that on the left remained normal. The right ulnar motor CMAPs (hypothenar and FDI) were now considerably lower in amplitude, and substantial slowing of the ulnar motor CV at the elbow was noted along the ulnar motor fibers supplying both muscles; NEE now revealed fibrillation potentials and substantially more MUAP loss in the right ulnar nerve-innervated hand muscles. Thus, it was obvious that the new right upper limb symptoms were caused by a superimposed ulnar neuropathy at the elbow, and not due to progression of his cervical syrinx.

Coexisting Spinal Cord and Peripheral Nerve Lesions

Plexopathies and mononeuropathies are found with some frequency in patients with SCDs. These may involve nerve fibers derived from spinal cord segments situated rostral or caudal to the involved segments, or they may originate from the damaged segments themselves (49, 60–62).

In regard to PNS lesions occurring superior to an SCD, brachial plexopathies and various mononeuropathies are found in the upper limbs in chronic paraplegic patients with some frequency. One example of this is crutch palsy: an infraclavicular plexopathy caused by excessive pressure placed on terminal nerves (most often the radial) in the axilla as the result of crutches that are ill fitted or used improperly. Similarly, ulnar neuropathies in the hand can result from the misuse of crutches and walkers (63). The more common situation, however, concerns mononeuropathies that develop in chronic wheelchair users. Hand symptoms suggestive of peripheral nerve compromise are surprisingly common in patients who are active wheelchair users, ranging from 45% to 74% (49, 60). Most often, the underlying nerve lesion is CTS. These probably are the result of chronic compression of the median nerve caused by the increased carpal canal pressure that occurs during the extremes of wrist flexion and wrist extension. In one series of 77 paraplegic patients, 38 (49%) had clinical changes suggestive of CTS (61). In two other series, consisting of 31 and 47 patients, the presence of CTS was confirmed by EDX examination in 55% to 64% of patients having these symptoms (49, 60). The percentages were much more diverse, however, in regard to the number of patients who had bilateral CTS: 13% in one series; 43% in another. The percentages also varied significantly in regard to the incidence of ulnar neuropathy in the same two groups of patients: 19% in one, 40% in another. In Aljure et al.'s series of 47 patients, 19 (40%) patients had combined CTS and ulnar neuropathy, and in 12 (25%) of them both of these PNS lesions were bilateral (60). Overall, there was very close agreement between the two series regarding the number of patients with one or more upper limb mononeuropathies: 66% to 68% (49, 60). Among the 47 patients studied by Aljure et al., although only 51% had symptoms or signs suggestive of median or ulnar mononeuropathies, 63% of them had EDX evidence of mononeuropathy (61). Whether the incidence of these upper limb mononeuropathies is related to the duration of the paraplegia is controversial; at least two studies have indicated that it can be (49, 60, 61). Because these mononeuropathies can compromise the independent functioning of these patients, whose activities of daily living are so dependent on their upper limbs, their early detection is of particular importance.

Plexopathies and mononeuropathies can involve nerve fibers that derive from the level of the SCD. These have two separate causes:

- They can develop at the same time as the focal SCD does, and for the same reason, thus brachial plexus fibers can be injured simultaneously with the cervical spinal cord by trauma. Similarly, ischemia caused by compromise of the abdominal aorta can simultaneously damage both the caudal spinal cord as well as the roots and plexuses derived from it.

- They can develop at various times after the SCD is established and for various reasons. Often the EDX examination can demonstrate or confirm that separate CNS and PNS lesions coexist.

Peripheral nerves that originate from spinal cord levels caudal to a focal SCD can manifest focal abnormalities. Thus, patients with SCDs involving the cervical or thoracic segments can develop focal mononeuropathies inferior to the level of the lesion in the paretic and paralyzed limbs caused by both traction and compression. Probably the nerves most commonly involved are the ulnar nerve along the elbow segment in quadriplegia and the common peroneal nerve at the fibular head in both quadriplegia and paraplegia. As noted in an earlier section, one of the alternate theories for the presence of fibrillation potentials being found in the muscles of hemiplegic, quadriplegic, and paraplegic limbs is that they are caused by one or more of such focal mononeuropathies (31).

SOME SPECIFIC SPINAL CORD DISORDERS

In this section, the EDX findings of three different SCDs will be discussed.

Anterior Horn Cell Disease

This category contains many distinct disorders, only a few of which will be reviewed.

Poliomyelitis and Post-polio Syndrome

Caused by one of three types of neurotrophic viruses, this disease occurred worldwide, often in epidemic form, until the introduction and widespread use of the Salk injectable vaccine between 1953 and 1956. Since that period, very few cases of acute poliomyelitis have occurred in developed countries. Consequently, most practicing electrodiagnosticians have never assessed patients with acute poliomyelitis. Instead, they are much more likely to have encountered patients with the residuals of remote poliomyelitis, to which their recent onset of symptoms may or may not be related. The EDX findings in patients with acute poliomyelitis consist of the following:

- The SNAPs are invariably normal (unless some superimposed mononeuropathy is present).
- The CMAPs are normal, low in amplitude, or unelicitable, depending on the specific spinal cord segment(s) involved and the particular muscles used for recording. Typically, when the cord segments supplying the recorded muscle are affected, the CMAP amplitudes are decreased in proportion to the degree of axon loss. The motor CVs, in contrast, usually are within the normal range.
- On NEE, fibrillation potentials and reduced MUAP recruitment are noted in muscles innervated by the involved segments. The severity of changes can vary substantially from one muscle to another and unilateral as opposed to bilateral changes at a given spinal cord level are typical. Fasciculation potentials and cramp potentials may or may not be seen. An important point is that any MUAPs present are normal in configuration, because the duration of the lesion is such that collateral sprouting has not had time to occur (6, 8).

With remote poliomyelitis (disorders of at least 12 months' duration and typically of many years), the EDX findings are substantially different from those described above, primarily because of the motor unit remodeling that has occurred as the result of collateral sprouting. Typically, the EDX examination reveals that the SNAPs are normal, unless a mononeuropathy (characteristically CTS) is superimposed, or unless the patient is more than 60 years of age, in which case the lower extremity SNAPs may be unelicitable. Concerning the motor NCS, in some instances the axon loss initially was so severe that the recorded muscle was totally or near totally denervated. Unelicitable or very low amplitude CMAPs result when attempts are made to record from them. In many cases, however, the CMAPs are within the normal range in amplitude, even when the recorded muscles, based on subsequent NEE, had undergone substantial denervation at the time of the acute attack. The CMAP amplitudes are misleading in this regard because they are indicative of the total number of muscle fibers in the recorded muscle responding to the stimulus rather than the total number of nerve fibers supplying the recorded muscles. Thus, they are reflecting the substantial amount of collateral sprouting that has occurred. On NEE, fibrillation potentials and occasionally fasciculation potentials may be seen in minimal to modest numbers in scattered muscles. Frequently the fibrillation potentials are very low in amplitude because they are being generated by very atrophic muscle fibers. Typically, reduced MUAP recruitment is seen in various amounts in different muscles, and the MUAPs show very prominent chronic neurogenic changes. MUAPs of three or more times normal duration and amplitude are commonly observed. Such so-called "giant" MUAPs (a term formerly in common use but now discouraged) are seen with such regularity in remote poliomyelitis and so infrequently in all other disorders that any time they are encountered during the NEE on a patient, immediate inquiry should be made regarding whether that patient ever had poliomyelitis. (This important fact very often is not mentioned by referring physicians, either because they themselves are not aware of it, or they do not consider it pertinent for the electrodiagnostician to know.) These grossly abnormal MUAPs frequently are found not only in clinically normal as well as abnormal muscles in the symptomatic limbs but also in muscles of the reputedly unaffected limb(s). Both patients and their physicians tend to seriously underestimate the extent of spinal cord involvement with poliomyelitis, often strikingly so. Occasionally, NEE of a muscle reveals only a marked mechanical resistance on needle insertion: no electrical activity at all seen in it. These findings indicate that the muscle was totally denervated at the time of the acute attack and was never reinnervated (6, 9).

As noted earlier, the most common reason for patients with poliomyelitis to be referred to the EDX laboratory is because they had an acute bout of the disease decades earlier and now are developing new neuromuscular symptoms. These new symptoms are attributed to their remote episode of poliomyelitis, a condition called post-polio syndrome. Although poliomyelitis produces impressive EDX findings, both acutely and as permanent residuals, post-polio syndrome per se causes no distinctive EDX changes: the EDX findings in patients with remote poliomyelitis who deny new symptoms are essentially indistinguishable from those who are experiencing them. Thus, the NEE changes are, for practical purposes, identical between the two groups. Because of this, the main reason EDX examinations are performed on patients with remote poliomyelitis is not to diagnose post-polio syndrome, but rather to confirm that the patient actually had poliomyelitis, or to detect some other disorder that may be responsible for their symptoms. In regard to the former reason, many middle-aged to elderly patients who, for most of their lives, have considered themselves victims of poliomyelitis as infants or young children have completely normal EDX examinations. Such findings are totally incompatible with their ever having had a bout of acute paralytic poliomyelitis, because poliomyelitis invariably leaves lifelong, often severe, EDX residuals, such as very prominent chronic neurogenic MUAP changes on NEE, even when the clinical abnormalities are minimal. Also, as noted earlier, because severe, widespread, permanent MUAP changes are characteristic of remote poliomyelitis, it can be exceedingly difficult, if not impossible, to identify any superimposed neuromuscular disorder whenever the diagnosis of the latter depends principally on detecting MUAP changes on NEE. In the presence of remote poliomyelitis, the MUAPs very often are so distorted that any additional alterations of them cannot be discerned. Among the disorders in the category are ALS, radiculopathies, and myopathies—the very ones most often included in the differential diagnosis of patients who have a history of remote poliomyelitis and who are now developing progressive weakness (6).

Amyotrophic Lateral Sclerosis

ALS is the most common type of AHC disease assessed in most EDX laboratories. It differs from all other AHC disorders in that it characteristically manifests UMN as well as LMN changes. The EDX findings in ALS vary considerably among patients, depending on the distribution, duration, and progression of the disease process. In a few patients, the disease appears to be almost generalized from onset. Frequently, in these patients, the process is rapidly progressive. Far more often, ALS begins in one or two spinal cord segments and then gradually spreads to involve others. Often it begins in the AHCs in the C8 and T1 segments, thereby presenting as unilateral or bilateral painless hand wasting. The L5 spinal cord segment also is commonly initially involved. Clinically, these produce a painless foot drop.

On EDX examination, the following typically are seen with ALS:

- The SNAPs are normal for age—although there are a few reports describing sensory NCS abnormalities with ALS (14–16).
- The CMAPs are normal or abnormal (i.e., low in amplitude or unelicitable), depending on whether the appropriate spinal cord segments are involved, and if they are, the severity of axon loss. Because the standard upper limb motor NCS (i.e., median, ulnar) are recorded from hand muscles innervated by the C8 and T1 spinal cord segments, one or more low-amplitude CMAPs are found with some frequency. If ulnar motor (recording FDI) NCS are added, in a significant number of patients a "split hand" is seen: the ulnar motor CMAP (FDI) is low in amplitude or unelicitable, whereas the ulnar motor CMAP (hypothenar) is normal, or only slightly low in amplitude. Often, in these circumstances, the median motor CMAP (recording thenar) also is affected. Why the muscles on the lateral aspect of the hand are

frequently much more severely denervated than those on the medial aspect of a hand is unclear, but this finding has diagnostic significance. In our experience, with proximal lesions, it is seen only with AHC disease (6, 9).

The diagnosis of ALS in the EDX laboratory, similar to that of all other AHC disorders, rests principally on the NEE findings. Typically, an extensive NEE is required, consisting of sampling at least one muscle innervated by every segment in the upper and lower limbs, as well as the mid to lower thoracic paraspinal muscles, and, if necessary, one or two muscles innervated by the cranial nerves. The goal is to find widespread fibrillation potentials and chronic neurogenic MUAP changes with at least some fasciculation potentials. The presence and density, if they are present, of fibrillation potentials in any given muscle tends to vary directly with the degree of clinical weakness it manifests. In contrast, fasciculation potentials, which often are even more widespread than the fibrillation potentials, tend to be more abundant in less affected muscles. (This is to be expected, because fasciculation potentials are generated by intact motor units, whereas fibrillation potentials are generated by muscle fibers of degenerated motor units.)

The chronic neurogenic MUAP changes typically seen with ALS usually are far less impressive than are those frequently observed with remote poliomyelitis. Thus, although MUAPs of increased duration are common, those of increased amplitude as well are relatively rare. This is because of the duration of the lesion; most patients with ALS are studied within a year or so of onset, long before they can develop, via extensive collateral sprouting, the unusually large MUAPs seen so often with remote poliomyelitis. Reduced MUAP recruitment typically is prominent also, at least in some muscles. However, as noted, ALS has a UMN component as well as an LMN one. When the UMN influence is great, reduced MUAP recruitment may not be seen because of incomplete MUAP activation; that is, the UMN lesion controls the MUAP firing pattern (9). In this regard, it is interesting to note that the fibrillation potentials seen in muscles of limbs that are obviously spastic (have hyperactive reflexes and positive Babinski sign) in ALS patients invariably are considered evidence of LMN damage and not UMN involvement. Thus, where ALS is concerned, the concept that fibrillation potentials can be seen with UMN disorders because of transsynaptic degeneration is ignored.

The EDX examination can be very helpful for distinguishing ALS from certain other generalized disorders with which it can be confused clinically, such as polymyositis or myasthenia gravis with prominent bulbar symptomatology. Unfortunately, however, it cannot distinguish a radiculopathy from early ALS, when the latter initially presents in a monosegmental distribution. Similarly, ALS restricted to the L5 and S1 spinal cord segments bilaterally cannot be distinguished from a cauda equina lesion by EDX examination. Thus, as noted previously, the EDX presentation of ALS is somewhat nonspecific, in that it is simply that of an intraspinal canal lesion. The diagnosis rests principally on the diffuse nature of the active and chronic denervation with ALS, and the presence of fasciculation potentials in at least some muscles. A pertinent note is that ALS cannot be diagnosed by EDX examination in a patient with remote poliomyelitis because the findings, for the most part, are identical. Although fibrillation potentials may be abundant with ALS, this feature is not diagnostic in itself.

Kennedy's Disease

This sex-linked recessive AHC disorder involves the sensory and motor neurons in both the bulbar and spinal cord segments. On EDX examination, a very unusual combination of changes typically is found. This consists of NCS abnormalities suggestive of a pure sensory polyneuropathy or neuronopathy (i.e., low amplitude or unelicitable SNAPs), along with NEE abnormalities indicative of a very chronic AHC disease (i.e., prominent chronic MUAP changes, with sparse numbers of fibrillation potentials), but often with abundant fasciculation potentials, especially in the face. In contrast to the sensory NCS and NEE, the motor NCS most often are normal, although they may be of low amplitude if the recorded muscles are substantially denervated (6).

Spinal Cord Injuries

Severe focal trauma to the spinal cord is "... one of the most catastrophic injuries—socially, economically, and physically—that can occur ..." (64). These lesions affect very predominantly males (more than 82% in one series) and those in younger age groups: 80% of patients are less than 45 years old. The median age of occurrence is 25 years and the most common age is 19 years. Fracture-dislocation of the spine, most often caused by sudden, violent flexion, is responsible for the majority of acute spinal cord injuries (SCI). The most common sites for these are the C5–C6, C6–C7, and the T12–L1 junctions. Whenever substantial spinal cord damage occurs without fracture-dislocation, usually it is the result of a hyperextension injury to the cervical spine in a patient with spondylosis. The most common causes for acute SCI are vehicular accidents, falls, gunshot and stab wounds, and diving accidents (64).

The EDX examination has a limited role in the initial assessment of patients with these injuries—far less of a role, for example, than that of neuroimaging studies. Nonetheless, at times EDX examinations can be quite helpful, especially by demonstrating the presence or absence of coexisting plexopathies. Moreover, later in the course, it can detect the presence of superimposed plexopathies and mononeuropathies, a task for which neuroimaging studies are of no benefit.

CASE REPORT. (D = digit; LAC = lateral antebrachial cutaneous nerve) A 20-year-old man sustained a cervical cord injury in a diving accident, which rendered him quadriplegic. The clinical findings were slightly asymmetrical from side to side, with those on the right being at a slightly higher cervical cord level. This asymmetry was confirmed on EDX examination. On NCS, all SNAPs were normal and equal bilaterally, including those that assess the C6 DRG (median, recording D1, LAC), the C7 DRG (median D2, median D3), both C6 and C7 DRG (radial, recording thumb base), and the C8 DRG (ulnar, recording D5). On motor NCS, the routine median (recording thenar) and ulnar (recording hypothenar) were normal bilaterally, as were axillary motor NCS (recording deltoid) bilaterally. The musculocutaneous (recording biceps) and radial motor (recording brachioradialis) CMAPs were asymmetrical, with those on the right being low in amplitude (4 mV vs. 12 mV, musculocutaneous; 5 mV vs. 13 mV, radial). On NEE on the right, the infraspinatus and deltoid appeared normal. Fibrillation potentials and severely reduced

MUAP recruitment were present in the biceps and brachioradialis with lesser but similar changes in the pronator teres; the flexor pollicis longus, extensor indicis proprius, first dorsal interosseous, and abductor pollicis brevis contain neither fibrillation potentials nor voluntary MUAPs. On the left, the infraspinatus, deltoid, biceps, and brachioradialis appeared normal; fibrillation potentials were present in the triceps, pronator teres, and flexor carpi radialis. In the triceps, no voluntary MUAPs could be activated, and in the remaining two muscles, markedly reduced MUAP recruitment was noted; in the flexor pollicis longus, extensor indicis proprius, abductor pollicis brevis, and first dorsal interosseous no voluntary MUAPs could be activated, but no fibrillation potentials were seen. Thus, the EDX examination confirmed the asymmetry of the cervical SCI; the lesion appeared to be at the level of the C6 cord segment on the right and the C7 segment on the left.

Intraspinal Canal Neoplasms

Neoplasms that involve the spinal cord portion of the CNS are considerably less frequent than those that involve the brain. In one series, the latter were almost seven times more common (2). Three types of intraspinal canal neoplasms are recognized:

- Intramedullary, which arise within the substance of the spinal cord, e.g., astrocytomas, ependymomas, and hemangioblastomas.
- Extramedullary-intradural, those situated outside the spinal cord in the meninges or roots, e.g., meningiomas, schwannomas, and filum terminale ependymomas.
- Extramedullary-extradural, those in the epidural tissues or the vertebral bodies. The latter include epidural tumors that are primary (multiple myeloma, osteogenic sarcoma, and chordomas), and those that are secondary (metastatic neoplasms). Prostate and breast cancer frequently metastasize to the vertebral column and epidural space.

The relative frequency of intraspinal canal neoplasms varies from one series to another but epidural tumors overall are the most frequent (2, 3).

Pain is probably the most common symptom with intraspinal canal neoplasms. It may be present for months before other symptoms or segmental signs appear. At some point in their course, these patients frequently have symptoms and signs in a "radicular" or "multiradicular" distribution, and for this reason many are referred to the EDX laboratory for assessment. Although the EDX findings typically are nonspecific in regard to etiology, their presence frequently initiates the appropriate neuroimaging studies (if they were not already planned). This is illustrated by the following case history; in this instance, the symptomatology was somewhat unusual in that pain was not present.

Case Report. (EDB extensor digitorum brevis; TA = tibialis anterior; AH = abductor hallucis) A 32-year-old man developed spontaneous weakness of plantar flexion and especially dorsiflexion of his right foot, which slowly progressed over the next year. He had no pain, paresthesias, or sphincter abnormalities. On clinical examination, atrophy and weakness of all the muscles distal to the right knee were present, most severely in the tibialis anterior; no abnormalities were noted on the left. Sensation was reduced in a right L5 dermatome distribution below the knee. The Achilles DTR was unelicitable on the right but normal on the left. The patient was referred to the EDX laboratory with a diagnosis of "multiple right lumbosacral radiculopathies." An EDX examination revealed the following. The sensory NCS (sural, superficial peroneal sensory) were normal in amplitude and equal bilaterally. The peroneal motor CMAPs (recording EDB) were normal on the left, but very low in amplitude on the right (9 mV vs. 0.9 mV); the peroneal motor CMAPs (recording TA) were normal on the left and low in amplitude on the right (7 mV vs. 2.4 mV). In contrast, the tibial motor NCS (recording AH) and the M-components of the H-wave test bilaterally were normal and equal in amplitude from side to side. The H-reflex was unelicitable on the right but low in amplitude (< 1 mV) on the left. On NEE, fibrillation potentials were present in moderate numbers in L5 and S1-innervated muscles on the right, and in some S1-innervated muscles on the left; reduced MUAP recruitment was noted in the right TA; in all the remaining muscles innervated by the L5 and S1 segments bilaterally, incomplete MUAP activation was seen. The MUAPs in all the L5 and S1-innervated muscles bilaterally were chronic neurogenic in appearance, particularly in the right TA and gluteus medius. The EDX findings were interpreted as showing evidence of a lumbar intraspinal canal lesion involving the L5 and S1 segments/roots bilaterally, more severe on the right, particularly for the L5 component. A subsequent MRI revealed changes suggestive of a lumbar intraspinal canal neoplasm, specifically a myxopapillary ependymoma of the filum terminale. This was subsequently verified at operation.

CONCLUSION

The EDX examination can be helpful in the assessment of suspected SCDs and of the complications arising from them, but its value varies substantially depending on a number of factors. All components of the EDX examination—NCS, NEE, and special studies—can be beneficial in this regard.

References

1. Clemente CD (ed.). *Gray's Anatomy,* 30th American ed., Philadelphia: Lea & Fibiger, 1985.
2. Adams RD, Victor M, Ropper AA. *Principles of Neurology,* 6th ed. New York: McGraw-Hill, 1997.
3. Byrne TN, Benzel EC, Waxman SG. *Disorders of the Spine and Spinal Cord.* New York: Oxford University Press, 2000.
4. Wilbourn AJ, Aminoff MJ. AAEM Minimonograph 32: The electrodiagnostic examination in patients with radiculopathies. *Muscle Nerve* 1998; 21:1612–1631.
5. Aminoff MJ. *Electromyography in Clinical Practice,* 3rd ed. New York: Churchill-Livingstone, 1998.
6. Wilbourn AJ, Ferrante MA. Clinical electromyography. In: Joynt RJ, Griggs RC, eds. *Baker's Clinical Neurology on CD-ROM.* Philadelphia, 2000.
7. Rosen JS, Lerner IM, Rosenthal AM. Electromyography in SCI. *Arch Phys Med Rehabil* 1969; 50:271–273.
8. Harmon RL, Agre JC. Electrodiagnostic findings in patients with poliomyelitis. *Phys Med Rehabil Clinics N Amer* 1994; 5:559–569.
9. Wilbourn AJ. Electrodiagnostic evaluation of the patient with possible ALS. In: Belch JM, Schiffman P, eds. *Amyotrophic Lateral Sclerosis: Diagnosis and Management for the Clinician.* Armonk NY: Futura, 1996:163–202.
10. Cole JL. Central nervous system physiology. In: DeLisa JA, Gans BM, eds. *Rehabilitation Medicine, Principles and Practice,* 3rd ed. Philadelphia: Lippincott-Raven, 1998:383–406.

11. Grundy BL, Friedman W. Electrophysiological evaluation of the patient with acute SCI. *Critical Care Clinics* 1983; 3:519–548.
12. Little JW, Stiens SA. Electrodiagnosis in SCI. *Phys Med Rehabil Clinics N Amer* 1994; 5:571–593.
13. Dumitru D. *Electrodiagnostic Medicine*. Philadelphia: Hanley Belfus Inc., 1995.
14. Shefner JM, Tyler HR, Krarup C. Abnormalities in the sensory action potential in patients with amyotrophic lateral sclerosis. *Muscle Nerve* 1991; 14:1242–1246.
15. Mondelli M, Rossi A, Passero S, Guazzi GC. Involvement of peripheral sensory fibers in amyotrophic lateral sclerosis: Electrophysiological study of 64 cases. *Muscle Nerve* 1993; 16:166–172.
16. Radtke RA, Erwin A, Erwin CW. Abnormal sensory evoked potentials in amyotrophic lateral sclerosis. *Neurology* 1986; 36:796–801.
17. Pullman SR, Rubin M. Large amplitude sensory nerve action potentials in myelopathy: an observation. *Muscle Nerve* 1991; 14:709–715.
18. Goldkamp O. Electromyography and nerve conduction studies in 116 patients with hemiplegia. *Arch Phys Med Rehabil* 1967; 48:59–63.
19. Aisen ML, Brown W, Rubin M. Electrophysiologic changes in lumbar spinal cord after cervical cord injury. *Neurology* 1992; 42:623–626.
20. Brown WF, Snow R. Denervation in hemiplegic muscles. *Stroke* 1990; 21:1700–1704.
21. Campbell JW, Herbison GJ, Chen YT, Jarveed M, Gussner CG. Spontaneous electromyographic potentials in chronic spinal cord injured patients: Relation to spasticity and length of nerve. *Arch Phys Med Rehabil* 1991; 72:23–27.
22. Johnson EW, Denny ST, Kelley JP. Sequence of electromyographic abnormalities in stroke syndrome. *Arch Phys Med Rehabil* 1975; 56:468–473.
23. Liberson WT, Yhu HL. Proximal-distal gradient in the involvement of the peripheral neurons in the upper extremities of hemiplegics. *Electromyogr Clin Neurophysiol* 1977; 17:281–286.
24. Spaans F, Wilts G. Denervation due to lesions of the central nervous system. *J Neurology Sciences* 1982; 57:291–305.
25. Spielholz NI, Sell GH, Goodgold J, Rusk HA, Greens SK. Electrophysiological studies in patients with spinal cord lesions. *Arch Phys Med Rehabil* 1972; 53:558–562.
26. Bhala RP. Electromyographic evidence of lower motor neuron involvement in hemiplegia. *Arch Phys Med Rehabil* 1969; 50:632–637.
27. Brandstater ME, Dinsdale SN. Electrophysiological studies in the assessment of spinal cord lesions. *Arch Phys Med Rehabil* 1976; 57:70–74.
28. Cruz Martinez AC. Electrophysiological study in hemiparetic patients. Electromyography, motor conduction velocity and response to repetitive nerve stimulation. *Electromyogr Clin Neurophysiol* 1983; 23:139–146.
29. DiBenetto M. Electrodiagnostic phenomena observed in patients with spinal cord lesions. *Electromyogr Clin Neurophysiol* 1977; 17:231–237.
30. Krueger KC, Waylonis GW. Hemiplegia: Lower motor neuron electromyographic findings. *Arch Phys Med Rehabil* 1973; 54:360–364.
31. Laurence TN, Pugel AV, Teasdall RD. Peripheral nerve involvement in SCI: An electromyographic study. *Arch Phys Med Rehabil* 1978; 59:309–313.
32. Nyboer VJ, Johnson HE. Electromyographic findings in lower extremities of patients with traumatic hemiplegia. *Arch Phys Med Rehabil* 1971; 52:256–259.
33. Onkelinx A, Chantraine A. Electromyographic study of paraplegic patients. *Electromyogr Clin Neurophysiol* 1975; 15:71–81.
34. Zalis AW, Lafratta CW, Fauls LB, Oester YT. Electrophysiological studies in hemiplegia: Lower motor neuron findings and correlates. *Electromyogr Clin Neurophysiol* 1976; 16:151–162.
35. Benecke R, Berthold A, Conrad B. Denervation activity in the EMG in patients with upper motor neuron lesions: Time course, local distribution, and pathogenetic aspects. *J Neurology* 1983; 230:143–151.
36. Alpert S, Idarraga S, Orbegozo J, Rosenthal AM. Absence of electromyographic evidence of lower motor neuron involvement in hemiplegic patients. *Arch Phys Med Rehabil* 1971; 52:179–181.
37. Alpert S, Jerrett S, Lerner IM, Rosenthal AM. Electromyographic findings in early hemiplegia. *Arch Phys Med Rehabil* 1973; 54:464–465.
38. Blaik Z, McGarry J, Daura R. Peripheral neuropathy in spinal cord injured patients. *Electromyogr Clin Neurophysiol* 1989; 29:469–472.
39. Chokroverty S, Medina J. Electrophysiological study of hemiplegia: Motor nerve conduction velocity, brachial plexus latency and EMG. *Arch Neurol* 1978; 35:360–363.
40. Petty J. Johnson EW. EMG in upper motor neuron conditions. In: Johnson EW, ed. *Practical Electromyography*. Baltimore: Williams & Wilkins, 1980:276–289.
41. Taylor RG, Laxman S, Kewalrumani LS, Fowler WM. Electromyographic findings in lower extremities in patients with high spinal cord injury. *Arch Phys Med Rehabil* 1974; 55:16–23.
42. Fisher MA. F-response latencies and durations in upper motor neuron syndromes. *Electromyogr Clin Neurophysiol* 1986; 26:327–332.
43. Sutton LR, Cohen BS, Krusen ML. Nerve conduction studies in hemiplegia. *Arch Phys Med Rehabil* 1967; 48:64–67.
44. Widener T, Cochran T, Gress RH, Fleming WC. Studies on velocity of nerve conduction in hemiplegics. *Southern Med J* 1967; 60:1194–1196.
45. Namba T, Schuman MH, Grob D. Conduction velocity in the ulnar nerve in hemiplegic patients. *J Neurol Sciences* 1971; 12:177–186.
46. Panin N, Paul BJ, Policoff LD. Nerve conduction velocities in hemiplegia: A preliminary report. *Arch Phys Med Rehabil* 1965; 46:467–471.
47. Panin N, Paul BJ, Policoff LD, Eson ME. Nerve conduction velocities in hemiplegia. *Arch Phys Med Rehabil* 1967; 48:606–610.
48. Takebe K, Narayan MG, Kukulka C, Basmajian JV. Slowing of nerve conduction velocity in hemiplegia: Possible factors. *Arch Phys Med Rehabil* 1975; 56:285–289.
49. Davidoff G, Werner R, Waring W. Compressive mononeuropathies of the upper extremity in chronic paraplegia. *Paraplegia* 1991; 29:17–24.
50. Hunter J, Ashby P. Secondary changes in segmental neurons below a spinal cord lesion in man. *Arch Phys Med Rehabil* 1984; 65:702–705.
51. Gooch JL, Griffin JB. Sensory nerve evoked response in SCI. *Arch Phys Med Rehabil* 1990; 71:975–978.
52. Eisen A, Odusote K. Amplitude of the F-wave: A potential means of documenting spasticity. *Neurology* 1979; 29:1306–1309.
53. Fisher MA, Shahani BT, Young RR. Assessing segmental excitability after acute rostral lesions. The F-response. *Neurology* 1978; 28:1265–1271.
54. Liberson WT, Yen Chen L-C, Fok SK, Patel KK, Yir G-H, Fried P. "H" reflexes and "F" waves in hemiplegia. *Electromyogr Clin Neurophysiol* 1977; 17:247–264.
55. Little JW, Halar EM. H-reflex changes following SCI. *Arch Phys Med Rehab* 1985; 66:19–22.
56. Segura RP, Sahgal V. Hemiplegic atrophy: Electrophysiological and morphological studies. *Muscle Nerve* 1981; 4:246–248.
57. Shemesh Y, Rozin R, Ohry A. Electrodiagnostic investigation of the motor neuron and spinal reflex arch (H-reflex) in SCI. *Paraplegia* 1977–8; 15:238–244.
58. Campbell WW. *Essentials of Electrodiagnostic Medicine*. Baltimore: Williams & Wilkins, 1999; 69.
59. Madalin K, Wilbourn AJ. The value of the electrodiagnostic studies with primary intraspinal canal neoplasms. *Muscle Nerve* 1988; 11:977 (abs).
60. Aljure J, Eltorar I, Bradley WE, Lin JE, Johnson B. Carpal tunnel syndrome in paraplegic patients. *Paraplegia* 1985; 23:182–186.
61. Gellman H, Chandler DR, Petrasek J, Sie I, Adkins R, Waters RL. Carpal tunnel syndrome in paraplegic patients. *J Bone Joint Surg* 1988A; 70:517–519.
62. Moskowitz E, Porter JJ. Peripheral nerve lesions in the upper extremity in hemiplegic patients. *N Engl J Med* 1963; 269:776–778.
63. Blankstein A, Shmueli R, Weingarden I. Hand problems due to prolonged use of crutches and wheelchairs. *Orthopedic Rev* 1985; 14:29–34.
64. Freed MM. Traumatic and congenital lesions of the spinal cord. In: Kottke FJ, Lehmann, JF, eds. *Krusen's Handbook of Physical Medical and Rehabilitation*. Philadelphia: WB Saunders, 1990:717–748.

7 Electrodiagnostic Evaluation of the Spinal Tracts

Mark A. Lissens

In various disorders of the spinal cord it is very important to obtain information of the neurophysiologic function of the spinal tracts, in diagnosis and prognosis as well as during treatment and rehabilitation. Both the sensory or ascending tracts and the motor or descending tracts can be evaluated electrodiagnostically, with somatosensory evoked potentials (SEPs) and with motor evoked potentials (MEPs) respectively.

SOMATOSENSORY EVOKED POTENTIALS

Methodology

SEPs are elicited with electrical stimulation delivered transcutaneously to a mixed or sensory nerve, or sometimes to the skin of the territory of an individual nerve or nerve root (dermatome). Especially the type Ia and II afferent nerve fibers are excited. Stimuli are monophasic rectangular pulses of short duration (100 to 300 μs) at a rate of 3 or 5 Hz and at an intensity that is two or three times above sensory threshold, or slightly above motor threshold if a mixed nerve is stimulated. To reduce the patient's discomfort, the skin contact impedance should be 5 kΩ or less.

In clinical settings the most commonly stimulated nerves are the median and ulnar nerve at the wrist and the posterior tibial nerve at the ankle, but any other accessible nerve can be stimulated.

SEP responses are recorded with either surface or needle electrodes, as well from the nerve proximal to the site of stimulation, as over the spine and scalp (mostly according to the international 10–20 system for the placement of EEG electrodes). Stimulus artifact is reduced by placement of a ground electrode on the stimulated limb. Muscle and movement artifacts can be reduced by sedation of the patient.

SEPs are extracted from background (cerebral) activity by means of computer averaging. The number of trials to be averaged depends on the quality of the recording, the amount of background noise, and the size of the signal of interest. Usually between 300 and 4,000 individual trials are required. At least two averages should be obtained to make sure that the SEP findings are reproducible. The clinically most used filter setting of the recording system is a bandpass of 30 to 3,000 Hz (Eisen and Aminoff, 1986; Cole and Pease, 1993; Maugière, 1996; Chiappa, 1997; Goldberg, 2000).

The SEP responses are characterized by a certain polarity at the active electrode with respect to the reference one and by a post-stimulus latency time. The voltage changes reflect the activation of sources within different parts of the central nervous system.

There are many variations in nomenclature, but the most typical labels for SEP studies use the polarity (P or N, for positive or negative) and expected latency (in milliseconds), for example P14 or N20.

When stimulating a nerve in the arm, it is mostly possible to consistently recognize an Erb's potential (N13/P13–14), reflecting the voltage difference recorded between the cervical spine and the midfrontal scalp (Fz), and an N20 in recordings made between the contralateral hand area of the scalp (C3' on the left scalp/C4' on the right scalp) and Fz. The cervical N13 probably reflects postsynaptic activity in the spinal cord, whereas P14 reflects activity in the medial lemniscus. The N20 is generated probably in the primary somatosensory cortex.

Similarly, P37 and N45 components are found in recordings over the vertex of the scalp (Cz) with respect to a cephalic reference following stimulation of the posterior tibial nerve in the lower extremities. The N20 and N45 components are followed by a number of different peaks, according to the site of recording over the scalp and probably reflecting distinct cortical generators (Eisen and Aminoff, 1986). Comparable to the cervical N13, a negative potential can be detected over the cauda equina and over the thoracolumbar spine, related predominantly to postsynaptic activity in the lumbar spinal cord (Seyal and Gabor, 1985).

Finally the central somatosensory conduction time (CSCT) can be determined as being the time interval between the major negative peak identified in the spine (e.g. N13 for the cervical spine) and the initial major negative peak of the cortical response (e.g. N20). It can be helpful in detecting slowed transmission through the central neuraxis, for example between the cervicomedullary junction and the cortex.

Absolute SEP component and intercomponent latencies as interside latency differences are also taken into account. Responses are considered to be abnormal if these exceed the mean value for control subjects by more than 2.5 or 3 standard deviations. Less stringent criteria may lead to high false-positive results. The presence or loss of specific components is also important in determining SEP abnormality. SEP amplitude and morphology changes, on the other hand, are less reliable because of the wide variability in normal subjects. Interside amplitude differences of more than 50%, however, may be of some significance.

Clinical Applications

Altered SEPs are not specific for the age or the nature of the underlying pathology and provide limited information on the exact location of the lesions proximal to the dorsal root ganglion. Although SEP abnormalities are etiologically nonspecific, they can be very helpful in several clinical conditions, in the diagnosis of numerous spinal disorders, in determining prognosis, in evaluating treatment, and in following-up patients, for instance during their recovery or rehabilitation.

Especially in spinal cord injury, spondylotic myelopathy, spinal cord compression, radiculopathy, multiple sclerosis, stroke, and in the critical care unit, SEPs can be applied clinically.

As well in spinal cord injury as in stroke patients, SEPs can have prognostic value in the acute and subacute stages (Spielholz et al., 1972; Chiappa, 1993; Maugière, 1996; Eisen and Aminoff, 1986; Curt and Dietz, 1999; Tzvetanov et al., 2005). Although less specific, SEPs seem to be rather sensitive in predicting outcome in the acute phase, meaning that when SEPs are absent, prognosis seems to be poor. When present, certainly if latency times are within normal limits, a better outcome can be expected. The specificity might increase when combining SEPs with MEPs (see next paragraph).

In cervical spondylytic myelopathy, SEPs can be helpful in the evaluation of the severity and level of the lesion, certainly if combined with other electrodiagnostic techniques, as well as in the follow-up of patients after surgery or other applied treatment or rehabilitation procedures (Perlik and Fisher, 1987; Maertens de Noordhout et al., 1991; Nakai et al., 2008).

In the intensive care unit, patients in coma are unlikely to recover from their condition when the cortical responses of the SEPs are bilaterally absent. This is especially true for atraumatic (e.g. anoxic) coma in adult patients (Goldberg, 2000).

In radiculopathy, the clinical application of SEPs is limited, certainly when SEPs are elicited by multisegmental nerve trunk stimulation. Therefore, dermatomal stimulation might have a higher diagnostic yield (Slimp et al, 1992). But even then scalp-recorded dermatomal SEPs have shown to be abnormal in only 20% to 25% of patients with lumbosacral compressive root lesions (Aminoff et al., 1985; Seyal et al., 1989), and in a similar or even lower number of cases with cervical radiculopathy (Leblhuber at al., 1988).

In multiple sclerosis, somatosensory evoked potentials can reflect the upper limb motor performance (Nociti et al., 2008).

MOTOR-EVOKED POTENTIALS

Historical Review

Fritsch and Hitzig in 1870 and Ferrier in 1873 already showed that the exposed motor cortex could be activated by electrical stimulation, and that this excitation was propagated along the descending motor tracts (Fritsch and Hitzig, 1870; Ferrier, 1873). This method offered an interesting alternative to studies of spontaneous and induced brain lesions to reconstruct the functional topography of the motor cortex (Penfield and Boldrey, 1937).

In 1954, Gualtierotti and Paterson tried to stimulate the unexposed cerebral cortex, which at that time was found to be very painful (Gualtierotti and Paterson, 1954). It was only in 1980 that Merton and Morton developed a technique for percutaneous delivery of individual electrical stimuli over the motor cortex of awake humans eliciting contralateral limb movements (Merton and Morton, 1980). This was probably the beginning of a new era in neurophysiological research and clinical neurophysiology.

In 1965, Bickford and Fremming developed a stimulator capable of producing powerful magnetic pulses, and demonstrated noninvasive peripheral nerve stimulation by pulsed magnetic fields (Bickford and Fremming, 1965). However, for technical reasons it remained impossible until 1982 to record the obtained muscle action potentials (Polson et al., 1982). The method was further refined, and in 1985 Barker et al. introduced a new type of magnetic cortical stimulator based on the principle of electromagnetic induction (Barker et al., 1985).

Electromagnetic induction—producing a current in a conductive object by using a moving or time-varying magnetic field—was first described by Michael Faraday in 1831 at the Royal Institute of Great Britain, and was the most relevant experimental observation for magnetic stimulation. Faraday wound two coils on an iron ring and found that whenever the coil on one side was connected with or disconnected from a battery, an electric current passed through the coil on the other side. The iron ring acted as a channel, linking the magnetic field from the first coil to the second. A change in the magnetic field, related to the changing current in the first coil, induced a current in the second coil. In fact, the iron ring only improved the coupling efficiency between the two coils, making the experiment more practical to perform, but the ring could be dispensed with if sufficient primary current was delivered. This is the case in noninvasive magnetic stimulation where the stimulating coil acts as one coil, space as the medium for the flow of the magnetic field, and the conductive living body as the second coil.

Mainly because transcranial magnetic stimulation (TMS) is less invasive and is painless, the number of clinical studies has increased over the last decade and many clinical applications have become available (Jarrat et al., 1990; Murray, 1990; Lissens, 1992; Cros and Chiappa, 1993). The technique provides reliable information about the functional integrity and conduction properties of the corticospinal tracts and motor control in the diagnostic and prognostic assessment of various neurological disorders. It allows doctors to follow the evolution of motor control and to evaluate the effect of different therapeutic procedures.

Principles of Magnetic Stimulation

A magnetic field is generated by passing an electric current through a coil of wire. A magnetic pulse produced from an electric current pulse will induce a current in an electrically conductive region, such as the human body. If the induced current is of sufficient amplitude and duration, it will stimulate neural tissue in its vicinity in exactly the same way as with conventional electrical stimulation.

Magnetic nerve stimulators typically consist of two distinct parts: a high-current pulse generator producing discharge currents of 5.000 A or more, and a stimulating coil producing magnetic field strengths of 1 Tesla or more with a pulse duration of about 1ms. The generator consists of a capacitor charge/discharge system together with the associated control and safety electronics. The stimulating coil, normally housed in molded plastic covers, consists of one or more tightly wound and well-insulated copper coils together with other electronic circuitry such as temperature sensors and safety switches. The main enclosure and the stimulating coil are interconnected by means of a flexible high-power cable.

Magnetic stimulators work by charging one or more energy storage capacitors and then rapidly transferring this stored energy from the capacitor(s) to the stimulating coil when the stimulus is required. The difficulty in producing magnetic nerve stimulators is related to the high discharge currents, voltages, and power levels involved in producing a brief magnetic pulse. Typically, 500 J of energy has to be transferred from the energy storage capacitor into the stimulating coil in about 100 μs. Power, measured in watts, is equivalent to joules per second. Consequently, the power output of a typical magnetic stimulator during the discharge phase is 5,000,000 watts (5 MW) sufficient to provide the electricity necessary for 1,000 homes for 1/1000th of a second. During the discharge, energy initially stored in the capacitor in the form of electrostatic charge is converted into magnetic energy in the stimulating coil in approximately 100ms. This fast rate of energy transfer produces a time-varying magnetic field build-up, which induces tissue currents in the vicinity of the coil in the order 1–20 mA/cm².

Because the magnetic field strength falls off as the distance from the stimulating coil increases, the stimulus strength is maximal close to the coil surface. The stimulation characteristics of the magnetic pulse, such as depth of penetration, strength, and accuracy depend on the rise time, peak magnetic energy transferred to the coil, and the spatial distribution of the field (Barker et al., 1990). The rise time and peak coil energy are governed by the electrical characteristics of the magnetic stimulator and stimulating coil, whereas the spatial distribution of the induced electrical field depends on the coil geometry and the anatomy of the region of induced current flow.

In 1985 the magnetic stimulators originally produced at Sheffield were equipped with circular coils of 90 mm mean diameter. These proved to be most effective for stimulation of the human motor cortex controlling the upper limbs with a large cortical representation, and also for stimulation of spinal nerve roots. To date, circular coils with a mean diameter of 80–100 mm are the most widely used in magnetic stimulation.

Nowadays, two types of magnetic stimulators are available: monophasic (such as the Magstim 200 stimulator) and polyphasic (such as the Cadwell stimulator), which modifies the way in which cerebral structures are excited.

Electrical and magnetic transcranial magnetic stimulation activate the brain at different sites (Day et al., 1987). Whereas the electrical stimulus excites the corticospinal neurons directly,

the magnetic stimulus excites these neurons transsynaptically, explaining the extra delay of a few milliseconds in magnetic stimulation as compared to electrical.

The physical characteristics of the frequently used 90-mm-diameter monophasic coil (Magstim Company, Whitland, UK) are an inside diameter of 66 mm, an outside diameter of 123 mm, a number of 14 turns, a peak magnetic field strength of 2.5 Tesla, and a peak electric field strength of 510 V/m.

Physiological Mechanisms

As previously mentioned, transcranial stimulation provides the first objective laboratory measurement of corticospinal tract function in humans without surgical exposure. The motor-evoked potential procedure consists of transcranial stimulation followed by measurement of the compound muscle action potential (CMAP) from different limb and trunk muscles.

Magnetic stimulation allows neurologists to safely, easily, and effectively stimulate most neural structures, unimpeded by fat and bone, and without discomfort to the patient. Until now, the technique has been mainly applied for stimulation of the peripheral and central motor pathways. Responses following magnetic stimulation can be recorded in a standard fashion from either the nerve or the muscle. Signal averaging is usually not necessary. Compound motor-evoked potentials from various muscles can be obtained in response to magnetic transcranial motor cortex stimulation, and nerve root, plexus, and peripheral nerve stimulation.

When the central nervous system is stimulated, the stimulation threshold can be reduced by approximately 30%, the response amplitude can be increased, and the response latency reduced by some 1–6 ms (usually about 1–2 ms) through pre-activation of the target muscle. This technique, referred to as "facilitation," has been described in considerable detail (Rothwell et al., 1987 and 1991; Day et al., 1987). The phenomenon of facilitation was noted in an early stage of the original transcutaneous electrical stimulation studies of Merton and Morton, and is equally prominent with magnetic brain stimulation (Hess et al., 1987).

The relationship between background force and CMAP amplitude is approximately linear with electrical stimulation, whereas a small background contraction of the order of 5% maximum has a striking facilitating effect with magnetic stimulation.

There are several different processes of facilitation. It is probable that facilitation occurs both at spinal and cortical levels. When attention is focused on accurate force production in a particular muscle, then facilitation occurs at small forces, which is likely to involve cortical mechanisms. Presumably during spinal facilitation more spinal motor neurons are recruited by an unchanged descending volley because their excitability is raised by the descending voluntary input, whereas the cortical facilitation depends on an actual increase in the descending volley caused by the magnetic stimulus.

Response latency shortening during voluntary contraction is likely to reflect application of the size principle of Henneman: the first corticomotoneuron cells to fire during a voluntary contraction are those that conduct most slowly, and with increasing contraction, larger, faster conducting neurons are recruited (Henneman et al., 1965). Moreover, single motor unit studies have demonstrated in humans that the first motor units to be stimulated magnetically are the first to fire under voluntary control, and are of relatively long latency (Hess et al., 1987). Later, larger units with faster conducting axons have shorter latencies.

With electrical stimulation however, an additional mechanism for the latency decrease is possible. To understand this, one must know that a series of positive waves is recordable from the contralateral corticospinal tract when an electrical stimulus is delivered to the exposed motor cortex of animals such as cat, baboon, or monkey (Patton and Amassian, 1954; Kernell and Chien-Ping, 1967). The first of these waves is termed the direct or D-wave, later descending volleys being indirect or I-waves. The D-wave is so called because its latency is too short to allow for an interposed synapse and it is therefore conducted directly in fast pyramidal tract axons. The D-wave is most probably produced by stimulation of proximal nodes of axons of larger corticospinal tract neurons, whereas I-waves appear at higher intensities of stimulation and are probably caused by synaptic activation of the same corticospinal neurons but through intracortical neural elements. There is only minimal temporal dispersion between the D- and I-waves, consistent with both being conducted in the fast corticospinal tract axons. Excitation of the alpha motor neuron cells of the spinal cord requires temporal and spatial summation of stimuli. A stimulus to the cortex will produce a volley of I-waves, possibly preceded by a D-wave according to the stimulus characteristics; anterior horn cell firing, and thus EMG activity will result. When comparing muscle responses to magnetic stimulation with those electrically induced, magnetic responses are of longer onset latency by around 2 ms (in hand muscles), are of simpler waveform, shorter duration, and larger amplitude. These differences suggest that electrical and magnetic stimulation activate the motor pathways at different sites. It is probable that electrical stimulation excites corticospinal neurons directly, causing an initial D-wave and subsequent I-wave volleys, and that magnetic stimulation acts transsynaptically, the better synchronized and longer latency response being due to a more homogeneous site of excitation resulting in I-waves, but no D-wave, impinging on the spinal motor neuron. Later studies, however, have shown that it is also possible to produce a D-wave in the pyramidal tract with magnetic stimulation when changing the current direction in certain (monophasic) coils.

Keeping these multiple descending volleys in mind, and coming back to the phenomenon of facilitation, an additional mechanism for the latency decrease is possible with electrical stimulation: when the muscle is relaxed, the initial D-wave may be insufficient to discharge the motor neuron and summation, with the following I-wave being required to fire the anterior horn cell, with a resultant longer latency response. During voluntary activity there are likely to be motor neurons near enough to threshold for activation to occur with the D-wave, causing a shorter latency with voluntary contraction. Whether summation of I-waves contributes in the same fashion with magnetic stimulation is uncertain, but it is probable that the variation in MEP onset latency observable when a series of brain stimuli are delivered, whether magnetic or electrical, is related at least in part to this phenomenon.

The synaptic delay for discharge by the motoneuron has two components: the excitatory postsynaptic potential (EPSP) delay (± 0.3 ms) and the delay for the EPSP to reach firing level. With strong stimulation of the motor cortex, the number of corticospinal neurons discharging and thus the amount of spatial summation of EPSP are increased, thereby shortening the delay

for motoneurons to attain firing level. When the muscle is relaxed, the motoneuron requires increased excitation to reach firing level, such as could be provided by temporal summation of motoneuron EPSPs elicited by direct and indirect corticospinal discharge. The need for indirect corticospinal discharge would impose an additional delay in the CMAP attributable to cortical synaptic delays and thus largely account for the difference observed (± 2 ms) in CMAP latency in contracted and relaxed muscle.

Another phenomenon (inhibitory) is the interruption of the ongoing voluntary muscle contraction produced by magnetic transcranial stimulation of the motor cortex. This phenomenon appears as a period of EMG silence lasting about 100–150 ms, which is defined as the "silent period" (Cantello et al., 1992; Inghilleri et al., 1993; Ziemann et al., 1993; Säisänen et al., 2008). This silent period is produced by a mixture of cortical and spinal inhibitory effects. Approximately the first 50 ms of the silent period are due to both cortical and spinal mechanisms. From this point onwards spinal mechanisms are progressively less important and the cortical inhibitory mechanisms act on the neural elements of the corticomotoneuronal system at the motor cortical level: a magnetic stimulus given during the second half of the silent period does not produce MEP, but electrical stimulation evokes almost unchanged muscle responses. In other words, the unexcitability of the motor cortex after a second magnetic stimulus indicates that the motor cortex per se is inhibited, whereas the excitability with electrical stimulation implies that corticospinal axons and spinal motoneurons are not inhibited (Cantello et al., 1992; Inghilleri et al., 1993; Schnitzler and Benecke, 1994).

Clinical Applications

Studies in normal subjects have shown that there is a somatotopic localization and preferential excitability of certain regions of the motor cortex, and that one has to take into account that the size, latency, and duration of the MEPs are critically dependent on the type, intensity, and localization of the stimulus, as well as on the excitability of the cortical and spinal motoneurons.

Depending on the purpose of the test there are many important parameters that can be measured in cortical stimulation, such as stimulation threshold, MEP-latency, MEP-amplitude, response morphology, central motor conduction time, silent period duration, fatigue, intracortical inhibitory and excitatory pathways, etc.

The central motor conduction time (CMCT) can be calculated by subtracting the latency in response to spinal root stimulation from the latency in response to cortical stimulation (Hugon et al., 1987; Claus, 1990). But it may be also calculated by using the F-wave latency (Robinson et al., 1988):

CMCT = Latency from cortex to muscle

$$-\frac{\text{F latency} - (\text{motor terminal latency} + 1)}{2}$$

CMCTs calculated using F-waves usually exceed those based on root stimulation, which stimulates the peripheral motor axons distal to the ventral roots.

CMCT can be affected by a number of factors at several levels, including the activation time of the pyramidal tract neurons, the transmission time between motor cortex and spinal motor neurons, the activation time of motor neurons, the time between motoneuron discharge and the site of stimulation of the motor root, and probably others (Komori and Brown, 1993).

The size of electromyographic responses to cortical stimulation or MEP-amplitude can be affected by the type of cortical stimulator (high-voltage electrical or magnetoelectrical) and by the stimulus intensity, as well as the activation of other muscles.

CMCT can be increased and MEP size reduced by several factors, such as reduced excitability of the motor cortex, slowed conduction between the motor cortex and spinal motor neurons, several factors at the motor neuron level, reduced conduction velocities in motor axons, and so on.

Clinical applications of transcranial stimulation include spinal cord injury, multiple sclerosis, anterior horn cell disorders (e.g., amyotrophic lateral sclerosis), spondylotic myelopathy, stroke, radiculopathy, various neuropathies, epilepsy (Tassinari and Michelucci, 1990; Hufnagel et al., 1990), degenerative ataxic disorders such as cerebellar ataxia and Friedreich's ataxia (Claus et al., 1988; Peretti et al., 1990; Murray, 1991), cranial nerve disorders (mainly the facial nerve: Maccabee et al., 1988; Schriefer et al., 1988), pathology of the respiratory muscles, and several others. It can also be used in the operating room during surgery, where monitoring motor conduction is a useful indicator of the integrity of the central motor pathways, especially during neurosurgical operations (Zentner, 1989; Jacobs et al., 2006; Macdonald et al., 2007), as well as in the intensive care unit (Firsching, 1992). Just like SEPs, MEPs can have prognostic value, mainly in spinal cord injury and stroke. Finally, it can be useful in follow-up of motor function during treatment and rehabilitation.

In multiple sclerosis (MS), most authors found clearly delayed CMCTs (Cowan et al., 1984; Mills and Murray, 1985; Hess et al., 1986; Ingram et al., 1988) in up to 79% of patients with definite MS (Hess et al., 1987). Absent MEPs were mostly seen in those MS patients with marked clinical disabilities. Increased CMCTs were often accompanied by dispersed and reduced size of MEPs, but no correlation was found between CMCT and duration of the disease. In MS patients with sexual dysfunction, prolonged CMCTs of pelvic floor muscles were seen (Opsomer et al., 1989). A higher rate of MEP abnormalities was found when an altered MRI signal was localized within the parietal cortex, centrum semiovale, and the internal capsule (Rossini at al., 1989).

In anterior horn cell disorders, more specifically in patients with amyotrophic lateral sclerosis, prolonged or absent MEPs were found, either with high-voltage electrical stimulation (Hugon et al., 1987; Beradelli et al., 1987; Ingram and Swash, 1987) or with magnetoelectrical stimulation (Eisen et al., 1990; Kohara et al., 1996). This was also shown in 1a subgroup of patients with primary lateral sclerosis (Brown et al., 1992). MEPs and cortical excitability can also be helpful in distinguishing anterior horn cell disease from other similar pathologies (Vucic at al., 2008; Attarian et al., 2008).

In spinal cord injury, a strong correlation was seen between MEP findings and motor function (Tegenthoff, 1992; Dimitrijevic et al., 1992; Lissens et al. 1992; Meyer et al., 1992). Decreased MEP amplitudes or absent MEP responses are more frequently seen in neoplastic than in inflammatory lesions, whereas in the latter more often increased latencies are seen (Linden et al., 1994). In high tetraplegic patients in whom the diaphragm is affected, MEPs can be recorded from the diaphragm as well as from other respiratory muscles in order to investigate the central motor conduction properties of this musculature (Lissens 1994; Zifko et al. 1996; Lissens et al., 1996).

In *spondylotic myelopathy*, CMCT has been reported to correlate well with clinical and radiological signs of cord compression (Kalupahana et al., 2008; Lo et al., 2006, Thompson et al., 1987; Abbruzzese et al., 1988; Masur et al., 1989; Maertens de Noordhout et al., 1991). CMCT is more often abnormal than amplitude or morphology of the MEPs. In cervical spondylosis, MEP abnormalities exceed those of SEPs, most probably because spondylosis and disc herniation are more likely to produce compression of the corticospinal tracts than of dorsal columns (Maertens de Noordhout et al., 1991). However, prolonged CMCT is not necessarily due to demyelination, but might also be the result from desynchronization of the descending volleys generated by cortical shocks (see also above: physiological mechanisms). Conduction block or axonal degeneration of the fastest-conducting fibers might also produce CMCT lengthening as well as desynchonization of the responses and reduction in amplitude (Thompson et al., 1987).

In the detection of lumbosacral radiculopathies, magnetoelectrical stimulation may have little practical place, whereas high-voltage electrical stimulation may turn out to be beneficial in the study of these radiculopathies. In the cervical region, however, both high-voltage electrical and magnetoelectrical stimulation are not so useful detectors of cervical radiculopathy, because they apparently stimulate the roots distal to the intervertebral foramen (Berger et al., 1987; Chokroverty et al., 1989; Britton et al., 1990; Weber et al., 2000).

In stroke, MEPs not only correlate well with clinical motor function, but can have prognostic value in the sub-acute stages. In some studies, abnormalities in central motor conduction were shown to be a better indicator of outcome than SEPs (Macdonell et al., 1989). MEPs seem to have a high specificity, but a much lower sensitivity in predicting functional outcome (Nascimbeni et al., 2006; van Kuijk et al., 2009). More specifically, when MEPs are present in the acute phase, outcome usually is favorable, whereas absent MEPs in the acute stages are often not correlated with poor outcome (Liepert, 2005; Piron et al., 2005; Dominkus et al., 1990; Chu et al., 1992; Lissens et al., 1992). Absent MEPs seem to be most characteristic of cortical-subcortical infarction (Macdonell et al., 1989).

Finally, MEPs can be useful in follow-up of motor function during treatment and rehabilitation, mainly in spinal cord injured and stroke patients, which not only is interesting for the therapeutic staff, but also for the patient's motivation (Liepert, 2005; Hummelsheim et al., 1995; Lissens et al., 1992).

References

1. Abbruzzese G, Dall'Agata D, Morena M, Simonetti S, Spandavecchia L, Severi P, Candriolli G, Favale E: Electrical stimulation of the motor cortex in cervical spondylosis. J Neurol Neurosurg Psychiatry, 1988, 51: 796–802.
2. Aminoff MJ, Goodin DS, Parry GJ, et al.: Electrophysiological evaluation of lumbosacral radiculopathies; electromyography, late responses and somatosensory evoked potentials. Neurology, 1985; 35: 1514–1518.
3. Attarian S, Vedel JP, Pouget J, Schmied A: Progression of cortical and spinal dysfunctions over time in amyotrophic lateral sclerosis. Muscle Nerve, 2008, 37: 364–375.
4. Barker AT, Jalinous R, Freeston IL: Non-invasive stimulation of the human motor cortex. Lancet, 1985, ii: 1106–1107.

5. Berardelli A, Inghilleri M, Formisano R, Accornero N: Stimulation of motor tracts in motor neurone disease. J Neurol Neurosurg Psychiatry, 1987, 50: 732–737.

6. Berger AR, Busis NA, Logigian EL et al.: Cervical root stimulation in the diagnosis of radiculopathy. Neurology, 1987, 37: 329–332.

7. Bickford RG, Fremming BD: Neuronal stimulation by pulsed magnetic fields in animals and man. Digest 6th Int Conf Med Electronics Biol Eng, 1965, p112.

8. Britton TC, Meyer BU, Herdmann J, Benecke R: Clinical use of the magnetic stimulator in the investigation of peripheral conduction time. Muscle Nerve, 1990, 13: 396–406.

9. Brown WF, Ebers GC, Hudson AJ et al.: Motor evoked responses in primary lateral sclerosis. Muscle Nerve, 1992, 15: 626–629.

10. Cantello R, Gianelli M, Civardi C, Mutani R: Magnetic brain stimulation: the silent period after the motor evoked potential. Neurology, 1992, 42: 1951–1959.

11. Chiappa KH, ed. Evoked potentials in clinical medicine. 3rd ed. Philadelphia, JB Lippincott-Raven, 1993.

12. Chokroverty S, Sachdeo R, Dilullo J, Duvoisin RC: Magnetic stimulation in the diagnosis of lumbosacral radiculopathy. J Neurol Neurosurg Psychiatry, 1989, 52: 767–772.

13. Chu NS, WU T: Motor response patterns and prognostic value of transcranial magnetic stimulation in stroke patients. In: Lissens MA (ed.): Clinical applications of magnetic transcranial stimulation. Leuven, Belgium, Peeters Press, 1992, 127–145.

14. Claus D, Harding AE, Hess CW, Mills KR, Murray NMF, Thomas PK: Central motor conduction in degenerative ataxic disorders: a magnetic stimulation study. J Neurol Neurosurg Psychiatry, 1988, 51: 790–795.

15. Claus D: Central motor conduction: Method and normal results. Muscle Nerve, 1990, 13: 1125–1132.

16. Cole JL, Pease W: Central nervous system electrodiagnostics. In: DeLisa J (ed.): Rehabilitation medicine: principles and practice. 2nd ed. Philadelphia, JB Lippincott-Raven, 1993.

17. Cowan JMA, Dick JPR, Day BL, Rothwell JC, Thompson PD, Marsden CD: Abnormalities in central motor pathways conduction in multiple sclerosis. Lancet, 1984, 2: 304–307.

18. Cros D, Chiappa KH: Clinical applications of motor evoked potentials. In: Devinsky O, Beric A, Dogali M (eds.): Electrical and magnetic stimulation of the brain and spinal cord. New York, Raven Press, 1993: 179–185.

19. Curt A, Dietz V: Electrophysiological recordings in patients with spinal cord injury: significance for predicting outcome. Spinal Cord, 1999, 37(3): 157–165.

20. Day BL, Thompson PD, Dick JP, Nakashima K, Marsden CD: Different sites of action of electrical and magnetic stimulation of the human brain. Neurosci Lett, 1987, 75(1): 101–106.

21. Day BL, Rothwell JC, Thompson PD, Dick JP, Cowan JM, Berardelli A, Marsden CD: Motor cortex stimulation in intact man. 2. Multiple descending volleys. Brain, 1987, 110: 1191–1209.

22. Dimitrijevic MR, Kofler M, McKay WB, Sherwood AM, Van der Linden C, Lissens MA: Early and late lower limb motor evoked potentials elicited by transcranial magnetic motor cortex stimulation. Electroenceph Clin Neurophysiol, 1992, 85: 365–373.

23. Dominkus M, Grisold W, Jelinek V: Transcranial electrical motor evoked potentials as a prognostic indicator for motor recovery in stroke patients. J Neurol Neurosurg Psychiatry, 1990, 53: 745–748.

24. Eisen A, Aminoff MJ. Somatosensory evoked potentials. In: Aminoff MJ (ed.): Electrodiagnosis in clinical neurology, 2nd ed. New York: Churchill Livingstone, 1986: 535–573.

25. Eisen A, Shtybel W, Murphy K, Hoirch M: Cortical magnetic stimulation in amyotrophic lateral sclerosis. Muscle Nerve, 1990, 13: 146–151.

26. Ferrier D: Experimental researches in cerebral physiology and pathology. West Riding Lunatic Asylum Medical Reports, 1873, 3: 30–96.

27. Firsching R: Clinical applications of magnetic TCS in comatose patients. In: Lissens MA (ed.): Clinical applications of magnetic transcranial stimulation. Leuven, Belgium, Peeters Press, 1992, 263–268.

28. Fritsch G, Hitzig E: Ueber die elektrische Erregbarkeit des Grosshirns. Arch Anat Physiol Wiss Med, 1870, 37: 300–332.

29. Goldberg G: Clinical neurophysiology of the central nervous system. Evoked potentials and other neurophysiologic techniques. In: Grabois M, Garrison SJ, Hart KA, Lehmkul LD (eds.): Physical medicine and rehabilitation. The complete approach. Malden, MA, Blackwell Science, 2000.

30. Gualtierotti T, Paterson AS: Electrical stimulation of the unexposed cerebral cortex. J Physiol, 1954, 125: 278–291.

31. Henneman E, Somjen G, Carpenter DO: Excitability and inhibitibility of motoneurones of different sizes. J Neurophysiol, 1965, 28: 599–620.

32. Hess CW, Mills KR, Murray NMF: Magnetic stimulation of the brain: facilitation of motor responses by voluntary contraction of ipsilateral and contralateral muscles with additional observations on an amputee. Neurosci Lett, 1986, 71: 235–240.

33. Hess CW, Mills KR, Murray NMF: Responses in small hand muscles from magnetic stimulation of the human brain. J Physiol, 1987, 388: 397–419.

34. Hess CW, Mills KR, Murray NMF, Schriefer TN: Magnetic brain stimulation: central motor conduction studies in multiple sclerosis. Ann Neurol, 1987, 22: 744–752.μ

35. Hufnagel A, Elger CE, Durmen HF, et al.: Activation of the epileptic focus by transcranial magnetic stimulation of the human brain. Ann Neurol, 1990, 27: 49–60.

36. Hugon J, Lubeau M, Tabaraud F, et al.: Central motor conduction in motor neuron disease. Ann Neurol, 1987; 22: 544–546.

37. Hummelsheim H, Hauptmann B, Neumann S: Influence of physiotherapeutic facilitation techniques on motor evoked potentials in centrally paretic hand extensor muscles. Electroencephalogr Clin Neurophysiol, 1995, 97: 18–28.

38. Inghilleri M, Berardelli A, Cruccu G, Manfredi M: Silent period evoked by transcranial stimulation of the human motor cortex and cervicomedullary junction. J Physiol, 1993, 161: 112–125.

39. Ingram DA, Swash M: Central motor conduction is abnormal in motor neuron disease. J Neurol Neurosurg Psychiatry, 1987, 50: 159–166.

40. Jacobs MJ, Mess W, Mochtar B, Nijenhuis RJ, Statius van Eps RG, Schurink GW: The value of motor evoked potentials in reducing paraplegia during thoracoabdominal aneurysm repair. J Vasc Surg, 2006, 43: 239–246.

41. Jarrat JA, Barker AT, Freeston IL, Jalinous R, Kandler RH, Jaskolski D: Magnetic stimulation of the human nervous system: clinical applications. In: Shokroverty S (ed.): Magnetic stimulation in clinical neurophysiology. Butterworths, Boston, 1990: 185–204.

42. Kalupahana NS, Weerasinghe VS, Dangahadeniya U, Senanayake N.: Abnormal parameters of magnetically evoked motor-evoked potentials in patients with cervical spondylotic myelopathy. Spine J, 2008, 8(4): 645–649. Epub 2007 Jan 22.

43. Kernell D, Chien-Ping WU: Responses of the pyramidal tract to stimulation of the baboon's motor cortex. J Physiol, 1967, 191: 653–690.

44. Kohara N, Kaji R, Kojima Y, Mills KR, Fujii H, Hamano T, Kimura J, Takamatsu N, Uchiyama T: Abnormal excitability of the corticospinal pathway in patients with amyotrophic lateral sclerosis: a single motor unit study using transcranial magnetic stimulation. Electroencephalogr Clin Neurophysiol, 1996, 101: 32–41.

45. Komori T, Brown WF: Central electromyography. In: Brown WF and Bolton CF (eds.): Clinical electromyography. Butterworth-Heinemann, Boston, 1993: 3–23.

46. Leblhuber F, Reisecker F, Boehm-Jurkovic H et al.: Diagnostic value of different electrophysiologic tests in cervical disc prolapse. Neurology 1988; 38: 1879–1881.

47. Liepert J.: Transcranial magnetic stimulation in neurorehabilitation. Acta Neurochir Suppl, 2005, 93: 71–74.

48. Linden D, Berlit P: Magnetic motor evoked potentials (MEP) in diseases of the spinal cord. Acta Neurol Scand, 1994, 90: 348–353.

49. Lissens MA (ed.): Clinical applications of magnetic transcranial stimulation. Leuven, Belgium, Peeters Press, 1992.

50. Lissens MA, McKay WB, Van der Linden C, Dimitrijevic MR: Transcranial motor cortex stimulation in patients with established spinal cord injury. In: Lissens MA (ed.): Clinical applications of magnetic transcranial stimulation. Leuven, Belgium, Peeters Press, 1992, 42–55.

51. Lissens MA, McKay WB: Value of motor evoked potentials elicited by magnetic transcranial motor cortex stimulation in the prognosis and follow-up during rehabilitation of stroke rehabilitation. In: Lissens MA (ed.): Clinical applications of magnetic transcranial stimulation. Leuven, Belgium, Peeters Press, 1992, 283–290.

52. Lissens MA: Motor evoked potentials of the human diaphragm elicited through magnetic transcranial brain stimulation. J Neurol Sci, 1994, 124: 204–207.

53. Lissens MA, Vanderstraeten GG: Motor evoked potentials of the respiratory muscles in tetraplegic patients. Spinal Cord, 1996, 34: 673–678.

54. Lo YL, Chan LL, Lim W, Tan SB, Tan CT, Chen JL, Fook-Chong S, Ratnagopal P: Transcranial magnetic stimulation screening for cord compression in cervical spondylosis. J Neurol Sci, 2006, 244:17–21. Epub 2006 Feb 14.

55. Maccabee PJ, Amassian VE, Cracco RQ, Cracco JB: Intracranial stimulation of facial nerve in humans with the magnetic coil. Electroencephalogr Clin Neurophysiol, 1988, 70: 350–354.

56. Macdonald DB, Al Zayed Z, Al Saddigi A: Four-limb muscle motor evoked potential and optimized somatosensory evoked potential monitoring with decussation assessment: results in 206 thoracolumbar spine surgeries. Eur Spine J, 2007, 16: S171–87. Epub 2007 Jul 19.

57. Maertens de Noordhout A, Remacle JM, Pepin JL et al.: Magnetic stimulation of the motor cortex in cervical spondylosis. Neurology, 1991, 41: 75–80.

58. Masur H, Elger CE, Render K, Fahrenhof G, Ludolf AC: Functional deficits of central sensory and motor pathways in patients with cervical spondylosis: a study of SEPs and EMG responses to non invasive brain stimulation. Electroencephalogr Clin Neurophysiol, 1989, 74: 450–457.

59. Maugière F: Clinical utility of somatosensory evoked potentials (SEPs): present debates and future trends. Electroencephalogr Clin Neurophysiol Suppl, 1996; 46: 27–33.

60. Merton PA, Morton HB: Stimulation of the cerebral cortex in the intact human subject. Nature, 1980, 285: 227.

61. Meyer B, Zentner J: Do motor evoked potentials allow quantitative assessment of motor function in patients with spinal cord lesions? Eur Arch Psychiatry Clin Neurosci, 1992, 241: 201–204.

62. Murray NMF: Magnetic stimulation of the brain: clinical applications. In: Shokroverty S (ed.): Magnetic stimulation in clinical neurophysiology. Boston, Butterworths, 1990: 205–231.

63. Murray NMF: The clinical usefulness of magnetic cortical stimulation. Electroencephalogr Clin Neurophysiol, 1991, 85: 81–85.

64. Nascimbeni A, Gaffuri A, Imazio P: Motor evoked potentials: prognostic value in motor recovery after stroke. Funct Neurol, 2006, 21(4): 199–203.

65. Nakai S, Sonoo M, Shimizu T.: Somatosensory evoked potentials (SEPs) for the evaluation of cervical spondylotic myelopathy: utility of the onset-latency parameters. Clin Neurophysiol, 2008, 119: 2396–2404. Epub 2008 Aug 31.

66. Nociti V, Batocchi AP, Bartalini S, Caggiula M, Patti F, Profice P, Quattrone A, Tonali P, Ulivelli M, Valentino P, Virdis D, Zappia M, Padua L: Somatosensory evoked potentials reflect the upper limb motor performance in multiple sclerosis. J Neurol Sci, 2008, 273(1–2): 99–102. Epub 2008 Aug 5.

67. Opsomer RJ, Caramia MD, Zarola F, Pesce F, Rossini PM: Neurophysiological evaluation of central-peripheral sensory and motor pudendal fibers. Electroenceph Clin Neurophysiol, 1989, 74: 260–270.

68. Patton HD, Amassian VE: Single and multiple unit analysis of cortical stage of pyramidal tract activation. J Neurophysiol, 1954, 17: 345–363.

69. Penfield W, Boldrey E: Somatic motor and sensory representation in the cerebral cortex of man as studied by electrical stimulation. Brain, 1937, 60: 389–443.

70. Peretti A, Caruso G, Lanzillo B, Madonna C, Filla A, Santoro L: Central motor conduction by different stimulation techniques: a study in Friedreich's ataxia patients. 1990.

71. Perlik SJ, Fisher MA: Somatosensory evoked response evaluation of cervical spondylotic myelopathy. Muscle Nerve, 1987; 10(6): 481–489.

72. Piron L, Piccione F, Tonin P, Dam M: Clinical correlation between motor evoked potentials and gait recovery in poststroke patients. Arch Phys Med Rehabil, 2005, 86(9): 1874–1878.

73. Polson MJR, Freeston IL, Barker AT: Stimulation of nerve trunks with time-varying magnetic fields. Med Biol Eng, UK, 1982, 20: 243–244.

74. Robinson LR, Jantra P, Maclean IC: Central motor conduction times using transcranial stimulation and F wave latencies. Muscle Nerve, 1988, 11: 174–180.

75. Rossini PM, Caramia M, Zarola F, Bernardi G, Floris R: Sensory (VEP, BAEP, SEP) and motor evoked potentials, liquoral and magnetic resonance findings in multiple sclerosis. Eur Neurol, 1989, 29: 41.

76. Rothwell JC, Thompson PD, Day BL, Dick JPR, Kachi T, Cowan JMA, Marsden CD: Motor cortex stimulation in intact man: 1.General characteristics of EMG responses in different muscles. Brain, 1987, 110: 1173–1190.

77. Rothwell JC, Ferbert A, Caramia MD, Kujirai T, Day BL, Thompson PD: Intracortical inhibitory circuits studied in humans. Neurology, 1991, 41(Suppl): 263P.

78. Rothwell JC, Thompson PD, Day BL, Boyd S, Marsden CD: Stimulation of the human motor cortex through the scalp. Exp Physiol, 1991, 76: 159–200.

79. Rothwell JC, Thompson PD, Day BL, Dick JPR, Kachi T, Cowan JMA, Marsden CD: Motor cortex stimulation in intact man: 1.General characteristics of EMG responses in different muscles. Brain, 1987, 110: 1173–1190.

80. Rothwell JC, Ferbert A, Caramia MD, Kujirai T, Day BL, Thompson PD: Intracortical inhibitory circuits studied in humans. Neurology, 1991, 41(Suppl): 263P.

81. Säisänen L, Pirinen E, Teitti S, Könönen M, Julkunen P, Määttä S, Karhu J: Factors influencing cortical silent period: optimized stimulus location, intensity and muscle contraction. J Neurosci Methods. 2008, 169: 231–238. Epub 2007 Dec 23.

82. Schnitzler A, Benecke R: Silent period after transcranial brain stimulation is of exclusive cortical origin: evidence from isolated cortical ischemic lesions in man. Neurosci Lett, 1994, 180(1): 33–41.

83. Schriefer TN, Mils KR, Murray NMF, Hess CW: Evaluation of proximal facial nerve conduction by transcranial magnetic stimulation. J Neurol Neurosurg Psychiatry, 1988, 51: 60–66.

84. Seyal M, Gabor AJ: The human posterior tibial somatosensory evoked potential: Synapse dependent and synapse independent spinal components. Electroencephalogr Clin Neurophysiol, 1985; 17: 171–176.

85. Seyal M, Sandhu LS, Mack YP: Spinal segmental somatosensory evoked potentials in lumbosacral radiculopathies. Neurology, 1989; 39: 801–805.

86. Slimp JC, Rubner DE, Snowden ML, Stolov WC: Dermatomal somatosensory evoked potentials: cervical, thoracic, and lumbosacral levels. Electroencephalogr Clin Neurophysiol, 1992, 84: 55–70.

87. Spielholz NI, Sell GH, Goodgold J, Rusk HA, Greens SK: Electrophysiological studies in patients with spinal cord lesions. Arch Phys Med Rehabil, 1972, 53(12): 558–562.

88. Tassinari CA, Michelucci R, Plasmati R et al.: Transcranial magnetic stimulation in epileptic patients: usefulness and safety. Neurology, 1990, 40: 1132–1133.

89. Tegenthoff M: Clinical applications of magnetic transcranial stimulation in acute spinal cord injury. In: Lissens MA (ed.): Clinical applications of magnetic transcranial stimulation. Leuven, Belgium, Peeters Press, 1992, 33–41.

90. Thompson PD, Dick JPR, Asselman P, Griffin GB, Day BL, Rothwell JC, Sheehy MB, Marsden CD: Examination of motor function in lesions of the spinal cord by stimulation of the motor cortex. Ann Neurol, 1987, 21: 389–396.

91. Tzvetanov P, Rousseff RT: Predictive value of median-SSEP in early phase of stroke: a comparison in supratentorial infarction and hemorrhage. Clin Neurol Neurosurg, 2005, 107: 475–481.

92. van Kuijk AA, Pasman JW, Hendricks HT, Zwarts MJ, Geurts AC: Predicting hand motor recovery in severe stroke: the role of motor evoked potentials in relation to early clinical assessment. Neurorehabil Neural Repair, 2009, 23(1): 45–51. Epub 2008 Sep 15.

93. Vucic S, Kiernan MC: Cortical excitability testing distinguishes Kennedy's disease from amyotrophic lateral sclerosis. Clin Neurophysiol, 2008, 119: 1088–1096. Epub 2008 Feb 29.

94. Weber F, Albert U: Electrodiagnostic examination of lumbosacral radiculopathies. Electromyogr Clin Neurophysiol, 2000, 40: 231–236.

95. Zentner J: Noninvasive motor evoked potential monitoring during neurosurgical operations on the spinal cord. Neurosurgery, 1989, 24: 709–712.

96. Ziemann U, Netz J, Szelényi A, Hömberg V: Spinal and supraspinal mechanisms contribute to the silent period in the contracting soleus muscle after transcranial magnetic stimulation of the human motor cortex. Neurosci Lett, 1993, 156: 167–171.

97. Zifko U, Remtulla H, Power K, Harker L, Bolton CF: Transcortical and cervical magnetic stimulation with recording of the diaphragm. Muscle Nerve, 1996, 19: 614–620.

8 Functional Assessment in Spinal Cord Injury Rehabilitation

Marcel P.J.M. Dijkers
Jeanne M. Zanca

Chronic disease and injury often result in difficulties performing day-to-day activities because of physical, cognitive, or emotional impairments. The process of determining the type and degree of such problems, or the ability to perform normal acts, activities, and roles is typically designated "functional assessment." This is a misnomer, in that "assessment of function" or "functioning assessment" more clearly expresses the nature of this activity. Terms that overlap with "functional assessment" (FA) to a considerable degree are health status assessment, disability assessment or measurement, geriatric assessment, and others (1, 2). All of these activities aim to measure to what degree the person in his or her functioning deviates from "normal," where normal may refer to typical functioning for persons without disabilities (either all persons, or persons of the same age, gender, education, etc.), or the person's own pre-injury status.

Assessment in this context refers to quantification, where the position of the person on a continuum ranging from unable (complete lack of function) to very able (on a level with or even better than "average" or pre-injury) is determined and expressed in a number. This is the meaning of the term FA as commonly used in health care and rehabilitation practice and research (3). However, the term assessment has a second meaning, referring to evaluation or valuation: the worth or meaning attached to the (amount of) function by the person involved or by others. Although the two types of "assessment" are strongly connected, the two are not synonymous. Whereas it is generally true that more able is considered "better" or "more valuable," people may differ in how they value one ability compared to another (walking vs. bathing), and in how they value one specific level of an ability compared to another level (4, 5). These inter-individual differences come into play more to the degree that FA shifts from basic human functions (e.g. grasping) to more complex ones (holding down a job). Traditional methods of FA deal exclusively with the quantification issues (which are far from simple by themselves), and not with the valuation question. However, it is

becoming increasingly clear that in order to assess with any level of adequacy what medical care and rehabilitation "produce," issues of valuation need to be dealt with (6).

FA in a narrow sense deals with Activities/Activity Limitations, and rehabilitation and other specialists have developed many measures to quantify self-care, mobility, everyday communication, and other types of activities. FA in a broad sense also includes measuring Impairments and Participation (7). In this chapter, we will give an overview of the concepts and techniques useful in understanding and evaluating FA instruments in all three categories, and of the issues involved in selecting them for clinical and research applications. An overview of available measures is provided, as are references to systematic reviews that discuss various groups of FA measures in detail.

THE DISABLEMENT CONTINUUM

As suggested above, "functioning" may cover an extremely broad area, from simple functions involving a single organ system to complex activities that are dependent on multiple physical and cognitive skills and are implemented in social interactions according to established social and cultural patterns. In Figure 1, the World Health Organization's (WHO) International Classification of Functioning, Disability, and Health (ICF) is used as a framework to delineate various concepts and terms encountered in the FA literature.

The WHO defines Impairment as "problems in body function or structure as a significant deviation or loss". In spite of the word "body," impairments include deficits in psychological functions (8, p. 12). The positive aspect is body functions, which are defined as the physiological functions of body systems. In a previous edition of the ICF, the International Classification of Impairments, Disabilities, and Handicaps (ICIDH [9]), the same term was used; the taxonomy offered, however, did not make a clear distinction between deficits of structure and deficits of function at the

This work was supported in part by a grant from the National Institute on Disability and Rehabilitation Research (NIDRR), Office of Special Education Services, U.S. Department of Education to Mount Sinai School of Medicine (H133N060027).

impairment level. In spinal cord injury (SCI), key measures of impairment include the motor and sensory scores of the International Standards for Classification of Spinal Cord Injury (10).

At the level of the person, Activity is characterized in the ICF as "execution of a task or action by an individual" (8, p. 14). Its negative aspect, Activity limitations, is defined as "difficulties an individual may have in executing activities" (8, p. 14). The ICIDH used the term "disability" for this concept, which was defined similarly to the current term "activity limitation." Within rehabilitation, the prototypical measure of activity limitations is the Functional Independence Measure (FIM [11]), but many other instruments have been used; in the SCI field, the Spinal Cord Independence Measure (SCIM) is employed increasingly, especially outside the United States (12).

Finally, the person in interaction with others may have Participation restrictions, which are defined as "problems an individual may experience in involvement in life situations" (8, p. 14); the positive counterpart, Participation, is characterized as "involvement in a life situation" (8, p. 14). In the ICIDH the term "handicap" was used for the negative aspect, which was defined in a manner quite different from the newer term. However, many of the measures developed to operationalize "handicap," such as the Craig Hospital Assessment and Reporting Technique (CHART [13]), are now used as measures of participation restrictions, including in the SCI literature.

Human activities range from simple acts such as stretching a leg to complicated pursuits such as running a household, and it is difficult to define the three concepts of Impairment, Activity (limitation) and Participation (restriction) in a clear and non-overlapping way (14–18). In some instances, it is not even simple to place any one act or activity in one of the three ICF baskets. Some measures of "functioning" overlap two or three of the concepts— intentionally or because the developers were not aware that the indicators they combined belonged to distinct conceptual classes.

Many terms developed prior to or outside the ICIDH/ICF framework can be placed on the same disablement continuum, as shown in Figure 8.1. The core interests of rehabilitation, activities of daily living (ADLs) (sometimes designated

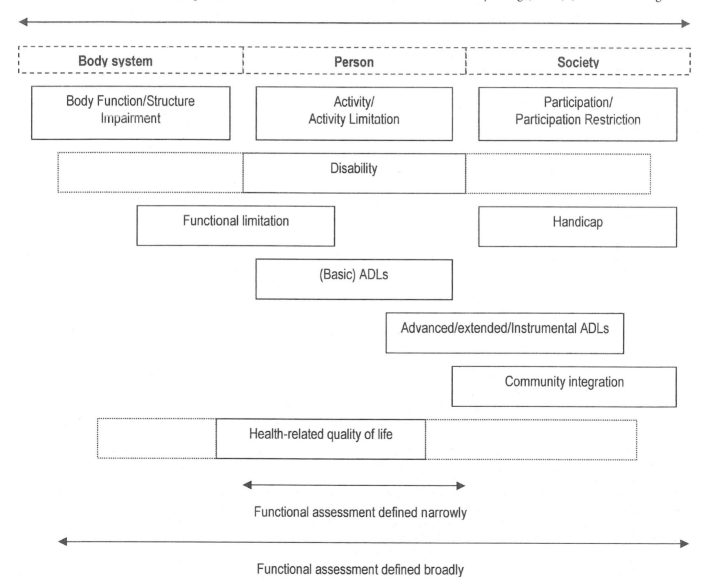

Figure 8.1 The continuum of functional assessment.

basic or personal ADLs) coincide with Activities. Extended (instrumental, advanced) ADLs are generally defined to straddle the activity-participation separation; on the other side of the continuum, Functional limitations typically represent activities such as grasping and lifting that cross the divide between Impairments and Activities (19). Community integration assessments may quantify aspects of IADLs, and other facets of participation, with emphasis on the social interactional components. Health status, a term used by health outcomes researchers, typically is defined and operationalized as combining elements of Impairment and Activity Limitations, although some measures (such as the well-known Short-Form 36)(SF-36 [20]) also include indicators of participation. The SF-36 is now increasingly used as a measure of quality of life (QOL). QOL has been defined in a number of ways (21, 22); most definitions and operationalizations of health-related QOL (HRQOL) overlap with Activities and Participation, and may even take in some aspects of Impairment.

THE STRUCTURE OF FUNCTIONAL ASSESSMENT INSTRUMENTS

At the simplest level, FA measures consist of a number of separate items, each one of which refers to a narrow or broad ability, skill, or activity—for instance, lifting overhead, transferring into a bathtub, or making telephone calls. On each item, anywhere from two to seven different levels or categories of "ability" are distinguished, which have quantitative values from 0 (or 1) to the highest. The lowest category corresponds to no ability/cannot do at all/need maximum help, and the highest to independence, "normal," or even above average. Additional metrics have been used, such as difficulty (23) and time needed (24). For measures of participation, metrics used include frequency of performing an activity (13), hours spent on an activity (25), share of activities performed (26), and others. The numbers a patient or subject receives on the constituent items typically are added together, and the total (with or without further arithmetical manipulation) reflects his or her functional status in the domain being measured. For some measures, the items all have the same number of categories (steps) and the same minimum and maximum value (e.g. FIM), but that is not necessarily the case—for instance, the Barthel Index (27) consists of some items with only two categories of ability, but the other items have three. Differential scoring of the categories from one item to the next can be used to express the relative weight (importance) of the constituent skills for overall functioning, according to the instrument's creator. A separate weighting step prior to addition can be used to achieve the same purpose.

The numeric values of the categories (item scale categories or steps) represent measurement on an ordinal scale—they only indicate relative order along the fully able/not able (or not participating at all/fully participating) continuum, but the differences between scale steps are not necessarily equivalent, and the values chosen for them are arbitrary. As a consequence, adding up the scores for the items to obtain the total score is not a legitimate operation. Therefore, total scores do not reflect the subject's/patient's position along a continuum that has a true zero point, and distances between scale points do not necessarily correspond to ability differences that exist in reality.

For instance, the difference between the FIM motor subscale scores of 20 and 40 is not necessarily the same as the difference between the scores of 40 and 60. (Equidistance between scale points and a true zero point constitute the definition of a ratio scale, which is what is required for calculating means for a group, or percentage improvement over time). One should be quite careful in interpreting FA instrument scores as applied to individuals and to groups. In particular, "percent improvement" and "change efficiency scores" should be considered as nothing but approximations of the mathematical precision they appear to offer. However, research has shown that if the item category values are chosen "reasonably," the sum of ordinal items corresponds quite well to values on a true ratio scale, at least for intermediate levels of the continuum of total scores (28). Rasch analysis (29), a mathematical procedure based on Item Response Theory (IRT) has been used to transform a set of scores on ordinal FA items into a score on an interval scale (13, 23, 28). (The theoretical assumptions and mathematical manipulations underlying Rasch-based FA instruments are beyond the scope of this chapter; good introductions to the technique and its application to FA may be found in Bond and Fox [29].)

ISSUES IN FUNCTIONAL ASSESSMENT

FA instruments seem simple to create and apply, and their apparent simplicity has led to developments of hundreds of measures, many of which have never seen more than one application. A number of issues need to be considered in their creation and application, many of which are linked to one another. Among some important concerns are the following:

Capacity and Performance

Two aspects of functioning are commonly distinguished: capacity and performance (8, 30) Capacity is what people can do under optimal circumstances—well rested, encouraged to do their best, in an environment with minimal barriers. Performance is what they do in everyday life. People who are capable of doing self-care may not always do it, for a variety of reasons. One of the most common is that their environment is not accommodating, or that the energy and time a task requires preferentially are spent on other, more worthwhile endeavors—whether that is employment or watching one's favorite soap opera. Studies with SCI patients have shown that many for whom self-care is a "marginal" skill prefer to have a personal care attendant or family member perform their care, so that they can get out of the house and get to their job (31).

At the Impairment end of the disablement continuum, measures of functional limitations tend to be capacity focused. The ASIA motor scale (32) is based on ability to contract key muscles, and the physician and patient are hardly interested in the patient's actual frequency of contracting those muscles. At the other end of the continuum, measures of participation or community integration without exception quantify performance. It is either impossible to test capacity (how could one test "ability to function as a brain surgeon"), or not of concern: it is actual performance that is of interest when evaluating the long-term outcome of rehabilitative efforts, not potential. It is in the middle ground, the domain of Activities, that a discrepancy between capacity and performance is most likely to be relevant, and where performance is modifiable with environmental and other interventions (30).

Testing, Observation, and Reporting on Performance

Three main methods are used to collect functional information. Testing involves requiring the patient or client (or research subject) to perform specific tasks or skills under the direct supervision of the test administrator, who times the test, assesses the amount of help from devices or aides that is needed, etc. This tends to occur in laboratory or clinical settings, but testing can also be done in the person's home or other locale where the activities involved are or should be performed (33). Depending on the degree to which the test situation approximates an optimal one, the resulting score quantifies optimal capacity, or capacity in the situation that is considered most relevant to the uses to which the functional information is to be put.

Observation of habitual behavior is the basis for quantifying what the person does do, rather than what he or she can do. Most functional assessments of Activity reported as part of inpatient or outpatient rehabilitation programs are observation-based—at least in theory. For instance, the Uniform Data System (UDS) FIM admission and discharge scores are based on what the patients do in the first three days after admission or the last three before discharge. In practice, there is continuous pressure on the patients to perform at their best, especially in treatment with Physical and Occupational Therapists, and the measure of performance turns into a measure of capacity. Research using the Level of Rehabilitation Scale (LORS), for instance, has shown that scores reported by therapists are systematically higher than those reported by nurses (34). Nurses presumably report on what they observe the patients doing when going about their life on the nursing unit, but therapists only see them during scheduled hours, where they cannot waste time observing what the patients do naturally—the therapists need to optimize the patients' performance.

A third way of collecting FA information is through report by the patient, or a proxy such as a family member. These reports can involve capacity (for instance, in the Capabilities of Upper Extremity instrument [19]), but more typically address performance. Questions are asked about how the person performs the various activities included in the FA measure in his or her daily routine. Using a standardized questionnaire, trained interviewers can reach a high level of inter-rater (inter-interviewer) reliability. This is how data are typically collected for follow-up assessments in the UDS and other program evaluation systems.

All three methods have their advantages and disadvantages, qua cost, personnel needed, required ability of the patient/subject to cooperate with the data collection, etc. If capacity data are of interest, testing is the preferred method; for true performance data, interviewing is the only feasible approach. Problems arise when the data obtained by two methods need to be linked. For instance, a typical question (clinically and in research) is whether the person manages to maintain or even improve on the skills he or she was discharged with from inpatient rehabilitation. The hospital data are typically collected using observation, in an environment that tends to be more accessible than the typical residence, and with

overt or covert pressure to perform one's best. The home follow-up data are normally collected using interviews and concern performance in a different environment in which there may be no incentive at all to use all the abilities taught in rehabilitation (35). If between hospital and home a change in functional performance is noted, is this due to the data collection method per se, or due to changes in the environment, or even because of changes in the true underlying capacity (continued neurological recovery)? This issue has hardly been studied, and we do not know enough about how scores on a given FA instrument may differ by data collection method to tease apart differences in scores (36).

The Nature of the Items in FA Instruments

In an IQ test, the person tested completes multiple arithmetic problems, similarities, and other items which in themselves are not of interest to the test administrator. The IQ score that results is of interest, because it gives an (approximate) indication of the person's overall intelligence. The focus is on the underlying trait—intelligence. In FA, however, the items most likely have intrinsic meaning to the person performing the assessment and to the individual assessed: they reflect activities that are of importance in and of themselves—whether it is stair climbing or communicating a simple idea. FA "tends to occur within a realistic setting that approximates the one in which the actual criterion behavior will occur" (2, p. 101). That does not mean that there is no underlying construct "functional ability" that is of interest—but the underlying ability is of concern mostly because it informs on the functional items that were part of the assessment, and possibly on those that were not part of it. Because the primary interest is in the items (tasks, activities) themselves, there always is a tendency to include in FA measures the full panoply of acts that are part of normal human functioning. The Patient Evaluation and Conference System (PECS) in one of its versions included 97 items, of which as many as applicable to the patient were to be completed by therapists (37, 38). Such an extensive menu is feasible when various staff report on patient status within their area of expertise (speech and language, neuropsychology, chaplaincy, etc.) but not in situations where subjects are tested or are required to report on their performance. Maintaining a balance between feasibility and inclusion of those functional tasks that are key to living has always been a balancing act for FA instrument developers. Measures that cover "all areas of life" (or at least all aspects of Activities and Participation) tend to consist of fairly broadly defined tasks (e.g. "dressing"), and limit the number to 10 to 20. Instruments developed for use by specific rehabilitation disciplines are apt to include more narrowly defined tasks ("putting on a pull-over") and include a large number: the Klein-Bell ADL Scale contains 170 items to cover just six areas: dressing, mobility, elimination, bathing/hygiene, eating, and emergency telephone use (39).

When the focus of FA shifts from performance of specific, individual tasks to the status of broad underlying abilities ("self care"; "motoric strength and coordination"), the need to include each and every possible item diminishes. Traditional psychometric methods can be used to show that the underlying construct can be measured with one set of items (indicators) as well as with another set, and that the resulting total scores will have high correlations with one another. For instance, some measures of functional limitations (the transition area between Impairments and Activities) do not attempt to "cover the waterfront"—they select activities that are representative of the entire universe of relevant items and use those to score, for instance, upper extremity functioning. After all, once it is known how much difficulty a subject has picking up a can of soup and how much with a ream of paper, it should be fairly clear how well she would do lifting a paperback book. To what degree this same reasoning applies at the other end of the disablement spectrum, Participation, is not yet known (17). The ICF distinguishes about 90 different aspects of "Participation," in 9 chapters covering communication, mobility, domestic life, etc. Is it necessary to obtain information on all of these to get a complete view of someone's level of Participation (18)? Or is it possible to extrapolate from three household tasks to all others, and also to know quite adequately how well the person does in the domain of civic responsibilities? That depends to a large degree on whether Participation is a single unidimensional construct or a large collection of items that all reflect Participation in some way, but do not even represent multiple dimensions of the same construct (40, 41). There presumably are key Participation components that no FA instrument would want to omit (work, social relations with family), but the need to collect information on all others is still not known. These and other problems involved in measuring Participation are discussed in greater detail elsewhere (18).

ISSUES IN MEASUREMENT: THE PSYCHOMETRIC CHARACTERISTICS OF FA INSTRUMENTS

Whenever we measure, error creeps into the resulting score, whether it is a small error in measuring simple concrete characteristics (for instance, the area of a room), or a large error in quantifying abstract concepts such as authoritarianism. FA is no exception, and the issue is not so much getting rid of the error (we never will be able to do that completely), but being sensitive to the amount of error our data may contain, and being aware what that means for any conclusions we draw and actions we

undertake based on those data. Metrology (the science of measuring) is a major concern in all science disciplines, and the developers and users of FA instruments have mostly relied on the metrological methodologies for instrument development originating in psychology, known as psychometrics. "Psychometrics" is a very technical and for most clinicians a very boring subject, but knowledge of some of the basics is necessary for the fruitful use of FA instruments. Additional information may be found in handbooks in this area (e.g. Streiner and Norman [42]) and didactic articles. The one by Johnston and Graves is not only focused on SCI, but addresses some issues in IRT approaches to measurement instrument development that are not touched upon here (43).

Traditionally, two aspects of the data reflecting the results of measurement have had most emphasis, validity, and reliability, but in clinical applications such issues as sensitivity and practicality are increasingly getting attention. In theory, reliability is an aspect of validity, but most people tend to think of them as separate characteristics of instruments (or, more properly, of the data produced by instruments), and the techniques for quantifying validity and reliability are separate. "Validity" refers to the question, is this instrument measuring what it purports to measure? If it is targeting characteristic X, do the numbers that result from the measurement operation (the "scores") actually reflect X, and not characteristic Y, or a little of X with a lot of trait Z? "Reliability" refers to the question, how reproducible is this measurement—if we repeated the measurement operation with the same or a similar "ruler," and we know that the person has not changed, would we get the same result? As illustrated in Figure 8.2, an instrument can be very reliable without being valid. If it is not reliable at all, it is by definition not valid. The goal we are aiming for is instruments that are both valid (they measure what we want to measure) and reliable (they give results that are reproducible).

Over the years, a great many techniques have been developed to estimate validity and reliability, each applicable to different situations. Unfortunately, psychologists and social scientists have fallen into the habit of "inventing" new types of validity and reliability, by naming them after the techniques. However, there is no such thing as test-retest reliability or construct validity.

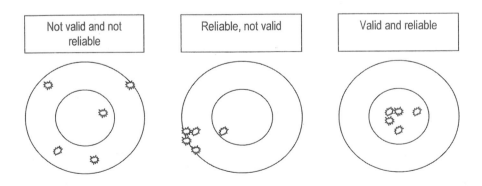

Only when all one's bullets (FA instrument items) hit the bull's eye (construct of interest) can it be said that the gun (measurement instrument) is true (valid). A concentration of hits somewhere else on the target suggests a flawed gun used by a steady-eyed shooter.

Figure 8.2   The relationship of reliability and validity.

There is only one validity and one reliability for each instrument, which are estimated using different techniques.

Reliability

Estimating the reliability of measures is the easiest to understand. All estimation methods are based on some form of repeat measurement. If two clinicians at the same time rate the ability of patient X on the FIM Grooming item, they should come up with the same number—or else one or both are wrong. We can estimate the reliability of the FIM grooming item as used by these two clinicians by having the two rate a few hundred patients, and calculate how often they agree—completely, or almost so. A statistical formula such as coefficient kappa (or weighted kappa) can be used to express the level of agreement. (Kappa also takes into account the fact that chance agreement may occur, especially if the number of categories is limited or one category is very "popular" with both raters.) All these formulas are constructed in such a way that the result, the reliability coefficient, varies between 0.00 (no reliability whatsoever) and 1.00 (perfect reliability). "Inter-rater reliability" can be estimated based on a few raters to represent all possible raters, so that we can have an idea as to how reliable this one-item instrument (FIM Grooming) is in the hands of the average clinician.

If the same patients are rated by the same clinician twice, we similarly can calculate "intra-rater reliability," the degree to which she agrees with her earlier ratings. There are two scenarios for this—either the patients' performance is videotaped, or the rater observes the patients twice. In the latter case, it is of course important that we are sure these patients have not changed in the mean time. In both instances, the clinician should "forget" about her rating the first time around—which is not that difficult if large numbers of ratings are to be made.

Functional status is a fairly broad and abstract entity (a "construct," in psychometrical parlance), and it is unlikely that a single item such as Grooming can represent the entire construct. Typically, we select multiple indicators (items), and combine them to adequately operationalize the theoretical definition we may have. Use of multiple indicators has another advantage—random measurement error in quantifying any one item is likely offset by the random error in another item. (For that reason, the more items there are in an instrument, the more reliable it will be, ceteris paribus, because the chance of random error being eliminated is increased. Any systematic error will remain, however, and practicality issues come into play if instruments are too long). Because each item in an FA instrument is a repeat measurement of the construct, like the two raters for Grooming are repeat measures, we can calculate the agreement between items as yet another estimate of reliability. A number of formulas to estimate "internal consistency reliability" exist, the most frequently used of which is (Cronbach's) coefficient alpha. "Split-half" and "parallel forms" reliability are related formulas. All of them take values between 0.00 and 1.00.

The minimal reliability a measure needs to have depends on the purpose to which the data are to be put. A minimum of 0.90 for situations where decisions on an individual patient need to be made (discharge Mrs. Jones or extend her stay another week?) is often quoted, but 0.70 or 0.80 is a typical minimum required for group applications, such as in program evaluation and research. Longer instruments tend to be more reliable, but the trend is toward the use of short forms, such as the SF-12 and the CHART-SF, rather than long ones, like their parents SF-36 and CHART. With better construction, new short instruments can offer reliability approximating that of older long ones. Another development is computer-adapted testing (CAT), in which only those questions that are targeted to the ability level of the person are being asked (44). For very simple instruments, paper-and-pencil adapted testing is possible (45, 46).

Validity

Validity cannot be estimated in such a simple way as reliability can, except in one unusual situation: there is an existing instrument that we are certain is perfectly valid and thus, perfectly reliable. In that case, we can administer this existing instrument and a newly proposed one to a sample, calculate the correlation between the two scores, and use that correlation as the estimate of the validity of the new measure. The issue of course is: if there is a perfectly good measure (a "gold standard"), why is there a need to develop a new one? The importance of having a shorter instrument may be the only acceptable reason. Less powerful methods to estimate validity are used in the more common situation: there is no existing measure, or the existing ones are problematic in themselves.

In the absence of a gold standard, correlations with existing measure(s) are used to validate a new one; it is assumed that the old and new measure will correlate strongly, providing evidence of "convergent validity." Sometimes correlations are also computed with characteristics that are seen as unrelated to the one the new measure is operationalizing; the expected low correlation is seen as evidence for "divergent validity."

"Face validity" is (in the eyes of most authorities) not a form of validity assessment, but an answer to the question, does the instrument "on the face of it" measure what those completing it expect to see—does a measure of trait X actually have questions about X that patients/subjects recognize as such? Some instruments have no or little face validity, but are perfectly valid—for instance, the Minnesota Multiphasic Personality Inventory (MMPI). However, instruments that lack face validity may not be completed, or not be completed correctly, because the patient fails to see their relevance. In the arena of FA, face validity is hardly an issue, because the activities that are used as indicators have a fairly low level of abstraction, and are recognized by patients as relevant to their life.

The closely related term "content validity" refers to a measure actually covering the entire construct the developer is targeting. It is generally determined by having experts draw up lists of necessary content for a measure of X, or checking the content of a draft measure against their unwritten expectations. Of course, this presumes there is a clear description (by the authors) of the concept they would like to operationalize—it makes no sense criticizing the veracity of a painted portrait if you don't know the person depicted. There are no standard formulas for calculating this validity aspect.

"Predictive validity" concerns the ability of a measure to predict a future state or event that is inherently linked to the characteristic being measured. A college entrance examination is said to have predictive validity if it can be used to accurately predict who in four (five, six) years will graduate. A parallel in FA would be the ability of a measure to predict for inpatient rehabilitation patients who will be successfully discharged home versus to a nursing home. One problem with predictive validity assessment is the fact that there are no hard and fast rules as to what should be the minimum level of success in predicting. We know that many factors affect successful independent living—the accessibility of the home, family, and other supports available, the person's determination and tolerance for risk, etc. Does an FA instrument have adequate predictive validity if predictions based on it are correct at least 50% of the time? At least 80%?

"Known group validity" is based on differences in scale scores between two groups that are known to differ in the characteristic the instrument aims to measure. The average score of persons with SCI on a measure of physical functioning should be lower than the average of persons with TBI; in case of a measure of cognitive functioning, the situation should be reversed. If the data do not parallel these expectations, it is quite likely the instrument is not measuring what we think it is. Alternatively, a lot of systematic error (bias) is reflected in the data. A similar problem as mentioned above occurs with determining known group validity: how much of the variation in the functional status of the overall group should be explained by diagnostic category, SCI vs. TBI? If every person with SCI is known to have a higher physical functioning level than every person with a TBI, things would be easy: the variation explained should be 100%, and everything lower than that would mean less than perfect validity. However, the distributions for functioning ability of the TBI and SCI groups overlap, and the variation explained in a t-test reflects both the difference between group means, the standard deviations around those means, and the random and systematic error in the measure we use. Stating that a good functional measure should explain between 1% and 100% of variance is not very helpful in selecting or developing an instrument.

Lastly, "construct validity" concerns the relationships between the measurement data of a (highly abstract) construct and data for other constructs. Sometimes we have a basis in theory to predict that construct K should be strongly related to (yet not identical with) construct L, and be independent of construct M. (For instance, "ADL ability is related to community integration, but unrelated to political party preference"). If the data bring this out, the operationalization of K should be valid (and similarly the operationalizations of L and M). If the predicted association between K and L is minimal or absent, however, we don't know if the problem is with the theory, or the operationalization of K, or the measurement of L. And it is an unusual theory that specifies the exact strength of the relationship between K and L, predicated on perfect measurement of the constructs involved. "Strong" or "very strong" is the best we get from theorists, and those are not very good starting points for evaluating the level of validity of the instruments involved.

The above discussion should make clear that estimating the validity of instruments is always less straightforward than the quantification of their reliability. Finding high values parallel to e.g., a 0.91 level of test-retest reliability just does not happen; validity coefficients are much lower because all methods of validity estimation are roundabout. In practice, it is necessary to use all possible methods of estimating validity, and based on multiple findings "patch together" evidence supporting validity—which never will be iron-clad. Finding encouraging levels of the various types of validity distinguished here, in multiple studies, with patterns of correlations that make sense based on expert knowledge, is what typically occurs. Fortunately, in the case of FA, the specialists involved have extensive knowledge of the determinants, correlates, intergroup differences, etc. of various aspects of functional status, making the issue of assessing the metrologic quality of specific measures less problematic than the preceding list of issues might suggest.

"Ecological validity" does not concern validity per se, but the relevance of assessment data to real-life situations outside the testing situation. Testing ambulation in situations that resemble the real world more than the parallel bars in the Physical Therapy gym provides data that are more "ecologically valid," but the standardization of testing might suffer. Standardization of testing has always been a keystone of psychometric methods of assessing reliability and validity of neuropsychological instruments, and of instruments of the abilities of individual patients or clients, all capacity measures. However, standardized environments tend to be dissimilar from the settings where people perform self-care, communicate, do work, and all other things captured under the umbrella of functioning. Testing in a standardized environment almost always means in an optimal environment (30), and the results tend therefore to be more indicative of capacity than of performance.

Sensitivity

It is easy to see that if an FA "measure" has just two categories, "able" and "unable," it lacks sensitivity: it cannot reflect fine distinctions in capacity/ability/performance, and it cannot be used to record minor but clinically significant changes in performance. Sensitivity refers to the ability of an instrument to capture distinctions that are clinically relevant or small enough to be of importance in research, across the full range of ability of the cases to be measured. When sensitivity is discussed in relation to change over time (from admission to discharge, for example), the term responsiveness is frequently used.

Floor effects and ceiling effects are one issue in sensitivity. The first terms refer to the lowest measurable level of performance on an FA instrument being higher than the status of the least able person to be measured. All individuals who have ability equal to the lowest measurable level or lower are clumped together and given the corresponding score. Vice versa, a ceiling effect means that the highest measurable level is lower than the performance level of at least some of the more able patients/clients/subjects. It should be noted that very often measures are developed for one population in which they have no floor or ceiling effects but then are applied to another in which they do. For instance, the FIM was designed to quantify functional status of rehabilitation inpatients, and any patient who achieves the maximum score on discharge probably was an inappropriate admission. However, a few years after onset of incomplete paraplegia (e.g. C4 or below, ASIA D), many persons will score at the maximum of the FIM Motor subscale. The FIM was never designed to distinguish between people with minimal deficits that do not affect functioning, other mere mortals, and superman. Thus, "lack of responsiveness" sometimes is a problem for which the instrument user is responsible, not the instrument developer.

Quantification of responsiveness is not done using formulas resulting in simple coefficients ranging from 0.0 (not responsive at all) to 1.0 (maximum responsiveness possible). All quantification methods are mostly useful for comparing the responsiveness of one measure with that of another, allowing one to select the most responsive one. A variety of indices are used, including effect sizes (the mean change between time 1 and time 2 divided by the standard deviation at time 1), the standardized response mean (the mean change between time 1 and time 2, divided by the standard deviation of change scores), receiver operating characteristic (ROC) analysis, and many others. Discussion of these indices is beyond the scope of this chapter; the reader is referred to the extensive literature (47–49). A particular subgroup of these indices involves the use of a global rating, typically by the patients themselves, that from time 1 to time 2 they have improved (or deteriorated) a little or a lot, or stayed the same. Score changes on any relevant FA measure should correspond to these subjective "transition ratings" (50, 51), or else it lacks responsiveness.

Other Psychometric Characteristics

Beyond validity, reliability, and sensitivity, there are a number of other characteristics of an FA measure that are relevant to its use in clinical, program evaluation, and research applications, most of which have to do with practicality:

- Language: Issues of wording are especially relevant to self-administered instruments such as the CUE (19), but may also be an issue with observational and other measures (52). Both the reading level and a translation in a language the user is familiar with are of concern. In SCI, the terms in standard instruments such as "walk" in the SF-36 may be problematic in that they are not applicable to those who use a wheelchair for mobility, and even may be interpreted as reflecting insensitivity on the part of the researcher (53).
- Training required: Many observational FA instruments and test-type measures require the user to be trained, and sometimes certified (33), in order to produce reliable data.
- Availability and costs: Some measures are copyrighted, and may not be available at all, or only for a one-time or per-use payment.
- Time and equipment required: Measures that take inordinate time on the part of the subjects or the administrator, or that use special equipment (in some test-type measures such as the Tufts Assessment of Motor Performance—TAMP [54]) may not be suitable outside research applications.
- Alternative versions: Availability of a proxy version may be useful for self-report measures used with children, adults with high tetraplegia, or individuals with cognitive-communicative deficits. Similarly, equivalent versions are of use in situations (e.g. psychological testing) where subjects may "learn the test," and would appear to gain in skills on repeat administration of a single version.
- Patient safety: If testing the ability to drive a car is disturbed by the tester's intervention every time there seems to be danger, the test result is not very realistic. On the other hand, not interfering at all is not to the benefit of the person tested—or the tester. Simulations such as virtual reality (see below) have been developed to make realistic testing in situations like this possible.
- Clinical utility: If administration and scoring of a measure does not add to the clinician's knowledge base, or if the

information does not help him or her to make decisions with respect to a particular patient or a class of patients, the instrument lacks clinical utility. Interpretability of the scores may contribute to clinical utility; availability of norms (for all persons with SCI, or preferably for subgroups who are comparable in terms of age, level and completeness of injury, etc.) is of benefit in some instances.

USES OF FUNCTIONAL ASSESSMENT

The origin of FA (defined narrowly as measurement of activity limitations) is in attempts by clinicians to express quantitatively the deficits patients had on admission to rehabilitation, and to monitor progress, or at least determine discharge status, so that there was some "proof" of the effectiveness of treatment, beyond the patient's simple report that he or she now could do things that were impossible or difficult before admission. The forerunners of instruments such as the Barthel Index (BI) (27) were simple checklists for recording (lack of) problems with performing self-care and mobility activities (2). From these simple early efforts, measurement instruments of sometimes great sophistication have grown. In addition, the range of applications of these instruments has expanded tremendously, so that we now can describe uses in the care of individual patients, in treatment programs as a whole, for reimbursement, and for research. The type of information needed in these various applications is somewhat different, and even when the basic instrument used is the same (the FIM is the "workhorse" of rehabilitation, and is used almost throughout all these types of applications), ideally there would be differences in scoring or other details.

Care of Individual Patients

Decisions on admission to inpatient and outpatient programs are often based on a formal FA, to see if the person has the types and degrees of deficits that the program is qualified and authorized to treat, either in general or for the specific person in question. The "baseline" assessment therefore is often communicated to the third-party payer, who may use it to approve program admission and a certain duration or intensity of treatment. The pre-admission or admission assessment is frequently the basis for a prognosis, which is communicated to the patient and the payer, and ideally underlies goal setting. Many programs use an FA instrument such as the FIM to set expected outcomes, either for classes of patients or for individual patients. Software applications have been developed to assist case managers to make such predictions; they are based in large part on a data base that contains information on many previous patients with the same rehabilitation diagnosis, age, gender, and co-morbidities.

Treatment monitoring using an FA measure is done in many rehabilitation programs, even if no explicit goal setting was done. Team rounds often consist of the reporting by "most responsible/knowledgeable therapies" (nursing for bladder; speech for expression, etc.) of the current status of the patient on the numeric items offered by the FA instrument used in the facility. Almost all rehabilitation programs quantify status on discharge, because that information is needed to document program results, and subsequently is used in program evaluation. Although treatment termination decisions are increasingly based on "external" criteria (e.g. a maximal length of stay approved by a third-party payer), ideally they are founded on either the accomplishment of goals or plateauing of the patient in terms of overall functional ability. In both instances, measurement of patient status should be performed using an instrument that has minimal error so that (lack of) change can be reliably determined. Decisions on treatment termination should be based on a number of factors that include not just functional status (achievement of treatment goal, plateauing) but also family factors, carry over, and continuation or generalization of functional skills learned in therapy to the home environment, to name a few.

FA information may also be used to communicate about progress and outcomes of treatment with persons who are not part of the team. Patients themselves, their family members, referral sources, and payers have a prime interest in the functional aspects of the patient's status, especially where it concerns Activities and Participation. One additional use of FA for individual cases is long-term monitoring of a patient's status. Especially in the case of progressive diseases, this type of information is important to make decisions on new treatments, changes in patient environments, etc. In fact, this use of FA has led to a designation of functional status information as a sixth (after the standard four and pain) vital sign (55).

Unfortunately, case managers and medical insurance companies may demand that improvement is measured using instruments that do not capture the extent of improvement that may be seen. An example is the use of the FIM in an SCI patient with high-level tetraplegia. This scale is unlikely to adequately document improvement due to the FIM's insensitivity in this group. In the outpatient setting, the FIM also may not capture higher-level improvements in function due to a ceiling effect. A broad understanding of the pitfalls of available scales allows the healthcare provider to best apply these measurements and educate insurers.

Program Administration and Evaluation

Most rehabilitation programs have as their overall goal something along the lines of "to improve quality of life by reducing impairments and increasing activities and participation." Program evaluation aims to assess to what degree a program indeed accomplishes what it sets out to do—improve the functional status of people with disablement. Basic questions are, do patients change for the better (program effectiveness), and if so, are resources used optimally in accomplishing this (program efficiency)? Program evaluation is required by the Commission on Accreditation of Rehabilitation Facilities (CARF)(http://www.carf.org), a widely recognized not-for profit that accredits rehabilitation organizations and programs.

Although change from program admission to discharge is common, it is unfortunately not easy to offer proof that the program deserves credit. For instance, a person with SCI may score higher on a post-test than on a pre-test for a number of reasons that have nothing to do with the selection, timing, quality, and quantity of services received. Positive change may be due to natural recovery, improved test-taking ability, and many other factors (56, 57). All rehabilitation programs face the same problem of proving effectiveness, and one (partial) solution that

has been found is to compare outcomes between programs, under the assumption that not all change in all programs can be explained by causes other than treatment received, and the "excess" change in the best programs is truly the result of interventions. Longitudinal evaluation of a program's outcomes is facilitated by the creation of a "minimum data set" for all programs that includes demographics, time since injury, and measures of injury severity, in addition to specific scales of functioning, selection of which depends on program type and time of follow-up (58). The UDS, in which many inpatient rehabilitation facilities in the United States participate, as well as some subacute facilities and nursing homes that offer rehabilitation, is one such data aggregator.

Comparisons between programs are only fair, of course, if their inputs (admission status) are the same; it may be much easier to bring an admit FIM score of 50 up to 100 for someone with SCI than for a patient with TBI. Thus, UDS and other aggregators produce reports that compare like with like, in terms of diagnostic group, co-morbidities, age, and other factors considered relevant to chances of program success—the relevant "case mix" (59). The focus of program evaluation tends to be on functional status change over time as the key indicator of program effectiveness. Because the better programs may achieve a certain level of change using far fewer resources than poorly organized ones, length of stay (LOS) is typically used as a gross indicator of resource use. Functional status change per day, then, is an indicator of program efficiency. (It may be worth repeating that a number of assumptions, including interval-level measurement of functional status, are made in calculating this index, assumptions that may not stand up to scrutiny.) There are other methods of evaluating a program's effectiveness, e.g. by calculating what percentage of the patients did achieve the goals that were set at admission. It is to be expected that a small percentage of patients do not progress as well as anticipated, e.g. due to intercurrent illness. But if a large percentage fails to achieve the standardized or individualized functional goals set for them, the program may be selecting patients who are inappropriate for its services, setting goals that are too high, or employing staff or utilizing treatments that are ineffective. Shifts in the program's admission and management policies or its processes may be needed. Unfortunately, routine program evaluation data tend to be insufficient to indicate where exactly the problem is and how it can be fixed; additional studies may be needed to obtain that information. Routine outcome data can and should be communicated to stakeholders, including current and future patients, third-party payers, and the local community. The Centers for Medicare and Medicaid Services (CMS) has started to post comparative functional outcomes for nursing homes and home health agencies on its Web site, and it is to be expected that similar "report cards" including FA information will be published in the future for many other facilities that offer rehabilitation of some type.

Choosing appropriate functional measures for the evaluation of an SCI program should be based on what point of the rehabilitation spectrum the program serves. Measures of Body Structure/Function would be apt for acute inpatient care. Activity measures are most appropriate for acute or subacute inpatient care; Participation measures are needed to assess the effectiveness and efficiency of outpatient services in the community, e.g. vocational rehabilitation services.

In addition to program evaluation and accreditation purposes, FA data are used in a variety of activities centering on improving the quality of program services. Whether called outcomes management, continuous quality improvement (CQI), or total quality management (TQM), they all involve considering the service-delivery organization as a system, with parts and subsystems that all should be studied continuously to reduce inefficiencies, improve administrative and clinical procedures, and reduce risks and adverse events (3). FA information almost by definition plays a key role in making decisions in programs that deal with individuals with SCI or other disabilities. For instance, an admission-to-discharge increase in functioning of less than a specified minimum could trigger an in-depth investigation into whether a problem (an "opportunity to improve processes") exists. FA information could also function as a monitor that is collected routinely to indicate performance of the program(s)—a vital sign for the organization.

Effective 2002, CMS has, under its Prospective Payment System (PPS), paid inpatient rehabilitation facilities (IRFs) fixed amounts for each patient discharged, rather than reimbursing (adjusted) charges, costs of operations, or some other formula used in earlier years and still used by some other payers. The fixed amounts are based in part on the functional status of the patient on admission, combined with diagnostic category (stroke, SCI, TBI, etc.) and age category. For functional status a minor variation on the FIM is used, which is embedded in the Inpatient Rehabilitation Facility-Patient Assessment Instrument (IRF-PAI [60]). The combination of diagnosis, status, category, and age defines a group of patients whose rehabilitation requires unique resources, as acknowledged in the payment amount for each case (61). (This payment is further adjusted for comorbidities ["tiers"], salary levels in the region the facility is located, etc.). The PPS has given IRFs financial incentive to hasten, if not improve functional improvement and other outcomes, and to perform more complete and accurate admission functional assessments. Nursing homes and home health agencies are paid on a similar basis as IRFs, but have their own forms. CMS is now (2009) developing an assessment instrument and payment system that would be applicable to all of post-acute care (62).

The National Committee on Vital and Health Statistics (NCVHS) has recommended capturing and classifying functional status information as part of routine health care transactions, so that administrative databases could be mined and used for a variety of purposes, including monitoring overall population health, health care management, public health planning, predicting costs and financial management, and policy development (63). At the moment, only limited information on functioning is available, mostly through Medicare files on special populations: those receiving inpatient rehabilitation, nursing home residents, and people receiving home health services. NCVHS suggested that, with modifications, the ICF might be a useful taxonomic system (a "uniform code") on which to base such data collection across the continuum of care. The uniform code would not prescribe how to measure functional status, but would only specify what data elements need to be reported. (In this sense, it would be comparable with e.g. the International Classification of Diseases (ICD), which does not specify how to diagnose a particular disease, only what the disorders of interest are and how they are related to one another).

A German group under the guidance of Stucki and associated with the WHO has begun the development of ICF "core sets"—listings of selected Impairments, Activity Limitations, and Participation Restrictions that are of particular relevance to the care and management of a particular diagnostic group (64), including SCI (65). The ICF allows coding of the severity of Impairments, Activity Limitations, and Participation Restrictions (66), but what is offered are very "primitive" methods of measurement. Presumably, productive use of the core sets, especially in applications beyond clinical care, requires FA measures.

Clinicians and researchers associated with the International Spinal Cord Society (ISCoS) have initiated a process of creating SCI "data sets." These data sets specify both the content and format of information that needs to be included in clinical records (basic data sets) and research records (basic and expanded data sets) in a particular area (67). To date, a core data set has been published (68), as well as data sets for pain (69), bowel function (70, 71), and urinary tract function and urodynamics (72, 73). Those focusing on FA as defined here are still under development.

Research

Program evaluation typically does not address what was done for individual patients to explain changes in functional status and link those interventions to outcomes (the "black box" aspect of rehabilitation) (74). It also does not systematically address alternative explanations for outcomes, and has no hard evidence for the effectiveness of traditional or innovative treatments. This is where research comes in. Per early March, 2009, Medline contained over 36,200 records marked with "Activities of Daily Living," which is the term used to classify papers on ADLs, (chronic) limitations of activity, independent living, and self care. FA papers are also indexed under other headings—for instance, "geriatric assessment" added another 8,700 unduplicated records. Of this total, only a small number address clinical application at the level of the individual (presumably less than 5%) and a slightly larger number (maybe 10%) concern the program level uses of FA measures. Most published research concerns the development of FA instruments, including assessing their reliability, validity, sensitivity, and practicality characteristics; the use of FA measures to evaluate the effects of rehabilitation or experimental rehabilitative treatments; screening subjects for such treatment programs; evaluating the links between Impairment, Activity, and Participation; describing the natural course of disablement; or assessing the financial and social impact of disability.

Because functioning is the central interest of rehabilitation providers, researchers, and their patients/clients, it is to be expected that much of their research uses FA information as either the "independent" (predictor) variable, the "dependent" (outcome) variable, or both. It is worthwhile to remember, though, that before any use is made of the results of this research, it needs to be assessed in terms of the applicability of the FA instruments selected, and their psychometric qualities. The conclusions of and recommendations by researchers are only as good as the FA instruments they used.

SUBJECTIVE VALUATION OF FUNCTIONAL PERFORMANCE

A major criticism of most of the FA measures used in SCI clinical care, program evaluation, and research is the fact that they do not reflect the subjective view of the person involved. "Normal functioning" may be a laudable goal, but not if that functioning detracts from the person's subjective QOL. Several studies have shown that measures of participation account for much more of the variance in life satisfaction or well-being than do measures of impairment or activity limitations (75–78). Thus, for at least some applications, the fit between functional activities and the person's values and preferences needs to be considered and reflected in some way in FA instruments, especially in Participation measures. The point of view of the insider, the person with SCI, to date has not been investigated with any degree of the attention it deserves.

Although most instruments designed to measure aspects of "functioning" have concentrated on the "how independent" and "how much" of acts, actions, and roles, a few have explored additional dimensions. Goal Attainment Scaling (GAS) and the Canadian Occupational Performance Measure (COPM) are semistructured approaches by which rehabilitation service recipients and clinicians formulate individualized goals for therapy and provide perceptions of the adequacy of their performance, their satisfaction with performance, and the importance of each goal to their lives (79–81). The choice of goals reflects individual valuation, as does the importance rating. An importance-weighted sum of outcome serves as the key evaluation measure. A number of other instruments with standardized content have included importance ratings such as the MACTAR (82) and many instruments traditionally classified as quality of life measures (83).

Versions of the Community Integration Questionnaire (CIQ) used principally in brain injury populations allow subjects to express their opinions and feelings about their participation (84, 85). Research with the Participation Objective Participation Subjective (POPS) indicates a similar disjunction between people's functional status and their satisfaction with that status, or interest in changing it (25). Several participation measures published in recent years incorporate an evaluative aspect of participation, including the Community Integration Measure (86), the Impact on Participation and Autonomy questionnaire (87), and the Keele Assessment of Participation (88); not all of these have seen use in SCI yet.

SELECTION OF A FUNCTIONAL ASSESSMENT MEASURE

The selection of an FA measure to apply in a clinical, administrative, or research situation is not straightforward. A first step always should be determining what one wants to measure: Activity (Limitation) only, or (aspects of) Impairment and Participation (Restriction) in addition. Although there are instruments such as the Disability Rating Scale used in TBI research that cover all three domains, they often do that poorly, and offer no separate scores for the two or three domains. As the correlations between Impairment, Activity Limitation, and Participation Restriction are typically low (89), using two or three separate instruments may be preferable. A second question is, what aspect of functioning is of interest, capacity or performance, and consequently what type of administration should be selected; testing in a laboratory or other setting, observation, or report by the patient or a proxy? This limits choices, and one's options might be even more restricted if the population one deals with has particular characteristics that make application of the most common instruments impossible—e.g. lack of English

proficiency. The resources available for administration—a special laboratory, administrator training, time availability of administrator and subject—typically play a major role in a decision. Lastly, metrologic characteristics—reliability, validity, sensitivity—should inform the selection, although in some situations the choice of instruments is so limited that one needs to accept a measure with less than stellar characteristics.

Over the years, a number of papers have been published that review FA measures, either in general (e.g., refs. 41, 79, 90–97) or specifically as applicable in SCI care and research (98–101). Recently, a number of systematic reviews of FA measures in SCI have been published that offer clinicians and researchers a simple way of identifying relevant measures and reviewing all (published) research relevant to psychometric characteristics. A systematic review is characterized by a protocol that is completed before the search for and abstracting of research papers is started. The protocol will specify the purpose and scope of the review, as well as the methods for identifying, qualifying, and abstracting papers. Thus, systematic reviews are more likely to include all relevant information, and offer recommendations that are less subjective than traditional (narrative) reviews.

As part of its review of interventions that have evidence for effectiveness in SCI rehabilitation, the Canadian SCIRE (Spinal Cord Injury Rehabilitation Evidence) initiative reviewed a number of outcome measures, including measures that operationalize components of functioning as traditionally defined in FA (102, 103). In the United States, a similar initiative has been developed under the aegis of the National Institute on Disability and Rehabilitation Research (NIDRR), involving SCI researchers and practitioners organized in the SCI Model Systems, the American Spinal Injury Association, and (more recently) ISCoS. Two of their systematic reviews involve FA issues (104, 105). Magasi and colleagues presented a review focusing on participation measures used in SCI studies (106). Lastly, Dawson et al. recently published a systematic review of FA outcome measures (107). Table 8.1 offers a listing of FA measures, most of which have been used in SCI research, in five categories: Impairments and functional limitations—entire body; impairments and functional limitations—upper extremity; impairments and functional limitations—lower extremity; activities/activity limitations; participation/participation restrictions. Assignment to these categories is based on the present authors' view of what construct each measure operationalizes; they concede that others might make different choices, and many measures could potentially be listed in more than one category. For each instrument, the most important references are provided; this includes generally the paper or papers in which the measure was first presented and/or in which the most important evidence for metrologic qualities (validity, reliability, etc.) was reported. Also provided is information on the SCI systematic review(s) in which the measure is included.

NEW(ER) TECHNOLOGIES IN FUNCTIONAL ASSESSMENT

The field of functional assessment, especially in its broad sense, is undergoing slow but certain change, resulting from the introduction of a number of technologies from other scholarly fields. This last section highlights some technologies already available, or about to move from prototype to useful means of collecting

Table 8.1 Functional Assessment Measures: Key References and Systematic Reviews

ABBREVIATION	MEASURE NAME	REFERENCE(S)	REFERENCES WITH SYSTEMATIC REVIEW
Impairments and Functional Limitations—Entire Body			
(ASIA)	International Standards for Neurological Classification of Spinal Cord Injury	10, 32, 132–139	102, 230
Impairments and Functional Limitations—Upper Extremity			
CUE	Capabilities of Upper Extremity	19	
THAQ	Tetraplegia Hand Activity Questionnaire	140	102
	van Lieshout Test of Hand Function	141, 142	
	Jebsen Hand Function Test	143–145	
Impairments and Functional Limitations—Lower Extremity			
WISCI II	Walking Index for Spinal Cord Injury	146–151	102, 105, 107
10 mWT	10 Meter Walk Test	152, 153	102, 105
50ftWT	50 feet Walk Test	154–157	105
6mWT	6 minute Walk Test	152, 158–164	105, 107
Activities/Activity Limitations			
BI	Barthel Index	2, 27	102, 104, 107
FIM	Functional Independence Measure	11, 165–170	102, 104, 107
QIF	Quadriplegia Index of Function	171–174	102, 104, 107
SCIM	Spinal Cord Independence Measure	12, 175–180	102, 104, 107
AM-PAC	Activity Measure—Post-Acute Care	181–185	
WC	Wheelchair Circuit	186–188	102
WST	Wheelchair Skills Test	189–192	102
NAC	Needs Assessment Checklist	193, 194	107
Participation/Participation Restrictions			
LIFE-H	Assessment of Life Habits	195–200	102, 106
CHART	Craig Handicap and Reporting Technique	13, 201–207	102, 106
CIQ	Community Integration Questionnaire	26, 208–212	
IPAQ	Impact on Participation and Autonomy Questionnaire	87, 213–219	102, 106
PM-PAC	Participation Measure—Post-Acute Care	40, 130, 220	
PARTS/M	Participation Survey/Mobility	221	102
POPS	Participation Objective, Participation Subjective	25	
GAS	Goal Attainment Scaling	81, 222–227	
COPM	Canadian Occupational Performance Measure	80, 228, 229	102

and processing FA information in routine clinical and research applications.

Ecological Momentary Assessment

Self-reports of feelings, experiences, and behaviors over a previous time period, unless part of a fixed daily routine, are notoriously unreliable. (Ask yourself: how often in the past month did you engage in small-talk with complete strangers? The CHART has this question.) Ecological momentary assessment (EMA) refers to a set of techniques to bring the reporting of information desired by a researcher closer to the time point the behavior or feeling occurs, and to have the report produced within the relevant setting rather than in a research office or over the telephone. At one extreme, EMA methods require the subject to complete a diary at the end of each day, in which the activities or moods of the day are recorded—the end-of-day (EOD) diary. Because even a distance of less than 24 hours may give play to random and systematic biases (memory, telescoping, latency effects, etc.), a more typical design is that the subject is alerted at multiple preset or random times a day, using a pager, special pre-programmed wrist-watch, or personal digital assistant (PDA), and then is

required to report a few key pieces of information, using a small carry-along diary, or a PDA or another type of palm-top computer. Because times are sampled, the method is also referred to as the experience sampling method (ESM), especially if the focus is on subjective experiences.

In the arena of FA, EMA could be used to answer questions like: in what activity are you currently engaged; how often in the past hour have you done activity X; with which people, if any, are you currently interacting? By means of appropriate methods of aggregating these discrete reports over a day, and individual days over a longer period, the researcher can obtain a more reliable overview of the person's Activities and Participation, provided compliance with completing the recordings is adequate (108). Compliance may be questionable, especially with paper-and-pencil methods, because EMA imposes quite a burden on subjects, and "for convenience" participants may complete all reports at the end of the day, or even just before turning the diary in to the researcher. PDAs can be used to date-stamp entries, so that at least the researcher is aware of falsification; in addition, they can be programmed to vary follow-up questions based on the answer to earlier ones ("branching"). To date, EMA methods have been used in FA research on a limited basis (109, 110).

Applications to SCI populations were not identified. Various books and articles are available that provide details on the method and present appropriate methods to process and analyze the complex and voluminous data that are produced (111–114).

Instrumented Recording

Pedometers can be used to track walking and other lower-extremity based physical activity; telemetry and other advanced technologies allow clinicians and researchers to have continuous information. Pedometers have been shown to correlate well with direct observation of activity, but less so with energy expenditure (115). Accelerometers can similarly record overall activity levels (116), but have potential to more specifically assess the frequency and duration of lower or upper extremity activity (117, 118), including tracking when, how intense, and for how long activity occurred (119). Using multiple one-axial or multi-axial accelerometers it is possible to determine time spent in different postures (sitting, lying, standing) and various physical activities (walking, cycling) (120). Further development of software algorithms may make it possible to make even more differentiation within the broad category of "activity" (121). A "data logger" attached to the spokes of a wheelchair will make it possible to determine the distance the user covers each day, and (using the Global Positioning System) what areas he or she frequented (122). Although pedometers and accelerometers are suitable for recording naturally occurring behavior, gait laboratories are more typically suited for testing a multitude of gait and wheelchair propulsion characteristics using walkways with built-in sensors, and videography (123).

Computer Administration of Tests

Traditionally, measurement of functional skills, whether by means of observation, testing, or subject or proxy report, has been predominantly a paper-and-pencil affair, where after the instrument has been administered, the data are scored for individual patients/clients in clinical applications, or for an entire group in research. In the latter case, the data typically are entered into computer files first, and scored using an algorithm. However, the wide availability of personal computers makes possible the administration of FA instruments using a computer. This can take the form of the client/research participant completing a questionnaire using a computer screen—a touch-sensitive screen to make it easiest on those with limited computer skills. Elimination of the costs and possible errors resulting from transcription of the data from paper to a computer file is one benefit; more important is the potential for branching—the capacity to offer different follow-up questions depending on the nature of the answer to an initial one. It is the equivalent of "skip" and "go to" instructions in self-administered paper and pencil questionnaires, but much more powerful, and is most fully exploited in CAT (see below). Similar benefits may be reaped in other administered interviews; Computer-Assisted Telephone Interviewing (CATI) has been a tool of public opinion polling for many years, ever since the door-to-door surveyor disappeared.

PDAs and other types of palmtop computers can also be used by clinicians and researchers to directly record and score observational data. Improving quality and ease of data entry comes at the cost of programming, which often is performed by commercial entities that sell a particular FA system. Lastly, testing may be completed using a computer, especially for tests that require timing, counting of errors, or other administrator functions that are arduous. It is expected that computer administration of FA instruments will become increasingly common in years to come, even for applications with small samples. "Authoring"-type software will make it possible to put together the user interfaces and underlying algorithms in limited time, even by clinicians or researchers lacking programming skills. In a sense, that time is here with such Web-based questionnaire design and administration services as Zoomerang (http://info.zoomerang.com). The completion of Web-based questionnaires and other instruments by patients/research subjects, with instant scoring of instruments and instant return of a total score or even an interpretive report, is another current application (124) that is expected to grow in importance (125).

Computer Adaptive Testing

Once it is known that a patient or research subject can walk two miles, it does not make much sense asking him if he can walk one mile, or get around in his own home. The answer will not provide any useful information, and it is more informative to ask next whether he can walk two miles on uneven ground carrying a ten-pound load. This is the premise underlying Computer Adaptive Testing (CAT): based on the known relative ordering of functional tasks in terms of difficulty, we can limit ourselves to asking only those questions that are informative as to the exact position of the person along the inability-ability continuum. In practice what is needed is prior analysis of the information on a sample of people who answer questions regarding all functional tasks included in a battery. Rasch analysis or another method of IRT then can be used to determine if the entire set defines a single dimension (e.g. physical ability), and the relative difficulty of the items. Then, for every new individual, we can use that information to determine his or her ability with a minimum set of questions. First, ability on a moderately difficult task is determined; based on the result, the questioning shifts to more difficult or to easier tasks, until her or his ability is known with a predetermined margin of error, or based on a preset number of items to be used (44, 126). In practice, computer algorithms are used to estimate ability level after each item has been completed, and to select the optimal next question to ask. It can be demonstrated that CAT creates sets of items that produce the same quantity and quality of information as the more expansive "item banks" from which these sets are drawn (44, 127, 128). To date, application of CAT to FA has been more demonstration of concept than use in daily clinical and research practice (129). However, the methodology has promise in more precise and more effective assessment of Impairments, Activity limitations, and possibly Participation (130).

Virtual Reality

Virtual Reality (VR) is the name for a collection of technologies allowing immersion of a person in an environment that is computer generated and interactive, in that it changes in response to behaviors and actions by the person—for instance, if in a virtual room projected using a head-mounted display (HMD) the person turns her head to the right, the right-hand wall rather than the front wall is displayed. The simulated world can be presented using a flat screen display, HMD, earphones or even 3D projection rooms, and the feedback is in response to gaze-tracking devices, gesture-sensing gloves, or other mechanisms to determine how the person interacts with the world she is presented. VR has been developed for treatment purposes, but more and more assessment opportunities are being realized.

Its unique capabilities in this area derive from the fact that VR is midway between the natural world and the testing laboratory. It is more real-life than the latter; it allows for the complexity of naturalistic settings, yet offers opportunities for the researcher or clinician to manipulate all aspects of that environment so as to afford clinical relevance and experimental control. Data can be collected on the client's/patient's/subject's response to the environment while that environment is made increasingly difficult (speed, number or order of stimulus presentations—e.g. cars on a virtual highway the person is required to cross) so as to challenge whatever skills and abilities (mobility, multitasking) are of interest to the test administrator (131).

References

1. Keith RA. Functional status and health status. *Arch Phys Med Rehabil.* 1994; 75:478–483.
2. Crewe NM, Dijkers M. Functional assessment. In: Scherer M, Cushman L, eds. *Psychological Assessment in Medical Rehabilitation Settings.* Washington DC: American Psychological Association, 1995:101–144.
3. Johnston MV, Eastwood E, Wilkerson DL, Anderson L, Alves A. Systematically assessing and improving the quality and outcomes of medical rehabilitation programs. In: Delisa JA, Gans BM, Walsh NE, eds. *Physical Medicine and Rehabilitation: Principles and Practice.* 4th ed. Philadelphia: Lippincott Williams Wilkins, 2005:1163–1192.
4. Stineman MG, Wechsler B, Ross R, Maislin G. A method for measuring quality of life through subjective weighting of functional status. *Arch Phys Med Rehabil.* 2003; 84:S15–22.
5. Ditunno PL, Patrick M, Stineman M, Ditunno JF. Who wants to walk? Preferences for recovery after SCI: A longitudinal and cross-sectional study. *Spinal Cord.* 2008; 46:500–506.
6. Brown M, Gordon WA. Empowerment in measurement: "muscle," "voice," and subjective quality of life as a gold standard. *Arch Phys Med Rehabil.* 2004; 85:S13–20.
7. Frey W. Functional assessment in the 80s: A conceptual enigma, a technical challenge. In: Halpern A, Fuhrer M, eds. *Functional Assessment in Rehabilitation.* Baltimore: Paul H. Brooks Publishing Co., 1984:11–43.
8. World Health Organization. *International Classification of Functioning, Disability and Health: ICF.* Geneva: World Health Organization; 2001.
9. World Health Organization. *International Classification of Impairments, Disabilities and Handicaps. A Manual of Classification Relating to the Consequenses of Disease.* Geneva: World Health Organization; 1980.
10. Marino RJ, Barros T, Biering-Sorensen F, et al. International standards for neurological classification of spinal cord injury. *J Spinal Cord Med.* 2003; 26 Suppl 1:S50–56.
11. Keith RA, Granger CV, Hamilton BB, Sherwin FS. The Functional Independence Measure: A new tool for rehabilitation. *Adv Clin Rehabil.* 1987; 1:6–18.
12. Itzkovich M, Gelernter I, Biering-Sorensen F, et al. The Spinal Cord Independence Measure (SCIM) version III: Reliability and validity in a multi-center international study. *Disabil Rehabil.* 2007; 29:1926–1933.
13. Whiteneck GG, Charlifue SW, Gerhart KA, Overholser JD, Richardson GN. Quantifying handicap: A new measure of long-term rehabilitation outcomes. *Arch Phys Med Rehabil.* 1992; 73:519–526.
14. Jette AM, Tao W, Haley SM. Blending activity and participation sub-domains of the ICF. *Disabil Rehabil.* 2007:1–9.
15. Jette AM, Haley SM, Kooyoomjian JT. Are the ICF activity and participation dimensions distinct? *J Rehabil Med.* 2003; 35:145–149.
16. Post MW, de Witte LP, Reichrath E, Verdonschot MM, Wijlhuizen GJ, Perenboom RJ. Development and validation of IMPACT-S, an ICF-based questionnaire to measure activities and participation. *J Rehabil Med.* 2008; 40:620–627.

17. Whiteneck GG, Dijkers MPJM. Measuring difficult to measure constructs: Participation and environmental factors. *Arch Phys Med Rehabil.* submitted.
18. Dijkers MP. Issues in the conceptualization and measurement of participation: An overview. *Arch Phys Med Rehabil.* submitted.
19. Marino RJ, Shea JA, Stineman MG. The Capabilities of Upper Extremity instrument: Reliability and validity of a measure of functional limitation in tetraplegia. *Arch Phys Med Rehabil.* 1998; 79:1512–1521.
20. Ware JE Jr, Sherbourne CD. The MOS 36-item short-form health survey (SF-36). I. Conceptual framework and item selection. *Med Care.* 1992; 30:473–483.
21. Dijkers M. Quality of life of individuals with spinal cord injury: A review of conceptualization, measurement, and research findings. *J Rehabil Res Dev.* 2005; 42:87–110.
22. Dijkers M. "What's in a name?" The indiscriminate use of the "quality of life" label, and the need to bring about clarity in conceptualizations. *Int J Nurs Stud.* 2007; 44:153–155.
23. Jette AM, Haley SM, Coster WJ, et al. Late life function and disability instrument: I. Development and evaluation of the disability component. *J Gerontol A Biol Sci Med Sci.* 2002; 57:M209–16.
24. Gerrity MS, Gaylord S, Williams ME. Short versions of the timed manual performance test. Development, reliability, and validity. *Med Care.* 1993; 31:617–628.
25. Brown M, Dijkers M, Gordon WA, Ashman T, Charatz H. Participation Objective, Participation Subjective: A measure of participation combining outsider and insider perspectives. *J Head Trauma Rehabil.* 2004; 19:459–481.
26. Dijkers M. Measuring the long-term outcomes of traumatic brain injury: A review of the Community Integration Questionnaire. *Journal of Head Trauma Rehabilitation.* 1997; 12:74–91.
27. Mahoney FI, Barthel DW. Functional evaluation: The Barthel index. *Md State Med J.* 1965; 14:61–65.
28. Linacre JM, Heinemann AW, Wright BD, Granger CV, Hamilton BB. The structure and stability of the Functional Independence Measure. *Arch Phys Med Rehabil.* 1994; 75:127–132.
29. Bond TG, Fox CM. *Applying the Rasch Model. Fundamental Measurement in the Human Sciences.* Mahwah, NJ: Erlbaum; 2001.
30. Marino RJ. Domains of outcomes in spinal cord injury for clinical trials to improve neurological function. *J Rehabil Res Dev.* 2007; 44:113–122.
31. Martin C, Dijkers M, DeSantis N. Self-care skills: Learning and abandoning. Chicago: American Spinal Injury Association; 1994.
32. Marino RJ, Ditunno JF, Donovan WH, et al, eds. *International Standards for Neurological and Functional Classification of Spinal Cord Injury.* Chicago: American Spinal Injury Association; 2000.
33. Park S, Fisher AG, Velozo CA. Using the assessment of motor and process skills to compare occupational performance between clinic and home settings. *Am J Occup Ther.* 1994; 48:697–709.
34. Malzer RL. Patient performance level during inpatient physical rehabilitation: Therapist, nurse, and patient perspectives. *Arch Phys Med Rehabil.* 1988; 69:363–365.
35. Dijkers MP, Yavuzer G, Ergin S, Weitzenkamp D, Whiteneck GG. A tale of two countries: Environmental impacts on social participation after spinal cord injury. *Spinal Cord.* 2002; 40:351–362.
36. Smith PM, Illig SB, Fiedler RC, Hamilton BB, Ottenbacher KJ. Intermodal agreement of follow-up telephone functional assessment using the Functional Independence Measure in patients with stroke. *Arch Phys Med Rehabil.* 1996; 77:431–435.
37. Jellinek HM, Torkelson RM, Harvey RF. Functional abilities and distress levels in brain injured patients at long-term follow-up. *Arch Phys Med Rehabil.* 1982; 63:160–162.
38. Harvey RF, Jellinek HM. Patient profiles: Utilization in functional performance assessment. *Arch Phys Med Rehabil.* 1983; 64:268–271.
39. Klein RM, Bell B. Self-care skills: Behavioral measurement with Klein-Bell ADL scale. *Arch Phys Med Rehabil.* 1982; 63:335–338.
40. Gandek B, Sinclair SJ, Jette AM, Ware JE Jr. Development and initial psychometric evaluation of the participation measure for post-acute care (PM-PAC). *Am J Phys Med Rehabil.* 2007; 86:57–71.
41. Dijkers MP, Whiteneck G, El-Jaroudi R. Measures of social outcomes in disability research. *Arch Phys Med Rehabil.* 2000; 81:S63–80.
42. Streiner DL, Norman GR. *Health Measurement Scales. A Practical Guide to their Development and use.* 3rd ed. Oxford: Oxford University Press; 2003.

43. Johnston MV, Graves DE. Towards guidelines for evaluation of measures: An introduction with application to spinal cord injury. *J Spinal Cord Med.* 2008; 31:13–26.

44. Dijkers MP. A computer adaptive testing simulation applied to the FIM instrument motor component. *Arch Phys Med Rehabil.* 2003; 84:384–393.

45. Bode RK, Heinemann AW, Semik P. Measurement properties of the Galveston Orientation and Amnesia Test (GOAT) and improvement patterns during inpatient rehabilitation. *Journal of Head Trauma Rehabilitation.* 2000; 15:637–655.

46. Cook KF, Roddey TS, Gartsman GM, Olson SL. Development and psychometric evaluation of the flexilevel scale of shoulder function. *Med Care.* 2003; 41:823–835.

47. Terwee CB, Dekker FW, Wiersinga WM, Prummel MF, Bossuyt PM. On assessing responsiveness of health-related quality of life instruments: Guidelines for instrument evaluation. *Qual Life Res.* 2003; 12:349–362.

48. Ward MM, Marx AS, Barry NN. Identification of clinically important changes in health status using receiver operating characteristic curves. *J Clin Epidemiol.* 2000; 53:279–284.

49. Diehr P, Chen L, Patrick D, Feng Z, Yasui Y. Reliability, effect size, and responsiveness of health status measures in the design of randomized and cluster-randomized trials. *Contemp Clin Trials.* 2005; 26:45–58.

50. Fischer D, Stewart AL, Bloch DA, Lorig K, Laurent D, Holman H. Capturing the patient's view of change as a clinical outcome measure. *JAMA.* 1999; 282:1157–1162.

51. Guyatt GH, Norman GR, Juniper EF, Griffith LE. A critical look at transition ratings. *J Clin Epidemiol.* 2002; 55:900–908.

52. Lawton G, Lundgren-Nilsson A, Biering-Sorensen F, et al. Cross-cultural validity of FIM in spinal cord injury. *Spinal Cord.* 2006; 44:746–752.

53. Meyers AR, Andresen EM. Enabling our instruments: Accommodation, universal design, and access to participation in research. *Arch Phys Med Rehabil.* 2000; 81:S5–9.

54. Gans BM, Haley SM, Hallenborg SC, Mann N, Inacio CA, Faas RM. Description and interobserver reliability of the Tufts Assessment of Motor Performance. *Am J Phys Med Rehabil.* 1988;67:202–210.

55. Bierman AS. Functional status: The sixth vital sign. *J Gen Intern Med.* 2001; 16:785–786.

56. Campbell DT, Stanley JC. *Experimental and Quasi-Experimental Designs for Research.* Chicago: Rand McNally and Company; 1963.

57. Johnston MV, Keith RA, Hinderer SR. Measurement standards for interdisciplinary medical rehabilitation. *Arch Phys Med Rehabil.* 1992; 73:S3–23.

58. Hall KM, Johnston MV. Outcomes evaluation in TBI rehabilitation. Part II: Measurement tools for a nationwide data system. *Arch Phys Med Rehabil.* 1994; 75:SC10–8; discussion SC 27–8.

59. Stineman MG, Escarce JJ, Goin JE, Hamilton BB, Granger CV, Williams SV. A case-mix classification system for medical rehabilitation. *Med Care.* 1994; 32:366–379.

60. Granger CV, Deutsch A, Russell C, Black T, Ottenbacher KJ. Modifications of the FIM instrument under the inpatient rehabilitation facility prospective payment system. *Am J Phys Med Rehabil.* 2007; 86:883–892.

61. Carter GM, Relles DA, Ridgeway GK, Rimes CM. Measuring function for Medicare inpatient rehabilitation payment. *Health Care Financ Rev.* 2003; 24:25–44.

62. Gage B, Stineman M, Deutsch A, et al. Perspectives on the state-of-the-science in rehabilitation medicine and its implications for Medicare postacute care policies. *Arch Phys Med Rehabil.* 2007; 88:1737–1739.

63. Iezzoni LI, Greenberg MS. Capturing and classifying functional status information in administrative databases. *Health Care Financ Rev.* 2003; 24:61–76.

64. Cieza A, Ewert T, Ustun TB, Chatterji S, Kostanjsek N, Stucki G. Development of ICF core sets for patients with chronic conditions. *J Rehabil Med.* 2004;(44 Suppl):9–11.

65. Biering-Sorensen F, Scheuringer M, Baumberger M, et al. Developing core sets for persons with spinal cord injuries based on the International Classification of Functioning, Disability and Health as a way to specify functioning. *Spinal Cord.* 2006; 44:541–546.

66. Ustun TB, Chatterji S, Kostanjsek N, Bickenbach J. WHO's ICF and functional status information in health records. *Health Care Financ Rev.* 2003; 24:77–88.

67. Biering-Sorensen F, Charlifue S, DeVivo M, et al. International spinal cord injury data sets. *Spinal Cord.* 2006; 44:530–534.

68. DeVivo M, Biering-Sorensen F, Charlifue S, et al. International spinal cord injury core data set. *Spinal Cord.* 2006; 44:535–540.

69. Widerstrom-Noga E, Biering-Sorensen F, Bryce T, et al. The international spinal cord injury pain basic data set. *Spinal Cord.* 2008; 46:818–823.

70. Krogh K, Perkash I, Stiens SA, Biering-Sorensen F. International bowel function basic spinal cord injury data set. *Spinal Cord.* 2009; 47:230–234.

71. Krogh K, Perkash I, Stiens SA, Biering-Sorensen F. International bowel function extended spinal cord injury data set. *Spinal Cord.* 2009; 47:235–241.

72. Biering-Sorensen F, Craggs M, Kennelly M, Schick E, Wyndaele JJ. International urodynamic basic spinal cord injury data set. *Spinal Cord.* 2008; 46:513–516.

73. Biering-Sorensen F, Craggs M, Kennelly M, Schick E, Wyndaele JJ. International lower urinary tract function basic spinal cord injury data set. *Spinal Cord.* 2008; 46:325–330.

74. DeJong G, Horn SD, Conroy B, Nichols D, Healton EB. Opening the black box of post-stroke rehabilitation: Stroke rehabilitation patients, processes, and outcomes. *Arch Phys Med Rehabil.* 2005; 86:S1–S7.

75. Heinemann AW, Whiteneck GG. Relationships among impairment, disability, handicap and life satisfaction in persons with traumatic brain injury. *Journal of Head Trauma Rehabilitation.* 1995; 10:54–63.

76. Pierce CA, Hanks RA. Life satisfaction after traumatic brain injury and the World Health Organization model of disability. *Am J Phys Med Rehabil.* 2006; 85:889–898.

77. Huebner RA, Johnson K, Bennett CM, Schneck C. Community participation and quality of life outcomes after adult traumatic brain injury. *Am J Occup Ther.* 2003; 57:177–185.

78. Dijkers M. Quality of life after spinal cord injury: A meta analysis of the effects of disablement components. *Spinal Cord.* 1997; 35:829–840.

79. Donnelly C, Carswell A. Individualized outcome measures: A review of the literature. *Can J Occup Ther.* 2002; 69:84–94.

80. Carswell A, McColl MA, Baptiste S, Law M, Polatajko H, Pollock N. The Canadian Occupational Performance Measure: A research and clinical literature review. *Can J Occup Ther.* 2004; 71:210–222.

81. Ottenbacher KJ, Cusick A. Goal Attainment Scaling as a method of clinical service evaluation. *Am J Occup Ther.* 1990; 44:519–525.

82. Tugwell P, Bombardier C, Buchanan WW, Goldsmith CH, Grace E, Hanna B. The MACTAR patient preference disability questionnaire—an individualized functional priority approach for assessing improvement in physical disability in clinical trials in rheumatoid arthritis. *J Rheumatol.* 1987; 14:446–451.

83. Dijkers MP. Individualization in quality of life measurement: Instruments and approaches. *Arch Phys Med Rehabil.* 2003; 84:S3–S14.

84. Johnston MV, Goverover Y, Dijkers M. Community activities and individuals' satisfaction with them: Quality of life in the first year after traumatic brain injury. *Arch Phys Med Rehabil.* 2005; 86:735–745.

85. Cicerone KD, Mott T, Azulay J, Friel JC. Community integration and satisfaction with functioning after intensive cognitive rehabilitation for traumatic brain injury. *Arch Phys Med Rehabil.* 2004; 85:943–950.

86. McColl MA, Davies D, Carlson P, Johnston J, Minnes P. The Community Integration Measure: Development and preliminary validation. *Arch Phys Med Rehabil.* 2001; 82:429–434.

87. Cardol M, de Haan RJ, van den Bos GA, de Jong BA, de Groot IJ. The development of a handicap assessment questionnaire: The Impact on Participation and Autonomy (IPA). *Clin Rehabil.* 1999; 13:411–419.

88. Wilkie R, Peat G, Thomas E, Hooper H, Croft PR. The Keele assessment of participation: A new instrument to measure participation restriction in population studies. Combined qualitative and quantitative examination of its psychometric properties. *Qual Life Res.* 2005; 14:1889–1899.

89. Weissscher N, de Haan RJ, Vermeulen M. The impact of disease-related impairments on disability and health-related quality of life: A systematic review. *BMC Med Res Methodol.* 2007; 7:24.

90. Cohen ME, Marino RJ. The tools of disability outcomes research functional status measures. *Arch Phys Med Rehabil.* 2000; 81:S21–S29.

91. Perenboom RJ, Chorus AM. Measuring participation according to the International Classification of Functioning, Disability and Health (ICF). *Disabil Rehabil.* 2003; 25:577–587.

92. Rust KL, Smith RO. Assistive technology in the measurement of rehabilitation and health outcomes: A review and analysis of instruments. *Am J Phys Med Rehabil.* 2005; 84:780–793.

93. Cardol M, Brandsma JW, de Groot IJ, van den Bos GA, de Haan RJ, de Jong BA. Handicap questionnaires: What do they assess? *Disabil Rehabil.* 1999; 21:97–105.

94. Eastwood EA. Functional status and its uses in rehabilitation medicine. *Mt Sinai J Med.* 1999; 66:179–187.

95. Moore DJ, Palmer BW, Patterson TL, Jeste DV. A review of performance-based measures of functional living skills. *J Psychiatr Res.* 2007; 41:97–118.

96. Thonnard JL, Penta M. Functional assessment in physiotherapy. A literature review. *Eura Medicophys.* 2007; 43:525–541.

97. Mortenson WB, Miller WC, Auger C. Issues for the selection of wheelchair-specific activity and participation outcome measures: A review. *Arch Phys Med Rehabil.* 2008; 89:1177–1186.

98. Ditunno JF Jr. Functional assessment measures in CNS trauma. *J Neurotrauma.* 1992; 9 Suppl 1:S301–S305.

99. Ditunno JF Jr, Burns AS, Marino RJ. Neurological and functional capacity outcome measures: Essential to spinal cord injury clinical trials. *J Rehabil Res Dev.* 2005; 42:35–41.

100. Steeves JD, Lammertse D, Curt A, et al. Guidelines for the conduct of clinical trials for spinal cord injury (SCI) as developed by the ICCP panel: Clinical trial outcome measures. *Spinal Cord.* 2007; 45:206–221.

101. Mulcahey MJ, Hutchinson D, Kozin S. Assessment of upper limb in tetraplegia: Considerations in evaluation and outcomes research. *J Rehabil Res Dev.* 2007; 44:91–102.

102. Miller WC, Curt A, Elliott S, et al. Outcome measures. In: Eng JJ, Teasell R, Miller WC, et al, eds. *SCIRE Spinal Cord Injury Rehabilitation Evidence.* 2007. Available at: http://www.icord.org/scire/pdf/SCIRE_CH22.pdf.

103. Lam T, Noonan VK, Eng JJ, SCIRE Research Team. A systematic review of functional ambulation outcome measures in spinal cord injury. *Spinal Cord.* 2008; 46:246–254.

104. Anderson K, Aito S, Atkins M, et al. Functional recovery measures for spinal cord injury: An evidence-based review for clinical practice and research. *J Spinal Cord Med.* 2008; 31:133–144.

105. Jackson AB, Carnel CT, Ditunno JF, Read MS, Boninger ML, Schmeler MR, Williams SR, Donovan WH; Gait and Ambulation Subcommittee. Outcome measures for gait and ambulation in the spinal cord injury population. *J Spinal Cord Med.* 2008; 31:487–499.

106. Magasi SR, Heinemann AW, Whiteneck GG, Quality of Life/Participation Committee. Participation following traumatic spinal cord injury: An evidence-based review for research. *J Spinal Cord Med.* 2008; 31:145–156.

107. Dawson J, Shamley D, Jamous MA. A structured review of outcome measures used for the assessment of rehabilitation interventions for spinal cord injury. *Spinal Cord.* 2008; 46:768–780.

108. Stone AA, Shiffman S. Capturing momentary, self-report data: A proposal for reporting guidelines. *Ann Behav Med.* 2002; 24:236–243.

109. Affleck G, Tennen H, Keefe FJ, et al. Everyday life with osteoarthritis or rheumatoid arthritis: Independent effects of disease and gender on daily pain, mood, and coping. *Pain.* 1999; 83:601–609.

110. Seekins T, Ipsen C, Arnold NL. Using ecological momentary assessment to measure participation: A preliminary study. *Rehabilitation Psychology.* 2007; 52:319–330.

111. Stone AA, Turkkan JS, Bachrach CA, Jobe JB, Kurtzman HS, Cain VS, eds. *The Science of Self-Report: Implications for Research and Practice.* Mahwah, NJ, US: Lawrence Erlbaum Associates, Publishers; 2000.

112. Reis HT, Gable SL. Event-sampling and other methods for studying everyday experience. In: Judd CM, Reis HT, eds. *Handbook of Research Methods in Social and Personality Psychology.* New York: Cambridge University Press, 2000:190–222.

113. Schwartz JE, Stone AA. Strategies for analyzing ecological momentary assessment data. *Health Psychol.* 1998; 17:6–16.

114. West SG, Hepworth JT. Statistical issues in the study of temporal data: Daily experiences. *J Pers.* 1991; 59:609–662.

115. Tudor-Locke C, Williams JE, Reis JP, Pluto D. Utility of pedometers for assessing physical activity: Construct validity. *Sports Med.* 2004; 34:281–291.

116. Busse ME, Pearson OR, Van Deursen R, Wiles CM. Quantified measurement of activity provides insight into motor function and recovery in neurological disease. *J Neurol Neurosurg Psychiatry.* 2004; 75:884–888.

117. Coronado M, Janssens JP, de Muralt B, Terrier P, Schutz Y, Fitting JW. Walking activity measured by accelerometry during respiratory rehabilitation. *J Cardiopulm Rehabil.* 2003; 23:357–364.

118. Uswatte G, Foo WL, Olmstead H, Lopez K, Holand A, Simms LB. Ambulatory monitoring of arm movement using accelerometry: An objective measure of upper-extremity rehabilitation in persons with chronic stroke. *Arch Phys Med Rehabil.* 2005; 86:1498–1501.

119. van den Berg-Emons HJ, Bussmann JB, Balk AH, Stam HJ. Validity of ambulatory accelerometry to quantify physical activity in heart failure. *Scand J Rehabil Med.* 2000; 32:187–192.

120. Tulen JH, Stronks DL, Bussmann JB, Pepplinkhuizen L, Passchier J. Towards an objective quantitative assessment of daily functioning in migraine: A feasibility study. *Pain.* 2000; 86:139–149.

121. Schasfoort FC, Bussmann JB, Stam HJ. Correlation between a novel upper limb activity monitor and four other instruments to determine functioning in upper limb complex regional pain syndrome type I. *J Rehabil Med.* 2005; 37:108–114.

122. Cooper RA, Thorman T, Cooper R, et al. Driving characteristics of electric-powered wheelchair users: How far, fast, and often do people drive? *Arch Phys Med Rehabil.* 2002; 83:250–255.

123. Koontz AM, Yang Y, Boninger DS, et al. Investigation of the performance of an ergonomic handrim as a pain-relieving intervention for manual wheelchair users. *Assist Technol.* 2006; 18:123–145.

124. Erlanger DM, Kaushik T, Broshek D, Freeman J, Feldman D, Festa J. Development and validation of a web-based screening tool for monitoring cognitive status. *J Head Trauma Rehabil.* 2002; 17:458–476.

125. Butcher JN, Perry J, Hahn J. Computers in clinical assessment: Historical developments, present status, and future challenges. *J Clin Psychol.* 2004; 60:331–345.

126. Gershon RC. Computer adaptive testing. *J Appl Meas.* 2005; 6:109–127.

127. Webster K, Cella D, Yost K. The Functional Assessment of Chronic Illness Therapy (FACIT) measurement system: Properties, applications, and interpretation. *Health Qual Life Outcomes.* 2003; 1:79.

128. Andres PL, Black-Schaffer RM, Ni P, Haley SM. Computer adaptive testing: A strategy for monitoring stroke rehabilitation across settings. *Top Stroke Rehabil.* 2004; 11:33–39.

129. Haley SM, Raczek AE, Coster WJ, Dumas HM, Fragala-Pinkham MA. Assessing mobility in children using a computer adaptive testing version of the Pediatric Evaluation of Disability Inventory. *Arch Phys Med Rehabil.* 2005; 86:932–939.

130. Jette A, Haley SM, Andres PL, Coster WJ. Development and initial testing of the Participation Measure for Post-Acute Care (PM-PAC). *Am J Phys Med Rehabil.*

131. Titov N, Knight RG. A computer-based procedure for assessing functional cognitive skills in patients with neurological injuries: The virtual street. *Brain Injury.* 2005; 19:315–322.

132. Maynard FM Jr, Bracken MB, Creasey G, et al. International standards for neurological and functional classification of spinal cord injury. *Spinal Cord.* 1997; 35:266–274.

133. Mulcahey MJ, Gaughan J, Betz RR, Johansen KJ. The international standards for neurological classification of spinal cord injury: Reliability of data when applied to children and youths. *Spinal Cord.* 2007; 45:452–459.

134. Cohen ME, Ditunno JF Jr, Donovan WH, Maynard FM Jr. A test of the 1992 international standards for neurological and functional classification of spinal cord injury. *Spinal Cord.* 1998; 36:554–560.

135. Marino RJ, Graves DE. Metric properties of the ASIA motor score: Subscales improve correlation with functional activities. *Arch Phys Med Rehabil.* 2004; 85:1804–1810.

136. Jonsson M, Tollback A, Gonzales H, Borg J. Inter-rater reliability of the 1992 international standards for neurological and functional classification of incomplete spinal cord injury. *Spinal Cord.* 2000; 38:675–679.

137. Graves DE, Frankiewicz RG, Donovan WH. Construct validity and dimensional structure of the ASIA motor scale. *J Spinal Cord Med.* 2006; 29:39–45.

138. Dasgupta AK. Post-traumatic epilepsy: Its complications and impact on occupational rehabilitation—an epidemiological study from India. *Occup Med (Lond).* 1998; 48:487–495.

139. Marino RJ, Jones L, Kirshblum S, Tal J, Dasgupta A. Reliability and repeatability of the motor and sensory examination of the international standards for neurological classification of spinal cord injury. *J Spinal Cord Med.* 2008; 31:166–170.

140. Land NE, Odding E, Duivenvoorden HJ, Bergen MP, Stam HJ. Tetraplegia hand activity questionnaire (THAQ): The development, assessment of arm-hand function-related activities in tetraplegic patients with a spinal cord injury. *Spinal Cord.* 2004; 42:294–301.

141. Post MW, Van Lieshout G, Seelen HA, Snoek GJ, Ijzerman MJ, Pons C. Measurement properties of the short version of the van lieshout test for arm/hand function of persons with tetraplegia after spinal cord injury. *Spinal Cord.* 2006; 44:763–771.

142. Spooren AI, Janssen-Potten YJ, Post MW, Kerckhofs E, Nene A, Seelen HA. Measuring change in arm hand skilled performance in persons with a cervical spinal cord injury: Responsiveness of the van lieshout test. *Spinal Cord.* 2006; 44:772–779.

143. Jebsen RH, Taylor N, Trieschmann RB, Trotter MJ, Howard LA. An objective and standardized test of hand function. *Arch Phys Med Rehabil.* 1969; 50:311–319.

144. Mikulic MA, Griffith ER, Jebsen RH. Clinical applications of a standardized mobility test. *Arch Phys Med Rehabil.* 1976; 57:143–146.

145. Beekhuizen KS, Field-Fote EC. Massed practice versus massed practice with stimulation: Effects on upper extremity function and cortical plasticity in individuals with incomplete cervical spinal cord injury. *Neurorehabil Neural Repair.* 2005; 19:33–45.

146. Ditunno JF Jr, Ditunno PL, Graziani V, et al. Walking Index for Spinal Cord Injury (WISCI): An international multicenter validity and reliability study. *Spinal Cord.* 2000; 38:234–243.

147. Dittuno PL, Dittuno JF Jr. Walking Index for Spinal Cord Injury (WISCI II): Scale revision. *Spinal Cord.* 2001; 39:654–656.

148. Morganti B, Scivoletto G, Ditunno P, Ditunno JF, Molinari M. Walking Index for Spinal Cord Injury (WISCI): Criterion validation. *Spinal Cord.* 2005; 43:27–33.

149. Ditunno JF, Scivoletto G, Patrick M, Biering-Sorensen F, Abel R, Marino R. Validation of the Walking Index for Spinal Cord Injury in a US and European clinical population. *Spinal Cord.* 2008; 46:181–188.

150. Ditunno JF Jr, Barbeau H, Dobkin BH, et al. Validity of the walking scale for spinal cord injury and other domains of function in a multicenter clinical trial. *Neurorehabil Neural Repair.* 2007; 21:539–550.

151. Kim MO, Burns AS, Ditunno JF Jr, Marino RJ. The assessment of walking capacity using the Walking Index for Spinal Cord Injury: Self-selected versus maximal levels. *Arch Phys Med Rehabil.* 2007; 88:762–767.

152. van Hedel HJ, Wirz M, Dietz V. Assessing walking ability in subjects with spinal cord injury: Validity and reliability of 3 walking tests. *Arch Phys Med Rehabil.* 2005; 86:190–196.

153. van Hedel HJ, Curt A. Fighting for each segment: Estimating the clinical value of cervical and thoracic segments in SCI. *J Neurotrauma.* 2006; 23:1621–1631.

154. Simmonds MJ, Olson SL, Jones S, et al. Psychometric characteristics and clinical usefulness of physical performance tests in patients with low back pain. *Spine.* 1998; 23:2412–2421.

155. Lee CE, Simmonds MJ, Novy DM, Jones S. Self-reports and clinician-measured physical function among patients with low back pain: A comparison. *Arch Phys Med Rehabil.* 2001; 82:227–231.

156. Reuben DB, Siu AL. An objective measure of physical function of elderly outpatients. The physical performance test. *J Am Geriatr Soc.* 1990; 38:1105–1112.

157. Dobkin B, Apple D, Barbeau H, et al. Weight-supported treadmill vs over-ground training for walking after acute incomplete SCI. *Neurology.* 2006; 66:484–493.

158. Butland RJ, Pang J, Gross ER, Woodcock AA, Geddes DM. Two-, six-, and 12-minute walking tests in respiratory disease. *Br Med J (Clin Res Ed).* 1982; 284:1607–1608.

159. Enright PL, Sherrill DL. Reference equations for the six-minute walk in healthy adults. *Am J Respir Crit Care Med.* 1998;158:1384–1387.

160. Cooper KH. A means of assessing maximal oxygen intake. Correlation between field and treadmill testing. *JAMA.* 1968; 203:201–204.

161. Steffen TM, Hacker TA, Mollinger L. Age- and gender-related test performance in community-dwelling elderly people: Six-minute walk test, berg balance scale, timed up & go test, and gait speeds. *Phys Ther.* 2002; 82:128–137.

162. Wirz M, Zemon DH, Rupp R, et al. Effectiveness of automated locomotor training in patients with chronic incomplete spinal cord injury: A multicenter trial. *Arch Phys Med Rehabil.* 2005; 86:672–680.

163. van Hedel HJ, Wirz M, Curt A. Improving walking assessment in subjects with an incomplete spinal cord injury: Responsiveness. *Spinal Cord.* 2006; 44:352–356.

164. Savci S, Inal Ince D, Arikan H, et al. Six-minute walk distance as a measure of functional exercise capacity in multiple sclerosis. *Disabil Rehabil.* 2005; 27:1365–1371.

165. Hamilton BB, Laughlin JA, Fiedler RC, Granger CV. Interrater reliability of the 7-level Functional Independence Measure (FIM). *Scand J Rehabil Med.* 1994; 26:115–119.

166. Nilsson AL, Sunnerhagen KS, Grimby G. Scoring alternatives for FIM in neurological disorders applying Rasch analysis. *Acta Neurol Scand.* 2005; 111:264–273.

167. Ottenbacher KJ, Hsu Y, Granger CV, Fiedler RC. The reliability of the Functional Independence Measure: A quantitative review. *Arch Phys Med Rehabil.* 1996; 77:1226–1232.

168. Ottenbacher KJ, Msall ME, Lyon NR, Duffy LC, Granger CV, Braun S. Interrater agreement and stability of the Functional Independence Measure (WeeFIM): Use in children with developmental disabilities. *Arch Phys Med Rehabil.* 1997; 78:1309–1315.

169. Ottenbacher KJ, Taylor ET, Msall ME, et al. The stability and equivalence reliability of the Functional Independence Measure for children (WeeFIM). *Dev Med Child Neurol.* 1996; 38:907–916.

170. Msall ME, DiGaudio K, Rogers BT, et al. The Functional Independence Measure for children (WeeFIM). conceptual basis and pilot use in children with developmental disabilities. *Clin Pediatr (Phila).* 1994; 33:421–430.

171. Gresham GE, Labi ML, Dittmar SS, Hicks JT, Joyce SZ, Stehlik MA. The Quadriplegia Index of Function (QIF): Sensitivity and reliability demonstrated in a study of thirty quadriplegic patients. *Paraplegia.* 1986; 24:38–44.

172. Yavuz N, Tezyurek M, Akyuz M. A comparison of two functional tests in quadriplegia: The Quadriplegia Index of Function and the Functional Independence Measure. *Spinal Cord.* 1998; 36:832–837.

173. Marino RJ, Huang M, Knight P, Herbison GJ, Ditunno JF Jr, Segal M. Assessing selfcare status in quadriplegia: Comparison of the Quadriplegia Index of Function (QIF) and the Functional Independence Measure (FIM). *Paraplegia.* 1993; 31:225–233.

174. Marino RJ, Goin JE. Development of a short-form Quadriplegia Index of Function scale. *Spinal Cord.* 1999; 37:289–296.

175. Catz A, Itzkovich M, Agranov E, Ring H, Tamir A. The Spinal Cord Independence Measure (SCIM): Sensitivity to functional changes in subgroups of spinal cord lesion patients. *Spinal Cord.* 2001; 39: 97–100.

176. Itzkovich M, Tripolski M, Zeilig G, et al. Rasch analysis of the Catz-Itzkovich Spinal Cord Independence Measure. *Spinal Cord.* 2002; 40:396–407.

177. Itzkovich M, Tamir A, Philo O, et al. Reliability of the Catz-Itzkovich Spinal Cord Independence Measure assessment by interview and comparison with observation. *Am J Phys Med Rehabil.* 2003; 82:267–272.

178. Catz A, Itzkovich M, Tesio L, et al. A multicenter international study on the Spinal Cord Independence Measure, version III: Rasch psychometric validation. *Spinal Cord.* 2007;45:275–291.

179. Wirth B, van Hedel HJ, Kometer B, Dietz V, Curt A. Changes in activity after a complete spinal cord injury as measured by the Spinal Cord Independence Measure II (SCIM II). *Neurorehabil Neural Repair.* 2008; 22:145–153.

180. van Hedel HJ, Dietz V, European Multicenter Study on Human Spinal Cord Injury (EM-SCI) Study Group. Walking during daily life can be validly and responsively assessed in subjects with a spinal cord injury. *Neurorehabil Neural Repair.* 2009; 23:117–124.

181. Haley SM, Coster WJ, Andres PL, et al. Activity outcome measurement for postacute care. *Med Care.* 2004; 42:I49–61.

182. Haley SM, Coster WJ, Andres PL, Kosinski M, Ni P. Score comparability of short forms and computerized adaptive testing: Simulation study with the Activity Measure for Post-Acute Care. *Arch Phys Med Rehabil.* 2004; 85:661–666.

183. Siebens H, Andres PL, Pengsheng N, Coster WJ, Haley SM. Measuring physical function in patients with complex medical and postsurgical conditions: A computer adaptive approach. *Am J Phys Med Rehabil.* 2005; 84:741–748.

184. Haley SM, Siebens H, Coster WJ, et al. Computerized adaptive testing for follow-up after discharge from inpatient rehabilitation: I. Activity outcomes. *Arch Phys Med Rehabil.* 2006;87:1033–1042.

185. Jette AM, Haley SM, Tao W, et al. Prospective evaluation of the AM-PAC-CAT in outpatient rehabilitation settings. *Phys Ther.* 2007; 87:385–398.

186. Kilkens OJ, Post MW, van der Woude LH, Dallmeijer AJ, van den Heuvel WJ. The wheelchair circuit: Reliability of a test to assess mobility in persons with spinal cord injuries. *Arch Phys Med Rehabil.* 2002; 83:1783–1788.

187. Kilkens OJ, Dallmeijer AJ, De Witte LP, Van Der Woude LH, Post MW. The wheelchair circuit: Construct validity and responsiveness of a test to assess manual wheelchair mobility in persons with spinal cord injury. *Arch Phys Med Rehabil*. 2004; 85:424–431.

188. Kilkens OJ, Dallmeijer AJ, Angenot E, Twisk JW, Post MW, van der Woude LH. Subject- and injury-related factors influencing the course of manual wheelchair skill performance during initial inpatient rehabilitation of persons with spinal cord injury. *Arch Phys Med Rehabil*. 2005; 86:2119–2125.

189. Kirby RL, Swuste J, Dupuis DJ, MacLeod DA, Monroe R. The wheelchair skills test: A pilot study of a new outcome measure. *Arch Phys Med Rehabil*. 2002; 83:10–18.

190. Kirby RL, Mifflen NJ, Thibault DL, et al. The manual wheelchair-handling skills of caregivers and the effect of training. *Arch Phys Med Rehabil*. 2004; 85:2011–2019.

191. Kirby RL, Dupuis DJ, Macphee AH, et al. The wheelchair skills test (version 2.4): Measurement properties. *Arch Phys Med Rehabil*. 2004; 85:794–804.

192. Mountain AD, Kirby RL, Smith C. The wheelchair skills test, version 2.4: Validity of an algorithm-based questionnaire version. *Arch Phys Med Rehabil*. 2004; 85:416–423.

193. Kennedy P, Hamilton LR. The Needs Assessment Checklist: A clinical approach to measuring outcome. *Spinal Cord*. 1999; 37:136–139.

194. Berry C, Kennedy P. A psychometric analysis of the Needs Assessment Checklist (NAC). *Spinal Cord*. 2003; 41:490–501.

195. Fougeyrollas P, Noreau L, Bergeron H, Cloutier R, Dion SA, St-Michel G. Social consequences of long term impairments and disabilities: Conceptual approach and assessment of handicap. *Int J Rehabil Res*. 1998; 21:127–141.

196. Rochette A, Desrosiers J, Noreau L. Association between personal and environmental factors and the occurrence of handicap situations following a stroke. *Disabil Rehabil*. 2001; 23:559–569.

197. Desrosiers J, Rochette A, Noreau L, Bravo G, Hebert R, Boutin C. Comparison of two functional independence scales with a participation measure in post-stroke rehabilitation. *Arch Gerontol Geriatr*. 2003; 37:157–172.

198. Desrosiers J, Bourbonnais D, Noreau L, Rochette A, Bravo G, Bourget A. Participation after stroke compared to normal aging. *J Rehabil Med*. 2005; 37:353–357.

199. Gagnon C, Mathieu J, Noreau L. Measurement of participation in myotonic dystrophy: Reliability of the LIFE-H. *Neuromuscul Disord*. 2006; 16:262–268.

200. Noreau L, Desrosiers J, Robichaud L, Fougeyrollas P, Rochette A, Viscogliosi C. Measuring social participation: Reliability of the LIFE-H in older adults with disabilities. *Disabil Rehabil*. 2004; 26:346–352.

201. Mellick D, Walker N, Brooks CA, Whiteneck G. Incorporating the cognitive independence domain into CHART. *J Rehabil Outcomes Meas*. 1999; 3:12–21.

202. Cusick CP, Gerhart KA, Mellick D, Breese P, Towle V, Whiteneck GG. Evaluation of the home and community-based services brain injury Medicaid waiver programme in Colorado. *Brain Inj*. 2003; 17:931–945.

203. Cusick CP, Brooks CA, Whiteneck GG. The use of proxies in community integration research. *Arch Phys Med Rehabil*. 2001; 82:1018–1024.

204. Cusick CP, Gerhart KA, Mellick DC. Participant-proxy reliability in traumatic brain injury outcome research. *J Head Trauma Rehabil*. 2000; 15:739–749.

205. Zhang L, Abreu BC, Gonzales V, Seale G, Masel B, Ottenbacher KJ. Comparison of the Community Integration Questionnaire, the Craig Handicap Assessment and Reporting Technique, and the Disability Rating Scale in traumatic brain injury. *J Head Trauma Rehabil*. 2002; 17:497–509.

206. Mellick D, Gerhart KA, Whiteneck GG. Understanding outcomes based on the post-acute hospitalization pathways followed by persons with traumatic brain injury. *Brain Inj*. 2003; 17:55–71.

207. Hall KM, Bushnik T, Lakisic-Kazazic B, Wright J, Cantagallo A. Assessing traumatic brain injury outcome measures for long-term follow-up of community-based individuals. *Arch Phys Med Rehabil*. 2001; 82:367–374.

208. Willer B, Ottenbacher KJ, Coad ML. The Community Integration Questionnaire. A comparative examination. *Am J Phys Med Rehabil*. 1994; 73:103–111.

209. Willer B, Rosenthal M, Kreutzer JS, Gordon WA, Rempel R. Assessment of community integration following rehabilitation for traumatic brain injury. *J Head Trauma Rehabil*. 1993; 8:75–87.

210. Willer B, Linn R, Allen K. Community integration and barriers to integration for individuals with brain injury. In: Finlayson MAJ, Garner SH, eds. *Brain Injury Rehabilitation: Clinical Considerations*. Baltimore: Williams and Wilkins, 1994: 355–375.

211. Sander AM, Seel RT, Kreutzer JS, Hall KM, High WM Jr, Rosenthal M. Agreement between persons with traumatic brain injury and their relatives regarding psychosocial outcome using the Community Integration Questionnaire. *Arch Phys Med Rehabil*. 1997; 78:353–357.

212. Sander AM, Fuchs KL, High WM Jr, Hall KM, Kreutzer JS, Rosenthal M. The Community Integration Questionnaire revisited: An assessment of factor structure and validity. *Arch Phys Med Rehabil*. 1999; 80:1303–1308.

213. Cardol M, de Haan RJ, de Jong BA, van den Bos GA, de Groot IJ. Psychometric properties of the Impact on Participation and Autonomy questionnaire. *Arch Phys Med Rehabil*. 2001; 82:210–216.

214. Cardol M, Beelen A, van den Bos GA, de Jong BA, de Groot IJ, de Haan RJ. Responsiveness of the Impact on Participation and Autonomy questionnaire. *Arch Phys Med Rehabil*. 2002; 83:1524–1529.

215. Vazirinejad R, Lilley JM, Ward CD. The 'Impact on Participation and Autonomy': Acceptability of the English version in a multiple sclerosis outpatient setting. *Mult Scler*. 2003; 9:612–615.

216. Sibley A, Kersten P, Ward CD, White B, Mehta R, George S. Measuring autonomy in disabled people: Validation of a new scale in a UK population. *Clin Rehabil*. 2006; 20:793–803.

217. Lund ML, Fisher AG, Lexell J, Bernspang B. Impact on Participation and Autonomy questionnaire: Internal scale validity of the Swedish version for use in people with spinal cord injury. *J Rehabil Med*. 2007; 39:156–162.

218. Kersten P, Cardol M, George S, Ward C, Sibley A, White B. Validity of the Impact on Participation and Autonomy questionnaire: A comparison between two countries. *Disabil Rehabil*. 2007; 29:1502–1509.

219. Franchignoni F, Ferriero G, Giordano A, Guglielmi V, Picco D. Rasch psychometric validation of the Impact on Participation and Autonomy questionnaire in people with Parkinson's disease. *Eura Medicophys*. 2007.

220. Haley SM, Gandek B, Siebens H, et al. Computerized adaptive testing for follow-up after discharge from inpatient rehabilitation: II. Participation outcomes. *Arch Phys Med Rehabil*. 2008; 89:275–283.

221. Gray DB, Hollingsworth HH, Stark SL, Morgan KA. Participation Survey/Mobility: Psychometric properties of a measure of participation for people with mobility impairments and limitations. *Arch Phys Med Rehabil*. 2006; 87:189–197.

222. Kiresuk TJ, Sherman RE. Goal Attainment Scaling: A general method for evaluating comprehensive community mental health programs. *Community Mental Health Journal*. 1968:4(6): 443–453.

223. Clark MS, Caudrey DJ. Evaluation of rehabilitation services: The use of Goal Attainment Scaling. *Int Rehabil Med*. 1983; 5:41–45.

224. Ottenbacher KJ, Cusick A. Discriminative versus evaluative assessment: Some observations on Goal Attainment Scaling. *Am J Occup Ther*. 1993; 47:349–354.

225. Malec JF. Goal Attainment Scaling in rehabilitation. *Neuropsychol Rehabil*. 1999; 9:253–275.

226. Cusick A, McIntyre S, Novak I, Lannin N, Lowe K. A comparison of Goal Attainment Scaling and the Canadian Occupational Performance Measure for paediatric rehabilitation research. *Pediatr Rehabil*. 2006; 9:149–157.

227. Tennant A. Goal Attainment Scaling: Current methodological challenges. *Disabil Rehabil*. 2007; 29:1583–1588.

228. Law M, Polatajko H, Pollock N, McColl MA, Carswell A, Baptiste S. Pilot testing of the Canadian Occupational Performance Measure: Clinical and measurement issues. *Can J Occup Ther*. 1994; 61:191–197.

229. Law M, Baptiste S, McColl M, Opzoomer A, Polatajko H, Pollock N. The Canadian Occupational Performance Measure: An outcome measure for occupational therapy. *Can J Occup Ther*. 1990; 57:82–87.

230. Furlan JC, Fehlings MG, Tator CH, Davis AM. Motor and sensory assessment of patients in clinical trials for pharmacological therapy of acute spinal cord injury: Psychometric properties of the ASIA standards. *J Neurotrauma*. 2008; 25:1273–1301.

9 Outcomes Following Spinal Cord Injury

Christina V. Oleson
Ien Sie
Robert L. Waters

Spinal cord injury (SCI) is one of the most devastating injuries an individual can sustain. In the United States, the incidence of SCI is approximately 11,000 cases per year with a prevalence of approximately 253,000 cases (1). Although the number of females with SCI is increasing as is the median age, victims remain predominantly young males, with the most common cause of injury being motor vehicle crashes (47%) (1). With the increasing number of older individuals, falls are now the second most common etiology for SCI (1). Regardless of cause, maximal return of function is one of the primary concerns for patients, their families, and clinicians. The dilemma for care providers is to encourage individuals with SCI to attain the highest functional level possible without offering false hope for performance of activities that may be impossible or impractical to achieve.

It is important for both clinicians and patients to have a reasonable expectation of functional outcomes following SCI. Clinicians must be able to prognosticate outcomes to plan a realistic, effective rehabilitation program. Knowledge of expected outcomes also helps to determine the effectiveness of various treatment interventions (pharmacologic and rehabilitation protocols). Finally, in the current healthcare system, with declining resources and a shift to managed care, it is essential to know expected outcomes so that the most cost-effective protocols to attain optimal function can be implemented in the shortest time possible. Just as it is inappropriate to deny or fail to provide essential and appropriate rehabilitation services, it is also inappropriate to provide valuable rehabilitation services and resources that will only minimally improve a patient's overall function or would be better utilized once barriers such as braces or pressure ulcers have been eliminated. Accurate prognostication following SCI will determine the treatment plan and minimize unnecessary interventions while justifying needed care and resources.

Patients and their families also must know what to expect in regard to functional outcomes so that they can plan ahead for the modifications or additional assistance that may be needed at discharge. For patients, the ability to walk is the primary functional outcome of interest. However, personal care needs, including the ability to continue independent living, sexuality, and occupational and recreational pursuits are also concerns.

Motor function is the primary determinant of overall function following SCI. Therefore, an accurate diagnosis of the level and completeness of SCI and a detailed assessment of neurologic function is essential for prognostication. A carefully performed neurologic examination performed immediately after injury is essential, not only to plan treatment interventions but also to provide a baseline to measure the rate of recovery over the days immediately following injury. Following an incomplete injury, rapid early recovery will likely be sustained over subsequent weeks and months, and the prognosis for long-term functional recovery is excellent. Various investigators have determined that a detailed neurologic examination performed at least 72 hours following traumatic SCI is a better prognostic tool for determining outcomes than an examination performed immediately following injury, because the results of an early examination may be compromised by pain, confusion, and associated injuries (2–4), including alcohol and drugs. Moreover, results of the neurologic examination can actually decline between 24 and 72 hours as postinjury swelling and cord edema reach a peak.

The accuracy of predicting recovery based on neurologic examination improves with a longer interval between onset of injury and the most recent neurologic examination. Whereas Waters and associates studied neurologic recovery in over 500 patients and found long-term motor recovery could be reliably predicted using the 1-month neurologic examination to predict recovery (5–8), Marino and colleagues found that a neurologic examination performed 1 week following injury had prognostic value for determining recovery (9). These investigators used the ASIA Impairment Scale (AIS) and the Frankel scale to predict neurologic recovery. Clearly, it is the responsibility of the rehabilitation practitioner to perform serial examinations on a frequent basis during the rehabilitation process, so that functional goals can be updated and modified appropriately. The authors recommend such examinations be performed on a weekly basis during initial rehabilitation, at a time when the patient is not fatigued and can provide full attention to the examiner. Burns and colleagues observed that among 11.3% of subjects that converted from complete to incomplete status during the first year, the majority had factors or conditions that compromised accuracy of the initial ASIA examination (10).

The International Standards for Neurologic and Functional Classification of SCI have been accepted as the most accurate and reliable instrument for documenting neurologic status following SCI (11). These standards require determination of both motor and sensory levels bilaterally, as well as determination of completeness of injury. To determine motor level of injury, ten key muscles representing specific spinal levels are tested bilaterally using the standard six-point (zero to five) manual muscle testing (MMT) scale. An individual with no neurologic deficit has an ASIA Motor Score (AMS) of 100 points (50 points each for left and right sides of the body or 50 points each for the bilateral upper extremities and the bilateral lower extremities). Sensory level is determined by testing key points in each of twenty-eight dermatomes on both the right and left sides of the body. Both pinprick and light-touch sensation are tested in each dermatome. Sensory function is scored on a three-point scale (zero to two). The total possible score for each of the sensory modalities is 112 points. Details of neurological assessment of SCI are covered in other chapters of this text.

Determining completeness of injury by the sacral sparing definition is the most important factor in determining recovery at neurologic levels distal to the lesion. A complete injury is one without any sensory or motor function in the lowest sacral segments. In an incomplete injury, there is partial preservation of motor and/or sensory function in the lowest sacral segments.

The differences in motor and sensory scores between successive neurologic examinations represent the recovery (or deterioration) that has occurred in the intervening period. By dividing the difference between scores by the number of days in the interval, the change per day can be calculated. Finally, by multiplying the change per day by 365 days, the annualized rate of change can be determined. The annualized rate represents the rate of change during a particular interval that could be expected if it were to continue for 1 year.

Once completeness of injury and level of injury (tetraplegia or paraplegia) have been determined, rate of recovery and individual muscle recovery data can be reviewed to predict recovery in a specific patient group. For the following discussion, patients are categorized as having complete or incomplete SCI, with the latter category then subdivided by the degree of sensory and/or motor preservation.

MOTOR RECOVERY

Complete SCI: ASIA Impairment Score (AIS) A

The majority of neurologic recovery after SCI is traditionally believed to occur in the first year after the injury. Fawcett et al. (12) recently summarized findings of several studies that examined conversion from complete (AIS A) to incomplete (AIS B–D) injury classification. Their analysis demonstrated that 80% of subjects initially classified as AIS A 3 to 28 days post-SCI remained complete at 1 year after injury. Twenty percent became incomplete, of which approximately half converted to AIS B and the other half to either AIS C or D. These statistics, which include

both paraplegic and tetraplegic individuals, represent study findings from before and after the 2000 Revision of the ASIA Classification of "motor incomplete" lesions. Prior to the year 2000, conversion of complete to incomplete status could be observed in persons with improvement of motor or sensory findings near the zone of injury. After 2000, a requirement of sacral sparing (sensation in S45, deep anal sensation, or volitional sphincter activity) was adopted in order for a patient to be considered incomplete. Moreover, for AIS C or D, the patient must have some degree of anal sensation *and* have sparing of motor function more than three levels below the motor level (11). Although some early studies that included persons with tetraplegia and paraplegia estimated a 20% conversion rate from complete to incomplete status, only 2%–3% improve to an AIS D classification (9). In addition, many among that small group of AIS D patients may not be ambulatory (9). Other studies estimate conversion rates from AIS A to B, C, or D at 4%–13% (5, 7, 9).

Although an early study by Maynard (13) reported a 1-year conversion rate of 19% for initially complete to incomplete injuries, 10% of patients in the sample had significant head injuries, thereby impairing subject participation and reliability. After eliminating subjects with head injuries, 103 cognitively intact participants remained, and no individuals with complete injuries in this subgroup regained ambulatory function at 1 year. The reader must also consider the data of Burns (10) that demonstrated that up to 9.3% of subjects initially considered to be AIS A at the 72-hour exam were reclassified as AIS B within the first week, due to challenges affecting the reliability of early ASIA examination in the group of 103 US Model System patients examined. In contrast, only 2.6% of subjects without factors impeding the accuracy of an early exam were reclassified. Among those with reliable early examinations indicating complete injuries at the 72-hour examination, only two of thirty (6.7%) converted to motor complete sensory incomplete (AIS B), but none converted to AIS C or D (motor and sensory incomplete).

Complete Tetraplegia

Only 10% of those with complete tetraplegia at 1 month following injury will convert to incomplete status. As in patients with complete paraplegia, motor recovery is minimal in those with conversion to incomplete status, but recovery of sacral function is enhanced. Recovery of motor strength is again independent of level of injury. Prediction of individual muscle recovery to functional strength will help in determining independent functioning. For example, 97% of wrist extensors with an initial strength of 1/5 will recover to at least 3/5 at 1 year following injury. Therefore, an individual who is initially dependent or needs assistance with tabletop activities and transfers can anticipate independence in these activities at 1 year following injury. With the exception of the triceps, all upper extremity muscles with an initial strength grade of at least 1/5 recovered to at least 3/5 by 1 year (Table 9.1). In cases of complete injury, these increases frequently occur at the level of injury and, if present, the adjacent zone of partial preservation.

Fawcett et al. (12) has illustrated the motor point average gains for AIS A, B, and C+D injuries over the first year for subjects in three large studies (US Model Systems, Sygen, and European

Table 9.1   Prediction of Lower Extremity Motor Recovery (23)

	PERCENTAGE WITH FUNCTIONAL STRENGTH >3/5 AT 1 YEAR		
MANUAL MUSCLE STRENGTH AT 1 MONTH*	COMPLETE PARAPLEGIA	INCOMPLETE PARAPLEGIA	INCOMPLETE TETRAPLEGIA
0/5	5%	26%	24%
1/5, 2/5	64%	85%	97%

*ASIA key muscles.

Multicenter Study about Spinal Cord Injury [EMSCI]). Their data, which encompass tetraplegic and paraplegic subjects, appear in Figure 9.1 (12). In cases of those with AIS D injuries with relatively good motor scores at the outset, one may see a smaller improvement due to a ceiling effect.

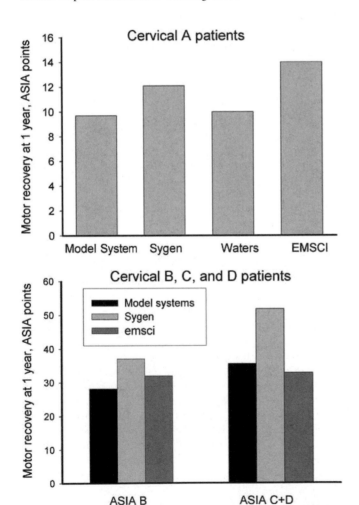

Figure 9.1 Motor recovery, measured in ASIA motor points, over the first year after SCI in AIS A, B, and C/D patients. The rates of recovery in the Model Systems, Sygen, and EMSCI studies are compared. (*Spinal Cord* 2007; 45(3):190–205.)

Complete Paraplegia (5)

In the overwhelming majority (96%) of patients with complete paraplegia as of 1 month postinjury, neurologic classification will remain complete. Recovery of motor function is related to level of injury. No patients with a neurologic level of injury (NLI) above T9 regained motor function 1 year following injury. At the more caudal levels of injury, there is a greater recovery of motor functions through recovered function in the zone of partial preservation.

Recovery of "functional" strength (3/5 or greater) is minimal in muscles with a grade of 0/5 at 1 month (Table 9.1). Only about 5% of these muscles will regain functional strength 1 year following injury. In contrast, 64% of muscles with either 1/5 or 2/5 strength at 1 month will have grade 3/5 strength at 1 year. Typically, muscles with motor strength of this magnitude occur in the zone of partial preservation. Improvement in this area may ultimately result in a change in the neurologic level of injury to a more caudal level, even though the overall grade of injury may remain complete. Fawcett's conversion data for both complete and incomplete levels of SCI are given in Figure 9.2. In studies by Waters of patients 1 year after injury, no complete tetraplegics (7) and only 5% of complete paraplegics (5) recovered adequate strength to ambulate.

Motor Complete Sensory Incomplete SCI (AIS B)

The category of motor complete sensory incomplete spinal cord injury represents only 11% of total SCI cases (1). Such persons have some sensory preservation in the lowest sacral segments but lack volitional motor function below the zone of injury. Two early studies by Foo (14) and Waters (6, 8) demonstrated better outcomes for motor recovery among those with initial pinprick sensation below the zone of injury. The above studies are limited by small numbers of subjects and use of the earlier Frankel scale. Applying the ASIA standards, Crozier et al. (15) found that among twenty-seven motor complete sensory incomplete subjects assessed at 72 hours postinjury, only two of eighteen (11%) ambulated at discharge from rehab if they lacked partial or complete pinprick below the injury at 72 hours. Conversely, eight of nine (89%) with some preserved pinprick below the zone of injury achieved community ambulation, defined as more than 200 feet, if pinprick below the injury was observed at initial evaluation.

Using the 72-hour ASIA examination, Oleson et al.(16) found that among 131 subjects with classification as AIS B, without regard to appreciation of pinprick, rates of ambulation were 48% at the level of at least Benzel V (able to ambulate 25 feet assisted or unassisted) and 24% for Benzel VI (able to walk 150 feet without a helper). However, success rates for the individual patient largely depended on preservation of pinprick sensation. Significant differences were observed for recovery of ambulation 1 year postinjury at a level Benzel V or better in 36% of persons with pinprick preservation in the lowest sacral segments 4 weeks postinjury versus just 4.4% of those without pinprick at S4–5. However no significant difference in ambulatory function 1 year later was seen for those with vs. without S4–5 pinprick preservation at the 72-hour exam. In contrast, lower extremity pinprick preservation in greater than 50% of lower extremity dermatomes L2-S1, observed at the 72-hour exam, was predictive of ambulation at a level of *greater than or equal to* Benzel V and for ambulation at

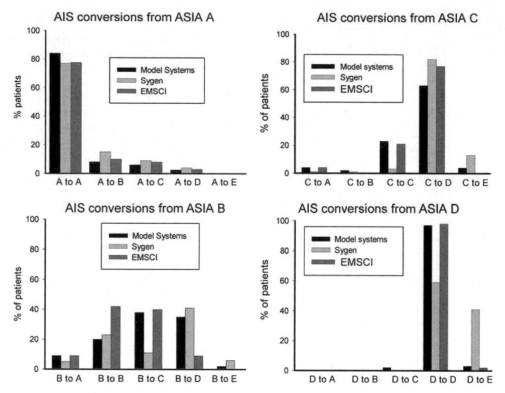

Figure 9.2 Percent AIS conversion from initial examination (within 3 days to 4 weeks of SCI) to the 1-year anniversary date after SCI. Data are from the US Model Systems, Sygen, and EMSCI databases. (*Spinal Cord* 2007; 45(3):190–205.)

or better than Benzel VI. This was true both for ambulatory function at the 6-month postinjury date and at 1 year. Overall, 66% of those with initial pinprick L2-S1 recovered ambulation at or better than Benzel grade V 1 year after SCI, and 40% recovered to a level at or better than Benzel grade VI. However, 44% of those lacking the threshold of 50% dermatomes L2–S1 with pinprick preservation achieved ambulation at least equal to Benzel V.

The reasoning that pinprick preservation may be prognostic for ambulation more than sensation of light touch or proprioception arises from the proximity within the spinal cord of the spinothalamic tract, carrying pinprick information, to the corticospinal track, responsible for motor function. In contrast, the dorsal columns located in the posterior cord carry light touch, proprioception, and vibratory sensation. The anterior cord syndrome predominantly affects spinothalamic, corticospinal, and other tracts located in the anterior two-thirds of the spinal cord, while sparing dorsal column function. Causes include anterior spinal artery lesions, aortic or cardiac surgical complications, or retroulsed disc or vertebral bony fragments from trauma or other degenerative condition (17). This syndrome carries a poor prognosis for motor recovery relative to other incomplete syndromes (14, 15).

Motor Incomplete and Sensory Incomplete SCI (AIS C and D)

For both incomplete paraplegia and tetraplegia, the majority of functional recovery is observed in the first 6–9 months, with little improvement seen after 12 months (6, 8). Persons with AIS grade C lack antigravity strength in the majority of myotomes below the neurologic level of injury (NLI) as defined by the International Standards for Classification of SCI (11). Persons with AIS grade D have at least a 3/5 in the majority of motor segments below the NLI.

For those with AIS C, persons under age 50 have a 91% chance of obtaining community ambulation upon discharge from rehabilitation, relative to only 42% of persons age 50 or older (18). Regardless of age, all those with AIS D ambulated following rehabilitation in this study (18). The previously described study by Burns and colleagues examined a variety of motor incomplete subtypes (central cord, Brown-Séquard, and mixed), but AIS C and D were separately analyzed. In a study by Penrod (19) limited to those with central cord syndrome, outcomes for ambulation differed significantly depending on the age of the participant. Ninety-seven percent of those under age 50, but only 41% of those age 50 or older, were able to ambulate at discharge from inpatient rehabilitation. However, authors did not separate those with AIS C and D. Both of the above studies examined ambulation at discharge from rehabilitation, with lengths of stay being anywhere from 3 to 6 months after injury in the early to mid-1990s. With changes in insurance coverage, discharge from both acute care and rehabilitation for incomplete tetraplegia in 2007 occurred in a fraction of that time (1), forcing long-term goals such as community ambulation to be met in an outpatient setting.

Central cord syndrome is the most common of incomplete syndromes. Seen commonly in the elderly, this condition has a profound effect on activities of daily living and self-care. Recovery occurs earlier and to a greater extent in the legs. Intrinsic hand function, essential to maintaining independence, is often the last impairment to improve and may not recover as well as the lower extremities (20). Brown-Séquard syndrome constitutes only 2%–4% of all traumatic spinal cord injuries but has among the best prognoses of all incomplete syndromes, with approximately 75% ultimately achieving community ambulation. This condition involves contralateral loss of pain and temperature, with ipsilateral loss of vibratory and proprioception function in addition to ipsilateral motor loss. This pattern of crossed sensory and motor findings results from hemisection of the spinal cord. Brown-Séquard SCI is also associated with an 80%–90% recovery of bowel and bladder function (21). Moreover, approximately 70% of patients achieve independence or modified independence with activities of daily living (21).

Figure 9.2 indicates that in three large clinical trials, a few patients initially rated as incomplete AIS C were classified as AIS A or B at 1 year. Although no explanation regarding the individual cases of regression could be offered due to the nature of the data collection, possible reasons for clinical decline after the first 72 hours are multiple. Possibilities include edema or inflammation leading to further nerve compression. Intra-operative or post operative complications following spinal stabilization, such as epidural hematoma, cord ischemia, or hardware failure, have also been observed (1).

Incomplete Tetraplegia

For patients with incomplete tetraplegia, recovery in the upper and lower extremities occurs concurrently, not sequentially. As with other categories of injury, the rate of motor recovery declines rapidly in the first 6 months following injury. Recovery of functional strength in individual muscles is favorable in patients with incomplete tetraplegia. All upper extremity muscles and 97% of lower extremity muscles with initial strength grades of 1/5 or 2/5 will recover to at least 3/5 by 1 year. In the upper extremity, 20% of muscles with an initial grade of 0/5 will recover functional strength (Tables 9.1 and 9.2). In the lower extremity, 24% of those with absent strength initially will recover to at least 3/5 by 1 year (Table 9.1).

Incomplete Paraplegia

In patients with incomplete paraplegia, motor recovery is independent of level of injury. The average increase in motor scores was twelve points at 1 year after injury. Among patients with incomplete paraplegia (includes AIS B, C, and D), 76% will attain community ambulation status at 1 year. Recovery of functional strength is also improved in those with incomplete paraplegia compared with complete paraplegia. For muscles with 0/5 strength at 1 month, 26% will recover functional strength at 1 year. Eighty-five percent of muscles with an initial strength of 1/5 or 2/5 will recover to 3/5 strength at 1 year (Table 9.1).

Timing of Motor Recovery: Early versus Late

Graphing the annualized rates of change against time since injury reveals the course of motor recovery. Regardless of level or completeness of injury, the majority of recovery occurs in the first 6 months following injury. The rate of change plateaus at approximately 9 months, but it does not equal zero (Figure 9.2). Although some motor recovery may continue 2 or more years after injury, the amount is generally small and not likely to significantly improve function. Mange and associates examined motor recovery in the zone of injury and compared recovery of motor complete and motor incomplete subjects. Their results suggest that patients with motor incomplete injuries recover earlier (22).

In studies by Waters, findings demonstrate that in the 4% of patients who undergo "late conversion" to incomplete status, motor recovery is limited. Late conversion is significant, however, for recovery of sacral functions. Approximately half of patients who undergo late conversions will regain volitional bowel and bladder function (5). Kirshblum et al. (23) examined rates of neurologic recovery between the first and fifth year postinjury. Among 539 subjects with AIS Grade A 1 year post injury, 3.5% improved to AIS grade B and 1.05% to each of grades C and D. The remaining 94.4% remained AIS grade A.

FUNCTIONAL RECOVERY

Ambulation

A primary concern of SCI patients (and their families) is whether they will be able to regain the ability to walk. Ambulation, like other functional outcomes, is dependent on many factors in addition to neurologic function. When the population of individuals with SCI is studied as a whole, experts generally agree that a minority of individuals are able to ambulate following SCI. Beyond the basic question of whether a patient will be able to ambulate or will rely solely on a wheelchair, there is the question of the degree of ambulatory function that can be attained.

Stauffer divided ambulatory status into four categories: community ambulatory, household ambulatory, exercise ambulatory, and nonambulatory (24). Community ambulators are able to transfer themselves out of bed or a wheelchair and walk reasonable distances in and out of the home without assistance from

Table 9.2 Prediction of Upper Extremity Motor Recovery (23)		
	PERCENTAGE WITH FUNCTIONAL STRENGTH >3/5 AT 1 YEAR	
MANUAL MUSCLE STRENGTH AT 1 MONTH*	COMPLETE TETRAPLEGIA	INCOMPLETE TETRAPLEGIA
0/5	20%	24%
1/5	90%	73%
2/5	100%	100%
*ASIA key muscles.		

another person. Household ambulators may or may not require assistance with transfers from bed or wheelchair; they are able to ambulate in the home with relative independence but are unable to ambulate outside of the home for any significant distance. These individuals frequently use a wheelchair for mobility outside the home. The exercise ambulator attains functional mobility with a wheelchair and can ambulate only under closely controlled conditions. Considerable physical assistance is also required to ambulate. Individuals who are nonambulators rely exclusively on a wheelchair. Both community and household ambulation are considered "functional" ambulation, whereas exercise ambulation is considered "nonfunctional."

The type of gait pattern utilized depends on the degree of neurologic loss. Waters (5) has determined that only 5% of individuals with complete paraplegia and no individuals with complete tetraplegia (7) will become community ambulators 1 year after injury. In the above studies, community ambulation was defined as ability to walk for more than 250 meters. Paraplegics lacking sufficient hip flexion for reciprocal gait pattern must utilize an energy intensive swing-through, crutch-assisted method (5). This technique requires arm and shoulder girdle strength sufficient to lift the weight of the entire body and swing it forward— impractical for routine mobility because this practice requires high rates of energy expenditure and results in a substantially slower walking speed (25). Thus, although an individual may utilize a swing-through gait pattern to negotiate architectural barriers or to walk for exercise or psychological reasons, few employ this manner of ambulation as their primary mode of mobility.

A reciprocal gait pattern can be utilized when there is pelvic control with at least 3/5 strength in the hip flexors and in one quadriceps (26). This form of gait allows for knee stability without the use of a knee-ankle-foot orthosis (KAFO). Although a reciprocal gait pattern requires less energy than a swing-through pattern, the rate of energy expenditure is still higher than that

demonstrated by able-bodied subjects. Those with incomplete injury are more likely to recover sufficient motor strength to permit reciprocal gait. Motor complete, sensory incomplete lesions have lesser probability of recovery than do motor incomplete lesions. Findings of several studies (15, 16, 18, 19) examining ambulation as the primary outcome measure are highlighted in Table 9.3. Although overall rates of community ambulation are 76% for incomplete paraplegia and 46% for incomplete tetraplegia, results are greatly influenced by ASIA grade and the modality of sensory sparing.

Hussey and Stauffer determined that there is a direct relationship between lower extremity strength and the ability to ambulate (26). They reported that pelvic control with at least fair hip extensor strength and fair strength in one knee extensor is required for community ambulation with a reciprocal gait pattern. In another study, Crozier and coworkers studied individuals with Frankel C ("motor useless") injuries (27). They studied recovery of the quadriceps muscle and reported that all patients who had achieved a quadricep strength of at least 3/5 at 2 months following injury progressed to become functional ambulators, whereas only two of eight patients who had not attained at least 3/5 by 2 months became functional ambulators. It is believed that strength of *greater than or equal to* 3/5 in the hip flexors on one side and *greater than or equal to* 3/5 quadriceps strength on the contralateral side allows successful community ambulation. This degree of function would permit use of one long leg brace with a fixed ankle in dorsiflexion and a locked knee and one short leg brace with a similarly dorsiflexed ankle. Proprioception, however, would also need to be largely intact.

Waters and colleagues measured energy expenditure during walking with instrumented crutches that measured axial loading. They found that the motor scoring system utilized by the American Spinal Injury Association (ASIA) was a simple clinical measure that also correlated strongly with walking ability (28). Individuals with ASIA lower extremity motor scores (LEMS) less

---

Table 9.3 Ambulation According to ASIA Grade

ASIA GRADE	BASELINE EXAM	RATES OF AMBULATION
ASIA A		
tetraplegia (ref. 7)	≤30 days	0% community at 1 year
paraplegia (ref. 5)	≤30 days	5% community at 1 year (no subjects above T9 level)
ASIA B		
with PP in ≥50% LE dermatomes (ref. 16)	<72 hours	40% community ambulation at 1 year
		67% only household ambulation at 1 year
with PP in <50% LE dermatomes	<72 hours	16% community ambulation at 1 year
		40% only household ambulation at 1 year
ASIA C		
under age 50 (ref. 18)	≤72 hours	91% at least household at rehab d/c
age 50 or older	≤72 hours	42% at least household at rehab d/c
ASIA D		
all ages (ref. 18)	≤72 hours	>95% community rehab d/c

than or equal to 20 were limited ambulators. These patients had slower average velocities, higher heart rates, subsequent greater energy expenditure, and greater axial loading exerted on assistive devices when compared to patients with LEMS of *greater than or equal to* 30 who attained community ambulation status. Individuals with LEMS of *greater than or equal to* 30 ambulated with physiologic parameters close to those demonstrated by able-bodied subjects.

Early determination of LEMS was also found to be predictive of ambulatory function 1 year following injury. Waters et al. determined that when patients were categorized by level and completeness of injury, the proportion of those who were ambulatory 1 year following injury increased as the initial LEMS increased (29). For example, among those with incomplete paraplegia, 33% with an initial LEMS of 0 ambulated, compared with 70% of those with LEMS between 1 and 9, and 100% for those with LEMS above 10. Because the LEMS represents strength in some of the key muscles involved in ambulation, it follows that a higher initial LEMS is predictive of successful ambulation.

Self-Care and Functional Mobility

Just as initial AIS grade can predict ability for ultimate ambulation, Functional Independence Measures (FIM) scores at discharge are also dependent on level and completeness of injury (30). Discharge FIM scores are strongly related to neurologic level for ASIA impairment grades A (motor complete), B (sensory incomplete), and C (motor incomplete with the majority of muscles below the NLI having muscle grades less than 3/5). However, individuals with motor incomplete lesions with the majority of muscles below the NLI having strength 3/5 or greater (AIS grade D) had relatively high FIM scores regardless of the neurologic level (30).

Graves and associates studied the effects of various rehabilitation indices, as well as neurologic measures on functional gains, and concluded that the ASIA Motor Score (AMS) was the most powerful predictor of gains in self-care activities and mobility (31). Furthermore, they determined that separating the AMS into upper extremity and lower extremity motor scores added to the predictive power.

Levels of function are dependent on patient motivation and training as well as on neurologic status. Because individuals with incomplete injuries can have vastly different motor and sensory function even at the same neurologic level of injury, it is not possible to predict functional outcomes based on NLI in incomplete patients. In patients with complete injuries, however, the motor and sensory function is fairly consistent within a given NLI. Guidelines for expected outcomes have been developed for these patients.

An expert panel of SCI professionals has developed a table of expected functional outcomes for various levels of motor complete SCI (Table 9.4). The panel emphasized that the outcomes are only generalizations of expected function under optimal conditions. They further stressed the importance of a careful evaluation of the unique circumstances and abilities of each patient in establishing goals for functional outcomes (30).

Outcomes are categorized into seven groups, representing activities of daily living (ADL), mobility concerns, and commu-

nication issues. Expected levels of assistance, based on FIM scores, and possible adaptations or specialized equipment needs are also presented.

Patients with injuries at the upper cervical levels (C1–C3) are typically dependent for all activities including respiration. Using a power wheelchair with head, chin, or breath control and a powered reclining chairback, they may become independent in pressure relief and positioning, and in wheelchair propulsion. These individuals may be independent in communication if specialized adaptive equipment is available (e.g., mouthstick, high-tech computers, environmental control units). Patients with a C4 NLI may be able to breathe without a ventilator. They are generally dependent for all other functional activities.

At the C5 NLI, individuals need less assistance for activities of daily living. For some activities, such as eating and upper extremity dressing, they may require assistance with setup but then are able to complete tasks. At this level, the use of specialized adaptive devices becomes critical in determining the level of assistance required to perform various dressing, eating, and grooming activities. The use of a manual chair with handrim projections is a possibility at this level, although some assistance will likely be required for propulsion outdoors, up inclines, or on rough surfaces.

At the lower cervical levels, C6 and C7–C8, individuals will still likely need assistance with bowel and bladder management, but they have the capability to be independent with nearly all other functional activities (with appropriate adaptive equipment). Although patients with a C6 level may still need a power wheelchair for community mobility, at the C7–C8 levels, a manual chair is typically used.

Individuals with paraplegia have the potential to be independent in all self-care activities, as well as with bowel and bladder management. The amount of assistance required for housekeeping declines with a more caudal NLI. Finally, ambulation is dependent on the level of NLI. Patients with NLI above T10 typically do not ambulate in a functional manner. At the T10–L2 levels, functional ambulation is possible but will probably entail a high energy cost if a swing-through gait pattern is required. Thus, at these levels, an individual capable of walking may still elect to use a wheelchair as a more efficient means of mobility.

Because these expected functional outcomes reflect generalities, it is important for providers and patients to be alert to individual circumstances that may limit their realization. Patient motivation and training play a large role in the ability to attain a certain functional level. Additionally, physical limitations or concomitant conditions may limit function. For example, patients with a NLI of C6 can typically attain independence in sliding board transfers. If, however, there is an elbow flexion contracture, independence will be delayed until full elbow extension is achieved. Similarly, whereas patients with paraplegia can become independent in dressing activities, they will be limited if they do not have adequate range of motion in the hamstrings. In addition to conditions that may limit range of motion (i.e., contractures, joint deformities, heterotopic bone), other factors that can affect achievement of optimal function include patient age, level of physical conditioning and potential for conditioning, length of time since injury, family support, spasticity, obesity, and other medical complications.

TABLE 9.4   Expected Functional Outcomes

LEVEL C1-3

Functionally relevant muscles innervated: Sternocleidomastoid; cervical paraspinal; neck accessories
Movement possible: Neck flexion, extension, rotation
Patterns of weakness: Total paralysis of trunk, upper extremities, lower extremities; dependent on ventilator
FIM/Assistance Data: Exp = Expected FIM score / **Med** = NSCISC median / **IR** = NSCISC interquartile range
NSCISC Sample Size: FIM = 15 / Assist = 12

	Expected Functional Outcomes	Equipment	FIM/Assistance Data		
			EXP	MED	IR
Respiratory	• Ventilator dependent • Inability to clear secretions	• 2 ventilators (bedside, portable) • Suction equipment or other suction management device • Generator/battery backup			
Bowel	Total assist	Padded reclining shower/commode chair (if roll-in shower available)	1	1	1
Bladder	Total assist		1	1	1
Bed Mobility	Total assist	Full electric hospital bed with Trendelenburg feature and side rails			
Bed/Wheelchair Transfers	Total assist	• Transfer board • Power of mechanical lift with sling			
Pressure Relief/Positioning	Total assist; may be independent with equipment	• Power recline and/or tilt wheelchair • Wheelchair pressure-relief cushion • Postural support and head control devices as indicated • Hand splints may be indicated • Specialty bed or pressure-relief mattress may be indicated			
Eating	Total assist		1	1	1
Dressing	Total assist		1	1	1
Grooming	Total assist		1	1	1
Bathing	Total assist	• Handheld shower • Shampoo tray • Padded reclining shower/commode chair (if roll-in shower available)	1	1	1
Wheelchair Propulsion	Manual: Total assist Power: Independent with equipment	• Power recline and/or tilt wheelchair with head, chin, or breath control and manual recliner • Vent tray	6	1	1–6
Standing/Ambulation	Standing: Total assist; Ambulation: Not indicated				
Communication	Total assist to independent, depending on work station setup and equipment availability	• Mouth stick, high-tech computer access; environmental control unit • Adaptive devices everywhere as indicated			
Transportation	Total assist	Attendant-operated van (e.g., lift, tie-downs) or accessible public transportation			
Homemaking	Total assist				
Assist Required	• 24-hour attendant care to include homemaking • Able to instruct in all aspects of care		24*	24*	12–24*

continued on next page

TABLE 9.4   *(Continued)*

LEVEL C4

Functionally relevant muscles innervated: Upper trapezius; diaphragm; cervical paraspinal muscles

Movement possible: Neck flexion, extension, rotation; scapular elevation; inspiration

Patterns of weakness: Paralysis of trunk, upper extremities, lower extremities; inability to cough, endurance and respiratory reserve low secondary to paralysis of intercostals

FIM/Assistance Data: **Exp** = Expected FIM score / **Med** = NSCISC median / **IR** = NSCISC interquartile range

NSCISC Sample Size: FIM = 28 / Assist = 12

	Expected Functional Outcomes	Equipment	FIM/Assistance Data		
			EXP	**MED**	**IR**
Respiratory	May be able to breathe without a ventilator	If not ventilator free, see C1-3 for equipment requirements			
Bowel	Total assist	Reclining shower/commode chair (if roll-in shower available)	1	1	1
Bladder	Total assist		1	1	1
Bed Mobility	Total assist	Full electric hospital bed with Trendelenburg feature and side rails			
Bed/Wheelchair Transfers	Total assist	• Transfer board • Power or mechanical lift with sling	1	1	1
Pressure Relief/Positioning	Total assist; may be independent with equipment	• Power recline and/or tilt wheelchair • Wheelchair pressure-relief cushion • Postural support and head control devices as indicated • Hand splints may be indicated • Specialty bed or pressure-relief mattress may be indicated			
Eating	Total assist		1	1	1
Dressing	Total assist		1	1	1
Grooming	Total assist		1	1	1
Bathing	Total assist	• Shampoo tray • Handheld shower • Padded reclining shower/commode chair (if roll-in shower available)	1	1	1
Wheelchair Propulsion	Power: Independent Manual: Total assist	• Power recline and/or tilt wheelchair with head, chin, or breath control and manual recliner • Vent tray	6	1	1–6
Standing/Ambulation	Standing: Total assist Ambulation: Not usually indicated	• Tilt table • Hydraulic standing table			
Communication	Total assist to independent, depending on work station setup and equipment availability	Mouth stick, high-tech computer access, environmental control unit			
Transportation	Total assist	Attendant-operated van (e.g., lift, tie-downs) or accessible public transportation			
Homemaking	Total assist				
Assist Required	• 24-hour care to include homemaking • Able to instruct in all aspects of care		24*	24*	16–24*

TABLE 9.4   *(Continued)*

LEVEL C5

Functionally relevant muscles innervated: Deltoid, biceps, brachialis, brachioradialis, rhomboids, serratus anterior (partially innervated)

Movement possible: Shoulder flexion, abduction, and extension; elbow flexion and supination; scapular adduction and abduction

Patterns of weakness: Absence of elbow extension, pronation, all wrist and hand movement; Total paralysis of trunk and lower extremities

FIM/Assistance Data: **Exp** = Expected FIM score / **Med** = NSCISC median / **IR** = NSCISC interquartile range

NSCISC Sample Size: FIM = 41 / Assist = 35

	Expected Functional Outcomes	Equipment	FIM/Assistance Data		
			EXP	**MED**	**IR**
Respiratory	Low endurance and vital capacity secondary to paralysis of intercostals; may require assist to clear secretions				
Bowel	Total assist	Padded shower/commode chair or padded transfer tub bench with commode cutout	1	1	1
Bladder	Total assist	Adaptive devices may be indicated (electric leg bag emptier)	1	1	1
Bed Mobility	Some assist	• Full electric hospital bed with Trendelenburg feature with patients control • Side rails			
Bed/Wheelchair Transfers	Total assist	• Transfer board • Power of mechanical lift	1	1	1
Pressure Relief/Positioning	Independent with equipment	• Power recline and/or tilt wheelchair • Wheelchair pressure-relief cushion • Hand splints • Specialty bed or pressure-relief mattress may be indicated • Postural support devices			
Eating	Total assist for setup, then independent eating with equipment	• Long opponens splint • Adaptive devices as indicated	5	5	2.5–5.5
Dressing	Lower extremity: Total assist Upper extremity: Some assist	• Long opponens splint • Adaptive devices as indicated	1	1	1–4
Grooming	Some to total assist	• Long opponens splint • Adaptive devices as indicated	1–3	1	1–5
Bathing	Total assist	• Padded tub transfer bench or shower/commode chair • Handheld shower	1	1	1–3
Wheelchair Propulsion	Power: Independent Manual: Independent to some assist indoors on noncarpet, level surface; some to total assist outdoors	Power: Power recline and/or tilt with arm drive control Manual: Lightweight rigid or folding frame with handrim modifications	6	6	5–6
Standing/Ambulation	Total assist	Hydraulic standing frame			
Communication	Independent to some assist after setup with equipment	• Long opponens splint • Adaptive devices as needed for page turning, writing, button pushing			
Transportation	Independent with highly specialized equipment; some assist with accessible public transportation; total assist for attendant-operated vehicle	Highly specialized modified van with lift			
Homemaking	Total assist				
Assist Required	• Personal care: 10 hours/day • Homecare: 6 hours/day • Able to instruct in all aspects of care		16*	23*	10–24*

continued on next page

TABLE 9.4   *(Continued)*

LEVEL C6

Functionally relevant muscles innervated: Clavicular pectoralis supinator; extensor carpi radialis longus and brevis; serratus anterior; latissimus dorsi

Movement possible: Scapular protractor; some horizontal adduction, forearm supination, radial wrist extension

Patterns of weakness: Absence of wrist flexion, elbow extension, hand movement; total paralysis of trunk and lower extremities

FIM/Assistance Data: **Exp** = Expected FIM score / **Med** = NSCISC median / **IR** = NSCISC interquartile range

NSCISC Sample Size: FIM = 43 / Assist = 35

	EXPECTED FUNCTIONAL OUTCOMES	EQUIPMENT	FIM/Assistance Data		
			EXP	MED	IR
Respiratory	Low endurance and vital capacity secondary to paralysis of intercostals; may require assist to clear secretions				
Bowel	Some total assist	• Padded tub bench with commode cutout or padded shower/commode chair • Other adaptive devices as indicated	1–2	1	1
Bladder	Some to total assist with equipment; may be independent with leg bag emptying	Adaptive devices as indicated	1–2	1	1
Bed Mobility	Some assist	• Full electric hospital bed • Side rails • Full to king standard bed may be indicated			
Bed/Wheelchair Transfers	Level: Some assist to independent Uneven: Some assist to total assist	• Transfer board • Mechanical lift	3	1	1–3
Pressure Relief/Positioning	Independent with equipment and/or adapted techniques	• Power recline wheelchair • Wheelchair pressure relief cushion • Postural support devices • Pressure-relief mattress or overlay may be indicated			
Eating	Independent with or without equipment; except cutting, which is total assist	Adaptive devices as indicated (e.g., u-cuff, tendenosis splint, adapted utensils, plate guard)	5–6	5	4–6
Dressing	Independent upper extremity; some assist to total assist for lower extremities	Adaptive devices as indicated (e.g., button; hook; loops on zippers, pants; socks, velcro on shoes)	1–3	2	1–5
Grooming	Some assist to independent with equipment	Adaptive devices as indicated (e.g., U-cuff, adapted handles)	3–6	4	2–6
Bathing	Upper body: Independent Lower body: Some to total assist	• Padded tub transfer bench or shower/commode chair • Adaptive devices as needed • Handheld shower	1–3	1	1–3
Wheelchair Propulsion	Power: independent with standard arm drive on all surfaces Manual: Independent indoors; some total assist outdoors	Manual: Lightweight rigid or folding frame with modified rims Power: may require power recline or standard upright power wheelchair	6	6	4–6
Standing/Ambulation	Standing: Total assist Ambulation: Not indicated	Hydraulic standing frame			

TABLE 9.4 *(Continued)*

LEVEL C6 *(Continued)*

Communication	Independent with or without equipment	Adaptive devices as indicated (e.g., tendenosis splint; writing splint for keyboard use, button pushing, page turning, object manipulation)			
Transportation	Independent driving from wheelchair	• Modified van with lift • Sensitized hand controls • Tie-downs			
Homemaking	Some assist with light meal preparation; total assist for all other homemaking	Adaptive devices as indicated			
Assist Required	• Personal care: 6 hours/day • Home care: 4 hours/day		10*	17*	8–24*

LEVEL C7–C8

Functionally relevant muscles innervated: Latissimus dorsi; sterna pectoralis; triceps; pronator quadrates; extensor carpi ulnaris; flexor carpi radialis; flexor digitorum profundus and superficialis; extensor communis; pronator/flexor/extensor/abductor pollicis; lumbricals [partially innervated]

Movement possible: Elbow extension; ulnar/wrist extension; wrist flexion; finger flexions and extensions; thumb flexion/extension/abduction

Patterns of weakness: Paralysis or trunk and lower extremities; limited grasp release and dexterity secondary to partial intrinsic muscles of the hand

FIM/Assistance Data: **Exp** = Expected FIM score / **Med** = NSCISC median / **IR** = NSCISC interquartile range

NSCISC Sample Size: FIM = 15 / Assist = 12

	Expected Functional Outcomes	Equipment	FIM/Assistance Data		
			EXP	MED	IR
Respiratory	Low endurance and vital capacity secondary to paralysis of intercostals; may require assist to clear secretions				
Bowel	Some to total assist	• Padded tub bench with commode cutout or shower commode chair • Adaptive devices as needed	1–4	1	1–4
Bladder	Independent to some assist	Adaptive devices as indicated	2–6	3	1–6
Bed Mobility	Independent to some assist	Full electric hospital bed or full to king standard bed			
Bed/Wheelchair Transfers	Level: Independent Uneven: Independent to some assist	With or without transfer board	3–7	4	2–6
Pressure Relief/Positioning	Independent	• Wheelchair pressure relief cushion • Postural support devices as indicated • Pressure-relief mattress/or overlay may be indicated			
Eating	Independent	Adaptive devices as indicated	6–7	6	5–7
Dressing	Independent upper extremities; Independent to some assist lower extremities	Adaptive devices as indicated	4–7	6	4–7
Grooming	Independent	Adaptive devices as indicated	6–7	6	4–7
Bathing	Upper body: Independent	• Padded transfer tub bench or shower/commode chair	3–6	4	2–6
	Lower extremity: Some assist to independent	• Handheld shower • Adaptive devices as needed			

continued on next page

TABLE 9.4   *(Continued)*

LEVEL C7–C8 *(Continued)*

Wheelchair Propulsion	Manual: Independent all indoor surfaces and level outdoor terrain; some assist with uneven terrain	Manual: Rigid or folding lightweight or folding wheelchair with modified rims	6	6	6
Standing/Ambulation	Standing: Independent to some assist Ambulation: Not indicated	Hydraulic or standard standing frame			
Communication	Independent	Adaptive devices as indicated			
Transportation	Independent car if independent with transfer and wheelchair loading/unloading; independent driving modified van from captain's seat	• Modified vehicle • Transfer board			
Homemaking	Independent light meal preparation and homemaking; some to total assist for complex meal prep and heavy housecleaning	Adaptive devices as indicated			
Assist Required	• Personal care: 6 hours/day • Homecare: 2 hours/day				

LEVEL T1–T9

Functionally relevant muscles innervated: Intrinsics of the hand including thumbs; internal and external intercostals; erector spinae; lumbricals; flexor/extensor/abductor pollicis

Movement possible: Upper extremities fully intact; limited upper trunk stability. Endurance increased secondary innervations of intercostals.

Patterns of weakness: Lower trunk paralysis. Total paralysis lower extremities.

FIM/Assistance Data: **Exp** = Expected FIM Score / **Med** = NSCISC Median / **IR** = NSCISC Interquartile Range

NSCISC Sample Size: FIM = 144 / Assist = 122

	EXPECTED FUNCTIONAL OUTCOMES	EQUIPMENT	FIM/Assistance Data		
			EXP	MED	IR
Respiratory	Compromised vital capacity and endurance				
Bowel	Independent	Elevated padded toilet seat or padded tub bench with commode cutout	6–7	6	4–6
Bladder	Independent		6	6	5–6
Bed Mobility	Independent	Full to king standard bed			
Bed/Wheelchair Transfers	Independent	May or may not require transfer board	6–7	6	6–7
Pressure Relief/Positioning	Independent	• Wheelchair pressure relief cushion • Postural support devices as indicated • Pressure-relief mattress or overlay may be indicated			
Eating	Independent		7	7	7
Dressing	Independent		7	7	7
Grooming	Independent		7	7	7
Bathing	Independent	• Padded tub transfer bench or shower/commode chair • Handheld shower	6–7	6	5–7
Wheelchair Propulsion	Independent	Manual rigid or folding lightweight wheelchair	6	6	6
Standing/Ambulation	Standing: Independent Ambulation: Typically not functional	Standing frame			

TABLE 9.4 *(Continued)*

LEVEL T1–T9 *(Continued)*

Communication	Independent				
Transportation	Independent in car, including loading and unloading wheelchair	Hand controls			
Homemaking	Independent with complex meal prep and light housecleaning; total to some assist with heavy housekeeping				
Assist Required	Homemaking: 3 hours/day		2*	3*	0–15*

LEVEL T10–L1

Functionally relevant muscles innervated: Fully intact intercostals; external obliques; rectus abdominis

Movement possible: Good trunk stability

Patterns of weakness: Paralysis of lower extremities

FIM/Assistance Data: Exp = Expected FIM Score / **Med** = NSCISC Median / **IR** = NSCISC Interquartile Range

NSCISC Sample Size: FIM = 71 / Assist = 57

	EXPECTED FUNCTIONAL OUTCOMES	EQUIPMENT	FIM/Assistance Data		
			EXP	**MED**	**IR**
Respiratory	Intact respiratory function				
Bowel	Independent	Padded standard or raised padded toilet seat	6–7	6	6
Bladder	Independent		6	6	6
Bed Mobility	Independent	Full to king standard bed			
Bed/Wheelchair Transfers	Independent		7	7	6–7
Pressure Relief/Positioning	Independent	• Wheelchair pressure-relief cushion • Postural support devices as indicated • Pressure-relief mattress or overlay may be indicated			
Eating	Independent		7	7	7
Dressing	Independent		7	7	7
Grooming	Independent		7	7	7
Bathing	Independent	• Padded transfer tub bench • Handheld shower	6–7	6	6–7
Wheelchair Propulsion	Independent all indoor and outdoor surfaces	Manual rigid or folding lightweight wheelchair	6	6	6
Standing/Ambulation	Standing: Independent Ambulation: Functional, some assist to independent	• Standing frame • Forearm crutches or walker • Knee, ankle, foot orthesis (KAFO)			
Communication	Independent				
Transportation	Independent in car, including loading and unloading wheelchair	Hand controls			
Homemaking	Independent with complex meal prep and light housecleaning; some assist with heavy housekeeping				
Assist Required	Homemaking: 2 hours/day		2*	2*	0–8*

continued on next page

TABLE 9.4   *(Continued)*

LEVEL L2–S5

Functionally relevant muscles innervated: Fully intact abdominals and all other trunk muscles; depending on level, some degree of hip flexors, extensors, abductors, adductors; knee flexors, extensors; ankle dorsi, flexors, plantar flexors

Movement possible: Good trunk stability. Partial to full control lower extremities.

Patterns of weakness: Partial paralysis lower extremities, hips, knees, ankle, foot

FIM/Assistance Data: Exp = Expected FIM Score / **Med** = NSCISC Median / **IR** = NSCISC Interquartile Range

NSCISC Sample Size: FIM = 20 / Assist = 16

	EXPECTED FUNCTIONAL OUTCOMES	EQUIPMENT	FIM/Assistance Data EXP	MED	IR
Respiratory	Intact function				
Bowel	Independent	Padded toilet seat	6–7	6	6–7
Bladder	Independent		6	6	6–7
Bed Mobility	Independent				
Bed/Wheelchair Transfers	Independent	Full to king standard bed	7	7	7
Pressure Relief/Positioning	Independent	• Wheelchair pressure-relief cushion • Postural support device as indicated			
Eating	Independent		7	7	7
Dressing	Independent		7	7	7
Grooming	Independent		7	7	7
Bathing	Independent	• Padded tub bench • Handheld shower	7	7	6–7
Wheelchair Propulsion	Independent on all indoor and outdoor surfaces	Manual rigid or folding lightweight wheelchair	6	6	6
Standing/Ambulation	Standing: independent Ambulation: Functional, independent to some assist	• Standing frame • Knee-ankle-foot orthosis or ankle-foot orthosis • Forearm crutches or cane as indicated			
Communication	Independent				
Transportation	Independent in car, including loading and unloading wheelchair	Hand controls			
Homemaking	Independent complex cooking and light housekeeping; some assist with heavy housekeeping				
Assist Required	Homemaking: 0–1 hour/day		0–1*	0*	0–2*

*Hours per day

Adapted from *Outcomes Following Traumatic SCI: Clinical Practice Guidelines for Health-Care Professionals* (ref. 12).

ALTERNATIVE FORMS OF NEUROLOGIC ASSESSMENT

Magnetic resonance imaging has proven to be a powerful tool in the assessment of intramedullary pathology subsequent to spinal cord injury. This modality provides far more information regarding the condition of the spinal cord in comparison to earlier technologies such as CT myelography. The latter technique, however, is used in cases of retained bullet fragments or other potentially ferromagnetic materials. Although the clinical evaluation, represented by the ASIA examination, is the single best predictor of neurological outcome (32), MRI findings can improve the ability of the clinician to provide an accurate prognosis (33), particularly in cases involving potentially unreliable or obtunded patients. Several reports (32, 34, 35) indicate that the presence of intramedullary hemorrhage at the time of initial SCI is indicative of a poor prognosis, and indeed suggests a complete (34) or at least a motor complete (36) SCI. Although the degree of bone or soft tissue injury did not correlate with injury severity, rostral limit of edema and total length of spinal cord edema was prognostic (34).

Marciello and associates (36) also examined recovery in upper and lower extremities by total motor index score (MIS) and found a median motor improvement in the upper extremities of 8 in the group with hemorrhage and 24 in the group without hemorrhage. Those without hemorrhage also had a median MIS change of 30 in the lower extremities, but all those with hemorrhage had scores of 0, both at the 72-hour initial assessment and at the 12- or 18-month follow-up. Boldin's investigation (37) supports evidence that the presence of extensive edema is associated with a poorer prognosis and that a hemorrhage longer than 4 mm appears to suggest poor neurological recovery at long-term reevaluation. Thus, smaller hemorrhages may be less damaging than larger ones in terms of overall recovery. Finally, a recent study by Miyanji and coauthors (38) found that maximal spinal cord compression was more predictive of neurologic outcome than spinal canal compromise. These authors also observed a correlation between spinal cord hemorrhage and cord swelling and unfavorable prognosis for recovery.

Presence of spinal cord edema and hemorrhage have also been compared to FIM scores (39). Overall, more dramatic improvement in self-care and mobility FIM subscores were observed in persons without hemorrhage relative to those with hemorrhage. Moreover initial and final FIM scores for all measures (self-care, sphincter, mobility/transfers, and locomotion/ambulation) were higher in subjects without hemorrhage. Edema length appeared unrelated to FIM outcomes, but rostral extent of edema had some influence on self-care skills. Although imaging findings can help estimate how much caregiver assistance an individual may ultimately require, MRI findings are less strongly associated with FIM scores than with motor scores, due to influences of age, cognition, motivation, physical endurance, and environment.

Electrodiagnostic testing has also been utilized for prognostic information and has proven useful in children under age 5 because children this young cannot reliably participate in the ASIA examination (40). Somatosensory-evoked potentials permit differentiation of complete vs. incomplete lesions and can be helpful in the unconscious patient (41). However, since this testing examines dorsal column function that carries only sensory fibers, presence of SSEP signals may not translate to motor function. Moreover, SSEPs are no more accurate than the clinical examination if the patient is able to communicate and cooperate fully in the ASIA examination (42). Calancie (43) observed that persons with motor incomplete cervical or thoracic SCI demonstrated large amplitude tendon responses on EMG testing. This finding, combined with presence of crossed adductor response to patellar tendon taps observed shortly after injury, predicted a better motor recovery. In contrast, those with complete SCI had small or absent amplitude responses and did not demonstrate a crossed adductor response to stimulation.

The question of interventions to improve neurologic or functional outcome, such as electrical stimulation or tendon transfers of the tetraplegic hand, have not been addressed in this chapter. The reader is referred to other sections of the book for this information.

CONCLUSION

Detailed neurologic examinations performed from 72 hours to 1 month following injury can provide data that can be used to reliably predict neurologic recovery at 1 year. Expected functional outcomes have been established for those with complete injuries at various neurologic levels of injury, whereas more variability is seen among those with incomplete injuries. When considering expected functional outcomes for both complete and incomplete subjects, it is crucial to consider the unique qualities of each patient, because individual differences can affect the actual level of function ultimately attained. Patient motivation and family support play a crucial role in achievement of expected motor and functional recovery. As time spent in the inpatient rehabilitation setting is continuing to decline because of pressure from third-party payers, it is essential that the clinician have a clear understanding of functional expectations. An awareness of what is possible and an understanding of the particular characteristics of each patient will enable the physician to provide optimal care. By anticipating factors that may hinder or facilitate recovery of function, the managing physician can strategically plan rehabilitation to maximize gains in an era of finite therapy, and often of limited financial resources.

References

1. The National SCI Statistical Center. *Spinal Cord Injury: Facts and Figures at a Glance*. Birmingham: University of Alabama at Birmingham National SCI Center, June 2007.
2. Brown PJ, Marino RJ, Herbison GJ, et al. The 72-hour examination as a predictor of recovery in motor complete quadriplegia. *Arch Phys Med Rehabil* 1991; 2:546–548.
3. Herbison GJ, Zerby SA, Cohen ME, et al. Motor power difference within the first two weeks post-SCI in cervical spinal cord quadriplegic subjects. *J Neurotrauma* 1991; 9:373–380.
4. Mange KC, Ditunno JF, Herbison GJ, et al. Recovery of strength at the zone of injury in motor complete and motor incomplete cervical spinal cord injured patients. *Arch Phys Med Rehabil* 1990; 71:562–565.
5. Waters RL, Yakura JS, Adkins RH, Sie I. Recovery following complete paraplegia. *Arch Phys Med Rehabil* 1992; 73:784–789.
6. Waters RL, Yakura JS, Adkins RH, Sie I. Motor and sensory recovery following incomplete paraplegia. *Arch Phys Med Rehabil* 1994; 75:67–72.
7. Waters RL, Yakura JS, Adkins RH, Sie I. Motor and sensory recovery following complete tetraplegia. *Arch Phys Med Rehabil* 1993; 4:242–247.
8. Waters RL, Yakura JS, Adkins RH, Sie I. Motor and sensory recovery following incomplete tetraplegia. *Arch Phys Med Rehabil* 1994; 75:306–311.
9. Marino RJ, Ditunno JF, Donovan WH, Maynard F. Neurologic recovery after traumatic spinal cord injury: Data from the model spinal cord injury systems. *Arch Phys Med Rehabil* 1999; 80:1391–1396.
10. Burns AS, Lee BS, Ditunno JF, Tessler A. Patient selection for clinical trials: The reliability of the early spinal cod injury examination. *J Neurotrauma*. 2003; 20:477–482.
11. American Spinal Injury Association/International Medical Society of Paraplegia (ASIA/IMSOP). *International Standards for Neurologic and Functional Classification of Spinal Cord Injury*, Revised 2000. Chicago: ASIA.
12. Fawcett JW, Curt LA, Steeves JD, et al. Guidelines for the conduct of clinical trials for spinal cord injury as develop by the ICCP panel: Spontaneous recovery after spinal cord injury and statistical power needed for therapeutic clinical trials. *Spinal Cord* 2007; 45:190–205.
13. Maynard FM, Reynolds GG, Fountain S, et al. Neurologic prognosis after traumatic quadriplegia. *J Neurosurg* 1979; 50:611–616.
14. Foo D, Subrahmanyan TS, Rossier AB. Post-traumatic acute anterior spinal cord syndrome. *Paraplegia* 1981; 19:201–205.
15. Crozier KS, Graziani V, Ditunno JF, Herbison GJ. Spinal cord injury: Prognosis for ambulation based on sensory examination in patients who are initially motor complete. *Arch Phys Med Rehabil* 1991; 72:119–121.

16. Oleson CV, Burns AS, Ditunno JF, Geisler FH, Coleman WP. Prognostic value of pinprick preservation in motor complete, sensory incomplete spinal cord injury. *Arch Phys Med Rehabil* 2005; 86:988–992.

17. Shepard MJ, Bracken MB. Magnetic resonance imaging and neurological recovery in acute spinal cord injury: Observations from the National Acute Spinal Cord Injury Study 3. *Spinal Cord* 1999; 37:833–837.

18. Burns SP, Golding DG, Rolle WA, Graziani V, Ditunno JF. Recovery of ambulation in motor incomplete tetraplegia. *Arch Phys Med Rehabil* 1997; 78:1169–1172.

19. Penrod LE, Hedge SK, Ditunno JF. Age effect on prognosis for functional recovery in acute, traumatic central cord syndrome. *Arch Phys Med Rehabil* 1990; 71:963–968.

20. Roth EJ, Lawler MH, Yarkony GM. Traumatic central cord syndromes: Clinical features and functional outcomes. *Arch Phys Med Rehabil* 1990; 71:18–23.

21. Roth EJ, Park T, Pang T, et al. Traumatic cervical Brown-Séquard and Brown-Séquard plus syndromes: The spectrum of presentations and outcomes. *Paraplegia* 1991; 29:582–589.

22. Mange KC, Ditunno JF, Herbison GJ, Jaweed MM. Recovery of strength at the zone of injury in motor complete and motor incomplete cervical spinal cord injured patients. *Arch Phys Med Rehabil* 1990; 71:562–565.

23. Kirshblum S, Millis S, McKinley W, Tulsky D. Late neurologic recovery after traumatic spinal cord injury. *Arch Phys Med Rehabil* 2004; 85:1811–1825.

24. Stauffer ES. *Study of 100 Paraplegics*. Rancho Los Amigos Papers, 1968.

25. Waters RL, Lunsford BR. The energy cost of paraplegic locomotion. *J Bone Joint Surg Br* 1985; 67A:1245–1250.

26. Hussey RW, Stauffer ES. Spinal Cord Injury: Requirements for ambulation. *Arch Phys Med Rehabil* 1973; 54:544–547.

27. Crozier, KS. Cheng LL, Graziani V, Zorn G, et al. Spinal cord injury: Prognosis for ambulation based on quadriceps recovery. *Paraplegia* 1992; 30:762–767.

28. Waters RL, Adkins R, Yakura J, Vigil D. Prediction of ambulatory performance based on motor scores derived from standards of the American Spinal Injury Association. *Arch Phys Med Rehabil* 1994; 75:756–761.

29. Waters RL, Yoshida GM. Prognosis of spinal cord injuries. In: Levine AM, ed. *Orthopaedic Knowledge Update, Trauma*. American Academy of Orthopaedic Surgeons, 1996:303–310.

30. *Outcomes Following Traumatic Spinal Cord Injury: Clinical Practice Guidelines for Health-Care Professionals*. Consortium for Spinal Cord Medicine. Paralyzed Veterans of America, 1999.

31. Graves DE, Frankiewicz RG, Carter E. Gain in functional ability during medical rehabilitation as related to rehabilitation process indices and neurologic measures. *Arch Phys Med Rehabil* 1999; 80:1464–1470.

32. Selden NR, Quint DJ, Patel N, D'Arcy HS, Papadopoulos SM. Emergency magnetic resonance imaging of cervical spinal cord injuries: Clinical correlation and prognosis. *Neurosurgery* 1999; 44:785–792.

33. Flanders AE, Spettell CM, Tartaglino LM, Friedman DP, Herbison GJ. Forecasting motor recovery following cervical spinal cord injury: Value of MR imaging. *Radiology* 1996; 201:649–655.

34. Flanders AE, Schaefer DM, Doan HT, Mishkin MM, et al. Acute cervical spine trauma: Correlation of MR imaging findings with degree of neurologic deficit. *Radiology* 1990; 177:25–33.

35. Schaefer DM, Flanders AE, Osterholm JL, Northrup BE. Prognostic significance of magnetic resonance imaging in the acute phase of cervical spine injury. *J Neurosurg* 1992; 76:218–233.

36. Marciello MA, Flanders AE, Herbison GJ, Schaefer DM, et al. Magnetic resonance imaging related to neurologic outcome in cervical spinal cord injury. *Arch Phys Med Rehabil* 1993; 74:940–946.

37. Boldin C, Raith J, Fankhauser F, Haunschmid C, et al. Predicting neurologic recovery in cervical spinal cord injury with postoperative MR imaging. *Spine* 2006; 31:554–559.

38. Miyanji F, Furlan JC, Aarabi B, Arnold PM, Fehlings MG. Acute cervical traumatic spinal cord injury: MR imaging findings correlated with neurologic outcome—prospective study with 100 consecutive patients. *Radiology* 2007; 243:820–827.

39. Flanders AE, Spettell CM, Friedman DP, Marino RJ, Herbison GJ. The relationship between the functional abilities of patients with cervical spinal cord injury and the severity of damage revealed by MR imaging. *Am J Neuroradiol* 1999; 20:926–934.

40. Mulcahey MJ, Gaughan J, Betz RR, Johansen KJ. The international standards for neurological classification of spinal cord injury: Reliability of data when applied to children and youths. *Spinal Cord* 2007; 45:452–459.

41. Houlden DA, Schwart ML, Klettke KA. Neurophysiological diagnosis in uncooperative trauma patients: Confounding factors. *J Trauma* 1992; 33:244–251.

42. Curt A, Dietz V. Ambulatory capacity in spinal cord injury: Significance of somatosensory evoked potentials and ASIA protocol in predicting outcome. *Arch Phys Med Rehabil* 1997; 78:39–43.

43. Calancie B, Molano MR, Broton JG. EMG for assessing the recovery of voluntary movement after acute spinal cord injury in man. *Clin Neurophysiol* 2004; 115:1748–1759.

II

ACUTE SPINAL CORD INJURY MANAGEMENT AND SURGICAL CONSIDERATIONS

10 Prehospital Management of Spinal Cord Injured Patients

William D. Whetstone

Management of the spinal cord injured (SCI) patient begins immediately post-injury by the first providers at the accident scene. Recent evidence-based guidelines from the American Association of Neurological Surgeons (AANS) are being used to improve techniques of prehospital management (1). It has been previously estimated that 3–25% of spinal cord injuries occur *after* the initial traumatic insult, either during transit or early in the course of treatment (2).

Over the last 20 years, there has been a dramatic improvement in prehospital management and thus an improvement in the neurologic prognosis of SCI patients arriving in the emergency department. During the 1970s, the majority of spinal cord injured patients arrived with complete cord lesions. This statistic, however, changed during the 1980s, when the majority of patients were found to have incomplete lesions (3).

In 1989 Garfin (4) stated that "no patient should be extricated from a crashed vehicle or transported from an accident scene without spinal stabilization." Stabilization of the cervical spine is credited as a key factor responsible for the decline of the percentage of complete spinal cord injury lesions from 55% in the 1970s to 39% in the 1980s, and for the significant reduction in mortality of multiple-injury patients with cervical spinal injuries (4). Unfortunately, there is no Class I or Class II medical evidence to support this claim.

On a practical basis, it is presumed that a large portion of spinal cord injury outcome improvement was the product of development of emergency medical services (EMS). EMS systems train providers in proper extrication techniques and coordinate expeditious transfer to a trauma center. In this chapter the five responsibilities of prehospital care (evaluation, resuscitation, immobilization, extrication, and transportation) will be defined and discussed (5).

EVALUATION

The evaluation phase consists of primary and secondary surveys as emphasized by ATLS guidelines (6). The "ABCDE" of the trauma primary survey are Airway maintenance with cervical spine control; Breathing and ventilation; Circulation with hemorrhage control; Disability assessment (e.g., neurologic status); and Exposure/environmental control (e.g., completely undressing the patient while preventing hyper- or hypothermia).

After completing the primary survey, the prehospital provider should perform an abbreviated secondary survey that consists of a more detailed head-to-toe evaluation of the injured patient. During this evaluation, it is of utmost importance to assume that the patient has not only a spinal cord injury, but also a potentially unstable spinal fracture. Thus, all evaluation must take place with full spinal immobilization.

The prehospital spinal cord evaluation attempts to quickly identify injured areas. It is important to note whether a patient is complaining of neck or back pain or has tenderness upon palpation in those areas. In order to better evaluate the spine, the patient should be log-rolled by three providers and the spine checked for bony tenderness or gross signs of trauma (Figures 10.1 and 10.2).

The effectiveness of the log-roll transfer technique has been questioned (7). Alternatives to the log-roll maneuver include the High Arm IN Endangered Spine (HAINES) method and the multi-hand, or fireman-lift, method. In the HAINES method, the patient is placed supine. With the upper portion of the "away" (contralateral) arm positioned in 180 degrees of abduction, the "near" (ipsilateral to the kneeling rescuer) arm is placed across the victim's chest. Both lower limbs are flexed. The rescuer's hands are used to stabilize the head and neck, and the patient is rolled away onto an extrication board or other transport device (8). The multi-hand, or fireman-lift, method involves several rescuers on either side of the patient; all rescuers slide their arms underneath the patient and lift the patient from one position to the other onto an extrication board or device.

Following evaluation, a succinct motor exam should be performed. A motor exam includes assessment of grip strength and foot dorsiflexion in addition to a gross sensory exam, which should alert the prehospital provider to the presence of a complete or partial cord injury. Signs of incontinence, urinary retention, priapism, or loss of anal sphincter tone should also be noted.

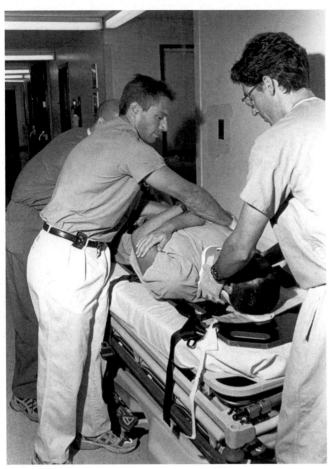

Figure 10.1   Log-roll technique. One provider (designated log-roll leader) at the head of the patient controls the head and cervical spine. Meanwhile, two assistants with interlinked arms control trunk and lower body.

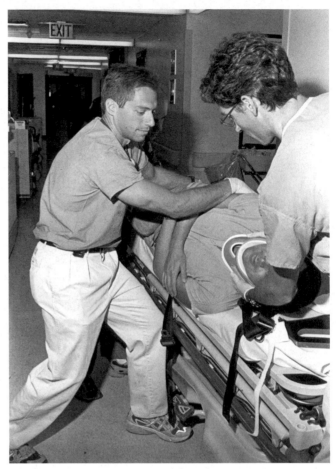

Figure 10.2   Log-roll technique. On leader's command, all three providers roll patient in a single, fluid motion (carefully avoiding any twisting motion). The fourth provider evaluates the thoracic and lumbar/sacral spine for tenderness.

Skin temperature and appearance should be evaluated. Warm, flushed skin suggests loss of sympathetic vascular tone below the injury level. Even in the absence of any of the above findings, the multiply injured or major trauma patient must be placed in a rigid collar and immobilized on a backboard for transport to a hospital.

RESUSCITATION

Resuscitation begins as early as during the evaluation and primary survey. Airway control is of the highest priority and should start with the immediate application of oxygen while the cervical spine is being immobilized. Initial airway management includes the basic maneuvers of chin lift, jaw thrust, and placement of a nasal or oral airway. Suction should be available in order to remove blood, secretions, and possible foreign bodies. If adequate oxygenation cannot be maintained and the paramedic crew is properly trained, the patient should be prepared for intubation. Either blind nasotracheal (presuming the patient has no evidence of midface trauma) or orotracheal intubation are considered appropriate, assuming they are performed with proper in-line cervical spine stabilization. Many studies have now demonstrated that orotracheal

intubation with in-line stabilization (Figure 10.3) is a safe method if performed by experienced personnel (9–11). In a cadaver model, Gerling et al. (12) showed that intubation with in-line stabilization did not cause any significant vertebral body movement. Intubation attempts with cervical collar immobilization, in contrast, did produce a significant amount of vertebral distraction. Thus, the cervical collar should always be opened prior to attempted intubation. If the airway cannot be secured following three intubation attempts, the prehospital provider should be prepared to perform a surgical airway.

Prehospital circulatory resuscitation consists of aggressive pursuit of intravenous access and proper fluid resuscitation. The cervical SCI patient may present with either neurogenic or hemorrhagic shock. Neurogenic shock is the result of a spinal cord injury at or above the fourth thoracic vertebra. These injuries cause a loss of sympathetic peripheral vascular tone and thus reduce central venous return. In contrast to hemorrhagic shock, in which there is compensatory tachycardia to hypovolemia, neurogenic shock is associated with bradycardia, the result of loss of sympathetic cardiac innervations leading to unopposed parasympathetic signals. Both hemorrhagic and neurogenic shock may be initially treated by placing the patient in a spine-immobilized

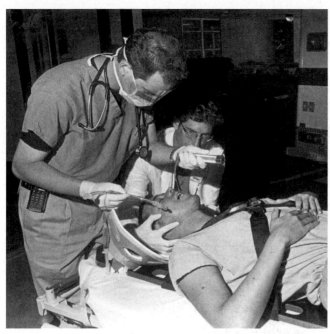

Figure 10.3 In-line stabilization. With rigid collar open, assistant prevents motion of head and neck while the patient is intubated.

Trendelenburg position (13). This maneuver will help decrease pooling of blood in the lower extremities and increase central venous return. Bleeding from the neck or spinal area should be controlled by direct pressure. Large-bore peripheral intravenous lines should be placed in anticipation of saline and blood infusion.

IMMOBILIZATION

To prevent further spinal cord injury, all prehospital personnel must be well trained in the techniques of immobilization. In most areas of the United States, all major trauma victims, patients complaining of neck pain or neurologic symptoms, and patients with altered mental status of uncertain cause are immobilized. With these liberal guidelines, cervical spine immobilization has become one of the most frequently performed prehospital procedures (14). It is estimated that nearly 5 million patients receive spinal immobilization annually at an average cost of $15 per person (15). In addition to the cost, overzealous immobilization can cause unneeded patient discomfort and increased paramedic scene time. There is some evidence that spinal immobilization increases the risk of pressure sores. Pressure sores were found as early as 2 hours after injury in one study (16). In another study, the length of time on a rigid spine board was significantly associated with the development of decubitus ulcers within 8 days of injury (17).

There is some debate about whether immobilization changes outcomes. Hauswald et al. (18) examined the effect of emergency out-of-hospital spinal immobilization on neurologic injury by comparing trauma patients in Malaysia, where no prehospital emergency medical services are available, to trauma patients in New Mexico, where prehospital spinal immobilization is routine. Interestingly, Malaysian patients were found to have a lower rate of neurologic disability. These data, however, have been criticized

because patients who died at the scene or during transport were excluded. Thus, it is difficult to apply these conclusions to the effectiveness of EMS in the United States (19).

Clinical criteria intended to identify a subset of patients that may not need immobilization have been studied. In a multicenter prospective study of 6,500 trauma patients, the application of clinical criteria—namely altered mental status, focal neurologic deficit, evidence of intoxication, spinal pain or tenderness, or suspected extremity fracture—predicted the majority of cervical spinal injuries that required immobilization. The predictive value was maintained with both high- and low-risk mechanisms of injury (20). The authors suggested that clinical criteria rather than the mechanism of injury be used as the standard by which spinal immobilization should be employed. Clinical criteria to select appropriate patients for spinal immobilization have also been studied in several emergency systems throughout the United States (21).

Recommendations regarding the adoption of EMS protocols for prehospital spinal immobilization await definitive studies of safety and efficacy. EMS personnel who make these assessments require intensive education and careful quality assurance scrutiny to ensure that trauma patients with potential spinal injuries are appropriately triaged and managed. The consensus opinion from the body of Class III clinical studies, anatomical and biomechanical data, and clinician experience is that all patients with cervical spinal column injuries or those with the potential for a cervical spinal injury following trauma should be treated with immobilization until injury has been excluded or definitive management has been initiated. Although there is insufficient evidence to support a treatment standard or a treatment guideline, practitioners are strongly encouraged to provide spinal immobilization to potentially spine-injured patients (1).

Technique of Immobilization

At the scene of the injury, the provider should place the patient in a neutral, supine position. With gentle traction applied by locking hands under the jaw and neck, the patient's head should be moved to be in vertical alignment with the body. This neutral position is critical in preventing any further damage to the cord. When removing a patient from a seated position, a cervical collar is first placed. One provider is responsible for the head and neck as the other personnel help move the patient's body in a coordinated movement while keeping the head and body in a neutral position. The patient is then placed on a backboard immediately while the person responsible for the head and neck continues to maintain in-line stabilization.

Because as many as 20% of spinal column injuries involve multiple noncontinuous vertebral levels, the entire spinal column is potentially at risk and should be immobilized (22). The best method is to use a rigid backboard. The neck is first secured with a rigid collar using a pre-fabricated immobilization kit with its own cushions and sandbag equivalent (Figure 10.4). Tape and Velcro straps are placed over the patient's forehead to prevent flexion of the neck. It is important to note that cervical collars alone are relatively ineffective in restricting neck motion (23). Collars must be combined with taping to limit both flexion and extension (24, 25). Following proper neck immobilization, the chest and abdomen are immobilized with seatbelts tightly fastened but allowing for inspiration (Figure 10.5).

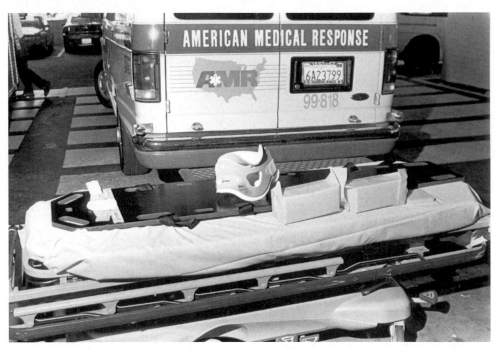

Figure 10.4   Immobilization equipment: rigid board, rigid collar, prefabricated immobilization kit with cushions and Velcro straps.

Helmet Removal

On-site management of the neck-injured helmeted patient differs from that for other traumatic cervical spine injuries. Although the helmet causes the patient's neck to be slightly flexed, particularly in the absence of shoulder pads, and may conceal life-threatening head injuries, its removal is not required in the field unless airway problems exist. If the helmet must be removed for airway access, the two-person technique recommended by the American College of Surgeons should be used: one provider maintains in-line immobilization while the other provider gently removes the helmet (26).

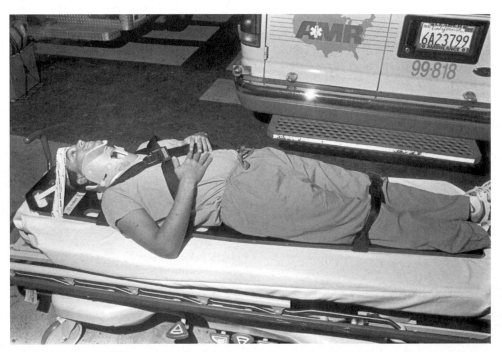

Figure 10.5   Properly immobilized patient.

The Injured Athlete

Unique management issues can arise when caring for an injured athlete. These include on-field evaluation, immobilization techniques, and removal of protective equipment. The first step in evaluating the athlete with a potential cervical spine injury is the on-field evaluation. The unconscious athlete should be carefully log-rolled into a supine position. The athlete's mouthpiece should be removed while the airway, breathing, and circulation are assessed. Protective equipment, such as a helmet or shoulder pads, should be left in place until adequate immobilization of the head and neck has occurred (27). Multiple studies have demonstrated that immobilizing the neck-injured football player with only the helmet or only the shoulder pads in place causes significant cervical spine malalignment (28–30). If protective equipment must be removed in the prehospital setting, the American College of Surgeons recommends using a team of three to four members, as detailed above (see Helmet Removal). The helmet should first be removed using the two-person technique (26). Shoulder pads must also be removed in an orderly manner while the head and neck are stabilized at the level of the torso. The anterior and axillary straps should be cut first. Then the head and thorax should be elevated as a unit as the shoulder pads are slid from under the athlete. Finally, the patient is lowered back down to the spine board and a cervical collar is applied (29).

EXTRICATION AND TRANSPORTATION

Accessibility of the accident site is the primary consideration in extricating a patient. Once the patient has been properly immobilized, the prehospital personnel must make a decision regarding the safest and fastest method of transportation. In remote rural regions, helicopter transport is an excellent option for direct evacuation to a trauma center. Although speed is important, the most important factor is transporting a patient safely to the emergency department with all systems stabilized in order to enhance the potential for maximum neurologic recovery.

References

1. Grabb P, Oyesiku N, Przybylski G, Resnick D, Ryken T. Pre-hospital cervical immobilization following trauma. AANS position paper 2001.
2. Podolsky S, Baraff LJ, Simon RR. Efficacy of cervical spine immobilization methods. *J Trauma* 1983; 23:461–465.
3. Green B, Eismont F, O'Heir J. Spinal cord injury as systems approach: prevention, emergency medical services and emergency room management. *Crit Care Clin* 1987; 3(3):471–493.
4. Garfin SR, Shackford SR, et al. Care of the multiply injured patient with cervical spine injury. *Clin Orthop Relat Res* 1989; 239:19–29.
5. Soderstrom CA, Brumback RJ. Early care of the patient with cervical spine injury. *Orthop Clin North Am* 1986; 17(1):3–13.
6. American College of Surgeons. Advanced trauma life support. Chicago: American College of Surgeons, 1993.
7. McGuire RA, Neville S, et al. Spinal instability and the log-rolling maneuver. *J Trauma* 1987; 27:525–531.
8. Gunn B, Eizenberg N, et al. How should an unconscious person with a suspected neck injury be positioned? *Prehosp Disaster Med* 1995; 10:239–244.
9. Suderman VS, Crosby ET. Occasional review: elective oral tracheal intubation in cervical spine-injured adults. *Can J Anesth* 1991; 38:785–791.
10. Shatney CH, Brunner RD, Nguyen TQ. The safety of orotracheal intubation in patients with unstable cervical spine fracture or high spinal cord injury. *Am J Surg* 1995; 170:676–680.
11. Criswell JC, Parr MJA, Nolan JP. Emergency airway management in patients with cervical spine injuries. *Anaesthesia* 1994; 49:900–903.
12. Gerling MC, Davis DP, Hamilton RS, Morris GF, Vilke GM, Garfin SR, Hayden SR. Effects of cervical spine immobilization technique and laryngoscope blade selection on an unstable cervical spine in a cadaver model of intubation. *Ann Emerg Med* 2000; 36:293–300.
13. Hockberger RS, Kirshenbaum KJ, Doris PE. Spinal injuries. In: Rosen, P, ed. *Emergency Medicine: Concepts and Clinical Practice.* 4th ed. vol. 1. St. Louis: Mosby, 1998:462–505.
14. DeLorenzo RA. A review of spinal immobilization techniques. *J Emerg Med* 1996; 14:603–613.
15. Orledge JD, Pepe PE. Out of hospital immobilization: is it really necessary? *Acad Emerg Med* 1998; 5:203–204.
16. Linares HA, Mawson AR, et al. Association between pressure sores and immobilization in the immediate post-injury period. *Orthopedics* 1987; 10:571–573.
17. Mawson AR, Biundo JJ Jr, et al. Risk factors for early occurring pressure ulcers following spinal cord injury. *Am J Phys Med & Rehabil* 1988; 67:123–127.
18. Hauswald M, Ong G, Tandberg D. Out-of-hospital spinal immobilization: its effect on neurologic injury. *Acad Emerg Med* 1998; 5:214–219.
19. Perry SD, McLellan B, et al. The efficacy of head immobilization techniques during simulated vehicle motion. *Spine* 1999; 24:1839–1844.
20. Domeier, RM. Indications for pre-hospital spinal immobilization. *Prehospital Emergency Care* 1999; 3:251–253.
21. San Mateo County, CA: EMS System Policy Memorandum #F-3A. 1991.
22. Forhna WJ. Emergency department evaluation and treatment of the neck and cervical spine injuries. *Emerg Med Clin North Am* 1999; 17:739–791.
23. Rosen P, McSwain N, Arata M. Comparison of two new immobilization collars. *Ann Emerg Med* 1992; 21:1189–1195.
24. McGuire R, et al. Spinal instability and the log-rolling maneuver. *J Trauma* 1987; 27:525–531.
25. Graziano A, Scheidel E, Cline J. A radiographic comparison of prehospital cervical immobilization methods. *Ann Emerg Med* 1987; 16:1127–1131.
26. McSwain N, Camelli R. Helmet removal from injured patients. *American College of Surgeons Committee on Trauma.* American College of Surgeons: Chicago, 1997, http://www.facs.org/trauma/publications/helmet.pdf (04T-0019).
27. Warren W, Bailes J. On the field evaluation of athletic neck injury. *Clin Sports Med* 1998; 17: 99–110.
28. Palumbo M, Hulstyn M, Fadale P. The effect of protective football equipment on alignment of the injured cervical spine—radiographic analysis in a cadaveric model. *Am J Sports Med* 1996; 24: 446–453.
29. Gastel J, Palumbo M, Hulstyn M. Emergency removal of football equipment: a cadaveric cervical spine injury model. *Ann Emerg Med* 1998; 32:411–417.
30. Donaldson W, Lauerman W, Heil B. Helmet and shoulder pad removal from a player with suspected cervical spine injury—a cadaveric model. *Spine* 1998; 23:1729–1733.

11 Management of Trauma Patients with Complex Injuries

Anil K. Kesani
Frank Anthony Liporace

The advent of modern medicine has greatly improved our understanding of the pathophysiology, clinical presentation, management, and prognosis of the multiply injured polytrauma patient. One often sees a multitude of injuries involving various organ systems in high-energy trauma patients. Treating physicians from various disciplines need to be adept in the care of trauma patients and have a basic understanding of the overall physiology, clinical presentation, management, pitfalls, and complications of the spectrum of injuries. This multidisciplinary approach allows the delivery of optimal care.

Polytrauma patients sustain injuries to multiple organ systems, which in turn results in a cascade of physiologic and immunologic systemic responses. While prompt resuscitative measures can help facilitate physiologic compensation and repair mechanisms, once severely injured trauma patients enter a severe shock state, the mortality rate escalates, with levels reported to be as high as 82% (26). Hence, the American College of Surgeons developed standardized advanced trauma life support (ATLS) protocols (57) to guide aggressive initial resuscitation of polytrauma patients in order to prevent the onset of this potentially irreversible condition (58).

Beyond acute hemodynamic stabilization maneuvers, the concept of "damage control surgery" has evolved to prevent further insult to an already traumatized patient by delaying or limiting the invasiveness of emergent or urgent operative interventions. Therefore, the trend has been to temporarily stabilize high-risk patients in the acute setting, allowing the peak inflammatory phase to resolve before definitive surgical treatment is performed (18, 38–40). In this chapter, we will discuss the pathophysiologic basis, clinical presentation, evaluation, and initial resuscitative measures, as well as emergent and delayed treatment of the polytrauma patient.

PATHOPHYSIOLOGY OF THE TRAUMA PATIENT

Physiologic Basis of High-Energy Injury

Injury to the human body from a traumatic insult starts a cascade of events initiated by a combination of circulatory volume loss and inflammatory mediators released by damaged tissues. The interplay between the circulatory volume loss and inflammatory mediator release dictates the timing and course of events, severity of injury, and the ultimate prognosis of the patient (18). Shock is a state in which the perfusion to tissues is sufficiently compromised that widespread cellular hypoxia occurs, potentially leading to systemic organ dysfunction (33). Shock is classified into several types: hypovolemic, cardiogenic, neurogenic, and septic (Table 11.1).

In the acute setting, the circulatory status is the primary issue. Initial circulatory volume loss can precipitate hypovolemic shock, which must be promptly detected. Failure to do so can lead to continued intravascular volume loss, hypotension, reduced tissue perfusion, increased sympathetic activity, tachycardia, and increased systemic vascular resistance (SVR). The increased SVR further decreases perfusion to tissues, resulting in release of inflammatory mediators such as TNF and IL-6 (41). If untreated, increased sympathetic tone results, which further propagates the cascade. As a result, decreased oxygen delivery to tissues, hypoxia, and accumulation of hydrogen ions secondary to anaerobic respiration from the breakdown of ATP to ADP-H$^+$ are pervasive. Cell death and mitochondrial degeneration occur throughout multiple organ systems, leading to the demise of the patient from multi-organ failure (32).

Hypovolemic Shock

Hypovolemic shock is related to circulatory volume loss. Hypovolemic shock has been classified by the ATLS into four groups

Table 11.1   Characteristic Features Present in Different Shock Types

	HYPOVOLEMIC SHOCK	CARDIOGENIC SHOCK	NEUROGENIC SHOCK	SEPTIC SHOCK
Heart rate	Tachycardia	Tachycardia	Bradycardia	Tachycardia
SVR	Increased	Increased	Decreased	Decreased
Peripheral circulation	Reduced	Reduced	Normal/increased	Increased

that are based on the volume of blood loss, pulse rate, blood pressure, pulse pressure, respiratory rate, urinary output, central nervous system/mental status, and fluid replacement requirements (Table 11.2).

The severity of hypovolemic shock can also be quantified by clinical parameters and laboratory findings, including arterial pH and base-deficit values obtained from blood gas analysis. Base deficit can be used to classify shock as mild, moderate, and severe (12, 13) (Table 11.3). Another important measure used to gauge the severity of hypovolemic shock is the lactate level (16). Lactate is produced as a byproduct of anaerobic respiration. Both base-deficit and lactate levels can be used to predict morbidity and mortality as well as to assess the adequacy of resuscitation (20).

Thoracic trauma can cause direct injury to the heart and precipitate cardiogenic shock due to pump failure. Neurogenic shock is seen in patients who have sustained a spinal cord injury. It leads to a shutdown of the autonomic nervous system and circulatory collapse. Neurogenic shock should not be confused with spinal shock. Discussed in more detail elsewhere, spinal shock is a transient phenomenon in which the spinal cord reflex arcs are absent. Heart rate is important in distinguishing between neurogenic, hypovolemic, and septic shock. Whereas tachycardia is typical for other types of shock, bradycardia is a hallmark finding of neurogenic shock. With systemic infection, septic shock results from release of endotoxins that cause vasodilation, subsequent loss of SVR, and resultant hypotension. A distinct feature of septic shock is the presence of warm extremities, as compared to cool extremities seen with hypovolemic or cardiogenic shock (53).

Inflammatory Host Response and Mediators

Localized injury usually results in a host response that is appropriate in magnitude and is ultimately self-limited. In contrast, severe multitrauma often cannot be managed by the patient's physiologic reserve and leads to systemic inflammatory response syndrome (SIRS) and possibly multiple organ failure (MOF). The initial response to injury is mediated primarily by norepinephrine and is directed toward preservation of circulation to the heart and brain at the expense of other tissues. With adequate resuscitative efforts, a hypermetabolic state can still persist, mediated by epinephrine, which is directed toward aiding in the reparative process of injured tissues by leukocytes.

In some cases, cytokine release may be overwhelming, leading to the systemic effects which may trigger remote inflammation (24). Many implicated inflammatory mediators have been reported to adversely affect trauma patients. These include IL-1, IL-6, IL-8, IL-10, TNF, TGF, and corticosterone (14, 25, 39, 42, 56). These mediators are produced during several stages: the initial traumatic insult, the body's resultant physiologic compensatory efforts, and delayed sepsis encountered during prolonged hospital stays.

A resultant secondary inflammatory reaction mediated by the release of chemokines, prostaglandins, leukotrienes, and reactive oxygen species can induce inflammatory cell migration into affected tissues (14). In turn, activation of procoagulatory and anticoagulatory factors may ultimately lead to disseminated intravascular coagulopathy (DIC) (14).

INJURY SCORING SYSTEMS AND THEIR UTILITY

Many scoring systems have been proposed to evaluate multiply injured trauma patients. These include the Glasgow Coma Scale (GCS), Abbreviated Injury Score (AISS), Injury Severity Score (ISS), Trauma Injury Severity Score (TISS), Revised Trauma Score (RTS), and Mangled Extremity Score. Scoring systems are

Table 11.2   Classification of Hypovolemic Shock Severity, Based on Clinical Parameters and Fluid Requirements

	CLASS I SHOCK	CLASS II SHOCK	CLASS III SHOCK	CLASS IV SHOCK
Blood loss (ml)	Up to 750	750–1,500	1,500–2,000	>2,000
Blood loss (% blood volume)	Up to 15%	15–30%	30–40%	>40%
Pulse rate (beats per minute)	<100	>100	>120	>140
Blood pressure	Normal	Normal	Decreased	Decreased
Pulse pressure (mmHg)	Normal or increased	Decreased	Decreased	Decreased
Respiratory rate (breaths per minute)	14–20	20–30	30–40	>35
Urine output (mL/h)	>30	20–30	5–15	Negligible
Central nervous system/mental status	Slightly anxious	Mildly anxious	Anxious, confused	Confused, lethargic
Fluid replacement (3:1 rule)	Crystalloid	Crystalloid	Crystalloid and blood	Crystalloid and blood

Source: Reference 42.

Table 11.3   Classification of Shock Severity and Volume Requirements Based on Base Deficit

		BASE DEFICIT GROUP			
	NUMBER OF PATIENTS	1 HOUR AFTER ADMISSION	2 HOURS AFTER ADMISSION	3 HOURS AFTER ADMISSION	4 HOURS AFTER ADMISSION
Mild (2 to −5)	70	2,966 ± 335	4,030 ± 520	5,881 ± 817	7,475 ± 786
Moderate (−6 to −14)	110	3,893 ± 322	7,522 ± 642	8,120 ± 718	13,007 ± 1,078
Severe (<−15)	29	6,110 ± 589 $P < 0.001$	9,800 ± 982 $P < 0.001$	10,909 ± 1,435 $P < 0.008$	16,396 ± 3,252 $P < 0.001$

Source: References 12, 13.

used to determine the severity of injury and to help guide management and prognosis. In addition, scoring systems are used for research and quality control purposes. Management decisions begin in the field. Paramedics can use scoring systems as a guide to determine which facility can provide the most appropriate level of care (i.e., whether a patient requires a level 1 trauma center). The scoring systems base their scores on the severity of injury to various anatomic and physiologic systems, as well as on age and on any preexisting conditions of the patients.

The GCS is one of the most popular and widely used systems. It is primarily used to quantify the severity of closed head injuries. The GCS grades three variables: the best motor response (which assesses overall central nervous system function), the best verbal response (which assesses cerebral function), and eye opening (which assesses brainstem function). GCS on admission is predictive of the severity of injury and mortality (37).

The AISS is based on obtaining individual scores between 0 and 6 for nine anatomic sites, including general, head, face, neck, thorax, spine, upper extremity, and lower extremity. With no injury, 0 is assigned; with maximal injury, 6. The scores from the various anatomic sites are added (6).

ISS is used primarily for research purposes; it is useful for retrospective analysis of different treatments. It is based on obtaining scores between 0 and 6 for six individual anatomic sites. With no injury, 0 is assigned; with maximal injury, 6. The highest three scores are squared and added. However, if any anatomic site obtains a score of six, mortality is likely to result, and therefore a score of seventy-five is assigned. ISS is a predictor of injury severity and mortality. ISS cannot predict outcomes in patients who have multiple injuries to the same anatomic site and long-term functional outcome predictions (17).

The RTS is based on the concept that death results from injury to critical systems, including the central nervous system, cardiovascular system, and respiratory system. Three variables (GCS, respiratory rate, and systolic blood pressure) are graded between 0 and 4, then added. Lower numbers indicate more severe injuries, with 97% of severely injured patients identified by a score of less than or equal to eleven. The RTS is useful in determining whether paramedics in the field should transfer a patient to a trauma center or less equipped site. Like the ISS, the RTS is unable to reliably predict outcome in patients with multiple severe injuries to the same anatomic area (11).

The trauma injury severity score (TISS) is derived from combining anatomical data from the ISS and physiologic data from the RTS systems. The TISS can identify unexpected survival and death in trauma patients, thereby allowing quality control and evaluation of new treatment protocols (23).

IN-THE-FIELD MANAGEMENT

Care of a polytrauma patient begins in the field with the rapid assessment and treatment of patients according to the ATLS protocol. Once the airway is secured, the patient should be ventilated in order to maintain adequate oxygenation. Some severely injured patients may require early intubation (within 2 hours), for this maneuver can improve clinical outcomes and reduce post-traumatic organ failure (55). The next priority is circulation. Blood pressure should be maintained via control of bleeding, intravenous (IV) fluid delivery, blood product administration, and external cardiac massage (i.e., chest compression) when indicated.

Next, attention should be directed to prevent further injury by removing the patient from ongoing injurious processes and proper immobilization with cervical collars and rigid spinal boards. Pediatric patients deserve special mention, for they require spinal boards with head cutouts or elevated trunk supports to prevent C-spine flexion when lying supine, because of their disproportionally larger heads. Athletes should have pads and helmets left in place until arrival at a hospital, where equipment removal can be performed in a controlled environment. However, importantly, face masks should be removed to aid in assessing and securing the airway. A quick examination of the extremities is prudent, followed by provisional alignment and splinting of recognized skeletal injuries. Meanwhile, in-field health care providers should decide the most appropriate facility to which to transport the patient.

PRIMARY SURVEY AND ACUTE MANAGEMENT IN-HOSPITAL

Patients who are unresponsive to in-field resuscitative measures need urgent evaluation for sources of hemodynamic compromise. Initial evaluation entails assessment by a multispecialty team that focuses on the chest, abdomen, and pelvis. Because it is an integral part of acute orthopedic management, intrapelvic bleeding secondary to pelvic fractures or dislocations must be recognized early. The most significant source of bleeding after fracture or dislocation is from intrapelvic venous disruption; less substantial arterial bleeding arises from the fracture surfaces (1).

Predictors of major hemorrhage include a systolic pressure of less than 90 mmHg, massive fluid requirements, ongoing transfusion requirements, hematocrit of less than 30, pulse rate of more than 130 beats per minute, displaced obturator ring fractures, and wide pubic symphyseal diastasis (7). Several options are available for those patients with unstable pelvic ring fractures, most commonly anteroposterior compression (APC, also known as "open book" injuries) and vertical shear injuries, with the goal of initial maneuvers to decrease the pelvic volume by achieving provisional fracture/dislocation reduction.

Acute Treatment Algorithm for Hemorrhagic Shock with Pelvic Fractures

The simplest and "lowest-tech" method of treating hemorrhagic shock with pelvic fractures is to apply a sheet or pelvic binder around the patient at the level of the greater trochanters to bring together the two halves of the hemipelvis, which are displaced with APC injuries. If this is unsuccessful, and arterial injury is suspected, arteriographic evaluation and embolization should be considered (2, 3). Burgess et al. demonstrated that 11% of patients required embolization for arterial bleeding after pelvic fractures, 20% of which had APC injuries (10). Furthermore, arteriography can help locate the site of the bleed, most commonly the pudendal/obturator arteries with anterior instability and the superior gluteal artery with posterior instability.

When these measures are not sufficient, external fixation of the pelvis should be considered; it has been demonstrated to decrease transfusion requirements, pain, and late deformity (61). Additional data have shown that mortality is reduced from 41% to 21% in patients admitted with SBP less than 100 mm and from 43% to 7% in those with head and pelvic injuries (48). In the next step in the algorithm, patients with persistent hypotension in whom external fixation of the pelvis has not been effective are most appropriately treated with an exploratory laparotomy, provided free fluid in abdomen has been detected on ultrasound (US) or diagnostic peritoneal lavage (DPL) (49, 50).

When FAST and DPL are negative (i.e., abdominal bleeding is not detected) and bleeding in the chest is ruled out, the pelvic injury is the likely source of hemodynamic instability. In these cases, more dramatic pelvic intervention should be considered. Ertel et al. demonstrated that pelvic packing with pelvic ring fixation with a C-clamp can effectively control severe hemorrhage in multiply injured patients (16). Beyond its proven efficacy in individual studies, as evidence of this algorithm's effectiveness in actual practice, enactment of institutional guidelines for pelvic trauma at trauma centers has been shown to reduce transfusion requirements and mortality rates (5).

Open pelvic fractures require emergency irrigation, debridement, and stabilization, for they have been associated with a high mortality of up to 50% (22). Thus, detection of open pelvic injuries is crucial, and relies on careful physical examination to look for sites of tenderness, open wounds (in the inguinal region, perineum, vagina, and rectum), instability on pelvic compression testing (only performed once to prevent intrapelvic clots disruption), and neurologic deficits. In one study, mortality risk was increased by the presence of a Gustillo grade III open fracture, among other factors. In another study that retrospectively reviewed thirty-nine patients with open pelvic fractures, pelvic sepsis occurred in 11% of patients, 60% of whom subsequently died (15).

Additional non-orthopedic procedures for concomitant injuries are frequently required following pelvic fractures. Large bowel and rectal injuries require early diverting colostomies to avoid sepsis and poor outcomes (22, 44). Vaginal lacerations require emergent irrigation and debridement in the operating room in collaboration with the gynecologic service. Bladder and urethral injuries may necessitate placement of a suprapubic catheter, followed by delayed repair.

Acute Management of the Spine

The spine, discussed in more detail elsewhere, should be systematically evaluated for injuries that can potentially lead to hemodynamic from neurogenic shock. In contrast to hemorrhagic shock, treatment typically consists of judicious fluid resuscitation with use of vasopressors to increase peripheral vascular tone. When spinal cord injury is suspected, maintaining oxygenation with supplemental oxygen and ensuring hemodynamic stability is paramount to minimizing secondary neurologic decline.

Extremities

Extremities should be evaluated for vascular injuries that can lead to ongoing blood loss. Stigmata for such injuries include brisk bleeding, an expanding hematoma, or absent pulses. Typically, vascular extremity injuries require urgent control of bleeding via vessel repair, ligation, temporary shunting, or, in severely unstable patients with mangled extremities, amputation. Grossly deformed extremities should be addressed by restoration of alignment via splinting or traction to help control bleeding and prevent further soft tissue damage.

SECONDARY SURVEY AND DECISION-MAKING

After hemodynamic stabilization, a more detailed secondary survey must be performed to detect and characterize the full spectrum of injuries. This entails a head-to-toe, systematic, anatomically based physical examination.

Imaging is an important part of the secondary survey. A CT scan of the head is mandatory in those patients who have impaired function on clinical assessment or are compromised by drug or alcohol intoxication. Intracranial bleeding, frank herniation, or impending herniation requires neurosurgical intervention. A plain radiograph of the chest should be obtained. If visceral injury is suspected, CT is usually performed. Pneumothorax and hemothorax should be appropriately addressed, if detected. A spiral CT scan of the abdominal cavity should also be obtained. Regardless of a negative abdominal CT, close clinical follow-up is warranted, for one study alone can miss up to 7% of injuries, most often small bowel perforations (51). Although they do not always require surgery, spleen and liver lacerations also command close observation. When substantial bleeding is found, exploratory laparotomy may be required. Bowel injuries, particularly those in the highly colonized large intestine, will require early diverting ostomies.

When assessing polytrauma patients, providers must assume that an injury to the spine exists and therefore immobilize the spine until injury can be ruled out. C-collars and log-roll precautions should also be used until spine "clearance." Because they are usually not life-threatening, extremity injuries are often overlooked, as are their impact on the ultimate functional status of trauma patients underestimated. Missed orthopedic extremity injuries can adversely affect immediate, as well as long-term, outcome. A recent meta-analysis of the literature has found a variable rate of 1.3–39% incidence for missed injuries and delayed diagnoses. Approximately 15–22.3% of patients with these had clinically significant missed injuries. Since the 1980s, the incidence of missed pelvic injuries has rapidly declined. Approximately 27–66% of unrecognized diagnoses in the studies within the meta-analysis were considered major injuries. Overall, the data suggest that approximately 10% of orthopedic injuries are missed during the acute hospitalization after trauma; most frequently, these are fractures of the hands and feet (45).

Evaluation of the extremity includes a detailed systematic physical exam looking for open wounds, deformity, tenderness, and crepitus, followed by careful evaluation of peripheral vascular perfusion and neural innervation of the extremity. When a neurovascular abnormality is associated with a deformity of the extremity, the limb should be immediately realigned and reexamined in hopes of an acute improvement. Nerve injuries are generally observed in the acute period, unless there is an obviously lacerated neural structure that can be repaired or another indication for surgery exists with a surgical incision placed in close proximity to the zone of suspected nerve injury (in which case the nerve can be explored).

When vascular injury is suspected, further investigations should be considered, including ankle-brachial pressure index and selective angiography. A recent prospective study by Stannard et al. found that physical examination had a positive predictive value of 90%, a negative predictive value of 100%, a sensitivity of 100%, and a specificity of 99% of arteriographically confirmed lesions (52). Moreover, Lynch et al. demonstrated that an ankle-brachial pressure index of <0.9 had a sensitivity of 87% and a specificity of 97% for arterial disruption when compared with the results of arteriography as the gold standard (28).

Vascular injuries mandate emergent surgical assessment and revascularization. Prophylactic fasciotomies should be considered, especially in cases with prolonged ischemia, for the resultant reperfusion injury can lead to compartment syndrome. Associated skeletal injuries are usually immobilized temporarily in an external fixator, with definitive internal fixation delayed until a later date (Figure 11.1).

Compartment syndrome is a potentially limb- and life-threatening condition, if not recognized and treated promptly. Heckman et al. demonstrated that irreversible muscle necrosis occurs after 8 hours of elevated compartment pressures (19). Missed compartment syndrome can locally lead to infection, contractures, and the need for amputation (31). Systemically, the resultant muscle necrosis can lead to release of myoglobin, as well as to inflammatory and toxic metabolites. The ensuing myoglobinuria, metabolic acidosis, and hyperkalemia can lead to renal failure, shock, hypothermia, and cardiac arrhythmias or failure (36). Hence, timely diagnosis and treatment is prudent to avoid poor outcome.

In an awake and alert patient, compartment syndrome can be detected with serial clinical evaluation. Patients typically complain of paresthesias and disproportional pain. On physical exam, pain on passive stretch is pathognomonic (29, 30, 35). However, intracompartmental pressure measurement is required in situations in which mental status impairment or sensory deficits exist (36). Compartment syndrome requires emergent intervention. Initially, casts and occlusive dressings must be released or removed. If these measures are unsuccessful, emergency fasciotomy (i.e., release of the affected muscular compartments) is performed to prevent tissue necrosis and long-term morbidity.

Open fractures can be classified from grade I to III according to the Gustillo and Anderson classification. Urgent I&D and skeletal stabilization is universally recommended (4). Of particular importance are open articular fractures. Whereas devitalized nonarticular bone fragments are routinely removed during debridement to avoid a nidus of infection, devitalized articular fragments are maintained to reapproximate the joint surface in hopes of minimizing long-term morbidity from joint incongruity.

DAMAGE-CONTROL SURGERY: TIMING OF TEMPORARY AND DEFINITIVE ORTHOPEDIC INJURY FIXATION

Originally, damage control surgery was developed to optimize the treatment of hemodynamically unstable patients with massive abdominal trauma. More recently, damage control surgery has been applied to the musculoskeletal and spinal care of polytrauma patients. Fundamental to the concept of damage control orthopedics is the understanding that injury to trauma patients occurs in two phases. In the first phase, injury is sustained from the index traumatic event. This sets in motion a variety of physiologic and inflammatory cascades that cannot be modified except by preventative measures. In the second phase, injury occurs by the exacerbation of physiologic and inflammatory reactions induced by surgical procedures to stabilize orthopedic injuries during the acute postinjury period. The physiologic and inflammatory insult that occurs in the second phase is potentially modifiable by performing more limited surgical procedures such as temporary external fixation in the acute injury period followed by delayed definitive fixation.

Review of the orthopedic trauma literature demonstrates that early stabilization of long bone fractures reduces morbidity (i.e., reduced incidence of pulmonary complications, faster rehabilitation, shorter ICU and hospital stays) and mortality in polytrauma patients (8, 9, 21). A recent prospective, randomized controlled multicenter trial demonstrated increased levels of inflammatory markers IL-6 and IL-8 in patients treated with primary intramedullary femoral stabilization within 24 hours of injury compared to a damage-control staged approach via initial external fixation with delayed conversion to an intramedullary nail (39). There is also evidence suggesting that extensive, immediate surgery to stabilize fractures (also known as "early total care"), particularly 2–4 days postinjury in hemodynamically unstable patients, can adversely affect patient outcomes (18, 38, 40). A study by Pape et al. demonstrated that early total care of orthopedic injuries in polytrauma patients during days 2–4 postinjury resulted in an increased risk of multiple organ failure, whereas definitive fracture stabilization during days 6–8 was associated with a lower risk of organ dysfunction (38). Another multicenter study reported a significantly higher incidence of ARDS (15.1%) in early total care patients receiving an initial IMN compared to damaged-control patients (9.1%) who received initial external fixation followed by delayed IMN (40).

In summary, definitive surgical fixation should be delayed until adequate resuscitation has been achieved. Some helpful parameters include base excess and lactate levels and a normalization of the inflammatory status of the patient, which typically occurs after 6 days from the initial traumatic insult.

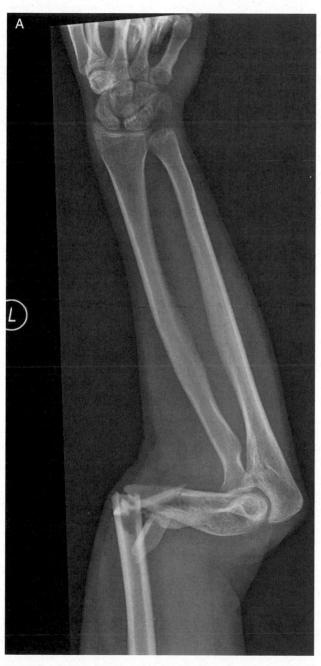

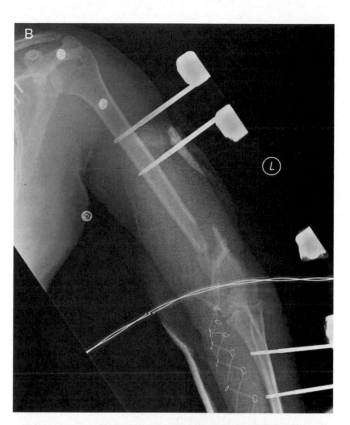

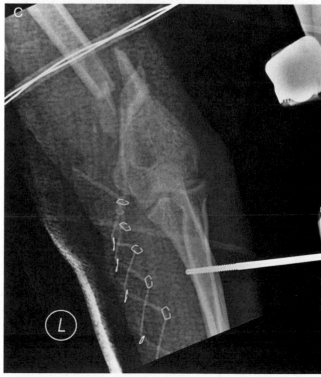

Figure 11.1 A patient with an open distal humerus fracture with brachial artery transection and maceration. Shown in **A** is an injury film. The patient underwent emergent brachial artery repair, spanning external fixation, and forearm fasciotomies shown in **B–D**. Two weeks later, the patient underwent open reduction and internal fixation of the humerus with removal of external fixation resulting in union, shown in **E** and **F**.

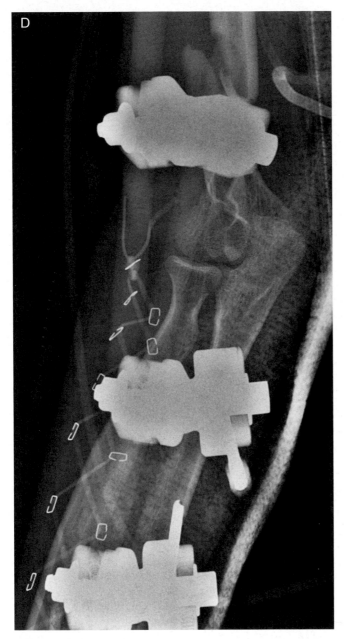

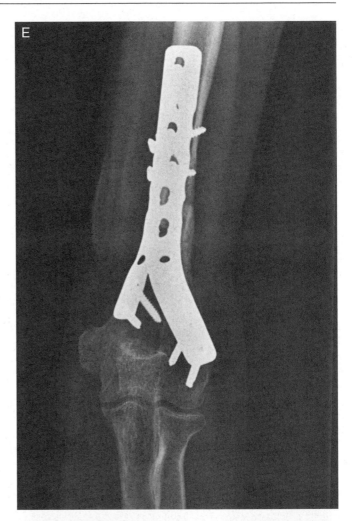

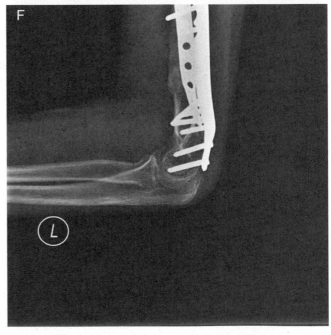

Figure 11.1 (Continued)

SUBACUTE SYSTEMIC COMPLICATIONS

Pulmonary Injury

Adult respiratory distress syndrome (ARDS) is unfortunately encountered all too often during the care of trauma patients. Risk factors for ARDS include direct lung contusion, aspiration of gastric contents, and the requirement of large quantities of transfused blood during resuscitation. Clinically, ARDS is characterized by dyspnea, tachypnea, and arterial hypoxemia that is unresponsive to oxygen therapy. Radiographically, it is characterized by bilateral pulmonary infiltrates. After trauma, mortality rate with ARDS is approximately 50%.

ARDS is a progressive condition consisting of several stages. The initial phase is an acute, exudative phase. During this phase, an inflammatory reaction, characterized by recruitment of neutrophils and macrophages, leads to disruption of the alveolar-capillary membrane, accumulation of proteinaceous material in the alveoli, alveolar epithelial disruption, inactivation of surfactant, and atelectasis. Atelectasis is not uniform, primarily affecting the dependent regions of the lungs. Ultimately, the above process leads to a ventilation-perfusion mismatch and arterial hypoxemia. By observing damage control principles as detailed above, further physiologic and immunologic insult, which can exacerbate the inflammatory reaction responsible for ARDS, can be lessened (40).

In those who survive the acute phase, progression into a chronic fibrotic stage is seen. This is characterized by fibrosing alveolitis, radiographic diffuse interstitial opacities, clinical signs of persisting hypoxemia, and increased alveolar dead space. These changes can lead to long-term morbidity, though most recover functionally despite sustaining chronic pulmonary changes.

Multiple Organ Failure and Sepsis

Multiple organ failure (MOF) and sepsis are delayed occurrences in trauma patients. MOF can be caused by an excessive, dysregulated inflammatory response. When hypotension is left untreated, it can be unresponsive to resuscitation, leading to coagulation disturbances and, ultimately, MOF. Clinical presentation includes hyperthermia, confusion, hypotension, and reduction in urine production. Mortality rates with MOF can be as high as 60% (27). In a review of 342 polytrauma patients, Regel et al. found that 11.4% developed MOF. Respiratory failure is the most frequent initial system to fail, which portends a poor prognosis compared to those presenting with failure of other organ systems such as the liver and cardiovascular systems. Risk factors for the development of MOF are severity, type, and distribution of injuries, and prolonged hemorrhagic shock. Therefore, experts recommend that the main thrust of therapeutic efforts should be effective treatment of hemorrhagic shock during the acute phase, with adequate resuscitation, optimal oxygenation, and early surgical treatment to avoid MOF (47).

MOF in combination with sepsis can result in even higher mortality rates. Sepsis leads to a strong immune response triggered by humoral and cellular elements. In turn, this leads to an increase in proinflammatory cytokines, including IL-6, IL-1, and TNF-α, which are released by mononuclear cells into the bloodstream (54). The cytokines induce a secondary inflammatory reaction by enhancing cell migration into tissues. The inflammatory reaction then leads to potent activation of procoagulatory and anticoagulatory pathways, which leads to disseminated intravascular coagulation, microvascular thrombosis, reduced tissue perfusion, tissue hypoxia, and end organ failure.

THROMBOEMBOLIC DISEASE

Venous thromboembolism (VTE) is a common and potentially fatal complication in trauma patients. VTE clinically manifests as deep vein thrombosis (DVT) or pulmonary embolism (PE). With DVT, patients clinically present with calf pain, tenderness, and possible erythema. Diagnosis of DVT is most commonly made by duplex ultrasound examination. Patients with PE present with dyspnea, pleuritic chest pain, and tachycardia. Diagnosis of PE is most often made with spiral chest CT with

contrast or a ventilation-perfusion scan. Particularly in the polytrauma setting, ventilation perfusion scans are often impractical, for patients are frequently mechanically ventilated. Untreated PE is associated with a mortality rate of approximately 30%. A recent meta-analysis suggests that spine fractures and spinal cord injuries are the strongest risk factors for DVT and PE (60). However, other risk factors include increased age, increased injury severity score, blood transfusions, long bone fractures, pelvic fractures, and head injuries (46).

Avoiding VTE complications is ideal. Of note, consensus on the optimal method of prophylaxis is lacking. Many trauma surgeons utilize a combination of mechanical DVT prophylaxis (in the form of pneumatic compression devices or foot pumps) in combination with low molecular weight heparin in high-risk, immobile patients. At the time of this writing, chemical prophylaxis is recommended for patients with spinal cord injuries, pelvic fractures, and complex lower extremity fractures requiring surgical fixation and prolonged bed rest. Types of chemical prophylaxis include aspirin, heparin, and low molecular heparin. However, a meta-analysis by Velmahos et al. demonstrated no evidence that any one method was clearly superior to another (59).

A recent study by Nathens et al. demonstrated a three-fold increase in DVT incidence (from 5 to 15%) in trauma patients who had chemical DVT prophylaxis administration delayed longer than 4 days (34). Therefore, if a high-risk patient has a contraindication to anticoagulation, such as a closed head injury, ISS of more than 9, or ongoing bleeding, insertion of a vena cava filter should be considered.

CONCLUSION

The management of polytrauma patients with multiple complex injuries often poses a considerable challenge requiring careful systematic evaluation, multidisciplinary management, and close clinical follow-up. Initially, ATLS protocols should be strictly followed in order to stabilize polytrauma patients, followed by carefully planned and executed multidisciplinary subacute definitive care. Once severely injured polytrauma patients are hemodynamically stable, musculoskeletal injuries can be temporarily stabilized according to damage control principles. Definitive treatment can then be undertaken when the overall medical condition of the patient is more favorable, as determined by interpretation of the physical examination, vitals, blood tests, laboratory markers of resuscitation (base deficit, lactate, and pH), and, possibly in the future, inflammatory markers such as cytokine levels. Notwithstanding survival of the acute injury, meticulous attention must be paid to prevent, detect, and treat subacute conditions that can present during prolonged hospital stays.

References

1. Agnew, S. G.: Hemodynamically unstable pelvic fractures. *Orthop Clin North Am*, 25(4): 715–21, 1994.
2. Agolini, S. F.; Shah, K.; Jaffe, J.; Newcomb, J.; Rhodes, M.; and Reed, J. F., 3rd: Arterial embolization is a rapid and effective technique for controlling pelvic fracture hemorrhage. *J Trauma*, 43(3): 395–9, 1997.
3. Allen, C. F.; Goslar, P. W.; Barry, M.; and Christiansen, T.: Management guidelines for hypotensive pelvic fracture patients. *Am Surg*, 66(8): 735–8, 2000.

4. Anderson, J. T.; Gustilo, R. B.: Immediate fixation in open fractures. *Orthop Clin North Am,* 11(3):569–78, 1980.

5. Balogh, Z.; Caldwell, E.; Heetveld, M.; D'Amours, S.; Schlaphoff, G.; Harris, I.; and Sugrue, M.: Institutional practice guidelines on management of pelvic fracture-related hemodynamic instability: do they make a difference? *J Trauma,* 58(4): 778–82, 2005.

6. Barancik, J. I., and Chatterjee, B. F.: Methodological considerations in the use of the abbreviated injury scale in trauma epidemiology. *J Trauma,* 21(8): 627–31, 1981.

7. Blackmore, C. C.; Cummings, P.; Jurkovich, G. J.; Linnau, K. F.; Hoffer, E. K.; and Rivara, F. P.: Predicting major hemorrhage in patients with pelvic fracture. *J Trauma,* 61(2): 346–52, 2006.

8. Bone, L., and Bucholz, R.: The management of fractures in the patient with multiple trauma. *J Bone Joint Surg Am,* 68(6): 945–9, 1986.

9. Bone, L. B.; Johnson, K. D.; Weigelt, J.; and Scheinberg, R.: Early versus delayed stabilization of femoral fractures. A prospective randomized study. *J Bone Joint Surg Am,* 71(3): 336–40, 1989.

10. Burgess, A. R.; Eastridge, B. J.; Young, J. W.; Ellison, T. S.; Ellison, P. S., Jr.; Poka, A.; Bathon, G. H.; and Brumback, R. J.: Pelvic ring disruptions: effective classification system and treatment protocols. *J Trauma,* 30(7): 848–56, 1990.

11. Champion, H. R.; Sacco, W. J.; Copes, W. S.; Gann, D. S.; Gennarelli, T. A.; and Flanagan, M. E.: A revision of the Trauma Score. *J Trauma,* 29(5): 623–9, 1989.

12. Davis, J. W.; Kaups, K. L.; and Parks, S. N.: Base deficit is superior to pH in evaluating clearance of acidosis after traumatic shock. *J Trauma,* 44(1): 114–8, 1998.

13. Davis, J. W.; Shackford, S. R.; Mackersie, R. C.; and Hoyt, D. B.: Base deficit as a guide to volume resuscitation. *J Trauma,* 28(10): 1464–7, 1988.

14. DeLong, W. G., Jr., and Born, C. T.: Cytokines in patients with polytrauma. *Clin Orthop Relat Res* (422): 57–65, 2004.

15. Dente, C. J.; Feliciano, D. V.; Rozycki, G. S.; Wyrzykowski, A. D.; Nicholas, J. M.; Salomone, J. P.; and Ingram, W. L.: The outcome of open pelvic fractures in the modern era. *Am J Surg,* 190(6): 830–5, 2005.

16. Ertel, W.; Keel, M.; Eid, K.; Platz, A.; and Trentz, O.: Control of severe hemorrhage using C-clamp and pelvic packing in multiply injured patients with pelvic ring disruption. *J Orthop Trauma,* 15(7): 468–74, 2001.

17. Harwood, P. J.; Giannoudis, P. V.; Probst, C.; Van Griensven, M.; Krettek, C.; and Pape, H. C.: Which AIS based scoring system is the best predictor of outcome in orthopaedic blunt trauma patients? *J Trauma,* 60(2): 334–40, 2006.

18. Harwood, P. J.; Giannoudis, P. V.; van Griensven, M.; Krettek, C.; and Pape, H. C.: Alterations in the systemic inflammatory response after early total care and damage control procedures for femoral shaft fracture in severely injured patients. *J Trauma,* 58(3): 446–52; discussion 452–4, 2005.

19. Heckman, M. M.; Whitesides, T. E., Jr.; Grewe, S. R.; Judd, R. L.; Miller, M.; and Lawrence, J. H., 3rd: Histologic determination of the ischemic threshold of muscle in the canine compartment syndrome model. *J Orthop Trauma,* 7(3): 199–210, 1993.

20. Husain, F. A.; Martin, M. J.; Mullenix, P. S.; Steele, S. R.; and Elliott, D. C.: Serum lactate and base deficit as predictors of mortality and morbidity. *Am J Surg,* 185(5): 485–91, 2003.

21. Johnson, K. D.; Cadambi, A.; and Seibert, G. B.: Incidence of adult respiratory distress syndrome in patients with multiple musculoskeletal injuries: effect of early operative stabilization of fractures. *J Trauma,* 25(5): 375–84, 1985.

22. Jones, A. L.; Powell, J. N.; Kellam, J. F.; McCormack, R. G.; Dust, W.; and Wimmer, P.: Open pelvic fractures. A multicenter retrospective analysis. *Orthop Clin North Am,* 28(3): 345–50, 1997.

23. Kilgo, P. D.; Meredith, J. W.; and Osler, T. M.: Incorporating recent advances to make the TRISS approach universally available. *J Trauma,* 60(5): 1002–8; discussion 1008–9, 2006.

24. Kim, P. K., and Deutschman, C. S.: Inflammatory responses and mediators. *Surg Clin North Am,* 80(3): 885–94, 2000.

25. Kobbe, P.; Vodovotz, Y.; Kaczorowski, D.; Mollen, K. P.; Billiar, T. R.; and Pape, H. C.: Patterns of Cytokine Release and Evolution of Remote Organ Dysfunction after Bilateral Femur Fracture. *Shock,* 2007.

26. Kuhne, C. A.; Ruchholtz, S.; Kaiser, G. M.; and Nast-Kolb, D.: Mortality in severely injured elderly trauma patients—when does age become a risk factor? *World J Surg,* 29(11): 1476–82, 2005.

27. Lehmann, U.; Grotz, M.; Regel, G.; Rudolph, S.; and Tscherne, H.: [Does initial management of polytrauma patients have an effect on the development of multiple organ failure? Evaluation of preclinical and clinical data of 1,112 polytrauma patients]. *Unfallchirurg,* 98(8): 442–6, 1995.

28. Lynch, K., and Johansen, K.: Can Doppler pressure measurement replace "exclusion" arteriography in the diagnosis of occult extremity arterial trauma? *Ann Surg,* 214(6): 737–41, 1991.

29. Matsen, F. A., 3rd; Winquist, R. A.; and Krugmire, R. B., Jr.: Diagnosis and management of compartmental syndromes. *J Bone Joint Surg Am,* 62(2): 286–91, 1980.

30. McQueen, M. M.; Christie, J.; and Court-Brown, C. M.: Acute compartment syndrome in tibial diaphyseal fractures. *J Bone Joint Surg Br,* 78(1): 95–8, 1996.

31. McQueen, M. M.; Gaston, P.; and Court-Brown, C. M.: Acute compartment syndrome. Who is at risk? *J Bone Joint Surg Br,* 82(2): 200–3, 2000.

32. Meade, P.; Shoemaker, W. C.; Donnelly, T. J.; Abraham, E.; Jagels, M. A.; Cryer, H. G.; Hugli, T. E.; Bishop, M. H.; and Wo, C. C.: Temporal patterns of hemodynamics, oxygen transport, cytokine activity, and complement activity in the development of adult respiratory distress syndrome after severe injury. *J Trauma,* 36(5): 651–7, 1994.

33. Fink, M. P.: *Shock: An overview.* Edited by Rippe, J. M., Irwin, R. S., Alpert, J. S., et al., Boston, MA, Little, Brown & Co., 1991.

34. Nathens, A. B. et al.: The practice of venous thromboembolism prophylaxis in the major trauma patient. *J Trauma,* 62(3): 557–62; discussion 562–3, 2007.

35. Olson, S. A., and Glasgow, R. R.: Acute compartment syndrome in lower extremity musculoskeletal trauma. *J Am Acad Orthop Surg,* 13(7): 436–44, 2005.

36. Ouellette, E. A.: Compartment syndromes in obtunded patients. *Hand Clin,* 14(3): 431–50, 1998.

37. Pal, J.; Brown, R.; and Fleiszer, D.: The value of the Glasgow Coma Scale and Injury Severity Score: predicting outcome in multiple trauma patients with head injury. *J Trauma,* 29(6): 746–8, 1989.

38. Pape, H.; Stalp, M.; v Griensven, M.; Weinberg, A.; Dahlweit, M.; and Tscherne, H.: [Optimal timing for secondary surgery in polytrauma patients: an evaluation of 4,314 serious-injury cases]. *Chirurg,* 70(11): 1287–93, 1999.

39. Pape, H. C. et al.: Impact of intramedullary instrumentation versus damage control for femoral fractures on immunoinflammatory parameters: prospective randomized analysis by the EPOFF Study Group. *J Trauma,* 55(1): 7–13, 2003.

40. Pape, H. C.; Hildebrand, F.; Pertschy, S.; Zelle, B.; Garapati, R.; Grimme, K.; Krettek, C.; and Reed, R. L., 2nd: Changes in the management of femoral shaft fractures in polytrauma patients: from early total care to damage control orthopedic surgery. *J Trauma,* 53(3): 452–61; discussion 461–2, 2002.

41. Pape, H. C.; van Griensven, M.; Rice, J.; Gansslen, A.; Hildebrand, F.; Zech, S.; Winny, M.; Lichtinghagen, R.; and Krettek, C.: Major secondary surgery in blunt trauma patients and perioperative cytokine liberation: determination of the clinical relevance of biochemical markers. *J Trauma,* 50(6): 989–1000, 2001.

42. Park, M. J.; Cooney, W. P., 3rd; Hahn, M. E.; Looi, K. P.; and An, K. N.: The effects of dorsally angulated distal radius fractures on carpal kinematics. *J Hand Surg [AM],* 27(2): 223–32, 2002.

43. Partrick, D. A.; Moore, F. A.; Moore, E. E.; Biffl, W. L.; Sauaia, A.; and Barnett, C. C., Jr.: Jack, A. Barney Resident Research Award winner. The inflammatory profile of interleukin-6, interleukin-8, and soluble intercellular adhesion molecule-1 in postinjury multiple organ failure. *Am J Surg,* 172(5): 425–9; discussed 429–31, 1996.

44. Pell, M.; Flynn, W. J., Jr.; and Seibel, R. W.: Is colostomy always necessary in the treatment of open pelvic fractures? *J Trauma,* 45(2): 371–3, 1998.

45. Pfiefer, R.; and Pape, H. C.: Missed injuries in trauma patients: a literature review. *Patient Saf Surg,* 23: 2–20, 2008.

46. Piotrowski, J. J.; Alexander, J. J.; Brandt, C. P.; McHenry, C. R.; Yuhas, J. P.; and Jacobs, D.: Is deep vein thrombosis surveillance warranted in high-risk trauma patients? *Am J Surg,* 172(2): 210–3, 1996.

47. Regel, G.; Grotz, M.; Weltner, T.; Sturm, J. A.; and Tscherne, H.: Pattern of organ failure following severe trauma. *World J Surg,* 20(4): 422–9, 1996.

48. Riemer, B. L.; Butterfield, S. L.; Diamond, D. L.; Young, J. C.; Raves, J. J.; Cottington, E.; and Kislan, K.: Acute mortality associated with injuries

to the pelvic ring: the role of early patient mobilization and external fixation. *J Trauma,* 35(5): 671–5; discussion 676–7, 1993.

49. Ruchholtz, S.; Waydhas, C.; Lewan, U.; Pehle, B.; Taeger, G.; Kuhne, C.; and Nast-Kolb, D.: Free abdominal fluid on ultrasound in unstable pelvic ring fracture: is laparotomy always necessary? *J Trauma,* 57(2): 278–85; discussion 285–7, 2004.

50. Sadri, H.; Nguyen-Tang, T.; Stern, R.; Hoffmeyer, P.; and Peter, R.: Control of severe hemorrhage using C-clamp and arterial embolization in hemodynamically unstable patients with pelvic ring disruption. *Arch Orthop Trauma Surg,* 125(7): 443–7, 2005.

51. Sorkey, A. J.; Farnell, M. B.; Williams, H. J., Jr.; Mucha, P., Jr.; and Ilstrup, D. M.: The complementary roles of diagnostic peritoneal lavage and computed tomography in the evaluation of blunt abdominal trauma. *Surgery,* 106(4): 794–800; discussion 800–1, 1989.

52. Stannard, J. P.; Sheils, T. M.; Lopez-Ben, R. R.; McGwin, G., Jr.; Robinson, J. T.; and Volgas, D. A.: Vascular injuries in knee dislocations: the role of physical examination in determining the need for arteriography. *J Bone Joint Surg Am,* 86-A(5): 910–5, 2004.

53. Tierney, L. M., M. P. S., Papadakis, M. A.: *Current Medical Diagnosis & Treatment.* Edited, Lange Medical Books, McGraw-Hill, 2007.

54. Tischendorf, J. J. et al.: The interleukin-6 (IL6)-174 G/C promoter genotype is associated with the presence of septic shock and the ex vivo secretion of IL6. *Int J Immunogenet,* 34(6): 413–418, 2007.

55. Trupka, A.; Waydhas, C.; Nast-Kolb, D.; and Schweiberer, L.: Early intubation in severely injured patients. *Eur J Emerg Med,* 1(1): 1–8, 1994.

56. Tschoeke, S. K.; Hellmuth, M.; Hostmann, A.; Ertel, W.; and Oberholzer, A.: The early second hit in trauma management augments the proinflammatory immune response to multiple injuries. *J Trauma,* 62(6): 1396–403; discussion 1403–4, 2007.

57. van Olden, G. D.; Meeuwis, J. D.; Bolhuis, H. W.; Boxma, H.; and Goris, R. J.: Advanced trauma life support study: quality of diagnostic and therapeutic procedures. *J Trauma,* 57(2): 381–4, 2004.

58. van Olden, G. D.; Meeuwis, J. D.; Bolhuis, H. W.; Boxma, H.; and Goris, R. J.: Clinical impact of advanced trauma life support. *Am J Emerg Med,* 22(7): 522–5, 2004.

59. Velmahos, G. C.; Kern, J.; Chan, L. S.; Oder, D.; Murray, J. A.; and Shekelle, P Prevention of venous thromboembolism after injury: an evidence-based report—part I: analysis of risk factors and evaluation of the role of vena caval filters. *J Trauma,* 49(1): 132–8; discussion 139, 2000.

60. Velmahos, G. C.; Kern, J.; Chan, L. S.; Oder, D.; Murray, J. A.; and Shekelle, P.: Prevention of venous thromboembolism after injury: an evidence-based report—part II: analysis of risk factors and evaluation of the role of vena caval filters. *J Trauma,* 49(1): 140–4, 2000.

61. Waikakul, S.; Harnroongroj, T.; and Vanadurongwan, V.: Immediate stabilization of unstable pelvic fractures versus delayed stabilization. *J Med Assoc Thai,* 82(7): 637–42, 1999.

12 Neuro-Critical Care Management of the Patient with an Acute Spinal Cord Injury

Dale Hoekema
H. Louis Harkey, III

Spinal cord injury (SCI) is a devastating condition that affects more young than elderly people. Fifty to sixty percent of those affected are between the ages of 16 and 30. Trauma is almost always the cause, with vehicular collisions and sports related injuries leading the list. In spite of the initial devastation, more than a quarter million survivors of SCI in the United States have resumed meaningful function in society (1). Given the opportunity, these young people can attain seemingly amazing instances of rehabilitation. The physiologic changes that occur with acute SCI are profound in nearly every organ system of the body. However, in the acute phase, respiratory, cardiovascular, gastrointestinal, and skin issues predominate. Guidelines for the care of the patient with acute SCI have been published and provide one of the fundamental resources in managing such patients (2, 3). Today, the standard for caring for such patients during the first several weeks following their injuries is being defined by designated Neuro-Critical Care Units (NCCU) (4–6). NCCU teams are familiar with the problems and pitfalls of such injuries and can efficiently employ neuro-protective strategies, stabilize the spine, and avoid some of the devastating consequences that may occur due to secondary injury.

SYSTEMIC RESUSCITATION AND SPINE STABILIZATION

Most areas of the United States now have either emergency medical systems (EMS) or paramedic systems that are the first responders to patients with SCI. They have been trained in spinal immobilization with a hard cervical collar and in techniques using a spine board to minimize motion and maximize alignment of the spinal column. They also have training in the management of the airway in the face of a suspected cervical spine injury (7). The quality of the care of these first responders is critical; hence, their training and maintenance of quality standards needs to be part of any regional trauma network.

When an SCI patient arrives at a medical center, physical examination based on the standard neurological classification endorsed by the American Spinal Injury Association (ASIA) should be performed (8). In addition, imaging studies with CT scanning of the spine with sagittal, coronal, and axial reconstruction have become the standard of care in evaluating the trauma patient with a suspected spinal cord injury. MRI of the spine gives superior information regarding the spinal cord and soft tissue structures. Obtaining an MRI may be considered in the initial evaluation because key injuries may be missed when CT scanning is used alone (9). If the patient is awake, cooperative, and hemodynamically stable, then the evaluation can be carried out quickly and definitively. However, if the patient has multiple other injuries, then the evaluation may be limited due to coma, severe traumatic brain injury (TBI), or the need for sedation. Even though CT imaging studies may be obtained as part of the trauma evaluation, even these may be delayed if the patient needs a trip to the operating room or interventional radiology to stop life-threatening bleeding (10).

The focus of the NCCU team during these first hours is to secure an airway and to resuscitate the patient hemodynamically. Lactic acidosis may develop and require aggressive volume replacement to clear the lactate. If blood loss is the problem, then transfusion of packed red blood cells (PRBC) and fresh frozen plasma must be infused, and the source of bleeding must be stopped. Because secondary neurological injury is most often related to hypoxemia and hypotension, great care is taken to avoid these occurrences. A major pitfall in the early efforts to resuscitate the patient with polytrauma and an SCI is to assume that hypotension is all due to volume loss. This can lead to missing the diagnosis of neurogenic hypotension (see Table 12.1), which has a distinctly different treatment. It is recommended, after the patient has received 8 to 10 liters of crystalloid in excess of observed fluid losses and is still hypotensive, that a central venous pressure (CVP) monitor or a pulmonary artery catheter (PAC) be placed to assist in guiding volume replacement in order to avoid iatrogenic pulmonary edema.

Pulmonary edema is the most likely complication of excessive fluid replacement in a patient with neurogenic shock versus hypovolemic shock. A bedside echocardiogram can also be helpful in making decisions at the bedside to determine if the

Table 12.1   Avoiding Pitfalls in the Care of the Patient with Acute Spinal Cord Injury in the Neuro-Critical Care Unit

PROBLEM	PITFALL	SOLUTION
1. Respiratory failure and the difficult airway	An incomplete SCI may become a complete injury if immobilization of the spine is inadequate with intubation. Onset of frank respiratory failure is often delayed 3–4 days following the SCI as secretions accumulate.	Early recognition of impending respiratory failure and proper management of the airway with an LMA, fiber-optic intubation, blind nasal intubation, OTI with in-line traction, or bedside tracheostomy is critical.
2. Hypotension	Neurogenic shock may not have been recognized in the polytrauma patient with multiple other injuries.	Volume loading to PAOP of 18 or an EDVI of 120, then pressors to MAP 85 (early hemodynamic monitoring!).
3. Pneumonia	Lack of good pulmonary secretion clearance and adequate lung expansion, inappropriate delays in oral tracheal intubation (OTI).	Aggressive respiratory care with IPPB, secretion clearance, high TV 12–15 cc/kg ventilation when mechanically ventilated, and early empiric antibiotics.
4. Atelectasis	Lack of good pulmonary secretion clearance and adequate lung expansion.	IPPB, bronchodilators, hyperinflation and suctioning, assisted cough, and mechanical ventilation if indicated.
5. DVT Pulmonary emboli	Lack of adequate prophylaxis and screening with Doppler ultrasound.	SCD stockings, LMWH to begin 24–48 hours postinjury unless contraindicated. Periodic screening for DVT with Doppler ultrasound.
6. Decubitus ulcers	The patient may have been left on a hard spine board and in hard C-collars longer than needed, not log rolling q 2 hr, poor nutritional support.	Remove spine board ASAP. Remove hard C-collar ASAP, initiate nutritional support early, log roll q 2 hr, early use of an air bed.
7. Malnutrition	Ileus is common with SCI; if unable to give enteral feedings in 48 hr, consider parenteral route; if pancreatitis is present, jejunal feedings are appropriate.	Follow prealbumin, and initiate nutritional support within 48 hr of admission.
8. Bradycardia Asystole	Suctioning or passing a feeding tube may worsen bradycardia and precipitate asystole and should be done with caution and anticipation.	Glycopyrolate, atropine, or isoproterenol may be needed temporarily for symptomatic bradycardia. Pacemakers are rarely indicated.
9. Anemia	Phlebotomy and hemodilution are common causes. Hemorrhage may be occult from other injuries and should not be overlooked. In most cases accepting a lower hematocrit is appropriate.	Erythropoietin may reduce transfusion needs by 50% but will not work without adequate substrate. Hence iron levels and B12 levels should be checked. If iron is low, it must be given intravenously.
10. Hypoxemia.	In the polytrauma patient with lactic acidosis many clinicians will avoid pressors and may cause iatrogenic pulmonary edema. Also consider neurogenic pulmonary edema.	Early and aggressive hemodynamic monitoring to avoid iatrogenic pulmonary edema. If ARDS is present, initiate appropriate treatment with PEEP early.

left ventricle is empty or full. Many clinicians caring for polytrauma patients with SCI tend to be overzealous with volume replacement because they are reluctant to use vasopressors if the lactate has not cleared, as pressors may prevent or slow clearing of the lactate (see Table 12.1). Furthermore, when a patient develops hypoxemia and diffuse pulmonary infiltrates, the tendency is to diagnose adult respiratory distress syndrome (ARDS), but this declaration is often premature. More precisely, the definition of ARDS is based on three criteria: diffuse infiltrates that are multi-lobar on a chest film, hypoxemia defined by a PaO_2/FIO_2 ratio of less than 200, and, most importantly, a pulmonary artery occlusion pressure (PAOP) of less than 18 or an end diastolic volume index (EDVI) of less than 120. Ideally, in the polytrauma patient with an acute SCI, the NCCU team will push fluids until

a PAOP of 18 and/or an EDVI of 120 is reached. Then, despite the fact that the lactate has not cleared, pressors should be started to normalize the blood pressure due to the presence of neurogenic shock (11, 12). This strategy will avoid iatrogenic pulmonary edema, accelerate rapid normalization of blood pressure, and help resolve lactic acidosis.

ARDS may develop due to a systemic inflammatory response syndrome (SIRS), or due to neurogenic pulmonary edema in the polytrauma patient with an acute SCI (13). The ARDS network demonstrated significantly lower mortality rates (30% rather than 40%) in patients ventilated with low tidal volumes of 5–6 cc/kg rather than the traditional tidal volumes of 10 cc/kg (14, 15). This strategy often results in passive hypercapnia that may be tolerated in the patient with an isolated spinal cord injury but not in a patient with an associated TBI. In the latter case, it is preferred to use pressure control ventilation with positive end expiratory pressure (PEEP) and higher tidal volumes while maintaining the total airway pressure under 35 to prevent barotrauma. This strategy allows adequate oxygenation and allows one to keep the PCO2 in the low 30s, which is often necessary to control the intracranial pressure (ICP).

Both inflammatory changes and edema in the spinal cord are the initial response to injury. This creates the setting for a potentially enlarging area of ischemia and progressive neurologic loss. Hence, it has now been proposed as an option in the guidelines for management of acute SCI to maintain a mean arterial pressure of 80–85 for the first week postinjury to assure adequate perfusion pressure and, at minimum, to avoid further neurologic loss due to relative hypotension (2, 16).

Initial immobilization of the spine in the NCCU may be accomplished with a variety of rigid collars. Cervical collars have a limitation; studies have shown that they allow up to 30% of flexion and extension, 45% of rotation, and 65% of lateral bending (17). Gardner Wells tongs with traction were introduced in 1973. They offer not only better stabilization but also the opportunity to reduce jumped facets and realign the spine, and thereby to reduce pressure on the acutely injured spinal cord. In 5% of cases, further neurologic loss may occur with the application of traction (18, 19). Most spine surgeons apply 5 to 10 pounds of traction per level above the level of injury in a graduated manner, along with performing repeated neurologic exams and taking lateral cervical spine films to see if the fracture or dislocation has been reduced. Thus, with a fracture dislocation at the C5/C6 level, this could mean that up to 50 pounds of traction might eventually be used. In exceptional situations, more than 10 pounds of traction per level may be applied under the direct supervision of the treating surgeon. If neurologic deterioration occurs or overdistraction is detected on the lateral radiographs, the weight is reduced or traction is discontinued. Patients with rigid spines due to ankylosing spondylitis or severe cervical spondylosis and those with atlanto-occipital dislocation should not undergo traction due to a higher risk of further neurologic deterioration (20).

Halo rings can be applied to the skull with four pins. The ring is then attached to four bars that are secured to a specially fitted vest that may limit motion of the spine to just 5 degrees. Halo devices became popular in the late 1960s (21). In a patient with a vertebral fracture and no spinal cord injury with excellent respiratory status, early placement of a halo vest may be appropriate. However, if the patient has an SCI and associated respiratory compromise, applying a halo vest should be delayed until the patient has either had a tracheostomy (to allow access for respiratory rescue) or until the patient has passed the high-risk period for respiratory failure. This crucial period will typically coincide with the time the patient is being transferred out of the NCCU. The vest itself further reduces chest compliance and impairs respiratory effort in a patient who is already suffering from respiratory compromise from a spinal cord injury. In addition, an emergent intubation in a patient with a halo vest is very difficult and puts the patient at risk of dying due to loss of the airway.

Surgical stabilization is indicated in many patients with SCI. Timing of surgery is dependent on the patient's overall condition and stability. In a patient with a TBI, spine stabilization often needs to be postponed until the period of intracranial hypertension due to brain swelling has resolved. In most cases, even with other injuries such as a hemo-pneumothorax or long bone fractures, spine stabilization takes priority and should be undertaken as soon as possible after the initial resuscitation is complete. In 2006 Fehlings et al. published an extensive review of the literature and reported that early decompression, in the first 24 hours following the injury, resulted in statistically overall better outcomes to both delayed decompression and conservative treatment. Both NCCU length of stay and medical complications were also reduced in the early surgery cohorts (22).

In contrast to the younger patients, who tend to sustain SCI from vehicular trauma or sports-related injuries, those over 50 years of age are more likely to sustain such an injury from a fall (23). Management in the NCCU is similar to that for younger patients, but complications, especially from respiratory failure and infection, are more common. Not surprisingly, an older patient with no comorbidities is likely to do significantly better than an elderly patient with multiple comorbidities. If an aggressive approach is taken, an early tracheostomy is often indicated (24). The long-term prognosis in a high complete cervical cord injury is significantly worse in the elderly. In these cases, timely discussion of end-of-life issues should be considered.

NEUROPROTECTIVE INTERVENTIONS

At the present time, there are no pharmaceutical agents that have met the strict criteria to be endorsed at the level of a "standard" or a "guideline" in the treatment of SCI by national societies in neurosurgery or other disciplines. Methylprednisolone (MPS) continues to be commonly used on the level of recommendation of an "option" in the management of acute SCI (2). Historically, a number of different agents seemed to show promise in the lab when used in animal models; however, none of the agents, including GM-1 ganglioside, Gacyclodine, and naloxone, have proven to be more effective than placebo in clinical trials. Tirilazad may be equivalent in efficacy with MPS when following a bolus of MPS as shown in NASCIS III. A number of agents are currently being tested in laboratory trials as the hope of discovering a novel neuroprotective pharmaceutical continues to be investigated (25).

It is important from several perspectives for clinicians caring for patients with SCI to know the history of the three National Acute Spinal Cord Injury Studies (NASCIS). First, MPS remains controversial among clinicians, though patients will ask about its efficacy. Second, no better pharmaceutical agent is available for recommendation in place of MPS. Third, the NASCIS trials have established the scientific method of prospective, randomized, placebo techniques that will remain the standard in future clinical trials regarding SCI.

The NASCIS I study was started in 1979 and published in 1984. It was the first large multicenter trial of SCI patients. MPS was chosen because of its ability to reduce inflammatory changes by stabilizing membranes and lysosomes in vitro. Animal models using MPS had shown benefits regarding neurologic recovery. Only two treatment arms were selected. There was no placebo arm included in the study. The two arms included a low-dose arm, in which patients were given MPS in a 100 mg IV loading dose, followed by 25 mg IV every 6 hours for 10 days. In the high-dose arm, patients were given MPS in a 1000 mg IV loading dose, followed by 250 mg IV every 6 hours for 10 days. A total of 330 patients were enrolled within 48 hours of SCI in nine study centers in the United States and Puerto Rico. The NASCIS I trial was the first to use motor and sensory index scores as primary outcome measurements. Both groups demonstrated similar improvement at 6 weeks and 6 months, but with a higher infection rate in the high-dose group. Several important conclusions were reached at the end of the trial. First, the question had to be raised: was MPS better than placebo? Hence, a placebo arm was included in NASCIS II. Second, would treatment sooner after the injury but for a shorter period of time show benefit but with fewer side effects compared to the NASCIS I study? Third, a large-scale clinical trial with SCI had been successfully carried out, and this trial became the model for all other clinical trials in SCI (26, 27).

The NASCIS II trial began in 1985; some important observations and conclusions from the laboratory influenced the protocol for this trial. It had been discovered that, in addition to MPS's classic and appreciated anti-inflammatory effect, it was also able to preserve spinal cord ultrastructure by inhibiting free radical–induced lipid peroxidation (28, 29). This effect, however, required higher doses, in the 15–30 mg/kg range. The treatment protocol in NASCIS II had three arms. The first was a placebo arm. A second arm used naloxone, an opiate antagonist that had shown promise in animal studies. It was given as a 5.4 mg/kg bolus over 15 minutes followed by a 45-minute pause and then an infusion of 4 mg/kg/hr over the next 23 hours. The third arm consisted of MPS given as a 30 mg/kg bolus over 15 minutes. This was followed by a 45-minute interval with no medication, followed by an infusion of MPS at 5.4 mg/kg/hr over the next 23 hours. NASCIS II included ten centers in the United States enrolling patients over a 3.5-year period. The NASCIS II trial enrolled 487 patients. The arm using MPS enrolled 162 patients; the arm using naloxone enrolled 154 patients, and the placebo arm enrolled 171 patients. The average time to enrollment was 8.7 hours; however, only 80% of patients had been enrolled in the 12-hour window set as the target at the beginning of the study. Sixty percent of the patients had a complete spinal cord injury. Between 5% and 8% of patients enrolled had normal motor exams with only sensory changes related to their SCI. This latter point became an issue for which the study was criticized. The arm treated with MPS did show a significant improvement in both sensory and motor function over the other two arms at 6 months but only in the subgroup treated within 8 hours of injury. Another criticism of the study is that the number in the subgroup treated within 8 hours was too small to conclude that neurologic improvement was statistically significant accept in the ASIA-A subgroup (30). Other criticisms included that the initial resuscitation protocols varied with each center, no functional assessment scale was used as an outcome measure, and no analysis of individual muscle group function to determine the region of drug-induced improvement was performed (31). Results of NASCIS II were first released in 1990 by the lay press, which began the controversy that lingers to the present time over the validity of the outcome of the study as claimed by the authors. Many clinicians were disturbed by the fact that the published results of the study lagged behind the introduction of MPS as a "new standard" in the management of SCI. Therefore, when the results were finally published, they were scrutinized and contested. A call for release of the raw data went unheeded and further undermined confidence in the conclusion of the study. Also, the U.S. Food and Drug Administration never approved MPS for the indication of its use

in SCI, ultimately reducing the recommendation for its use to an "option."

When the NASCIS III trial was started in 1991, the intention was to address some of the shortcomings of the NASCIS II trial. A functional outcomes assessment was added. A closer look at time to treatment was included, and a longer high-dose infusion was added to assess the benefits and risks of this strategy. Sixteen centers participated in North America, and primary outcomes measured were neurologic improvement and safety data. In the NASCIS III trial, 499 patients were randomized to three treatment arms within 6 hours of injury. The first arm consisted of 166 patients randomized to MPS given in a bolus and infusion over 24 hours as in the NASCIS II protocol. The second arm consisted of a similar number of patients randomized to receive the same loading dose of MPS but followed by tirilazad mesylate given as a bolus infusion at 2.5 mg/kg every 6 hours for 48 hours. The third arm consisted of 167 patients who received NASCIS II standard MPS treatment for 24 hours, but in addition, the MPS infusion of 5.4 mg/kg/hr was continued for a second 24 hours. There was no placebo arm. Efficacy outcome measurement was similar to that of the NASCIS II protocol with the addition of the Functional Independence Measurement (FIM) to assess the functional impact of the therapy. As in the prior NASCIS trials, assessment was carried out at 6 weeks and 6 months following treatment. Interestingly, in NASCIS III, a higher percentage of patients had normal exams on entry into the trial compared with NASCIS I and II (24.7% of the 24-hour MPS group, 10.8% of the 48-hour tirilazad group, and 13.9% of the 48-hour MPS group). All three groups had similar functional improvement if treated within 3 hours of injury. More functional motor and sensory improvement was noted in those participants treated between 3 and 8 hours with the 48-hour MPS infusion. This was statistically significant. Also, the FIM scores were better for this group. Although mortality was similar in all three groups, the group that received the 48-hour infusion of MPS had a higher incidence of severe pneumonia. Although severe sepsis was more common in the 48-hour MPS group, it did not reach statistical significance. The authors published their results in 1997 and concluded that if a patient with SCI could be treated within 3 hours, he/she should receive the 24-hour infusion of MPS protocol used in NASCIS II and III. If a patient presented between 3 and 8 hours of injury, the authors recommended the 48-hour infusion of MPS used in the NASCIS III protocol (25, 32).

Although controversial, these landmark studies were the first to apply the scientific method of a prospective, randomized, placebo-controlled, and double-blinded technique to such a large number of SCI patients. Measurable end points had been developed and improved upon in the subsequent NASCIS trials. Further studies using MPS have been performed since the NASCIS trials with some suggesting benefit and others finding no difference from placebo. However, these subsequent trials had even more flaws in design and methodology than the NASCIS trials (33–35). Penetrating injuries to the spinal cord were excluded from the NASCIS trials, but other studies have looked at this subset of patients and have shown no benefit from MPS regarding neurologic improvement, and in fact have shown a higher infection rate (36).

The use of MPS in the NCCU remains selective. If the patient is young and healthy and presents within 3 hours of injury, the risks of treatment are minimal, and the 24-hour infusion protocol should be initiated. On the other hand, if the patient is older and has comorbidities, even if he/she presents within 3 hours, the risk of infection may offset any potential benefit, and MPS should probably not be used. Patients between these two extremes should be judged by the clinician based on the potential benefit compared to the potential risk. No clinician should be compelled any longer to use MPS due to fear of litigation. The compelling reasons to use it at a level other than an "option" can no longer be supported.

Two other neuroprotective strategies include avoidance of hyperthermia and maintenance of euglycemia. Van Den Berghe et al. demonstrated a decreased mortality and morbidity rate in a surgical ICU population with tight glycemic control. Others have suggested benefit from tight glycemic control in specific neurologic disorders (37, 38). The literature reports ample evidence of neuroprotection in animal models for hypothermia as well as similarly favorable evidence in stroke, in TBI, and for anoxic brain insults following cardiac arrest in humans (39). As of yet, no convincing evidence justifies the use of therapeutic hypothermia to treat humans with acute SCI. Some studies, however, report evidence that fever or hyperthermia may be damaging to injured neurons and that the use of aggressive measures to maintain normothermia in the patient with an acute SCI are justified (40, 41).

Psychological issues in dealing with the patient with acute SCI and his or her family are very important. A reactive depression is common among patients and some family members even during the first weeks following injury. Appropriate assessment and treatment of the patient is imperative, and referral of family members for similar care may also be indicated (42).

RESPIRATORY FAILURE

In addition to optimizing the neurologic outcome for a patient with acute SCI, the foremost critical responsibility of the NCCU clinician is to recognize that a complete injury at the cervical level, especially above C4, indicates that progressive respiratory failure is likely to occur and must be addressed appropriately. In some instances of complete injuries above C4, patients will already have been intubated in the field or the emergency department because of respiratory failure or due to other injuries. Bach demonstrated that in complete injuries of the cervical spine between C5 and C7, tidal volume (TV), vital capacity (VC), and negative inspiratory force (NIF) all dropped to less than one-third of normal following the injury (43). When the patient suffers an ASIA-A injury in the cervical region, all intercostal muscles lose their innervation and cease to function. In addition, the abdominal muscles that play a key role in splinting the chest to allow a patient to have an effective cough have also been lost. Ironically, the classic SCI patient who arrives in the NCCU from the emergency department with an isolated but complete C5 tetraplegia does not appear to be in respiratory distress despite having lost more than 50% of TV and VC. The careful observer will note paradoxical movement of the chest wall, which may fall with inspiration instead of rising due to the loss of the intercostal muscles. If the patient is asked to cough, it will be extremely weak. Most patients, however, speak with no difficulty. Expiratory muscles are preferentially lost, and hence expiratory reserve volume (ERV) is markedly reduced. Functional residual capacity (FRC) is also notably reduced. Thus, the acute tetraplegic patient who breathes spontaneously suffers from an acute restrictive lung defect. Small tidal volumes and the inability to cough effectively

in order to adequately clear secretions result in progressive ventilation-perfusion (VQ) mismatching, atelectasis, and hypoxemia. Monitoring the patients respiratory status is critical and should include bedside pulmonary mechanics every 6 hours consisting of spontaneous VC, TV, minute ventilation (VE), rapid shallow breathing index (RSBI), and NIF. At least daily, ABGs or pulse oximetry combined with end tidal CO_2 measurements and daily chest films should be obtained. If the VC falls below 15 cc/kg, the NIF is between 20 and zero, the PCO2 rises above 45, and the RSBI is approaching 100, the patient will probably require intubation and mechanical ventilatory support (44, 45). How well the patient does from a respiratory point of view depends on a number of factors. If the patient is young, strong, healthy, not obese, and is motivated to cooperate with the respiratory therapist, then the patient might easily avoid the need for mechanical ventilation and attain the goal of 50%–60% of the normal predicted VC. The skill of the NCCU physician, and particularly the respiratory therapist, is critically important. Goals for proper respiratory management include prevention of atelectasis and establishment of an effective cough to clear secretions. Tools that are helpful in accomplishing this include intermittent positive airway pressure (IPPB), bronchodilators, and an abdominal binder combined with appropriate coaching in the assisted cough technique. The Emerson "Cough Assist In-exsufflator" has also proven to be a valuable tool to remove airway secretions in acute SCI patients. It works with high flows of air in both inspiration and expiration in quick bursts and is effective in actually lifting secretions from the lower airways to the mouth or tracheostomy without causing pulmonary injury (46). Other tools have also been developed and are being marketed for this purpose; they include easily applied positive air pressure (EZPAP), intrapulmonary percussive ventilation (IPV), and transtracheal augmented ventilation (TTAV) using transtracheal catheters (Cadence) (47, 48). Chest physiotherapy also plays a role in the management of these patients when they have developed a consolidation. High frequency chest wall oscillation (HFCWO) performed with a vest and special ICU beds with a built-in ability to rotate the patient and perform chest physiotherapy with high frequency performed through the mattress on a timed basis may also be beneficial in patients with consolidations (49).

Noninvasive ventilation (NIV) may be appropriate for some of these patients, especially at night, when they tend to take smaller tidal volumes while they sleep and are more prone to atelectasis. The bi-level positive airway pressure (BIPAP) machine, built and marketed by Respironics, is widely used for this purpose. BIPAP has certain limitations and pitfalls the clinician should be familiar with. First, BIPAP requires a cooperative and awake patient. Second, because NIV may result in blowing some air into the stomach, these patients should not be allowed to eat because of concern about vomiting and aspiration. Third, BIPAP cannot be used for prolonged periods because of the risk of skin breakdown under the face mask. Finally, fourth and most importantly, BIPAP should not be used in the severely compromised, who should be intubated. Although BIPAP may work temporarily, if the patient's condition worsens, less reserve remains, and acute deterioration might occur after removing the BIPAP mask and before the endotracheal tube can be placed (43). NIV is also contraindicated in patients with significant bulbar dysfunction who have difficulty swallowing and handling their secretions.

Many NCCUs now offer bedside tracheostomy placement using a modified percutaneous dilational technique (PDT). Patients with high cervical injuries that are classified ASIA-A should undergo this procedure in the first few days following their injury because they will require a prolonged course of mechanical ventilation. For patients at the C4 level and below, an early tracheostomy may be appropriate depending on the age of the patient, other injuries, and comorbidities. This procedure, using the modified percutaneous dilatory technique, has proven to be safe and cost effective. The complications are similar to the open surgical technique and include tracheal stenosis as the most concerning long-term complication, although this occurs only rarely (50). Also to be considered for an early tracheostomy are SCI patients being treated with a halo vest that have an injury above the C4 level or below and whose respiratory status is particularly compromised.

Pneumonia is the most likely infection to occur in the NCCU during the care of the patient with an acute SCI (44). These patients are prone to develop pneumonia due to the marked reduction in VC and TV and to the difficulty they have mobilizing secretions. The key to prevention is early and appropriate lung expansion and secretion clearance. In selected patients, this may best be accomplished with intubation or tracheostomy placement. When based on a clinical diagnosis of fever, infiltrates, sputum production, and leukocytes, early empiric treatment of pneumonia prevents the development of more severe infection. A series of tracheal aspirate or bronchialalveolar ravage sputum cultures may be taken. Although a predominate organism might be helpful if grown, cultures are inconclusive in nearly 50% of cases. Empiric therapy with antibiotics should be narrowed at 48 hours, if possible, based on cultures; otherwise, the regimen should be limited to a 5–7 day course. The trend in treating nosocomial pneumonia is to treat early and aggressively but to shorten the course of antibiotics to avoid the development of resistant organisms (51).

If a pleural effusion or pneumothorax occurs and is significant in size, it should be treated with appropriate chest tube placement or thoracentesis. Because these patients are already suffering from a severe drop in respiratory reserve evacuation, even a mild- to moderate-sized effusion or pneumothorax may make a substantial difference in improving their respiratory status. Pleural fluid should always be sent for analysis to rule out a potential empyema (44). Mechanical ventilation of the patient with a high cervical SCI is poorly understood and executed in most non neuro-critical care units. Because the ARDS network results were published in 2000, the general trend in most intensive care units has been to ventilate patients with lower tidal volumes, in the 5–6 cc/kg range (14). Although this strategy focused on the prevention of barotrauma in the study that was only applied to patients with ARDS, most clinicians have inappropriately extrapolated this approach to all ICU patients. For decades now, SCI centers, such as Craig Hospital in Englewood, Colorado, have been advocating the use of higher tidal volumes (15–20 cc/kg or more) in patients with acute SCI. They have published several studies that have suggested that this strategy in this patient population results in a lower incidence of atelectasis, pneumonia, and shorter times to weaning from mechanical ventilation (52). The larger tidal volumes are achieved slowly by raising the TV only 100 cc per day. Plateau pressures are kept below 35, and peak pressures are kept below

40 to prevent barotrauma. With the larger tidal volumes, static compliance is actually improved, and airway pressures remain low. It must be understood that in the patient with an acute ASIA-A cervical spine injury it takes about 5 weeks for the intercostal muscles to become spastic. Until spasticity in these muscles develops, the chest wall is not stiff enough to give the diaphragms the mechanical advantage they need to generate higher tidal volumes and vital capacities (44). During this 4–6 week period, the best strategy is to increase the tidal volume slowly to a target of 12–15 cc/kg, using a volume control mode and a rate of about ten breaths per minute. The higher tidal volumes help prevent atelectasis and pneumonia, thereby allowing these patients time for their own pulmonary mechanics to improve substantially so that they can again breathe spontaneously (see Figures 12.1 through 12.3). Astute NCCU physicians consider premature attempts to wean these patients from mechanical ventilation to be inappropriate; such attempts ignore the evolution of chest wall physiology, thus increasing the risk of pneumonia and putting patients through unneeded periods of respiratory distress. Although this methodology is still widely unused and unaccepted, it has a sound physiologic basis and a proven track record at nationally recognized model SCI centers. Therefore, the National Institute on Disability and Rehabilitation Research (NIDRR) has funded an ongoing study being performed at Craig Hospital comparing high and low tidal volume ventilation in a prospective randomized fashion. One arm is randomized to a TV of 20 cc/kg, and the other arm to a TV of 10 cc/kg (using calculated ideal body weights). End points of the study include incidence of atelectasis, pneumonia, and time to weaning from mechanical ventilation (53).

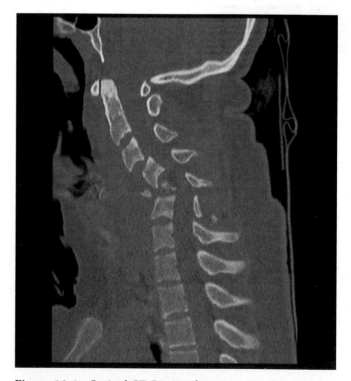

Figure 12.1 Sagittal CT C-spine demonstrating a C2/C3 subluxation and C4/C5 fracture dislocation in a 16-year-old female with an ASIA-A C4-level of tetraplegia.

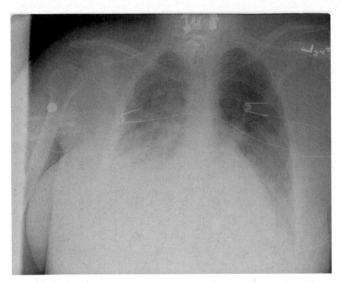

Figure 12.2   Chest film of a 16-year-old female with an ASIA-A C4-level tetraplegia, demonstrating bibasilar pneumonia while being ventilated with traditional small tidal volume ventilation of 7–8 cc/kg.

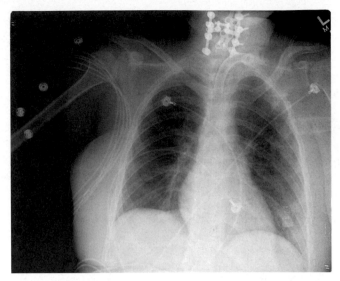

Figure 12.3   Chest film of a 16-year-old female with an ASIA-A C4-level tetraplegia, demonstrating improved lung expansion and clearing of prior infiltrates while now being ventilated with high tidal volume ventilation 12–15 cc/kg.

Management of the airway in a patient with a cervical SCI can be challenging. Of greatest concern is the patient with an incomplete injury and a fracture dislocation that is unstable. Manipulation of the neck in this patient may result in further cord damage, thus changing an incomplete injury to a complete one. Early clinical recognition of respiratory failure begins with the identification of the neurologic level of injury. If the neurologic level is above C4, then intubation is likely to be needed and should be anticipated. An awake, blind nasal intubation allows control of the airway without need for manipulating the neck. A fiber optically guided intubation is also a good choice but requires time to anesthetize the patient's airway with laryngeal nerve blocks, nebulized lidocaine, and transtracheal application of lidocaine; it also requires a cooperative patient. If the patient has favorable anatomy for oral tracheal intubation and securing the airway is urgent, then inline axial traction may be used with a relatively low risk of worsening the neurologic exam. However, if the patient has unfavorable anatomy for intubation, then a laryngeal mask airway (LMA) may serve as a bridge until the patient may be fiber optically intubated through the LMA or until a bedside tracheostomy can be performed. An NCCU should have personnel trained, immediately available, and comfortable in performing a bedside tracheostomy or cricothyrotomy in the patient with a difficult airway (50, 54).

CIRCULATORY FAILURE AND NEUROGENIC SHOCK

Spinal shock is the loss of all or most sympathetic mediated physiologic reflexes below the level of the spinal cord injury. These reflexes are mediated through the spinal cord between T1 and L1. Hence, any injury above T1 may result in profound spinal shock, but injuries that are complete in the lower thoracic levels may also exhibit a degree of spinal shock. Spinal shock is manifested by flaccid extremities and areflexia. Neurogenic shock, which is a component of spinal shock, applies specifically to the

loss of sympathetically mediated peripheral vascular tone and hypotension as a result. Spinal shock may last for a day or two, or it may last for days following the injury. In addition, unopposed parasympathetic activity is manifested by increased vagal tone with bradycardia and increased oral and bronchial secretions. Initially, both pre-load and after-load are reduced. Patients with a blunt SCI will have hypotension two-thirds of the time due to neurogenic shock alone, with the remainder having shock due to both a neurogenic basis and to hemorrhage associated with other injuries. Neurogenic shock is readily responsive to catecholamine pressors, which should be instituted to prevent secondary injury due to spinal cord ischemia due to hypotension (2, 55). The events related to acute SCI are a dynamic process. In a subset of patients, at the time of the acute injury, there may be a brief catecholamine outpouring, resulting in a short but severe rise in pre-load and after-load, contributing to the development of pulmonary edema. Hemodynamic monitoring may be very helpful in these patients to assist in differentiating between ARDS and volume overload as the etiology of a worsening hypoxemic respiratory failure and to optimize volume resuscitation and use of pressers.

Bradycardia occurs in more than half of the patients with acute SCI due to unopposed vagal tone. It is critical to monitor these patients' cardiac rhythms closely because medical therapy may be required if the patient becomes symptomatic. Rarely, asystole can occur, and infrequently, a temporary pacemaker may be indicated. Permanent pacemakers are rarely indicated. If symptomatic bradycardia occurs, the use of glycopyrolate, atropine, or isoproterenol may be beneficial (see Table 12.1). Significant bradycardia can last up to 6 weeks but usually resolves after the first week following acute SCI. Tracheal suctioning and passing a feeding tube, both of which may increase vagal tone, can be the precipitating factor leading to asystole and should be performed with caution and anticipation in these patients (56).

Shock from sepsis, hemorrhage, pulmonary embolism, and cardiac sources (myocardial infarction, cardiac contusion, pericardial tamponade, and acute valvular failure) are not rare in the NCCU. Hence, when new hypotension occurs, all should be considered. Unexplained hypotension should be evaluated with appropriate studies, including blood cultures, electrocardiogram, cardiac enzymes, echocardiography, chest CT, and serial hematocrits. The evaluation should be tailored to the findings on exam, and clues should be based on the history and clinical course. Adrenal insufficiency should also be considered and evaluated with a random cortisol level or an ACTH stimulation test followed by physiologic doses of hydrocortisone until the adrenal status is ascertained. In a patient with septic shock, in addition to appropriate cultures, identification of the source and removal of the focus of infection (i.e., central line), and initiation of appropriate antibiotics and pressors, one should consider the use of drotrecogin alpha as an adjunct, as it clearly reduces mortality in the subset of patients who are more severely ill (57).

DEEP VENOUS THROMBOSIS PREVENTION

Prophylaxis to prevent deep venous thrombosis (DVT) and pulmonary emboli (PE) should be performed with standing orders aggressively in all SCI patients. Most patients with an acute SCI are transiently hypercoagulable due to tissue factors released from their traumatic injuries (58). Aito reported a 2% incidence of DVT in a cohort of patients with SCI when low molecular weight heparin (LMWH), compression stockings, and sequential calf compressors were employed early, compared to historical controls with a 26% incidence when these measures were not used consistently (59). LMWH should be used 48–72 hours postsurgery or postinjury, unless contraindicated (see Table 12.1). Support hose and sequential calf compressors are also helpful adjuncts. Prophylactic inferior vena cava filters should not be used routinely but may be indicated in selected high-risk trauma patients who cannot be anticoagulated or who have failed anticoagulation (60). Surveillance duplex ultrasound is noninvasive and simple to use at the bedside and is beneficial for periodically screening SCI patients in the NCCU for DVT (61).

RENAL FAILURE AND SIADH

Acute renal failure (ARF) is not an uncommon problem in the patient with acute SCI during his or her stay in the NCCU. When it occurs, the first sign may be low urine output rather than a rising creatinine. Evaluation includes examination of the urine for casts and cellular components as well as urine electrolytes to calculate the fractional excretion of sodium (62). Pre-renal azotemia is the most common cause of renal insufficiency in the hospitalized patient. Hence, if the fractional excretion of sodium is less than 1, and central venous pressure is less than 5, a volume challenge is in order. If the patient does not respond to these measures but has been adequately volume loaded, then a renal ultrasound to rule out hydronephrosis should be performed, and the urinary catheter should be irrigated to rule out the possibility of bladder outlet obstruction. Renal toxic drugs should be considered, and the medication administration record reviewed. Aminoglycoside antibiotics continue to a frequent offender. Ace inhibitors may contribute to a drop in glomerular filtration rate, and if in use, should be stopped. Acute interstitial nephritis is often due to antibiotics or nonsteroidal anti-inflammatories. This diagnosis may be made if the urine stain for eosinophils is positive.

If the patient has sustained a significant soft tissue injury, then rhabdomyolysis should be suspected. In this case, serum creatinine phophokinase and a urine myoglobin test should be ordered (62). Many polytrauma patients receive large and repeated doses of intravenous contrast agents with their radiographic studies as well as numerous blood products; both could be potentially the cause of ARF. Continuous renal replacement therapy performed through a dialysis catheter may be temporarily needed if ARF develops. Fortunately, most cases of ARF are reversible, and in this setting, dialysis is only required as a bridge to recovery. The syndrome of inappropriate antidiuretic hormone (SIADH) is most common in patients with TBI or pneumonia but may also be seen occasionally in the patient with an isolated acute SCI. The diagnosis of SIADH suggests that the brain inappropriately releases too much of the ADH hormone. A basic assumption in making the diagnosis is that the patient is euvolemic. If the patient is hypovolemic, then the brain may be appropriately releasing excessive ADH in an attempt to restore the intravascular volume by hanging on to water at the distal renal tubule. Hence, accurate assessment of the patient's volume status is critical because, if the patient is hypovolemic, then the diagnosis of SIADH cannot be made. If the patient is euvolemic and hyponatremic (sodium 130), then the patient should be excreting very dilute urine in order to bring his/her serum sodium back to the normal range of about 140. The normal range of urine osmolality spans from 50 to 1200. If the patient's urine osmolality in this setting is 400–600, it is still too high, and the diagnosis of SIADH can be made. Treatment of SIADH begins with free water restriction but may also include hypertonic saline depending on the overall clinical picture. If the patient has a TBI with elevated ICP, then it becomes more urgent to maintain the sodium above 140, and the use of hypertonic saline becomes justified. Other agents, including arginine vasopressin receptor antagonists, may be useful in treating the SIADH syndrome. Care should be taken to monitor the serum sodium frequently enough that large swings in the serum sodium may be prevented. If rapid and large swings in the serum sodium occur, central pontine mylenolysis may occur (63). Urinary tract infections (UTI) may occur in the NCCU associated with an indwelling urinary catheter. However, the best means of preventing UTIs is to ultimately remove the catheter and perform intermittent catheterization. Most acute SCI patients' stay in the NCCU is limited to 2 weeks. Hence UTIs become much more of a problem and concern during the rehabilitation phase. Urine cultures should be sent if the patient has pyuria, fever, or cloudy urine. Intermittent catheterization is usually instituted by week 3 if the patient with acute SCI has a prolonged stay in the NCCU (64).

GASTROINTESTINAL FAILURE

Spinal shock results in gastric distention and decreased bowel motility, which may culminate in a paralytic ileus. The result can be devastating in the patient with an acute SCI because marked respiratory compromise has already occurred. The ileus results in further loss of diaphragmatic function with hydrostatic pressure pushing the diaphragm cephalad and further decreasing overall lung compliance, with an additional decrease in VC and TV and progressive impairment of the patient's ability to cough. Intubation may be required as a result. Decompression with nasal-gastric suctioning will help decrease intra-abdominal pressure. Because the clinical exam is limited due to the lack of sensation and pain, appropriate studies such as abdominal/pelvic CT scanning may be needed to exclude a bowel perforation, mechanical bowel obstruction, or volvulus. Pancreatic enzymes should be checked to rule out the possibility of pancreatitis. Given time, the ileus generally resolves spontaneously. Prokinetic agents such as erythromycin and metoclopromide have been shown to be helpful. Avoidance of drugs that depress bowel motility, such as narcotics and drugs with anti-cholinergic side effects, is also important.

Early nutritional support has been shown to play a critical role in the care of the acutely hypercatabolic injured trauma patient (65). Enteral feeding has also been shown to be superior to parenteral feeding, particularly because of the lower risk of infection seen with enteral feedings (66). Studies have demonstrated an obligatory negative nitrogen balance in SCI patients due paralysis of a significant muscle mass and associated atrophy. SCI patients have less metabolic expenditure than patient without SCI. Because they are less active, caloric intake and predicted energy expenditure (PEE) will be lower than expected, and appropriate adjustments using the Harris-Benedict equation should be made in calculating caloric needs (67). The nutritional status may be followed by checking periodic prealbumin, albumin, and transferrin levels, as well as anthropometric measurements, but muscle loss due to the SCI must be factored into this assessment. Negative skin tests suggest an anergic state and may be an indication of malnutrition. For the intubated patient or for the patient with a tracheostomy, a nasal-gastric or nasal-jejuna tube is the preferred mode of delivery of tube feeding (68). Because many SCI patients will be able to eat by mouth with or without a tracheostomy soon after their NCCU stay, it is appropriate to try to avoid the risks associated with a gastrostomy tube. Although a subset of patients will require a gastrostomy tube, there has been a concerning trend in our opinion of an overuse of this intervention. There is a definite complication rate of peritonitis frequently associated with sepsis and sometimes death; hence, the implementation of this procedure should be limited to patients who have clear cut indications (69).

A special bowel program should be instituted in every spinal cord-injured (SCI) patient due to decreased bowel motility following spinal cord injury. This may include stool softeners, fiber, and gentle oral cathartics combined with digital stimulation. Diarrhea is not uncommon in the NCCU and most frequently is related to the bowel flora being destroyed by broad-spectrum antibiotics. Pseudomembranous colitis may occur as a complication of antibiotic use, and the clinician should have a low threshold to send stool for a *Clostridium difficile* toxin assay because early identification and treatment with metronidazole or oral vancomyacin may prevent the development of toxic megacolon (70).

Since the advent of proton pump inhibitors that have been used prophylactically in the NCCU, the incidence of gastric stress ulcers and upper gastrointestinal bleeding has become negligible. Routine use of these agents is an important part of preventive management in the NCCU (71). Pancreatitis may occur in the patient with SCI in the NCCU. The tip off is usually the development of a paralytic ileus. In this setting, pancreatic enzymes should be sent and, if elevated, should be followed on a daily basis. Nutritional therapy should be continued with jejunal feedings. A new jejunal tube, referred to a as a "tiger tube," is now commercially available and is self propelled due to its unique design; it will

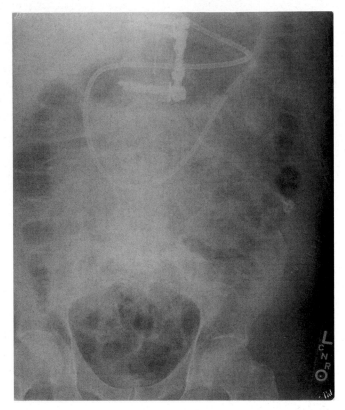

Figure 12.4   This 45-year-old man with an L1 burst fracture has developed postoperative pancreatitis and is being nourished through a self-propelled jejunal feeding tube known as a "tiger tube."

pass into the jejunum without fluoroscopic guidance in most cases (see Figure 12.4) (68). Studies have indicated a lower morbidity rate in pancreatitis when nutritional support is administered enterally compared with total parenteral nutrition (TPN) (72). A triglyceride level should be checked to exclude hyperlipidemia as the cause of pancreatitis, and an abdominal ultrasound should be performed to rule out "gall stone" pancreatitis. Some medications can be the source of pancreatitis, and one of the most common ones implicated in the NCCU is ace inhibitors. They should be discontinued if in use. If the clinician is forced to use TPN for some reason, intralipid should be avoided because it may worsen the pancreatitis. Propofol is a lipid-rich drug commonly used in the NCCU that should be avoided in the setting of pancreatitis.

ANEMIA

Anemia is almost universally a problem in the NCCU. This is mostly due to phlebotomy, for blood samples sent to the clinical laboratory may be numerous, but it also may be in part due to hemorrhage from the initial traumatic event or related to surgery. Anemia may also be related to hemodilution related to aggressive rehydration. During the first week following injury, most clinicians prefer to maintain a hematocrit in the 30% range in TBI or acute SCI to optimize oxygen delivery to the damaged neural tissue, although good clinical studies are lacking to support this strategy. In subsequent weeks, the threshold may be lowered to a hematocrit of 24%. The use of erythropoietin has allowed the neuro-critical care clinician to reduce transfusion requirements by nearly one-half, along with their attendant risks of hepatitis and associated immunosuppressive effects. If erythropoietin is to be used, however, both iron levels and a B-12 level should be checked because erythropoietin is not effective without adequate substrate (73, 74).

If the iron level is low, it should be raised with intravenous iron. Sodium ferric gluconate complex (Ferrlecit) at a dose of 125 mg a day for 7 days will completely restore the body's iron stores. In comparison to older forms of intravenous iron, Ferrlecit has an excellent safety profile.

DECUBITUS ULCERS

The old axiom "an ounce of prevention is worth a pound of cure" certainly applies to the prevention of decubitus or pressure-related skin breakdown in patients with SCI. A model NCCU will excel at decubitus ulcer prevention. Some of the key factors in prevention include turning the patient every two hours beginning at the time of admission, cleansing the skin with appropriate bathing techniques, and implementing specialized mattresses early on that distribute the pressure on the skin. Also, it is very important to initiate nutritional support early to avoid the development of a malnourished state. Prevention and judicious management of diarrhea also improves skin care. The Braden scale and modified Braden scale have been developed to identify patients at greater risk and should be implemented (75). Hard cervical collars should be removed as soon as possible, and collars such as the Aspen that distribute pressure more evenly on the skin should be used when a cervical collar must be part of the patient's care plan.

CONCLUSION

During the first several weeks after the initial injury, SCI patients present the NCCU clinician the opportunity to smoothly transition them to an appropriate rehabilitation facility and to avoid many of the common pitfalls that have plagued their management in the past (see Table 12.1). Appropriate neuroprotective interventions, immobilization, and early surgical stabilization of the spine offer the best opportunities to avoid further neurologic loss. Early recognition of spinal and neurogenic shock, especially in the polytrauma SCI patient, may be critical in preventing secondary injury due to both hypotension and hypoxemia by judicious volume resuscitation and timely use of presser agents. Respiratory failure to some degree occurs in all cervical SCI patients. Many patients will be able to avoid intubation and mechanical ventilation if the NCCU team is aggressive in respiratory care and monitoring for worsening respiratory failure. If the patient does require intubation and mechanical ventilation, then this should be performed in a timely basis, and electively, rather than waiting for a crisis to develop. The difficult airway should be recognized and dealt with appropriately to avoid loss of the airway or inappropriate manipulation of the fractured spine. Early bedside tracheostomy is indicated, particularly for the high and complete cervical spine injury. Pneumonia in the past has been all too common in the patient with the high cervical cord injury ventilated with small tidal volumes. Clinicians caring for the patient with the high cervical cord injury must recognize the value and safety of using higher tidal volume ventilation and of recognizing and treating pneumonia early with empiric antibiotics (see Figures 12.1 through 12.3). Development

of resistant organisms may be avoided by shortening the duration of antibiotic use. Deep venous thrombosis, decubitus ulcers, and malnutrition are almost always avoidable by using aggressive interventions to prevent them. Bradycardia must be recognized as not uncommon in the patient with an acute SCI. However, treatment is rarely indicated, and if required, is limited to medications. Blood transfusions should be minimized by accepting a lower hematocrit as a threshold for transfusion and by reducing phlebotomy and using erythropoietin along with appropriate substrates.

ACKNOWLEDGMENT

I would like to thank Daniel Lamberts MD, Director of Craig Hospital, for much help in supplying needed references and for reviewing this manuscript.

References

1. Lin V, Devisor MJ. *Spinal Cord Medicine.* 1st ed. Vol. 1. Chapter 4: Epidemiology of spinal cord injury. New York: Demos, 2003:79–85.
2. Hadley MN, et al. Guidelines for the management of acute cervical spine and spinal cord injuries. *Clin Neurosurg* 2002; 49:407–498.
3. Guidelines for management of acute cervical spinal injuries. Introduction. *Neurosurgery* 2002; 50(3 Suppl):S1.
4. Aito S. Complications during the acute phase of traumatic spinal cord lesions. *Spinal Cord* 2003; 41(11):629–635.
5. Diringer MN, Edwards DF. Admission to a neurologic/neurosurgical intensive care unit is associated with reduced mortality rate after intracerebral hemorrhage. *Crit Care Med* 2001; 29(3):635–640.
6. Ball PA. Critical care of spinal cord injury. *Spine* 2001; 26(24 Suppl): S27–30.
7. Sanchez AR II, Sugalski MT, LaPrade RF. Field-side and prehospital management of the spine-injured athlete. *Curr Sports Med Rep* 2005; 4(1):50–55.
8. ASIA. *International Standards for Neurological Classification of Spinal Cord Injury.* Chicago: American Spinal Injury Association, 2002.
9. Lammertse D, et al. Neuroimaging in traumatic spinal cord injury: an evidence-based review for clinical practice and research. *J Spinal Cord Med* 2007; 30(3):205–214.
10. Harris MB, Sethi RK, The initial assessment and management of the multiple-trauma patient with an associated spine injury. *Spine* 2006; 31(11 Suppl):S9–15, S36.
11. Jardin F, et al. Improved prognosis of acute respiratory distress syndrome 15 years on. *Intensive Care Med* 1999; 25(9):936–941.
12. Rosenberg AL. Fluid management in patients with acute respiratory distress syndrome. *Respir Care Clin N Am* 2003; 9(4):481–493.
13. Baumann A, et al. Neurogenic pulmonary edema. *Acta Anaesthesiol Scand* 2007; 51(4):447–455.
14. Ventilation with lower tidal volumes as compared with traditional tidal volumes for acute lung injury and the acute respiratory distress syndrome. The Acute Respiratory Distress Syndrome Network. *N Engl J Med* 2000; 342(18):1301–1308.
15. Wheeler AP, Bernard GR. Acute lung injury and the acute respiratory distress syndrome: a clinical review. *Lancet* 2007; 369(9572):1553–1564.
16. Ishizawa K, et al. Hemodynamic infarction of the spinal cord: involvement of the gray matter plus the border-zone between the central and peripheral arteries. *Spinal Cord* 2005; 43(5):306–310.
17. Pringle RG. Early management of the severely injured patient. *J R Soc Med* 1998; 91(4):233.
18. Marshall LF, et al. Deterioration following spinal cord injury: a multicenter study. *J Neurosurg* 1987; 66(3):400–404.
19. Gardner WJ. The principle of spring-loaded points for cervical traction. Technical note. *J Neurosurg* 1973; 39(4):543–544.
20. Fried LC. Cervical spinal cord injury during skeletal traction. *JAMA* 1974; 229(2):181–183.
21. Waters R, Adkins RH, Nelson R. Cervical spinal cord trauma: evaluation and nonoperative treatment with halo-vest immobilization. *Contemp Orthop* 1987; 14:35–45.

22. Fehlings MG, Perrin RG. The timing of surgical intervention in the treatment of spinal cord injury: a systematic review of recent clinical evidence. *Spine* 2006; 31(11 Suppl):S28–36.

23. Kannus P, et al. Alarming rise in the number and incidence of fall-induced cervical spine injuries among older adults. *J Gerontol A Biol Sci Med Sci* 2007; 62(2):180–183.

24. Harrop JS, et al. Tracheostomy placement in patients with complete cervical spinal cord injuries: American Spinal Injury Association Grade A. *J Neurosurg* 2004; 100(1 Suppl Spine):20–23.

25. Lammertse DP. Update on pharmaceutical trials in acute spinal cord injury. *J Spinal Cord Med* 2004; 27(4):319–325.

26. Bracken MB, et al. Efficacy of methylprednisolone in acute spinal cord injury. *JAMA* 1984; 251(1):45–52.

27. Bracken MB, et al. Methylprednisolone and neurological function 1 year after spinal cord injury: results of the National Acute Spinal Cord Injury Study. *J Neurosurg* 1985; 63(5):704–713.

28. Bracken MB, et al. A randomized, controlled trial of methylprednisolone or naloxone in the treatment of acute spinal-cord injury: results of the Second National Acute Spinal Cord Injury Study. *N Engl J Med* 1990; 322(20):1405–1411.

29. Hall ED, Braughler JM. Glucocorticoid mechanisms in acute spinal cord injury: a review and therapeutic rationale. *Surg Neurol* 1982; 18(5):320–327.

30. Nesathurai S. Steroids and spinal cord injury: revisiting the NASCIS 2 and NASCIS 3 trials. *J Trauma* 1998; 45(6):1088–1093.

31. Geisler FH, Dorsey FC, Coleman WP. Recovery of motor function after spinal-cord injury—a randomized, placebo-controlled trial with GM-1 ganglioside. *N Engl J Med* 1991; 324(26):1829–1838.

32. Bracken MB, Shepard MJ, Holford TR. Methylprednisolone for 24 or 48 hours or tirilazad mesylate for 48 hours in the treatment of acute spinal cord injury: results of the third NASCIS randomized controlled trial. *JAMA* 1997; 277:1597–1604.

33. Gerhart KA Jr, et al. Utilization and effectiveness of methylprednisolone in a population based sample of spinal cord injury patients. *Paraplegia* 1995; 33:316–321.

34. George ER, et al. Failure of methylprednisolone to improve the outcome of spinal cord injury. *Am Surg* 1995; 61:659–664.

35. Otani K., Abe H, et al. Beneficial effects of methylprednisolone in the treatment of acute spinal cord injury. *Sekisui Sekisui* 1994; 7:633–647.

36. Levy M, Gans W, et al. Use of methylprednisolone as an adjunct in the management of patients with penetrating spinal cord injury: outcome analysis. *Neurosurgery* 1996; 39:1141–1149.

37. Van Den Berghe G, Wouters P, et al. Intensive insulin therapy in critically ill patients. *N Engl J Med* 2001; 345:1359–1367.

38. Ferro J, et al. Other neuroprotective therapies on trial in acute stroke. *Cerebrovasc Dis* 2006; 21(Suppl 2):127–130.

39. Axelrod Y, Diringer MN. Temperature management in acute neurologic disorders. *Crit Care Clin* 2007; 22:767–785.

40. Tokutomi T, Morimoto K, et al. Optimal temperature for the management of severe traumatic brain injury: effect of hypothermia on intracranial dynamics and metabolism. *Neurosurgery* 2003; 52:102–112.

41. Suz P, Vavilala MS, et al. Clinical features of fever associated with poor outcome in severe pediatric traumatic brain injury. *J Neurosurg Anesthesiol* 2006; 18:5–10.

42. Dryden D, Saunders LD, et al. Depression following traumatic spinal cord injury. *Neuroepidemiology* 2005; 25:55–61.

43. Bach JR. Continuous noninvasive ventilation for patients with neuromuscular disease and spinal cord injury. *Semin Respir Crit Care Med* 2002; 23(3):283–292.

44. Peterson W, Kirshblum S. *Spinal Cord Medicine*. Chapter 9: Pulmonary management of spinal cord injury. Lippincott, Williams, & Wilkins, 2002: 135–154.

45. Chao DC, Scheinhorn DJ. Determining the best threshold of rapid shallow breathing index in a therapist-implemented patient-specific weaning protocol. *Respir Care* 2007; 52(2):159–165.

46. Winck JC, et al. Effects of mechanical insufflation-exsufflation on respiratory parameters for patients with chronic airway secretion encumbrance. *Chest* 2004; 126(3):774–780.

47. Brack T, et al. Transtracheal high-flow insufflation supports spontaneous respiration in chronic respiratory failure. *Chest* 2005; 127(1):98–104.

48. Deakins K, Chatburn RL. A comparison of intrapulmonary percussive ventilation and conventional chest physiotherapy for the treatment of atelectasis in the pediatric patient. *Respir Care* 2002; 47(10): 1162–1167.

49. Tecklin J. High frequency chest wall oscillation (HFCWO) for neuromuscular patients with airway clearance needs. *Respir Ther* 2005; 1:28–33.

50. Browd SR, MacDonald JD. Percutaneous dilational tracheostomy in neurosurgical patients. *Neurocrit Care* 2005; 2(3):268–273.

51. Singh N, et al. Short-course empiric antibiotic therapy for patients with pulmonary infiltrates in the intensive care unit: a proposed solution for indiscriminate antibiotic prescription. *Am J Respir Crit Care Med* 2000; 162(2, Part 1):505–511.

52. Peterson P, Whiteneck G. *The Management of High Quadraplegia: Pulmonary Physiology and Medical Management*. New York: Demos, 1989:35–50.

53. http://www.craighospital.org/InfoResources/2007-2012%20Research %20at%20Craig%20Hospital.pdf.

54. Criswell JC, Parr MJ, Nolan JP. Emergency airway management in patients with cervical spine injuries. *Anaesthesia* 1994; 49(10):900–903.

55. Atkinson PP, Atkinson JL. Spinal shock. *Mayo Clin Proc* 1996; 71(4): 384–389.

56. Winslow EB, et al. Spinal cord injuries associated with cardiopulmonary complications. *Spine* 1986; 11(8):809–812.

57. Bernard GR. Drotrecogin alfa (activated) (recombinant human activated protein C) for the treatment of severe sepsis. *Crit Care Med* 2003; 31(1 Suppl):S85–93.

58. Petaja J, et al. Fibrinolysis and spinal injury: relationship to post-traumatic deep vein thrombosis. *Acta Chir Scand* 1989; 155(4–5):241–246.

59. Aito S, et al. Primary prevention of deep venous thrombosis and pulmonary embolism in acute spinal cord injured patients. *Spinal Cord* 2002; 40(6):300–303.

60. Maxwell RA, et al. Routine prophylactic vena cava filtration is not indicated after acute spinal cord injury. *J Trauma* 2002; 52(5):902–906.

61. Kadyan V, et al. Surveillance with duplex ultrasound in traumatic spinal cord injury on initial admission to rehabilitation. *J Spinal Cord Med* 2003; 26(3):231–235.

62. Anderson RJ, Barry DW. Clinical and laboratory diagnosis of acute renal failure. *Best Pract Res Clin Anaesthesiol* 2004; 18(1):1–20.

63. Patel GP, Balk RA. Recognition and treatment of hyponatremia in acutely ill hospitalized patients. *Clin Ther* 2007; 29(2):211–229.

64. Trautner BW, Darouiche RO. Prevention of urinary tract infection in patients with spinal cord injury. *J Spinal Cord Med* 2002; 25(4):277–283.

65. Hasenboehler E, et al. Metabolic changes after polytrauma: an imperative for early nutritional support. *World J Emerg Surg* 2006; 1:29.

66. Moore FA, et al. Early enteral feeding, compared with parenteral, reduces postoperative septic complications: the results of a meta-analysis. *Ann Surg* 1992; 216(2):172–183.

67. Rodriguez DJ, Benzel EC, Clevenger FW. The metabolic response to spinal cord injury. *Spinal Cord* 1997; 35(9):599–604.

68. Davies AR, Bellomo R. Establishment of enteral nutrition: prokinetic agents and small bowel feeding tubes. *Curr Opin Crit Care* 2004; 10(2): 156–161.

69. Aschl G, et al. [Indications and complications of percutaneous endoscopic gastrostomy]. *Wien Klin Wochenschr* 2003; 115(3–4):115–120.

70. Russmann H, et al. Evaluation of three rapid assays for detection of *Clostridium difficile* toxin A and toxin B in stool specimens. *Eur J Clin Microbiol Infect Dis* 2007; 26(2):115–119.

71. Devlin JW. Proton pump inhibitors for acid suppression in the intensive care unit: formulary considerations. *Am J Health Syst Pharm* 2005; 62(10 Suppl 2):S24–30.

72. Abou-Assi S, O'Keefe SJ. Nutrition support during acute pancreatitis. *Nutrition* 2002; 18(11–12):938–943.

73. Corwin HL, et al. Efficacy of recombinant human erythropoietin in the critically ill patient: a randomized, double-blind, placebo-controlled trial. *Crit Care Med* 1999; 27(11):2346–2350.

74. Hebert PC, Tinmouth A, Corwin HL. Controversies in RBC transfusion in the critically ill. *Chest* 2007; 131(5):1583–1590.

75. Fife C, et al. Incidence of pressure ulcers in a neurologic intensive care unit. *Crit Care Med* 2001; 29(2):283–290.

13 Factors Affecting Surgical Decision Making

Patrick J. Connolly
Robert J. Nascimento

Spine injuries in the United States number more than a million cases per year. The vast majority of these injuries are benign soft tissue injuries that do not require surgical treatment or prolonged immobilization. In the United States, there are approximately 50,000 spine fractures each year, 11,000 of which involve injury to the spinal cord with associated neurologic deficit (1, 2). Although spine fractures are most often secondary to motor vehicle accidents, falls, or diving accidents, recent reports indicate a disturbing increase in the incidence of spine injuries related to firearms (3).

Most often, the patient who has sustained a spinal column injury is a young male between the ages of 15 and 35. The injury to the spinal column frequently occurs at either the cervicothoracic or the thoracolumbar junction.

An increased awareness by emergency personnel has allowed earlier spine stabilization both at the scene of the accident and in the emergency room. Rapid stabilization of the spine can contribute to a reduction in the progression of an incomplete spinal cord injury (SCI) to a complete SCI. Despite this heightened awareness of spine injuries, a number of cervical spine fractures are still missed early in the evaluation process. Evaluation for spine injury requires complete history-taking from the patient or emergency medical technicians (EMTs), as well as a comprehensive orthopedic and neurologic examination (4).

PATIENT EVALUATION

Patients with spine injuries may present as victims of multiple trauma or with an isolated injury to the spine. At the time of admission to the hospital, EMT personnel are invaluable in relaying information concerning the scene of the accident.

The physician should initially survey the vital signs, airway, breathing, and circulation. Following this, a brief examination of the patient's level of consciousness and neurologic status should be performed. At completion of the initial resuscitation efforts and primary survey for life-threatening injuries, the spine trauma evaluation may proceed. In a multitrauma setting, a patient should be considered to have a cervical spine injury until completion of the secondary physical examination and thorough radiographic assessment. Noncontiguous spinal injuries occur in 5% to 20% of those with spine fractures. As many as 15% of patients have associated major visceral involvement (5).

A complete examination first involves inspection for evidence of head injury, abdominal contusion, or skin lacerations. Severe facial and scalp injuries can be associated with cervical spine injury and may help the examiner deduce the mechanism of injury. Abdominal contusion is a diagnostic clue for flexion-distraction (lap belt) injuries to the spine. In a cooperative patient, palpation of the spine from the skull to the coccyx for areas of localized tenderness is extremely helpful to localize a spinal injury. Root-specific muscle strength testing of the upper and lower extremities and rectal examination for tone and sensation are extremely important in determining the anatomical level of injury. Cranial nerve examination, sensory response to pin and light touch, deep tendon, and plantar reflexes complete the spine injury assessment. Finally, careful documentation of the initial examination is essential.

GENERAL PRINCIPLES OF TREATMENT

The important components of treating patients who have sustained a spine injury are immobilization, medical stabilization, restoration of spinal alignment, neural decompression, and spinal stabilization.

Initial immobilization should be performed in the field using a rigid cervical collar as well as a spinal board and sandbags. Immobilization should be maintained until the patient has been evaluated and cleared by the treating physician. If the patient has not been stabilized in the field, cervical spinal stabilization should be one of the first steps taken by the evaluating physician in the emergency room.

Medical stabilization follows the basic principles of trauma care. This requires continuous monitoring of the patient's respiratory and cardiovascular status and is generally conducted in the emergency room or intensive care unit setting. Patients with spinal cord injuries and *neurogenic shock* present with hypotension and bradycardia as a result of the traumatic sympathectomy. *Spinal shock* is different from neurogenic shock and is defined as the absence of spinal reflex activity below an SCI. The significance of spinal shock is that it limits the ability to both classify the extent of paralysis and predict recovery of cord function. Spinal shock should be considered resolved with the return of the bulbocavernosus reflex (BCR) after 48 hours from injury. In a small percentage of patients, the BCR never returns.

Realignment of the injured cervical spine is usually accomplished with skeletal traction via a halo ring or cranial tongs. Although recently there has been some concern about the necessity of MRI or myelography before the reduction of a cervical spine dislocation, this is generally not needed in a setting where the patient is being placed in traction while awake and is subjected to repeat neurologic and radiographic evaluation.

IMAGING

The open-mouth anteroposterior (AP) view of the spine is essential for evaluation of the upper cervical spine. The standard AP view of the spine allows evaluation of lateral mass and sagittal plane fractures. Lateral cervical spine radiographs are an essential part of the evaluation. Although 85% of significant injuries will be detected with a lateral cervical spine radiograph that allows visualization of C7, an injury at the cervical thoracic junction may escape detection. Consequently, current spine trauma protocol should require complete cervical spine radiographs with full visualization of the body of Tl. If this is not possible, a swimmer's view or CT scan is required.

MRI is extremely helpful in the evaluation of patients with SCI or neurologic deficit. It may complement, but does not replace, CT. A thin-section CT scan of the spine provides greater bone detail and remains the gold standard for demonstrating fracture pattern and canal compromise in spinal injuries.

Technetium bone scanning is occasionally helpful in ruling out occult injuries of the spine in patients with prolonged symptoms and an otherwise negative radiographic evaluation.

MECHANISM OF INJURY AND STABILITY OF THE FRACTURE

Spine fractures can be classified on the basis of the mechanism of injury (6–10). Injuries to the spine may occur secondary to the forces of flexion, extension, lateral rotation, axial loading, or a combination of these forces. The forces that most often cause injury to the spinal cord are a combination of flexion and axial loading. The specific fracture that these forces produce varies according to the age of the patient, preexisting medical conditions (i.e., osteoporosis, ankylosing spondylitis, etc.), and the level of injury.

Spine fracture classification, along with personal experience and training, enable the surgeon to develop a treatment plan. The degree of stability or instability of an SCI will change with time as the osseous elements heal. Therefore, an injury that might initially be considered unstable may well be stable 12 weeks after injury. Conversely, an injury that involves primarily ligamentous structures may become less stable with time. Most spine fracture classification systems are designed to evaluate acute injuries.

Holdsworth (9) is credited with developing the first spine fracture classification that included specific recommendations

for treatment. Denis (7) modified this system by adding the concept of the three columns of the thoracic and lumbar spine. Allen and Ferguson (6) developed a mechanistic classification of closed, indirect fractures and dislocations of the lower cervical spine. In each system, the goal of fracture classification is to determine whether the fracture is stable or unstable. The transitional zones of the spine, specifically the cervicothoracic junction and the thoracolumbar junction, are often affected. The explanation of this phenomenon is twofold: a change in rigidity associated with the rib cage and thoracic spine, and a change in the sagittal alignment that occurs at the thoracic spine (cervical lordosis, thoracic kyphosis, lumbar lordosis). The location of a fracture can be just as important as the fracture pattern in regard to stability. Specifically, fractures in the mid-thoracic region are inherently more stable in the presence of an intact rib cage than are similar fractures at the thoracolumbar junction. Although the specifics of spinal stabilization are beyond the scope of this chapter, in general, a patient who has been realigned with traction or postural reduction, and does not have significant canal compromise, is often treated with posterior stabilization and fusion alone. In injuries that are treated with an anterior decompressive procedure, anterior bone grafting alone does not provide immediate internal fixation, and anterior or posterior stabilization is required.

In the authors' view, fractures associated with SCI are, by definition, unstable and are usually best treated with surgical stabilization. Immediate stabilization allows for early mobilization and rehabilitation. These benefits must be weighed against the potential risks of surgery, such as infection and inadequate fracture stabilization. Each fracture has a so-called personality of its own, and the method of spinal stabilization depends on the personality of the fracture as well as the ability of the surgeon. If surgery will not provide immediate improved spinal stability, then it should probably not be performed.

CLASSIFICATION OF SPINAL CORD INJURY

SCI can be broadly classified as complete or incomplete (4). The diagnosis of complete SCI cannot be made until spinal cord shock resolves. If the BCR is present and there is no motor or sensory function below the level of injury, then by definition the injury is complete. If, following the return of the BCR, the patient has some sensation below the level of injury, then he or she is considered to be sensory incomplete. If the BCR has returned and the patient has some motor function and sensation below the level of injury, the he or she is considered to be sensory and motor incomplete.

There are four incomplete SCI syndromes. *Anterior cord syndrome* is characterized by injury to the anterior cord at the level of spinal injury, with relative sparing of the dorsal column sensory pathways. The mechanism of injury is usually a compression or flexion type injury. Clinically, there is paralysis in portions of the upper limbs. In the lower extremities, deep pressure and position sense are preserved, with no motor function below the area of injury. The prognosis for anterior cord syndrome is the worst of all incomplete syndromes.

Posterior cord syndrome is rare. In this injury, there is preservation of motor function with loss of sensory function below the level of injury.

Central cord syndrome is common. The mechanism of injury is usually an extension injury that occurs in an older patient with preexisting cervical spondylosis and/or stenosis. Clinically, the patient has a greater loss of function in the upper extremities than in the lower extremities. Perianal sensation is often preserved. Historically, this has been ascribed to the somatotopic organization of the corticospinal tract (CST), as the arm fibers are centrally located and the lower extremity fibers are located more peripherally. However, more recent investigations show that the CST in higher primates is not somatotopically organized and that the clinical syndrome may be secondary to the disproportionate influence of the CST on hand and upper extremity motor function versus lower extremity function.

Brown-Séquard syndrome is produced by a predominant injury to a lateral half of the spinal cord. Motor paralysis and proprioception loss are greater on the side of the injury. Pain and temperature sensory loss are greater contralateral to the side of the SCI. This syndrome has a fair prognosis for functional recovery.

In the clinical setting, there often arises confusion in the so-called labeling of cord injury syndromes. In an incomplete SCI, the caudal segments of the spinal cord are either stronger, weaker, or the same. Caudal loss is consistent with an anterior cord syndrome. A patient with better caudal motor strength than cranial motor strength has a central cord-type lesion. Patients with isolated nerve root injuries should be classified as having neurologic deficit without SCI.

SPINAL CORD INJURY

Most spinal cord deficit is attributed to contusion and/or compression rather than to complete transection. The initial blunt injury leads to a secondary sequence of molecular and cellular events that result in ischemia, tissue hypoxia, and secondary tissue degeneration. The extent of tissue damage and the resulting neural injury can be related to the magnitude of the initial force. Whether the initial blunt insult or the effect of continued pressure on the damaged neural elements is of greater consequence in causing persistent neural deficits remains a topic of controversy. The microvasculature can be disrupted by mechanical deformation and propagated by edema, thrombosis, or further vasoconstriction induced by local and circulating factors. Although the initial insult to the spinal cord is currently irreversible, maintenance of perfusion at the cellular level of the spinal cord, if possible, is important to protect the remaining living, healthy tissue and to possibly improve recovery.

PHARMOCOLOGIC TREATMENT OF SPINAL CORD INJURY

The goal of pharmacologic intervention is to decrease secondary neurologic damage following the initial mechanical injury (1, 2, 11, 12). To understand the rationale of pharmacologic treatment of SCI, a brief discussion of secondary SCI is necessary.

Numerous theories exist regarding secondary SCI. Overall, the SCI site becomes an area of ischemia, hypoxia, and edema. The free-radical theory suggests that, because of depletion of antioxidants, free radicals accumulate and attack membrane lipids. Lipid peroxides are produced, and the cell membranes fail. In the calcium theory, there is an influx of extracellular calcium into the nerve cell. This, in turn, activates phospholipases, causing a resultant interruption of mitochondrial activity and a disruption of the cell membrane.

The explanation for the observed effects of methylprednisolone is that it suppresses the breakdown of cell membranes by inhibiting lipid peroxidation and hydrolysis at the site of injury. The high doses required are those shown to be most effective in inhibiting lipid peroxidation and the breakdown of neurofilaments in laboratory-induced SCI.

Because the beneficial effects of methylprednisolone on SCI are believed to be unrelated to its glucocorticoid effects, interest has developed in the utilization of 21-aminosteroids for SCI. Tirilazad is a lazeroid (synthetic 21-aminosteroid). It is a potent antioxidant without the glucocorticoid effects of methylprednisolone. GM 1 gangliosides are complex glycolipids of an acid nature that are present in high concentrations in central nervous system (CNS) cells. Although their functions are not entirely clear, there is experimental evidence that suggests they augment neurite outgrowth, induce regeneration and sprouting of neurons, and restore neurologic function after injury. GM-1 may be effective in treating SCI even if administration is delayed for 48 hours. In a recent multicenter trial, it was shown that patients with a motor incomplete injury had a more rapid time course of neurologic recovery. However, it failed to show a long-term difference in achieving "marked neurologic recovery" (13). Unfortunately, the one major drawback of GM-1 is that it may have an antagonistic effect on the neuroprotective role of methylprednisolone. This may become quite cumbersome in the design of further clinical trials.

Current recommendations are a result of the third National Acute Spinal Cord Injury Study (NASCIS-III). The recommended guideline for patients who receive treatment within 3 hours of injury is the administration of methylprednisolone as a bolus (30 mg/kg body weight) followed by an infusion (5.4 mg/kg/hr) for 23 hours. For those patients in which methylprednisolone is initiated within 3 to 8 hours of injury, the infusion should continue for 48 hours.

ROLE OF ANATERIOR DECOMPRESSION

Direct anterior spinal cord decompression (14, 15) should be considered when there is significant residual anterior compression of the spinal cord following realignment. In the past, concern existed about the further injury and destabilization by anterior procedures, but recent work has shown a significant benefit for patients with both complete and incomplete quadriplegia. Although the exact timing of anterior decompressive procedures is not entirely clear, animal studies indicate that the effect of spinal cord compression is inversely related to the duration of compression. In the authors' practice, patients with SCI, both complete and incomplete, undergo imaging assessment following their initial stabilization and realignment. If significant anterior cord compression remains following realignment with traction, then an anterior decompressive procedure should be considered in both the incomplete and complete SCI patient to maximize the recovery of cord injury and root return, respectively.

In general, because of the relative size of the upper cervical spine, a decompressive procedure of the upper cervical spine is rarely, if ever, indicated. In the lower cervical spine, the vast majority of patients can be successfully stabilized by a posterior procedure alone. If significant canal compromise by disc or bony fragments occurs following reduction, then an anterior decompression along with surgical stabilization is usually performed. The benefits of anterior cervical decompression with residual canal compromise are twofold: it provides a biomechanically sound fusion environment and provides an optimal environment for neurologic recovery and root return.

In thoracic and lumbar injuries, realignment and posterior stabilization provides an indirect decompression of the spinal canal that often eliminates the requirement for anterior decompression. If significant canal compromise (often defined as greater than 50% canal compromise) remains following posterior reduction and stabilization, then an anterior decompression may be necessary. In most clinical situations, an anterior thoracic or lumbar decompression is not urgently or emergently required. The decision to perform an anterior decompression in the acute setting, via a thoracotomy or a thoracolumbar approach, requires careful consideration. The potential benefit of anterior decompression is often outweighed by the deleterious effect that a thoracotomy may have on a multitrauma patient.

TIMING OF SURGERY

When a progressive neurologic deficit exists in the presence of malalignment and spinal canal compromise, emergency decompression is indicated. In all others with SCI, the timing of surgery is controversial (1, 14, 15). Some authors recommend treatment as soon as the patient is medically stable, whereas others advocate a delay of 4 or more days to allow for posttraumatic swelling to resolve. A recent review suggested that there is emerging evidence that surgery within 24 hours may reduce length of intensive care unit stay as well as postinjury medical complications (16).

Delamarter evaluated the effect of the timing of spinal cord decompression in a canine SCI model. In his study, a constriction band was utilized to create controlled paraplegia. In the group that was decompressed at 1 hour following injury, the animals recovered neurologic function. In the group that was decompressed at 6 hours following injury, there was no neurologic recovery. The results of his study suggested that not all of the injury to the spinal cord occurred at the initial trauma and that early decompression had a significant role in neurologic recovery.

Whether early decompression and reduction of neural structures enhances neurologic recovery continues to be debated. Although animal studies suggest a benefit with early decompression, this hypothesis has not been clinically proven. Indeed, significant functional recovery has been observed following anterior decompression of the spinal cord in patients whose initial injury was up to 20 years old. Currently, a reasonable approach would be to treat nonprogressive neurologic deficits on a semi-urgent basis, when the patient's systemic condition is medically stable.

GUNSHOT WOUNDS

Over the last 15 years, there has been fluctuation in the incidence of spinal cord injury related to violence and, in particular, to gunshot wounds. Statistics from 2000 to June 2006 show that 11.2% of SCI is related to violence. The 1990s held the highest percentage of injuries related to violence with an incidence of approximately 22% (2, 17). Data from 1991 reported that a staggering 52% of total admissions for SCI at one regional SCI center were related to gunshot wound trauma (4). Whether the current trend of a decrease in SCI secondary to violence will continue well into the twenty-first century will remain to be seen. These astounding numbers are certainly alarming.

These injuries rarely cause sufficient bone or ligamentous injury to warrant surgical treatment. Immobilization with a halo vest or rigid cervical orthosis usually provides adequate stability for healing. The issue of removing a bullet from the spinal canal remains controversial. The argument for bullet removal revolves around diminishing the risk of CSF leak, meningitis, lead toxicity, pain, neurological decline, and bullet fragment migration. The argument for the nonoperative approach is that retention of bullet fragments does not routinely lead to complications and that the risks of surgical intervention outweigh the potential benefits of fragment removal.

Overall, these cases are never straightforward. They must be evaluated on a case-by-case basis. If the bullet fragment is creating compressive pathology, its removal may benefit the patient. Likewise, bullet migrations in the spinal canal or progression of neurologic deficit are indications for surgical intervention. Recent studies evaluated the impact of bullet removal in SCI patients. The conclusion of the studies was that removal of the bullet did not affect the incidence of pain. Bullet removal from the canal between T1 and T11 had no significant effect on motor recovery, but when bullets were removed from the cauda equina region, patients did receive some benefit.

PATHOLOGIC BONE

Fractures associated with minimal trauma are most often associated with pathologic bone. Osteoporosis, metastatic disease, and ankylosing spondylitis are associated with spine fractures. Each disease presents its own challenges in the treatment of spine fractures (18–23).

Osteoporosis is the most prevalent metabolic bone disease. Osteoporotic compression fractures often occur in the elderly. Most often, these fractures are stable in nature and do not require surgical intervention. Unstable fractures associated with SCI, when they do occur, require careful surgical planning. The usual methods of surgical stabilization often fail to provide adequate surgical stabilization in light of this soft bone. The judicious use of polymethylmethocroylate is often necessary.

Metastatic spinal lesions are an important consideration in the evaluation of low-impact spine fractures. Metastatic lesions are identified at autopsy in 40% to 80% of patients who die of cancer. Spinal cord compression occurs in 20% of patients with spinal metastases. In treating patients with metastatic spine fractures, the surgeon must consider the overall health of the patient, the degree of pain, and the biology of the primary tumor, as well as the integrity and stability of the spinal column.

Patients with ankylosing spondylitis have a 3.5-times greater incidence of cervical spine injury than the normal population. Seventy-five percent of the spine fractures sustained by patients with ankylosing spondylitis occur in the cervical spine. The diagnosis is often delayed. Patients typically present with complaints of neck pain following minimal trauma. The mechanism of injury is most often a hyperextension injury. Because of the disease process, the spine breaks like a solid long bone. These fractures are highly unstable, and patients are at a high risk for neurologic complications.

Traditional treatment for this type of fracture is rigid immobilization with a halo cast or a vest, paying careful attention to alignment and to maintenance of the patient's pre-injury alignment. Recent development in spinal instrumentation has allowed for rigid internal fixation; in the hands of some experienced spine surgeons, early stabilization with a combined anterior and posterior procedure is now the treatment of choice for fractures in patients with ankylosing spondylitis.

CONCLUSION

When treating patients with SCI, the physician must look at the individual needs of the patient. Age, level of injury, fracture pattern, preexisting medical conditions, and associated traumatic injuries are factors that influence the treatment plan. If early mobilization of the patient through surgical stabilization is realistic, then early surgical intervention should be performed.

References

1. Delamarter RB, Coyle J. Acute management of spinal cord injury. *J Am Acad Orthop Surg* 1999; 7:166–175.
2. Inamasu J, Guiot BH. Initial evaluation and management of spinal trauma. Orthopedic Knowledge Update. *Spine 3.* 2006; 179–187.
3. Waters RL, Adkins RH. The effects of removal of bullet fragments retained in the spinal canal. *Spine* 1991; 16:934–939.
4. Connolly PJ, Yuan HA. Cervical Trauma. *Orthopaedic Knowledge Update V (OKU-V).* AAOS Publications, 1996.
5. Vaccaro AR, An HA, Lin SS. *J Spinal Disord* 1992; 5:320–329.
6. Allen BL, Ferguson RL, Lehmann TR, O'Brien RP. Mechanistic classification of closed indirect fractures and dislocations of the lower cervical spine. *Spine* 1982; 7:1–27.
7. Denis F. The three column spine and its significance in the classification of acute thoracolumbar spinal injuries. *Spine* 1983; 8:817–831.
8. Gertzbein SD. Spine update. Classification of thoracic and lumbar fractures. *Spine* 1994; 19:626–628.
9. Holdsworth FW. Fractures, dislocations, and fracture-dislocations of the spine. *J Bone Joint Surg Br* 1963; 45B:6–20.
10. McCormack T, Karaikovic E, Gaines RW. The load sharing classification of spine fractures. *Spine* 1994; 19:1741–1744.
11. Bracken MD, et al. A randomized controlled trial of methylprednisolone or naloxone in the treatment of acute spinal cord injury. *N Engl J Med* 1990; 322:1405–1411.
12. Geisler FH, Dorsey FC, Coleman WP. Recovery of motor function after spinal cord injury: a randomized placebo-controlled trial with GM-1 ganglioside. *N Engl J Med* 1991; 324:1829–1838.
13. Geisler, FH, et al. The sygen multicenter acute spinal cord injury study. *Spine* 2001; 26 (24S):S87–98.
14. Anderson, PA, Bohlman, HH. Anterior decompression and arthrodesis of the cervical spine: long-term motor improvement. Improvement in complete traumatic quadriplegia. *J Bone Joint Surg Br* 1991; 74A:683–692.
15. Bohlman, HH, Anderson PA. Anterior decompression and arthrodesis of the cervical spine: long-term motor improvement. Improvement in incomplete traumatic quadriparesis. *J Bone Joint Surg Br* 1992; 74A: 671–682.
16. Fehlings, MG, Perrin, RG. The timing of surgical intervention in the treatment of spinal cord injury: a systematic review of the recent clinical evidence. *Spine* 2006; 31(11 Suppl):S28–35.
17. National Spinal Cord Injury Statistical Center. *Spinal Cord Injury: Facts and Figures at a Glance.* Last updated June 2006. http://www.spinalcord.uab.edu/show.asp?durki=21446
18. Faciszewski T, McKierman FE, Rao R. Management of osteoporotic vertebral compression fractures. Orthopaedic Knowledge Update. *Spine 3.* 2006; 377–386.
19. Cronen GA, Emery SE. Benign and Malignant Lesions of the Spine. Orthopaedic Knowledge Update. *Spine 3.* 2006; 351–366.
20. Patel NM, Jenis LG. Inflammatory Arthritis of the Spine. Orthopaedic Knowledge Update. *Spine 3.* 2006; 342–346.
21. Broom MJ, Raycroft JF. Complications of fractures of the cervical spine in ankylosing spondylitis. *Spine* 1988; 13:763–766.
22. Foo D, Sarkarati M, Marcelino V. Cervical spinal cord injury complicating ankylosing spondylitis. *Paraplegia* 1985; 23:358–363.
23. Taggard DA, Traynelis VC. Management of cervical spinal fractures in ankylosing spondylitis with posterior fixation. *Spine* 2000; 25:2035–2039.

Bibliography

LD Anderson, RT D'Alonzo. Fractures of the odontoid process of the axis. *Bone Joint Surg* 1974; 56A:1663–1674.

HH Bohlman. Acute fractures and dislocations of the cervical spine. *J Bone Joint Surg* 1979; 61A:1119–1142.

HH Bohlman, JS Kirkpatrick, RB Delamarter, M Leventhal. Anterior decompression for late pain and paralysis after fractures of the thoracolumbar spine. *Clin Orthop* 1994; 24–29.

DP Chan, NK Seng, KT Kaan. Nonoperative treatment in burst fractures of the lumbar spine (L2–L5) without neurologic deficits. *Spine* 1993; 18:320–325.

JR Chapman, PA Anderson. Thoracolumbar spine fractures with neurologic deficit. *Orthop Clin North Am* 1994; 25:595–612.

JC Clohisy, BA Akbarnia, RD Bucholz, JK Burkus, RJ Backer. Neurologic recovery associated with anterior decompression of spine fractures at the thoracolumbar junction (T12–L1). *Spine* 1992; 17:5325–330.

LA Davis, SA Warren, DC Reid, K Oberle, LA Saboe, MG Grace. Incomplete neural deficits in thoracolumbar and lumbar spine fractures. Reliability of Frankel and Sunnybrook scales. *Spine* 1993; 18:257–263.

CA Dickman, MA Yahiro, HT Lu, MN Melkerson. Surgical treatment alternatives for fixation of unstable fractures of the thoracic and lumbar spine. A meta-analysis. *Spine* 1994; 19:22665–22735.

TA Duff. Management of cervical spine fractures. *Neurosurg* 1990; 73:478–479.

DK Ebelke, MA Asher, JR Neff, DP Kraker. Survivorship analysis of VSP spine instrumentation in the treatment of thoracolumbar and lumbar burst fractures. *Spine* 1991; 16:5428–5432.

FJ Eismont, MJ Arena, BA Green. Extrusion of an intravertebral disc associated with traumatic subluxation or dislocation of cervical beets. *J Bone Joint Surg* 1991; 73A:1555–1560.

TA Garvey, FJ Eismont, LJ Roberti. Anterior decompression, structural bone grafting, and Caspar plate stabilization for unstable cervical spine fractures and/or dislocations. *Spine* 1992; 17:5431–5435.

KI Ha, SH Han, M Chung, BK Yang, GH Youn. A clinical study of the natural remodeling of burst fractures of the lumbar spine. *Clin Orthop* 1996; 210–214.

JG Heller, FX Pedlow. Tumors of the spine, orthopaedic knowledge update. *Spine* 1997; 235–256.

RJ Huler, SI Esses, and DJ Botsford. Work status after posterior fixation of unstable but neurologically intact burst fractures of thoracolumbar spine. *Paraplegia* 1991; 29:600–606.

H Kinoshita, Y Nagata, H Ueda, K Kishi. Conservative treatment of burst fractures of the thoracolumbar and lumbar spine. *Paraplegia* 1993; 31:58–67.

GR Klein, AR Vaccaro, TJ Albert, M Schweitzer, D Deely, D Karasick, JM Coder. Efficacy of magnetic resonance imaging in the evaluation of posterior cervical spine fractures. *Spine* 1999; 24:771–774.

JM Lane, HA Sandhu. Osteoporosis of the spine. Orthopaedic Knowledge Update. *Spine* 1997; 227–234.

RW Lindsey, W Dick. The fixateur interne in the reduction and stabilization of thoracolumbar spine fractures in patients with neurologic deficit. *Spine* 1991; 16:5140–145.

RW Lindsey, W Dick, S Nunchuck, G Zach. Residual intersegmental spinal mobility following limited pedicle fixation of thoracolumbar spine fractures with the fixateur interne. *Spine* 1993; 18:474–478.

DC Mann, BW Bruner, JS Keene, AB Levin. Anterior plating of unstable cervical spine fractures. *Paraplegia* 1990; 28:564–572.

C Olerud, S Andersson, B Svensson, J Bring. Cervical spine fractures in the elderly: factors influencing survival in 65 cases. *Acta Orthop Scand* 1999; 70:509–513.

DR Ripa, MG Kowall, PR Myer, JJ Russin. Series of 92 Traumatic Cervical Spine Injuries Stabilized with Anterior ASIF Plate Fusion Technique. *Spine* 1991; 16 (Suppl): 46–55.

RC Sasso, HB Cotler, JD Reuben. Posterior fixation of thoracic and lumbar spine fractures using DC plates and pedicle screws. *Spine* 1991; 16:S134–139.

RC Sasso, HB Cotler. Posterior instrumentation and fusion for unstable fractures and fracture-dislocations of the thoracic and lumbar spine. A comparative study of three fixation devices in 70 patients. *Spine* 1993; 18:450–460.

E Sim, PM Stergar. The fixateur interne for stabilising fractures of the thoracolumbar and lumbar spine. *Int Orthop* 1992; 16:322–329.

AM Star, AA Jones, JM Cotler, RA Balderson, R Sinha. Immediate Closed Reduction of Cervical Spine dislocations using traction. *Spine* 1990; 15:1068–1072.

JS Torg, H Pavlov, SE Genuraio, B Sennett, RJ Wisniewski, BH Robi, C Jahre. Neuropraxia of the cervical spinal cord with transient quadraplegia. *J Bone Joint Surg* 1986; 68A:1354–1370.

JS Torg, SG Glasgow. Criteria for return to contact activities after cervical spine injury. *Athletic Injuries to the Head, Neck, and Face.* 2nd ed. New York: Mosby 1991: 589–608.

AR Vaccaro. Combined anterior and posterior surgery for fractures of the thoracolumbar spine. *Instr Course Lect* 1999; 48:443–449.

JN Weinstein. Differential diagnosis and surgical treatment of pathologic spine fractures. *Instr Course Lect* 1992; 41:301–315.

M Yazici, B Atilla, S Tepe, A Calisir. Spinal canal remodeling in burst fractures of the thoracolumbar spine: A computerized tomographic comparison between operative and nonoperative treatment. *Spinal Disord* 1996; 9:409–413.

14 Cervical Injuries: Indications and Options for Surgery

Jared Toman
Christopher M. Bono
Mitchel B. Harris

Despite advances in motor vehicle safety devices and accident prevention, fractures of the cervical spine still occur with substantial frequency, being present in 2%–6% of all trauma patients. Moreover, nearly half of all cervical spine fractures will involve concurrent injury to the spinal cord or nerve roots (11). Considering the potential consequences of these lesions, fractures of the cervical spine often require surgical intervention. However, the choice of procedure is contingent upon a number of factors (5–7, 19, 38, 47, 51).

The main objectives of surgery are neural decompression, spinal realignment, and stabilization. The optimal approach may be anterior, posterior, or a combination of the two. In some cases, external stabilization techniques such as cranial tongs or halo immobilization are useful preoperative adjuncts. Operative stabilization of the cervical spine can be effected by an array of instrumentation options that include wires, plates, and screws (19, 28, 47). These techniques have been applied in both anterior and posterior surgery.

Cervical spinal instrumentation is most commonly used to realign and stabilize two or more spinal segments with the ultimate long-term goal being solid bony fusion (5, 19). Less frequently, screws can be used to maintain reduction and potentiate healing of a single fractured vertebra. A common example is a compression screw used to treat an odontoid fracture; this facilitates healing of the fracture but is not a fusion procedure. Following a cervical fracture or dislocation, surgical stabilization via an appropriate surgical approach is often the crucial step in allowing the injured patient to be mobilized and begin rehabilitation (3).

PREOPERATIVE EVALUATION

Injury Mechanism

Cervical injury can occur from either blunt or penetrating trauma (1, 34). Penetrating trauma rarely produces mechanically unstable injuries (34). Therefore, this chapter will focus on those injuries resulting from blunt force. Blunt trauma can give rise to a variety of forces that can lead to bony or ligamentous failure.

Fractures and dislocations can be the product of abrupt flexion, extension, axial load, lateral bending, or combinations of these injury mechanisms (1). Theoretically, pure acceleration causes extension-type injuries, whereas pure deceleration leads to flexion-type injuries. Actual injury mechanisms are more complex. For example, extension force vectors are usually followed by recoiling hyperflexion of the head and neck. Abrupt rotation of the head on the body or vice versa can also be a primary mode of cervical injury.

Most commonly, the victim undergoes a sudden acceleration or deceleration force, which causes the head to be propelled in relation to the body. The body is the usual point of contact at which this sudden change in velocity occurs. For example, a seatbelt restrains the body during a head-on collision, causing the head to be thrust forward. It is therefore important to recognize that forces applied remotely to the head or neck, such as from movement of the chest, abdomen, or even appendicular skeleton, can be associated with cervical spine injury. Illustrating this point, as many as 3% of victims with blunt abdominal trauma have concurrent cervical cord injuries (59).

Less commonly, but not infrequently, the head or neck itself sustains a direct trauma. Examples include diving injuries or spear tackling in football, in which the force is delivered to the head. These often lead to axial loading injuries, though flexion and extension injuries can also occur (64).

Mechanism Influences Injury Type

Understanding the mechanism of injury can help determine the optimal treatment and aid in preoperative decision-making. Flexion injuries of the subaxial spine (below C2) can produce fractures of the vertebral body or dislocations and separations of the posterior elements. Which of these occurs is dependent on the location of the instantaneous axis of rotation

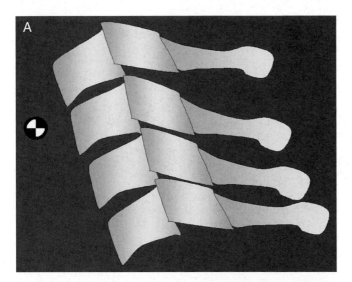

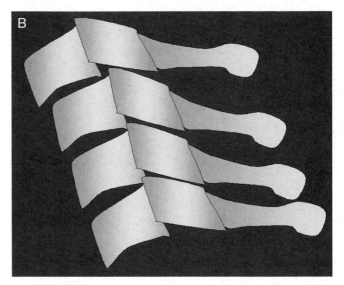

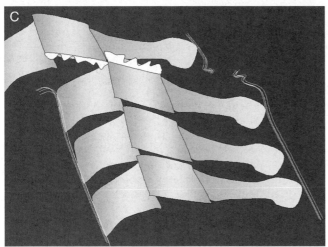

Figure 14.1 A flexion-distraction mechanism rotates around an axis anterior to the cervical spine causes tension failure within the anterior and posterior elements (**A**). Further energy leads to gross instability with facet subluxation (**B**) or frank dislocation of the articular surfaces (**C**). Severe cases are associated with circumferential ligamentous disruption.

It is important to appreciate that one mechanism of injury does not have an exclusive relationship with a single vertebral injury pattern. Rather, the failure of osseous or ligamentous structures in the cervical spine is the result of a complex and incompletely understood interplay between the temporal response of cervical elements to an applied force and the relative positions of those elements at the time of trauma (49). This has been demonstrated most eloquently by the work of Torg et al.

during the time of injury. For example, if the axis of rotation is anterior to the vertebral body, then the posterior ligaments, facet capsules, and discs will be subjected to distractive forces. This is the mechanism that produces bilateral facet dislocations (Figure 14.1A–C). If the spine acutely rotates around an axis within the facet joints, then the vertebral body will be compressed while the posterior ligaments are stretched. This is the mechanism thought to produce flexion-type teardrop fractures and compression fractures (Figure 14.2) (63). In many cases, these are associated with a disruption of the posterior spinal ligamentous complex, which may not be readily apparent on plain radiographs. Thus, further evaluation using magnetic resonance imaging (MRI) can reveal injury or frank disruption indicating a highly unstable lesion not readily appreciated by plain films alone (20).

Recognition of the mechanism of injury also plays a key role in the management of upper cervical injuries such as C2 traumatic spondylolistheses (or hangman's fractures). The majority of these fractures arise from an extension force and are reduced with axial traction (Figure 14.3) (38). In contrast with other patterns, the flexion-type fracture (IIa) (Figure 14.4) is exaggerated with cervical traction, necessitating axial compression for adequate reduction.

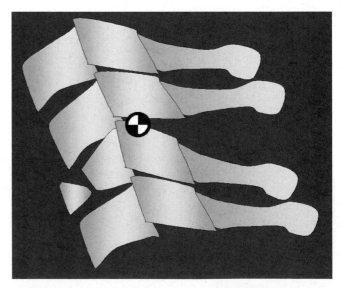

Figure 14.2 A flexion-compression mechanism rotates around an axis within or near the facet joints. This leads to distraction of the posterior elements and compression of the anterior elements (i.e., vertebral body). This often leads to the characteristic teardrop vertebral body fragment.

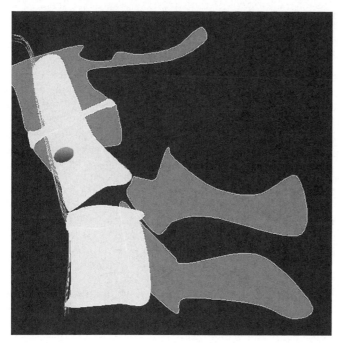

Figure 14.3 Understanding injury mechanism is also important with upper cervical injuries. A type II hangman's injury is caused by an extension force that leads to angulation and displacement that occurs around an intact ALL. This injury is reduced with longitudinal traction.

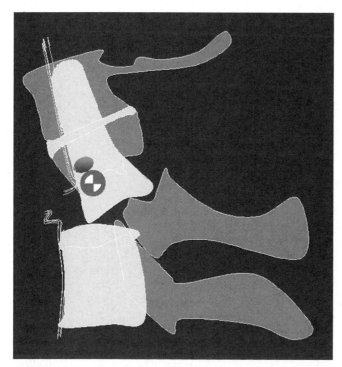

Figure 14.4 A type IIa hangman's injury is caused by a hyperflexion force that leads to angulation but minimal displacement. This injury is reduced by compression and can be made worse by traction.

(64), in that a single mechanism of documented axial load to the top of football players' helmets resulted in cervical burst fractures, flexion teardrop fractures, and facet dislocations.

Imaging

Selection of appropriate radiological studies is predicated on both clinical evaluation as well as predetermined imaging protocols. After a higher energy trauma, most trauma center protocols call for some method of cervical spine imaging. This can be a lateral cervical radiograph or a computerized tomogram (CT) with sagittal and coronal reformations. In recent years, the latter has become a first-line imaging modality in high-volume trauma centers, largely as a result of advances in high-speed image acquiescence using helical CT scanners. Despite this trend, high-quality plain radiographs remain an acceptable imaging modality for initial cervical evaluation. Practitioners should be aware of the 5%–20% chance of missing an injury with plain X-rays alone (24, 35, 38).

Plain radiographs can also be considered a component of the secondary general trauma survey, which is performed once the patient's airway and hemodynamic status have been stabilized. However, obtaining acceptable plain films can be difficult, especially in the setting of concomitant injuries that might preclude manipulation of the jaw or upper extremities. For this reason, helical CT has become a popular method of secondary radiographic evaluation of the spine. Once a cervical injury has been detected, plain films are important in preoperative planning and fracture follow-up, even in the presence of a CT scan (22). These should include an anteroposterior (AP) and a lateral view, at minimum. Open-mouth and swimmer's views are helpful in imaging the atlanto-axial and cervicothoracic junctions, respectively.

CT images of the cervical spine are more sensitive than plain films for detecting fractures (10, 14, 31, 57). They can demonstrate subtle, nondisplaced fractures as well as injuries in the occipitocervical and cervicothoracic junctions that can be difficult to detect with plain radiographs (33). Advances in sagittal and coronal reformations have made CT a useful method for assessing alignment; a drawback of using axial images alone is that they can miss dislocations or translational deformities in the transverse plane. CT is an excellent method of evaluating and quantifying the degree of canal compromise from bony encroachment and is superior to MRI in delineating fracture lines (12).

MRI is the modality of choice for evaluation of the spinal cord, nerve roots, discs, and ligaments. It can demonstrate soft tissue or bone edemas, which are more subtle signs of injury. Images of patients with spinal cord injury can show intra-parenchymal cord hemorrhage or edema (70). MRI has led to the extinction of the so-called spinal cord injury without radiographic abnormality (SCIWORA). For example, it readily demonstrates cord injury in patients with underlying cervical spondylosis with no obvious fracture or dislocation. MRI offers unique information regarding the integrity of the ligamentous structures, including the anterior longitudinal ligament (ALL), alar and transverse ligaments, and posterior ligamentous complex (PLC) (20, 63). MRI is considered mandatory by some surgeons to detect herniated discs prior to closed reduction of a facet dislocation (20, 22, 29). Magnetic resonance arteriography

(MRA) is an effective noninvasive means of evaluating the patency of the vertebral arteries, which are often traumatically injured with cervical injuries, particularly those that communicate with the foramen transversarium (23).

SPINAL STABILITY

Restoration of stability is a paramount objective of cervical spine surgical intervention. Determining whether a cervical injury is stable or unstable can sometimes be challenging and is subject to widely variable criteria and interpretations (45, 55).

The concept of stability can refer to both mechanical and neurological status. Mechanical stability refers to the relative motion of vertebral segments under the physiologic demands of usual activity. This has been defined as greater than normal motion at a spinal segment under physiologic stresses (77). Neurological stability denotes a state in which no further neural damage will be caused under the physiologic stresses that are imposed. For example, an unconscious, ventilator-dependent patient who has a well-aligned but mechanically unstable cervical fracture will be placing few demands on his spine. Thus, as long as he remains relatively immobile and on logroll precautions, he is at little risk for causing further fracture displacement or additional neurological injury. Neurological instability would only be realized if the patient were mobilized or seated upright, whereby the weight of his head would be borne through his "biomechanically unstable neck." As long-term recumbency is associated with numerous complications, surgical stabilization is usually recommended so that the patient can be safely mobilized. This would restore mechanical stability and maintain neurological stability. Stabilization of the spine facilitates nursing care and respiratory, physical, and occupational therapy for these patients.

Many systems to assess mechanical stability have been proposed. Denis et al. (13) introduced a three-column system, initially developed for the thoracolumbar spine. Effectively, the columns can be considered longitudinal members that span the length of the spine. The anterior column consists of the anterior longitudinal ligament (ALL), the anterior aspect of the intervertebral disc, and the anterior half of the vertebral body. Likewise, the middle column is made up of the posterior longitudinal ligament (PLL) and the respective posterior aspects of the disc and vertebral body. The posterior column refers to all remaining structures including the pedicles, laminae, transverse processes, facet joint, and PLC (which includes the ligamentum flavum, interspinous ligaments, and supraspinous ligaments). It is important to note that the junction of the middle and posterior columns forms the spinal canal. Normally, the spine rotates around an axis within the spinal canal, ensuring as little motion as possible in the region of the neural elements (27). Others have proposed two-column theories that considers Denis's anterior and middle column as one, while the components of the posterior column remain the same. In recent years, the latter system has become more popular.

A column can be compromised by a fracture or ligamentous disruption. By Denis's definition, disruption of two or more columns imparts instability (13). In the two-column theory of stability, PLC integrity (posterior column) is the key to mechanical spinal stability. Exceptions are gunshot wounds to the cervical spine that, because of the projectile-induced injury mechanism, can be stable even with fractures of all columns (34).

White and Panjabi proposed a scoring system to quantify stability of the cervical spine (77). One of the key features of this system is measurement of translation and angular deformity at the site of the injury. More than 3.5 mm of translation or 11 degrees of kyphosis compared to the uninjured level above or below is considered a criterion for mechanical instability. Despite its popularity, clinical studies have yet to confirm the validity of this system in predicting the need for operative stabilization. In practice, spinal stability is determined by collation of information gleaned from the history, physical examination, plain radiography, CT, and MRI on an individualized, case-by-case basis.

Ruling out a cervical spine injury in a patient with neck pain and negative imaging studies is a common situation. In the awake, neurologically intact, cooperative patient, dynamic flexion-extension lateral radiographs can reveal abnormal motion between vertebral segments. Flexion-extension lateral radiographs should be deferred for two to three weeks after injury. Pain and muscle spasm limit neck excursion and lead to false-negative studies (74).

SURGICAL TREATMENT OPTIONS

Goals of Surgery

The potential goals of surgery for cervical spine injuries are to correct traumatic deformities, restore mechanical stability, and decompress the neural elements. Not all injuries require all three goals to be addressed. For example, a transverse ligament disruption will lead to C1–C2 instability. In these cases, the surgical goal is to reduce the atlantodens interval and stabilize the segments. Although realignment can be considered indirect decompression, there is no formal removal of bone or soft tissue required. In contrast, a cervical burst fracture with fragment retropulsion in a patient with a spinal cord injury requires anterior corpectomy for decompression, strut grafting for fusion, and plate stabilization. These injuries can occur without significant kyphotic deformity. In a final example, a central cord injury in a spondylotic spine may require decompression, though no stabilization, fusion, or realignment is necessary, as these can occur without fracture or dislocation. These surgical goals can be met by a variety of methods, including skeletal traction, anterior surgery, and posterior surgery.

Surgical Timing

The optimal timing of surgery in patients with neurological deficits is unclear. Early practitioners believed that surgery should be delayed to allow the patient to be medically stabilized and the initial spinal cord swelling to resolve. In fact, they hypothesized that early surgery might be potentially detrimental (42). More recent studies have demonstrated that surgery performed as soon as 8 hours does not appear to increase the rate of complications or lead to neurologic decline (48, 75).

The two most commonly proposed benefits of earlier versus later surgery are improved rates of neurologic recovery and improved ability to mobilize the patient without concern of spinal displacement. Good evidence that early surgery for thoracic and lumbar fractures decreases medical complications, specifically respiratory failure, has only recently become available (44). Similar evidence in the cervical spine could not be found.

Animal studies have suggested a significant benefit to earlier decompression after acute spinal cord injury (17). However, there is little clinical evidence to support that early surgical decompression and stabilization improves neurologic recovery rates. In the only randomized, prospective, controlled trial found in the literature, surgery performed for cervical spinal cord injuries less than 72 hours versus more than 5 days from the injury demonstrated no significant difference in motor scores at final follow-up (67). Supportively, other nonrandomized prospective studies have demonstrated that surgery performed within 8 hours or within 24 hours from injury did not result in better neurologic outcomes (72). In one interesting report, performing surgery within 8 hours from the time of injury was feasible in only 10% of cases (48, 75).

Anterior Decompression and Stabilization

Anterior exposure of the spine can be achieved through a longitudinal or transverse incision. The incision is made at the approximate level of the injured segment(s). Palpable surface landmarks include the cricoid cartilage (C6), thyroid cartilage (C4–C5), the hyoid bone (C3), and the carotid tubercle (C6). Superficial dissection proceeds between the medial border of the sternocleidomastoid and the anterolateral aspect of the strap muscles. Deeper dissection is carried medial to the carotid sheath and lateral to the trachea and esophagus. The vertebral bodies and discs are finally exposed by sweeping away the alar and prevertebral fasciae. The longus colli muscles are elevated off of the lateral aspects of the vertebral bodies. Self-retaining retractors are placed underneath the medial borders of these muscles to maintain exposure (52, 65). Anatomical dangers are the recurrent laryngeal nerve, more variably located on the right side than the left, and the sympathetic chain, which is at risk with lateral dissection on top of the longus colli (18).

Anterior surgery of the cervical spine can be used to achieve all three surgical goals (2, 7, 63). It is considered ideal for subaxial fractures that involve the vertebral body, such as burst fractures and teardrop fractures (65). In such cases, the injured discs and fractured bones are removed in piecemeal fashion until the spinal canal is entered. This is called a corpectomy. The PLL, if intact, is a useful posterior limit to bone and disc removal. If this ligament is torn, greater care must be taken during this process. At all times, clear visualization of the neural elements must be maintained when working in the spinal canal, and exiting nerve roots should be inspected and decompressed over the involved segments.

Corpectomy leaves a void between the cranial and caudal end-plates of the uninjured segments. Traditionally, this is filled with a structural bone graft (2, 7). However, synthetic materials such as titanium mesh cages filled with a morcelized bone graft can also be used (Figure 14.5). The purpose of the graft or cage is twofold. First, it acts as a strut to maintain the height of the anterior column. For this reason, cortical bone must be used, as softer cancellous bone cannot sustain the large imposed forces and tends to subside over time. Most commonly, a tricortical autograft from the patient's anterior iliac crest is used, although an allograft can also be placed (56, 58, 66). The second purpose of the graft is to fuse the vertebrae across the injured segments to lend long-term stability. When using cages, this occurs in and around the cage.

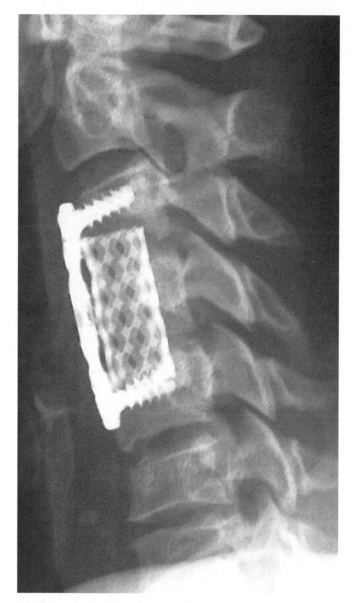

Figure 14.5 In lieu of autograft or allograft struts, titanium mesh cages can be filled with morcelized bone to reconstruct the anterior spine after corpectomy for a fracture.

A bone graft strut or cage lends some intrinsic stability with neck flexion. With neck extension, however, these compressive forces at the end-plates are diminished. Normally, the ALL acts as the check-rein to limit these distraction forces. This structure is obligatorily removed during anterior cervical surgery. Anterior cervical plates can help restore stability in extension. Plates should span the injured segments and are anchored into uninjured cranial and caudal vertebral bodies with bone screws. In some circumstances, anterior instrumentation can obviate the need for external postoperative orthoses, shorten the length of time they are worn postoperatively, or allow for less rigid immobilization (54).

An anterior approach can also be used to treat upper cervical injuries. Odontoid screws are placed under fluoroscopic visualization through an incision made at the C5–C6 level. The C1–C2 junction is rarely approached anteriorly (2, 52). The mandible and its associated structures are an obstruction to a traditional anterior approach. In rare cases, a transoral approach is indicated to access the odontoid process or the C1–C2 lateral mass joints (43). This is accomplished by incising the posterior pharyngeal mucosa at the approximate level of the hard palate. Stabilization procedures are difficult and dangerous to perform through this approach, but have been described. At present, this approach is best utilized for pure excisional procedures, as instrumentation or graft placement through the oral cavity carries a high risk of infection. If stability of the upper cervical spine is compromised, a posterior fusion and/or instrumentation is recommended (6).

Posterior Decompression and Stabilization

The posterior approach can be used to access the cervical spine from the occiput down to the cervicothoracic junction. Utilizing a midline incision, the paraspinal muscles are elevated off of the bony elements to expose the spinous processes, laminae, lateral masses, and facet joints. At C1, lateral dissection is limited by the vertebral artery, which lies between 1.5 and 2 cm from the midline. Dissection should not extend beyond the posterolateral aspects of the facet joints in the subaxial spine, as this can lead to inadvertent injury to the vertebral arteries.

Posterior cervical decompression involves laminectomy. This is less frequently indicated than anterior decompression for cervical trauma. Canal compromise with fractures and dislocations are usually the result of vertebral body fragment retropulsion and misalignment, respectively. The former is best addressed with anterior surgery; the latter is best addressed with reduction, which can be achieved by closed methods or by anterior or posterior open manipulation. Laminectomy is an ineffective means of decompressing the spinal canal with burst fractures. It removes a potentially intact posterior column, which can cause further instability. Laminectomy is rarely indicated to retrieve posterior bone or bullet fragments.

Posterior surgery for cervical fractures and dislocations is most useful for performing open reductions and stabilization procedures. Some facet dislocations are not reducible by closed means. Although open anterior reductions are possible, they are technically challenging. The posterior approach allows direct visualization and open reduction of the dislocated joints. It is considered a so-called bailout technique for failed attempts at anterior reduction. The spinous processes and laminae can be manipulated using lamina spreaders or towel clips. In particularly stubborn cases, a portion of the superior articular process of the caudal segment can be removed to facilitate reduction. A preoperative MRI to rule out a herniated disc fragment is indicated prior to open posterior reduction (20).

Stabilization and fusion are readily achieved through a posterior approach. Instrumentation methods have advanced significantly over the past decade. Lateral mass screw-rod fixation (Figure 14.6A–B) has largely replaced older and less stable methods of fixation such as interspinous wiring, facet wiring, and hook constructs in the subaxial spine. Posterior fusion provides long-term stability to the injured segments. It is effected by placing a morcelized bone graft over decorticated regions that should include the facet joints, lateral masses, and laminae. Sublaminar wiring is still considered a viable option for C1–C2 fixation. Newer techniques of C1 lateral mass and C1–C2 transarticular

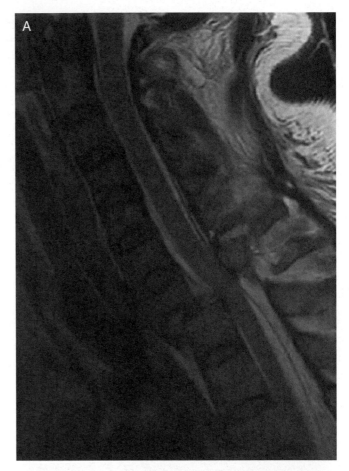

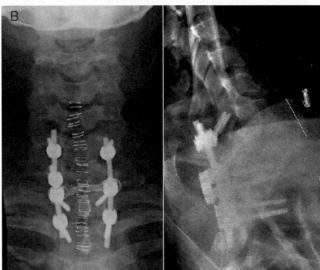

Figure 14.6 A sagittal T2-weighted MRI of a patient with a bilateral C7–T1 facet dislocation that was not reducible by closed methods (**A**). The MRI does not demonstrate a herniated disc fragment at the level of the dislocation. A posterior open reduction with lateral mass fixation at C6 and C7 (and pedicle screws in T1 and T2) was performed. Postoperative radiographs (**B**) show anatomical alignment.

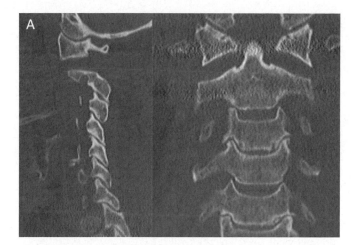

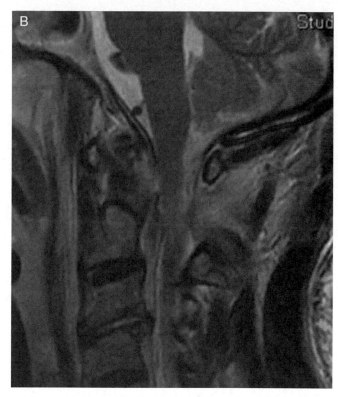

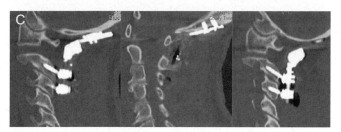

Figure 14.7 Sagittal and coronal CT reconstructions of a patient with an occipitocervical dissociation (**A**). In this case, gross ligamentous failure occurred through the C1–C2 junction, as seen in the MRI (**B**). The injury was stabilized using an occipital plate that was attached to C2 and C3 lateral mass screws (**C**).

screw fixation provide superior stability and fusion rates but are technically more demanding. The development of occipital screws and plates has revolutionized the treatment of occipito-cervical injuries (Figure 14.7A–C).

SPECIFIC INJURIES

Bony Anatomy

C1, also known as the atlas, is a bony ring that rotates around the dens, also known as the odontoid process of axis (or C2). It has broad inferior articular surfaces that allow rotation while providing stability. The atlas articulates with the occiput through its two superior articular surfaces. The posterior ligaments between C1 and C2 are sufficiently lax to allow a large range of motion. Conversely, the anterior ligaments, including the transverse and alar ligaments, are thicker, as they are the primary stabilizers of C1 on C2 and are located closer to the axis of rotation. The dens is a cephalad projection of the C2 body, though embryologically, it is derived from the centrum of C1. This leaves an arterial watershed area at the waist of the dens, predisposing it to nonunion after fracture. The transverse ligament extends from the posterior aspect of the dens to the posterior aspect of the anterior arch of C1. The alar ligaments span from the anterior tip of the dens to the anterolateral aspect of the foramen magnum. The axis intimates with C3 through inferior articular surfaces that are posteriorly offset. This offset places the intervening region (pars interarticularis) at particular risk for fracture with flexion, axial compression, or extension moments (i.e., hangman's fractures).

This change also marks the transition into the more uniform lower cervical spine morphology. Vertebrae in the subaxial spine (C3–C7) share similar anatomical arrangements as thoracic and lumbar regions that include intervertebral discs, vertebral bodies, pedicles, facet joints, laminae, and spinous processes. The vertebral body is connected to the posterior arch via two pedicles. At the pedicle–lamina junction, superior and inferior processes project to articulate with adjacent levels. The transverse processes in the cervical spine are distinct from those of the thoracic and lumbar spines. They cradle the exiting nerve root and have a foramen that transmits the vertebral artery as it passes superiorly.

Occipitocervical Injuries (C0–C1)

Occipitocervical injuries can vary widely. Most occipital condyle fractures can be treated by closed methods, either in hard collar or halo vest. The presence of an occipital condyle fracture should raise the practitioner's suspicion for more serious injuries, such as occipitocervical dissociations or dislocations. In the past, these injuries were thought to be inconsistent with survival. Advances in in-field life support, critical care, and injury recognition have seen an increasing number of survivors. Classification systems have been proposed that distinguish injuries based on the direction of displacement. However, these injuries should be considered highly unstable lesions that require operative stabilization. Current methods of rigid internal fixation of the occipitocervical junction using plates, screws, and rods have largely obviated the need for postoperative halo vest immobilization.

Atlas (C1) Injuries

The majority of injuries to the atlas can be treated nonsurgically with either halo vest or cervical collar (32, 73). With a spacious spinal canal, cord injury is generally less likely to involve the C1–C2 region than with subaxial trauma. Injuries can be divided into two groups: posterior ring fractures and lateral mass fractures. Moreover, the stability of these lesions depends in large part on the competence of the transverse ligament, and thus an MRI is a critical imaging study in the preoperative period (26).

Posterior Ring Fractures

Most posterior ring fractures of the atlas are stable and heal well with a hard collar or halo vest. The mechanism of injury is usually axial load with hyperextension and results in a burst-type pattern of fracture. Importantly, however, these fractures are associated with concomitant cervical spinal injuries in 50% of cases (38). The most frequently encountered associated lesion is a type II dens fracture, which may be displaced or nondisplaced. In this situation, the dens fracture should be stabilized. It is the authors' preference to place an odontoid screw to stabilize the fracture (30). This can preserve motion of the atlanto-axial joint, and it obviates a larger posterior fusion procedure. With the odontoid fixed, a halo vest or hard collar can be used postoperatively to protect the fixation in light of a disrupted posterior ring.

C1 Bursting (Jefferson) Fractures

The term lateral mass refers to the articular complex of the atlas and its supporting structures. Unique among other vertebrae in its anatomy, the superior and inferior joint surfaces are paired bilaterally and situated directly on top of one another. In addition to transmitting all applied axial loads, the columns between these articulations act as the junctions between the anterior and posterior rings. Thus, the mechanism of injury is usually axial load with varying degrees of flexion or extension. Given the resultant forces experienced by these osseous columns, fractures can develop anterior to, across, or posterior to the articular surfaces (4).

Fracture of the lateral mass can be unilateral or bilateral, and both types can be stable or unstable with varying degrees of ligamentous damage. Bilateral fractures of the anterior and posterior arches are colloquially referred to as Jefferson fractures (36). Distinct to injury at this level, stability is assessed by the amount of lateral displacement. On an open-mouth anteropos-

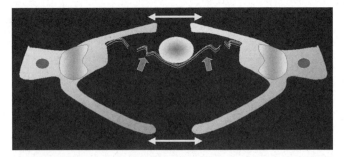

Figure 14.9 Biomechanical studies have shown that C1 bursting (Jefferson) fractures can lead to transverse ligament disruption as the two halves of the ring displace laterally.

terior radiograph, this can be measured as the bilateral total millimeters of lateral overhang of the C1 lateral mass on the C2 lateral mass (Figure 14.8). More than 7 to 10 mm of combined displacement implies disruption of the transverse ligaments and instability (Figure 14.9) (38, 61); however, the ligament can also be assessed directly with MRI (15). Stable lateral mass fractures can be treated in a hard cervical orthosis (73). Unstable fractures are reduced with an initial period of traction followed by halo vest immobilization. Because the transverse ligament will likely not heal, flexion-extension views should be obtained after radiographic bony union; this will unmask a subluxation of C1 on C2. If atlanto-axial instability is present, or if the transverse ligament is found to be disrupted on MRI, then posterior C1–C2 fusion is indicated.

C1–C2 Injuries

C1–C2 Instability (Transverse/Alar Ligament Disruption)

C1–C2 instability can occur. It is detected by widening of the atlanto-dens interval (ADI) (Figure 14.10). The ADI in adults is

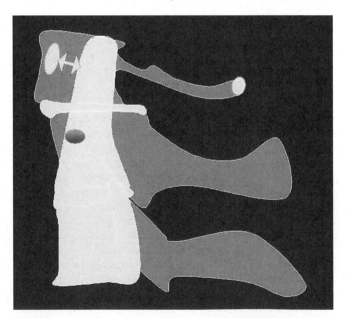

Figure 14.10 The atlantodens interval (ADI, **double arrow**) is widened if sagittal C1–C2 instability is present. Normally, this distance should measure less than 2–3 mm in adults.

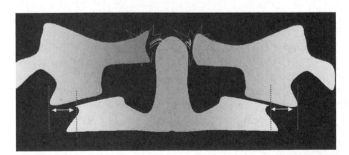

Figure 14.8 The lateral mass C1–C2 overhang can be measured. If the combined distance is greater than 7–8 mm, then transverse ligament disruption is strongly suspected.

normally less than 3 mm (77), whereas in children, it can be up to 4 mm. Disruption of the transverse ligament alone results in an ADI of no greater than 5 mm. Only with further injury to the alar ligaments can greater degrees of instability occur. Careful flexion-extension radiographs can demonstrate occult instability in an awake, neurologically intact patient. If frank widening is noted on a static lateral film, CT, or MRI, then flexion-extension radiographs are not indicated. High-quality MR images obtained with powerful magnets can detect anatomical discontinuity of the ligaments. Flexion-extension radiographs should also be obtained after C1 ring or dens fractures have healed to detect occult transverse ligament injury. Treatment of C1–C2 instability is usually surgical (73). Posterior C1–C2 fusion and stabilization is preferred (38). There are various methods of stabilization available. Historically, sublaminar wires using a so-called Gallie or Brooks method have been advocated. More rigid methods include placing screws into the C1 lateral mass and using C2 pedicle screws, or inserting screws that cross the C1–C2 lateral mass joints (transarticular or Magerl's screws [16]).

C1–C2 Rotatory Subluxation

Rotatory subluxation occurs most commonly in children. It is often the sequela of nontraumatic processes such as retropharyngeal infection (i.e., Grisel's syndrome). Less commonly, it occurs after trauma from abrupt rotational forces. Presentation can include a so-called cock-robin posture of the neck, in which the head is rotated away and tilted toward the side of the injury. Dynamic CT scans that compare axial images of the head rotated to the left and to the right are diagnostic. If identified early, gentle traction leads to a complete reduction in most cases, after which the patient can be successfully treated in collar or halo vest. Stable unreducible lesions may also be treated nonoperatively; they do not produce functional limitation. Unstable injuries are open-reduced, stabilized, and fused using a posterior approach (38, 46).

Axis (C2) Injuries

Odontoid (Dens) Fracture

Odontoid fractures tend to occur from flexion or extension mechanisms. Though it is not a hard-and-fast rule, flexion injuries are more common in younger people, whereas extension injuries are more common in older people. Spinal cord injuries are uncommon because of the capacious spinal canal in this region. Odontoid injuries can be classified according to anatomic location. Type I fractures arise at the tip or apex of the process and most probably represent a bony avulsion of the apical ligament (Figure 14.11). They can herald more significant injuries, such as occipitocervical dissociations, though alone, type I fractures are adequately treated in a soft collar (26).

Type II fractures are the most problematic (Figure 14.12). The aforementioned watershed area of blood supply compromises bone healing. Identified risk factors for nonunion include advanced age (older than 55 to 65 years old), more than 4 to 5 mm of displacement, and angulation of more than 10 or 11 degrees (38). Suspected risk factors are smoking and diabetes. Closed reduction can be achieved with traction and varying degrees of neck flexion or extension depending on the deformity. In younger

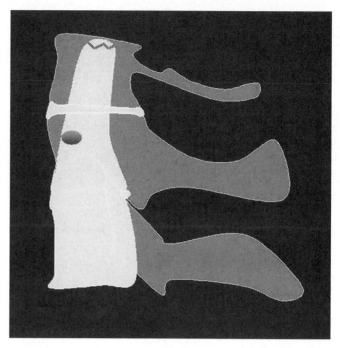

Figure 14.11 Type I odontoid fractures are avulsion injuries from the tip of the process. By themselves, they are stable, but they can be a sign of more significant injury, such as an occipitocervical dissociation.

patients, halo fixation or surgical stabilization is recommended. Surgery can include a posterior C1–C2 fusion. Alternatively, an anteriorly placed odontoid lag screw can result in restoration of stability and can promote fracture healing without fusion. In older patients, the optimal treatment is less clear. Recent authors have documented a high complication and mortality rate with halo use in the elderly. In contrast, osteoporosis and medical comorbidities can make surgery risky in this population. A growing number of surgeons have therefore opted to treat even markedly displaced Type II and III fractures in elderly patients with hard collar alone, provided there is no neurologic deficit. Fibrous unions with little residual instability often result in no clinical manifestations.

In the original description, Type III fractures occur through the C2 vertebral body (2). A more recent study found that interobserver agreement is improved if type III injuries are

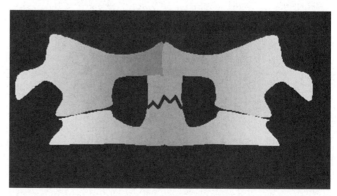

Figure 14.12 Type II odontoid fractures occur through the watershed region at the waist of the process.

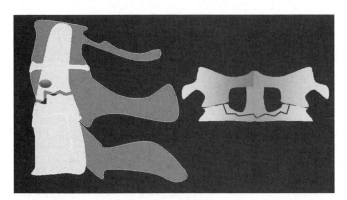

Figure 14.13 Type II fractures occur through the C2 vertebral body (left). A more contemporary definition notes that the fracture line must extend into the C1–C2 lateral mass joint (right).

defined as those in which the fracture line extends into the C2 superior articular surfaces (Figure 14.13) (25). Blood supply is rich in the primarily cancellous bone of the C2 body. Thus, healing is much more reliable than with type II fractures. Nondisplaced fractures can be treated in a hard cervical collar. Displaced fractures should be reduced and treated in a halo. Surgery can also be performed. If operative management is undertaken, posterior C1–C2 stabilization and fusion is preferred over odontoid screw fixation (41).

Traumatic Spondylolisthesis (Hangman's Fractures)

Traumatic spondylolisthesis of C2 is a bit of a misnomer. Although it is an appropriate term for type III injuries, less severe lesions are perhaps better termed pars interarticularis fractures. The fracture

typically occurs in the region between the more anterior cranial articular process and the posterior situated caudal articular surface. Type I injuries are fractures with less than 3 mm of displacement. They are typically stable and can be treated in a hard collar until fracture union. Type Ia variants have a fracture line that extends into the posterior C2 body (Figure 14.14). In contrast to most other types of hangman's fractures, they are not canal expanding fractures. Thus, they are associated with a higher rate of neurological deficit and should be distinguished from type I or II fractures. Type II injuries exhibit displacement and angulation. They radiographically appear as if the proximal C2 fragment has tilted anteriorly around an axis about the C2–C3 disc. Reduction is readily achieved with halo traction and slight hyperextension. Definitive treatment includes halo vest application for 8 to 12 weeks. Predictors of successful halo treatment include less than 11 degrees of initial angulation and/or less than 6 mm of displacement (71). Type IIa fractures exhibit angulation but no or minimal translation. They are flexion-type injuries that worsen with traction (37, 62). Reduction is achieved by compression and extension in a halo vest. The hallmark of Type III fractures is dislocation of one or both C2–C3 facet joints (Figure 14.15). They exhibit the highest rate of neurologic injury and mechanical instability among hangman's fractures. In most cases, treatment is open reduction, stabilization, and posterior fusion of C2–C3 (37). An interfragmentary compression screw placed into the C2 pars interarticularis is another option.

Subaxial Spine (C3–C7)

With a comparatively smaller spinal canal and a propensity for larger displacements, subaxial cervical spine fractures and

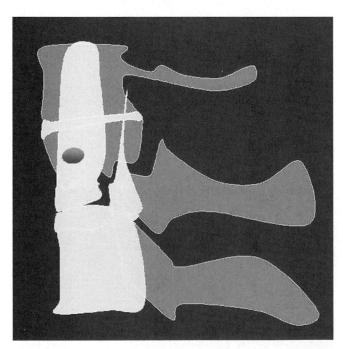

Figure 14.14 The pars fragment is attached to a shell of the posterior vertebral body with a type Ia hangman's fracture. They are associated with a higher rate of neurologic injury than standard type I fractures.

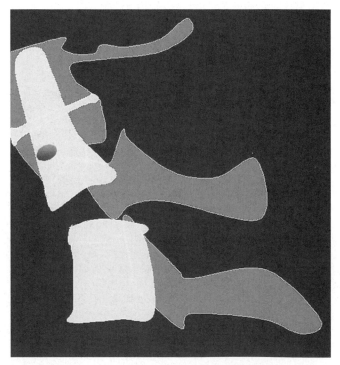

Figure 14.15 Type III hangman's fractures, by definition, exhibit dislocation of the C2–C3 facet joint. They are highly unstable and require surgical stabilization.

dislocations are associated with a higher rate of neurologic injury than upper cervical trauma (2, 7, 63). As such, they often benefit from decompression and stabilization procedures.

Lateral Mass (Facet/Pedicle Fractures) without Dislocation

Lateral mass fracture is a nonspecific category that has been used to refer to a variety of injuries that include facet fractures, pedicle fractures, lateral lamina fractures, and the so-called floating lateral mass (pedicle and lamina fracture at the same level). The common link is that they are thought to occur from a rotational injury mechanism. Facet fractures, which are more accurately described as articular process fractures, are the most common (Figure 14.16). Treatment is somewhat controversial. Some surgeons aggressively treat all injuries with surgical stabilization. This decision is based on the unpredictable fracture personality. Some unilateral, nondisplaced, seemingly stable fractures can allow progressive subluxation, whereas others with similar fracture patterns heal with anatomical alignment. With the availability of MRI, the importance of disc integrity and the ALL have been highlighted as predictors of stability (Figure 14.17) (39). More recently, the size of the fracture fragment has been suggested as a predictor of late displacement (9, 60). In the authors' practice, non- or minimally displaced fractures are initially treated in a hard collar. An MRI is obtained to examine the ALL and intervertebral disc. If these are injured, then surgical treatment is considered. Anterior discectomy and fusion has resulted in better postoperative alignment than posterior surgery (39).

Facet Dislocations and Subluxations

Dislocation of a facet joint implies that the articular surfaces of the joint are no longer apposed. Subluxation refers to a situation in which joint has slipped but some portion of the articular surfaces are still apposed. Pathoanatomically, the inferior articular process of the cranial vertebra (which normally lies posterior to the superior articular process of the caudal vertebra) is pulled over the superior articular process of the caudal segment

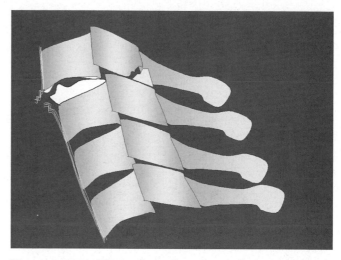

Figure 14.17 Figure of a unilateral articular process (facet fracture) with low-grade anterolisthesis. Note that the disc and ALL are disrupted.

(Figure 14.18) (55, 63). Injuries can be unilateral or bilateral. Bilateral dislocations are associated with higher energy mechanisms, higher rates of spinal cord injury, and massive posterior ligamentous disruption (70). The injury mechanism is flexion-distraction about an axis of rotation that lies anterior to the spine. This leads to tension failure of the posterior ligaments, the facet capsules, and the intervertebral disc. Usually, the only ligament structure that remains intact is the ALL. Of note, variations of this mechanism are responsible for the majority of injuries to the subaxial spine. Treatment of bilateral facet dislocations is reduction and operative stabilization/fusion. The role of prereduction MRI is controversial. Controversy is centered around the risk of neurologic decline from reducing a dislocation with a herniated disc. Studies have shown that closed reduction with cranial tong traction in an awake, cooperative, and examinable patient is safe in that it is not associated with worsening neurologic injury in patients with herniated disc fragments (68, 69). Some surgeons feel that a prereduction MRI is compulsory, and they recommend

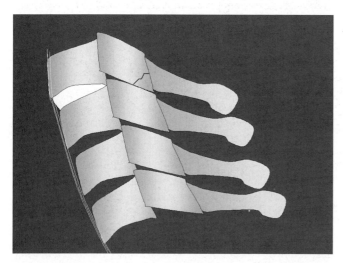

Figure 14.16 Figure of a nondisplaced unilateral articular process (facet) fracture. Note that the disc and ALL are intact.

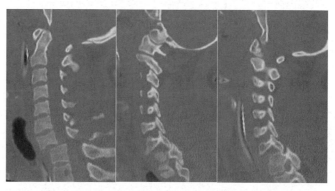

Figure 14.18 Left paramedian (left), sagittal (center), and right paramedian (right) CT images showing the orientation of a dislocated facet joint. The inferior articular process of the cranial (dislocated) segment is located anterior to the superior articular process of the caudal segment. Bilateral facet dislocation is shown; this usually results in greater than or equal to 50% anterior translation.

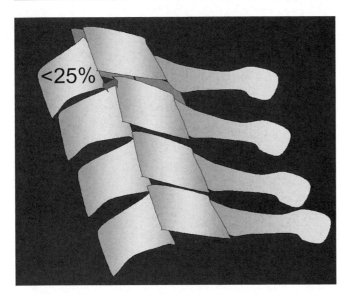

Figure 14.19 Diagram of a unilateral facet dislocation. This usually does not result in more than 25% anterior translation.

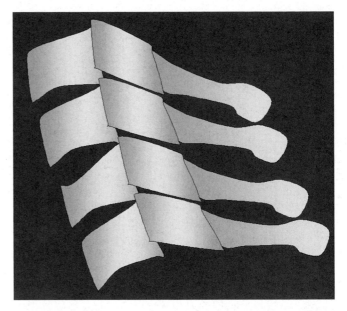

Figure 14.20 Diagram of a simple compression fracture. Fractures with minimal height loss, little or no kyphosis, and no translation usually have an intact PLC; these are considered stable injuries.

open anterior removal of the disc fragment before reduction of the dislocation. Provided that there are no herniated disc fragments after reduction as detected by a postreduction MRI, an anterior or posterior approach can be used to treat the injury. Anterior surgery can consist of discectomy, fusion, and plating. Posterior surgery includes lateral mass fixation of the injured levels.

Unilateral facet dislocations can occur with less ligamentous disruption than bilateral dislocations (Figure 14.19). As such, they are more difficult to reduce by closed methods. Most advocate operative treatment of these injuries, with similar options as described above for bilateral dislocations. Some unilateral facet dislocations are mechanically stable and can be treated nonoperatively. However, persistent unilateral dislocation can limit motion, can cause chronic pain, and may lead to radiculopathy (63). For these reasons, nonoperative management is not the current authors' preference. Similar controversy exists concerning the role of prereduction MRI. In the current authors' algorithm, anterior discectomy and fusion with plating is performed if a closed reduction can be achieved. If the injury is not reducible by closed methods and there is no disc fragment, then posterior surgery is preferred.

Compression Fractures

Compression fractures of the subaxial cervical spine are usually stable injuries (Figure 14.20). They represent the early stages of a more severe injury called a teardrop fracture that occurs from a flexion-compression mechanism (discussed below). PLC disruption is rare. PLC injury should be suspected if there is marked kyphosis (greater than 11 degrees). An MRI is invaluable in evaluating the posterior ligaments in equivocal cases. Stable injuries are treated in a hard collar for 3 months.

Teardrop Fractures

Teardrop fractures result from a flexion-compression mechanism. Hyperflexion occurs about an axis of rotation located near

or at the facet joints. Compression of the vertebral body results in shearing of the anteroinferior aspect of the bone to create the characteristic triangular-shaped fragment. Further injury can result in retrolisthesis (posterior subluxation) of the fractured vertebra on the level below. This feature leads to canal compromise. A sagittal fracture line is often seen, which leads to misclassification of these injuries as burst fractures. Retrolisthesis implies that the facet capsules have failed and that the injury is likely to be unstable. Spinal cord injuries are not uncommon. Treatment can include a halo vest, anterior surgery, or posterior fixation. One study demonstrated equivalent clinical and neurologic outcomes between halo vest and anterior surgery; however, radiographic results (i.e., correction of kyphosis) were superior with anterior surgery (21). Anterior surgery usually consists of corpectomy of the fractured bone followed by strut grafting and anterior plate fixation. Posterior surgery is less popular and is usually reserved for neurologically intact patients with injuries that are well reduced in traction prior to surgery (8).

Burst Fractures

Abrupt axial loading of the cervical spine column can lead to burst fractures. By definition, these are comminuted vertebral body fractures that involve the posterior vertebral body (Figure 14.21). Fragment retropulsion into the spinal canal is common, which leads to a high rate of spinal cord injury. PLC injury may or may not be present. Strong indicators of PLC injury are marked kyphosis at the fracture site (Figure 14.22). Cranial tong traction can be used to restore alignment. In addition, ligamentotaxis can partially reduce the retropulsed fragments to effect some indirect canal decompression. Operative treatment is almost always recommended. This usually includes anterior corpectomy to decompress the canal, strut grafting, and plate fixation. The integrity of the PLC can influence a surgeon's decision to plan additional posterior stabilization surgery.

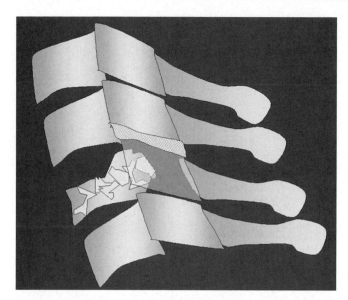

Figure 14.21 Cervical burst fractures have comminuted body fractures that often have fragments protruding into the spinal canal.

Nonoperative care is reserved for rare cases in which a burst fracture shows minimal retropulsion, normal alignment, no signs of PLC injury, and no neurologic deficit.

Miscellaneous Fractures

There is a wide array of cervical spine fractures that garner little attention in the literature. They are usually stable fractures that do not require surgery. Transverse process fractures do not compromise mechanical stability of the spine. They can, however, be associated with vertebral artery injuries. Many centers require MR arteriography of the neck if a transverse process fracture or one that communicates with the foramen transversarium has been detected. Isolated spinous process fractures are inherently stable and typically can be managed with a hard collar. Spinous

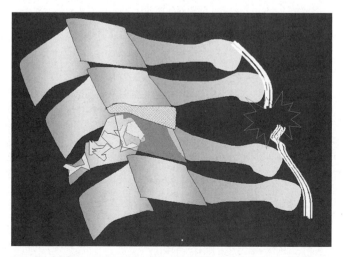

Figure 14.22 Diagram of an unstable cervical burst fracture. PLC disruption is strongly suggested by marked kyphosis at the injured segment.

process fractures are often associated with other more significant injuries such as facet dislocations or teardrop fractures. By themselves, transverse process and spinous process fractures can be treated in a hard collar for 6 weeks.

POSTOPERATIVE CARE

Postoperative care is influenced by the surgical procedure, concomitant injuries, and surgeon preference. Wound care includes daily dressing changes until the incision is dry. With stable fixation, patients can be mobilized as needed. Prophylactic antibiotics are continued for 48 hours after surgery. Deep vein thrombosis (DVT) prophylaxis can include lower extremity sequential compression devices and thromboembolic stockings for the first 72 to 96 hours after surgery. Chemical DVT prophylaxis can be started after 96 hours. A hard collar is kept in place. However, diligent skin care is required to avoid pressure breakdown along the occiput or upper back. Although there are no concrete guidelines with regard to early orthosis removal, most surgeons maintain the collar in place for 3 months following surgery. The type and extent of the instrumentation procedure may also alter the degree to which collar wear is found necessary. Plain radiographs are obtained at regular intervals (2 weeks, 1 month, 3 months, 6 months, 1 year) until solid union is seen.

COMPLICATIONS

Surgical management in trauma patients is frequently challenged by concomitant conditions such as open wounds, burns, head injury, sepsis, and cardiopulmonary compromise. Long stays in the intensive care unit, prolonged periods of immobilization, and nutritional depletion can increase the chances for a variety of complications (40). Patients with cervical spinal cord injury have difficulty with pulmonary toilet, increasing the chance for pneumonia and other respiratory complications.

Postoperative complications can vary widely. Wound infection is reportedly more frequent after urgent/emergent surgery for spine thoracic and lumbar spine fractures than elective spine surgery for degenerative disorders (40, 53). Although a similar study has not examined cervical fractures, a similar trend might be expected. In general, anterior cervical procedures have a lower incidence of wound infections than do posterior approaches (7, 54). Definitive treatment of wound infections usually involves open surgical debridement, intraoperative cultures, and appropriate antibiosis. Instrumentation is generally left in place (76). One study found the presence of a tracheostomy did not increase the rate of postoperative infection following anterior cervical surgery (50).

Postoperative airway complications can occur in the immediate postoperative period. These are more common with anterior procedures. Risk factors include multilevel surgery, upper cervical approach, and longer operative duration. Approach-related nerve injuries include recurrent laryngeal nerve palsy, superior laryngeal nerve palsy, Horner's syndrome from sympathetic plexus injury, and (rarely) hypoglossal nerve palsy. Iatrogenic neurologic injury can be caused by implant misplacement, intraoperative displacement, or hypoxemia. Importantly, one must recognize that up to 6% of patients with spinal cord injuries will have neurologic progression from the injury itself, which can be difficult to discern from an insult caused by surgery. Immediate postoperative imaging studies should be obtained to check spinal alignment and hardware placement.

SUMMARY

The goals of surgical treatment of cervical fractures and dislocations are to restore mechanical stability, relieve pressure on the neural elements, and prevent late deformity. Each of these goals has distinct indications and can be met by various operative techniques. Operative plans represent a coalescence of many considerations tailored to the individual patient, injury, and clinical scenario.

References

1. Allen B, Ferguson R, Lehmann T, et al. A mechanistic classification of closed, indirect fractures and dislocations of the lower cervical spine. *Spine* 1982; 7:1982.
2. Anderson P, Bohlman H. Anterior decompression and arthrodesis of the cervical spine: long-term motor improvement. *J Bone Joint Surg* 1992; 74A:683–692.
3. Anderson P, Bryniarski M, McMahom J. Posterior stabilization of sub-axial cervical spine trauma: indications and techniques. *Injury* 2005; 36(S):B36–43.
4. Anonymous. Management of combination fractures of the atlas and axis in adults. *Neurosurgery* 2002; 50:140–147.
5. Apfelbaum R. The use of anterior caspar plate fixation in acute cervical spine injury. *Surg Neurol* 1992; 38:162–163.
6. Bohler J. Anterior stabilization for acute fractures and non-unions of the dens. *J Bone Joint Surg* 1982; 64A:18–26.
7. Bohlman H, Anderson P. Anterior decompression and arthrodesis of the cervical spine: long-term motor improvement. Part I: Improvement in incomplete traumatic quadriparesis. *J Bone Joint Surg* 1992; 74A: 671–682.
8. Bono C. Opinion: posterior fixation. *J Orthop Trauma* 2004; 18:641–642.
9. Bono C, Vaccaro A, Fehlings M, et al. Measurement techniques for lower cervical spine injuries: consensus statement of the Spine Trauma Study Group. *Spine* 2006; 31:603–609.
10. Brown C, Antevil J, Sise M, et al. Spiral computed tomography for the diagnosis of cervical, thoracic, and lumbar spine fractures: its time has come. *Journal of Trauma-Injury Infection & Critical Care* 2005; 58:890–896.
11. Burney R, Maio R, Maynard F. Incidence, characteristics and outcome of spinal cord injury at trauma centers in North America. *Arch Surg* 1993; 128:596–599.
12. Carter J, Mirza S, Tencer A. Canal geometry changes associated with axial compressive cervical spine fractures. *Spine* 2000; 2000:1.
13. Cybulski G, Douglas R, Meyer P, et al. Complications in three-column cervical spine injuries requiring anterior-posterior stabilization. *Spine* 1992; 17:253–256.
14. Diaz J, Gillman C, Morris J. Are five-view plain films of the cervical spine unreliable? A prospective evaluation in blunt trauma patients with altered mental status. *J Trauma* 2003; 55:658–663.
15. Dickman C, Sonntag V. Injuries involving the transverse atlantal ligament: classification and treatment guidelines based upon experience with 39 injuries. *Neurosurgery* 1997; 40:886–887.
16. Dickman C, Sonntag V. Posterior C1–C2 transarticular screw fixation for atlantoaxial arthrodesis. *Neurosurgery* 1998; 43:275–280.
17. Dimar J, Glassman S, Raque G. The influence of spinal canal narrowing and timing of decompression on neurologic recovery. *Spine* 1999; 24:1623–1623.
18. Ebraheim N, Lu J, Yang H. Vulnerability of the sympathetic trunk during the anterior approach to the lower cervical spine. *Spine* 2000; 13.
19. Ebraheim N, Rupp R, Savolaine E, et al. Posterior plating of the cervical spine. *J Spinal Disord* 1995; 8:111–115.
20. Eismont F, Arena M, Green B. Extrusion of an intervertebral disc associated with traumatic subluxation or dislocation of cervical facets: case report. *J Bone Joint Surg* 1991; 73A:1555–1560.
21. Fisher C, Dvorak M, Leith J, et al. Comparison of outcomes for unstable lower cervical flexion teardrop fractures managed with halo thoracic vest versus anterior corpectomy and plating. *Spine* 2002; 27:160–166.
22. France J, Bono C, Vaccaro A. Initial radiographic evaluation of the spine after trauma: when, what, where, and how to image the acutely traumatized spine. *J Orthop Trauma* 2005; 19:640–649.
23. Friedman D, Flanders A, Thomas C. Vertebral artery injury after acute cervical spine trauma: rate of occurrence as detected by MR angiography and assessment of clinical consequences. *Am J Roent* 1995; 164:443–447.
24. Goldberg W, Mueller C, Mower W. Distribution and patterns of blunt traumatic injury to the cervical spine. *Ann Emerg Med* 2001; 38:17–21.
25. Grauer J, Shafi B, Hilibrand A, et al. Proposal of a modified, treatment-oriented classification of odontoid fractures. *Spine* 2005; 5:123–129.
26. Greene K, Dickman C, Marciano F. Acute axis fracture: analysis of management and outcome in 340 consecutive cases. *Spine* 1997; 22: 1843–1854.
27. Haher T, O'Brien M, Felmly W, et al. Instantaneous axis of rotation as a function of the three columns of the spine. *Spine* 1992; 17:149–154.
28. Hamilton A, Webb J. The role of anterior surgery for vertebral fractures with and without cord compression. *Clin Orthop* 1994; 300:79–89.
29. Hart R, Vaccaro A, Nachwalter R. Cervical facet dislocation: when is magnetic resonance imaging indicated? *Spine* 2002; 27:116–118.
30. Henry A, Bohly J, Grosse A. Fixation of odontoid fractures by an anterior screw. *J Bone Joint Surg* 1999; 81B:472–477.
31. Katz M, Beredjiklian P, Vresilovic E, et al. Computed tomographic scanning of cervical spine fractures: does it influence treatment? *J Orthop Trauma* 1999; 13:338–343.
32. Kontautas E, Ambrozaitis K, Kalesinskas R, et al. Management of acute traumatic atlas fractures. *Eur Spine J* 2005; 18:402–405.
33. Korres D, Papageloupoulos P, Mavrogenis A, et al. Multiple fractures of the axis. *Orthopedics* 2004; 27:1096–1099.
34. Kupcha P, An H, Cotler J. Gunshot wounds to the cervical spine. *Spine* 1990; 15:1058–1063.
35. Kwon B, Vaccaro A, Grauer J, et al. Subaxial cervical spine trauma. *J Am Acad Orthop Surg* 2006; 14:78–89.
36. Lee T, Green B, Petrin D. Treatment of stable burst fracture of the atlas (Jefferson fracture) with rigid cervical collar. *Spine* 1998; 23:1963–1967.
37. Levine A, Edwards C. The management of traumatic spondylolisthesis of the axis. *J Bone Joint Surg Am* 1985; 3:217–226.
38. Levine A, Edwards C. Treatment of injuries in the C1–C2 complex. *Orthop Clin North Am* 1986; 17:31–44.
39. Lifeso R, Colucci M. Anterior fusion for rotationally unstable cervical spine fractures. *Spine* 2000; 25:2028–2034.
40. Lim M, Lee J, Vaccaro A. Surgical infections in the traumatized spine. *Clin Orthop Relat Res* 2006; 444:114–119.
41. Maak T, Grauer J. The contemporary treatment of odontoid injuries. *Spine* 2006; 31:S53–60.
42. Marshall L, Knowlton S, Garfin S. Deterioration following spinal cord injury. *J Neurosurg* 1987; 66:400–404.
43. McAfee P, Bohlman H, Riley L. The anterior retropharyngeal approach to the upper part of the cervical spine. *J Bone Joint Surg Am* 1987; 69:1371–1383.
44. McHenry T, Mirza S, Wang J, et al. Risk factors for respiratory failure following operative stabilization of thoracic and lumbar spine fractures. *J Bone Joint Surg Am* 2006; 88:997–1006.
45. Mirza S, Bellabarba C, Chapman J. Principles of Spine Trauma Care. In: Bucholz R, Beckman J, Court-Brown C, eds. *Principles of Spine Trauma Care*. 6th ed. New York: Lippincott, Williams, and Wilkins, 2006: 1403–1433.
46. Mummaneni P, Haid R. Atlantoaxial fixation: overview of all techniques. *Neurol India* 2005; 53:408–415.
47. Murphy M, Daniaux H, Southwick W. Posterior cervical fusion with rigid internal fixation. *Orthop Clin North Am* 1986; 17:55–65.
48. Ng W, Fehlings M, Cuddy B. Surgical treatment of acute spinal cord injury pilot study #2: evaluation of protocol for decompressive surgery within 8 hours after injury. *Neurosurg Focus* 1999; 6:3.
49. Nightingale R, McElhaney J, Richardson W. Experimental impact injury to the cervical spine: relating motion of the head to mechanism of injury. *J Bone Joint Surg* 1996; 78:412–421.
50. Northrup B, Vaccaro A, Rosen J. Occurrence of infection in anterior cervical fusion for spinal cord injury after tracheostomy. *Spine* 1995; 20: 2449–2453.

51. Osti O, Fraser R, Griffiths E. Reduction and stabilization of cervical dislocations. *J Bone Joint Surg* 1989; 71B:275–282.
52. Perez-Cruz M, Samartzis D, Fessler R. Anterior cervical discectomy and corpectomy. *Neurosurgery* 2006; 58:355–359.
53. Rechtine G, Bono P, Cahill D, et al. Postoperative wound infection after instrumentation of thoracic and lumbar fractures. *J Orthop Trauma* 2001; 15:566–569.
54. Rhee J, Park J, Yang J, et al. Indications and techniques for anterior cervical plating. *Neurol India* 2005; 53:433–439.
55. Rizzolo S, Vaccaro A, Colter J. Cervical spine trauma. *Spine* 1994; 19: 2288–2298.
56. Ryu S, Mitchell M, Kim D. A prospective randomized study comparing a cervical carbon fiber cage to the Smith-Robinson technique with allograft and plating: up to 24 months follow-up. *Eur Spine J* 2006; 15: 157–164.
57. Schenarts P, Diaz J, Kaiser C. Prospective comparison of admission computed tomographic scan and plain films of the upper cervical spine in trauma patients with altered mental status. *J Trauma* 2001; 51:663–668.
58. Siddiqui A, Jackowski A. Cage vs tricortical graft for cervical interbody fusion: a prospective, randomized study. *J Bone Joint Surg Br* 2003; 85: 1019–1025.
59. Soderstrom C, McArdle D, Ducker T. The diagnosis of intraabdominal injury in patients with cervical cord trauma. *J Trauma* 1983; 23: 1061–1065.
60. Spector L, Kim D, Affonso J, et al. Use of computed tomography to predict failure of nonoperative treatment of unilateral facet fractures of the cervical spine. *Spine* 2006; 31:2827–2835.
61. Spence K, Decker S, Sell K. Bursting atlantal fracture associated with rupture of the transverse ligament. *J Bone Joint Surg* 1970; 52A:543–549.
62. Starr J, Eismont F. Atypical hangman's fractures. *Spine* 1993; 18: 1954–1957.
63. Stauffer E. Management of spine fractures: C3 to C7. *Orthop Clin North Am* 1986; 17:45–53.
64. Torg J, Pavlov H, O'Neill M. The axial teardrop fracture: a biomechanical, clinical and roentgenographic analysis. *Am J Sports Med* 1991; 19: 355–364.
65. Ulrich C, Arand M, Nothwang J. Internal fixation on the lower cervical spine: biomechanics and clinical practice of procedures and implants. *Eur Spine J* 2001; 10:88–100.
66. Vaccaro A, Cirello J. The use of allograft bone and cages in fractures of the cervical, thoracic, and lumbar spine. *Clin Orthop Relat Res* 2002; 394: 19–26.
67. Vaccaro A, Daugherty R, Sheehan T. Neurologic outcome of early versus late surgery for cervical spinal cord injury. *Spine* 1997; 22.
68. Vaccaro A, Falatyn S, Flanders A. Magnetic resonance imaging of the intervertebral disc, spinal ligaments, and spinal cord before and after closed tracture reduction of cervical spine dislocations. *Spine* 1999; 24:1210–1217.
69. Vaccaro A, Kreidl K, Pan W, et al. Usefulness of MRI in isolated upper cervical spine fractures in adults. *J Spinal Disord* 1998; 11:289–294.
70. Vaccaro A, Madican L, Albert T. Magnetic resonance imaging analysis of soft tissue disruption after flexion-distraction injuries of the subaxial cervical spine. *Spine* 2001; 26:1866–1872.
71. Vaccaro A, Madigan L, Bauerle W, et al. Early halo immobilization of displace traumatic spondylolisthesis of the axis. *Spine* 2005; 27: 2229–2233.
72. Vale F, Burns J, Jackson A. Combined medical and surgical treatment after acute spinal cord injury: results of a prospective pilot study to assess the merits of aggressive medical resuscitation and blood pressure management. *J Neurosurg* 1997; 87:239–246.
73. Vieweg U, Schultheiss R. A review of halo vest treatment of upper cervical spine injuries. *Arch Orthop Trauma Surg* 2001; 121:50–55.
74. Wang J, Hatch J, Sandhu H, et al. Cervical flexion and extension radiographs in acutely injured patients. *Clin Orthop* 1999; 365:111–116.
75. Waters R, Adkins R, Yakura J. Effect of surgery on motor recovery following spinal cord injury. *Spinal Cord* 1996; 34:188–192.
76. Weinstein M, McCabe J, Cammisa F. Postoperative spinal wound infection: a review of 2,391 consecutive index procedures. *J Spinal Disord* 2000; 13:422–426.
77. White A, Panjabi M. *Clinical Biomechanics of the Spine.* 2nd ed. Philadelphia: Lippincott-Raven, 1990.

15 Thoracolumbar Fractures

Andrew K. Simpson
Peter G. Whang
Joseph Hong
Avraam Ploumis
Alexander R. Vaccaro

Approximately 3%–6% of all skeletal fractures involve the spinal column, with nearly 90% localizing to the thoracic or lumbar vertebrae (1). The majority of these injuries are known to occur between T11 and L2 at the so-called thoracolumbar junction. With their attachments to the rib cage and the coronal orientation of their facet joints, the thoracic vertebrae are much more rigid than the lumbar segments; because these transitional levels link fixed kyphotic and mobile lordotic regions of the spine, the thoracolumbar junction encounters greater biomechanical stresses and is therefore particularly susceptible to traumatic disruption.

The development of standardized treatment protocols for thoracolumbar injuries has proven to be a daunting task. Many individuals with stable fractures who are neurologically intact may be managed conservatively with activity modification and bracing techniques. Alternatively, surgical intervention consisting of spinal fusion and/or decompression is routinely recommended for patients who exhibit unstable injuries or significant neurologic deficits, in order to facilitate their early mobilization and avoid the numerous complications that may arise during a period of prolonged recumbency. Unfortunately, the optimal therapeutic strategy for patients who present with spinal fractures associated with moderate deformity, canal compromise, or an incomplete neurologic injury is still controversial because there is very little Class I data at this time, and the evidence reported by existing studies is somewhat contradictory. The indications for any treatment modality are largely influenced by the mechanism of injury and the neurologic status of the patient, both of which serve to define the concept of spinal stability. By taking into account these and other critical factors, it may be possible for practitioners to optimize the long-term clinical outcomes of individuals who sustain these potentially devastating fractures.

PREVALENCE AND SOCIAL IMPACT OF THORACOLUMBAR FRACTURE

The incidence of thoracolumbar injuries has been shown to demonstrate a bimodal distribution, affecting at least 1 in 20,000 individuals living in the United States. In younger adults, these fractures require high-energy forces that are typically imparted during traumatic events including motor vehicle collisions, falls from a height, and sports-related accidents (2). However, these injuries are also commonly observed within the geriatric population following relatively minor incidents such as a fall from a standing position. Up to 50% of thoracolumbar fractures will also give rise to neurologic deficits, which clearly increase the morbidity experienced by these patients (3–6); in cases of paraplegia or other catastrophic spinal cord injuries, the mortality rate may be as high as 7% in the first year alone (7).

MECHANISMS OF INJURY

Thoracolumbar fractures may be broadly categorized as compression, burst, flexion-distraction (i.e., Chance), or fracture-dislocation, according to their primary mechanisms of injury. This information is not only essential for elucidating the pathogenesis of these fractures but may also be helpful for predicting their overall stability and for guiding subsequent treatment. One of the most popular mechanistic classification systems was proposed by Denis in 1983, based on his seminal paradigm of spinal stability (3). In this model, the spine is composed of three distinct columns consisting of discrete anatomic structures: anterior (anterior longitudinal ligament, anterior half of the vertebral body, and intervertebral disc), middle (posterior half of the vertebral body and disc, posterior longitudinal ligament), and posterior column (posterior bony elements, remaining posterior ligaments).

Compression injuries are produced when axial loads are applied to the flexed spine, resulting in failure of the anterior vertebral body with preservation of the middle column. Because the zone of injury is limited to the anterior portion of the vertebrae, these wedge fractures are generally considered to be stable; nevertheless, concomitant damage to the posterior ligamentous complex (PLC) is suggestive of a more severe injury that has further compromised the integrity of the spine (Figure 15.1).

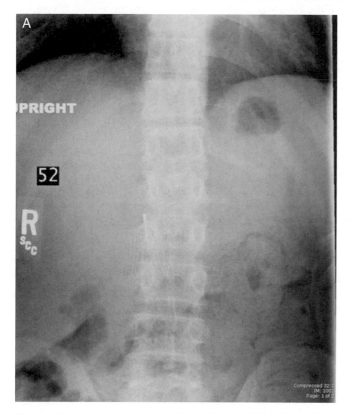
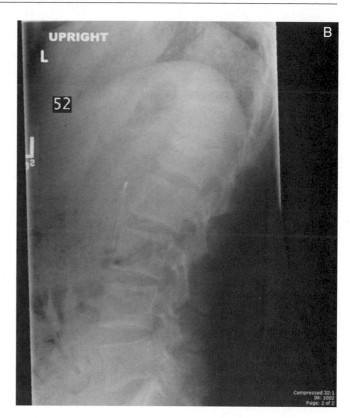

Figure 15.1 Anteroposterior (**A**) and lateral (**B**) radiographs demonstrate an L1 compression fracture with minimal compression of anterior vertebral body.

More substantial axial forces may lead to the disruption of both the anterior and middle columns, which is characteristic of burst fractures. Unlike compression injuries, where the posterior aspect of the vertebral body is not affected, burst fractures are more likely to bring about compression of the neural elements secondary to retropulsion of osseous fragments into the spinal canal (Figure 15.2).

With Chance or "seat belt"-type injuries, the spine is subjected to a combined flexion-distraction moment, which may pass through either bone or soft tissues (i.e., the disc space). With

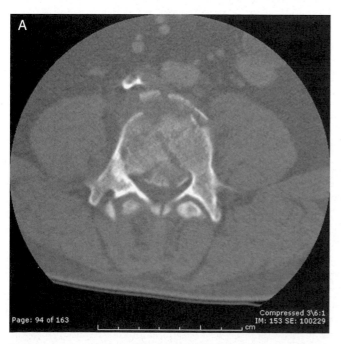
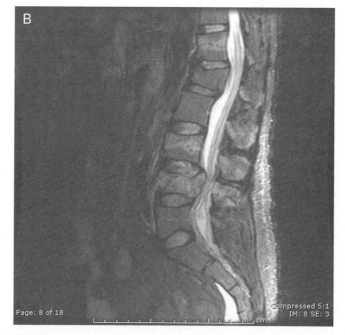

Figure 15.2 Axial CT (**A**) and sagittal MRI STIR (**B**) images of an L4 burst fracture reveal retropulsed bony fragments in the spinal canal and damage to the posterior ligamentous complex, which are indicative of a biomechanically unstable injury.

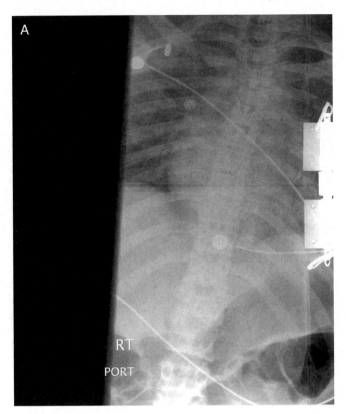
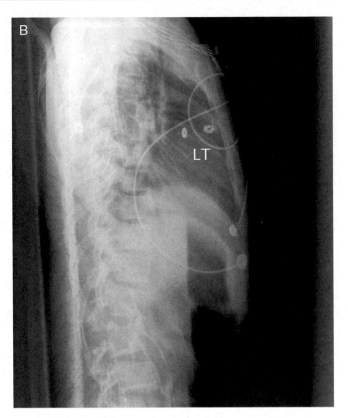

Figure 15.3   Anteroposterior (**A**) and lateral (**B**) radiographs demonstrate a "seat-belt" flexion-distraction injury at L1–L2 level.

flexion-distraction fractures, the specific pattern of injury is contingent upon the location of the rotational axis. If the center of rotation is located between the anterior and middle columns, then the vertebral body will be compressed, whereas the posterior elements will undergo distraction; in contrast, all of these structures will fail in tension when the axis is anterior to the spine. Because a large proportion of these patients are victims of motor vehicle accidents, it is imperative that the treating physician maintain a high index of suspicion for other nonspinal injuries during the initial evaluation of these individuals because associated intra-abdominal conditions have been shown to occur in as many as 45% of these cases (Figure 15.3) (8). Fracture-dislocations represent a collection of extremely unstable injuries that usually require a high-energy traumatic insult. By definition these fractures extend through the entire spine (both anteriorly and posteriorly) and are frequently accompanied by extensive sagittal and/or coronal plane deformities. Given the dire consequences of this pathologic translation, it is not surprising that this class of thoracolumbar injuries demonstrates the highest rate of neurologic deficits (Figure 15.4) (5, 6).

HISTORY AND PHYSICAL EXAM

Any individual who presents with a history of a significant trauma to the axial skeleton should be assumed to have a thoracolumbar spinal injury until proven otherwise. Thoracolumbar fractures, especially those without attendant neurologic deficits, may be easily overlooked in the acute setting, when the attention

of the patient is often diverted away from the spine. In fact, nearly half of this population will ultimately be diagnosed with injuries to other organs (30%—1 system, 20%—2 systems, 5%—3+ systems) (9).Whenever feasible, a thorough history should be obtained from both the patient and any other witnesses who were in attendance at the scene because certain details of the incident may help to establish the diagnosis of a thoracolumbar injury. For automobile accidents, these include the speed and trajectory of the vehicle, whether restraints were in place, and whether any air bags were deployed; similarly, it is useful to know the height and the point of impact of those who have fallen. Patients with acute thoracolumbar injuries consistently complain of a constellation of symptoms such as back pain and restricted range of motion. Depending on the status of the neural elements, they may also be aware of new-onset weakness, numbness, and other neurologic changes.

During the physical examination, the spine should be carefully inspected for any gapping or malalignment of the posterior elements. Tenderness to palpation directly over a spinous process may be evident at the fracture site, and the locations of any ecchymoses, lacerations, and swelling are often indicative of the mechanism of injury. For instance, an abdominal contusion created by a lap belt may be observed in conjunction with a flexion-distraction fracture (10–12). A comprehensive neurologic evaluation should be performed at once, and all the relevant findings should be meticulously documented in order to identify the level of injury and assess the functional integrity of the neural elements. Moreover, serial examinations are required to ensure that any evolving neurologic deterioration is not missed over

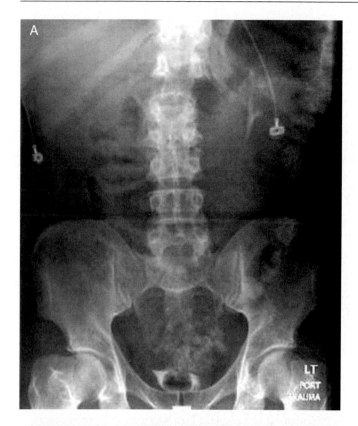

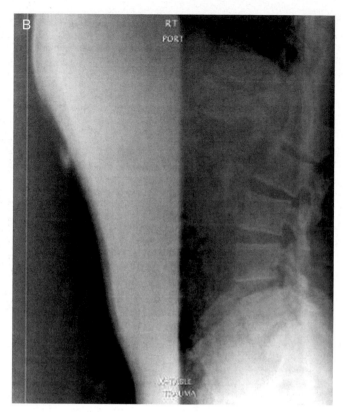

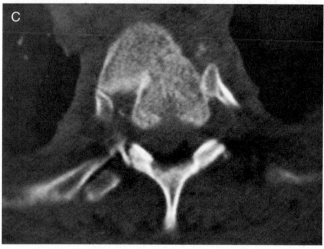

Figure 15.4 Anteroposterior (**A**) and lateral (**B**) radiographs demonstrate a fracture dislocation of the thoracolumbar junction with complete dissociation of the T12 and L1 vertebral bodies. An axial CT image (**C**) at the level of the injury exhibits a "double vertebral body sign" with obvious compression of the spinal cord.

symptoms of spinal shock. The resolution of this transient period of spinal cord dysfunction may be signaled by a return of the bulbocavernosus reflex and sacral sensory sparing, at which time the true extent of the impairment may be confirmed, and the long-term prognosis of the individual may be predicted with greater accuracy (13).

DIAGNOSTIC IMAGING

A complete battery of radiographic studies should be obtained as part of the initial workup of patients with thoracolumbar injuries. With few exceptions, plain X-rays are the most readily available method for imaging the spine, so anteroposterior and lateral views of the fracture should be acquired as soon as possible. Adequate visualization of the rest of the spinal column must also be achieved because the prevalence of noncontiguous vertebral fractures may be as high as 20% in these situations (14). Based on the presumed mechanism of injury, additional diagnostic examinations of the appendicular skeleton or other major organ systems may also be warranted (e.g., radiographs of the knee and calcaneus with burst fractures, arteriogram or ultrasound of the abdomen with flexion-distraction injuries).

The Spine Trauma Study Group recently published a review of the current literature, which emphasized what they recognized

time. Because the spinal cord normally terminates behind the L1 vertebral body, a fracture in this region may harm any number of anatomic structures. Injury to the nerve roots may give rise to altered sensation in a dermatomal distribution, myotomal weakness, or hyporeflexia. Traumatic insults to the spinal cord may bring about a spectrum of abnormalities ranging from incomplete sensory and motor disturbances in the lower extremities to frank paraplegia, whereas damage to the conus medullaris or cauda equina is more likely to result in isolated urinary or fecal incontinence.

Patients who appear to have suffered complete spinal cord injuries must undergo further testing to determine whether they are simply exhibiting the temporary neurologic signs and as the three key parameters that reflect the biomechanical stability of the injured spinal column—sagittal alignment, amount of vertebral body compression, and dimensions of the spinal canal (15). According to this analysis, the values that should be calculated on biplanar X-rays of the spine include the Cobb angle, sagittal-to-transverse canal diameter ratio, and percentages of vertebral body translation, anterior compression, and canal occlusion. An AP view of a fractured vertebra may reveal changes in the coronal alignment as well as widened interpedicular or interspinous distances, all of which imply that considerable displacement may have occurred at the level of injury. Likewise, a lateral radiograph may depict instability in the sagittal plane and allow for the measurement of any loss in vertebral body height or focal deformity that may exist with compression or burst fractures; with anterior column injuries, a kyphosis greater than 30 degrees has been shown to correlate with a torn PLC (16–21). Computed tomography (CT) is another imaging technique that is regularly employed for the evaluation of thoracolumbar injuries because it provides axial views and multiplanar reconstructions of the anatomy so that the fracture pattern and the patency of the spinal canal may be assessed with greater precision. Using CT scans, Vaccaro et al. demonstrated that smaller mid-sagittal and larger transverse canal diameters were associated with an increased prevalence of neurologic deficits among individuals with thoracolumbar injuries (22). Thin-slice spiral CT is widely accepted as the study of choice for diagnosing these fractures in the setting of polytrauma because its enhanced sensitivity may lead to both improved clinical outcomes and lower costs (23, 24).

Most practitioners would agree that magnetic resonance imaging (MRI) is obligatory for cases in which there is evidence of neurologic decline so that any ongoing compression of the spinal cord or other neural structures may be clearly visualized. However, even in the absence of any apparent deficits, this modality is also beneficial for identifying other pathologic conditions that may be present, such as an epidural hematoma, myelomalacia, or posterior ligamentous disruption.

CLASSIFICATION SYSTEMS

Although various paradigms for categorizing thoracolumbar fractures have been proposed in the past, there remains little consensus among spine specialists regarding the most expedient method for stratifying these injuries. Besides exhibiting excellent validity and reproducibility, the ideal classification scheme should also be based on objective clinical and radiographic criteria so that it is both comprehensive and easy to use. It is equally as important that this algorithm be able to direct subsequent treatment and predict patient outcomes.

Historically, the two most popular approaches for classifying thoracolumbar fractures were the Denis and AO (Magerl) systems. Both of these schemes incorporate multiple levels of organization, requiring injuries to be sequentially segregated into numerous subcategories. The inter- and intraobserver reliabilities of these two models have been examined by several different authors. Blauth et al. reported that the mean interobserver reliability of the AO method was only 67% with a kappa (κ) value of 0.33, corresponding to only fair agreement (25). In their comparison of these algorithms, Oner et al. noted that the Denis system was more reproducible than the AO scheme ($\kappa = 0.60$ and 0.35, respectively) (26). These findings were corroborated by Wood et al., who also

concluded that the interobserver agreement of the Denis algorithm was superior to that of the AO system ($\kappa = 0.606$ and 0.475, respectively) (27). Collectively, these studies suggest that the AO method is inclusive of all types of thoracolumbar injuries but may be difficult to implement because its complicated alphanumeric scoring protocol diminishes its reproducibility; conversely, the more reliable Denis scheme may be too broad, such that it excludes any atypical fracture configurations.

In response to the limitations of these traditional classification systems, Vaccaro et al. introduced a novel paradigm known as the Thoracolumbar Injury Severity Score (TLISS) (28). Originally conceived by a panel of experts in the field of spinal trauma, the TLISS model integrates three primary variables: (1) mechanism of injury as derived from appropriate radiographic images, (2) status of the posterior ligamentous complex (PLC), and (3) neurologic examination of the individual. The specific point values assigned to these categories are combined to generate a total score, which may serve as an effective tool for guiding the subsequent management of these fractures. In an attempt to make this process less subjective, this algorithm was later modified so that the mechanism-of-injury parameter was replaced by fracture morphology, giving rise to the Thoracolumbar Injury Classification and Severity Score (TLICS, Table 15.1). Although each of these schemes has demonstrated excellent overall reproducibility and reliability in prospective investigations, the interrater correlation of the TLISS system has been shown to be greater than that of the TLICS model, which indicates that the mechanism of trauma may be a more critical parameter than fracture morphology for the classification of thoracolumbar injuries (29). Nevertheless, it is assumed that both of these issues will need to be considered in order to facilitate the diagnosis and treatment of these complex fractures.

Table 15.1   Thoracolumbar Injury Classification and Severity Score (TLICS) (29)

Parameter	Points
Morphology	
Compression	1
Burst	2
Translational/rotational	3
Distraction	4
Neurologic Status	
Intact	0
Nerve root injury	2
Spinal cord/conus medullaris injury	
Complete	2
Incomplete	3
Cauda equina	3
Posterior Ligamentous Complex	
Intact	0
Indeterminate	2
Disrupted	3

Treatment Recommendations
Total score < 3: Nonoperative treatment
Total score = 4: Nonoperative vs. operative treatment
Total score > 5: Operative treatment

NEUROPROTECTIVE AGENTS

In individuals with spinal cord injuries, the rapid initiation of certain medical therapies may play a crucial role in mitigating the acute neurologic insult and maximizing the degree of functional recovery. Any impairment of the spinal cord may be attributed to the initial mechanical contusion of the neural tissues, which triggers a complex series of molecular and cellular events resulting in local edema, microvascular insufficiency, and the release of inflammatory mediators that are known to be neurotoxic (30–32). The major goal of these pharmacologic strategies is to impede any progression of the injury by counteracting the detrimental effects of this secondary cascade. First and foremost, the neurologic status may be improved with aggressive fluid resuscitation and arterial pressure support in an effort to maintain spinal cord perfusion and avoid prolonged ischemia (33). The intravenous administration of corticosteroids may also theoretically protect the neural elements following these types of catastrophic injuries by decreasing the production of neurotoxic cytokines, stabilizing cellular membranes, reducing edema, and buffering electrolyte imbalances (13, 43–44). The second National Acute Spinal Cord Injury Study (NASCIS II) demonstrated superior long-term neurologic outcomes associated with steroid therapy so that many spinal cord injury patients are now given a 30 mg/kg bolus of methylprednisone over the first hour; the treatment is continued at a rate of 5.4 mg/kg/hr (34). The NASCIS III affirmed that individuals whose infusions are started within 3 hours may be treated for only 24 hours, whereas those who present between 3 and 8 hours after the time of the injury should receive a total of 48 hours of steroid therapy (35). Unfortunately, high-dose steroid therapy is not without its hazards, and the use of these medications in patients who are already immunocompromised as a consequence of the significant trauma they have sustained may increase their risks of contracting pneumonia or sepsis. Even though a growing number of critics have expressed their reservations about the validity of the NASCIS II and III trials, these recommendations have been largely adopted as the standard of care so that in this litigious medical environment many physicians may feel compelled to adhere to these guidelines despite the lack of any definitive evidence confirming their efficacy (36). Other pharmacologic agents currently under investigation for this purpose include opiate receptor antagonists, calcium channel blockers, free radical scavengers, lipid peroxidase inhibitors, and glycolipids (37, 38).

NONOPERATIVE TREATMENT

The manner in which a thoracolumbar fracture is addressed may be influenced by a range of patient-related characteristics such as neurologic status, biomechanical integrity of the spinal column, medical comorbidities, and associated traumatic injuries. Regardless of the approach that is selected, the goals of treatment are the same: restoration of physiologic spinal stability with correction of any deformity, amelioration of neurologic deficits, pain control, and early rehabilitation.

Nonoperative measures may be a viable option for patients with stable fracture patterns and a normal neurologic examination who are unlikely to develop any changes in alignment or delayed loss of function. For example, the majority of patients with compression injuries will experience symptomatic relief when placed in a molded thoracolumbosacral orthosis or a Jewitt hyperextension brace, which, in most cases, will bring about successful fracture healing within 12 weeks (39–41). Caution must be exercised with compression fractures that exhibit more than 50% vertebral body height loss, greater than 15–20 degrees of kyphosis, or disruption of the posterior ligamentous structures because these injuries may not be able to be managed solely with external immobilization due to failure of the supporting posterior tension band, which may precipitate even further segmental collapse.

Burst fractures also arise from axial loading of the spine but are inherently less stable than simple compression injuries because the fracture extends from the anterior portion of the vertebral body to the posterior cortex. The indications for the conservative treatment of burst injuries are analogous to those that have been established for compression fractures. Thus, it may be reasonable to advocate a trial of bracing for individuals who are neurologically intact and whose imaging studies demonstrate no significant compromise of the posterior ligamentous complex, but close follow-up of these patients is mandatory to ensure that there is no progression of deformity or decline in neurologic function (42, 43). Although immobilization alone may be sufficient for stable burst injuries (44, 45), a prospective, randomized, multicenter study demonstrated that surgical intervention may actually lead to improved outcomes. In this series, short-segment posterior fusions gave rise to a decreased incidence of late deformity, better functional scores, and a higher percentage of subjects who returned to work compared to a nonoperative regimen consisting of bed rest followed by the use of a Jewitt orthosis (46). Nonoperative treatment is rarely employed for flexion-distraction injuries or fracture-dislocations. In certain situations, it may be acceptable to immobilize a bony Chance fracture in a hyperextension brace, but the secure fixation of purely soft tissue injuries is difficult to achieve in the absence of spinal instrumentation. Fracture-dislocations also exhibit substantial translational and rotational instability that virtually always requires open reduction and the placement of metal implants.

Up to 95% of patients with incomplete spinal cord injuries will improve by at least one Frankel grade with nonsurgical protocols as the inflammatory response affecting the neural tissues resolves and the severity of any cord impingement decreases secondary to remodeling of bony fragments (47, 48). Similarly, satisfactory results may also be obtained by bracing fractures associated with complete cord-level injuries. However, late kyphotic deformities, either with or without any accompanying neurologic deficits, may be observed in as many as 21% of individuals with thoracolumbar fractures who are managed conservatively (48–50).

OPERATIVE MANAGEMENT

For many thoracolumbar injuries, an operative procedure may be performed in an attempt to optimize clinical outcomes and avoid many of the complications that are known to occur with nonoperative methods. The decision to pursue surgical intervention is influenced by multiple factors such as the fracture pattern and biomechanical properties of the spinal column as well as the neurologic function and hemodynamic status of the patient. In general, most practitioners would agree that any individual who presents with an incomplete deficit in the setting of marked canal compromise, signs of neurologic decline, or a grossly unstable injury may benefit from surgery. By restoring the normal alignment of the spine and relieving any persistent compression of the neural elements, either directly or indirectly, these operative techniques have the potential to engender meaningful neurologic recovery in patients with incomplete deficits (4, 51). The surgical fixation of thoracolumbar fractures may also enhance the rehabilitation of individuals with complete spinal cord injuries and minimize the incidence of posttraumatic deformities and other adverse events (52–54). The importance of the timing of surgery for cases in which there is a documented neurologic deficit remains a matter of some debate. In animal models, rapid decompression of neural structures has been found to yield superior functional outcomes compared to procedures conducted in a delayed fashion (55). Whereas several clinical studies have emphasized the need for urgent treatment (i.e., within 24 hours of the injury), the only prospective, randomized trial comparing patients with thoracolumbar fractures who underwent early versus late decompression failed to detect any significant differences between these two cohorts (55, 56). Anterior, posterior, or circumferential approaches have all been described for the operative management of thoracolumbar pathology, but the preferred surgical technique for any given fracture may be dependent on the objective neurologic findings of the patient, the amount of kyphosis or evidence of disruption of the posterior ligamentous complex on spinal images, and the existence of other nonspinal injuries (Figure 15.5). Neurologic deficits normally arise when bony fragments are displaced posteriorly from the fractured body, so an anterior procedure may be ideal for an individual with an incomplete injury who demonstrates substantial canal occlusion (i.e., greater than 67% of the total area) because it offers an unobstructed view of the dura and allows for a more meticulous decompression of the spinal cord and nerve roots. An anterior approach may also be mandatory in instances where there is extensive vertebral comminution that may require the insertion of a load-sharing interbody implant. Anterior surgeries are often combined with posterior fixation since standalone constructs may not confer enough stability to adequately treat fracture-dislocations or other injuries where the posterior ligamentous complex is no longer intact.

A posterior operative strategy may also be employed to decompress the neural elements, either directly through a laminectomy, costotransversectomy, transpedicular, or extracavitary approach or indirectly by applying distractive forces across the injured segment. A laminectomy is often performed to release nerve roots that may be trapped within posterior element fractures, to repair traumatic durotomies, or to evacuate an epidural hematoma; in the upper thoracic spine, a formal decompression may also be necessary if the fracture may not be accessible through a thoracotomy (57–60). Alternatively, any impingement of the neural structures may be addressed through a number of posterolateral approaches including costotransversectomy, transpedicular, lateral extracavitary, and lateral extrapleural parascapular techniques (61–65). For an individual with moderate canal stenosis, indirect reduction of thoracolumbar fractures may be accomplished posteriorly by taking advantage of distraction and ligamentotaxis, which shifts these retropulsed pieces away from the thecal sac. Nevertheless, this method appears to be less effective in cases where there is greater than 67% canal compromise or when the operation has been delayed more than 3 days (66–68). In addition to facilitating the reduction of thoracolumbar fractures, posterior procedures may also

be utilized to stabilize these injuries. With the advent of modern pedicle screw systems, the surgeon is able to place instrumentation across the entire vertebral body, thus increasing the rigidity of these constructs. This approach is particularly well suited for unstable burst, Chance, or fracture-dislocation injuries where the posterior implants may serve to reinforce the absent posterior tension band. An isolated fusion may be sufficient for patients who are neurologically intact or those with complete spinal cord injuries in whom a decompression is likely to be of little value. Finally, a posterior approach may be the only option for individuals with pulmonary disease, morbid obesity, or thoracoabdominal injuries who cannot tolerate an extensile anterior exposure.

There continues to be a paucity of Class I data conclusively proving the superiority of one surgical approach over the others. Although multiple studies have shown that posterior techniques may give rise to clinical and radiographic outcomes equivalent to anterior or circumferential operations (67, 69–71), others have reported that an anterior decompression may promote greater recovery of motor strength and sphincter function relative to posterior indirect reduction methods (16, 72). In one of the few published prospective, randomized clinical trials comparing the results of thoracolumbar fractures treated with either an anterior or a posterior procedure, patients who were treated anteriorly demonstrated lower complication and reoperation rates (73). Anterior fixation may also maintain sagittal alignment better than short-segment posterior fusions, which may be predisposed to developing progressive kyphosis (74). Clearly, additional well-designed studies must be completed in order to determine which of these surgical approaches is most appropriate for a given thoracolumbar injury.

SUMMARY

The junctional anatomy of the thoracolumbar spine increases the susceptibility of this region to injury. In younger patients these fractures typically occur as a result of motor vehicle collisions and other accidents that impart significant forces to the spine, whereas older individuals more often sustain these injuries after relatively lower energy trauma. The proper evaluation of these fractures is predicated upon a thorough history and physical examination as well as a complete set of radiographs and cross-sectional imaging studies. Although there is some evidence to suggest that neuroprotective agents may serve to improve neurologic function in patients with incomplete deficits, the administration of high-dose steroids remains a controversial topic. Regardless of the therapeutic strategy that is implemented, the goals of treatment are to preserve or restore spinal stability, correct any associated deformity, maximize neurologic function, relieve pain, and promote the early rehabilitation of these patients. Based on the mechanism and morphology of the injury, certain types of these fractures may be adequately managed with external immobilization, whereas others are more effectively addressed through surgical means. At this time, the well-accepted indications for operative intervention include incomplete spinal cord injuries brought about by ongoing compression of the neural elements, evidence of progressive neurologic deterioration, or fractures that are considered to be unstable. Unfortunately, in many cases the optimal method for treating thoracolumbar injuries is still unknown, and a universal treatment algorithm has yet to be

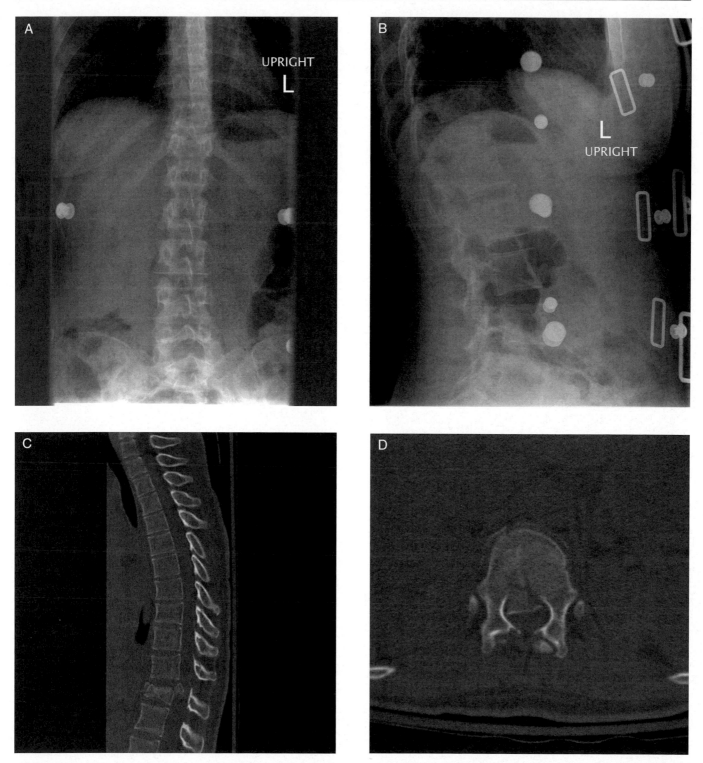

Figure 15.5   Imaging studies of a patient who presented with an incomplete neurologic deficit secondary to a T12 burst fracture. Anteroposterior (**A**) and lateral (**B**) radiographs demonstrate an obvious deformity involving the thoracolumbar junction with loss of vertebral body height and focal kyphosis. Sagittal (**C**) and axial (**D**) CT images reveal retropulsion of a bony fragment into the spinal canal resulting in compression of the neural elements.

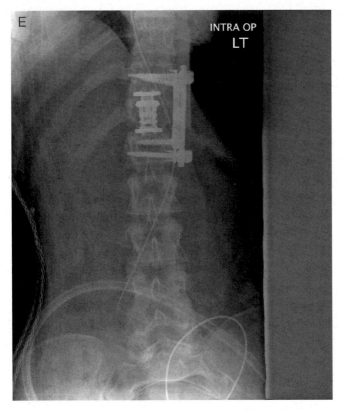
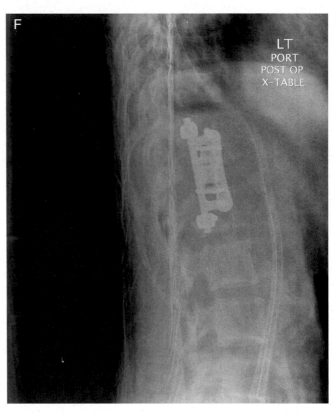

Figure 15.5   *(continued)* Postoperative anteroposterior (**E**) and lateral (**F**) X-rays were obtained following T12 corpectomy with insertion of an expandable cage and placement of anterior instrumentation from T11 to L1.

established because of challenges associated with defining the concept of spinal stability. Clearly, validated classification systems like the Thoracolumbar Injury Severity Score (TLISS) will likely prove to be a reliable technique for stratifying these fractures and directing subsequent therapy. In the future, it is imperative that multiple prospective, randomized, controlled clinical trials be performed to assess the long-term outcomes of both conservative and operative modalities as well as to compare the various surgical approaches that may be utilized for the treatment of these fractures.

*R*eferences

1. Dewald RL. Burst fractures of the thoracic and lumbar spine. *Clin Orthop Relat Res* 1984; 189:150–161.
2. Gertzbein SD. Scoliosis Research Society. Multicenter spine fracture study. *Spine* 1992; 17:528–539.
3. Denis F. The three columns of the spine and its significance in the classification of acute thoracolumbar spine injuries. *Spine* 1983; 8:817–831.
4. McEvoy RD, Bradford DS. The management of burst fractures of the thoracic and lumbar spine: experience in 53 patients. *Spine* 1985; 10:631–637.
5. Denis F, Burkus J. Shear fracture-dislocation of the thoracic and lumbar spine associated with forceful hyperextension (lumberjack paraplegia). *Spine* 1992; 17:156–161.
6. Liu YJ, Chang MC, Wang ST, Yu WK, et al. Flexion-distraction injury of the thoracolumbar spine. *Injury* 2003; 34:920–923.
7. Shikata J, Yamamuro T, Lida H, Shimizu K, Yoshikawa J. Surgical treatment for paraplegia resulting from vertebral fractures in senile osteoporosis. *Spine* 1990; 15:589–591.
8. Anderson PA, Rivera FP, Maier RV, Drake C. The epidemiology of seatbelt-associated injuries. *J Trauma* 1991; 31:61–67.
9. Savitsky E, Votey S. Emergency department approach to acute thoracolumbar spine injury. *J Emerg Med* 1997; 15(1):49–60.
10. Gumley G, Taylor TKF, Ryan MD. Distraction fractures of the lumbar spine. *J Bone Joint Surg Br* 1982; 64(5):520–525.
11. Chapman JR, Agel J, Jurkovich GJ, Bellabarba C. Thoracolumbar flexion-distraction injuries: associated morbidity and neurological outcomes. *Spine* 2008; 33:648–657.
12. Gertzbein S, Count-Brown C. Flexion-distraction injuries of the lumbar spine. *Clin Orthop Relat Res* 1988; 227: 50–52.
13. Stauffer ES. Spinal cord injury syndromes. *Semin Spine Surg* 1991; 3: 87–91.
14. Albert TJ, Levine MJ, Ann HS, Cotler JM, Balderston RA. Concomitant noncontiguous thoracolumbar and sacral fractures. *Spine* 1993; 18(10):1285–1291.
15. Keynan O, Fisher CG, Vaccaro A, Fehlings MG, et al. Radiographic measurement parameters in thoracolumbar fractures: a systematic review and consensus statement of the Spine Trauma Study Group. *Spine* 2006; 31:E156–E165.
16. Bradford D, McBride G. Surgical management of thoracolumbar spine fractures with incomplete neurologic deficits. *Clin Orthop Relat Res* 1987; 218:201–215.
17. Denis F. Thoracolumbar injuries. *Instr Course Lect* 1988; 230.
18. Esses SI. The placement and treatment of thoracolumbar spine fractures: an algorithmic approach. *Orthop Rev* 1988; 17:571–584.
19. Jacobs RR, Asher MA, Snider RK. Thoracolumbar spinal injuries: a comparative study of recumbent and operative treatment in 100 patients. *Spine* 1980; 5:463–477.
20. Jacobs RR, Casey MP. Surgical management of thoracolumbar spinal injuries. *Clin Orthop Relat Res* 1984; 189:22–35.
21. Weitzman G. Treatment of stable thoracolumbar spine compression fractures by early ambulation. *Clin Orthop Relat Res* 1971; 176:116–122.
22. Vaccaro AR, Nachwalter RS, Klein GR, Sewards JM, et al. The significance of thoracolumbar spinal canal size in spinal cord injury patients. *Spine* 2001; 26: 371–376.
23. Wintermark M, Mouhsine E, Theumann N, Mordasini P, et al. Thoracolumbar spine fractures in patients who have sustained severe trauma: depiction with multi-detector row CT. *Radiology* 2003; 227: 681–689.

24. Blackmore CC, Ramsey SD, Mann FA, Deyo RA. Cervical spine screening with CT in trauma patients: a cost-effectiveness analysis. *Radiology* 1999; 212:117–125.

25. Blauth M, Bastian L, Knop C, Lange U, Tusch G. Inter-observer reliability in the classification of thoraco-lumbar spinal injuries [in German]. *Orthopade* 1999; 28:662–681.

26. Oner FC, Ramos LM, Simmermacher RK, Kingma PT, et al. Classification of thoracic and lumbar spine fractures: problems of reproducibility. A study of 53 patients using CT and MRI. *Eur Spine J* 2002; 11:235–245.

27. Wood KB, Khanna G, Vaccaro AR, Arnold PM, et al. Assessment of two thoracolumbar fracture classifications systems as used by multiple surgeons. *J Bone Joint Surg Am* 2005; 87:1423–1429.

28. Vaccaro AR, Zeiller SC, Hulbert RJ, Anderson PA, et al. The thoracolumbar injury severity score: a proposed treatment algorithm. *J Spinal Disord Tech* 2005; 18:209–215.

29. Whang PG, Vaccaro AR, Poelstra KA, Patel AA, et al. The influence of fracture mechanism and morphology on the reliability and validity of two novel thoracolumbar injury classification systems. *Spine* 2007; 32:791–795.

30. Bracken MB, Shephard MJ, Collins WF. A randomized, controlled trial of methyl-prednisolone or naloxone in the treatment of acute spinal-cord injury: results of the Second National Acute Spinal Cord Study. *N Engl J Med* 1990; 322:1405–1411.

31. Delamarter RB, Sherman J, Carr JB. Pathophysiology of spinal cord injury: recovery after immediate and delayed decompression. *J Bone Joint Surg Am* 1995; 77:1042–1049.

32. Salzman SK, Betz RR. Experimental treatment of spinal cord injuries. In: Betz RR, Mulcaheny MJ, eds. *The Child with a Spinal Cord Injury.* Rosemont, IL: American Academy of Orthopaedic Surgeons, 1996:63.

33. Vale FL, Burns J, Jackson AB. Combined medical and surgical treatment after acute spinal cord injury: results of a prospective pilot study to assess the merits of aggressive medical resuscitation and blood pressure management. *J Neurosug* 1997; 87(2):239–246.

34. Bracken MB, Shepard MJ, Collins WF, Holford TR, et al. A randomized, controlled trial of methylprednisone or naloxone in the treatment of acute spinal-cord injury: results of the Second National Acute Spinal Cord Injury Study. *N Engl J Med* 1990; 322:1405–1411.

35. Bracken MB, Shepard MJ, Holford TR, Leo-Summers L, et al. Administration of methylprednisone for 24 or 48 hours or tirilized mesylate for 48 hours in the treatment of acute spinal cord injury: results of the Third National Acute Spinal Cord Injury Randomized Controlled Trial. *JAMA* 1997; 277:1597–1604.

36. Hall ED, Springer JE. Neuroprotection and acute spinal cord injury: a reappraisal. *NeuroRx* 2004; 1:80–100.

37. Baptiste DC, Fehlings MG. Pharmacological approaches to repair the injured spinal cord. *J Neurotrauma* 2006; 23:318–334.

38. Baptiste DC, Fehlings MG. Update on the treatment of spinal cord injury. *Prog Brain Res* 2007; 161:217–233.

39. Argenson C, Boileau P. Specific injuries and management. In: Floman Y, Farcy JP, Argenson C, eds. *Thoracolumbar Spine Fractures.* New York: Raven Press Ltd., 1993:195–214.

40. Patwardhan AG, Li S, Gavin T. Orthotic stabilization of thoracolumbar injuries. *Spine* 1990; 15:654–661.

41. Hitchon PW, Turner JC, Haddad SF. Management options in thoracolumbar burst fractures. *Surg Neurol* 1998; 49(6):619–626.

42. Fredrickson BE, Yuan HA, Bayley JC. The nonsurgical treatment of thoracolumbar injuries. *Semin Spine Surg* 1990; 2:70–78.

43. Reid DC, Hu R, Davis LA. The nonsurgical treatment of burst fractures in the thoracolumbar spine. *J Trauma* 1988; 28:1188–1194.

44. Shen WJ, Liu TJ, Shen YS. Nonoperative treatment versus posterior fixation for thoracolumbar junction burst fractures without neurologic deficit. *Spine* 2001; 26:1038–1045.

45. Wood K, Buttermann G, Mehbod A, Garvey T, et al. Operative compared with nonoperative treatment of a thoracolumbar burst fracture without neurologic deficit: a prospective, randomized study. *J Bone Joint Surg Am* 2003; 85:773–781.

46. Siebenga J, Leferink VJ, Segers MJ, Bakker FC, et al. Treatment of traumatic thoracolumbar spine fractures: a multicenter prospective randomized study of operative versus nonsurgical treatment. *Spine* 2006; 31:2881–2890.

47. de Klerk LW, Fontijne WP, Stijnen T. Spontaneous remodeling of the spinal canal after conservative management of thoracolumbar burst fractures. *Spine* 1998; 23(9):1057–1060.

48. Fredrickson BE, Yuan HA, Miller HM. Burst fractures of the fifth lumbar vertebra. *J Bone Joint Surg Am* 1982; 64(7):1088–1093.

49. Denis F, Armstrong GW, Searls K. Acute thoracolumbar burst fractures in the absence of neurologic deficit. *Clin Orthop Relat Res* 1984; 189:142–149.

50. Mumford J, Weinstein JN, Spratt KF. Thoracolumbar burst fractures, the clinical efficacy, and outcome of nonoperative management. *Spine* 1993; 18:955–970.

51. Jacobs RR, Asher MA, Snider RK. Thoracolumbar spinal injuries. *Spine* 1980; 5(5):463–477.

52. Bohlman HH, Freehafer A, Dejak J. The results of treatment of acute injuries of the upper thoracic spine with paralysis. *J Bone Joint Surg Am* 1985; 67:360–369.

53. Schlegel J, Yuan H, Fredrickson B. Timing of surgical decompression and fixation of acute spinal fractures. *Ortho Trans* 1992; 16:688.

54. Wilmont CB, Hall KM. Evaluation of acute surgical intervention in traumatic paraplegia. *Paraplegia* 1986; 24:71–76.

55. Carlson GD, Minato Y, Okada A. Early time-dependent decompression for spinal cord injury: vascular mechanisms of recovery. *J Neurotrauma* 1997; 14(12):951–962.

56. Gaebler C, Maier R, Kutscha-Lissberg F. Results of spinal cord decompression and thoracolumbar pedicle stabilization in relation to the time of operation. *Spinal Cord* 1999; 37(1):33–39.

57. An HS, Vaccaro AR, Cotler JM. Low lumbar burst fractures: comparison among body cast, Harrington rod, Luque rod, and Steffe plate. *Spine* 1991; 16:440–444.

58. Garfin SR, Mowery CA, Guerra J. Confirmation of the posterolateral technique to decompress and fuse thoracolumbar spine burst fractures. *Spine* 1985; 10(3):218–223.

59. Whitesides TE. Traumatic kyphosis of the thoracolumbar spine. *Clin Orthop Relat Res* 1977; 128:78–92.

60. Cammisa FP, Eismont FJ, Green BA. Dural laceration occurring with burst fractures and associated laminar fractures. *J Bone Joint Surg Am* 1989; 71:1044–1052.

61. Hardaker WT, Cook WA, Friedman AH. Bilateral transpedicular decompression and Harrington rod stabilization in the management of severe thoracolumbar burst fractures. *Spine* 1992; 17(2):162–171.

62. Ahlgren BD, Herkowitz HN. A Modified posterolateral approach to the thoracic spine. *J Spinal Disord* 1995; 8(1):69–75.

63. Maiman DJ, Larson SJ. Lateral extracavitary approach to the thoracic and lumbar spine. In: Rengachary SS, Wilkins RH, eds. *Neurosurgical Operative Atlas.* Philadelphia: Williams and Wilkins, 1992:153–161.

64. Graham AW, MacMillan M, Fessler RG. Lateral extracavitary approach to the thoracic and thoracolumbar spine. *Orthopedics* 1997; 20(7):605–610.

65. Fessler RG, Dietz DD Jr, Millan MM, Peace D. Lateral parascapular extrapleural approach to the upper thoracic spine. *J Neurosurg* 1991; 75:349–355.

66. Crutcher JP Jr, Anderson PA, King HA, Montesano PX. Indirect spinal canal decompression in patients with thoracolumbar burst fractures treated by posterior distraction rods. *J Spinal Disord* 1991; 4:39–48.

67. Gertzbein SD, Crowe PL, Fazl M, Schwartz M, Rowed D. Canal clearance in burst fractures using the AO internal fixator. *Spine* 1992; 17:558–560.

68. Willen J, Lindahl S, Irstam L, Nordwall A. Unstable thoracolumbar fractures: a study by CT and conventional roentgenology of the reduction effect of Harrington instrumentation. *Spine* 1984; 9:214–219.

69. Danisa OA, Shaffrey CI, Jane JA, Whitehall R, et al. Surgical approaches for the correction of unstable thoracolumbar burst fractures: a retrospective analysis of treatment outcomes. *J Neurosurg* 1995; 83:977–983.

70. Been HD, Bouma GJ. Comparison of two types of surgery for thoracolumbar burst fractures: combined anterior and posterior stabilization vs. posterior instrumentation only. *Acta Neurochir* 1999; 141:349–357.

71. Esses SI, Botsford DJ, Kostuik JP. Evaluation of surgical treatment for burst fractures. *Spine* 1990; 15:667–673.

72. McAfee PC, Bohlman HH, Werner FW. Anterior decompression of traumatic thoracolumbar fractures with incomplete neurologic deficit using a retroperitoneal approach. *J Bone Joint Surg Am* 1985; 67:89–104.

73. Wood KB, Bohn D, Mehbod A. Anterior versus posterior treatment of stable thoracolumbar burst fractures without neurologic deficit: a prospective, randomized study. *J Spinal Disord Tech* 2005; 18(Suppl): S15–23.

74. Sasso RC, Renkens K, Hanson D, Reilly T, et al. Unstable thoracolumbar burst fractures: anterior-only versus short-segment posterior fixation. *J Spinal Disord Tech* 2006; 19:242–248.

III

MEDICAL MANAGEMENT

16 Respiratory Dysfunction in Spinal Cord Disorders

Ahmet Baydur
Catherine S.H. Sassoon

Data from the U.S. National Spinal Cord Injury Statistical Center reveal that the mortality rates for individuals with neurologically incomplete and complete cervical cord lesions are nine and eighteen times higher, respectively, than for those of the same age in the general population (1). Diseases of the respiratory system are the leading cause of death in patients with *cervical* spinal cord injuries (SCIs). Overall, 20% of deaths during the first 15 years after injury are caused by respiratory illnesses. Several factors adversely affect mortality, including the level of cord injury, age, preexisting cardiopulmonary disease, concomitant injuries, and delayed recognition of and attention to pulmonary problems (1–3). The level and the duration of cord injury have a significant impact on the function of the respiratory system and its defenses. To understand the extent of respiratory dysfunction in these patients, it is necessary to review the pathophysiology of respiratory dysfunction that causes alterations in the respiratory pump and respiratory system control mechanisms.

PATHOPHYSIOLOGY

Respiratory Muscles

The degree of respiratory impairment in patients with SCI depends on the level of the injury, although partially functioning segments may contribute to improved function. High cervical cord lesions (C1–C4) are associated with the greatest respiratory muscle dysfunction. Patients with lesions at C1 and C2 cannot maintain effective spontaneous ventilation. Low cervical cord lesions (C5–C8) affect the intercostal, parasternal, scalene, and abdominal muscles but leave the diaphragm, trapezii, sternocleidomastoid, and the clavicular portion of the pectoralis major muscles intact. Lesions at the thoracic level affect the intercostal and abdominal muscles, whereas lesions at lumbar levels cause little, if any, respiratory compromise.

Most studies on respiratory muscle function have been performed, in the seated position, in patients with chronic injury (defined as an injury of 1 year duration or longer) (4). Hopman and coworkers (5) showed that in patients with cord lesion at C4–C7, global respiratory muscle strength decreased when compared to that of control subjects matched for age and body mass.

In the study by Sinderby and coworkers (6), approximately 80% of patients with low cervical cord injury (C5–C8) had diaphragm muscle strength within the range of that of normal subjects (mean, 120 cm H_2O). Diaphragm muscle strength was measured as the maximum transdiaphragmatic pressure (PDI_{max}). Subjects achieved this maximum pressure using a visual feedback method in which the subject was encouraged to generate a target transdiaphragmatic pressure displayed on an oscilloscope (7). Despite the maintenance of inspiratory muscle and diaphragm muscle strength, both global inspiratory and diaphragm muscle endurance is limited in these patients. When they breathed against an incremental threshold load, the ratio of the pressure generated at the maximum load to the maximum inspiratory pressure (PI_{max}) was significantly lower than that of the control subjects (49% versus 82%), suggesting that the inspiratory muscles have limited capacity to generate pressure against the load (5). These findings indicate early development of inspiratory muscle fatigue (5). During resting breathing, the tension–time index of the diaphragm (TTDI), defined as the product of the ratio of mean transdiaphragmatic pressure (PDI) and PDI_{max}, and the duty cycle (TI/Ttot: the ratio of inspiratory time to total breath cycle duration, respectively) is higher than that of normal subjects (0.7 versus 0.4, respectively). This provides further evidence of diaphragm muscle fatigue (6, 8). In fact, during arm or leg ergometer exercises, seven of the ten patients with low cervical cord injury were observed to develop diaphragm muscle fatigue at low workloads, preceding the development of task failure (9). Despite the development of diaphragm muscle fatigue, those patients were still capable of increasing the PDI associated with increasing tidal volume (VT) and respiratory frequency (fr) until task failure. Furthermore, conditioning of the diaphragm with inspiratory resistive training (10) or phrenic nerve stimulations appears to improve strength and endurance of the diaphragm (11) and lung function (12).

In patients with low cervical cord injury, the diaphragm not only functions as the major inspiratory muscle, but also as a trunk extensor muscle (13). When performing forward trunk flexion, these patients exhibit continuous and augmented diaphragm electrical activity and abdominal pressures (14). During posture imbalance, the postural needs temporarily override the respiratory function, but this postural loading to the diaphragm risks the development of diaphragm muscle fatigue (13).

Paralysis of the abdominal muscles in patients with SCI results in ineffective cough and impaired clearance of airway secretions. To assist in cough, during forced expiration, patients with tetraplegia can recruit the clavicular portion of the pectoralis major to deflate the rib cage (15). Repetitive isometric contraction training of the pectoralis major for 6 weeks improves the expiratory function in these patients (16). Estenne and coworkers (17) demonstrated that the abdominal muscles retain their force-generating ability if they are stimulated by paired magnetic stimulation to the abdominal muscles. In these patients, abdominal muscle strength is 60% less than in healthy control subjects (14). Abdominal muscles also demonstrate phasic electrical activity when ventilatory demand increases; such activity is absent during tidal breathing (18). Its effect decreases the compliance of the abdominal wall, allowing the diaphragm to generate a greater intra-abdominal pressure during inspiration and causing improved inflation of the lower rib cage.

With paralysis of both the major inspiratory and expiratory muscles, as in patients with high spinal cord injury (C1–C2), De Troyer and coworkers (19) demonstrated that these patients can use the sternocleidomastoid muscles, as well as other neck muscles (trapezii, platysma, sterno, and mylohyoid) to sustain brief periods of spontaneous breathing. Contraction of these muscles expands the upper rib cage anteriorly, decreases pleural pressure, and is accompanied by a fall in intra-abdominal pressure, thus causing inward displacement of the lateral walls of the lower rib cage. Thus, the benefit of recruiting the accessory muscles to augment spontaneous breathing can be negated by the paradoxical movement of the lower rib cage.

Respiratory Mechanics

Lung Mechanics

During acute injury, the forced vital capacity (FVC) of patients with tetraplegia is markedly reduced, with no expiratory reserve volume detectable (20). Ledsome and Sharp (20) showed that 1 week after injury, the FVC of patients with tetraplegia (C5–C6) was 30%, and the forced expiratory volume in 1 sec (FEV1) was 27% of predicted normal value (20). Both FVC and FEV1 improve significantly at 5 weeks (45% and 42% of predicted, respectively) and continue to improve at 5 months after the injury (58% and 59% of predicted, respectively) (20). Gains in ventilatory parameters are small thereafter (4, 21). In the Ledsome and Sharp (20) study, five patients with injury to the lowest functional segment of C4 showed a mean FVC of 24% of predicted, and all of these patients required mechanical ventilatory support for 2 to 3 weeks. Three months postinjury, their FVC increased to 44% of predicted (range 18% to 62%).

The impaired function of the diaphragm in the acute stage of injury is attributable to the mechanical inefficiencies associated with paradoxical rib cage movement and unfavorable changes in thoracoabdominal compliance as a result of inspiratory muscle paralysis. The improvement of lung function over

time could be related to improved neurologic function in the cord segments at and above the injury level. The development of spasticity and reflex contraction of the intercostal and abdominal muscles may cause the rib cage to become more stable (22). In the acute stage, the degree of lung function impairment and the level of the injury are not predictive of the recovery of lung function (21).

In the chronic stage of injury, the level and completeness of injury, combined with tobacco smoking history, serve as predictors of lung function impairment (23, 24). Almenoff and coworkers (23) studied 165 patients with SCI. Patients with high complete cervical tetraplegia had lower FVC, FEV1, and peak expiratory flow (PEF) than those with incomplete lesions of the same and lower levels of injury. In the patients with low tetraplegia or high and low paraplegia, the extent of the motor lesion did not affect the degree of lung function impairment. Tobacco smoking played a significant role. The FEV1 and PEF in current smokers were markedly reduced compared with ex-smokers and those who never smoked.

Posture affects lung function in patients with SCI (24) (Figure 16.1). With the exception of vital capacity (VC), the direction of changes in total lung capacity (TLC) and functional residual capacity (FRC) is similar to that of healthy subjects: that is, both TLC and FRC decrease in the supine posture when compared to the seated posture (25, 26). In healthy subjects, VC decreases when changing from the upright to the supine posture (27). In contrast, patients with tetraplegia and high paraplegia exhibit VC increases when changing from the upright to the supine posture (24–26). Estenne and De Troyer (26) described supine position increases of 16% in tetraplegic subjects and 11% in paraplegic subjects (Figure 16.2). This increase in VC in the supine posture results primarily from the reduction in residual volume (RV) caused by the effect of gravity on the abdominal contents (Figure 16.3). The application of an abdominal binder helps to maintain the RV in the seated posture by compressing the abdominal contents into the diaphragm, thus improving thoracoabdominal compliance and placing the diaphragm at a more efficient, stretched, resting posture. This effect appears to be independent of changes in intrathoracic blood volume (26).

The lung compliance (CstL) of patients with acute and chronic tetraplegia is markedly reduced: approximately 52% of that of control healthy subjects (28). This reduction in CstL plateaus 1 month after the injury and does not change significantly over time. When CstL is corrected for lung volume, the mean value falls to near 70% of predicted value for healthy subjects (28). This suggests that the decrease in CstL is partly attributable to reduced lung volume and partly to the altered mechanical properties of the lung. De Troyer and Heilporn (29) demonstrated similar findings in their patients with chronic tetraplegia (CstL of 60% of predicted value for healthy subjects) in whom intercostal muscle activity was completely absent. Conversely, in the two patients in whom intercostal muscle electrical activity was detected, CstL was within normal limits (93% of predicted). The authors concluded that the intercostal muscles help to stabilize the chest wall and prevent lung collapse.

Chest Wall Mechanics

The chest wall compliance of patients with tetraplegia is also reduced. Estenne and De Troyer (30) studied thoracoabdominal

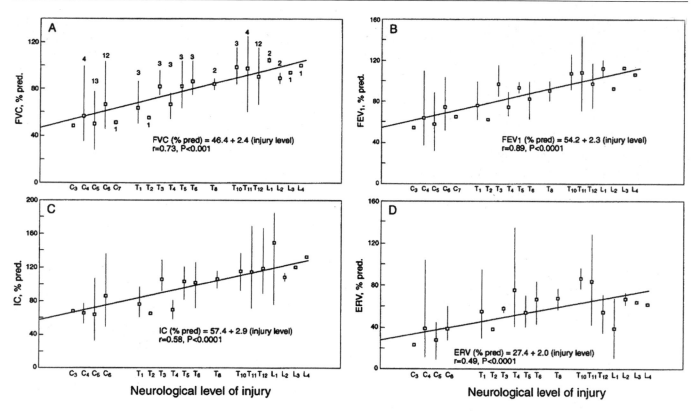

Figure 16.1   Spirometric variables in seated spinal cord–injured subjects distributed according to lesion level. (**A**) forced vital capacity (FVC; $n = 74$); (**B**) forced expiratory volume in 1 second (FEV$_1$; $n = 74$); (**C**) inspiratory capacity (IC; $n = 73$); (**D**) expiratory reserve volume (ERV; $n = 73$). Values are means and ranges of percent predicted (% pred.) values for healthy persons. Numbers above squares in A are number of subjects at each injury level and are the same for B–D. The individual with C7 tetraplegia did not have IC and ERV measured. (From Figure 1, reference 24, with permission.)

compliance in twenty patients with chronic tetraplegia. The thoracic compliance decreased to an average of 55% of normal, whereas the abdominal compliance increased to 170% of normal. Thus, the decreased chest wall compliance is primarily caused by the abnormally stiff rib cage in the chronic stage of injury (Table 16.1). The stiffened rib cage in these patients is likely caused by alterations in the elastic properties of the rib cage itself. These compliance changes result in greater abdominal

contribution to tidal volume, when compared to healthy subjects (31). In addition, when abdominal contents fall toward the pelvis as an upright posture is achieved, the diaphragm lacks a fulcrum; diaphragm contraction results in reduced lower rib cage expansion and further reduces tidal volume. The use of binders while

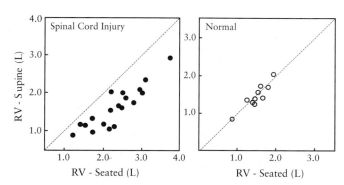

Figure 16.3   The effect of the supine and seated posture on residual volume (RV) in patients with SCI and in healthy subjects. The markedly reduced residual volume (RV) in the supine posture is responsible for the elevated vital capacity (see Figure 16.1) and is caused by the effect of gravity on the abdominal contents in those patients with paralyzed abdominal muscles. The dashed line is line of identity. (From reference 26, with permission.)

Figure 16.2   The effect of the supine and seated posture on vital capacity (VC) in patients with SCI and healthy subjects. In contrast to healthy subjects, the VC of patients with SCI (C4–T7) is higher in the supine than in the seated posture. The dashed line is line of identity. (From reference 26, with permission.)

Table 16.1   Static Lung and Chest Wall Compliance and Its Rib Cage and Abdominal Components in Patients with Quadriplegia

	L/cm H$_2$O	% Predicted
Static lung compliance	0.215 ± 0.010	73.4 ± 3.4
Static chest wall compliance	0.132 ± 0.009	72.1 ± 4.5
Rib cage compliance	0.085 ± 0.005	55.1 ± 3.4
Abdominal compliance	0.047 ± 0.004	170.7 ± 15.0

Values are mean ±SE; n = 20. (From reference 30 with permission.)

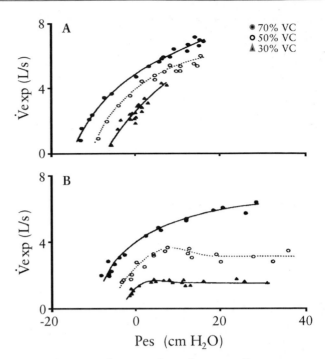

Figure 16.4 Isovolume esophageal pressure-flow curves computed at 70% (**closed circles**), 50% (**open circles**), and 30% (**closed triangles**) of vital capacity in representative patients with quadriplegia. (**A**) Patient without dynamic compression of the airways. (**B**) Patient with dynamic compression of the airways, as indicated by the flow plateau at 50% and 30% of vital capacity. (From reference 34, with permission.)

the patient is supine is not recommended, because restriction of the lower rib cage by this practice reduces tidal volumes.

Airway Mechanics

During cough, healthy subjects develop peak pleural pressures of greater than 100 cm H$_2$O (32). This induces dynamic compression of the intrathoracic airways, which causes the linear velocity and kinetic energy of the flowing gas to increase markedly (33), thus accelerating mucus secretions mouthward. Because of paralysis of the abdominal muscles, the cough effort is impaired in patients with SCI, particularly in patients with tetraplegia. Despite paralysis of the expiratory muscles, Estenne and coworkers (34) recently demonstrated evidence of dynamic airway compression in six of the twelve patients studied. Patients who demonstrated dynamic airway compression show an obvious flow plateau at lower lung volumes on the isovolume esophageal pressure flow curves (Figure 16.4). Direct observation with videoendoscopy confirms the dynamic compression of the airways in those patients. The results of this study suggest that contraction of the clavicular portion of the pectoralis major is capable of producing dynamic compression of the airways. For this reason, strength-training of the pectoralis major to enhance its pressure generating capacity will potentially enhance cough effort, particularly when combined with the application of an abdominal binder (34).

Although patients with tetraplegia demonstrate dynamic airway collapse, one study of patients with chronic tetraplegia demonstrated a significant bronchodilation effect with the administration of inhaled bronchodilator (35) and airway hyperreactivity to inhaled metacholine (36). The mechanism of this airway hyperresponsiveness is thought to be caused by the unopposed cholinergic tone, because the inhaled anticholinergic agent, ipatropium bromide, blocks the response (36–38). Similarly, the metacholine hyperresponsiveness is also blocked by baclofen, a gamma-aminobutyric acid (GABA) agonist. Through interaction with GABA receptors, baclofen inhibits the release of acetylcholine from the postganglionic cholinergic neurons that innervate the airway smooth muscle (39).

Control of Breathing

Pattern of Breathing

The resting breathing pattern in patients with tetraplegia is characterized by a small VT, an increased respiratory rate, and a VE

similar to that of age-matched healthy controls (40). The inspiratory time (TI) is the same as in controls, whereas the expiratory time (TE) is significantly shortened, thus accounting for the increase in respiratory frequency. Mean inspiratory flow rate (VT/Ti) is smaller than in controls. In the seated position, when VT is partitioned between the rib cage and abdominal compartments, expansion of the abdomen is associated with expansion of the lower rib cage. However, rib cage expansion is greater in the transverse than in the anteroposterior diameter. In addition, many of these patients have a reduced anteroposterior diameter of the upper rib cage (paradoxical rib cage motion) (41–43) (Figure 16.5). This paradoxical rib cage motion is predominantly seen in the supine rather than in the seated posture and is caused by a paralysis of the rib cage inspiratory muscles, particularly the parasternal intercostals and the scalenes. This paradoxical rib cage motion is less frequently seen in SCI patients with injury at or below C7, because of the persistent activity of the scalene muscles (41).

Ventilatory Drive

Studies on the control of breathing in patients with tetraplegia have shown conflicting results (43–46). The drive to breathe can be assessed as the ventilatory or occlusion pressure response to hypercapnia during CO$_2$ rebreathing. The occlusion pressure is the airway or mouth pressure measured at 0.1 seconds when the subject breathes against an occlusion; this is commonly called P0.1. P0.1 reflects the neuromuscular drive, unaffected by

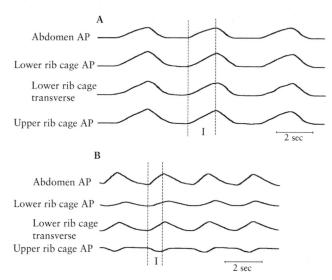

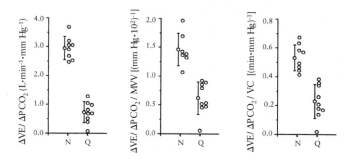

Figure 16.6 Left panel: Ventilatory response to hypercapnia ($\Delta VE/\Delta PCO_2$) in nine patients with quadriplegia (Q) and eight normal (N) subjects. **Middle panel**: The ventilatory response to hypercapnia normalized for maximum voluntary ventilation (MVV). **Right panel**: The ventilatory response to hypercapnia normalized for vital capacity (VC), respectively. The ventilatory response to hypercapnia in patients with Q is significantly less than in N subjects ($p < 0.001$), even when normalized for indices of respiratory muscle performance. **Circles** are mean values; **bars** are standard deviation. (From reference 46, with permission.)

Figure 16.5 The pattern of breathing in a healthy control subject (**A**) and in a patient with C5 SCI (**B**) partitioned into the abdominal and rib cage compartments. The figure shows the respiratory changes in anteroposterior (AP) diameter of the abdomen, lower rib cage (at the fifth costal cartilage), and upper rib cage (at manubrium sterni). Changes in the transverse diameter of the lower rib cage are shown with an upward deflection indicating an increase, and a downward deflection indicating a decrease in diameter. I indicates the duration of inspiration. In the healthy subject, the abdomen and the rib cage diameters increase uniformly and synchronously. In the patient with quadriplegia, the lower ribcage expands more in the transverse than in the AP diameter, and the upper rib cage AP diameter decreases rather than increases (paradoxical motion of the upper rib cage). (From reference 42, with permission.)

alterations in respiratory system mechanics. One study in patients with chronic tetraplegia (C4–C7) noted that the slope of the ventilatory and P0.1 responses to hypercapnia were similar to those of the control subjects (43). This finding was attributed to the incomplete nature of the spinal injury and the relatively low ventilatory response in the control subjects. In other studies, depression of the ventilatory and P0.1 responses to hypercapnia was found after SCI. This was attributed to respiratory muscle weakness (44), decreased compliance (44), and/or altered geometry of the chest wall (45). Manning and coworkers (46) demonstrated that tetraplegic patients (C5–C8) having complete cord injury for at least 1 year had blunting of the ventilatory and P0.1 responses to hypercapnia. The slope of the ventilatory response to hypercapnia was significantly less than in control subjects, and the P0.1 response to CO_2 was lower in the patients than in the control group. Even after normalizing the above values with indices of respiratory muscle function—that is, maximal voluntary ventilation and vital capacity (VC)—the responses remained low (Figure 16.6). The blunting of the hypercapnic response does not seem to be mediated by endogenous opioids, because the administration of naloxone did not improve the response (46). The authors also studied two subjects with acute cord injury in whom sequential measurements were obtained over 7 to 8 months. The blunted hypercapnic response persisted despite a 50% increase in VC, a 67% increase in PI_{max}, and a marked

increase in expiratory reserve volume (ERV) (Figure 16.7). This suggests that, in patients with tetraplegia, respiratory muscle weakness alone does not explain the blunted hypercapnic response and that these patients have impairment in chemoreceptor function. In contrast to respiratory center response to hypercapnia, information regarding the respiratory center response to hypoxia after tetraplegic injury is limited and inconclusive (43).

Individuals with SCI have a reduced ability to regulate body temperature due to impaired innervation of sweat glands and cutaneous blood vessels (47, 48). A recent study of ten patients with C4–L5 spinal injuries showed that such individuals displayed a greater ventilatory frequency response than able-bodied subjects to an equivalent heat stress (a heated water-perfusion garment) (49). Subjects with a greater reduction in heat loss capacity displayed a more pronounced ventilatory response, although the authors believed that this was too modest a response to represent a thermal adaptation in humans with spinal cord injury. The ventilatory response could have been a result of changes in carbon dioxide sensitivity with heating, catecholamine production, hypothalamus interaction with respiratory control centers, or a combination of these factors.

Load Compensation

Despite the blunted response to hypercapnia, tetraplegic patients free of hypoxemia have the ability to compensate for an increased mechanical load, such as breathing against added inspiratory resistance (43). An added inspiratory resistive load results in an increase in the P0.1 response to hypercapnia when compared to that of the unloaded condition (43). Neural inspiratory drive, estimated as the rate of rise of the moving average of the diaphragmatic electromyogram (EMG), also increased with an added load (45). These responses were similar to those seen in normal subjects. Likewise, the ventilatory and P0.1 responses to hypercapnia remain unchanged with change in posture from the supine position to a 60-degree tilted position (50) or seated position (51)

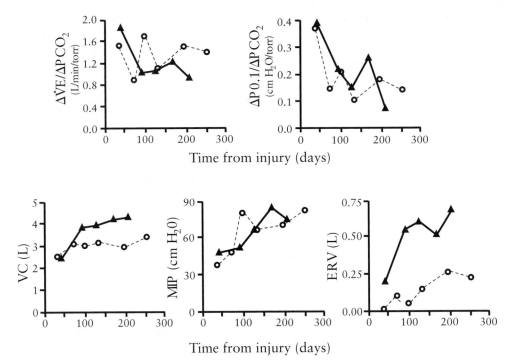

Figure 16.7   Upper panel: Sequential measurements of the ventilatory ($\Delta VE/\Delta PCO_2$) and occlusion pressure ($\Delta P0.1/\Delta PCO_2$) responses to hypercapnia and respiratory muscle function in two patients with acute quadriplegia. **Lower panel**: Improvement in respiratory muscle function, vital capacity (VC), and maximum inspiratory pressure (MIP) was not associated with an increase in the ventilatory or occlusion pressure response to hypercapnia. The circles and triangles represent each of the two patients. (From reference 46, with permission.)

(which foreshortens the diaphragm and places it at a mechanical disadvantage). Sassoon et al. (52) noted that the rate of rise of the diaphragmatic electromyogram response to hypercapnia was significantly higher in the seated than in the supine position, a change that was not observed in a control group. Hence, the compensatory increase in diaphragmatic activation with ventilatory loading or change in posture remains intact, despite disrupted afferent feedback from rib cage mechanoreceptors.

When tetraplegic patients are challenged with an inspiratory resistive load, VT is preserved through the use of defenses similar to those employed by healthy controls (53). However, the inspiratory duration is significantly less than in controls (54). In control subjects, the prolonged inspiratory duration during breathing against inspiratory resistive load serves to minimize peak pressure, a variable directly proportional to the sensation of dyspnea (53, 55). This is achieved at the expense of the increased energy requirements of the inspiratory muscles (53). Thus, under loaded condition, the intensity of central neural output in patients with SCI is maintained to achieve adequate VT, but the respiratory timing component is altered, partly as a result of chest wall receptor activity, perhaps in an attempt to minimize energy requirements (56).

Sensation of Dyspnea

In healthy subjects, the sensation of dyspnea that is perceived as "air hunger" can be distinguished from dyspnea perceived as increased "work and effort" (57). Perceived "air hunger" is consistently associated with changes in PCO_2, whereas perceived

"work and effort" is associated with changes in ventilation. The sensation of "air hunger" arises as a result of chemoreceptor afferent activity or medullary corollary discharge (57, 58). Conversely, the sensation of "work and effort" arises from respiratory muscle mechanoreceptors, awareness of cortical motor drive to respiratory muscles, or both (57). In patients with SCI, the perception of "air hunger" to increased PCO_2 or reduced tidal volume is intact. Manning and coworkers (59) studied the sensation of "air hunger" in ventilator-dependent patients with C2–C3 quadriplegia. In this study, first VT and the respiratory frequency of the ventilator were maintained constant at baseline ventilator settings while end-tidal CO_2 ($P_{ET}CO_2$) was increased. Then, VT was reduced to 40% to 70% of baseline VT, while $P_{ET}CO_2$ was maintained constant. The sensation of "air hunger" correlated significantly with the mean $P_{ET}CO_2$. Similarly, there was a correlation between VT and the sensation of "air hunger," although the sensation of "work or effort" was not evaluated. Nevertheless, these findings suggest that the sensation of "air hunger" in patients with tetraplegia is intact, and its modification is independent of afferent information from the chest wall.

MANAGEMENT OF RESPIRATORY COMPLICATIONS

Respiratory Complications

Respiratory failure following acute SCI may occur because of partial or complete respiratory muscle paralysis, fatigue of remaining intact muscles, or in association with pleuropulmonary pathology. Jackson and Groomes (60), in their study of 205 patients with high quadriplegia (C1–C4), found the most common complications were atelectasis in 40% and pneumonia in 63% of the patients. These findings are similar to those in Fishburn's study (61), which showed a 50% incidence of atelectasis or pneumonia in spinal cord–injured patients with injury level from C3 to T11.

The occurrence of respiratory complications in patients with acute SCI contributes significantly to both length of stay and hospital costs during the initial admission. In a study of 413 cervically injured patients, Winslow et al. (62) found that mechanical ventilation, occurrence of pneumonia, need for surgery, and use of tracheostomy account for nearly 60% of the variance in hospital costs. Each of these variables, when considered independently, was a better predictor of hospital costs than was the level of injury. The authors concluded that the number of complications experienced during the initial acute care hospitalization was a more important determinant of length of stay and hospital costs than was level of injury.

Low cervical SCI can also pose a major risk for potentially fatal airway and pulmonary complications. In a retrospective study of 186 patients with C5–T1 cord injuries (58% complete), the overall pneumonia rate was 50%, and mortality was 15% (66% and 26%, respectively, in those with complete lesions), with 68% requiring intubation, of which two-thirds needed tracheostomy (50% of incomplete SCI required tracheostomy for intractable respiratory failure) (63). Complications requiring long-term support are common following lower cervical SCI, especially in those with complete lesions. Early intubation is mandatory for complete SCI patients, and also for incomplete SCIs at the first signs of respiratory failure.

Anterior cervical spine surgery may result in regional edema or hematoma and upper airway, carotid artery, recurrent laryngeal nerve, vertebral artery, or stellate ganglion injury if dissection occurs at the C7–T2 level (64). These complications can lead to airway compromise and predispose the patient to postextubation respiratory complications. The overall complication rate following anterior cervical surgery is approximately 6% (65). Exposure of three or more vertebral levels, exposure involving C2 through C4, and an intraoperative time of more than 5 hours are risk factors associated with airway complications. About one-third of the airway complications require reintubation (65). Many of these reintubations may be difficult. In the presence of cervical spine abnormalities, fiberoptic intubation is the preferred means of intubation.

The use of the halo vest to provide stability to the spine in the management of patients with SCI has been shown to produce as much as a 9% decrease in forced vital capacity in supine cervical and high thoracic-injured patients (66). However, this decline in VC is not clinically significant in comparison to the decline in VC (13%) when changing from the supine to seated posture. Maloney et al. (67) and Goldman et al. (68) have reported that an abdominal binder can support the abdomen, forcing the diaphragm cephalad, and thus improving VC in the sitting position in quadriplegics.

Many patients with high cervical cord injury will recover substantial respiratory function following the acute insult (20, 69, 70). Ledsome and Sharp (20) measured the vital capacity (VC) sequentially in patients still breathing spontaneously after cervical spinal damage and demonstrated a progressive improvement

from 31% to 58% of predicted VC between the first and 20th week. In a retrospective study, Carter et al. (69) showed that of the twenty-two patients with injury level at and below C4 with unilateral diaphragmatic paralysis, sixteen (73%) had improvement of VC after a mean interval of 76 days, with the longest duration for recovery being 14 months. Even patients with a C2–C3 level of injury can expect a significant recovery of diaphragmatic function. Oo et al. (70) found that 25% of patients with a VC of 15 ml/kg could be weaned off ventilatory support between 93 and 430 (mean 246) days after injury; those with a VC of 10 ml/kg weaned later, after an average of 290 days. The weaning time is likely to be influenced by the duration of paralysis because those recovering after prolonged paralysis have to regain diaphragmatic function.

Cough Effort and Secretion Clearance

Patients with neuromuscular disorders have diminished cough capacity, primarily because of expiratory muscle weakness (71). When these patients, including those who have SCI, contract an upper respiratory infection, they often produce airway secretions that they cannot clear because of an ineffective cough (72). The most difficult problem is in the acute phase of the cord injury, when large amounts of secretions are produced because of unopposed vagal tone (73). This leads to acute respiratory distress, hypoxemia, worsening hypercapnia (which may be superimposed on chronic alveolar hypoventilation), and the need for intubation for ventilatory support and airway suctioning. When the expiratory muscles are assisted to help eliminate secretions, these events can often be avoided.

Cough flows will be diminished when (a) the patient cannot inhale at least 1.5 L because of weak inspiratory muscles; (b) inadequate thoracic abdominal pressures cannot be generated because of weak abdominal muscles or loss of glottic control; (c) weakened bulbar muscles or tracheostomy preclude firm glottic closure or upper airway stability during the cough; or (d) irreversible airway obstruction occurs, such as with tracheal stenosis or chronic obstructive pulmonary disease. To prevent pneumonia and respiratory failure, these patients more often receive supplemental oxygen and physical therapy to clear airway secretions, rather than modalities to assist their respiratory muscles.

Kang et al. (74) described three assisted cough techniques in forty cervical SCI patients as generating higher values of VC, MIP, and MEP than during unassisted cough efforts. The MIP showed a more significant correlation with the voluntary or assisted cough capacity than the MEP.

Assisted Cough Techniques

As a rule, anyone with a VC below 1.5 L should receive a maximal insufflation delivered by a manual resuscitator or portable volume ventilator to achieve adequate cough flows. This action alone can more than double peak cough flows (75). Once an optimal volume is reached, the expiratory muscles can either be self-assisted or manually assisted by one of several methods that require care-provider assistance (76). Manually assisted coughing techniques include the *costophrenic assist*, the *Heimlich-type* or abdominal thrust assist, the *anterior chest compression* assist, and the *counterrotation* assist (75, 76). Most individuals with inadequate vital capacities but good bulbar muscle function can also be taught glossopharyngeal breathing to obtain optimal volume (77).

Mechanically Assisted Coughing

Mechanical insufflation-exsufflation involves the delivery of a maximal insufflation followed immediately by a decrease in pressure of about 80 cm H_2O. It is indicated if the individual cannot maintain a spontaneous VC of at least 1.5 L because of weak oropharyngeal muscles. Mechanical insufflation-exsufflation can generate as much as 600 L/min of expiratory flow that exsufflates (sucks out) the airways. Insufflation-exsufflation can be applied through a full-face mask, a simple mouthpiece, or a translaryngeal or tracheostomy tube (Figure 16.8). It is most effective when bulbar muscle function and airway patency are adequate to permit manually assisted peak cough flows of 160 L/min or greater. The ability to generate adequate peak cough flows is more important than the ability to breathe in, because it permits the long-term management of individuals with high cervical cord injuries (78). Mechanical insufflation-exsufflation can be simpler and easier than manually assisted coughing, which requires a cooperative patient, good coordination between the patient and caregiver, and adequate physical effort and frequent application.

A weaning approach, emphasizing noninvasive inspiratory and expiratory muscle aids, can eliminate the need for indwelling tracheostomy tubes and tracheal suctioning in appropriate SCI individuals. In addition to the cost reduction, ventilator users who are converted from tracheostomy to predominantly noninvasive positive pressure ventilation (NPPV) for long-term ventilatory support prefer it for safety, convenience, comfort, speech, swallowing, sleep, and appearance (79). Evidence also suggests that noninvasively supported 24-hour ventilator users with functional bulbar musculature have significantly fewer respiratory complications than tracheostomy-supported patients (78).

Fiberoptic bronchoscopy (FOB) should be reserved for atelectasis resulting from large mucus plugs, which cannot be removed by manual or mechanical coughing measures. Because FOB may cause tracheobronchial irritation, edema, hypoxemia, and aspiration, this technique is usually reserved for patients who have not responded to more conservative measures, such as use of curved-tip suction catheters for left lower lobe atelectasis (80), prone positioning, bronchodilators, and careful hydration to ensure liquid secretions.

Another device shown to be effective in the clearance of secretions is high-frequency chest wall oscillation (HFCWO), which consists of an inflatable vest connected by tubes to a generator. During therapy, the vest inflates and deflates rapidly, applying gentle pressure to the chest wall, facilitating the loosening and removal of thin mucus to move it toward the larger airways, where it can be cleared by coughing or suctioning (81–83) (Figure 16.9). There have been no studies comparing outcome in manual and machine-assisted cough techniques with HFCWO in patients with SCI.

Ventilatory Assistance

Tracheostomy-assisted Intermittent Positive Pressure Ventilation (T-IPPV)

Tracheostomy and T-IPPV have been the mainstay in the long-term management of the high-level SCI patient. The tracheostomy is also maintained in patients using electrophrenic stimulation because of the tendency of these patients to experience upper airway collapse during sleep (84) and as a safety measure in the event of phrenic pacer failure. Indications for assisted ventilation in the SCI individual are listed in Table 16.2. Because of an increased incidence of sleep-disordered breathing in SCI individuals, periodic evaluation of lung function and nocturnal monitoring of oxyhemoglobin saturation and end-tidal PCO_2 should be done to determine the need for assisted ventilation (77).

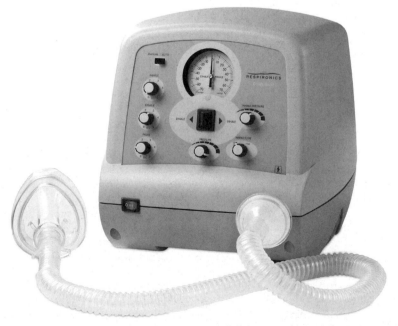

Figure 16.8 Mechanical insufflation-exsufflation device with tubing and full-face mask used to assist in expelling secretions from lungs. (Image courtesy of Philips Respironics, Murrysville, PA.)

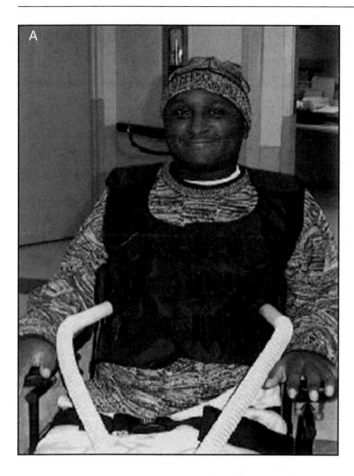

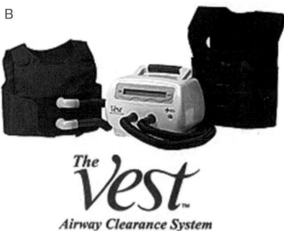

The Vest ™

Airway Clearance System

Figure 16.9 (**A**) A cervical cord–injured individual receiving high-frequency chest wall oscillation by means of a Chest Vest™ system. After being hospitalized for pneumonia a year and a half earlier, the patient has remained infection free, and out of the hospital. He was able to have his tracheostomy removed soon after he started treatments (30 minutes each morning). After discharge from the hospital, he has maintained independence in the community, continuing his rehabilitation program. (**B**) Components of the Vest™ system. (© 2006 Hill-Rom Services, Inc. Reprinted with permission—all rights reserved.)

Table 16.2 Indications for Assisted Ventilation in Individuals with Quadriplegia and Respiratory Failure

A. Signs and Symptoms:
- Clinical evidence of inspiratory muscle fatigue: Dyspnea, tachypnea . 30 breaths/min, paradoxical breathing (chest-abdomen asynchrony)
- Sleep dysfunction [frequent nocturnal awakenings (> 3), difficult arousals, morning or continuous headaches]
- Hypersomnolence
- Difficulty with concentration
- Irritability, anxiety
- Impaired intellectual function
- Cor pulmonale
- Polycythemia

B. Physiologic Criteria:
- FVC < 10 ml/kg or 25 percent predicted
- MVV < 25 percent predicted (< 40 L/min in males, < 25 L/min in females)
- PI_{max} < 50 cm H2O
- Daytime PaCO2 > 50 mm Hg

Abbreviations: FVC, forced vital capacity; MVV, maximum voluntary ventilation; PI_{max}, maximal inspiratory mouth pressure.

Morbidity and mortality are high with T-IPPV. Whiteneck et al. (85) reported that 55% of ventilator-dependent SCI patients experienced yearly pulmonary problems with an average hospital stay of 22 days per year. The survival rate in this study was 40% at 5 to 9 years postinjury (85). Splaingard (86) reported 37% mortality in 3 years for twenty-six traumatic SCI patients on T-IPPV, including twenty patients with C1–C3 quadriplegia. Carter et al. (87) reported a 49% mortality rate in thirty-five respirator-dependent tetraplegic patients on T-IPPV or electrophrenic respiration at a mean of 1.5 years postinjury or 4 years after pacemaker placement, respectively. Late ventilator weaning can occur months to years postinjury (88, 89).

Continuous ventilation at high volumes can help prevent the development of atelectasis, a common problem in the acute setting. When it is used judiciously, the risks of complications from bronchopleural air leak, alveolar damage (volutrauma, pulmonary edema), and altered hemodynamics can be minimized. Peterson and colleagues (90) compared the weaning ability of twenty-three individuals with C3–C4 quadriplegia receiving low VT ventilation (<20 ml/kg body weight) with nineteen individuals who received high VT ventilation (>20 ml/kg body weight). Although the two groups were equivalent in neurologic level and completeness, muscular function, initial spontaneous VC, the weaning method used (T-piece), and final spontaneous VC, those in the large VT group successfully weaned an average of 21 days faster than the lower VT group (38 days versus 59 days, $p = 0.02$). Complications (mostly pneumonia) were few and occurred at about the same rate in both groups.

With the widespread use of endotracheal methods, complications related to tracheostomy and long-term T-IPPV are numerous. These include nosocomial pneumonia, mucus plugging, cardiac arrhythmias, accidental disconnection, chronic purulent bronchitis, granulation tissue formation, stomal infections, sinusitis, tracheomalacia, tracheal perforation, hemorrhage, stenosis, fistula, vocal cord paralysis, and hypopharyngeal muscle dysfunction (2). The tracheostomy tube requires special attention, including regular bronchial suctioning, site care, and cannula changes. Swallowing difficulties may occur as a result of impediment to the strap muscles, glottic closure and cricopharyngeal sphincter function, and compression of the esophagus. Tracheal suctioning may cause irritation, bleeding, the formation of granulation tissues, increased secretions, and hypoxia. Suctioning often misses the left main bronchus (61).

Critical pathways have been espoused as effective means to improve outcomes in SCI patients. In a retrospective study of ninety-eight patients with cervical spinal injury, Nates et al. (91) demonstrated a significant and consistent decrease in length of hospital stay, ventilator days, and costs in the neurotrauma intensive care unit over a period of 27 months when compared to a historical unit data preceding the implementation of the spinal cord pathway. There were also significant advantages of admitting patients to the neurotrauma unit when compared to admission to other specialty intensive care units.

Noninvasive Ventilation

Noninvasive (i.e., nontracheostomy-assisted) positive pressure ventilation (NPPV) is increasingly used as an alternative for patients with chronic respiratory insufficiency. Such techniques have been described mostly in the management of patients with muscular dystrophy and poliomyelitis (77, 92, 93). Until the early 1980s, the literature concerning these methods was mostly limited to the application of body (negative pressure, "iron lung") ventilators (77, 93). Upper airway collapse and aspiration are

potential complications, and many patients are unable to tolerate this method of ventilation over an extended period. Respiratory support by intermittent positive pressure via a variety of nasal or oral interfaces has been used to support individuals with various neuromuscular and chest wall disorders (77, 89, 94). Bach and Alba (89) showed that twenty-three of twenty-five ventilated patients with traumatic tetraplegia could be converted from tracheostomies to noninvasive ventilation through a carefully monitored sequence of manual and mechanical coughing techniques, progressive tracheostomy cuff deflation, and adjustment of delivered ventilator volumes for adequate insufflation and speech. Some patients can master the use of mouth IPPV or learn glossopharyngeal breathing to supplement tidal volumes.

The biphasic positive airway pressure system (BiPAP) is a simple, mechanical system that provides noninvasive respiratory pressure support via nasal mask (Figure 16.10). Unlike continuous positive airway pressure, it has the ability to provide different levels of inspiratory and expiratory positive airway pressure. The latter also provides positive end-expiratory pressure. Tromans et al. (95) were able to apply BiPAP successfully in twenty-eight patients. This technique was shown to be useful in preventing respiratory failure and as a means of facilitating weaning from full-time ventilation.

Of the ventilator devices available for home use, the pneumobelt (a cyclically inflated corset) may have advantages as an option for interim or permanent ventilation of high SCI individuals without severe bulbar dysfunction. Miller et al. (96) described their experience using the pneumobelt in high tetraplegic patients. Twelve subjects were able to progress within days to up to 4 hours of continuous use, and thereafter to 12-hour

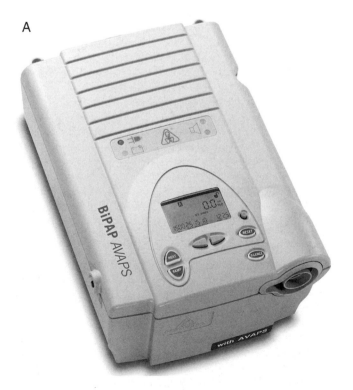

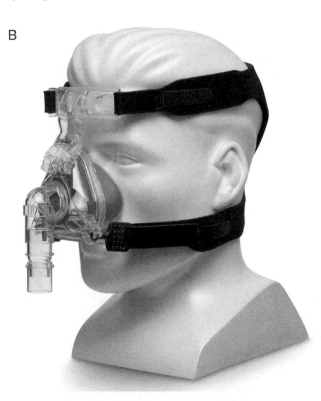

Figure 16.10 **(A)** A compact and lightweight bilevel airway pressure unit with a user interface and an integrated heated humidifier. This device can be used in patients with other neuromuscular disorders and in selected patients with advanced chronic obstructive lung disease. **(B)** An example of a nasal interface used in noninvasive ventilation. (Images courtesy of Philips Respironics, Murrysville, PA.)

or all-day use. The major advantages included improved appearance (no tracheostomy), speech, and mobility. Disadvantages included pump noise, promotion of stomach gas, and positioning difficulties. By placing the corset's horizontal upper border approximately two finger breadths below the costophrenic junction, one can avoid the paradoxical expansion of the chest caused by enclosure of the lower thorax, as described by Hill (97). The pneumobelt's major limitation is that individuals must be sitting upright to use it. This device employs the same principle as the rocking (oscillating) bed in displacing abdominal contents.

Electrophrenic Pacing

The main indications for electrophrenic stimulation are ventilatory insufficiency caused by disruption of central control over phrenic nerve motoneurons and malfunction of the respiratory control center (84). Diaphragmatic pacemakers cannot be used in patients with respiratory muscle paralysis resulting from phrenic nerve (cell body) damage, parenchymal lung disease, or acute respiratory failure. High cervical cord injuries are treatable by diaphragmatic pacing, provided that the lower motoneurons of the phrenic nerves (C3–C5) are intact (98). In addition, SCI individuals should be neurologically stable for at least 3 months, and long-term access to technological and clinical support services must be present. Full time ventilatory support can often be achieved with progressive conditioning of the diaphragm, usually after 3 to 4 months of bilateral pacing (98).

Ventilation by phrenic pacing provides certain advantages to the user (99, 100). It circumvents the need for positive pressure ventilation and attendant potential problems with the tracheostomy. It can improve the ability to speak and smell more normally, reduce the risk of accidental interruption of ventilation, provide greater independence, and reduce costs and time for ventilatory care (101). It can, however, increase the risk of upper airway collapse and aspiration of secretions. Fodstadt (102) reported the outcomes in forty patients using diaphragm pacing unilaterally, on alternate sides or on both sides simultaneously, 8 to 24 hours daily. Five tetraplegics used their pacers at different time intervals during sleep and intermittently during wakefulness. Six tetraplegics stopped pacing after intermittent phrenic nerve stimulation for 1 month to 3 years. By lengthening the pulse duration, adjusting the threshold ramp, and changing the inspiratory time, it was possible to increase tidal volumes, decrease upper airway resistance, and achieve smoother diaphragmatic contractions.

A permanent tracheostomy is usually a necessity with fulltime pacing to keep the upper airway unobstructed. There is a lack of coordination between the paced diaphragm, the upper airway muscles, and the accessory respiratory muscles in these patients. Upper airway resistance is augmented by diaphragmatic contraction or diminished inspiratory upper airway muscular activity and may be induced by diaphragmatic pacing during sleep in patients with SCI (103).

Quality-of-Life Issues in Ventilated Individuals

The incidence of traumatic SCI in the United States varies between 7,000 and 10,000 cases annually. Although 41% of all SCI individuals require mechanical ventilation at some time during the initial hospitalization, far fewer patients require ventilatory support at discharge. Despite this, more patients with ventilator-dependent tetraplegia are surviving; 2% of patients were discharged utilizing ventilators in 1973, compared to 6% through 1986 (104). Although substantial personal care needs are required for all individuals with tetraplegia, there is a widely held belief that being dependent on a ventilator is inconsistent with a high quality of life. Most of the literature on the quality of life in this population has focused on the mentally incompetent or terminally ill individuals for whom ventilator use does not prolong meaningful life (105). Bach and Tilton (106) evaluated the effects of complete traumatic tetraplegia on the life satisfaction and well-being of eighty-seven persons, forty-two of whom were ventilator supported 2 or more years after injury. The ventilator-assisted individuals with tetraplegia were significantly more satisfied with their housing, family life, and employment (when applicable) than were the spontaneously breathing tetraplegics. Only 24% of the ventilator-assisted tetraplegic patients expressed general dissatisfaction with their lives, compared with 36% of the spontaneously breathing individuals.

Another longitudinal study by Krause (107) found that an SCI individual's life satisfaction continued to improve over a 15-year period, which started at least 2 years after injury. The ventilator-dependent individuals, with more limited functional abilities than spontaneously breathing SCI patients, seem to place more importance on their family lives and personal relationships in evaluating their quality of life.

Ventilatory Muscle Training in Quadriplegia

One of the first clinical applications of respiratory muscle training was diaphragm training in tetraplegic patients (10). Some patients are dyspneic in the upright position (while performing daily activities). This is caused by the caudal displacement of the diaphragm, which results in a shortening of its resting length. In these patients, respiratory infections can increase respiratory load and reduce breathing reserves. Gross et al. (10) thought it reasonable to train the diaphragm for increased strength and endurance under heavy loads at near-normal ventilations. The method chosen was voluntary eupneic inspiratory resistive training in tetraplegic patients. These authors demonstrated a significant and progressive increase in PI_{max} at FRC and in the critical inspiratory mouth pressure that developed in each inspiration below which electromyographic changes of diaphragmatic fatigue (i.e., a decrease in the ratio of high to low amplitude of the diaphragmatic electromyogram) did not develop.

Other training programs have been described in tetraplegia. Huldtgren et al. (108) assessed lung volumes and PI_{max} in patients who were treated 15 minutes a day for 6 weeks by lung insufflation using a manually operated pump and performing forced voluntary expirations and inspirations against a resistance. TLC, ERV, and VC all improved significantly upon treatment. Maximum expiratory pressure (PE_{max}) and PI_{max} more than doubled after 6 weeks of treatment. Interestingly, however, Huldtgren et al. (108) found that although lung volumes remained well preserved in five patients who were reassessed 5 years after treatment, PI_{max} values had deteriorated toward pretreatment values. These findings are consistent with the spontaneous improvement (without muscle training) in VC and other lung volumes seen several weeks following injury in SCI individuals, but also the near return to baseline of muscle force generation after cessation of nonresistive ventilatory muscle endurance training in subjects with cystic fibrosis (109). Similar improvements in respiratory function were found by Rutchik et al. (110), who employed inspiratory resistive training over 8 weeks. By contrast, however, these authors found that in seven subjects in whom measurements were obtained 6 months later, both FVC and PI_{max} remained preserved.

The endurance-type challenge offered by inspiratory resistive breathing is compatible with the predominant recruitment of Type I (slow) fibers (111). Endurance training has previously been shown to reprogram the genetic expression pattern of skeletal muscle, transforming its components to make it more resistant (112). Recently Gea et al. (113) showed that breathing against moderate levels of inspiratory resistance quickly induces an increase in expression of the genes encoding the slow isoform of myosin-heavy chain (MyHC) in canine respiratory muscles. Thus, even transient respiratory overloads affect the phenotypic characteristics of muscles. The type of MyHC is the main factor that determines the velocity of muscle contraction, ATPase activity, and hence, the rate of muscle fatigue. Fibers consisting of slow MyHC isoforms produce slow, economic contractions, whereas fast MyHC isoforms are adapted to producing rapid, powerful movements. An interesting implication of the study of Gea et al. (113) is the possibility of inducing a phenotypic adaptation of respiratory muscles in humans through the use of a training protocol designed to increase endurance.

De Troyer et al. (15) demonstrated the expiratory activity generated by the clavicular portion of the pectoralis major during voluntary expiratory efforts in tetraplegic subjects (see above). This was demonstrated by an expiratory reserve volume that averaged 0.5 L in the seated position. Because the pectoralis major has a motor innervation from C5 to C7, its function is at least partly preserved after transection of the lower cervical cord, and its insertion on the medial half of the clavicle enables it to pull down the manubrium and upper ribs. This action results in the compression of the upper portion of the rib cage and partial deflation of the lungs. Thus, cough in tetraplegic patients results from more than just passive elastic recoil of the respiratory system (114). By binding the abdomen with a nonelastic strap and strengthening the clavicular portion of the pectoralis major through an appropriate training program (16), patients with SCI can increase their cough effort and clear bronchial secretions. They might also be able to generate higher intrathoracic pressures and expiratory flows using techniques described by Bach (75).

Pharmacologic Therapy

In addition to the restrictive respiratory impairment described in individuals with SCI, it has been recently reported that approximately 40% of otherwise healthy tetraplegics undergoing routine pulmonary function testing demonstrate a significant bronchodilator response (>12%) following inhalation of metaproterenol (35) or ipatropium bromide (38). These findings suggest that many individuals with SCI, in addition to their restrictive impairment, have an obstructive ventilatory impairment characterized by an increase in airway tone. Furthermore, such individuals also demonstrate airway hyperresponsiveness with methacholine challenge testing, a response that is completely blocked by ipatropium bromide (37). These findings support the

hypothesis that airway hyperresponsiveness in tetraplegic patients represents loss of sympathetic innervation of the lung, thereby leaving intact unopposed bronchoconstrictor cholinergic activity. However, the reduced lung volumes in these subjects also suggest the possibility that airway hyperresponsiveness is caused by the loss of the ability to stretch airway smooth muscle by deep breathing (115, 116). Not only do patients with SCI experience atelectasis and pneumonia as major causes of morbidity and mortality, but many also complain of chronic cough (18% to 23%), sputum production (24% to 50%) and wheeze (37% to 50%) (35, 117). Some subjects in these studies were current or former smokers, indicating that, despite variable respiratory muscle loss, associated respiratory symptoms do not mask those caused by smoking (i.e., sputum production and wheezing). Thus, chronic inhaled bronchodilator use and smoking cessation programs are potentially useful approaches to decrease the incidence of mucus retention and respiratory complications. Recently, it was shown that iptratropium improves specific conductance in SCI patients, although it does not change thoracic gas volume (118).

BASES FOR FUTURE RESEARCH

Little data are available describing the risks for late respiratory failure or the potential effectiveness of treatments to delay or prevent it. Contrary to prevailing belief, the long-term perceived quality of life and well-being are similar in ventilator-dependent and spontaneously breathing patients with SCI. The evidence base for the management of respiratory issues in SCI encompasses only a few aspects of this field. In addition, there are few randomized clinical trials or other designs to decrease bias. Most studies of quadriplegia are of the retrospective observational variety. Many studies fail to describe interventions in detail and lack appropriate controls. More prognosticating data are needed regarding level of injury, completeness, and time since injury, as they relate to respiratory complications and recovery. Cohort sizes are small, limiting statistical power.

The U.S. Model Spinal Cord Injury Systems program is a network designed to maintain a database, provide continuing education, and participate in collaborative research relating to SCI (119). The "Model Systems" database has added to our knowledge of the prevalence, nature, cost, and sequelae of SCI. The data have demonstrated improvement in survival of patients with SCI since the 1970s. The database is used to provide guidelines in the respiratory care of patients. Still, further information regarding ventilator settings, frequency and type of respiratory therapy, and other specific details on day-to-day management practices is needed to correlate clinical practice with health outcomes already in the Model Systems data. The Department of Veteran Affairs (VA) network has developed a national registry of veterans with SCI, but its clinical data remains insufficiently detailed for effective outcomes research, particularly in the area of respiratory management.

The Model Systems data should also provide information on the prevalence of respiratory illnesses and complications in the course of care following SCI. Such data can be useful in estimating the burden of illness and for analysis of cost-effectiveness. A clinical research network would provide opportunities for implementing respiratory management protocols across multiple institutions, and to compare clinical outcomes associated with different protocols (119). The effects on outcomes of newer respiratory interventions such as noninvasive ventilation, manual and mechanical cough-assist techniques, and HFCWO should be assessed.

Most published research on respiratory complications in SCI deals with those of acute injury. As long-term survival increases, the prevalence of patients with chronic SCI and respiratory complications grows larger. Currently, there is little data on the occurrence of late respiratory failure or on preventive measures. Data from the Model Systems facilities and the Veterans Administration SCI Centers (119) could provide valuable information in this regard.

References

1. DeVivo MJ. Life expectancy and causes of death for persons with spinal cord injuries: research update. UAB Station, Spain Rehabilitation Center, University of Alabama at Birmingham, 1990.
2. Bellamy R, Pitts RW, Stauffer S. Respiratory complications in traumatic quadriplegia. *J Neurosurg* 1973; 39:596–600.
3. Hachen HJ. Idealized care of the acutely injured spinal cord in Switzerland. *J Trauma* 1977; 17:931–936.
4. Haas F, Axen K, Pineda H, Gandino D, Haas A. Temporal pulmonary function changes in cervical cord injury. *Arch Phys Med Rehabil* 1985; 66:139–144.
5. Hopman MTE, Van der Woude LVH, Dallmeijer AJ, Snock G, Folgering HTM. Respiratory muscle strength and endurance in individuals with tetraplegia. *Spinal Cord* 1997; 35:104–108.
6. Sinderby C, Weinberg J, Sullivan L, Borg J, et al. Diaphragm function in patients with cervical cord injury or prior poliomyelitis infection. *Spinal Cord* 1996; 34:204–213.
7. Laporta D, Grassino A. Assessment of transdiaphragmatic pressure in humans. *J Appl Physiol* 1985; 58:1469–1471.
8. Bellemare F, Grassino A. Effect of pressure and timing of contraction on human diaphragm fatigue assessed by phrenic nerve stimulation. *J Appl Physiol* 1982; 53:1190–1195.
9. Sinderby C, Weinberg J, Sullivan L, Lindstrom L, Grassino A. Electromyographical evidence for exercise-induced diaphragm fatigue in patients with chronic cervical cord injury or prior poliomyelitis infection. *Spinal Cord* 1996; 34:594–601.
10. Gross D, Ladd HW, Riley ZJ, Macklem PT, Grassino A. The effect of training on strength and endurance of the diaphragm in quadriplegia. *Am J Med* 1980; 68:27–35.
11. Nochomovitz ML, Hopkins M, Brodkey J, Montenegro H, et al. Conditioning of the diaphragm with phrenic nerve stimulation after prolonged disuse. *Am Rev Respir Dis* 1984; 130:685–688.
12. Zupan A, Savrin R, Erjavee T, Kralj A, et al. Effects of respiratory muscle training and electrical stimulation of abdominal muscles on respiratory capability in tetraplegic patients. *Spinal Cord* 1997; 35:540–545.
13. Sinderby C, Ingvarsson P, Sullivan L, Wickstrom I, Lindstrom L. The role of the diaphragm in trunk extension in tetraplegia. *Paraplegia* 1992; 30:389–395.
14. Sinderby C, Ingvarsson P, Sullivan L, Wickstrom I, Lindstrom L. Electromyographic registration of diaphragmatic fatigue during sustained trunk flexion in cervical cord injured patients. *Paraplegia* 1992; 30:669–677.
15. De Troyer A, Estenne M, Heilporn A. Mechanism of active expiration in tetraplegic subjects. *N Engl J Med* 1986; 314:740–744.
16. Estenne M, Knoop C, Vanvaerenbergh J, Heilporn A, De Troyer A. The effect of pectoralis muscle training in tetraplegia subjects. *Am Rev Respir Dis* 1989; 139:1218–1222.
17. Estenne M, Pinet C, De Troyer A. Abdominal muscle strength in patients with tetraplegia. *Am J Respir Crit Care Med* 2000; 161:707–712.
18. Goldman JM, Silver JR, Lehr RP. An electromyogram study of the abdominal muscles of tetraplegic patients. *Paraplegia* 1986; 24:241–246.
19. De Troyer A, Estenne M, Vincken W. Rib cage motion and muscle use in high tetraplegics. *Am Rev Respir Dis* 1986; 133:1115–1119.
20. Ledsome JR, Sharp JM. Pulmonary function in acute cervical cord injury. *Am Rev Respir Dis* 1981; 124:41–44.
21. Bluechardt MH, Wiens M, Thomas SG, Plyley MJ. Repeated measurements of pulmonary function following spinal cord injury. *Paraplegia* 1992; 30:768–774.
22. Guttman L, Silver JR. Electromyographic studies on reflex activity of the intercostal and abdominal muscles in cervical cord lesions. *Paraplegia* 1965; 3:1–22.
23. Almenoff PL, Spungen AM, Lesser M, Bauman WA. Pulmonary function survey in spinal cord injury: influences of smoking and level and completeness of injury. *Lung* 1995; 173:297–306.
24. Baydur A, Adkins RH, Milic-Emili J. Lung mechanics in individuals with spinal cord injury: effects of injury level and posture. *J Appl Physiol* 2001; 90:405–411.
25. Ali J, Qi W. Pulmonary function and posture in traumatic quadriplegia. *J Trauma* 1995; 39:334–337.
26. Estenne M, De Troyer A. Mechanism of the postural dependence of vital capacity in tetraplegic subjects. *Am Rev Respir Dis* 1987; 135:367–371.
27. McMichael J, McGibbon JP. Postural changes in the lung volume. *Clin Sci* 1940; 4:175–183.
28. Scanlon PD, Loring SH, Pichurko BM, McCool FD, et al. Respiratory mechanics in acute quadriplegia: lung and chest wall compliance and dimensional changes during respiratory maneuvers. *Am Rev Respir Dis* 1989; 139:615–620.
29. De Troyer A, Heilporn A. Respiratory mechanics in quadriplegia. The respiratory function of the intercostal muscles. *Am Rev Respir Dis* 1980; 122:591–600.
30. Estenne M, De Troyer A. The effects of tetraplegia on chest wall statics. *Am Rev Respir Dis* 1986; 134:121–124.
31. Mortola JP, Sant'Ambrogio G. Motion of the rib cage and the abdomen in tetraplegics patients. *Clin Sci Mol Med* 1978; 54:25–32.
32. Milic-Emili J, Orzalesi M, Cook CD, Turner JM. Respiratory thoracoabdominal mechanics in man. *J Appl Physiol* 1964; 19:217–223.
33. Knudson RJ, Mead J, Knudson DE. Contribution of airway collapse to supramaximal expiratory flows. *J Appl Physiol* 1974; 36:653–667.
34. Estenne M, Van Muylem A, Gorini M, Kinnear W, et al. Evidence of dynamic airway compression during cough in tetraplegic patients. *Am J Respir Crit Care Med* 1994; 150:1081–1085.
35. Spungen AM, Dicpinigaitis PV, Almenoff RL, Dauman WA. Pulmonary obstruction in individuals with cervical spinal cord lesions unmasked by bronchodilator administration. *Paraplegia* 1993; 31:404–407.
36. Dicpinigaitis PV, Spungen AM, Bauman WA, Absgarten A, Almenoff PL. Bronchial hyperresponsiveness after cervical spinal cord injury. *Chest* 1994; 105:1073–1076.
37. Singas E, Lesser M, Spungen AM, Baumann WA, Almenoff PL. Airway hyperresponsiveness to methacholine in subjects with spinal cord injury. *Chest* 1996; 110:911–915.
38. Almenoff PL, Alexander LR, Spungen AM, Lesser MD, Bauman WA. Bronchodilatory effects of ipatropium bromide in patients with tetraplegia. *Paraplegia* 1995; 33:274–277.
39. Dicpinigaitis PV, Spungen AM, Bauman WA, Absgarten A, Almenoff PI. Inhibition of bronchial hyperresponsiveness by the GABA-agonist baclofen. *Chest* 1994; 106:758–761.
40. Loveridge BM, Dubo HI. Breathing pattern in chronic quadriplegia. *Arch Phys Med Rehabil* 1990; 71:495–499.
41. Estenne M, De Troyer A. Relationship between respiratory muscle electromyogram and rib cage motion in tetraplegia. *Am Rev Respir Dis* 1985; 132:53–59.
42. De Troyer A, Estenne M. The respiratory system in neuromuscular disorders. In: Roussos C, ed. *The Thorax*. Part C. New York: Marcel Dekker, Inc., 1995:2177–2212.
43. Pokorski M, Morikawa T, Takaishi S, Masuda A, et al. Ventilatory response to chemosensory stimuli in quadriplegic subjects. *Eur Respir J* 1990; 3:891–900.
44. Bergofsky EH. Mechanism for respiratory insufficiency after cervical cord injury. *Ann Intern Med* 1964; 61:435–447.
45. Adams L, Frankel H, Garlick J, Guz A, et al. The role of spinal cord transmission in the ventilatory response to exercise in man. *J Physiol (Lond)* 1984; 355:85–97.
46. Manning HL, Brown R, Scharf SM, Leith DE, et al. Ventilatory and P0.1 response to hypercapnia in quadriplegia. *Respir Physiol* 1992; 89:97–112.
47. Sawka MN, Latzka WA, Pandolf KB. Temperature regulation during upper body exercise: able-bodied and spinal cord injured. *Med Sci Sports Exerc* 1989; 21:S132–S140.

48. Muraki S, Yamasaki M, Ishii K, Kikuchi K, Seki K. Relationship between core temperature and skin blood flux in lower limbs during prolonged arm exercise in persons with spinal cord injury. *Eur J Appl Physiol* 1996; 72:330–334.

49. Wilsmore BR, Cotter JD, Bashford GM, Taylor NAS. Ventilatory changes in heat-stressed humans with spinal-cord injury. *Spinal Cord* 2006; 44:160–164.

50. Kelling JS, DiMarco AF, Gottfried SB, Altose MD. Respiratory responses to ventilatory loading following low cervical spinal cord injury. *J Appl Physiol* 1985; 59:1752–1756.

51. McCool FD, Brown R, Mayewski RJ, Hyde RW. Effects of posture on stimulated ventilation in quadriplegia. *Am Rev Respir Dis* 1988; 138: 101–105.

52. Sassoon CSH, Laurente-Tjoa F, Rheeman C, Gruer S, Mahutte CK. Neuromuscular compensation with changes in posture during hypercapnic ventilatory and occlusion pressure responses in quadriplegia (abstract). *Chest* 1993; 103:165S.

53. Im Hof V, West P, Younes M. Steady-state response of normal subjects to inspiratory resistive load. *J Appl Physiol* 1986; 60:1471–1481.

54. Im Hof V, Dubo H, Daniels V, Younes M. Steady-state response of quadriplegic subjects to inspiratory resistive load. *J Appl Physiol* 1986; 60:1482–1492.

55. Burdon JGW, Killian KJ, Stubbing DG, Campbell EJM. Effect of background loads on the perception of added loads to breathing. *J Appl Physiol* 1983; 54:1222–1228.

56. Axen K, Haas SS. Effect of thoracic deafferentation on load-compensating mechanisms in humans. *J Appl Physiol* 1982; 52:757–767.

57. Lansing RW, Im BSH, Thwing JI, Legedza ATR, Banzett RB. The perception of respiratory work and effort can be independent of the perception of air hunger. *Am J Respir Crit Care Med* 2000; 162:1690–1696.

58. Banzett RB, Lansing RW, Reid MB, Adams L, Brown R. "Air hunger" arising from increased PCO_2 in mechanically ventilated quadriplegics. *Respir Physiol* 1989; 76:53–68.

59. Manning HL, Shea SA, Schwartzstein RM, Lansing RW, et al. Reduced tidal volume increases "air hunger" at fixed PCO_2 in ventilated quadriplegics. *Respir Physiol* 1992; 90:19–30.

60. Jackson A, Groomes TE. Incidence of respiratory complications following spinal cord injury. *Arch Phys Med Rehabil* 1994; 75:270–275.

61. Fishburn MJ, Marino RJ, Ditunno JF. Atelectasis and pneumonia in acute spinal cord injury. *Arch Phys Med Rehabil* 1990; 71:197–200.

62. Winslow C, Bode RK, Felton D, Chen D, Meyer PR. Impact of respiratory complications on length of stay and hospital costs in acute cervical spine injury. *Chest* 2002; 121:1548–1554.

63. Hassid VJ, Schinco MA, Tepas JJ, Griffen MM, et al. Definitive establishment of airway control is critical for optimal outcome in lower cervical spinal cord injury. *J Trauma* 2008; 65:1328–1332.

64. Nazon D, Abergel G, Hatem CM. Critical care in orthopedic and spine surgery. *Crit Care Clin* 2003; 19:33–53.

65. Sagi HC, Beutler W, Carroll E, et al. Airway complications associated with surgery on the anterior cervical spine. *Spine* 2002; 27:949–953.

66. Maeda CJ, Baydur A, Waters RL, Adkins RH. The effect of the halovest and body position on pulmonary function in quadriplegia. *J Spinal Disord* 1990; 3:47–51.

67. Maloney FP. Pulmonary function in quadriplegia: effects of a corset. *Arch Phys Med Rehabil* 1979; 60:261–265.

68. Goldman JM, Rose LS, Williams SJ, Silver JR, Denison DM. Effect of abdominal binders on breathing in tetraplegic patients. *Thorax* 1986; 41:940–945.

69. Carter RE. Unilateral diaphragmatic paralysis in spinal cord injury patients. *Paraplegia* 1980; 18:267–273.

70. Oo T, Watt JWH, Soni BM, Sett PK. Delayed diaphragm recovery in 12 patients after high cervical spinal cord injury: a retrospective review of the diaphragm status of 107 patients ventilated after acute spinal cord injury. *Spinal Cord* 1999; 37:117–122.

71. Johnson K, Grant T, Peterson P. Ventilator weaning for the patient with high-level paraplegia. *Top Spinal Cord Inj Rehabil* 1997; 2:11–20.

72. Bach JR, et al. Neuromuscular ventilatory insufficiency: the effect of home mechanical ventilator use vs. oxygen therapy on pneumonia and hospitalization rates. *Am J Phys Med Rehabil* 1998; 77:8–19.

73. Bhaskar KR, Brown R, O'Sullivan DD, Melia S, et al. Bronchial mucus hypersecretion in acute quadriplegia: macromolecular yields and glycoconjugate composition. *Am Rev Respir Dis* 1991; 143:640–648.

74. Kang SW, Shin JC, Park CI, Moon JH, et al. Relationship between inspiratory muscle strength and cough capacity in cervical spinal cord injured patients. *Spinal Cord* 2006; 44:242–248

75. Bach JR. Mechanical insufflation-exsufflation: comparison of peak expiratory flows with manually assisted and unassisted coughing techniques. *Chest* 1993; 104:1553–1562.

76. Massery M. Manual breathing and coughing aids. *Phys Med Rehabil Clin N Am* 1996; 7:407–422.

77. Bach JR. Update and perspectives on noninvasive respiratory muscle aids. *Chest* 1994; 105:1230–1240.

78. Bach JR, Saporito LR. Criteria for extubation and tracheostomy tube removal for patients with ventilatory failure: a different approach to weaning. *Chest* 1996; 110:1566–1571.

79. Bach JR. A comparison of long-term ventilatory support alternatives from the perspective of the patient and care giver. *Chest* 1993; 104:1702–1706.

80. Freedman AP, Goodman L. Suctioning the left bronchial tree in the intubated adult. *Crit Care Med* 1982; 10:43–45.

81. Anbar RD, Powell KN, Ianuzzi DM. Short-term effect of ThAIRapy® Vest on pulmonary function of cystic fibrosis patients. *Am J Respir Crit Care Med* 1998; 157(Suppl):A130.

82. Arens R, Gozal D, Omlin KJ, Vega J, et al. Comparison of high frequency chest compression and conventional chest physiotherapy in hospitalized patients with cystic fibrosis. *Am J Respir Crit Care Med* 1994; 150:1154–1157.

83. Castagnino M, Vojtova J, Kaminski S, Fink R. Safety of high-frequency chest wall oscillation in patients with respiratory muscle weakness. *Chest* 1996; 110:S65.

84. Glenn WWL, Sairenji H. Diaphragm pacing in the treatment of chronic ventilatory insufficiency. In: Roussos C, Macklem PT, eds. *The Thorax.* Part B. New York: Marcel Dekker, 1985:1407–1440.

85. Whiteneck GG, Carter RE, Hall K, Menter RR, et al. Collaborative study of high quadriplegia (abstract). *Arch Phys Med Rehabil* 1985; 66:575.

86. Splaingard ML, Frates RC, Jefferson LS, Rosen CL, Harrison GM. Home negative pressure ventilation: report of 20 years of experience in patients with neuromuscular disease. *Arch Phys Med Rehabil* 1985; 66:239–242.

87. Carter RE, Donovan WH, Halstead L, Wilkerson MA. Comparative study of electrophrenic nerve stimulation and mechanical ventilatory support in traumatic spinal cord injury. *Paraplegia* 1987; 25:86–91.

88. Lamid S, Reaglie GF, Welter K. Respirator-dependent quadriplegic: problems during the weaning period. *J Am Paraplegia Soc* 1985; 8:33–37.

89. Bach JR, Alba AS. Noninvasive options for ventilatory support of the traumatic high level quadriplegic patient. *Chest* 1990; 98:613–619.

90. Peterson WP, Barbalata L, Brooks CA, Gerhart KA, et al. The effect of tidal volumes on the time to wean persons with high tetraplegia from ventilators. *Spinal Cord* 1999; 37:284–288.

91. Nates J, Aravindan N, Berner DK, Snedeker C, Luther KM. Critical pathways help to improve outcomes in spinal cord injury patients. *Crit Care Med* 2003; 31(12) (Suppl):A87.

92. Leger P, Jennequin J, Gerard M, Robert D. Home positive pressure ventilation via nasal mask for patients with neuromuscular weakness or restrictive lung or chest wall deformities. *Respir Care* 1989; 37:73–77.

93. Baydur A, Layne E, Aral H, Krishnareddy N, et al. Long-term noninvasive ventilation in the community for patients with musculoskeletal disorders: 46 year experience and review. *Thorax* 2000; 55:4–11.

94. Bach JR, Alba AS, Saporito LR. Intermittent positive pressure ventilation via the mouth as an alternative to tracheostomy for 257 ventilator users. *Chest* 1993; 103:174–182.

95. Tromans AM, Mecci M, Barrett FH, Ward TA, Grundy DJ. The use of the biphasic positive pressure system in acute spinal cord injury. *Spinal Cord* 1998; 36:481–484.

96. Miller HJ, Thomas E, Wilmot CB. Pneumobelt use among high quadriplegic population. *Arch Phys Med Rehabil* 1988; 69:369–372.

97. Hill NS. Clinical application of body ventilators. *Chest* 1986; 90:897–905.

98. Glenn WWL, Hogan JF, Loke JSO, Cieselski TE, et al. Ventilatory support by pacing of the conditioned diaphragm in quadriplegia. *N Engl J Med* 1984; 172:755–773.

99. Marcus CL, Jansen MT, Poulsen MK, et al. Medical and psychosocial outcome of children with congenital central hypoventilation syndrome. *J Pediatr* 1991; 119:888–895.

100. Ilbawi MN, Idriss FS, Hunt CE, Brouillete RT, DeLeon SY. Diaphragmatic pacing in infants: techniques and results. *Ann Thorac Surg* 1985; 40:323–329.
101. Creasey G, Elefteriades J, DiMarco A, Talonen P, et al. Electrical stimulation to restore respiration. *J Rehabil Res Dev* 1996; 33:123–132.
102. Fodstadt H. Phrenicodiaphragmatic pacing. In: Roussos C, ed. *The Thorax.* Part C. New York: Marcel Dekker, 1995:2597–2617.
103. Danon J, Druz WS, Goldberg NB, Sharp JT. Function of the isolated paced diaphragm and the cervical accessory muscles in C1 quadriplegics. *Am Rev Respir Dis* 1979; 119:909–919.
104. DeVivo MJ, Rutt RD, Black KJ, Go BK, Stover SL. Trends in spinal cord injury demographics and treatment outcomes between 1973 and 1986. *Arch Phys Med Rehabil* 1992; 73:424–430.
105. Freed MM. Quality of life: the physician's dilemma. *Arch Phys Med Rehabil* 1984; 65:109–111.
106. Bach JR, Tilton MC. Life satisfaction and well-being measures in ventilation assisted individuals with traumatic tetraplegia. *Arch Phys Med Rehabil* 1994; 75:626–632.
107. Krause JS. Longitudinal changes in adjustment after spinal cord injury: a 15-year study. *Arch Phys Med Rehabil* 1992; 73:564–568.
108. Huldtgren AC, Fugl-Meyer AR, Jonasson E, Bake B. Ventilatory rehabilitation in posttraumatic quadriplegia. *Eur J Respir Dis* 1980; 61:347–356.
109. Keens TG, Krastins IRB, Wannamaker EM, Levison H, et al. Ventilatory muscle endurance training in normal subjects and patients with cystic fibrosis. *Am Rev Respir Dis* 1977; 116:853–860.
110. Rutchik A, Weissman AR, Almenoff PL, Spungen AN, et al. Resistive inspiratory muscle training muscle training in subjects with chronic cervical spinal cord injury. *Arch Phys Med Rehabil* 1998; 79:293–297.
111. Leeuw T, Pette D. Coordinate changes in the expression of troponin subunit and myosin heavy-chain isoforms during fast-to-slow transition of low-frequency-stimulated rabbit muscle. *Eur J Biochem* 1993; 213:1039–1046.
112. Sharon RS, Karopondo DL, Kraemer WJ, Fry AC, et al. Skeletal muscle adaptations during early phase of heavy-resistance training in men and women. *J Appl Physiol* 1994; 76:1247–1255.
113. Gea J, Hamid Q, Czaika G, Zhu E, et al. Expression of myosin heavy-chain isoforms in the respiratory muscles following inspiratory resistive breathing. *Am J Respir Crit Care Med* 2000; 161:1274–1278.
114. Siebens AA, Kirby NA, Poulos DA. Cough following transection of spinal cord at C6. *Arch Phys Med Rehabil* 1964; 45:1–8.
115. Skloot G, Permutt S, Togias A. Airway hyperresponsiveness in asthma: a problem of limited smooth muscle relaxation with inspiration. *J Clin Invest* 1995; 96:2393–2403.
116. Pliss LB, Ingenito EP, Ingram RH. Responsiveness, inflammation, and effects of deep breaths on obstruction in mild asthma. *J Appl Physiol* 1989; 66:2298–2304.
117. Ashba J, Garshick E, Tun CG, Lieberman SL, et al. Spirometry: acceptability and reproducibility in spinal cord injured subjects. *J Am Paraplegia Soc* 1993; 16:197–203.
118. Mateus SRM, Beraldo PSS, Horan TA. Cholinergic bronchomotor tone and airway caliber in tetraplegic patients. *Spinal Cord* 2006; 44:269–274.
119. Agency for Healthcare Research and Quality, U.S. Department of Health and Human Services. AHRQ Publication No. 01-E014, September 2001, http://www.ahrq.gov/clinic/tp/spinaltp.htm

17 Sleep Disorders in Spinal Cord Injury

Lawrence J. Epstein
Robert Brown

S leep is a time of rest for most people and is associated with reductions in cardiovascular and neuromuscular activity and the resolution of somnolence. Those with sleep disorders do not get the restorative benefits of sleep. Their sleep time may be shortened or their sleep fragmented, and they can awaken feeling as sleepy as when they went to bed. The available studies on sleep in spinal cord injury (SCI) patients suggest high rates of sleep disorders. In one questionnaire study of medical problems in SCI, 34% of 353 individuals reported sleep disturbance in the week prior to the survey, and 30% complained of fatigue (1). In another study of patients with nontraumatic spinal cord lesions undergoing inpatient rehabilitation, 14.5% of 297 individuals reported disturbed sleep (2). These surveys did not directly compare SCI patients to an able-bodied control group. However, Hyppa et al. found that SCI patients had more sleep complaints than patients with different chronic illnesses, specifically type-2 diabetes and myocardial infarction (3), and Biering-Sorensen et al. found that SCI patients had reduced sleep quality, measured by the Nordic Sleep Questionnaire, compared to able-bodied controls (4). And in a study of individuals living in the community, 312 men with SCI were found to spend a significantly greater portion of their day sleeping than a comparison group of 3,617 able-bodied men (5). The data suggest that the high prevalence of fatigue in SCI is caused in large part by disordered sleep. In this chapter, we describe the information available on sleep disorders in SCI and how the injury contributes to the development of those sleep disorders.

NORMAL SLEEP

To understand the disorders that occur during sleep, it is important to have an understanding of normal sleep. Despite its external appearance, sleep is a dynamic state, progressing through multiple stages in a relatively predictable manner. During sleep there are two states that are as distinct from each other as each is from wakefulness. Dreaming occurs during rapid eye movement (REM) sleep and is defined by an activated electroencephalographic (EEG) pattern (low-voltage, high-frequency wave activity), muscle atonia, and episodic bursts of eye movements (6). Non–rapid eye movement (NREM) sleep has a higher voltage, lower frequency EEG that reflects the synchrony of cortical activity. NREM is divided into three stages, representing a rough continuum of depth of sleep. Stages 1 and 2 represent lighter sleep. Stage 3 is referred to as slow-wave sleep because of its characteristic low-frequency, high-voltage EEG (6). Although stage 2 is restorative, slow-wave sleep is more so, being replaced first after sleep deprivation (7).

There is a typical progression of sleep stages throughout the night. The normal adult spends a short time in stages 1 and 2 before progressing rapidly to slow-wave sleep (see Figure 17.1). The first third of the night is dominated by slow-wave sleep. Within the sleep period there is a NREM/REM cycle that determines the order of, and amount of time in, the various sleep stages. A complete NREM/REM cycle occurs every 90 to 110 minutes. The first REM period is usually brief. The subsequent REM periods become progressively longer and predominate in the last third of the sleep period. Overall, adults spend 45% to 60% of sleep time in stages 1 and 2 NREM sleep, 13% to 23% in stage 3 (slow-wave) sleep, and 20% to 25% in REM sleep (8).

The likelihood of falling asleep at a particular time is a function of two processes: the drive to sleep and the phase of the circadian rhythm (9). The drive to fall asleep increases during wakefulness and the likelihood of sleeping increases with time since the last sleep period. The drive is relieved by sleeping, which is a homeostatic process. The human circadian rhythm regulator, located in the hypothalamic suprachiasmatic nuclei (SCN) (10), controls the sleep-wake cycle and influences many physiologic processes, including core body temperature, hormone secretion, blood pressure, and renal function (11). The phase of the circadian rhythm affects the likelihood of falling asleep as well as the distribution of sleep stages. Figure 17.2 shows one model of the interaction between the homeostatic and circadian rhythm tendency to sleep. Sleep is most likely to occur when the circadian-controlled propensity to fall asleep coincides

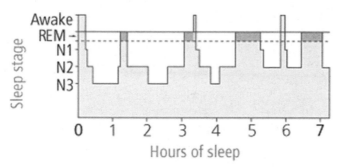

Figure 17.1 This idealized hypnogram illustrates the usual progression of sleep stages in the normal young adult. This is a dynamic process, with progression through multiple stages throughout the night. Sleep is initially entered through non–rapid eye movement (NREM) sleep, and the first third of the night is dominated by slow-wave sleep (stage 3). Rapid eye movement (REM) sleep occurs after about 90 minutes, then recurs with a periodicity of 90 to 110 minutes. The first REM episode is typically short. With subsequent cycles, REM periods are longer, and slow-wave sleep tends not to occur. (Reprinted with permission from Epstein LJ, ed. *Improving Sleep: A Guide to a Good Night's Rest.* Boston: Harvard Health Publications, 2007.)

with a prolonged time since the last sleep period. Typically this occurs at night (9).

The usual sleep pattern can be disrupted for many reasons, such as aging, shift work, medical problems, medications, and environmental factors such as noise and temperature (12–14). A complaint of difficulty sleeping, fragmented sleep, or excessive daytime sleep or sleepiness requires a thorough evaluation

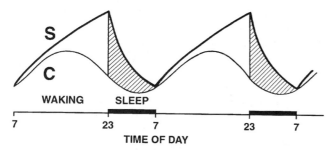

Figure 17.2 This is a graphical representation of the two-process model of sleep regulation. S represents the homeostatic sleep drive, which rises during waking and declines during sleep. As S increases, the likelihood of sleeping increases. C represents the circadian rhythm cycle as measured by body temperature. The greatest tendency to sleep occurs during the trough of body temperature. The optimal time for sleep occurs when S is at its peak and C is in its trough, which coincides with the typical nighttime sleep period. Wake up typically occurs where C and S intersect. (Reprinted with permission from Borbely AA. Sleep homeostasis and models of sleep regulation. In: Kryger MH, Roth T, Dement WC, eds. *Principles and Practice of Sleep Medicine.* 2nd ed. Philadelphia: WB Saunders Co., 1994:316.)

of the patient's sleep-wake pattern, sleep environment, bedtime routine, medical history, and medication use (15).

SLEEP PATTERNS IN SCI

Sleep patterns in SCI can be disrupted both by the injury itself and by the consequences and treatment of the injury. Fragmentation of sleep leads to sleep deprivation and the symptoms of fatigue and hypersomnolence.

SCI patients commonly report disrupted sleep in survey studies. Respondents describe that their sleep is disturbed by physical discomfort (pain, spasticity, paresthesias), emotional distress, and interventions necessary to manage their condition (bladder management, turning in bed) (3, 4). Patients reported more difficulty falling asleep, more awakenings from sleep, daytime sleepiness, and greater use of sleeping medications in one survey utilizing the Nordic Sleep Questionnaire (4). Budh et al. examined the contributors to poor sleep (16). In addition to the Nordic Sleep Questionnaire, they administered concurrent questionnaires about pain and mood. They found that anxiety, along with pain intensity and depression, were predictors of poor sleep. Those reporting continuous pain had more difficulty falling asleep, less restful sleep, and poorer quality sleep than those with no pain or only intermittent pain. In a follow-up study, the same group of investigators enrolled twenty-seven patients with SCI and neuropathic pain into a chronic pain management program and compared their responses to eleven SCI controls without pain (17). The program used cognitive behavioral therapy, a multidimensional approach utilizing educational sessions, cognitive therapy, relaxation training, stretching, light exercise, and body awareness training. At the end of the 10-week program, the treatment group showed reductions in depression, reductions in use of pain medication, a decrease in reported sleep problems, and a tendency toward better sleep.

In SCI, standard care can produce fragmented sleep. The prevention and treatment of pressure sores requires frequent turning that disrupts sleep (18). Bladder catheterization and bowel management programs often require disruption of normal sleep patterns (19). For inpatients, a nonconducive sleep environment is created by the timing of vital signs measurement, medication administration, physician visits, meals, and the noise and lighting of the hospital environment.

Investigators have looked into whether SCI itself disrupts the normal sleep pattern. Esteves et al. evaluated sleep changes with SCI in an animal model (20). They compared the sleep of Wistar rats with a T9 surgical transection with a group that had undergone sham back surgery. Over the 15 days studied, the SCI rats experienced reductions in sleep efficiency, increased sleep fragmentation, and change in the usual sleep stage distribution and circadian timing of sleep and wakefulness. The investigators felt this study supported the hypothesis that the SCI is a key factor, along with others such as inactivity, in altering sleep patterns.

Adey et al. (21) examined nighttime EEG sleep patterns in seventeen individuals with SCI (fourteen with high cervical lesions, two with upper thoracic lesions, and one with a lower thoracic lesion). Individuals with high cervical injuries had a significant increase in the amount of light sleep and a reduction in the amount of deep sleep and REM sleep. The change was more pronounced in those with a longer time since injury. Subjects with thoracic lesions had sleep stage proportions similar to the able-bodied. This study was limited in many respects. The sample size was small, the patients were not evaluated for the presence of other sleep disorders, and there were no controls for those medications, commonly used in SCI, which can change sleep stage presentation. For example, REM is suppressed with antidepressants (22), and slow-wave sleep is reduced by benzodiazepines (23). McEvoy et al. also reported an increase in light sleep and a reduction in REM sleep compared to able-bodied controls in their study of forty SCI patients (24). However, they did not separate out the sleep of the 27.5% of their patients with obstructive sleep apnea, which can alter sleep stage distribution, from those without sleep-disordered breathing. Scheer et al. did not find any differences in sleep stage distribution in five SCI subjects (two thoracic, three cervical) (25). However, they did find reduced total sleep duration and reduced sleep efficiency as well as a prolonged REM sleep latency in those with cervical SCI. The cervical SCI subjects spent double the amount of time awake after sleep onset as those with thoracic SCI and healthy controls. The authors concluded that the sleep disruption was likely due to abnormal melatonin secretion related to the cervical SCI.

The impact of SCI on melatonin secretion and circadian rhythm has been more extensively studied. The length of the circadian rhythm cycle corresponds approximately to the 24-hour day-night period. The maintenance of appropriate timing of the circadian clock, called *entrainment,* is controlled by several factors, the most potent of which is exposure to light (26). The pathway by which the SCN controls the secretion of endocrine hormones is shown in Figure 17.3. Melatonin is produced in single nightly episodes by the pineal gland, with the onset occurring just before bedtime and terminating soon after waking. Melatonin is not typically produced during the daytime and can be suppressed at night by exposure to bright light (27). Light mediates SCN activity, and thus melatonin secretion, through the retinohypothalamic pathway. Unlike pituitary hormones, the SCN is thought to control melatonin secretion through an efferent neural pathway that loops through the cervical spinal cord and innervates the pineal gland via the superior cervical ganglia (28). This pathway, and therefore melatonin secretion, is at risk in SCI above the nerve roots that innervate the superior cervical ganglia. Melatonin may be involved in the regulation of the circadian pattern (29), which, in turn, affects the control of sleep and wakefulness. Thus, whether melatonin secretion is abnormal is essential to the study of sleep in SCI.

There have been several studies evaluating melatonin secretion in SCI. Kneisley et al. (30) measured urinary melatonin excretion in six tetraplegics and one paraplegic at multiple times over a 24-hour day. They found that the tetraplegics did not exhibit the normal day-night variation in melatonin levels when compared to able-bodied controls or the paraplegic. Of note, basal melatonin levels throughout the 24-hour period were elevated. However, compared to current assays, the melatonin assay available at that time was insensitive. Li et al. (31) studied serum melatonin levels over 12 hours in eight subjects with cervical SCI, three with upper thoracic SCI and nine with low thoracic or lumbar SCI. Again, no diurnal melatonin rhythm was present in the subjects with upper SCI, whereas rhythmicity of secretion was preserved in subjects with lower lesions. However, they found that basal melatonin levels were low in those with cervical lesion.

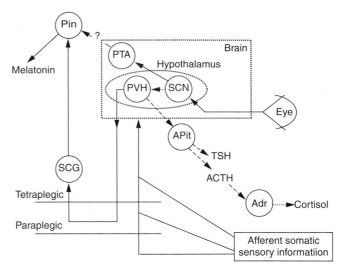

Figure 17.3 Diagram of the putative pathways involved in the generation of circadian rhythmicity in TSH, cortisol, and melatonin. The pathways that would be interrupted by a neurologically complete injury to the lower cervical (tetraplegic) and upper thoracic (paraplegic) spinal cord are also shown. In tetraplegia, peripheral sympathetic innervation of the pineal gland is abolished, whereas in paraplegia, peripheral sympathetic innervation of the pineal gland remains intact. In both paraplegia and tetraplegia, afferent somatic sensory information does not reach the brain. (Adr, adrenal cortex; APit, anterior pituitary; Pin, pineal; PTA, pretectal area; PVH, paraventricular nucleus of the hypothalamus; SCG, superior cervical ganglion.) (Reprinted with permission from Zeitzer JM, Ayas NT, Shea SA, Bown R, Czeisler CA. Absence of detectable melatonin and preservation of cortisol and thyrotropin rhythms in tetraplegia. *J Clin Endocrinol Metab* 2000; 85:2189–2196.)

To resolve the conflicting results of these two studies, Zeitzer et al. (32) studied melatonin, cortisol, and thyrotropin (TSH) levels in three neurologically complete tetraplegic and two neurologically complete paraplegic subjects exposed to a rigorous constant routine protocol. The output of the circadian timing system can be masked by multiple variables, including activity, body position, food intake, temperature, and light levels. The constant routine protocol holds these variables constant (26). Subjects participated in a 4-day study in rooms free from time cues, with temperature constant and lights dim. After an 8-hour sleep period, the subjects began a 46-hour period of enforced wakefulness in the semirecumbent position with liquid and meals given in hourly aliquots. Serum was sampled three times an hour through an indwelling catheter. The tetraplegics had no detectable basal melatonin levels and demonstrated no rhythmicity of melatonin secretion. Both paraplegic subjects demonstrated normal melatonin rhythmicity (see Figure 17.4). In contrast, the rhythmic production of cortisol and TSH was intact in all subjects regardless of level. These findings support the hypothesis that, to produce melatonin, the human pineal gland must be stimulated by the sympathetic nervous system via a neural pathway through the cervical spinal cord.

The neural pathway from the retina to the pineal gland that controls melatonin secretion travels closely with the oculosympathetic pathway that descends from the hypothalamus, through

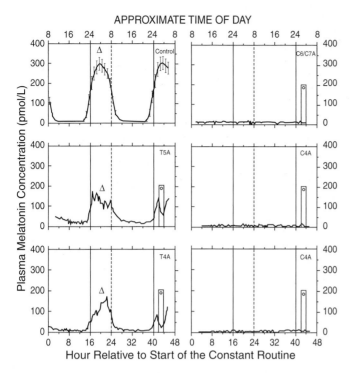

APPROXIMATE TIME OF DAY

Figure 17.4 Melatonin waveforms in a group of able-bodied control subjects (average + SEM; *n* = 24; **upper left**) and in T4A paraplegic (**lower left**), T5A paraplegic (**middle left**), C6/7A tetraplegic (**upper right**), C6A tetraplegic (**middle right**), and C4A tetraplegic (**lower right**) patients during a 46-hour constant routine. Included in the figure are the time of the melatonin maximum (**open triangle**), the times of habitual bed (**solid line**) and wake time (**dashed line**), and the time of a 2-hour episode of brighter light (**open box**). (Reprinted with permission from Zeitzer JM, Ayas NT, Shea SA, Bown R, Czeisler CA. Absence of detectable melatonin and preservation of cortisol and thyrotropin rhythms in tetraplegia. *J Clin Endocrinol Metab* 2000; 85:2189–2196.)

the cervical spinal cord, then ascends to the superior cervical ganglion. Injury to this pathway results in oculosympathetic paresis (OSP) syndrome, also called Horner's syndrome, consisting of miosis, ptosis, and anhidrosis. Because the two neural pathways travel together, SCI that interferes with melatonin secretion would be expected to also cause OSP. Zeitzer et al. showed this association in five SCI patients (33). The two individuals with thoracic SCI, below the level of the two pathways, did not have abnormal melatonin secretion or OSP. Bilateral OSP and absence of melatonin production occurred in the three subjects with cervical SCI. The presence of bilateral OSP on examination can be used to predict loss of melatonin production.

SLEEP DISORDERS IN SPINAL CORD INJURY

Sleep-Disordered Breathing

Obstructive sleep apnea (OSA) is a disorder of breathing during sleep characterized by repetitive collapse of the upper airway. OSA is common in the able-bodied population and has significant health consequences. Risk factors for OSA in the able-bodied include increased age, obesity, increased neck circumference,

sedative or alcohol use, and a family history of OSA (34–38). Several studies suggest that the SCI population may be at greater risk for OSA than the general population.

During inhalation, pressure in the pharyngeal airway decreases because of the combination of contraction of the muscles of inhalation and the flow-resistant properties of the airway. This negative pressure tends to collapse the airway. Because individuals with OSA typically have smaller than normal pharyngeal airways (39), flow-resistive pressure drops are greater, and therefore, their pharyngeal airways are particularly vulnerable to collapse. During wakefulness, reflex and behavioral mechanisms activate dilator muscles and maintain patency of the upper airway (40), called neuromuscular compensation. During sleep, these mechanisms diminish and, in OSA, are inadequate to prevent marked narrowing or even complete collapse of the upper airway. Complete collapse causes apnea: that is, total cessation of airflow (see Figure 17.5). The event terminates with a brief arousal from sleep and the reestablishment of neuromuscular compensation to open the airway. Hypopnea is the term for a significant but not complete airway collapse that substantially diminishes airflow and triggers associated arousal and hypoxemia.

The clinical consequences of OSA are the direct result of abnormalities occurring during sleep. The repetitive arousals cause fragmentation of sleep and loss of its restorative function. The arousals are also associated with increased sympathetic nervous system activity. Hypoxemia, hypercapnia, acidemia, marked swings in pulmonary and systemic blood pressure, and cardiac dysrhythmias occur during and immediately following the apneic episodes. The end result is excessive sleepiness, performance decrements, systemic and pulmonary hypertension, and higher than expected rates of cardiovascular events such as stroke and myocardial infarction (41).

Snoring is a cardinal symptom of OSA, caused by the partial collapse of the upper airway. Ayas et al. studied the prevalence and predictors of snoring in an SCI cohort (42). Subjects responding to a questionnaire on respiratory function in SCI were asked about the occurrence and frequency of snoring. In the cohort of 197 men with chronic stable SCI, 43% reported snoring. Obesity, being married, and using antispasticity medications were predictors of habitual snoring with the highest risk for snoring (odds ratio 7.0, 95% C.I. 2.71–18.09, *p* = 0.001) occurring in those individuals who were overweight (BMI ≥ 25.3) and used antispasticity medications, specifically baclofen, diazepam, or the combination.

The prevalence of OSA in 30- to 60-year-old able-bodied males, defined by an apnea + hypopnea index (AHI) of greater than or equal to fifteen events per hour of sleep, is 9% (34). Initial attempts to study this in SCI were inadequate because only pulse oximetry was used (43–45). Such studies do not provide any information on the nature or architecture of sleep or the cause of the desaturation.

Studies of the prevalence of OSA in SCI have found rates ranging from 15% to 83% (24, 46–51); these rates are much higher than those found in the able-bodied population. Part of the variation is caused by differing definitions of OSA and the use of different methods for studying sleep and breathing (see Table 17.1). Five studies used overnight polysomnography, the most sensitive and accurate method for monitoring sleep and breathing, and an AHI of greater than or equal to 15 as a

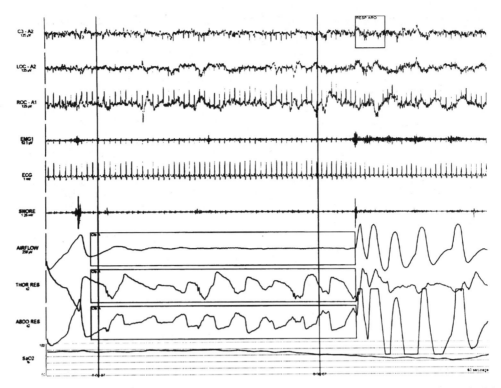

Figure 17.5 A polysomnographic tracing from an SCI patient with obstructive sleep apnea. The top channel of this 60-second tracing is a central electroencephalogram lead (C3–A2). With the onset of sleep, the upper airway collapses, and airflow stops. Ventilatory effort continues in an attempt to overcome the obstruction, shown by the continued movement in the effort channels (THOR RES = chest wall movement; ABDO RES = abdominal wall movement). The apnea continues until arousal from sleep occurs (RESP ARO), at which time the airway opens and breathing resumes. The lack of airflow causes hypoxemia, shown by the drop in oxyhemoglobin saturation (SaO2). (LOC-A2 = left eye lead; ROC-A1 = right eye lead; EMG1 = chin electromyogram; ECG = electrocardiogram; SNORE = snore microphone.)

Table 17.1   Studies of the Prevalence of Obstructive Sleep Apnea (OSA) in SCI

AUTHOR (REFERENCE)	STUDY TYPE	OSA CRITERIA	N	OSA PREVALENCE
Short et al. (48)	PSG	SaO$_2$ dips >4% at a rate >15/hr	22	6 (26%)
		>5/hr	22	10 (45%)
Flavell et al. (44)	Oximetry	10% of study spent at <90% SaO$_2$	10	3 (30%)
Cahan et al. (45)	Oximetry in all, PSG in 7/16	SaO$_2$ profile below the normal range	16	6 (38%)
		AHI>10	7	3 (43%)
Klefbeck et al. (49)	Oximetry + respiratory movement monitoring	ODI>6 + 45% periodic respiration time	33	5 (15%)
McEvoy et al. (24)	PSG	AHI>15	40	11 (28%)
		AHI>5	40	12 (30%)
Burns et al. (53)	Respiratory monitoring	AI>5 + abnormal sleepiness	20	8 (40%)
Ayas et al. (51)	PSG	AHI >15	42	13 (31%)
Stockhammer et al. (52)	PSG	AHI>15	50	31 (62%)
Berlowitz et al. (60)	PSG	AHI>10	23	19 (83%)
		AHI>15	23	15 (65%)
Le Duc et al. (55)	Unattended home PSG	AHI≥5 + clinical symptoms	41	22 (53%)

PSG = polysomnography; SaO$_2$ = oxyhemoglobin saturation; AHI = Apnea/Hypopnea Index; AI = Apnea Index; ODI = Oxygen Desaturation Index = average number of SaO$_2$ drops>4%/hour of sleep.

Table 17.2 Reason for Sleep Apnea Evaluation According to Survey Respondents

	N	%
Witnessed apnea events	15	44
Severe snoring	5	15
Sleepiness	4	12
Fatigue	3	9
Poor sleep	3	9
Evaluation of associated medical disorder	2	6
Other	2	6
Unknown to participant	6	NA

NA = not applicable.
Total number of respondents = 34.
Adapted from Burns et al. *Am J Phys Med Rehabil* 2005;84:620–625.

Multiple studies have evaluated potential factors associated with the development of OSA in SCI, often with conflicting results. The most consistent factors associated with OSA are measures of increased weight (presence of obesity, high BMI, increased neck circumference) (24, 50–52, 55, 60) and complaints of daytime sleepiness (52, 55). Although the presence of sleepiness is associated with OSA, the majority of patients with OSA do not complain of excessive sleepiness (61) (see Table 17.2). The level of injury, ASIA scores and pulmonary function tests are consistently not predictive of OSA (24, 45, 48–52). Age has been associated with OSA in some studies (51, 52) but not others (45, 48, 50, 53). Similarly, use of antispasticity medication has been predictive of OSA in some studies (50–52) but not others (45, 55). Time since injury was predictive in one study (52) but not in three others (45, 48, 49). The assorted risks for OSA in SCI are summarized in Table 17.3. Larger studies are needed to clarify the risk groups.

A reason for the differences in identified risk factors may be the different timeframes in the course of SCI that sleep and breathing are evaluated. One group monitored breathing and sleep for the first year following acute SCI (60). They studied tetraplegics immediately postinjury and then five times over the subsequent year. OSA was not present immediately after the injury but developed in 60% after 2 weeks, with a peak of 83% at 6 months. Neck and abdominal girth both dropped in the first few weeks after injury, but after that point, there was a steady rise. The likelihood of developing OSA was associated with the increase in neck circumference and abdominal girth. The AHI dropped in almost all patients following the withdrawal of benzodiazepine medications. Only a small portion of the patients, who were not intubated, were able to be studied immediately postinjury, and not all patients were studied at each testing period. However, this study suggests that OSA is a result of the SCI and develops postinjury in association with increased neck and abdominal girth.

Based on data available currently, it appears that individuals with SCI are at increased risk for developing OSA. Information is not available on whether the long-term clinical consequences of OSA are similar in SCI and the able-bodied, though one study found that SCI patients with OSA had higher rates of cardiac medication use compared to those without OSA (52). This may reflect a greater tendency to cardiac complications in the OSA group, similar to that seen in the able-bodied. This is also an area that needs more study.

definition of OSA (24, 48, 51–53). The OSA rates ranged from 26% to 65%, which is markedly higher than the 9% estimate in the general able-bodied population. The current clinical definition of OSA is an AHI of greater than or equal to 5 plus symptoms suggestive of sleep apnea, such as sleepiness, gasping for air, snoring, or witnessed apnea (54). The prevalence of OSA in the able-bodied using this definition is 2% in women and 4% in men. The two SCI studies using this definition found a prevalence of 40% and 53% (53, 55).

There are many possible reasons for increased OSA rates in SCI. In the able-bodied, the best independent predictors of OSA are increased BMI and neck circumference (34, 35). Sedentary lifestyles might lead to increased body fat after injury. An increase in neck size, independent of weight gain, has been demonstrated in tetraplegics (56). The level and completeness of injury might influence the likelihood of OSA. This is because higher level injuries lead to reduced lung volumes. At lower lung volumes, upper airway diameter is reduced, thus predisposing a person to airway collapse (57). Medications used commonly in SCI might contribute to the high rate of OSA. For example, benzodiazepines promote airway collapse through selective reduction of upper airway dilator muscle activity (58). Last, those with SCI spend a greater amount of time in the supine position (24), a position that causes a decrease in the cross-sectional size of the airway (59).

Table 17.3 Comparison of Risk Factors for OSA between SCI and Able-Bodied

ASSOCIATED WITH OSA IN ABLE-BODIED	ASSOCIATED WITH OSA IN SCI	NOT ASSOCIATED IN SCI	POSSIBLY ASSOCIATED IN SCI
Increased BMI	Increased BMI	Level of injury	Age
Increased neck circumference	Increased neck circumference	ASIA scores	Antispasticity medication
Daytime sleepiness	Daytime sleepiness	Pulmonary function tests	
Increased age			
Male gender			
Family history of OSA			
Alcohol or sedative use			

BMI = body mass index; ASIA = American Spinal Injury Association.

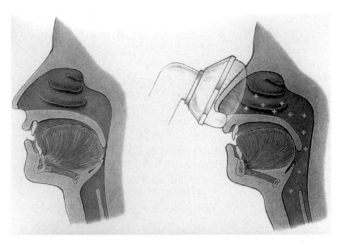

Figure 17.6 Nasal continuous positive airway pressure (CPAP) prevents the collapse of the upper airway. Occlusion of the upper airway during an obstructive apnea is shown in the left panel, with collapse occurring behind the soft palate and the base of the tongue. CPAP provides a pneumatic stent that keeps the upper airway open (right panel). (Reproduced from the slide set entitled "Sleep Apnea: Diagnosis and Treatment," used with permission from the American Academy of Sleep Medicine.)

Continuous positive airway pressure (CPAP) is the treatment of choice for OSA (62). CPAP is applied to the upper airway via a mask that covers the nose or nose and mouth. The pressure acts as a pneumatic stent to prevent the narrowing and closure of the upper airway (Figure 17.6). The device is highly effective, but limited by tolerance and compliance. In a case-control study of SCI patients previously diagnosed with OSA, only 47% were receiving treatment. The majority had been unable to tolerate CPAP therapy or did not accept treatment (50). In another study, daytime sleepiness was predictive of acceptance of CPAP therapy (52). Only sixteen of the thirty-one SCI patients diagnosed with OSA agreed to treatment with CPAP, and five discontinued therapy after a few weeks. However, ten of eleven patients with daytime sleepiness symptoms continued with therapy. Burns et al. further investigated CPAP use (61). They evaluated compliance with CPAP therapy in forty individuals with OSA and SCI who answered a mail survey on sleep habits. Twenty of thirty-two (63%) patients who tried CPAP were continuing to use it and reported high levels of usefulness and improvement in symptoms. Reasons for stopping CPAP were inability to fall asleep while wearing CPAP (63%), lack of improvement in symptoms (25%), or belief that treatment was unnecessary (8%). Side effects included nasal congestion (60%), mask discomfort (40%), dryness (30%), frequent awakenings (30%), and complaints from bed partner (5%), which are similar in type and number to the able-bodied using CPAP (62). Intensive support in the early treatment period has been shown to improve compliance in the able-bodied with similar complaints (63). SCI patients with OSA may face additional barriers to treatment with CPAP because of inability to manipulate the CPAP mask by themselves to relieve discomfort or improve fit. Otherwise, SCI does not limit use of this device.

Other treatment options include oral appliances that move either the tongue or mandible forward to open the posterior airspace, or upper airway surgery. One group proposed a 6-week resistive inspiratory muscle training program for tetraplegia patients (64). At the end of the program, measures of respiratory muscle strength and endurance were improved, and nocturnal oxyhemoglobin desaturation was reduced. However, they did not measure sleep and breathing directly, so it is not clear if the patients had OSA or if the improvement was due to a reduction in obstruction or change in respiratory muscle function. There is currently no information available regarding the efficacy of the alternative OSA treatments in the SCI population.

Nocturnal Movement Disorders

Spasticity is common after SCI and can present as hyperactive tendon jerks, clonus, increased muscle tone, and spontaneous muscle spasms. These movements can cause the fragmentation of sleep. In one survey, 65% of respondents reported that spasms, most commonly extensor spasms, interfered with their sleep (65). The usual treatment is antispasticity medication, typically baclofen and/or diazepam. Two studies used intrathecal baclofen to reduce leg spasms and found that, compared to oral baclofen, postawakening muscle activity was reduced, and sleep continuity improved without impairment of respiratory function (66, 67). It is unclear how much of this benefit was caused by the antispasticity effects or by the purely sedative properties of the medication.

Periodic limb movements of sleep (PLMS) are stereotyped repetitive movements that occur during sleep. Also called nocturnal myoclonus (although by definition they are longer than myoclonic movements), they typically occur in clusters of movements lasting 0.5 to 5 seconds, with a periodicity of 5 to 90 seconds, and repeat for several minutes to hours (see Figure 17.7). The movements may occur in one or both lower limbs and typically are more numerous during the first half of the night. A range of movement amplitudes can be seen, from simple dorsiflexion of the foot to a triple flexion response. They are most common in stages 1 and 2 sleep and are unusual in REM sleep (54). The movements can cause arousal from sleep and lead to sleep fragmentation, nonrestorative sleep, and daytime sleepiness. In the able-bodied, the risk factors for PLMS include diabetes mellitus, anemia, uremia, peripheral neuropathy, and iron deficiency. PLMS can be exacerbated by antidepressants and lithium, as well as by withdrawal from suppressive medications such as benzodiazepines and anticonvulsants (68). The pathophysiology of PLMS is unknown; however, there is evidence that the leg movements result from a central nervous system (CNS) dopamine deficiency. Drugs that increase dopamine, such as levodopa, decrease PLMS, whereas those that block dopamine release, like gamma-hydroxybutyrate, increase the movements (69). Opioids are also potent inhibitors of PLMS (70). Successful treatment of PLMS with dopamine agonists and opioid derivatives has led to hypotheses that there are dopamine- and opiate-dependent pathways that are involved in the regulation of reflex limb movements. Increasing central nervous system dopamine or endorphin levels decreases the reflex movements.

These repetitive lower limb movements are increased in SCI. Yokota et al. (71) first noted involuntary leg movements in ten patients with myelopathies, two of whom had SCI. The movements were stereotyped repetitive movements of the legs consisting of flexion of the ankle, knee, and hip (triple flexion), with a duration of 0.5 to 5 seconds. In the SCI patients, the

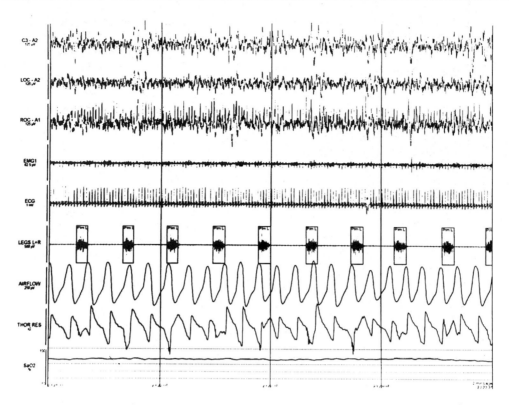

Figure 17.7 A polysomnographic tracing of an SCI patient with periodic limb movements of sleep (PLMS). The top channel of this 2-minute tracing is a central electroencephalogram lead (C3–A2). The PLMS can be seen in the leg electromyogram channel (LEGS L+R), which monitors movements in either leg. Note the repetitive chain of movements occurring during NREM sleep. There is no evidence of sleep-disordered breathing. (LOC-A2 = left eye lead; ROC-A1 = right eye lead; EMG1 = chin electromyogram; ECG = electrocardiogram; THOR RES = chest wall movement; SaO2 = oxyhemoglobin saturation.)

movements persisted during wakefulness and sleep, including REM sleep in one. The clinical and polysomnographic presentations were identical to those described for PLMS in the able-bodied. Because the movements occurred in patients with neurologically complete SCI, the data suggested that PLMS were generated in the spinal cord. Other authors have described stereotyped movements identical to PLMS in SCI subjects (72, 73). The PLMS continued in REM sleep with even more regularity than in NREM and caused arousals from sleep. The authors postulated that PLMS were generated in the spinal cord and were usually under inhibition from the CNS site involved in the motor inhibition that occurs during REM sleep. Their data suggest that SCI released the spinal generator from inhibitory control, allowing the movements to occur. Others found that, in SCI, the number of PLMS was reduced by physical activity (74, 75). They postulated that the endorphins produced by exercise were responsible for the reduction in movements in a manner similar to the reduction seen with the use of opioids.

Physical exercise raises central endorphin levels (76). De Mello et al. conducted a series of studies to evaluate the effect of physical exercise on frequency of PLMS in SCI. They measured PLMS after exercise using a hand-cranked bicycle ergometer. The rate of PLMS was measured during overnight polysomnography 12 and 36 hours after exercise and after a 45-day exercise program. The rate of PLMS was reduced significantly in all

conditions after exercise (77). In another study, they compared the effects of a dopamine agonist with physical exercise to treat PLMS in SCI (78). In a placebo controlled trial, thirteen subjects with T7–T12 complete SCI underwent trials with 30 days of L-DOPA and a three-times-per-week exercise program for 45 days. Both treatment paradigms resulted in a significant reduction in the frequency of PLMS measured by polysomnography. There was no difference between the two treatment groups. The authors concluded that dopamine agonists and physical exercise were effective in reducing PLMS and should be used to treat PLMS in paraplegics.

An animal model of PLMS has been developed in rats using a surgical T9 SCI. Wistar rats were studied for 7 days after a surgical SCI, and rates of PLMS were compared with rats undergoing sham surgery. Ten of eleven rats developed PLMS 3–7 days following the SCI, whereas none of the rats in the sham group demonstrated PLMS (79). In a similar study observing rats with surgical SCI for 15 days, the number of animals developing PLMS was significantly greater than in the sham surgery group (20). These studies suggest that the movements are generated in the spinal cord without cortical involvement.

Complaints of fragmented sleep, daytime sleepiness, and repetitive spasms should prompt an examination for PLMS. The current literature does not address whether standard treatments in the able-bodied, such as dopamine agonists, sedative/hypnotics, and opioids, are effective in the SCI population. This is an area also in need of research.

Other Sleep Disorders

Insomnia, the most common sleep disorder in able-bodied persons, is estimated to occur chronically in as many as 60 million Americans (80). In SCI, factors that may promote insomnia include disruption of normal sleep patterns, chronic pain or discomfort, depression or adjustment disorders, temperature dysregulation, and chronic medication use. An additional factor, perhaps related to the disruption of normal melatonin rhythmicity in cervical SCI, may be disorders of circadian rhythm (32). However, there is not any information on the prevalence or presentation of these disorders in SCI.

Evaluating Sleep and Sleep Disorders

SCI patients frequently complain about the quality of their sleep (1) but often don't present with the typical symptoms of sleep disorders. For instance, the majority of SCI patients with OSA do not complain of sleepiness (61). This makes it essential to assess sleep patterns during routine SCI evaluations. Patients should be specifically asked about their sleep-wake routine, whether their sleep was restorative, if they are sleepy during the daytime, and whether they have symptoms of sleep disorders such as snoring and gasping at night (OSA), difficulty getting to sleep or staying asleep (insomnia), or frequent leg kicking (PLMS) (15). A positive answer to any of these questions should elicit a more thorough sleep evaluation (see Table 17.4). Questionnaires have been developed to look for sleep disorders, but many of these

are limited by questions not applicable to those with SCI. Although not specifically developed for SCI, the reproducibility of the Basic Nordic Sleep Questionnaire (81) has been tested in SCI (82). Positive responses suggestive of a sleep fragmentation disorder on a questionnaire or during examination should prompt testing with a sleep study to establish the diagnosis and determine severity. The severity of the symptoms and the sleep disorder will determine appropriate therapy.

CONCLUSION

In SCI, sleep disorders occur as a consequence of the injury and its treatment. Awakenings, so that individuals can receive specialized care such as turning to prevent decubitus ulcers, disrupt sleep. The injury itself disrupts the function of the circadian rhythm system, appears to facilitate PLMS, and may promote the development of OSA. The data reviewed in this chapter show that a sleep assessment should be included in the evaluation of all individuals with SCI.

R*eferences*

1. Levi R, Hultling C, Nash MS, Seiger A. The Stockholm spinal cord injury study: medical problems in a regional SCI population. *Paraplegia* 1995; 33:308–315.
2. Nair KPS, Taly AB, Maheshwarappa BM, Kumar J, et al. Nontraumatic spinal cord lesions: a prospective study of medical complications during in-patient rehabilitation. *Spinal Cord* 2005; 43:558–564.
3. Hyyppa MT, Kronholm E. Quality of sleep and chronic illness. *J Clin Epidemiol* 1989; 42:633–638.
4. Biering-Sorensen F, Biering-Sorensen M. Sleep disturbances in the spinal cord injured: an epidemiological questionnaire investigation, including a normal population. *Spinal Cord* 2001; 39:505–513.
5. Pentland W, Harvey AS, Smith T, Walker J. The impact of spinal cord injury on men's time use. *Spinal Cord* 1999; 37:786–792.
6. The AASM Manual for the Scoring of Sleep and Associated Events: Rules, Terminology and Technical Specification.
7. Berger RJ, Oswald I. Effects of sleep deprivation on behavior, subsequent sleep, and dreaming. *J Ment Sci* 1962; 108:457–465.
8. Carskadon MA, Dement WC. Normal human sleep: an overview. In: Kryger MH, Roth T, Dement WC, eds. *Principles and Practice of Sleep Medicine.* 4th ed. Philadelphia: W.B. Saunders, 2005; 19.
9. Daan S, Beersma DGM, Borbely AA. Timing of human sleep: recovery process gated by a circadian pacemaker. *Am J Physiol* 1984; 246: R161–R178.
10. Reppert SM, Weaver DR, Rivkees SA, Stopa EG. Putative melatonin receptors in a human biological clock. *Science* 1988; 242:78–81.
11. Kryger MH, Roth T, Carskadon M. Circadian rhythms in humans: an overview. In: Kryger MH, Roth T, Dement WC, eds. *Principles and Practice of Sleep Medicine.* 2nd ed. Philadelphia: W.B. Saunders, 1994; 301–308.
12. Carskadon MA, Brown ED, Dement WC. Sleep fragmentation in the elderly: relationship to daytime sleep tendency. *Neurobiol Aging* 1982; 3:321–327.
13. Czeisler CA, Moore-Ede MC, Coleman RM. Rotating shift work schedules that disrupt sleep are improved by applying circadian principles. *Science* 1982; 217:460–463.
14. Ancoli-Israel S, Kripke DF, Mason W, Messin S. Sleep apnea and nocturnal myoclonus in a senior population. *Sleep* 1981; 4:349–358.
15. Strollo PJ. Sleep disorders in primary care. In: Poceta JS, Mitler MM, eds. *Sleep Disorders: Diagnosis and Treatment.* Ottawa: Humana Press, 1998; 1–20.
16. Budh CN, Hultling C, Lundeberg T. Quality of sleep in individuals with spinal cord injury: a comparison between patients with and without pain. *Spinal Cord* 2005; 43:85–95.
17. Budh CN, Kowalski J, Lundeberg T. A comprehensive pain management programme comprising educational, cognitive and behavioural interventions for neuropathic pain following spinal cord injury. *J Rehabil Med* 2006; 38:172–80.

Table 17.4   Components of Sleep History

Sleep/wake cycle	Time to bed/time out of bed
	Time to fall asleep
	Weekend changes to routine
	Daytime naps
The sleep period	Awakenings and ability to return to sleep
	Cause of awakenings
	Snoring, breath stops, gasping for air
	Leg kicking
	Pain, trouble breathing, reflux
Daytime functioning	Excessive sleepiness
	Attention, memory, concentration problems
	Motor vehicle or work accidents
	Drowsy driving problems
Sleep habits	Bedroom conducive to sleep
	Caffeine, alcohol, drug use
	Timing of exercise
	Appropriate pre-sleep routine
Medical problems that disrupt sleep	Hyper/hypothyroidism, angina, heart failure, stroke, Parkinson's disease, COPD, chronic pain syndromes, diabetes
Medications	Stimulants, sedatives, medications that affect sleep

18. Krouskop TA, Noble PC, Garber SL, Spencer WA. The effectiveness of preventive management in reducing the occurrence of pressure sores. *J Rehabil Res Dev* 1983; 20:74–83.

19. Kilinc S, Akman MN, Levelnoglu F, Ozker R. Diurnal variation of antidiuretic hormone and urinary output in spinal cord injury. *Spinal Cord* 1999; 37:332–335.

20. Esteves AM, Mello MT, Squarcini CFR, Lancellotti CLP, et al. Sleep patterns over 15-day period in rats with spinal cord injury. *Spinal Cord* 2007; 45:360–366.

21. Adey WR, Bors E, Porter RW. EEG sleep patterns after high cervical lesions in man. *Arch Neurol* 1968; 19:377–383.

22. Jobert M, Jahnig P, Schulz H. Effect of two antidepressant drugs on REM sleep and EMG activity during sleep. *Neuropsychobiology* 1999; 39:101–109.

23. Gaillard JM, Blois R. Effect of the benzodiazepine antagonist Ro 15–1788 on flunitrazepam-induced sleep changes. *Br J Clin Pharmacol* 1983; 15:529–536.

24. Evoy RD, Myketyn I, Sajkov D, Flavell H, et al. Sleep apnea in patients with quadriplegia. *Thorax* 1995; 50:612–619.

25. Scheer FAJL, Zeitzer JM, Ayas, NT, Brown R, et al. Reduced sleep efficiency in cervical spinal cord injury: association with abolished night time melatonin secretion. *Spinal Cord* 2006; 44:78–81.

26. Czeisler CA, Kronauer RE, Allan JS, Duffy JF, et al. Bright light induction of strong (type 0) resetting of the human circadian pacemaker. *Science* 1989; 244:1328–1332.

27. Shanahan TL, Czeisler CA. Light exposure induces equivalent phase shifts of the endogenous circadian rhythms of circulating plasma melatonin and core body temperature in men. *J Clin Endocrinol Metab* 1991; 73:227–235.

28. Vollrath L. Functional anatomy of the human pineal gland. In: Reiter RJ, ed. *The Pineal Gland*. New York: Raven Press, 1984; 285–382.

29. Cassone VM. Effects of melatonin on vertebrate circadian systems. *Trends Neurosci* 1990; 13:457–464.

30. Kneisley LW, Moskowitz, MA, Lynch HJ. Cervical spinal cord lesions disrupt the rhythm in human melatonin excretion. *J Neural Transm* 1978; 13(S):311–323.

31. Li Y, Jiang DH, Wang ML, Jiao DR, Pang SF. Rhythms of serum melatonin in patients with spinal lesions at the cervical, thoracic, or lumbar region. *J Clin Endocrinol* 1989; 30:47–56.

32. Zeitzer JM, Ayas NT, Shea SA, Brown R, Czeisler CA. Absence of detectable melatonin and preservation of cortisol and thyrotropin rhythms in tetraplegia. *J Clin Endocrinol Metab* 2000; 85:2189–2196.

33. Zeitzer JM, Ayas NT, Wu AD, Czeisler CA, Brown R. Bilateral oculosympathetic paresis associated with loss of nocturnal melatonin secretion in patients with spinal cord injury. *J Spinal Cord Med* 2005; 28:55–59.

34. Young TT, Palta M, Dempsey J, Skatrud J, et al. The occurrence of sleep-disordered breathing among middle-aged adults. *N Engl J Med* 1993; 32:1230–1235.

35. Davies RJ, Stradling, JR. The relationship between neck circumference, radiographic pharyngeal anatomy, and the obstructive sleep apnoea syndrome. *Eur Respir J* 1990; 3:509–514.

36. Berry RB, Kouchi K, Bower J, Prosise G, Light RW. Triazolam in patients with obstructive sleep apnea. *Am J Respir Crit Care Med* 1995; 151:450–454.

37. Issa FG, Sullivan CE. Alcohol, snoring and sleep apnea. *J Neurol Neurosurg Psychiatry* 1982; 45:353–359.

38. Redline S, Tishler PV, Tosteson TD, et al. The familial aggregation of obstructive sleep apnea. *Am J Respir Crit Care Med* 1995; 151:682–687.

39. Isono S, Remmers JE, Tanaka A, Sho Y, et al. Anatomy of the pharynx in patients with obstructive sleep apnea and in normal subjects. *J Appl Physiol* 1997; 82:1319–1326.

40. Mezzanotte WS, Tangel DJ, White DP. Waking genioglossal EMG in sleep apnea patients versus normal controls (a neuromuscular compensatory mechanism). *J Clin Invest* 1992; 89:1571–1579.

41. Epstein LJ, Weiss JW. Clinical consequences of obstructive sleep apnea. *Semin Respir Crit Care Med* 1998; 19:123–132.

42. Ayas NT, Epstein LJ, Lieberman SL, Tun CG, et al. Predictors of loud snoring in spinal cord injury. *J Spinal Cord Med* 2001; 24:30–34.

43. Braun SR, Giovannoni R, Levin AB, Harvey RF. Oxygen saturation during sleep in patients with spinal cord injury. *Am J Phys Med* 1982; 61:302–309.

44. Flavell H, Marshall R, Thornton AT, Clements PL, et al. Hypoxia episodes during sleep in high tetraplegia. *Arch Phys Med Rehabil* 1992; 73:623–627.

45. Cahan C, Gothe B, Decker MJ, Arnold JL, Strohl KP. Arterial oxygen saturation over time and sleep studies in quadriplegic patients. *Paraplegia* 1993; 31:172–179.

46. Bonekat HW, Andersen G, Squires J. Obstructive disordered breathing during sleep in patients with spinal cord injury. *Paraplegia* 1990; 28:393–398.

47. Biering-Sorenson M, Norup PW, Jacobsen E, Biering-Sorenson F. Treatment of sleep apnea in spinal cord injured patients. *Paraplegia* 1995; 33:271–273.

48. Short DJ, Stradling JR, Williams SJ. Prevalence of sleep apnea in patients over 40 years of age with spinal cord lesions. *J Neurol Neurosurg Psychiatry* 1992; 55:1032–1036.

49. Klefbeck B, Sternhag M, Weinberg J, Levi R, et al. Obstructive sleep apneas in relation to severity of spinal cord injury. *Spinal Cord* 1998; 36:621–628.

50. Burns SP, Kapur V, Yin KS, Buhrer R. Factors associated with sleep apnea in men with spinal cord injury: a population-based case-control study. *Arch Phys Med Rehab* 2001; 39:15–22.

51. Ayas NT, Epstein LJ, Brown R, Hibbert AM, Garshick E. Baclofen use and age predict obstructive sleep apnea in spinal cord injury. *Sleep* 1999; 22:S294.

52. Stockhammer E, Tobon A, Michel F, Eser P, et al. Characteristics of sleep apnea syndrome in tetraplegic patients. *Spinal Cord* 2002; 40:286–294.

53. Burns P, Little JW, Hussey JD, Lyman P, Lakshminarayanan S. Sleep apnea syndrome in chronic spinal cord injury: associated factors and treatment. *Arch Phys Med Rehabil* 2000; 81:1334–1339.

54. American Academy of Sleep Medicine ICSD-2. *International Classification of Sleep Disorders*. 2nd ed. Westchester, IL: American Academy of Sleep Medicine, 2005.

55. Leduc BE, Dagher JH, Mayer P, Bellemare F, Lepage Y. Estimated prevalence of obstructive sleep apnea-hypopnea syndrome after cervical cord injury. *Arch Phys Med Rehabil* 2007; 88:333–337.

56. Frisbie JH, Brown R. Waist and neck enlargement after quadriplegia. *J Am Paraplegia Soc* 1994; 17:177–178.

57. Hoffstein V, Zamel N, Phillipson EA. Lung volume dependence of pharyngeal cross-sectional area in patients with obstructive sleep apnea. *Am Rev Respir Dis* 1984; 130:175–178.

58. Leiter JC, Knuth SL, Krol RC, Bartlett D. The effect of diazepam on genioglossal muscle activity in normal human subjects. *Am Rev Respir Dis* 1985; 132:216–219.

59. Pevernagie DA, Stanson AW, Sheedy PF II, Daniels BK, Shepard JW Jr. Effects of body position on the upper airway of patients with obstructive sleep apnea. *Am J Respir Crit Care Med* 1995; 152:179–185.

60. Berlowitz DJ, Brown DJ, Campbell DA, Pierce RJ. A longitudinal evaluation of sleep and breathing in the first year after cervical spinal cord injury. *Arch Phys Med Rehabil* 2005; 86:1193–1199.

61. Burns SP, Yavari RM, Bryant S, Kapur V. Long term treatment of sleep apnea in persons with spinal cord injury. *Am J Phys Med Rehabil* 2005; 84:620–625.

62. Engleman HM, Asgari-Jirhandeh N, McLeod AL, Ramsay CF, et al. Self-reported use of CPAP and benefits of CPAP therapy. *Chest* 1996; 109:1470–1476.

63. Hoy CJ, Vennelle M, Kingshott RN, Engleman HM, Douglas NJ. Can intensive support improve continuous positive airway pressure use in patients with the sleep apnea/hypopnea syndrome? *Am J Respir Crit Care Med* 1999; 159:1096–1110.

64. Wang TG, Wang YH, Tang FT, Lin KW, Lien IN. Resistive inspiratory muscle training in sleep-disordered breathing of traumatic tetraplegia. *Arch Phys Med Rehabil* 2002; 83:491–496.

65. Little JW, Micklesen P, Umlauf R, Britell C. Lower extremity manifestations of spasticity in chronic spinal cord injury. *Am J Phys Med Rehabil* 1989; 68:32–36.

66. Kravitz HM, Corcos DM, Hansen G, Penn RD, et al. Intrathecal baclofen: effects on nocturnal leg muscle spasticity. *Am J Phys Med Rehabil* 1992; 71:48–52.

67. Bensmail D, Quera Salva MA, Roche N, Benyahia S, et al. Effect of intrathecal baclofen on sleep and respiratory function in patients with spasticity. *Neurology* 2006; 67:1432–1436.

68. Montplaisir J, Godbout R, Pelletier G, Warnes H. Restless legs syndrome and periodic limb movements during sleep. In: Kryger MH, Roth T, Dement WC, eds. *Principles and Practice of Sleep Medicine*. 2nd ed. Philadelphia: W.B. Saunders, 1994; 589–597.

69. Brodeur C, Montplaisir J, Godbout R, Marinier R. Treatment of restless legs syndrome and periodic movements during sleep with L-dopa: a double blind, controlled study. *Neurology* 1988; 38:1845–1848.

70. Kavey N, Walters AS, Hening W, Gidro-Frank S. Opioid treatment of periodic movements in sleep in patients without restless legs. *Neuropeptides* 1988; 11:181–184.

71. Yokota T, Hirose K, Tanabe H, Tsukagoshi H. Sleep-related periodic leg movements (nocturnal myoclonus) due to spinal cord lesion. *J Neurol Sci* 1991; 104:13–18.

72. Dickel MJ, Renfrow SD, Moore PT, Berry RB. Rapid eye movement sleep periodic leg movements in patients with spinal cord injury. *Sleep* 1994; 17:733–738.

73. Lee MS, Choi YC, Lee SH, Lee SB. Sleep-related periodic leg movements associated with spinal cord lesions. *Mov Disord* 1996; 11:719–722.

74. de Mello ME, Lauro FAA, Silva AC, Tufik S. Incidence of periodic leg movements and of the restless legs syndrome during sleep following acute physical activity in spinal cord injury subjects. *Spinal* 1996; 34:294–296.

75. de Mello MT, Silva AC, Rueda AD, Poyares D, Tufik S. Correlation between K complex, periodic leg movements (PLM), and myoclonus during sleep in paraplegic adults before and after an acute physical activity. *Spinal Cord* 1997; 35:248–252.

76. Goldfarb AH, Jamurtas AZ, Kamimori GH, Hegde S, et al. Gender effect on beta-endorphin response to exercise. *Med Sci Sports Exerc* 1998; 30:1672–1676.

77. de Mello MT, Silva AC, Esteves AM, Tufik S. Reduction of periodic leg movement in individuals with paraplegia following aerobic physical exercise. *Spinal Cord* 2002; 40:646–649.

78. de Mello MT, Esteves AM, Tufik S. Comparison between dopaminergic agents and physical exercise as treatment for periodic limb movements in patients with spinal cord injury. *Spinal Cord* 2004; 42:218–221.

79. Esteves AM, de Mello MT, Lancelotti CLP, Natal CL, Tufik S. Occurrence of limb movement during sleep in rats with spinal cord injury. *Brain Res* 2004; 1017:32–38.

80. Report of the National Commission on Sleep Disorders Research. *Wake Up America: Executive Summary and Executive Report*, Vol. 1. Department of Health and Human Services, January 1993:36–37.

81. Partinen M, Gislason T. Basic Nordic Sleep Questionnaire (BNSQ): a quantitated measure of subjective sleep complaints. *J Sleep Res* 1995; 4(S1):150–155.

82. Biering-Sorensen F, Biering-Sorensen M, Hilden J. Reproducibility of Nordic Sleep Questionnaire in spinal cord injured. *Paraplegia* 1994; 32:780–786.

18 Cardiovascular Dysfunction in Spinal Cord Disorders

Sunil Sabharwal

Cardiovascular function is altered in individuals with spinal cord injury SCI (1–14). Impairment of autonomic function after SCI is a major contributory factor (14–22). In cervical and high thoracic injuries in particular, interruption to the sympathetic outflow plays a key role in cardiovascular dysfunction. Loss of supraspinal regulatory control of the sympathetic nervous system results in reduced overall sympathetic activity below the level of injury and causes problems such as hypotension, bradycardia, and a blunted cardiovascular response to exercise (14, 15). Morphologic changes occur in sympathetic preganglionic neurons distal to the injury (23, 24). Peripheral alpha-adrenergic hyper-responsiveness may occur, and probably contributes to the excessive pressor response seen in autonomic dysreflexia (25, 26). In addition to autonomic abnormalities, there are indirect effects of reduced physical activity, altered metabolic function, and other SCI-related conditions on cardiovascular function (6, 8, 22, 27, 28).

Various cardiovascular issues of concern after SCI are discussed in the subsequent section, and the major manifestations are summarized in Table 18.1.

Table 18.1 Cardiovascular Issues in SCI

Hypotension
    Low baseline blood pressure
    Orthostatic hypotension
Bradycardia, arrhythmias, cardiac arrest
Autonomic dysreflexia
Reduced cardiovascular fitness and altered exercise capacity
Influence on coronary and peripheral artery disease
    Impact on risk factors
    Silent ischemia, atypical presentations
    Special diagnostic and treatment considerations
Venous thromboembolism
Cardiovascular effects of medications in SCI

LOW BASELINE BLOOD PRESSURE

Low blood pressure is commonly found in acute and chronic SCI primarily after cervical or high thoracic injury (14, 29). An inverse relationship has been described between the level of lesion and reduced blood pressure (10, 12, 14). Patients with complete cervical injury have lower than normal blood pressure; those with lower thoracic or lumbar lesions have normal resting pressures. The lowered baseline blood pressure seen with higher spinal cord lesions is thought to be caused by reduced sympathetic activity below the level of injury that results in reduced vasomotor tone (14).

ORTHOSTATIC HYPOTENSION

Orthostatic hypotension (OH) has been arbitrarily defined as a fall of more than 20 mmHg systolic blood pressure on assuming the upright position (30). However, a smaller drop in blood pressure may be equally important when associated with relevant symptoms that indicate impaired perfusion. Some have defined OH simply as a symptomatic fall in blood pressure in the upright posture (31). OH following SCI is common and well documented (30–35).

Pathophysiology

The major underlying abnormality in SCI-related OH is a lack of sympathetically mediated reflex vasoconstriction, especially in large vascular beds, such as those supplying the splanchnic region and skeletal muscle (14, 30–37). The gravitational effects of venous pooling in the lower extremities, accompanied by a lack of compensatory changes in other vascular beds, leads to the fall in blood pressure. Venous pooling results in reduced filling pressure at the heart, and decrease in the end-diastolic filling volume and stroke volume. Tachycardia may occur due to reflex vagal inhibition, but is not sufficient to compensate for the reduced sympathetic response. Symptoms are less likely to occur in SCI below the origin of the major splanchnic outflow at T6 and with incomplete injuries (31, 37). The prevalence of OH as well as the degree of fall in blood pressure are higher with cervical than with thoracic injuries (32). Low plasma volume, hyponatremia, and cardiovascular deconditioning may be additional contributing factors in some instances of OH after SCI (30). OH has been reported to be more common after traumatic than nontraumatic SCI (38).

OH often, but not always, improves over time (31, 37). Compensatory changes in other vascular beds may contribute to blood pressure homeostasis. Reduced blood flow to the kidneys may activate afferent glomerular dilatation and result in the stimulation of the renin-angiotensin aldosterone system (39–41). Other potential mechanisms for improvement over time include vascular wall receptor hypersensitivity, some recovery of postural reflexes at the spinal level, and increased skeletal muscle tone (39, 41–44). Tolerance to symptoms of OH often develops over time even with continued evidence of postural reduction in blood pressure in the upright position. It has been suggested that autoregulation of cerebral blood flow, rather than systemic blood pressure, may play a dominant role in the adaptation to OH (45).

Clinical Features

Many of the key manifestations of OH occur as a result of cerebral hypoperfusion (37, 39). These include dizziness, loss of consciousness, and visual disturbances such as blurred vision, scotoma, tunnel vision, graying out, and color defects. Pallor, auditory deficits, and nonspecific weakness and lethargy may also occur. Excess sweating may occur above the level of injury. OH may hinder participation in rehabilitation therapies due to occurrence of symptoms with mobilization treatments that involve sitting up or standing (35).

Postural hypotension may be influenced by several factors (Table 18.2), many of which are reversible (30, 39, 46). These include rapid changes in position and prolonged recumbency. Hypotension may be worse in the morning on rising. Heavy meals may exacerbate fall in blood pressure in response to shunting of blood to the splanchnic circulation after a meal (47, 48). Physical exertion, alcohol intake, or a hot environment can precipitate hypotension by promoting vasodilatation (39, 49). Sepsis and dehydration can worsen symptoms. Several medications can induce or worsen postural hypotension. Tricyclic antidepressants (TCA), antihypertensives, diuretics, and narcotic analgesics can precipitate this response. The late development or worsening of OH months or years after injury may be a sign of posttraumatic

syringomyelia and should prompt suspicion of this condition and appropriate diagnostic studies (50).

Management

No single treatment for OH in SCI is consistently effective. Success may be increased by trying various measures in combination and by individualizing management (51–54). The goal of treatment is to alleviate the disability caused by symptoms, rather than to achieve an optimal target blood pressure reading.

A number of practical nonpharmacologic measures (Table 18.3) can be taken to minimize the hypotensive effects (51), although evidence of effectiveness in SCI is limited for most. Small, frequent meals may minimize postprandial symptoms (48). Patients may have greater functional capacity before a meal than in the hour following a meal and may be able to adjust their activities accordingly. If blood pressure is higher later in the day, physical exertion, such as exercise programs or physical therapy, may be better tolerated in the afternoon rather than the early morning (49). The nocturnal diuresis that sometimes occurs in SCI may lead to inadequate blood volume. Elevating the head of the bed (reverse Trendelenberg position) may reduce nocturnal diuresis, morning postural hypotension, hypovolemia, and supine hypertension, although patients may not be able to tolerate more than a few degrees of head-up tilt during the night (51). Rapid changes in position should be avoided, as should excessive exertion in hot environments. A review of patient medications is mandatory and modification may be indicated to minimize hypotensive side-effects. If vasoactive medications are being administered with meals, that may be particularly disabling. Liberalizing salt and water intake may improve blood volume, although benefit of salt loading has not been sufficiently proven in people with SCI (30). Abdominal binders and compressive stockings can be used in an attempt to increase venous pressure and reduce venous pooling through decreased capacitance of leg and abdominal vascular beds (55). However, donning these may present practical problems for people with SCI and there is conflicting evidence of effectiveness (30, 56, 57). Repeated

---

Table 18.2   Reversible Factors Exacerbating Symptomatic Postural Hypotension in SCI

Prolonged recumbency
Rapid position change
Heavy meals
Physical exertion
Hot environment
Dehydration (diarrhea, viral illness)
Sepsis
Medications: Diuretics, antidepressants, alpha blockers, narcotics

---

Table 18.3   Management of Orthostatic Hypotension in SCI

Identify and minimize exacerbating factors (Table 18.2)
Increase salt intake
Compression stockings, abdominal binder
Tilt table, progressive postural challenges
Head-up tilt during sleep
Elevating wheelchair leg rests
Reclining or tilt-in-space wheelchair
Functional electrical stimulation
Biofeedback
Body-weight–supported treadmill training
Pharmacological treatment
    Fludrocortisone
    Sympathomimetic amines
        Ephedrine
        Midodrine
    Other medications (little reported use for SCI-related OH)

and gradual increase in postural challenges, such as with the use of a tilt-table, may be useful in the acute stages (31, 37). A tilt-in-space or reclining wheelchair is beneficial for accommodating to a progressive increase in the sitting angle and also allows reclining in response to symptoms. Evidence for use of body weight-supported treadmill training to improve orthostatic tolerance (58) is currently insufficient.

There is some evidence to support a role for functional electrical stimulation (FES) in the treatment of OH in SCI (59, 60). FES-induced contraction of leg muscles may increase venous return and increase cardiac output and stroke volume, which can increase blood pressure and decrease hypotension-related symptoms. The response appears to be dose-dependent and independent of the site of stimulation. Further research in this area is warranted. Biofeedback has also been tried for the management of OH in SCI (61).

Pharmacologic Management

Several drugs have been used to treat OH (Table 18.3), though many are of limited benefit (51–54, 62–74). The drugs for which there has been the most experience in use for SCI-related OH include fludrocortisone (62, 63), ephedrine (65, 66), and midodrine (68–73). Of these, only Midodrine is FDA approved for the treatment of neurogenic OH and has established effectiveness through randomized controlled trials (69, 70).

Fludrocortisone is a potent mineralocorticoid with little glucocorticoid activity. It has been used to manage the OH related to autonomic dysfunction for more than 40 years (62, 63). The pressor action of fludrocortisone is a result of sodium retention, which occurs over several days (51, 62). This delayed action should be clear to the patient as well as provider to avoid expectations of immediate benefit. For the same reason, doses should be altered no faster than on a weekly or biweekly interval. In addition to enhancing renal sodium conservation, fludrocortisone increases the sensitivity of arterioles to norepinephrine (51). Many patients have received benefit with a once-daily regimen. However, it has been suggested that a twice-daily regimen may be more efficacious, because the drug has been demonstrated to have a relatively short half-life of 2 to 3 hours (51). The usual starting dose is 0.1 mg/day given orally. Doses lower than 0.05 mg daily are rarely of any benefit. The dose can be increased by 0.1 mg increments at intervals of 1 to 2 weeks. Few patients need more than 0.4 mg daily, although there are reports in the literature of higher doses being used. No significant glucocorticoid effect is seen at these doses, but ACTH suppression, manifested by reduced cortisol level, may occur at higher doses. Fludrocortisone treatment can be associated with several side effects (31, 37, 51). Because fluid retention is critical to the beneficial effect, patients often gain between 5 to 8 pounds before optimal effect is seen, although higher weight gain than that should be avoided. Fludrocortisone should be avoided in patients who are unable to tolerate an increased fluid load, such as those with congestive heart failure. Electrolyte imbalance can also occur with fludrocortisone treatment, and periodic checking of serum electrolytes is advisable. Hypokalemia is especially common and may occur in as many as 50% of patients within 2 weeks. It should be treated with concomitant potassium supplementation. Hypomagnesemia may occur in 5% of patients and usually responds secondarily to correction of hypokalemia, although some patients may

need small doses of magnesium sulfate. Headache is another relatively common side effect of fludrocortisone, although it may be more of a problem in healthy, young adults than in sick or elderly patients. Potential drug interaction with warfarin may require patients on this drug to increase warfarin dose to maintain previous protimes after starting fludrocortisone.

Ephedrine was the first available orally active sympathomimetic drug. It has been used for the treatment of hypotension for many years (37, 66). It acts primarily through the release of stored catecholamines and has additional direct action on adrenoreceptors. It is nonselective and mimics epinephrine in its spectrum of effects (51). The usual oral dose is 25 to 50 mg repeated every 4 hours as needed. Its use is often individualized to maximize efficiency; for example, administering it 15 to 30 minutes prior to arising. Side effects include risk of supine hypertension, tremulousness, palpitations, and occasionally cardiac arrhythmias in susceptible patients (51, 66). Sympathomimetic effects on the bladder sphincter may increase urinary retention. Insomnia may occur, because it is a CNS stimulant. Tachyphylaxis may occur with repetitive dosing, especially among patients taking three or more doses per day over several weeks. The stimulant properties of this drug present the possibility of abuse and dependence.

Midodrine is an alpha1-adrenoreceptor agonist that has well-established effectiveness in patients with neurogenic OH (68–70). It has been used with some success to treat the OH associated with SCI (71, 73), with demonstrated improvement in systolic blood pressure during exercise as well as exercise tolerance (73). Midodrine directly increases blood pressure by arteriolar and venous constriction. It is a prodrug that is metabolized to desglymidodrine after absorption. It is 93% absorbed following oral administration and its bioavailability is not affected by food. Its half-life is 30 minutes, and the half-life of its active metabolite, desglymidodrine, is about 3 hours. The use of this drug must be individualized to attain maximum therapeutic benefit. Typically midodrine is initiated at a dose of 2.5 mg with breakfast and lunch, but the dose is rapidly increased at 2.5 mg increments until a satisfactory response is achieved, to a maximum of 30 mg a day (72). Patients are often maintained on a dose of 5 to 10 mg on arising, a second dose mid-morning, and a third dose mid-afternoon. The use of midodrine early in the day provides the maximum effect when the patient most needs it and avoids the side effect of excessive supine hypertension at night. Supine hypertension is the potentially most serious adverse effect, and it is essential to monitor both supine and sitting blood pressure in patients maintained on midodrine. Sleeping with the head elevated and taking the last dose at least 4 hours before bedtime may help minimize supine hypertension. Other side effects of midodrine are also predominantly related to its alpha1-adrenoreceptor agonist activity. Stimulation of the piloerector muscles results in patients commonly experiencing the sensation of gooseflesh, paresthesia of the scalp, or pruritis. These symptoms are often mild and may even be a welcome sign that the drug is functioning, but a few patients find these troublesome enough to discontinue treatment. Action on the alpha-receptors in the bladder may exacerbate urinary retention.

Other agents have been used to treat OH with variable success (51), but there is little to no published experience of their use in SCI-related OH. Nonsteroidal anti-inflammatory drugs, such as indomethacin or ibuprofen, act through inhibition of prostaglandin-induced vasoconstriction (51). Clonidine has been reported to cause a paradoxical beneficial increase in blood pressure in some patients with OH (74). Ergot alkaloids, recombinant human erythropoietin, the vasopressin analog desmopressin (DDAVP), and the somatostatin analog octreotide (51) have also been used. Long- or short-term treatment of OH with desmopressin minimizes fluid loss (51). Single intranasal doses at bedtime have been used to prevent nocturia and morning postural hypotension. Octreotide inhibits the release of gut peptides, thus producing vasodilating and hypotensive effects. Because many of these peptides are released after a meal, octreotide has been suggested for managing postprandial hypotension (48).

BRADYCARDIA AND CARDIAC ARREST

The imbalance of the autonomic nervous system caused by a decrease in sympathetic activity and a relative predominance of parasympathetic activity results in bradycardia (14, 75). This is a particular problem with cervical injuries and may even be life threatening in the acute stage, but usually resolves after the first 2 to 6 weeks after injury. The tracheal stimulation that occurs during suctioning or bronchial toilet can precipitate reflex bradycardia and even cardiac arrest in recently injured patients by increasing the unopposed vagal stimulation (75, 76). Management consists of ensuring adequate oxygenation, prompt treatment of factors such as respiratory infections that can contribute to hypoxia, and the administration of atropine about 10 minutes prior to tracheal suction, if needed. Temporary cardiac pacemakers have been used in patients with severe recurrent episodes (77). There is no evidence of a significant increase in cardiac arrhythmias in patients with chronic SCI (78).

AUTONOMIC DYSREFLEXIA

SCI at the thoracic level T6 or above (i.e., above the major splanchnic outflow) predisposes the patient to autonomic dysreflexia (AD), although occurrence with injuries as low as T8 is possible (79–80). AD results from noxious stimuli, which in turn trigger sympathetic hyperactivity. Inhibitory impulses that arise above the level of injury are blocked so that there is unopposed sympathetic outflow. Denervation hypersenstivity of peripheral adrenergic receptors below the level of injury may also contribute to the pathophysiology. Bladder problems are the most common precipitating cause, followed by bowel distension or impaction, but any noxious stimulus below the level of injury can precipitate AD (79). The pathogenesis, clinical features, and management of autonomic dysreflexia are also discussed in detail elsewhere in this textbook (see Chapter 41, Autonomic Dysfunction in Spinal Cord Disease).

Signs and symptoms of autonomic dysreflexia (AD) are summarized in Table 18.4 (79). The feature of most concern with autonomic dysreflexia is the significant and potentially life-threatening elevation in blood pressure. Blood pressure of 20–40 mm Hg above baseline may be a sign of AD. It reflects increased sympathetic outflow, which can also result in pallor and piloerection. Compensatory parasympathetic response with vasodilation above the level of injury may cause pounding headache, nasal congestion, flushed skin above the level of injury, constricted pupils, and sometimes a relative bradycardia. Life-threatening complications may include cardiac arrhythmias, seizures, or intracranial bleeding.

Table 18.4   Symptoms and Signs of Autonomic Dysreflexia
Sudden, significant increase in blood pressure
Pounding headache
Flushing of the skin above the level of the SCI, or possibly below
Blurred vision, appearance of spots in the patient's visual fields
Nasal congestion
Profuse sweating above the level of the SCI, or possibly below the level
Piloerection or goose bumps above the level of SCI, or possibly below
Bradycardia (may be a relative slowing only and still within normal range)
Cardiac arrhythmias
Feelings of apprehension or anxiety
Minimal or no symptoms, despite a significantly elevated blood pressure

The Consortium for Spinal Cord Medicine has published clinical practice guidelines for the acute management of autonomic dysreflexia (79). Autonomic dysreflexia (AD) is a life-threatening emergency and persons with tetraplegia can be at life-long risk. Prompt identification and management is critical. If the patient has signs and symptoms of dysreflexia, the blood pressure is elevated, and the individual is supine, immediately sit the person up. Loosen any clothing or constrictive devices. Monitor the blood pressure and pulse frequently. Quickly survey for instigating causes, beginning with the urinary system. If an indwelling urinary catheter is not in place, catheterize the individual. Prior to inserting the catheter, instill lidocaine jelly (if readily available) into the urethra. If the individual has an indwelling urinary catheter, check the system along its entire length for kinks, folds, constrictions, or obstructions, and for correct placement of the indwelling catheter. If a problem is found, correct it immediately. Avoid manually compressing or tapping on the bladder. If the catheter is not draining and the blood pressure remains elevated, remove and replace the catheter. If the catheter cannot be replaced, consult a urologist. If acute symptoms of autonomic dysreflexia persist, including a sustained elevated blood pressure, suspect fecal impaction. If the elevated blood pressure is at or above 150 mm Hg systolic, consider pharmacologic management to reduce the systolic blood pressure without causing hypotension prior to checking for fecal impaction. Use an antihypertensive agent with rapid onset and short duration (e.g., nifedipine bite and swallow, 2% nitroglycerin ointment, or prazosin) while the causes of autonomic dysreflexia are being investigated, and monitor the individual for symptomatic hypotension. If fecal impaction is suspected, check the rectum for stool. If precipitating cause of AD is not yet determined, check for other less frequent causes. Monitor the individual's symptoms and blood pressure for at least 2 hours after resolution of the AD episode to make sure that it does not recur. If there is poor response to the treatment specified above and/or if the cause of the dysreflexia has not been identified, strongly consider admitting the individual to the hospital to be monitored, to maintain pharmacologic control of the blood pressure, and to investigate other causes of the dysreflexia. Document the episode in the individual's medical record. Once the individual with spinal cord injury has been stabilized, review the precipitating causes with the individual and care givers, and provide education as necessary. Individuals with tetraplegia and their caregivers should be able to recognize and treat AD and be taught to seek emergency treatment if it is not promptly resolved (79).

REDUCED CARDIOVASCULAR FITNESS AND ALTERED EXERCISE CAPACITY

The available muscle mass under voluntary control is reduced after SCI (81). In addition, reduced sympathetic efferent output in people with high complete SCI results in a loss of the normal mechanisms that compensate for the cardiovascular stresses induced by active physical exercise (14, 81–83). Thus, exercise capacity as measured by the attainable VO_{2max} is reduced, and exercise intolerance leads to general deconditioning. Neither sympathetically mediated vasoconstriction with increased venous return nor increased heart rate and myocardial contractility is available in response to aerobic and anaerobic activities in these patients, although partial tachycardia may occur through a reduction in vagal activity and possibly through humeral mechanisms. Studies have shown that individuals with tetraplegia have a significantly lower maximal heart rate compared with able-bodied controls or those with paraplegia (83). In spite of these limitations, various potentially effective options for exercise in SCI have been described (84–95). Detailed discussion addressing exercise options after SCI is included in other sections of this textbook. (See Chapter 64.)

CORONARY HEART DISEASE

It has been suggested that the prevalence of coronary heart disease (CHD) is increased after SCI compared to the general population (6, 22, 96–100). However, the evidence for this is relatively weak (101) and there are other reports that suggest no significant difference in CHD prevalence between patients with SCI and otherwise comparable untrained able-bodied adults (101, 102). The small number of subjects, inadequate control for confounding variables, and differences in patient populations and outcomes studied may account for the discrepancy in results among different studies (101). Although cardiovascular diseases are among leading causes of death in chronic SCI, some have suggested that this may be attributable more to effect of aging than to the injury itself (101). In any case, heart disease is now a major cause of mortality and morbidity in patients with SCI, and with the aging of the population with SCI, CHD-related issues have become increasingly important in the care of these patients (103–107). Information from the SCI model system database suggests that heart disease is a leading cause of mortality in patients with spinal cord injury (103, 104). Cardiovascular disease was the leading cause of death in persons with SCI duration of 30 years or more (106). Although CHD was not separated out in this group because of lack of autopsy data, it likely comprises the major proportion of deaths. The importance of heart disease as a cause of mortality in people with SCI is also supported by other databases (105). It is therefore important for SCI care providers to be aware of the risk factors and prevention strategies for CHD, and to be familiar with unique issues in the diagnosis and management of CHD in patients with SCI.

Table 18.5 Potentially Increased Cardiovascular Risk Factors after SCI

Decreased physical activity
Low HDL cholesterol
Impaired glucose tolerance, insulin resistance
Increased proportion of body fat
Psychosocial factors
    Depression
    Social isolation
Hypothesized effects of SCI on emerging risk factors

Risk Factors and Prevention Strategies

Risk factors for atherosclerosis and CHD have been extensively studied and well described in the general population (108, 109). Long-term epidemiologic studies, such as the Framingham study, have provided important information on the establishment of these factors (108). Nonmodifiable risk factors include increasing age, male sex, and a positive family history of CHD. A history of early onset of CHD in first-degree relatives is especially significant, and these patients should be carefully identified and screened for CHD. The major modifiable risk factors, where interventions have been shown to be successful, include hypertension, cigarette smoking, lipid disorders (high LDL cholesterol, low HDL cholesterol), physical inactivity, obesity, and diabetes or impaired glucose tolerance (109–120). In addition to established risk factors, there are several emerging risk factors being studied. There may be an increased prevalence of some risk factors in patients with chronic SCI (Table 18.5) (90–95).

Motivation both on the part of the patient and the provider is critical for the successful preventive interventions to reduce risk of CHD (109). Prevention begins with a discussion of risk factors with the patient. Risk factor screening and global estimation of risk of CHD is indicated in all adults (109). The key intervention goals are listed in Table 18.6 (109, 110).

Table 18.6 Key Prevention Targets for Coronary Heart Disease (CHD)

Smoking cessation
Lipid management to goal
Blood pressure control
Weight management
Physical activity
Diabetic management to goal
Additional components of secondary prevention with known CHD:
    Antiplatelet agents (aspirin), anticoagulants
    Renin-angiotensin aldosterone system blockers
    Beta blockers

Hypertension

There is a consistent and continuous association of blood pressure levels with cardiovascular disease and excellent evidence that treatment of hypertension decreases morbidity and mortality from cardiac disease (114). In patients with SCI, a low rather than high baseline blood pressure is typical (14, 37). However, there are reports that suggest a significant prevalence of hypertension in these patients (121). This hypertension is often idiopathic, although it can be related to renal disease in some cases (122). Hypertension is common when SCI is the result of aortic disease or complications of aortic repair. At this time, there is no substantive evidence that episodic autonomic dysreflexia predisposes to chronic heart disease. Autonomic dysreflexia in people with SCI above thoracic level 6 is clinically distinguishable from essential hypertension by its presentation, course, and episodic nature. (79, 80)

Key lifestyle modifications in those with hypertension are the restriction of sodium intake, limitation of alcohol to 1 to 2 drinks a day, increased physical activity, and appropriate weight control (114). Drug management is very effective if compliance is maintained. Joint National Committee guidelines (JNC 7) recommend a blood pressure of less than 140/90 mmHg as a general target, less than 130/80 mm Hg with diabetes or chronic renal disease, and less than 120/80 mm Hg with left ventricular dysfunction (114). At this time it is not established if target blood pressure levels for people with SCI should be different from those for the general population. SCI-related considerations may impact choice of medications. Thiazide diuretics, which are recommended as first line options for the general population (114), may not be practical for those on an intermittent catheterization schedule for bladder management because of the associated diuresis.

Cigarette Smoking

The link between smoking and CHD is well established (113, 123, 124). There is a significant decrease in risk for myocardial infarction shortly after smoking cessation (123). A systematic process to identify all smokers is crucial (109, 110). Smoking cessation requires frequent single or group intervention sessions, with an attempt to set a date to quit smoking, as well as follow-up visits (125–126). Providers should ask about tobacco use at every visit, advise every tobacco user to quit, assist by counseling and developing a plan for quitting and arranging follow-up, and consider referral to special programs and/or pharmacotherapy, including nicotine replacement and bupriopion. Nicotine patches (21 mg, 14 mg, 7 mg, in decreasing steps over 10 to 12 weeks) or nicotine gum (2 mg or 4 mg) can be used. Nicotine spray, lozenges, or inhalers are other options. Various behavioral practices may be effective for individual patients, such as switching to a lower-nicotine brand (cigarette fading), attempts to have the patient place cigarettes in inaccessible places, and smoking the first cigarette later in the day. Because tobacco dependence may be characterized by relapses and remissions, clinicians should be ready to engage smokers and reengage relapsed smokers with options for new medication strategies and additional counseling resources (125). Avoidance of exposure to second-hand smoke at home or work should be encouraged (109).

Lipid Abnormalities

Elevated LDL-C level is a proven risk factor for CHD (127). There is convincing evidence that significant reduction of LDL cholesterol reduces the rate of CHD progression (109, 110, 128, 129). HDL cholesterol is a strong protective factor, and high HDL levels are inversely related to the risk of CHD (128). There is evidence to suggest that HDL levels are lower in the population with chronic SCI as compared to the general population (97, 130, 131). About 24% to 40% of people with SCI were reported to have HDL cholesterol of less than 35 mg/dl, compared to only 10% of the general population (96, 97). The relationship, if any, to completeness or level of injury is not established. Levels of LDL cholesterol in people with SCI are similar to those of the general population (96, 97).

The first step in selection of therapy for lipid abnormalities is to assess a person's risk status (128). All adults should have a complete lipoprotein profile at least once every 5 years (128, 129). Causes of secondary dyslipidemia (e.g. diabetes, hypothyroidism, certain drugs such as anabolic steroids) should be ruled out in those with abnormal results. Intensity of risk reduction therapy should be adjusted to a person's absolute risk. A value of LDL cholesterol over 160 mg/dl is considered high. LDL-C goal for those with 2 or more risk factors is below 130 mg/dl. For secondary prevention in those with known CHD or in those with CHD equivalents (other atherosclerotic heart disease, diabetes, or multiple risk factors that confer a 10-year risk of CHD greater than 20%), an LDL level of less than 100 mg/dl is the target, and a goal of less than 70 mg/dl may be reasonable with known CHD or other atherosclerotic disease (109, 110, 129). Although caution may be required when extrapolating findings from studies in able-bodied adults due to the physiological differences in SCI, current evidence does not suggest using a different threshold to define or treat abnormal lipid and carbohydrate measures for people with SCI compared to able-bodied adults (101).

Therapeutic lifestyle changes include reduced intake of saturated fats, increased intake of plant stanols/sterols and soluble fiber, appropriate weight reduction, and increased physical activity (109, 128, 129). Fat intake recommendations are more stringent in those with known CHD (110). Drug treatment should be started if lifestyle changes alone don't suffice, usually with a statin, although bile acid resins or niacin may also be considered (128, 129). Dose is advanced to bring LDL-C to goal range, and combination therapy may be required if goal is not achieved with monotherapy. At this time, there is no consensus regarding drug treatment for isolated low HDL cholesterol levels, and effective lifestyle modifications are the key for HDL cholesterol intervention (109, 128, 129). These include smoking cessation, weight reduction for overweight patients, and increased activity for sedentary patients. Although alcohol intake in moderation may increase HDL cholesterol levels, initiation of alcohol for this purpose is not warranted, considering the other medical, cognitive, and drug-interaction risks of alcohol use in the SCI patient population.

Physical Activity

There is strong evidence that a sedentary lifestyle is an independent risk factor for CHD (132). Several possible mechanisms for the beneficial effects of physical activity have been suggested (120). These include an antiatherogenic effect through increased HDL cholesterol and decreased LDL cholesterol and triglycerides, favorable effects on platelet adhesiveness and blood viscosity, increased insulin sensitivity, more effective cardiac use of oxygen with conditioning, and reduction of blood pressure. American Heart Association (AHA) guidelines for prevention of CHD recommend that physical activity be performed for at least 30 minutes on most days of the week (109). Flexibility training should complement this regimen.

People with SCI often lead a sedentary lifestyle as a result of their impaired mobility, lack of access, limited exercise options, and stress-related musculoskeletal injuries; additionally, they have an altered physiologic response to exercise due to loss of exercising muscle mass as well as altered autonomic function (5, 22, 27, 133–135). Physical exertion from activities of daily living and everyday mobility with SCI is not adequate for cardiovascular fitness (22, 91). Although cardiovascular fitness and work capacity may be improved with aerobic exercise in people with SCI (22), optimal exercise interventions for improving cardiovascular fitness remain to be determined, and data about the impact of exercise on cardiovascular risk in SCI is limited (22, 101, 134). It is still not known if physical activity confers the same level of risk reduction in those with SCI as in the general population (22). Individuals with SCI should be encouraged to use some of several available exercise options (135–141). These are further discussed elsewhere in this textbook (see Chapter 64), and include arm ergometry, wheelchair ergometry, and swimming (135). FES training may improve exercise tolerance, endurance, and cardiovascular fitness (140–141). Very limited data exists regarding changes in cardiovascular fitness with body-weight supported treadmill training in persons with incomplete SCI (22, 58, 137).

Obesity and Excessive Weight

Obesity adversely affects cardiac function, increases the risk factors for coronary heart disease, and is an independent risk factor for cardiovascular disease (117, 118). Once the acute injury phase is over, persons with SCI generally have lower energy expenditure than able-bodied people (142). Rates for those with chronic tetraplegia are generally lower than in those with paraplegia. As a result, excessive weight gain is not uncommon. Traditional measures of obesity (such as weight or body mass index) may not be reliable after SCI due to loss of muscle mass and higher percent of body fat making it difficult to estimate obesity prevalence in SCI (101). Patients with chronic quadriplegia have a decreased lean body mass and an increased percentage of body fat (101, 142, 143). Excess body fat contributes to insulin resistance and increases the risk for CHD (27, 117, 118). Because energy needs decrease with chronic SCI, a reduction in calories consumed is appropriate, as is regular exercise. People with SCI often have suboptimal dietary intake, so nutritional counseling and intervention are especially important (144, 145). It has been suggested that depending on the level of injury, basal energy requirements should be reduced from those calculated for able-bodied individuals by a factor ranging from 10% for those with low paraplegia to 25% for those with high tetraplegia (145). Because of decreased lean muscle mass, ideal body weights may

be 10 to 20 pounds lower than those recommended in the general population, depending on the level of SCI.

Diabetes, Impaired Glucose Tolerance, and Hyperinsulinemia

The risk for CHD is especially high for individuals with diabetes (119). Much of this risk is caused by lipid abnormalities, but factors such as insulin levels and blood glucose also appear to have an independent role (119, 128, 146–150). A positive association between insulin levels and the subsequent risk for cardiovascular disease has been demonstrated (149). The constellation of risk factors constituting the metabolic syndrome includes abdominal obesity, atherogenic dyslipidemia, raised blood pressure, insulin resistance, and prothrombotic and proinflammatory states (110, 128). Spinal cord injured veterans with diabetes mellitus (DM) had much higher rates of CHD, myocardial infarction, and other co-morbidities than those without DM (151). The prevalence of impaired glucose tolerance, insulin resistance, and hyperinsulinemia in individuals with chronic SCI has been reported to be increased (152); however the data is weak and inconclusive (101, 153). Prevalence is highly dependent on the demographics of the population studied, and definitive conclusions about a causal relationship with SCI cannot be made from current data (101). One study reported higher rate of DM in veterans with SCI compared to the general population, but rates were similar when compared to other veterans (151), suggesting that demographic factors other than SCI may be contributing. Suggested determinants of increased insulin resistance in SCI include changes in insulin sensitivity after denervation of skeletal muscle, prolonged inactivity, and increased adiposity (131, 152). Weight management, dietary modifications, physical exercise, and blood glucose control are important interventions in these patients (110, 154, 155). Focused attention to diabetic measures has been shown to be associated with significant improvement in these conditions in a population with SCI and DM (156).

Psychosocial Factors

There is evidence that psychosocial factors may contribute to the risk of CHD (157–160). Some of the identified factors for which there is convincing evidence include depression, social isolation, and chronic life stresses. Epidemiological studies have demonstrated a graded relationship between the degree of depression and the predictability of coronary events (162). Depression is an independent risk factor for mortality with acute MI or unstable angina (159). The presumed mechanisms involve evidence of impaired platelet function in depression and the promotion of atherogenesis through hormonal changes such as an increased cortisol level. Social isolation is measured by the lack of family, friends, or group activities as a regular part of an individual's life. Such social isolation or a low level of emotional support has been associated with a three-fold risk for subsequent cardiac events after myocardial infarction (160). Although estimates of prevalence vary, there is evidence that depression and social isolation are more common in people with SCI than in the general population (163–165). Assessment of depressive symptomology and the social support system should be a routine part of the evaluation of these patients, followed by appropriate medical and psychosocial interventions (165).

Emerging Risk Factors

In addition to the classically identifiable risk factors described, studies have identified a diverse group of additional possible risk factors for CHD, although at present there are no conclusive guidelines regarding the significance or intervention strategies for many of these (161, 166). Some of these factors include oxidants, platelet activators, elevated plasma homocysteine, lipoprotein, and inflammatory markers such as C-reactive protein and other prothrombotic and proinflammatory markers (161, 166–171). Whereas most of the reported studies for these are in the general population, there are a few reports relating to the SCI population. Some reports have suggested platelet abnormalities in SCI, including abnormalities of aggregation, resistance to inhibition by prostacyclin, and the presence of a prostacyclin receptor antibody (97, 172). The significance of these findings is not clear at present. Other studies have suggested elevated CRP levels in the SCI population (173, 174). A hypothesis relating to the effect of recurrent urinary tract infections with a resultant increase in inflammatory markers such as C-reactive protein (CRP) has also been presented as a factor increasing the risk of CHD in SCI (173). However, there is no conclusive proof for this theory at this time and CRP may be a marker of coronary inflammation in patients with CHD rather than a significant etiologic factor by itself in CHD pathogenesis (166). Studies of homocysteine levels in SCI are small and demonstrate elevated levels with increasing age and in smokers (175, 176). Data related to prevalence compared to able-bodied individuals is inconclusive. The role of folate or vitamin B12 supplementation in the management of those with increased homocysteine levels is not clear at this time.

Symptoms and Signs

Cardiac pain impulses travel in the afferent sympathetic nerves through the upper five thoracic segments, through the spinal cord via the spinothalamic tract, to the thalamus and then to the cortex (177). Individuals with SCI above the T5 level may not perceive chest pain with angina or even with acute myocardial infarction (178–180) because of the interruption of cardiac sympathetic afferent input. Jaw or neck pain or toothache may be prominent in these patients. It has been suggested that vagal afferent nerves may play a role in the radiation of cardiac pain to the jaw and neck, based on observations of persistence of this aspect of angina in people who have undergone thoracic sympathectomy (177). These vagal afferents are typically intact after SCI. Other atypical presentations of coronary episodes may include autonomic dysreflexia, changes in baseline spasticity, nausea, episodic shortness of breath, and fatigue. Because of the lack of typical chest pain, the diagnosis may be delayed or missed by both the patient and provider (178–180). Conversely, gastroesophageal reflux, which is common after SCI, may be mistaken for angina (181). There may also be confusion in the interpretation of physical signs in differentiating congestive heart failure from lung crackles caused by atelectasis or dependent edema, both of which are common in SCI (180).

Diagnostic Testing

An EKG may reveal evidence of current or past ischemic disease, which should be differentiated from the nonspecific ST-segment and T-wave changes that have been reported after SCI (182).

Table 18.7   Unique Issues in the Diagnosis of CHD after SCI

Atypical presentations, lack of chest pain
Underdiagnosis of coronary heart disease (CHD)
Delayed treatment
Inadequate secondary prevention
Confusing physical signs
    Dependent edema versus heart failure
    Atelectasis versus left ventricular failure
Nonspecific ST-segment and T-wave changes in SCI
Cardiac stress testing
    Inability to perform traditional treadmill test
    Suboptimal sensitivity of arm versus leg exercise
    Difficulty in interpreting significance of exercise induced hypotension
    Indication for pharmacologic stress testing

Traditional treadmill exercise stress tests or bicycle ergometry cannot be performed because of the physical limitations after SCI (180). Arm ergometry can be performed in patients with paraplegia, but not tetraplegia, using either wheelchairs or upper extremity ergometers (183). However, maximal arm exercise produces less cardiovascular stress than leg exercise so latent cardiac abnormalities may be missed (180, 184). The significance of hypotension with physical exercise may be difficult to interpret in SCI in the absence of accompanying signs of ischemia (180). For these reasons, pharmacologic stress testing is often the most practical option in patients with SCI (185). These tests consist of the administration of a pharmacologic agent such as dobutamine, adenosine, or dipyridamole to induce cardiac stress, in combination with a form of cardiac imaging (185, 186). Examples include dobutamine echocardiography and dipyridamole scintigraphy. Defects in wall motion by echocardiography or perfusion by scintigraphy indicate the presence and severity of cardiac disease. Special issues relating to the diagnosis of CHD in patients with SCI are summarized in Table 18.7.

Management

The principles of management of CHD in SCI are essentially the same as for those in the general population (180, 187), as are those for secondary prevention in those with known cardiovascular disease (110). The spectrum of interventions, including lifestyle changes, medications, angioplasty, and cardiac revascularization, should be available to people with SCI as appropriate (180). People with SCI may not be able to tolerate traditional antianginal medication doses because of low blood pressure, so the introduction of medications at lower doses with careful blood pressure monitoring may be needed (37). Aspirin and beta-blockers are routinely recommended for patients with atherosclerotic cardiovascular disease and post-myocardial infarction unless contraindicated (110, 188–190). Because of the use of sildenafil and other phosphodiesterase-5 (PDE-5) inhibitors for SCI-related erectile dysfunction (191, 192), patients should be specifically questioned about their use if considering nitrate therapy for angina to avoid potential life-threatening hypotension with concurrent use of these drugs. Angiotensin-converting enzyme

(ACE) inhibitors have been shown to reduce the risk of further coronary events after myocardial infarction (193). These drugs should be used cautiously, with careful monitoring of electrolytes, blood urea nitrogen, and creatinine if there is underlying renal insufficiency due to SCI-related urologic problems. Additionally, because of the potentially significant role of the renin-angiotensin system in maintaining blood pressure in people with tetraplegia, severe hypotension may occur with ACE inhibitors in these patients (194, 195), so caution and low initial dose is prudent when starting these drugs (196). Cardiac rehabilitation programs follow the same principles as in able-bodied individuals (187), and patients with SCI can be easily integrated into cardiac rehabilitation group classes (180). Adaptations to address mobility limitations may be needed. For example, progressive wheelchair propulsion may be substituted for a traditional progressive walking program, although success may be limited by musculoskeletal complications in shoulders, elbows, and wrists. The energy requirements for wheelchair propulsion on a level surface by paraplegic individuals have been shown to be equivalent to those needed for able-bodied ambulation (197). Patients may need retraining in the use of energy conservation techniques during activities of daily living.

VENOUS THROMBOEMBOLISM

Thromboembolism is a major problem in the initial weeks after SCI (198–201), although the reported incidence varies significantly depending on the surveillance technique used. Potentially life threatening pulmonary embolism is the most serious complication (198). Venostasis due to impairment of the venous muscle pump and a transient hypercoagulable state are contributory factors (200). Venous Thromboembolims (VTE) following SCI is also discussed elsewhere in this textbook in detail (See Chapter 19.).

The Consortium for Spinal Cord Medicine's Clinical Practice Guidelines on "Prevention of Thromboembolism in Spinal Cord Injury" provide evidence-based recommendations for prevention (200). Compression hose or pneumatic devices should be applied to the legs of all patients for the first two weeks following injury. Anticoagulant prophylaxis with either low-molecular weight heparin or adjusted dose unfractionated heparin should be initiated within 72 hours after SCI, provided there is no active bleeding or coagulopathy. The recent switch from unfractionated heparin to low molecular weight heparin for the prevention of VTE may account for a decrease in the frequency of this complication in patients with spinal cord injury (201). The duration of anticoagulant prophylaxis is controversial and should be individualized depending on the need, medical condition, functional status, and the risk to the patient. Anticoagulants should be continued until discharge in patients with incomplete injuries, for 8 weeks in patients with uncomplicated complete motor injury, and for 12 weeks or until discharge for those with complete motor injury and other risk factors (e.g., lower limb fractures, history of thrombosis, cancer, heart failure, obesity, or age over 70). Vena cava filter placement is indicated in patients with SCI who have failed anticoagulants prophylaxis or who have a contraindication to anticoagulation (such as CNS or GI bleeding). Filters should also be considered in patients with complete motor paralysis due to high cervical cord injury (C2, C3), or with poor cardiopulmonary reserve. However, filter placement is not a

substitute for thromboprophylaxis. In symptomatic patients, ultrasound of legs and/or ventilation/perfusion lung scanning is indicated. If clinical suspicion is strong but tests are negative or indeterminate, consider venography of the legs, lung spiral CT, or pulmonary angiography. With documented DVT, mobilization and exercise of the lower extremity should be withheld 48 to 72 hours until appropriate medical therapy is implemented.

Risk for thrombo-embolism is much lower in chronic SCI. However, patients with SCI who have acute medical illnesses or require surgical procedures are at similar or increased risk for DVT as any other patient, and reinstitution of prophylactic measures should be considered, depending on the clinical situation (200).

PERIPHERAL ARTERIAL DISEASE

With aging, there is increasing comorbidity from complications of peripheral vascular disease, especially in diabetics and smokers (202, 203). The prevalence of this condition in the SCI population is not well established. Some reports suggest a relatively high incidence of limb amputation because of vascular disease in patients with SCI (204), and reduced arterial circulation to the legs has been reported in SCI (205–207). Factors that may increase the predisposition to arterial disease in these patients include those for atherosclerosis, such as lipid abnormalities, smoking, and glucose intolerance (208).

Clinical Evaluation

A delay in diagnosis of peripheral arterial disease (PAD) may occur in patients with SCI because of the lack of the cardinal symptom of intermittent claudication (203, 208–210). Symptoms of more advanced limb ischemia, such as rest pain or numbness, may also be absent, and patients may first present with gangrenous changes or other signs of advanced disease. Peripheral vascular disease may present with nonhealing skin ulcers in SCI (205). Examination of peripheral pulses and foot examination for ischemic skin changes should be performed routinely as part of the periodic evaluation of patients with SCI (209). However, skin discoloration and cool temperature in the feet may occur in SCI even without evidence of significant peripheral vascular disease, and the dependent leg edema that occurs in SCI may make the palpation of foot pulses difficult.

Diagnostic Testing

Because of the limitations of history and physical evaluation of arterial disease in these patients, vascular testing may be indicated for diagnosis, assessment of disease severity, and the monitoring of disease progression or regression (203, 208). Specific arterial tests include continuous-wave Doppler, segmental pressures, transcutaneous oximetry, and imaging studies (202, 208–209). Continuous-wave Doppler or duplex scanning detects blood motion. In the normal artery, the pulsatile waveform is usually triphasic. With mild stenosis, there is dampening of the signal. As severity worsens, the signal becomes monophasic. Segmental pressures can be measured by sequentially inflating and deflating pneumatic cuffs around the limb or digit and using the continuous-wave Doppler to determine the systolic pressure at which arterial flow resumes during cuff deflation. The most commonly reported segmental pressure is an ankle-brachial index (ABI). An ABI of greater than 1.0 is considered normal, 1.0 to 0.8 reflects mild disease, 0.8 to 0.5 moderate disease, and less than 0.5 severe disease (208–209). ABI may prove to be a useful screening tool for PAD in individuals with SCI (211). This measurement cannot be used when blood vessels walls are noncompressible due to calcification, as occurs commonly in diabetics. Transcutaneous oximetry is used to evaluate skin blood flow by using oxygen-sensitive electrodes. This measurement is also useful in determining the adequacy of skin perfusion for healing at a given amputation site. Values above 40 mmHg are generally adequate, whereas those below 20 mmHg are not. Imaging modalities such as 2-D real-time ultrasound, computed tomography (CT), and magnetic resonance angiography are being increasingly used instead of invasive angiography.

Management

Minimizing risk factors such as smoking, diabetes, and hyperlipedemia is a key component of management (110, 202, 208, 209). Because CHD is a common comorbidity in those with peripheral vascular disease and a frequent cause of death in these patients, primary and secondary prevention measures for CHD are indicated. Limb revascularization for the relief of claudication may not be an issue because of the lack of this symptom in patients with SCI. Arterial reconstruction for occlusive disease may be difficult because of small and atrophic arteries in SCI (212). Consideration of amputation for patients with advanced disease should be a team decision that should include the patient and SCI physician in addition to the surgeons. The effect of amputation on balance and transfers, weight redistribution with new pressure areas, and skin breakdown of the insensate stump are some factors that should be included in the deliberations (204, 213). After amputation, patients should be evaluated by the rehabilitation team. They often need a new wheelchair and retraining for transfers and wheelchair mobility, in addition to education for stump and skin care.

DRUG-RELATED CARDIOVASCULAR ADVERSE EFFECTS

SUCCINYLCHOLINE-INDUCED CARDIAC ARREST The rapid development of hyperkalemia leading to cardiac arrest has been reported in patients with thoracolumbar spinal cord injuries who have lower motor neuron injury with denervated muscles (214). The presumed mechanism involves the spread of the acetylcholine- and succinylcholine-sensitive area from the myoneural junction to more of the muscle membrane, so that with depolarization, a large potassium efflux may occur (214, 215). Patients with thoracolumbar injuries must receive alternative nondepolarizing muscle relaxants instead of succinylcholine for anesthesia during surgical procedures.

EFFECTS OF MEDICATIONS USED FOR SCI-RELATED DYSFUNCTION Many of the drugs used for treating problems directly or indirectly related to SCI have significant cardiovascular effects. The vulnerability of people with SCI to the hypotensive side effects of medications was discussed in the previous section on OH (37). This may be a significant problem with medications used to treat problems such as spasticity, pain, or depression in SCI, and may affect the choice of drugs used to treat these conditions. As previously mentioned, sildenafil and other PDE-5 inhibitors are now often used to treat SCI-related erectile dysfunction (191, 192). Most patients can tolerate these drugs without significant problems, but hypotension may necessitate a lower starting dose and caution in upgrading the dosage in some. The major concern with sildenafil use in SCI is its interaction with nitrates. Concomitant use of the two drugs can cause catastrophic, even fatal, hypotension (191, 192). Because topical nitroglycerin ointment is often used to treat autonomic dysreflexia, patients with cervical and thoracic injuries above T6 should be strongly cautioned against the concurrent use of these medications. Providers should inquire about PDE-5 inhibitor use prior to initiating topical nitrates or using intravenous nitroglycerin for emergency treatment of high blood pressure in dysreflexia.

References

1. Krassioukov A, Claydon VE. The clinical problems in cardiovascular control following spinal cord injury: an overview. *Prog Brain Res* 2006; 152:223–229.
2. Lavis TD, Scelza WM, Bockenek WL. Cardiovascular health and fitness in persons with spinal cord injury. *Phys Med Rehabil Clin N Am* 2007 May; 18(2):317–31
3. Bravo G, Guizar-Sahagun G, Ibarra A, et al: Cardiovascular alterations after spinal cord injury: an overview. *Curr Med Chem* 2004; 2:133–48
4. Mathias CJ, Frankel HL: Cardiovascular control in spinal man. *Ann Rev Physiol* 1988; 50:577–92
5. Dela F, Mohr T, Jensen CMR et al. Cardiovascular Control During Exercise: Insights From Spinal Cord–Injured Humans. *Circulation* 2003; 107:2127
6. Myers J, Lee M, Kiratli J. Cardiovascular disease in spinal cord injury: an overview of prevalence, risk, evaluation, and management. *Am J Phys Med Rehabil* 2007 Feb; 86(2):142–52.
7. Groah SL, Weitzenkamp D, Sett P, et al: The relationship between neurological level of injury and symptomatic cardiovascular disease risk in the aging spinal injured. *Spinal Cord* 2001; 39:310–7
8. Bauman WA, Kahn NN, Grimm DR, et al: Risk factors for atherogenesis and cardiovascular autonomic function in persons with spinal cord injury. *Spinal Cord* 1999; 37:601–16
9. Jacobs PL, Mahoney ET, Robbins A. Hypokinetic circulation in persons with paraplegia. *Med Sci Sports Exerc* 2002; 34(9):1401–1407.
10. Lehman KG, Lane JG, Piepmeier JM, et al. Cardiovascular abnormalities accompanying acute spinal cord injury in humans: Incidence, time course and severity. *J Am Coll Cardiol* 1987; 10:46–52.
11. McKinley WO, Jackson AB, Cardenas DD, DeVivo MJ. Long-term medical complications after traumatic spinal cord injury: A regional model systems analysis. *Arch Phys Med Rehabil* 1999; 80:1402–1410.
12. Kessler KM, Pina I, Green B, et al. Cardiovascular findings in quadriplegic and paraplegic patients and in normal subjects. *Am J Cardiol* 1986; 58:525–530.
13. Glenn MB, Bergman SB. Cardiovascular changes following spinal cord injury. *Top Spinal Cord Inj Rehabil* 1997; 2:47–53.
14. Teasell RW, Arnold MO, Krassioukov A, et al. Cardiovascular consequences of loss of supraspinal control of the sympathetic nervous system after spinal cord injury. *Arch Phys Med Rehabil* 2000; 81(4):506–516.
15. Claydon VE, Krassioukov AV. Orthostatic hypotension and autonomic pathways after spinal cord injury. *J Neurotrauma* 2006 Dec; 23(12): 1713–25.
16. Wallin BG, Stjernberg L. Sympathetic activity in man after spinal cord injury. *Brain* 1984; 107:183–198.
17. Stjernberg L, Blumberg H, Wallin BG. Sympathetic activity in man after spinal cord injury. Outflow to muscle below the lesion. *Brain* 1986; 109:695–715.
18. Claus-Walker J, Halstead LS. Metabolic and endocrine changes in spinal cord injury: II (section 1). Consequences of partial decentralization of autonomic nervous system. *Arch Phys Med Rehabil* 1982; 63: 569–575.

19. Wallin BG, Stjernberg L. Sympathetic activity in man after spinal cord injury. *Brain* 1984; 107:183–198.
20. Claydon VE, Hol AT, Eng JJ, Krassioukov AV. Cardiovascular responses and postexercise hypotension after arm cycling exercise in subjects with spinal cord injury. *Arch Phys Med Rehabil* 2006 Aug; 87(8):1106–1114.
21. Mathias CJ, Frankel HL. Autonomic disturbances in spinal cord lesions. In: Bannister R, Mathias CJ, eds. *Autonomic Failure: A Textbook of Clinical Disorders of the Autonomic Nervous System*. Oxford: Oxford University Press; 1992:839–881.
22. Warburton DER, Sproule S, Krassioukov A, Eng JJ. Cardiovascular Health and Exercise Following Spinal Cord Injury. In: Eng JJ, Teasell RW, Miller WC, Wolfe DL, Townson AF, Aubut J, Abramson C, Hsieh JTC, Connolly S, eds. *Spinal Cord Injury Rehabilitation Evidence*. Vancouver, 2006; 7.1–7.28.
23. Krassioukov AC, Weaver LC. Morphological changes in sympathetic preganglionic neurons after spinal cord injury in rats. *Neuroscience* 1996; 70:21 1–26.
24. Krassioukov AV, Bunge RP, Puckett WR, Bygrave M. The changes in human spinal cord sympathetic preganglionic neurons after spinal cord injury. *Spinal Cord* 1997; 37:6–3.
25. Arnold JM, Feng QP, Delaney GA, Teasell RW. Alpha adrenoceptor hyperresponsiveness in quadriplegic patients with autonomic dysreflexia. *Clin Auton Res* 1995; 5:267–270.
26. Naftchi NE. Mechanism of autonomic dysreflexia. Contributions of catecholamines and peptide neurotransmitters [review]. *Ann NY Acad Sci* 1990; 579:133–148.
27. Washburn RA, Figoni SF: Physical activity and chronic cardiovascular disease prevention in spinal cord injury: a comprehensive literature review. *Top Spinal Cord Inj Rehabil* 1998; 3:16–32
28. Deitrich JE, Whedon JD, Shorr F. Effects of immobilization upon various metabolic and physiological functions of normal man. *Am J Med* 1948; 4:3–36.
29. Mathias CI, Christensen NI, Frankel HL, Spalding IMK. Cardiovascular control in recently injured tetraplegics in spinal shock. *Q J Med* 1979; 48:273–287.
30. Krassioukov A, Warburton DER, Teasell RW, Eng JJ. Orthostatic Hypotension Following Spinal Cord Injury. In: Eng JJ, Teasell RW, Miller WC, Wolfe DL, Townson AF, Aubut J, Abramson C, Hsieh JTC, Connolly S, editors. *Spinal Cord Injury Rehabilitation Evidence*. Vancouver, 2006; 16.1–16.17. Also available at www.icord.org/scire.
31. Nobunaga AI. Orthostatic hypotension in spinal cord injury. *Top Spinal Cord Inj Rehabil* 1997; 4(1):73–80.
32. Claydon VE, Steeves JD, Krassioukov A. Orthostatic hypotension following spinal cord injury: understanding clinical pathophysiology. *Spinal Cord* 2006; 44:341–351.
33. Cariga P, Ahmed S, Mathias CJ, Gardner BP. The prevalence and association of neck (coathanger) pain and orthostatic (postural) hypotension in human spinal cord injury. *Spinal Cord* 2002; 40:77–82.
34. Faghri PD, Yount JP, Pesce WJ, Seetharama S, Votto JJ. Circulatory hypokinesis and functional electric stimulation during standing in persons with spinal cord injury. *Arch Phys Med Rehabil* 2001; 82:1587–1595.
35. Illman A, Stiller K, Williams M. The prevalence of orthostatic hypotension during physiotherapy treatment in patients with an acute spinal cord injury. *Spinal Cord* 2000; 38:741–747
36. Yardley CP, Fitzsimons CL, Weaver LC. Cardiac and peripheral vascular contributions to hypotension in spinal cats. *Am J Physiol* 1989; 257:H1347–H1353.
37. Blackmer J. Orthostatic hypotension in spinal cord injured patients. *J Spinal Cord Med* 1997; 20(2): 212–217.
38. McKinley WO, Jackson AB, Cardenas DD, DeVivo MJ. Long-term medical complications after traumatic spinal cord injury: a regional model systems analysis. *Arch Phys Med Rehabil* 1999; 80:1402–1410.
39. Mathias CJ. Orthostatic hypotension: causes, mechanisms, and influencing factors. *Neurology* 1995; 45(Suppl 5):S6–S11.
40. Houtman S, Colier WN, Oeseburg B, et al. Systemic circulation and cerebral oxygenation during head-up tilt in spinal cord injured individuals. *Spinal Cord* 2000; 38(3):158–163.
41. Mathias CJ, Christensen NJ, Corbett JL, et al. Plasma catecholamines, plasma renin activity and plasma aldosterone in tetraplegic man, horizontal and tilted. *Clin Sci Molec Med* 1975; 49:291–299.
42. Guttman L, Munro AF, Robinson R et al. Effect of tilting on the cardiovascular responses and plasma catecholamine levels in spinal man. *Paraplegia* 1963; 1:4–18.
43. Johnson RH, Park DM. Effect of change of posture on blood pressure and plasma renin concentration in men with spinal transections. *Clin Sci* 1973; 44:539–546.
44. Poole CJM, Williams TDM, Lightman SL, et al. Neuroendocrine control of vasopressin secretion and its effect on blood pressure in subjects with spinal cord transection. *Brain* 1987; 110:727–735.
45. Gonzalez F, Chang JY, Banovac K, et al. Autoregulation of cerebral blood flow in patients with orthostatic hypotension after spinal cord injury. *Paraplegia* 1991; 29(1):1–7.
46. Lopes P, Figoni SF, Perkash I. Upper limb exercise effect on tilt tolerance during orthostatic training of patients with spinal cord injury. *Arch Phys Med Rehabil* 1984; 65:251–253.
47. Baliga RR, Catz AB, Watson LD, et al. Cardiovascular and hormonal responses to food ingestion in humans with spinal cord transection. *Clin Auton Res* 1997; 7(3):137–141.
48. Jansen RW, Lipsitz LA. Postprandial hypotension: Epidemiology, pathophysiology, and clinical management. *Ann Intern Med* 1995; 1222:286.
49. King ML, Lichtman SW, Pellicone JT, et al. Exertional hypotension in spinal cord injury. *Chest* 1994; 106: 1166–1171.
50. Maynard FM. Posttraumatic cystic myelopathy in motor incomplete quadriplegia presenting as progressive orthostasis. *Arch Phys Med Rehabil* 1984; 65(1):30–32.
51. Robertson D, Davis TL. Recent advances in the treatment of orthostatic hypotension. *Neurology* 1995; 45(Suppl 5):S26–S31.
52. Freeman R. Treatment of orthostatic hypotension. *Semin Neurol* 2003; 23:435–442.
53. Onrot J, Goldberg MR, Hollister AS, et al. Management of chronic orthostatic hypotension. *Am J Med* 1986; 80:454–464.
54. Treatment of postural hypotension. A review. *Drugs* 1990; 39:74–85.
55. Kerk JK, Clifford PS, Snyder AC, Prieto TE, O'Hagan KP, Schot PK, Myklebust JB, Myklebust BM. Effect of an abdominal binder during wheelchair exercise. *Med Sci Sports Exerc* 1995; 27:913–919.
56. Hopman MT, Monroe M, Dueck C, Phillips WT, Skinner JS. Blood redistribution and circulatory responses to submaximal arm exercise in persons with spinal cord injury. *Scand J Rehabil Med* 1998; 30:167–174.
57. Hopman MT, Groothuis JT, Flendrie M, Gerrits KH, Houtman S. Increased vascular resistance in paralyzed legs after spinal cord injury is reversible by training. *J Appl Physiol* 2002; 93:1966–1972.
58. Ditor DS, Macdonald MJ, Kamath MV, Bugaresti J, Adams M, McCartney N, Hicks AL. The effects of body-weight supported treadmill training on cardiovascular regulation in individuals with motor-complete SCI. *Spinal Cord* 2005; 43:664–673.
59. Raymond J, Davis GM, van der Plas M. Cardiovascular responses during submaximal electrical stimulation-induced leg cycling in individuals with paraplegia. *Clin Physiol Funct Imaging* 2002; 22:92–98.
60. Sampson EE, Burnham RS, Andrew BJ. Functional electrical stimulation effect on orthostatic hypotension after spinal cord injury. *Arch Phys Med Rehabil* 2000; 81(2):139–143.
61. Brucker BS, Ince LP. Biofeedback as an experimental treatment for postural hypotension in a patient with a spinal cord lesion. *Arch Phys Med Rehabil* 1977; 58(2):49–53.
62. Groomes TE, Huang CT. Orthostatic hypotension after spinal cord injury: Treatment with fludrocortisone and ergotamine. *Arch Phys Med Rehabil* 1991; 72(1):56–58.
63. Chobanian AV, Volicer L, Tifft CP, et al. Mineralocorticoid-induced hypertension in patients with orthostatic hypotension. *N Engl J Med* 1979; 301:68–73.
64. Chobanian AV, Tifft CP, Faxon DP, et al. Treatment of orthostatic hypotension with ergotamine. *Circulation* 1983; 67:602–609.
65. Hoeldtke RD, Cavanaugh ST, Hughes JD. Treatment of orthostatic hypotension: Interaction of pressor drugs and tilt table conditioning. *Arch Phys Med Rehabil* 1988; 69:895–898.
66. Davies B, Bannister R, Sever P. Pressor amines and monoamine oxidase inhibitors for treatment of postural hypotension in autonomic failure. Limitations and hazards. *Lancet* 1978; 1:172–175.
67. Schatz IJ. Orthostatic hypotension: II. Clinical diagnosis, testing, and treatment. *Arch Intern Med* 1984; 144:1037–1041.
68. McTavish D, Goa KL. Midodrine: A review of its pharmacological properties and therapeutic use in orthostatic hypotension and secondary hypotensive disorders. *Drugs* 1989; 38:757–777.
69. Jankovic J, Gilden JL, Hiner BC, et al. Neurogenic orthostatic hypotension: A double-blind placebo controlled study with midodrine. *Am J Med* 1993; 95:38–48.

70. Low PA, Gilden JL, Freeman R, et al. Efficacy of midodrine vs. placebo in neurogenic orthostatic hypotension: a randomized double-blind multicenter study. *JAMA* 1997; 277(13):1046–1051.

71. Barber DB, Rogers SJ, Fredrickson MD, et al. Midodrine hydrochloride and the treatment of orthostatic hypotension in tetraplegia: two cases and a review of literature. *Spinal Cord* 2000; 38(2):109–111.

72. Wright RA, Kaufmann HC, Perera R, Opfer-Gehrking TL, McElligott MA, Sheng KN, Low PA. A double-blind, dose-response study of midodrine in neurogenic orthostatic hypotension. *Neurology* 1998; 51:120–124.

73. Nieshoff EC, Birk TJ, Birk CA, Hinderer SR, Yavuzer G. Double-blinded, placebo-controlled trial of midodrine for exercise performance enhancement in tetraplegia: a pilot study. *J Spinal Cord Med* 2004; 27:219–225.

74. Robertson D, Goldberg MR, Hollister AS, et al. Clonidine raises blood pressure in severe orthostatic hypotension. Am J Med 1983; 74:193–200.

75. Frankel HL, Mathias CJ, Spalding JM. Mechanisms of reflex cardiac arrest in tetraplegic patients. *Lancet* 1975; ii:1183–1195.

76. Dollfus P, Frankel HL. Cardiovascular reflexes in tracheostomised tetraplegics. *Paraplegia* 1965; 2:227–235.

77. Gilgoff IS, Ward SLD, Hohn AR. Cardiac pacemaker in high spinal cord injury. *Arch Phys Med Rehabil* 1991; 72:601–603.

78. Leaf DA, Bahl RA, Adkins RH. Risk of cardiac dysrhythmias in chronic spinal cord injury patients. *Paraplegia* 1993; 31:571.

79. Consortium for Spinal Cord Medicine. *Acute Management of Autonomic Dysreflexia: Individuals with Spinal Cord Injury Presenting to Health-Care Facilities.* 2nd Ed. Paralyzed Veterans of America, 2001.

80. Bycroft J, Shergill IS, Chung EA, Arya N, Shah PJ. Autonomic dysreflexia: a medical emergency. *Postgrad Med J* 2005 Apr; 81(954):232–5

81. Figoni SF. Perspectives on cardiovascular fitness and SCI. *J Am Paraplegia Soc* 1990; 13:63–71.

82. Hooker SP, Wells CL. Effects of low- and moderate-intensity training in spinal cord-injured persons. *Med Sci Sports Exerc* 1989; 21:18–22.

83. Coutts KD, Rhodes EC, McKenzie DC. Maximal exercise responses of tetraplegics and paraplegics. *J Appl Physiol* 1983; 55:479–482.

84. Hooker SP, Figoni SF, Rodgers MM, et al. Physiologic effects of electrical stimulation leg cycle exercise training in spinal cord injured persons. *Arch Phys Med Rehabil* 1992; 73:470–476.

85. Hooker SP, Scremin AM, Mutton DL, Kunkel CF, Cagle G. Peak and submaximal physiologic responses following electrical stimulation leg cycle ergometer training. *J Rehabil Res Dev* 1995; 32:361–366.

86. Laskin JJ, Ashley EA, Olenik LM, et al. Electrical stimulation-assisted rowing exercise in spinal cord injured people: a pilot study. *Paraplegia* 1993; 31:534–541.

87. Nash MS, Jacobs PL, Montalvo BM, Klose KJ, Guest RS, Needham-Shropshire BM. Evaluation of a training program for persons with SCI paraplegia using the Parastep 1 ambulation system: part 5. lower extremity blood flow and hyperemic responses to occlusion are augmented by ambulation training. *Arch Phys Med Rehabil* 1997; 78:808–814.

88. Cowell LL, Squires WG, Raven PB. Benefits of aerobic exercise for the paraplegic: a brief review. *Med Sci Sports Exerc* 1986; 18:501–508.

89. Davis GM, Shephard RJ, Leenen FH. Cardiac effects of short term arm crank training in paraplegics: echocardiographic evidence. *Eur J Appl Physiol* 1987; 56:90–96.

90. Gass GC, Watson J, Camp EM, Court HJ, McPherson LM, Redhead P. The effects of physical training on high level spinal lesion patients. *Scand J Rehabil Med* 1980; 12:61–65.

91. Hoffman MD. Cardiorespiratory fitness and training in quadriplegics and paraplegics. *Sports Med* 1986; 3:312–330.

92. Knutsson E, Lewenhaupt-Olsson E, Thorsen M. Physical work capacity and physical conditioning in paraplegic patients. *Paraplegia* 1973; 11:205–216.

93. Cooney MM, Walker JB. Hydraulic resistance exercise benefits cardiovascular fitness of spinal cord injured. *Med Sci Sports Exerc* 1986; 18:522–525.

94. Nilsson S, Staff PH, Pruett ED. Physical work capacity and the effect of training on subjects with long-standing paraplegia. *Scand J Rehabil Med* 1975; 7:51–56.

95. Hjeltnes N, Aksnes AK, Birkeland KI, Johansen J, Lannem A, Wallberg-Henriksson H. Improved body composition after 8 weeks of electrically stimulated leg cycling in tetraplegic patients. *Am J Physiol* 1997; 273:1072–1079.

96. Bauman WA, Kahn NN, Grimm DR, et al. Risk factors for atherogenesis and cardiovascular autonomic function in persons with spinal cord injury. *Spinal Cord* 1999; 37(9): 601–616.

97. Bauman WA, Spungen AM. Metabolic changes in persons after spinal cord injury. *Phys Med Rehabil Clin North Am* 2000, 11(1):109–140.

98. Krum H, Howes L, Brown D, et al. Risk factors for cardiovascular disease in chronic spinal cord injury patients. *Paraplegia* 1992, 30:381.

99. Yekutiel M, Brooks ME, Ohry A, Yarom J, Carel R. The prevalence of hypertension, ischaemic heart disease and diabetes in traumatic spinal cord injured patients and amputees. *Paraplegia* 1989; 27(1):58–62.

100. Szlachcic Y, Carrothers L, Adkins R, Waters R. Clinical significance of abnormal electrocardiographic findings in individuals aging with spinal injury and abnormal lipid profiles. *J Spinal Cord Med* 2007; 30(5):473–6

101. Wilt TJ, Carlson FK, Goldish GD, et al. *Carbohydrate & Lipid Disorders & Relevant Considerations in Persons with Spinal Cord Injury.* Evidence Report/Technology Assessment No. 163 (Prepared by the Minnesota Evidence-based Practice Center under Contract No. 290–02–0009.) AHRQ Publication No. 08-E005. Rockville, MD. Agency for Healthcare Research and Quality. January 2008.

102. Cardus D, Ribus-Cardus F, McTaggart WG. Coronary risk in spinal cord injury: Assessment following a multivariate approach. *Arch Phys Med Rehabil* 1992; 73:930–933.

103. DeVivo MJ, Black KJ, Stover SL. Causes of death during the first 12 years after spinal cord injury. *Arch Phys Med Rehabil* 1993; 74:248–254.

104. DeVivo MJ, Krause JS, Lammertse DP. Recent trends in mortality and causes of death among persons with spinal cord injury. *Arch Phys Med Rehabil* 1999; 80:1411–1419.

105. Soden RJ, Walsh J, Middleton JW, et al. Causes of death after spinal cord injury. *Spinal Cord* 2000; 38:604–610.

106. Whiteneck GG, Charlifue SW, Frankel HL, Fraser MH, Gardner BP, Gerhart KA, et al. Mortality, morbidity, and psychosocial outcomes of persons spinal cord injured more than 20 years ago. *Paraplegia* 1992; 30(9):617–30.

107. Garshick E, Kelley A, Cohen SA, et al: A prospective assessment of mortality in chronic spinal cord injury. *Spinal Cord* 2005; 43:408–16

108. Kannel WB. Contribution of the Framingham study to preventive cardiology. *J Am Coll Cardiol* 1990; 62: 515–523.

109. Pearson TA, Blair SN, Daniels SR, et al: American Heart Association Guidelines for Primary Prevention of Cardiovascular Disease and Stroke: 2002 Update: Consensus Panel Guide to Comprehensive Risk Reduction for Adult Patients without Coronary or Other Atherosclerotic Vascular Diseases. American Heart Association Science Advisory and Coordinating Committee. *Circulation* 2002; 106:388–391.

110. AHA; ACC; National Heart, Lung, and Blood Institute, Smith SC Jr, Allen J, Blair SN, Bonow RO, Brass LM, Fonarow GC, Grundy SM, Hiratzka L, Jones D, Krumholz HM, Mosca L, Pearson T, Pfeffer MA, Taubert KA. AHA/ACC guidelines for secondary prevention for patients with coronary and other atherosclerotic vascular disease: 2006 update endorsed by the National Heart, Lung, and Blood Institute. *J Am Coll Cardiol* 2006 May 16; 47(10):2130–2139.

111. Smith SC Jr, Jackson R, Pearson TA, Fuster V, Yusuf S, Faergeman O, Wood DA, Alderman M, Horgan J, Home P, Hunn M, Grundy SM. Principles for national and regional guidelines on cardiovascular disease prevention: a scientific statement from the World Heart and Stroke Forum. *Circulation* 2004; 109:3112–3121.

112. McGovern PG, Pankow JS, Shahar E, Doliszny KM, Folsom AR, Blackburn A, Luepter RV. Recent trends in acute coronary heart disease: mortality, morbidity, medical care, and risk factors: the Minnesota Heart Survey Investigators. *N Engl J Med* 1996; 334:884–890.

113. U.S. Department of Health and Human Services. The Health Consequences of Smoking: A Report of the Surgeon General. Washington, DC: US Department of Health and Human Services, Centers for Disease Control and Prevention, National Center for Chronic Disease Prevention and Health Promotion, Office on Smoking and Health; May 27, 2004. Available at http://www.surgeongeneral.gov/library/smokingconsequences.

114. Chobanian AV, Bakris GL, Black HR, Cushman WC, Green LA, Izzo JL Jr, Jones DW, Materson BJ, Oparil S, Wright JT Jr, Roccella EJ; Joint National Committee on Prevention, Detection, Evaluation, and Treatment of High Blood Pressure. National Heart, Lung, and Blood Institute; National High Blood Pressure Education Program Coordinating Committee. Seventh report of the Joint National

Committee on Prevention, Detection, Evaluation, and Treatment of High Blood Pressure. *Hypertension* 2003; 42:1206–1252.

115. Expert Panel on Detection, Evaluation, and Treatment of High Blood Cholesterol in Adults. Executive Summary of the Third Report of The National Cholesterol Education Program (NCEP) Expert Panel on Detection, Evaluation, And Treatment of High Blood Cholesterol in Adults (Adult Treatment Panel III). *JAMA* 2001; 285:2486–2497.

116. Thompson PD, Buchner D, Pina IL, Balady GJ, Williams MA, Marcus BH, Berra K, Blair SN, Costa F, Franklin B, Fletcher GF, Gordon NF, Pate RR, Rodriguez BL, Yancey AK, Wenger NK; American Heart Association Council on Clinical Cardiology Subcommittee on Exercise, Rehabilitation, and Prevention; American Heart Association Council on Nutrition, Physical Activity, and Metabolism Subcommittee on Physical Activity. Exercise and physical activity in the prevention and treatment of atherosclerotic cardiovascular disease: a statement from the Council on Clinical Cardiology (Subcommittee on Exercise, Rehabilitation, and Prevention) and the Council on Nutrition, Physical Activity, and Metabolism (Subcommittee on Physical Activity). *Circulation* 2003; 107:3109–3116.

117. Klein S, Burke LE, Bray GA, Blair S, Allison DB, Pi-Sunyer X, Hong Y, Eckel RH; American Heart Association Council on Nutrition, Physical Activity, and Metabolism. Clinical implications of obesity with specific focus on cardiovascular disease: a statement for professionals from the American Heart Association Council on Nutrition, Physical Activity, and Metabolism: endorsed by the American College of Cardiology Foundation. *Circulation* 2004; 110(18):2952–2967.

118. National Institutes of Health; National Heart, Lung, and Blood Institute. Clinical guidelines on the identification, evaluation, and treatment of overweight and obesity in adults: the evidence report. National Institutes of Health; National Heart, Lung, and Blood Institute; September 1998. Publication No. 98–4083. Available at http://www.nhlbi.nih .gov/guidelines/obesity/ob_gdlns.pdf.

119. Kannel WB, McGee DL. Diabetes and glucose tolerance as risk factors for cardiovascular disease: The Framingham study. *Diabetes Care* 1979; 2:120–126.

120. Warburton DE, Nicol CW, Bredin SS. Health benefits of physical activity: the evidence. *CMAJ* 2006; 174(6):801–809.

121. Frankel H, Michaelis L, Golding D, et al. The blood pressure in paraplegia. *Paraplegia* 1972; 10:193.

122. Talbot H. Renal disease and hypertension in paraplegics and quadriplegics. *Med Serv J Canada* 1966; 22:570.

123. Rosenberg L, Kaufman DW, Helmrich SP, et al. The risk of myocardial infarction after quitting smoking in men under 55 years of age. *N Engl J Med* 1985; 313: 1511–1514.

124. Ockene IS, Miller NH. Cigarette smoking, cardiovascular disease and stroke: A statement for healthcare professionals from the American Heart Association. *Circulation* 1998; 96:3243–3247.

125. Burke MV, Ebbert JO, Hays JT. Treatment of tobacco dependence. *Mayo Clin Proc* 2008 Apr; 83(4):479–483.

126. Kottke TE, Battista R, DeFriese GH, et al. Attributes of successful smoking cessation interventions in medical practice. A meta-analysis of 39 controlled trials. *JAMA* 1988; 259:2882–2889.

127. Pekkanen J, Linn S, Heiss G, et al. Ten-year mortality from cardiovascular disease in relation to cholesterol level among men with and without pre-existing cardiovascular disease. *N Engl J Med* 1990; 322:1700–1707.

128. National Cholesterol Education Program (NCEP) Expert Panel on Detection, Evaluation, and Treatment of High Blood Cholesterol in Adults (Adult Treatment Panel III). Third Report of the National Cholesterol Education Program (NCEP) Expert Panel on Detection, Evaluation, and Treatment of High Blood Cholesterol in Adults (Adult Treatment Panel III) final report. *Circulation* 2002; 106:3143–3421

129. Grundy SM, Cleeman JI, Merz CN, Brewer HB Jr, Clark LT, Hunninghake DB, Pasternak RC, Smith SC Jr, Stone NJ. Implications of recent clinical trials for the National Cholesterol Education Program Adult Treatment Panel III guidelines. *Circulation* 2004; 110(2):227–239.

130. Bauman WA, Adkins RH, Spungen AM, et al. Is immobilization associated with an abnormal lipoprotein profile? Observations from a diverse cohort. *Spinal Cord* 1999; 37:485–493.

131. Bauman WA, Spungen AM. Disorders of carbohydrate and lipid metabolism in veterans with paraplegia or quadriplegia: A model of premature aging. *Metabolism* 1994; 43:749–756.

132. Berlin JA, Colditz GA. A meta-analysis of physical activity in the prevention of coronary heart disease. *Am J Epidemiol* 1990; 132:612–628.

133. Figoni SF. Exercise responses and quadriplegia. *Med Sci Sports Exerc* 1993; 25:433–441.

134. Fernhall B, Heffernan K, Jae SY, Hedrick B. Health implications of physical activity in individuals with spinal cord injury: a literature review. *J Health Hum Serv Adm* 2008; 30(4):468–502.

135. Jacobs PL, Nash MS. Exercise recommendations for individuals with spinal cord injury. *Sports Med* 2004; 34(11):727–751.

136. Jacobs PL, Beekhuizen KS. Appraisal of Physiological Fitness in Persons with Spinal Cord Injury. *Topics Spinal Cord Inj* 2005; 10(4):32–50.

137. Nash MS, Jacobs PL, Johnson BM, Field-Fote E. Metabolic and cardiac responses to robotic-assisted locomotion in motor complete tetraplegia: A case report. *J Spinal Cord Med* 2004; 27(1):78–82.

138. Nash MS, Jacobs PL. Cardiac structure and function in exercise trained and sedentary persons with paraplegia. *Med Sci Sports Exerc* 1998; 30:1336–1337.

139. Thijssen DH, Heesterbeek P, van Kuppevelt DJ, Duysens J, Hopman MT. Local vascular adaptations after hybrid training in spinal cord-injured subjects. *Med Sci Sports Exerc* 2005; 37(7):1112–1118.

140. Wheeler GD, Andrews B, Lederer R, Davoodi R, Natho K, Weiss C, et al. Functional electric stimulation-assisted rowing: Increasing cardiovascular fitness through functional electric stimulation rowing training in persons with spinal cord injury. *Arch Phys Med Rehabil* 2002; 83(8):1093–1099.

141. Newham DJ, Donaldson N. FES cycling. *Acta Neurochir Suppl* 2007; 97(Pt 1):395–402.

142. Mollinger L, Spurr G, et al. Daily energy expenditure and basal metabolic rates of patients with spinal cord injury. *Arch Phys Med Rehabil* 1985; 66:420.

143. Spungen AM, Adkins RH, Stewart CA, Wang J, Pierson RN Jr, Waters RL, et al. Factors influencing body composition in persons with spinal cord injury: a cross-sectional study. *J Appl Physiol* 2003; 95(6):2398–2407.

144. Tomey KM, Chen DM, Wang X, Braunschweig CL. Dietary intake and nutritional status urban community-dwelling men with paraplegia. *Arch Phys Med Rehabil* 2005; 86:664–671.

145. Peiffer S, Blust P, Leyson J. Nutritional assessment of the spinal cord injured patient. *J Am Diet Assoc* 1981; 78:501.

146. Grundy SM, Benjamin IJ, Burke GL, et al. Diabetes and cardiovascular disease: A statement for healthcare professionals from the American Heart Association. *Circulation* 1999; 100:1134–1146.

147. American Diabetes Association. Standards of medical care in diabetes. *Diabetes Care* 2004; 27(suppl 1):S15–S35.

148. Grundy SM, Cleeman JJ, Daniels SR, et al. and American Heart Association; National Heart, Lung, and Blood Institute. Diagnosis and management of the metabolic syndrome an American Heart Association/National Heart, Lung, and Blood Institute Scientific Statement, *Circulation* 2005; 112:2735–2752

149. Ruige JB, Assendelft WJ, Decker JM, et al. Insulin and the risk of cardiovascular disease: a meta-analysis. *Circulation* 1998; 97:996–1001.

150. Despres JP, Lamarche B, Mauriege P, et al. Hyperinsulinemia as an independent risk factor for ischemic heart disease. *N Engl J Med* 1996; 334:952–957.

151. Lavela SL, Weaver FM, Goldstein B, Chen K, Miskevics S, Rajan S, Gater DR Jr. Diabetes mellitus in individuals with spinal cord injury or disorder. *J Spinal Cord Med* 2006; 29(4):387–395.

152. Duckworth WC, Solomon SS, Jallepalli P, Heckemeyer C, Finnern J, Powers A. Glucose intolerance due to insulin resistance in patients with spinal cord injuries. *Diabetes* 1980; 29:906–910.

153. Liang H, Chen D, Wang Y, Rimmer JH, Braunschweig CL. Different risk factor patterns for metabolic syndrome in men with spinal cord injury compared with able-bodied men despite similar prevalence rates. *Arch Phys Med Rehabil* 2007 Sep; 88(9):1198–1204.

154. American Diabetes Association. Standards of medical care in diabetes. *Diabetes Care* 2004; 27(suppl 1):S15–S35.

155. Bolen S, Feldman L, Vassy J, Wilson L, Yeh HC, Marinopoulos S, Wiley C, Selvin E, Wilson R, Bass EB, Brancati FL. Systematic review: comparative effectiveness and safety of oral medications for type 2 diabetes mellitus. *Ann Intern Med* 2007 Sep 18; 147(6):386–399.

156. Rajan S, Hammond MC, Goldstein B. Trends in diabetes mellitus indicators in veterans with spinal cord injury. *Am J Phys Med Rehabil* 2008 Jun; 87(6):468–474.

157. Rozanski A, Blumenthal JA, Kaplan J. Impact of pyschological factors on the pathogenesis of cardiovascular disease and implications for therapy. *Circulation* 1999; 99:2192–2197.

158. Strike PC, Steptoe A. Psychosocial factors in the development of coronary artery disease. *Prog Cardiovasc Dis* 2004 Jan-Feb; 46(4): 337–347.

159. Zellweger MJ, Osterwalder RH, Langewitz W, Pfisterer ME. Coronary artery disease and depression. *Eur Heart J* 2004 Jan; 25(1):3–9.

160. Kaplan GA, Keil JE. Socioeconomic factors and cardiovascular disease: A review of the literature. *Circulation* 1993; 88:1973–1998.

161. Liebson PR, Amsterdam EA. Prevention of coronary heart disease: part II. secondary prevention, detection of subclinical disease, and emerging risk factors. *Disease-a-Month* 2000; 46(1):1–124.

162. Pratt LA, Ford DE, Crum RM, et al. Depression, psychotropic medication, and risk of myocardial infarction: Prospective data from the Baltimore ECA follow-up. *Circulation* 1996; 94:3123–3129.

163. Brown PJ, Stass WE. Suicide in the spinal cord injury population. *Arch Phys Med Rehabil* 1988; 69:702.

164. Macleod AD. Self-neglect of spinal injured patients. *Paraplegia* 1988; 26:340–349.

165. Consortium for Spinal Cord Medicine. Clinical Practice Guidelines: Depression Following Spinal Cord Injury. Washington, D.C.: Paralyzed Veterans of America, 1998.

166. Ridker PM. Evaluating novel cardiovascular risk factors: Can we better predict heart attacks? *Ann Intern Med* 1999; 130:933–937.

167. Force T, Miani R, Hibberd P, et al. Aspirin-induced decline in prostacyclin production in patients with coronary artery disease is due to decreased endoperoxide shift. *Circulation* 1991; 84:2286–2293.

168. Ridker PM, Glynn RJ, Hennekens CH. C-reactive protein adds to the predictive value of total and HDL cholesterol in determining risk of first myocardial infarction. *Circulation* 1998; 97:2007–2011.

169. Eikelbloom JW, Lonn E, Genest JJ Jr, et al. Homocysteine and cardiovascular disease: A critical review of the epidemiological evidence. *Ann Intern Med* 1999; 131:363–375.

170. Undas A, Brozek J, Szczeklik A. Homocysteine and thrombosis: from basic science to clinical evidence. *Thromb Haemost* 2005 Nov; 94(5): 907–915.

171. Yu R, Yekta B, Vakili L, Gharavi N, Navab M, Marelli D, Ardehali A. Proatherogenic high-density lipoprotein, vascular inflammation, and mimetic peptides. *Curr Atheroscler Rep* 2008 Apr; 10(2):171–176.

172. Kahn NN, Bauman WA. Prostacyclin receptor antibody in SCI and persons with associated cardiovascular risk factors [abstract]. *J Spinal Cord Med* 2000; 23(3):202–203.

173. Vaidyanathan S, Soni BM, Singh G, et al. Recurrent urinary infection, raised serum levels of C-reactive protein, and the risk of cardiovascular disease in patients with spinal cord injury: a hypothesis. *Spinal Cord* 1998; 36(12):868–869.

174. Liang H, Mojtahedi MC, Chen D, Braunschweig CL. Elevated C-reactive protein associated with decreased high-density lipoprotein cholesterol in men with spinal cord injury. *Arch Phys Med Rehabil* 2008 Jan; 89(1):36–41.

175. Bauman WA, Adkins RH, Kemp BJ, et al. Vasculotoxic plasma homocysteine levels in a population with SCI [abstract]. *J Spinal Cord Med* 2000; 23(3):201–202.

176. Ramasamy M, Schmitt J, Midha M. Serum homocysteine level: Is it a major coronary risk factor in spinal cord injury patients [abstract]. *J Spinal Cord Med* 2000; 23(3):202.

177. Malliani A, Lombard F. Considerations of fundamental mechanisms eliciting cardiac pain. *Am Heart J* 1982; 103(4):575.

178. Walker W, Khokhar M. Silent cardiac ischemia in cervical spinal cord injury: Case study. *Arch Phys Med Rehabil* 1992; 73(1):91.

179. Sanford P, Sabharwal S. Diagnosis of myocardial infarction in a patient with complete tetraplegia [abstract]. *J Spinal Cord Med* 2000; 23(Suppl 1):47.

180. Stiens SA, Johnson MC, Lyman PJ. Cardiac rehabilitation in patients with spinal cord injuries. In: Halar EM (ed.), Cardiac rehabilitation: Part II. *Phys Med Rehabil Clin North Am* 1995, 6(2):263–296.

181. Price N, Schubert ML, Vijay MR. Gastrointestinal disease in the spinal cord injury patient. *Physical Medicine and Rehabilitation: State of the Art Reviews* 1987; 1:3, 475–488.

182. Blocker WP, Merrill JM, Krebs MA, et al. An electrocardiographic survey of patients with spinal cord injury. *Am Correct Ther J* 1983; 37:101.

183. Drory Y, Ohry A, Brooks ME, et al. Arm crank ergometry in chronic spinal cord injured patients. *Arch Phys Med Rehabil* 1990, 71:389.

184. VanLoan M, McCluer 5, Lofton JM, Boileau RA. Comparison of maximal physiological responses to arm exercise among able-bodied paraplegics and quadriplegics. *Med Sci Sports Exerc* 1985; 17:250.

185. Bauman W, Raza M, Chayes Z, et al. Tomographic thallium-201 myocardial perfusion imaging after intravenous dipyridamole in asymptomatic subjects with quadriplegia. *Arch Phys Med Rehabil* 1993, 74(7):740.

186. Geleijnse ML, Fioretti PM, Roelandt JR. Methodology, feasibility, safety and diagnostic accuracy of dobutamine stress echocardiography. *J Am Coll Cardiol* 1997; 30:595–606.

187. Wenger NK. Current status of cardiac rehabilitation. *J Am Coll Cardiol* 2008 Apr 29; 51(17):1619–1631.

188. Willard JE, Lange RA, Hillis LD. The use of aspirin in ischemic heart disease. *N Engl J Med* 1992; 327:175–181.

189. U.S. Preventive Services Task Force. Aspirin for the primary prevention of cardiovascular events: recommendations and rationale. *Ann Intern Med* 2002; 136:157–160.

190. Phillips KA, Shlipak MG, Coxson P, et al. Health and economic benefits of increased beta blocker use following myocardial infarction. *JAMA* 2000; 284:2748–2754.

191. Derry FA, Dinsmore WW, Fraser M, et al. Efficacy and safety of oral sildenafil (Viagra) in men with erectile dysfunction caused by spinal cord injury. *Neurology* 1998; 51(6):1629–1633.

192. Soler JM, Previnaire JG, Denys P, Chartier-Kastler E. Phosphodiesterase inhibitors in the treatment of erectile dysfunction in spinal cord-injured men. *Spinal Cord* 2007; 45(2):169–173.

193. E. Braunwald, M.J. Domanski, S.E. Fowler et al. and PEACE Trial Investigators. Angiotensin-converting-enzyme inhibition in stable coronary artery disease. *N Engl J Med* 2004; 351:2058–2068.

194. Schmitt JK, Koch KS, Midha M. Profound hypotension in a tetraplegic patient following angiotensin-converting enzyme inhibitor, lisinopril. *Paraplegia* 1994; 32: 871874.

195. Alam M, Unwin RJ, Frankel HL, Peart WS, Mathias CJ. Cardiovascular and hormonal effects of captopril in tetraplegia. *Clin Auton Res* 1992; 2:59.

196. Wecht JM, Radulovic M, Weir JP, Lessey J, Spungen AM, Bauman WA. Partial angiotensin-converting enzyme inhibition during acute orthostatic stress in persons with tetraplegia. *J Spinal Cord Med* 2005; 28(2): 103–108.

197. Fisher S, Gullickson G. Energy cost of ambulation in health and disability: A literature review. *Arch Phys Med Rehabil* 1978; 59:124.

198. Green D. Diagnosis, prevalence, and management of thromboembolism in patients with spinal cord injury. *J Spinal Cord Med* 2003; 26(4):329–334.

199. Miranda AR, Hassouna HI. Mechanisms of thrombosis in spinal cord injury. *Hematol Oncol Clin North Am* 2000; 14(2):401–416.

200. Consortium for Spinal Cord Medicine. *Clinical Practice Guidelines: Prevention of Thromboembolism in Spinal Cord Injury.* 2nd ed. Washington, D.C.: Paralyzed Veterans of America, 1999.

201. Green D, Sullivan S, Simpson J, Soltysik RC, Yarnold PR. Evolving risk for thromboembolism in spinal cord injury (SPIRATE Study). *Am J Phys Med Rehabil* 2005; 84(6):420–422.

202. Aronow WS. Peripheral arterial disease. *Geriatrics* 2007; 62(1): 19–25.

203. Yokoo KM, Kronon M, Lewis VL Jr, McCarthy WJ, McMillan WD, Meyer PR Jr. Peripheral vascular disease in spinal cord injury patients: a difficult diagnosis. *Ann Plast Surg* 1996; 37(5):495–499.

204. Grundy DJ, Silver JR. Amputation for peripheral vascular disease in the paraplegic and tetraplegic. *Paraplegia* 1983; 21:305–311.

205. Deitrick G, Charalel J, Bauman W, Tuckman J. Reduced arterial circulation to the legs in spinal cord injury as a cause of skin breakdown lesions. *Angiology* 2007; 58(2):175–184.

206. Nash MS, Montalvo BM, Applegate B. Lower extremity blood flow and responses to occlusion ischemia differ in exercise-trained and sedentary tetraplegic persons. *Arch Phys Med Rehabil* 1996; 77: 1260–1265.

207. Taylor PN, Ewins DJ, Fox B, Grundy D, Swain ID. Limb blood flow, cardiac output and quadriceps muscle bulk following spinal cord injury and the effect of training for the Odstock functional electrical stimulation standing system. *Paraplegia* 1993; 31:303–310.

208. Hankey GJ, Norman PE, Eikelboom JW. Medical Treatment of Peripheral Arterial Disease. *JAMA* 2006; 295(5): 547–553.

209. Lee BY. Management of peripheral vascular disease in the spinal cord injured patient. In: *Comprehensive Management of the Spinal Cord Injured Patient.* Philadelphia: WB Saunders 1991; 1–11.
210. Sabharwal S. Limb amputations in patients with spinal cord injury [abstract]. *Arch Phys Med Rehabil* 1996; 77:940.
211. Grew M, Kirshblum SC, Wood K, Millis SR, Ma R. The ankle brachial index in chronic spinal cord injury: a pilot study. *J Spinal Cord Med* 2000; 23(4):284–288.
212. Sobel M, McNeil P, Hussey RW, et al. Vascular surgery in spinal cord injured patients. *J Am Paraplegia Soc* 1990; 13:108–109.
213. Ohry A, Heim M, Steinbach TV, et al. The needs and unique problems facing spinal cord injured persons after limb amputation. *Paraplegia* 1983; 21:260–263.
214. Brooke MM, Donovan WH, Stolov WC. Paraplegia: succinylcholine-induced hyperkalemia and cardiac arrest. *Arch Phys Med Rehabil* 1978; 59:306–309.
215. Martyn JA, Richtsfeld M. Succinylcholine-induced hyperkalemia in acquired pathologic states: etiologic factors and molecular mechanisms. *Anesthesiology* 2006 Jan; 104(1):158–169.

19 Thromboembolism in Spinal Cord Disorders

David Chen

Thromboembolism, which includes deep vein thrombosis (DVT) and pulmonary embolism (PE), remains a common complication of spinal cord injury (SCI), and continues to be a major cause of morbidity and mortality in this patient population.

Despite a greater awareness of this potentially life-threatening condition and improved preventive measures, thromboembolism continues to occur with significant frequency, especially in the acute period following injury. The recent experience of the Model Systems SCI Program has found that since 1996, DVT occurred in 9.8% of persons during acute rehabilitation and PE in 2.6% (1). In comparison, prior to 1992, it was reported that the incidence of DVT was 13.6% and PE was 3.8% during acute care or rehabilitation (1).

Although it is generally accepted that the risks for thromboembolism decrease with time post-injury, one must recognize that the potential for developing this complication still exists even in the chronic period following injury. McKinley et al. found in the Model Systems SCI experience that the incidence of DVT reported at first year follow-up was 2.1%, and even at year 2 was 1.0% (2). The incidence of PE at year 1 follow-up was 0.5%, and remained at that rate at years 2, 5, 10, and 20 (2).

The true incidence and frequency of this complication, however, are not entirely known. A review of the literature reveals varying incidence figures from a number of investigators. This is probably attributable to the differences in diagnostic techniques or assessment criteria used in their studies.

Some of the earliest studies were based on autopsy reports or clinical presentation and findings. In one of the earliest published studies, Tribe reported that the cause of death in the first 3 months following SCI was pulmonary emboli in 37% of patients (3). In a later report, Walsh and Tribe reported a 13.2% incidence of thromboembolism in a population of 500 patients (4). In a review of 431 persons with SCIs, Watson reported a 12% incidence of DVT and a 5% incidence of PE (5). In a later study, Watson further found that in those persons who developed thromboembolism, 85% of cases occurred within the first month post-injury (6). In these studies, it is important to recognize that

in many of the reported episodes of PE there was no clinical evidence of DVT.

In recent years, the availability of more advanced diagnostic techniques has improved the diagnostic accuracy for DVT. Interestingly, the greater sensitivity of these techniques has resulted in the reports of higher incidence of DVT and PE by more recent investigators. Using I^{125}-fibrinogen leg scanning, Todd et al. reported a 100% incidence of DVT in the SCI patients studied. However, in 40% of these individuals, the positive findings could not be confirmed by venography (7). Myllynen et al. similarly reported a 100% incidence of DVT when using fibrinogen scanning (8). Other investigators have also reported on the high incidence of DVT when utilizing fibrinogen scanning as the diagnostic criteria, whereas others have recently reported similar higher incidences utilizing venography, which many believe to be the gold standard in diagnosing DVT. In summarizing these more recent reports that utilize diagnostic techniques that are theoretically more accurate, the incidence of DVT in SCI individuals ranges from 23% to 100% (9–12).

Although the incidence of clinically significant thromboembolism appears to be generally less than recently reported incidence rates that utilize more sensitive diagnostic techniques, it is still imperative that our understanding of those risk factors that predispose this patient population to development of DVTs and PEs improve so that effective prophylactic measures may be utilized, given the potentially devastating consequences of this condition.

PATHOPHYSIOLOGY AND RISK FACTORS

In examining the risk for developing thromboembolism in any medical condition, it is often helpful to recall Virchow's Triad (13), which describes three factors that may contribute to the development of thrombogenesis. These three factors are the blood vessel wall, blood flow, and blood constituents.

The blood vessel wall, more specifically the venous endothelium, may be injured by extrinsic pressure on the paralyzed extremity in the neurologically impaired patient. In addition, the acute course of a spinal cord injured person is frequently complicated by sepsis or other infections, which result in the creation of an inflammatory state. This often results in the production and exposure of the vessel walls to free oxygen radicals or endotoxins, which may damage the endothelium and provoke thrombosis.

Altered blood flow results in a venous stasis that predisposes the individual to the development of thrombus. Contributions to the reduced venous flow include failure of the venous muscle pump in the paralyzed limb, increased blood viscosity secondary to dehydration, transudation of fluid into the interstitial spaces of the paralyzed limb, and hyperfibrinogenemia (14, 15).

Alterations in blood constituents may result in alterations in hemostasis and a transient hypercoagulable state in persons with SCI (16). Several investigators have shown that there are increased levels and activity of factor VIII and vonWillebrand factor in acute SCI (17, 18). It has also been shown that increases of these factor levels begin soon after injury and reach maximum values—often two to three times normal—about a week after injury. This coincides with the peak incidence of venous thrombosis in the group studied (18). In addition to raised levels of clotting factors, changes in the inhibitors of coagulation and fibrinolysis after acute SCI also increase the risk of thrombus development. Decreases in antithrombin III have been found in persons following trauma or surgery, and a reduction in fibrinolytic activity has also been shown after acute SCI (15, 19.) Diminished fibrinolysis may occur through three mechanisms: a decrease in the release of tissue plasminogen activator caused by the lack of muscle contraction in the paralyzed limb (20, 21); inhibition of plasminogen binding to fibrin by high concentrations of fibrinogen (22); and increases in plasma levels of plasminogen activator-1 (19).

A number of clinical factors have been suggested to be associated with a higher risk for development of thromboembolism in persons with SCI. In a review of 2,186 persons with acute SCI, Ragnarsson et al. found a higher rate of occurrence of DVT among those with motor complete injuries, a greater risk for DVT in paraplegics than tetraplegics, and a higher rate of occurrence in males (23). It was further noted that the incidence of PE was not influenced by degree or level of injury. Age was not a factor in the development of DVT, but PE was noted to be higher in persons aged 61 to 75 years. Green et al. reported that in an analysis of 243 persons with acute SCI, a higher incidence of venous thromboembolism was seen in persons who were over the age of 35 years, obese, with flaccid paralysis, or a history of cancer (24).

CLINICAL PRESENTATION AND DIAGNOSTIC MODALITIES
Deep Vein Thrombosis

In the able-bodied population, the early diagnosis of DVT is often delayed by the nonspecific nature of the clinical signs and symptoms usually associated with DVT (swelling, warmth, discoloration). The fact that many of these signs and symptoms occur in other disorders associated with SCI further complicates diagnosis in these patients. For example, heterotopic ossification in persons with SCI is often heralded by the development of swelling, erythema, and increased warmth in the affected extremity. In fact, it is well recognized that the clinical diagnosis of DVT in the SCI population is low in accuracy and specificity (25). Of even greater

concern are those individuals who were found to have DVT by objective tests, yet presented no specific clinical signs or symptoms, or had very general, nonspecific signs such as fever (26). This fact emphasizes that the clinical suspicion for DVT must be high in this patient population, and underscores the importance of objective testing for making the proper diagnosis.

Impedance plethysmography (IPG) measures the rapid decrease in electrical resistance of a limb when an occlusive tourniquet is deflated, after taking into account the venous capacitance. Occlusion of a proximal vein, for example by a new DVT, significantly reduces the rate of venous outflow after the tourniquet is released, and accordingly reduces the change in electrical resistance.

It should be emphasized, however, that this test is unable to differentiate whether an occlusion is caused by a thrombosis or an extrinsic compression of the vessel. It has also been suggested that the specificity of IPG in spinal cord patients is lower because of the decreased venous outflow and capacitance found in most persons with SCI (27). In addition, IPG has very low sensitivity for DVT below the popliteal vein.

Duplex ultrasound or scanning is probably the most frequently used noninvasive diagnostic modality for DVT. There are actually two components to the ultrasound study, the Doppler and the scan. The Doppler component indirectly measures the flow velocity in the vessel. The ultrasound beam is reflected from the column of venous blood at a frequency proportional to the flow velocity. The scan component of the ultrasound is made possible by the ability to visualize venous flow by reconstructing the reflected waves to provide anatomic detail. Scanning along the entire length of an accessible vein may locate a thrombus. In addition, experienced technicians will look for variations in flow caused by respiration with Valsalva's maneuver, or vein compression. Observing vein compression is a valuable technique, because noncompressibility is characteristic of an obstructed vessel.

The limitations of this diagnostic modality include an inability to clearly image particular veins, such as the iliacs and profunda femoris, and an inability to distinguish interrupted venous flow caused by turbulent flow and extrinsic compression of the vein from an occluding thrombus. In symptomatic individuals, the sensitivity and specificity of ultrasound is high; however, in asymptomatic persons, the sensitivity of this modality has been found to be quite low, thus making it a poor screening tool for DVT (28).

Venography remains the gold standard for the detection and localization of DVT. This invasive procedure requires the injection of a contrast medium, usually into a dorsal foot vein, followed by a series of radiographs taken to visualize the network of veins in the lower extremities. The presence of a thrombus may be identified in several ways, including a constant intraluminal filling defect seen in more than one view, cutoff of the contrast medium at a constant site below a nonfilled segment with reappearance above the site, or persistent nonfilling of the deep venous system above the knee despite adequate dye infusion (29). Because it is an invasive procedure, venography may produce pain at the site of injection. In addition, the procedure itself can produce phlebitis, and hypersensitivity reactions may occur with the contrast media.

In general, a patient in whom there is a clinical suspicion for DVT should be initially evaluated with venous ultrasound. If the results are equivocal or negative, but clinical suspicion is high, venography should be performed.

Pulmonary Embolism

As is similar in DVT, the diagnosis of PE in the individual with SCI is often delayed because of the nonspecific symptoms that commonly accompany its presentation. Presenting symptoms may include dyspnea, tachypnea, tachycardia, fever, or chest pain; these are also symptoms found with pneumonia or atelectasis. Less commonly, PE may initially present as syncope, hypotension, and arrhythmia. Unfortunately, in some individuals, the initial presentation of PE is sudden death. With the lack of specific symptoms and frequent silent clinical presentation, it is important to have a high index of suspicion, especially because of the potentially devastating consequences, such as death.

If there is a clinical suspicion of PE, the initial diagnostic procedure commonly performed is the ventilation-perfusion (V/Q) lung scan. In this procedure, macroaggregated albumin particles labeled with technetium-99m are infused intravenously to display the distribution of lung blood flow. This part of the procedure is combined with the inhalation of xenon-127 gas or technetium-99m sulfur colloid aerosol to image the airways. When interpreting the study, one compares the blood flow portion with the airway study, looking for areas of the lung that have reduced blood flow, but adequate ventilation of the airways. V/Q lung scans are interpreted in terms of the probability of PE—low, intermediate, or high. It has been shown that in persons with a high clinical suspicion of PE and high-probability scans, or low clinical suspicion and low-probability scans, accuracy of the study exceeds 90% (30). Additionally, it was found that if clinical suspicion was high, the presence of PE was found in 66% of persons with intermediate probability scans, and 40% with low probability scans. Conversely, if clinical suspicion was low, PE was found in 16% of persons with intermediate probability scans, and 4% with low probability scans.

Like venography in DVT, pulmonary angiography is currently the gold standard for the diagnosis of PE. This study involves the injection of a radiographic contrast medium into the main pulmonary outflow tract and taking multiple radiographic images. Pulmonary emboli may be visualized as intraluminal filling defects, sharp cutoffs, or absence of filling despite multiple injections of contrast.

At the present time, the use of single-detector and multidetector spiral computed tomography (spiral CT or ultrafast CT) has been advocated for the diagnosis of PE, especially in situations where pulmonary angiography is not available or there is an intermediate probability V/Q scan and the avoidance of an invasive contrast study is desired (31). Ultrafast CT uses X-rays produced by a magnetically steered electron beam that strike a stationary tungsten target. Ultrafast CT allows for scan times of 50 and 100 ms (compared with scan times of 1 s for conventional CT), very few motion artifacts, and a more reliable degree of contrast enhancement. This procedure also has the advantage of requiring only about 20 minutes to complete (32).

TREATMENT AND MANAGEMENT OF THROMBOEMBOLISM

In the past, the standard treatment for established venous thromboembolism has been anticoagulation with unfractionated heparin, given by constant intravenous infusion, followed immediately by oral warfarin for a specified number of months. The objective of this initial treatment is to prevent new thrombus formation and the extension of existing thrombus. Standard anticoagulation will not prevent embolization from existing thrombus or induce dissolution of the thrombus.

Treatment is generally initiated by the administration of an intravenous bolus of heparin. Various protocols or regimens have been studied and recommended for the administration of intravenous heparin in patients with venous thromboembolism. Hull et al. suggest an initial intravenous heparin bolus of 5000 U (33), whereas Raschke et al. recommend an initial bolus dose based on body weight, 80 IU/kg (34). Both well-recognized regimens then include the constant infusion of intravenous heparin, with the goal of achieving an activated partial thromboplastin time (aPTT) of at least 1.5 times the mean normal control value. Both protocols involve periodically obtaining the aPTT and adjusting the heparin dose. It is important that an aPTT of at least 1.5 times control be achieved within 24 to 72 hours of initiating treatment; otherwise effectiveness is reduced and the risk of recurrent thrombosis is increased (33, 35, 36).

Today, a number of low molecular weight heparin (LMWH) preparations are available and have been studied as an initial anticoagulant treatment for acute thromboembolism. A number of clinical trials have examined the use of subcutaneous unmonitored LMWH compared with continuous intravenous heparin for the treatment of proximal venous thrombosis and have shown that LMWH is at least as effective and safe (less major bleeding and mortality) as unfractionated heparin (37–42). Several studies have also shown the equivalent effectiveness of LMWH when compared to unfractionated heparin in the treatment of acute pulmonary embolism (42, 43).

LMWHs differ from unfractionated heparins in a number of advantageous ways: (a) increased bioavailability (greater than 90% after subcutaneous injection); (b) prolonged half-life and predictable clearance, which enables once or twice daily injection; and (c) a predictable antithrombotic response based on body weight, which permits treatment without the need for laboratory monitoring (44–47). In addition, LMWHs appear to have fewer serious complications such as bleeding, osteoporosis, and heparin-induced thrombocytopenia when compared to unfractionated heparin (48–50).

After initiation of treatment with either unfractionated or low molecular weight heparin, oral anticoagulation with warfarin follows and should be continued long term. The purpose of long-term anticoagulant therapy is to prevent recurrent thromboembolic disease. It is generally recommended that heparin and warfarin treatment should overlap by 4 to 5 days.

Warfarin is administered at an initial dosage of 5 to 10 mg/day for the first 2 days. The daily dose is then adjusted according to the International Normalized Ratio (INR), which was developed by the World Health Organization and has become the accepted standardization of the prothrombin time (PT) for monitoring oral anticoagulant therapy. Heparin therapy is discontinued on the fourth or fifth day following initiation of warfarin therapy, provided the INR is in the recommended therapeutic range of 2 to 3 (51). It should be emphasized that individuals metabolize warfarin at different rates, so that selection of the correct dosage of warfarin must be individualized. Therefore, frequent INR determinations are often required early on to establish therapeutic anticoagulation.

Once the anticoagulant effect and warfarin dosage are stable, the INR should be monitored every 1 to 3 weeks at regular intervals. If any factors exist that may produce an unpredictable response to warfarin or the possibility of an alteration in dosage (e.g., concomitant drug therapy such as antibiotics), the INR should be monitored more frequently (51).

Although the optimal duration of treatment for thromboembolism is not entirely clear, it is generally recommended that treatment of a first episode with warfarin in the general population should be at least 3 months, and possibly as long as 6 months. This regimen probably holds true for persons with reversible or time-limited risk factors, however, in persons with chronic conditions, such as SCI, the optimal duration is not known (52–54).

PREVENTIVE MANAGEMENT OF THROMBOEMBOLISM

Given the significant risk, morbidity, and mortality of thromboembolism in the SCI population, it is clear that methods to prevent the development of this medical complication should be strongly considered and implemented.

Various nonpharmacologic modalities and pharmacologic agents are available and frequently utilized in trying to prevent the development of DVTs. These are discussed below in greater detail, including their effectiveness in the SCI population.

Nonpharmacologic Modalities

Early Mobilization

Minimizing immobility and initiating out-of-bed activity at the earliest possible time is desirable and believed to be beneficial in preventing thromboembolism in the hospitalized patient. It has been shown that early ambulation of patients following acute myocardial infarction significantly reduced the incidence of DVT (55).

However, for a number of obvious reasons, ranging from the presence of other associated injuries, to respiratory complications, to instability of the spine and the neurologic deficits themselves, early mobilization and ambulation are frequently not possible or practical in the acute SCI patient. For these individuals, passive range-of-motion (ROM) exercises are often initiated by physical and occupational therapists in the intensive care setting. In addition to preventing joint contractures and skin complications, there have been suggestions that this activity may also contribute to the prevention of DVT. Unfortunately, there are no studies that have examined the effectiveness of passive or active exercises in preventing DVTs.

Compression Stockings

Graduated elastic or compression stockings are frequently used in hospitalized persons who are immobilized for prolonged periods of time. These commercially available items, which may be calf- or thigh-length, apply firm pressure to the extremity in a graduated fashion (greater distally than proximally) and reduce the venous capacitance of the extremity. Compression stockings have been shown to be effective in reducing the incidence of DVT in low-risk surgical patients; however, their effectiveness in SCI patients is not known (56).

Pneumatic Compression Sleeves

Pneumatic compression sleeves (PCSs) are commercially available devices that are applied to the lower limbs to exert rhythmic, sequential compression of the calves and thighs. These devices are readily available and frequently used in the general hospital population for DVT prophylaxis, and have been found to be effective in persons at moderate risk for DVT, such as persons with malignant disease or those undergoing general surgery (57). Their effectiveness may be attributed to their better ability to augment lower extremity venous return, improve flow velocity and volume flow rate, and stimulate fibrinolysis (58).

In the SCI population, PCS have been found in clinical studies to be variably effective in preventing DVT. Green et al. demonstrated a reduction in DVT in persons with new motor-complete SCI with PCS alone compared to persons in which no prophylaxis was used, and an even greater reduction in persons where PCS were used in combination with aspirin and dipyridamole (59). Merli et al. also reported a reduction in DVT in persons with SCI utilizing a combination therapy consisting of PCS, compression stockings, and low-dose unfractionated heparin (60).

Although they provide some benefit, it appears that they are not sufficient alone in preventing DVT in the SCI population. In addition, drawbacks with these devices include the need to don and doff the sleeves to allow the patient in the rehabilitation setting to participate in therapeutic activities. Occasionally, an inability to tolerate the sleeves occurs in individuals with extreme sensory hypersensitivity and dysesthetic pain caused by their neurologic injuries.

Vena Cava Filter

In recent years, placement of vena cava filters has become an increasingly performed procedure in trauma and other high-risk patient populations to prevent PE (61). It should be emphasized that the presence of a filter itself does not prevent the development of venous thrombosis. In the past, vena cava filter placement was usually reserved for those patients in whom anticoagulant prophylaxis was contraindicated or in those with established DVT in whom anticoagulation was contraindicated (e.g., active or potential bleeding complications).

Although no large-scale studies have examined the use of filters specifically in SCI patients, examination of a small series of SCI individuals and several studies of high-risk trauma patients (which have included persons with SCI) have reported the effectiveness of vena cava filters in reducing the incidence of symptomatic PE (62–65).

The effectiveness of vena cava filters in preventing PE must be weighed against any potential adverse effects when considering their use. Potential complications include cava thrombosis, filter migration, and vena cava perforation. Filter migration and malposition are usually the result of poor insertion technique or anatomic anomalies of the vena cava or renal veins, and can be avoided by obtaining preinsertion inferior vena cavagrams and insertion of the filter under fluoroscopic guidance. After placement of the filter, a follow-up abdominal film should be performed to confirm filter placement and position (64).

The increasing use of vena cava filters as prophylaxis for PE in the SCI population has raised concerns regarding potential long-term complications. The recent development and availability of temporary or removable vena cava filters may address these concerns. However, at the present time, data and literature on its indications, criteria for use and removal, and outcomes in this population are limited, and therefore require further study (66).

It bears repeating that the use of vena cava filters does not prevent the development of DVT and its potential comorbidities. In fact, it has been suggested that even with the concomitant use of low-dose heparin, the risk of recurrent DVT is higher in persons with filters than in those without filters (67).

Pharmacologic Agents

Warfarin

As a means of prophylaxis, the use of warfarin has the advantage of being orally effective. However, it has the disadvantage of requiring close monitoring of the prothrombin time or INR, and the increased risk of bleeding complications. The close monitoring of the coagulation times and need for frequent dose adjustment is commonly necessary in the acute SCI patient, who may be receiving other medications that may potentiate or inhibit the anticoagulant effects of warfarin. These patients' nutritional status may be poor, thus potentially enhancing the effects of the anticoagulant agent; or, in those undergoing surgery, patients often will require the temporary withholding and restarting of warfarin.

When used as a prophylactic agent, warfarin is commonly used in smaller dosages with the goal of achieving minimal prolongation of the prothrombin time (4 seconds above control;

INR of 1.5–2.0). Using this approach, an effective prophylactic benefit may be attained while minimizing the potential bleeding risks (68).

Unfractionated Heparin

Unfractionated heparin (UFH) has been and continues to be a commonly used pharmacologic agent for the prevention of DVT in the general medical population. Low doses of 5,000 U administered subcutaneously 2 to 3 times daily are used for most medical patients, and for those undergoing general abdominal, urologic, and gynecologic surgery (68). For those patients at higher risk for DVT (e.g., persons with hip or knee replacement, or SCI), the use of adjusted-dose heparin with the goal of achieving a slightly prolonged aPTT has been found to be effective, although bleeding complications are higher (69, 70). In persons with acute SCI, the use of adjusted-dose heparin is one of the recommended options for prophylaxis of thromboembolism (71).

Low Molecular Weight Heparin

The benefits and increased effectiveness of LMWH for the prevention of thromboembolism in a variety of patient populations has been increasingly reported in recent years (57, 72). Currently, there are a number of LMWH preparations commercially available; these have been approved by the U.S. Food and Drug Administration (FDA) for use in the prophylaxis of DVT in patients undergoing abdominal, pelvic, hip, and knee surgical procedures.

Table 19.1   Guidelines for the Prevention of Thromboembolism in SCI: Clinical Decision Table

LEVEL OF RISK	MOTOR INCOMPLETE	MOTOR COMPLETE	MOTOR COMPLETE WITH OTHER RISK[a]
Intensity of Prophylaxis			
Low	Compression hose Compression boots and	Compression hose Compression boots and	Compression hose Compression boots and
Intermediate	UH[b]:5000 U q12h; or LMWH+++	UH+: Dose adjusted to high normal high normal aPTT[c]; or LMWH[d]	UH+: Dose adjusted to high normal high normal aPTT[c]; or LMWH[d] and
High	—	—	Inferior vena cava filter in certain situations
Duration of Prophylaxis	Compression boots: 2 weeks; Anticoagulants: While in hospital for ASIA class D and up to 8 weeks for ASIA class C	Compression boots: 2 weeks; Anticoagulants: at least 8 weeks	Compression boots: 2 weeks; Anticoagulants: 12 weeks or until discharge from rehabilitation

[a]Other risk factors: lower limb fracture, previous thrombosis, cancer, heart failure, obesity, age over 70.
[b]UH = unfractionated heparin.
[c]aPTT = activated partial thromboplastin time.
[d]LMWH = low molecular weight heparin, prophylactic dose as recommended by the manufacturers.
(Reproduced with permission from Consortium for Spinal Cord Medicine. *Prevention of Thromboembolism in Spinal Cord Injury*, 2nd edition. Washington, DC: Paralyzed Veterans of America.)

Although no LMWH preparations are currently FDA approved for prophylaxis specifically in the acute SCI population, there are a number of published studies and reports of the increased effectiveness of LMWH in decreasing the incidence of DVT in this patient group (73–77), and it has been suggested and recommended by the Consortium for Spinal Cord Medicine as one of the more effective forms of DVT prophylaxis in persons with acute SCI (71).

Duration of Preventive Management

The duration of DVT prophylaxis in persons with acute SCI has been and remains controversial. Prolonging the administration of any anticoagulant agent unnecessarily exposes the individual to the increased risk of bleeding complications and adds to the cost of health care, yet discontinuing any treatment prematurely may expose the patient to the increased risk of developing a thromboembolus. It has been recommended that the duration of prophylaxis be individualized, depending on the risk factors, need, medical condition, functional status, and care and support services of the individual (71). Recommended guidelines for the prevention of thromboembolism in persons with SCI have been developed by the Consortium for Spinal Cord Medicine and are shown in Table 19.1.

R*eferences*

1. Chen D, Apple DA, Hudson LM, Bode R. Medical complications during acute rehabilitation following spinal cord injury—current experience of the model systems. *Arch Phys Med Rehabil* 1999; 80:1397–1401.
2. McKinley WO, Jackson AB, Cardenas DD, DeVivo MJ. Long-term medical complications after traumatic spinal cord injury: A regional model systems analysis. *Arch Phys Med Rehabil* 1999; 80:1402–1410.
3. Tribe CR. Causes of death in early and late stages in paraplegia. *Paraplegia* 1963; 1:19–47.
4. Walsh JJ, Tribe C. Phlebo-thrombosis and pulmonary embolism in paraplegia. *Paraplegia* 1965; 3:209–213.
5. Watson N. Anticoagulation therapy in prevention of venous thrombosis and pulmonary embolism in spinal cord injury. *Paraplegia* 1968; 6:113–121.
6. Watson N. Anticoagulant therapy in the treatment of venous thrombosis and pulmonary embolism in acute spinal cord injury. *Paraplegia* 1974; 12:197–201.
7. Todd JW, Frisbie JH, Rossier AB, et al. Deep venous thrombosis in acute spinal cord injury: comparison of 125 I fibrinogen leg scanning, impedance plethysmography and venography. *Paraplegia* 1976; 14:50–57.
8. Myllynen P, Kammonen M, Rokkanen P, et al. Deep venous thrombosis and pulmonary embolism in patients with acute spinal cord injury: a comparison with non-paralyzed patients immobilized due to spinal fractures. *J Trauma* 1985; 25:541–546.
9. Merli G, Herbison G, Ditunno J, et al. Deep vein thrombosis: Prophylaxis in acute spinal cord injured patients. *Arch Phys Med Rehabil* 1988; 69:661–664.
10. Petaja J, Myllynen P, Rokkanen P, et al. Fibrinolysis and spinal injury: relationships to posttraumatic deep vein thrombosis. *Acta Chiruga Scandinavica* 1989; 155: 241–246.
11. Yelnik A, Dizien O, Bussel B, et al. Systemic lower limb phlebography in acute spinal cord injury in 147 patients. *Paraplegia* 1991; 29:253–260.
12. Gunduz S, Ogur E, Mohur H, et al. Deep vein thrombosis in spinal injured patients. *Paraplegia* 1993; 31:606–610.
13. Virchow R. Phlogose und thrombose in gefabsystem. In: Virchow R, ed. *Gesammelte Abdhandlunhen zur Wissenschaftlicgen Medicin.* Frankfurt: Meidinger Sohn, 1856:458.
14. Seifert J, Stoephasius E, Probst J, et al. Blood flow in muscles of paraplegic patients under various conditions measured by a double isotope technique. *Paraplegia* 1972; 10:185–191.
15. Green D, Chen D. Spinal cord injury: Pathophysiology of hypercoagulability and clinical management. In: Seghatchian MJ, Samama MM, Hecker SP, eds. *Hypercoagulable States: Fundamental Aspects, Acquired Disorders, and Congenital Thrombophilia.* Boca Raton, FL.: CRC Press, 1996; 293–302.
16. Rossi E, Green D, Rosen J. Sequential changes in factor VIII and platelets preceding deep vein thrombosis in patients with spinal cord injury. *Br J Haematology* 1980; 45:143–151.
17. Myllynen P, Kammonen M, Rokkanen P, et al. The blood F VIII:Ag/F VIII:C ratio as an early indicator of deep venous thrombosis during posttraumatic immobilization. *J Trauma* 1987; 27:287–290.
18. Green D, Rossi EC, Yao JST, et al. Deep vein thrombosis in spinal cord injury: effect of prophylaxis with calf compression, aspirin, and dipyridamole. *Paraplegia* 1982; 20:227–234.
19. Petaja J, Myllynen P, Rokkanen P, et al. Fibrinolysis and spinal injury: Relationships to posttraumatic deep vein thrombosis. *Acta Chiruga Scandinavica* 1989; 155: 241–246.
20. Wiman B, Ljungberg B, Chmielewska J, et al. The role of the fibrinolytic system in deep vein thrombosis. *J Lab Clin Med* 1985; 105:265–270.
21. Katz RT, Green D, Sullivan T, Yarkony G. Functional electric stimulation to enhance systemic fibrinolytic activity in spinal cord injury patients. *Arch Phys Med Rehabil* 1987; 68:423–426.
22. McDonagh J. Suppression of plasminogen binding to fibrin by high fibrinogen: A mechanism for how high fibrinogen enhances the risk of thrombosis. *Bull Sanofi Assn Thromb Res* 1994; 4:2–20.
23. Ragnarsson K, Hall KM, Wilmot CB, et al. Management of pulmonary, cardiovascular, and metabolic conditions after spinal cord injury. In: Stover S, DeLisa JA, Whiteneck GG (eds.), *Spinal Cord Injury: Clinical Outcomes from the Model Systems.* Gaithersburg, MD: Aspen Publishers, 1995:79–99.
24. Green D, Hartwig D, Chen D, et al. Spinal cord injury risk assessment for thromboembolism (SPIRATE Study). *Am J Phys Med Rehabil* 2003; 82:950–956.
25. Hirsh J, Hull RD. *Venous Thromboembolism: Natural History, Diagnosis, and Management.* Boca Raton, FL: CRC Press, 1987.
26. Weingarden DS, Weingarden SI, Belen J. Thromboembolic disease presenting as fever in spinal cord injury. *Arch Phys Med Rehabil* 1987; 68:176–177.
27. Frieden RA, Ahn JH, Pineda HD, et al. Venous plethysmography values in patients with spinal cord injury. *Arch Phys Med Rehabil* 1987; 169:427–429.
28. Davidson BL, Elliott CG, Lensing AWA. Low accuracy of color Doppler ultrasound in the detection of proximal leg vein thrombosis in asymptomatic high-risk patients. *Ann Int Med* 1992; 117:735–738.
29. Williams JE, Marshall MW. Vascular radiology. In: Brant WE, Helms CA, eds. *Fundamentals of Diagnostic Radiology,* 2nd ed. Philadelphia: Lippincott, 1999:571–613.
30. The PIOPED Investigators. Value of the ventilation/perfusion scan in acute pulmonary embolism. Results of the prospective investigation of pulmonary embolism diagnosis (PIOPED). *JAMA* 1990; 263:2753–2759.
31. McRae SJ, Ginsberg JS. Update in the diagnosis of deep-vein thrombosis and pulmonary embolism. *Curr Opin Anaesthesiol* 2006; 19:44–51.
32. Pulmonary embolism: diagnosis with ultrafast CT. *Mayo clinical update* 1996; 12:1–2.
33. Hull RD, Raskob GE, Rosenbloom DR, et al. Optimal therapeutic level of heparin therapy in patients with venous thrombosis. *Arch Intern Med* 1992; 152:1589–1595.
34. Raschke RA, Reilly BM, Guidry JR, et al. The weight-based heparin dosing nomogram compared with a 'standard care' nomogram. *Ann Intern Med* 1993; 119:874–881.
35. Hull RD, Raskob GE, Brant RF, et al. The importance of initial heparin treatment on long-term clinical outcomes of antithrombotic therapy. *Arch Intern Med* 1997; 157:2317–2321.
36. Hull RD, Raskob GE, Brant RF, et al. Relation between the time to achieve the lower limit of the aPTT therapeutic range and recurrent venous thromboembolism during heparin treatment for deep vein thrombosis. *Arch Intern Med* 1997; 157:2562–2568.
37. Hull RD, Raskob GE, Pineo GF, et al. Subcutaneous low molecular weight heparin compared with continuous intravenous heparin in the treatment of proximal vein thrombosis. *N Engl J Med* 1992; 326:975–988.
38. Prandoni P, Lensing AW, Buller HR, et al. Comparison of subcutaneous low molecular weight heparin with intravenous standard heparin in proximal deep vein thrombosis. *Lancet* 1992; 339:441–445.

39. Lopaciuk S, Meissner AJ, Filipecki S, et al. Subcutaneous low molecular weight heparin versus subcutaneous unfractionated heparin in the treatment of deep vein thrombosis. A Polish multicentre trial. *Thromb Haemost* 1992; 68:14–18.

40. Simonneau G, Charbonnier B, Decousus H, et al. Subcutaneous low molecular weight heparin compared with continuous intravenous unfractionated heparin in the treatment of proximal deep vein thrombosis. *Arch Intern Med* 1993; 153:1541–1546.

41. Lindmarker P, Holmstrom M, Granqvist S, et al. Comparison of once-daily subcutaneous Fragmin with continuous intravenous unfractionated heparin in the treatment of deep venous thrombosis. *Thromb Haemost* 1994; 72:186–190.

42. Simonneau G, Sors H, Charbonnier B, et al. A comparison of low molecular weight heparin with unfractionated heparin for acute pulmonary embolism. *N Engl J Med* 1997; 337:663–669.

43. The Columbus Investigators. Low molecular weight heparin in the treatment of patients with venous thromboembolism. *N Engl J Med* 1997; 337:657–662.

44. Andersson LO, Barrowcliffe TW, Holmer E, et al. Molecular weight dependency of the heparin potentiated inhibition of thrombin and activated factor X: effect of heparin neutralization in plasma. *Thromb Res* 1979; 15:531–541.

45. Barrowcliffe TW, Curtis AD, Johnston EA, et al. An international standard for low molecular weight heparin. *Thromb Haemost* 1988; 60:1–7.

46. Fareed J, Walenga JM, Racanelli A, et al. Validity of the newly established low molecular weight heparin standard in cross referencing low molecular weight heparins. *Haemostasis* 1988; 3 (Suppl):33–47.

47. Hirsh J, Levine MN. Low molecular weight heparin. *Blood* 1992; 79:1–17.

48. Lensing AW, Prins MH, Davidson BL, et al. Treatment of deep venous thrombosis with low molecular weight heparins. *Arch Intern Med* 1995; 155:601–607.

49. Shaughnessy SG, Young E, Deschamps P, Hirsh J. The effects of low molecular weight and standard heparin on calcium loss from fetal rat calvaria. *Blood* 1995; 86: 1368–1373.

50. Warkentin TE, Levine MN, Hirsh J, et al. Heparin induced thrombocytopenia in patients treated with low molecular weight heparin or unfractionated heparin. *N Engl J Med* 1995; 332:1330–1335.

51. Hirsh J, Dalen JE, Anderson DR, et al. Oral anticoagulants: Mechanism of action, clinical effectiveness and optimal therapeutic range. *Chest* 1998; 114(5):445S–469S.

52. Research Committee of the British Thoracic Society. Optimum duration of anticoagulation for deep vein thrombosis and pulmonary embolism. *Lancet* 1992; 340:873–876.

53. Schulman S, Rhedin AS, Lindmarker P, et al. A comparison of six weeks with six months of oral anticoagulation therapy after a first episode of venous thromboembolism. *N Engl J Med* 1995; 332:1661–1665.

54. Levine MN, Hirsh J, Gent M, et al. Optimal duration of oral anticoagulant therapy: a randomized trial comparing four weeks with three months of warfarin in patients with proximal deep vein thrombosis. *Thromb Haemost* 1995; 74:606–611.

55. Miller RR, Lies JE, Carretta RF, et al. Prevention of lower extremity venous thrombosis by early mobilization. *Ann Intern Med* 1976; 84:700–703.

56. Wells P, Lensing A, Hirsh J. Graduated compression stockings in the prevention of postoperative venous thromboembolism: a meta-analysis. *Arch Intern Med* 1994; 154:67–72.

57. Geerts WH, Pineo GF, Heit JA, et al. Prevention of venous thromboembolism: the seventh ACCP conference on antithrombotic and thrombolytic therapy. *Chest* 2004; 126:338S-400S.

58. Salzman E, McManama G, Shapiro A, et al. Effect of optimization of hemodynamics on fibrinolytic activity and antithrombotic efficacy of external pneumatic calf compression. *Ann Surg* 1987; 206:636–641.

59. Green D, Rossi E, Yao J, et al. Deep vein thrombosis in spinal cord injury: Effect of prophylaxis with calf compression, aspirin, and dipyridamole. *Paraplegia* 1982; 20:227–234.

60. Merli G, Crabbe S, Doyle L, et al. Mechanical plus pharmacological prophylaxis for deep vein thrombosis in acute spinal cord injury. *Paraplegia* 1992; 30:558–562.

61. Stein PD, Kayali F, Hull RD. Spiral computed tomography for the diagnosis of acute pulmonary embolism. *Thromb Haemost* 2007; 98:713–720.

62. Wilson JT, Rogers FB, Wald SI, et al. Prophylactic vena cava filter insertion in patients with traumatic spinal cord injury: Preliminary results. *Neurosurg* 1994; 35:234–239.

63. Khansarinia S, Dennis JW, Veldenz HC, et al. Prophylactic Greenfield filter placement in selected high-risk trauma patients. *J Vasc Surg* 1995; 22:231–236.

64. Rogers FB, Strindberg G, Shackford SR, et al. Five-year follow-up of prophylactic vena cava filters in high-risk trauma patients. *Arch Surg* 1998; 133:406–411.

65. Wojcik R, Cipolle MD, Fearen I, et al. Long-term follow-up of trauma patients with a vena caval filter. *J Trauma* 2000; 49:839–843.

66. Johns JS, Nguyen C, Sing RF. Vena cava filters in spinal cord injuries: evolving technology. *J Spinal Cord Med* 2006; 29:183–190.

67. Decousus H, Leizoravicz A, Parent F, et al. A clinical trial of vena caval filters in the prevention of pulmonary embolism in patients with proximal deep-vein thrombosis. *N Engl J Med* 1998; 338:409–415.

68. Green D. Venous Thromboembolism. In: Green D, ed. *Medical Management of Long-Term Disability*, 2nd ed. Boston: Butterworth-Heinemann, 1996:199–216.

69. Green D, Lee MY, Ito VY, et al. Fixed- versus adjusted-dose heparin in the prophylaxis of thromboembolism in spinal cord injury. *JAMA* 1988; 260:1255–1258.

70. Hirsh J, Raschke R. Heparin and low-molecular-weight heparin: the seventh ACCP conference on antithrombotic and thrombolytic therapy. *Chest* 2004; 126:188S–203S.

71. Consortium for Spinal Cord Medicine. *Prevention of Thromboembolism in Spinal Cord Injury*, 2nd ed. Washington, D.C.: Paralyzed Veterans of America, 1999.

72. Green D, Hirsh J, Heit J, et al. Low molecular weight heparin: A critical analysis of clinical trials. *Pharmacol Rev* 1994; 46:89–109.

73. Green D, Lee MY, Lim AC. Prevention of thromboembolism after spinal cord injury using low molecular weight heparin. *Ann Intern Med* 1990; 113:571–574.

74. Green D, Chen D, Chmiel JS, et al. Prevention of thromboembolism in spinal cord injury: role of low molecular weight heparin. *Arch Phys Med Rehabil* 1994; 75:290–292.

75. Harris S, Chen D, Green D. Enoxaparin for thromboembolism prophylaxis in spinal injury. *Am J Phys Med Rehabil* 1996; 75:1–3.

76. Geerts WH, Jay RM, Code KI, et al. A comparison of low-dose heparin with low-molecular-weight heparin as prophylaxis against venous thromboembolism after major trauma. *N Engl J Med* 1996; 335: 701–707.

77. Spinal Cord Injury Thromboprophylaxis Investigators. Prevention of venous thromboembolism in the rehabilitation phase after spinal cord injury: prophylaxis with low dose heparin or enoxaparin. *J Trauma* 2003; 54:1111–1115.

20 Infection and Spinal Cord Injury

Rabih O. Darouiche

More than a quarter of a million Americans suffer from the consequences of spinal cord injury (SCI), and with an annual incidence of 40 cases per million population, over 11,000 new cases of SCI occur in the United States each year (1). As the life expectancy of patients with SCI increases, the number of patients who experience the consequences of this ailment escalates. This distinct population of patients is prone to unique and quite complex medical problems, including infection, that require multidisciplinary input from a large sector of healthcare providers, including physiatrists, internists, infectious disease physicians, urologists, neurologists, plastic surgeons, and orthopedic surgeons.

Although most infections that occur in spinal cord-injured persons also affect able-bodied patients, the frequency and clinical characteristics of infections vary between these populations. The objectives of this chapter are to (1) assess the relationship between infection and SCI, (2) address the most common infections and their unique aspects, and (3) discuss the impact of multiresistant organisms in this healthcare setting.

RELATIONSHIP BETWEEN INFECTION AND SCI

The most common infectious cause of SCI is spinal epidural abscess, which most commonly is due to *Staphylococcus aureus* (2). The rising incidence of spinal epidural abscess contributes to the expanding population of patients with SCI (3). Not only can infection cause SCI, but it frequently occurs subsequent to the injury and results in major morbidity and mortality. Excluding pain, urinary tract infection (UTI) is the most common complication after both traumatic (4) and nontraumatic (2) SCI, and its frequency even exceeds that of spasticity. Although infections can occur both in the acute and chronic settings after SCI, the vast majority of infections occur long after the injury, taking into consideration that spinal cord-injured patients can live almost as long as able-bodied counterparts.

There exists no strong scientific evidence that injury to the spinal cord in and by itself depresses host immunity. For instance, the function of T and B lymphocytes in infection-free patients with SCI is reportedly normal (5). Although patients with SCI usually have higher levels of inflammatory markers (including complement, C-reactive protein, and cytokines like interleukin-6 and tumor necrosis factor-alpha) than able-bodied cohorts, this difference can be attributed to unrecognized inflammation or occult infection (6, 7). However, patients with SCI may receive medications (such as high-dose glucocorticosteroids in the acute setting of injury) or suffer from complicating conditions (including malnutrition and renal failure long after the injury) that can impair immune response to infection. Additionally, there exist bodily system-specific factors that predispose spinal cord-injured patients to infection of the corresponding systems. For instance, both urinary stasis and bladder catheterization of the neurogenic bladder predispose to frequent episodes of UTI. Not only does urinary stasis greatly impair the washout effect of voiding that would naturally protect against infection of the urinary tract, but it also interferes with the phagocytic ability of bladder epithelial cells. Even though some techniques of bladder catheterization could be less infection-prone than others (for instance, intermittent bladder catheterization vs. indwelling bladder catheters), none can be carried out without any risk of introducing organisms into the urinary tract. In the context of respiratory infections, both paralytic ileus and abnormal state of consciousness due to associated head injury and/or illicit drug use predispose to aspiration pneumonia in the acute stage of SCI. Additionally, in persons with cervical or high thoracic cord lesions, weakness of the intercostal and diaphragmatic muscles impairs the capacity to clear respiratory secretions, thereby enhancing bacterial presence. Likewise, the combination of tissue breakdown in anesthetic and paralyzed areas, urinary leakage, and fecal contamination promote infection of pressure sores.

Patients with SCI generally have a higher rate of hospital-acquired infections than other groups of hospitalized patients (8). About one-third of patients with SCI develop infection during hospitalization, with an overall incidence of 35 episodes of hospital-acquired infection per 1,000 hospital-days (8). Frequent insertion in spinal cord-injured patients of urologic, vascular, respiratory, gastrointestinal, orthopedic, and neurosurgical devices predispose to a variety of device-related infections. This helps explain why hospital-acquired infections most commonly affect the urinary tract, bloodstream, and bone and joint (8). In addition to causing serious medical complications, hospital-acquired infections increase the length of stay and incur major additional costs.

URINARY TRACT INFECTIONS

This is the most common infection in patients with SCI, as it occurs at a rate of 2.5 episodes per patient per year (9). Very importantly, UTI can manifest differently in these subjects than in the general population. Unlike able-bodied subjects with UTI who usually complain of dysuria, frequency, urgency, suprapubic discomfort, and flank pain or tenderness, these signs and symptoms are often absent in infected patients with SCI. Instead, UTI in patients with SCI frequently manifests with urinary leakage, change in voiding habits, worsening muscle spasm, increasing autonomic dysreflexia, and fever. These rather unusual manifestations are not specific to UTI as they may be caused by a number of other conditions, including urologic (such as obstruction of bladder catheter and urinary stones) and nonurologic (such as heterotopic bone ossification, osteomyelitis, pressure sores, and ingrown toenails) conditions.

The lack of specific urinary symptoms in insensate patients is the single most important impediment to the diagnosis of UTI in this population. Another potential obstacle to diagnosing UTI is the ubiquitous presence in this population of bacteriuria, which constitutes the cornerstone for diagnosing this infection. Almost all patients with chronic indwelling bladder catheters and about two-thirds of subjects who undergo intermittent bladder catheterization are bacteriuric. Most cases of bacteriuria in patients with SCI represent asymptomatic bladder colonization, which, in turn, may or may not progress to symptomatic infection (10). Pyuria, which can reflect inflammation of the uromucosal lining and signal the progression from bladder colonization to symptomatic UTI, is also not specific for UTI, thereby further impeding the ability to diagnose infection. In fact, UTI in catheter-dependent patients is not the most common cause of pyuria, which can also be caused by a variety of noninfectious conditions, including catheter manipulation, renal stones, urologic intervention, and interstitial nephritis. Other abnormal laboratory findings that are commonly reported in urinalysis, including nitrite and leukocyte esterase, are also not specific for UTI (11). Another diagnostic limitation is that about two-fifths of patients with SCI incorrectly attribute their bouts of illness to UTI (12).

Not unexpectedly, the nonspecific nature of clinical manifestations and laboratory findings of UTI in patients with SCI often results in overdiagnosis of this infection. In clinical studies of this population of patients, the most commonly used definition of UTI comprises significant bacteriuria ($>10^5$ CFU/ml), pyuria ($>10^4$ WBC/ml of uncentrifuged urine or >10 WBC/hpf for spun urine), clinical manifestations of fever ($>100°F$), suprapubic or flank discomfort, bladder spasm, change in voiding habits, increased spasticity, and/or worsening dysreflexia, provided that no other potential etiologies for these clinical manifestations could be identified (13–15).

Because asymptomatic bacteriuria can potentially progress to symptomatic infection, it is theoretically possible that prevention of asymptomatic bacteriuria could decrease the rate of symptomatic UTI. However, studies have reported conflicting efficacy

(16–18). Although preventative use of an antibiotic could decrease the rate of UTI due to organisms susceptible to that particular antibiotic, the overall incidence of UTI caused by all organisms (including organisms susceptible or resistant to that particular antibiotic) is not significantly altered (16, 17). Because of the lack of overall efficacy, possibility of drug-adverse events, and potential emergence of antibiotic resistance, preventative use of systemic antimicrobials is usually not justified (19). Possible exceptions include the presence of struvite urinary stones in association with urea-splitting organisms, such as *Proteus mirabilis* (20) and *Providentia stewartii*, and clinical scenarios where asymptomatic bacteriuria might be associated with complications, as is the case in pregnant patients and those embarking on urologic procedures (21). Although there exist some clinical data regarding the ability of some antimicrobial-modified, short-term, indwelling bladder catheters to reduce the rate of bacteriuria in non-SCI patients, there is no evidence so far that such catheters can prevent UTI in SCI patients with long-term indwelling bladder catheters. By limiting the movement of the indwelling bladder catheter and resulting injury to the uroepithelium, the use of a catheter-securement device was found in a prospective, randomized, multicenter clinical trial in patients with SCI to protect against catheter-related UTI as compared with traditional catheter care (22).

Notwithstanding the limitations of using antibiotic-based measures for prevention of UTI, there exists an emerging interest in examining the role of novel preventative approaches. The most innovative approach has been bacterial interference, which is based on the principal that nonpathogenic organisms can adversely impact the presence of urinary pathogens (23). Pilot data from both nonrandomized open-label (13, 14) and randomized double-blinded (15) clinical trials indicated that intentional colonization of the neurogenic bladder with a nonpathogenic strain of *E. coli* 83972 significantly reduces the rate of symptomatic infection in spinal cord-injured patients with history of frequent episodes of UTI. Another potentially protective approach that has recently attracted much attention is the use of cranberry supplement in an attempt to inhibit bacterial adherence to the uroepithelium and reduce the biofilm formarion by urinary pathogens without altering the urine PH (24). However, the clinical efficacy of this approach in patients with SCI remains rather controversial, as some studies demonstrated benefit (24) whereas others did not (25).

The vast majority of episodes of UTI in patients with SCI are caused by commensal bowel flora, primarily Gram-negative bacilli and enterococci, that may also exist in the perineum (26). The microbiology of organisms residing in the bladder can be affected by many factors, including patient's gender and level of SCI. For instance, *Klebsiella pneumoniae* is a very common cause of urinary tract infection in hospitalized patients (10, 27), but *Escherichia coli* and *Enterococcus* species cause more than two-thirds of bouts of UTI in female patients undergoing intermittent bladder catheterization (28). Although growth of more than one organism in urine cultures obtained from the general population is usually regarded as clinically irrelevant and prompts a repeat urine culture, this finding cannot be routinely ignored in patients with SCI in whom about half of all positive urine cultures yield polymicrobial flora (29). Even in patients who have pyelonephritis in association with polymicrobial bacteriuria, growth of only one organism from blood cultures may not negate the contribution by other organisms grown in urine cultures to UTI. Because it is difficult to accurately differentiate between isolated organisms that are pathogenic and those that do not contribute to clinical infection, it may be reasonable to treat all potentially pathogenic organisms grown from urine cultures.

Asymptomatic bacteriuria in catheter-dependent patients should not be treated with systemic antibiotics (30) or bladder irrigation (31). The duration of therapy for symptomatic UTI is usually based on the site of infection. Laboratory techniques that theoretically could help distinguish between upper and lower UTI, including evaluation of urine samples obtained via ureteral catheterization, sequential analysis of urine specimens after irrigation of the bladder (bladder washout), and examination for antibody coating of urinary bacteria are cumbersome and are almost never utilized in the clinical setting. That is why most healthcare providers localize the site of UTI on the basis of clinical findings. For example, the presence of high fever, chills, systemic toxicity, and/or leukocyte casts in urinary sediment generally points to infection of the upper urinary tract. Pyelonephritis is particularly likely to occur in patients with vesicoureteral reflux and is usually treated with a 2-week course of antibiotics. A longer duration of antibiotic therapy (4 to 6 weeks) is advocated in patients with persistent infection, documented relapse of infection, or prostatitis. Although studies in otherwise healthy individuals indicate that a single dose or a 3-day course of oral antibiotics may eradicate uncomplicated lower UTI in women (32), these short courses of treatment may not be applicable in the catheter-dependent SCI population, at least in part because of the concern about the ability of systemic antibiotics to eradicate bacteria embedded within the biofilm around infected catheters (33). A prospective, randomized, double-blind, placebo-controlled trial showed a significantly better response to a 14-day vs. 3-day course of ciprofloxacin for treatment of lower UTI in spinal cord-injured patients, but that study excluded subjects with long-term indwelling bladder catheters (34). At the present time, most cases of UTI in catheter-dependent patients with SCI are being treated with a 10-day course of antibiotics.

Because the urinary tract frequently becomes colonized with other organisms during or after treatment for a specific urinary pathogen, follow-up urine cultures should not be routinely obtained in the presence of adequate clinical response to antibiotic therapy. Likewise, there is no need to monitor the regression of pyuria in patients who clinically respond to treatment (35). In these neurologically impaired patients with persistent or recurrent UTI, the urinary tract should be assessed for anatomic (abscess, stone, excessive sediment, obstruction, and stricture) and functional (vesicoureteral reflux, and high residual volume of urine in bladder) abnormalities (36).

RESPIRATORY TRACT INFECTIONS

Pneumonia is the leading cause of death by infection in patients with acute or chronic SCI and is the most common pulmonary complication in the immediate post-injury period (37). In addition to escalating mortality and resulting in serious morbidity, pneumonia drastically prolongs the length of hospital stays and augments healthcare costs (38). Pneumonia is particularly likely to evolve among older persons and during the first few months after cervical or high thoracic injuries that cause weakness of the diaphragmatic and intercostal muscles, thereby impairing the capacity to clear respiratory secretions. Aspiration pneumonia often follows injury in persons who have an abnormal state of consciousness that is caused by an associated head injury and/or illicit drug ingestion that can further worsen paralytic ileus. Community-acquired aspiration pneumonia is largely caused by anaerobes, whereas gram-negative and anaerobic bacteria are the usual culprit among hospitalized persons. The presence of an endotracheal or tracheostomy tube predisposes both to pneumonia and tracheitis that are commonly caused by methicillin-resistant *Staphylococcus aureus* (MRSA) and *Pseudomonas aeruginosa*. Like in able-bodied persons and absent aspiration and respiratory devices, community-acquired respiratory tract infections in spinal cord-injured patients are commonly caused by *Streptococcus pneumoniae*, *Haemophilus influenzae*, and *Branhamella catarrhalis* (39).

Patients with cervical or thoracic SCI may have no or altered sensations of dyspnea and chest pain, but they also may not be able to adequately cough because of weakness in their diaphragmatic and intercostal muscles. In the absence of voiced respiratory complaints, one may rely on certain physical findings (distressed appearance, fever, tachypnea, tachycardia, etc.) and abnormal test results (leukocytosis, hypoxemia, and infiltrates on chest radiographs) to diagnose pneumonia. In that regard, pneumonia can be clinically confused with a number of noninfectious pulmonary complications, including atelectasis, pulmonary embolism, fat embolism, and chemical pneumonitis. For instance, atelectasis, like pneumonia, can cause fever and commonly occurs in patients with cervical or high thoracic SCI who retain pulmonary secretions. Unfortunately, the location of pulmonary involvement may not help distinguish atelectasis from pneumonia because both conditions predominantly affect the left lung. Because of ineffective cough, quadriplegic patients may not be able to provide adequate sputum samples. If tracheal secretions are not available for microbiologic examination, bronchoscopy may be required for both diagnostic and therapeutic purposes. Another potentially confounding diagnosis is pulmonary embolism. This is particularly troublesome because the majority of patients with SCI disclose no thrombotic source for pulmonary embolism, and some may have baseline roentgenographic lung abnormalities that make it difficult to discern the cause of acute pulmonary disease. Although a definitive diagnosis of pulmonary embolism may require a pulmonary angiogram, this condition can be reasonably ruled out if the blood d-dimer test is negative. Fat embolism to the lungs may also mimic pneumonia. It can occur acutely after SCI in association with fractures of the long bones and can be clinically differentiated from pneumonia in the presence of petechiae and cerebral dysfunction. Chemical pneumonitis due to aspiration can also be confused with bacterial pneumonia. Microbiologic examination of adequate samples of respiratory secretions can help distinguish between these two conditions by demonstrating in infected patients the presence of a plethora of organisms (along with inflammatory white blood cells).

The mainstay measure for prevention of respiratory infections is aggressive respiratory care, including adequate pulmonary toilet and frequent suctioning. The use of systemic antibiotics for the prevention of pneumonia in high-risk patients with SCI is not advocated. Because pneumonia can either occur more frequently or result in more serious complications in patients with SCI than in the general population, eligible patients should be immunized against potentially preventable causes of pneumonia. In that regard, about two-thirds of patients with SCI are eligible for vaccination against *S. pneumoniae* and influenza virus by virtue of old age, chronic respiratory disease, and/or residence in chronic-care facilities. The antibody responses to the pneumococcal (40) and influenza vaccination (41) in spinal cord-injured persons are reportedly adequate. Although there have been no prospective studies that examined the clinical benefit of these vaccinations in patients with SCI, it is generally recommended that patients at risk receive the pneumococcal vaccine every 5 years and the influenza vaccine annually.

In the absence of prospective, randomized clinical trials that assessed the optimal type and duration of antibiotic therapy for respiratory tract infections in patients with SCI, one may rely on management guidelines that have been established in the general population (42). In general, pneumonia and tracheitis in patients with SCI are usually treated with a 10- to 14-day course of antibiotic therapy that is initially chosen based on the knowledge of the likely infecting organisms and subsequently guided by the results of antimicrobial susceptibilities. For example, a quinolone or a combination of a macrolide and a cephalosporin are adequate for empiric treatment of community-acquired respiratory infections in the absence of aspiration or respiratory devices (43). However, coverage for anaerobes and gram-negative bacteria is required for therapy of hospital-acquired aspiration pneumonia, whereas agents effective against MRSA and multidrug resistant *P. aeruginosa* should be empirically considered in patients with respiratory devices. The reported observation that most prescriptions for antibiotics, including broad-spectrum agents, are given to patients with SCI for acute respiratory conditions that do not require antibiotic therapy underscores the essential role of education in preventing antibiotic abuse and potential antibiotic resistance (44).

INFECTIONS OF SOFT TISSUE AND BONE

Although UTI and pneumonia are the most common and life-threatening infections respectively, in patients with SCI, infections of pressure sores are the most problematic. Factors that contribute to skin and soft tissue infection in the vicinity of pressure sores include breaks in skin integrity and bacterial contamination due to soiling of the ulcer by feces or urine. The former factor predisposes to infection by skin organisms including staphylococci and streptococci, whereas the latter promotes infection by gram-negative bacilli and anaerobic bacteria. Patients with SCI are more likely than the general population to develop Fournier gangrene, the most fearsome form of necrotizing fasciitis that affects the perineal and genital regions and usually results from polymicrobial infection (45).

The majority of pressure sores in patients with SCI develop in areas adjacent to the ischium, sacrum, and greater trochanter. Because these patients usually have absent or altered sensations in the area of the pressure ulcer and cannot directly visualize the affected body area, the provided history is usually incomplete and infection is already advanced at the time of presentation. The diagnostic quandary caused by the patients' deficient history is further augmented by the expression of neurogenic or referred pain that may have no relation to the infection. Another limiting historical factor is that many pressure ulcers are chronic or recurrent and have previously been treated differently for undocumented infections by different healthcare providers. Physical findings, including fever and local inflammatory changes (purulent drainage, erythema, swelling, and warmth) are mostly relied upon to clinically diagnose infection of pressure sores.

Laboratory-based diagnosis of infection of pressure sores is quite problematic. Because of the universal bacterial colonization of pressure sores, swab cultures of open ulcers and sinus tracts should not be obtained unless infection is clinically evident. Needle aspiration is sometimes attempted, but cultures of obtained material tend to overestimate the number of bacterial isolates (46). Biopsy of deep soft tissue is the most reliable means for determining the microbiologic cause of infection. Another diagnostic problem centers around the ability to delineate the extent and depth of infection in association with pressure sores. Deep soft tissue abscesses may exist below apparently healed pressure sores in patients with unexplained fever or bacteremia. Although nuclear scans are highly sensitive for detecting soft tissue abscesses, these tests can yield false positive results in patients who have an infected pressure sore without an associated abscess. In general, soft tissue abscesses in association with an infected pressure sore are more accurately diagnosed by CT scan or MRI than by nuclear scans. Because pressure necrosis affects subcutaneous and muscular tissues more so than the skin, the visualized opening of a sinus tract onto the skin may seem deceptively small. Although generally helpful, probing of the sinus tract may still not reveal the full depth of the sinus tract. Sinography constitutes the gold-standard technique for delineating the full depth of the sinus tract and any potential communication with bone, joint, visceral organs, or deep-seated abscesses. In patients with nonhealing moist pressure sores, injection of dye into the bladder or bowel may detect viscerocutaneous fistulas.

Diagnosis of osteomyelitis beneath pressure ulcers, the most common form of osteomyelitis in patients with SCI, is even more tedious than diagnosis of soft tissue infection. Neither clinical evaluation (duration of ulcer, bone exposure, purulent drainage, fever, peripheral WBC count, and erythrocyte sedimentation rate) nor radiologic examination (plain roentgenogram and technetium bone scan) correlates well with the likelihood of finding histopathologic evidence for bone infection beneath deep nonhealing pressure sores (47). Both bone scan (an extremely misused imaging test that commonly yields confusing results) and indium scan are very sensitive but poorly specific (due to sequestration of technetium molecules in areas of bone with pressure-induced changes and in foci of heterotopic bone ossification) tools for diagnosing osteomyelitis beneath pressure sores (48). Therefore, these nuclear scans should be used primarily for their high negative predictive value (i.e. to rule out osteomyelitis and obviate the need for performing bone biopsy) rather than their low positive predictive value (i.e. to diagnose osteomyelitis).

Definitive diagnosis of osteomyelitis beneath pressure sores is made by histopathologic examination of bone tissue (47). Although failure of pressure sores to heal can be due to underlying osteomyelitis, it is more likely caused by noninfectious systemic (malnutrition) or local (pressure-related changes, heterotopic bone ossification, and spasticity) conditions. This helps explain why percutaneous needle bone biopsy yields histopathologic evidence for osteomyelitis beneath nonhealing pressure sores in only the minority of biopsied patients (47). Because percutaneous bone biopsy may fail to sample the truly infected focus, intraoperative bone biopsy can be more sensitive in diagnosing osteomyelitis beneath pressure sores.

Although patients with complete SCI are at risk for vertebral osteomyelitis (49), the vast majority of cases of osteomyelitis in this population occur beneath pressure sores. Not only is it difficult to determine if bone beneath a pressure sore is infected, but it may also be cumbersome to accurately discern which organisms are responsible for bone infection. Swab cultures of overlying ulcers usually do not predict the organisms causing osteomyelitis. Furthermore, because fibrotic tissue adherent to bone is usually colonized with bacteria, bone cultures are frequently positive in patients in whom histopathologic examination of bone tissue is incompatible with osteomyelitis. Therefore, in patients with histopathologic evidence of osteomyelitis, it may be reasonable to treat all organisms that grow from bone cultures, except those that are usually considered as colonizers, such as *S. epidermidis* and diphtheroids. Diagnostic limitations are particularly prominent in patients with multiple pressure sores because results from one bone site may not accurately predict if bone beneath the other pressure sores is infected and by which organism(s). Osteomyelitis beneath pressure sores can be either mono- or polymicrobial and can be caused by a variety of organisms, including gram-positive cocci (particularly *S. aureus* and *Streptococcus* species), gram-negative bacilli (particularly by organisms belonging to the *Enterobacteriaceae* group), and anaerobes bacteria (mainly *Bacteroides* species).

Optimal management of infected pressure sores usually requires a combination of antibiotic therapy and surgical intervention. A lack of response to seemingly adequate treatment may be due to inadequate antibiotic therapy, unrecognized soft tissue abscess, undiagnosed osteomyelitis, or fistulous communication with the urinary or gastrointestinal tract. A 10- to 14-day course of antibiotics is usually adequate for treatment of infected soft tissue in patients without underlying osteomyelitis. Although organisms that were not discovered in initial cultures subsequently appear in the pressure sore even after observing an adequate clinical response to antibiotic therapy, this phenomenon often reflects clinically irrelevant bacterial colonization of open wounds. Although the ideal duration and route of antibiotic therapy for osteomyelitis beneath pressure sores has not been demonstrated, most patients receive 4 to 6 weeks of intravenous antibiotics; in cases of chronic osteomyelitis, this is often followed by a few months of oral antibiotic therapy. If all infected bone is surgically removed, a shorter course of antibiotic therapy may be adequate.

Surgical debridement of necrotic tissue and drainage of purulent collections are essential for establishing cure of the infection. Musculocutaneous flap surgery is superior to debridement alone because the transposition of a well-vascularized muscle provides better vascular supply to facilitate healing, enhances host defense against infection, and allows for more extensive removal of devitalized tissue. When clinically indicated, a pre- or intraoperative bone biopsy should be done before embarking on plastic reconstructive surgery (50). Should postoperative myocutaneous flap wound infection evolve, it can impair the viability of the musculocutaneous flap, require further surgical intervention, and lead to amputation (51).

BLOODSTREAM INFECTIONS

The most common identifiable sources of bloodstream infection in this population are the urinary tract, vascular access, pressure sores, bone, deep-seated purulent collections, and vascular catheters (52). Although staphylococci are the usual cause of bacteremia arising from infection of short-term vascular catheters or pressure sores, gram-negative bacilli are more likely to seed the bloodstream from an infected urinary tract or a long-term hemodialysis catheter (53, 54). Because vascular catheter-related bacteremia is several-fold more likely to be caused by gram-negative bacteria in patients with SCI than in the general population (55), consideration should be given to inclusion of gram-negative coverage when giving empiric antibiotic therapy for this potentially life-threatening infectious condition in spinal cord-injured patients.

MULTIRESISTANT BACTERIA IN THE SCI SETTING

Although multiresistant organisms can exist in all areas of the hospital, they are particularly prominent in particular units that house critically ill persons or specific groups of patients, including those with SCI. The four major groups of multiresistant bacteria that have a predilection to affect SCI units more so than general nursing wards include MRSA, vancomycin-resistant *Enterococcus* (VRE), gram-negative bacilli that produce extended-spectrum beta lactamase (ESBL), and *Clostridium difficile*. Unfortunately, roommate contacts of patients colonized or infected by any of these multiresistant bacteria are at increased risk for acquiring those organisms (56).

Of the above-listed multiresistant organisms, MRSA is the most common culprit, as it has become a major cause of not just nosocomial but also community acquired infections (57, 58). Although routine decolonization is not necessary, hospital surveillance and strict adherence to basic infection control guidelines can blunt MRSA spread and potentially reduce the risk of developing infection by this organism (57, 59). Unlike MRSA, which could potentially exist in almost every bodily system, VRE is cultured mostly from the urine, particularly catheter-dependent patients. Although most episodes of growth of VRE from urine cultures represent asymptomatic bacteriuria and do not require antibiotic treatment, VRE colonization and residence in a long-term facility increase the risk for subsequent bacteremia (60). Catheter-dependent patients with SCI are predisposed to develop UTI due to ESBL-producing gram-negative bacilli, including *E. coli*, *Klebsiella pneumoniae*, and others that are resistant to at least beta-lactam antibiotics and often are susceptible to only aminoglycosides and/or carbapenems (61, 62). In addition to causing UTI, these pathogens that colonize the "reservoir" of stools also infect adjacent bodily sites such as pressure sores. Because of the relatively high incidence of infection in spinal cord-injured patients and frequent administration of antibiotics, these patients, who often have asymptomatic presence of *C. difficile* in stools, have an alarming likelihood of developing clinical infection by this opportunistic organism (63, 64). In patients with neurogenic bowel and defective sensations, *C. difficile*-associated gastrointestinal disease can remain clinically undetected until a catastrophe such as toxic megacolon or bowel perforation evolves.

References

1. Spinal cord facts and figures, June 2006 update. National Spinal Cord Injury Statistical Center. *J Spinal Cord Med* 2007; 30:539–540.
2. McKinley W, Merrell C, Meade M, Brooke K, DiNicola A. Rehabilitation outcomes after infection-related spinal cord disease: a retrospective analysis. *Am J Phys Med Rehabil* 2008; 87:275–280.
3. Darouiche RO. Spinal epidural abscess. *N Engl J Med* 2006; 355: 2012–2020.

4. Tauqir SF, Mirza S, Gul S, Ghaffar H, Zafar A. Complications in patients with spinal cord injuries sustained in an earthquake in Northern Pakistan. *J Spinal Cord Med* 2007; 30:373–377.

5. Lyons M. Immune function in spinal cord injured males. *J Neurosci Nurs* 1987; 19:18–23.

6. Wang TD, Wang YH, Huang TS, Su TC, Pan SL, Chen SY. Circulating levels of markers of inflammation and endothelial activation are increased in men with chronic spinal cord injury. *J Formos Med Assoc* 2007; 106:919–928.

7. Davies AI, Hayes KC, Dekaban GA. Clinical correlates of elevated serum concentrations of cytokines and autoantibodies in patients with spinal cord injury. *Arch Phys Med Rehabil* 2007; 88:1384–1393.

8. Evans CT, LaVela SL, Weaver FM, et al. Epidemiology of hospital-acquired infections in veterans with spinal cord injury and disorder. *Infect Control Hosp Epidemiol* 2008; 29:234–242.

9. Siroky MB. Pathogenesis of bacteriuria and infection in the spinal cord injured patient. *Am J Med* 2002; 113 (Suppl. 1A):67S–79S.

10. Darouiche R, Cadle R, Zenon G, Markowski J, et al. Progression from asymptomatic to symptomatic urinary tract infection in patients with SCI: a preliminary study. *J Am Paraplegia Soc* 1993; 16:221–226.

11. Hoffman JM, Wadhwani R, Kelly E, Dixit B, et al. Nitrite and leukocyte dipstick testing for urinary tract infection in individuals with spinal cord injury. *J Spinal Cord Med* 2004; 27:128–132.

12. Linsenmeyer TA, Oakley A. Accuracy of individuals with spinal cord injury at predicting urinary tract infections based on their symptoms. *J Spinal Cord Med* 2003; 26:352–357.

13. Hull RA, Rudy DC, Donovan WH, Wieser IE, et al. Virulence properties of *Escherichia coli* 83972, a prototype strain associated with asymptomatic bacteriuria. *Infect Immun* 1999; 67:429–432.

14. Hull RA, Rudy DC, Donovan WH, et al. Clinical outcome of intentional bladder colonization with *E. coli* 83972. *J Urol* 2000; 163:872–877.

15. Darouiche RO, Thornby JI, Cerra-Stewart C, Donovan WH, Hull RA. Bacterial interference for prevention of urinary tract infection: a prospective, randomized, placebo-controlled, double-blind pilot trial. *Clin Infect Dis* 2005; 41:1531–1534.

16. Sandock DS, Gothe BG, Bodner DR. Trimethoprim-sulfamethoxazole prophylaxis against urinary tract infection in the chronic spinal cord injury patient. *Paraplegia* 1995; 33:156–160.

17. Morton SC, Shekelle PG, Adams JL, et al. Antimicrobial prophylaxis for urinary tract infection in persons with spinal cord dysfunction. *Arch Phys Med Rehabil* 2002; 83:129–138.

18. Salomon J, Denys P, Merle C, et al. Prevention of urinary tract infection in spinal cord-injured patients: safety and efficacy of a weekly oral cyclic antibiotic (WOCA) programme with a 2 year follow-up—an observational prospective study. *J Antimicrob Chemother* 2006; 57:784–788.

19. Jayawardena V, Midha M. Significance of bacteriuria in neurogenic bladder. *J spinal Cord Med* 2004; 27:102–105.

20. Hung EW, Darouiche RO, Trautner BW. *Proteus* bacteriuria is associated with significant morbidity in spinal cord injury. *Spinal Cord* 2007; 45:616–20.

21. Pannek J, Nehiba M. Morbidity of urodynamic testing in patients with spinal cord injury: is antibiotic prophylaxis necessary? *Spinal Cord* 2007; 45:771–774.

22. Darouiche RO, Goetz L, Kaldis T, Cerra-Stewart C, et al. Impact of StatLock securing device on symptomatic catheter-related urinary tract infection: a prospective, randomized, multicenter clinical trial. *Am J Infect Control* 2006; 34:555–560.

23. Darouiche RO, Hull RA. Bacterial interference for prevention of urinary tract infection: an overview. *J Spinal Cord Med* 2000; 23:136–141.

24. Hess MJ, Hess PE, Sullivan MR, Nee M, Yalla SV. Evaluation of cranberry tablets for the prevention of urinary tract infections in spinal cord injured patients with neurogenic bladder. *Spinal Cord* 2008, April 8 [Epub ahead of print].

25. Lee B, Haran MJ, Hunt LM, et al. Spinal-injured neuropathic bladder antisepsis (SINBA) trial. *Spinal Cord* 2007; 45:542–550.

26. Waites KB, Canupp KC, DeVivo MJ. Microbiology of the urethra and perineum and its relationship to bacteriuria in community-residing men with spinal cord injury. *J Spinal Cord Med* 2004; 27:448–452.

27. Kil KS, Darouiche RO, Hull RA, Mansouri MD, Musher DM. Identification of a *Klebsiella pneumoniae* strain associated with nosocomial urinary tract infection. *J Clin Microbiol* 1997; 35:2370–2374.

28. Bennett CJ, Young MN, Darrington H. Differences in urinary tract infection in male and female spinal cord injury patients on intermittent catheterization. *Paraplegia* 1995; 33:69–72.

29. Darouiche RO, Priebe M, Clarridge JE. Limited vs. full microbiological investigation for the management of symptomatic polymicrobial urinary tract infection in adult spinal cord-injured patients. *Spinal Cord* 1997; 35:534–539.

30. Nicolle LE, Bradley S, Colgan R, et al. Infectious Diseases Society of America guidelines for the diagnosis and treatment of asymptomatic treatment in adults. *Clin Infect Dis* 2005; 40:643–654.

31. Waites KB, Canupp KC, Roper JF, Camp SM, Chen Y. Evaluation of 3 methods of bladder irrigation to treat bacteriuria in persons with neurogenic bladder. *J Spinal Cord Med* 2006; 29:217–226.

32. McCarty JM, Richard G, Huck W, et al. A randomized trial of short-course ciprofloxacin, ofloxacin, or trimethoprim/sulfamethoxazole for the treatment of acute urinary tract infection in women. Ciprofloxacin Urinary Tract Infection Group. *Am J Med* 1999; 106:292–299.

33. Reid G, Potter P, Delaney G, Hsieh J, et al. Ofloxacin for the treatment of urinary tract infections and biofilms in spinal cord injury. *Int J Antimicrob Agents* 2000; 13:305–307.

34. Dow G, Rao P, Harding G, et al. A prospective, randomized trial of 3 or 14 days of ciprofloxacin treatment for acute urinary tract infection in patients with spinal cord injury. *Clin Infect Dis* 2004; 39:658–664.

35. Joshi A, Darouiche RO. Regression of pyuria during the treatment of symptomatic urinary tract infection in patients with spinal cord injury. *Paraplegia* 1996; 34:742–744.

36. Deck AJ, Yang CC. Perinephric abscesses in the neurologically impaired. *Spinal Cord* 2001; 39:477–481.

37. Burns SP. Acute Respiratory infections in persons with spinal cord injury. *Phys Med Rehabil Clin N Am* 2004; 42:450–458.

38. Winslow C, Bode RK, Felton D, Chen D, Meyer PR Jr. Impact of respiratory complications on length of stay and hospital costs in acute cervical spine injury. *Chest* 2002; 121:1548–1554.

39. Chang HT, Evans CT, Weaver FM, Burns SP, Parada JP. Etiology and outcomes of veterans with spinal cord injury and disorders hospitalized with community-acquired pneumonia. *Arch Phys Med Rehabil* 2005; 86:262–267.

40. Darouiche RO, Groover J, Rowland J, Musher D. Pneumococcal vaccination for patients with spinal cord injury. *Arch Phys Med Rehabil* 1993; 74:1354–1357.

41. Trautner BW, Atmar RL, Hulstrom A, Darouiche RO. Inactivated influenza vaccination for people with spinal cord injury. *Arch Phys Med Rehab* 2004; 85:1886–1889.

42. Burns SP, Weaver FM, Parada JP, et al. Management of community-acquired pneumonia in persons with spinal cord injury. *Spinal Cord* 2004; 42:450–458.

43. Lodise TP, Kwa A, Cosler L, Gupta R, Smith RP. Comparison of beta-lactam and macrolide combination therapy versus fluoroquinolone monotherapy in hospitalized Veterans Affairs patients with community-acquired pneumonia. *Antimicrob Agents Chemother* 2007; 51:3977–3982.

44. Evans CT, Smith B, Parada JP, Kurichi JE, Weaver FM. Trends in antibiotic prescribing for acute respiratory infection in veterans with spinal cord injury and disorder. *J Antimicrob Chemother* 2005; 55:1045–1049.

45. Nambiar PK, Lander S, Midha M, Ha C. Fournier gangrene in spinal cord injury: a case report. *J Spinal Cord Med* 2005; 28:121–124.

46. Rudensky B, Lipschits M, Isaacsohn M, et al. Infected pressure sores: Comparison of methods for bacterial identification. *South Med J* 1992; 85:901–903.

47. Darouiche RO, Landon GC, Klima M, Musher DM, Markowski J. Osteomyelitis associated with pressure sores. *Arch Intern Med* 1994; 154:753–758.

48. Melkun ET, Lewis VL Jr. Evaluation of (111) indium-labeled autologous leukocyte scintigraphy for the diagnosis of chronic osteomyelitis in patients with grade IV pressure ulcers, as compared with a standard diagnostic protocol. *Ann Plast Surg* 2005; 54:633–636.

49. Frisbie JH, Gore RL, Strymish JM, Garshick E. Vertebral osteomyelitis in paraplegia: incidence, risk factors, clinical picture. *J Spinal Cord Med* 2000; 23:15–22.

50. Han H, Lewis VL Jr, Wiedrich TA, Patel PK. The value of Jamshidi core needle bone biopsy in predicting postoperative osteomyelitis in grade IV pressure ulcer patients. *Plast Reconstr Surg* 2002; 110:118–122.

51. Garg M, Rubayi S, Montgomerie JZ. Postoperative wound infections following mycocutaneous flap surgery in spinal injury patients. *Paraplegia* 1992; 30:734–739.

52. Mylotte JM, Graham R, Kahler, et al. Epidemiology of nosocomial infection and resistant organisms in patients admitted for the first time to an acute rehabilitation unit. *Clin Infect Dis* 2000; 30:425–432.

53. Montgomerie JZ, Chan E, Gilmore D, et al. Low mortality among patients with spinal cord injury and bacteremia. *Rev Infect Dis* 1991; 13:867–871.

54. Wall BM, Mangold T, Huch KM, Corbett C, Cooke CR. Bacteremia in the chronic spinal cord injury population: risk factors for mortality. *J Spinal Cord Med* 2003; 26:248–253.

55. Hussain R, Cevallos ME, Darouiche RO, Trautner BW. Gram-negative intravascular catheter-related bacteremia in patients with spinal cord injury. *Arch Phys Med Rehabil* 2008; 89:339–342.

56. Zhou Q, Moore C, Eden S, Tong A, McGeer A, Mount Sinai Hospital Infection Control Team. Factors associated with acquisition of vancomycin-resistant enterococci (VRE) in roommate contacts of patients colonized or infected with VRE in a tertiary care hospital. *Infect Control Hosp Epidemiol* 2008; 29:398–403.

57. Thom JD, Wolfe V, Perkash I, Lin VW. Methicillin-resistant *Staphylococcus aureus* in patients with spinal cord injury. *J Spinal Cord Med* 1999; 22:125–131.

58. Kappel C, Widmer A, Geng V, et al. Successful control of methicillin-resistant *Staphylococcus aureus* in a spinal cord injury center: a 10-year prospective study including molecular typing. *Spinal Cord* 2008; 46:438–444.

59. Mylotte JM, Kahler L, Graham R, Young L, Goodnough S. Prospective surveillance for antibiotic-resistant organisms in patients with spinal cord injury admitted to an acute rehabilitation unit. *Am J Infect Control* 2000; 28:291–297.

60. Olivier CN, Blake RK, Steed LL, Salgado CD. Risk of vancomycin-resistant Enterococcus (VRE) bloodstream infection among patients colonized with VRE. *Infect Control Hosp Epidemiol* 2008; 29:404–409.

61. Apisarnthanarak A, Bailey TC, Fraser VJ. Duration of stool colonization in patients infected with extended-spectrum beta-lactamase-producing *Escherichia coli* and *Klebsiella pneumonia*. *Clin Infect Dis* 2008; 46:1322–1323.

62. Waites KB, Chen Y, DeVivo MJ, Canupp KC, Moser SA. Antimicrobial resistance in gram-negative bacteria isolated from the urinary tract in community-residing persons with spinal cord injury. *Arch Phys Med Rehabil* 2000; 81:764–769.

63. Marciniak C, Chen D, Stein AC, Semik PE. Prevalence of *Clostridium difficile* colonization at admission to rehabilitation. *Arch Phys Med Rehabil* 2006; 87:1086–1090.

64. Mylotte JM, Graham R, Kahler L, Young BL, Goodnough S. Impact of nosocomial infection on length of stay and functional improvement among patients admitted to an acute rehabilitation unit. *Infect Control Hosp Epidemiol* 2001; 22:83–87.

21 The Immune System and Inflammatory Response in Persons with Spinal Cord Injury

Frederick S. Frost
Lily C. Pien

Through thousands of years of recorded human history, spinal cord injury (SCI) has been described as a fatal condition. Prior to the era of effective antibiotic medications, most patients who survived their initial injury died soon thereafter as a result of recurrent infectious illnesses and their sequelae—cachexia, dehydration, and renal failure, often from secondary amyloidosis. Despite the remarkable gains in survival and life expectancy in this population, which became possible with the advent of modern antibiotics, infectious illness remains a major cause of mortality and morbidity. To this day, the highest ratio of actual to expected deaths after spinal cord injury comes from sepsis (1).

In this chapter, a brief summary of the innate and acquired immune response in the normal host is presented, along with a description of the soluble mediators of inflammation and immunity. An overview of basic clinical and research laboratory testing is provided as background for discussion of the studies that deal with alterations in these responses, as documented after SCI. This information also serves as the basis for understanding a fertile area of current research on curative therapies. Researchers hope to reduce neurological damage by modifying the patient's immunological response to acute spinal cord injury.

INFLAMMATORY AND IMMUNOLOGIC RESPONSES IN THE NORMAL HOST

In normal individuals, the innate immune response is comprised of cellular and soluble components that lack memory: these components remain unchanged even with repeated exposures to foreign material or pathogens (2). This response is carried out through the interaction of cells (Table 21.1) and soluble inflammatory mediators. Macrophages recognize foreign molecules via their carbohydrate membrane receptors, as well as by surface receptors for the complement proteins and antibodies that bind to foreign microorganisms. Both macrophages and neutrophils engulf foreign material by phagocytosis and subject internalized microorganisms to a wide

range of toxic intracellular substances. Other cells, the interdigitating dendritic cells, recognize the complex molecular patterns present on the cell walls of yeasts, gram-positive, and gram-negative bacteria. These cells normally carry out endocytosis of circulating extracellular foreign material and are activated by endogenous danger signals. These signals might include the release of interferon from cells infected with a virus or an increase in circulating acute phase proteins (APPs) present in areas of necrotic cell death. Eosinophils offer an innate defense against parasites, mainly through the release of toxic proteins and oxygen metabolites into the extracellular fluid. Like eosinophils, basophils and mast cells secrete leukotrienes, prostaglandins, and cytokines, but differ from eosinophils in their high-affinity surface receptors for immunoglobulin (IgE), which triggers the release of histamine. Histamine, in turn, brings about localized contraction of smooth muscle and changes vascular permeability.

Natural killer (NK) cells, derived from the lymphocyte cell line, kill virally infected cells and cells whose surface markers have been transformed to signal distress. NK cells do not require previous exposure to the pathogen or foreign material. These cells form a powerful line of defense against infection, malignancy, and toxic debris, recognizing their targets by their disordered expression of several cell surface receptor subgroups. These cells are capable of differentiating between self and non-self material and receive inhibitory signals from host-specific major histocompatability complex (MHC) molecules on potential target cells. Infected, distressed, or malignant cells lose their MHC surface molecules, marking them for destruction by NK cells.

The production of a variety of soluble proteins that modulate immunologic activity is carried out, mainly in the liver, in response to circulating cell breakdown products, foreign carbohydrates and proteins, and antibodies in the bloodstream. These molecules, collectively termed acute phase proteins (APPs), modulate response to infection and inflammation. These proteins play a wide range of physiologic roles. The complement proteins, albumin, fibrinogen, haptoglobin, and other coagulation proteins

Table 21.1   Differentiation of Hematopoietic Stem Cells

Pleuripotent stem cells differentiate into lymphoid stem cells or myeloid stem cells. T lymphocytes, natural killer (NK) cells, and B lymphocytes are derived from lymphoid stem cells. Myeloid stem cells differentiate into lineage-specific precursors or colony forming units (CFUs). Examples of cell functions are given.

		GENERATION			
1	**2**	**3**	**4**	**5**	**FUNCTIONS**
	Lymphoid stem cell line	T lymphocyte (thymus)			Helper T cells Destroy virus-infected cells Activate phagocytes Control immune response
		NK lymphocyte			Kill non-sensitized target cells
		B lymphocyte (bone marrow)	Plasma cell		Produce antibodies
Pleuripotent stem cell	Myeloid stem cell line	CFU-GM	Neutrophil monocyte	Macrophage	Engulf and break down pathogens, antigens, and debris
		CFU-Eo	Eosinophil		Regulate inflammation, kill parasites
		CFU-E	Erythrocyte		Carry oxygen
		CFU-Meg	Megakaryocyte		Parent cell of platelets
		CFU-Baso	Basophil		Produce inflammatory mediators
		CFU-MC	Mast cell		Produce inflammatory mediators, prostaglandins, leukotrienes

fall into this group and have important clinical implications in the development and propagation of septic, thrombotic, and autoimmune responses. The activation of the circulating complement cascade in response to the presence of foreign molecules brings about a number of important responses to infection. The C3B complement molecule binds to the cell surface of invading microorganisms, thus enhancing phagocytosis. Other complement proteins have the ability to attract neutrophils. Through interaction and cross linkage, complement proteins can form a membrane attack complex, perforating the membrane of targeted cells. Other complement proteins trigger mast cells to release histamine.

Cytokines, a group of soluble molecules produced by macrophages, lymphocytes, NK cells, and cells infected by viruses, are immunologically active. They convey signals between cells of the immune system. This group (Table 21.2) includes the interferons, the interleukins, and tumor necrosis factors (TNFs). The interaction between cytokines, APPs, hormones, and neurotransmitters is complex and allows for an integrated network aimed at regulating the response to infection and injury. Better understanding of the manner by which these substances govern inflammation and the response to infection has allowed for improved methods of measuring clinical disease processes, and for the development of novel therapies for a variety of disease conditions, including atherosclerosis, rheumatoid arthritis, multiple sclerosis, and sepsis.

The Acquired Immune Response

The acquired immune response involves the proliferation of lymphocytes from primordial stem cells of the fetal liver and

Table 21.2   Major Classes of Cytokines

CLASS	FUNCTION	CYTOKINES
Immunoregulatory lymphocyte function	Activation, growth, differentiation of lymphocytes and monocytes	IL-2 IL-4 TGFβ
Proinflammatory	Response to infection	IL-1 TNFα IL-6 Chemokines
Immunoregulatory leukocyte function	Regulates immature leukocyte growth and differentiation	IL-3 IL-7 GM-CSF

in the bone marrow, which are programmed to recognize specific molecules, known as antigens (3). The development of these cells is governed by cytokines and by the influence of stromal cells, such as fibroblasts. Two types of lymphocytes, B-cells and T-cells, carry out a variety of discrete functions aimed at eliminating foreign antigens. Communication and interaction between these two cell types amplify and target a full immunologic response.

The Normal B-Cell Response

B-cells secrete immunoglobulins, the antigen-specific antibodies used in eliminating microorganisms. These antibodies possess a C-terminal (the constant region), which identifies the antibody as either IgG, IgA, IgM, IgD, or IgE. Each of these has different functions. These antibodies can be found in the circulation, or bound to B-cell membranes, where they serve to bind the B-cell to an antigen. Each antibody also contains an N-terminal, a variable region that is specially constructed to match the cell surface molecules of target cells and foreign material. Through the cutting, splicing, and modifying of less than 400 genes that code the variable N-terminal of the antibody, more than 10^{15} different antibody responses are possible. Each B-cell line expresses only one of a huge number of potential antibodies on its surface. Most pathogens, however, bear multiple different antigenic sites, called *epitopes*, on their cell surfaces. B-cells with surface antibody receptors that match these epitopes bind to the pathogen and are activated. This activation results in a proliferation of multiple clones of B-cells, which express and secrete antibodies specific to the bound pathogen.

Two types of B-cells offer different types of defense against foreign antigens. Primitive B_1 cells secrete short active IgM, which has low specificity and affinity toward antigens and binds to commonly encountered antigens. More difficult challenges to the immune system require B_2 cells. Initially expressing low-affinity IgM and IgD on their surfaces, these cells switch to the use of high-affinity IgG, IgA, and IgE receptors after exposure to an antigen. These long-lived lymphocytes are activated to clone themselves and produce an accelerated response, or memory, to a previously encountered antigen with the help of cytokines and complement. Finally, in the secondary lymphoid tissues (spleen, lymph nodes, and mucosa), some B_2 cells differentiate into plasma cells, which secrete soluble antibodies into the blood stream that bind to pathogens and facilitate removal by macrophages, neutrophils, monocytes, and T-cells.

The Normal T-Cell Response

T-cells, derived from stem cells originating in the bone marrow, develop in the thymus throughout life. Like B-cells, T-cells bear surface receptors with constant and variable components. Unlike B-cells, however, these receptors bind with short peptides on other cell surfaces, which are produced as a result of antigen processing inside the distressed cell. Intracellular processing combines an MHC molecule with a preprocessed antigen peptide. In the thymus, the exposure of populations of T-cells with a variety of surface receptors with different affinities to both self- and non-self-surface proteins allows preferential selection and export of populations of T-cells that have only weak affinity to self-MHC complexes. Outside the thymus, these cells are unlikely to generate autoimmune damage, but retain the ability to become activated if a complex of foreign surface peptide plus self-MHC molecules is encountered.

The activation of T-cells occurs when the affinity of its receptors for a given antigen or MHC combination exceeds a certain threshold. This activation results in a proliferation of T-cell clones, thus generating effector T-cells (cytotoxic and helper T-cells) and memory T-cells. Memory cells can be distinguished from naïve T-cells by the presence of the CD45RO molecule on the surface. These cells are primed, when faced with a later antigen challenge, to rapidly clone large numbers of antigen-specific lymphocytes.

The differentiation of T-cell surface protein expression in the thymus allows us to identify subsets of T-cells based on their expression of cluster of differentiation (CD) molecules on the cell surfaces. Two important classes of these, the CD4 and CD8 surface molecules, help distinguish T-cells with varying functions. CD4 T-cells usually are helper T-cells, which secrete the powerful pro-immunologic cytokines when exposed to MHC Class II molecules on B-cells and activated macrophages. CD8 cells recognize MHC Class I molecules, which are present on all nucleated cells. These T-cells are cytotoxic; thus, any virus-infected cell can be recognized and eliminated by inserting proteolytic enzymes into the cell. As opposed to NK cells, these highly evolved cytotoxic T-cells are antigen specific and allow rapid amplification of a targeted immune response. CD8 cells also secrete cytokines, including TNF and interferon, thus reinforcing antiviral defenses in adjacent cells that are not yet infected.

Clinical Assessment of the Immune Response and Inflammatory States

Soluble Markers of Inflammation

Within minutes of an injury or infectious insult, altered levels of soluble serum proteins and cytokines can be detected in the serum of humans (4). The erythrocyte sedimentation rate (ESR), a laboratory test used for over seven decades, measures the rate at which erythrocytes fall through serum, and is largely determined by the amount of soluble fibrinogen present in the sample. The use of the ESR represented a great scientific advance when introduced in the 1920s, but it is an indirect measurement of APPs and can be influenced by red-cell morphology, age, and the concentration of serum immunoglobulins. Newer tests allow the direct measurement of the acute phase response. Two APPs, C-reactive protein (CRP) and serum amyloid A, exhibit rapid changes in plasma concentration as the patient's condition worsens or improves, and have been shown to be sensitive markers for inflammatory disease. The physiologic actions of these proteins are protean, but involvement with the immune response to infection and injury is unquestioned. CRP binds phosphocholine on foreign cell walls, activates the complement system, and promotes attachment to phagocytic cells. Serum amyloid A influences cholesterol metabolism during stress and causes adhesion and chemotaxis of immune cells (5). Serum amyloid A is the precursor of amyloid A, the principal component of secondary amyloidosis deposits in the kidney and skin. The serum concentration of other APPs, including haptoglobin and fibrinogen, increases days later, whereas other serum protein concentrations, most notably those of serum albumin and transferrin, decrease during the days after exposure to infection (4, 6).

The measurement of cytokine levels provides an invaluable research tool in the study of disease pathogenesis and may someday allow clinicians the opportunity to gauge disease activity, predict outcomes, and monitor treatment efficacy. Their presence in the blood stream is strongly associated with tissue damage and inflammation, indicating activation of the immune system. The measurement of these regulatory molecules in the clinical setting is limited, however, by their rapid degradation in vivo, the presence of multiple cytokine forms (e.g. a, b) binding to serum proteins, and presence of soluble cytokine receptors (7). A wide array of new treatments that alter disease states through their impact on circulating cytokines have been made possible through increased understanding of the cytokine response to inflammation and infection.

Laboratory Testing of Cellular Immunity

Several useful laboratory tests are available to measure cellular immune function. A preliminary workup for immunodeficiency includes a complete blood cell count (CBC), differential count, and platelet count (8). Those with abnormal neutrophil, eosinophil, or lymphocyte numbers; abnormal granulocyte, erythrocyte, or platelet morphology; and Howell–Jolly bodies should be considered for further evaluation (9). In most cases, sophisticated testing should be carried out in a medical center specializing in the care of patients with rare immunologic disorders. Antibody deficiencies can be detected by quantitative immunoglobulin testing, as well as by assessment of antibody titers to previous immunizations (diphtheria, tetanus, H. flu). Primary T-cell deficiencies are suggested by lack of a thymic shadow on chest x-ray, skin test anergy to *Candida albicans*, or by the measurement of T-cell subset populations. An abnormal neutrophil count can suggest phagocyte deficiency, whereas complement assays can assess for abnormalities in the production of these soluble cofactors in the cellular response.

THE INFLAMMATORY AND IMMUNE RESPONSE AFTER SCI

Many patients with SCI are suspected to have deficits in immune function, primarily on the basis of multiple recurrent infections. The frequency of infections alone is a very poor indicator of impairment in immune function. In many cases, recurrent infections in this population are precipitated by impairment in integument and mucosal barrier defenses associated with neurologic injury.

Some special circumstances may exist that raise the clinical suspicion that impairment in immunity may exist and warrant further testing (4). Recurrent fungal infections, although usually related to quinolone antibiotic use, may also herald a granulocyte or T-cell defect. Persistent sinopulmonary infections are seen in those with impaired B-cell immunity. Although many patients with SCI exhibit chronic urinary colonization with pseudomonas and staphylococci bacteria, the presence of a granulocyte defect might be considered in patients with clinical

Table 21.3   Systemic Effects of Chronic Inflammation

Metabolic changes: Loss of muscle and negative nitrogen balance, decreased gluconeogenesis, osteoporosis, increased hepatic lipogenesis, increased lipolysis in adipose tissue, decreased lipoprotein lipase activity in muscle and adipose tissue, cachexia
Hematopoetic changes: Anemia of chronic disease, leukocytosis, thrombocytosis
Neuroendocrine changes: Fever; somnolence; anorexia; increased secretion of corticotropin-releasing hormone, corticotropin, and cortisol; increased secretion of arginine vasopressin; decreased production of insulin-like growth factor 1; increased adrenal secretion of cathecholamines; impaired growth; reduced testosterone

infections that are life threatening, infections that persist for long periods, or in those with multiple recurrences that don't respond to standard therapy.

Forty years ago, clinicians treating persons with SCI had an intimate awareness of the cumulative, long-term health effects of recurrent infections and inflammation. Secondary renal amyloidosis was a frequent cause of renal failure and death in this population. The danger associated with chronically high circulating levels of the APP serum amyloid A have been well described (10). Damage to the lungs and kidneys related to activation of circulating inflammatory cells is easily demonstrated in animal models (11, 12). Thankfully, amyloidosis and renal failure are now rarely seen. Over the last three decades, advances in the general medical care of persons with SCI, most notably in the field of antibacterial therapy and bladder care, have resulted in longer life expectancies. Despite this, virtually all of the systemic phenomena known to be associated with chronic inflammation are seen in persons with longstanding SCI (Table 21.3). Although infections are the most notable precipitants of an inflammatory response in these patients, other processes (subsequent trauma, burns, stress, strenuous exercise, bone fractures, childbirth, autoimmune disease) may also trigger an acute phase response that, in the presence of chronic disease, becomes persistent, self-perpetuating, and detrimental.

The impairments in barrier defense against infection precipitated by SCI are well recognized. Lung, bladder, and gastrointestinal mucosal barriers are rendered vulnerable by the withdrawal of normal neurologic innervation. In the lungs, mucous hypersecretion accompanies acute SCI, probably because of the effects of unopposed vagal innervation on the airway submucosal glands (13). Impaired bladder emptying and the need for artificial drainage methods result in chronic inflammation and erosive changes in the bladder mucosa, thus reducing the powerful antimicrobial effect of mucosal enzymes that usually prevent bacterial adherence to urinary tract structures. Hemorrhoids and rectal fissures are common after SCI and provide another route of invasion for colonic pathogens (14).

Multiple changes in skin morphology have been documented after SCI. Similarities in skin biopsies between SCI and scleroderma patients provide evidence that these changes may be autoimmune in nature (15). Primary neurologic factors are certainly important as well. Pressure ulcers afflict over

60 percent of SCI patients in the community setting (8), but are very rare in patients with amyotrophic lateral sclerosis (ALS), implicating the absence of normal autonomic and sensory nerve function to the skin in the SCI population (16). Although cellular and humoral immune responses to infection weaken somewhat with aging, accelerated aging effects on the skin and mucosal barriers account for substantial morbidity in older individuals with SCI.

The pathogens that have breached the ectodermal and endodermal obstacles made vulnerable by SCI are met with two additional levels of defense, the innate and acquired immune responses. With the advancement of laboratory techniques aimed at the study of the immune system and the inflammatory response, researchers have been able to delineate the mechanisms of these responses, and data are available to detail changes that occur after SCI (Table 21.4).

Deficits in global immune function and the presence of a chronic inflammatory state have been documented in the acute and chronic phases of spinal cord injury (17–26). Cruse (27, 28) noted an initial decline in NK and T-cell function shortly after injury. These abnormalities improved toward normal levels as the patients were studied at 6 months post-injury. Whether these changes came about as a result of rehabilitation exercise treatment as opposed to a time-dependent recovery after an initial trauma is difficult to ascertain.

The level of neurological injury likely impacts the degree to which the immune system is altered after spinal cord injury.

Table 21.4 Disordered Immune and Inflammatory Response after Spinal Cord Injury	
Frost FS (18)	Elevated CRP but not cytokines in chronic SCI—highest levels in those with indwelling urinary catheters
Huang TS (40)	Elevated serum leptin
Campagnolo (32)	DHEA and NKCC higher in tetraplegia, but not in paraplegia
Iverson PO (29)	Impaired proliferation of progenitor cells in complete SCI
Campagnolo (31, 35)	Reduced NK cell counts, impaired neutrophil phagocytosis
Cruse JM (21)	Reduced levels of cellular adhesion molecules on leukocytes of patients with pressure ulcers
Segal JL (17, 25)	IL-6, IL2r, and ICAM-1 elevated in all SCI patients, highest in those with pressure ulcers—IL2 receptors high in tetraplegia, not paraplegia
Kleisch (22)	Depressed T-cell function and activation
Nash (23)	Reduced helper-to-suppressor cell ratio after SCI
Cruse JM (24)	Depressed NK cytotoxicity and lymphocyte transformation
Cruse JM (24, 27, 28)	Reduced NK function after acute SCI improved with time and rehabilitation
Rebhun J (20)	Elevated complement and acute phase proteins in acute and chronic SCI

The presence of a more profound suppression of immune function in patients with tetraplegia and complete spinal cord transection, in contrast to that found in those with less severe SCI has been demonstrated (29–32). These findings support the theory that alterations in immune response after SCI can be attributed, at least in part, to impairment of the neurologic systems that influence the inflammatory and immune response. Nash, in his comprehensive review of this topic (19), detailed the evidence found in animal and human studies supporting this influence. Adrenergic receptors are found on immune cells in the animal model, and there is documentation of direct innervation of the primary and secondary lymphoid tissues by adrenergic efferents. Chemical sympathectomy, as well as manipulation of the autonomic nervous system, is known to alter lymphocyte-dependent immunity. The deleterious impact of stress, whether physical or emotional, on the immune system is well described. The stress induced by autonomic dysregulation after SCI, and especially by episodes of autonomic dysreflexia, may well be an important cause of immune suppression in this group. In his 1993 study, Nash noted a suppression of monocyte counts and an inhibition of the lymphocyte proliferative response associated with tetraplegic micturition (33).

Neurologic trauma is known to affect immunologic function indirectly, through the pituitary adrenal axis, and through endocrine and neuropeptide regulation (34). Stress induces the release of adrenocorticotrophic hormone from the pituitary gland. This induces the release of immunosuppressive glucocorticoids. In addition, the adrenal medulla releases catecholamines that alter leukocyte migration and lymphocyte responsiveness. Other hormones, including insulin, thyroxin, growth hormones, somatostatin, and the sex hormones, modulate T- and B-cell functions in complex ways. A number of abnormalities in endocrine function accompany SCI. Abnormal endocrine physiology involving sex hormones, aldosterone, catecholamines, and methylhydoxymandelic acid have been described (35). Levels of dehydroepiandrosterone and dehydroepiandrosterone sulfate (hormones that participate in interleukin-2 synthesis—a potent immunosuppressant) are higher in persons with tetraplegia than in control subjects (29). These findings offer a direction for future research into treatments for immune dysfunction (36). The administration of synthetic hormones has been considered as a promising treatment for diseases with autoimmune characteristics, such as the use of androgens for multiple sclerosis.

It is reasonable to implicate several comorbid conditions that depress immune function in able-bodied individuals as important factors in the development of immune abnormalities after SCI. Diabetes, glucose intolerance, insulin resistance, and abnormal serum leptin levels are associated with impaired cellular immunity and clinical infections (37, 38). All of these laboratory findings are present in disproportionate frequency after SCI (39, 40). Other clinical conditions frequently seen in those with SCI (chronic pain, muscle wasting, sedentary lifestyle, nutritional deficits, psychologic stress) are associated with in vitro and in vivo measures of depressed immune function (19, 41). Cause-and-effect relationships, however, are difficult to determine. In addition, many drugs commonly used by persons with SCI (opiates, diazepam, nonsteroidal anti-inflammatory drugs) are known to influence soluble and cellular-mediated immune responses (19). It is unclear whether the presence of pain, or the use of large doses of pain medication, has the greatest immunosuppressant effect. Clinicians, long aware of the strong immunosuppressive effects of methylprednisolone, nonetheless utilize this drug's strong anti-inflammatory properties, in hopes of reducing secondary neurologic damage after acute SCI. Whether the strong immunosuppressive qualities of this drug are of clinical importance in this setting is a topic of debate. The use of lazeroid preparations such as tirilizad, which has much less glucorticoid activity than methylprednisolone, may obviate these potential drawbacks of steroid use (42).

Although SCI patients show multiple abnormalities in the laboratory testing of the immune and inflammatory response, the clinical relevance of these abnormalities is unclear. These responses to injury, insult, and infection may vary widely with age, gender, and comorbid conditions. The measurement of acute phase proteins is a good predictor of the extent and severity of inflammation in some diseases (e.g., rheumatoid arthritis) but not in others (e.g., lupus) (4). Powerful new therapies have been developed that alter the serum levels of soluble mediators and affect changes in immunologic response. Two drugs, etanercept and infliximab, which lower the levels of the pro-inflammatory cytokine TNF, are now in common use for the treatment of rheumatoid arthritis. Another drug, recombinant activated protein C, has been shown to reduce proinflammatory cytokine levels and reduce mortality from sepsis in humans (43). The judicious clinical use of therapies that alter the cytokine and immune response demands that the acute phase response to a variety of disease states, in a variety of different hosts, be clearly defined.

It is convenient to assume that the laboratory abnormalities seen in SCI patients represent a loss of homeostasis that might benefit from therapies that alter the chronic inflammatory response. Elevated levels of CRP and evidence of endothelial activation are found in persons with spinal cord injury, and are consistent with the American Heart Association classification of high risk for cardiovascular disease in the able-bodied (44-46). This is certainly concordant with the increased risk of atherogenic disease found in patients with long-standing SCI. But assuming that persons with spinal cord injury have identical risk factors as able-bodied individuals is a precarious notion. Other persons with chronic diseases are known to have subclinical and clinical conditions that drastically change the associations between risk factors and outcomes seen in the general population. For example, dialysis patients who are obese and have "unfavorable" lipid profiles survive the longest (47). When examining the laboratory profiles and health risks after spinal cord injury, the difference between clinical disease association and causation is important to delineate.

Experience has shown that some of these laboratory abnormalities could represent a protective immune and inflammatory phenomena, or adaptive response to stress, injury, or chronic infection. Blocking this response may not necessarily be a good idea. For example, the use of anti-inflammatory medication appears to promote immune suppression and to prolong symptoms of the common cold (48). The complex immunological and metabolic responses to SCI are just being elucidated.

Like renal failure, AIDS, and rheumatoid arthritis, chronic human SCI presents another experimental model for the study of the mechanisms and effects of inflammation and recurrent infections in long-standing, chronic illness. Treatments now used to modify the inflammatory and immunologic effects (e.g., anemia, nutritional wasting, osteoporosis) of these diseases represent promising therapeutic opportunities for physicians treating patients with chronic SCI. Patients with SCI will benefit from research into the disease mechanisms and treatment of these other chronic illnesses.

THE IMMUNE SYSTEM AND SPINAL CORD CURE

The immunological privileges of the central nervous system provide protection against autoimmune injury to nerve cells. Although thousands of immune cells are viewed in every peripheral blood smear, the presence of a few leukocytes in a sample of cerebrospinal fluid is cause for grave concern. Injured peripheral nerves may recover over time, but recovery in the central nervous system injury is much more limited. The immune system plays a role in this difference. Macrophages carry out the removal of debris and promote recovery in peripheral nerve injuries. Mice that are bred to be deficient in macrophages lack the capacity to repair peripheral nervous system injuries (49). Although damage to the spinal cord by direct tissue destruction at the moment of injury may be substantial, the cytokine cascades and humoral immune responses that are demonstrated in the days and weeks after injury may underlie much of the secondary damage to the spinal cord that occurs after the initial trauma—damage that induces scarring, reduction of regeneration potential, and disability. These immune mechanisms provide a fertile field of research for those investigating strategies for spinal cord injury repair (26), as researchers attempt to modify the timing and select the participants in the immune response to injury (50).

Hours after SCI, invasion of the injury site by neutrophils has been demonstrated in humans, a phenomenon that has been associated with poor cell survival (51). The microglia that constitute the resident immune protection of the central nervous system are activated just days after injury, but these cells do not have the intrinsic ability to create a microenvironment sufficient for the survival of damaged nerves. Recruitment of adaptive immune cells to the area (e.g., T and B lymphocytes) is demonstrated as well. High levels of circulating autoantibodies to GM-1 (against myelin-associated glycoprotein) are found in humans after spinal cord injury (52).

These concepts led to the phase I and phase II human research trials carried out in Israel and the United States, arising out of the work of many researchers, notably Michal Schwartz (53). Patients with complete cervical cord injuries underwent injection of their damaged spinal cord with autologous macrophages, which had been harvested from their peripheral blood and activated against the patient's dermal cells. Less than a dozen subjects were enrolled, so conclusions about efficacy could not be drawn, but the treatments were generally well tolerated. These carefully controlled and monitored trials were carried out with great effort and at expense, owing to the substantial logistical and scientific hurdles that were encountered. Phase II spinal cord injury trials were subsequently halted, mainly due to financial reasons, although studies engaging these techniques for other neurological diseases continue. Results of these studies are likely to hold high relevance and interest for the field of spinal cord injury research (54). It has been suggested that future trials need not involve direct injection of activated immune cells into the spinal cord. There is evidence that activated cells are likely to pass through a damaged blood brain barrier at the site of neurological injury, and that local migration of these cells could be accomplished more simply, by re-infusing them into the bloodstream of injured patients.

Even more intriguing is the possibility of developing an immunization against secondary spinal cord damage. In the rabbit model, immunoglobulin responses can be generated through immunization against proteins that are known to block neurological recovery in the CNS. These immunoglobulins have been demonstrated to reduce secondary damage at the nerve injury site (55). If a more immediate response is needed, generating passive immunity by injection with immune globulin is a possibility, much as we treat human rabies exposure with equine immune globulin. As we gain a better understanding of what constitutes the best local milieu for nerve repair, we learn about the cytokines and proteins that are beneficial, and which cells can manufacture these substances. Getting the right cells to the area of the neurological damage, at the right time, and subsequently removing them at the right time, is an essential element of multi-modality cure research.

References

1. DeVivo MJ, Kartus PL, Stover SL, Rutt RD, Fine PR. Cause of death for patients with spinal cord Injuries. *Arch Intern Med* 1989; 149:1761–1766.
2. Delves PJ, Roitt IM. The immune system: First of two parts. *N Engl J Med* 2000; 343(1) 37–49.
3. Delves PJ, Roitt IM. The immune system: Second of two parts. *N Engl J Med* 2000; 343(2)108–117.
4. Gabay C, Kushner I. Mechanisms of disease: Acute phase proteins and other systemic responses to inflammation. *N Engl J Med* 1999; 340(6):448–454.
5. Malle E, DeBeer FC. Human serum amyloid A protein: A prominent acute phase reactant for clinical practice. *Eur J Clin Invest* 1996; 26:427–435.
6. Gitlin JD, Colten HR. Molecular biology of the acute phase plasma proteins. In: Pick E, Landy M, eds. *Lymphokines* Vol 14. San Diego, CA: Academic Press 1987; 123–153.
7. Rossio JL, Rager HC, Goundry CS, Crisp EA. Cytokine testing in clinical trial monitoring. In: Rose N, Friedman H, eds. *Manual of Clinical Immunology*, 4th ed. Washington D.C.: American Society for Microbiology 942–947.
8. Fleisher TA, Tomar RH. Introduction to diagnostic laboratory immunology. *JAMA* 1997; 278, 22:1823–1834.
9. Puck JM. Primary immunodeficiency diseases. *JAMA* 1997; 278: 1835–1841.
10. Urieli-Shoval S, Linke RP, Matznery. Expression and function of serum amyloid A, a major acute phase protein in normal and disease states. *Current Opinion in Hematology* 2000; 7(10):64–69.
11. Gris D, Hamilton EF, Weaver LC. The systemic inflammatory response after spinal cord injury damages lungs and kidneys. *Exp Neurol* 2008; 211(1): 259–70.
12. Riegger T, Conrad S, Liu K, et al. Spinal cord injury induced immune depression syndrome. *Eur J Neurosci* 2007; 25(6):1743–7.
13. Bhaskar KR, Brown R, O'Sullivan DD, et al. Bronchial mucus hypersecretion in acute quadriplegia. *Am Rev Respir Dis* 1991; 143:630–638.
14. Stone JM, Nino-Murcia M, Wolfe UA. Chronic gastrointestinal problems in spinal cord injury patients: A prospective analysis. *Am J Gastroenterol* 1990; 85: 1114–1119.
15. Stover SL, Gay RE, Koopman W, Sahgal V, Gale LL. Dermal fibrosis in spinal cord injury patients: A scleroderma variant? *Arthritis & Rheumatism* 1980; 23(11):1312–1317.
16. Watanabe S, Yamada K, Ono S, et al. Skin changes in patients with amyotrophic lateral sclerosis: Light and electron microscopic observations. *J Am Acad Dermatol* 1987; 17:1006–1012.
17. Segal JL, Brunnemann SR. Circulating levels of soluble interleukin 2 receptors are elevated in the sera of humans with spinal cord injury. *J Am Paraplegia Soc* 1993; 16:30–33.
18. Frost FS, Schreiber P, Kushner I. Assessment of chronic inflammation after spinal cord injury using measurements of C-reactive protein and cytokines. *Arch Phys Med Rehabil* 2003; In press.
19. Nash MS. Known and plausible modulators of depressed immune functions following spinal cord injuries. *J Spinal Cord Med* 2000; 23:2,111–120.
20. Rebhun J, Madorsky JGB, Glovsky M. Proteins of the complement system and acute phase reactants in sera of patients with spinal cord injury. *Ann Allergy* 1991; 66:335–338.
21. Cruse JM, Lewis RE, Bishop GR, Lampton JA, Mallory MD, Bryant ML, Keith JC. Adhesion molecules and wound healing in spinal cord injury. *Pathobiology* 1996; 64(4):193–197.
22. Kleisch WF, Cruse JM, Lewis RE, Bishop GR, et al. Restoration of depressed immune function in spinal cord injury patients receiving rehabilitation therapy. *Paraplegia* 1996; 34(2):82–90.
23. Nash MS. Immune responses to nervous system decentralization and exercise in quadriplegia. *Med Sci Sports Exerc* 1994; 26(2):164–171.
24. Cruse JM, Lewis RE, Bishop GR, et al. Decreased immune reactivity and neuroendocrine alterations related to chronic stress in spinal cord injury and stroke patients. *Pathobiology* 1993; 61(3–4):183–192.
25. Segal JL, Gonzales E, Yousefi S, et al. Circulating levels of IL-2R, ICAM-1, and IL6 in spinal cord injuries. *Arch Phys Med Rehabil* 1997; 78(1):44–47.
26. McTigue DM, Popovich PG, Jakeman LB, Stokes BT. Strategies for spinal cord injury repair. *Prog Brain Res* 2000; 128:3–8.
27. Cruse JM, Lewis RE, Bishop GR, et al. Neuroendocrine immune interactions associated with loss and restoration of immune system function in spinal cord injury and stroke patients. *Immunol Res* 1992; 11:104–116.
28. Cruse JM, Lewis RE, Dilioglou S. Review of immune function, healing of pressure ulcers, and nutritional status in patients with spinal cord injury. *J Spinal Cord Med* 2000; 23(2):129–135.
29. Iversen PO, Hjeltnes N, Holm B, et al. Depressed immunity and impaired proliferation of hematopoietic progenitor cells in patients with complete spinal cord injury. *Blood* 2000; 96(6):2081–2083.
30. Campagnolo DI, Dixon D, Schwartz J, et al. Altered innate immunity following spinal cord injury. *Spinal Cord* 2008; 46(7): 477–481.
31. Campagnolo DI, Bartlett JA, Keller SE, et al. Impaired phagocytosis of staphylococcus aureus in complete tetraplegics. *Am J Phys Med Rehabil* 1997; 76(4):276–280.
32. Campagnolo DI, Bartlett JA, Keller SE. Influence of neurological level on immune function following spinal cord injury: A review. *J Spinal Cord Med* 2000; 23:2,121–128.
33. Nash MS, Vandenakkar CB, Fletcher MA, et al. Catecholamine influences of micturition on phenotypic and functional indices of host defense in a quadriplegic. *J Am Soc Paraplegia* 1993; 16(2):135.
34. Male D. *Immunology.* 3rd ed. London: Mosby, 1999.
35. Campagnolo DI, Bartlett JA, Chatterton R, et al. Adrenal and pituitary hormone patterns after spinal cord injury. *Am J Phys Med Rehabil* 1999; 78(4):361–366.
36. Giltay EJ, Fonk JC, Blomberg BM, et al. In vivo effects of sex steroids on lymphocyte responsiveness and immunoglobulin levels in humans. *J Clin Endocrin Metabolism* 2000; 5(4):1648–1657.
37. Jones RI, Peterson CM. Hematologic alterations in diabetes mellitus. *Am J Med* 1981; 70(2):339–352.
38. Pomposelli JJ, Baxter JK, Babineau TJ, et al. Early postoperative glucose control predicts nosocomial infection rate in diabetic patients. *J Parenter Enteral Nutr* 1998; 22(2):77–81.
39. Bauman WA. Carbohydrate and lipid metabolism in individuals after spinal cord injury. *Top Spinal Cord Injury Rehabil* 1977; 2(4):1–22.
40. Huang TS, Wang YH, Chen SY. The relation of serum leptin to body mass index and to serum cortisol in men with spinal cord injury. *Arch Phys Med Rehabil* 2000; 81(12):1582–1586.
41. DeLeo JA, Yezierski RP. The role of neuroinflammation and neuroimmune activation in persistent pain. *Pain* 2001; 90:1–6.
42. Bracken MB, Shepard MJ, Holford TR, et al. Administration of methylprednisolone for 24 or 48 hours or tirilazad mesylate for 48 hours in the treatment of acute spinal cord injury. *JAMA* 1997; 277:1597–1604.
43. Bernard GR, Vincent JL, Laterre PF, et al. Efficacy and safety of recombinant human activated protein C for severe sepsis. *N Engl J Med* 2001; 344, 10:699–709.

44. Davies AL, Hayes KC, Dekaban GA. Clinical correlates of elevated serum concentrations of cytokines and autoantibodies in patients with spinal cord injury. *Arch Phys Med Rehabil* 2007; 88(11):1384–1393.

45. Gibson AE, Buchholz AC, Martin Ginnis KA. C-Reactive protein in adults with chronic spinal cord injury: increased chronic inflammation in tetraplegia vs paraplegia. *Spinal Cord* 2008; 46(9): 616–621.

46. Wang TD, Wang YH, Huang TS, et al. Circulating levels of markers of inflammation and endothelial activation are increased in men with chronic spinal cord injury. *J Formos Med Assoc* 2007; 106(11):919–928.

47. Tsirpanlis G, Boufidou F, Zoga M. Low cholesterol along with inflammation predicts morbidity and mortality in hemodialysis patients. *Hemodial Int* 2009; 13(2):197–204.

48. Graham NM, Burrell CJ, Dougles RM, Debelle P, Davies L. Adverse effects of aspirin acetaminophen, and ibuprofen on immune function, viral shedding and clinical status in rhinovirus-infected volunteers. *J Infectious Dis* 1990; 162(6):1277–1282.

49. Sanders VM, Jones KJ. Role of immunity in recovery from a peripheral nerve injury. *J Neuroimmune Pharmacol* 2006 March; 1(1):11–19.

50. Ziv Y, Avidan H, Pluchino S, et al. Synergy between immune cells and adult neural stem/progenitor cells promotes functional recovery from spinal cord injury. *Proc Natl Acad Sci USA* 2006 Aug 29; 103(35): 13174–13179.

51. Fleming JC, Norenberg MD, Ramsay DA, et al. The cellular inflammatory response in human spinal cords after injury. *Brain* 2006; 129 (Pt 12):3249–3269.

52. Davies AL, Hayes KC, Dekaban GA. Clinical correlates of elevated serum concentrations of cytokines and autoantibodies in patients with spinal cord injury. *Arch Phys Med Rehabil* 2007; 88(11):1384–1393.

53. Schwartz M, Yoles E. Immune-based therapy for spinal cord repair: autologous macrophages and beyond. *J Neurotrauma* 2006; 23(3–4):360–370.

54. Knoller N, Auerbach G, Fulga V, et al. Clinical experience using incubated autologous macrophages as a treatment for complete spinal cord injury: phase I study results. *J Neurosurg Spine* 2005; 3(3):171–172.

55. David S. Recruiting the immune response to promote long distance axon regeneration after spinal cord injury. *Prog Brain Res* 2002; 137:407–414.

22 Endocrine and Metabolic Consequences of Spinal Cord Injuries

James K. Schmitt
Diane L. Schroeder

Spinal cord injury (SCI) has an impact on the endocrine system in several ways. The diagnosis and treatment of common endocrine disorders present unique challenges in the spinal cord injured patient population. Neurologic injury can predispose patients to the development of endocrine disorders. This chapter serves as a guide to the diagnosis and treatment of common endocrine disorders and places a special focus on the features of endocrinopathy in SCI patients.

EFFECTS OF SYMPATHETIC DENERVATION

Sympathetic fibers coming from the T5–T12 region innervate the pancreas, adrenal medulla, and juxtaglomerular apparatus of the kidney (1). As a result, cord lesions above T12 can affect these organ systems. Sympathetic stimulation inhibits insulin secretion. Conversely, the parasympathetic nervous system stimulates insulin secretion. A lack of sympathetic activity, as might be present during the spinal shock phase of injury, results in unopposed parasympathetic activity from a fully functional vagus nerve outflow. Basal and stimulated insulin secretion, therefore, will tend to be higher in tetraplegic persons after acute injury. Compensatory mechanisms that suppress insulin secretion, such as hypoglycemia, depend on sympathetic tone and will be less effective in acute tetraplegic persons.

Sympathetic activity inhibits the juxtaglomerular apparatus. The reduced sympathetic tone found in acute SCI results in elevation of plasma renin, angiotensin II, and aldosterone. Angiotensin II is a potent vasoconstrictor, which acts to raise blood pressure and stimulates thirst. Aldosterone stimulates sodium retention and potassium wasting by the kidney. The effects of angiotensin II and aldosterone tend to reverse the hypotensive effects of diminished sympathetic output.

Sympathetic denervation is very rare and short lived after SCI. This is a problem mainly during the brief period of spinal shock after SCI. Within weeks, sympathetic activity recovers, although this activity is unpredictable and disorganized. Remember, the sympathetic chain is not injured, and the cord still functions below the level of injury, after spinal shock resolves.

Lack of sympathetic input to the adrenal medulla results in impaired release of catecholamines. The adrenal medulla, as the only source of epinephrine, is unable to mount an appropriate pressor response in the acute injury phase.

THE SPECTRUM OF ENDOCRINE ABNORMALITIES AFTER SCI

As a chronic disease process, longstanding SCI can produce a variety of nonspecific effects on endocrine function. Chronic pyelonephritis may cause renal failure, which results in phosphate retention, hypocalcemia, and secondary hyperparathyroidism. SCI patients are predisposed to pneumonia and other infections, which may result in increased antidiuretic hormone levels and hyponatremia. The physical inactivity associated with SCI has a profound effect on metabolic function. Decreased energy expenditure causes an increase in adiposity. Muscle atrophy occurs below the level of the cord lesion. Resistance to insulin occurs as a result of these effects. Insulin resistance can result in diabetes mellitus, hyperlipidemia, low HDL levels, and hypertension (2). Endocrinopathy, by producing bony overgrowth (acromegaly) or weakening (osteoporosis), may rarely be a cause of spinal cord compression (3).

PITUITARY DISORDERS

The secretion of pituitary hormones does not require an intact spinal cord (4). The most important pituitary hormone for survival is adrenocorticotrophic hormone (ACTH). With stress (e.g., acute SCI, infections, trauma) ACTH stimulates cortisol production by the adrenal cortex. Cortisol works in concert with catecholamines to maintain the blood pressure. This cortisol response constitutes the major adaptive response to the injury or illness. Subtle abnormalities in the hypothalamic-pituitary-adrenal axis have been noted in SCI patients (5–8). However, these studies suggest that the ACTH and cortisol responses to stressors, such as pyrogens, are normal.

Stress, such as that caused by injury or illness, results in impaired growth hormone (GH) secretion, thus reducing the intrinsic stimuli for the growth and maintenance of muscle mass. In addition, stress and chronic illness result in suppression of follicle stimulating hormone (FSH) and luteinizing hormone (LH). Suppressed gonadotropins result in low testosterone and estrogen levels, which can be detrimental.

Antidiuretic hormone is secreted in response to hypovolemia and increased serum osmolality. In normal subjects, antidiuretic hormone is secreted in a diurnal rhythm, with the highest levels occurring at night and therefore decreasing nocturnal urine production. However, in tetraplegic patients, the diurnal rhythm is absent (Figure 22.1). Some authorities have attributed the nocturnal increase in urine production found in tetraplegics to the lack of the nocturnal surge in antidiuretic hormone (ADH) and recommend nocturnal ADH therapy (9). The inappropriate secretion of antidiuretic hormone (SIADH) occurs with increased frequency in SCI patients. SIADH is often associated with tumors such as bronchogenic carcinoma, central nervous system disorders such as subdural hematoma, drugs such as chlorpropamide, and pulmonary processes such as pneumonia and respiratory failure. The diagnosis of SIADH is suggested by low serum osmolality and sodium levels, with an inappropriate elevation of urine osmolality. SIADH is treated by fluid restriction. Occasionally, pharmacologic treatment is required. The agent of choice is demeclocycline, which causes a nephrogenic form of diabetes insipidus.

Hypopituitarism is a deficiency of one or more pituitary hormones. Causes of hypopituitarism include radiation, trauma

(such as may occur during SCI), and infiltrative processes, such as amyloidosis, tuberculosis, and tumors. Signs of hypopituitarism relate to resultant hormonal deficiencies. ACTH deficiency results in decreased serum cortisol, causing weakness, hyponatremia, and hypotension. Gonadotropin deficiency results in decreased testosterone and sperm production in the male, and decreased estrogen and ovulation in the female. Thyroid stimulating hormone (TSH) deficiency results in hypothyroidism. Growth hormone deficiency in prepuberal patients results in impaired growth.

Diabetes insipidus can be caused by damage to the pituitary gland or hypothalamus, such as may occur during trauma (central diabetes insipidus) or because of damage to the renal tubules, or such as may occur with lithium use (nephrogenic diabetes insipidus). The diagnosis of diabetes insipidus is suspected if the patient passes large amounts of dilute urine, which fails to concentrate with fluid restriction. Diabetes insipidus is treated with desmopressin, a vasopressin agonist. Desmopressin is administered intranasally in doses of 2.5 to 20 micrograms. Desmopressin may be also administered parenterally. Certain oral medications, such as chlorpropamide and carbamazepine, enhance the effectiveness of vasoprossin at the renal tubule.

Patients with hypopituitarism exhibit decreased target hormone levels and decreased trophic hormone levels. The treatment of hypopituitarism involves determining the underlying cause and replacing the deficient hormones. For persons with hypopituitarism secondary to trauma, gradual improvement in hormone levels can be expected after recovery. Patients with persistent ACTH deficiency must be treated with stress-dose glucocorticoids (e.g., 100 mg of hydrocortisone IV every six hours) at times of stress, such as infection.

Hyperpituitarism is rare after SCI; symptoms suggestive of hyperpituitarism warrant a workup for pituitary tumors. Increased ACTH results in Cushing's syndrome (central obesity, hypertension, peripheral muscle wasting, striae). Increased growth hormone results in gigantism and acromegaly. Increased TSH causes hyperthyroidism. Increased serum prolactin causes galactorrhea and hypogonadism. Large pituitary tumors will, in addition, present with mass effects such as headaches and visual field effects. The treatment of most pituitary tumors is resection or irradiation of the tumor. The exception is prolactinomas, which often respond to bromocriptine and other dopamine agonists.

Because head trauma can be present in as many as 47% of persons with SCI, dysfunction of the pituitary-hypothalamic axis must be suspected, especially when multi-trauma patients present with polyuria and low specific gravity urine. Diabetes insipidus can be treated with pitressin, and coexistent adrenal insufficiency must be addressed. Endocrine testing for ACTH, TSH, FSH, LH, cortisol, free thyroxine, and estrogen/testosterone can help direct further hormone replacement.

THYROID DISORDERS

Thyroid hormone is necessary for muscle function, body growth, and energy production (10). Patients who are hyperthyroid complain of weight loss, anxiety, and hyperthermia. Examination signs of hyperthyroidism include hyperactive reflexes, enlarged thyroid glands, and tremors. Hyperthyroidism is usually caused by Graves disease (diffuse enlargement of the thyroid gland

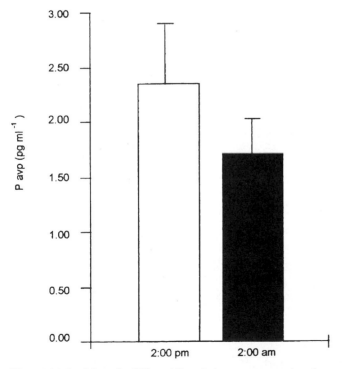

Figure 22.1 Mean (± SE) antidiuretic hormone secretion during the day in 27 tetraplegic patients. Figure shows absence of nocturnal increase in ADH level. (Reprinted with permission. Zollar et al., Nocturnal polyuria and antidiuretic hormone in spinal cord injury. *Arch Phys Med Rehabil* 1997; 78:455–458.)

secondary to thyroid stimulating immunoglobin [TSI]) or by thyroid hormone secreting nodules. In most cases of hyperthyroidism, Free T4 (thyroxine) and Free T3 (triiodothyronine) levels are both elevated, and the TSH is suppressed.

The signs of hyperthyroidism may be difficult to interpret in SCI patients. Thyrotoxicosis is treated with medication such as beta blockers to slow the pulse, thioureas (propylthiouracil or methimazole) to inhibit thyroid hormone synthesis, and iodides to inhibit thyroid hormone release. The treatment of choice for most causes of hyperthyroidism is radioactive iodine, which ablates the thyroid gland. Surgery is rarely indicated.

Patients having hypothyroidism may present with weight gain, hypothermia, impaired mental capacity, constipation, hair loss, and delayed relaxation phase of deep tendon reflexes. Hypothyroidism is also difficult to diagnose in SCI patients. These patients may be hypothermic from the impaired thermoregulation of SCI, constipation is ubiquitous, and pathologic reflexes are difficult to evaluate. Hypothyroidism is treated with levothyroxine. The average replacement dose is 0.1 to 0.15 mg/day. In patients with severe hypothyroidism or coronary disease, replacement is initiated at a low dose (0.025 to 0.05 mg/day) and increased at monthly intervals until the TSH level is normalized. Tetraplegics may have silent myocardial ischemia. Therefore, thyroid hormone replacement in middle-aged and elderly patients with cardiac risk factors should be performed cautiously.

SICK EUTHYROID SYNDROME

SCI patients are at risk for a variety of chronic and acute illnesses, which can result in the sick euthyroid syndrome (11). In less-severe illness, deiodination of T4 to T3 and deiodination of reverse T3 are both impaired. As a result T3 is low and reverse T3 is elevated. (Figure 22.2)

In life-threatening illnesses, such as sepsis, proteins are produced that displace T4 from its protein binding sites. As a result, TSH is depressed and the total T4 is decreased. In critically ill patients, a low T4 level correlates with a poor prognosis. In the sick euthyroid syndrome, the TSH level is not elevated, but subtle enzyme changes exist that indicate that hypothyroidism may be present. Thyroid hormone replacement in the sick euthyroid syndrome does not improve the prognosis (11).

Prakash et al. (12) found that the T3 level correlated with the level and duration of SCI, with the lowest levels found in new tetraplegics and the highest levels in ambulatory paraplegics.

These findings suggest that in acute SCI, conversion of T4 to T3 is impaired.

Case Study

A 30-year-old man who had been tetraplegic for 10 years following a knife wound was evaluated for pressure sores, chronic osteomyelitis of the hips, secondary amyloidosis, and renal failure. Because of lethargy, the diagnosis of hypothyroidism was considered. Thyroid function testing revealed serum T4 1.5 μl/dL (normal 4.5–10.5) and RT3μ 45% (N-23–35%). Serum TSH was less than 4 microunits/dL (normal less than 7). Free thyroxine index was normal.

Discussion

The combination of low T4 and high RT3U suggests that the abnormality in thyroid function testing is caused by a decrease in thyroid hormone binding proteins. The normal TSH confirms that the patient is euthyroid. The serum albumin was found to be 2.3 g/dl (normal 3.5 to 5.5 g/dl), and 24-hour urinary protein excretion was 13 g. The abnormality in thyroid function tests was caused by nephrotic syndrome secondary to systemic amyloidosis.

ADRENOCORTICAL HORMONES

The major hormones secreted by the adrenal cortex are cortisol, aldosterone, and dehydroepiandrosterone (13). Cortisol is under control of the hypothalamic-pituitary axis and is secreted in a negative feedback mode (see Figure 22.3). Stress results in the release of corticotrophin-releasing hormone (CRH) from the hypothalamus, which stimulates ACTH secretion from the pituitary. ACTH in turn stimulates cortisol release from the adrenal gland. Cortisol stimulates gluconeogenesis and is necessary for the body's response to stress. Without cortisol, SCI patients having other medical conditions such as sepsis and myocardial infarction face the likelihood of irreversible shock.

Aldosterone, the major mineralocorticoid of the body, stimulates sodium reabsorption and potassium excretion by the kidney. Aldosterone is primarily under control of the renin-angiotensin system. Hypovolemia and hyperkalemia stimulate renin release by the juxtaglomerular apparatus of the kidney. Renin secretion is inhibited by the sympathetic nervous system. As a result of disordered sympathetic inhibition after SCI, renin,

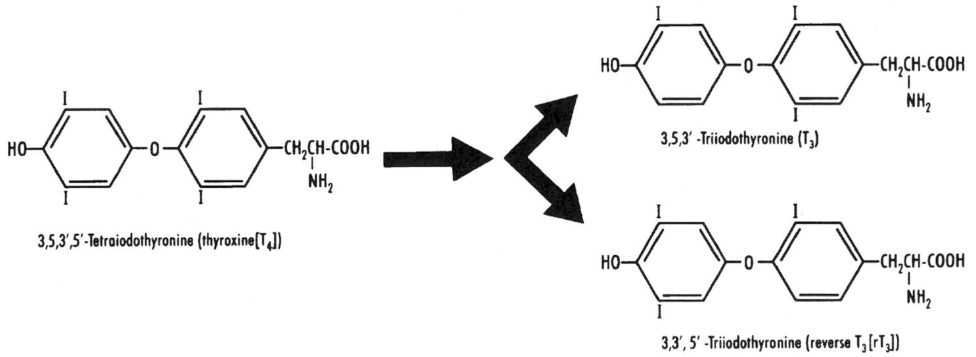

Figure 22.2   Deiodination of thyroxine (T4) to triiodothyronine (T3) and reverse T3.

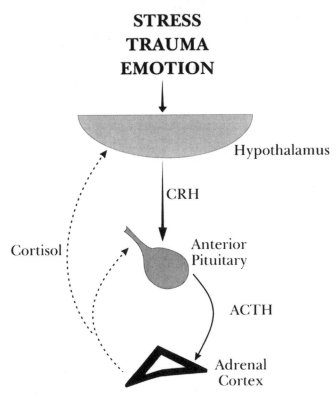

**STRESS
TRAUMA
EMOTION**

Hypothalamus

CRH

Cortisol

Anterior
Pituitary

ACTH

Adrenal
Cortex

Figure 22.3 Hypothalamic-pituitary-adrenal axis. High levels of serum cortisol suppress ACTH and CRH. With low levels of cortisol, CRH and ACTH become elevated.

angiotensin II, and aldosterone can be elevated in tetraplegic patients. Dehydroepiandrosterone, the major adrenal androgen, can also be elevated.

Cushing's syndrome, characterized by increased glucocorticoid levels, can occur with pituitary tumors, adrenal adenomas, and in the setting of exogenous glucocorticoid production. Patients with Cushing's syndrome present with hypertension, truncal obesity, carbohydrate intolerance, and peripheral wasting. The obesity that occurs in some sedentary SCI patients can mimic Cushing's syndrome. The initial screening test for Cushing's syndrome is an overnight dexamethasone suppression test: one milligram of dexamethasone (a synthetic steroid that is not detected by the cortisol assay) is administered at 11 p.m. At 8 a.m., a serum cortisol level is drawn. In normal subjects the morning cortisol is suppressed below 5 micrograms per ml. If the morning cortisol level is not suppressed, further testing, including 24-hour urine cortisol secretion, is done. In normal subjects, the 24-hour urinary cortisol secretion is below 70 micrograms. In almost all patients with Cushing's syndrome, the 24-hour urine cortisol is elevated.

Patients with Cushing's syndrome caused by an adrenal adenoma will have a depressed ACTH level, whereas patients with a pituitary cause will have inappropriately elevated ACTH levels. Cushing's syndrome, depending on the cause, is treated by the removal of the pituitary tumor or adrenal tumor.

Primary adrenal insufficiency occurs with damage to the adrenal cortex from causes such as autoantibodies or infiltrative diseases such tuberculosis, cancer, and amyloidosis (which occurs with increased frequency in patients with SCI). Secondary

adrenal insufficiency is caused by lack of ACTH. Some causes of secondary adrenal insufficiency are pituitary tumors, radiation of the pituitary gland, and chronic suppression with exogenous glucocorticoids. Secondary adrenal insufficiency may also occur from brain trauma associated with SCI (14). Patients with primary adrenal insufficiency or Addison's disease will lack cortisol and aldosterone. As a result, these patients will be hypotensive, hyperkalemic, and hyponatremic. It may be difficult to differentiate the orthostatic hypotension of tetraplegia from that of adrenal insufficiency.

Patients with Addison's disease often are hyperpigmented from increased melanocyte stimulating hormone levels. The major concern with adrenal insufficiency is the possibility that these patients will go into shock when stressed. SCI patients may be treated with glucocorticoids for a variety of conditions, including COPD. Patients who have been treated with glucocorticoids for 2 weeks or more within the preceding year may be at risk for adrenal insufficiency. The most convenient way of evaluating adrenal function is the cortrosyn (synthetic ACTH) test: At 8:00 a.m., a baseline serum cortisol is obtained. Then 0.25 milligrams of cortrosyn are administered intramuscular or intravenously. Serum cortisol levels are obtained at 30, 45, and 60 minutes. A normal test is a basal serum cortisol above 7 micrograms per ml, which increases to above 18 micrograms per ml during the test. If acute adrenal insufficiency is suspected (e.g. hypotension is present), patients should be treated with intravenous saline and 300 mg of hydrocortisone per day, given intravenously in divided doses. Patients with chronic adrenal insufficiency are treated with 25 mg of cortisone acetate, given in the morning, and 12.5 mg of cortisone acetate, given in the afternoon, or 20 mg of hydrocortisone in the morning and 10 mg in the afternoon. Patients with Addison's disease lack aldosterone as well as cortisol. Mineralocorticoid may be replaced with 0.1 mg of fludrocortisone per day. This dose of fludrocortisone is often used to treat postural hypotension in tetraplegic patients.

Case Study

A 24-year-old soldier was injured by a roadside bomb while on duty in Iraq. In addition to a C7 spinal cord injury, penetrating wounds to the head were present. Polyuria of dilute urine consistent with the diagnosis of diabetes insipidus was noted. Because of the possibility of an injury to the pituitary, the patient was treated with stress dose steroids. Subsequent endocrine testing revealed hypopituitarism.

Discussion

The presence of diabetes insipidus in the polytrauma patient alerted the medical team to the possibility of adrenal insufficiency, and lifesaving glucocorticoid replacement was administered

ADRENAL MEDULLA

Pheochromocytomas are catecholamine secreting tumors of the adrenal medulla (15, 16). Patients with pheochromocytomas have manifestations of increased catecholamine levels, including hypertension, tachycardia, headache, and sweating. Autonomic dysreflexia also produces these symptoms, so it is important to distinguish the two disorders. Table 22.1 compares the clinical

Table 22.1   Clinical Characteristics of Autonomic Dysreflexia and Pheochromocytoma

SYMPTOM/SIGN	AUTONOMIC DYSREFLEXIA	PHEOCHROMOCYTOMA
Hypertension	Present intermittently	Present (may be intermittent)
Headache	Often present	Sometimes
Provoked by visceral stimulation (e.g., bladder)	Usually	Rarely
Vasodilation above cord lesion	Present	Absent
Sweating	Localized to upper body, or unilateral	Diffuse
Bradycardia during paroxysm	Often	Absent
Unilateral Horner syndrome	Occasionally present	Absent

Modified from Ref. (1).

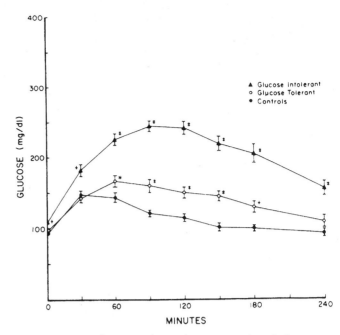

Figure 22.4 Glucose values after 100 g of oral glucose in glucose-tolerant and glucose-intolerant SCI patients versus control subjects. *p < .05, +p < .01 ± p <. 001. (From Duckworth WL, et al. Glucose intolerance due to insulin resistance in patients with spinal cord injuries. *Diabetes* 1980; 906–910. Reproduced with permission from the American Diabetes Association, Inc.)

characteristics of autonomic dysreflexia and pheochromocytoma. Basal catecholamine secretion in pheochromocytomas is elevated; however, serum and urinary catecholamine levels in tetraplegics are less than those in normal subjects. Although serum catecholamine levels increase during paroxysms of autonomic dysreflexia, they do not exceed the baseline levels found in able-bodied persons. If the catecholamine levels are obtained during a period when the paroxysms of autonomic dysreflexia are not occurring, they will be normal. If the diagnosis is still uncertain, clonidine can be administered. Clonidine will not decrease the blood pressure or catecholamine levels in pheochromocytoma, but will in autonomic dysreflexia. Autonomic dysreflexia is common in SCI patients, occurring in 66 to 85% of tetraplegic patients. However, pheochromocytoma is rare, occurring in fewer than 1 of 1,000 hypertensive patients.

Diabetes Mellitus

Diabetes Mellitus (17) is defined as a fasting serum glucose of 126 mg/dl or a random glucose of over 200 mg/dl. There are two major forms of diabetes mellitus. About 10% of diabetics are Type I (insulin dependent, IDDM) who have essentially no insulin secretion and are therefore ketoacidosis prone. Type I diabetes mellitus is due to autoimmune destruction in the islet cells. Type II diabetes mellitus has attained epidemic levels in the United States. This is because of an increasing proportion of obesity in the population. The initial factor in the genesis of Type II diabetes mellitus is insulin resistance.

Duckworth et. al. (18) found that 23 of 41 of SCI patients had abnormal glucose tolerance (see Figure 22.4). Even in SCI patients with normal glucose tolerance, serum glucose exceeded levels in controls. In those patients, insulin levels exceeded those in controls (Figure 22.5). Thus the diabetes mellitus of spinal cord injury is caused by insulin resistance. Multiple characteristics of

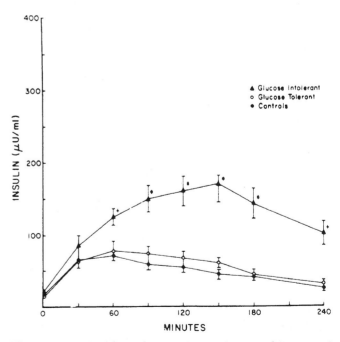

Figure 22.5 Insulin values in SCI patients and in control subjects during oral glucose tolerance test. +p < .01, ± p < .001 (From Duckworth WL, et al. Glucose intolerance due to insulin resistance in patients with spinal cord injuries. *Diabetes* 1980; 24:906–910. Reprinted with permission from the American Diabetes Association, Inc.)

SCI patients can predispose to insulin resistance, including muscle wasting, adiposity, and inactivity (2).

Because Type II diabetes mellitus is usually related to obesity, weight reduction is often the initial therapy. The American Diabetes Association's recommendations tie caloric intake to target body weight (19). In this plan carbohydrates comprise 55–60% of calories, proteins comprise 0.85 g/kg body weight, and fat intake accounts for ≤30% of total calories. Cholesterol is restricted to <300 mg/day. An SCI patient's ideal body weight is corrected in proportion to the type of injury. For a paraplegic patient the ideal body weight is 80% of that of an ambulatory patient of the same size. For a tetraplegic patient the ideal body weight is 60% of that of an ambulatory patient of the same height.

The metabolic requirements and the ability to exercise are both reduced in spinal cord injury patients. Therefore, the ability to treat and prevent diabetes mellitus by nonpharmacologic means is reduced in spinal cord injury patients. The initial pharmacological treatment of diabetes mellitus often includes agents that reverse insulin resistance such as biguanides (metformin) and thiazolidinediones (e.g. pioglitazone) (20). Because of the risk of lactic acidosis, metformin is contraindicated in renal failure. Use of long-acting medications such as glucophage XR decreases side effects. Whereas metformin may produce weight loss, thiazolidinediones are associated with weight gain. When the hemoglobin AIC is not brought below 7%, additional agents are added. Agents that increase insulin secretion such as sulfonylureas and meglitinides are used. A final type of oral agent is acarbose, which inhibits the digestion of oligosaccharide in the small intestine, thereby reducing postprandial hypoglycemia. Side effects include abdominal pain, diarrhea, and flatulence, which may be especially troublesome in SCI patients.

Major oral agents used in the treatment of Type II diabetes mellitus are shown in Table 22.2.

With the passage of time, beta cell exhaustion occurs and insulin is required to maintain diabetic control (21). In many patients, especially those who are obese, there is benefit from adding insulin to oral agents. Addition of an intermediate or long-acting insulin such as NPH or glargine at bedtime normalizes the fasting glucose level, thereby reducing the glucose level throughout the day. The initial insulin dose in units may be calculated by dividing the fasting blood glucose (mg/dl) by 18 or the body weight in kilograms by 10.

As insulinopenia progresses, the patient's insulin requirements may resemble those of a Type I diabetic. A basal insulin level is produced by one or two shots a day of intermediate-acting insulin such as NPH, or by a single dose of glargine insulin. The postprandial increase in glucose is prevented by short-acting insulin such as regular or lispro.

The classic regimen consists of 0.5 to 1 unit per kilogram of insulin per day with 2/3 of the dose given before the morning meal and 1/3 before the evening meal. Intermediate-acting insulin such as NPH is combined with short-acting insulin such as regular in a 2 to 1 ratio. More recently, rapidly acting insulins such as lispro have been developed that may be given at the time of a meal, thus decreasing the risk of hypoglycemia if a later meal is missed. A typical regimen is to provide a basal level of insulin by giving glargine at bedtime, and to mimic the mealtime insulin surge by administering lispro one unit per 8 grams of carbohydrate before meals.

Rapidly acting insulins given immediately before meals have an advantage in SCI patients who cannot feed themselves or give insulin. The caretaker can inject the patient immediately before the meal, thus increasing convenience and decreasing risk of hypoglycemia.

Premixed insulins are available such as a Humalog mix 75/25, which is a fixed ratio mixture of 25% rapid-acting lispro-based and 75% protamine-based immediately acting insulin. Such insulins given twice a day provide a basal insulin level and prevent postprandial hyperglycemia. Commonly used insulin preparations are shown in Table 22.3.

The use of insulin in SCI patients poses problems. The absorption of insulin is increased in an exercising extremity (22, 23). Increased absorption of insulin may result in hypoglycemia. These effects may be especially important in the SCI patient who has some upper extremity function. Insulin should be injected below the sensory level to avoid this problem. Diabetic control is assessed by home glucose monitoring and hemoglobin AIC (an index of glycemic control during the preceding 8–12 weeks). Home glucose monitoring is especially important in SCI patients who may have erratic glucose levels and may be unable to sense hypoglycemia.

Table 22.2 Oral Agents Used in Type II Diabetes Mellitus

Drug	Daily Dose	Duration of Action (hr)
Metformin	500–2000 mg	24
Pioglitazone	15–45 mg	24
Rosiglitazone	2–8 mg	24
Glyburide	2.5–20 mg	>24
Glipizide	2.5–20 mg	>24
Glimepiride	1–8 mg	>24
Repaglinide	1–4 mg w/every meal	5–6
Nateglinide	60–120 mg w/every meal	3–4
Acarbose	25–150 mg	10

Table 22.3 Insulin Preparations

Preparation	Onset (hr)	Peak (hr)	Effective Duration (hr)
Short-Acting			
Lispro	<.25	0.5–1.5	3–4
Insulin Aspart	<.25	0.5–1.5	3–4
Regular	0.5–1	2–3	3–6
Intermediate-Acting			
NPH	2–4	6–10	10–16
Lente	3–4	6–12	12–18
Long-Acting			
Ultralente	6–10	10–16	18–20
Glargine	4	No peak	24

Adapted from Powers A. "Diabetes Mellitus II." In: Kasper D, et al. (eds.). *Harrison's Principles of Internal Medicine.* McGraw Hill, New York 2005. pp. 2152–2180.

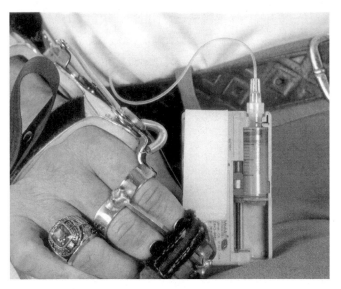

Figure 22.6   C6 tetraplegic with insulin infusion pump.

Wide swings in serum glucose and hypoglycemia unawareness can result in impaired mental status and confusion, placing the paralyzed patient at special risk. An insulin infusion pump, which normalizes serum glucose (Figure 22.6), delivers a basal amount of insulin to control glycemia in the fasting state. Before meals, the rate of infusion is increased. Such pumps improve diabetic control and can prevent wide swings in glucose (24).

Diabetic Control and Complications

Diabetes mellitus results in both microvascular and macrovascular complications. Microvascular complications include diabetic retinopathy, neuropathy, and nephropathy. Diabetics are also at increased risk for the macrovascular complications of coronary disease and strokes.

The Diabetes Control and Complications Trial (DCCT) investigated whether intensive diabetic control could prevent complications (25). The test included 1444 Type I diabetics who were randomly assigned to either intense insulin (3 or more injections per day or an insulin infusion pump) or standard treatment (one or two shots per day). Hemoglobin AIC levels and serum glucose levels were 1.5 to 2% lower and 60 to 80 mg/dl lower respectively in those receiving intensive therapy than in those receiving conventional care. There was a significant reduction in retinopathy (76%), proteinuria (54%), and clinical neuropathy (60%) in patients receiving intensive therapy. Although this study was conducted on Type I diabetics, it seems likely that the conclusions are valid for Type II diabetics as well.

The complications of diabetes mellitus may be difficult to diagnose in SCI patients. Myocardial ischemia may be silent because of the destruction of sensory pathways. Peripheral neuropathy may likewise be silent or difficult to distinguish from the effects of the cord lesion. The only sign that the peripheral neuropathy is present may be a decrease in the magnitude of reflexes in the lower extremity. It may be difficult to distinguish the autonomic neuropathy of diabetes mellitus from the effects of a high cord lesion. In situations where the cord lesion is partial, the effects of autonomic neuropathy add to those on the cord

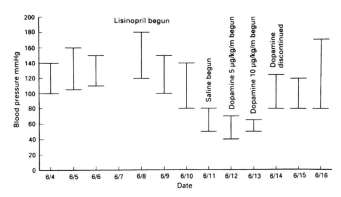

Figure 22.7   Effect of lisinopril on blood pressure of a C6 tetraplegic. (Reprinted with permission, *Paraplegia* 1994; 32: 871–875.)

lesion. Likewise, it may be difficult to distinguish the effects of diabetic nephropathy from renal failure from other causes, such as amyloidosis or chronic pyelonephritis. A combination of diabetic nephropathy and renal amyloidosis is especially problematic, because both conditions cause proteinuria. Angiotensin-converting enzyme inhibitors protect the kidney. They are recommended for the treatment of hypertension in diabetics and of elevated urinary albumin. However, angiotensin-converting enzyme inhibitors may cause life-threatening hypotension in tetraplegic patients in whom the renin-angiotensin axis is utilized to support blood pressure to compensate for the lack of sympathetic input. (Figure 7.7) These agents should be used cautiously or not at all with tetraplegic patients (26).

Metabolic Syndrome

The metabolic syndrome is a collection of cardiovascular risk factors that are due to insulin resistance (27). The presence of any three of the five characteristics of abdominal obesity, elevated triglycerides, low HDL cholesterol, elevated blood pressure, and elevated fasting glucose constitute the metabolic syndrome, placing the patient at increased cardiovascular risk. Several of these factors occur commonly in SCI patients. The treatment of the metabolic syndrome is diet and exercise, which is often difficult in SCI patients.

HYPOGLYCEMIA

Hypoglycemia (28) is classified as fasting, reactive or postprandial. SCI patients may be at risk for both forms of hypoglycemia. Fasting hypoglycemia is caused by a lack of glucose production during gluconeogenesis, and can be seen in the increased uptake of glucose into insulin-sensitive tissues. Fasting hypoglycemia occurs in the setting of end-stage liver disease, large mesenchymal tumors (which may consume glucose or produce substances with insulin-like activity), hypoglycemic agents, the use of certain medications (such as pentamidine), and insulinomas. The signs and symptoms of hypoglycemia in ambulatory persons include sweating, hunger, palpitations, anxiety, and mental confusion.

Mathias et al. (29) studied the physiologic responses to hypoglycemia in tetraplegic persons and in normal controls. In the tetraplegic group, the usual signs and symptoms of hypoglycemia did not occur. Instead, most of the tetraplegic subjects had symptoms of impaired glucose delivery to the brain, such as drowsiness and altered mentation (neuroglycopenia). Gerich et al. (30) stated that adrenalectomized patients were not able to increase epinephrine levels following hypoglycemia, but found that their recovery from hypoglycemia was normal. However, when the glucagon response to hypoglycemia was abolished by somatostatin, prolonged hypoglycemia resulted. Palmer et al. (31) found that the glucagon response was not affected by cervical cord transection in humans, although the catecholamine response to hypoglycemia was decreased (see Figures 22.8 and 22.9). This indicates that a normal sympathetic nervous system is not required for glucagon secretion. These data suggest that glucagon is a critical hormone for the recovery from hypoglycemia in the tetraplegic patient. The use of medications that inhibit glucagon action (such as indomethacin) might therefore impair recovery from hypoglycemia in tetraplegics (32).

Mathias et al. (29) found that fish insulin-induced hypoglycemia in tetraplegic patients failed to suppress serum insulin levels. In normal subjects, alpha adrenergic blockade, by allowing unopposed parasympathetic activity, has been shown to cause increased serum insulin levels and impair suppression of

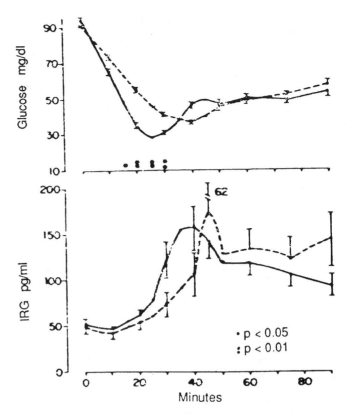

Figure 22.9 Plasma glucose and glucagon response (mean ± SEM) to intravenous insulin in five tetraplegic patients (- - - -) and six controls (——). (From Palmer JP, et al. Glucagon response to hypoglycemia in sympathectomized man. *J Clin Invest* 1976; 57:522–525. Reproduced by copyright permission of the American Society for Clinical Investigation.)

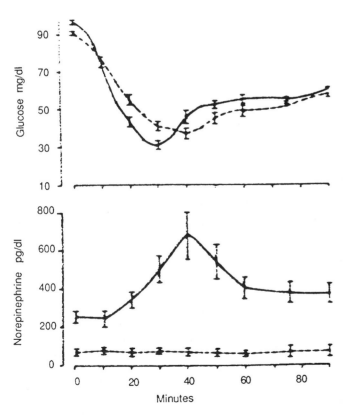

Figure 22.8 Plasma glucose and norepinephrine response (mean ± SEM) to insulin-induced hypoglycemia in five tetraplegic patients (- - - -) and seven controls (——). (From Palmer JP et al, Glucagon response to hypoglycemia in sympathectomized man. *J Clin Invest* 1976; 57:522–525. Reprinted by copyright permission of the American Society for Clinical Investigation.)

insulin by hypoglycemia. Impaired sympathetic tone may result in elevated serum insulin levels in tetraplegic patients.

A major substrate for gluconeogenesis is amino acids. The brain is the major glucose-requiring organ in the fasting state. SCI patients have muscle atrophy, thereby increasing the ratio of brain mass to muscle mass. As described above, tetraplegic persons can have elevated fasting serum insulin levels. These patients can be pre-disposed to fasting hypoglycemia. In normal subjects, the catecholamine response to exercise stimulates gluconeogenesis and impairs glucose uptake by muscles, thereby protecting from hypoglycemia. Tetraplegic persons, who often cannot exercise, lack a normal catecholamine response to hypoglycemia. The use of newer exercise techniques, such as functional electrical stimulation (FES), may predispose these patients to exercise-induced hypoglycemia. (33)

REACTIVE HYPOGLYCEMIA

A carbohydrate-containing meal stimulates insulin secretion. Sometimes the serum insulin level is elevated after the blood glucose has returned to normal. This may cause hypoglycemia 1 to 5 hours after meals. SCI patients, who have an increased insulin response to carbohydrates, can be predisposed to reactive hypoglycemia (17). The treatment of reactive hypoglycemia is the avoidance of large, carbohydrate-rich meals. Reactive hypoglycemia may be also seen in prediabetic states. In this case, the treatment is weight reduction, exercise, and sometimes the institution of oral agents. By reducing insulin resistance, hyperinsulinism will be reduced, thereby preventing reactive hypoglycemia. Acarbose, an alpha glucosidase inhibitor, may be useful in the treatment of reactive hypoglycemia in tetraplegic patients (34). Acarbose, by decreasing glucose absorption, prevents hyperinsulinism and reactive hypoglycemia.

Treatment of Hypoglycemia

Mild hypoglycemia can be treated with oral glucose solution or juice. In more severe hypoglycemia, or in situations where oral administration of glucose is not possible, parenteral therapy must be given. High tetraplegics may need assistance in the treatment of hypoglycemia. Glucagon 1 mg is available in kits. The powder can be quickly reconstituted in diluent and administered IV, IM, or SQ. For glucagon to be effective, there must be adequate liver stores of glycogen. The standard parenteral therapy of hypoglycemia is intravenous glucose. Fifty cc of 50% dextrose is administered IV over 5 minutes. Then an infusion of 5% or 10% dextrose may be started. The duration of parenteral glucose treatment depends on the cause of hypoglycemia. Hypoglycemia caused by regular insulin and a missed meal may require only a few hours therapy. If the hypoglycemia is caused by a long-acting medication, such as chlorpropamide or glargine, especially in an SCI patient with impaired renal function, parenteral treatment may be required for days.

LIPID DISORDERS

Lipoproteins are complex macromolecules that transport non-polar lipids through the aqueous environment of plasma (35). Each lipoprotein particle has on its surface one or more apoproteins that have a variety of structural and functional roles. The major apoproteins are A, B, C, and E. Apoprotein B is the major apoprotein of the triglyceride-rich lipoproteins secreted by the liver (very low-density lipoprotein, VLDL). Dietary triglyceride is carried in chylomicrons. Low-density lipoprotein (LDL) transports cholesterol into the arterial wall. High-density lipoprotein (HDL) removes cholesterol from the vessel wall. If a fasting or random serum cholesterol is elevated, a fasting lipid profile should be ordered. The recommended level of LDL cholesterol depends on the concomitant cardiac risk factors, which include male gender, age greater than 45, hypertension, HDL cholesterol below 35, diabetes mellitus, history of smoking, and a family history of coronary disease. If fewer than two risk factors are present, the LDL cholesterol goal is below 160. If two or more risk factors are present, the LDL cholesterol goal is below 130. If there is documented coronary disease, diabetes mellitus, or kidney disease the LDL cholesterol goal is below 100 mg/dl. With extreme cardiovascular risk such as occurs in patients with vascular disease and diabetes mellitus, the metabolic syndrome, or smoking the LDL cholesterol goal is below 70 mg/dl. SCI patients often have low HDL cholesterol levels. Brenes et al (36) found that HDL cholesterol levels in SCI patients correlated with their degree of activity (Figure 22.10)

SCI patients are also predisposed to diabetes mellitus. Furthermore, Yekutiel (37) found that the incidence of hypertension was increased in paraplegic patients. Because of these risk factors

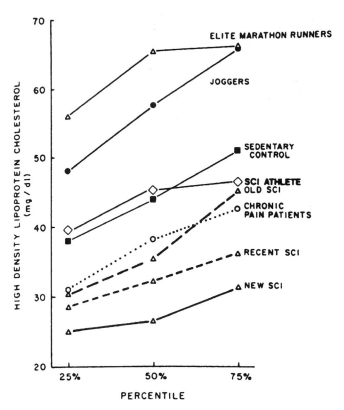

Figure 22.10   High-density lipoprotein cholesterol in subjects who perform various levels of physical activity. (From Brenes G, et al. High density lipoprotein cholesterol concentrations in physically active and sedentary spinal cord injury patients. *Arch Phys Med Rehabil* 1986; 67:445.)

for coronary disease, the LDL cholesterol should be aggressively lowered in SCI patients.

Treatment of Hyperlipidemia

Weight loss results in the lowering of total and LDL cholesterol. The ideal weight of an SCI patient is lower than that of an ambulatory patient of the same height; caloric intake is based on ideal weight. By using a wheelchair aerobic fitness trainer that allows arm exercise 2 or 3 times a week, paraplegic and low tetraplegic patients can significantly decrease their serum cholesterol level (38). Exercise also increases HDL cholesterol. Exercise may be difficult in tetraplegic patients; however, FES may be a useful modality (33, 38).

If diet and exercise fail to lower lipid levels, medication is indicated. HMG coA reductase inhibitors are in common use for the control of serum cholesterol. The side effects of these agents include myopathy and elevated liver function tests. Myopathy may be difficult to diagnose in SCI patients. Nicotinic acid lowers serum cholesterol and triglycerides, and raises HDL cholesterol, which is often low in SCI patients. Side effects of nicotinic acid include the elevation of liver enzymes, worsening of carbohydrate tolerance, and flushing. Flushing from nicotinic acid might be mistaken for autonomic dysreflexia in tetraplegic patients. Fibrates lower serum triglycerides and cholesterol and raise HDL cholesterol. Fibrates are most useful in patients with elevated serum triglycerides. Myopathy is also a potential side effect of these agents. Bile acid binding resins, such as cholestyramine, produce a moderate reduction of serum cholesterol. Bile acid binding resins are contraindicated when there is a significant elevation of serum triglycerides, because they will elevate serum triglycerides further. Bile acid sequestrants increase the risk of cholelithiasis and constipation, which are already common in SCI patients.

SCI patients are predisposed to multiple forms of hyperlipidemia because of their tendency to glucose intolerance. These patients are at risk for the lipid disorders associated with diabetes mellitus, including hypertriglyceridemia, low HDL, and small dense LDL particles. Small dense LDL particles are especially atherogenic. SCI patients are at increased risk for renal failure and the nephrotic syndrome. Patients with uremia often have hypertriglyceridemia and low HDL cholesterol levels, and nephrotic syndrome results in increased VLDL production by the liver. There is evidence that regardless of the level of LDL cholesterol in diabetics, statins are beneficial in preventing cardiovascular events (39). Statins should be part of the treatment regimen in all diabetics. The evaluation of lipid profiles is a key component in the long-term medical care of SCI patients.

Calcium Disorders

In healthy individuals, serum calcium is maintained within narrow physiologic limits (40, 41). The major hormone involved in calcium homeostasis, parathyroid hormone, is secreted by the parathyroid glands in response to a decrease in ionized serum calcium. Vitamin D_2 (7-dehydrocholesterol) is converted to vitamin D_3 in the skin under the influence of sunlight (Figure 22.11). Vitamin D3 is hydroxylated to 25-hydroxyvitamin D in the liver. The best index of stored vitamin D is the 25-hydroxy-vitamin D level (Figure 22.12). Bauman et. al (42) found that 25-hydroxyvitamin D levels were decreased in SCI patients and that there was an inverse correlation between vitamin D levels and PTH levels. This finding of secondary hyperparathyroidism is likely to result in the development of progressive osteoporosis in SCI patients. Parathyroid hormone causes osteoclasts to release calcium from bone and increases renal phosphate excretion. Parathyroid hormone also stimulates the conversion of 25-hydroxyvitamin D to 1, 25-dihydroxyvitamin D in the kidney. 1, 25-dihydroxyvitamin D causes calcium absorption by the renal tubules. Patients with SCI have been found to have suppressed PTH and 1, 25-dihydroxyvitamin D levels and increased serum phosphate and prolactin in the setting of normal Ca++ levels (43). The degree of PTH suppression correlates with the degree of neurologic impairment.

Primary hyperparathyroidism is an inappropriate elevation of parathyroid hormone due to adenoma, carcinoma, or hyperplasia of the parathyroid glands. These conditions produce elevated ionized serum calcium and low serum phosphate levels. A critical element in the diagnosis of primary hyperparathyroidism is an inappropriate elevation of the PTH level. In other forms of hypercalcemia, the PTH level is suppressed. Primary hyperparathyroidism is treated by resection of the adenoma or subtotal resection of the hyperplastic parathyroid glands. Secondary hyperparathyroidism is most commonly caused by renal failure, low calcium intake, or reduced exposure to

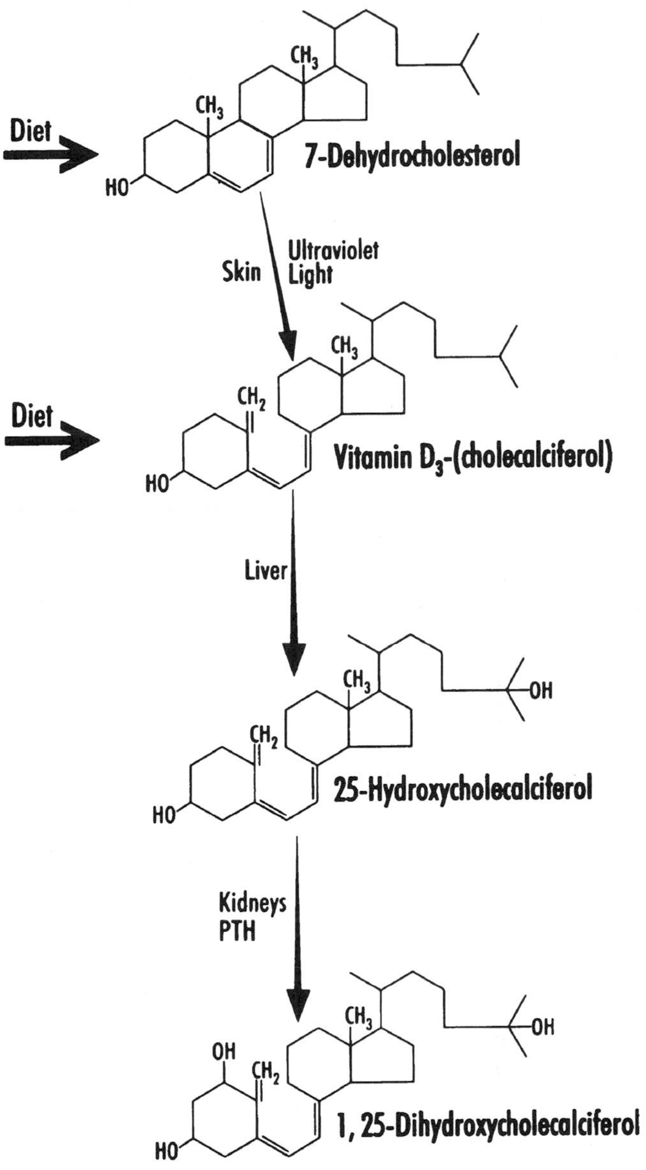

Figure 22.11   Metabolism of vitamin D.

sunlight—common scenarios in SCI patients. Impaired renal function results in phosphate retention. Phosphate binds ionized calcium and also decreases the renal production of 1, 25-dihydroxyvitamin D. Secondary hyperparathyroidism results in the worsening of osteoporosis, which further decreases the low bone density of SCI patients and results in an even greater fracture risk. Hypoparathyroidism is manifest by low serum calcium and high serum phosphate levels.

The most common causes of hypoparathyroidism are thyroid surgery and autoimmune destruction of the parathyroid glands. Because 50% of extracellular calcium is bound to protein, patients with low serum albumin, such as may occur in SCI patients with renal amyloidosis and nephrotic syndrome, will exhibit decreased serum calcium. In these patients, an ionized serum calcium level should be obtained. Hypocalcemia produces the physical findings of muscular irritability, such as tetany.

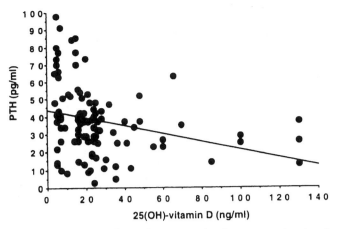

Figure 22.12 Correlation between 25(OH)-vitamin D level and parathyroid hormone level in spinal cord injury patients. (From Bauman et al. Vitamin D deficiency in veterans with chronic spinal cord injury. *Metabolism* 1995; 44:1612.)

The physical findings of hypocalcemia may be difficult to elicit in SCI patients.

Hypercalcemia occurs in the setting of hyperparathyroidism, hypervitaminosis D, immobilization, and other causes. Immobilization increases osteoclast activity and decreases osteoblast activity, thus resulting in hypercalcemia, especially in young people, where the bones are already in a high turnover state. Signs and symptoms of hypercalcemia include mental confusion, frequent urination, and thirst. The treatment of hypercalcemia is hydration with normal saline, which increases renal calcium excretion. Various drugs decrease osteoclast activity, including calcitonin, mithramycin, and bisphosphonates. The use of pamidronate, a bisphosphonate, has been advocated for the treatment of immobilization hypercalcemia (44). Between 60 and 90 mg are administered intravenously. Bisphosphonates cannot be used in children because of the risk of precipitating a rachitis syndrome.

Hypocalcemia is treated by the infusion of intravenous calcium: 94 mg (one ampule) of calcium gluconate can be added to a liter of D5W (5% glucose in water) and administered over 6 to 8 hours. In situations in which the serum phosphate is elevated, it is important that the serum phosphate be lowered prior to the administration of calcium to prevent precipitation of calcium phosphate. The administration of glucose stimulates insulin release. Insulin mediated glucose uptake into cells lowers serum phosphate.

Hypoparathyroidism may result in chronic hypocalcemia and hyperphosphatemia. Hypoparathyroidism is treated with 1 to 2 grams of elemental calcium per day and vitamin D. Between 50 and 100,000 units of Vitamin D2 (ergocalciferol) are administered per day. Alternatively, a more active metabolite such as 1, 25 (OH) D3 (calcitriol) may be administered. The standard dose is 0.25 micrograms per day, which is increased at 4- to 8-week intervals to 1 microgram per day. The target serum calcium in the treatment of hypoparathyroidism is 8 to 9 mg/dl. Patients with hypoparathyroidism lack the hypocalciuric effect of PTH. Therefore, higher levels of serum calcium may result in hypercalciuria and renal stones.

The high bone turnover state that occurs in the first several months after spinal cord injury reduces bone density significantly (45). Pearson et al. (46) found that patients who ambulate and receive etidronate therapy can preserve their bone density. Ambulation and bisphosphonates seem to work synergistically to maintain bone mass. Bisphosphonates, such as alendronate, produce esophageal irritation and erosions. To reduce this side effect, the patient sits upright for 30 minutes after the medication is taken. This may be difficult in tetraplegic patients. An alternate treatment is intravenous pamidronate given once a month (47).

REPRODUCTIVE FUNCTION IN SPINAL CORD INJURY PATIENTS

The pulsatile secretion of gonadotropin releasing hormone (GnRH) from the hypothalamus stimulates the release of luteinizing hormone (LH) and follicle stimulating hormone (FSH) from the pituitary gland (48, 49). In males, LH stimulates the differentiation of the Leydig cells of the testis and promotes the conversion of cholesterol to testosterone and the secretion of testosterone. Testosterone is largely bound to sex hormone binding globulin (SHBG). FSH stimulates sperm production by the seminiferous tubules. The seminiferous tubules secrete inhibin, a peptide that exists in a closed-loop feedback with FSH. When seminiferous tubules are damaged, inhibin decreases and FSH increases. In the female, FSH stimulates the ovarian production of both androgens and estrogens.

Sex hormones in the female are also largely bound to circulating plasma proteins. Sex hormones exist in a closed-loop feedback with the hypothalamus. Therefore, in patients with impaired gonadal function, FSH and LH increase. Nance et al. (50) studied FSH and LH levels in SCI males having varying degrees of injury. Those patients having the most severe neurologic deficits had elevated gonadotropin levels and an exaggerated response to GnRH. It is theorized that trauma and impaired thermogulation (which is most pronounced in the high cord lesions) results in damage to the testes.

Semen analysis in SCI patients shows a decreased number and motility of spermatozoa and abnormal morphology (51). The carnitine level of spermatozoa, which is an index of epididymal function, is decreased in SCI patients. Biopsies of the testes of patients with paraplegia and tetraplegia show a lack of spermatogenesis and atrophy (Figure 22.13).

Ovarian function is less affected in the female SCI patient than is testicular function in the male. The internal location of the ovaries, compared to the external location of the testes, may be protective, because the effects of temperature extremes can be reduced. In addition, testicular infections, seeded from the contiguous urinary structures, likely bring about chronic damage to the reproductive structures.

Reflex erectile function occurs in as many as 80% of SCI patients, especially in those with incomplete lesions. Fewer patients experience ejaculation and orgasm. With sexual counseling and newer techniques for augmenting erectile dysfunction, many male patients enjoy a satisfactory sex life. Although significant differences have been found between able-bodied women and women with disabilities, no significant differences in sexual desire have been found between the groups. The severity of disability was not significantly related to level of sexual activity and orgasm in SCI women with intact sexual reflexes (52).

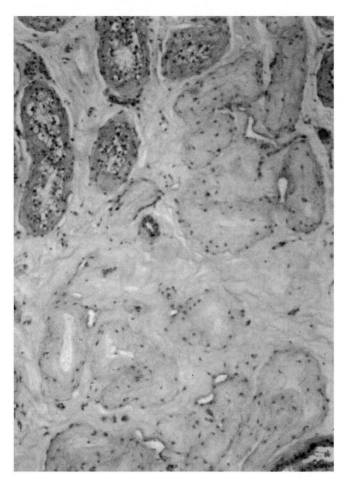

Figure 22.13 Seminiferous tubule atrophy in a tetraplegic man (×400) (autopsy specimen). (Courtesy of Dr. B. Kipreos. Department of Pathology, Hunter Holmes McGuire Veterans Medical Center, Richmond, Virginia.)

Sex Hormone Replacement

Estrogen replacement (49) probably affects women with SCI more than it does ambulatory patients. Estrogen improves the lipid profile by lowering the LDL cholesterol and raising the HDL cholesterol, which may be decreased in the SCI patient. Estrogen also prevents osteoporosis, which is accelerated in the paralyzed areas. Premarin®, given at a daily dose of 0.625 mg daily from the first through 25th days of the month prevents osteoporosis and flushing. Oral estrone sulfate (.625 to 1.25 mg), estradiol (1 mg), or transdermal estrogen programmed to deliver 0.05 mg/day of estradiol may be used. Estrogen treatment increases the risk of endometrial cancer. The addition of a progestin such as medroxyprogesterone acetate (5–10 mg) on the 14th to 25th day of the month reduces the risk of endometrial cancer.

However, in the Heart and Estrogen/Progestin Replacement Study (HERS), treatment of post-menopausal women with established coronary disease with estrogen plus progesterone was found to increase the risk of thromboembolic and gall bladder disease (53), both of which are more common in SCI patients. The risk of coronary artery disease was not decreased. Estrogen treatment is therefore not recommended for secondary prevention of coronary disease. The Women's Health Initiative Group (54) found that even in healthy women, estrogen/progesterone replacement increased cardiovascular risk, pulmonary embolism, and breast cancer. Therefore, routine estrogen replacement is not recommended.

In the male, androgen may be replaced with testosterone enanthate or cypionate 200 mg IM q2 weeks or 300 g IM q3 weeks. More recently the testosterone patch has been found to provide effective replacement. Hypogonandal men are predisposed to osteoporosis and anemia. Androgen replacement may have valuable secondary effects in men with SCI. Before androgen therapy is instituted, risk counseling and screening for prostate neoplasm are appropriate.

Anabolic steroids increase muscle mass and aid in healing. Spungen et. al (55) have found that treatment of spinal cord injury patients with the androgen oxandrolone improves ventilatory function. A negative aspect of androgen treatment is abnormalities in liver function and reduction in HDL cholesterol.

CONCLUSION

SCI affects the endocrine system, primarily through unpredictable sympathetic nervous system function and the effects of inactivity. The usual nocturnal increase in ADH secretion does not occur with increased frequency in SCI. Both hypothyroidism and hyperthyroidism are more difficult to diagnose in SCI patients than in ambulatory patients. Type II diabetes mellitus, caused by insulin resistance, occurs with increased frequency in SCI patients. The metabolic syndrome occurs commonly and is more difficult to treat. The usual signs of hypoglycemia, such as anxiety and sweating, may not be present in insulin-treated patients. Autonomic dysreflexia may mimic pheochromocytoma. Immobilization hypercalcemia may occur, especially in acutely injured teenagers with tetraplegia. Although some SCI patients have depressed PTH levels, SCI patients are at increased risk for hypovitaminosis D, which increases osteoporosis risk. Ambulation works synergistically with bisphosphonates to decrease osteoporosis. Hypogonadism, especially in males, is more common in SCI patients than in ambulatory patients. Androgens may improve muscle mass in SCI patients.

ACKNOWLEDGMENTS

The authors are indebted to Ms. Alice B. Johnson and Ms. Sonya M. Matthews for their excellent administrative assistance.

References

1. Schmitt JK, Adler RA. Endocrine-metabolic consequences of spinal cord injury. *Phys Med Rehab State Art Rev* 1987; 1:425–440.
2. Bauman W, Spungen A. Disorders of carbohydrate and lipid metabolism in veterans with paraplegia or quadriplegia: a model of premature aging. *Metabolism* 1994; 43:749–756.
3. Schmitt, J. Endocrine-metabolic causes of spinal cord injury. 2009 *Nova Scientific Publications* (in press).
4. Melmed S, Jameson J. "Disorders of the anterior pituitary and hypothalamus". In: Kasper D, ed. *Harrison's Principles of Internal Medicine* 16th ed. New York: McGraw-Hill 2005:2076–2097.
5. Claus-Walker J, Halstead LS. Metabolic and endocrine changes in spinal cord injury. II(Section 1): Consequences of partial decentralization of the autonomic nervous system. *Arch Phys Med Rehabil* 1982; 63:569–573.

6. Claus-Walker J, Halstead LS. Metabolic and endocrine changes in spinal cord injury. II (Section 2): partial decentralization of the autonomic nervous system. *Arch Phys Med Rehabil* 1982; 63:576–580.

7. Claus-Walker J, Halstead LS. Metabolic and endocrine changes in spinal cord injury. III. Less quanta of sensory input plus bedrest and illness. *Arch Phys Med Rehabil* 1982; 63:628–631.

8. Claus-Walker J, Halstead LS. Metabolic and endocrine changes in spinal cord injury. IV. Compound neurologic dysfunctions. *Arch Phys Med Rehabil* 1982; 63:632–631.

9. Szollar S, Dunn K, Brandt S, Fincher J. Nocturnal polyuria and antidiuretic hormone levels in spinal cord injury. *Arch Phys Med Rehabil* 1997; 78:455–458.

10. Jameson J, Weetman AP. "Disorders of the thyroid gland". In: Kasper, D, ed. *Harrison's Principles of Internal Medicine.* 16th ed. New York: McGraw-Hill 2005:2104–2127.

11. Zaloga GP, Smallridge RC. Thyroid hypofunction in acute illness. *Semin Respir Med* 1985; 7:95–107.

12. Prakash V, Lin M, Song C, Perkash I. Thyroid hypofunction in spinal cord injury patients. *Paraplegia* 1980; 1856–1863.

13. Williams G, Dluhy R. "Disorders of the adrenal cortex". In: Kasper, D, ed. *Harrison's Principles of Internal Medicine 16th Edition, New York, McGraw-Hill* 2005; 2127–2148.

14. Webster J, Bell K. Primary adrenal insufficiency following traumatic brain injury: a case report and review of the literature. *Arch Phys Med Rehabil* 1997; 78:314–318.

15. Naftchi N, Wooten G, Lowman E, et al. Relationship between serum dopamine-beta hydroxylase activity, catecholamine metabolism and hemodynamic changes during paroxysmal hypertension in quadriplegics. *Circ Res* 1974; 35:850–861.

16. Landsberg L, Young J. "Pheochromocytoma." In: Kasper, D, ed. *Harrison's Principles of Internal Medicine.* New York McGraw-Hill 2005:2148–2153.

17. Defronzo, R. Pathogenesis of type II diabetes mellitus. *Med Clinics NA* 2004; 88:787–835.

18. Duckworth WC, Solomon SS, Jallepalli P, et al. Glucose intolerance due to insulin resistance in patients with spinal cord injuries. *Diabetes* 1980; 29:906–910.

19. American Diabetes Association Clinical Practice Recommendations 2003. *Diabetes Care* 2004; 27:51.

20. Lebovitz, H. Oral antidiabetic agents. *Med Clin NAM.* 2004;88:847–863.

21. Davis, T, Edlemon, S. Insulin therapy in type II diabetes *Med Clin NAM.* 2004; 88:865–895.

22. Koivisto VA, Felig P. Effects of leg exercise on insulin absorption in diabetic patients. *N Engl J Med* 1978; 298:79–83.

23. Koivisto VA, Felig P. Alterations in insulin absorption and in blood glucose control associated with varying insulin injection sites in diabetic patients. *Ann Intern Med* 1980; 298:79–83.

24. Barlascini C, Schmitt J, Adler R. Insulin pump treatment of type I diabetes mellitus in a patient with C6 quadriplegia. *Arch Phys Med Rehabil* 1989; 70:58–60.

25. Diabetes Control and Complications Trial Research Group. The effect of intensive treatment of diabetes on the development and progression of long-term complications of insulin-dependent diabetes mellitus. *N Engl J Med* 1993; 329:976–986.

26. Schmitt JK, Koch KS, Midha M. Profound hypotension in a tetraplegic patient following angiotensin-converting enzyme inhibitor lisinopril. Case report. *Paraplegic* 1994; 32:871–875.

27. Garber A. The metabolic syndrome. *Med Clin NAM* 2004; 88:837–847

28. Cryer P. "Hypoglycemia." In: Kasper, D, ed. *Harrison's Principles of Internal Medicine.* 16th ed. New York: McGraw-Hill 2005:2180–2185.

29. Mathias C, Frankel H, Turner R, et al. Physiological responses to insulin hypoglycaemia in man. *Am J Physiol* 1979; 236(4):380–385.

30. Gerich J, Davis J, Lorenzi M, et al. Mechanisms of recovery from insulin-induced hypoglycemia in man. *Am J Physiol* 1979; 236(4):380–385.

31. Palmer JP, Henry DP, Benson JW, et al. Glucagon response to hypoglycemia in sympathectomized man. *J Clin Invest* 1976; 57:522–525.

32. Barlascini D, Schmitt J. Indomethacin, hypoglycemia, quadriplegia. *Arch Phys Med Rehabil* 1987; 69:746.

33. Scott T, Peckham P. Functional electrical stimulation and its application to the management of spinal cord injury. In: Young R, Woolsey R, eds. Philadelphia: WB Saunders, 1995:377–396.

34. Schmitt J, Koch K, Midha M. Prevention of reactive hypoglycemia in a C6 tetraplegic with the glucosidase inhibitor acarbose. Proceedings of the 46th Annual Meeting of the American Paraplegia Society, Las Vegas, Nevada, 2000.

35. Witztum J, Steinberg D. "The hyperlipoproteinemias." In: Bennett D, Plum F, eds. *Cecil Textbook of Medicine.* Philadelphia: WB Saunders, 1996:1086–1095.

36. Brenes G, Dearwater M, Sharpera R, et al. High density lipoprotein cholesterol concentrations in physically active and sedentary spinal cord injury patients. *Arch Phys Med Rehabil* 1986; 1964:445–450.

37. Yekutiel M, Brooks M, Ohry A, et al. The prevalence of hypertension, ischemic heart disease and diabetes in traumatic spinal cord injured patients and amputees. *Paraplegia* 1986; 27:58–62.

38. Midha M. Schmitt J, Sclater M. Exercise effect with the wheelchair aerobic fitness trainer on conditioning and metabolic function in disabled persons, A pilot study. *Arch Phys Med Rehabil* 1999; 80:258–261.

39. Colhoun H, Betteridge J, Durrington P et. al. Primary prevention of cardiovascular disease with atorvastatin in type 2 diabetes in the collaborative atorvastatin diabetes study (CARDS): multicentre randomized placebo-controlled trial *Lancet* 2004; 364:685–696.

40. Dawson-Hughes B. "Vitamin D." In: Bennett D, Plum F, eds. *Cecil Textbook of Medicine.* Philadelphia: WB Saunders, 1996:1357–1359.

41. Spiegel A. The parathyroid glands, hypercalcemia and hypocalcemia. In: Bennett D, Plum F, eds. *Cecil Textbook of Medicine.* Philadelphia: WB Saunders, 1996:1365–1373.

42. Bauman W, Zhong Y, Schwartz E. Vitamin D deficiency in veterans with chronic spinal cord injury. *Metabolism* 1995; 44:1612–1616.

43. Mechanik J, Pomerantz F, Flanagan S. Parathyroid hormone suppression in spinal cord injury patients is associated with the degree of neurologic impairment and not the level of injury. *Arch Phys Med Rehabil* 1997; 78:642–646

44. Kedlaya D, Brandstater M, Lee J. Immobilization hypercalcemia in incomplete paraplegia: Successful treatment with pamidronate. *Arch Phys Med Rehabil* 1998; 79:222–225.

45. Kaya K, Aybay C, Ozel, S. Evaluation of bone mineral density in patients with spinal cord injury. *J Spinal Cord Med.* 2006; 29:346–401

46. Pearson E, Nance P, Leslie W, et al. Cyclical etidronate: Its effect on bone density in patients with acute spinal cord injury. *Arch Phys Med Rehabil* 1998; 79:269–272.

47. Nance P, Schryvers O, Leslie W, Ludwig S, Krahn J, et. al Intravenous pamidronate attenuates bone density loss after acute spinal cord injury. *Arch Phys Med Rehabil* 1999; 80:243–251.

48. Bhasin S. "Testicular disorders". In: Kronenberg, M, ed. *Williams Textbook of Endocrinology* 11th ed. Philadelphia: Saunders, 2008:645–694.

49. Bulun S, Adushi E. "The physiology and pathology of the female reproductive axis". In: Kronenberg, M, ed. *Williams Textbook of Endocrinology,* 11th ed. Philadelphia: Saunders, 2008:541–614.

50. Nance P, Shears A, Givne H, et al. Gonadal regulation in men with flaccid paraplegia. *Arch Phys Med Rehabil* 1985; 66:757–759.

51. Monga M, Bernie J, Rajasekaran M. Male infertility and erectile dysfunction in spinal cord injury—a review. *Arch Phys Med Rehabil* 1999; 80:1331–1339.

52. Nosek M, Rintala D, Young M, Howland C, et al. Sexual functioning among women with physical disabilities. *Arch Phys Med Rehabil* 1996; 77:107–115.

53. Hulley, S, Grady D, Bush T, et al. Randomized trial of estrogen plus progestin for secondary prevention of coronary heart disease in post menopausal women. *JAMA* 1998; 280:605–613.

54. Writing Group for the Women's Health Institute Investigators. Risks and benefits of estrogen plus progestin in healthy post menopausal women. *JAMA* 2002; 288:321–333.

55. Spungen A, Grimm D, Strakhan M, et al. Treatment with an anabolic steroid is associated with improvement in respiratory function in person with tetraplegia. *Mt. Sinai J Med* 1999; 66:201–205.

23 Primary Care for Persons with Spinal Cord Injury

James K. Schmitt
John David McGurl
Meena Midha

The medical care of an individual can be likened to the performance of an orchestra, with each instrument representing a healthcare provider. When we are young, the number of instruments is relatively few and may consist only of a pediatrician and a nurse. As we grow older, the orchestra enlarges, and in our old age may include such members as a cardiologist, rheumatologist, oncologist, and geriatrician. The conductor of the orchestra is the primary care provider who determines which other providers the patient requires. The primary care provider is usually the first one whom the patient sees when he is ill. This individual may be an internist, family practitioner, or nurse practitioner. The care of the spinal cord injury (SCI) patient is usually more complex than that of the ambulatory patient and requires an orchestra of rehabilitation specialists, nurses, neurologists, social workers, and many others. The work of the primary care provider of the SCI patient is therefore more complicated than that of the provider of care for ambulatory patients. Many people with disabilities have difficulty finding a physician who is knowledgeable about their healthcare needs (1).

The primary care provider for an SCI patient varies. It may be a neurologist, rehab physician, internist, family practitioner, nurse practitioner, or physician assistant in private practice. However, because of the complexity of SCI patients, a large proportion of SCI patients receive their primary care in SCI centers, such as exist in Veterans' Affairs medical centers. The provider is usually a physician specifically trained in the care of SCI patients. In 48% of patients with SCI, their rehabilitation physician is considered their primary care provider (2). SCI patients are often at a disadvantage in managed care systems (3). Managed care favors the care of patients who are basically well. Such patients require only preventive medicine, such as blood pressure and serum cholesterol determinations. Patients with chronic disabling processes, such as spinal cord disease, are at increased risk for deterioration in their health. Managed care organizations often underestimate the healthcare needs of such patients, inappropriately limiting their length of stay in hospitals and providing fewer resources than are necessary for optimum

medical care. In this regard, federally sponsored institutions such as VA SCI centers seem to be more patient-friendly than private institutions.

Spinal cord disease often has a devastating impact on the physical, psychological and social well being of its victims. SCI increases many of the risk factors for disease, and its victims have a narrower margin of health than the general population (4, 5). Impaired ventilation and cough in tetraplegics predisposes these patients to pneumonia, mucus plugging, and ventilatory failure. Injuries to the thoracic cord may result in impaired cough and a predisposition to pneumonia.

The loss of mobility results in pressure sores, osteomyelitis, osteoporosis, and heterotopic ossification. Increased reliance on the upper extremities may result in the upper extremity overuse syndrome. (5) Inactivity predisposes to obesity, which results in low HDL cholesterol and diabetes mellitus (6). Cardiovascular disease is the major cause of death in SCI patients. (7) Impaired sensation results in a propensity to injury from a variety of sources including foreign bodies, trauma, and burns. Silent myocardial ischemia in the tetraplegic may delay the diagnosis of coronary disease (7). The first manifestation of coronary disease may be congestive heart failure. The disruption of the autonomic nervous system is close to being unique to spinal cord injury. Autonomic dysreflexia results in paroxysms of hypertension, which may be life threatening. Autonomic dysreflexia may mimic conditions ranging from essential hypertension to pheochromocytoma (8). Impaired micturition results in infection and vesicoureteral reflux, which in turn results in chronic renal failure (9). Chronic indwelling catheters predispose to bladder stones and malignancy. Impaired sexual performance and fertility are common complaints in the SCI population. Prolonged recumbency, obesity, delayed gastric emptying, and use of medications such as diazepam and anticholinergics results in gastroesophageal reflux disease. Cholelithiasis occurs more commonly in patients with SCI, as may gastrointestinal pseudo-obstruction. SCI patients are on more medications (10) than ambulatory patients, which results in an increased risk for drug interactions. SCI patients have a relative increase in body water, resulting in an increased volume of distribution for water-soluble drugs such as gentamycin. The increased volume of distribution means that larger loading doses are required, and clearance may be delayed in patients who may already have impaired clearance from chronic renal failure.

Sir Ludwig Guttman stated that "of the many forms of disability which can beset mankind, a severe injury or disease of the SCI undoubtedly constitutes one of the most devastating calamities of human life." SCI patients are commonly depressed, have chronic pain, and are unemployed. Sometimes these problems can be managed by the primary care provider. However, often psychiatrists, psychologists, social workers, and other professionals may be required. The diagnosis and treatment of the many conditions seen by the primary care provider is described in other chapters of this book.

One of the primary duties of the primary care provider is encouragement of behavior that prevents disease. The SCI patient and his provider may falsely assume that the patient is already too infirm for preventive medicine to make a difference. The most important health promoting behaviors are proper nutrition, weight control, smoking cessation, stress management, physical fitness, elimination of drug and alcohol abuse, disease and injury prevention, development of social support, and surveillance (11).

PERIODIC EVALUATION OF THE SPINAL CORD INJURY PATIENT

At the time of the annual evaluation, a complete physical examination should be performed, including a dental exam and tonometry to screen for glaucoma. The neurologic examination of spinal cord disease is described in another chapter.

US Recommended Adult Immunization Schedule

VACCINE	AGE GROUP		
	19-49 years	50-64 years	>65 years
Tetanus, diphtheria, pertussis (Td/Tdap)	1 dose Td booster every 10 years		
	Substitute 1 dose of Tdap for Td		
Human papillomavirus (HPV)	3 doses (females)		
Measles, mumps, rubella (MMR)	1 or 2 doses	1 dose	
Varicella	2 doses (0, 4-8 wks)	2 doses (0, 4-8 wks)	
Influenza	1 dose annually	1 dose annually	
Pneumococcal (polysaccharide)	1-2 doses		1 dose
Hepatitis A	2 doses, (0, 6-12 mos, or 0, 6-18 mos)		
Hepatitis B	3 doses (0, 1-2, 4-6 mos)		
Meningococcal	1 or more doses		

 For all persons in this category who meet the age requirements and who lack evidence of immunity (e.g., Lack documentation of vaccination or have no evidence of prior infection).

Recommended if some other risk factor is present (e.g., On the basis of medical, occupational, lifestyle or other indications).

Figure 23.1 U.S. Recommended Adult Immunization Schedule, modified from the recommendations of the Advisory Committee on Immunization Practices, the American College Obstetricians and Gynecologists, and the American Academy of Family Physicians, October 1, 2006.

Immunizations

Primarily because of respiratory compromise and impaired cough, SCI patients are at increased risk for pulmonary infections. When pneumonia occurs, it is more likely to be fatal. Immunization is probably the most cost-effective health measure provided for SCI patients. The standard recommendation for pneumococcal vaccination is that it be given to adults with cardiovascular disease, pulmonary disease, diabetes mellitus, alcoholism, cirrhosis, asplenia, chronic renal failure, HIV, hematologic malignancies, and to high-risk populations such as some native Americans, institutionalized patients, and all adults aged 65 or over (12, 13). SCI patients often fall into one or more of the above categories, and it is the authors' opinion that pneumococcal vaccination should be performed in the majority of SCI patients. A second dose of pneumococcal vaccine should be considered 6 or more years later for adults at high risk of disease and in patients who lose antibody rapidly (nephrotic syndrome, renal failure, transplant recipients). Influenza vaccination should be given annually to patients at high risk for complications such as pneumonia, and to institutionalized patients and healthcare workers.

High-risk patients include patients with chronic cardiopulmonary disorders and patients with chronic diseases, such as diabetes mellitus and chronic renal disease. Hepatitis B immunization is achieved through three doses given over a 6-month period. Hepatitis A immunization should be administered to high-risk populations such as international travelers, intravenous drug users, and homosexuals. A schedule of immunizations is shown in Figure 23.1 (13). TB skin testing should be performed at least annually in high-risk patients. These include residents and staffs of long-term care facilities, individuals with chronic diseases such as renal failure and diabetes mellitus, patients taking steroids or immunosuppressive agents, alcoholics and users of intravenous drugs, and the contacts of infectious TB cases.

PULMONARY EVALUATION

Routine chest X-rays are not recommended. Only if a patient has symptoms of pneumonia, congestive heart failure, or other pulmonary problems, is chest X-ray indicated. Of all cancer deaths, 30% are from lung cancer. (14) Screening chest X-rays for lung cancer in smokers have not been shown to significantly increase survival and are not recommended. Likewise, routine spirometry is not recommended. In patients with COPD or other chronic pulmonary diseases, spirometry should be done to follow the course of the disease (4).

The spiral CT scan has the ability to detect pulmonary lesions at an early stage, thereby improving survival from lung cancer (14, 15). Even though the cost of screening with spiral CT increases; it seems to be cost effective. However, this technique has not yet attained widespread acceptance.

Dermatological Examination

The pressure sore is the most common cutaneous problem encountered in the SCI patient. As the longevity of SCI patients has increased, the incidence of pressure ulcers has increased (16, 17) A major source of morbidity and mortality is pressure ulcers, which should be searched for at each clinic visit. See Chapter 49 for further details.

Skin infections, such as cellulitis and intertrigo, are common in the SCI patient and require vigilant examination. Condom catheters may cause contact dermatitis, erosions, and maceration.

Malignancies such as melanoma and squamous cell and basal cell carcinoma should be searched for, especially in sun-exposed areas.

CARDIOVASCULAR DISORDERS

The risk factors for coronary artery disease include smoking, male gender over 45, hypertension, diabetes mellitus, chronic renal disease, and low HDL cholesterol. Family history of coronary events should be evaluated (2, 3). Diabetes mellitus and low HDL are more common in SCI patients than in the general population. A normal blood pressure for an SCI patient is 140/90 or below. A fasting lipid profile should be obtained yearly. The target LDL cholesterol is 160 mg/dl if one or fewer risk factors are present. With two or more risk factors, the target LDL cholesterol is below 130 mg/dl. If the patient has known coronary disease, diabetes mellitus, or chronic renal disease, the target LDL cholesterol is l00 mg/dl. In view of the potential for multiple risk factors for coronary disease, the determination of the lipid profile is a key part of annual screening. If diet fails, drugs such as HMG COA reductase inhibitors should be used to achieve cholesterol goals.

An ECG should be done annually to provide a baseline. ECG screening is more important in the SCI patient than in the ambulatory patient because the SCI patient may have silent myocardial ischemia. If the ECG suggests coronary disease, or the patient has symptoms such as chest pain or dyspnea, a full cardiac evaluation should be done. A chest X-ray may show cardiomegaly and pulmonary congestion secondary to silent infarction. Exercise tolerance testing can be done in paraplegics with arm crank ergometry. However, nuclear studies such as persantin-thallium scans can be used to assess risk for ischemia in tetraplegics and paraplegics. Catheterization is the gold standard for assessing coronary artery patency.

Case Study

A 58-year-old C6 tetraplegic was noted to have pedal edema and bibasilar rales at his periodic evaluation. He denied chest pain but he noted that he was a little more dyspneic than usual. An ECG showed Q-waves in V1—V4 consistent with an old anterior wall myocardial infarction. A chest X-ray showed cardiomegaly and pulmonary congestion. A cardiac catheterization was performed and showed extensive four-vessel coronary disease and an ejection fraction of 15%. Percutaneous transcoronary angioplasty (PTCA) was performed. A fasting lipid profile showed a total cholesterol of 240 mg/dl, with an LDL cholesterol of 180 mg, an HDL cholesterol of 20 mg/dl, and a VLDL cholesterol of 40 mg/dl. He was placed on furosemide 40 mg and lisinopril 10 mg to control his congestive heart failure and lovastatin 20 mg/per day to control serum lipids. His symptoms improved and his serum cholesterol declined to 110 mg/dl.

Discussion

This man's sensory deficit prevented chest pain, thus resulting in a silent myocardial infarction with subsequent congestive heart failure. The high LDL cholesterol and low HDL cholesterol put him at high risk for coronary disease.

HYPERTENSION

Hypertension is usually treated by the primary care practitioner rather than by a subspecialist (18, 19). The presence of hypertension compounds the damage done by other cardiovascular risk factors. Tetraplegics are somewhat protected from the development of hypertension by sympathetic underactivity. However, obesity and inactivity result in an increase in the incidence of hypertension in paraplegics. Yekutiel and others (19) found that 34% of patients with SCI had hypertension, as compared to 18.6% of ambulatory control subjects. Hypertension in patients with an intact neuroaxis may be defined as a diastolic blood pressure of greater that 85 to 90 mmHg or systolic blood pressure greater than 140 mmHg. It seems reasonable to accept this value as the upper limit of normal blood pressure for a paraplegic subject. The baseline blood pressure in tetraplegic persons is 90 to 110/56 to 70 mmHg. However, there is no evidence that the level of blood pressure requiring treatment in a tetraplegic should be lower than that in a paraplegic or ambulatory person. The goal of treatment in most patients is to bring the blood pressure below 140/85 to 90 mmHg. However, in certain patients (diabetic patients, patients with renal insufficiency, and patients with congestive heart failure), the goal blood pressure is 130/80 mmHg. These conditions often occur in SCI patients.

Hypertension is divided into stages (18). Patients with Stage 1 hypertension have diastolic blood pressure of 90 to 99 mmHg. Patients with Stage 2 hypertension have a diastolic blood pressure of 100 to 109 mmHg, and patients with diastolic blood pressures above 109 have Stage 3 hypertension. However, there is increasing evidence that an elevated systolic blood pressure imparts a greater cardiovascular risk than elevated diastolic blood pressure. (18) The pulse pressure, which is the difference between systolic and diastolic blood pressure, seems to be a major predictor of risk for conditions such as congestive heart failure. Obviously, the more severe the hypertension, the more aggressive the treatment must be. For example, a patient with a blood pressure of 145/89 mmHg could be initially treated with diet and exercise and seen at 3-month intervals. A patient with a blood pressure of 188/110 mmHg may need to be started on medication immediately and reevaluated in 1 to 2 weeks. Paraplegics whose sympathetic nervous systems are largely spared are most likely to be hypertensive. The algorithm for treatment of hypertension in these patients is therefore similar to that in ambulatory patients (18). Before treatment of hypertension is initiated, secondary causes, including autonomic dysreflexia, renal artery stenosis, chronic renal failure, hyperaldosteronism, and pheochromocytoma should be ruled out. Reduction of caffeine and alcohol intake, and cessation of tobacco use may decrease blood pressure.

Treatment of hypertension should be initiated with restriction of sodium, weight reduction in overweight individuals, and if possible, exercise. Remember that the ideal weight of a paraplegic is 80% that of an ambulatory patient of the same height, and that of a tetraplegic is only 60% of his ambulatory counterpart. Arm exercise can be performed in paraplegic and low tetraplegic persons. In persons with complete cord lesions above C5, functional electrical stimulation may be used to facilitate exercise. Moderate sodium restriction (120 meq/day) for 6

months lowers systolic blood pressure in ambulatory persons by an average of 8 mmHg and diastolic blood pressure by an average of 5 mmHg (20). Diet and exercise would seem to be less useful measures for lowing blood pressure in SCI patients than in ambulatory patients.

If several months of nonpharmacologic therapy fail to control blood pressure, medication should be initiated. Available data prove that lowering blood pressure with thiazide diuretics, beta blockers, and calcium channel blockers reduces overall mortality and morbidity for strokes and heart attack (18). Furthermore, thiazides and beta blockers are relatively inexpensive. Low-dose diuretics are as effective or more effective as first line therapy in prevention of cardiovascular events (21). Therefore, if there is no indication for other agents, these agents should be used initially to control hypertension in SCI patients. Renal failure found commonly in SCI patients makes thiazides ineffective as antihypertensives. A recent meta-analysis has found that beta blockers were less effective in preventing stroke than other medications (22).

Hydrochlorthiazide or chlorthalidone dosed at 12.5 to 50 mg per day may be begun. Alternatively, a beta blocker may be started, such as metoprolol (50 mg per day; maximum dose 300 mg/day) or propranolol (40 mg per day; maximum dose 480 mg/day). Thiazide diuretics may worsen diabetes mellitus. SCI patients are at risk for hyponatremia, especially when placed on thiazide diuretics (23). Beta blockers are contraindicated in asthma and COPD, because they may cause bronchospasm. Certain types of patients may have compelling indications for specific classes of drugs. Diabetics, especially those with proteinuria, require ACE inhibitors for renal protection, which may be even more important in the SCI patient whose renal function may be compromised by conditions such as chronic pyelonephritis. Patients with a history of myocardial infarction require beta blockers. However, beta blockers may exacerbate bradycardia and impair recognition of and recovery from hypoglycemia in insulin-treated diabetics. Peripheral alpha blockers, such as prazosin, have the advantage of reducing urethral sphincter tone, but may also cause postural hypotension.

Calcium channel blockers, which were initially introduced as antianginal agents, may in theory provide special benefits to SCI patients (18). Dihydropyridine calcium channel blockers are predominantly vasodilators. The first-generation agents, such as nifedipine, have a modest effect on cardiovascular contractility. Second-generation agents, such as amlodipine, have essentially no effect on myocardial contractility. SCI patients may have decreased cardiac output secondary to myocardial ischemia, which is often silent. Dihydropyridine calcium channel blockers have the advantage of improving cardiac output while lowering blood pressure. Nondihydropyridine calcium channel blockers, such as diltiazem, decrease myocardial contractility. By impairing cardiac contractility and inhibiting atrioventricular conduction, they may be cardioprotective. Short-acting calcium channel blockers (such as nifedipine) increase cardiovascular events when used to treat hypertension (24). However, long-acting calcium channel blockers (such as amlodipine and verapamil) do not share these possible dangers.

If there is no response to the medication, or troublesome side effects occur, another medication should be substituted. If there is an inadequate response to medication, but the medication is well tolerated, a second agent should be added. If the initial drug is not a diuretic, a diuretic should be added. Diuretics work synergistically with other agents. For example, diuretics decrease plasma volume, thereby making the patient more sensitive to the effects of ACE inhibitors.

When hypertension is noted in a tetraplegic patient, autonomic dysreflexia should be considered before a commitment is made to chronic pharmacologic treatment. Loss of sympathetic tone results in increased reliance on the renin-angiotensin system to maintain blood pressure, especially when hypovolemia has been induced by a diuretic. Angiotensin-converting enzyme inhibitors may therefore induce profound hypotension in tetraplegic subjects and should be avoided or used with extreme caution in these patients (25).

LABORATORY VALUES

A complete blood count (CBC) should be ordered to detect processes such as anemia, infection, and drug-related thrombocytopenia. Electrolytes, blood urea nitrogen (BUN), and creatinine should be measured and a fasting lipid profile should be determined. Blood levels of medications such as digoxin and phenytoin should be determined when indicated, and liver function tests should be performed with use of medications such as the statins. SCI patients are at increased risk for carbohydrate intolerance (8). A fasting serum glucose should be obtained yearly. Diabetes mellitus is defined by fasting serum glucose of 126 mg/dl or higher or a random glucose of 200 mg/dl or higher.

The medical literature suggests that elevation of homocysteine levels predicts coronary events. However, there is no evidence that reducing homocysteine levels with folic acid reduces coronary events. Routine determination of the serium homocysteine level is therefore not recommended. (26)

A body of evidence suggests that coronary events are in part due to inflammation. However, no well-conducted study has found that treatment of infection with an antibiotic reduces risk of cardiovascular events. The routine measurement of C-Reactive Protein (CRP) is therefore not recommended (26). Routine HIV testing is cost-effective (27). However, the test requires time spent counseling, especially if it is positive.

DIABETES MELLITUS

In diabetic patients, the hemoglobin A1C level should be measured at each clinic visit. Ideally, the hemoglobin AlC should be below 7 mg/dl. Fundoscopic examination by an ophthalmologist, optometrist, or retinal photos should be performed annually. A complete foot exam should be performed and referral to a podiatrist made when indicated. In ambulatory diabetics, foot sensation is evaluated with a monofilament to detect neuropathy. This is often not possible in SCI patients.

For a detailed analysis of diabetes mellitus in the SCI patient, please see Chapter 22.

DEPRESSION

Depression occurs with increased frequency in SCI patients (28). Depressed people are more likely to develop myelopathy from mechanisms such as suicide attempts, and SCI often results in depression. Depressed mood, despondency, and grief are common reactions to serious illness. Grief includes depressed mood, anger, guilt, anxiety, hopelessness, and despair. Grief may last 2 years or more.

For further details, see Chapter 77.

Case Study

A 28-year-old C5 tetraplegic noted difficulty concentrating and failing college grades. Psychologic testing revealed impaired recent memory. A further interview revealed that he met the DSM IV criteria for major affective disorder. He had a strong family history of depression. He was placed on antidepressant medication and improved.

Discussion

The symptom that prompted attention was impaired cognitive functioning. However, careful questioning revealed other criteria for the diagnosis of depression.

COLORECTAL CANCER SCREENING

SCI patients are probably not at increased risk for colorectal cancer, but symptoms such as constipation are more difficult to interpret. The American Cancer Society recommends fecal occult blood testing to be done annually for all asymptomatic individuals beginning at age 50 (29, 30). This has been reported to reduce mortality from colon cancer by one-third. The American Cancer Society and the American College of Physicians recommend that patients of normal risk be screened with sigmoidoscopy every 3 to 5 years beginning at 50 years of age (A 35-cm flexible sigmoidoscopy can reach 45% to 50% of cancers and a 60-cm sigmoidoscope can reach 50% to 60%). The American College of Physicians states that performance of an air-contrast barium enema (ACBE) every 5 years is an alternative to sigmoidoscopy. However, barium enema has low sensitivity for detecting large polyps. When fecal hemoccult is positive, flexible sigmoidoscopy combined with ACBE should be done. The sigmoidoscope can better evaluate the rectum, which may be obscured in the ACBE. Alternatively, colonoscopy should be performed.

Colonoscopy is increasingly recommended as the screening procedure of choice for colorectal malignancy (30, 31). Colonoscopy allows visualization of the entire colon and is superior to ACBE in detecting polyps. First-degree relatives of victims of colon cancer at age 50 or younger should have colonoscopy or ACBE every 5 years beginning at 35 to 40 years of age. Virtual colonoscopy, which may be more convenient for the spinal cord injury, involves a computerized image of the colon. The sensitivity for detecting lesions larger than 1cm is high. However, the false positive rate is also high, although with improving technology the false positive rate is declining (31).

Case Study

A 58-year-old C6 tetraplegic underwent yearly evaluation using flexible sigmoidoscopy. Tests performed every three years for the preceding nine years had been normal. Fecal occult blood tests, which had previously been negative, became positive. Colonoscopy was performed and a constricting adenocarcinoma was found at 70 cm. The cancer was removed at laparotomy.

Discussion

Fecal occult blood testing was negative for years despite the presence of cancer. The tumor was beyond the range of the flexible sigmoidoscope, so that colonoscopy would probably have allowed earlier diagnosis of the malignancy.

GENITOURINARY SYSTEM

The SCI patient is at increased risk for deterioration of renal function, which is a major cause of death in these patients (5, 9). The most important cause of renal complications is impaired voiding, resulting in increased bladder pressure and vesicoureteral reflux. Other factors, such as infection, renal stones, and increased use of nephrotoxic medication, also contribute. The serum creatinine level is a poor predictor of renal function, especially in the SCI patient. The Cockcroft-Gault equation (32) estimates the creatinine clearance:

$$\text{Creatinine clearance} = \frac{(140 - \text{age}) \times \text{body wt (kg)}}{72 \times \text{serum creatinine (mg/dl)}}$$

The use of nomograms developed for the SCI patient improves the estimation of creatinine clearance, because the creatinine clearance can be directly determined. The timed renal excretion of creatinine over several hours estimates the 24-hour creatinine clearance with reasonable accuracy.

The annual assessment of renal function should include 24-hour creatinine clearance, or radioisotope renal scan. Renal ultrasound or KUB should be performed annually to assess the size and morphology of kidneys. Enlarged kidneys indicate acute renal disease or postrenal obstruction. Small kidneys indicate chronic renal disease.

Intravenous pyelograms are not required unless there is a specific indication, such as the localization of a renal stone. Patients with indwelling catheters are at increased risk for bladder cancer (33, 34). Cystoscopy is therefore recommended after 10 years of use of an indwelling catheter. Other indications for cystoscopy are the presence of risk factors such as smoking, frequent urinary tract infections, or hematuria or other evidence of cancer. Prostate cancer occurs with no higher frequency in SCI patients than in ambulatory patients, but is the most common cancer in older men (35).

A digital rectal exam should be performed annually in males over 40. At the time of the digital rectal exam, the prostate should be examined for nodularity and size.

The utility of prostate specific antigen (PSA) screening for the diagnosis of prostate cancer is uncertain. The presence of prosthetic devices or indwelling catheters, which are common in SCI patients, increases the PSA. The determination of PSA has not been shown to decrease mortality from prostate cancer. Many elderly patients who have subclinical prostate cancer die of other causes. The surgical treatment of prostate cancer has a high incidence of the complications of impotence and urinary incontinence, although these complications may be less of an issue in SCI patients. The patient should be counseled about prostate cancer yearly at age 50 and PSA testing should be offered. An elevated PSA and/or a nodule on digital rectal exam must prompt a GU referral. In patients with colostomies whose rectums are closed, digital exam of the prostate can't be performed.

Case Study

A 53-year-old T4 paraplegic was found to have a decreased creatinine clearance of 40 cc/min at annual screening (the prior creatinine clearance had been 90 cc per min). The patient emptied his bladder by reflex voiding. Urinalysis showed many WBCs, RBCs, protein, and RBC casts. Renal ultrasound showed kidneys increased in size with no evidence of reflux. Post-void residual urine volume was 20 cc.

Antistreptolysin O titer was elevated and the diagnosis of post-streptococcal glomerulonephritis was made. The patient then recalled that several months earlier he had had a throat infection. He was placed on prednisone and renal function rapidly improved.

Discussion

The relatively sudden decline in creatinine clearance signaled a problem. Postvoiding residual volume was normal, making vesicoureteral reflux unlikely. Enlarged kidneys on ultrasound and red cell casts in the urine sediment suggested intrinsic renal disease. For a detailed discussion of the genitourinary problems of SCI patients, see appropriate chapters.

SUBSTANCE ABUSE

SCI patients are probably at increased risk for substance abuse (36, 37). Indeed, substance abuse, such as alcoholism, may cause the injury through events such as drunk driving. Chronic pain increases the risk of substance abuse. Smoking is the leading cause of preventable death in the United States. Smoking cessation is the single most important counseling topic. The health risk of tobacco smoking is greater in SCI patients, especially tetraplegics, than in the general population. Impaired ventilation and cough predispose to pneumonia, and the risk is made even greater by smoking. Obstructive lung disease superimposed on the restrictive disease in tetraplegics accelerates the progression to ventilator dependence and death. Second-hand smoke is probably a greater risk to SCI patients than to ambulatory patients.

Smoking cessation should be discussed at each visit that the patient makes. If the patient wishes to quit, nicotine patches and gum or drugs such as bupropion may be prescribed and referral to a smoking cessation clinic made. Obtaining a urine drug screen at the time of a clinic provides proof that the patient is not using elicit drugs and is using the medication that is prescribed.

The substance abuse history begins with questions about nonthreatening subjects. Then the subject moves to questions about legal and illegal substances, such as the number of drinks taken per day. There are several questionnaires available to aid in this process. The briefest of the instruments is the CAGE Questionnaire, which has 85% sensitivity and 89% specificity (37):

1. Have you ever felt you ought to Cut down on drinking?
2. Have people Annoyed by you criticized your drinking?
3. Have you ever felt bad or Guilty about your drinking?
4. Have you ever had a drink first thing in the morning to steady your nerves or get rid of a hangover (Eye-opener)?

One yes response should raise the suspicion of alcohol abuse. More than one "yes" response should be considered a strong indicator that alcohol abuse exists. Other screening questionnaires include the CAGE AID Questionnaire, the Alcohol Use Disorders Identification Test, the Michigan Alcoholism Screening Test (MAST), and the Drug Abuse Screening Test (DAST). If screening for alcohol or other drug abuse is positive, referral for rehabilitation should be considered. Obtaining a urine drug screen at the time of a clinic visit provides proof that the patient is not using elicit drugs and is using the medication that is prescribed.

Case Study

A 38-year-old C7 complete tetraplegic was noted to be tremulous and tachycardic to 120 beats per minute at his primary care visit. Blood pressure was 160/80. The diagnosis of autonomic dysreflexia was considered. However, upon questioning, the patient reported that he consumed two six-packs of beer per day for the past several months and had stopped drinking only two days before his clinic visit.

The diagnosis of alcohol withdrawal syndrome was made. He was placed on diazepam and referred for alcohol rehab.

Discussion

Alcoholics occasionally stop drinking before a clinic visit, or at the time of hospitalization, so that the alcohol withdrawal syndrome results. This can be mistaken for sepsis, myocardial infarction, or other acute illness, or, in the case of tetraplegics, autonomic dysreflexia. Other clues that alcoholism is present include abnormal liver function tests and a high mean red blood cell volume.

WOMEN'S HEALTH ISSUES

Women with SCI have a higher incidence of amenorrhea and infertility than ambulatory women. The death rate from cervical cancer has dropped dramatically since the advent of the Pap smear. The American Cancer Society (29) recommends that all women have annual Pap smears at the onset of sexual activity or at 18 years of age. After a woman has had three or more consecutive normal annual examinations, the Pap test may be performed less frequently. The American College of Physicians recommends that sexually active women between the ages of 25 and 65 years be screened with a Pap smear every 3 years.

The pelvic examination in women with SCI is technically more difficult and for that reason may be neglected. At the time of the pelvic exam, a rectal exam and bimanual exam of the pelvis should be performed. Enlargement of an ovary may mean a cyst, or, especially in the post-menopausal patient, cancer.

Breast cancer is the most common cancer among American women. Major risk factors are age over 50 and a first-degree relative with breast cancer. The early detection of breast cancer significantly decreases the mortality. Recommendations vary, but yearly breast examination seems appropriate. Mammography is the most effective means of the early detection of breast cancer, with sensitivities of 70% to 90% and specificity of 90% to 95%.

Most major authorities (38) recommend annual mammography screening for women 50 and older. The American Cancer Society and American College of Obstetricians and Gynecologists recommend a screening mammogram every 1 to 2 years in women 40 to 49 years of age.

If menopause is present, the woman may be considered for estrogen replacement. From theoretical considerations, estrogen replacement may be even more important in women with SCI than in ambulatory women. Estrogen prevents bone loss, which may be accelerated in SCI. Estrogen also increases the HDL level, which may be low in women with SCI. However, prospective studies have failed to show a cardio-protective effect of estrogen-progesterone. In fact, the risk of cardiac events was increased (39, 40). Estrogen treatment is not recommended for the prevention of coronary artery disease.

NUTRITIONAL EVALUATION

SCI patients are at increased risk for nutritional problems (8, 41). Inactivity promotes muscle wasting and adiposity. The daily caloric requirement for a paraplegic should be based on an ideal body weight that is 5% to 10% below standard. The ideal body weight for a tetraplegic is 10% to 15% less than standard. Diets that don't take this into account may cause obesity. If obesity is present, diet and increased exercise, if feasible, should be initiated.

The SCI patient may also be at risk for malnutrition. The reduced ability to buy food, the inability to feed oneself, and even caretaker abuse may cause malnutrition. The SCI patient is at greater risk for illness, which increases catabolism. At the time of the periodic evaluation, the patient should be asked if he is following any prescribed diet. A recent weight loss or gain of 10 pounds or more should prompt a search for the cause. The most useful element of the physical examination for assessing nutrition is body weight. By using the height, the ideal body weight can be determined from tables. The Body Mass Index, which is weight in kilograms divided by the height in meters squared, is useful because it is independent of height and gender. The loss of subcutaneous fat and muscle is difficult to interpret in SCI patients. The use of skinfold thickness calipers to define triceps skinfold (TSF) thickness is the most practical technique to estimate body fat. From the triceps skinfold thickness, the arm muscle circumference may be calculated from the following formula:

$$AMC \ (cm) = Arm \ circumference - TSF \ (cm)$$

The AMC and TSF may be used to estimate nutritional status. The AMC and TSF are useful in defining marasmic type malnutrition or mixed disorders. Although tissue wasting below the level of injury may be difficult to interpret in SCI patients, the AMC and TSF provide useful information in patients whose lesions spare the arm musculature. Hypoalbuminema is a marker for malnutrition. Reduced levels of other proteins such as transferrin, prealbumin, and retinol-binding protein also are associated with malnutrition, but the levels of these proteins don't predict risk for malnutrition any better than serum albumin.

PAIN

Pain is now regarded as the fifth vital sign. Two-thirds of SCI patients complain of pain (42). Pain is classified as nociceptive pain, which is caused by a noxious impulse, and neuropathic pain, which is caused by damage to a nerve. Local pain at the level of spinal injury is nociceptive in nature. Diffuse burning or aching pain below the level of injury, which is the most common type of pain in patients with SCI, is neuropathic. See Chapter 38 for more information on pain management.

SPASTICITY

More than 75% of SCI patients have spasticity one year after discharge (5). An increase in spasticity may signal the presence of an exacerbating factor such as syringomyelia, infection, or decubitus ulcer. Spasticity may be treated with stretching exercises and medication including baclofen, benzodiazepines, and dantroline. For more information on treating spasticity in the SCI patient, see Chapter 40.

MUSCULOSKETAL DISORDERS

SCI patients are prone to the same rheumatologic and orthopedic disorders as ambulatory patients (43, 44). Disorders coming from overuse of the lower extremities are reduced in incidence, but overuse of the upper extremities is more common in the SCI patient.

Underuse results in osteoporosis and predisposes to fracture (43). Osteoporosis may, in part, be prevented by calcium and vitamin D supplements, and by bisphosphonates such as pamidronate. Periodic bone mineral density determination is useful, especially in post-menopausal women.

Heterotopic ossification (HO) involves only areas below the neurologic defect (45). It most commonly involves areas that are adjacent to the hips and knees. It begins with localized swelling and inflammation, which progresses to ossification and calcification. HO may be mistaken for thrombophlebitis, cellulitis, and joint infection. HO may be prevented by range-of-motion exercises and bisphosphonates.

The shoulder is the primary joint for transfer or ambulation by wheelchair or crutches. Shoulder pain and limitation of motion may signal the development of subdeltoid bursitis, bicipital tendonitis, and rotator cuff tear (45). The major goals of management are preservation of function and pain reduction. Reduction of work through the use of devices, such as electric wheelchairs, and the use of nonsteroidal anti-inflammatory drugs (NSAIDs) and steroid injections can reduce inflammation and prevent functional loss.

Case Study

A 56-year-old man with C6–C7 tetraplegia from a fall 1 year earlier presented for his annual evaluation. He complained of swelling and pain in his hands during the prior 2 months. Radiographs of the hands and wrists revealed cystic changes, and a bone scan demonstrated increased uptake in both wrists and hands. The diagnosis of reflex sympathetic dystrophy was made. Upon further questioning, the patient informed his provider that physical therapy following his injury had been delayed because of pneumonia.

Reflex sympathetic dystrophy presents as pain and swelling in an extremity, trophic skin changes, and the signs and symptoms of vasomotor instability. It may be prevented by early physical therapy.

PREVENTION OF ACCIDENTS AND VIOLENCE

Accidents and violence cause most spinal cord injuries. At their periodic evaluation, SCI patients should be questioned and counseled on the prevention of accidents. The wearing of seatbelts and the safe handling of firearms are important subjects for such discussions.

THE GERIATRIC SPINAL CORD INJURY PATIENT

The lifespan of the spinal cord injury patient is lengthening (46). This is due to improved treatment of and prevention of complications of spinal cord injury such as renal failure and ventilatory failure. In addition, there are advances that have improved the longevity of the American population as a whole. Some of these measures are use of statins, early intervention in the acute coronary syndrome by thrombolytics and percutaneous coronary angiography (PTCA), newer antibiotics, and improved treatment of cancer. The population explosion of "Baby Boomer Elderly" will be paralleled by increase in the numbers of "spinal cord elderly." The effects of aging on physiology will add to the impairments of spinal cord injury. Both conditions have an impact on cardiac, renal, neuromuscular, endocrine, rheumatologic, and other aspects of body function. The Primary Care provider must assess the ability of the patient to perform activities of daily living (ADLs) at each clinic visit.

The interacting effects of aging and spinal cord injury make care of the elderly spinal cord injury patient especially challenging.

CONCLUSION

The primary care of SCI patients is more complicated than that of ambulatory patients. SCI immediately impairs mobility, and ventilatory and autonomic function. Later, spinal injury affects the heart, kidneys, skin, and musculosketal system. The SCI patient has a narrower margin of health than ambulatory patients have. For this reason, preventive measures such as immunization to prevent influenza and pneumonia are more important in the SCI patient. Because of impaired sensation, the diagnosis of conditions such as the acute abdomen and myocardial infarction may be delayed. The primary care of SCI patients presents a continuing challenge. The providers of primary care to the SCI patient must be ever vigilant.

ACKNOWLEDGMENT

The authors are indebted to Mrs. Debbie Elder for her excellent secretarial work.

References

1. Batavia AJ, Dejong G, Burns TJ, Burns QW, Smith SM, Butler D. A managed care program for working age persons with physical disabilities: A feasibility study. Washington, D.C.: NRH Research Center, Robert Wood Johnson Foundation, 1989.
2. Bockenek WL, Bluzn JM. Health care needs assessment in a population with severe disability. Am J Phys Med Rehabil 1994; 73:144.
3. DeLisa JA, Kirshblum S. A review: Frustrations and needs in clinical care of SCI patients. J Spinal Cord Med 1997; 20:384—390.
4. Schmitt JK, Midha M, McKenzie N. Medical complications of spinal cord disease. In: Young R, Woolsey R, eds. Diagnosis and Management

of Disorders of the Spinal Cord. Philadelphia: WB Saunders, 1995; 297—316.

5. Ditunno JF, Formal CS. Chronic spinal cord injury. NEJM 1994; 33:550—556.

6. Brenes G, Dearwater MS, Shapero R., et al. High density lipoprotein cholesterol concentrations in physically active and sedentary spinal cord injured patients. Arch Phys Med Rehabil 1986; 76:445–450.

7. Walker WC, Khokar MS. Silent cardiac ischemia in cervical spinal cord injury. Case study. Arch Phys Med Rehabil 1992; 73:91.

8. Armenti-Kapros B, Nambiar P, Lippman H, et al. An unusual cause of autonomic dysreflexia; pheochromocytoma in an individual with tetraplegia. Spinal Cord Med 2003; Summer, 26:172–5.

9. Mayo ME, Bradley WE. The urinary bladder in spinal cord disease. In: Young R, Woolsey R, eds. Diagnosis and Management of Disorders of the Spinal Cord. Philadelphia: WB Saunders, 1995; 211–243.

10. Segal JL. Clinical pharmacology of spinal cord injury. In: Young R, Woolsey R, eds. Diagnosis and Management of Disorders of the Spinal Cord. Philadelphia: WB Saunders, 1995; 441–438.

11. Bockenek WI, Mann N, Lanig I, Dejong G, Beatty L, Delisa JA, Gaus BM, eds. Primary care for persons with disability. Philadelphia: Lippincott, 1998; 905–928.

12. Keusch G, Bart K, Miller M. Immunization principles and vaccine use. In Kasper G, ed. Harrison's Principles of Internal Medicine, 16th ed. New York: McGraw Hill, 2005; 713–725.

13. Recommended Adult Immunization Schedule United States, Oct 2006–Sep 2007. Approved by the Advisory Committee on Immunization Practices, the American College of Obstetricians and Gynecologists and the American Academy of Family Physicians.

14. Survival of patients with stage I lung cancer detected on CT screening. The International Early Lung Cancer Action Program. Investigators NEJM 2006; 355:1763–1771.

15. American College of Chest Physicians. Diagnosis and Management of Lung Cancer. ACCP evidence-based guidelines. Chest 2003; 123:15.

16. Krause J, Vines C, Farley T, Sniezek J, Coker J. An exploratory study of pressure ulcers after spinal cord injury. Relationship to protective behaviors and risk factors. Arch Phys Med Rehabil 2001; 82:107–113.

17. Garber S, Rintala D, Hart K, Fuhrer M. Pressure ulcer risk in spinal cord injury. Predictors of ulcer status over 3 years. Arch Phys Med Rehabil 2000; 81:465–471.

18. Chobanian A, Bakris G, Black H, et al. The Seventh Report of the Joint National Committee on Prevention of High Blood Pressure. The JNC 7 Report JAMA 2003; 289:2560–2572.

19. Yekutiel M, Brooks ME, Ohry A, et al. The prevalence of hypertension, ischemic heart disease, and diabetes in traumatic spinal cord injured patients and amputees. Paraplegia 1989; 27:58–62.

20. Omvik P, Myking OL. Unchanged central dynamics after six months of moderate sodium restriction with or without potassium supplementations in essential hypertension. Blood Pressure 1995; 4:32–41.

21. Psaty B, Lumley T, Furberg L. Health outcomes associated with various antihypertensives used as first line agents: a network metaanalysis. JAMA 2003; 284:2534–44.

22. Lindholm L, Carlberg B, Samuelsson, O. Should beta blockers remain the choice in the treatment of primary hypertension? A meta-analysis. Lancet 2005; 366:1543–53.

23. Stacy W, Midha M. The kidney in the spinal cord injury patient. Phys Med Rehabil 1987; 1:415–423.

24. Psaty BM, Heckbert SR, Koepsell TD, et al. The risk of myocardial infarction associated with antihypertensive drug therapy. JAMA 1995; 274:620–625.

25. Schmitt JK, Koch KS, Midha M. Profound hypotension in a tetraplegic patient following angiotensin-converting enzyme inhibitor, lisinopril. Paraplegia 1994; 32:871–874.

26. Libby P. Prevention and treatment of atherosclerosis. In Kasper, D et al., eds. Harrison's Principles of Internal Medicine, 16th ed. New York: McGraw Hill, 2005; pp1425–1433.

27. Sanders G, Bayoumi A, Sundaram V, et al. Cost-effectiveness of screening for HIV in the era of highly active antiretroviral therapy. N Eng J Med 2005; 352:570–585.

28. Kennedy P, Rogers B. Anxiety and depression after spinal cord injury: A longitudinal analysis. Arch Phys Med Rehabil 2000; 81:932–937.

29. American Cancer Society Guidelines for Early Detection of Cancer. American Cancer Society, Atlanta, Georgia, 2008.

30. Ransohoff D, Sandler R. Screening for colorectal cancer, NEJM 2002; 346:40–44.

31. Ransohoff D. Virtual colonoscopy—what it can do vs. what it will do. JAMA 2004; 291:1772–1774.

32. Cockroft DW, Gault MH. Prediction of creatinine clearance from serum creatinine. Nephron 1976; 16:31–41.

33. Navon JD, Soliman H, Khonsari F, et al. Screening cystoscopy and survival in spinal cord injury patients with squamous cell cancer of the bladder. J Urol 1997; 157:2109–2111.

34. Stonehil WH, Goldman HB, Dmochouski RR. The use of urine cytology for diagnosing bladder cancer in spinal cord injury patients. J Urol 1997; 157:2112–2114.

35. Nelson W, DeMarzo A, Isaacs W. Prostate Cancer. N Eng J Med 2003; 349:366–381.

36. U.S. Department of Health and Human Services. The Health Consequences of Tobacco Abuse: A Report of the Surgeon General. National Center for Chronic Disease Prevention and Health Promotion Office on Smoking and Health, 2003.

37. Fleming F, Mundt M, French M, et al. Brief physician advice for problem drinkers: long term efficacy and benefit—cost analysis. Alcohol Clin Exp Res 2002; 26:36–43.

38. Smith RA, Saslow D, Sawyer KA, et al. American Cancer Society Guidelines for Breast Cancer Screening: update 2003. CA Cancer J Clin 2003; 53:141–164.

39. Hulley S, Grady D, Bush T, et al. Randomized trial of estrogen plus progestin for secondary prevention of coronary disease in post menopausal women. JAMA 1998; 280:605–613.

40. Writing Group for the Women's Health Initiative Investigating risks and benefits of estrogen plus progestin in healthy post menopausal women. Principle results from the Women's Health Initiative Randomized Controlled Trial. JAMA 2002; 288:231–333.

41. Halsted C, Looksey K, Kohlmeier C, et al. Clinical nutrition education relevance and roles models. Am J Clin Nutrition 1998; 67:192–196.

42. Woolsey RM. Pain in spinal cord injury disorders. In: Young R, Woolsey RM, eds. Diagnosis and Management of Disorders of the Spinal Cord. Philadelphia: WB Saunders, 1995; 354–362.

43. Garland DE, Stewart CA, Adkins RA (eds.). Osteoporosis after spinal cord injury. J Orthop Res 1992; 10:371–379.

44. Garland DE. A clinical perspective on common forms of acquired heterotopic ossification. Clin Ortho 1991; 263:13–29.

45. Gellman H, Sie, IH, Waters RL. Late complications of the weight bearing upper extremity in the paraplegic patient. Clin Orthop 1988; 233:132–135.

46. Krause J, Coker J. Aging after spinal cord injury: a 35 year longitudinal study. JSCM 2006; 24:371–376.

24 The Role of Pharmacokinetics in Optimizing Drug Therapy in Patients with Spinal Cord Injury

J. Steven Richardson
Jack L. Segal

Among the many factors contributing to successful drug therapy, perhaps second in importance only to selecting the right drug is maintaining appropriate concentrations of that drug in the patient's blood. If blood levels are too low, the patient is deprived of the therapeutic benefits of the drug. If too high, the hazards of drug toxicity are added to the list of the patient's problems. Most drugs have a fairly wide range of acceptable blood concentrations. This range, from just above the ineffective level to just below the toxic level, is referred to as the therapeutic window of the drug. Some drugs, such as digoxin, lithium, and phenytoin, have very narrow therapeutic windows, and a dose that is just a little too high for a particular patient can result in toxic blood levels. Pharmacodynamics (i.e., what the drug does to the patient's body or to the offending organism) determine the appropriate drugs for the disease. Pharmacokinetics (i.e., what the patient's body does to the drug) determine the dose and dosing frequency needed to maintain drug blood levels within the therapeutic window. The recommended dose of a drug is calculated to ensure that enough drug molecules are absorbed into the bloodstream and distributed to the target organ to bring about the desired therapeutic response at the site of action. The recommended dosing schedule is selected to maintain the drug concentration within the therapeutic window by ensuring that enough new drug molecules are added to the patient's bloodstream to replace those that the patient's body has eliminated. Typically, the standard dose and dosing schedule of a drug are based on observations of how that drug is handled by able-bodied young adult volunteers. Subsequent modifications are based on clinical experience with the drug in patients with the target disease, and with subgroups of patients who have difficulty handling the standard doses. Some of these subgroups, whose pharmacokinetic parameters differ from the majority, are the very young, the very old, and those with spinal cord injury (SCI) (1). Although the special dosing requirements for pediatric and geriatric patients are now widely available and thoroughly discussed in the clinical literature, the changes needed for SCI patients and the rationale for those changes are not. In addition, with the dramatic rise in the life expectancy of SCI patients and of the population in general, the provision of appropriate health care for geriatric SCI patients will become increasingly important (2, 3, 4). This chapter reviews the basic principles of pharmacokinetics, outlines some of the physiologic changes induced by SCI that render standard dosing regimes problematic for SCI patients, and to illustrate the application of these principles to clinical situations, discusses the rationale for the dosing changes needed for drugs used to treat infections and to control spasticity, two common problems in SCI patients.

PHARMACOTHERAPY

In the clinical setting, decisions involved in the use of a specific drug to treat a specific patient with a specific ailment are usually rather straightforward: administer the drug of choice at the recommended dose and frequency. However, the decisions involved in identifying "the drug of choice," and in establishing the "recommended dose and frequency," reflect extensive research on the pharmacodynamic and pharmacokinetic properties of the drug. Most of the time, following standard procedures results in maintaining an appropriate concentration of the drug in the target organ for a sufficient length of time to bring about the successful treatment of the patient's condition. However, for some patients, standard dosing is not enough (5, 6), and so they do not improve. For other patients, standard dosing is too much, and they suffer the consequences of toxic overdose. These opposite reactions of different individuals to identical drug doses are due to pharmacokinetic differences among people (7, 8).

Pharmacokinetics

When a patient is given a drug, the drug molecules are absorbed into the bloodstream, distributed by the blood to the target organ (and throughout the rest of the body), metabolized, and excreted. Hence, the pharmacokinetic parameters are absorption, distribution, metabolism, and excretion—A, D, M, E.

Absorption

Most drugs are fat soluble, and whether they are given orally, transcutaneously, subcutaneously, or intramuscularly, they are absorbed into the bloodstream by passive diffusion down a concentration gradient. The rate of diffusion/absorption is determined by the molecular size, lipophilicity, and ionization of the drug; the permeability, thickness, and surface area of the absorptive surface; and the concentration difference between the site of administration and the blood. The rate of absorption is fastest for a small, highly fat-soluble, nonionized drug, being absorbed across a highly permeable, thin, large-area membrane that has a high rate of blood flow to carry off drug molecules as soon as they enter the blood, thereby maintaining the concentration gradient. All drugs given orally are absorbed better from the small intestine than from the stomach because of the greater surface area and the greater blood flow of the small intestine. Some drugs, such as weak acids or very weak bases, which would be mostly nonionized in the acidic stomach fluid, are absorbed from the stomach too, but the bulk of drug absorption occurs in the small intestine.

BIOAVAILABILITY   The oral bioavailability of a drug is the percentage of the oral dose of that drug that ends up in the systemic circulation (5, 9). Relatively few drugs have complete oral bioavailability. All of the molecules of oral doses of diazepam, valproic acid, sulfamethoxazole, and trimethoprim end up in the systemic blood (i.e., 100% bioavailability), and so do almost all of the molecules of oral doses of amoxicillin, cephalexin, clonidine, enalapril, indomethacin, theophylline, and warfarin (bioavailabilities of 90% to 100%). These drugs are both lipophilic and hydrophilic, are mostly nonionized at the pHs found in the gastrointestinal (GI) tract, and are not metabolized by enzymes in the gut or on their first pass through the liver in the liver portal blood flow. Among the drugs with low oral bioavailability are propranolol (26%), morphine (24%), acyclovir (23%), cyclosporine (23%), terbutaline (14%), and the aminoglycoside antibiotics (essentially 0%). Drugs with low bioavailabilities tend to be drugs that are either highly ionized in the gut (morphine), or highly hydrophilic and poorly lipophilic (the aminoglycosides), or highly metabolized in the gut or on first pass through the liver (propranolol). The majority of clinically relevant drugs have oral bioavailabilities ranging from 40% to 80%.

Distribution

Drug distribution is the movement of a drug from one location in the body to another. Drug distribution, like drug absorption, is generally by passive diffusion down the concentration gradient. As long as blood levels are higher than tissue levels, the drug moves out of the blood and into the tissues. When blood levels fall below tissue levels, the drug leaves the tissues and returns to the blood. While in the blood, drugs bind to plasma proteins: acidic drugs bind to several different sites on albumin, and basic drugs bind to lipoproteins or to alpha-1 acid glycoprotein. The degree of plasma protein binding of different drugs varies from none (acetaminophen and lithium) to 99% (diazepam, furosemide, and warfarin); many drugs are in the 80–98% range. For any particular drug, there is a constant equilibrium between the percentage of the drug that is bound, and the percentage that is free in the plasma. Drug molecules that are bound to plasma proteins are not able to leave the blood. Only the unbound molecules are free to diffuse out of the blood to provide the therapeutic concentration in the target organ or to be removed from the body. The plasma protein binding sites may become saturated at high drug concentrations, and competition occurs between drugs that bind to the same site on plasma proteins.

VOLUME OF DISTRIBUTION   The volume of distribution is the theoretic volume of water into which a known dose of a drug must be dissolved to achieve the concentration observed in the patient's blood. To emphasize the theoretic nature of this term, it is also known as the apparent volume of distribution. Comparing the volume of distribution (Vd) of a drug to the physiologic volumes of the various water compartments of the human body gives some indication of how extensively the drug is distributed throughout the body and how much of it is bound to storage sites in the tissues. Furosemide (Vd about 8 L) is found mostly in the blood (about 5 L for a 70-kg person); amoxicillin (Vd 15 L) mostly in the extracellular fluid (14 L); prazosin (Vd 42 L) in total body water (42 L); and diltiazem (Vd 220 L) is stored in tissues.

Metabolism

Drug metabolism, perhaps more correctly referred to as drug biotransformation, is an enzymatic process in which the drug molecule is usually made more polar, and therefore less lipophilic. A molecule of the lipophilic parent drug may be filtered or excreted by the kidney into the lumen of the nephron, but because the drug molecule is lipophilic, it diffuses back into the bloodstream and only a small fraction of the drug dose actually leaves the body in the urine. The less lipophilic polar metabolite of the drug may be excreted in the urine, or it may be acted on by other enzymes that make it even more polar and easier to excrete. Thus, drug metabolism is a crucial step in removing lipophilic compounds from the body. In general, the metabolites of a drug lack its pharmacodynamic properties, and drug metabolism usually terminates the desired therapeutic action. However, this is not always the case. Some drugs are metabolized into compounds that share the pharmacologic actions of the parent drug; other medications are given as inactive prodrugs that require metabolism into an active form to provide the therapeutic benefit. Consequently, drug metabolism should not be considered to be drug "detoxification."

CYTOCHROME P450 ISOZYMES   Although liver cells perform the bulk of drug metabolism, cells in other organs can do so as well. The actual metabolic transformation of drugs, and a wide variety of endogenous and food-derived lipophilic compounds, is carried out by a large number of mixed-function oxidase enzymes, collectively referred to as the cytochrome P450 isozymes. They are structurally-related enzymes located in the membranes of the smooth endoplasmic reticulum of cells in the liver and other tissues. The cytochrome P450s are a superfamily of iron-containing enzymes that add a functional group, usually a hydroxyl (10), to the structure of hormones, bile acids, and other endogenous lipophilic molecules, and to exogenous lipophilic molecules such as drugs, nutrients, and environmental chemicals that have entered the body. This facilitates the excretion of these compounds by making them more polar and less lipophilic. In addition to assisting the removal of lipophilic compounds from the body, cytochrome P450 enzymes are also involved in the synthesis of hormones, eicosanoids and bile acids, and in the regulation of cholesterol levels in the body (11).

The individual members of the cytochrome P450 superfamily are referred to using the nomenclative CYP (for the superfamily) plus a number identifying a family grouping of isozymes with a more than 40% homology of amino acid sequences (e.g., CYP2). An additional letter identifies a subfamily grouping with more than 55% homology with each other (CYP2D), and another number identifies one specific enzyme (CYP2D6). Of the 57 different CYP isozymes that have been found in mammals, 95% of drugs are metabolized by five of them: CYP1A2, CYP2C9, CYP2C19, CYP2D6, or CYP3A4 (12). Although most drugs are metabolized by more than one CYP isozyme, the metabolism of a particular drug may be done more efficiently by a particular isozyme. The simultaneous or sequential administration of two or more compounds that are preferred substrates for the same isozyme will alter the metabolism of both drugs, and unless dosing is adjusted, will result in undesired blood concentrations of the drugs. If one of the drugs induces the shared isozyme, metabolism of the second drug will be increased and its blood levels will fall, possibly to subtherapeutic concentrations. Conversely, if one of the drugs inhibits the shared isozyme, metabolism of the second drug will be slowed and its blood levels rise, possibly to toxic or lethal concentrations. The prudent practitioner would be well advised to determine and to take into account changes in CYP isozyme activity due to smoking, diet, or other drugs before prescribing any drug to a patient. The inactivation of CYP isozymes by a wide variety of drugs, herbal preparations, and chemicals in foods and in the environment has been recently reviewed by Johnson (12).

Because preliminary investigations suggest that SCI reduces liver drug metabolism (13) and gene activity (14), and alters drug side-effect and overdose profiles in unexpected ways, the consequences of drug–drug and food–drug interactions at the level of cytochrome P450 metabolism may be particularly problematic for patients with SCI.

Excretion

Drug excretion, or more usually the excretion of the nonlipophilic metabolites of the drug, is accomplished primarily by the kidneys. For most drugs, the drug or the metabolites are filtered or secreted by the nephron and removed from the body in the urine. For some drugs, the drug or the metabolites are secreted into the bile and may leave the body in the feces. In the case of the biliary excretion of the original drug, the drug may be reabsorbed into the blood stream. In other cases, enzymes in the gut convert the nonlipophilic, inactive metabolites back into the original lipophilic active drug, which is then reabsorbed and given another opportunity to express its pharmacodynamic action. This process of enterohepatic recirculation of a drug can dramatically prolong the length of time needed to eliminate the drug, and can complicate the task of determining the dosing frequency needed to maintain drug levels within the therapeutic window.

CLEARANCE AND HALF-LIFE   Two related concepts that are important when considering pharmacokinetic principles are drug clearance and drug half-life. Drug clearance is measured as the volume of blood or plasma from which a compound is irreversibly removed per unit time; it is usually expressed as milliliters per minute. Lipophilic compounds are cleared by being metabolized in the liver. Nonlipophilic compounds are cleared by being filtered and/or secreted in the kidney. Dosing frequency is designed to replace the drug molecules that have been cleared from the blood. The plasma half-life of a drug is the length of time required for the concentration of that drug in the plasma to be cut in half. For most drugs, this is also the time needed to eliminate half of the drug molecules from the body. Some drugs, such as aspirin, omeprazole, hydralazine, and the aminoglycoside antibiotics, are tightly or irreversibly bound to their receptors or to other sites within the cells, or are sequestered within tissues, and continue to exert their effects long after unbound molecules of the drug are no longer detectable in the plasma. Repeated administration of such drugs can result in enhanced toxicity, even though plasma levels are within the "normal" range. The half-life of a drug is roughly proportional to the volume of distribution of that drug.

Drugs with a large volume of distribution tend to have longer half-lives than do drugs with a small volume of distribution. Following a single dose, or when a drug has been discontinued, it generally takes three half-lives for the blood levels of that drug to fall below the therapeutic window, and five half-lives for blood levels of that drug to reach zero. When switching a patient to a new drug, to avoid unwanted drug interactions at the CYP enzymes or at the receptors, a useful rule of thumb is to wait three to five times the half-life of the discontinued drug before starting the new drug. This rule of thumb is a little more complicated when dealing with drugs such as diazepam and fluoxetine, which have metabolites with the same pharmacologic activity as the parent drug. Although all of the molecules of the discontinued drug may be gone from the blood in five of its half-lives, the original drug effect will continue until the concentrations of all of the active metabolites fall below the therapeutic window. It is the biologic half-life of the drug, which is the half-life of the persistence of the initial drug effect, rather than the plasma half-life of the prescribed drug alone that is of primary clinical importance when discontinuing a drug with active metabolites or a drug whose effect persists after blood levels are no longer measurable.

For example, the plasma half-life of diazepam is around 30 hours, but its active metabolites make its biologic half-life well over 100 hours. The plasma half-life of fluoxetine is around 50 hours, and the biologic half-life of fluoxetine and its active metabolites is around 10 days. Omeprazole has a plasma half-life of less than 1 hour, but it continues to block the proton pump in parietal cells, and gastric acid secretion remains suppressed for about 3 days. Consequently, to reduce the chances of untoward drug interactions, it may be clinically prudent to wait a week or more after diazepam and a month or more after fluoxetine before starting a new drug.

Pharmacokinetic Changes Induced by Spinal Cord Injury

As a group, people with SCI have varying degrees of disruption of numerous physiologic processes controlling organ function and homeostasis that not only endow them with unique pharmacokinetic characteristics (1, 5, 6), but also result in the expression of the symptoms of disease states (15, 16) and the signs of drug toxicity and adverse effects in unusually subtle or exaggerated ways. These physiologic changes include functions controlled directly or indirectly by the autonomic nervous system such as delayed gastric emptying, reduced GI motility, impaired blood flow to muscles, skin, and liver, edema, loss of blood pressure and body temperature regulation, and impaired immune system activity (17), as well as functions seemingly independent of the autonomic nervous system such as lowered plasma proteins and anemia (Figure 24.1).

Although there is a rough correlation between the spinal level of the lesion, the extent of the lesion, and the physiologic changes induced by the lesion, there are also wide individual differences among people with SCI, and the specific changes present can differ between people with seemingly identical lesions. Needless to say, this makes precise predictions of drug response in a given patient problematic, but until the needed basic research has been done, the following considerations will help in attaining pharmacotherapeutic goals while avoiding drug toxicity and therapeutic misadventures in patients with SCI.

Absorption

Among those physiologic changes that alter drug absorption are delayed gastric emptying (18, 19), reduced GI motility (20), and reduced blood flow to the skin, the muscles (21, 22), and internal organs. Although all of these will alter the absorption of orally administered drugs, the direction of the effect will differ for different drugs. For instance, in the acid environment of the stomach (pH less than 3), basic drugs (usually drugs whose generic or chemical name ends in "ine") become ionized, which makes them polar. This reduces their lipophilicity and therefore reduces their absorption and bioavailability. Conversely, the

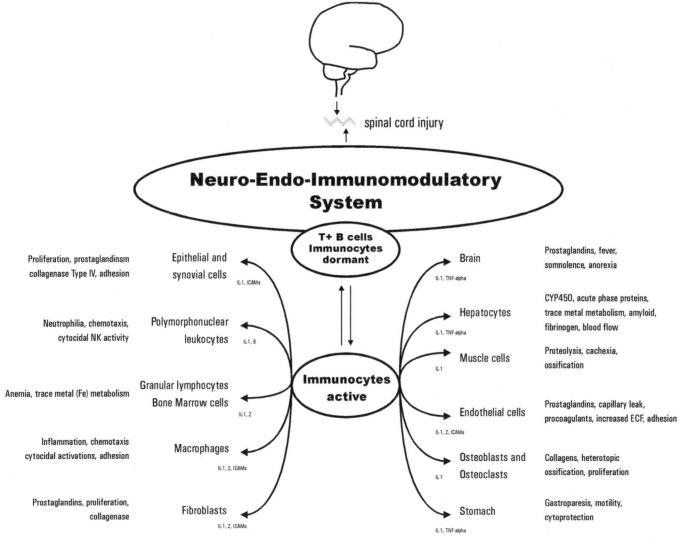

Figure 24.1 The effects of selected immunomodulatory compounds on various cells and tissues. Spinal cord injury disrupts the homeostatic control of the neuroendocrine-immunomodulatory system, and alters the activity of mediators of immune function. In the figure, IL-1, IL-2, and IL-6 are interleukin-1, interleukin-2, and interleukin-6, respectively; ICAMs is intercellular adhesion molecules; and TNF-α is tumor necrosis factor-α.

acidity of the stomach increases the nonionized, nonpolar fraction of acidic drugs (usually drugs that do not end in "ine"), thus increasing their lipophilicity, absorption and bioavailability. Consequently, basic drugs tend not to be absorbed until they reach the small intestine (pH around 5), whereas acidic drugs start entering the blood while still in the stomach. Because of their delayed gastric emptying, patients with SCI experience a rapid therapeutic effect with acidic drugs, such as aspirin or acetaminophen, and a delayed response with basic drugs, such as codeine or meperidine. Reduced intestinal motility, by prolonging the contact of the drug molecules with the large absorptive surface area of the small intestine, may even out the overall absorption of basic and acidic drugs, but when speed of onset of drug action is desired, an acidic drug should act faster in SCI patients than a basic drug with the same therapeutic indication.

Another consequence of reduced GI motility is the increased exposure of orally administered drugs to the contents of the gut. Some drugs, such as digoxin, are destroyed by bacteria in the gut and have reduced bioavailability in SCI patients. On the other hand, drugs that undergo enterohepatic recirculation, such as lorazepam, have greatly prolonged half-lives in SCI patients (23). Reduced blood flow to the GI tract, the skin, and the muscles of SCI patients may not alter the total bioavailability of a drug given orally, transcutaneously, or by subcutaneous or intramuscular injection, but the reduced blood flow does reduce the rate of absorption and the peak blood concentration. Moreover, the further reduction of blood perfusion in paralyzed muscles would suggest that drugs given by transcutaneous patch (e.g., heparin, testosterone, estrogen, clonidine, nicotine, scopolamine), or by subcutaneous or intramuscular injection, would be more reliably absorbed and more likely to produce the desired therapeutic effect when administered to sensate, nonparalyzed limbs.

Distribution

Those physiologic changes induced by SCI that alter drug distribution include reduced blood volume, reduced hemoglobin, reduced blood flow and organ perfusion (24), reduced plasma proteins (25), reduced lean body mass, and increased extracellular fluid/edema (25–27). Just as lowered blood flow retards drug absorption, it also impairs drug distribution. The reduced delivery of drug molecules to the target tissues would be expected to slow the attainment of therapeutically effective drug concentrations at the site of action. The increase in body fat and in extracellular water expands the total volume into which the drug must distribute and lowers drug concentrations in the blood. This further impairs the delivery of drug molecules to the site of action and further compromises the therapeutic response.

The resolution of these difficulties in attaining therapeutically effective drug concentrations at the target organ can also be complicated by the reduction of plasma proteins in the SCI patient. Fewer plasma protein binding sites means that less drug is needed to saturate all of the sites. Once all of the binding sites with affinity for the administered drug are saturated, the free fraction of the drug increases, and more molecules of the drug are free to leave the blood and enter the tissues. Depending on the individual patient's plasma protein profile, this increased free fraction may compensate for the impaired drug distribution so that therapeutic concentrations of the drug are achieved at the site of action after all. Conversely, in a patient with reduced

plasma protein binding sites, standard dosing may produce toxic drug levels. Among the numerous potentially toxic drugs prescribed to patients with SCI, the extent of binding of only a single aminoglycoside antibiotic, amikacin, has been experimentally determined in people with SCI (28).

Metabolism

Those changes in SCI patients that have a bearing on drug biotransformation are altered liver activity caused by reduced catecholamine metabolism (13, 29), reduced hepatic blood flow, impaired GI and gall bladder motility (30), reduced plasma proteins (25), and although convincing evidence is currently lacking, possibly altered CYP isozyme activities (14). It is an obvious truism that the liver can metabolize only what is brought to it by the blood. Decreased blood perfusion of the liver can reduce the clearance of drugs by metabolism and may prolong drug plasma half-life. If plasma proteins are reduced, then a greater fraction of the drug molecules that are delivered to the liver will be unbound and free to enter the liver cells for metabolism. Although the pre-systemic metabolism of drugs is usually considered as reducing bioavailability, the enzymes of the gut also play a clinically significant role in the metabolism of many drugs. Basic drugs are typically nonionized at the blood pH of 7.4. If such a molecule should happen to diffuse into the stomach (pH less than 3) or the intestine (pH around 5), it will become ionized and unable to diffuse back out into the bloodstream. Once the drug is trapped in the gut, the reduced GI motility of the SCI patient provides ample opportunity for the drug to be metabolized by enzymes in the mucosal cells and in the lumen of the gut. As discussed above, we usually refer to the CYP isozymes as drug metabolizing enzymes, but their original purpose (in the eons of life before drugs were invented) was to contribute to the survival of the organism by synthesizing hormones, prostaglandins, lipids, and other useful compounds, and by helping the organism get rid of endogenous and exogenous lipophilic compounds that were harmful or no longer needed. The wide-spread changes seen in the lipid (31, 32), protein (25), endocrine (33–35) and neural (36, 37, 40–42) profiles of SCI patients, may, since CYP isozymes contribute to all of these, be due to altered CYP isozyme activity. However, as of the writing of this chapter, information on CYP isozymes in SCI patients has not yet been published.

Excretion

The final step in removing drugs from the body is excretion in the urine or in the feces. As with the liver, renal blood flow may be diminished in SCI patients. Drugs such as digoxin and aminoglycoside antibiotics such as gentamicin and amikacin are almost exclusively excreted intact (unmetabolized) by the kidneys. Traditionally, in both SCI and in able-bodied patients, the adequacy of kidney function is routinely clinically assessed by measuring the clearance of endogenous creatinine; this correlates highly with the glomerular filtration rate (GFR). For those drugs eliminated more or less intact by the kidney, an accurate measure of GFR is critically important. Unfortunately, the measurement of endogenous creatinine clearance in patients with SCI is often unreliable and gives an erroneous GFR. For a variety of reasons, such as a sedentary life style, impaired skeletal muscle turnover, and diminished endogenous production of creatinine, the clinical assessment and direct measurement of creatinine clearance can, even in SCI patients with normal kidney function, give a misleading estimate of GFR with potentially dire consequences for the patient, namely death in the case of digoxin, and permanent hearing loss and kidney damage in the case of the aminoglycosides. Several authors have addressed the problem of determining an accurate GFR in SCI patients. Mirahmadi et al. (43) suggested that a good approximation of creatinine clearance, and thus of GFR, could be obtained for SCI patients simply by recalculating the standard equation for the renal clearance of creatinine in able-bodied humans. Mohler et al. (44) constructed easy-to-use nomograms derived from the experimental measurement of creatinine clearance in patients with SCI. Segal and colleagues, following their studies on the pharmacokinetics of the aminoglycoside antibiotic gentamicin, recognized that the direct measurement of the total body clearance of a drug that is removed from the body exclusively by the kidneys, such as gentamicin, should give an accurate measure of the GFR. Their method of calculating GFR (45) is a multifactorial model incorporating the patient's gentamicin clearance and SCI population-specific patient identifiers and demographic data, and is shown in Figure 24.2 and in Table 24.1. Comparatively speaking, the Segal Method seems to provide the best estimate of GFR in SCI patients.

In SCI patients, the elimination of drugs or drug metabolites that are excreted or secreted by the kidneys or are excreted

in the bile can be impaired, with the result that the elimination half-lives of these drugs are increased. The half-lives of drugs that undergo enterohepatic recirculation, such as lorazepam, are further prolonged in SCI patients (23). Due to the increased half-life of drugs in SCI patients, standard drug doses and/or dosing intervals must be altered to avoid increasing blood levels of the drug into the toxic range.

Pharmacokinetics and Pharmacotherapy in Two Common Clinical Problems in SCI Patients

The clinical management of specific medical conditions in SCI patients is thoroughly covered in other chapters in this text. However, the following brief discussion of the drug treatment of infections and spasticity in SCI patients is presented to demonstrate the application of pharmacokinetics and pharmacodynamics in predicting drug response, making therapeutic decisions, and understanding the reactions of SCI patients to drugs.

Infectious Diseases

Patients with SCI have an increased incidence of a wide variety of infections in general, and are at particular risk of developing life-threatening complications of infections of skin pressure ulcers, the urinary tract, and the lungs. The treatment of these

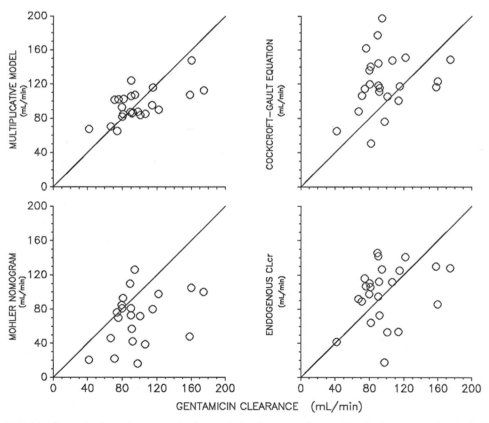

Figure 24.2 The individual panels show the strength of association between the total body clearance of a single intravenous dose of gentamicin and four methods for predicting glomerular filtration rate (GFR) in spinal cord injured patients. The best linear correlation ($r = 0.79$, $p < .05$, $n = 24$) was found between measured gentamicin clearance and the Multiplicative Model developed by Segal and colleagues. See Table 24.1 for the equations derived from this model.

Table 24.1   Clearance Predictor Equations in SCI Multiplicative Model

---

Equation A and Equation B are nearly identical Multiplicative Models (i.e., mathematical expressions) that provide very accurate estimates of gentamicin clearance, and therefore glomerular filtration rate, in spinal cord injured patients. These models incorporate spinal cord injured population specific variables and the Cockcroft-Gault equation. Each model was derived from a multivariate, nonlinear, all-subsets regression analysis. Both models correlate highly with creatinine clearance measured directly in spinal cord injured patients, and provide a more precise, less biased prediction of glomerular filtration rate than measured creatinine clearance, the method of Cockcroft and Gault, or the spinal cord injury nomograms (44).

CLEARANCE PREDICTOR EQUATIONS IN SCI MULTIPLICATIVE MODEL

A. $CL_{gent} = e^{-0.5746} \times (Age)^{0.7202} \times (\text{C-G } CL_{cr})^{0.5870} \times (INJDUR + 1)^{-0.1284}$

B. $CL_{gent} = e^{-0.3092} \times (Age)^{0.6729} \times (\text{C-G } CL_{cr})^{0.5758} \times (INJDUR + 1)^{-0.1129} \times (INJLVL + 1)^{-0.0912}$

Where:

   CL_{gent} is gentamicin clearance in patients with SCI in mL/min

   Age is in years

   C-G CL_{cr} Cockcroft-Gault CL_{cr} in mL/min

   INJDUR is injury duration in years

   INJLVL is level of spinal cord injury

---

conditions is complicated not only by the physiologic changes and the resulting pharmacokinetic alterations induced by SCI, but also by the deficiencies in immune system function that have been demonstrated in SCI patients (17, 39, 40, 41, 42, 46, 47). A clinically important implication of the impaired immune system in SCI patients is that those antibiotics that actually kill bacteria, such as the penicillins, cephalosporins, quinolones, aminoglycosides, or vancomycin, would be better choices for treating infections in SCI patients than antibiotics, such as the macrolides, sulfonamides, and tetracyclines, which stop bacterial replication but depend on the immune system to kill to existing bacteria. It has long been known that hearing loss and kidney damage are the toxic consequences of excessive, or even therapeutic, blood levels of the aminoglycosides. As discussed above, extra caution with the use of these agents in SCI patients may be warranted (48, 49, 50, 51) in light of the potential reduction in renal clearance induced by SCI. This reduced clearance prolongs the half-life of aminoglycosides, and unless the time between doses is increased, may result in elevated plasma levels and an increased risk of hearing loss and kidney damage. In contrast to the aminoglycosides, the penicillins and cephalosporins are not, except for people who are allergic to them, hazardous to humans, and so standard dosing can be used for all.

The quinolone antibiotics are also relatively benign, but do have adverse reactions that are relevant to spinal cord medicine. The quinolones interfere with collagen metabolism, which in addition to causing arthropathy, can weaken tendons and ligaments, thus increasing the risk of rupture. Because weight-bearing structures in the shoulder such as the rotator cuff are overly stressed by wheelchair propulsion and other activities engaged in by SCI patients, the risk of tendon rupture and rotator

cuff tears should be considered before using a quinolone in these patients (52). A second concern with the quinolones is that ciprofloxacin is a strong inhibitor of CYP1A2. Because theophylline and tizanidine are metabolized by CYP1A2, if ciprofloxacin (other quinolones are less of a concern) is given to a patient taking theophylline or tizanidine, the metabolism of the latter drugs will be reduced, and unless their doses are reduced, their blood levels will rise to the toxic range. Patients on theophylline may develop hyperreflexia, diarrhea, tachypnea, arrhythmias, seizures, circulatory failure, and respiratory arrest leading to death. Patients on tizanidine may develop somnolence, fatigue, hypotension, coma, and respiratory depression. The quinolone antibiotics also reduce GABA-mediated neuronal inhibition in the central nervous system. This not only lowers the seizure threshold and increases the risk of seizures induced by theophylline and other drugs, but also may induce or exacerbate spasticity in SCI patients. These pharmacodynamic and pharmacokinetic interactions suggest caution with the use of quinolone antibiotics in people with SCI.

Spasticity Reduction

Spasticity, a motor syndrome characterized by increased muscle tone, exaggerated tendon jerks, and flexor spasms, is a common result of lesions to the upper motor neurons. Baclofen, diazepam, tizanidine, gabapentin, clonidine, and dantrolene are the pharmacologic agents currently used to reduce the disruptive impact of spasticity on the lives of SCI patients (53). The equivocal results of antispasticity drugs given to SCI patients (54) may reflect the idiosyncratic pharmacokinetic profiles of these patients caused by the physiologic changes induced by their SCI.

Following standard dosing recommendations in these patients results in some of them having subtherapeutic blood levels while others are exposed to excessively high toxic levels.

Baclofen, a structural analog of the inhibitory neurotransmitter GABA, is excreted unchanged by the kidneys. It acts as an agonist at GABA-B receptors on presynaptic nerve terminals, and reduces the release of a variety of neurotransmitters in the brain and in the spinal cord. Stimulation of the GABA-B receptor hyperpolarizes the presynaptic nerve membrane and prevents the release of the neurotransmitter from that nerve terminal. Diazepam facilitates the GABA-mediated opening of the chloride channels linked to GABA-A receptors. This also hyperpolarizes neural membranes, blocks action potentials, and reduces the release of neurotransmitters from their nerve terminals. It seems that the antispastic actions of both baclofen and diazepam are due to their inhibition of the release of excitatory neurotransmitters in the motor horn of the spinal cord. In the able-bodied, baclofen produces less sedation than diazepam and does not reduce muscle strength, as may be the case with dantrolene. In addition to having unpredictable antispasticity effects, oral baclofen has an unusual, albeit uncommon, withdrawal syndrome that includes hallucinations and seizures. The neurochemical basis for this involves both receptor changes induced by chronic baclofen and baclofen's short half-life of 3 to 4 hours (55). Being an agonist, chronic baclofen downregulates (i.e., makes subsensitive) GABA-B receptors. By inhibiting the release of numerous neurotransmitters in the brain, chronic baclofen upregulates (i.e., makes supersensitive) downstream receptors for dopamine, norepinephrine, serotonin, glutamate, and other neurotransmitters. When baclofen is discontinued, it is completely cleared from the body in five half-lives, i.e., about 20 hours. However, it takes the subsensitive GABA-B receptors and supersensitive downstream receptors two to three weeks to return to their pre-baclofen level of sensitivity. As soon as the baclofen is gone, neurotransmitter release returns to normal, but the released transmitters are now acting on supersensitive receptors that overdrive their respective neural pathways. Over-driving dopamine produces a paranoid state similar to that seen in amphetamine overdose. Overdriving glutamate produces seizures. These brain-related complications of baclofen withdrawal can be avoided by gradually reducing the dose of baclofen over a 4- to 6-week period, or by administering baclofen intrathecally directly into the spinal cord via implantable programmable infusion pumps. The intrathecal administration of baclofen is, however, an invasive, complex procedure that has met with variable success in selected patients (56).

An alternative to baclofen is the orally active agent tizanidine (57). Tizanidine is a structural analog of clonidine and, like clonidine, is an agonist at norepinephrine alpha-2 receptors and at imidazoline receptors in the CNS. Also like clonidine, tizanidine reduces spasticity, but unlike clonidine does so at doses having little effect on blood pressure. Tizanidine facilitates both presynaptic and postsynaptic inhibition in the spinal cord and also inhibits transmission in pain pathways in the spinal cord. Whether these actions are mediated by alpha-2 receptors or by imidazoline receptors remains to be established. As discussed above, tizanidine is metabolized by CYP1A2, and in the presence of compounds that alter the activity of CYP1A2, changes to the patient's dosing regimen are required. In addition to ciprofloxacin as mentioned previously, CYP1A2 is also potently inhibited by fluoxamine (58), and to a lesser extent by other antidepressant drugs. These drugs reduce the metabolism of tizanidine, prolong its half-life and increase its level in the patient's blood. Conversely, the activity of CYP1A2 is induced by carbamazepine, phenytoin, and the barbiturates and polycyclic aromatic hydrocarbons in cigarette smoke (59). These compounds speed up the metabolism of tizanidine, reduce its half-life and decrease its level in the patient's blood. Tizanidine has a narrow therapeutic window and attaining appropriate therapeutic plasma levels in specific patients has been problematic (60). Taking into account factors altering the pharmacokinetics of tizanidine may greatly improve the successful control of spasticity in SCI patients with this agent. Although there do not appear to be any adverse interactions between baclofen and tizanidine (61), existing studies have been done with healthy, able-bodied subjects. Comparable studies with SCI patients remain to be performed. Other compounds, such as gabapentin (62) and 4-aminopyridine (63, 64), also show promise in reducing spasticity in SCI patients, but as with so many other aspects of spinal cord medicine, more research is needed.

CONCLUSION

As a consequence of the disruption of central neural pathways, spinal cord-injured humans have a wide range of altered or absent physiologic processes. These changes present complex challenges to the optimal use of drugs in treating the medical problems of SCI patients. Unfortunately, at the present time, a complete understanding of the physiologic changes and the resulting alterations in pharmacokinetic parameters induced by SCI await future investigations. The development of a comprehensive formulary of drugs of choice and rational dosing schedules, based on information from population studies of biomarkers and pharmacokinetic characteristics specific for treating medical diseases in SCI patients, would contribute greatly to improving the quality of life of patients with spinal cord injuries (65, 66, 67). In the meantime, adjusting drug dosing in light of the known characteristics of spinal cord injured humans, and in anticipation of their unique responses to drugs, will help to ensure the delivery of optimal, cost-effective healthcare to this population of patients. Incorporating pharmacokinetic principles into planning decisions when considering drug therapy for people with SCI will assist in maintaining plasma drug levels within the therapeutic range, and in attaining the appropriate response for these patients.

References

1. Segal JL, Rosenzweig IB. Therapeutic drug monitoring and treatment of spinal cord injury. *Therapeutic Drug Monitoring and Toxicology* 2000; 21:37–52.
2. Adkins RH. Research and interpretation perspectives on aging related physical morbidity with spinal cord injury and brief review of systems. *Neuro Rehabil* 2004; 19:3–13.
3. Capoor J, Stein AB. Aging with spinal cord injury. *Phys Med Rehabil Clin N Am* 2005; 16: 129–161.
4. Branco F, Cardenas DD, Svircev JN. Spinal cord injury: A comprehensive review. *Phys Med Rehabil Clin N Am* 2007; 18:651–679.
5. Segal JL, Hayes KC, Brunnemann SR, Hsieh JTC, Potter PJ, Pathak MS, Tierney DS, Mason D. Absorption characteristics of sustained-release 4-aminopyridine (Fampridine SR) in patients with chronic spinal cord injury. *J Clin Pharmacol* 2000; 40:402–409.
6. Campbell B, Brien JE. Pharmacokinetics in spinal cord injured patients. *Aust J Hosp Pharm* 1995; 25:327–332.

7. Derendorf H, Lesko LJ, Chaikin P, Colburn WA, et al. Pharmacokinetic/pharmacodynamic modeling in drug research and development. *J Clin Pharmacol* 2000; 40:1399–1418.

8. Stowe CD, Lee KR, Storgion SA, Phelps SJ. Altered phenytoin pharmacokinetics in children with severe, acute traumatic brain injury. *J Clin Pharmacol* 2000; 40:1452–1461.

9. Gilman TM, Segal JL, Brunnemann SR. Metoclopramide increases the bioavailability of dantrolene in spinal cord injury. *J Clin Pharmacol* 1996; 36:64–71.

10. Coon MJ. Omega oxygenases: Nonheme-iron enzymes and P450 cytochromes. *Biochem Biophys Res Commun* 2005; 338:378–385.

11. Luoma PV. Cytochrome P450—physiological key factor against cholesterol accumulation and the atherosclerotic vascular process. *Ann Med* 2007; 39:359–370.

12. Johnson WW. Cytochrome P450 inactivation by pharmaceuticals and phytochemicals: Therapeutic relevance. *Drug Metab Rev* 2008; 40:101–147.

13. Segal JL, Brunnemann SR. Altered catecholamine levels are associated with changes in hepatic oxidative metabolism in humans with spinal cord injury. Abstract. *J Clin Pharmacol* 1991; 31:844.

14. Segal JL, Brunnemann SR, Casteñeda-Hernádez G, Guizar-Sahagun G. Altered hepatocyte gene expression in a rat model of chronic spinal cord injury. *J Clin Pharmacol* 2000; 40:1045–1065.

15. Bauman WA, Spungen AM. Coronary heart disease in individuals with spinal cord injury: Assessment of risk factors. *Spinal Cord* 2008; advance online publication 8 January: 11 pages.

16. Finnie AK, Buchholz AC, Martin Ginis, KA, SHAPE SCI Research Group. Current coronary heart disease risk assessment tools may underestimate risk in community-dwelling persons with chronic spinal cord injury. *Spinal Cord* 2008; advance online publication 11 March: 8 pages.

17. Segal JL. Immunoactivation and altered intercellular communication mediate the pathophysiology of spinal cord injury. *Pharmacotherapy* 2005; 25:145–156.

18. Segal JL, Milne N, Brunnemann SR. Gastric emptying is impaired in patients with spinal cord injury. *Am J Gastroenterol* 1995; 90:466–470.

19. Enck P, Greving I, Klosterhalfen S, Wietek B. Upper and lower gastrointestinal motor and sensory dysfunction after human spinal cord injury. *Prog Brain Res* 2006; 152:373–384.

20. Krogh K, Mosdal C, Laurberg S. Gastrointestinal and segmental colonic transit times in patients with acute and chronic spinal cord lesions. *Spinal Cord* 2000; 38:615–621.

21. Seifert J, Lob G, Stoephasius E, Probst J, Brendal W. Blood flow in muscles of paraplegic patients under various conditions measured by a double isotope technique. *Paraplegia* 1972; 10:185–191.

22. Deitrick G, Charalel J, Bauman W, Tuckman J. Reduced arterial circulation to the legs in spinal cord injury as a cause of skin breakdown lesions. *Angiology* 2007; 58:175–184.

23. Segal JL Brunnemann SR, Eltorai IM, Vulpe M. Decreased systemic clearance of lorazepam in humans with spinal cord injury. *J Clin Pharmacol* 1991; 31:651–656.

24. Houtman S, Oeseburg B, Hopman MT. Blood volume and hemoglobin after spinal cord injury. *Am J Phys Med Rehabil* 2000; 79:260–265.

25. Lipetz JS, Kirshblum SC, O'Conner KC, Voorman SJ, Johnson MV. Anemia and serum protein deficiencies in patients with traumatic spinal cord injury. *J Spinal Cord Med* 1997; 20:335–340.

26. Nuhlicek DN, Spurr GB, Barboriak JJ, Rooney CB, et al. Body composition of patients with spinal cord injury. *European J Clin Nutrition* 1988; 42:765–773.

27. McDonald CM, Abresch-Meyer AL, Nelson MD, Widman LM. Body mass index and body composition measures by dual x-ray absorptiometry in patients aged 10 to 21 years with spinal cord injury. *J Spinal Cord Med* 2007; 30(Suppl 1):S97–S104.

28. Brunnemann SR, Segal JL. Amikacin serum protein binding in spinal cord injury. *Life Sciences* 1991; 49: PL1–PL5.

29. Dimova-Apostolova G, Angelova A, Vaptzarova K. Catecholamine concentration in rat liver after high level transection of the spinal cord. *Life Sciences* 1999; 64:2375–2381.

30. Milne N, Segal JL, Rypins EB, Brunnemann SR, Lyons KP. Biliary kinetics in spinal cord injury. Abstract. *J Nuclear Med* 1987; 28:688.

31. Schmid A, Halle M, Stützle C, König D, Baumstark MW, Storch M-J, Schmidt-Trucksäß A, Lehmann M, Berg A, Keul J. Lipoproteins and free plasma catecholamines in spinal cord injured men with different injury levels. *Clin Physiology* 2000; 20:304–310.

32. Segal JL, Tayek, JA. Effects of a potassium channel blocker, 4-aminopyridine, on lipid profiles and cardiovascular risk factors in patients with spinal cord injury. *Am J Clin Med* 2006; 3: 11–15 .

33. Mechanik JI, Pomerantz F, Flanagan S, Stein A, et al. Parathyroid hormone suppression in spinal cord injury patients is associated with the degree of neurologic impairment and not the level of injury. *Arch Phys Med Rehabil* 1997; 78:692–696.

34. Segal JL, Thompson JF, Tayek, JA. Effects of long-term 4-aminopyridine therapy on glucose tolerance and glucokinetics in patients with spinal cord injury. *Pharmacotherapy* 2007; 27:789–792.

35. Maruyama Y, Mizuguchi M, Yaginuma T, Kusaka M, et al. Serum leptin, abdominal obesity and the metabolic syndrome in individuals with chronic spinal cord injury. *Spinal Cord*, 2008; advance online publication 22 January: 6 pages.

36. Bunten DC, Warner AL, Brunnemann SR, Segal JL. Heart rate variability is altered following spinal cord injury. *Clin Autonomic Res* 1998; 8:329–334.

37. Segal JL, Warner AL, Brunnemann SR, Bunten DC. 4-aminopyridine influences heart rate variability in long-standing spinal cord injury. *Am J Therapeutics* 2002; 9:29–33.

38. Isoda WC, Segal JL. Effects of 4-aminopyridine on cardiac repolarization, PR interval, and heart rate in patients with spinal cord injury. *Pharmacotherapy* 2003; 23:133–136.

39. Segal JL. Spinal cord injury: Are interleukins a molecular link between neuronal damage and ensuing pathobiology? *Perspect Biol Med* 1993; 36:222–240.

40. Nash MS. Known and plausible modulators of depressed immune functions following spinal cord injuries. *J Spinal Cord Med* 2000; 23:111–120.

41. Cruse JM, Lewis RE, Roe DL, Dilioglou S, et al. Facilitation of immune function, healing of pressure ulcers, and nutritional status in spinal cord injury patients. *Exp Mol Pathol* 2000; 68:38–54.

42. Segal JL, Gonzales E, Yousefi S, Jamshidipour L, Brunnemann SR. Circulating levels of IL-2R, ICAM-1, and IL-6 in spinal cord injuries. *Arch Phys Med Rehabil* 1997; 78:44–47.

43. Mirahmadi MK, Byrne C, Barton C, Penera N, et al. Prediction of creatinine clearance from serum creatinine in spinal cord injury patients. *Paraplegia* 1983; 21:23–29.

44. Mohler JL, Barton SD, Blouin RA, Cowen DL, Flanigan RC. The evaluation of creatinine clearance in spinal cord injury. *J Urol* 1986; 136:366–369.

45. Segal JL, Gilmen TA, Thompson JF. Single-dose gentamicin clearance is a predictor of creatinine clearance in spinal man. *AM J Ther* 2009; advance online publication. Epub ahead of print, 13 June: 6 pages.

46. Lucin KM, Sanders VM, Jones TB, Malarky WB, Popovich PG. Impaired antibody synthesis after spinal cord injury is level-dependent and is due to sympathetic nervous system dysregulation. *Exp Neurol* 2007; 207:75–84.

47. Campagnolo DI, Dixon D, Schwartz J, Bartlett JA, Keller SE. Altered innate immunity following spinal cord injury. *Spinal Cord* 2008; advance online publication 12 February: 5 pages.

48. Segal JL, Brunnemann SR, Gordon SK, Eltorai, IM. Amikacin pharmacokinetics in patients with spinal cord injury. *Pharmacotherapy* 1988; 8:79–81.

49. Segal JL, Brunnemann SR, Gray DR. Gentamicin bioavailability and single-dose pharmacokinetics in spinal cord injury. *Drug Intell Clin Pharm* 1988; 22:461–465.

50. Segal JL, Brunnemann SR, Eltorai, IM. Pharmacokinetics of amikacin in serum and in tissue contiguous with pressure sores in humans with spinal cord injury. *Antimicrob Agents Chemother* 1990; 34:1422–1428.

51. Vaidyanathan S, Peloquin C, Wyndaele J-J, Buczynski AZ, et al. Amikacin dosing and monitoring in spinal cord injury patients: Variation in clinical practice between spinal injury units and differences in experts' recommendations. *The Scientific World Journal* 2006; 6:187–199.

52. Alfaham M, Holt ME, Goodchild MC. Arthropathy in a patient with cystic fibrosis taking ciprofloxacin. *Br Med J* 1987; 295(6600):699.

53. Nance PW, Young RR. Antispasticity medications. *Phys Med Rehabil Clin N Am* 1999; 10:337–355.

54. Tarrico M, Pagliacci MC, Telaro E, Adone R. Pharmacological interventions for spasticity following spinal cord injury: Results of a Cochrane systematic review. *Europa Medicophysica* 2006; 42:5–15.

55. Keegan DL, Richardson JS, Kirby AR. A possible neurochemical basis for the neuropsychiatric aspects of baclofen therapy. *Internat J Neuroscience* 1983; 20:249–254.

56. Kamensek J. Continuous intrathecal baclofen infusions. An introduction and overview. *Axone* 1999; 20:67–72.

57. Kamen L, Henney HR, Runyan JD. A practical overview of tizanidine use for spasticity secondary to multiple sclerosis, stroke, and spinal cord injury. *Curr Med Res Opin* 2008; 24:425–439.

58. Granfors MT, Backman JT, Neuvonen M, Ahonen J, Neuvonen PJ. Fluoxamine drastically increases concentrations and effects of tizanidine: A potentially hazardous interaction. *Clin Pharmacol Ther* 2004; 75:331–341.

59. Backman JT, Schröder MT, Neuvonen PJ. Effects of gender and moderate smoking on the pharmacokinetics and effects of the CYP1A2 substrate tizanidine. *Eur J Clin Pharmacol* 2008; 64:17–24.

60. Henney HR, Runyan JD. A clinically relevant review of tizanidine hydrochloride dose relationships to pharmacokinetics, drug safety and effectiveness in healthy subjects and patients. *Internat J Clin Pract* 2008; 62:314–324.

61. Schellenberger MK, Groves L, Shah J, Novak GD. A controlled pharmacokinetic evaluation of tizanidine and baclofen at steady state. *Drug Metab Dispos* 1999; 27: 201–204.

62. Gruenthal M, Mueller M, Olson WL, Priebe MM, et al. Gabapentin for the treatment of spasticity in patients with spinal cord injury. *Spinal Cord* 1997; 35:686–689.

63. Segal JL, Pathak MS, Hernandez JP, Himber PL, et al. Safety and efficacy of 4-aminopyridine in humans with spinal cord injury: A long-term, controlled trial. *Pharmacotherapy* 1999; 19:713–723.

64. Segal JL, Brunnemann SR. 4-Aminopyridine alters gait characteristics and enhances locomotion in spinal cord injured humans. *J Spinal Cord Med* 1998; 21:200–204.

65. Segal JL, Pathak MS. Optimal drug therapy and therapeutic drug monitoring after spinal cord injury: A population-specific approach. *Am J Therapeutics* 2001; 8:451–463.

66. Ette EI, Williams P, Sun H, Fadiran E, Ajayi FO, Onyiah LC. The process of knowledge discovery from large pharmacokinetic data sets. *J Clin Pharmacol* 2001; 41:25–34.

67. Colburn WA, Lee JW. Biomarkers, validation and pharmacokinetic-pharmacodynamic modelling. *Clin Pharmacokinet* 2003; 42:997–1022.

25 Nutrition in Spinal Cord Injury

Heather Lynn Powell
Fredrick S. Frost

IMPORTANCE OF NUTRITION IN SPINAL CORD INJURY

Good nutrition is essential to good health. Dietary intake provides the constituents necessary for optimal mental and physical health, and for aiding resistance to infections, skin breakdown, and other common conditions in spinal cord injury (SCI). Conversely, a poor diet can contribute to morbidity and mortality, playing a major role in development of chronic illnesses such as hypertension, diabetes, and atherosclerosis (1). Malnutrition in the setting of acute injury or disease also contributes to co-morbidities, poor outcomes, and longer hospital lengths of stay (2–6). The importance of a proper nutritional care plan in the treatment of acute illness and the prevention or treatment of chronic diseases has been well documented, accentuating the role of the nutritional assessment in identifying malnourished persons, or those at risk for malnutrition, for such intervention. Though a standard method for evaluating nutrition status does not currently exist, a complete nutritional assessment includes history, physical examination, laboratory assessments, anthropometric measurements, and dietary evaluation.

Individuals living with SCI need to be monitored more closely for proper nutrition than the able-bodied population, as they are more susceptible to many disease processes responsive to nutrition. After spinal cord injury, changes occur in muscle mass, body habitus, activity level, metabolism, and gastrointestinal motility and function (see Table 25.1). In addition, myelopathy and associated denervation produces insulin resistance, unfavorable alterations in lipid profiles, and inflammation—as evidenced by increased levels of high-sensitivity C-reactive protein (7–9). These factors contribute to an increased risk for weight gain and metabolic syndrome, and subsequently diabetes mellitus and cardiovascular disease (10, 11). Electrolyte abnormalities can occur after SCI as well, particularly hyponatremia and both hypercalcemia (acute injury) and hypocalcemia (chronic injury) (12–16). Finally, multiple vitamin deficiencies are common and well-documented in persons with chronic SCI,

as will be discussed later in this chapter. These factors result in the need for at least annual history/ physical examinations, with weight trends and laboratory assessments of nutrional status.

NUTRITION BASICS

Fat-Soluble Vitamins

The fat-soluble vitamins A, D, E, and K are stored in the liver and adipose tissue until utilized, but excess amounts cannot be excreted; thus, toxicity may occur. Vitamin A has an important role in cellular differentiation and proliferation, in addition to vision, collagen synthesis, and immune function. Vitamin A deficiency may result in delayed wound healing and an increased susceptibility to infections, both common concerns in SCI. However, replacement therapy must be administered cautiously due to risk of toxicity. Excellent naturally occurring sources of vitamin A include spinach, cantaloupes, carrots, sweet potatoes, and liver. Vitamin E acts as an antioxidant, protecting cells from the damaging effects of free radicals, which are implicated in the development of cardiovascular disease and cancer. Vitamin E also plays a role in immunocompetence, particularly in the elderly. Vitamin K is essential for normal coagulation. It is stored in the liver, where vitamin K–dependent coagulation factors are synthesized. In persons with severe hepatic dysfunction, lower serum levels of these coagulation factors result in increased bleeding time and risk for hemorrhage. Vitamin K is produced by the normal flora of the GI tract, and is found in cabbage, cauliflower, spinach, and other green leafy vegetables, cereals, and soybeans.

The importance of vitamin D and calcium in bone growth and remodeling is evident in diseases such as rickets, osteomalacia, osteopenia, and osteoporosis. Vitamin D increases calcium absorption from 10–15% to 30–40% of dietary intake, likewise increasing uptake of phosphorus from 60% to 80%. Also, most tissues and cells have vitamin D receptors, suggesting a more pervasive role for this vitamin than the skeletal system. Vitamin D modulates many genes encoding proteins

Table 25.1 Nutritional Implications in Acute and Chronic SCI	
FACTORS CONTRIBUTING TO NUTRITIONAL RISK	CONSEQUENCES OF SCI

• Immobilization
  – Hypercalcemia
  – Hypercalciuria
 	
• Dysphagia (Cervical SCI)
 	
• Paralytic ileus/constipation
• Neurogenic bowel
• Neurogenic bladder
  – Restricted fluid intake
 	
  – Risk of renal disease
  – UTIs
• Decreased skeletal muscle mass
 	
• Pulmonary dysfunction
  – Loss of appetite
• Depression/grief
  – Loss of appetite
• Pressure ulcers
  – Protein and fluid loss
  – Impaired access to healthy foods
	• Anemia
	• Glucose intolerance
	• Negative nitrogen balance
	• Decreased energy expenditure
	• Osteoporosis
	• Pulmonary dysfunction
	  – Difficulty weaning from mechanical ventilation
	• Pressure ulcers
	• Poor wound healing
	• Impaired immune function

important for cell proliferation, differentiation, and cell death, in addition to neuromuscular and immune functions. Recent evidence indicates that vitamin D might play some role in reduction of inflammation and the prevention and treatment of many chronic diseases, such as hypertension, glucose intolerance, type 1 and type 2 diabetes, and multiple sclerosis. In addition, vitamin D supplementation has been associated with a significant reduction in all-cause mortality. Unfortunately, vitamin D deficiency is common, particularly in colder climates. An excellent source of vitamin D is sunlight exposure. In the United States, many foods are fortified with vitamin D, such as milk, yogurt, fruit juices, and cereals, but few naturally contain this vitamin. The best sources of vitamin D are fish— i.e. salmon, tuna, and mackerel—and fish liver oils, though small amounts of vitamin D are found in beef liver, cheese, egg yolks, and some mushrooms.

Water-Soluble Vitamins

The body readily excretes and cannot store appreciable concentrations of the water-soluble vitamins B and C (with the exception of B vitamins pyridoxine and cyanocobalamin), necessitating frequent consumption. The B vitamins—thiamine (B1), riboflavin (B2), niacin (B3), pantothenic acid (B5), pyridoxine (B6), biotin (B8), folate (B9), and cyanocobalamin (B12)—act as coenzymes or cofactors for many essential enzymes, including those necessary for the breakdown of carbohydrates, proteins, and fats for energy. Folate and vitamin B12 act as coenzymes in DNA and RNA synthesis. Vitamin B12 also protects myelin sheaths of nerve cells from degeneration. After binding to intrinsic factor—a protein produced by acid-secreting parietal cells in

the gastric mucosa—vitamin B12 is absorbed in the ileum. Vitamin B12 deficiency can result in pernicious anemia and neurologic symptoms, such as paresthesias, balance difficulties, and dementia. Vitamin B12 is found in meat, fish, poultry, eggs, and dairy products. Vegan diets, gastric bypass surgeries, or damage to or removal of the ileum place individuals at particular risk for B12 deficiency. Vitamin C has many important roles as an antioxidant, in the immune system, in production and maintenance of collagen, and in the synthesis of epinephrine, serotonin, thyroxine, and adrenal steroid hormones. All fruits and vegetables contain some vitamin C, but the highest levels are found in citrus fruits, broccoli, strawberries, and leafy green vegetables.

Minerals

Calcium, the most abundant mineral in the human body, is largely stored in the bones and teeth (99% of body stores), supporting skeletal structural integrity. Calcium is needed for smooth and skeletal muscle contraction, as a cofactor for many enzymes, and for neurotransmitter release. Circulating calcium levels are tightly regulated, and demineralization of bone occurs if dietary intake is inadequate. High sodium and high protein diets contribute urinary excretion of calcium. Dairy is the primary source of calcium in most American diets; other calcium-containing foods include beans, cabbage, broccoli, spinach, and kale.

Zinc is an essential trace element required for the activity of over 300 enzymes. Wound healing and immune function are impaired in zinc deficiency, which may occur via wound drainage, chronic diarrhea, or a protracted low dietary intake. Oysters contain more zinc per serving than any other food, but red meat and poultry are the primary dietary sources in the United States. Other options are beans, nuts, crab and lobster, whole grains, fortified breakfast cereals, and dairy products. Use of zinc supplementation in persons without zinc deficiency should be monitored closely, as high levels of zinc my actually impair wound healing, phagocytosis, and copper metabolism. Long-term supplementation with high doses of zinc is discouraged secondary to possible adverse effects, such as impaired copper metabolism.

Protein-Calorie Malnutrition

Protein-calorie malnutrition (PCM) is common in elderly persons and in patients with chronic diseases, and may be present in up to 50% of hospitalized patients (17). The presence of PCM increases morbidity, mortality, and risk of infection. For more severe types of PCM, kwashiorkor, or marasmus, it is useful to separate body protein stores into somatic (muscle) proteins and visceral (non-muscle) proteins (18). In the case of protein deprivation with adequate caloric intake, as seen in kwashiorkor, visceral protein levels may be well below normal with relatively normal anthropometric assessments. The severe hypoalbuminemia in kwashiorkor results in extravascular fluid accumulation and marked edema, and alterations in hormone levels, such as insulin, somatotropin, vasopressin, and cortisol. Adult kwashiorkor is commonly seen in persons with inadequate protein intake in the presence of a catabolic state, as with major trauma or severe burns. Conversely, emaciation with relatively normal visceral protein levels may occur in the setting of calorie/energy deprivation, such as marasmus. A third form of PCM is marasmic kwashiorkor—a condition that has features of both. Some have suggested that PCM is a spectrum of a single disease separated by adaptation to starvation, with mounting of an appropriate response in marasmus and failure to adapt in kwashiorkor. Kwashiorkor carries a worse prognosis than marasmus.

LABORATORY ASSESSMENT

Visceral Proteins

Synthesized by the liver and released into the serum, visceral protein levels decrease in the setting of protein malnutrition and are thus used as surrogate markers for nutrition status. Examples of visceral proteins include albumin, prealbumin, transferrin, and retinol-binding protein. This group largely serves in the plasma as binding, transport, and immunologically active proteins. Visceral proteins are negative acute phase reactants, with decreased hepatic production in the presence of inflammatory cytokines in exchange for positive acute phase reactants, such as C-reactive protein, fibrinogen, ceruloplasmin, and complement factors C3 and C4. Furthermore, inflammation results in transcapillary leakage of albumin and prealbumin, decreasing plasma concentrations.

Albumin

For many years, albumin levels have been used as an indicator of visceral protein stores and thus nutrition status, backed by evidence to support the correlation between low albumin levels and an increased risk of overall morbidity and mortality (4, 19, 20). Albumin functions as the major contributor to the osmotic pressure of intravascular fluid, also binding to various substances in the blood, such as bilirubin, cortisol, fatty acids, metals, and some medications. Serum levels are a component of routine hepatic function testing and inexpensive to assess in the laboratory. Unfortunately, albumin levels are relatively insensitive to changes in nutrition status, with a half-life of 20 days and a large body pool (21). In addition, albumin levels are influenced by hydration status and renal function (21). To further complicate the picture, an increased elimination rate of serum albumin has been documented in persons with SCI, showing greater loss with higher levels of injury and in inflammatory status, as seen with chronic pressure ulcers (22–25). Thus, serum albumin levels have been replaced by similar proteins with shorter half-lives as indicators of recent nutrition status or response to nutritional intervention.

Prealbumin

Thyroxine-binding prealbumin, also known as transthyretin, has emerged in recent years as the preferred marker for laboratory assessment of malnutrition, correlating well with patient outcomes (21, 26, 27). Several properties of serum prealbumin (PAB) make it a good indicator of protein and nutrition status, such as its short half-life (2 days), ease of testing, and high ratio of essential to nonessential amino acids (21). With adequate protein supplementation in severe protein-calorie malnutrition, prealbumin levels should increase up to 2 mg/dL per day if no nutritionally confounding factors are present. In otherwise

healthy children with severe PCM, PAB levels increased within the first 48 hours of appropriate nutritional intervention, reaching normal levels within 8 days (5, 21). Increases in PAB concentrations of >4 mg/dL per week are thought to indicate a switch from a catabolic to anabolic state (2). However, serum PAB levels are quite sensitive to inflammatory conditions, with a strong inverse correlation to CRP levels. In fact, suppression of inflammation with corticosteroid therapy increases PAB levels. Unfortunately, reliable PAB levels may be difficult to obtain in the presence of the chronic inflammation and CRP elevation frequently seen in the SCI population. In acute inflammatory conditions, increasing prealbumin levels may indicate an improvement in nutritional *or* metabolic status with improvements in the systemic inflammatory response (2). Hence, obtaining a CRP level with initial prealbumin testing is recommended. To assess trends or response to nutritional and other treatment interventions, CRP and PAB may be analyzed serially at intervals more than 3 days apart (2).

Other markers traditionally used in the assessment of nutritional status, such as transferrin, lymphocyte count, cholesterol level, retinol-binding protein, and fibronectin are described in Tables 25.2 and 25.3.

Transferrin plays a large role in the absorption, transportation, and release of iron into the general circulation. Transferrin is typically saturated to about 1/3 of its total iron-binding capacity, but in iron deficiency anemia, transferrin levels increase in proportion to the deficiency of iron stores. It has a half-life of 8–10 days, making it more responsive than albumin to recent changes in nutrition. However, transferrin lacks specificity and sensitivity to nutrition status. The total lymphocyte count (TLC) has also been used as a marker for nutrition status, but it too has been criticized for its lack of specificity and sensitivity. Lymphocytes function as a primary source of viral defense and antibody production. Obviously, the lymphocyte count increases with certain infections and decreases with immune suppression, as with steroid administration or malnutrition. Total cholesterol levels decrease in the presence of malnutrition, and low cholesterol levels (<175 mg/dl) have been linked to increased mortality in the elderly (28). Retinol-binding protein is the primary transport protein for vitamin A (retinol), binding to one molecule of prealbumin and one molecule of retinol, protecting it from oxidation. In vitamin A deficiency, the concentration of retinol-binding protein in the liver rises and the serum levels fall, indicating that retinol is necessary for hepatic release of this protein. Finally, fibronectin is the only serum protein marker not solely synthesized by hepatocytes, but also produced by epithelial cells, fibroblasts, and macrophages. Fibronectin is particularly important in wound healing and in decreasing vascular permeability. In the presence of tissue injury or inflammation, fibronectin deposition occurs, decreasing serum levels (29). Thus, as is the case with other negative acute phase reactants, fibronectin levels are not reliable in the presence of inflammation, and low levels are often present in SCI (30).

ANTHROPOMETRIC MEASUREMENTS

The ideal weight can be difficult to reach and maintain in the SCI population, due to reduced energy requirements, activity restrictions, and lack of access to healthy foods. However, the impact of

Table 25.2   Commonly Used Laboratory Markers of Nutritional Status

Serum Marker	Normal Range*; Level of Nutritional Risk	Half-life	Factors Altering Level
Prealbumin	15 to 35 mg/dL • 11–15 mg/dL: Increased risk of malnutrition • 5–11 mg/dL: High risk • <5 mg/dL: Poor prognosis In dialysis patients, PAB of <30 mg/dL indicates an increased risk of malnutrition.	2–3 days	Decrease: Acute or chronic inflammation, acute stress, zinc deficiency, liver failure, overhydration. Increase: Renal insufficiency, glucocorticosteroid therapy, progestational agents, acute alcohol intoxication.
Albumin	4 to 6 g/dl; <3.5 g/dL • 2.8–3.5 g/dL: Mild visceral protein depletion • 2.1–2.7 g/dL: Moderate visceral protein depletion • <2.1 g/dL: Severe visceral protein depletion	21 days	Decrease: Overhydration, increased excretion, acute stress, acute or chronic inflammation, age, liver failure. Increase: Dehydration, reduced plasma volume, exogenous administration.
Transferrin	250–300 mg/dL • 150–250 mg/dl: mild depletion • 100–150 mg/dl: moderate depletion • <100 mg/dl: severe depletion	7–10 days	Decrease: Liver failure, increased excretion, acute stress, acute or chronic inflammation, possible decrease with high-dose antibiotic therapy. Increase: Iron deficiency anemia, oral contraceptives, pregnancy, viral hepatitis, chronic blood loss, dehydration.
Retinol-Binding Protein	20–80 mg/L	10–12 hours	Decreased: Vitamin A deficiency**, Cadmium poisoning, hyperthyroidism, chronic liver disease, cystic fibrosis, acute stress. Increased: Estrogens, renal failure.
Fibronectin (FN)	0.3–0.35 mg/mL	15–22 hours	Decreased: Burns, trauma, sepsis, and binding to actin, fibrin, DNA, or *staphylococcus aureus*. Increased: FN-rich cryoprecipitate or blood products.
Total Lymphocyte Count	<1500/mm³		Increased: Acute viral infection, Connective tissue disease, hyperthyroidism, Addison's Disease, splenomegaly Decreased: AIDS, bone marrow suppression, aplastic anemia, neoplasms, steroids, adrenocortical hyperfunction, multiple sclerosis, myasthenia gravis, Guillain-Barre syndrome
Total Cholesterol	<160 mg/dl		Increased: High fat diet, primary hyperlipoproteinemia, acute myocardial infarction, obstructive liver disease, hypothyroidism, nephrotic syndrome, diabetes mellitus, anabolic steroids, progestins, thiazides Decreased: Abetalipoproteinemia, severe liver disease, malnutrition

* Reference values may vary by laboratory.

**In vitamin A deficiency, the hepatic levels of retinol-binding protein rise and the serum levels fall, suggesting that the presence of retinol is necessary for hepatic release.

excessive weight gain or loss can be significant in this population. On either end of the spectrum, problems with skin and deep tissue breakdown are paramount. If too thin, the risk for tissue breakdown over bony prominences is high; if too large, additional weight (typically in the abdominal region) applies increased forces to loaded tissues, causing damage from mechanical deformation and vascular compression, resulting in ischemia. In addition, small weight gains can negatively impact transfers and other activities of daily living, and thus the independence of persons with SCI.

Ideal Body Weight

The ideal body weight (IBW) for persons with SCI can be calculated depending on level of injury, derived from traditional height-weight equations (23). No universally accepted IBW equation exists for the general population, but the most commonly used equations yield similar results, derived from the same height-weight tables (31). The equation used in the chart below was loosely translated into pounds and inches from

Table 25.3   General Indicators of Nutrition Status

Visceral protein	Prealbumin, albumin, transferrin, retinol-binding protein
Overall protein utilization	Nitrogen balance
Somatic protein	Creatinine height index
Protein deficiency	Total lymphocyte count
Protein-calorie malnutrition (moderate to severe)	Skin antigen testing—cellular immune function anergy

Broca's index. For IBW in paraplegia, 5–10% is subtracted from the calculated standard IBW. In tetraplegia, 10–15% is subtracted from the standard IBW. In addition, deductions are made from these IBW calculations for those with the following amputations: about 6–7.1% reduction for a transtibial amputation, 10% for a transfemoral amputation, and 16–18.6% for a hip disarticulation (29).

Standard Ideal Body Weight

Males: 110 lb for the first 5 ft in ht + 5 lb for each inch over 5 ft

Females: 100 lb for the first 5 ft in ht + 5 lb for each inch over 5 ft

Conversion for SCI

Paraplegia: Standard IBW − 5% to 10%
Tetraplegia: Standard IBW − 10% to 15%

Body Mass Index

Many persons with SCI are classified as overweight or obese using standard body mass index calculations, unadjusted for loss of lean body mass. Fat mass correlates with level of spinal cord injury, with increasing fat percentages in higher lesions (32). Greater quantities of total body fat are also associated with older age and longer duration of injury (8). In a sample of 95 men with chronic paraplegia, 57% were "overweight" using the standard calculations for body mass index unadjusted for SCI (BMI ≥ 25 kg/m (2)), with 19% classified as "obese" (BMI ≥ 30 kg/m²) (33). Only 7% were considered underweight (BMI < 18.5 kg/m²), leaving only 36% of participants within the ideal BMI range. A chart review of 408 veterans (401 male and 7 female) revealed 27.9% of subjects had a normal BMI, 3.6% were underweight, and 65.8% were overweight with 29.9% considered obese (34). Unfortunately, although many persons with SCI are classified as overweight or obese using standard BMI calculations, this grossly underestimates the percentage of persons with SCI who meet criteria for overweight/obesity considering loss of lean body mass (11, 35). In fact, comparison of SCI and able-bodied subjects at a given BMI revealed 9.4 kg more fat mass in persons with SCI (36). In 2007, a review of anthropometric data of 7959 veterans with SCI was published, classifying 33% of subjects as overweight and 20% as obese, using standard BMI values (37). When using BMI ranges adjusted for SCI—overweight 23–27 kg/m² and obesity >28 kg/m²—the prevalence of overweight and obesity increased to 37%, and 31%, respectively. Higher BMIs correlated with paraplegia, being white, and with age greater than 50 years.

A recent assessment of percentage fat mass in comparison to BMI in SCI patients revealed that about 74% of subjects who were clinically obese had a BMI < 30 kg/m², whereas if the BMI cutoff for obesity in SCI were lowered to 25 kg/m², only 26% of obese subjects were missed. These investigators also found that subjects with a BMI as low as 22kg/m² were at elevated risk for obesity-related illnesses using percentage of fat mass and CRP. These investigators concluded that in persons with chronic SCI, BMI values greater than 22 kg/m² should herald increased risk for obesity and obesity-related chronic diseases (38).

Skinfold Thickness and Mid-Arm Muscle Circumference

Other methods to estimate body fat composition are skinfold thickness and mid-arm muscle circumference (MAMC) measurements, particularly in patients with unaffected upper extremities. Skinfold thickness is a measure of subcutaneous fat stores, measured at various body sites, such as over the triceps, subscapular, suprailiac, and abdominal areas. The triceps skin fold thickness (TSF) is measured midway between the acromion process and olecranon of the non-dominant arm by gently pulling the skin and subcutaneous tissue away from the muscle, and measuring the thickness with a caliper. In men, thickness less than 12.5 mm implies undernutrition, whereas over 20 mm suggests excess body fat stores. Likewise, in women less than 16.5 mm is indicative of undernutrition and greater than 25 mm is indicative of excess fat reserves. This is a relatively insensitive method of measuring fat stores, as a number of variables influence skin fold thickness, including fluid shifts, age, and ethnic background (18). Skin fold thickness measurements are best reserved for measuring subcutaneous adipose stores in chronic conditions over a period of months to years (29). The MAMC reflects both caloric adequacy and muscle mass, calculated from the mid arm circumference (MAC) and the TSF thickness using the following formula:

$$MAMC = MAC - \pi \times (TSF \text{ in mm})$$

This measurement has questionable validity in the SCI population, however, and low inter-observer reliability in non-SCI patients (23, 39).

Waist-to-Hip Ratio

Finally, the waist-to-hip circumference ratio measures the distribution of subcutaneous and intra-abdominal fat. The ratio tends to increase with age and excess weight, and may be falsely elevated with denervation of trunk musculature, as seen in spinal cord injuries above the lowest thoracic levels. To determine the waist-to-hip ratio, first measure waist circumference at the midpoint between the inferior portion of the lateral rib cage and the iliac crest, then the hip circumference at its widest point. The ratio is then calculated as follows:

$$\text{Waist-to-hip ratio} = (\text{Waist circumference})/(\text{Hip circumference})$$

In persons without SCI, waist-to-hip ratios of greater than 0.95 for men and 0.80 for women indicate increased risk for heart disease and metabolic syndrome, whereas ratios below these values confer decreased risk for obesity-related health problems (40). The validity of this tool has not been established in the SCI population (35).

ACUTE NUTRITION CONSIDERATIONS

Nutritional Care Plan for Acute Spinal Cord Injury

The nutritional care plan for patients after acute SCI begins with a thorough nutritional assessment and continues with close monitoring of nutritional status, to include weekly weights. Weight loss is common initially, often with a >10% reduction of pre-injury weight within the first month (41). On average, persons with tetraplegia sustain greater weight loss (30–50 lb) than paraplegia (10–35 lb) (25). A majority of the early weight loss (> 85%) can be attributed to loss of lean body mass from denervation atrophy of muscles below the level of the lesion (41). Despite expected acute weight losses, many clinicians suggest investigation of any significant (>10%) weight reduction with patient/family interview, evaluation for iatrogenic or medical causes, and dietary assessment with calorie count. Exacerbating loss of body mass from denervation, gastrointestinal motility is markedly decreased, and often enteral feeds are held secondary to the presence of a neurogenic ileus. Nutritional status and dietary adequacy should be aggressively monitored in the acute setting, requiring consultation with a registered dietician. Assessment of protein nutrition should be performed via serial prealbumin levels (ideally with CRP) in addition to other labs, as previously mentioned.

Initiation of Early versus Late Feeding

Dvorak et al. (42) compared outcomes of initiating early (<72hrs) versus late (>120hrs) enteral feeding in 23 patients with acute cervical SCI, citing similar studies performed in other patient populations with worse outcomes in the early feeding groups, or with no difference in outcomes in early or late feeding groups (43–45). They found no difference in incidence of infections, nutritional status, feeding tolerance, average ventilator hours, or length of acute-care hospital stay. Interestingly, only one subject had no infectious complications. The frequency of feeding intolerance was non-significantly higher in the late group; nausea and diarrhea represented the majority of these complications. The authors concluded from this pilot study that early enteral nutritional support may not be as critical for persons sustaining acute cervical SCI secondary to the metabolic differences in this population in the acute post-injury period.

Dysphagia

Although dysphagia is a known complication of cervical spinal cord injury (CSCI), the incidence and mechanism of this pathology has not been well-studied. Dysphagia is a well-known complication of anterior spine stabilization and tracheotomy placement, both commonly performed procedures after CSCI. Also, the risk of severe dysphagia is higher with concomitant lower cranial nerve injury. In a sample of 51 patients with acute CSCI and respiratory insufficiency, Wolf and Meiners (46) reported that 21 (41%) experienced moderate to severe dysphagia, 20 (39%) had mild dysphagia from laryngeal edema or mild aspiration, and 10 (20%) patients exhibited no evidence of dysphagia. Of the patients with severe dysphagia acutely, only 3 out of 21 (14%) had severe dysphagia on follow-up. Thus, persons with cervical spinal cord lesions are at risk for aspiration and should be screened for dysphagia. If a feeding tube must be placed for long-term enteral access, then jejunostomy might be preferred over a gastrostomy placement to decrease the risk of aspiration. In a 2002 publication, the American Association of Neurological Surgeons and the Congress of Neurological Surgeons reviewing nutrition after SCI observed that no recommendations have been issued for the composition of feeds after SCI, though literature on patients with head injury supports at least 15% of calories from protein (high nitrogen), less than 15% glucose/dextrose, at least 4% from essential fatty acids, and supplementation with vitamins, essential elements, and trace minerals (47).

Negative Nitrogen Balance and Metabolism

Patients with severe trauma, but without SCI, will enter a hypermetabolic state acutely after injury with elevations in urinary nitrogen excretion. This resolves within 1–3 weeks after injury, with nitrogen balance moving from negative to normal or positive. However, in the setting of denervation from SCI, it is nearly impossible to establish a positive nitrogen balance during the acute phase of injury, and the duration of the negative nitrogen balance is longer (41). Approximately 85–100% of this nitrogen deficit is attributed to loss of lean body mass (41). Rodriquez et al. (48) studied 10 SCI patients and 20 trauma patient controls. In the seven week study period, none of the SCI patients achieved a neutral or positive nitrogen balance. In fact, they found that the peak negative balance in SCI occurs during a phase when energy expenditure is decreasing, and thus it does not respond to increases in calorie or protein intake. However, in order to prevent accelerated protein breakdown during the acute injury phase, administration of 2 grams of protein/kilogram of IBW is recommended.

In a subsequent publication (49), Rodriquez measured the nitrogen balance and predicted energy expenditure (PEE) and actual energy expenditures (MEE) in 12 subjects with acute SCI (10 complete SCI, 2 incomplete) for 4 weeks, or until the initiation of oral nutrition. The PEE was calculated using the Harris-Benedict equation for Basal Energy Expenditure (BEE), with an activity factor of 1.2 for bedrest and an injury factor of 1.6 for major trauma.

Nitrogen Balance

NB = (24-hr protein intake in g/6.25) − (24-hr urinary urea nitrogen in grams + 4 g*)

[*4 g added to account for miscellaneous nitrogen losses]

Harris-Benedict equation

Men: BEE = 66 + (13.8 × wt in kg) + (5 × ht in cm) − (6.8 × age)

Women: BEE = 655 + (9.6 × wt in kg) + (1.8 × ht in cm) − (4.7 × age)

Predicted Energy Expenditures

$$PEE = BEE \times 1.2 \text{ (bedrest)} \times 1.6 \text{ (major trauma)}$$

Measurements were not recorded if any inconsistencies in nutrition administration or fluctuations in FiO2 were found. During week 1, 4 of 10 subjects had a positive nitrogen balance, followed by persistent negative nitrogen balances in all subjects except one with incomplete injury. As for energy requirements, comparisons of predicted and measured expenditures are as follows: week 1, MEE < PEE in 7 of 9 subjects; week 2, MEE < PEE in 4 of 7 subjects; week 3, 2 of 2 subjects with MEE > PEE; and week 4, MEE < PEE in 3 of 4 subjects. The complex interplay of acute post-traumatic hypermetabolism and hypercatabolism and decreased energy expenditures from flaccid paralysis make it difficult to anticipate the energy requirements of this population during this period. The authors concluded that the use of the standard activity and stress factors with the Harris-Benedict equation overestimate caloric needs, and reliance on nitrogen balance assessments to calculate dietary needs in this population will most likely lead to overfeeding. Other investigators have found that the Harris-Benedict equation, with and without activity and injury factors, is inaccurate in acute SCI, recommending indirect calorimetry for assessment of energy expenditure (41, 47, 50).

Constipation and Appetite

Initially after admission to acute inpatient rehabilitation, most patients do not maintain proper dietary intake for a variety of reasons. Constipation generally causes nausea and poor appetite, and it is unfortunately quite common upon admission to a rehabilitation facility, particularly if the patient was previously not on a proper bowel program and/or had very limited activity on the acute ward. Also pain, depression/grief, and other medical conditions and medications, i.e. narcotics, may adversely affect oral intake. As the patient becomes more active and involved in therapies in addition to maintenance of a proper bowel regimen and simplification of his or her medications, appetite typically improves.

CHRONIC NUTRITION CONSIDERATIONS

Dietary Evaluations in Community-Dwelling Subjects

Long-term nutritional recommendations for SCI individuals are similar to that of the general population. The same nutrients are necessary, but the caloric need is diminished due to activity limitations, muscular atrophy, and higher fat composition (51–53). Buchholz et al. estimated the resting metabolic rate is 14–27% lower in persons with chronic SCI compared to non-injured subjects, resulting in an overestimation of energy requirements in individuals with SCI by 5–32% using standard equations (54, 55). Levine et al. (56) analyzed the dietary intake of 33 healthy subjects with chronic SCI (24 male, 9 female). Although overall caloric intake was 75% of that recommended for able-bodied persons by the gender-specific 1989 Recommended Dietary Allowances (RDA), the total energy intake was high in fat calories (7.6 and 1.5% above recommended percentage for males and females, respectively), low in carbohydrate calories (average of 16.5% below recommended levels), and slightly above recommended calories from protein. In addition to excessive fat intake, the ratio of polyunsaturated to saturated fat was about half of the AHA target of 1.0. For micronutrients, comparison of the average intake of the subjects' diets to the RDA for males and females is represented in Table 25.4. Average fiber intake was only 25% of recommend levels for the general population. Cholesterol intake of the SCI subjects was lower than that of the general population and below American Heart Association (AHA) guidelines. Levine concluded that the involvement of a registered dietician and nutritional education was needed for persons with SCI.

Table 25.4   Identified Nutrient Deficiencies

ASSESSMENT	PEIFFER ET AL. 1981 (REF. 23)	LEVINE ET AL. 1992 (REF. 56)	WALTERS ET AL. 2008 (REF. 57)	PETCHKRUA ET AL. 2003 (REF. 59)
Macronutrient	*Paraplegia* No deficiencies in kcal or protein intake—fat not assessed* *Tetraplegia* Inadequate kcal intake*	*Males & Females* Low-calorie intake: Low carbohydrate, slightly high protein, high fat*	*Males & Females* Appropriate macronutrient percentages: *Carbohydrate* M: 52%, F: 53%; *Protein* M: 16%, F: 17%; *Fat* M: 30%, F: 28%*	N/A
Micronutrient	*Paraplegia* Vitamin A *Tetraplegia* Vitamin A, thiamin, calcium, iron	*Males* Vitamin A, thiamin, riboflavin, pyridoxine, vitamin E, calcium, magnesium, zinc, potassium, pantothenate, copper *Females* Pyridoxine, calcium, iron, magnesium, zinc, copper	*Males & Females* Vitamin A, magnesium, folate, zinc, vitamin C, vitamin B12, thiamin, vitamin B6, riboflavin, potassium, calcium, vitamin D	Vitamin B12 by: • Subnormal vitamin B12: 5.7% • Supranormal MMA: 19% • Both subnormal/low normal vitamin B12 and supranormal MMA: 13.3%

*These studies based their assessments on recommendations established for the general population, not accounting for the decreased energy requirements in persons with SCI.

In comparison, a dietary analysis of a Canadian cohort of community-dwelling persons with SCI showed an adequate energy intake with appropriate average percentages of macronutrients in both males and females for both paraplegia and tetraplegia (57). Fiber intake was below recommended levels, as well as many micronutrients (See Table 25.4). Interestingly, calcium intake was significantly higher in persons with complete versus incomplete injury. Use of dietary supplementation was assessed during 2 visits, revealing 25–26% consumed multivitamins, 19–29% calcium, 12–22% vitamin D, and 6–9% vitamin C. The investigations in this chapter involving macronutrient assessments in persons with SCI did not adjust for the diminished energy needs in this population, but compared the subjects' intake to the recommendations available for the able-bodied persons.

Vitamins A, C, and E

Mossavi et al. (58) examined the serum levels of vitamins A, C, and E in 110 persons (79 male/31 female) with chronic SCI in the community. These three micronutrients were examined for their antioxidant properties and role in the prevention of cardiovascular disease, cancer, and pressure ulcers. They found that 16.4% of these subjects had serum vitamin A levels below reference range, 37.3% were deficient in vitamin C, and 30.0% were deficient in vitamin E. Older persons and persons who were older at time of SCI had higher levels of vitamins A and E, though no correlation was found with time since injury, gender, or race. Correlations were found between serum vitamin A levels and the completeness and level of injury, in that lower levels of vitamin A corresponded with more severe neurologic impairment, i.e. lower levels associated with tetraplegia than paraplegia or with ASIA grade A, B, or C than ASIA D. Persons with at least one pressure ulcer in the preceding year had lower levels of vitamin A, which may have caused disruption of collagen metabolism in this group. The positive relationship between age and levels of vitamins A and E were thought to be related to education and compliance with a healthy, balanced diet as compared to the younger subjects. Note that serum vitamin A levels may remain normal despite fluctuations in oral intake and deficiency in certain tissues.

Vitamin B12

Another study evaluating the prevalence of vitamin B12 deficiency in the SCI population analyzed fasting blood samples for serum B12, methylmalonic acid (MMA), folic acid, and homocysteine levels (59). In vitamin B12 deficiency, MMA and homocysteine are elevated, though the most sensitive marker of B12 deficiency is a high MMA. In this sample of 105 men with chronic SCI, serum B12 levels were subnormal and MMA levels supranormal in 5.7% (6 of 105) of subjects. Including these six subjects, MMA levels were supranormal in 19% (20 of 105) overall. The true prevalence of vitamin B12 deficiency was likely within this range (5.7–19%). Laboratory profiles with an elevated MMA and a low or low-normal serum B12 existed in 13.3% of the study sample, which was thought by investigators to most strongly correlate with B12 deficiency in persons with SCI. No subjects had low folate levels by laboratory criteria. Vitamin B12 deficiency was most common in persons with more severe spinal cord injury (more complete, higher levels), ages 40–59, and with longer duration of injury. The higher prevalence of B12 deficiency in middle-aged males with

SCI differs from the general population, which holds higher prevalence in the elderly. Interestingly, although a substantial number of false-positive MMA levels existed in this study, false-positive elevations of MMA rarely occur in non-SCI populations without renal insufficiency. Regularly prescribed medications may also contribute to B12 deficiency in this population by altering its absorption, notably H_2-blockers, proton pump inhibitors, and metformin, in addition to vitamin C supplementation (60). These investigators (59) recommended regular laboratory screening for B12 deficiency in SCI patients, though the frequency of this testing is not yet established.

Calcium and Vitamin D

Recent studies have shown that use of vitamin D supplements was associated with a reduction in overall mortality, with implications of a preventative role in insulin resistance, diabetes, and hypertension. Unfortunately, vitamin D deficiency is quite common in the SCI population (61–63). Zhou et al. found that 25-hydroxyvitamin D and total serum calcium levels were significantly lower in 92 men with spinal cord injury as compared to 28 able-bodied controls (62). The 25-hydroxyvitamin D levels in individuals with tetraplegia were lower than those with paraplegia, though this difference did not reach statistical significance. The lowest vitamin D and calcium levels were found in subjects with pressure ulcers and low activity levels. Investigators concluded that these decrements in vitamin D levels could be partially attributed to reduced sunlight exposure from hospitalizations and greater physical disability. In another comparison of SCI subjects (n = 100) to able-bodied controls (n = 50), the incidence of vitamin D and calcium deficiencies was significantly higher in the SCI group—32% were vitamin D deficient and 17% had low total calcium levels (63). However, the mean levels for both nutrients were similar in the SCI and control groups. The low total calcium levels in these studies could be attributed to hypoalbuminemia, altered vitamin D metabolism, or inadequate calcium intake—all of which are common in SCI.

To determine the appropriate dose of replacement therapy for vitamin D deficiency, Bauman et al. (64) studied replacement therapy in vitamin D-deficient subjects with chronic SCI and the effects of vitamin D supplementation on SCI subjects with and without low levels of serum 25-hydroxyvitamin D. In the replacement therapy branch of the study, 10 subjects were given 50 micrograms of vitamin D3 twice a week for 14 days, and in the supplementation branch, 40 subjects received 20 micrograms of vitamin D3 daily for 12 months. All subjects received supplemental calcium. In both groups, serum 25-hydroxyvitamin D levels increased significantly, though in the replacement group, 8 or 10 subjects still had subnormal levels by day 14, and in the supplementation group 9 subjects had subnormal and 23 had low-normal levels at one year (compared to 33 and 6, respectively, at baseline). The authors concluded that higher doses of vitamin D therapy for longer duration were required to adequately replace deficient vitamin D stores.

Lipid Profiles

Unfortunately, spinal cord injury has a negative impact on the fasting lipid profiles, resulting in elevated levels of low-density lipoprotein (LDL), low levels of high-density lipoprotein, and elevated triglycerides (TG), favoring atherosclerosis and accelerated development of cardiovascular disease (9, 11). The severity of injury appears to influence cholesterol levels, with lower HDL values in persons with a higher level or degree of injury (65). Total cholesterol was higher in those with paraplegia, but TC/HDL ratios were higher in subjects with tetraplegia. Jones (66) and Manns et al. (8) reported an association between low HDL, elevated post-load insulin, and low activity levels in individuals with SCI. Comparison of men and premenopausal women with the same level of lesion showed higher levels of HDL and lower TC/HDL ratios in women, with no significant difference between the sexes in TC, LDL, and TG levels (67). However, subjects with tetraplegia had significantly higher TG levels than those with paraplegia. Others have reported a strong negative correlation between HDL and TG concentrations in the SCI population (9).

Environmental Factors

Unfortunately, it is far easier and cheaper to obtain processed foods high in fat and sugar than healthy foods, such as fresh produce, lean meat, and whole grains in today's society. With the addition of impaired mobility, environmental barriers add greatly to difficulties in acquiring healthy foods on a regular basis. Moreover, poverty is more prevalent in persons with physical disabilities, further hindering access to the more expensive nutrient-rich and low-fat foods, such as fresh fruits and vegetables. In 2008, two low-income neighborhoods of similar size, one urban and one suburban, were compared for selection of healthy food choices and wheelchair accessibility of local grocery and convenience stores (68). The urban stores were more abundant (48 compared to 34 suburban), but fewer had entrances manageable with a wheelchair (46% versus 88%). Within the stores, factors such as aisle width, product height, counter height, ease of opening refrigerator doors, etc. did not differ significantly between the two regions, nor did the low availability of healthy affordable foods.

Community Nutrition Knowledge

Many experts, particularly those involved in analyzing the dietary intakes of persons with chronic SCI, recommend consultation with a dietician to outline proper food choices in this group. Some recommend annual performance of such an evaluation (60). Although many patients are seen by a dietician during their acute rehabilitation stay, information received during this time period may not be retained or considered significant compared to other factors faced during transition into the community. Assessment of the nutrition knowledge and dietary intake of 95 men with paraplegia for over one year in the Chicago area revealed a significant correlation between diet quality (as per the Healthy Eating Index-f) and competency on a nutrition questionnaire, though this significance may have been overpowered by the effect of overall education and income (33). This assessment also showed relationships between poor diet and anthropometric measures (BMI), poverty, smoking, and living alone. No correlation was found between depression and diet quality. In keeping with other mentioned investigations, overall calorie intake was low, cholesterol intake was low (only two-thirds of participants met recommended consumption), fiber intake was lacking (12% meeting recommended intake), and diets included too much total fat (18% compliance with recommendations) and saturated fat (33% in compliance

with recommendations). In addition, less than 35% of subjects consumed recommended sodium, fruit, and vegetable intake, and only 16% complied with suggested daily dairy servings. This study supports the need for more diet and nutrition education in the SCI community.

Energy Expenditure with Ambulation

In 1978, Fisher and Gullickson reviewed energy costs of different methods of ambulation (69). Compared to walking at 5 km/hr in able-bodied subjects, wheelchair ambulation resulted in a 9% increase in calories per meter, whereas ambulation with braces and crutches in persons with paraplegia at a much slower rate (1.28 km/ hr) resulted in over 5 times the calorie expenditure. For persons with paraplegia, the high energy demands and slow pace of ambulation with braces and crutches makes wheelchair ambulation the preferred method of ambulation. For its fitness benefits, manual wheelchair mobility is recommended for as long as possible, though most long-term wheelchair users must convert to powered mobility with age and chronic overuse injuries in the upper extremities at some point.

After incomplete SCI, muscle fibers below the level of the lesion convert to fast-twitch glycolytic fibers, resulting in loss of endurance and early fatigue. In 2007, Nash et al. published a study on nutrient supplementation in three persons with incomplete SCI after ambulation to fatigue, to determine the effects of immediate carbohydrate and protein administration after intense exercise for recovery and performance on subsequent trials (70). Subjects received 5 days of experimental (maltodextrin and whey protein) or control (slowly digested soy protein) drinks within 5 minutes of ambulation to fatigue, followed by a weekend rest period, and another 5 days of the same. A two-week wash-out period ensued, and the process was then repeated with the supplement not yet received. Both subjects and data collectors were blinded to the composition of the supplement. All subjects walked longer time periods, farther distances, and with greater energy expenditure during experimental supplementation compared to control. The immediate administration of liquid carbohydrate was thought to enhance recovery by rapidly replenishing depleted glycogen stores, with whey protein stimulating an insulin response and delaying post-exercise protein catabolism by supplying amino acids. The investigators concluded that the effects seen on exercise performance with carbohydrate and whey supplementation supported the reliance of partially denervated muscles on glycogen.

Pressure Ulcers and Nutrition

Aggressive nutritional support, adequate hydration, and consultation with a dietician are recommended for all patients with a Stage III or IV pressure ulcer or deep tissue injury. For healing of advanced pressure sores, approximately 30–35 calories/kg/day and 1.25–1.50 grams of protein/kg/day is recommended (71). The protein and calorie requirements for wound healing are higher than in chronic SCI and less than in the acute post-injury period. The increased protein requirements for wound healing are necessary to replace the large protein losses occurring at the wound site, and to achieve a positive nitrogen balance. Dehydration may also easily occur secondary to fluid losses in draining pressure ulcers. Any vitamin deficiencies, particularly subnormal levels of vitamin C, vitamin A, and zinc should be corrected. Many experts recommend supplementation with vitamin C (500–1000 mg/day) and zinc (50 mg/day) in the presence of Stage III or IV pressure ulcers, regardless of the serum levels (71). Finally, anticoagulants and corticosteroids should be discontinued if possible.

According to the "Pressure Ulcer Prevention and Treatment Following SCI: A Clinical Practice Guideline for Health-Care Professionals," published in 2000 (30), evaluation of nutritional status of persons with SCI should include dietary intake analysis, anthropometric measurements, and biochemical parameters such as prealbumin, albumin, hemoglobin, hematocrit, transferrin, and total lymphocyte count. Serial measurements to assess for trends may be more helpful than single assessments. Some references suggested that low albumin levels may contribute to pressure ulcer development by causing interstitial edema, thus interfering with oxygen and nutrient transport to the tissues, resulting in damage (72, 73). Albumin infusions are not recommended, but maximization of nutritional support is. Anemia could contribute to the reduced oxygen supply to tissues, but iron replacement is not necessarily recommended, as the low hemoglobin and hematocrit levels may not stem from iron deficiency, but from an inability to use iron stores appropriately. Hematochromatosis may result from unnecessary iron supplementation. Finally, the Consortium for SCI Medicine recommended ensuring adequate intake of calories, protein, micronutritents (zinc, vitamin C, vitamin A, and vitamin E), and fluids to aid wound healing (30). To help achieve these nutritional goals, it may be helpful to increase feeding frequency to six small meals a day. If dietary goals cannot be met with oral intake, enteral or parenteral supplementation is required. Total parenteral supplementation should be reserved for persons with severe GI dysfunction unable to tolerate enteral feeds.

Though nutritional interventions for the prevention and treatment of pressure ulcers are generally accepted as standard care, few studies have shown clinical benefit from any particular supplement (74), particularly in the SCI population. The 2008 Cochrane Review "Nutritional interventions for preventing and treating pressure ulcers," examined 8 randomized controlled trials (RCTs) analyzing the effects of adding mixed nutritional supplements, vitamin C, zinc, or protein to the dietary regimen of surgical, elderly, or critically ill patient populations (75). Most of these publications were too small and of poor quality and/or were plagued with high drop-out rates—frequently encountered complications in dietary-based studies. Of four RCTs using mixed nutritional supplements for the prevention of pressure ulcers in non-SCI at-risk populations, only one was of adequate size to reach statistical significance in support of such intervention, though in the other three studies fewer pressure ulcers developed in the supplement groups. In the pressure ulcer treatment trials, two RCTs using vitamin C supplementation yielded contradictory results, and one study examining the effects of zinc was far too small to show clinical effectiveness or statistical significance, with considerable dropout before completion. Interestingly, analyses of zinc levels in persons with protein-energy malnutrition showed a significant correlation in presence of skin lesions and zinc deficiency, with pressure ulcers only present in the malnourished subjects with low zinc levels (76, 77). More research on this subject is imperative to develop evidence-based dietary regimens for the prevention and treatment of pressure ulcers.

Finally, the scales for assessing pressure ulcer risk validated in the general population are not particularly helpful in SCI. The widely-used Braden scale is divided into six categories: sensory perception, moisture, activity, mobility, nutrition, and friction and shear. Obviously, the presence of SCI generates a low score (high risk for pressure ulcer development), with altered sensation, bowel/bladder dysfunction contributing to skin maceration, impaired mobility and limited activity, and increased friction and shear. Thus, the Braden scale is not routinely used on the SCI unit.

RECOMMENDATIONS

Diet

There is a general agreement that people with and without SCI should consume a diet rich in fruits, vegetables, and whole-grain products low in total fat, saturated fat, cholesterol, and sodium. Fruit and vegetable intake inversely relate to risk of metabolic syndrome, diabetes, and cardiovascular disease. Conversely, diets high in saturated fat increase serum cholesterol more than any other single nutrient, with elevations of apolipoproteins named as a principle causative factor in cardiovascular disease. Unfortunately, persons with SCI tend to consume diets low in fruits and vegetables and many necessary minerals and vitamins, and high in total and saturated fat. Also, persons with SCI are often erroneously advised to avoid calcium and dairy products secondary to hypercalcemia observed in the acute post-injury period (78). To prevent or correct poor dietary habits, consultation with a registered dietician should be considered for community-dwelling persons with SCI. If proper nutrition cannot be met by diet, deficiencies should be addressed by the use of supplements. Exercise should be encouraged whenever possible to counter the effects of low physical activity in paraplegia and tetraplegia, namely decreased HDL, higher triglycerides, higher fasting glucose, larger abdominal girth, and higher markers of chronic inflammation (elevated CRP)—all key components of metabolic syndrome (8).

Protein and Calorie Requirements

The gold standard for determining energy expenditure and caloric needs is indirect calorimetry. Once only practical in the inpatient setting using a metabolic cart, advancements in the portability and ease of use of these machines have made them useful in the outpatient setting as well. However, due to the expense and limited availability of this technology, most clinicians rely on calculations to estimate energy needs.

The energy requirements in persons with chronic tetraplegia are approximately 22.7 kcal/kg/day, and 27.9 kcal/kg/day in those with paraplegia. This suggested caloric intake falls well below the recommended calories for maintenance as calculated by body weight in the same person non-injured (79). If attempting to lose weight, then the above calculation should be performed on the desired or ideal body weight—which is also lower in those with SCI due to loss of muscle mass. As in the general population, calorie deductions based on advanced age and sedentary lifestyle should be considered, whereas allowances for the increased caloric requirements of athletes and otherwise active persons should be made. Unfortunately, the "typical" easily accessible, affordable American diet is high in fat and refined sugar, with inadequate intake of fiber, complex carbohydrates, and many vitamins and minerals, making it difficult to comply with the low energy needs in SCI while maintaining appropriate intake of recommended nutrients.

In chronic SCI, protein requirements match that of the general population—0.8 g/kg. However, larger amounts are required during the acute post-injury phase or when pressure ulcers are present. The recommended daily protein intake is 1.25–1.50 g/kg/day for healing of Stage III or IV pressure ulcers, and in the hypercatabolic state of acute injury it is 2 g/kg/day. Because only certain amounts of protein can be processed before additional intake is converted into fat, it is important to include a serving of protein with each meal or with snacks, instead of attempting to consume the daily requirements in one meal, e.g. a large steak with dinner.

Fiber

The suggested fiber intake in patients with SCI is unclear. In the able-bodied population, fiber has been shown to decrease mouth to anus transit time and assist with weight and blood sugar control. It has also been implicated in decreasing the incidence of cancer and cardiovascular diseases. In persons with SCI levels C4–T12 and neurogenic bowel, Cameron et al. studied the effects of increasing baseline dietary fiber intake on gastrointestinal transit time and stool weight (80). Increasing fiber consumption from 25 g/day to 31 g/day resulted in a significant increase in mean colonic transit time (28.2 to 42.2 hr) and rectosigmoid transit time (7.9 to 23.3 hr), whereas mouth to anus transit time, right and left colon transit time, and stool weight remained unchanged. The investigators recommended further studies to elucidate optimal dietary fiber intake in persons with neurogenic bowel from SCI.

The 1998 Paralyzed Veterans of America (PVA) Clinical Practice Guidelines on Neurogenic Bowel Management in Adults with Spinal Cord Injury (81) discourages placing all persons with SCI on similar high-fiber diets. Instead, the consortium recommends assessing the existing fiber content of each individual's diet and making adjustments to optimize his or her bowel program as needed, with an initial daily fiber intake of least 15 g/day. If more dietary fiber is required, additional fiber should come from variety of sources and increases made gradually. Excellent sources of fiber include whole grains, bran products, leafy greens, and raw vegetables.

Nutritional Assessments for Persons with SCI

In 1981, Peiffer et al. developed a set of indicators of nutritional risk in persons with SCI, as shown in Table 25.5 (23). Since that time no formal guide for routine nutrition screening in SCI has been established, though major advancements in our understanding of metabolism and nutrition in SCI have occurred.

A 2008 review of obesity in SCI provided a set of recommendations for clinicians involved in SCI care in the outpatient setting (35). This publication suggested checking weights at every clinic visit and tracking trends, discussing these trends with the patient and determining his or her personal goals, and assessing the need for intervention based on this data. The health care provider should be familiar with exercise options for persons with SCI based on completeness and level of injury, initiating a prescription for physical or recreational therapy as needed. In addition, diet should be discussed and dietary recommendations

Table 25.5 Guidelines for Identifying Nutritional Risk in SCI Patients (Ref. 23)

Body Weight	>10% below recommended IBW*
Serum albumin	<3.0 g/dL
Caloric intake	<Calculated maintenance or anabolic requirement
Protein intake	<Calculated maintenance or anabolic requirement
Hemoglobin	<12 g/dL
Hematocrit	<37%
Creatinine-ht index	<60% of standard

*IBW: Ideal body weight as adjusted for paraplegia or tetraplegia.

made, with referral to a nutritionist or dietician if indicated. As mentioned, registered dieticians are important members of the acute care and rehabilitation teams, and regular consultation with these clinicians are recommended in the inpatient and outpatient setting (60).

CONCLUSION

Unfortunately, it is difficult to practice evidence-based medicine in the realm of nutrition, because much more is assumed than has been proven. Randomized controlled trials are difficult to perform on this subject, secondary to the low compliance and high dropout rate. In particular, the effects of dietary requirements on wound healing are difficult to assess for such a multifactorial issue. More research is necessary on the topic of nutrition in spinal cord injury before further guidelines can be established.

References

1. Danaei G, Ding EL, Mozaffarian D, et al. The preventable causes of death in the United States: comparative risk assessment of dietary, lifestyle, and metabolic risk factors. PLoS Med 2009; 6(4):e1000058.
2. Shenkin A. Serum prealbumin: Is it a marker of nutritional status or of risk of malnutrition? Clin Chem 2006; 52(12):2177–2179.
3. Kaufman HH, Rowlands BJ, Stein DK, Kopaniky DR, Gildenberg PL. General metabolism in patients with acute paraplegia and quadriplegia. Neurosurgery 1985; 16(3):309–313.
4. Dempsey DT, Mullen JL, Buzby GP. The link between nutritional status and clinical outcome: can nutritional intervention modify it? Am J Clin Nutr 1988; 47(2 Suppl):352–356.
5. Spiekerman AM. Nutritional assessment (protein nutriture). Anal Chem 1995; 67(12):429R–436R.
6. Klein JD, Hey LA, Yu CS, et al. Perioperative nutrition and postoperative complications in patients undergoing spinal surgery. Spine 1996; 21(22):2676–2682.
7. Frost F, Roach MJ, Kushner I, Schreiber P. Inflammatory C-reactive protein and cytokine levels in asymptomatic people with chronic spinal cord injury. Arch Phys Med Rehabil 2005; 86(2):312–317.
8. Manns PJ, McCubbin JA, Williams DP. Fitness, inflammation, and the metabolic syndrome in men with paraplegia. Arch Phys Med Rehabil 2005; 86(6):1176–1181.
9. Bauman WA, Spungen AM. Disorders of carbohydrate and lipid metabolism in veterans with paraplegia or quadriplegia: a model of premature aging. Metabolism 1994; 43(6):749–756.
10. Banerjea R, Sambamoorthi U, Weaver F, Maney M, Pogach LM, Findley T. Risk of stroke, heart attack, and diabetes complications

among veterans with spinal cord injury. Arch Phys Med Rehabil 2008; 89(8):1448–1453.

11. Bauman WA, Spungen AM. Metabolic changes in persons after spinal cord injury. Phys Med Rehabil Clin N Am 2000; 11(1):109–140.

12. Peruzzi WT, Shapiro BA, Meyer PR, Jr., Krumlovsky F, Seo BW. Hyponatremia in acute spinal cord injury. Crit Care Med 1994; 22(2):252–258.

13. Leehey DJ, Picache AA, Robertson GL. Hyponatraemia in quadriplegic patients. Clin Sci (Lond) 1988; 75(4):441–444.

14. Soni BM, Vaidyanthan S, Watt JW, Krishnan KR. A retrospective study of hyponatremia in tetraplegic/paraplegic patients with a review of the literature. Paraplegia 1994; 32(9):597–607.

15. Massagli TL, Cardenas DD. Immobilization hypercalcemia treatment with pamidronate disodium after spinal cord injury. Arch Phys Med Rehabil 1999; 80(9):998–1000.

16. Biyani A, Inman CG, el Masry WS. Hyponatraemia after acute spinal injury. Injury 1993; 24(10):671–673.

17. Haider M, Haider SQ. Assessment of protein-calorie malnutrition. Clin Chem 1984; 30(8):1286–1299.

18. Sardesai VM. Introduction to clinical nutrition. 2nd ed. New York: Marcel Dekker; 2003.

19. Reinhardt GF, Myscofski JW, Wilkens DB, Dobrin PB, Mangan JE, Jr., Stannard RT. Incidence and mortality of hypoalbuminemic patients in hospitalized veterans. JPEN J Parenter Enteral Nutr 1980; 4(4):357–359.

20. Doweiko JP, Nompleggi DJ. The role of albumin in human physiology and pathophysiology, Part III: Albumin and disease states. JPEN J Parenter Enteral Nutr 1991; 15(4):476–83.

21. Beck FK, Rosenthal TC. Prealbumin: a marker for nutritional evaluation. Am Fam Physician 2002; 65(8):1575–1578.

22. Ring J, Seifert J, Lob G, Stephan W, Probst J, Brendel W. Elimination rate of human serum albumin in paraplegic patients. Paraplegia 1974; 12(2):139–144.

23. Peiffer SC, Blust P, Leyson JF. Nutritional assessment of the spinal cord injured patient. J Am Diet Assoc 1981; 78(5):501–505.

24. Laven GT, Huang CT, DeVivo MJ, Stover SL, Kuhlemeier KV, Fine PR. Nutritional status during the acute stage of spinal cord injury. Arch Phys Med Rehabil 1989; 70(4):277–282.

25. Cloninger MC. Nutritional management of patients with spinal injury: paraplegia versus quadriplegia. Arch Phys Med Rehabil 1980; 61:489.

26. Bernstein LH, Leukhardt-Fairfield CJ, Pleban W, Rudolph R. Usefulness of data on albumin and prealbumin concentrations in determining effectiveness of nutritional support. Clin Chem 1989; 35(2):271–274.

27. Robinson MK, Trujillo EB, Mogensen KM, Rounds J, McManus K, Jacobs DO. Improving nutritional screening of hospitalized patients: the role of prealbumin. JPEN J Parenter Enteral Nutr 2003; 27(6):389–395; quiz 439.

28. Schupf N, Costa R, Luchsinger J, Tang MX, Lee JH, Mayeux R. Relationship between plasma lipids and all-cause mortality in nondemented elderly. J Am Geriatr Soc 2005; 53(2):219–226.

29. Matarese LE, Gottschlich MM. Contemporary nutrition support practice: a clinical guide. 2nd ed. Philadelphia: Saunders, 2003.

30. Pressure ulcer prevention and treatment following spinal cord injury: a clinical practice guideline for health-care professionals. J Spinal Cord Med 2001; 24 Suppl 1:S40–101.

31. Pai MP, Paloucek FP. The origin of the "ideal" body weight equations. Ann Pharmacother 2000; 34(9):1066–1069.

32. Nuhlicek DN, Spurr GB, Barboriak JJ, Rooney CB, el Ghatit AZ, Bongard RD. Body composition of patients with spinal cord injury. Eur J Clin Nutr 1988; 42(9):765–773.

33. Tomey KM, Chen DM, Wang X, Braunschweig CL. Dietary intake and nutritional status of urban community-dwelling men with paraplegia. Arch Phys Med Rehabil 2005; 86(4):664–671.

34. Gupta N, White KT, Sandford PR. Body mass index in spinal cord injury—a retrospective study. Spinal Cord 2006; 44(2):92–94.

35. Rajan S, McNeely MJ, Warms C, Goldstein B. Clinical assessment and management of obesity in individuals with spinal cord injury: a review. J Spinal Cord Med 2008; 31(4):361–372.

36. Jones LM, Legge M, Goulding A. Healthy body mass index values often underestimate body fat in men with spinal cord injury. Arch Phys Med Rehabil 2003; 84(7):1068–71.

37. Weaver FM, Collins EG, Kurichi J, et al. Prevalence of obesity and high blood pressure in veterans with spinal cord injuries and disorders: a retrospective review. Am J Phys Med Rehabil 2007; 86(1):22–29.

38. Laughton GE, Buchholz AC, Martin Ginis KA, Goy RE. Lowering body mass index cutoffs better identifies obese persons with spinal cord injury. Spinal Cord 2009.

39. Bishop CW, Pitchey SJ. Estimation of the mid-upper arm circumference measurement error. J Am Diet Assoc 1987; 87(4):469–473.

40. Canoy D, Boekholdt SM, Wareham N, et al. Body fat distribution and risk of coronary heart disease in men and women in the European Prospective Investigation Into Cancer and Nutrition in Norfolk cohort: a population-based prospective study. Circulation 2007; 116(25): 2933–2943.

41. Kearns PJ, Thompson JD, Werner PC, Pipp TL, Wilmot CB. Nutritional and metabolic response to acute spinal-cord injury. JPEN J Parenter Enteral Nutr 1992; 16(1):11–15.

42. Dvorak MF, Noonan VK, Belanger L, et al. Early versus late enteral feeding in patients with acute cervical spinal cord injury: a pilot study. Spine 2004; 29(9):E175–80.

43. Ibrahim EH, Mehringer L, Prentice D, et al. Early versus late enteral feeding of mechanically ventilated patients: results of a clinical trial. JPEN J Parenter Enteral Nutr 2002; 26(3):174–181.

44. Minard G, Kudsk KA, Melton S, Patton JH, Tolley EA. Early versus delayed feeding with an immune-enhancing diet in patients with severe head injuries. JPEN J Parenter Enteral Nutr 2000; 24(3):145–149.

45. Eyer SD, Micon LT, Konstantinides FN, et al. Early enteral feeding does not attenuate metabolic response after blunt trauma. J Trauma 1993; 34(5):639–43; discussion 643–644.

46. Wolf C, Meiners TH. Dysphagia in patients with acute cervical spinal cord injury. Spinal Cord 2003; 41(6):347–353.

47. Nutritional support after spinal cord injury. Neurosurgery 2002; 50(3 Suppl):S81–84.

48. Rodriguez DJ, Clevenger FW, Osler TM, Demarest GB, Fry DE. Obligatory negative nitrogen balance following spinal cord injury. JPEN J Parenter Enteral Nutr 1991; 15(3):319–322.

49. Rodriguez DJ, Benzel EC, Clevenger FW. The metabolic response to spinal cord injury. Spinal Cord 1997; 35(9):599–604.

50. Young B, Ott L, Rapp R, Norton J. The patient with critical neurological disease. Crit Care Clin 1987; 3(1):217–233.

51. Rice HB, Ponichtera-Mulcare JA, Glaser RM. Nutrition and the spinal cord injured individual. Clin Kines 1995; 49(1):21–27.

52. Sedlock DA, Laventure SJ. Body composition and resting energy expenditure in long term spinal cord injury. Paraplegia 1990; 28(7):448–454.

53. Zurlo F, Larson K, Bogardus C, Ravussin E. Skeletal muscle metabolism is a major determinant of resting energy expenditure. J Clin Invest 1990; 86(5):1423–1427.

54. Buchholz AC, McGillivray CF, Pencharz PB. Differences in resting metabolic rate between paraplegic and able-bodied subjects are explained by differences in body composition. Am J Clin Nutr 2003; 77(2):371–378.

55. Buchholz AC, Pencharz PB. Energy expenditure in chronic spinal cord injury. Curr Opin Clin Nutr Metab Care 2004; 7(6):635–639.

56. Levine AM, Nash MS, Green BA, Shea JD, Aronica MJ. An examination of dietary intakes and nutritional status of chronic healthy spinal cord injured individuals. Paraplegia 1992; 30(12):880–889.

57. Walters JL, Buchholz AC, Martin Ginis KA. Evidence of dietary inadequacy in adults with chronic spinal cord injury. Spinal Cord 2009; 47(4):318–322.

58. Moussavi RM, Garza HM, Eisele SG, Rodriguez G, Rintala DH. Serum levels of vitamins A, C, and E in persons with chronic spinal cord injury living in the community. Arch Phys Med Rehabil 2003; 84(7): 1061–7.

59. Petchkrua W, Burns SP, Stiens SA, James JJ, Little JW. Prevalence of vitamin B12 deficiency in spinal cord injury. Arch Phys Med Rehabil 2003; 84(11):1675–1679.

60. Barber D, Foster D, Rogers S. The importance of nutrition in the care of persons with spinal cord injury. J Spinal Cord Med 2003; 26(2):122–123.

61. Vaziri ND, Pandian MR, Segal JL, Winer RL, Eltorai I, Brunnemann S. Vitamin D, parathormone, and calcitonin profiles in persons with long-standing spinal cord injury. Arch Phys Med Rehabil 1994; 75(7):766–769.

62. Zhou XJ, Vaziri ND, Segal JL, Winer RL, Eltorai I, Brunnemann SR. Effects of chronic spinal cord injury and pressure ulcer on 25(OH)-vitamin D levels. J Am Paraplegia Soc 1993; 16(1):9–13.

63. Bauman WA, Zhong YG, Schwartz E. Vitamin D deficiency in veterans with chronic spinal cord injury. Metabolism 1995; 44(12):1612–1616.

64. Bauman WA, Morrison NG, Spungen AM. Vitamin D replacement therapy in persons with spinal cord injury. J Spinal Cord Med 2005; 28(3):203–207.

65. Bauman WA, Adkins RH, Spungen AM, Kemp BJ, Waters RL. The effect of residual neurological deficit on serum lipoproteins in individuals with chronic spinal cord injury. Spinal Cord 1998; 36(1):13–17.

66. Jones LM, Legge M, Goulding A. Factor analysis of the metabolic syndrome in spinal cord-injured men. Metabolism 2004; 53(10):1372–1377.

67. Schmid A, Knoebber J, Vogt S, et al. Lipid profiles of persons with paraplegia and tetraplegia: sex differences. J Spinal Cord Med 2008; 31(3):285–289.

68. Mojtahedi MC, Boblick P, Rimmer JH, Rowland JL, Jones RA, Braunschweig CL. Environmental barriers to and availability of healthy foods for people with mobility disabilities living in urban and suburban neighborhoods. Arch Phys Med Rehabil 2008; 89(11):2174–2179.

69. Fisher SV, Gullickson G, Jr. Energy cost of ambulation in health and disability: a literature review. Arch Phys Med Rehabil 1978; 59(3):124–133.

70. Nash MS, Meltzer NM, Martins SC, Burns PA, Lindley SD, Field-Fote EC. Nutrient supplementation post ambulation in persons with incomplete spinal cord injuries: a randomized, double-blinded, placebo-controlled case series. Arch Phys Med Rehabil 2007; 88(2):228–233.

71. Niedert KC, Dorner B. Nutrition care of the older adult: a handbook for dietetics professionals working throughout the continuum of care. 2nd ed. Chicago: American Dietetic Association; 2004.

72. Krouskop TA, Noble PC, Garber SL, Spencer WA. The effectiveness of preventive management in reducing the occurrence of pressure sores. J Rehabil R D 1983; 20(1):74–83.

73. Strauss EA, Margolis DJ. Malnutrition in patients with pressure ulcers: morbidity, mortality, and clinically practical assessments. Adv Wound Care 1996; 9(5):37–40.

74. Thomas DR. Nutritional factors affecting wound healing. Ostomy Wound Manage 1996; 42(5):40–42, 44–46, 48–49.

75. Langer G, Knerr A, Kuss O, Behrens J, Schlömer GJ. Nutritional interventions for preventing and treating pressure ulcers. Cochrane Database of Systematic Reviews 2003; (4).

76. Goel R, Misra PK. Study of plasma zinc protein energy malnutrition. Indian Pediatr 1980; 17(11):863–867.

77. Scheinfeld NS, Mokashi A, Lin A. Protein-Energy Malnutrition. In: eMedicine from WebMD [serial online].

78. Cassidy J. Nutritional health issues in people with high-level tetraplegia. Top Spinal Cord Inj Rehabil 1997; 2(3):64–69.

79. Cox SA, Weiss SM, Posuniak EA, Worthington P, Prioleau M, Heffley G. Energy expenditure after spinal cord injury: an evaluation of stable rehabilitating patients. J Trauma 1985; 25(5):419–423.

80. Cameron KJ, Nyulasi IB, Collier GR, Brown DJ. Assessment of the effect of increased dietary fibre intake on bowel function in patients with spinal cord injury. Spinal Cord 1996; 34(5):277–83.

81. Clinical practice guidelines: Neurogenic bowel management in adults with spinal cord injury. Spinal Cord Medicine Consortium. J Spinal Cord Med 1998; 21(3):248–293.

26 Spinal Cord Injury and Aging

Amitabh Jha
Susan B. Charlifue
Daniel P. Lammertse

Spinal cord injury (SCI) can change a person's life instantaneously. Within the first few years following such an injury, various degrees of neurologic recovery may occur, followed by a prolonged period of apparent stability. Life expectancy in recent decades has improved for people with SCI (1), though much of this improvement may be attributed to improved survival in the first 2 years postinjury (2). However, as these individuals age, they are increasingly likely to experience changes in their once-stable health and functional abilities. Therefore, it is important that clinicians understand the theoretical and practical issues of human aging to better address the consequences of aging in this unique population.

This chapter describes many of the processes associated with aging in people with SCI with a body system-by-body system discussion of how aging in SCI has an impact on both physical and psychosocial health, now and in the future.

THE GENITOURINARY SYSTEM

Diminished bladder capacity and urethral compliance, an increase in uninhibited detrusor contractions and residual bladder volumes, and a gradual decline in kidney function are some of the findings associated with normal human aging in the general population (3–5). In addition, age-related changes in the diurnal output of urine result in an increase in nocturia. Another finding is that elderly individuals appear to be at increased risk for urinary tract infections (UTIs), presumably related to the decline in immune function, postmenopausal changes, and the effects of prostatism (6).

Following SCI, the physiologic disruption of genitourinary function is characterized by the loss of volitional control over micturition as well as the loss of coordination of detrusor and sphincter reflexes. Once these reflexes have recovered, there is a tendency to sphincter-detrusor dyssynergia and elevated lower urinary tract pressure over time. This can lead, ultimately, to hypertrophy of the detrusor muscle and decreased bladder compliance. The cumulative effect of these changes can also result in the development of hydronephrosis and upper tract deterioration (6).

Urinary tract complications have been declining as a cause of death in SCI over the past 30 years (7) and now account for only 2.3% of deaths (1). This improved urinary tract-related mortality rate is likely due to clinical advances in urologic management and modern antibiotic treatment. It is important, however, to note that SCI-related alterations in urinary tract physiology pose significant risks to health and that urologic complications continue to be common among people living with SCI (8, 9). Data from the U.S. Spinal Cord Injury Model Systems show that the incidence of abnormal renal function testing increases with both age and duration of injury, and that removal of urinary tract stones, most common in persons using indwelling catheters, increased from 3.1% at 5 years to 10.8% at 20 years postinjury.

The method of bladder management appears to be associated with certain urinary complications and frequently changes with both aging and years postinjury (10, 11). Typically, studies have documented higher rates of bladder stones, UTIs, and bladder cancer associated with the use of indwelling catheters. For individuals who are managed with an indwelling catheter, anticholinergic medication used routinely may improve health outcomes (12, 13). Individuals using long-term intermittent catheterization may be at an increased risk for developing urethral stricture and epididymo-orchitis (14).

Cancer of the bladder appears to be increased by the presence of SCI in many studies (15–18), though such findings are not universal (19, 20). Risk factors for the development of bladder cancer that are related to SCI include recurrent UTI as well as the use of indwelling catheters (21, 22). It appears that malignant degeneration requires the cumulative effects of exposure to various risk factors (such as recurrent infections, indwelling catheter management, urinary tract stones, cigarette smoking, etc.) over a long period of time. People with SCI who develop bladder carcinoma typically present with hematuria. Unfortunately, hematuria is not a reliable indicator of bladder cancer in people with SCI, because it also commonly occurs with UTI, bladder stones, and catheter changes.

These tumors are commonly metastatic and invasive at the time of diagnosis in people with SCI, highlighting the importance of developing effective screening methods. Urine cytology and biochemical markers of urinary tract malignancy do not appear to be appropriate screening tools at present, because of their high false-positive rate, which can be caused by concomitant UTI and related hematuria. Although the effectiveness of screening cystoscopy to detect these tumors in chronically catheterized spinal cord individuals has been questioned by some, most clinicians feel that this method remains the best option for early detection of bladder cancer in persons with SCI (21, 23, 24). In addition, because of the risk of chronic prostatitis related to recurrent UTI, it is reasonable to speculate that there may be some added risk of prostate cancer in males with chronic SCI, although there is no evidence to date that such an association exists. In fact, one study found a lower incidence of carcinoma of the prostate in those spinal cord injured individuals who were more disabled, suggesting that, at the very least, there is no added risk of this cancer associated with SCI (25). However, when detected, it is often at a more advanced stage and grade (26), highlighting that males aging with SCI should be considered at risk and be provided with the age-specific prostate cancer screening that is recommended for their general population counterparts (27).

Guided by an awareness of these issues, the long-term follow-up for people with SCI should include attention to the potential for functional deterioration and the development of urinary tract cancers. The clinical approach is based on prevention and early detection. The person with SCI should be educated regarding the fundamentals of bladder management in an effort to reduce the risk of recurrent UTI. This includes education regarding adequate hydration, hygienic bladder management techniques, and regular urologic follow-up. Individuals who elect to use indwelling catheter methods of bladder management should receive adequate information regarding the accompanying risk of bladder cancer. Cigarette smoking has also been identified as a significant risk factor for bladder cancer; therefore, smoking cessation programs should also be encouraged for those who smoke.

THE GASTROINTESTINAL SYSTEM

The consequences of aging on gastrointestinal physiology in the general population are well described, showing that a generalized decline in gut motility accompanies the aging process (28). Acid secretion in the stomach is also diminished with increasing years, and the stomach exhibits diminished emptying of fluid meals but relatively unimpaired emptying of solid food. The small bowel shows little, if any, specific change related to aging; however, the colon and rectum exhibit diminished motility and an increase in diverticular disease (29). Surveys of people with SCI have documented a variety of gastrointestinal complications that accompany the aging process and have been associated with an increased need for ADL assistance (30).

In the gastrointestinal system, colorectal function is significantly altered by SCI and would be expected to be a substantial source of problems in the person aging with SCI. It is known that colonic transit time is prolonged in persons with spinal cord injury, especially in the left colon and rectum (31–33). This finding correlates with the common report of constipation in this population. Specifically, a British study of persons more than 20 years postinjury showed that 42% of the subjects had difficulties with constipation, whereas 27% reported problems with fecal incontinence, and 35% had gastrointestinal pain (34, 35). Those with tetraplegia were more likely to report fecal incontinence, whereas constipation was more likely to be reported by people with paraplegia and those who used digital stimulation, manual evacuation, or valsalva for their bowel routines. Furthermore, megacolon may be associated with being over 50 years of age or 10 years postinjury (36).

The most profound alteration in gastrointestinal physiology resulting from SCI is the loss of volitional control over bowel emptying. This requires the adoption of an individualized bowel evacuation regimen that incorporates a variety of reflex stimulation maneuvers, laxatives, and dietary interventions. It is believed that constipation manifested by difficulties in producing reflex bowel evacuation is commonly the result of the anorectal dyssynergia or inadequate rectal expulsive force caused by SCI gut motility impairment (37). The primary treatment approach is based on an assessment of the existing bowel routine, with suggestions for alterations based on common sense. Many people with SCI have chosen excessively long intervals between bowel programs for their convenience. They should be encouraged to maintain a bowel program frequency of daily or every other day. The use of laxatives or enemas should be avoided or kept to a minimum. Suppository use is considered supplemental to digital stimulation and evacuation when necessary. For some individuals with refractory bowel dysfunction characterized by excessively long bowel programs or frequent fecal incontinence, opting for an elective colostomy may significantly improve quality of life (38).

Hemorrhoids and periodic rectal bleeding are also common accompaniments to chronic SCI, with a majority of individuals reporting these conditions (39). For minor symptomatic lesions, topical therapy may be sufficient. For more severe hemorrhoids, banding is commonly required. In the most severe refractory cases presenting with abundant hemorrhoid tissue and recurrent significant bleeding, operative hemorrhoidectomy may be necessary.

No evidence exists to date to suggest that persons with SCI are at added risk of colon cancer. However, it is safe to assume that this population is at risk equal to the general population for this common cancer. For that reason, periodic SCI follow-up should include screening for colorectal cancer (40). Fecal occult blood may not be a reliable screening tool because of the frequent presence of hemorrhoids, rectal prolapse, and other distal rectal pathology in the SCI population. Therefore, people with SCI in the at-risk age group should be endoscopically screened periodically. The endoscopist should be familiar with the risk of autonomic dysreflexia and be prepared to treat blood pressure elevation or other sequelae during the procedure.

There has been speculation about an increased incidence of gastroesophageal reflux disease (GERD) in people with SCI. However, one study showed no significant difference in the overall incidence of reflux disease, although there was a higher prevalence of more severe esophagitis in the SCI subjects (41). It has been suggested that changes in gastric motility may be implicated in chronic abdominal distention in long-term SCI, but the underlying cause of gastric dilatation remains poorly understood (40). Evidence suggests that gallstone disease is up to seven times more prevalent in the SCI population than in the general population (42, 43). It does not appear that the formation of gallstones in SCI is specifically related to aging (44), and the added risk of gallstone disease appears to be restricted to individuals with lesions above T10, with the increased incidence of stones generally occurring within the first year postinjury. Nonetheless, clinicians should be aware of the increased incidence of this condition with age in general, when evaluating abdominal complaints in the long-term follow-up population. In addition, despite an increased risk for the development of gallstones in people with SCI, the risk of biliary complications was not of sufficient magnitude in this group to warrant prophylactic cholecystectomy (45–47).

Because of the high frequency of gastrointestinal problems in the aging SCI population, specific attention to bowel symptoms should be incorporated into routine follow-up procedures. Regular assessment of the bowel program should be done, and ongoing education regarding bowel program performance, ways to manage and/or modify the bowel routine, and a bowel-friendly diet should be emphasized.

THE INTEGUMENT

Multiple factors result in the aging of human skin. Normal aging results in atrophy and changes in the histologic structures that comprise the dermis (48). Elasticity and vascularity of the dermis, and collagen content are diminished, predisposing aging skin to injury. Flattening of the dermal-epidermal junction and thinning of the epidermis result in a decreased tolerance to shear and a greater likelihood of epidermal detachment and blister formation. Diminished vascularity and sweating also may heighten the risk of thermal injury. People with SCI are known to be at risk for skin trauma resulting in pressure ulcers, commonly related to immobility, lack of sensory protection, and spasticity. Data from the United States Model Spinal Cord Injury Systems showed the incidence of pressure ulcers increasing from 15% at 1 year following SCI to nearly 30% at 20 years postinjury (49, 50), and the incidence may be increasing in recent years (51). The risk is highest in those with complete tetraplegia, who demonstrated a 40% prevalence of pressure ulcers at the 20-year follow-up. The basic principles of pressure relief, debridement, and asepsis are still the foundation of successful conservative management (52, 53). Large and deep skin sores will commonly require myocutaneous flap closure. Local infection necessitates treatment with appropriate antibiotics, and deep wounds should raise the suspicion of contiguous osteomyelitis. In these instances, a bone biopsy should be performed for the purposes of diagnosis and identification of the causative organisms, to guide antibiotic therapy.

Chronic open skin sores of long duration have been associated with the development of Marjolin's ulcer, and the development of squamous carcinoma in the sore (52), with one study recommending biopsy of chronic ulcers of more than 10 years duration (54). Because of the high frequency of skin sore occurrence in the chronic SCI population, periodic assessment should include a thorough evaluation of the integument and a reinforcement of skin sore prevention education. The clinical approach to managing skin sores in SCI is primarily prevention through patient education. This involves instruction on skin protection, pressure relief, hygiene, and routine surveillance.

If initiated promptly and performed diligently, conservative treatment of pressure sores is commonly effective.

THE NERVOUS SYSTEM

Changes related to the nervous system in the aging general population have been reported to include loss of vibratory sensation, muscle mass, and strength; slower reaction time; decreased fine coordination and agility; decreased deep tendon reflexes; and deteriorating stability in station and gait (55–60). The aging spinal cord histologically shows loss of myelinated tracts as well as a loss of anterior horn cells. However, significant changes may not occur until after the fifth decade (61). A study of persons aging with SCI of more than 20 years duration showed that 12% reported some sensory loss, and more than one in five individuals reported increasing motor deficits over the years (62). Without further study, it is not possible to state with certainty that an age-related loss of myelinated tracts and dropout of anterior horn cells may contribute to these reported symptoms.

In studies of people with long-term SCI, a high incidence of upper extremity entrapment neuropathies has been reported, with up to 63% of people with paraplegia showing evidence of these, both on electrodiagnostic testing and on symptom surveys (63, 64). The most frequent site of involvement is the median nerve at the wrist, but ulnar nerve entrapments at the elbow and wrist are also common. Because of repeated hand contact with wheelchair rims, as well as positioning of the wrist during transfer activities and pressure relief, individuals with SCI are clearly at risk for nerve entrapments in the upper extremities. It is suspected that the incidence of significant entrapment increases with duration of injury, although this has not been conclusively proven. Treatment for this condition should include assessing the mechanics of mobility and daily living activities to determine any underlying sources of repetitive trauma. For some individuals, the resolution of symptoms may necessitate a modification of activities. In addition, education regarding techniques to conserve and protect wrist function may be beneficial for some individuals. Other modalities include wrist splinting to reduce repetitive trauma at the extremes of wrist flexion and extension, which are known to contribute to carpal tunnel symptomatology. Although corticosteroid injection therapy has been tried as a conservative measure for people with carpal tunnel syndrome, the benefit may be only temporary. Although ulnar entrapments at the wrist may prompt consideration of surgical treatment, SCI survivors with these neuropathies are usually successfully treated with activity and equipment modification and rarely require surgical intervention. However, when conservative measures fail to provide a relief of symptoms in people with significant entrapments, surgical release of the entrapped nerve is often recommended. Individuals undergoing such surgery should anticipate a period of restricted activity after the surgery, which may temporarily necessitate an increased need for assistance from others. Postoperative activity restrictions have been reduced with some recent advances in surgical techniques, including the percutaneous endoscopic approach to transverse carpal ligament section.

When individuals with chronic SCI experience neurologic deterioration, it is most commonly the result of progressive posttraumatic cystic myelopathy (65, 66). This condition is also referred to as posttraumatic syringomyelia, and is characterized by the progressive enlargement of a cystic cavity originating at the site of injury and extending in either a cephalad or caudal direction in the spinal cord. More recently, the concept of progressive cystic myelopathy has been broadened to include progressive noncystic or myelomalacic myelopathies. These conditions are thought to be a part of a pathophysiologic continuum. The onset of this neurologic complication may vary from several months to several decades after injury, but it most commonly occurs within the first 5 to 10 years postinjury. Signs and symptoms of late progressive neurologic deterioration include losses of sensory and/or motor function, increasing spasticity, neurologic pain, increasing autonomic dysreflexia, increasing sweating, and the development of a variable, positional Horner's syndrome. Confirmation of this diagnosis includes a combination of the typical history and physical findings and magnetic resonance imaging (MRI) of an abnormality of an enlarging syrinx cavity or myelomalacic spinal cord. Arachnoid scarring that interferes with spinal fluid flow and spinal cord mobility appears to be the underlying mechanism of progressive spinal cord pathology. When neurologic deterioration is progressive, surgical treatment, including untethering of the arachnoid scar and, in some cases, the shunting of cyst cavity fluid, is warranted (67, 68). All individuals with SCI have the potential for late neurologic change; therefore, the assessment of motor and sensory function, as well as a neurologic review of systems, should be included in periodic follow-up. Appropriate electrodiagnostic and imaging studies are indicated in the presence of signs or symptoms of neurologic deterioration (68, 69).

THE MUSCULOSKELETAL SYSTEM

In the general population, musculoskeletal system aging is characterized by deterioration of articular cartilage function. This ultimately leads to degenerative arthritic changes, both in the spine and in joints of the appendicular skeleton (70). Because of the unique physical stresses required in people with SCI during mobility activities, it is not surprising that overuse syndromes of the upper extremities are common in this population.

More than 50% of SCI survivors have been shown to report upper extremity pain (71, 72) with shoulder discomfort being the most frequent complaint, followed by pain at the wrist. Transfer activities, wheelchair propulsion, and pressure relief maneuvers most commonly produce upper extremity discomfort. Although acromioclavicular degenerative changes may be seen on X-ray, plain radiographs commonly are of limited value in assessing shoulder pain in these individuals. In symptomatic individuals with SCI who report shoulder pain, arthrography and MRI imaging have better diagnostic yield, commonly showing impingement syndrome and rotator cuff tears (73, 74). Most studies demonstrate that the prevalence and severity of upper extremity overuse problems are correlated with both age and duration of injury. These problems can be managed conservatively, including conducting a periodic review of daily activities and mobility mechanics, which may result in suggestions for activity modification in an effort to avoid pain-causing maneuvers (75). Individuals with overuse syndrome at the shoulders may have a muscular imbalance across the glenohumeral joint, with anterior musculature development being significantly greater than that posterior to the shoulder. Muscular balance

across the joint to restore optimal glenohumeral geometric relationships may be facilitated with an exercise regimen specifically designed to address the posterior shoulder girdle (72). Surgery for impingement or rotator cuff tears has been suggested when conservative measures are unsuccessful. Individuals with SCI who contemplate operative treatment for impingement or rotator cuff tears should anticipate a prolonged and possibly difficult postoperative rehabilitation period as well as a temporary impact on independence, with additional personal care assistance commonly being required (76, 77).

Osteoporosis is a common accompaniment to the aging process. This condition is most typically associated with postmenopausal elderly women, but it also occurs in aging men (78, 79). Osteoporosis caused by paralysis and disuse is commonly felt to be the underlying risk factor for pathologic fractures following SCI. Lower extremity osteoporosis develops rapidly in the first year postinjury, with about one-third of the original bone mass being lost by 16 months postinjury before relative stability is achieved (80). Of note, an extremity fracture rate of over 30% for individuals followed for several decades has been reported (81). In addition, data from the U.S. Model Spinal Cord Injury Systems indicate that women are more likely to develop long bone fractures in the lower extremities as the time postinjury increases (49). Various interventions have been proposed, including standing, functional electrical stimulation (FES), and treatment with biphosphonates. However, no treatment has yet been shown to provide long-term prevention of osteoporosis and protection from fracture risk (82). Preliminary trials of pamidronate showed some promise (83), although more recent evidence suggested less efficacy in preventing bone loss (84). SCI clinicians should incorporate a thorough symptom review and examination as a part of a periodic reassessment to identify musculoskeletal complaints at their earliest onset.

THE IMMUNE SYSTEM

The normal immune system declines with age, and the risk of infection increases (85, 86). In addition, the function of the immune system is known to be influenced by factors such as depression, deterioration of social support systems, chronic pain, neuroendocrine changes, and the influence of medications (87). There is evidence of a diminished immune function in people with SCI above the T10 level, which is manifest by impaired bacterial phagocytosis (88). A longitudinal study of people with SCI of more than 20 years duration showed a dramatic increase in urinary tract infections (UTIs) among those aged 60 and over, and a slight increase in the frequency of infection between the 10th and 30th postinjury year (34). Because factors such as depression, diminished psychosocial support, polypharmacy, and chronic pain may coexist in people with SCI, it would appear safe to assume that those aging individuals will have an increased likelihood of immune impairment when compared to their nondisabled counterparts, and recent evidence suggests that aging with SCI is in fact associated with immunological changes (89).

Studies have suggested that exercise and rehabilitation therapies are associated with improved cellular immunity in persons with SCI (90, 91); conversely, indwelling urinary catheters and skin ulcers may be associated with an ongoing systemic inflammatory response (92). It is hoped that further research in immunology, immunologic assessment, and treatment will result

Table 26.1 Aging Effects on Organ Systems

Body System	Usual Aging	Aging with SCI
Genitourinary system	• Diminished bladder capacity • Diminished urethral compliance • Increased uninhibited detrusor contractions • Increased residual bladder volumes • Gradual decline in kidney function • Increased UTIs	Intermittent catheterization • sphincter–detrusor dyssynergia • hypertrophy of the detrusor muscle and decreased bladder compliance • hydronephrosis and upper tract deterioration • urethral stricture • epididymitis Indwelling catheter • increased UTIs • incidence of abnormal renal function testing increases • urinary tract stones • bladder cancer
Gastrointestinal system	• Decline in gut motility • Diminished acid secretion • Increase in diverticular disease • Increased colon cancer risk	• Constipation • Incontinence • Gastrointestinal pain • Hemorrhoids • Gallstones (?)
Integument system	• Decreased elasticity, vascularity, and collagen content of dermis • Decreased shear tolerance • Increased blisters	• Increased pressure ulcer risk • Squamous cell carcinoma (Marjolin's ulcer)
Nervous system	• Loss of vibratory sensation, muscle mass and strength • Slower reaction time • Decreased fine coordination and agility • Decreased stability in station and gait.	• Entrapment neuropathies • Posttraumatic syringomyelia
Musculoskeletal system	• Deterioration of articular cartilage • Osteoporosis	• Upper extremity overuse injuries • Muscle imbalance • Disuse osteoporosis
Immune system	• Declines with age	• More frequent UTIs

in interventions designed to improve immune defenses in people with chronic SCI.

A summary of the effects of age on each body system is shown in Table 26.1.

PSYCHOSOCIAL ASPECTS

Although it is clear from the previous section of this chapter that there may be numerous age-related physical changes that can further limit function and independence for people with SCI as they grow older, this is not necessarily true for the psychosocial aspects of a person's life.

Independence

Aging individuals may experience increasing generalized fatigue, muscle weakness, sensory loss, and arthritic changes, all of which may lead to diminished physical independence and quality of life (93–100). Recent data from the National Center for Health Statistics showed that nearly 20% of the civilian community-dwelling population of the United States aged 55–64 and more than 34% of those aged 65 and older reported some degree of activity limitation (101).

With spinal cord injury, aging may magnify dependency issues as an individual's needs and abilities change over time. Indeed, functional decline or decreasing physical independence has been identified as an adverse outcome of long-term spinal cord injury. Research has shown both cross-sectional and longitudinal significant increases in the need for assistance among older individuals (30, 102, 103). Fortunately, rehabilitation provides health practitioners a wealth of well-established techniques to help preserve functional ability and maintain independence for people aging with SCI and other disabilities. Therapeutic re-education regarding various transfer and mobility activities and modifying existing equipment or using different durable medical equipment and assistive devices may help an individual retain independence. When assistance from others does increase or become necessary, efforts to incorporate this help into an individual's life in such a way that still enables him or her to maintain maximal independence is critical. Independence, when not possible physically, is still intellectually realistic, allowing the individual with SCI to make decisions and be the key player in all health and care-related issues such as having the power to hire, train, and even fire helpers.

Community Integration, Life Satisfaction, and Depression

Community integration goes beyond physical functioning, focusing on an individual's involvement in community and family activities and social roles (104–106). Studies of individuals with SCI have summarized the finding that individuals with less severe neurologic injuries, of younger age, of Caucasian ethnicity, and with more education will achieve greater community integration (107, 108). In turn, greater community participation is associated with better life satisfaction (109). Environmental factors, such as attitudinal, architectural, and policy barriers, do not appear to be significant predictors of community participation, but they are major predictors of life satisfaction (108).

Depression and life satisfaction may be related to how well a person copes with changes that occur as a result of aging. Studies have demonstrated that depression is common among individuals with SCI (110–112) and is more severe for individuals who are older and with longer durations of SCI (113). When the factor of aging is considered in life satisfaction, research results have not been consistent. Some studies indicate that life satisfaction for people with SCI is not necessarily negatively impacted by aging (102), whereas others find mixed patterns of change over time (114, 115). Studies that do find negative effects of aging report significant differences in self-perceived quality of life, with younger individuals and those having been injured for shorter periods of time rating their quality of life better than older individuals (34, 116, 117). This variation in findings may be a consequence of the differences in how older and younger individuals assess quality of life. It is clear, however, that aging is only one aspect of quality of life, and life satisfaction following spinal cord injury can also be related to overall general health, social support, community integration, and personal factors, as well as level of injury and expectations about functional abilities (118–120). Research has also demonstrated that the presence of not only certain health conditions such as pressure sores or pain, but also diminished life satisfaction, is often the best predictor of that same condition in later years (50). Nonetheless, in general, it does appear that individuals with SCI maintain relatively good and reportedly stable life satisfaction over time—even after many years of living with SCI (121).

Clearly, the concept of life satisfaction (or happiness, well-being, or quality of life) is multidimensional and complex, incorporating a combination of biological, psychological, interpersonal, social, economic, and cultural dimensions, all worthy of further study in the population of individuals aging with SCI. Ultimately, it is the responsibility of both healthcare providers and people with SCI and their families to work cooperatively in an attempt to identify the underlying factors that may negatively influence community participation and quality of life. This involves a careful look at the person with SCI, the living situation, the available resources, and the environment. Successful aging is the result of a well-integrated assessment of these multiple areas and of making adjustments or

recommendations to benefit as effectively as possible the person aging with SCI.

Looking to the Future

Numerous studies attest to the finding that long-term survival following spinal cord injury has improved in recent years (34, 122), with life expectancies often extending into the sixth and seventh decades of life. In spite of these improvements, however, life expectancy for the person with SCI is still much lower than that of the general population (2). Survival following SCI is impacted not only by level and severity of injury (2, 122), but also by age at injury (123) and decade of injury (124, 125). Although it is an encouraging finding that people with SCI are surviving longer, they consequently may be at greater risk to develop chronic health conditions typically associated with aging. In addition, many of these conditions, especially when complicated by SCI, may lead to death. Those who provide healthcare and services to this unique population will therefore encounter new challenges when attempting to facilitate successful aging of these individuals. Working together with members of the gerontologic sciences community will help those who are providing services to people aging with spinal cord injuries understand the additional complexities associated with the aging process.

The long-term management of individuals aging with SCI is not limited to clinical follow-up. Efforts should also be focused on education, both for the growing population of individuals aging with SCI and for clinicians. Through a multifaceted approach, effective strategies designed to minimize conditions and complications that occur with aging can be identified and implemented. Regular physical assessments should attend not only to the SCI-specific health issues, but also to those problems associated with aging in general. It is also important to recognize any conditions that appear to be changing, such as pain, fatigue, spasticity, and bowel or bladder programs, as these may herald more serious health consequences over time.

In addition to regular clinical monitoring of aging and SCI-specific conditions, pertinent and timely educational materials for the person aging with SCI should be made available. It should be emphasized and reemphasized that continued rehabilitation or equipment modifications may be necessary as the years pass. Aging need not be a topic to be avoided or one that raises concerns or fears. It is simply another facet of living with SCI. With an integrated approach to addressing aging issues, we can gain a greater understanding of this important segment of life, develop pathways to more successful outcomes, and, ideally, help minimize the fears and stigma often associated with aging.

References

1. DeVivo MJ, Krause JS, Lammertse DP. Recent trends in mortality and causes of death among persons with spinal cord injury. *Arch Phys Med Rehabil* 1999; 80:1411–1149.
2. Strauss DJ, DeVivo MJ, Paculdo DR, Shavelle RM. Trends in life expectancy after spinal cord injury. *Arch Phys Med Rehabil* 2006; 87:1079–1085.
3. Resnick NM, Yalla SV. Aging and its effect on the bladder. *Semin Urol* 1987; 5:82–86.
4. Madersbacher S, Pycha A, Klingler CH, et al. Interrelationships of bladder compliance with age, detrusor instability, and obstruction in elderly men with lower urinary tract symptoms. *Neurourol Urodyn* 1999; 18:3–15.

5. Pfisterer MH, Griffiths DJ, Schaefer W, Resnick NM. The effect of age on lower urinary tract function: a study in women. *J Am Geriatr Soc* 2006; 54:405–412.

6. Madersbacher G, Oberwalder M. The elderly para- and tetraplegic: special aspects of the urological care. *Paraplegia* 1987; 25:318–323.

7. National Spinal Cord Injury Statistical Center. Spinal cord injury: facts and figures at a glance. *J Spinal Cord Med* 2005; 28:379–380.

8. Vaidyanathan S, Soni BM, Gopalan L, et al. A review of the readmissions of patients with tetraplegia to the Regional Spinal Injuries Centre, Southport, United Kingdom, between January 1994 and December 1995. *Spinal Cord* 1998; 36:838–846.

9. Cardenas DD, Hoffman JM, Kirshblum S, McKinley W. Etiology and incidence of rehospitalization after traumatic spinal cord injury: a multicenter analysis. *Arch Phys Med Rehabil* 2004; 85:1757–1763.

10. Drake MJ, Cortina-Borja M, Savic G, Charlifue SW, Gardner BP. Prospective evaluation of urological effects of aging in chronic spinal cord injury by method of bladder management. *Neurourol* 2005; 24:111–116.

11. Hansen RB, Biering-Sorensen F, Kristensen JK. Bladder emptying over a period of 10–45 years after a traumatic spinal cord injury. *Spinal Cord* 2004; 42:631–637.

12. O'Leary M, Erickson JR, Smith CP, McDermott C, et al. Effect of controlled-release oxybutynin on neurogenic bladder function in spinal cord injury. *J Spinal Cord Med* 2003; 26:159–162.

13. Bennett N, O'Leary M, Patel AS, Xavier M, et al. Can higher doses of oxybutynin improve efficacy in neurogenic bladder? *J Urol* 2004; 171:749–751.

14. Ku JH, Jung TY, Lee JK, Park WH, Shim HB. Influence of bladder management on epididymo-orchitis in patients with spinal cord injury: clean intermittent catheterization is a risk factor for epididymo-orchitis. *Spinal Cord* 2006; 44:165–169.

15. Melzak J. The incidence of bladder cancer in paraplegia. *Paraplegia*. 1966; 4:85–96.

16. Kaufman JM, Fam B, Jacobs SC, et al. Bladder cancer and squamous metaplasia in spinal cord injury patients. *J Urol* 1977; 118:967–971.

17. El-Masri WS, Fellows G. Bladder cancer after spinal cord injury. *Paraplegia* 1981; 19:265–270.

18. Stonehill WH, Dmochowski RR, Patterson AL, Cox CE. Risk factors for bladder tumors in spinal cord injury patients. *J Urol* 1996; 155:1248–1250.

19. Pannek J. Transitional cell carcinoma in patients with spinal cord injury: a high risk malignancy? *Urology* 2002; 59:240–244.

20. Subramonian K, Cartwright RA, Harnden P, Harrison SC. Bladder cancer in patients with spinal cord injuries. *BJU Int* 2004; 93:739–743.

21. Yang CC, Clowers DE. Screening cystoscopy in chronically catheterized spinal cord injury patients. *Spinal Cord* 1999; 37:204–207.

22. Groah SL, Weitzenkamp DA, Lammertse DP, Whiteneck GG, et al. Excess risk of bladder cancer in spinal cord injury: evidence for an association between indwelling catheter use and bladder cancer. *Arch Phys Med Rehabil* 2002; 83:346–351.

23. Navon JD, Soliman H, Khonsari F, Ahlering T. Screening cystoscopy and survival of spinal cord injured patients with squamous cell cancer of the bladder. *J Urol* 1997; 157:2109–2111.

24. Shokeir AA. Squamous cell carcinoma of the bladder: pathology, diagnosis and treatment. *BJU Int* 2004; 93:216–220.

25. Frisbie JH, Binard J. Low prevalence of prostatic cancer among myelopathy patients. *J Am Paraplegia Soc* 1994; 17:148–149.

26. Scott PA Sr, Perkash I, Mode D, Wolfe VA, Terris MK. Prostate cancer diagnosed in spinal cord–injured patients is more commonly advanced stage than in able-bodied patients. *Urology* 2004; 63:509–512.

27. Wyndaele JJ, Iwatsubo E, Perkash I, Stohrer M. Prostate cancer: a hazard also to be considered in the aging male patient with spinal cord injury. *Spinal Cord* 1998; 36:299–302.

28. Hall KE, Proctor DD, Fisher L, Rose S. American Gastroenterological Association future trends committee report: effects of aging of the population on gastroenterology practice, education, and research. *Gastroenterology* 2005; 129:1305–1338.

29. Whiteway J, Morson BC. Pathology of the aging—diverticular disease. *Clin Gastroenterol* 1985; 14:829–846.

30. Liem NR, McColl MA, King W, Smith KM. Aging with a spinal cord injury: factors associated with the need for more help with activities of daily living. *Arch Phys Med Rehabil* 2004; 85:1567–1577.

31. Krogh K, Mosdal C, Laurberg S. Gastrointestinal and segmental colonic transit times in patients with acute and chronic spinal cord lesions. *Spinal Cord* 2000; 38:615–621.

32. Leduc BE, Spacek E, Lepage Y. Colonic transit time after spinal cord injury: any clinical significance? *J Spinal Cord Med* 2002; 25:161–166.

33. Valles M, Vidal J, Clave P, Mearin F. Bowel dysfunction in patients with motor complete spinal cord injury: clinical, neurological, and pathophysiological associations. *Am J Gastroenterol* 2006; 101:2290–2299.

34. Whiteneck GG, Charlifue SW, Frankel HL, et al. Mortality, morbidity, and psychosocial outcomes of persons spinal cord injured more than 20 years ago. *Paraplegia* 1992; 30:617–630.

35. Menter R, Weitzenkamp D, Cooper D, Bingley J, et al. Bowel management outcomes in individuals with long-term spinal cord injuries. *Spinal Cord* 1997; 35:608–612.

36. Harari D, Minaker KL. Megacolon in patients with chronic spinal cord injury. *Spinal Cord* 2000; 38:331–339.

37. Nino-Murcia M, Stone JM, Chang PJ, Perkash I. Colonic transit in spinal cord–injured patients. *Invest Radiol* 1990; 25:109–112.

38. Rosito O, Nino-Murcia M, Wolfe VA, Kiratli BJ, Perkash I. The effects of colostomy on the quality of life in patients with spinal cord injury: a retrospective analysis. *J Spinal Cord Med* 2002; 25:174–183.

39. Stone JM, Nino-Murcia M, Wolfe VA, Perkash I. Chronic gastrointestinal problems in spinal cord injury patients: a prospective analysis. *Am J Gastroenterol* 1990; 85:1114–1119.

40. Cosman BC, Stone JM, Perkash I. The gastrointestinal system. In: Whiteneck GG, Charlifue SW, Gerhart KA, et al., eds. *Aging with Spinal Cord Injury*. New York: Demos Publications, 1993; 117–127.

41. Singh G, Triadafilopoulos G. Gastroesophageal reflux disease in patients with spinal cord injury. *J Spinal Cord Med* 2000; 23:23–27.

42. Apstein MD, Dalecki-Chipperfield K. Spinal cord injury is a risk factor for gallstone disease. *Gastroenterology* 1987; 92:966–968.

43. Rotter KP, Larrain CG. Gallstones in spinal cord injury (SCI): a late medical complication? *Spinal Cord* 2003; 41:105–108.

44. Xia CS, Han YQ, Yang XY, Hong GX. Spinal cord injury and cholelithiasis. *Hepatobiliary Pancreat Dis Int* 2004; 3:595–598.

45. Moonka R, Stiens SA, Eubank WB, Stelzner M. The presentation of gallstones and results of biliary surgery in a spinal cord injured population. *Am J Surg* 1999; 178:246–250.

46. Moonka R, Stiens SA, Resnick WJ, et al. The prevalence and natural history of gallstones in spinal cord injured patients. *J Am Coll Surg* 1999; 189:274–281.

47. Moonka R, Stiens SA, Stelzner M. Atypical gastrointestinal symptoms are not associated with gallstones in patients with spinal cord injury. *Arch Phys Med Rehabil* 2000; 81:1085–1089.

48. Fenske NA, Lober CW. Structural and functional changes of normal aging skin. *J Am Acad Dermatol* 1986; 15:571–585.

49. McKinley WO, Jackson AB, Cardenas DD, DeVivo MJ. Long-term medical complications after traumatic spinal cord injury: a regional model systems analysis. *Arch Phys Med Rehabil* 1999; 80:1402–1410.

50. Charlifue S, Lammertse DP, Adkins RH. Aging with spinal cord injury: changes in selected health indices and life satisfaction. *Arch Phys Med Rehabil* 2004; 85:1848–1853.

51. Chen Y, DeVivo MJ, Jackson AB. Pressure ulcer prevalence in people with spinal cord injury: age-period-duration effects. *Arch Phys Med Rehabil* 2005; 86:1208–1213.

52. Yarkony G.M. Aging skin, pressure ulcerations, and spinal cord injury. In: Whiteneck GG, Charlifue SW, Gerhart KA, et al., eds. *Aging with Spinal Cord Injury*. New York: Demos Publications, 1993; 39–52.

53. Consortium for Spinal Cord Medicine Clinical Practice Guidelines. Pressure ulcer prevention and treatment following spinal cord injury: a clinical practice guideline for health-care professionals. *J Spinal Cord Med* 2001; 24(Suppl 1):S40–101.

54. Eltorai IM, Montroy RE, Kobayashi M, Jakowatz J, Gutierrez P. Marjolin's ulcer in patients with spinal cord injury. *J Spinal Cord Med* 2002; 25:191–196.

55. Pathy M. The central nervous system: clinical presentation and management of neurologic disorders in old age. In: Brocklehurst JC, ed. *Textbook of Geriatric Medicine and Gerontology*. 2nd ed. Edinburgh: Churchill-Livingstone, 1985.

56. Hatzitaki V, Amiridis IG, Arabatzi F. Aging effects on postural responses to self-imposed balance perturbations. *Gait Posture* 2005; 22:250–257.

57. Lauretani F, Bandinelli S, Bartali B, et al. Axonal degeneration affects muscle density in older men and women. *Neurobiol Aging* 2006; 27:1145–1154.

58. Olafsdottir H, Yoshida N, Zatsiorsky VM, Latash ML. Elderly show decreased adjustments of motor synergies in preparation to action. *Clin Biomech (Bristol, Avon)* 2007; 22:44–51.

59. Olafsdottir H, Zhang W, Zatsiorsky VM, Latash ML. Age-related changes in multifinger synergies in accurate moment of force production tasks. *J Appl Physiol* 2007; 102:1490–1501.

60. Shaffer SW, Harrison AL. Aging of the somatosensory system: a translational perspective. *Phys Ther* 2007; 87:193–207.

61. Morrison R. *The Effect of Advancing Age upon the Human Spinal Cord.* Cambridge, MA: Harvard University Press, 1959.

62. Lammertse DP. The nervous system. In: Whiteneck GG, Charlifue SW, Gerhart KA, et al., eds. *Aging with Spinal Cord Injury.* New York: Demos Publications, 1993; 129–137.

63. Gellman H, Sie I, Waters RL. Late complications of the weight-bearing upper extremity in the paraplegic patient. *Clin Orthop Relat Res* 1988; 233:132–135.

64. Davidoff G, Werner R, Waring W. Compressive mononeuropathies of the upper extremity in chronic paraplegia. *Paraplegia* 1991; 29:17–24.

65. Edgar R, Quail P. Progressive post-traumatic cystic and non-cystic myelopathy. *Br J Neurosurg* 1994; 8:7–22.

66. Falci S, Holtz A, Akesson E, et al. Obliteration of a posttraumatic spinal cord cyst with solid human embryonic spinal cord grafts: first clinical attempt. *J Neurotrauma* 1997; 14:875–884.

67. Lee TT, Arias JM, Andrus HL, Quencer RM, et al. Progressive posttraumatic myelomalacic myelopathy: treatment with untethering and expansive duraplasty. *J Neurosurg* 1997; 86:624–628.

68. Falci SP, Lammertse DP, Best L, et al. Surgical treatment of posttraumatic cystic and tethered spinal cords. *J Spinal Cord Med* 1999; 22:173–181.

69. Bursell JP, Little JW, Stiens SA. Electrodiagnosis in spinal cord injured persons with new weakness or sensory loss: central and peripheral etiologies. *Arch Phys Med Rehabil* 1999; 80:904–909.

70. Waters RL, Sie IH, Adkins RH. The musculoskeletal system. In: Whiteneck GG, Charlifue SW, Gerhart KA, et al., eds. *Aging with Spinal Cord Injury.* New York: Demos Publications, 1993; 53–71.

71. Dalyan M, Cardenas DD, Gerard B. Upper extremity pain after spinal cord injury. *Spinal Cord* 1999; 37:191–195.

72. Paralyzed Veterans of America Consortium for Spinal Cord Medicine. Preservation of upper limb function following spinal cord injury: a clinical practice guideline for health-care professionals. *J Spinal Cord Med* 2005; 28:434–470.

73. Bayley JC, Cochran TP, Sledge CB. The weight-bearing shoulder: the impingement syndrome in paraplegics. *J Bone Joint Surg Am* 1987; 69:676–678.

74. Escobedo EM, Hunter JC, Hollister MC, Patten RM, Goldstein B. MR imaging of rotator cuff tears in individuals with paraplegia. *AJR Am J Roentgenol* 1997; 168:919–923.

75. Boninger ML, Koontz AM, Sisto SA, et al. Pushrim biomechanics and injury prevention in spinal cord injury: recommendations based on CULP-SCI investigations. *J Rehabil R D* 2005; 42:9–19.

76. Robinson MD, Hussey RW, Ha CY. Surgical decompression of impingement in the weightbearing shoulder. *Arch Phys Med Rehabil* 1993; 74:324–327.

77. Goldstein B, Young J, Escobedo EM. Rotator cuff repairs in individuals with paraplegia. *Am J Phys Med Rehabil* 1997; 76:316–322.

78. Wright VJ. Osteoporosis in men. *J Am Acad Orthop Surg* 2006; 14:347–353.

79. Gennari L, Bilezikian JP. Osteoporosis in men. *Endocrinol Metab Clin North Am* 2007; 36:399–419.

80. Garland DE, Stewart CA, Adkins RH, et al. Osteoporosis after spinal cord injury. *J Orthop Res* 1992; 10:371–378.

81. Frisbie JH. Fractures after myelopathy: the risk quantified. *J Spinal Cord Med* 1997; 20:66–69.

82. Giangregorio L, McCartney N. Bone loss and muscle atrophy in spinal cord injury: epidemiology, fracture prediction, and rehabilitation strategies. *J Spinal Cord Med* 2006; 29:489–500.

83. Nance PW, Schryvers O, Leslie W, Ludwig S, et al. Intravenous pamidronate attenuates bone density loss after acute spinal cord injury. *Arch Phys Med Rehabil* 1999; 80:243–251.

84. Bauman WA, Wecht JM, Kirshblum S, et al. Effect of pamidronate administration on bone in patients with acute spinal cord injury. *J Rehabil R D* 2005; 42:305–313.

85. Ershler WB. Biomarkers of aging: immunological events. *Exp Gerontol* 1988; 23:387–389.

86. Weksler ME. Immune senescence. *Ann Neurol* 1994; 35(Suppl):S35–37.

87. Nash MS, Fletcher MA. The immune system. In: Whiteneck GG, Charlifue SW, Gerhart KA, et al., eds. *Aging with Spinal Cord Injury.* New York: Demos Publications, 1993; 159–181.

88. Campagnolo DI, Bartlett JA, Chatterton R Jr, Keller SE. Adrenal and pituitary hormone patterns after spinal cord injury. *Am J Phys Med Rehabil* 1999; 78:361–366.

89. Kahn NN, Bauman WA, Sinha AK. Appearance of a novel prostacyclin receptor antibody and duration of spinal cord injury. *J Spinal Cord Med* 2005; 28:97–102.

90. Nash MS. Immune responses to nervous system decentralization and exercise in quadriplegia. *Med Sci Sports Exerc* 1994; 26:164–171.

91. Kliesch WF, Cruse JM, Lewis RE, Bishop GR, et al. Restoration of depressed immune function in spinal cord injury patients receiving rehabilitation therapy. *Paraplegia* 1996; 34:82–90.

92. Frost F, Roach MJ, Kushner I, Schreiber P. Inflammatory C-reactive protein and cytokine levels in asymptomatic people with chronic spinal cord injury. *Arch Phys Med Rehabil* 2005; 86:312–317.

93. Bear-Lehman J, Albert SM, Burkhardt A. Cutaneous sensitivity and functional limitation. *Topics in Geriatric Rehabilitation* 2006; 22: 61–69.

94. Song J, Chang RW, Dunlop DD. Population impact of arthritis on disability in older adults. *Arthritis Rheum* 2006; 55:248–255.

95. Couture M, Lariviere N, Lefrancois R. Psychological distress in older adults with low functional independence: a multidimensional perspective. *Arch Gerontol Geriatr* 2005; 41:101–111.

96. Rejeski WJ, Fielding RA, Blair SN, et al. The lifestyle interventions and independence for elders (LIFE) pilot study: design and methods. *Contemp Clin Trials* 2005; 26:141–154.

97. Collins K, Rooney BL, Smalley KJ, Havens S. Functional fitness, disease and independence in community-dwelling older adults in western Wisconsin. *WMJ* 2004; 103:42–48.

98. Corti MC, Rigon C. Epidemiology of osteoarthritis: prevalence, risk factors and functional impact. *Aging Clin Exp Res* 2003; 15:359–363.

99. Kee CC. Older adults with osteoarthritis: psychological status and physical function. *J Gerontol Nurs* 2003; 29:26–34.

100. Dutta C. Significance of sarcopenia in the elderly. *J Nutr* 1997; 127:992S–993S.

101. National Center for Health Statistics. *Health, United States, 2006 with Chartbook on Trends in the Health of Americans.* Hyattsville, MD: US Department of Health and Human Services, 2006.

102. Charlifue SW, Weitzenkamp DA, Whiteneck GG. Longitudinal outcomes in spinal cord injury: aging, secondary conditions, and well-being. *Arch Phys Med Rehabil* 1999; 80:1429–1434.

103. Amsters DI, Pershouse KJ, Price GL, Kendall MB. Long duration spinal cord injury: perceptions of functional change over time. *Disabil Rehabil* 2005; 27:489–497.

104. Boschen KA, Tonack M, Gargaro J. Long-term adjustment and community reintegration following spinal cord injury. *Int J Rehabil Res* 2003; 26:157–164.

105. Charlifue S, Gerhart K. Community integration in spinal cord injury of long duration. *Neurorehabilitation* 2004; 19:91–101.

106. Forchheimer M, Tate DG. Enhancing community re-integration following spinal cord injury. *Neurorehabilitation* 2004; 19:103–113.

107. Whiteneck G, Tate D, Charlifue S. Predicting community reintegration after spinal cord injury from demographic and injury characteristics. *Arch Phys Med Rehabil* 1999; 80:1485–1491.

108. Whiteneck G, Meade MA, Dijkers M, Tate DG, et al. Environmental factors and their role in participation and life satisfaction after spinal cord injury. *Arch Phys Med Rehabil* 2004; 85:1793–1803.

109. Carpenter C, Forwell SJ, Jongbloed LE, Backman CL. Community participation after spinal cord injury. *Arch Phys Med Rehabil* 2007; 88:427–433.

110. Kemp BJ, Kahan JS, Krause JS, Adkins RH, Nava G. Treatment of major depression in individuals with spinal cord injury. *J Spinal Cord Med* 2004; 27:22–28.

111. Dryden DM, Saunders LD, Rowe BH, et al. Depression following traumatic spinal cord injury. *Neuroepidemiology* 2005; 25:55–61.

112. Osteraker AL, Levi R. Indicators of psychological distress in postacute spinal cord injured individuals. *Spinal Cord* 2005; 43:223–229.

113. Krause JS, Kemp B, Coker J. Depression after spinal cord injury: relation to gender, ethnicity, aging, and socioeconomic indicators. *Arch Phys Med Rehabil* 2000; 81:1099–1109.

114. Krause JS, Broderick L. A 25-year longitudinal study of the natural course of aging after spinal cord injury. *Spinal Cord* 2005; 43:349–356.

115. Krause JS, Coker JL. Aging after spinal cord injury: a 30-year longitudinal study. *J Spinal Cord Med* 2006; 29:371–376.

116. Charlifue SW, Gerhart KA, Whiteneck GG. Conceptualizing and quantifying functional change: an examination of aging with spinal cord injury. *Topics in Geriatric Rehabilitation* 1998; 13:35–48.

117. Post MW, de Witte LP, van Asbeck FW, van Dijk AJ, Schrijvers AJ. Predictors of health status and life satisfaction in spinal cord injury. *Arch Phys Med Rehabil* 1998; 79:395–401.

118. McColl MA, Walker J, Stirling P, Wilkins R, Corey P. Expectations of life and health among spinal cord injured adults. *Spinal Cord* 1997; 35:818–828.

119. Weitzenkamp DA, Gerhart KA, Charlifue SW, Glass CA, Kennedy P. Ranking the criteria for assessing quality of life after disability: evidence for priority-shifting among long-term spinal cord injury survivors. *Br J Health Psychol* 2000; 5:57–69.

120. McColl MA, Arnold R, Charlifue S, Glass C, et al. Aging, spinal cord injury, and quality of life: structural relationships. *Arch Phys Med Rehabil* 2003; 84:1137–1144.

121. Charlifue S, Gerhart K. Changing psychosocial morbidity in people aging with spinal cord injury. *Neurorehabilitation* 2004; 19: 15–23.

122. Krause JS, DeVivo MJ, Jackson AB. Health status, community integration, and economic risk factors for mortality after spinal cord injury. *Arch Phys Med Rehabil* 2004; 85:1764–1773.

123. Alander DH, Parker J, Stauffer ES. Intermediate-term outcome of cervical spinal cord-injured patients older than 50 years of age. *Spine* 1997; 22:1189–1192.

124. DeVivo MJ, Ivie CS III. Life expectancy of ventilator-dependent persons with spinal cord injuries. *Chest* 1995; 108:226–232.

125. Frankel HL, Coll JR, Charlifue SW, et al. Long-term survival in spinal cord injury: a fifty year investigation. *Spinal Cord* 1998; 36: 266–274.

IV

MANAGEMENT OF THE BLADDER, BOWEL, SEXUAL DYSFUNCTION, AND WOMEN'S HEALTH

27 Normal and Abnormal Micturition

John S. Wheeler, Jr.
Cynthia S. Fok

Normal micturition is a process that involves both bladder and urethral function. Urinary continence requires a normal compliant bladder and an active competent urethral sphincter, whereby any increase in bladder and abdominal pressure is offset by an even greater increase in urethral pressure. The normal micturition process includes passive filling of the bladder that uses these continent mechanisms, and bladder emptying that requires relaxation of the urethra and its sphincters in conjunction with a well-coordinated voluntary bladder contraction. This whole process occurs under the control of the central nervous system, which integrates the sympathetic and parasympathetic nervous systems with the somatic nervous system to provide normal micturition (1). Furthermore, this process also depends on the normal integrity of the anatomic and physiologic structures of the male and female pelvis.

Voiding dysfunction, especially urinary incontinence, is caused by any one or a number of defects in the micturition system that can result in the inability of the urethra and its sphincters to increase pressure in response to increasing bladder pressure. Abnormalities in the neurologic anatomy and physiology, alone or along with defects in pelvic anatomy or physiology, can cause voiding dysfunction and/or urinary incontinence.

BASIC NEUROUROLOGY (1)

The basic neuroanatomy and neurophysiology of the lower urinary tract must be understood and evaluated before considering management. Anatomically, the bladder is divided into the bladder base, which includes the trigone and bladder neck, which are intimately connected to the pelvic floor, and the bladder body, the bladder dome, the superior part of the bladder adjacent to the other pelvic viscera. The urinary outlet has two urethral sphincters: the internal smooth muscle sphincter at the proximal urethra and bladder neck and the external striated muscle that encompasses the membranous urethra and is attached integrally to the pelvic floor (Figure 27.1). Females have a poorly defined, less complex sphincter than males, surrounding a shorter urethra.

Males have a prostate gland located between the two sphincter regions.

The parasympathetic nervous system provides motor supply to the bladder and mediates bladder contractions via the pelvic nerve that originates in the S2 and S4 sacral cord level, the conus medullaris. The preganglionic nerve arises from the sacral cord detrusor nucleus, courses along the rectum and bladder base, and terminates in postganglionic nerves, which are contained within the bladder wall. A branch of the parasympathetic nerve also interacts with the sympathetic nerves to modulate its response, which will promote bladder contractility. The sympathetic nerves originate from the T11 to L2 spinal cord level, course along the great vessels, and synapse at the inferior mesenteric and hypogastric plexuses. The postganglionic hypogastric nerve supplies the bladder neck and proximal urethra, including the prostate gland (in the male), and indirectly affects the parasympathetic function. This nerve system mediates bladder storage primarily. The somatic nerve originates from the S2 to S4 pudendal nucleus (in the ventral horn of the spinal cord) and courses along the autonomic nerves to innervate the external striated muscle sphincter and mediate bladder storage by increasing urethral resistance (Figure 27.1).

Neurotransmitters, released at the neuromuscular junction, are received by appropriate neuroreceptors (2). Cholinergic receptors are located in the bladder base and body and mediate bladder contraction, activated by the acetylcholine released by the parasympathetic nerves. The adrenergic receptors are activated by norephinephrine released by the sympathetic nerves. Beta-adrenergic receptors are located in the bladder body and mediate bladder inhibition, promoting bladder storage and continence. Alpha-adrenergic receptors are located in the bladder base and proximal urethra (and the prostate) at the internal sphincter and mediate bladder neck contraction, promoting continence, by increasing urethral resistance (Figure 27.2). Acetylcholine is also released at the pudendal neuromuscular junction and mediates external sphincter contraction, also promoting continence. Other potential neurotransmitters such as adenosine triphosphate, vasoactive peptides, enkephalins, substance P, and

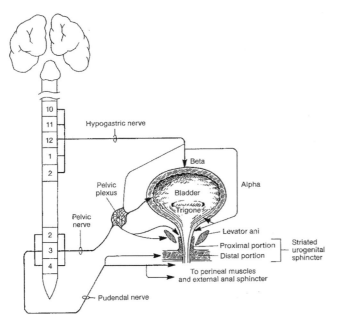

Figure 27.1 Innervation of the lower urinary tract. (Reproduced with permission from Walters MD, Karram MM. *Urogynecology and Reconstructive Pelvic Surgery.* Mosby Inc.)

nitric oxide have been identified in the lower urinary tract and may be deemed useful in future bladder management if they can be appropriately manipulated (2). In addition, estrogens help maintain urethral tone in females via local estrogen receptors located in and around the vessels of the spongy urethral tissue. Estrogen also helps maintain pelvic muscle tone.

Sensory innervation occurs through the pelvic nerve mediating bladder wall stretch reception during filling of the bladder. The hypogastric nerve is responsible for mediating bladder mucosal pain and temperature.

The central nervous system normally controls and coordinates micturition. During micturition, afferent sensory nerve activation results from bladder filling and pressure, travels to the sacral cord, and ascends from the sacral cord to the rostral pontine reticular formation, the micturition center. This center coordinates urethral sphincter relaxation just before a normal

detrusor contraction and initiates and sustains detrusor contraction during voiding. The Pontine Micturition Center is controlled by the prefrontal cortex via the anterior cingulate gyrus (3). This gyrus receives input from the limbic system and afferent input from the periaqueduct gray area—all to net inhibit the pontine center that is normally faciatory to micturition (3). With the normal onset of micturition, the cingulate gyrus is less active and disinhibits the pontine center that facilitates micturition (3). With an increase in bladder volume, sensory information goes to the prefrontal cortex, and the anterior cingulate gyrus increases activity to suppress the pontine center (3).

Voluntary control of the detrusor is from the frontal cortex to the pons and down the reticulospinal tract of the spinal cord to the detrusor nucleus and is net inhibitory. Without this control the bladder would have involuntary, uninhibited contractile activity. The frontal cortex also has direct corticospinal tract connections to the pudendal nucleus to help voluntarily control the external sphincter (Figure 27.3).

Knowledge of this neuroanatomy enables one to understand bladder function associated with certain lesions (1). For example, a stroke in the frontal cortex may cause a loss of cortical inhibition to the pons, resulting in uninhibited detrusor activity (detrusor hyperreflexia), but coordination between bladder and sphincter would be preserved due to the intact pontine sacral axis. A lesion below the pons (i.e., spinal cord injury) would result in the lack of coordinated bladder sphincter activity (bladder sphincter dyssynergia) owing to the disrupted pontine sacral axis.

A summary of normal voluntary micturition includes bladder filling, storage, and emptying of the bladder (1). During bladder filling, pressure in the bladder rises slowly with a compliant bladder wall and minimal cholinergic activity. Urethral resistance also increases at this time. At a critical pressure and volume (the micturition threshold), sympathetic nerve activity increases, causing contraction of the internal sphincter via alpha reception, promoting continence. Also, pudendal nerve activity increases involuntarily (and voluntarily) to contract the external urethral sphincter, promoting continence. Bladder filling occurs at low intravesical pressure, with normal sensation and no involuntary bladder activity.

Eventually, bladder distension leads to coordinated micturition. Voluntary inhibition of somatic discharge to the external sphincter decreases urinary outlet resistance.

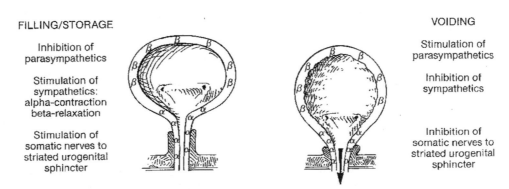

Figure 27.2 Autonomic neurotransmission of the bladder during filling and emptying. (Reproduced with permission from Walters MD, Karram MM. *Urogynecology and Reconstructive Pelvic Surgery.* Mosby Inc.)

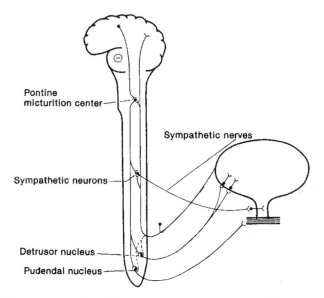

Figure 27.3 Central nervous system innervation of the lower urinary tract. (Reproduced with permission from Krane RJ, Siroky, MB. *Clinical Neurourology.* Little, Brown.)

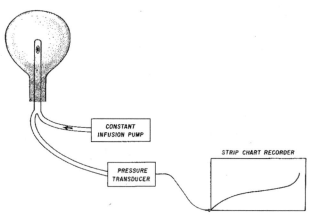

Figure 27.4 One channel cystometry. (Reproduced with permission from Raz S. *Female Urology.* WB Saunders Co.)

Sympathetic activity decreases, causing bladder neck relaxation and facilitation of parasympathetic nerve activity, promoting a bladder contraction. The pons, modulated by the frontal cortex, coordinates this activity to allow normal voiding with decreased urethral sphincter resistance, no urinary outlet obstruction, and a well-functioning bladder.

NEUROUROLOGIC EVALUATION

To assess the function of the bladder and/or urethra, an appropriate evaluation is made that includes a basic patient history, including a questionnaire and voiding diary to document the micturition pattern and a physical examination, especially to evaluate the pelvic anatomy and neurologic system. Pelvic anatomy is assessed by examining for pelvic prolapse or other defects in the female and prostate disease in the male. The focus of the neurourologic examination includes an assessment of the pelvic and lower extremity sensation, tone, and reflexes, especially the bulbo-synaptic reflex. The bulbo-synaptic reflex is a monosynaptic reflex of the sacral cord, which is performed by providing an afferent stimulus (penile, clitoral, or pubic stimulation, or foley catheter tug) simultaneously with the examiner's finger in the rectum to sense a reflex pelvic muscle contraction caused by the stimulus. The reflex is present in most patients with an intact sacral cord.

A urinalysis and urine culture is done to rule out any obvious pathologic processes (i.e., urinary tract infection and tumor). A cystoscopy should be done if such processes are found. Next, an assessment of urinary function is done. Micturition is best defined by the urodynamic evaluation, which includes urinary flow rate, bladder cystometrogram (CMG), sphincter electromyography (EMG), leak point pressure (LPP) measurement, and urethral pressure profile (UPP). The flow rate evaluation is a noninvasive quantification of urinary flow that depends on volume and speed of the voided stream. A poor flow rate may indicate urinary outlet obstruction or ineffective detrusor

activity. After determining the flow rate, a catheter is passed into the bladder, and a postvoid residual urine amount is recorded. A large volume (>100 ml) is also usually secondary to an obstruction or to an ineffective detrusor. A cystometrogram (CMG) will assess the efficacy of the detrusor and further differentiate these problems.

The CMG monitors bladder pressure during bladder filling and emptying by use of a catheter in the bladder that is connected to a pressure transducer (Figure 27.4). Gas (carbon dioxide) or water is infused at a controlled rate, often 30–60 ml/min, which is usually faster than physiologic filling. The CMG assesses bladder compliance, sensation, volume, and presence or absence of normal or uninhibited bladder activity (detrusor instability). Total CMG includes both bladder and abdominal pressure measurements. The true detrusor CMG can be determined by subtracting the abdominal pressure (measured by a rectal or intravaginal pressure transducer) from the total CMG pressures. The latter requires at least a four-channel CMG (Figure 27.5).

The pressure flow study will more accurately indicate the presence or absence of urinary outlet obstruction (4). This is the recorded bladder pressure at the point of maximal urinary flow. The recorded values can be plotted against a standard nomogram to assess the relative value of the obstruction. This is important because a low urinary flow rate does not necessarily indicate urinary obstruction unless it is associated with a high bladder pressure. Also, a high urinary flow rate does not rule out urinary obstruction unless it is associated with a low bladder pressure.

EMG is an assessment of pudendal nerve function with the use of a recording electrode on the perineum or the rectal or vaginal wall, or the use of needle electrodes placed into the external sphincter via the perineum. Nerve depolarization of the muscle membrane results in electrical potentials that are received by the electrodes and recorded. The total EMG reflects activity of the urinary outlet by recording pelvic floor striated muscle and external sphincter activity. Increased EMG activity usually indicates increased urethral resistance, and decreased EMG activity usually indicates decreased urethral resistance. Furthermore, EMG recorded simultaneously with detrusor activity (CMG) assesses the detrusor sphincter interaction. In addition, decreased EMG

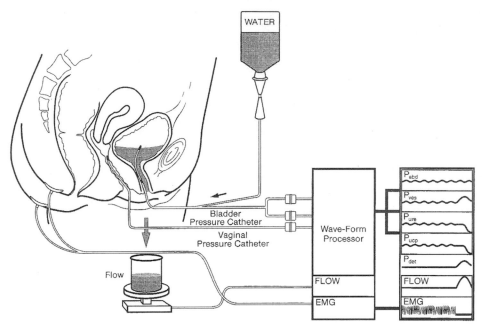

Figure 27.5 Multichannel urodynamics measuring intravesical, intraabdominal, and intraurethral pressures, subtracted true detrusor pressure, uroflow, and electromyography. (Reproduced with permission from Walters MD, Karram MM. *Urogynecology and Reconstructive Pelvic Surgery.* Mosby Inc.)

activity may be indicative of pudendal neuropathy and, again, decreased urethral resistance.

Assessment of the proximal urethral sphincter can be done by voiding cystourethrography; the patient voids radiographic contrast under radiographic monitoring. It also can be assessed by the UPP, which measures urethral pressure at points along the urethral length by use of a small catheter that is slowly withdrawn along the urethra and connected to a pressure transducer. A decreased urethral length or pressure may indicate weak pelvic floor muscles and correlate with stress urinary incontinence.

Leak point pressure measurements are the most recent parameters that have been popularized (5). The CMG leak point pressure is the detrusor pressure measured at which point the bladder, usually an unstable (overactive) or poorly compliant bladder, leaks. Generally, a persistent CMG pressure over 40 cm H_2O places the upper urinary tract at risk for hydronephrosis, reflux and infection (6). The stress (valsalva, cough) leak point pressure is the bladder pressure measured at which point the patient leaks with stress during filling CMG (usually at 150- to 200-cm filling volume). It is also equivalent to the bladder pressure needed to drive urine across the urethra (5). Basically, it is a quantification of the Marshall test that is performed with a full bladder, under stress, during the pelvic examination.

The normal CMG and EMG start with low bladder pressure, at zero volume, and as bladder filling increases to 300 to 400 ml, with the bladder pressure increasing slightly, the patient feels a sensation of fullness (Figure 27.6). The EMG increases as the patient feels the sensation to void (the guarding reflex). At the micturition threshold (the patient's bladder volume limit and the point at which the patient is ready to void), the EMG silences, urethral resistance diminishes, and there is a rapid bladder contraction, as noted by a rapid increase in detrusor

pressure, with sphincteric relaxation. Here, the patient has a normal, well-controlled and coordinated void, as recorded by flow rate.

The above basic urodynamics will generally provide a urologic diagnosis as to the etiology of the voiding dysfunction and will help classify it (7). If the patient had a more complex history or had failed previous treatments, more sophisticated urodynamic studies would probably be needed. Combination voiding cystourethrography with concomitant urodynamic pressure measurements will provide a more exact diagnosis, if needed. However, even though this method of lower urinary tract monitoring is state of the art, it is not universally available.

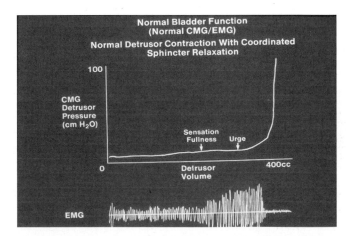

Figure 27.6 Basic representative normal CMG and EMG pattern.

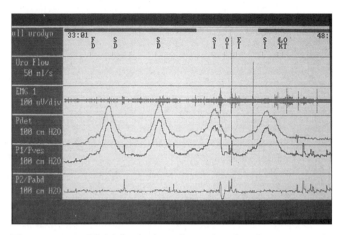

Figure 27.7 Multichannel urodynamics showing neurogenic overactive bladder or detrusor hyperreflxia.

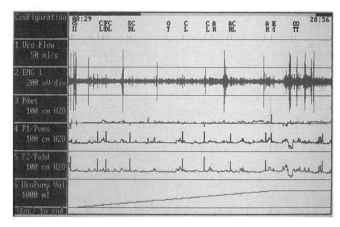

Figure 27.9 Multichannel urodynamics showing neurogenic noncontractile bladder or detrusor areflexia.

The first pattern in the classification is detrusor instability, which is the involuntary detrusor activity (detrusor overactivity) with bladder pressure changes over 15 cm of water during bladder filling that cannot be suppressed (Figure 27.7). There is a short latency between the urge to void and the detrusor contraction at usually low volumes. The patient can have irritative voiding symptoms, frequency, urgency, and nocturia, and he or she can have obstructive symptoms (i.e., decreased force of stream, hesitancy, straining) if it is related to obstruction. If the etiology of the instability is neurologic in nature, then the problem is termed detrusor *hyperreflexia* (7) (or neurogenic detrusor overactivity [8]). Detrusor hyperreflexia can occur with coordinated urethral sphincter relaxation, typical of suprapontine lesions, such as a cerebral vascular accident. Detrusor hyperreflexia also can occur with discoordinated sphincter activity (vesicosphincter dyssynergia), in which the sphincter contracts abnormally during the bladder contraction, causing increased bladder pressure (Figure 27.8). This pattern is typical of patients with spinal cord injury (SCI). In patients without neurogenic cause, the detrusor instability can be caused by urinary tract inflammations, urinary obstruction, or bladder lesions, or it can be idiopathic or functional.

The second pattern is the "acontractile detrusor," which is the lack of detrusor contraction during CMG (Figure 27.9). It can be a normal finding, probably owing to test inhibition or functional causes, or it can be neurogenic in origin. If so, it is termed *detrusor areflexia* (7) (or noncontractile detrusor [8]). To differentiate neurogenic from nonneurogenic detrusor areflexia, a Bethanechol test can be done (9). The Bethanechol test is based on Cannon's law of a denervated organ being supersensitive to its neurotransmitter (9). A supersensitive response to Bethanechol (urecholine) during CMG (bladder pressure change over 15 cm H_2O at 100 cc volume) can usually confirm a neuropathic bladder (9).

NEUROUROLOGIC TREATMENT

If voiding function results from a normal micturition reflex of bladder filling and urinary storage and emptying, then the voiding dysfunction can result from either a failure of urinary storage or a failure of urinary emptying (1). Urinary retention is an extreme consequence of failure to empty the bladder, whereas urinary incontinence is an extreme consequence of failure to store urine (1). Therefore, treatment of urinary incontinence must focus on the improvement of urinary storage capabilities (1). Failure to store urine can be caused either by defects in the bladder's ability to hold urine (i.e., bladder instability or poor compliance) or by defects in the urethra's ability to withhold bladder pressure (i.e., poor urethral resistance). Also, treatment of urinary retention must focus on the improvement of urinary emptying capabilities (1). Failure to empty the bladder can be caused either by defects in the bladder's ability to empty urine because of poor bladder contraction or by the urethra's inability to allow urine flow because of urethral obstruction (1).

To improve storage of urine, bladder overactivity must be suppressed by medication (primarily anticholinergics), electrical stimulation (via feedback inhibition), or possibly even surgical augmentation of the bladder (1). Furthermore, urethral resistance must be improved to improve incontinence via

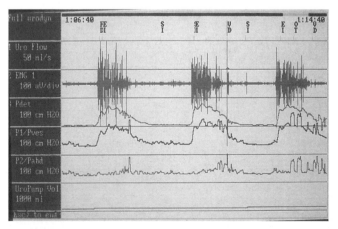

Figure 27.8 Multichannel urodynamics showing neurogenic overactive bladder with sphincter dyssynergia.

medication (alpha adrenergics), electrical stimulation, or Kegel exercises, or by surgical means that increase resistance (urethropexy or urethral sling, artificial sphincter, or urethral bulking agents) (1).

To improve emptying of urine, bladder underactivity can possibly be treated with medication (cholinergics, although these usually do not work) or (more typically) by intermittent catheterization (1). Additionally, urethral resistance can be lowered by either medication (primarily alpha adrenergic blockers) or surgery (transurethral resection of the obstruction) (1).

A new treatment, botulinum toxin (Botox), can be injected into the external sphincter to minimize sphincter dyssynergia or into the bladder wall (muscle) to suppress overactive detrusor (10). However, it has not been approved by the FDA for use as such, even though multiple reports have supported its benefit in these situations.

In summary, knowledge of the neuroanatomy and physiology of the normal and abnormal lower urinary tract can be enhanced and better understood by urodynamics. Urodynamic tests will define the problem and then help guide appropriate therapy, especially in patients who have voiding dysfunction and a complex neurologic history, such as SCI.

References

1. Wein AJ. Classification of voiding dysfunction: a simple approach. In: Barrett DM, Wein AJ, eds. *Controversies in Neuro-Urology.* New York: Churchill Livingstone, 1984.
2. deGroat WC, Kawatani M. Neuro control of the urinary bladder. *J Neurol Urodyn* 1985; 4:285–300.
3. Griffiths D, Tadic S. Bladder control, urgency, and urge incontinence: evidence from functional brain imaging. *J Neurol Urodyn* 2008; 27:466–474.
4. Griffiths DJ. Pressure flow studies of micturition. *Urol Clin North Am* 1996; 23(31):279.
5. McGuire EJ, Cespedes RD, O'Connell, H. Leak point pressures. *Urol Clin North Am* 1996; 23(2):253.
6. McGuire EJ, Woodside JR, Border TA, Weiss RM. Prognostic value of urodynamic testing in myelodysplastic patients. *J Urol* 1981; 126:205–209.
7. Krane RT, Siroky MB. Classification of neurourologic disorders. In: *Clinical Neurourology.* Krane RT, Siroky MB, eds. Boston: Little, Brown, 1979.
8. Abrams P, Cardoza L, Fall M, Griffiths D, et al. The standardisation of terminology of lower urinary tract function. *Neurourol Urodyn* 2002; 21:167–178.
9. Lapides J, Frend CR, Ajemian EP, Reus WF. A new test for neurogenic bladder. *J Urol* 1962; 88:245.
10. Smith CP, Chancellor MB. Emerging role of botulinum toxin in the management of voiding dysfunction. *J Urol* 2004; 171:2128–2137.

28 Chronic Renal Insufficiency

Cyril H. Barton

Chronic renal disease is defined as either kidney damage or decreased kidney function (decreased GFR <60 mL/min/ 1.73 m²) for 3 or more months, irrespective of cause. This is accompanied by symptoms and signs of uremia when nearing end stage disease, hypertension in the majority, isosthenuria and broad casts, and atrophic kidneys on renal sonogram (1). It affects approximately 26 million Americans, the majority of whom are unaware of the disease process until it has progressed significantly. A recent cross-sectional analysis of the National Health and Nutrition Examination Surveys (NHANES 1988–1994 and NHANES 1999–2004) revealed that the prevalence of chronic kidney disease in the United States in 1999–2004 is higher than it was in 1988–1994. This rise in the prevalence is partly explained by a rise in diabetes and hypertension as shown in the data collected through surveillance programs (2–5).

Chronic renal insufficiency remains a serious complication of longstanding spinal cord injury (SCI), and it causes substantial morbidity and mortality in this setting. In a large necropsy series reported by Tribe and Silver in 1969, renal insufficiency was the primary cause of death in the great majority (75%) of cases studied (6). In a subsequent report published in 1977 by Hackler (7) (involving a cohort of World War II and Korean War veterans with traumatic SCI), chronic renal failure was found to be the principal cause of death in 45% of patients. An additional report by Borges and Hackler (involving a group of Vietnam War veterans with SCI) demonstrated a further reduction in the percentage of deaths from renal causes (20%) (8), and in 1982 Price reported a renal-related mortality rate of only 14% in a long-term follow-up study (involving a large group of civilian SCI patients) (9). More recent studies continue to demonstrate this trend. DeVivo et al., through a process of merging survival data (from the National Database, available collaborative studies, and the Social Security Administration), have shown that kidney and urinary tract diseases account for only a small percentage (3.5%) of all deaths in SCI patients (10, 11). However, diseases of the urinary system were found to be the most frequent secondary contributing cause of death in SCI patients. Much of the progress in the prevention of renal insufficiency and the reduction of

urinary tract disease–related mortality in SCI patients has been achieved through a combination of intensive patient education, the prevention and control of infection, the prevention of reflux, and most importantly, special attention to the maintenance of urine flow and bladder drainage (10–14).

Pathogenesis

Tubulointerstitial diseases, characterized by progressive renal insufficiency (with associated pyuria but only minimal proteinuria) have been generally described as the predominant type of kidney disease occurring in SCI patients. However, it has been our experience that moderate to heavy proteinuria, indicative of glomerular disease, is frequently present in SCI patients with moderate to advanced renal insufficiency. It would therefore appear that both tubulointerstitial and glomerular injury are involved in the development of chronic renal failure in patients with longstanding SCI. This concept is consistent with a growing body of evidence indicating that multiple predisposing factors and at least several pathophysiologic processes are likely involved in the genesis of chronic renal insufficiency in patients with longstanding SCI. These include chronic pyelonephritis, nephrolithiasis, obstructive nephropathy, reflux nephropathy, amyloidosis, and hypertensive nephrosclerosis (10, 12, 14–21).

In a study by our group, chronic UTI with pyelonephritis contributed to renal failure in 100% of 43 SCI patients with end-stage renal disease (22), which is similar to the experience reported by other investigators (6). In SCI patients, bacteria may gain easy access to the bladder via an indwelling catheter or as a complication of intermittent catheterization. Fecal contamination, as well as the dampness associated with absorbent garments, may also increase the frequency and rate of bacterial colonization and subsequent infection. Also, in patients with decubitus ulcers, there is often cross infection between infected pressure sores and the urinary tract (22). Moreover, in SCI patients, UTIs are frequently perpetuated by impaired urinary drainage, the presence of urinary calculi, or the use of indwelling catheters (12, 14, 20, 22, 23). Furthermore, the combination of active infection and functional obstruction often leads to vesicoureteral reflux, along with a progressive destructive pyelonephritis. In addition to causing tubulointerstitial injury and predisposing to pyelonephritis, reflux nephropathy has been associated with the development of focal glomerulosclerosis (24). This condition generally presents with proteinuria and hypertension, and may cause or contribute to progressive renal failure in SCI patients. The mechanism by which vesicoureteral reflux leads to glomerulosclerosis is thought to involve the development of glomerular capillary hypertension with subsequent hyperfiltration injury. It should be noted, however, that the development of glomerular capillary hypertension (in the remaining functioning nephrons) is nonspecific and appears to be part of a maladaptive response to progressive nephron loss irrespective of cause (i.e., reflux, infection, or other causes).

The incidence of stone formation in spinal cord injury patients has not changed over the years despite the major breakthroughs in urological care (25). Nephrolithiasis is a frequent finding in patients with longstanding SCI, occurring most often in patients with persistent or recurrent UTI; however, a number of factors may be involved in the genesis of this abnormality (25–30). Although hypercalciuria caused by immobilization is common during the early phase of SCI, it is usually absent or less pronounced during the more chronic phases of this condition (31). In fact, urinary calcium excretion may be reduced in those patients with chronic renal impairment because of an associated impairment in vitamin D metabolism or by the development of secondary hyperparathyroidism. In addition, we have noted substantial hyperoxaluria in a group of spinal cord injured patients with varying degrees of renal insufficiency that may be caused by increased intestinal absorption of oxalate occasioned by the associated impairment of bowel motility (32). We have also noted reductions in urinary citrate in SCI patients, and other investigators have confirmed this observation (33–35). Consequently, a reduction in the urinary content of citrate, which is a potent inhibitor of stone formation, may be a causal factor in the genesis of urolithiasis in this population. Recent studies involving *Oxalobacter formigenes* have shown its role in the etiopathogenesis of hyperoxaluria, hypocitraturia, and subsequent nephrolithiasis. Oxalate homeostasis is partly controlled by this gram-negative anaerobic bacterium, and its loss from the gut flora (from prolonged and widespread use of antibiotics in SCI patients) have been associated with an increased absorption of oxalate, thereby increasing the risk for hyperoxaluria and recurrent calcium oxalate urolithiasis (36–39). Experimental probiotic treatments using *O. formigenes* or its enzyme analog *oxalyl-CoA decarboxylase* have shown to reduce the level of oxalate in the urine, thus decreasing oxalate stone formation (40–44). However, UTI caused by urease-producing organisms is probably the most important predisposing factor with regard to urolithiasis (23, 34). Such infections can facilitate the formation of struvite stones by providing an abundance of ammonium while also greatly increasing the urinary pH. Urinary stasis, related to functional obstruction, and the increased excretion of inflammatory debris associated with infection, also facilitate stone formation in SCI patients. The development of urolithiasis, in turn, can contribute to renal deterioration by causing urinary obstruction and/or by providing a nidus for infection, thus prolonging the duration and complicating the management of UTI. Sequential studies have also revealed significant reductions

in renal plasma flow in SCI patients following the development of nephrolithiasis (45). Moreover, infection stones substantially increase the risk for complications such as pyonephrosis and urosepsis in SCI patients.

The development of amyloidosis is an important cause of renal insufficiency in patients with long-standing SCI (16, 18, 21). In addition, amyloidosis is a major cause of heavy proteinuria in this population. According to the results of autopsy studies reported by Tribe and Silver, 50% of patients studied had evidence for renal amyloidosis (6). In a study involving 43 spinal cord injured patients with end-stage renal disease, we confirmed the presence of renal amyloidosis in 81% (46). The higher incidence of renal amyloidosis in our patients was thought to be a function of greater longevity made possible by the availability of maintenance hemodialysis. Infected pressure sores, osteomyelitis, and UTIs complicated by pyelonephritis appear to be the major causal factors in the genesis of secondary amyloidosis.

As a final consideration, hypertensive nephrosclerosis may contribute to the progression of renal failure in SCI patients (particularly in those patients with underlying renal insufficiency) (13, 16). This observation is based on clinical experience as well as autopsy data and underscores the importance of maintaining good blood pressure control.

Prevention

Current preventive care practices include maintaining good control and stringent management of diabetes and blood pressure. Complications from chronic kidney disease increase at lower GFR levels as shown by the data from NHANES III, providing a strong basis for using GFR to classify the stage of severity of chronic kidney disease. The 5-stage system (Table 28.1) developed as a guideline by the National Kidney Foundation—Kidney Disease Outcome Quality Initiative (NKF K/DOQI) allows for the formulation of an appropriate plan of care for individuals with chronic kidney disease (47, 48).

Chronic renal insufficiency is a potentially preventable complication of SCI. This is evidenced by the steady decline in mortality from renal causes, which parallels our better understanding of the causal mechanisms involved in renal injury as well as improvements in technology and education. Specifically, improvements in the diagnosis and management of urinary tract obstruction and infection have played a pivotal role in reducing the incidence of renal disease and the related morbidity and mortality.

This begins with good bladder management, which includes the maintenance of a low voiding pressure; the provision of a relatively large-capacity low-pressure storage system; and prevention of infection (14). Ideally, good bladder management will be achievable via reflex voiding. Gentle suprapubic tapping helps initiate reflex voiding. If this is successfully accomplished, post-void residual volumes should be less that 100 ml, and bladder pressures (during storage and while voiding) should be below 35 to 40 cm H_2O. In some patients, high voiding pressures can be ameliorated with the use of either alpha-adrenergic blocking drugs or antispasticity agents, whereas the administration of musculotropic relaxants, tricyclic antidepressants, anticholinergic agents (oral and intravesical) (49–51), intravesical vanilloids (e.g., resiniferatoxin), and the newer muscarinic receptor specific agents can improve bladder storage capacity

Table 28.1 Chronic Kidney Disease: A Clinical Action Plan

Numbered stages identify patients who have chronic kidney disease; unnumbered stage indicates patients who have increased risk for chronic kidney disease. Chronic kidney disease is defined as kidney damage or GFR < 60 mL/min/ 1.73 m² for ≥3 months. Kidney damage is defined as pathologic abnormalities or markers of damage, including abnormalities in blood or urine tests or imaging studies.

STAGE	DESCRIPTION	GFR (ML/MIN/ 1.73 M²)	ACTION*
	At increased risk	≥60 (with CKD risk factors)	Screening CKD risk reduction
1	Kidney damage with normal or ↑ GFR	≥90	Diagnosis and treatment
			Treatment of comorbid conditions Slowing progression CVD risk reduction
2	Kidney damage with mild or ↓ GFR	60–89	Estimating progression
3	Moderate ↓ GFR	30–59	Evaluating and treating complications
4	Severe ↓ GFR	15–29	Preparation for kidney replacement therapy
5	Kidney failure	<15 (or dialysis)	Replacement (if uremia present)

*Includes actions in preceding stages.
Abbreviations: GFR = glomerular filtration rate; CKD = chronic kidney disease; CVD = cardiovascular disease.

(7, 52–56). Intravesical vanilloids (e.g., capsaicin and resiniferatoxin) have also been studied in patients who present with high voiding pressures and incontinence from detrusor hyperreflexia (57–59). When reflex voiding is not feasible, the utilization of intermittent bladder catheterization provides a viable option. A clean technique should be used (regarding catheterization), and bladder overdistention must be avoided through the use of frequent or timely catheterization. Furthermore, the adjunctive use of medication may be effective in both increasing bladder capacity and reducing intravesical pressure (12, 14). Placement of a chronic indwelling catheter, however, is less desirable because of the increased risk for UTI, calculous disease, dysreflexia, and bladder cancer (12, 14, 20). In male patients, external sphincterotomy may be useful in lowering the intravesicular pressure and in ameliorating vesicoureteral reflux as well as allowing a catheter-free status in patients with detrusor–sphincter dyssynergia (14). More recent studies have shown the utility of Botulinum toxin A as a chemical neurolytic agent in the management of detrusor hyperreflexia with or without dyssynergia,

especially in patients who cannot tolerate the side effects from the oral medications (60, 61).

It is recommended that assessment of the urinary tract be performed annually to screen for bladder changes, vesicoureteral reflux, and calculous disease (12, 14). This can usually be accomplished with a cystogram, ultrasonography, excretory urography (if renal function is normal), videourodynamics, and cystoscopy if needed. Renal scintigraphy has also been used to screen the upper tracts and has particular advantages: it is non–user dependent, with a decreased exposure to radiation and to the contrast dye. It is preferred by some SCI urologists as shown in a more recent survey of clinical practices regarding surveillance testing for patients with neurogenic bladders (62, 63).

Prevention or effective management of urolithiasis is also very important in SCI patients. Measures that effectively prevent or reduce the frequency and severity of UTIs, as well as treatment designed to minimize obstruction and maintain satisfactory urine flow, are essential in reducing urolithiasis risk (12, 14, 23, 29). Such measures are particularly important in preventing the formation of struvite stones, which are the most common type of renal calculi seen in SCI patients and the most problematic. In addition, the use of urease inhibitors may prove to be useful in the management of struvite stones (64, 65). Patients who form calcium oxalate stones may benefit from a reduction in dietary oxalate, improved bowel care, and oral pyridoxine supplementation, which decreases endogenous oxalate production. In addition, increasing oral calcium intake can reduce oxalate absorption by chelating dietary oxalate in the intestine. Also, patients should be advised against consuming large quantities of vitamin C, which acts as an oxalate precursor and increases the production of endogenous oxalate (66–68). As a final consideration, the administration of inhibitors of stone formation (e.g., magnesium supplements and/or potassium citrate) may prove useful in SCI patients, although to our knowledge, such therapy has not been evaluated in this setting.

Because secondary amyloidosis is a consequence of chronic infection and suppuration, its prevention is predicated on either the prevention or effective management of infection. SCI patients are at high risk for a number of infections, including UTIs with pyelonephritis, that may be further complicated by abscess formation (renal and perinephric) and sepsis. Pressure ulcers are also common, having an annual incidence of approximately 23% (13,17,69,70). Moreover, these lesions often become infected and may be further complicated by the development of cellulitis or osteomyelitis. Respiratory complications, however, are the leading cause of mortality in SCI patients, with atelectasis and pneumonia being particularly problematic in patients who have high cervical lesions (10, 11, 17, 71). With further progress in the area of infectious disease management, both mortality and morbidity rates should continue to improve in SCI patients.

Clinical and Laboratory Features

Progression of renal disease causes not only a reduction in excretory function but also results in renal-related metabolic and endocrine dysfunction. Diminished excretory function is manifested by a reduction in the glomerular filtration rate with associated elevations in BUN and serum creatinine levels. As noted, because of reduced muscle mass, the magnitude of serum creatinine elevation in SCI patients may be considerably less than in able-bodied individuals with comparable renal insufficiency. For the same reason, the serum concentration and urinary excretion of creatinine are proportionately lower in quadriplegics when compared with paraplegics having comparable levels of renal function (72). However, it should be noted that the measurement of creatinine clearance can be reliably used to assess glomerular filtration rate in SCI patients. This is because the clearance of a substance measures the efficiency of excretion (i.e., the greater the excretion of creatinine per unit concentration in plasma, the higher the clearance). Consequently, the clearance of creatinine would not be affected by differences in muscle mass or creatinine production. Calculation of creatinine clearance however, requires a timed urine collection (usually for a period of 12 or 24 hours) with concurrent measurements of the urinary creatinine concentration (Ucr), plasma creatinine concentration (Pcr), and urinary flow rate (V); as well as the use of the following clearance formula:

$$\text{Creatinine clearance} = \text{UcrV/Pcr}$$

where *Ucr* and *Pcr* are generally measured in mg/dl, and *V* is measured in ml per minute. However, in SCI patients, one should avoid using standard formulas or nomograms that estimate (rather than measure) creatinine clearance and are based on the assumed presence of a normal muscle mass. We compared creatinine clearance measurements obtained from urine and serum collections with those calculated from the serum creatinine concentration using an equation popularized by Cockroft and Gault (72, 73):

$$Ccr = \frac{(140 - \text{age}) \times \text{wt (kg)}}{72 \times \text{Scr (mg/dl)}}$$

for men. and for women:

$$Ccr = \frac{(140 - \text{age}) \times 0.85 \text{ wt (kg)}}{72 \times \text{Scr (mg/dl)}}$$

where *Ccr* represents creatinine clearance (ml/min), wt stands for body weight, and Scr represents serum creatinine concentration (mg/dl). In this study, we found that, whereas the measured and calculated values closely approximated one another (in the able-bodied group), the Cockroft and Gault formula substantially overestimated the true (measured) creatinine clearance in SCI patients. Specifically, the calculated creatinine clearance overestimated the measured value by 20% in paraplegics and 40% in quadriplegics, necessitating the use of correction factors (0.8 in quadriplegics and 0.6 in paraplegics) (72, 73).

In contrast to serum creatinine, the BUN concentration in SCI patients has been shown to be comparable to values obtained from able-bodied persons with similar levels of renal function, dietary protein intake, and metabolic status (74). It should be noted, however, that BUN levels are usually affected to a greater extent than serum creatinine by factors such as dietary protein intake, catabolic rate, and state of hydration. Because moderate to advanced renal insufficiency in SCI is often caused by a combination of glomerular and tubulointerstitial disease, urinary findings typically include proteinuria, hematuria, and pyuria. The presence of heavy proteinuria or development of the nephrotic syndrome (i.e., >3.5 grams of urinary protein per 24 hours) usually signifies glomerular involvement with either secondary amyloidosis or focal glomerulosclerosis. Evidence for tubulointerstitial disease would include the presence of polyuria, impaired urinary concentrating ability, impaired urinary sodium reabsorption, renal tubular acidosis, or hyporeninemic hypoaldosteronism. Although the ability to conserve sodium and water is usually impaired in most SCI patients with renal disease, problems related to sodium-volume overload will also occur in patients with moderate to severe renal failure, which may be manifested by the development of hypertension, cardiac failure, and pulmonary edema.

The kidneys are the principal organs involved in potassium excretion, and in response to progressive nephron loss, tubular secretion of potassium is increased in the remaining functional nephrons. Increased potassium secretion by colonic mucosa also helps maintain potassium homeostasis in patients with impaired renal function. However, in the presence of severe renal insufficiency, these adaptive mechanisms often fail in the prevention of hyperkalemia. Severe hyperkalemia can also occur in patients with moderate renal insufficiency, wherein large amounts of potassium enter the extracellular fluid compartment from an exogenous source (i.e., with the ingestion of potassium-rich food or the intravenous administration of fluids containing potassium). In addition, the excessive release of potassium from the intracellular compartment caused by hemolysis, rhabdomyolysis, tissue necrosis, or hypercatabolic states can cause severe hyperkalemia in patients with impaired renal function. Furthermore, any condition or agent capable of adversely affecting the renal tubular secretion of potassium (i.e., reduced distal sodium delivery, oliguria, hyporeninemia, and hypoaldosteronism, or the use of potassium-sparing diuretics, ACE-Is, ARBs, and/or NSAIDs) will substantially increase the risk for hyperkalemia in CRF patients, even those having only mild to moderate renal insufficiency. Likewise, constipation increases the risk for hyperkalemia in CRF patients by limiting the colonic excretion of potassium. This is of particular significance in SCI patients, who frequently suffer from impaired colonic motility and anal sphincter dysfunction. Hyperkalemia, in turn, predisposes patients to severe electrophysiologic disorders that can cause life-threatening arrhythmias, cardiac conduction defects, and cardiac arrest, as well as muscle weakness or paralysis. Accordingly, hyperkalemia represents one of the most critical complications of renal insufficiency.

Patients with renal insufficiency also have a compromised capacity for magnesium excretion, and consequently they are at risk for hypermagnesemia. This condition can cause skeletal muscle weakness or paralysis, the loss of deep tendon reflexes, cardiac conduction defects, as well as alterations in mental status. Therefore, the use of magnesium-containing antacids and laxatives should be generally avoided in patients with renal insufficiency.

Endocrinologic Disorders

The metabolic and endocrine functions of the kidneys are multifaceted and include the production of specific hormones (e.g., erythropoietin, 1,25(OH)$_2$D$_3$, and prostaglandins) and regulation of the renin-angiotensin-aldosterone system. In addition, the kidneys participate in the metabolism and excretion of various polypeptide and steroid hormones, and also serve as target organs for a number of hormones (e.g., aldosterone, parathormone, atrial natriuretic peptide, and antidiuretic hormone). In chronic renal failure, parallel losses involving both the excretory and endocrine functions of the kidney are compounded by profound biochemical abnormalities (induced by renal insufficiency) that can adversely affect the function of other endocrine glands. Accordingly, severe renal insufficiency is associated with multiple endocrinopathies, the discussion of which is beyond the scope of this chapter. One additional consideration regarding SCI patients with end-stage renal disease is the high incidence of amyloidosis involving various endocrine organs, which may further contribute to endocrine dysfunction in this setting (75).

Hematologic Complications

One of the most constant and disabling consequences of end-stage renal disease is anemia, which is primarily related to erythropoietin deficiency (76). However, impaired iron utilization, a shortened erythrocyte life span, nutritional deficiencies, and blood loss are also involved in the genesis of anemia in chronic renal failure (77). In a study involving the hematopoietic system in end-stage renal disease (ESRD) we found anemia to be of greater severity in SCI patients treated with hemodialysis compared to able-bodied hemodialysis patients (78). In addition, we noted a high incidence of amyloid deposition in the bone marrow of SCI patients with ESRD, which may also be a contributing factor in the development of anemia.

Another complication of severe renal insufficiency is platelet dysfunction, which can predispose to bleeding problems. In our studies involving coagulation and fibrinolytic pathways, patients with longstanding SCI and ESRD have revealed numerous abnormalities in both the intrinsic and extrinsic pathways (79–82). There was also an increased prevalence of antithrombin III deficiency, along with decreased protein C anticoagulant activity (in the presence of increased protein C antigen concentration) (82). In addition, significant alterations were noted in the fibrinolytic system, including a marked reduction in tissue plasminogen activator activity (82). Overall the coagulation and fibrinolytic abnormalities observed in this population suggest a predisposition for thrombophilic diathesis.

DISORDERS OF BONE AND MINERAL METABOLISM

The kidneys are the principal producer of $1,25(OH)_2D_3$ (the biologically active metabolite of vitamin D), which is essential in calcium absorption and normal bone metabolism. Advanced renal insufficiency causes $1,25(OH)_2D_3$ deficiency, which in turn can result in a negative calcium balance and osteomalacia. Furthermore, the combination of $1,25(OH)_2D_3$ deficiency, hypocalcemia, and hyperphosphatemia (the latter a consequence of reduced renal phosphate excretion) stimulates parathyroid activity, which often results in secondary hyperparathyroidism. Moreover, the complications of secondary hyperparathyroidism, including high-turnover bone disease, metastatic calcifications, and osteitis fibrosa cystica, substantially contribute to morbidity and mortality in ESRD (83–85). Recent studies have shown that risk for metastatic soft tissue calcification is significantly increased when the serum calcium phosphate (Ca X P) product exceeds 60 to 70 mg^2/dL^2 (83, 86). Bone disease (in SCI-ESRD) may be further complicated by demineralization, related to chronic acidosis and reduced physical activity. In addition, aluminum-related bone disease can occur in patients who are receiving aluminum-containing compounds (usually in the form of antacids or phosphate binders) (87). Aluminum overload has also been reported in patients inadvertently dialyzed with aluminum-contaminated water (88). Aluminum toxicity (which can cause bone disease, dementia, myopathy, and anemia) has been substantially curtailed with the use of better water purification techniques in dialysis and by the diminished use of aluminum-containing phosphate binders. The latter has been accomplished by the substitution of effective nonaluminum containing phosphate binders (e.g., calcium carbonate, calcium acetate, and Sevelamer (Renagel®). A newer nonaluminum, noncalcium phosphate binder, Lanthanum carbonate (Fosrenol®), has recently been approved for the treatment of hyperphosphatemia in patients with end-stage renal disease (89). More recent studies of Lanthanum showed efficacy in lowering serum phosphorus levels along with decreased PTH levels. Further studies are ongoing to determine safety with prolonged exposure to the drug (90, 91).

Finally, a peculiar type of amyloidosis has been described in long-term dialysis patients, where there is deposition of amyloid fibrils (containing beta-2-microglobulin) in collagen tissue, particularly in the synovia of joints and tendons, as well as in subchondral bone (92). The most common clinical manifestations of this disease are carpal tunnel syndrome and a destructive spondyloarthropathy typically involving the shoulders, knees, hips, and axial skeleton. Characteristic radiographic findings include erosions and defects involving the margins of affected bone, particularly at tendon insertion sites, as well as the presence of radiolucent cystic lesions within subchondral bone. The pathophysiology of this dialysis-related amyloidosis involves tissue accumulation of beta-2-microglobulin (a low-molecular weight protein expressed by nucleated cells), which is normally filtered and degraded by the kidneys. Although beta-2-microglobulin is removed with dialysis (up to 400 to 600 mg/wk with high-flux dialysis), accumulation continues because of the high rate of production (approximately 1,500 mg/wk). Consequently, the only known effective treatment for this condition is successful kidney transplantation (21, 93).

Neurologic Consequences

Both the central nervous system (CNS) and peripheral nervous system (PNS) are affected by uremia. Some of the major CNS manifestations include the reversal of normal sleep patterns, reduction in cognitive function, asterixis, confusion, obtundation, and coma. Uremic peripheral neuropathy can involve both sensory and motor modalities (often more severe in the legs than in the arms) (94–96). CNS manifestations readily improve with the institution of adequate dialysis therapy. However, once significant uremic neuropathy develops, the response (if any) to dialysis therapy is slow and incomplete. For this reason, dialytic therapy should be initiated prior to the development of clinically significant peripheral neuropathy. Because the superimposed neurologic manifestations of uremia can compound and greatly magnify disability in SCI patients, the early institution of renal replacement therapy should be considered in this setting.

Cardiovascular and Pulmonary Complications

Severe renal insufficiency predisposes patients to fluid overload, congestive heart failure, pulmonary edema, and hypertension (97–101). However, a combination of dietary fluid and sodium restriction, dialysis, and the use of antihypertensive agents can effectively control these problems.

Nevertheless, the most common cause of death in CRF patients is cardiovascular disease (i.e., myocardial infarction, stroke, cardiomyopathy, and congestive heart failure) (98, 102, 103). Moreover, in ESRD the relative risk for cardiovascular death is approximately 17 times that of the general population (103). Although not fully understood, the increased risk for cardiovascular disease in CRF patients appears to be multifactoral, involving conventional risk factors (e.g., hypertension, dyslipidemia, hypercoagulability, sedentary lifestyle, obesity, and smoking), as well as other causes or risk factors more specifically related to CRF (e.g., abnormal calcium and phosphorous, metabolism, hyperparathyroidism, vascular calcification, oxalate retention, hyperhomocystinemia, increased carbamylation and glycation of macromolecules, increased oxidative stress, and endothelial dysfunction) (98–101). Furthermore, ESRD patients are shown to have a high prevalence of left ventricular hypertrophy as well as high serum levels of inflammatory mediators (i.e., C-reactive protein), which are also considered markers for cardiovascular risk and mortality. Therefore, given the very high cardiovascular event rate associated with renal failure, SCI patients with CRF should be placed in the highest risk stratum with respect to both the management of risk factors and decisions regarding treatment. This would include the early detection and control of hypertension, dyslipidemia, and obesity, the avoidance of tobacco, and if possible, the implementation of an aerobic exercise program. Because of the increased risk of gastrointestinal bleeding in patients with CRF, aspirin therapy is generally not recommended as primary prevention; however, as secondary prevention (i.e., in patients with established cardiovascular disease) we recommend low-dose aspirin (81 to 150 mg daily) unless otherwise contraindicated. In addition, the use of antioxidants (e.g., vitamin E, ascorbic acid, or probucol) may be beneficial in reducing cardiovascular risk, as evidenced by a recent report showing vitamin E to be effective in reducing LDL-oxidation in dialysis patients (104, 105). Again, it should be noted that when ascorbic acid is administered to CRF patients, the daily dose should not exceed 100 mg because of the risk for increased oxalate production. With regard to hyperhomocystinemia, there is evidence that treatment with folic acid (1 to 15 mg/d), pyridoxine (50 to 100 mg/d), and vitamin B12 (1 mg/d) can lower serum homocysteine levels in CRF patients (106, 107). In addition, there are recent data indicating that a combination of intravenous folinic acid and pyridoxine may be even more effective in lowering serum homocysteine levels in ESRD patients (108).

Additional measures that may be beneficial in reducing cardiac risk in CRF patients include early treatment of anemia with erythropoietin targeted to maintain the hematocrit between 33% and 36%; prevention of hyperphosphatemia; aggressive treatment of secondary hyperparathyroidism; the timely initiation

and maintenance of adequate dialysis; and the maintenance of adequate nutrition (101, 107–111).

Pericarditis is generally a late manifestation of untreated uremia, which can be complicated by cardiac tamponade (97, 101, 109, 112). The presence of uremic pericarditis signifies the need for the prompt institution of dialytic therapy. Patients already receiving "adequate dialysis" may occasionally develop dialysis-associated pericarditis that does not appear to be uremic-related. However, an assessment of dialysis adequacy is indicated in all dialysis patients presenting with pericarditis, because an inadequate dialysis regimen may be an underlying factor in the genesis of this condition (107, 109, 112, 113). Patients should also be evaluated for other potential triggering factors or causes of pericarditis, including intercurrent infection, hyperparathyroidism, hyperuricemia, chronic volume overload, and malnutrition. Additionally, the occurrence of pericarditis may be a manifestation of an underlying systemic disease (e.g., systemic lupus erythematosus) or related to the use of a drug (e.g., minoxidil). Acute pericarditis should be suspected in patients who present with chest pain and fever; the diagnosis is confirmed by the presence of a pericardial friction rub. Echocardiography is also useful in detecting and monitoring the progress of pericardial effusions. It should be noted, however, that small asymptomatic pericardial effusions (<100ml) are routinely present on ultrasonography in dialysis patients and probably have no clinical relevance. Patients with acute pericarditis should be hospitalized and closely monitored for arrhythmias, as well as for signs of impending tamponade (e.g., pulsus paradoxus or unexplained dialysis-associated hypotension) (107, 112). The management of dialysis-associated pericarditis includes

- Intensifying the dialysis regimen by increasing the frequency of dialysis, usually to five treatments per week for a period of 2 to 4 weeks.
- Avoidance of anticoagulation (to reduce the risk of tamponade, heparin-free dialysis should be used).
- Avoidance of volume depletion; and patients should not be excessively ultrafiltrated below their targeted dry weight.
- Attainment of adequate pain control using either acetaminophen, codeine, hydrocodone, or, in extreme cases, morphine sulfate. It should be noted that neither the use of NSAIDs, systemic steroids, nor intrapericardial steroids has been shown to be particularly beneficial in the management of pericarditis-related pain (112).
- Timely surgical attention to cardiac tamponade with drainage, preferably via subxiphoid pericardiostomy. Blind-needle pericardiocentesis should only be used as emergency treatment for life-threatening tamponade. Although most patients recover from pericarditis with conservative management, this disease still accounts for 3% to 4% of all deaths in dialysis patients, and constrictive pericarditis can occasionally occur as a delayed complication.

There is a large body of data demonstrating an increased prevalence of various cardiac abnormalities in CRF patients (e.g., ischemic heart disease, cardiomyopathy, and pericarditis) (98, 99, 113, 114). Not surprisingly, cardiac disease also appears to be highly prevalent in SCI patients with CRF. This is evident from sequential autopsy data analyzed at our center, where all 48 of the SCI-ESRD patients who were examined demonstrated one or more cardiac abnormalities (115). These included fibrinous pericarditis (50%), left and right ventricular hypertrophy (45% and 20%, respectively), left and right ventricular dilation (40% and 30%, respectively), cardiac amyloidosis (25%), myocardial fibrosis (45%), and coronary arteriosclerosis (45%). In addition to pulmonary congestion and edema (thought to be the result of uncontrolled hypervolemia), a number of pulmonary abnormalities were also noted in the majority of patients examined. These included pneumonia, pulmonary interstitial and pleural fibrosis, and pulmonary arteriosclerosis (116).

Infections

Bacterial infections are also highly prevalent in SCI patients with advanced renal failure. Furthermore, chronic infections involving the urinary tract, pressure wounds, and osteomyelitis may be contributing factors in the development and progression of renal disease. In a survey of 43 SCI-ESRD patients, practically all had evidence for chronic, active UTI, whereas the majority were noted to have infected pressure ulcers (some with associated osteomyelitis) (22). In addition, vascular access infection, respiratory infection, peritonitis (mainly occurring in those patients treated with peritoneal dialysis), and sepsis were encountered with considerable frequency. Cross-infection between pressure sores, urinary tract, and the blood access or peritoneal access site was also frequently observed. Fever and significant leukocytosis were either absent or disproportionately mild, considering the severity of the associated infection, and in more than 50% of cases, septicemia was the immediate cause of death.

Gastrointestinal Complications and Related Disease

Gastrointestinal (GI) complications (which are common in SCI-ESRD patients) may be related to a variety of factors, including SCI per se, the effects of chronic renal failure, medication side effects, as well as the side effects and complications of renal replacement therapy. With regard to SCI, during the first month post-injury, adynamic ileus and gastric ulcerations are the most frequently reported GI complications, whereas in patients with chronic SCI, fecal impaction is the most frequent GI-related problem (117). Gastroesophageal reflux disease (GERD) is also commonly seen in SCI patients. This condition may be exacerbated by associated recumbency, immobilization, and irregular mealtime patterns. Furthermore, impaired gastric emptying (more common in patients with lesions above T1) may also exacerbate GERD and increase the risk for related complications such as gastritis, esophagitis, and GI bleeding (118). Additional factors that predispose to GI bleeding in this setting include stress ulcers, malnutrition, hypovolemic shock, and increased exposure to medications such as NSAIDs, corticosteroids, and anticoagulants (119, 120). Another common problem in SCI patients is intestinal obstruction that may occur during the initial post-injury period either because of adynamic ileus or pseudo-obstruction related to trauma, surgery, anesthesia, or severe medical illness (e.g., pneumonia or sepsis). Because of the loss of both autonomic nervous system stimulation and central control of the act of defecation, constipation with fecal impaction may be problematic in patients with chronic SCI. Moreover, the superimposition of renal failure can adversely affect the frequency,

severity, and nature of gastrointestinal complications in SCI patients. For example, some of the most common symptoms of uremia per se are gastrointestinal (e.g., anorexia, nausea, and vomiting), whereas stomatitis, gastritis, duodenitis, and colitis with associated GI bleeding are frequent complications of uncontrolled uremia. Characteristically, uremic-related GI manifestations should rapidly improve following the institution of dialysis. Therefore, the persistence of any symptoms or manifestations of GI disease in a patient receiving adequate dialysis therapy should prompt further evaluation to identify the cause of the persisting symptomatology.

A second concern involves the apparent increased risk for GI disease in "nonuremic" ESRD patients on maintenance dialysis, where a higher prevalence of gastritis, GERD, duodenitis, hiatal hernia, pancreatitis, and gallbladder disease is reported (121–124). Furthermore, GI disease related to beta-2-microglobulin amyloid infiltration has been reported in long-term chronic dialysis patients; our group observed a high incidence of gastrointestinal pathology in SCI-ESRD patients related to secondary amyloidosis, with involvement of both the liver and alimentary tract (21, 125).

Also reported in dialysis patients is an increased incidence of GI angiodysplasia, a condition that can cause life-threatening, difficult-to-manage recurrent episodes of GI bleeding (126, 127). Other conditions that increase the risk for GI bleeding in ESRD include esophagitis, gastritis, duodenitis, and colitis, as well as the occurrence of single discrete ulcerations, usually located in the cecum or ascending colon (122, 128, 129). In addition, the use of medications such as aspirin, NSAIDs, prednisone, and oral iron has been associated with upper GI bleeding in dialysis patients. Furthermore, underlying platelet dysfunction (commonly present in uncontrolled uremia) can reoccur as a consequence of inadequate dialysis, and should therefore be ruled out as a causal factor with regard to GI bleeding in ESRD patients. If present, qualitative platelet dysfunction (as evidenced by a prolonged IV bleeding time) should improve following the restoration of adequate dialysis therapy. When indicated, a more rapid improvement in platelet function (within one to two hours) can be accomplished with desmopressin (DDAVP) administration (0.3 µg/kg IV or SC); however, this effect is of short duration (lasting only six to eight hours) and repeat dosing may be ineffective (130). The intravenous administration of estrogen (0.6 mg/kg/day for five days) may also be effective in improving abnormal bleeding times (its onset of action is approximately six hours, whereas duration of effect is approximately 30 days) (131). Moreover, in patients who are at increased risk for bleeding, hemodialysis should be performed using a heparin-free protocol (132).

Of additional concern in able-bodied hemodialysis patients is the disproportionately high incidence of acute abdominal disease, including acute pancreatitis, diverticulitis, spontaneous colonic perforation, bowel infarction, and strangulated abdominal wall hernia (124, 133–135). Because SCI is also associated with increased risk for acute abdominal disease, it would be logical to assume that SCI-ESRD patients have at least a similar, if not greater risk for life-threatening acute abdominal disease. Moreover, because visceral sensation is generally impaired in SCI patients, many of the signs and symptoms that would normally facilitate an early diagnosis of acute abdominal disease are obscured. For example, after bowel perforation, abdominal discomfort may not be apparent until inflammation has reached the upper abdominal peritoneum, which receives innervation from high cervical cord segments. Because early diagnosis of life-threatening acute abdominal disease is often difficult in SCI patients, even vague or apparently mild symptomatology must be taken seriously.

Other GI-related problems reported to occur with increased frequency in chronic hemodialysis patients include constipation, ascites, liver disease, and rarely GI disease related to beta-2-microglobulin amyloid infiltration (121, 136–139). Constipation (already problematic in SCI patients) may be further aggravated with the development of ESRD as a result of factors such as the implementation of a "renal diet" and the related fluid restriction, or from the use of medications (e.g., calcium-containing phosphate binders, oral iron preparations, and calcium antagonists). To minimize constipation and prevent fecal impaction, patients should be maintained on a good bowel management program that ensures regular and complete evacuation. Meals should be given at regular times, the intake of high-fiber foods encouraged, physical activity should be encouraged, and fluid intake should be as liberal as possible, considering the severity of renal insufficiency and the related volume of urine output. The use of bulk-forming laxatives and stool softeners (emollient laxatives) is also helpful in establishing and regulating bowel programs, and the intermittent use of a stimulant laxative may be useful in moving stool that has impacted proximal to the rectum.

An idiopathic form of ascites is associated with renal failure and dialysis. However, in patients who develop ascites, underlying causes such as liver disease, abdominal malignancies, heart failure, and constrictive pericarditis should be ruled out, because hemodialysis-associated ascites is a diagnosis of exclusion (136). Although the pathogenesis of this condition is not fully understood, it is thought to result from a combination of chronic fluid-volume overload and increased capillary permeability. Support for this comes from the observation that most patients diagnosed with hemodialysis-associated ascites have a history of chronic volume overload and large interdialytic weight gains as a consequence of dietary indiscretion. Because anorexia, progressive malnutrition, and life-threatening cachexia often complicate this condition, aggressive management is warranted. This includes a combination of achieving strict patient compliance regarding dietary salt and fluid restriction and increasing fluid removal during dialysis with an aggressive regimen of ultrafiltration.

Liver disease in dialysis patients may result from infection with either hepatitis B (HBV) or C (HCV) virus (137–142). However, because of a combination of factors, including better serologic techniques used in screening blood products, reduced blood transfusion requirements in dialysis patients (related to the routine use of erythropoietin), and the implementation of vaccination programs, the incidence of HBV infection has progressively declined. Consequently, HCV has now emerged as the most common type of viral hepatitis in hemodialysis patients, having a reported prevalence rate (for anti-HCV positivity) ranging from 1% to 20% (138–140, 142, 143).

Dialysis patients are also at increased risk for drug-induced or toxic hepatitis, which can occur in association with a variety of different types of drug exposures, including allopurinol, methyldopa, fluoxymesterone, diazepam, ampicillin, indomethacin, and iron dextran (144, 145). In patients suspected of having drug-induced hepatitis, discontinuation of the offending agent is generally followed by improvement in liver function. Iron overload with hemosiderosis can occur in patients who have received large amounts of iron (usually in the form of parenterally administered iron or as a result of multiple blood transfusions). A presumptive diagnosis of hepatic siderosis can be made in patients exhibiting a combination of elevated transaminases (ALT and AST), high serum ferritin levels (>1000 µg/L), and a history compatible with iron overload. Treatment should include the elimination of any exogenous source of iron as well as mobilization of iron from tissue stores. The latter can be accomplished with the administration of erythropoietin, wherein the resulting increase in red blood cell formation and iron utilization facilitates the mobilization of iron from tissue stores. In severe cases, where serum ferritin levels exceed 2000 µg/L, the combination of phlebotomy and erythropoietin administration is shown to be both safe and efficacious in the management of hepatic siderosis (144).

Another consideration is that GI symptomatology may be caused by or related to some aspect of the dialysis procedure per se (i.e., cytokine release, an electrolyte imbalance, or possibly a dialysate contaminant). Moreover, the development of GI symptomatology during dialysis may be indicative of a potentially serious dialysis-related complication. For example, the occurrence of nausea or vomiting during hemodialysis is usually an early manifestation of volume depletion (related to excessive ultrafiltration). Consequently, these symptoms often herald the onset of hypotension and are also frequently accompanied by weakness, light-headedness, and muscle cramps (146). On the other hand, nausea and vomiting occurring toward the end of a dialysis treatment, or shortly thereafter, may be an early manifestation of the dialysis disequilibrium syndrome (DDS) (147–150). However, this syndrome primarily occurs in severely azotemic patients following the initiation of a hemodialysis regimen that is overly efficient with regard to the rate and magnitude of solute removal. DDS is characterized by a constellation of signs and symptoms ranging from nausea, vomiting, agitation, and headache in mild cases to stupor, seizures, and coma in severe cases. Although most cases of DDS occur within the first 6 months of hemodialysis therapy, this syndrome can occur virtually any time in association with a highly efficient dialysis, especially in patients who have been previously underdialyzed; for example, when a long-duration, high-efficiency hemodialysis treatment is performed as compensation for one or more missed treatments. In addition, DDS is more likely to occur in pediatric and elderly dialysis patients as well as in patients undergoing twice-weekly dialysis as opposed to three-times-a-week dialysis. Although its pathogenesis remains controversial, DDS is thought to result from a rapid increase in brain cell water, which causes brain edema. This pathophysiologic shift in water content from the extracellular fluid into the cells is caused by a transient reduction in extracellular fluid osmolality of sufficient magnitude to allow the rapid movement of water into cells along an osmolar gradient. Apparently, the combination of an underlying uremic-related increase in brain osmolality, caused by an increase in idiogenic osmoles, and a dialysis-related rapid reduction in plasma solute content, caused by the removal of urea and other readily dialyzable solutes, results in the development of a transient, but substantial, osmolar gradient between the brain and the extracellular fluid compartment. Because the increased brain osmolality is related to an increase in idiogenic osmoles and not to urea per se, the rapid reduction in plasma urea (with high-efficiency dialysis) disproportionately lowers plasma and extracellular fluid osmolality despite the fact that urea freely crosses cell membranes and is cleared from both brain and plasma at essentially the same rate. DDS can be avoided by prescribing an initial series of low-efficiency dialysis treatments. When initiating hemodialysis, the following is recommended:

- Avoid exceeding a 30% reduction in BUN during the initial two-dialysis treatments. This can be accomplished by using a small surface area dialyzer, maintaining a relatively low blood flow rate (not to exceed 250 ml/min), and limiting the duration of dialysis to 2 hours.
- Use dialysate with a sodium concentration approximately equal to the patient's serum sodium concentration and containing at least 200 ml/dL of glucose. It is noteworthy that DDS has not been described with peritoneal dialysis (PD). This is probably a function of the relative inefficiency of PD in clearing small-molecular weight solutes.

Nutritional Disorders

Many patients with ESRD have evidence of protein-energy malnutrition as defined by various biochemical and anthropometric parameters (151–153). Moreover, both the prevalence and severity of malnutrition appear to be even greater in SCI patients with chronic renal failure. This was demonstrated in a study involving dialysis patients with and without spinal cord injury. The SCI group exhibited a higher incidence of suboptimal dry body weight along with reduced values (regarding measurements of mid-arm muscle circumference, triceps skin fold thickness, serum albumin concentration, serum transferrin level, and total lymphocyte counts) when compared with the group of able-bodied dialysis patients (154). A variety of factors are thought to be operative in the genesis of protein–energy malnutrition in this population, including chronic infection, amyloidosis, depression, anorexia, and prescribed or self-imposed protein restriction. In addition, factors related to the dialysis procedure per se may adversely affect nutrition. These include the release of proinflammatory cytokines, an increased catabolic effect, and the loss of nutrients that can occur in association with either hemodialysis or peritoneal dialysis (substantial losses of protein can also occur with peritoneal dialysis). In turn, malnutrition has been shown to be an important risk factor for increased morbidity and mortality in ESRD patients (86). Consequently, every effort should be made to maintain a good state of nutrition in SCI patients.

Management

The management of SCI patients with chronic renal disease should begin with the identification and correction of any potentially reversible components of renal insufficiency, such as urinary obstruction (functional or mechanical), active infection, renal hypoperfusion, and/or severe hypertension. In CRF patients with significant residual renal function (i.e., glomerular filtration rates greater than 10 ml/min.), every effort should be made to delay further progression of renal disease. This can be achieved by maintaining satisfactory urinary flow, along with effective treatment of urolithiasis and control of infection (e.g., urinary tract, pressure wounds, and osteomyelitis). Additional renal protective measures include the maintenance of normal blood pressure and the avoidance of nephrotoxin exposure. Furthermore, the administration of an angiotensin-converting enzyme inhibitor (ACE-I) or angiotensin-II receptor blocking drug (ARB) may be beneficial in reducing the rate of progression of renal failure in selected patients (e.g., those with hypertension and/or proteinuria, with mild to moderate renal insufficiency). These agents can prevent the development of glomerular capillary hypertension and hyperfiltration, which is a maladaptive process shown to accelerate the progression of nephron loss in patients with underlying renal disease (155, 156). Mild protein restriction (approximately 0.8 g/kg/day with high biologic value protein) has also been shown to reduce glomerular capillary pressure and slow the rate of progression of renal disease (157). Although both of the aforementioned treatments effectuate renal protection by the same putative mechanism (a reduction in glomerular capillary pressure), this is accomplished via different actions on the glomerular microcirculation. In the case of ACE-Is and ARBs, the reduction in glomerular capillary pressure is the result of efferent arteriolar dilatation, caused by inhibition of angiotensin II-mediated vasoconstriction. In protein restriction, however, glomerular capillary pressure reduction is caused by afferent arteriolar vasoconstriction, apparently related to the inhibition of vasodilatory prostaglandins (158, 159).

As previously noted, SCI patients with renal insufficiency often exhibit an inability to conserve sodium and water. Consequently, they are at increased risk for dehydration and volume depletion, which can occur as the result of increased gastrointestinal fluid losses, increased insensible losses, or enhanced renal losses. Conversely, other SCI patients, particularly those with more advanced renal insufficiency, also develop an inability to normally excrete sodium and volume, which accordingly places them at risk for volume overload and related complications (e.g., hypertension and pulmonary edema). Therefore, close attention should be given to the fluid-volume and electrolyte status in SCI patients with renal insufficiency, especially in the event of an intervening illness. Moreover, when glomerular filtration falls irreversibly (below 8 to 10 ml/min.), renal replacement therapy should be instituted with hemodialysis, peritoneal dialysis, or possibly renal transplantation. Published data regarding the use of dialysis in SCI patients are still very limited, whereas information concerning renal transplantation in this setting is practically nonexistent.

Hemodialysis

With the development and implementation of dialysis, the mortality associated with acute renal failure has been reduced, and death as a direct consequence of ESRD has been virtually eliminated. Moreover, the noted beneficial effects of dialysis (reported in able-bodied ESRD patients) are for the most part achievable in SCI-ESRD patients. However, because of the increased prevalence of pneumonia, pulmonary embolism, nonischemic heart disease, septicemia, amyloidosis, and malnutrition, the mortality rate in SCI patients on maintenance dialysis is expectedly higher than that observed in able-bodied patients (160–162).

As in all extracorporeal systems, hemodialysis requires the establishment of an adequate vascular access: selection of the specific type and anatomical location of the access is generally determined both by the patient's needs as well as by practicality.

For example, a short-term or temporary access is appropriate for use in the treatment of potentially reversible acute renal failure or for temporary use in an ESRD patient who has a failed permanent access. A number of double-lumen catheters are currently available for use in either the femoral, subclavian, or jugular vein; however, the internal jugular vein is the preferred site for catheter placement. This is because subclavian catheters are associated with an increased risk for subclavian vein stenosis, whereas femoral catheters both restrict lower extremity movement and have a high infection rate when left in place for more than 2 days (163–165). Additional complications shared by all transcutaneous catheters include hemorrhage, thrombosis, and infection. Furthermore, hemothorax or pneumothorax can immediately complicate placement of internal jugular and subclavian vein catheters; therefore, a post-procedure chest radiograph must be obtained (163, 166).

A long-term or permanent blood access should be placed in patients requiring chronic hemodialysis. Currently, the most commonly used permanent vascular accesses are the arteriovenous (AV) fistula and the arteriovenous (AV) graft (163, 166, 167). These devices are subcutaneous and may be created or placed in either an upper or lower extremity. The preferred site for an AV fistula is the distal (nondominant) forearm, where the anastomosis is usually created between the radial artery and cephalic vein; however, if this is not feasible, upper arm vessels can be used (e.g., an elbow brachiocephalic anastomosis). If it is not possible to create an AV fistula, an adequate blood access can almost always be established with either an AV graft or a transposed brachial-basilic vein fistula (163, 167). The most widely used AV grafts are composed of synthetic material (polytetrafluoroethylene [PTFE]). The currently recommended sites and types of AV grafts in order of preference are (a) a forearm curved looped brachial cephalic graft, (b) an upper arm straight graft, (c) a forearm straight radial cephalic graft, and (d) a looped thigh graft (163, 166, 168). A final option (for vascular access) is the placement of a subcutaneously tunneled, cuffed central venous catheter. The use of this type of catheter should be reserved for patients who are unsuitable for peritoneal dialysis, and where either the lack of adequate blood vessels or the presence of complications, such as distal limb ischemia, precludes the use of an AV vascular access.

Important complications of vascular access devices include infection with or without sepsis, access stenosis or thrombosis, formation of an aneurism or pseudoaneurysm, access rupture with hemorrhage, and limb ischemia distal to the access (163, 166, 169, 170). Overall, the preferred type of vascular access is the AV fistula, which has proven to be the safest and longest lasting type of permanent access. AV fistulas, however, must be created at least 4 to 6 weeks (preferably 2 to 3 months) before they are suitable for use in hemodialysis. Furthermore, the size and condition of the patient's peripheral blood vessels can limit their application. Although AV (PTFE) grafts have certain advantages (e.g., the variety of potential placement sites, the ability to bridge distant vessels, and an excellent capacity for high blood-flow rates) they are overall less desirable than AV fistulas because of a higher incidence of complications, particularly infection, stenosis, and thrombosis (mainly attributable to the foreign nature of the AV conduit) (163, 166). The subcutaneously tunneled, cuffed central venous catheter, however, is the type of access most frequently complicated by infection;

the relative risk of bacteremia is reported to be 7.6%, compared with AV fistulae (171).

Dialysis centers should have in place a team of trained personnel, including a nephrologist, vascular surgeon, and interventional radiologist, as well as nurses and technicians who are responsible for the planning, placement, and maintenance of vascular accesses and who are experienced in managing the related complications. When a patient is initially diagnosed with chronic renal failure, every effort should be made to protect the cephalic veins, especially in the nondominant arm. This vein should not be subjected to venipuncture or the placement of an indwelling catheter; however, veins in the dorsum of the hand may be used for this purpose.

Hemodialysis Treatment in Spinal Cord Injury

Although limited, the clinical experience would indicate that standard dialysis procedures are generally well tolerated in SCI patients (160, 162, 172,173). However, one potentially problematic area regarding hemodialysis in SCI patients involves the type of buffer used (the two buffers currently in use are bicarbonate and acetate). Acetate, which is a congener of bicarbonate, is metabolized to bicarbonate primarily by skeletal muscle. Consequently, patients with reduced muscle mass (i.e., SCI patients) are more susceptible to acetate accumulation and toxicity (174). The adverse effects of acetate accumulation include arterial hypoxemia (related to associated hypocapnia and hypoventilation), peripheral vasodilation, decreased myocardial contractility, metabolic acidosis, vasomotor instability, nausea, vomiting, headache, and fatigue. Therefore, in view of the increased potential for acetate accumulation in patients with reduced muscle mass, bicarbonate buffered dialysate should be preferentially used in SCI patients (175). Fortunately, the vast majority of dialysis facilities currently utilize or have the capability of utilizing bicarbonate buffered dialysate.

A second problematic area concerns the relative biocompatibility of the artificial membrane used in hemodialysis. Of the four membrane types currently in use (cellulose, substituted cellulose, cellulose synthetic, and synthetic) the least biocompatible is cellulose (148). Artificial membranes made from unsubstituted cellulose on contact with blood can both activate the complement system and stimulate the activation of phagocytic cells. This, in turn, can result in numerous adverse effects including the activation of proinflammatory cytokines, the generation of reactive oxygen species, cell lysis, hypoxemia, and tissue injury (176–178). In contrast, dialyzers utilizing membranes made from substituted cellulose (e.g., cellulose acetate) or synthetics (e.g., polyacrylonitrile, polysulfone, polycarbonate, and polyamine) are associated with considerably less complement activation. Furthermore, in experimental animal models of ARF, an inverse relationship between the rate of recovery from ARF and the complement-activating potential of the dialysis membrane has been recently demonstrated (179, 180). Furthermore, studies in humans with ARF have demonstrated both a reduction in mortality as well as an increased rate in the recovery of renal function when dialysis was performed using synthetic biocompatible membranes compared with dialysis using nonbiocompatible membranes (181, 182). Therefore, in the management of ARF, compelling data support the preferential use of biocompatible dialyzers. Data in chronic hemodialysis patients also indicate that the use of nonbiocompatible dialyzers may adversely affect patients by increasing lipid peroxidation and the generation of reactive oxygen species (176–178). In addition, the use of non-biocompatible membranes has been shown to cause or aggravate hypoxemia in patients undergoing hemodialysis (148, 169). One of the proposed mechanisms for this involves increased leukocyte sequestration in pulmonary capillaries, producing "leukocyte microthrombic," which is thought to be mediated via enhanced expression of leukocyte adhesion molecules. However, it should be noted that dialysis-associated hypoxemia appears to be multifactorial, involving a number of mechanisms that include

- Hypocapnia-induced compensatory alveolar hypoventilation (observed with acetate-buffered dialysate), as a consequence of intradialytic losses of CO_2
- Compensatory hypoventilation caused by alkalemia (observed with bicarbonate-buffered dialysate), when high concentrations of bicarbonate (>35 mEq/L) are used
- Histamine-mediated abnormalities that affect ventilation and perfusion (resulting from complement-induced mast cell degranulation) (148, 169)

Peritoneal Dialysis

Before the advent of indwelling peritoneal catheters, peritoneal dialysis was used only as a temporary modality in the treatment of acute renal failure. However, during the past two decades peritoneal dialysis has emerged as one of the major therapeutic modalities for the treatment of ESRD (167, 183). Furthermore, several variations of peritoneal dialysis are now available for use in the management of renal failure. These include intermittent peritoneal dialysis (IPD), continuous cycler-assisted peritoneal dialysis (CCPD), and continuous ambulatory peritoneal dialysis (CAPD). Because IPD is usually performed at night while the patient is asleep (via an automated delivery system) it is often referred to as nocturnal intermittent peritoneal dialysis (NIPD). CCPD is identical to NIPD except that in the former, the patient performs at least one additional long-dwell daytime exchange. With CAPD, usually four intermediate-dwell exchanges (approximately six hours per exchange) are performed daily, on a continuous basis.

Although each of these modalities (CAPD, CCPD, NIPD) has been proved to be effective as renal replacement therapy in able-bodied patients, published data regarding the practicality and efficacy of peritoneal dialysis in SCI-ESRD patients are very limited. It has been our experience, however, that long-term IPD is as effective as hemodialysis in SCI patients in regard to controlling azotemia, volume, serum electrolytes, and acid–base balance (173). Moreover, a study of SCI patients treated with IPD exhibited greater hemodynamic stability compared to those receiving hemodialysis; however, serum albumin levels were substantially lower in IPD-treated patients because of losses from the peritoneal cavity (173). This recognized complication of peritoneal dialysis might compound the problem of protein–energy malnutrition that is frequently present in SCI-ESRD patients. In our experience, the incidence of peritonitis is not increased in SCI-ESRD patients, compared to able-bodied ESRD patients. However, in patients who develop peritonitis, the infecting organism is often concomitantly present in

the urine and/or a decubitus ulcer, indicative of cross-contamination.

With improvements in peritoneal catheter design, method of placement, and maintenance, as well as the implementation of more effective aseptic procedures and improved catheter connection technology, the overall incidence of peritonitis has markedly decreased in patients treated with peritoneal dialysis (183). It is, therefore, our opinion that CAPD, CCPD, or NIPD can provide a viable alternative form of renal replacement therapy in selected SCI-ESRD patients. However, there are a number of important issues that require careful consideration regarding the use of peritoneal dialysis in SCI-ESRD patients.

- Because protein loss (associated with peritoneal dialysis) may compound pre-existing protein–calorie malnutrition, the patient's nutritional status should be carefully evaluated and frequently monitored. Furthermore, in our opinion, preexisting hypoalbuminemia should be considered a relative contraindication to peritoneal dialysis (184).
- The observation that the bacteria infecting or colonizing pressure sores or the urinary tract are likely to contaminate the peritoneal cavity via the PD catheter underscores the importance of meticulous observance of aseptic technique during catheter disconnect–reconnect procedures (e.g., necessitated by dialysate bag exchanges or during hook up with an automated system). In our opinion, the presence of infected pressure sores is another relative contraindication to peritoneal dialysis.
- A further consideration involves the increased frequency of respiratory diseases, which are currently the leading cause of mortality in patients with SCI (10, 11). We have also observed a high incidence of acute and chronic pulmonary disorders in SCI patients with advanced renal disease (116). Consequently, there is understandable concern that instillation of large volumes of fluid into the peritoneal cavity may further compromise both respiratory function and the resistance to pulmonary infection. In such circumstances, the use of multiple small-volume exchanges (approximately 1 liter) with shorter dwell times (1 to 2 hours), which can be easily accomplished with a programmable automated cycler, may substantially diminish the risk for pulmonary compromise. However, the use of hemodialysis (with biocompatible dialyzers) may be more appropriate in pulmonary-compromised patients.
- High concentrations of glucose are required to provide the osmotic force for ultrafiltration in peritoneal dialysis. Consequently, the absorption of glucose from the peritoneal cavity can cause hyperglycemia during the procedure and can also occasionally result in delayed reactive hypoglycemia. This issue is of further concern in view of the reported high incidence of glucose intolerance among spinal cord injured patients (185).
- Abdominal muscle weakness, impaired intestinal motility, and related constipation, which are often present in SCI patients, can occasionally interfere with peritoneal dialysis efficiency (particularly dialysate drainage). In turn, incomplete drainage of dialysate from the peritoneal cavity can cause abdominal distention and bloating, and can also result in suboptimal solute and water clearances. Therefore, patients undergoing peritoneal dialysis require proper bowel

care as well as appropriate positional changes to optimize dialysate drainage.

Dietary Considerations

The primary objective of dietary regimens in SCI patients receiving dialysis is to provide adequate nutrition while preventing fluid overload, hypertension, hyperkalemia, and hyperphosphatemia. Protein–energy malnutrition is a common complication of CRF, and in turn, a poor nutritional state predisposes ESRD patients to impaired wound healing, increased susceptibility to infection, difficulties with rehabilitation, and increased mortality (86, 151, 154). The cause of malnutrition in CRF is often multifactorial, involving medical, psychosocial, economic, and possibly cultural factors (186).

The nutritional status of patients on maintenance dialysis can be assessed routinely by a combination of valid, complementary measures. These measures provide clinically useful characterization of the protein–energy nutritional status of these patients (187).

Anorexia, which is commonly present in patients with CRF, may be a manifestation of uremia per se, or caused by other factors associated with ESRD (e.g., an intercurrent illness, infection, depression, medications, dialysis, or an altered sensation of taste) (151, 152, 186). Anorexia, nausea, and vomiting are well-known complications of uremia that should resolve with adequate dialysis. However, in certain patients, the dialysis procedure itself may cause or contribute to anorexia. With peritoneal dialysis, abdominal distention related to the instillation of dialysate can cause sensations of fullness and satiety, with resulting anorexia (183, 186). Side effects of hemodialysis such as nausea, vomiting, fatigue, and malaise can also contribute to malnutrition (169, 186). These symptoms may be related to excessive ultrafiltration or to dialysis-associated cytokine release. Limiting interdialytic weight gain to approximately 1 liter (by strict adherence to dietary salt and fluid restriction) obviates the necessity for large-volume or excessive ultrafiltration with dialysis. For example, in anuric patients, recommended sodium and water restriction is 2 grams and 1 liter per day, respectively. If the patient is being dialyzed with a poorly biocompatible cellulosic membrane dialyzer, changing to a more biocompatible dialyzer may also improve symptoms such as nausea and anorexia. Some losses of nutrients invariably occur during dialysis, including water-soluble vitamins, amino acids, and intact proteins. Using peritoneal dialysis, protein losses average 9 grams/day. Protein losses during hemodialysis are negligible, however; polypeptide and amino acid losses can average 10 to 13 grams per treatment (183, 186). Ghrelin is a recently discovered orexigenic hormone that stimulates food intake and energy metabolism. The hormone has been analyzed in individuals undergoing dialysis, and thus may play a role in anorexia seen in these patients. Further studies are ongoing to determine appropriateness of therapy using this gastric hormone (189).

In the management of malnutrition, it is important to recognize and treat comorbid conditions (e.g., chronic infection or depression) that are often present in this setting. Gastroparesis,

Table 28.2   Recommended Measures for Monitoring Nutritional Status of Maintenance Dialysis Patients (188)

CATEGORY	MEASURE	MINIMUM FREQUENCY OF MEASUREMENT
I. Measurements that should be performed routinely in all patients	1. Predialysis or stabilized serum albumin	Monthly
	2. Percent of usual postdialysis (MHD) or post-drain (CPD) body weight	Monthly
	3. Percent of standard (NHANES II) body weight	Every four months
	4. Subjective global assessment	Every six months
	5. Dietary interview and/or diary	Every six months
	6. nPNA	Monthly for MHD; every three to four months for CPD
II. Measures that can be useful to confirm or extend the data obtained from the measures in Category I	1. Predialysis or stabilized serum pre-albumin	As needed
	2. Skinfold thickness	As needed
	3. Mid-arm muscle area, circumference, or diameter	As needed
	4. Dual-energy X-ray absorptiometry	As needed
III. Clinically useful measures, which, if low, might suggest the need for a more rigorous examination of protein-energy nutritional status	Predialysis or stabilized serum • Creatinine • Urea nitrogen • Cholesterol	As needed
	Creatinine index	As needed

Source: From the National Kidney Foundation Chronic Kidney Disease 2006: A Guide to Select NKF-KDOQI Guidelines and Recommendations.
Abbreviations: CPD = chronic peritoneal dialysis; MHD = maintenance HD; nPNA = protein equivalent of total nitrogen appearance normalized to body weight; NHANES = National Health and Nutrition Evaluation Survey.

which is often related to ANS dysfunction in SCI patients, usually responds to metoclopramide (administered 15 to 30 minutes prior to meals and at bedtime). The altered sensation of taste in ESRD patients has been attributed to zinc deficiency; consequently, this condition may improve with oral zinc supplementation (20 mg/day) (190–192). Medications most likely to cause anorexia, nausea, and dyspepsia in dialysis patients are the aluminum- or calcium-containing phosphate binders and the oral iron preparations. The substitution of Renagel® as a phosphate binder or the use of an intravenous iron dextran preparation in place of oral iron are effective in minimizing these side effects.

It is also important to recognize that ESRD is associated with numerous hormonal and metabolic disturbances, including insulin resistance, decreased biologic effects of insulin-like growth factors, increased plasma levels of catabolic hormones (e.g., cortisol and glucagon), a high prevalence of secondary hyperparathyroidism, defective erythropoietin production, chronic metabolic acidosis, and abnormal carbohydrate, fat, and protein metabolism. Individually or in combination, these abnormalities are no doubt responsible for a wide variety of uremic manifestations. In aggregate, they also adversely affect nutritional status by inducing a state of hypercatabolism (152, 169, 186). Moreover, therapeutic modalities that ameliorate uremic-induced hormonal and metabolic dysfunction also improve nutritional status in ESRD patients. These include adequate dialysis therapy, effective treatment of anemia (using erythropoietin), correction of metabolic acidosis, and effective control of hyperparathyroidism (186, 193, 194). Furthermore, there is evidence that the administration of recombinant human growth hormone and the use of intradialytic parenteral nutrition can increase protein anabolism and improve overall nutritional status in malnourished dialysis patients (195, 196).

Dietary recommendations for stable chronic dialysis patients include the following:

- Protein intake should be approximately 1.2 g/kg/day, with at least 50% being of high biologic value.
- Because dialysis patients have impaired cell energy metabolism, caloric intake for sedentary, nonobese patients should be approximately 35 kcal/kg/day, with carbohydrate providing 40% to 50% of the total calories. Higher caloric intakes are required in patients who are underweight, in patients who routinely engage in strenuous activity, and in hypercatabolic patients (i.e., related to trauma, surgery, or infection).
- Protein and caloric intake should be based not on the patient's actual body weight, but instead on the average body weight for healthy subjects of the same age, sex, height, and body frame as that of the patient.
- Sodium and water restriction (in anuric patients on hemodialysis) should be 1–2 g/day (40–80 mEq/day) and 1 liter/day, respectively. Compliance with sodium restriction is necessary to control excessive thirst, hypervolemia, and hypertension. In anuric patients receiving peritoneal dialysis, sodium and water intake can usually be liberalized to 3–4 g/day (130–170 mEq/day) and 2–2.5 liters/day, respectively.
- Hyperkalemia is a common and potentially life-threatening problem in ESRD patients. Therefore, in most patients, dietary potassium intake should not exceed 2–3 g/day (50–75 mEq/day). However, in patients with significant

residual renal function, only mild potassium restriction may be necessary.
- Because of the presence of renal failure–related vitamin D deficiency, dietary calcium requirements in CRF patients generally exceed the recommended 1 g/day for healthy nonuremic adults. To help achieve positive calcium balance, a higher dialysate calcium concentration (3.5 mEq/L) or calcitriol (vitamin D) supplementation may be required in some patients. However, it should be noted that the majority of ESRD patients receive moderate to large quantities of calcium carbonate or calcium acetate as phosphate binders, and consequently, hypercalcemia may be problematic (197, 198).
- In ESRD, dietary phosphate should be restricted to 0.8 g/day to reduce the risk for hyperphosphatemia, which plays a major role in the associated disturbances in calcium and bone metabolism. For example, hyperphosphatemia inhibits the 1-hydroxylation of vitamin D (exacerbating 1,25 dihydroxy vitamin D deficiency). Hyperphosphatemia also stimulates parathyroid hormone (PTH) secretion, which often leads to the development of secondary hyperparathyroidism. Furthermore, a reduction in serum ionized calcium, usually resulting from a combination of hyperphosphatemia and vitamin D deficiency, is an additional stimulus for PTH secretion. Hyperphosphatemia is also commonly associated with metastatic soft tissue calcifications, which is usually seen in patients with high Ca X P products (i.e., >60–70 mg²/dL²). Moreover, mortality rates are shown to be higher in ESRD patients (when Ca X P products exceed 72 mg²/dL², or serum phosphate levels are >6.6 mg/dL) (181). The control of serum phosphate, to levels of 6.5 mg/dL or lower but ideally in the range of 4.5–5.5 mg/dL, usually requires a combination of dietary phosphate restriction (approximately 800 mg/day), adequate dialysis therapy, and the administration of phosphate binders with meals (e.g., calcium acetate, calcium carbonate, and/or Renagel®). In addition, calcimimetic agents (e.g., Cinacalcet hydrochloride) have been used for secondary hyperparathyroidism of renal failure. The mechanism of action involves binding to calcium receptors in the parathyroid gland to increase their affinity for extracellular calcium, leading to a reduction in PTH secretion. Use of this agent at doses of 30–50 mg twice a day has been shown to decrease serum PTH levels to <250 pg/mL in 41% of patients on dialysis (199).
- Dialysis patients are also at greater risk for developing deficiencies involving water-soluble vitamins and certain minerals, which may occur as a consequence of reduced dietary intake, diminished absorption, altered metabolism, or from losses related to dialysis per se. Therefore, the following daily vitamin/mineral prescription is recommended: folic acid (1 mg), pyridoxine (20 mg), thiamin (30 mg), and zinc (20 mg), plus the usual daily allowance of other B vitamins (186, 200). Although plasma levels of selenium are reported to be low in dialysis patients, the effects or possible benefits of administering this important antioxidant have not been studied in this setting (201–203). Likewise, the potentially beneficial effects of vitamin E have not been studied in dialysis patients; however, there are preliminary data indicating that vitamin E may ameliorate the oxidative damage associated with both lipid peroxidation and iron therapy

(104). As previously discussed, the administration of vitamin C should be limited to 150 mg/day because higher doses can cause hyperoxalemia (186). Finally, the administration of vitamin A should be avoided, as serum vitamin A levels are generally already elevated in CRF because of the combination of decreased renal catabolism and increased serum levels of retinal A binding protein (186).

Medication and Pharmacologic Considerations

In addition to vitamins, trace elements, and phosphate binders, the majority of ESRD patients also require medication for the management of anemia and hypertension. The recommended range of 33% to 36% for target hematocrits can be achieved with the use of erythropoietin, which is generally administered intravenously (thrice weekly) with hemodialysis or subcutaneously administered (twice weekly) in peritoneal dialysis patients (111, 113, 204, 205). However, for erythropoietin to be effective, folate, vitamin B_{12}, and iron stores must be replete. Low serum levels of iron and ferritin and/or a low transferrin saturation value (<20%) are indicative of iron deficiency. Iron-deficient patients should be evaluated for blood loss, including occult losses from the GI tract. However, it should be recognized that hemodialysis patients have an increased risk for iron-deficiency anemia because of unavoidable losses of small quantities of blood with dialysis (retained in the extracorporeal circulation). In addition to iron deficiency and chronic blood loss, other causes of erythropoietin-resistant anemia include hemolysis, aluminum intoxication, underlying infection or inflammation, secondary hyperparathyroidism, and bone marrow disease.

In the treatment of iron-deficiency anemia, oral iron preparations (e.g., ferrous sulfate, ferrous fumarate, or ferrous sulfate) may be used in doses providing 100 to 200 mg daily of elemental iron. In patients intolerant or refractory to oral iron, intravenous preparations (e.g., iron dextran, ferric gluconate, or ferric hydroxysaccharate) may be used. Intravenous iron administration is generally required for correction of anemia in hemodialysis patients (caused by the associated increased iron losses), whereas with peritoneal dialysis, oral iron therapy is usually effective in correcting anemia (111). Currently there are three preparations of intravenous iron—iron dextran (INFeD® or Dexferrum®, can be given intramuscularly), iron gluconate (Ferrlecit®), and iron sucrose (Venofer®). In iron-deficient patients, a total dose of approximately 1,000 mg of intravenous iron will usually replete iron stores. When using iron dextran in hemodialysis patients, it is our preference to administer this in 100-mg infusions (diluted in 50 ml of normal saline), which is given incrementally over 10 consecutive dialysis treatments. When using iron gluconate, we follow the protocol recommended by Nissenson et al., wherein 125 mg of iron gluconate, diluted in 200 ml of normal saline, is infused over two hours during eight consecutive hemodialysis treatments (206). In the United States Iron Sucrose (Venofer®) Clinical Trials Group, iron sucrose was given in two dosing regimens: 100 mg of iron sucrose is given over 10 consecutive dialysis sessions in iron deficient patients; iron replete patients were given 100 mg of iron sucrose weekly for 10 weeks (maintenance regimen) (207).

When peritoneal dialysis patients require parenteral iron therapy for practical reasons, we administer larger individual doses of iron dextran (i.e., 250–500 mg diluted in 250–500 ml of normal saline infused over 30–60 minutes); consequently, 1,000 mg of iron can be given in two to four sessions. Because of the risk for anaphylactic reactions (occurring in approximately 0.7% of patients treated with iron dextran) a test dose of 0.5 ml of iron dextran (25 mg/ml) is recommended (208). Delayed milder reactions with fever, myalgia, and lymphadenopathy have also been reported in association with iron dextran administration. Furthermore, these reactions are more common when individual doses exceed 250 mg (208). The therapeutic efficacy of iron therapy can be evaluated by the hemoglobin/hematocrit response that usually occurs within 3 to 4 weeks, whereas the serum iron, ferritin, and transferrin saturation percentage are useful in monitoring iron stores. However, a period of approximately 3 to 4 weeks is also required (post–iron therapy) for these tests to accurately reflect iron stores.

Hypertension in patients with ESRD often has a volume-related component, which may respond to a combination of dietary sodium restriction and fluid removal with dialysis. However, many ESRD patients with hypertension also require medication for blood pressure control, and most antihypertensive agents can be safely and effectively used in the management of hypertension in SCI-ESRD patients. These include calcium channel antagonists, angiotensin-converting enzyme inhibitors (ACE-Is), angiotensin II receptor blockers (ARBs), alpha-blockers, beta-blockers, central sympatholytics, and vasodilators (209–212). Diuretics, however, are generally ineffective in patients with ESRD, although large doses of loop diuretics (e.g., furosemide) have been used with some success in the management of hypertension and volume overload in selected ESRD patients (i.e., those with a GFR > 5–10 ml/min).

SCI patients with advanced renal disease are usually exposed to a wide variety of medications. However, because of the pathophysiologic effects of both SCI and renal insufficiency, the bioavailability, distribution, and metabolism of pharmacologic agents are often altered. For example, drug bioavailability can be affected by the alterations in GI motility and absorption commonly present in SCI-ESRD patients. Furthermore, increased gastric alkalinization in uremic patients (resulting from the action of gastric urease on urea) may reduce the bioavailability of agents dependent on acid hydrolysis for absorption (213). Uremia is also associated with alterations in first-pass hepatic metabolism that can have opposing effects on drug bioavailability (214). For example, uremic-associated inhibition of hepatic biotransformation could function to increase drug bioavailability, whereas uremic-associated reduction in protein binding could decrease drug bioavailability by increasing the availability of unbound drug for hepatic metabolism.

The apparent volume of drug distribution (a mathematical construct useful in estimating the drug dose necessary to achieve therapeutic plasma levels) is also affected in SCI-ESRD patients (214, 215). For example, drugs that are water soluble or highly protein bound tend to be restricted to the extracellular fluid compartment, and consequently have relatively small volumes of distribution. In contrast, lipid-soluble drugs that can readily enter cells and tissue have comparatively large volumes of distribution. Therefore, conditions that result in decreased drug–protein binding (e.g., uremia and hypoproteinemia) cause the apparent volume of distribution of protein-bound drugs to increase. The relationship between the apparent volume of distribution of a drug and its degree of binding is demonstrated by the following:

$$Vd = VB + VT\,(FB/FT)$$

where Vd is the apparent volume distribution, VB and VT are the actual volumes of blood and water in tissues, respectively, and FB and FT are the fractions of free drug in blood and tissue, respectively. In addition, the presence of edema or ascites increases the Vd of water-soluble and protein-bound drugs, whereas muscle wasting (which is highly prevalent in SCI-ESRD) decreases Vd (215, 216). Because Vd, after completion of drug absorption, is equal to the fractional absorption of the dose (fxD) divided by the plasma concentration (c) of the drug, Vd can also be calculated using the following:

$$Vd = \frac{fxD}{c}$$

The most important consideration, however, is that the metabolism and excretion of a wide variety of drugs are profoundly affected by renal insufficiency per se. Although certain drugs are excreted in the urine essentially unaltered, most drugs undergo biotransformation prior to their excretion. Hepatic biotransformation, in turn, involves a number of reactions, including oxidation, reduction, and hydrolysis, as well as synthetic processes (i.e., conjugation and acetylation) by which the parent drug or agent is transformed into various metabolites. In the presence of renal failure, the reaction rates for both hydrolysis and reduction are reduced, whereas the oxidation rate of various drugs is accelerated (215, 216). Thus, in addition to its profound influence on drug excretion, renal insufficiency can affect drug metabolism via alterations in hepatic biotransformation.

Of further consideration is that total body clearance or elimination of a drug is determined by the summation clearance of all involved organ systems (i.e., renal, hepatic, pulmonary, and others). Also, for convenience and practicality, most drug assays are obtained from plasma, and accordingly, reflect the plasma concentration of the respective drug rather than total body concentration. Therefore, both the terminology and the concept of plasma drug clearance should be used in place of total body drug clearance; nevertheless, both terms are frequently used interchangeably. The concept of plasma clearance (Clp) is described by the following expression:

$$Clp = Clr + Clnr$$

where Clr and $Clnr$ represent renal and nonrenal clearances, respectively.

The renal clearance of a drug is determined not only by its rate of glomerular filtration but also by the net effect of tubular modulation (i.e., tubular secretion and/or reabsorption of the drug). In general, the kidneys do not readily clear drugs that have a large volume of distribution or are extensively bound in tissue. Likewise, drugs that are highly protein bound are not cleared very well by glomerular filtration because of their poor filterability; however, their renal excretion may be substantially increased by proximal tubular secretion. Obviously, with progressive renal failure, the capacity for filtration and tubular secretion is lost. Furthermore, because the plasma clearance of such a

wide variety of pharmaceutic agents is affected by renal failure, the physician must have access to a comprehensive source regarding drug dosing guidelines in renal failure. Fortunately, there are a number of excellent publications available for this purpose (215–218). For drug-dose adjustments in SCI patients with renal insufficiency (assuming the serum creatinine is stable), the GFR can be estimated, preferably from measurement of creatinine clearance or from the clearance of an exogenously administered radionuclide (219, 220). Alternatively, the GFR can be estimated using the empiric formula developed by Cockcroft and Gault, along with the appropriate correction factors for paraplegia and quadriplegia (72, 73):

(In males) GFR = (140 − age in years) × (wgt in kg) ÷ 72 × (serum Cr in mg/dL)
(In females) GFR = value for males × 0.85
(In paraplegia) GFR = value for males × 0.60
(In quadriplegia) GFR = value for males × 0.40

Regarding the administration of drug loading doses in patients with renal insufficiency, in general, a similar loading-dose equivalent as that administered to patients with normal renal function can be safely given in renal failure in situations that require the rapid achievement of therapeutic drug levels. If the loading dose of the drug is not known, it can be calculated using the following formula:

$$\text{Loading dose} = Vd \times IBW \times Cp$$

where Vd is the apparent volume of distribution of the drug (in liters/kg), IBW refers to the patient's ideal body weight (in kg), and Cp represents the desired steady-state plasma concentration of the drug. However, in SCI patients with reduced muscle mass, we recommend using the measured body weight (in kg) rather than IBW.

There are basically two methods by which maintenance drug dosing can be accomplished in renal failure patients. The first is to administer a smaller dose at standard dose intervals, and the second method is to administer the standard dose at prolonged intervals. In the first method, the appropriate dose reduction (or fractional dose) can be calculated using the following formula:

$$Df = t\,{}^{1}/_{2}\ normal \div t\,{}^{1}/_{2}\ renal\ failure$$

where Df is the fractional dose; $t\,{}^{1}/_{2}\ normal$ is the elimination half-life of the drug with normal renal function, and $t\,{}^{1}/_{2}\ renal\ failure$ is the elimination half-life of the drug with renal insufficiency. If it is deemed advantageous to maintain normal dosing intervals (e.g., when administering a drug with a narrow therapeutic range and short plasma half-life), the amount of drug per dose can be estimated by the following expression:

$$\text{Dose in renal impairment} = \text{Normal dose} \times Df$$

However, when prolonged dose intervals are more advantageous, either for convenience or in cases where the drug has a broad therapeutic range and long plasma half-life, the dosing interval can be estimated using the following expression:

$$\text{Dose interval in renal impairment} = \text{Normal dose interval} \div Df$$

Moreover, when drug toxicity is correlated with high trough levels (i.e., aminoglycosides), long dosing intervals are beneficial in reducing toxicity. Additionally, various combinations of drug dose reduction and interval prolongation have been successfully used in patients with renal insufficiency.

In summary, the approach to drug therapy in SCI patients with renal insufficiency should begin with an estimation of residual renal function. This can be accomplished by several methods designed to estimate GFR, including the measurement of creatinine clearance, the use of clearance measurements from exogenously administered radionuclide markers, or the use of the Cockcroft and Gault formula with appropriate modifications for paraplegia and quadriplegia (72, 219, 220). Once the degree of renal insufficiency is known, a number of sources can be referred to for drug dosing guidelines in renal failure, including the *Physicians' Desk Reference* (215–218). Alternatively, drug-dosing schedules can be derived or modified using the formulas and concepts provided herein. Moreover, particularly when toxicity is an issue, the appropriate measurements of plasma or serum drug levels should be utilized in the determination of dosing schedules.

An additional consideration in dialysis patients is that some drug removal may occur during dialysis, thus necessitating further dosing adjustments. In fact, substantial amounts of certain drugs can be removed from plasma, especially with hemodialysis. This occurs mainly by diffusion, wherein the drug or its metabolites cross the dialysis membrane, from plasma to dialysate, along a concentration gradient. However, a number of factors function to minimize drug removal by dialysis. These include the molecular size of the drug/metabolite, the degree of protein binding, the apparent volume of drug distribution, the rate at which the drug/metabolite is transported between plasma and other fluid compartments, and the extent to which the drug/metabolite is eliminated from the body by nonrenal mechanisms. Consequently, the removal from plasma of a drug/metabolite by hemodialysis is not very efficient when (a) the molecular mass (i.e., drug/metabolite) exceeds 500 daltons; (b) when protein binding exceeds 90%; (c) when the apparent volume of distribution is large (i.e., V_d of drug/metabolite > 1 liter/kg body weight); (d) when the distribution of the drug from plasma to other body compartments occurs rapidly; or (e) when extensive tissue binding occurs.

The hemodialysis clearance of a drug/metabolite can be estimated by the following formula:

$$Cl\, HD = Cl\, urea \times \frac{60}{MW\, drug}$$

where $Cl\, HD$ and $Cl\, urea$ are the dialysis clearances of the drug and urea, respectively, and MW drug is the molecular weight of the respective drug. Therefore, for a drug/metabolite to undergo substantial clearance by hemodialysis (in the range of 15–100 ml/min), it must be relatively small (i.e., MW < 500 daltons), essentially confined to plasma or in ready equilibrium with plasma, and present in sufficient concentration (unbound to protein). This added capacity for drug removal by dialysis patients is expressed by the following:

$$Clp = Clr + Clnr + Cld$$

where Clp represents total plasma (drug/metabolite) clearance, Clr and $Clnr$ refer to renal and nonrenal clearance, respectively, and Cld represents (drug/metabolite) clearance by dialysis. With respect to hemodialysis, drug/metabolite clearance may be increased with the use of high-efficiency, high-flux dialyzers in conjunction with high dialysate and blood flow rates.

Regarding drug removal in patients undergoing peritoneal dialysis, the same basic principles applicable in hemodialysis also apply here. Therefore, as a general rule, if a drug/metabolite is cleared with hemodialysis, it will also be cleared with peritoneal dialysis. However, with peritoneal dialysis, drug/metabolite clearance is far less efficient. For specific recommendations regarding drug dosing in both hemodialysis and peritoneal dialysis patients, the reader is referred to Aronoff et. al (218).

CONCLUSION

As a final consideration, it is important to acknowledge that our understanding of drug bioavailability and pharmacokinetics in the setting of renal failure is essentially based on data from studies involving able-bodied patients with renal insufficiency. Consequently, the validity of inferentially basing recommendations regarding the use of pharmacologic agents in SCI-ESRD patients on data extrapolated from studies in able-bodied ESRD patients and supported only by limited clinical experience is questionable. Although SCI-ESRD patients share many similarities with their able-bodied counterparts, on balance they should be viewed as a distinct and unique group of patients. Accordingly one must be concerned with the possibility that some unforeseen factor or factors may be present in this population that could affect drug bioavailability and/or pharmacokinetics in an unpredictable way. Moreover, the virtual absence of hard data in this area indicates the need for studies designed to systematically evaluate the bioavailability, pharmacokinetics, and pharmacodynamics of selected drugs in SCI patients with renal insufficiency.

References

1. Levey A, Coresh J, Balk E, Kausz A, Levin A, Steffles M, Hogg R, Perrone R, Lau J, Eknoyan G. National Kidney Foundation Practice Guidelines for Chronic Kidney Disease: Evaluation, classification, and stratification. *Ann Intern Med.* 2003; 139:137–147.
2. Coresh J, Selvin E, Stevens LA, Manzi J, Kusek JW, Eggers PO, Van Lente F, Levey AS. Prevalence of chronic kidney disease in the United States. *JAMA* 2007 Nov 7; l298(17):2038–2047.
3. United States Renal Data System. *USRDS 2007 Annual Data Report: Atlas of End-Stage Renal Disease in the United States.* Bethesda, MD: National Institutes of Health, National Institute of Diabetes and Digestive and Kidney Diseases; 2007. Available from: URL: http://www.usrds.org/atlas_2007.htm.
4. Coresh J, Astor BC, Greene T, Eknoyan G, Levey AS. Prevalence of chronic kidney disease and decreased kidney function in the adult US population: Third National Health and Nutrition Examination Survey. *Am J Kidney Dis;* 2003; 41(1):1–12.
5. Coresh J, Byrd-Holt D, Astor B, Briggs J, Eggers P, Lacher D, Hostetter T. Chronic kidney disease awareness, prevalence, and trends among U.S. adults, 1999–2000. *J Am Soc Nephrol.* 2005:16:180–188.
6. Tribe CR, Silver JR. *Renal Failure in Paraplegia.* London: Pitman Medical, 1969; 13–89.
7. Hackler RH. A 25-year prospective mortality study in the spinal cord injured patient: comparison with the long-term living paraplegic. *J Urol* 1977; 117(4):486–488.
8. Borges PM, Hackler RH. The urologic status of the Vietnam war paraplegic: A 15-year prospective followup. *J Urol* 1982; 127(4):710–711.

9. Price M. Some results of a fifteen year vertical study of urinary tract function in spinal cord injured patients: A preliminary report. *J Am Paraplegia Soc* 1982; 5:31.

10. DeVivo MJ, Black KJ, Stover SL. Causes of death during the first 12 years after spinal cord injury. *Arch Phys Med Rehabil* 1993; 74(3):248–254.

11. DeVivo MJ, Kartus PL, Stover SL, Rutt RD, Fine PR. Cause of death for patients with spinal cord injuries. *Arch Intern Med* 1989; 149(8): 1761–1766.

12. Ditunno JF, Jr. Formal CS. Chronic spinal cord injury. *N Engl J Med* 1994; 330(8):550–556.

13. Imai K, Kadowaki T, Aizawa Y, Fukutomi K. Problems in the health management of persons with spinal cord injury. *J Clin Epidemiol* 1996; 49(5):505–510.

14. Lightner DJ. Contemporary urologic management of patients with spinal cord injury. *Mayo Clin Proc* 1998; 73(5):434–438.

15. Vaziri ND. Pathophysiology of end-stage renal disease in spinal cord injury. *Mt Sinai J Med* 1993; 60(4):302–304.

16. Barton CH, Vaziri ND, Gordon S, Tilles S. Renal pathology in end-stage renal disease associated with paraplegia. *Paraplegia* 1984; 22(1):31–41.

17. Whiteneck GG, et al. Mortality, morbidity, and psychosocial outcomes of persons spinal cord injured more than 20 years ago. *Paraplegia* 1992; 30(9):617–630.

18. Dalton JJ Jr, Hackler RH, Bunts RC. Amyloidosis in the paraplegic; Incidence and significance. *J Urol* 1965; 65:553–555.

19. Wall BM, Huch KM, Mangold TA, Steere EL, Cooke CR. Risk factors for development of proteinuria in chronic spinal cord injury. *Am J Kidney Dis* 1999; 33(5):899–903.

20. Lamid S. Long-term follow-up of spinal cord injury patients with vesicoureteral reflux. *Paraplegia* 1988; 26(1):27–34.

21. Merlini G, Bellotti V. Molecular mechanisms of amyloidosis. *N Eng J Med.* 2003; 349(6):583–596.

22. Vaziri ND, Cesario T, Mootoo K, Zeien L, Gordon S, Byrne C. Bacterial infections in patients with chronic renal failure: Occurrence with spinal cord injury. *Arch Intern Med* 1982; 142(7):1273–1276.

23. Kohli A, Lamid S. Risk factors for renal stone formation in patients with spinal cord injury. *Br J Urol* 1986; 58(6):588–591.

24. Kincaid-Smith PS, Bastos MG, Becker GJ. Reflux nephropathy in the adult. *Contrib Nephrol* 1984; 39:94–101.

25. Ost MC, Lee BR. Urolithiasis in patients with spinal cord injuries: risk factors, management and outcomes. *Curr Opin Urol* 2006 Mar; 16(2):93–9.

26. Burr RG. Calculosis in paraplegia. *Int Rehabil Med* 1981; 3(3):162–167.

27. DeVivo MJ, Fine PR, Cutter GR, Maetz HM. The risk of renal calculi in spinal cord injury patients. *J Urol* 1984; 131(5):857–860.

28. Lloyd LK. New trends in urologic management of spinal cord injured patients. *Cent Nerv Syst Trauma* 1986; 3(1):3–12.

29. Hall MK, Hackler RH, Zampieri TA, Zampieri JB. Renal calculi in spinal cord-injured patient: Association with reflux, bladder stones, and foley catheter drainage. *Urology* 1989; 34(3):126–128.

30. Hansen RB, Biering-Sorensen F, Kristensen JK. Urinary calculi following traumatic spinal cord injury. *Scand J Urol Nephrol.* 2007; 41(2): 115–119.

31. Claus-Walker J, Campos RJ, Carter RE, Vallbona C, Lipscomb HS. Calcium excretion in quadriplegia. *Arch Phys Med Rehabil* 1972; 53(1):14–20.

32. Vaziri ND, Nikakhtar B, Gordon S. Hyperoxaluria in chronic renal disease associated with spinal cord injury. *Paraplegia* 1982; 20(1):48–53.

33. Burr RG, Nuseibeh I. Biochemical studies in paraplegic renal stone patients. 1. Plasma biochemistry and urinary calcium and saturation. *Br J Urol* 1985; 57(3):269–274.

34. Nikakhtar B, Vaziri ND, Khonsari F, Gordon S, Mirahmadi MD. Urolithiasis in patients with spinal cord injury. *Paraplegia* 1981; 19(6):363–366.

35. Burr RG, Nuseibeh I, Abiaka CD. Biochemical studies in paraplegic renal stone patients. 2. Urinary excretion of citrate, inorganic pyrophosphate, silicate and urate. *Br J Urol* 1985; 57(3):275–278.

36. Kaufman DW, Kelly JP, Curhan GC, Anderson TE, Dretler SP, Preminger GM, Cave DR. Oxalobacter formigenes may reduce the risk of calcium oxalate kidney stones. *J Am Soc Nephrol* 2008; 19(6):1197–1203.

37. Sidhu H, Schmidt ME, Cornelius JG, Thamiselvan S, Kahn SR, Hesse A, Peck AB. Direct correlation between hyperoxaluria/oxalate stone disease and the absence of the gastrointestinal tract-dwelling bacterium Oxalobacter formigenes: possible prevention by gut recolonization or

38. Allison MJ, Cook HM, Milne DB, Gallagher S, Clayman RV. Oxalate degradation by gastrointestinal bacteria from humans. *J Nutr* 1986; 116(3):455–460

39. Allison MJ, Dawson KA, Mayberry WR, Foss JG. Oxalobacter formigenes gen. nov., sp. nov: oxalate-degrading anaerobes that inhabit the gastrointestinal tract. *Arc Microbiol* 1985; 141(1):1–7.

40. Vaidyanathan S, von Unruh GE, Watson ID, Laube N, Willet S, Sone BL. Hyperoxaluria, hypocitraturia, hypomagnesiuria, and lack of intestinal colonization by *Oxalobacter formigenes* in a cervical spinal cord injury patient with suprapubic cystostomy, short bowel, and nephrolithiasis. *Scientific World J* 2006 6; 6:2403–2410.

41. Hatch M, Cornelius J, Allison M, Sidhu H, Peck A, Freel RW. *Oxalobacter sp.* reduces urinary oxalate excretion by promoting enteric oxalate secretion. *Kidney Int* 2006; 69(4):691–698.

42. Troxel SA, Sidhu H, Kaul P, Low RK. Intestinal *Oxalobacter formigenes* colonization in calcium oxalate stone formers and its relation to urinary oxalate. *J Endourol* 2003; 17(3):173–176.

43. Duncan SH, Richardson AJ, Kaul P, Holmes RP, Allison MJ, Stewart CS. *Appl Environ Microbiol* 2002; 68(8):3841–3847.

44. Sidhu H, Allison MJ, Chow JM, Clark A, Peck AB. Rapid reversal of hyperoxaluria in a rat model after probiotic administration of *Oxalobacter formigenes*. *J Urol* 2001; 166(4):1487–1491.

45. Kuhlemeier KV, Huang CT, Lloyd LK, Fine PR, Stover SL. Effective renal plasma flow: Clinical significance after SCI. *J Urol* 1985; 133(5):758–761.

46. Vaziri ND, Mirahmadi MK, Barton CH, Eltorai I, Gordon S, Byrne C, Paul MV. Clinicopathological characteristics of dialysis patients with spinal cord injury. *J Am Paraplegia Soc* 1983; 6(1):3–6.

47. Levey AS: National Kidney Foundation: National Kidney Foundation Practice Guidelines for chronic kidney disease; evaluation, classification, and stratification. *Ann Intern Med* 2003; 139:137

48. K/DOQI clinical practice guidelines for chronic kidney disease: evaluation, classification, and stratification. Kidney Disease Outcome Quality Initiative. *Am J Kidney Dis* 2002; 39:S1–246.

49. Ethans KD, Nance PW, Bard RJ, Casey AR, Schryvers OI. Efficacy and safety of tolterodine in people with neurogenic detrusor overactivity. *J Spinal Cord Med* 2004; 27(3):214–218.

50. Combined intravesical and oral Oxybutynin chloride in adult patients with spinal cord injury. *Urology* 2000; 55(3):358–362.

51. Vaidyanathan S, Soni BM, Brown E, Sett P, Krishnan KR, Bingley J, Markey S. Effect of intermittent urethral catheterization and oxybutynin bladder instillation on urinary continence status and quality of life in a selected group of spinal cord injury patients with neuropathic bladder dysfunction. *Spinal Cord* 1998; 36(6):409–414.

52. Amend B, Hennenlotter J, Schäfer T, Horstmann M, Stenzl A, Sievert KD. Effective treatment of neurogenic detrusor dysfunction by combined high dose antimuscarinics without increased side effects. *Eur Urol* 2008; 53(5):1021–1028.

53. O'Leary M, Erickson JR, Smith CP, McDermott C, Horton J, Chancellor MB. Effect of controlled-release oxybutynin on neurogenic bladder function in spinal cord injury. *J Spinal Cord Med* 2003; 26(2):159–162.

54. Chapple CR, Yamanishi T, Chess-Williams R. Muscarinic receptor subtypes and management of the overactive bladder. *Urology* 2002; 60I(5 Suppl 1):82–88.

55. Pannek J, Sommerfeld HJ, Bötel U, Senge T. Combined intravesical and oral Oxybutynin chloride in adult patients with spinal cord injury. *Urology* 2000; 55(3):358–362.

56. Vaidyanathan S, Soni BM, Brown E, Sett P, Krishnan KR, Bingley J, Markey S. Effect of intermittent urethral catheterization and oxybutynin bladder instillation on urinary continence status and quality of life in a selected group of spinal cord injury patients with neuropathic bladder dysfunction. *Spinal Cord* 1998; 36(6):409–414.

57. Silva C, Silva J, Ribiero MJ, Avelino A, Cruz F. Urodynamic effect of intravesical resiniferatoxin in patients the neurogenic detrusor overactivity of spinal origin: results of a double blind randomized placebo-controlled trial. *Eur Urol* 2005; 48(4)650–655.

58. Kuo HC. Effectiveness of intravesical resiniferatoxin in treating detrusor hyperreflexia and external sphincter dyssynergia in patients with chronic spinal cord lesions. *BJU Int* 2003; 92(6):597–601.

59. Kim JH, Rivas DA, Shenot PJ, Green B, Kennelly M, Erickson JR, O'Leary M, Yoshimura N, Chancellor MB. Intravesical resiniferatoxin for

refractory detrusor hyperreflexia: a multicenter, blinded, randomized, placebo-controlled trial. *J Spinal Cord Med* 2003; 26(4):358–363.

60. Ehren I, Volz D, Farrelly E, Berglund L, Brundin L, Hultling C, Lafolie P. Efficacy and impact of botulinum toxin A on quality of life in patients with neurogenic detrusor overactivity: a randomized, placebo-controlled, double blind study. *Scand J Urol Nephrol* 2007; 41(4): 335–340.

61. MacDonald R, Fink HA, Huckabay C, Monga M, Wilt TJ. Botulinum toxin for treatment of urinary incontinence due to detrusor overactivity: A systematic review of effectiveness and adverse effects. *Spinal Cord* 2007; 45(8):535–541.

62. Consortium for Spinal Cord Medicine. *Bladder Management for Adults with Spinal Cord Injury: A Clinical Practice Guideline for Health-Care Providers.* 2006:15–16.

63. Razdan S, Leboeuf L, Meinbach DS, Weinstein D, Gousse AE. Current practice patterns in the urologic surveillance and management of patients with spinal cord injury. *Urology* 2003; 61(5):893–896.

64. Griffith DP, Gleeson MJ, Lee H, Longuet R, Deman E, Earle N. Randomized, double blinded trial of Lithostat (acetohydroxamic acid) in the palliative treatment of infection-induced urinary calculi. *Eur Urol* 1991; 20(3):243–247.

65. Griffith DP, Khonsari F, Skurnick JH, James KE. A randomized trial of acetohydroxamic acid for the treatment and prevention of infection-induced urinary stones in spinal cord injury patients. *J Urol* 1988; 140(2):318–324.

66. Chai W, Liebman M, Kynast-Gales S, Massey L. Oxalate absorption and endogenous oxalate synthesis from ascorbate in calcium oxalate stone formers and non-stone formers. *Am J Kidney Dis* 2004; 44(6):1060–1069.

67. Traxer O, Huet B, Poindexter J, Pak CY, Pearle MS. Effect of ascorbic acid consumption on urinary stone risk factors. *J Urol* 2003; 170(2Pt1): 397–401.

68. Herbert V. Risk of oxalate stones from large doses of vitamin C. *N Engl J Med* 1978; 298(15):856.

69. Cardenas DD, Hoffman JM, Kirschblum S, McKinley W. Etiology and incidence of rehospitalization after traumatic spinal cord injury: a multicenter analysis. *Arch Phys Med Rehabil* 2004; 85(11):1757–1763.

70. McKinley WO, Jackson AB, Cardenas DD, DeVivo MJ. Long-term medical complications after traumatic spinal cord injury: a regional model systems analysis. *Arch Phys Med Rehabil* 1999; 80(11):1402–1410.

71. DeVivo MJ, Krause J, Lammertse D. Recent trends in mortality and causes of death among persons with spinal cord injury. *Arch Phys Med Rehabil* 1999; 80(11):1411–1419.

72. Mirahmadi MK, Byrne C, Barton C, Penera N, Gordon S, Vaziri ND. Prediction of creatinine clearance from serum creatinine in spinal cord injury patients. *Paraplegia* 1983; 21(1):23–29.

73. Cockcroft DW, Gault MH. Prediction of creatinine clearance from serum creatinine. *Nephron* 1976; 16(1):31–41.

74. Vaziri ND, Bruno A, Mirahmadi MK, Golji H, Gordon S, Byrne C. Features of residual renal function in end-stage renal failure associated with spinal cord injury. *Int J Artif Organs* 1984; 7(6):319–322.

75. Barton CH, Vaziri ND, Gordon S, Eltorai I. Endocrine pathology in spinal cord injured patients on maintenance dialysis. *Paraplegia* 1984; 22(1):7–16.

76. Eschbach JW. The anemia of chronic renal failure: pathophysiology and the effects of recombinant erythropoietin [clinical conference]. *Kidney Int* 1989; 35(1):134–148.

77. Vaziri ND. *Current Dialysis Therapy.* Philadelphia: Hanley and Belfus, 1986; 158–161.

78. Vaziri ND, Byrne C, Mirahmadi MK, Golji H, Nikakhtar B, Alday B, Gordon S. Hematologic features of chronic renal failure associated with spinal cord injury. *Artif Organs* 1982; 6(1):69–72.

79. Vaziri ND, Winer RL, Alikhani S, Danviryasup K, Toohey J, Hung E, Gordon S, Eltorai I, Paule P. Antithrombin deficiency in end-stage renal disease associated with paraplegia: Effect of hemodialysis. *Arch Phys Med Rehabil* 1985; 66(5):307–309.

80. Vaziri ND, Winer RL, Alikhani S, Toohey J, Paule P, Danviryasum K, Gordon S, Eltorai I. Extrinsic and common coagulation pathways in end-stage renal disease associated with spinal cord injury. *Paraplegia* 1986; 24(3):154–158.

81. Vaziri ND, Winer RL, Toohey J, Danviriyasup K, Alikhani S, Eltorai I, Gordon S, Paule P. Intrinsic coagulation pathway in end-stage renal disease associated with spinal cord injury treated with hemodialysis. *Artif Organs* 1985; 9(2):155–159.

82. Vaziri ND, Patel B, Gonzales AE, Winer RL, Eltorai I, Gordon S, Danviryasup K. Protein C abnormalities in spinal cord injured patients with end-stage renal disease. *Arch Phys Med Rehabil* 1987; 68(11):791–793.

83. Block GA, Hulbert-Shearon TE, Levin NW, Port FK. Association of serum phosphorus and calcium x phosphate product with mortality risk in chronic hemodialysis patients: a national study. *Am J Kidney Dis* 1998; 31(4):607–617.

84. Rostand SG, Sanders C, Kirk KA, Rutsky EA, Fraser RG. Myocardial calcification and cardiac dysfunction in chronic renal failure. *Am J Med* 1988; 85(5):651–657.

85. Massry SG, Smogorzewski M. Mechanisms through which parathyroid hormone mediates its deleterious effects on organ function in uremia. *Semin Nephrol* 1994; 14(3):219–231.

86. Lowrie EG, Lew NL. Death risk in hemodialysis patients: The predictive value of commonly measured variables and an evaluation of death rate differences between facilities. *Am J Kidney Dis* 1990; 15(5): 458–482.

87. Wills MR, Savory J. Aluminium poisoning: Dialysis encephalopathy, osteomalacia, and anaemia. *Lancet* 1983; 2(8340):29–34.

88. Alfrey AC, Hegg A, Craswell P. Metabolism and toxicity of aluminum in renal failure. *Am J Clin Nutr* 1980; 33(7):1509–1516.

89. Finn WF, Joy MS, Hladik G; Lanthanum Study Group. Efficacy and safety of lanthanum carbonate for reduction of serum phosphorus in patients with chronic renal failure receiving hemodialysis. *Clin Nephrol* 2004; 62(3):193–201.

90. deFreitas D, Donne RL, Hutchison AJ. Lanthanum carbonate—a first line phosphate binder? *Semin Dial* 2007; 20(4):325–328.

91. Finn WF; SPD 405-307 Lanthanum Study Group. Lanthanum carbonate versus standard therapy for the treatment of hyperphosphatemia: safety and efficacy in chronic maintenance hemodialysis patients. *Clin Nephrol* 2006; 65(3):191–202.

92. Koch KM. Dialysis-related amyloidosis [clinical conference]. *Kidney Int* 1992; 41(5):1416–1429.

93. National Kidney Foundation. K/DOQI clinical practice guidelines for bone metabolism and diseases in chronic kidney disease. *Am J Kidney Dis* 2003; 42:S1–S202. Available at http://www.kidney.org/professionals/kdoqi/guidelines_bone/index.htm.

94. Hailpern SM, Melamed ML, Cohen HW, Hostetter TH. Moderate chronic kidney disease and cognitive function in adults 20-59 years of age: Third National Health and Nutrition Examination Survey (NHANES III). *J Am Soc Nephrol* 2007; 18(7):2205–2213.

95. Murray AM, Tupper DE, Knopman DS et al. Cognitive impairment in hemodialysis is common. *Neurology* 2006; 67:216–223.

96. Ifudu O. Care of patients undergoing hemodialysis. *N Engl J Med* 1998; 339(15):1054–1062.

97. Rostand SG, Brunzell JD, Cannon ROd, Victor RG. Cardiovascular complications in renal failure [editorial]. *J Am Soc Nephrol* 1991; 2(6):1053–1062.

98. London G, Parfrey PS. Cardiac disease in chronic uremia: Pathogenesis. *Adv Renal Replac Ther* 1997; 4:194–211.

99. Bloembergen WE. Cardiac disease in chronic uremia: Epidemiology. *Adv Renal Replac Ther* 1997; 4:185–193.

100. Parfrey PS, Foley RN, Harnett JD, Kent GM, Murray DC, Barre PE. The outcome and risk factors for left ventricular disorders in chronic uremia. *Nephrol Dial Transpl* 1996; 11:1277–1285.

101. Tomson CRV. *Comprehensive Clinical Nephrology.* London: Mosby, 2000; 70.1–70.14.

102. US Renal Data System: USRDA 1991 *Annual Report.* Bethesda, MD: The National Institute of Diabetes and Digestive and Kidney Diseases, 1991.

103. Raine AEG, Magreiter R, Brunner FP. Report on management of renal failure in Europe, XXII, 1991. *Nephrol Dial Transplant* 1992; (Suppl 2):7–35.

104. Islam KN. Alpha-tocopherol supplementation decreases the oxidative susceptibility of LDL in renal failure patients on dialysis therapy. *Atherosclerosis* 2000; 150:217–224.

105. Uzum A, Toprak O, Gumustas MK, Ciftci S, Sen S. Effect of vitamin E therapy on oxidative stress and erythrocyte osmotic fragility in patients on peritoneal dialysis and hemodialysis. *J Nephrol* 2006; 19(6):739–745.

106. Bostom AG, Shemin D, Lapane KL, Hume AL, Yoburn D, Nadeau MR, Bendich A, Selhub J, Rosenberg IH. High dose B-vitamin treatment of hyperhomocysteinemia in dialysis patients. *Kidney Int* 1996; 49:147–152.

107. Nicholls AJ. *Handbook of Dialysis*, 3rd ed. Philadelphia: Lippincott, Williams and Wilkins, 2000; 583–600.

108. Touam M. Effective correction of hyperhomocysteinemia in hemodialysis patients by intravenous folinic acid and pyridoxine therapy. *Kidney Int* 1999; 56:2292–2296.

109. Parfrey PS, Lameire N. *Complications of Dialysis*. New York: Marcel Decker, 2000; 269–302.

110. U.S. Renal Data System: *USRDS 2007 Annual Data Report: Atlas of End Stage Renal Disease in the United States*. Bethesda, MD. National Institutes of Health, National Institute of Diabetes and Digestive and Kidney Diseases, 2007.

111. National Kidney Foundation: K/DOQI Clinical Practice Guidelines and Clinical Practice Recommendations for Anemia in Chronic Kidney Disease. *Am J Kidney Dis* 2006; 47:S1–S146 (Suppl 3); available at http://www.kidney.org/professionals/kdoqi/guidelines_anemia/index.htm.

112. Ventura SC, Garella S. The management of pericardial disease in renal failure. *Semin Dial* 1990; 3:21.

113. Alpert MA, Ravenscraft MD. Pericardial involvement in end-stage renal disease. *Am J Med Sci* 2003; 325(4):228–236.

114. Parfrey PS, Harnett JD, Barre PE. The natural history of myocardial disease in dialysis patients. *J Am Soc Nephrol* 1991; 2(1):2–12.

115. Pahl MV, Vaziri ND, Gordon S, Tuero S. Cardiovascular pathology in dialysis patients with spinal cord injury. *Artif Organs* 1983; 7(4):416–419.

116. Fairshter RD, Vaziri ND, Gordon S. Frequency and spectrum of pulmonary diseases in patients with chronic renal failure associated with spinal cord injury. *Respiration* 1983; 44(1):58–62.

117. Gore RM, Mintzer RA, Calenoff L. Gastrointestinal complications of spinal cord injury. *Spine* 1981; 6(6): 538–544.

118. Fealey RD, Szurszewski JH, Merritt JL, DiMagno EP. Effect of traumatic spinal cord transection on human upper gastrointestinal motility and gastric emptying. *Gastroenterology* 1984; 87(1):69–75.

119. Kewalramani LS. Neurogenic gastroduodenal ulceration and bleeding associated with spinal cord injuries. *J Trauma* 1979; 19(4):259–265.

120. Kiwerski J. Bleeding from the alimentary canal during the management of spinal cord injury patients. *Paraplegia* 1986; 24(2):92–96.

121. Adams PL, Rutsky EA, Rostand SG, Han SY. Lower gastrointestinal tract dysfunction in patients receiving long-term hemodialysis. *Arch Intern Med* 1982; 142(2):303–306.

122. Ala-Kaila K, Paronen I, Paakkala T. Increased incidence of duodenitis in chronic renal failure. *Ann Clin Res* 1988; 20(3):154–157.

123. Avram MM. High prevalence of pancreatic disease in chronic renal failure. *Nephron* 1977; 18(1):68–71.

124. Milito G, Taccone-Gallucci M, Brancaleone C, Nardi F, Cesca D, Boffo V, Casciani CU. The gastrointestinal tract in uremic patients on long-term hemodialysis. *Kidney Int Suppl* 1985; 17:S157–S160.

125. Meshkinpour H, Vaziri N, Gordon S. Gastrointestinal pathology in patients with chronic renal failure associated with spinal cord injury. *Am J Gastroenterol* 1982; 77(8):562–564.

126. Marcuard SP, Weinstock JV. Gastrointestinal angiodysplasia in renal failure. *J Clin Gastroenterol* 1988; 10(5):482–484.

127. Gilmore PR. Angiodysplasia of the upper gastrointestinal tract. *J Clin Gastroenterol* 1988; 10(4):386–394.

128. Posner GL, Fink SM, Huded FV, Dunn I, Calderone PG, Joglekar SS. Endoscopic findings in chronic hemodialysis patients with upper gastrointestinal bleeding. *Am J Gastroenterol* 1983; 78(11):720–721.

129. Mills B, Zuckerman G, Sicard G. Discrete colon ulcers as a cause of lower gastrointestinal bleeding and perforation in end-stage renal disease. *Surgery* 1981; 89(5):548–552.

130. Mannucci PM, Remuzzi G, Pusineri F, Lombardi R, Valsecchi C, Mecca G, Zimmerman TS. Deamino-8-D-arginine vasopressin shortens the bleeding time in uremia. *N Engl J Med* 1983; 308(1):8–12.

131. Livio M, Mannucci PM, Vigano G, Mingardi G, Lombardi R, Mecca G, Remuzzi G. Conjugated estrogens for the management of bleeding associated with renal failure. *N Engl J Med* 1986; 315(12):731–735.

132. Caruana RJ. Heparin-free dialysis: Comparative data and results in high-risk patients. *Kidney Int* 1987; 31:1351–1357.

133. Diamond S, Emmet M, Henrich W. Bowel infarction: A common occurrence in dialysis patients (abstract). *Kidney Int* 1986; 29:212.

134. Bartolomeo RS, Calabrese PR, Taubin HL. Spontaneous perforation of the colon. A potential complication of chronic renal failure. *Am J Dig Dis* 1977; 22(7):656–657.

135. Diamond SM, Emmett M, Henrich WL. Bowel infarction as a cause of death in dialysis patients. *JAMA* 1986; 256(18): 2545–2547.

136. Popli S, Daugirdas JT, Ing TS. Dialysis ascites [editorial]. *Int J Artif Organs* 1980; 3(5):257–258.

137. Harnett JD, Parfrey PS, Kennedy M, Zeldis JB, Steinman TI, Guttmann RD. The long-term outcome of hepatitis B infection in hemodialysis patients. *Am J Kidney Dis* 1988; 11(3):210–213.

138. Da Porto A, Adami A, Susanna F, Calzavara P, Poli P, Castelletto MR, Amici GP, Teodoni T, Okolicsanyi L. Hepatitis C virus in dialysis units: A multicenter study. *Nephron* 1992; 61(3):309–310.

139. Malaguti M, Capece R, Marciano M, Arena G, Luciani MP, Striano M, Biagini M. Antibodies to hepatitis C virus (anti-HCV): prevalence in the same geographical area in dialysis patients, staff members, and blood donors. *Nephron* 1992; 61(3):346.

140. Conway M, Catterall AP, Brown EA, Tibbs C, Gower PE, Curtis JR, Coleman JC, Murray-Lyon IM. Prevalence of antibodies to hepatitis C in dialysis patients and transplant recipients with possible routes of transmission [see comments]. *Nephrol Dial Transplant* 1992; 7(12):1226–1229.

141. Fabrizi F, Messa P, Martin P. Hepatitis B virus infection and the dialysis patient. *Semin Dial* 2008; Apr 6.

142. Baid-Agrawal S, Pascual M, Moradpour D, Frei U, Tolkoff-Rubin N. Hepatitis C virus infection in HD and kidney transplant pts, *Rev Med Virol* 2008; 18(2):97–115.

143. Rahnavardi, M, Moghaddam, SMH, Alavian, SM. Hepatitis C in hemodialysis patients: Current global magnitude, natural history, diagnostic difficulties, and preventive measures. *Am J Nephrol* 2008; 28:628–640 (DOI: 10.1159/000117573).

144. Eijgenraam FJ, Donckerwolcke RA. Treatment of iron overload in children and adolescents on chronic haemodialysis. *Eur J Pediatr* 1990; 149(5):359–362.

145. Simon P, Meyrier A. Drug-induced liver cytolysis in hemodialyzed patients. *Kidney Int* 1979; 15:453.

146. Daugirdas JT. Dialysis hypotension: A hemodynamic analysis (editorial review). *Kidney Int* 1991; 39:233–245.

147. Silver SM, DeSimone JA, Jr., Smith DA, Sterns RH. Dialysis disequilibrium syndrome (DDS) in the rat: Role of the "reverse urea effect." *Kidney Int* 1992; 42(1):161–166.

148. Bergman H, Daugirdas JT, Ing TS. *Handbook of Dialysis*, 3rd ed. Philadelphia: Lippincott, Williams and Wilkins, 2001; 102–120.

149. Brouns R, De Deyn PP. Neurological complications in renal failure: a review. Clin Neurol Neurosurg 2004 Dec; 107 (1):1–16.

150. Silver SM, Sterns RH, Halperin ML. Brain swelling after dialysis: old urea or new osmoles? *Am J Kidney Dis* 1996; 28(1):1–13.

151. Alvestrand A. Protein metabolism and nutrition in hemodialysis patients. *Contrib Nephrol* 1990; 78:102–118.

152. Blagg CR. Importance of nutrition in dialysis patients [editorial]. *Am J Kidney Dis* 1991; 17(4):458–461.

153. Blumenkrantz MJ, Kopple JD, Gutman RA, Chan YK, Barbour GL, Roberts C, Shen FH, Gandhi VC, Tucker CT, Curtis FK, Coburn JW. Methods for assessing nutritional status of patients with renal failure. *Am J Clin Nutr* 1980; 33(7):1567–1585.

154. Mirahmadi MK, Barton CH, Vaziri ND, Gordon S, Penera N. Nutritional evaluation of hemodialysis patients with and without spinal cord injury. *J Am Paraplegia Soc* 1983; 6(2):36–40.

155. Hostetter TH, Olson JL, Rennke HG, Venkatachalam MA, Brenner BM. Hyperfiltration in remnant nephrons: A potentially adverse response to renal ablation. *Am J Physiol* 1981; 241(1):F85–93.

156. Giatras I, Lau J, Levey AS. Effect of angiotensin-converting-enzyme inhibitors on the progression of non-diabetic renal disease: A meta-analysis of randomized trials. *Ann Intern Med* 1997; 127:337–345.

157. Pedrini MT, Levey AS, Lau J, Chalmers TC, Wang PH. The effect of dietary protein restriction on the progression of diabetic and non-diabetic renal diseases: A meta-analysis. *Ann Intern Med* 1997; 124:627–632.

158. Meyer TW, Anderson S, Rennke HG, Brenner BM. Reversing glomerular hypertension stabilizes established glomerular injury. *Kidney Int* 1987; 31(3):752–759.

159. Lafayette RA, Mayer G, Park SK, Meyer TW. Angiotensin II receptor blockade limits glomerular injury in rats with reduced renal mass. *J Clin Invest* 1992; 90(3):766–771.

160. Mirahmadi MK, Vaziri ND, Ghobadi M, Nikakhtar B, Gordon S. Survival on maintenance dialysis in patients with chronic renal failure

associated with paraplegia and quadriplegia. *Paraplegia* 1982; 20(1):43–47.

161. Stacy WK, Falls WF, Hussey RW. Chronic hemodialysis of SCI patients. *J Am Paraplegia Soc* 1983; 6(1):7–9.

162. Vaziri ND, Bruno A, Byrne C, Mirahmadi MK, Nikakhtar B, Gordon S, Zeien L. Maintenance hemodialysis in end-stage renal disease associated with spinal cord injury. *Artif Organs* 1982; 6(1):13–16.

163. Ethier JH, Lindsay RM, Barre PE, Kappel JE, Carlisle EJ, Common A. Clinical practice guidelines for vascular access. Canadian Society of Nephrology. *J Am Soc Nephrol* 1999; 10(Suppl 13):S297–S305.

164. Bander SJ, Schwab SJ. Central venous angioaccess for hemodialysis and its complications. *Semin Dial* 1992; 5:121–128.

165. Schillinger F, Schillinger D, Montagnac R, Milcent T. Post catheterization vein stenosis in haemodialysis: comparative angiographic study of 50 subclavian and 50 internal jugular accesses. *Nephrol Dial Transplant* 1991; 6(10):722–724.

166. Besrab A, Raja RM. *Handbook of Dialysis*, 3rd ed. Philadelphia: Lippincott, Williams and Wilkins, 2001; 67–101.

167. National Kidney Foundation. KDOQI Clinical Practice Guidelines and Clinical Practice Recommendations for 2006 Updates: Hemodialysis Adequacy, Peritoneal Dialysis Adequacy and Vascular Access. *Am J Kidney Dis* 2006; 48:S1–S322.

168. Harland RC. Placement of permanent vascular access devices: Surgical considerations. *Adv Ren Replace Ther* 1994; 1(2):99–106.

169. Denker BM, Chertow GM, Owen WF Jr. *The Kidney*, vol II, 6th ed. Philadelphia: WB Saunders Company, 2000; 2373–2453.

170. Valji K, Bookstein JJ, Roberts AC, Davis GB. Pharmacomechanical thrombolysis and angioplasty in the management of clotted hemodialysis grafts: early and late clinical results. *Radiology* 1991; 178:243–247.

171. Hoen B, Paul-Dauphin A, Hestin D, Kessler M. EPIBACDIAL: A multicenter prospective study of risk factors for bacteremia in chronic hemodialysis patients. *J Am Soc Nephrol* 1998; 9(5):869–876.

172. Vaziri ND. Long-term haemodialysis in spinal cord injured patients. *Paraplegia* 1984; 22(2):110–114.

173. Vaziri ND, Lopez G, Nikakhtar B, Gordon S, Penera N. Peritoneal dialysis in renal failure associated with spinal cord injury. *J Am Paraplegia Soc* 1984; 7(4):63–65.

174. Vinay P, Prud'Homme M, Vinet B, Cournoyer G, Degoulet P, Leville M, Gougoux A, St-Louis G, Lapierre L, Piette Y. Acetate metabolism and bicarbonate generation during hemodialysis: 10 years of observation. *Kidney Int* 1987; 31(5):1194–1204.

175. Mastrangelo F, Rizzelli S, Corliano C, Montinaro AM, De Blasi V, Alfonso L, Aprile M, Napoli M, Laforgia R. Benefits of bicarbonate dialysis. *Kidney Int Suppl* 1985; 17:S188–S193.

176. Himmelfarb J, Ault KA, Holbrook D, Leeber DA, Hakim RM. Intradialytic granulocyte reactive oxygen species production: A prospective, crossover trial. *J Am Soc Nephrol* 1993; 4(2):178–186.

177. Loughrey CM, Young IS, Lightbody JH, McMaster D, McNamee PT, Trimble ER. Oxidative stress in haemodialysis. *QJM* 1994; 87(11):679–683.

178. Toborek M, Wasik T, Drozdz M, Klin M, Magner-Wrobel K, Kopieczna-Grzebieniak E. Effect of hemodialysis on lipid peroxidation and antioxidant system in patients with chronic renal failure. *Metabolism* 1992; 41(11):1229–1232.

179. Schulman G, Fogo A, Gung A, Badr K, Hakim R. Complement activation retards resolution of acute ischemic renal failure in the rat. *Kidney Int* 1991; 40(6):1069–1074.

180. Harris KP, Schreiner GF, Klahr S. Effect of leukocyte depletion on the function of the postobstructed kidney in the rat. *Kidney Int* 1989; 36(2):210–215.

181. Schiffl H, Lang SM, Konig A, Strasser T, Haider MC, Held E. Biocompatible membranes in acute renal failure: Prospective case-controlled study [see comments]. *Lancet* 1994; 344(8922):570–572.

182. Hakim RM, Wingard RL, Parker RA. Effect of the dialysis membrane in the treatment of patients with acute renal failure [see comments]. *N Engl J Med* 1994; 331(20):1338–1342.

183. Burkhart JM, Nolph KD. *The Kidney*, vol II, 6th ed. Philadelphia: WB Saunders Company, 2000; 2455–2517.

184. Tzamaloukas AH, Raj DS, Onime A, Servilla KS, Vanderjagt DJ, Murata GH. The prescription of peritoneal dialysis. *Semin Dial* 2008; 21(3):250–257.

185. Duckworth WC, Jallepalli P, Solomon SS. Glucose intolerance in spinal cord injury. *Arch Phys Med Rehabil* 1983; 64(3):107–110.

186. Rocco MV, Blumenkrantz MJ. *Handbook of Dialysis*, 3rd ed. Philadelphia: Lippincott, Williams and Wilkins, 2001; 420–445.

187. National Kidney Foundation. Kidney Disease Outcomes Quality Initiative (K/DOQI) Clinical Practice Guidelines for Nutrition in Chronic Renal Failure. *Am J Kidney Dis* 2000; 35:S1–140 (Suppl 2). Available at http://www.kidney.org/professionals/kdoqi/guidelines_updates/doqi_nut.htm.

188. Tribe CR, Silver JR. *Renal Failure in Paraplegia*. London, England: Pittman Medical, 1969; 35–90.

189. Bossola M, Tazza L, Giungi S, Luciani G. Anorexia in hemodialysis patients: an update. *Kidney Int* 2006; 70(3):417–422.

190. Chevalier CA, Liepa G, Murphy MD, Suneson J, Vanbeber AD, Gorman MA, Cochran C. The effects of zinc supplementation on serum zinc and cholesterol concentrations in hemodialysis patients. *J Ren Nutr* 2002; 12(3):183–189.

191. Mahajan SK, Prasad AS, Lambujon J, Abbasi AA, Briggs WA, McDonald FD. *Am J Clin Nutr* 1980; 33(7):1517–1521.

192. Atkin-Thor E, Goddard BW, O'Nion J, Stephen RL, Kolff WJ. Hypogeusia and zinc depletion in chronic dialysis patients. *Am J Clin Nutr* 1978; 31(10):1948–1951.

193. Kaupke CJ, Vaziri ND. Nutritional implications of erythropoietin therapy in dialysis patients. *Semin Dial* 1992; 5:254.

194. Mitch WE, May RC, Maroni BJ, Druml W. Protein and amino acid metabolism in uremia: Influence of metabolic acidosis. *Kidney Int Suppl* 1989; 27:S205–S207.

195. Ziegler TR, Rombeau JL, Young LS, Fong Y, Marano M, Lowry SF, Willmore DW. Recombinant human growth hormone enhances the metabolic efficacy of parenteral nutrition: A double-blind, randomized controlled study. *J Clin Endocrinol Metab* 1992; 74(4):865–873.

196. Goldstein DJ, Strom JA. Intradialytic parenteral nutrition: Evolution and current concepts. *J Renal Nutr* 1991; 1:9.

197. Andress DL. Vitamin D in chronic kidney disease: A systemic role for selective Vitamin D receptor activation. *Kidney Int* 2006; 69(1):33–43.

198. Andress DL. Vitamin D treatment in chronic kidney disease. *Semin Dial* 2005; 18(4):315–321.

199. Block GA. Cinacalcet for secondary hyperPTH in patient receiving hemodialysis. *N Engl J Med* 2004; 350:1516.

200. Descombes E, Hanck AB, Fellay G. Water soluble vitamins in chronic hemodialysis patients and need for supplementation. *Kidney Int* 1993; 43(6):1319–1328.

201. Heaf J, Jakobsen U, Tvedegaard E, Kanstrup IL, Fogh-Andersen N. Dietary habits and nutritional status of renal transplant pts. *J Ren Nut* 2004; 14(1):20–25.

202. Kalantar-Zadeh K, Kopple JD. Trace elements and vitamins in maintenance dialysis patients. *Adv Ren Replace Ther* 2003; 10(3):170–182.

203. Sher L. Role of Selenium in the effects of dialysis on mood and behavior. *Med Hypotheses* 2002; 59(1):89–91.

204. NKF-DOQI clinical practice guidelines for the treatment of anemia of chronic renal failure. National Kidney Foundation-Dialysis Outcomes Quality Initiative. *Am J Kidney Dis* 1997; (4 Suppl 3): S192–S240.

205. Fishbane S, Paganini EP. *Handbook of Dialysis*, 3rd ed. Philadelphia: Lippincott, Williams and Wilkins, 2001; 477–494.

206. Nissenson AR, Lindsay RM, Swan S, Seligman P, Strobos J. Sodium ferric gluconate complex in sucrose is safe and effective in hemodialysis patients: North American Clinical Trial. *Am J Kidney Dis* 1999; 33:471–482.

207. Aronoff GR, Bennett WM, Blumenthal S, Charytan C, Pennell JP, Reed J, Rothstein M, Strom J, Wolfe A, Van Wyck D, Yee J; United States Iron Sucrose (Venofer®) Clinical Trials Group. Iron Sucrose in hemodialysis patients: safety of replacement and maintenance regimens. *Kidney Int* 2004; 66(3):1193–1198.

208. Vanwyck DB. Iron dextran in chronic renal failure. *Semin Dial* 1991; 4:112–114.

209. Hou FF, Zhang X, Zhang GH. Efficacy and safety of benazepril for advanced chronic renal insufficiency. *N Engl J Med* 2006; 354:131–140.

210. Wolf G, Ritz E. Combination therapy with ACE inhibitors and angiotensin II receptor blockers to halt progression of chronic renal disease: pathophysiology and indications. *Kidney Int* 2005; 67:799–812.

211. Bianchi S, Bigazzi R, Caiazza A, Campese A, Campese VM. A controlled, prospective study of the effects of Atorvastatin on proteinuria and progression of kidney disease. *Am J Kidney Dis* 2003; 41:565–570.

212. Hebert LA, Wilmer WA, Falkenhain ME, Ladson-Wofford SE, Nahman NS Jr, Rovin BH. Renoprotection: one or many therapies? *Kidney Int* 2001; 59:1211–1226.

213. Anderson RJ, Gambertoglio JG, Schrier RW. *Clinical Use of Drugs in Renal Failure*. Springfield, IL: Charles C. Thomas, 1976.

214. Aronoff GR, Erbeck KM. *Principles and Practice of Dialysis*, 2nd, ed. Baltimore: Williams and Wilkins, 1999; 125–140.

215. Cutler RE, Forland SC, St John Hammond, PG. *Textbook of Nephrology*, vol 2, 3rd ed. Baltimore: Williams & Wilkins, 1995; 1597–1625.

216. Olyaei AJ, De Mattos AM, Bennett WM. *The Kidney*, vol II, 6th ed. Philadelphia: WB Saunders Company, 2000; 2606–2653.

217. Aronoff GR, Erbeck K, Brier ME. *Principles and Practice of Dialysis*, 2nd ed. Baltimore: Williams & Wilkins, 1999; 125.

218. Aronoff GR, Berns JS, Brier ME, Golper TA, Morrison G, Singer I, Swan SK, Benner WM. *Drug Prescribing in Renal Failure*, 4th ed. American College of Physicians, 1999.

219. Gaspari F, Mosconi L, Vigano G, Perico N, Torre L, Virotta G, Bertcchi C, Remuzzi G, Ruggenenti P. Measurement of GFR with a single intravenous injection of nonradioactive iothalamate. *Kidney In*t 1992; 41(4):1081–1084.

220. Sanger JJ, Kramer EL. Radionuclide quantitation of renal function. *Urol Radiol* 1992; 14(2):69–78.

29 Urologic Management in Spinal Cord Injury

Mandeep Singh
Inder Perkash
Donald R. Bodner

The annual incidence of spinal cord injury (SCI) is estimated to be between 30 and 50 per million and may actually be higher, because those with minimal impairment may not be included. There are approximately 250,000 individuals with SCI in the United States, and an additional about 11,000 new injuries occur each year. The urologic management of individuals with SCI has changed dramatically in the last century. Mortality related to renal complications after SCI has decreased from 80% for those injured in World War I, to 25% during the Korean War, to minimal numbers during the Vietnam War (1, 2). In the relatively short time since World War II, physicians have begun to better understand the management of the neurogenic bladder. With improvement in urodynamic techniques and a better understanding of their significance, along with the development of intermittent catheterization and newer-generation antibiotics, renal failure is no longer the leading cause of death in SCI patients. The leading causes of death today are respiratory failure, pulmonary emboli, septicemia, and neoplasms (3). Urologic causes of death, including urosepsis, genitourinary complications, and renal failure, have decreased to less than 6% with the adoption of regular urologic surveillance and proper bladder management (4, 5). For these favorable outcomes to be maintained, the urologist should be an integral member of the multidisciplinary SCI team, and lifelong routine urologic follow-up should be performed for the well-being of SCI patients.

The primary goal in the urologic management of the SCI patient is to maintain renal function. The main causes of renal failure include bladder sphincter dyssynergia, urinary tract infections (UTIs), and amyloidosis resulting from chronic pressure sores. Urologic testing identifies those patients at risk for upper urinary tract morbidity, and early intervention can prevent or minimize these complications. A basic understanding of the neuroanatomy and neurophysiology of micturition and the changes that occur after SCI is an essential foundation for individuals caring for patients with a neurogenic bladder.

NEUROLOGIC CONTROL OF MICTURITION

The spinal cord carries messages to and from the brain to accomplish voluntary control over micturition. Diseases of the central nervous system (CNS) affect control over micturition. The extent of bladder and sphincter function is also affected by the level of the spinal cord lesion. The micturition reflex center has been localized in the pontine-mesencephalic reticular formation in the brainstem. There are interconnections from the micturition reflex center to the frontal lobes and other areas in the cortex and subcortical areas. The reticular spinal tracts are in close proximity to the pyramidal tracts in the lateral columns of the spinal cord.

The portions of the brain involved with bladder control, urgency, and urge incontinence have been mapped using positron emission tomography (PET) scans as well as functional MRI (6–8). Bladder control depends on extensive regions of the brain. Urethral afferents mapped in the pariaqueductal gray are mapped in the insula, forming the basis of sensation, whereas the anterior cingulated gyrus provides monitoring and control, and voiding decisions are made in the prefrontal cortex (7).

Efferent fibers from the micturition center connect to the detrusor motor nuclei, located in the gray matter of the second through fourth spinal cord roots (9). The S3 and S4 segments have the primary parasympathetic enervation to the bladder via the pelvic splanchnic nerve. When activated, the primary role of the parasympathetic enervation to the bladder is detrusor contraction and bladder emptying. The S2 segment, via the pudendal nerve, provides the main enervation for voluntary control of the external striated urinary sphincter. Sympathetic enervation to the bladder and sphincter mechanism originates from the thoracolumbar (T12–L2) segments of the spinal cord and travels via the hypogastric ganglia to synapse in the bladder neck and bladder body. Stimulation of alpha fibers at the bladder neck and proximal urethra (smooth muscle urinary sphincter) causes the bladder neck and proximal urethra to contract, whereas stimulation of the beta fibers in the bladder body causes it to relax. The net effect of sympathetic stimulation is urine storage (Figure 29.1).

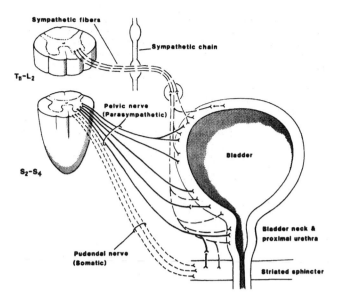

Figure 29.1 Schematic showing nerve enervation to the bladder for micturition and storage. (From Bodner DR. Urologic management of the spinal cord injured patient. In: Resnick MI, ed. *Current Trends in Urology,* Vol. 4. Baltimore: Williams and Wilkins, 31 [with permission].)

Intracranial lesions above the pons result in bladder hyper-reflexia, with preserved coordination of the bladder and urinary sphincter. Lesions below the pons, but above the conus, will often produce bladder sphincter dyssynergia. Lesions at the conus itself can render the bladder areflexic.

For micturition to occur in a neurologically intact individual, signals from the micturition center are sent to the spinal cord to initiate voiding. A voluntary relaxation of the external striated urinary sphincter is followed by the opening of the bladder neck, and then by reflex contractrion of the detrusor. The bladder empties with negligible residual. Once voiding is complete, bladder pressure decreases, the urethral pressure increases, and the bladder neck closes. External sphincter electromyographic activity increases with bladder filling. Because of the viscoelastic properties of the smooth muscle of the bladder, large volumes of urine can be accommodated at low pressure. There should be no leakage of urine during the storage phase, and the bladder pressure should remain low, without bladder contractions occurring. At a certain point, when it is again appropriate to void, the cycle repeats itself.

CHANGES WITH SPINAL CORD INJURY

SCI can result in significant changes to the function of the urinary bladder and the bladder outlet. Initially, after SCI, there is often a period of spinal shock when the bladder is areflexic. During this period, the patient is first managed with an indwelling catheter until medically stable, and intermittent catheterization is then instituted when possible. The bladder's function can be anticipated by the level of the injury. Lower thoracic and lumbar injuries that involve the conus may injure the parasympathetic nerve roots to the bladder and render the bladder areflexic. Injuries to the spinal cord above the conus frequently result in a bladder that will contract spontaneously and result in incontinence. Injuries below

the pons and above the conus are prone to bladder sphincter dyssynergia. When this occurs, the outlet (external striated sphincter and/or bladder neck) becomes spastic and closes as the bladder contracts to empty. The net effect is increased bladder pressure and incomplete bladder emptying. Over time, chronically elevated pressures in the bladder can lead to vesicoureteral reflux, hydronephrosis, and renal deterioration. Identifying and treating bladder sphincter dyssynergia, and maintaining low resting bladder pressures, is an important part of the urologic management of SCI patients.

Individuals with neurogenic bladder are prone to bacterial colonization of the urinary tract, especially when indwelling catheters are used, but even with intermittent catheterization or reflex voiding. These individuals are more susceptible to symptomatic UTIs. Basic urologic management requires an understanding of when it is appropriate to treat bacteria in the urinary tract and when reevaluation with urinary tract imaging and urodynamics is necessary to treat recurrent infections or unexplained autonomic dysreflexia.

UROLOGIC EVALUATION

Renal Imaging

Trauma severe enough to cause SCI can affect other organ systems, including the kidneys. For renal imaging, contrast-enhanced computerized tomography (CT) has become the current gold standard, replacing intravenous pyelography (IVP). CT scanning provides accurate staging of urologic and nonurologic injuries. Supplementary use of IVP, angiography, ultrasonography, nuclear scintigraphy, and magnetic resonance imaging (MRI) may be complementary to conventional modalities. If there is suspected urethral or bladder injury, a retrograde urethrogram along with a CT, conventional cystogram, or CT cystogram should be performed (10).

Baseline imagining of the urinary tract is performed after injury once the patient is medically stabilized. Follow-up upper tract imaging including ultrasound of the kidneys, ureters, and bladder should be obtained yearly and become part of the patient's annual history and physical examination. Routine follow-up studies also include blood urea nitrogen (BUN) and serum creatinine levels along with urinalysis and urine cultures. Nuclear renal scans and creatinine clearances are also regularly performed in some centers. Changes in upper tract imaging should be a signal to the urologist to reevaluate the bladder management being used. For example, the development of bladder or kidney stones in an individual who manages the bladder with an indwelling catheter would be a compelling argument for alternative, catheter-free bladder management. Understanding how the urinary bladder and sphincters work together is an important part of the urologic evaluation and is tested with urodynamics.

Urodynamic Evaluation

The urodynamic evaluation of the bladder and urinary sphincter is fundamental to the urologic evaluation of the SCI patient. Testing of the bladder and sphincter function should be done shortly after injury once the individual is out of the spinal shock period. Spinal shock can last for several days to several months following injury. Once the bladder begins to contract spontaneously, urodynamics should be obtained. In an individual with an injury to the conus or cauda equina, in which there is a lower motor neuron injury to the bladder (the bladder remains areflexic), or in an individual with an upper motor injury (above the conus), in which no spontaneous voiding has occurred by 3 months, baseline urodynamics should be obtained to evaluate the bladder and sphincter. This urodynamic analysis helps define the status of bladder (i.e., contractile bladder, areflexic bladder, and/or bladder sphincter dyssynergia). Without urodynamics in this circumstance, an individual can develop unrecognized hydronephrosis and upper tract pathology. Urodynamics should be repeated once the individual is voiding or at least 1 year after injury, and then as needed. Recurrent UTIs, the development of bladder or kidney stones, and unexplained autonomic dysreflexia are indications for repeating urodynamic tests along with upper tract imaging studies.

Urodynamics consist of a multitude of tests designed to evaluate the bladder and urinary sphincter during both bladder storage and bladder emptying. The most basic tests consist of cystometrics (CMG), external urinary sphincter electromyography (EMG), and uroflowmetry. These can be performed while simultaneously imaging the bladder and bladder outlet with fluoroscopy (videourodynamics), which is helpful in identifying and differentiating more complicated neurourologic voiding problems. The urine should be sterile prior to performing these tests to prevent bacteremia.

Cystometrics are performed using either CO_2 or water. Water tests are favored, because they are more reproducible. A small triple-lumen catheter (6–9 F) is placed in the bladder and used to fill the bladder and simultaneously record the pressures. Abdominal pressure is obtained simultaneously by placing a catheter in the rectum or vagina and recording pressure. True bladder pressure is then determined by subtracting the abdominal pressure from the recorded bladder pressure. Residual volume is noted along with bladder capacity and compliance, and any uninhibited bladder contractions are recorded. Patients are asked to tell when they have a feeling of bladder filling and a strong urge to urinate. The patient is then instructed to void. Male paraplegic and quadriplegic patients cannot stand and void, as ambulatory patients can. Gentle suprapubic tapping with the fingers can often elicit a bladder contraction, and voiding pressures can then be determined. Simultaneous blood pressure helps diagnose potential for autonomic dysreflexia (25).

In neurologically normal individuals, the first sensation of bladder filling occurs around 100 ml. A desire to void occurs when there is about 300 to 500 ml of fluid in the bladder. During filling, bladder pressures are generally around 20 cm of water. With fibrosis of the bladder, the pressure may rise quickly; these bladders are considered noncompliant. The bladder pressure during voiding is recorded. The residual bladder volume is recorded prior to beginning the study and after voiding. Residuals of less than 100 ml in patients with neurogenic bladder are generally acceptable.

Urinary sphincter activity is observed during bladder contraction. Simultaneous urinary sphincter contraction and detrusor contraction is found with detrusor-sphincter dyssynergia. Videourodynamics, when available, permit observation of the bladder and the outlet both during bladder storage and emptying and help to differentiate internal (smooth muscle of the bladder neck and proximal urethra) from external (striated muscle) sphincter dyssynergia.

Urethral Pressure Profile

The urethral pressure profile represents the lateral closure pressure along the length of the urethra. It is usually studied with a multichannel catheter. Profilometry with a pull-through catheter provides a graphic representation of the lateral pressure along the length of the urethra. The bladder is generally empty for these studies (11). For static urethral pressure profiles, a triple-lumen catheter is used, with one of the holes meant for sensing pressure positioned in the posterior urethra. (The first hole in the catheter is generally 1 cm from the tip of the catheter, to measure bladder pressure, and the second hole is placed laterally 10 cm distally, to measure pressure in the urethra.) In patients with SCI, increased urethral pressure, along with increased EMG activity during a rise in bladder pressure, is consistent with bladder sphincter dyssynergia.

Transrectal Linear Ultrasound

Bladder neck obstruction is easily visualized via transrectal linear sonography. Simultaneous cystometrics, along with transrectal linear ultrasonography, have the advantage over cine radiography of avoiding radiation. Secondary bladder neck obstruction, secondary to a ledge in patients with SCI, has been reported (12). The recognition of this obstruction may be important for explaining difficulties in intermittent catheterization. A coude tip catheter is most effective in this setting.

BLADDER MANAGEMENT

Every attempt must be made to achieve a balanced bladder. In this setting, the bladder contracts at relatively low pressures (less than 50 to 60 cm of water), and voiding results in low residuals (approximately 100 ml or less). For men, external condom catheters can be considered for urine collection. Care in using these devices must be taught to patients to ensure that the catheters are not applied too tightly and are sized properly. Problems can occur with external condom catheters. If the condom catheter falls off and clothing becomes wet, it may lead to skin breakdown and pressure sores. Catheters that are applied too tightly may lead to strangulation injuries. Individual sensitivity to adhesives used in some of the appliances may cause skin irritation and abrasions.

No external urinary collection devices for women are ideal, and alternative therapies include chronic catheters, anticholinergic medication with intermittent catheterization, botulinum toxin injection, bladder augmentation, and posterior sacral rhizotomies. These alternatives are considered when incontinence remains a problem for these individuals.

Recently, the Consortium for Spinal Cord Medicine produced evidence-based clinical practice guidelines regarding bladder management in adults with SCI. These guidelines are an excellent resource in the care of patients with SCI and bladder dysfunction (13).

Intermittent Catheterization

Intermittent catheterization is the preferred bladder management technique after acute injury, once the patient is medically stabilized. Catheterization should be performed at a frequency that keeps bladder residual below 400 cc. Individuals are generally started at a 4- to 6-hour frequency of catheterization. A sterile catheterization technique is performed by nursing personnel, but once an individual is able to perform self-catheterization at home, a clean technique is employed. Urine should be routinely cultured. The bladders of patients on intermittent catheterization, as well as those using chronic indwelling catheters, will be colonized, and cultures will show bacteriuria. Individuals should not routinely be treated with antibiotics for asymptomatic bacteriuria, because overtreatment leads to the emergence of resistant bacteria. Those signs and symptoms that may require treatment include an elevation in temperature, suprapubic or flank pain, new onset incontinence, increased spasticity, autonomic dysreflexia, cloudy urine with increased odor, malaise, lethargy, or sense of unease (14). An increased number of white blood cells in the urine (usually greater than 5 to 10 WBC/HPF) is associated with tissue penetration. Patients may need anticholinergics to have full continence in between catheterizations. If an individual has a symptomatic UTI, antibiotic therapy should be instituted based on prior culture and susceptibility testing, while awaiting new cultures (15, 16). If recurrent infections continue despite optimal clean intermittent catheterization technique, considerations should be given to instituting a sterile intermittent catheterization program (13).

Chronic Indwelling Catheters

Chronic indwelling catheters have the convenience of draining the bladder without requiring manual dexterity or an attendant to perform intermittent catheterization. An indwelling catheter does not have the risk of incontinence, as occurs when an external condom catheter falls off. However, indwelling catheters are associated with bladder stones, kidney stones, and UTIs. Concretions and calcifications can form on the balloon and break off into the bladder, forming a nidus for UTI and bladder stone formation. The urine becomes colonized with bacteria from chronic catheters. Although both indwelling catheterization and intermittent catheterization increase the risk of symptomatic lower tract infection, epididymitis, recurrent symptomatic UTI, and pyelonephritis seem to be elevated in relation to indwelling catheter use (17). Urethral trauma from pulling on the catheter, urethral erosion, strictures, bladder fibrosis, and a higher incidence of bladder cancer occur with the use of chronic indwelling catheters. Trauma to the urethra from the catheter can result in erosion of the urethra, thus leading to traumatic hypospadias formation. Patients should be encouraged to seek alternative methods of bladder management in an attempt to remain catheter free. For those individuals with indwelling catheters for more than 8–10 years, surveillance of the bladder should be performed routinely to rule out bladder tumor occurrence. Options for surveillance include cystoscopy, urine cytology, fluorescence in situ hybridization (FISH), and random bladder biopsy. Most of the patients would need anticholinergics to prevent upper tract changes.

Bladder Sphincter Dyssynergia

Bladder sphincter dyssynergia is a potential cause of renal failure in patients with SCI below the level of the micturition center in the pons and above the conus medularis. The striated sphincter becomes spastic, and instead of remaining open during micturition, it may close and block off the urinary stream (Figure 29.2).

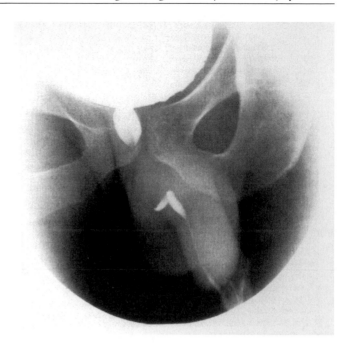

Figure 29.2 Voiding cystourethrogram consistent with detrusor–external sphincter dyssynergia. Note the closed external sphincter and dilated prostatic urethra.

Bladder sphincter dyssynergia results in high pressure voiding, inefficient bladder emptying, and increased postvoid residuals. If unrecognized, this can lead to bladder hypertrophy, vesicoureteral reflux, and upper tract deterioration. Urodynamics should be performed shortly after SCI once the patient is voiding spontaneously or within 3 months of injury to identify those at risk for bladder sphincter dyssynergia. Silent hydronephrosis has been reported as early as 6 months after SCI in patients who were not yet voiding and were thought to still be in spinal shock.

Pharmacologic Management of Bladder Sphincter Dyssynergia

The primary goal in the urologic management of the SCI patient is to maintain renal function. It has been shown that sustained high pressures in the bladder lead to upper tract damage. Bladder-relaxant drugs (anticholinergic, antimuscarinic, antispasmodic) are used to decrease bladder voiding pressure, reduce or eliminate reflex incontinence, reduce the frequency of intermittent catheterization, keep an individual dry between catheterizations, and decrease uninhibited contractions in individuals with chronic indwelling catheters.

The first line in the medical treatment of bladder sphincter dyssynergia is the use of anticholinergic medications (oxybutynin, propanthelene, darfenacin, solfenacin, trospium) to lower detrusor pressure, in combination with alpha blockers (phenoxybenzamine, prazosin, terazosin, doxazosin, alfuzosin, tamsulosin), which are used to lower outlet resistance by blocking smooth muscle alpha receptors at the bladder neck and proximal urethra. Complications of alpha blocker therapy include orthostatic hypotension. Depending on the clinical setting and urodynamic findings, pharmacologic management may be used in combination with reflex voiding or intermittent catheterization. When intermittent catheterization is used, anticholinergics are the primary adjunctive medications employed in an attempt to keep the individual dry between catheterizations. Side effects of anticholinergics include dry mouth, constipation, double vision, and occasionally confusion in older patients. The undesired side effects of the medications can lead an individual to become noncompliant in taking the anticholinergics.

Another treatment modality that has been used to treat detrusor sphincter dyssynergia is transurethral or transperineal injection of botulinum toxin. The toxin is injected directly into the sphincter mechanism and has been shown to be effective in decreasing urethral pressures and postvoid residual volumes (18). The toxin generally loses its effectiveness within 3 to 6 months, and repeat injections are usually necessary.

Botulinum toxin can also be injected into the bladder wall to treat overactive bladder in those on intermittent catheterization to achieve continence (19–21). A systematic literature review of eighteen articles evaluating the efficacy or safety of Botox in neurogenic detrusor overactivity concluded that Botox injected into the detrusor muscle provided clinically significant improvement in adults with neurogenic detrusor overactivity (NDO) and incontinence refractory to antimuscarinics (19). It was noted that the amount of Botox used was typically 300 U, injected at 1-cc volumes in thirty separate sites in the bladder, avoiding the trigone and dome (19). Kuo reported that quality of life satisfaction improved for urinary incontinence and bladder dysfunction in 78% of patients in one series with spinal cord lesions and detrusor sphincter dyssynergia who received detrusor botulinum toxin A injections (20). In another small series of nineteen patients, with a 6-year follow-up, fifteen patients (88.2%) were completely continent, and renal pelvis dilatation and vesicoureteral reflux were resolved in all cases (21). Apostolidis et al. reported no histologic changes in the urothelium of human overactive bladder following intradetrusor injections of botulinum neurotoxin type A for the treatment of neurogenic or idiopathic detrusor overactivity (22).

Surgical Management of Bladder Sphincter Dyssynergia

When pharmacologic management is insufficient or not tolerated, and in patients with limited hand function, transurethral sphincterotomy is considered (23). The sphincter can be cut with electrocautery at the 12 o'clock position to make the sphincter incompetent. Complications of the procedure include bleeding, incomplete destruction of the sphincter, and stricture formation. Impotence was observed more frequently when the sphincter was cut at the 5 and 7 o'clock positions. Today, impotence following transurethral sphincterotomy occurs only in a small percentage of patients. Following sphincterotomy, the patient uses an external condom catheter, and the risk for upper tract deterioration is lessened. Excellent long-term results have been reported using contact laser surgery for sphincterotomy, with few long-term complications and a low reoperation rate. Laser sphincterotomy is therefore the procedure of choice, depending upon the availability of laser equipment. Holmium laser (HO:YAG) has been used with minimal to no bleeding, both at surgery and perioperatively. The usual setting is 1.5 joules × 10 or 15 hertz (24–26).

As an alternative to sphincterotomy, the UroLume® prosthesis, a braided wire mesh stent, can be implanted in the urethra to hold the external sphincter open (Figure 29.3). The surgery required to place the stent is minimally invasive and reversible. Migration of the stent is possible until it is well epithelialized. Complications of stricture, significant bleeding, and impotence

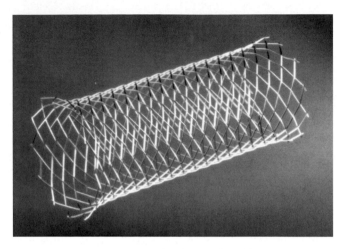

Figure 29.3 UroLume® stent. This is placed by cystoscopy to keep the external urinary sphincter open.

can be avoided (27). Several studies have been conducted on the use of different stents for the treatment of detrusor sphincter dyssynergia (28). Potential complications of urethral stents include stone encrustation, difficulty with stent removal, and tissue growth into the stent, causing obstruction.

Anterior Sacral Root Stimulation for Bladder Emptying

Electrical stimulation of the anterior sacral roots is an effective alternative for producing micturition on demand with low residuals in individuals with suprasacral spinal cord injuries (29). Posterior sacral rhizotomy abolishes reflex incontinence and increases bladder capacity and compliance. It also renders the rectum areflexic and can create serious problems with bowel evacuation. It has not been widely accepted in the United States. Bladder sphincter dyssynergia and autonomic dysreflexia originating from a bladder etiology are eliminated. Posterior sacral rhizotomy abolishes reflex erection and ejaculation in the male, along with any preserved sensation, and potential candidates should be counseled in this regard. Urination is achieved with poststimulus voiding (Figure 29.4). The bladder smooth muscle and striated urethral sphincter contract

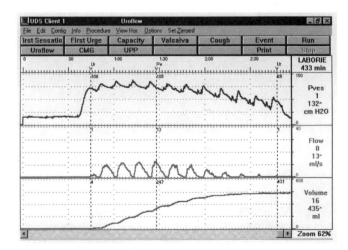

Figure 29.4 Vocare® anterior sacral root stimulation producing poststimulus voiding. The voiding pattern is interrupted, with urination occurring during the gaps in stimulation.

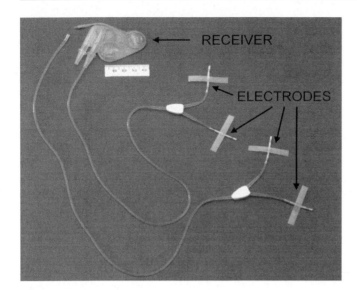

Figure 29.5 The components of the Vocare® anterior sacral root stimulator, showing the implanted receiver and extradural electrodes.

with electrical stimulation. When the stimulation is turned off, the external sphincter relaxes more quickly than the bladder, and post-stimulus voiding is achieved. By fine tuning the stimulating parameters of bursts and gaps, the controller is individualized to optimize voiding for each patient.

Ideal candidates for anterior sacral stimulation are female SCI patients who are incontinent despite medication and can self-transfer because they have to the potential to be continent and because they will not suffer from a loss of erections or ejaculation. The posterior sacral rhizotomy renders them continent, and the bladder is then emptied with electrical stimulation. The Vocare® (Finetech-Brindley) anterior sacral root stimulator (Figure 29.5) has been extensively implanted in patients in Europe and around the world. The first Finetech-Brindley anterior sacral root stimulator was implanted in the United States at the Cleveland Veterans Administration Medical Center in 1992. Since that time, over 100 patients in the United States with SCI have had the device implanted. UTIs have decreased, and upper tracts have been preserved using this technique. A laminectomy is required. Vesicoureteral reflex is improved or eliminated in nearly all patients implanted with the Vocare® device. Combined posterior and anterior sacral root nerve stimulation is also under investigation in an attempt to eliminate the need for posterior sacral rhizotomy (30).

Reconstructive Surgery and Urinary Diversion

For small fibrotic bladders, augmentation cystoplasty can be performed to increase bladder capacity and decrease bladder storage pressure. Individuals who are considered for this procedure should have adequate hand function to perform intermittent catheterization of the augmented bladder, if required. When combined with a continent abdominal stoma, bladder neck closure may be required to prevent incontinence.

If it is not feasible to augment the native bladder, a continent urinary diversion can be considered using a segment of bowel for the urinary pouch. Again, adequate hand function is required for

catheterization. Alternatively, when primary methods of bladder management have failed, diversion of the urine from the bladder can be performed via an intestinal segment, most commonly the ileal conduit.

AUTONOMIC DYSREFLEXIA

A chapter on the urologic management of SCI patients is not complete without a discussion of autonomic dysreflexia. Patients with SCI at T6 and above are prone to autonomic dysreflexia, which is characterized by unopposed sympathic discharge that results in severe hypertension, sweating, piloerection, and bradycardia. Lesions above T5 lead to sympathetic denervation of the splanchnic bed, which is supplied by the greater splanchnic nerve. Visceral activity, such as a distended bladder or full rectum, produces peripheral vasoconstriction that is normally countered by vasodilation in the splanchnic bed through the greater splanchnic nerve. The baroreceptors in the carotid body sense the hypertension and attempt to compensate by stimulating the vagus nerve, which leads to bradycardia. Treatment consists of elevating the bed and eliminating the noxious stimulus. If the bladder is distended, draining the bladder or irrigating a plugged catheter is often sufficient to stop the reflex. Sublingual nifedipine helps to reduce the blood pressure when required. The use of a nitroglycerine patch is also effective in lowering the blood pressure. When autonomic dysreflexia occurs during procedures in the operating room, those medications to lower blood pressure preferred by the anesthesiologist can be administered. Spinal anesthesia is also effective in preventing the response. Significant long term relief in autonomic dysreflexia (AD) has been reported following a successful transurethral sphincterotomy (TURS) (25).

CONCLUSION

Lifelong routine urologic follow-up remains a key component to the well-being of individuals with SCI. Follow-up every 6 to 12 months helps to ensure that renal function is preserved. Ideally, the urologist is part of a multidisciplinary team, and follow-up can be performed in an SCI unit during the annual physical examination. Urinalysis and urine cultures are routinely followed, along with a renal panel. Upper tract imaging studies are repeated yearly. Urodynamics are obtained more frequently initially until the patient is stabilized and then as needed. For patients experiencing urologic complications or problems, such as recurrent bladder infections, autonomic dysreflexia, or stone formation, repeat urodynamics should be performed, and a change in bladder management should be considered. Bladder management should be individualized to optimize the patient's personal preferences and well-being. For example, reflex voiding with an external collection device may not be the best choice for a young paraplegic male who wants to wear short pants during the summer and have no collection device on his leg. In this setting, intermittent catheterization and anticholinergics may be preferred. Preserving renal function is the primary goal of urologic care. Finding a bladder management regime that is best accepted and least offensive to an individual will produce the greatest likelihood of success.

References

1. Donnelly J, Hackler RH, Bunts RC. Present urologic status of the World War II paraplegic: 25-year follow-up: comparison with the status of the 20-year Korean War paraplegic and the 5-year Vietnam paraplegic. *J Urol* 1972; 108:558.

2. Borges PM, Hackler RH. The urologic status of the Vietnam War paraplegic: a 15 year prospective follow-up. *J Urol* 1982; 127:710.

3. Samsa GP, Patrick CH, Feussner JR. Long-term survival of veterans with traumatic spinal cord injury. *Arch Neurol* 1993; 50:904–914.

4. Hartkopp A, Bronnum-Hansen H, Seidenshchnur AM, Biering-Sorensen F. Survival and cause of death after traumatic spinal cord injury: a long-term epidemiological survey from Denmark. *Spinal Cord* 1997; 35:76–85.

5. National Spinal Cord Injury Statistical Center. *Spinal Cord Injury: Facts and Figures at a Glance.* Birmingham, AL.

6. Takao T, Tsujimura A, Miyagawa Y, Kiuchi H, et al. Brain responses during the first desire to void: a positron emission tomographic study. *Int J Urol* 2008; 15(8):724–728.

7. Griffith D, Tadic SC. Bladder control, urgency, and urge incontinence: evidence from functional brain imaging. *Neurourol Urodyn* 2008; 27(6):466–474.

8. Griffith D, Tadic SC, Schaefer W, Resnick NW. Cerebral control of the bladder in normal and urge-incontinent women. *Neuroimage* 2007; 37(1):1–7.

9. Bradley WE, Teague CT. Spinal cord organization of micturition reflex afferents. *Exp Neurol* 1968; 22:504.

10. Kuan JK, Porter J, Wessells H. Imaging for genitourinary trauma. *AUA Update Series* 2006; 25(4):21–32.

11. Brown M, Wickham J. The urethral pressure profile. *Br J Urol* 1969; 41:211.

12. Perkash I, Friedland GW. Real-time gray-scale transrectal linear array ultrasound in urodynamic evaluation. *Semin Urol* 1985; 3(1):49–59.

13. Linsenmeyer TA, Bodner DR, Creasey, GH, et al. Bladder management for adults with spinal cord injury: a clinical practice guideline for healthcare providers. *J Spinal Cord Med* 2006; 29(5):527–573.

14. National Institute on Disability and Rehabilitation Research Consensus Statement. The prevention and management of urinary tract infections among people with spinal cord injuries. *J Am Paraplegia Soc* 1992; 15:194–204.

15. Garner JS, Jarvis WR, Emori TG. CDC definitions for nosocomial infections. In: Olmsted RN, ed. *APIC Infection Control and Applied Epidemiology: Principles and Practice.* St. Louis: Mosby, 1996:A1–A20.

16. Mylotte JM, Kahler L, Graham R, et al. Prospective surveillance for antibiotic resistant organisms in patients with spinal cord injury admitted to an acute rehabilitation unit. *Am J Infect Control* 2000; 28: 291–297.

17. Weld KJ, Dmochowski, RR. Effect of bladder management on urological complications in spinal cord–injured patients. *J Urol* 2000; 163:768–772.

18. Schurch B, Hauri D, Rodic B, et al. Botulinum-A toxin as a treatment of detrusor sphincter dyssynergia: a prospective study in 24 spinal cord injury patients. *J Urol.* 1996; 155:1023–1029.

19. Karsenty G, Denys P, Amarenco G, De Seze M, et al. Botulinum toxin A (Botox) intradetrusor injections in adults with neurogenic detrusor overactivity/neurogenic overactive bladder: a systematic literature review. *Eur Urol* 2008; 53(2):240–241.

20. Kuo HC. Therapeutic satisfaction and dissatisfaction in patients with spinal cord lesions and detrusor sphincter dyssynergia who received detrusor botulinum toxin A injection. *Urology* 2008; 72(5):1056–1060.

21. Giannantoni A, Mearini E, Del Zingaro M, Porena M. Six-year follow-up of Botulinum Toxin A intradetrusorial injections in patients with refractory neurogenic detrusor overactivity: clinical and urodynamic results. *Eur Urol* 2008.

22. Apostolidis A, Jacques TS, Freeman A, Kalsi V, et al. *Eur Urol* 2008;53(6):1245–1253.

23. Perkash I. Detrusor-sphincter dyssynergia and dyssynergia responses: recognition and rationale for early modified transurethral sphincterotomy in complete spinal cord injury lesions. *J Urol* 1978; 120:469.

24. Perkash I. Contact laser sphincterotomy: further experiences and longer follow-up. *Spinal Cord* 1996; 34:227.

25. Perkash I. Transurethral sphincterotomy provides significant relief in autonomic dysreflexia in spinal cord injured male patients: long-term follow up results. *J Urol* 2007;177(3):1026–1029.

26. Perkash I. Donald Munro Lecture 2003. Neurogenic bladder: past, present, and future. *J Spinal Cord Med* 2004; 27(4):383–386.

27. Chancellor MB, et al. Sphincteric stent versus external sphincterotomy in spinal cord injured med: prospective randomized multicenter trial. *J Urol* 1999; 161:1893.

28. Denys PI, Thiry-Escudie N, Ayoub A, et al. Urethral stent for the treatment of detrusor sphincter dyssynergia: evaluation of the clinical, urodynamic, endoscopic, and radiological efficacy after more than 1 year. *J Urol* 2004; 172(2):605–607.

29. Creasey GH, Ho CH, Triolo RJ, et al. Clinical applications of electrical stimulation after spinal cord injury. *J Spinal Cord Med* 2004; 27(4):365–375.

30. Kirkham AP, Knight SL, Craggs MD, et al. Neuromodulation through sacral nerve roots 2 to 4 with a Finetech-Brindley sacral posterior and anterior root stimulator. *Spinal Cord* 2002; 40(6):272–281.

30 Urolithiasis in Spinal Cord Disorders

Daniel J. Culkin
Ikechukwu Oguejiofor

The spinal cord injured (SCI) patient is unique and presents the clinician with significant challenges. This is especially true regarding renal and urinary tract stone disease. Detection and treatment of urinary tract stones has seen great advances in recent years. In addition, better understanding of micturition physiology and the availability of less invasive treatments have greatly reduced the incidence and recurrence of stone disease and associated morbidity in this population (1, 2). This chapter reviews urolithiasis in the SCI population; pathogenesis of stone formation; and the complications, diagnosis, treatment, and prevention of stone disease.

HISTORY OF UROLITHIASIS IN THE SCI POPULATION

The mortality of SCI patients following World War I was very high, as represented by the fact that none of these patients was alive at the beginning of World War II (3). However, SCI survival increased to 80% for post–World War II and Korean War veterans. Renal disease, including urosepsis, renal failure, and stone disease accounted for 40% of the mortality in this post–World War II SCI population (4, 5). Continued advances in the care of these patients were also evident in the 15-year follow-up analysis of Vietnam War SCI veterans. This data showed that, although the overall mortality of SCI patients stayed the same, deaths from renal disease decreased.

Later in the twentieth century, several advancements further reduced morbidity and improved survival of the SCI stone patient. These included a greater understanding of lower urinary tract physiology and dysfunction, as well as developments in the technology to identify lower urinary tract pathology. The introduction of urodynamics allowed for early detection of lower urinary tract dysfunction, reestablishment of low-pressure storage and emptying, and prevention of upper tract deterioration (1). The prevention of infections, such as cystitis and pyelonephritis, and the introduction of ureteral stents allowed the emergent drainage of obstructed and/or infected urinary tracts. Also, the development of broad-spectrum antibiotics, as

well as antibiotics with excellent sensitivity to genitourinary tract organisms, has decreased the incidence of life-threatening urosepsis. A 2006 report from the National Spinal Cord Injury Database shows that the causes of death that appear to have the greatest impact on reduced life expectancy for the SCI population are pneumonia, pulmonary emboli, and septicemia, as compared to renal failure in decades past (6).

Other advancements in endourology have obviated the need for open surgery and facilitated emergent drainage, thereby greatly reducing morbidity and mortality. Anticholinergics and clean intermittent catheterization allow low-pressure storage and emptying (1). Finally, improved imaging techniques, especially the helical computed tomography (CT) scan, allow prompt and accurate diagnosis (7–9).

These advancements have improved the care of both SCI and ambulatory patients with stones. The impact of these advances can be seen by a shift in the presentation of SCI patients with advanced stone disease with renal deterioration, renal failure, and high mortality to patients with survival rates approaching that of the ambulatory population (2).

NATURAL HISTORY AND EPIDEMIOLOGY

There has not been an overall incidence study of SCI in the United States since the 1970s. However, the estimated annual incidence of SCIs in the United States is 40 per million, which is extrapolated to 11,000 SCIs per year (6). As of June 2006, approximately 253,000 people in America are living with SCI with a range of between 225,000 and 296,000 people (6). The average age of injury is 38 years (6). Although the total number of patients is low, the number of years of impairment is high. The male-to-female ratio is 4:1 (6). Motor vehicle accidents account for the majority of postwar SCI, followed by acts of violence, falls, and injuries from recreational sports. Sports injuries have decreased over time, whereas injuries due to falls have increased. Acts of violence caused 13.3% of spinal cord injuries prior to 1980, and peaked between 1990 and 1999 at 24.8%, before declining to only 13.7% since 2000 (6).

The incidence of stone formation in the general population is 0.4%, with an incidence of 0.6% and 0.18% in men and women, respectively (10). The prevalence is 10.1% among males and 5.8% among females (10). The average recurrence rate is 30% to 40%, with 30% of stone formers having more than three recurrences (10).

A longitudinal study by Chen et al. showed that 7% of SCI patients develop kidney stones within 10 years of injury, but the greatest risk period is within the first 3 months after injury (11). A positive correlation between severity of injury, bladder instrumentation for emptying, and kidney stones was demonstrated after the first year postinjury (11).

The incidence of stone disease in SCI patients remains unchanged in the last 25 years (12).

Historical reports suggested that renal calculi in SCI patients was mostly composed of struvite stones (magnesium ammonium phosphate) and carbonate apatite stones, likely as a result of urea splitting organisms and chronic bacteriuria (13). Struvite stones have a tendency to form staghorn calculi, and they are of great concern. They usually require multiple procedures to rid the patient of the stones. Contemporary work by Matlaga et al. demonstrated metabolic etiology as the most common cause of renal calculi in patients with neurogenic bladder (14). The shift in the composition of stones in neurogenic bladder patients is most likely due to better lower urinary tract management, for example clean intermittent catheterization. All SCI patients need metabolic workups with stone analysis in order to institute stone prevention.

Despite great advances made in the care of SCI patients and in the management of urolithiasis, there is still significant morbidity and mortality associated with stone disease. Renal deterioration due to vesicoureteral reflux, stasis, obstruction, and infection are possible complications of stone disease in general. The goal in SCI patients should be prevention of stone disease. A high index of suspicion is needed for early diagnosis and definitve management.

RISK FACTORS

Emphasis on prevention of stones requires identification and elimination of risk factors that lead to stone disease. Risk factors include immobilization, impaired bladder function, alkaline urine, chronic indwelling catheterization, the level and completeness of injury, chronic UTIs, and the presence of foreign bodies (see Table 30.1).

Immobilization following injury predisposes SCI patients to immbolization hypercalciuria. Hypercalciuria occurs approximately 2–3 days postinjury and normalizes in about 5–8 months (15). This can contribute to the formation of calcium stones.

Impaired bladder function is a risk for the development of both bladder and kidney stones. Neuropathic bladders can lead to urinary stasis, high-pressure bladder for both storage and/or emptying, vesicoureteral reflux, and hydronephrosis (16). Urinary stasis due to poor bladder emptying will lead to bacterial colonization and infection. Urodynamics can identify those patients at risk for bladder dysfunction and allow the initiation of early bladder management.

Alkaline urine predisposes one to the formation of magnesium ammonium phosphate and calcium phosphate stones. Infections produced by urease-producing organisms create alkaline urine. Magnesium ammonium phosphate and calcium phosphate stones form in alkaline urine because of their high pKa value (17).

Bladder management methods also affect the risk of stone formation. Chronic indwelling catheter management of the bladder carries a substantially increased risk of stone formation and renal deterioration (18). The risk is independent of sex, age, and level of injury (19). Suprapubic or urethral catheterization has no effect on this risk (19). Clean intermittent catheterization (CIC) shows the least risk of stone formation, at approximately 0.2% per year (19).

The level and completeness of the SCI may affect stone development. There is debate over whether upper tract stone formation is associated with the level of SCI (20). The use of chronic indwelling catheters (i.e., urethral Foley and/or suprapubic tube urinary diversion) is not uncommon in those patients who do not have use of their hands and fingers. However, these catheters may potentiate stone development. It is not surprising that a patient with a suprasacral cord lesion has a 67% chance of developing a stone (21).

Because tetraplegic SCI patients typically have difficulties with independent living, they cannot perform decatheterization strategies such as CIC or use external fitting catheters. Spontaneous voiding between catheterization can be problematic with CIC. Difficulties with external fitting catheters include chronic penile skin changes, catheter dislodgment, and autonomic dysreflexia. For these reasons, a suboptimal form of lower urinary tract drainage, such as chronic indwelling catheters, may be utilized. Chronic indwelling catheters lead to recurrent bacteriuria, UTIs, and, eventually, stones.

ETIOLOGIES OF STONE FORMATION

Theories of Stone Formation

There are four theories to explain the formation of a urinary calculus. These include supersaturation, crystallization or nucleation, inhibitor absence, and anatomic abnormalities. Some or all of these processes contribute to the development of a clinically significant stone (Table 30.2).

The *supersaturation theory* is based on the binding of salts, which occurs after a certain concentration is obtained. A compound's thermodynamic solubility product (ksp) defines the

---

Table 30.1 Risk Factors for Stones

Alkaline urine
Recurrent urinary tract infections
Neurogenic bladder
Level and extent of injury

Table 30.2 Theories of Stone Formation

Supersaturation
Crystallization/nucleation
Reduction of inhibitors
Anatomical abnormalities

saturation of a compound in a solution. The ksp of a compound is equal to the product of a pure chemical in equilibrium between a solid and solvent in solution. If the salt concentration is less than the ksp, then the compound remains in solution. However, if the salt concentration exceeds the ksp, then the compound precipitates. Temperature and the pH of a solution also affect solubility.

The *crystallization* or *nucleation theory* states that when ions or molecules in a dissociated state bind, crystals form. These crystals cluster to form lattice structures. Crystals are nucleated from preexisting structures, epithelial cells, cellular debris, red blood cell cast, and other crystals. These crystals grow by aggregation. Epitaxy is a form of crystallization in which one type of crystal aggregates around the lattice of a different crystal (2, 22).

Inhibitors are substances that modify or alter crystal growth, thus preventing stone formation. Although urine may be supersaturated with a salt, these inhibitors can prevent stone formation. These molecules work by forming complexes with active surface compounds, which reduces the binding of calcium to oxalate. Citrate is the most important urinary stone inhibitor (23). Magnesium, pyrophosphate, nephrocalcin, glycosamine, RNA fragments, and Tamm-Horsfall glycoproteins are other important stone formation inhibitors (23). The absence or reduction of these inhibitors can aid in the production of stone formation.

Although crystals may form, they generally do not become very large, and they "wash out" before they become clinically significant, because of their short transit time within the urinary tract. However, an anatomic or functional abnormality can cause an obstruction to the flow of urine, and thus the retention of urinary crystals. These crystals anchor to epithelium and cause further crystals to aggregate into stones.

The clinically evident stones have gone through several processes: beginning as ions in solution, they become supersaturated and more concentrated. Once their concentration exceeds their solubility, they form crystals and become a nidus for nucleation, aggregation, and further growth. If inhibitors are present, stone formation may be prevented. Conversely, if there is an absence or reduction in key inhibitors in the urine, then further growth may occur.

Pathophysiology of Stone Formation in SCI Patients

Two phases of stone development follow SCI. The first phase occurs within the first 3 months following the injury (11). This corresponds to the period following injury when the patient is immobile. These are usually calcium stones. Immobility causes bone demineralization and an increase in calcium turnover and excretion, leading to hypercalciuria. The hypercalciuric state may lead to precipitation of calcium stones in the urine.

The second phase of stone disease occurs after the acute period, when deterioration of bladder function occurs. Stasis of urine can lead to high postvoid residuals, high voiding pressures, vesicoureteral reflux, and recurrent UTIs, all of which may cause urinary stones.

Stone Classification

Stones are classified into various types, including de novo stones and stones that antedate the SCI. The chemical composition, as well as the location of stones and the various metabolic and nonmetabolic causes of stone formation, is briefly discussed. (Refer to Table 30.3.)

Table 30.3 Stone Classifications

COMPOSITION	MORPHOLOGY	LOCATION
Calcium	Partial staghorn	Kidney
Uric acid	Complete staghorn	Bladder
Cystine		Calyceal
Struvite		Ureteropelvic junction
Matrix		
Other		

Calcium Stones

Calcium stones are heterogenous in composition and pathophysiology (24). Calcium oxalate and calcium phosphate are the most frequently encountered compounds. Hypercalciuria, hypercalcemia, and hyperoxaluria are three common metabolic disorders that lead to calcium stone formation.

Hypercalciuria

This common metabolic abnormality is encountered in 60% of stone formers in the ambulatory population (24) and also occurs in the SCI population. There are several metabolic causes of hypercalciuria that lead to stone formation. *Absorptive hypercalciuria* is caused by an increased intestinal calcium absorption. This causes an increase in renal filtered calcium and produces hypercalciuria. Another problem often encountered is that renal calcium loss can produce a hypocalcemiac state, which causes a secondary hyperparathyroidism. Parathyroid hormone causes intestinal absorption and bone resorption of calcium, which leads to further calcium wasting and hypercalciuria. *Resorptive hypercalciuria* is caused by excessive bone resorption of calcium, primarily from hyperparathyroidism. A *renal phosphate leak* creates hyperphosphaturia, which can produce the excess $1,25\text{-}(OH)_2$-vitamin D that produces hypercalciuria (24). Citrate is the most important inhibitor of calcium binding to oxalate and phosphate, because citrate complexes with calcium ions in the urine. Metabolic acidosis and hypokalemia, not uncommon in clinical presentations, can cause hypocitriuria (24).

Hypercalcemia produces a 33% chance of developing a renal stone (25). Hypercalcemia is caused by hyperparathyroidism, sarcoidosis, steroids, malignancy, idiopathic causes, and immobilization (26). Immobilization is the second most common cause of stone disease in the SCI population. Immobilization causes the increased bone resorption of calcium, which, in turn, increases renal filtration. This creates hypercalciuria and the precipitation of calcium oxalate and calcium phosphate stones.

Hyperoxaluria

Hyperoxaluria leads to calcium oxalate formation by increasing the urinary saturation of calcium oxalate (24). Primary hyperoxaluria is caused by an autosomal recessive disorder in oxalate biosynthesis that causes an increase in the hepatic production of oxalate. Secondary hyperoxaluria (i.e., enteric oxaluria) is caused by intestinal hyperabsorption of oxalate (24). Only this condition is clinically significant in the SCI population. It is caused by intestinal malabsorption of bile acids and fats. The bile acids and fats within the lumen of the bowel bind to calcium, hence reducing the amount of free calcium left to bind to oxalate in the bowel lumen. This will lead to increased oxalate absorbtion from the intestine and excretion in the urine. Oxalate complexes with calcium within the renal tubules, precipitates, and aggregates to form stones.

Uric Acid Stones

Uric acid stones are produced in acidic urine (i.e., pH below 5.5). The pH is less than the dissociation constant of uric acid in acidic urine, thus causing an increase in undissociated uric acid and leading to uric acid stone formation. Gout, myeloproliferative disorders, and chemotherapy are common causes of these stones. They are radiolucent on plain X-ray but can be visualized on CT scan. Once again, this metabolic abnormality is usually coincidental with SCI but may be of clinical significance.

Cystine Stones

An autosomal recessive disorder causes the abnormal transport of cystine. This defect in cystine transport causes cystinuria. Cystine crystals are usually hexagonal in shape. They are generally present in young children and appear as multiple stones or a staghorn calculus on radiography. They appear as a coincidental abnormality in the SCI patient.

Struvite Stones

Struvite stones are infectious stones composed of magnesium ammonium phosphate. Struvite stones are common stones seen in the SCI population, and they are caused by urease-producing bacteria. The most common are *Proteus, Pseudomonas, Klebsiella, Providentia, E. coli, Staphylococcus epidermis,* and *Ureaplasm* (17). Urease catalyzes the breakdown of urea and water to ammonium and bicarbonate, thus leading to very alkaline urine:

$$NH_2—CO—NH_2 + H_2O + (urease) \rightarrow 2NH_4 + HCO_3$$

The bicarbonate produces alkaline urine having a pH level generally greater than 7.2 (23). Alkaline urine facilitates the precipitation and crystallization of magnesium ammonium phosphate, calcium carbonate, and calcium phosphate (17). Struvite stones develop following a UTI, which causes tissue damage and inflammatory debris. This serves as a nidus for stone precipitation and facilitates further stone growth.

Chronic indwelling catheters lead to struvite stones because they cause the bacterial colonization of urine. Dysfunctional voiding and poor emptying can lead to urinary stasis and large postvoid residuals, which can also enhance bacteria growth, infections, and bladder calculi. If the patient has concomitant vesicoureteral reflux or high voiding pressures, the upper urinary tract can be seeded with these bacteria, causing upper tract infections and subsequent renal damage. Struvite stones generally have

bacteria within the interstices of the stone. Once a struvite stone forms, it can continue to progress until it forms a staghorn.

Matrix Stones

Matrix calculi are composed of coagulated mucoids with little crystalline component. They are predominantly found in individuals with recurrent infections of urease-producing organisms. They are radiolucent and may be mistaken for uric acid stones, although the association with alkaline urine and infection is certainly helpful in this distinction. These stones, because of their lack of crystalline structure and proteinaceous texture, are not amenable to extracorporeal techniques and usually require endourologic interventions, such as percutaneous nephrolithotomy and extraction.

MORPHOLOGY AND LOCATION

Staghorn Calculus

The term "staghorn" describes the appearance of the stone on radiograph. A staghorn calculus occupies the renal pelvis with an extension into two or more infundibula; these may be partial or complete (27). See Figure 30.1. Staghorns are commonly composed of struvite stones.

Bladder Calculus

Bladder stones are seen in endemic underdeveloped areas of the world and are caused by malnutrition (23). In developed countries, they are caused by bladder outlet obstruction and/or the presence of a foreign body. The obstruction in an SCI patient

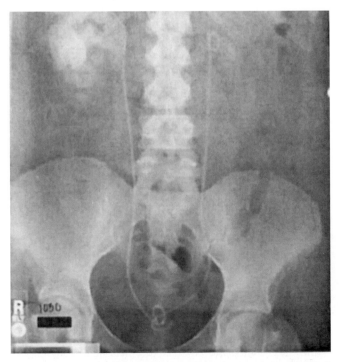

Figure 30.1   KUB film showing right staghorn calculus and left renal calculus.

may be functional, caused by a neuropathic bladder, or occasionally pieces of a catheter (such as the balloon) may be retained, thus providing a nidus for stone formation. An indwelling Foley may act as a foreign body. Bladder stones can also originate from stones in the upper urinary tract and are usually uric acid or struvite (23). These stones provide a persistent supply of bacteria and, if not removed, may predispose a patient to stones in the upper urinary tract.

Diverticular Calyceal Stones

The renal calyx diverticulum is a transitional, lined, cystic cavity that abuts and may communicate with the renal calyx through a diverticular neck. These diverticula may drain poorly, leading to bacterial colonization and possibly to infections that predispose one to stone formation. Even though approximately 10% of all calyceal diverticula contain stones, this is an unusual finding and should be considered coincidental rather than primarily related to the SCI.

CLINICAL PRESENTATION

A lack of familiarity with the SCI population patterns of presentation in stone disease may lead to delays or errors in diagnosis and management that could prove to be morbid and sometimes even lethal. Symptoms related to stones in the SCI population vary according to the level and degree of completeness of the injury (28).

In the ambulatory population, an obstructing stone can produce acute renal colic or intense spasmodic pain located in the flank or ipsilateral abdomen. Stones obstruct in four places in the urinary tract: the renal calyces, the ureteropelvic junction, the ureter where it crosses the iliac vessels, and the ureterovesical junction. Each of these locations has a typical referred pain: flank, side, lower quadrant, and testicle or labia, respectively. The ambulatory patient usually complains of the inability to find a comfortable position. Gross hematuria and/or UTI may also coexist.

However, patients with sensory deficits from SCI have subtle symptoms (2). These patients may or may not have pain, or they may present with nausea and vomiting, which can be mistaken for gastrointestinal (GIT) disease (2). They may have bacteriuria and UTI that are refractory to antibiotics (2). The refractory UTI is the most common presentation (16), and symptoms may include fever, tachycardia, hypotension, tachypnea, and abdominal and/or flank tenderness. A palpable flank mass indicating pyonephrosis and possible xanthogranulomatous pyelonephritis may occur (26). The clinical presentation is quite variable and subtle. An SCI patient may only perceive fatigue and anorexia without any localizing symptoms. A high index of suspicion is frequently required to make the diagnosis by radiologic assessment.

DIAGNOSIS

An organized and systematic workup is the key to a timely and proper diagnosis. This begins with a thorough history and physical examination including vital signs. The classic signs of upper urinary tract obstruction are rarely present in the SCI population, and only vague systemic signs and symptoms may be present. Complaints that may be voiced include "not feeling quite right,"

having a loss of appetite, or having a UTI that does not clear with antibiotics. The appropriate laboratory and radiographic studies will substantiate clinical suspicions.

Laboratory Tests

Laboratory testing should include serum electrolytes, blood urea nitrogen (BUN), creatinine (Cr), a complete blood count (CBC), and urinalysis (UA) with dipstick analysis and a microscopic assessment of spun sediment. An elevated white blood count with a shift to the left indicates the possibility of a serious infection. The UA may identify very alkaline urine (i.e., pH 8), which could indicate an infection with a urea-splitting organism. Elevated BUN and Cr indicate the possibility of renal insufficiency from post-renal obstruction. This laboratory assessment is an important first step in selecting the indicated imaging test to confirm the diagnosis of stone.

Electrolyte abnormalities must be identified and corrected. These can occur in association with vomiting, diarrhea, and fluid overhydration. The presence of white blood cells (WBC), red blood cells (RBC), or bacteria in the urine are also important in prioritizing intervention and/or diagnostics because infection and obstruction place the SCI patient at risk for urosepsis and mandate immediate drainage of the obstruction. Hematuria also suggests that a stone is present.

Imaging

The goal of imaging is to identify pathology (i.e., stone), to evaluate the size and location of the stone, and to evaluate the presence and degree of obstruction (17). Several radiographic tools are commonly used to diagnose and treat urolithiasis (Table 30.4).

X-Rays

The KUB film or flat plate is an X-ray that includes the kidneys, ureters, and bladder. It is excellent for identifying calcific densities that may overlie the urinary tract. However, this is a two-dimensional picture, and another type of imaging is required to localize the calcification to the urinary tract. Also, radiolucent stones made up of uric acid, matrix, or xanthine may not be visualized. Struvite and cystine stones are also less dense and may be obscured by GI material within the colon.

Intravenous Pyelogram (IVP)

The IVP has traditionally been the imaging test of choice for the diagnosis of stones. It provides a gross assessment of renal function and includes a vascular, nephrographic, and excretory phase.

Table 30.4   Radiographic Imaging
Flat plate (KUB) of abdomen
Intravenous pyelogram
Helical CT scan
Ultrasound
Retrograde pyelogram

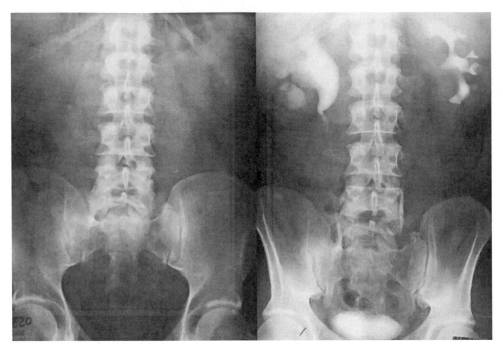

Figure 30.2 An IVP with a stone at the right UPJ and a stone in the left kidney on the scout film. There is obstruction to flow with hydronephrosis on the left on the 10-minute film.

It provides confirmation of a calcified stone within the collecting system, with the addition of oblique films or the identification of a radiolucent filling defect that may represent a uric acid stone. This does require the intravenous infusion of a contrast agent with potential nephrotoxicity. Contraindications include renal insufficiency and allergy to the contrast. Patients at risk can undergo chemoprevention for anaphylaxis with oral steroids and Benadryl®, with close monitoring for allergy. (See Figure 30.2.)

Computed Tomography (CT)

Unenhanced helical CT is an excellent imaging tool that offers the advantages of rapid scan time, safety, high accuracy, minimal invasiveness, and the identification of radiolucent stones. Many experts believe that this is the modality of choice for diagnosing stones in the acute setting. It can be used with patients who are allergic to contrast. It has an 81% chance of visualization, 100% sensitivity, and 94% specificity (7). The noncontrast films can identify extra-urinary structures (7). Perhaps its greatest utility is that it does not require intravenous infusion of contrast and also has the diagnostic capability to visualize gastrointestinal tract diseases and other pathologies within the retroperitoneum and abdomen. For this reason, in emergent and urgent clinical situations, it has become the diagnostic test of choice (see Figures 30.3 and 30.4).

Ultrasonography

Ultrasound is a good screening tool that is noninvasive, although it is limited by its low specificity. It can demonstrate renal and bladder stones but is less effective with ureteral stones. It has minimal toxicity, and it is useful in identifying hydronephrosis

and perinephric fluid collection, as found in perirenal abscesses (see Figures 30.5 and 30.6).

Retrograde Pyelography

Pyelography uses nonionic contrast and can be given to patients with contrast allergies. It is performed at the time of cystoscopy and is used to define the urinary tract anatomy. This approach offers the advantage of confirmation of the stone and its location and simultaneous relief of obstruction or removal of stone with endourological techniques.

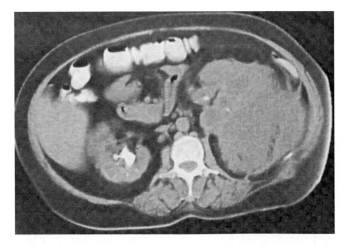

Figure 30.3 CT scan demonstrates a xanthogranulomatous pyelonephritis of the left kidney. This kidney shows chronic inflammatory changes with a stone in the center of the inflammatory process.

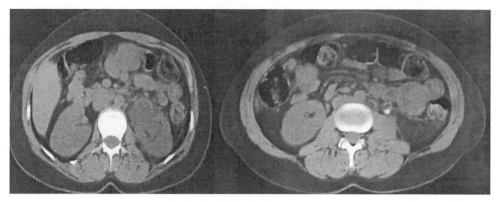

Figure 30.4   Helical CT scan without contrast demonstrating hydronephrosis with stranding around left kidney.

TREATMENT

SCI is a devastating event that results in multisystem impairment, and the resultant morbidity dramatically affects the patient, the family, and the community. The clinical complexity of the SCI patient is apparent when one considers the high prevalence of comorbidities. SCI patients are predisposed to having impaired primary and secondary muscles of respiration, deep vein thrombosis, pressure sores or ulcers, and impaired response to infection and wound healing. Impaired muscles of respiration can cause respiratory insufficiency, a weakened cough response, and an inability to clear airway secretions, which, in turn, may result in atelectasis or pneumonia. The reported incidence of deep venous thrombosis ranges from 47% to 72%. The death rate from pulmonary emboli is noted to be as high as 37% in the presence of an existing deep vein thrombosis (DVT). It is important that the clinician have a strong index of suspicion and promptly treat any comorbid conditions. These problems may be subtle in their clinical presentation. However, the very low reserve strength of this patient population can cause a patient to quickly slide into a critical prognosis. An associated occurrence of chronic indolent infection can also drain the patient's reserve.

The stone patient can have either "medical" or "surgical" stone disease. Medical stones are calculi without evidence of infection, obstruction, or deteriorating renal function, and are

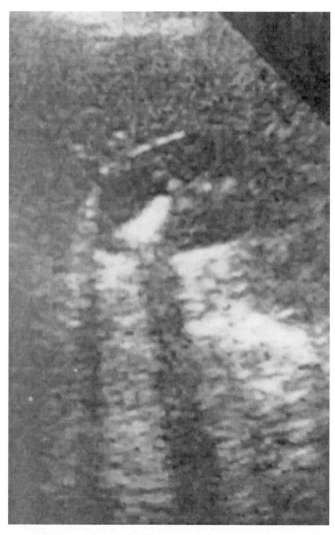

Figure 30.6   Ultrasound shows stone in the upper pole of the kidney.

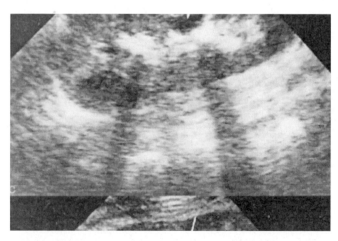

Figure 30.5   Ultrasound represents a right kidney with two stones. There is a hyperechoic area in the superior and middle pole of the kidney with shadowing behind each stone.

Table 30.5   Indications for Surgery

Pain
Recurrent infections
Increasing size
Recurrent hematuria
Deterioration of renal function
Failure of medical management

---

nonenlarging on serial X-rays (2). Surgical stone disease refers to calculi that are associated with an increase in size on serial X-rays, the presence of an obstruction, gross hematuria, recurrent UTIs, pain, and progressive renal insufficiency (2). Surgical treatment may require emergent drainage, urinary diversion, or surgical removal (see Table 30.5).

Surgical Treatment

The goal of treatment is complete stone removal. Close attention needs to be paid to coexistent pathologies such as UTIs, neuropathic bladder, and potential metabolic abnormalities. These must be addressed to prevent stone recurrence. Emergent relief of obstruction with an infection should be performed immediately to prevent sepsis and renal damage (29). Acutely, the patient should be hydrated, and the symptoms of pain, nausea, and vomiting should be treated as well. If infection is suspected, then broad-spectrum antibiotic treatment should be initiated, and the urine should be strained to obtain the stone for analysis (2). If a patient has a surgical stone, then it must be removed to prevent infection, preserve renal function, and decrease symptoms (2). Percutaneous nephrostolithotomy, extracorporeal shock wave lithotripsy, ureteroscopy, and open nephrolithotomy are the surgical modalities reviewed (see Table 30.6 and Appendix 1).

Endourology

Urinary Diversion: Stent or Percutaneous Nephrostomy Tube

The identification of infection in the presence of a stone with obstruction is an emergency and requires emergent surgical

---

Table 30.6   Surgical Treatment of Stone Disease

BLADDER STONES	URETERAL STONES	RENAL STONES
Cystoscopy Cystolithalopexy Energy sources: electrohydraulic, lithotripsy, ultrasound, Holmium laser	Distal ureter *Ureteroscopy and lithotripsy Proximal and mid-ureter *ESWL	ESWL (size <2 cm stone) Percutaneous nephrostolithotomy (>2 cm stone) Energy sources: lithotripsy: EHL, lithoclast, Holmium laser

*Preferred.

---

intervention to relieve this obstruction. Cystoscopy and the retrograde placement of a ureteral catheter or a JJ stent can accomplish this. This technique diverts the infected urine around the obstructing calculus, whether it is located in the ureter or the renal pelvis. If retrograde techniques are unsuccessful, then the urologist and/or radiologist must be prepared to provide percutaneous antegrade drainage with either ultrasound-directed, CT scan–guided, and/or fluoroscopic-visualized placement of a percutaneous nephrostomy tube. The presence of perirenal fluid collection (i.e., abscess) necessitates percutaneous drainage as well. These techniques are frequently life saving. Once drainage is obtained, and the infection is treated with appropriate antibiotic therapy, subsequent surgical intervention is elective.

Endourologic Surgical Techniques

Ureteroscopy

Ureteroscopy can be performed through either an antegrade or a retrograde approach. This section focuses on retrograde approaches; the antegrade approach is discussed in the "Percutaneous Nephrostolithotomy" section. Access to the kidney is gained by placing a flexible wire into the kidney through a cystoscope. Retrograde ureteroscopy can be performed with either a flexible or rigid ureteroscope. Once the stone is located, it can be removed with a stone basket or be fragmented using a pulse laser (Holmium) or electrohydraulic lithotripsy. After stone removal, reevaluation of the ureter is performed to look for retained fragments or ureter injury. Smaller rigid and flexible instrumentation with fiberoptic scopes has greatly widened the indications for this approach. Ureteroscopy in SCI patients usually involves the use of flexible ureterscopes due to problems associated with retrograde instrumentation in these patients in the dorsal lithotomy position (12). Due to musculoskeletal contractures, rigid instruments are sometimes very difficult to use, and positioning is usually challenging.

Ureteroscopy is an invasive procedure requiring a general anesthetic or conscious sedation. It also may require an energy source for lithotripsy of stones (i.e., laser, ultrasonic, electrohydraulic) (Figure 30.7). There is a risk of ureteral injury with laser and electrohydrolic lithotripsy. Furthermore, if a ureteral stent is placed at the time of surgery, then a second procedure is required for removal. Ureteroscopy offers an advantage, in that it allows immediate treatment of a stone with minimal hospitalization and can be performed as an outpatient procedure. This approach provides significant cost savings and can result in a stone-free status without the inconvenience of spontaneous passage of fragments. Finally, ureteroscopy offers excellent stone-free rates of greater than 90% in appropriately selected patients.

The criteria for selection include the location and size of the ureteral stone. A retrospective review by Krambeck et al. shows that stones located anywhere in the urinary tract can be treated with ureteroscopy and either laser or electrohydraulic lithotripsy. They show that ureteroscopic procedures achieve equivalent stone-free rates as extracorporeal shock wave lithotripsy (ESWL) (overall = 91.7%, proximal stone-free rate = 87.3%, and distal stone-free rate = 94.2%) (30). The overall complication rate was 1.9%, with a 0.2% stricture rate, a 1.5% ureteral perforation rate, and no avulsions (30). These rates are

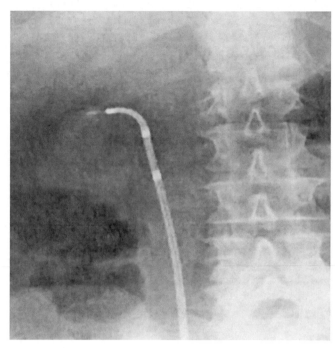

Figure 30.7 A flexible ureteroscope adjacent to a lower pole stone.

lower compared to previous complication rates and could be due to advances made in equipment and technique. Outcomes of ureteroscopically managed stone disease in SCI patients only and their clearance rates are not published.

Percutaneous Nephrostolithotomy

Prior to starting the percutaneous nephrostolithotomy (PCNL), the urine must be sterilized. The patient undergoes general or local anesthesia. The patient is placed in the prone position. Localization of entry is through a posterior calyx with biplanar C-arm fluoroscopy. Visualization can be assisted by injection of contrast through an external ureteral catheter (2). Sequential dilation is performed through a nephrostomy tract to 34 French (2). The renal collecting system is inspected with a nephroscope. If a stone is less than 1 cm, then the stone can be grasped with forceps. However, if the stone is greater than 1 cm, the stone will need fragmentation with an energy source (i.e., electrohydraulic lithotripsy, ultrasonic lithotripsy, or pulsed laser) in order to be extracted (Figure 30.8).

Multiple access sites may be necessary to remove all stones. Nephrostograms and nephrotomograms should be done in 24 to 48 hours to determine if there are any residual stones. PCNL is recommended for upper and middle pole stones larger than 2 cm, cystine stones larger than 1.5 cm, lower pole kidney stones larger than 1 cm, and staghorn calculi. It is also indicated for stones smaller than 1 cm, if there is a narrow infundibulum, acute infundibular pelvic angle (>90 degrees), or a stone of hard composition. Furthermore, PCNL can be used as a salvage procedure on ureteral stones, if ESWL or ureteroscopy has failed (27, 31, 32). Finally, PCNL is indicated for densely impacted stones, stones proximal to a ureteral stent, or an obstructed ureter without proximal hydronephrosis. *Antegrade ureteroscopy* can be used in

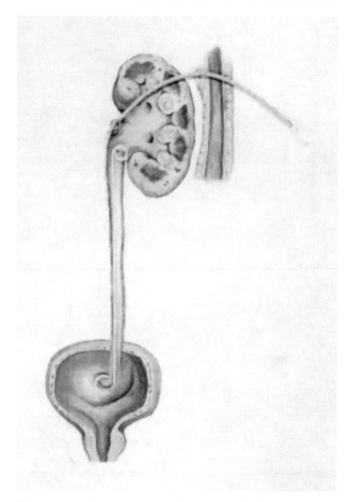

Figure 30.8 Percutaneous nephrostomy tube drainage.

conjunction with PNCL. After access is gained, a flexible ureteroscope or cystoscope can be manipulated into the ureter, thus allowing stones to be extracted or ablated with an energy source, EHL, or Holmium laser. Visualization of the ureter down to the bladder can performed. Overall, percutaneous nephrostolithotomy has an 80% to 85% stone-free rate and approaches 95% to 100% with repeat procedures. In the SCI population, stone-free rates are similar. More recent studies support this findings. The success of PCNL is limited by dense fascia scars, immobile kidneys, distorted intrarenal architecture, bulky stones, scoliosis, kidney malrotation, ectopia, and obesity (27).

The complications of PCNL are enhanced by the complexity of medical problems inherent to SCI patients (33, 34). Fevers can occur if the urine is not sterile. This can lead to perirenal abscesses. Pneumonia and atelectasis are common because of poor inspiratory effort. Bleeding, retained stones, ureteral edema and perforation, pneumothorax, hemothorax, nephrointestinal fistulas, and urosepsis are encountered complications.

An advantage of PCNL over open surgery is that a local anesthetic can be used or that less general anesthesia time is required. PCNL does not produce large, poor healing wounds. There is less convalescence time, and fewer blood transfusions are required. Finally, the cost is less. Open lithotomy is not always

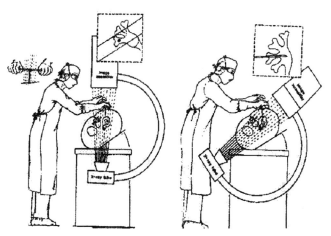

Figure 30.9 Setup for percutaneous access and intrarenal surgery for stone disease.

successful for complete stone removal and may necessitate repeat procedures. Repeat PCNL is safer, more effective, and costs less than a repeat open lithotomy (Figure 30.9).

Extracorporeal Shock Wave Lithotripsy

The advent of extracorporeal shock wave lithotripsy (ESWL) in the early 1980s provided a noninvasive mode of therapy for renal and upper ureteral calculi (35). ESWL utilizes a high-energy spark that causes an explosive vaporization of water. Recent developments include a reduction in the size of the equipment, decreased space requirements, portability, and reduced requirements for anesthesia. Shock waves are created and transmitted to a second focal point—the stone—which is blasted and fragmented. Biplane C-arm fluoroscopy is used to localize the stone. Repeat procedures might be necessary. Stones that are fragmented either pass spontaneously or are extracted (Figure 30.10).

SCI patients can have large stones with large fragments. ESWL has a stone fragmentation rate of 89% in ambulatory patients and 73% in the SCI population (32). The stone clearance rate is between 80% and 92% (36). The retreatment rate is between 5% and 10%. SCI patients have poor clearance with ESWL because of a large stone burden and poor mobility (Figure 30.11).

The advantages of ESWL are that it has minimum morbidity and mortality; local anesthetic can be used with intravenous sedation; and it offers some advantage over ureteroscopy for distal ureteral stone because it is noninvasive, offers minimum risk of ureteral injury or stricture, and may not require a general anesthetic. The most frequent complication of ESWL is retained fragments. The morbidity arises mainly from obstruction caused by the accumulation of stone fragments (36), and there is a 15% chance of requiring an adjunctive procedure. Bleeding, sepsis, and hypertension are other common complications. Less frequent complications include mucosal abrasions, ureteral perforations, ureteral stricture, and sepsis. The major restriction to ESWL is pregnancy, bleeding diathesis, anatomic impediment, and a weight limit of the lithotriptor table (32). ESWL has been safely performed on SCI patients with cardiac pacemakers (37) and baclofen pumps (38).

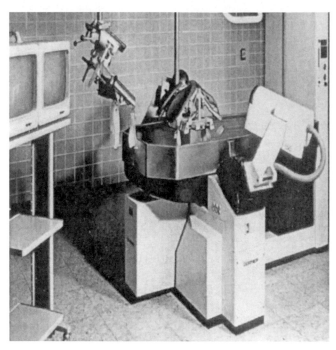

Figure 30.10 HM3 Dornier lithotripter: large bath fixed biplanar fluoroscopy and large space.

Combination or *sandwich therapy* combines the success of percutaneous nephrostolithotomy with the low morbidity of ESWL. The PCNL debulks the stone, the ESWL fragments any residual stone, and the PCNL clears any residual fragments with either a flexible or a rigid nephroscope (27). This is a very effective regimen. Combination therapy has a stone clearance rate of between 80% and 90% (39).

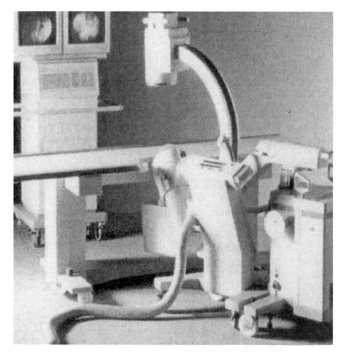

Figure 30.11 Lithotron small water balloon transportable and minimal anesthesia.

Open Surgery

Open surgery for urolithiasis is an historical form of surgery for stone disease that is rarely performed today. It was indicated for patients with anatomic abnormalities of fusion and/or ascent (e.g., horseshoe kidney and kidneys with vascular abnormalities).

A *simple nephrectomy* is indicated in the presence of advanced renal deterioration (26). A partial nephrectomy may be indicated when severe atrophic changes exist (26). This is essential to assure that the salvage of a renal unit (which may require multiple procedures) has sufficient clearance ability to justify a salvage strategy. Otherwise, a nephrectomy may be the least morbid procedure and may provide the greatest long-term success.

PHARMACOLOGIC THERAPY

Although urease inhibitors, such as acetohydroxamic acid (AHA) and hydroxyurea (HU), block stone growth (40), they are ineffective in dissolving stones. Stone recurrences after treatment with AHA and HU range between 18% and 45%. These compounds decrease the urine ammonia levels that lower the urine pH to less than 5 (41). AHA therapy is associated with serious adverse events in 22% to 68% of cases, with reported rates of stone growth or recurrence at 17% and 42%, respectively (42, 43). Side effects include DVTs, phlebitis, tremors, and intolerable headaches (17, 43, 44). The high risk of complications with these oral urease inhibitors must be weighed against the high success of the various minimally invasive surgical procedures (e.g., PCNL, ESWL) (Table 30.7).

Chemolysis using Renacidin or Hemacidin is used as an intracavitary irrigation with accesses such as a nephrostomy tube or a ureteral catheter to remove or dissolve stone(s) (41, 45). Chemolysis lowers urine pH to around 3.9. These mixtures of anhydrides, lactones, and magnesium salts dissolve struvite and calcium phosphate stones. Bladder calculi can also be dissolved with these chemolytic agents through a three-way continuous irrigation Foley catheter drainage system. Chemolysis may be used to dissolve small retained fragments post-ESWL or PCNL. Chemolysis has also been used for patients who are poor surgical candidates (46). Chemolysis must be performed with antibiotics on board and continuous monitoring for signs of sepsis. If the patient develops a fever, increases in white cell count, SGOT or magnesium, or pain, then the irrigation must be discontinued

immediately (17). Potential adverse events include urosepsis and life-threatening complications, such as hypermagnesia, a condition which is commonly manifested as seizures. This mandates close monitoring of the patient by nursing or medical staff. Because of the great success obtained with surgical interventions, chemolysis is primarily of historical interest.

Increased fluid intake should be prescribed to all stone formers. Fluid intake to keep urine output at 2 to 3 liters per day is desired. This increased fluid intake creates a dilute urine, which, in turn, decreases the concentration of ions in the urine.

Acidification of the urine is not useful. Ammonia chloride (NH_4Cl) has been used, but it is very difficult and dangerous to obtain a pH sufficient to prevent stone formation.

CONCLUSION

SCI patients are a special group with complex problems. The goals of treatment are to improve lower tract function, treat UTIs, and completely clear the urinary tract of stones. An emphasis on identifying risk factors and preventing stones has led to a decrease in the incidence of stones in the SCI population. New and less invasive modalities have made open surgery historic. Failure to treat stones in SCI patients may lead to recurrent UTIs, renal failure, and even death.

The future of stone management, diagnosis, and prevention in the SCI population will be derived from several strategies. The most rational direction is the prevention of SCI. Improved safety in automobiles, the prevention of driving while impaired, appropriate risk management in industry, and the prevention of violent crime are areas that will significantly reduce the incidence of SCI. Advances will also come in the development of less invasive surgical techniques such as laparoscopy, improvements in ESWL, and further miniaturization of endoscopes. In addition, developments in biotechnology, such as nerve regeneration, may one day allow the repair of the neurologic injury with full recovery of function.

*R*eferences

1. McGuire EJ, Woodside JR, et al. Prognostic value of urodynamic testing in myelodysplastic patients. *J Urol* 1981; 126(2):205–209.
2. Culkin DJ, Wheeler JS. Current management of urolithiasis in the spinal cord injury patient. *J Am Paraplegia Soc* 1987; 10(2):23–27.
3. Mattera CJ. Spinal trauma: new guidelines for assessment and management in the out of hospital environment. *J Emerg Nurs* 1998; 24(6):523–534; quiz 535–538.
4. Donnelly J, Hackler RH, et al. Present urologic status of the World War II paraplegic: 25-year followup. Comparison with status of the 20 year Korean War paraplegic and 5 year Vietnam paraplegic. *J Urol* 1972; 108(4):558–562.
5. Wadewitz P, Langlois PJ, et al. Present urologic status of the World War 2 paraplegic: 20-year follow-up comparison with status of the 10-year Korean War paraplegic. *J Urol* 1967; 98(6):706–715.
6. National Spinal Cord Injury Statistical Center. *Spinal Cord Injury: Facts and Figures at a Glance.* 2006. www.spinalcord.uab.edu
7. Chen MY, Zagoria RJ. Can non-contrast helical computed tomography replace intravenous urography for evaluation of patients with acute urinary tract colic? *J Emerg Med* 1999; 17(2):299–303.
8. Katz DS, Lane MJ, et al. Unenhanced helical CT of ureteral stones: incidence of associated urinary tract findings. *AJR Am J Roentgenol* 1996; 166(6):1319–1322.
9. Liu W, Stevenson G. Low dose nonenhanced helical CT scan of renal colic: assessment of ureteric stone detection and measurement of effective dose equivalent. *Radiology* 2000; 215(1):51–54.

Table 30.7 Pharmacologic Treatment for Struvite Stones
Urease inhibitors
• acetohydroxamic acid
• hydroxy urea
Urine acidifier
• Renacidin
• Hemacidin
Antibiotics
Diet modification
• decrease protein
• decrease vitamin C
• no adjustment to calcium
Increase fluid intake

10. Trinchieri A, Pisani E. Increase in the prevalence of symptomatic upper urinary tract stones during the last ten years. *Urology* 2000; 37(1):23–25.

11. Chen Y, DeVivo MJ, Roseman JM. Current trend and risk factors for kidney stones in persons with spinal cord injury: a longitudinal study. *Spinal Cord* 2000; 38:346–353.

12. Ost MC, Lee BR. Urolithiasis in patients with spinal cord injuries: risk factors, management and outcomes. *Curr Opin Urol* 2006; 16:1693–1699.

13. Burr RG. Urinary calculi composition in patients with spinal cord lesions. *Arch Phys Med Rehabil* 1978; 59:84.

14. Matlaga BR, Kim SC, Watkins SL, Kuo RL, et al. Changing composition of renal calculi in patients with neurogenic bladder. *J Urol* 2006; 175:1716–1719.

15. Vaidyanathan S, Watson ID, et al. Recurrent vesical calculi, hypercalciuria, and biochemical evidence of increased bone resorption in an adult male with paraplegia due to spinal cord injury: is there a role for intermittent oral disodium etidronate therapy prevention of calcium phosphate bladder stones? Clinical Case Discussion. *Spinal Cord* 2005; 43:269–277.

16. Donnellan SM, Bolton DM. The impact of contemporary bladder management techniques on struvite calculi associated with spinal cord injury. *BJU Int* 1999; 84(3):280–285.

17. Shortliffe LM, Spigelman SS. Infection stones: evaluation and management. *Urol Clin North Am* 1986; 13(4):717–726.

18. Hall MK, Hackler RH, et al. Renal calculi in spinal cord–injured patient: association with reflux, bladder stones, and foley catheter drainage. *Urology* 1989; 34(3):126–128.

19. Ord J, Lunn D, Reynard J. Bladder management and risk of bladder stone formation in spinal cord injured patients. *J Urol* 2003; 170(5):1734–1737.

20. Levy DA, Resnick MI. Management of urinary stones in the patient with spinal cord injury. *Urol Clin North Am* 1993; 20(3):435–442.

21. DeVivo MJ, Fine PR, et al. The risk of renal calculi in spinal cord injury patients. *J Urol* 1984; 131(5):857–860.

22. Khan SR. Calcium phosphate/calcium oxalate crystal association in urinary stones: implications for heterogeneous nucleation of calcium oxalate. *J Urol* 1997; 157(1):376–383.

23. Menon M, Parulkar B, et al. Urinary lithiasis: etiology, diagnosis, and management. In: Walsh P, ed. *Campbell's Urology*. Philadelphia: WB Saunders, 1998; 3:2659–2734.

24. Pak CY. Etiology and treatment of urolithiasis. *Am J Kidney Dis* 1991; 18(6):624–637.

25. Tori JA, Kewalramani LS. Urolithiasis in children with spinal cord injury. *Paraplegia* 1979; 16(4):357–365.

26. Vargas A, Mendex R. Staghorn calculus: its clinical presentation, complication, and management. *J Urol* 1982; 127:860–862.

27. Kahnoski RJ, Lingeman JE, et al. Combined percutaneous and extracorporeal shock wave lithotripsy for staghorn calculi: an alternative to anatrophic nephrolithotomy. *J Urol* 1986; 135(4):679–681.

28. Vaidyanathan S, Soni BM, et al. Recurrent bilateral renal calculi in a tetraplegic patient. *Spinal Cord* 1998; 36(7):454–462.

29. Vaidyanathan SB, Soni M, et al. Pathophysiology of autonomic dysreflexia manifesting recurrent dysreflexic episodes. *Spinal Cord* 1998; 36(11): 761–770.

30. Krambeck AE, Murat FJ, et al. The evolution of ureteroscopy: a modern single-institution series. *Mayo Clin Proc* 2006; 81(4):468–473.

31. Spirnak JP, Bodner D, et al. Extracorporeal shock wave lithotripsy in traumatic quadriplegic patients: can it be safely performed without anesthesia? *J Urol* 1988; 139(1):18–19.

32. Lazare JN, Saltzman B, et al. Extracorporeal shock wave lithotripsy treatment of spinal cord injury patients. *J Urol* 1988; 140(2):266–269.

33. Culkin DJ, Wheeler JS Jr, et al. Percutaneous nephrolithotomy in the spinal cord injury population. *J Urol* 1986; 136(6):1181–1183.

34. Culkin DJ, Wheeler JS, et al. Percutaneous nephrolithotomy: spinal cord injury vs. ambulatory patients. *J Am Paraplegia Soc* 1990; 13(2):4–6.

35. Ehreth JT, Drach GW, et al. Extracorporeal shock wave lithotripsy: multicenter study of kidney and upper ureter versus middle and lower ureter treatments. *J Urol* 1994; 152(5 Pt 1):1379–1385.

36. Constantinides C, Recker F, et al. Extracorporeal shock wave lithotripsy as monotherapy of staghorn renal calculi: 3 years of experience. *J Urol* 1989; 142(6):1415–1418.

37. Vaidyanathan S, Hirst R, Parsons KF, et al. Bilateral extracorporeal shock wave lithotripsy in a spinal cord injury patient with a cardiac pacemaker. *Spinal Cord* 2001; 39:286–289.

38. Vaidyanathan S, Johnson H, Singh G, et al. Extra corporeal shock wave lithotripsy of calculi located in lower calyx of left kidney in a spinal cord injury patient who has implantation of baclofen pump in the ipsilateral loin. *Spinal Cord* 2002; 40:94–95.

39. Niedrach WL, Davis RS, et al. Extracorporeal shock-wave lithotripsy in patients with spinal cord dysfunction. *Urology* 1991; 38(2):152–156.

40. Safani MM, Tatro DS. Acetohydroxamic acid-dissolution of urinary stones? *Drug Intell Clin Pharm* 1981; 15(11):886.

41. Gleason M, Griffith DP. Infection stones. In: Resnick M, Pak CYC, eds. *Urolithiasis: A Medical and Surgical Reference*. Philadelphia: WB Saunders, 1990:113–132.

42. Griffith DP, Khonsari F, et al. A randomized trial of acetohydroxamic acid for the treatment and prevention of infection-induced urinary stones in spinal cord injury patients. *J Urol* 1988; 140(2):318–324.

43. Williams JJ, Rodman JS, et al. A randomized double-blind study of acetohydroxamic acid in struvite nephrolithiasis. *N Engl J Med* 1984; 311(12):760–764.

44. Gleason M, Griffith DP. *Infection Stones*. Philadelphia: WB Saunders, 1990.

45. Dretler SP, Pfister RC. Primary dissolution therapy of struvite calculi. *J Urol* 1984; 131(5):861–863.

46. Puppo P, Germinale F, et al. Propionhydroxamic acid in the management of struvite urinary stones. *Contrib Nephrol* 1987; 58:201–206.

APPENDIX 1

```
┌─────────────────────────────────┐
│   Spinal Cord Injury Patient with│
│     Suspected Kidney Stone       │
└─────────────────────────────────┘

┌─────────────────────────────────┐
│   KUB (Abdominal X-Ray)          │
│   Noncontrast Helical CT Scan    │
│   UA and Urine Culture           │
└─────────────────────────────────┘
         Stone Diagnosed
┌─────────────────────────────────┐
│          Location                │
│            Size                  │
│        ± Infection               │
│   ± Hydronephrosis or Obstruction│
└─────────────────────────────────┘
```

+ Infection & − Hydronephrosis	+ Infection & + Hydronephrosis	− Infection & − Hydronephrosis
↓	↓	↓
Antibiotics 1st	Antibiotics with Ureteral Stent *or* Percutaneous Nephrostomy Tubes	Treatment Options

Kidney

Upper and Middle Pole	Lower Pole
↓	↓
ESWL (<2 cm) PCNL Ureteroscopy	PCNL Ureteroscopy ESWL (<2 cm)

Ureteral

Distal Ureter	Mid-Ureter	Proximal Ureter
↓	↓	↓
Ureteroscopy	Ureteroscopy ESWL	Ureteroscopy ESWL PCNL

Bladder

Bladder
↓
Cystolithalopaxy (Holmium Laser or EHL) Open Surgery

ESWL = extracorporeal shockwave lithotripsy
PCNL = percutaneous nephrolithotomy
EHL = electrohydraulic lithotripsy

31 The Gastrointestinal System after Spinal Cord Injury: Assessment and Intervention

Steven A. Stiens
Ashwani K. Singal
Mark Allen Korsten

THE NEUROGENIC GASTROINTESTINAL SYSTEM

Spinal cord injury interrupts the functional coordination of many body systems. This challenges the patient and the interdisciplinary rehabilitation team to construct effective patient-centered plans for adaptation (1, 2). The gastrointestinal system is not exempt from involvement. Fortunately, autonomic and intrinsic nervous systems of the gut preserve some coordination. Traditionally, attention has been focused on neurogenic colonic dysfunction, but increasingly it is evident that there are significant effects of SCI throughout the gastrointestinal (GI) tract.

GASTROINTESTINAL DYSFUNCTION AND DISABLEMENT: SYMPTOMS, IMPAIRMENTS, ACTIVITY LIMITATIONS, AND BARRIERS TO PARTICIPATION

The pervasive effect of SCI on the person extends through involvement of many systems, resulting in a variety of impairments that limit adaptive compensation with SCI. The personal impact of GI dysfunction and specifically colonic dysfunction after SCI can be particularly life limiting. Symptoms of gastrointestinal dysfunction detract from quality of life as observed by many investigators (3–5). Symptoms are quite varied from one person with SCI to another. Table 31.1 outlines some of the common symptoms. Specifically, neurogenic bowel dysfunction produces impediments to self-concept and personal relationships. Fecal incontinence occurs in up to 75% of patients with a predominant frequency of between a few times a month and once a year (6). Free time and family life are significantly impacted (3). In addition, the cost of equipment, medications, and attendant care increase the burden of care after SCI.

Particular impairments that result from SCI include sensory deficits and paralysis of the pelvic floor musculature. In addition, paralysis and sensory deficits of the limbs can limit independence in the adaptive habits required to compensate for the neurogenic bowel. As with all aspects of spinal cord medicine, the practice must include both biopsychosocial and disablement perspectives (7).

Gastrointestinal dysfunction after SCI has many potential effects on the person.

Biopsychosocial perspectives of SCI include not only the gastrointestinal system dysfunction but also necessarily relate this system's function to the person as a whole, and to his or her family, work, and community. From a disablement perspective, limitations in organ dysfunction (i.e., colonic peristalsis) are viewed as impairments. Human tasks such as willful defecation are affected, resulting in specific activity limitations. Constipation and difficulty with evacuation affect up to 80% of people with SCI (6). Finally, the impact of gastrointestinal dysfunction on life activity results in what had been termed handicaps, but what are now referred as barriers to participation (8).

ORAL CAVITY: TARTAR, CARIES, AND OCCLUSION PROBLEMS

In the early stages of spinal cord injury management, physiological as well as psychological considerations preclude all but emergency dental treatment (9). However, as the patient recovers from the initial injury, issues concerning oral health maintenance and prevention arise. The etiology of dental disease is multifactorial, with factors including failure of the patient to maintain plaque control, diet, production of saliva, smoking, and occlusal traumatism (10).

Possibly the single most important factor contributing to the growth and accumulation of plaque is the failure or inability of the patient to maintain adequate daily mechanical plaque removal. Persons with SCI, particularly tetraplegics, who are dependent on caregivers for daily oral care, tended to have poorer oral hygiene, more severe gingivitis, and more periodontal disease than those who performed home self-care independently (11).

Table 31.1 Gastrointestinal Symptoms of Persons with Spinal Cord Injury

Dysphagia	Constipation
Heartburn	Difficulty with passing flatus
Sour eructations	Perineal burning
Epigastric bloating	Abdominal distention
Early satiety	Abdominal cramping

Saliva, a secretion that is rich in antibodies, especially IgA, provides a flushing action that helps clear bacteria from the mouth (12). Xerostomia is a clinical condition where salivary secretion is decreased either as a result of disease or as a side effect of a particular drug or treatment (e.g., radiotherapy). It is postulated that a low salivary secretion rate allows oral flora associated with development of caries to overgrow and cause periodontal disease (13). In this regard, a variety of drugs that may reduce salivary flow are commonly administered to persons with SCI. Specifically, drugs that reduce spasticity, such as tizanidine and baclofen, can produce xerostomia (14, 15). Anticholinergic medications such as amitriptyline and oxybutynin can produce a dry mouth as well.

Persons with SCI have been advised that a high fiber diet and a large liquid intake level are useful in preventing constipation (16). This type of diet has additional advantages, including prevention of periodontal disease, facilitation of weight loss, reduction in cancer risk, and prevention of coronary artery disease. In this respect, a number of studies in animals have shown that the consistency of the diet, rather than the composition, has a more important effect on the formation of plaque and development of gingivitis. Indeed, a soft diet, one that is mashed and mixed with liquid, leads to an increased rate of periodontal disease (17). This study may lead one to conclude that a soft mashed diet places SCI patients at risk for periodontal disease. However, other than illustrating such an effect, a specific diet (e.g., raw uncooked vegetables) recommendation that prevents periodontal disease could not be substantiated by the literature.

Smoking is a particularly harmful habit in persons with SCI, given the inherent fire hazard, danger of burns, and increased risk for cardiovascular disease (18). Within the oral cavity, smoking is known to cause mucositis of the palate, and tobacco smoke has been demonstrated to have a deleterious effect on the periodontium. The mechanism by which tobacco affects the oral cavity has been linked to its inhibitory effect on the salivary leukocytes that prevent plaque formation (19).

Occlusal traumatism refers to unphysiologic or excessive forces applied to the teeth. When excessive, these forces may lead to trauma and result in periodontitis (10). This is particularly pertinent for persons with spinal cord injury because they may depend on their mouths for purposes other than mastication (20–26). A mouthpiece can be attached to mouth sticks, for example, which produces a lever arm that can translate high torque forces to the teeth. For example, the use of a mouthpiece provides the person with high tetraplegia control over many facets of her or his environment. However, prolonged use of tools like mouth sticks, in theory, may lead to dental damage. Mouthpieces should be tried and individually fit to each user. Patients should be queried about pain with use. Patients who use mouthpieces should bring them to their dentists for check of fit and oral examination for signs of dental damage from use.

THE ESOPHAGUS: DYSPHAGIA AND REFLUX

During the acute phase of spinal cord injury, the esophagus may be involved directly or indirectly (27). Thoracic or abdominal esophageal perforation is a common consequence of both penetrating and blunt trauma (28–31). A high index of suspicion is required for its early diagnosis and for avoiding complications. In suspected cases, endoscopic or radiographic confirmation is essential (31). Iatrogenic contributions to swallowing problems include forced supine position, tong traction, and halo vest immobilization. Positioning up at 30 degrees or more for all drinking and eating can be helpful.

Dysphagia after acute cervical spinal cord injury occurs in up to 20% of cases, and half of the patients are asymptomatic. Predictors include age, tracheostomy, and anterior approach cervical spinal surgery (32). Early specific diagnosis can be accomplished with bedside examination by a speech pathologist, a fiberoptic endoscopic examination of swallowing (FEES), or a videofluoroscopic study of swallowing (VFSS). Positioning up at 30 degrees or more for all drinking and eating can be helpful. Interdisciplinary treatment of severe dysphagia can reduce up to 90% of symptoms and can prevent pneumonias (33). A controlled manometric study of the pharyngeal and lower esophageal sphincters revealed abnormally high relaxing pressures (18.4 vs. 3.9) and abnormally high bolus prepulsion pressures (23.8 vs. 2.2) after SCI in comparison to controls (34). Swallowing studies demonstrate poor pharyngeal stripping, sluggish opening of the cricopharyngeal muscle, excessive pooling in the pyriformis sinus, delayed pharyngeal elevation, and some frank aspiration (32). These findings have been historically associated with the need for a tracheostomy, continued use of ventilator dependence, and cervical spine surgery (34). Pharyngeal dysphasia increases the risk for pneumonia, and in some series, myotomy has been used to reduce cricopharyngeal outflow resistance.

The increased incidence of upper gastrointestinal tract pathology among patients with spinal cord injury has been demonstrated in several studies (27, 35, 36). A number of factors predispose these patients to esophageal disease, particularly gastroesophageal reflux. Reduced diaphragmatic strength results in chronic elevation and reduced lower esophageal sphincter pressures. SCI patients, especially tetraplegics, spend a greater proportion of their time in the supine or semi-upright position. In lower thoracic SCI, abdominal muscles are used more frequently to increase intra-abdominal pressure for a Valsalva maneuver as a result of chronic constipation, which could lead to transient relaxation of the lower esophageal sphincter and to subsequent reflux of gastric contents in the esophageal lumen. There is evidence of esophageal dysmotility, which may increase the risk for reflux esophagitis (37).

The characteristic symptom of gastroesophageal reflux disease (GERD) (i.e., heartburn) may not be present in tetraplegics. Those whose lesions are below T7 would be expected to present with similar complaints as the spinally intact. This may explain why fewer SCI patients present for evaluation of esophageal disorders. Many of these patients may be initially treated with PPIs or H2 receptor antagonists, and if symptoms persist, endoscopic or manometric studies should be pursued. However, persons who have lesions at higher levels (above T7) may only experience waterbrush, an acidic aftertaste, and may fail to experience typical heartburn. Unfortunately, esophageal disease may not be recognized until the patient complains of dysphagia or develops GI bleeding. Then, a diagnostic procedure can confirm the cause and help to determine appropriate treatment (Figure 31.1). As stated, the prevalence of high-grade esophagitis is higher after SCI. With this in mind, it could be argued that patients with SCI, especially those who have higher lesions, should be screened for esophageal disease.

Once identified, therapy for GERD in individuals with SCI is similar to that in other patients and can be either medical (Figure 31.1) or surgical. Nonpharmacologic therapies include lifestyle modifications, such as reduction of caffeine, chocolate, peppermint, and alcohol intake, along with smoking cessation. Staying upright after meals and avoiding meals immediately before bedtime may also improve symptoms (38). Treatment is generally directed toward acid suppression and improvement in motility within the limits of available medications. Antacids, histamine-2 receptor antagonists (H_2RAs), and proton pump inhibitors (PPIs) are the agents most commonly used in controlling acid secretion. PPIs have been shown to be superior to H_2RAs and are the most effective agents for initial acute therapy of GERD, as they provide more complete acid control (39).

Medications promoting gastrointestinal motility include bethanechol, metoclopramide, and cisapride. Cisapride has been shown to be safe and well tolerated in a population of patients with mild-to-moderate gastroesophageal reflux disease (40), but the possibility of fatal arrhythmias (41) has resulted in its withdrawal from the market. The use of metoclopramide and bethanechol is also limited due to their prominent side effects, especially the extrapyramidal symptoms with which they are associated (42, 43).

There are a number of reasons for the failure of medical therapy for GERD, including noncompliance, recurrent symptoms when medications are stopped or reduced, intractable symptoms despite medication use, and occurrence of complications such as esophageal stricture, aspiration, or laryngitis. In such instances, surgery is an effective and useful option. Most operations can now be performed laparoscopically, an approach that considerably reduces the postoperative recovery time. Surgical approaches re-approximate the stomach and the esophagus to the natural position and approximate the crura of the diaphragm. Fundoplication techniques that include partial wrapping of the gastric fundus around the base of the esophagus prevent reflux and are less likely to result in dysphagia (44).

STOMACH AND DUODENUM: INCOMPLETE EMPTYING AND PEPTIC ULCER DISEASE

During the first few weeks after SCI, impairment in gastric emptying is common especially in patients with lesions above T1. Prolongation of gastric emptying persists into chronic SCI (45).

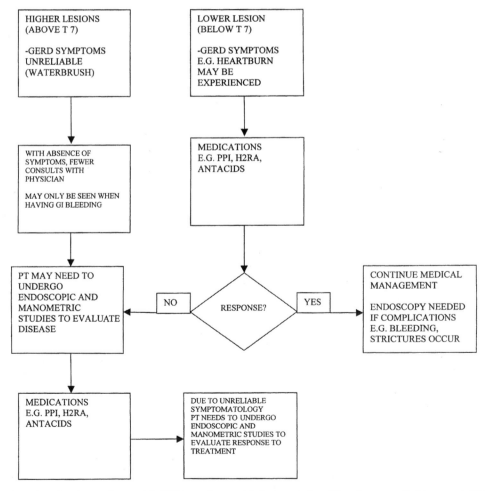

Figure 31.1   The algorithm divides patients with SCI into those with lesions below T7, who can reliably report GERD symptoms, and those with lesions above T7, who may not report symptoms.

Treatment with intravenous metoclopramide at 5–10 mg per dose or with bethanechol at 25 mg, 30 minutes before meals, is effective. During the acute period, there is also an increased risk for gastric erosions, gastroduodenal ulcerations, and perforation. These risks have been attenuated with the empiric use of H2 blockers, proton pump inhibitors, and stool guaiac surveillance for gastrointestinal bleeding.

The risk for ulcers after SCI is being evaluated in animal models. Animal studies have shown that there is a direct relationship between the onset of the injury and the degree of ulceration (46). A single cause for the pathogenesis of gastroduodenal ulceration and hemorrhage has not been substantiated. Several mechanisms have been proposed, including acute ischemia of the gastric mucosa and an imbalance between the parasympathetic and sympathetic activity governing digestive function (35). In fact, in rats, cervical cord transection alone does not increase gastric acid output or plasma gastrin levels. However, addition of vagal stimulation enhances gastric acid output in rats with cervical cord transection. However, the characteristics of gastric ulceration are not similar to what is seen acutely after spinal cord injury in humans (47). Further research is necessary.

Superior Mesenteric Artery Syndrome: Duodenal Obstruction with the "Nutcracker"

Superior mesenteric artery syndrome (SMAS) is a condition attributed to intermittent functional obstruction of the third segment of the duodenum between the superior mesenteric artery and the aorta (48). This is also known as Wilkie's syndrome, or body cast syndrome. The Wilkie series of seventy-five cases remains the largest review (49). Symptoms that are part of the classic presentation are persistent epigastric pain and postprandial fullness, followed by nausea and vomiting. The syndrome is more common in tetraplegics after SCI (50). The four diagnostic categories that predispose one to SMAS are wasting diseases (burns, cancer, endocrine disorders), severe injuries (head

trauma, abdominal injuries, spinal fractures with casting), dietary disorders (anorexia nervosa, malabsorption syndrome), and the postoperative state (51).

The diagnosis is confirmed with a barium upper GI series (51). Findings include dilatation of the proximal duodenum and a "cut off" of the transverse duodenum blocking barium flow. The superior mesenteric artery (SMA) comes off the aorta at the L1 level and traverses the root of the mesentery of the small intestine over the duodenum in a ventral and caudal direction. (Figure 31.2) The angle between the small bowel mesentery and the aorta is most acute when patients are supine. Closure of this angle over the duodenum has been termed the "nutcracker effect."

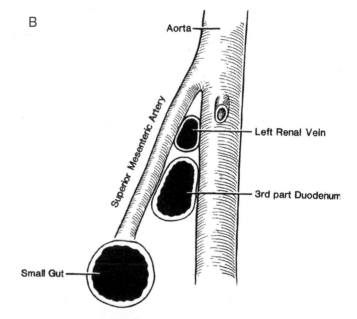

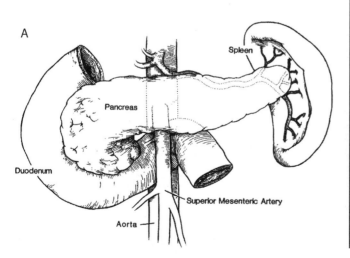

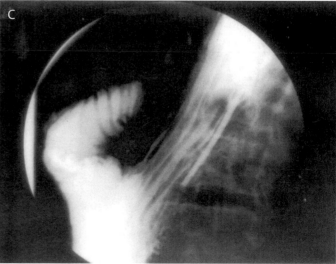

Figure 31.2 Superior mesenteric artery syndrome. (**A**) The anatomic relation of the duodenum, superior mesenteric artery, and aorta in the anterior frontal view. (**B**) The lateral view of the third segment of the duodenum and the renal view, as they laterally traverse the posterior abdomen. The weight of the small intestine on the superior mesenteric artery tethers these structures like a "nutcracker." (From Roth E, Fenton L, Gaebler-Spira D, Frost F, Yarkony G. Superior mesenteric artery syndrome in acute traumatic quadriplegia: case reports and literature review. *Arch Phys Med Rehabil* 1991; 72:417–420, with permission.) (**C**) Radiograph of the duodenum after oral administration of contrast. Partial obstruction is demonstrated.

In spite of the risk, the actual clinical incidence of SMAS among patients with SCI is rather low and was estimated to be 0.53% in a cohort of 567 patients (27). Other conditions that may mimic SMAS include poor gastric emptying seen frequently in tetraplegics, peptic ulcer disease, gastroesophageal reflux, ileus, and colonic impaction. Initial screening should include flat and upright abdominal films, electrolytes, a complete blood count, and serum amylase.

Treatment starts with a constellation of conservative measures, which almost always improve symptoms while attempts are being made to eliminate the causes. Sitting the patient up reduces the forces on the duodenum and facilitates gravity flow in the gut. All meals should be taken sitting upright. Lying down in the right lateral recumbent position for 1 hour facilitates bolus transfer from the stomach through the duodenum into the jejunum (51). A recommended surgical option is duodenojejunostomy from the second portion of the duodenum to the jejunum (52). Other surgical options include gastrojejunostomy and Roux-en-Y duodenojejunostomy (53).

THE PANCREAS: INCREASED RISK FOR PANCREATITIS

The pancreas is affected in the acute phase of the spinal injury as well (27). It has been hypothesized that, due to the spinal cord trauma, sympathetic-parasympathetic imbalance may result in hyperstimulation of the sphincter of Oddi, which may lead to stasis of secretions and pancreatic damage (54). Pancreatitis may appear as early as 3 days after injury, but its presence may be masked because of the loss of sensory, motor, and reflex functions (55).

The diagnosis of pancreatitis is supported by increases in amylase and lipase in excess of three times the upper limit of normal, although lipase level is the preferred indicator, as other conditions besides pancreatic inflammation (e.g., macroamylasemia, parotitis, some carcinomas) can also lead to amylase elevation. Several criteria have been formalized to determine the severity of pancreatitis in its initial presentation. Among these are Ranson's criteria (Table 31.2), the APACHE II severity of disease classification system, the Balthazar-Ranson Grading System, and the CT severity index. These are used in spinally intact persons, and their utility in SCI patients has not been validated. Among the imaging

---

Table 31.2   Ranson's Criteria to Determine Severity of Pancreatitis

At Admission
- Age > 55 Years
- WBC > 16,000/mm²
- Glucose > 200 mg/dl
- LDH > 350 iu/L
- AST > 250 u/L

During Initial 48 h
- HCT decrease of > 10 vol%
- BUN increase of > 5 mg/dl
- Calcium < 8 mg/dl
- PaO_2 < 60 mm Hg
- Base deficit > 4 meq/L
- Fluid sequestration > 6 L

Table 31.3   Severe Acute Pancreatitis

Early Prognostic Signs
- Ranson's signs ≥ 3
- Apache II score ≥ 8

Organ Failure
- Systolic bp < 90 mm Hg
- PaO_2 ≤ 60 mm Hg
- Creatinine > 2 mg/dl
- GI bleeding > 500 ml/24 h

Local Complications
- Necrosis
- Abscess
- Pseudocyst

---

studies, an abdominal ultrasound should be performed initially to determine whether the cause is gallstones and whether any pancreatic pseudocysts are present. A contrast CT should be performed on patients who show evidence of severe pancreatitis (Table 31.3) to delineate interstitial from necrotizing pancreatitis.

The goals of medical therapy include supportive care, limitation of systemic complications, prevention of pancreatic necrosis, and prevention of pancreatic infection once necrosis has taken place. Supportive care includes use of narcotics if pain is present, fluid resuscitation to prevent hypovolemia caused by third space losses and vomiting, and parenteral nutritional support if oral nutrition is to be withheld for more than 7 days. Oral feedings may resume once pain has subsided. Patients who have severe pancreatitis caused by gallstones should undergo urgent endoscopic retrograde cholangiography, and stones in the common bile duct should be removed. Although several factors may lead to pancreatic necrosis, impairment of the microcirculation may be the most important. Thus, vigilance in maintaining fluid hydration may be beneficial in limiting pancreatic necrosis. In patients with necrotizing pancreatitis associated with organ failure, it is reasonable to initiate treatment with antibiotics with a broad spectrum of activity against aerobic and anaerobic bacteria.

THE GALL BLADDER: STASIS AND INCREASED STONE INCIDENCE

It has been demonstrated that gallstones are more prevalent in persons with spinal cord injury (56–58). The pathophysiologic mechanisms that contribute to the increased incidence of cholelithiasis after SCI have not yet been conclusively defined. Cholelithiasis has been observed to affect between 5% and 17.5% of men in developed Western countries (59). Prevalence studies that have focused on persons with SCI have demonstrated prevalence rates of 17% (58), 21%–30% (60), 29% (56), and 31% (57).

The changes in parasympathetic and sympathetic nervous system innervation modulation of gallbladder activity after SCI may alter contractibility and cholestasis. The gallbladder receives sympathetic innervation from T7 through T10. Decreases in gallbladder motility have been associated with a variety of diagnoses such as diabetes mellitus that also include a higher prevalence of gallstones.

Gallbladder dysmotility is the most studied mechanism for higher prevalence of gallstones. The gallbladder receives sympathetic innervation from T7 to T10. The contributions from the parasympathetic and sympathetic nervous systems to the modulation of gallbladder activity after SCI alter its contractibility. It has been hypothesized that impaired gallbladder motility results in stasis, thus predisposing one to gallstone formation (56). However, some gallbladder contractility studies show that contractility is normal and that the cause of low gallbladder ejection fraction is due to a smaller baseline gallbladder resting volume (61). Tandon et al. attempted to document the formation of gallstones soon after SCI by prospective ultrasonographic study of the gallbladders of persons with SCI and controls (62). They found an increased volume of biliary sludge in patients with SCI above T10 and a reduced gallbladder fasting volume in the same group. None of the subjects developed any gallstones. This increased incidence of biliary sludge was shown in subjects with SCI, despite normal contractility (62). The authors evaluated the gallbladder contractility by measuring the gallbladder volume in the fasting and the postprandial states. However, using hepatobiliary imaging with technium 99m-labeled iminodiacetic acid analogue (99Tcm-DISIDA) in eighteen normal controls, sixteen trauma controls, and forty-five SCI subjects, abnormal filling fraction and abnormal ejection fraction of gallbladder was shown in 52% and 59%, respectively, among SCI cases (63). These abnormalities were particularly noted in females with high and severe SCI (63). It also remains possible that the pathogenesis of gallstones after spinal cord injury may simply be due to an increase in the incidence of conventional risk factors commonly associated with the disease, primarily obesity (60). The occurrence of cholelithiasis during acute SCI has been related to the following factors: acute trauma, decreased gut motility, reduction in food intake, intravenous hyperalimentation, parenteral nutrition, rapid weight loss, and mobilization of peripheral fat stores (56, 61). Acute acalculous cholecystitis after spinal cord injury has also been described (64). As with pancreatitis, acute cholecystitis in persons with spinal cord injury may not be readily apparent because pain and tenderness in the right upper quadrant of the abdomen may be absent. Nausea, vomiting, and fever may occur but are, of course, quite nonspecific. When these symptoms persist, however, an abdominal ultrasound and CT scan should be obtained. Delayed diagnosis of acute cholecystitis may lead to gangrene of the gallbladder, a serious complication with a high mortality rate. Given the inherent difficulties in the diagnosis of cholecystitis, some have suggested routine ultrasonographic screening for gallstones in persons with spinal cord injury and elective laparoscopic cholecystectomy if gallstones are detected.

Due to the high incidence of gallstones after SCI and the potential risk for higher morbidity should cholecystitis occur, may clinicians have deliberated on the need for and timing of cholecystectomy. The sensory deficits that result from SCI have been considered to mask symptoms that would prevent timely diagnosis. Despite this, the majority of patients with SCI and cholelithiasis present with biliary colic and chronic abdominal pain (58). In their retrospective review of thirty-five patients who had cholecystectomy 1 year after SCI, 63% had presented with chronic abdominal pain and biliary colic, and thirteen patients (37%) had acute presentation (acute cholecystitis in nine, cholangitis in two, and acute pancreatitis in two). The authors also showed that symptoms are not necessarily obscured by SCI regardless of the level of injury (58). Similar results were reported in a survey and chart review (57) of the patients at one SCI cen-

ter, revealing forty-five SCI patients from a population of approximately 500 who had cholecystectomy. Twenty of these patients presented with biliary colic, four had nonspecific symptoms, and two underwent prophylactic cholecystectomy. Nine patients had acute cholecystitis; eight of the nine had right upper quadrant or epigastric pain as well as elevated white blood cell counts.

A retrospective study of the rate of cholecystectomy after SCI revealed an annual rate of 6.3% that included both symptomatic patients and prophylactic operations. This cholecystectomy rate of 6.3% is slightly higher than the combined rate of 3.7% to 5.1% observed in the general population (65). This higher incidence of cholecystectomy after SCI is partly due to the high number of prophylactic gallbladder resections. Adjusted rates show that need for cholecystectomy after SCI was not substantially different than in the general population (58).

Biliary surgery, when performed on persons with SCI, has a similar morbidity as compared with the general population. A review of the surgical procedures and operative courses of the SCI patients revealed outcomes that were comparable to the general population. Patients with high lesions did not show a greater propensity to develop cholecystitis or advanced biliary disease versus biliary colic than those with low lesions. Spinal cord–injured patients were less likely to present with cholecystitis or advanced biliary disease than were general patients. Furthermore, comparisons of operative times, conversions from laparoscopic to open procedures, estimated blood loss, morbidity, and mortality did not substantially differ between SCI and the general population (65).

THE ILEUM AND JEJUNUM: ILEUS ADYNAMIC

During the first few days to weeks after spinal cord injury, abdominal distention is common. This is often attributed to nonmechanical intestinal obstruction or paralytic adynamic ileus. People with SCI have many risk factors for this, including major trauma, surgery, anesthesia, and severe medical illness (66). Evaluation requires a careful check for the presence of bowel sounds. Confirmation comes from an abdominal radiograph (upright and supine films) that will reveal dilated loops of intestine with air fluid levels. Management includes replacement of fluids and electrolytes using an intravenous route. The intestines can be decompressed by placing a nasogastric tube. After the first few months after SCI, the symptoms are rarely attributed to the small intestine, although there have been reports of delayed procecal transit times using the noninvasive hydrogen breath test (67). One study (67) reported procecal transit times averaging 180 minutes versus mean control values of 98 minutes. These values could potentially be affected by the volume of colonic contents. Further investigation is needed to determine if this promotes bacterial overgrowth or has any other clinical significance.

MANAGEMENT OF ACUTE ABDOMEN IN PATIENTS WITH SCI

Patients with neurological diseases may not be able to perceive abdominal pain, which is the most common complaint of acute abdomen in able-bodied persons (68). Patients with SCI above T7 have flaccidity and paralysis of the abdominal wall, with loss of visceral sensations (55). Acute abdomen in patients with SCI may present with other gastrointestinal symptoms such as ileus, nausea, vomiting, diarrhea, jaundice, hematemesis, and melena or with atypical symptoms such as anorexia, weight loss, fever, confusion, or hypotension (69). Sometimes, the presentation is confined to abnormalities on abdominal examination with abdominal distension, visible peristalsis, hypo- or hyperactive bowel sounds, or abnormal laboratory values such as leucocytosis and increased levels of amylase/lipase. Rarely, features of autonomic dysreflexia such as sweating, palpitations, and hypertension may be the only manifestations of an underlying acute abdomen in these individuals. Moreover, fever and leucocytosis are unreliable signs due to autonomic dysfunction and stress in these patients (70). The most important step in diagnosing acute abdomen during spinal shock is simply recognizing the possibility that it might exist (55). A thorough history and physical examination is a must for proper diagnosis and management.

Preliminary Evaluation

In patients with vomiting, the presence of stale food particles suggests gastric outlet obstruction or impaired gastric emptying. Bile in the vomitus indicates that the lesion is distal to the second portion of the duodenum. Questioning about the use of nonsteroidal anti-inflammatory drugs (NSAIDs) is essential, as they frequently cause gastric irritation and have a potential to cause GI bleeding. Hemorrhoids and anal fissures are common in SCI patients as a cause of lower GI bleeding (LGIB). Acute diarrhea in patients with SCI could be due to overflow as a result of fecal impaction or due to clostridium difficile colitis, especially in patients transferred from SCI units or nursing homes. Even urinary tract infection (UTI) may occasionally present as an acute abdomen.

A detailed physical examination should be done looking for dehydration, evidence of sepsis (tachycardia, hypotension, tachypnea, altered mental status), visible gastric (left to right in upper quadrant) or intestinal (stepladder) peristalsis, succussion splash (indicates gastric stasis), altered bowel sounds, abdominal tenderness and/or rigidity, and any abdominal masses. Rectal examination is important for ruling out fecal impaction, masses, and GI bleeding. A basic laboratory workup should be carefully assessed for any drop in hematocrit or leucocytosis, for electrolyte abnormalities such as hypokalemia and hyponatremia, for acid base abnormalities with anion gap, and increased amylase/lipase levels. Urine analysis, culture, and microscopic examination are done to exclude a UTI. Erect and supine films of the abdomen should be viewed for air-fluid levels or free air under the diaphragm (indicating perforation of a hollow viscus). Ultrasonography (USG) is useful for evaluating the gallbladder; however, it is limited for assessment of the pancreas in obese persons and in those with abdominal distention. In these cases, a contrast enhanced CT scan of the abdomen is done to assess the pancreas. One should make sure that the renal function is normal before administering contrast.

Patients with acute abdomen are kept nil per oral (NPO). Intravenous (IV) fluids and electrolytes are replaced. Pain medications are provided as needed. Opiates should be avoided in patients with intestinal obstruction, and NSAIDs in those with GI bleeding. PPI by the IV route is given for patients with acute upper GI bleeding and gastric outlet obstruction. Nasogastric suction is done for patients with recurrent vomiting and with perforated viscus. Antibiotics are given (after drawing relevant blood and urine cultures) to patients with acute cholecystitis, intestinal obstruction, perforation, and severe pancreatitis.

Further Evaluation

If, despite the aforementioned measures, the patient is not getting better, then a GI or surgical consult is mandatory. Further workup is dependent upon the likely diagnosis (Figures 31.3 and 31.4).

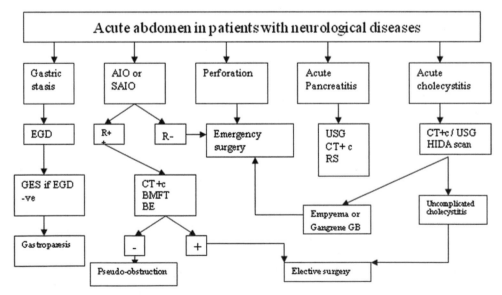

Figure 31.3 Algorithm for the workup of neurologically impaired patients with suspected acute abdomen. USG = ultrasonogram; AIO = acute intestinal obstruction; SAIO = subacute intestinal obstruction; R+ = response to conservative treatment; R− = no response to conservative treatment; EGD = esophagogastroduodenoscopy; GES = gastric emptying study; CT+c = contrast-enhanced CT scan; BMFT = barium meal follow-through; BE = barium enema; RS = Ranson's scoring; HIDA = hepatic iminodiacetic acid.

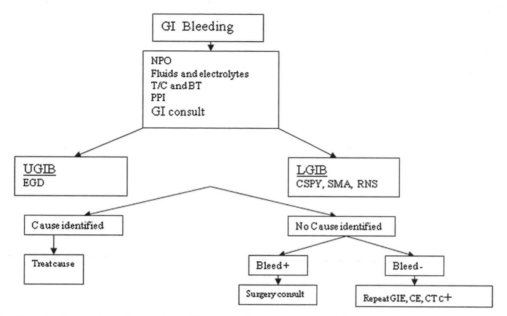

Figure 31.4   Algorithm for the workup of neurologically impaired patients with GI bleeding. NPO = nil per oral; T/C = type and cross match; BT = blood transfusion; PPI = proton pump inhibitor; EGD = esophagogastrodudenoscopy; UGIB = upper GI bleeding; LGIB = lower GI bleeding; CSPY = colonoscopy; SMA = superior mesenteric angiography; RNS = radionuclide study; GIE = GI endoscopy; CE = capsule endoscopy; CTc+ = contrast-enhanced CT scan.

Patients with pancreatitis should be assessed for its severity using a contrast-enhanced CT scan. Magnetic resonance cholangio-pancreatogram (MRCP) is done in patients with biliary obstruction or dilated biliary ducts on USG. Stones in the common bile duct can be removed endoscopically (ERCP). A HIDA scan with nonvisualization of the gallbladder suggests cystic duct obstruction and can diagnose acute cholecystitis with a sensitivity of 97% and a specificity of 90% (71). Patients with acute abdomen may require emergency surgery for unrelieved obstruction, perforated viscus, complicated cholecystitis, or undiagnosed acute GI bleeding despite endoscopic and other assessments.

THE COLON: FECAL STORAGE, DESICATION, AND ELIMINATION

Colon Anatomy and Physiology: The Works

The human colon receives a largely liquid suspension from the small bowel. Over a period that may last 1–3 days, the colon is capable of extracting water from that non-digestible waste, and it moves the increasingly solid stool toward the rectum for ultimate evacuation. Both of these functions require coordinated contractions of the inner circular and outer longitudinal muscle layers of the colon. These contractions produce movements of two basic types: those that impede propulsion to permit mixing and water absorption from colonic contents (segmental contractions) and those that produce caudad motion of the luminal contents toward the rectum (high pressure peristaltic waves). The peristaltic smooth muscle contractions are believed to be autonomous, arising as a result of stimulation from nerves that reside within the wall of the colon. The term enteric nervous system has been applied to this neural network (72). It consists of Meissner's submucosal plexus and Auerbach's intra-

muscular plexus and the neurons that interconnect them. Together, they comprise an independent nervous system for the gut that orchestrates inherent automaticity. In fact, recent investigations have identified interstitial cells of Cajal, in the submucosal as well as in the intramuscular layer of the gut with particular prominence in the right colon (73). These have been suggested to be "pacemaker cells" that modulate colonic contraction and affect smooth muscle excitability. This aspect of colon physiology remains largely intact after SCI. However, propulsive contraction as well as the act of defecation function best with neural input from outside the colon. These extrinsic influences involve sacral parasympathetic nerves as well as somatic nerves. Not unexpectedly, these latter pathways are often altered after both upper and lower neuron injuries to the spinal cord.

The colon receives parasympathetic and sympathetic innervation (Figure 31.5). The vagus nerve (parasympathetic) descends from the brainstem, innervating from the distal two-thirds of the esophagus to end at the splenic flexure of the colon. Sympathetic supply comes from the *mesenteric* (T5–T12) and the *hypogastric* (T12–L3) nerves. The pelvic floor is innervated by the mixed somatic *pudendal nerve* (S2–S4).

With intact neural circuitry, normal colonic peristalsis and defecation occur under combined autonomic and voluntary somatic control (74). Colonic peristalsis consists of mixing segmental contractions on the right and more propulsive patterns on the left. Giant migratory contractions (GMC) of the colon actively propel stool toward the rectum. Cecum-to-anus colonic transport typically takes 12 to 20 hours (75). GMCs occur more frequently in the morning and with the *gastrocolonic reflex*.

The *gastrocolonic reflex* is an increase in colonic motility induced by feeding. The motility starts in minutes, peaks in less than an hour, and may last for a few hours. The term

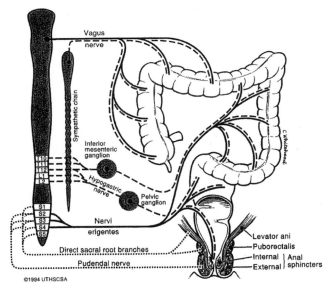

Figure 31.5 Autonomic and somatic innervation of the colon, anal sphincters, and pelvic floor. Spinal cord segments and nerve branches are illustrated. Dashed lines represent sympathetic pathways with prevertebral ganglia. Solid black lines depict parasympathetic pathways that synapse with ganglia in the myenteric nervous system within the colon wall. The vagus originates from the medulla, and the nervi erigentes (also called the pelvis splanchnic nerve) come from the conus. Dotted lines represent mixed nerves supplying somatic musculature of the external anal sphincter and the pelvic floor. (From King JC, Stiens SA. In: Brandon R, ed. *Neurogenic Bowel Management in Physical Medicine and Rehabilitation.* 2nd ed., 2000:579–591, with permission.)

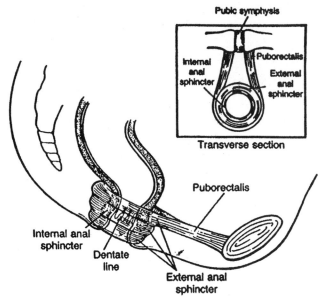

Figure 31.6 Sagittal and transverse views of the rectum and sphincters. Sagittal view of the rectum, anal canal, and surrounding muscles. The puborectalis muscle forms a sling posteriorly around the rectum at the anorectal junction. The external anal sphincter (skeletal muscle) surrounds the anal canal and is closely associated with the puborectalis muscle. The internal anal sphincter (smooth muscle) lies within the ring of external sphincter muscles and is a continuation of the inner circular layer of the smooth muscles of the rectal wall. (From Madoff RD, Williams JG, Caushaj PF. Fecal incontinence. *N Engl J Med* 1992; 326:1002–1007, with permission.)

gastrocolonic is used because the mechanism is not conclusively defined and may be vagal, intrinsic neural pathways in the colon or hormonal effects via gastrin (76), motilin (77), or cholecystokinin. Fatty foods and proteins provide the best stimulus. Spinal cord injury may interfere with the strength of the response (78, 79).

Continence is maintained by the *internal anal sphincter* (IAS) (smooth muscle), the *external anal sphincter* (somatic muscle), and the *puborectalis muscles* (80). Together, they make up the *anal sphincter mechanism* (Figure 31.6). The IAS is the major contributor to pressure in the anal canal at rest, which averages 50 to 100 mm Hg and is not altered by SCI (80, 81). The external anal sphincter (EAS) is somatic musculature with continuous contraction that increases in response to mechanical stimulation or challenges to continence (82). The EAS contracts to retain stool if the rectum is rapidly dilated. This is referred to as the *holding reflex.*

Voluntary defecation begins with the sensation of rectal dilatation from stool advancement (Table 31.4). This stretches the puborectalis muscle (Figure 31.7) and the rectal wall, which signals the urge to defecate (83). As stool approaches the internal sphincter, it automatically relaxes (*recto-anal inhibitory reflex*), and the external anal sphincter is voluntarily contracted to maintain continence.

When the situation is socially appropriate, voluntary defecation occurs (Figure 31.7). Sitting straightens the rectum and

makes the anorectal angle less acute. To initiate defecation, the external anal sphincter and the puborectalis muscle are relaxed. Then, the glottis is closed, the diaphragm descends, and abdominal muscles contract to raise intra-abdominal pressure via the Valsalva maneuver. Sigmoid peristalsis mediated by longitudinal muscle layer contractions and gravity then propel the stool out.

Table 31.4   The Sequence of Events in Normal Defecation

Involuntary activity

a. *Giant migratory contractions* (GMC) advance stool through the colon to the rectum.

b. Stool distends the rectum and stretches the puborectalis muscle as the internal sphincter relaxes—*recto-anal inhibitory reflex.* This triggers a conscious urge to defecate.

c. External anal sphincter and puborectalis muscle contraction retains stool—*holding reflex.*

Voluntary activity

a. Relaxation of the external anal sphincter and the puborectalis.

b. Contraction of the levator ani, external abdominals, and diaphragm combined with glottis closure elevates intra-abdominal pressure and aids peristalsis in propelling stool out.

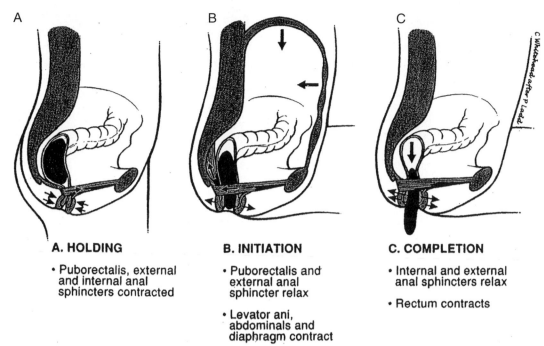

A	B	C
A. HOLDING	**B. INITIATION**	**C. COMPLETION**
• Puborectalis, external and internal anal sphincters contracted	• Puborectalis and external anal sphincter relax • Levator ani, abdominals and diaphragm contract	• Internal and external anal sphincters relax • Rectum contracts

Figure 31.7 Sphincter relaxation and increase in intra-abdominal pressure during defecation. (**A**) Defecation is prevented by a statically increased tone of the internal anal sphincter and puborectalis, as well as by the mechanical effects of the acute anorectal angle. Dynamic responses of the external anal sphincter and puborectalis to rectal distention reflexes or increased intra-abdominal pressures further impede defecation. (**B**) To initiate defecation, the puborectalis muscle and external anal sphincter relax, while intra-abdominal pressure is increased by a Valsalva maneuver, which is facilitated by squatting. The levator ani helps reduce the acute anorectal angle to open the distal anal canal to receive the stool bolus. (**C**) Intrarectal reflexes result in continued internal anal sphincter relaxation and rectal propulsive contractions, which help expel the bolus through the open canal. (Modified from Shiller LR. Fecal incontinence. In: Sleisenger MH, Fordtran JS, eds. *Gastrointestinal Disease: Pathophysiology, Diagnosis, Management.* 4th ed. Philadelphia: WB Saunders, 1989, with permission.)

Colon and Pelvic Floor Impairments: Pathophysiology That Contributes to Activity Limitations in Storage and Defecation

The term *neurogenic bowel* is used to refer to colon and pelvic floor dysfunction resulting from any nervous system damage or developmental defect (central peripheral, autonomic, or enteric). Neurogenic bowel as a term is quite general and includes a variety of types of dysfunction that are related to neural lesions located along the spinal cord, along the peripheral nerves, and within the enteric nervous system of the colon. The response patterns associated with these various lesions can be reviewed by starting at the muscle layers of the colon and working toward the spinal cord and supra-spinal centers (84). Potential impairments include lack of perception of need to defecate, increased transit time, constipation, incontinence, and discoordination of fecal elimination. All of these limit the human task of socially appropriate and efficient defecation, producing significant limitations in social activity. Constipation is difficult to define in a population that often requires assistance for bowel care; however, less than three bowel movements per week, incomplete evacuation, and chronic abdominal distention are criteria that are frequently used (85). A quantitative study of a heterogeneous group of patients with SCI estimated that 58% had constipation and that 33% had abdominal discomfort (86). Chronic visceral pain has been reported to affect between 3% and 10% of the SCI population, with the onset occurring months to years after injury (87).

Autonomic nervous system lesions that denervate the gut have little sustained effect on function. Fortunately, the gut enteric nervous system remains functionally intact after spinal cord damage, although, microscopic findings of ganglion cell loss and Schwann cell proliferation within the colon wall have been attributed to trans-synaptic effects of central and peripheral nerve lesions (88, 89). Gut wall neuroplastic changes such as branching and neural circuit remodeling are expected to occur in response to spinal lesions, but the actual effects on enteric nervous control of gut function are yet to be elucidated. There are two basic patterns of colonic and pelvic floor dysfunction: lower motor neuron and upper motor neuron (84).

Lower Motor Neuron Neurogenic Bowel

This condition presents a pattern of colonic dysfunction that results from a lesion affecting parasympathetic cell bodies within the spinal cord at the conus, their axons in the cauda equina, parasympathetic axons in the inferior splanchnic nerve, and somatic motor axons in the pudendal nerve (90). This pattern of colonic and pelvic floor dysfunction is common in patients with SCI lesions at vertebral level T10 and below. After lesions to the inferior splanchnic nerves or conus, the descending colon wall has a lower resting tone with no spinal cord–mediated reflex peristalsis. Slow stool propulsion with segmental colonic peristalsis is coordinated by the myenteric plexus alone, while water absorption continues. The predominant mixing peristaltic pattern segmental and excess absorption produces a dryer and rounder stool shape referred to as *scybalous* (84). The external anal sphincter (EAS) is frequently denervated due to pudendal nerve damage, preventing reflex EAS sphincter contraction and increasing the risk for incontinence. In addition, the pelvic floor laxity and decreased puborectalis tone contribute to a loss of anorectal angle and the absence of a holding reflex. Unfortunately, the rectal-anal inhibitory reflex is retained even in lesions of the conus medullaris or cauda equina (88, 91). This further contributes to the risk for incontinence by reflex relaxation of the internal sphincter on rectal distention as stool advances. Furthermore, the levator ani muscles and external anal sphincter lack tone, allowing the sigmoid and rectum to descend into the pelvis and the perineum to sag. This further reduces and opens the rectal angle and the rectal lumen (92). Therefore, stool is more apt to slip out during pressure releases or contraction of innervated abdominal musculature.

Upper Motor Neuron Neurogenic Bowel

This condition is produced by a spinal cord lesion anywhere above the conus medullaris. The spinal cord below the lesion usually retains perfusion that spares the gray matter in order to preserve conal reflex function at levels S1 through S4. Stool transit times through the colon are slower after SCI. Transit time remains a very significant clinical measure of colonic function (93), although findings must be interpreted with consideration of the frequency of bowel care. Stool transit times can be increased with standardized bowel programs that include an increase in bowel care frequency (94). Excessive rectosigmoid distention can occur with infrequent or ineffective evacuation. Distention of the rectum alone can slow intestinal transit (95). Cervical spinal cord lesions are associated with prolonged mouth-to-cecum transit (MCTT). Many people with prolonged gastric emptying (96) and paraplegia exhibit MCTTs that are comparable to normal. In vivo studies of the UMN colon have demonstrated excessive colonic wall and external anal sphincter tone (97).

The external anal sphincter (EAS) is included in the striated muscle that makes up the pelvic floor. This musculature becomes spastic after UMN lesions and can obstruct defecation (97). Recent perfusion manometry studies have shown resting anal sphincter pressures that are comparable to controls without SCI, but SCI patients with lower than normal resting anal sphincter pressures tended to have more severe bowel symptoms (98). This may be due to chronic overdistention of the rectum.

Colonic mucosal surface electromyographic studies have demonstrated that persons with UMN SCI have a higher basal colonic activity than do members of the general population (78, 89). This may contribute to imbalance of innervation, overactive segmental peristalsis, underactive propulsive peristalsis, and a hyperactive holding reflex with spastic EAS constriction, producing megacolon and rectal impaction (85, 99). Cervicothoracic spinal cord injury interrupts cortical inhibitory pathways, creating excessive sympathetic stimulation and increased smooth muscle tone throughout the colon (79). This constellation of problems responds to an upper motor neuron bowel program and bowel care technique with a mechanical (100), chemical, or electrical stimulus to trigger and sustain reflex defecation (84).

Intracolonic pressures have been investigated with pressure monitors with gradual distention from continuous infusion.

Initial studies of colonic compliance of the UMN colon were reported in the 1940s using water manometry (101). Steep rises in intracolonic pressures up to 40 mmHg (normal 5–15 mmHg) were observed in subjects with UMN SCI, at infusion volumes as low as 400–600 ml (79). Some of these studies (100, 102) have proposed a hyperreflexic response of the left colon that is analogous to that of the UMN bladder. Other investigators (103) have utilized colometrograms, in which water was infused into the rectum at a slower rate of 100 ml/min with continuous intracolonic pressure measurement. These and other subsequent studies with gradual or intermittent rectal infusion have demonstrated gradual increases in intracolonic pressure and adaptation to distention with colonic compliances that have approached normal (104, 105). Single pressure measurements using a hydraulic system may not reliably reflect actual pressures throughout the colon because segmental constriction may artifactually raise pressures close to the monitor while more proximal pressures are lower.

A variety of other methodologies have been utilized in the study of colonic pressure transport after SCI (75, 88, 91, 106). A review of methods by Wald has suggested that these techniques could be useful for clinical evaluation of colonic and anorectal motility (107). However, studies of colonic motility that involve pressure-sensing catheters being placed in the colon are short term, and patients are prone to catheter displacement during the recording period. To overcome these limitations of colonic motility, studies described a technique wherein the motility catheter is tethered to the bowel wall using endoscopically deployed clips (108). This new approach is employed to study the effect of UMN SCI on colon motility. Colonic pressures and motility are recorded with four pressure transducers located at different levels in the left colon (Figure 31.8). In a study on eight subjects with SCI (four paraplegics and four tetraplegics), the effect of food on colonic motility (using the catheter with pressure transducers and tethered to the colonic wall with endoscopic clips) was evaluated, and patients were compared with able-bodied individuals (109). The baseline colonic motility was reduced in SCI subjects. Although the colonic motility was reduced in response to meals, this was noticed only in the descending colon and not in the

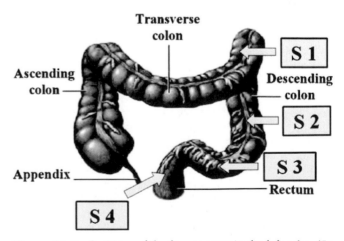

Figure 31.8 Positions of the four sensors in the left colon (S1 = splenic flexure; S2 and S3 = descending colon; S4 = rectum). The sensors are separated by 10 cm.

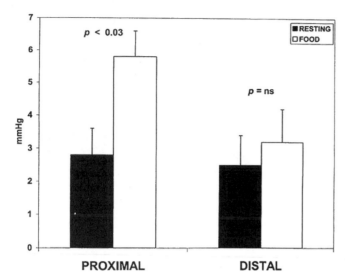

Figure 31.9 Regional variation in colonic motility after meals in SCI subjects. The colonic motility index was significantly higher in the descending colon and not in the rectosigmoid colon.

rectosigmoid colon (Figure 31.9) (109). Previously, investigators have also suggested that the gastrocolonic response after complete SCI is less robust or is absent (78, 79). Using the same technique, the colonic motility index (product of mean amplitude of colonic contraction and percentage of activity) was shown to be reduced in subjects with SCI during sleep as compared to able-bodied subjects (1.5 vs. 5.8, $p < 0.02$) (110). Within the SCI group, the colonic motility during sleep (111) was reduced as compared to motility pre-sleep (1.5 vs. 2.8, $p < 0.02$) and post-sleep (1.5 vs. 4.3, $p < 0.03$) (110).

Colonic transit time can also be measured with sequentially swallowed markers that are followed through the colon with serial radiographs (111, 112). Investigations applying this technique in UMN SCI have illustrated markedly delayed left colon and rectal transit times in persons with UMN SCI as compared with controls (75, 91). A recent study demonstrated prolonged ascending, transverse, and descending transit times with supraconal UMN SCI and prolonged rectosigmoid transit times in conal LMN/cauda equina lesions (111). Technetium (113) and Indium-111 Amberlite scintigraphy have also been utilized to investigate colonic transport in subjects with UMN SCI (106). An isotope Amberlite IR-120-P was encapsulated in gelatin and coated with methacrylate to allow release at a higher pH in the colon. In scintigraphic imaging of the colon after oral ingestion of the isotope capsule, the emptying half time of the colon was increased in subjects with SCI in comparison to controls (29 ± 27 hr vs. 6.81 ± 3.03 hr, $p < 0.01$ for ascending colon and 42 ± 12 hr vs. 15.3 ± 7.16 hr, $p < 0.01$ for ascending and transverse colon). These and other transit studies suggest that abnormalities of colonic function after UMN SCI can involve the entire colon and may require oral agents in addition to rectal medications and reflex stimulation in order to get effective defecation (84).

In conclusion, the lower motor neuron pattern of dysfunction results from lesions to the inferior splanchnic nerve to the descending colon and the pelvic nerve to the pelvic floor. This results in sluggish propulsion, dry stool and rounder stool shape,

and a high risk of incontinence due to low tone of the external anal sphincter. The upper motor neuron pattern of dysfunction results from a spinal cord lesion above the conus resulting in hypersegmentation in colonic peristasis, less propulsion, and stool retention with a tight (spastic) external sphincter.

Interdisciplinary Rehabilitation Interventions: Minimize Disablement Associated with Neurogenic Bowel Dysfunction

Interventions directed toward problems associated with the neurogenic bowel are managed similar to other issues that confront the patient in the rehabilitation process (84). Neurogenic bowel is listed as a problem under diagnoses and is grouped with other impairments. The problem should be stated as succinctly as possible but should include a designation of the upper motor neuron (UMN) or lower motor neuron (LMN) pattern. The rehabilitation database must include a comprehensive accurate neurologic examination and diagnoses that could impact colonic function or methods for compensation. Impairments of colonic function must be derived from history, examination, and appropriate laboratory and functional studies (84). Findings from the history and physical examination are related, and diagnoses and treatment plans are developed. Specific difficulties such as constipation, difficulty with evacuation, and fecal incontinence must be understood and quantified (84, 114). The full variety of pathology, impairments, and activity limitations that interact to prevent ability to maintain continence and willfully defecate must be assessed from the perspective of the entire person. Next, limitations in functional mobility, as well as assets, such as strength for transfers, sitting balance, and residual colonic reflex function, which can be utilized in bowel care procedures through education task modification or use of medications, must be sought out. Finally, barriers to full life participation need to be addressed with careful consideration of the person's life goals and role expectations, particularly with regard to cultural, sexual, and vocational roles.

The design of the entire rehabilitation process is to overcome the patient's problems from neurogenic bowel; therefore, knowledge of the individual person and his/her limitations in disablement is required (84). Strengths for adaptation and derivation of person-centered goals are elicited (84, 114). Typically, a particular interdisciplinary team member coordinates this effort. Usually this member is the primary nurse in close association with the physiatrist, occupational therapist, and social worker. In the inpatient setting, scheduling can be especially difficult because of the time-consuming nature of bowel care, as well as the number of individuals on the rehabilitation unit who require bowel care assistance (16). Evening bowel care often allows for more predictable attendance of daily therapies (84). Incontinence episodes seem to be more common during the few hours after bowel care. Evening bowel care allows for positioning and draping in bed to allow for the possibility of further involuntary incontinence of stool (84).

The goals and needs projected by the individual after the acute rehabilitation process is complete must derive from an entire bowel program that is compatible with the post-rehabilitation lifestyle (115). The scheduling and technique of the new bowel care procedure are particularly important. The demands for work or school, the duration of bowel care, and the needs of other members of the household must all be considered in creating individualized scheduling (84, 116). Should attendant care be needed on an intermittent basis, early morning bowel care and evening bowel care can often fit into part-time intermittent schedules. The cost of attendant care and equipment must be figured into the life care plan (116).

A patient-centered approach is essential for the design of each bowel program. Individual bowel programs are derived from patterns of bowel function from the patient's past and are practically adapted to the patient's role performance and resources (114, 115). The challenge to the interdisciplinary team is to educate the patient about altered physiology after SCI and to empower the patient to design a bowel program and a bowel care technique that is effective and that supports his or her lifestyle (84).

Patient History: A Survey of the Past to Design a New Bowel Program

The history should start with a classic gastrointestinal review of systems that includes identification of pertinent related diagnoses that predate the SCI. Key questions to ask in the initial interview are summarized in Table 31.5. Previous bowel conditions and habits must be related to current function, support resources, and life demands.

The patterns of pre-morbid bowel function lay the foundation for the postinjury bowel program (84). Factors to consider include timing of bowel movement frequency, volume, and consistency of bowel movements, as well as the amount of time needed to complete bowel care. Pre-morbid symptoms, especially of constipation, may be modified. Otherwise, pre-morbid routines should be replicated as closely as possible in order to take advantage of well-established patterns. Scheduling elimination shortly after a meal takes advantage of the gastrocolonic response, although as noted above, this may be somewhat blunted after SCI.

Any gastrointestinal conditions that were present before SCI could complicate the bowel program. Conditions such as laxative dependency, diabetes, irritable bowel syndrome, or inflammatory bowel disease may prolong or accelerate transit time, affect the responsiveness of the gut to bowel care medications, and even predispose the individual to life-threatening complications, such as toxic megacolon, should the bowel program be ineffective (84).

Table 31.5 Baseline Medical History for Neurogenic Bowel

A. **Premorbid history**: daily fluid intake, diet (fiber, meal frequency, spice preferences, amounts), bowel movements (frequency, duration, difficulties), stool (consistency color, mucus, blood), medications.

B. **Current status**: injury level, daily fluid intake, diet, medications, patient's understanding of SCI's effect on elimination, bowel care (frequency, duration, digital stimulation frequency/technique), bowel incontinence (time of day, frequency, relationships to eating).

C. **Lifestyle goals**: schedules for work or school, availability of assistance if needed, amount of time needed to complete bowel care regime.

SCI individuals need to be very compliant with bowel programs. For example, potentially constipating drugs were used by 39.5% of a sample of patients with SCI for depression and detrusor hyper-reflexia (117). Patients need to understand the relationship between their previous gastrointestinal problems and their post-SCI bowel dysfunction. The history and physical examination is an opportunity for the clinician to demonstrate these effects and to educate the patient and caregivers.

Physical Examination: Survey for Pathology, Impairments, Activity Limitations, and Complications

A comprehensive perspective is necessary, as capabilities of many body systems interact to compensate for impairments in stool storage and elimination. The purpose of the examination is to identify pathologies and functional deficits as well as functional capabilities and methods for compensation. To accomplish this, an examination that includes the nervous, gastrointestinal, musculoskeletal, and integumentary systems is most likely to yield the information required to plan a successful bowel program (115).

The abdominal examination is a practical place to start (84). Inspection for asymmetry and abdominal distention is done first. Auscultation for bowel sounds and bruits in all four quadrants precedes palpation. Abdominal muscle spasticity can be minimized by supporting the flexed knees with a pillow. The colon should be palpated in a clockwise direction starting at the right lower quadrant, following its course as it encircles the abdomen (115). The ascending and transverse colon have varied positions in the abdomen. The descending colon reliably follows the left lateral abdomen and becomes retroperitoneal as the colon descends toward the pelvis (84). Masses, organomegaly, or high colonic impaction can be detected with superficial and deep palpation (118). Should inflammation or organ distention be present, palpation may not trigger pain perception, spastic rigidity, or local tenderness.

The rectal examination can provide much useful information. Anal contraction with cutaneous contact demonstrates *anocutaneous reflex* function. To start the rectal examination, the tip of the lubricated examining finger should be held gently against the anal verge, thus allowing gradual relaxation of anal tone. Sphincter tone and response of gradual dilatation reveals innervation and the presence of spasticity. Voluntary contraction demonstrates motor incomplete SCI. As the sphincter opens, the examining finger should be directed toward the umbilicus in order to follow the anal canal and approach the rectal angle at the puborectalis muscle. At the puborectalis, gentle pressure toward the sacrum is applied to assess the puborectalis for tone and spasticity (84). The voluntary strength of the EAS, puborectalis, and bulbocavernosus can be graded, and endurance can be assessed. Stool consistency and caliber should be noted. A stool specimen should be tested for occult blood.

The neurologic examination will yield information about the level of spinal cord injury, the completeness of the injury, and whether the bowel function would be expected to be an upper motor neuron or lower motor neuron pattern. This requires a complete assessment of the various sacral reflexes. These reflexes include anocutaneous reflex, anal tone, bulbocavernosus reflex, and the internal anal sphincter reflexes. The *anocutaneous reflex* consists of contraction of the external anal sphincter in response to perianal skin stimulation; this should be elicited with a pin in four quadrants surrounding the anal verge (84). This reflex is mediated by the inferior hemorrhoidal branch of the pudendal nerve (S2–S5). *Anal tone* is the resistance to introduction of the examining finger and the squeeze presented in the anal canal. The *bulbocavernosus reflex* is the contraction of the anal sphincter in response to a squeeze of the head of the penis (S3 dermatomal level) or clitoral pressure. The bulbocavernosus reflex is elicited by pinching or pricking the dorsal glans penis (S3) or by applying light pressure over the clitoris while simultaneously palpating for bulbocavernosus and EAS for contraction (S2, S3) with a gloved lubricated finger in the anal canal. A few trials should be completed to reliably attribute EAS contraction to the glans penis or clitoral pressure (84). The response frequently extinguishes after an initial strong anal contraction. Contraction of the IAS with the stimulation of digital introduction to the rectum beyond the EAS constitutes the *internal anal sphincter reflex.* The IAS closes immediately upon withdrawal. This reflex is sympathetically mediated through the hypogastric plexus.

The physical examination of the colon and pelvic floor can be complimented by a few laboratory tests. A stool guaiac test is utilized to detect the presence of fecal blood. Unfortunately, this test has a high false positivity rate due to hemorrhoidal bleeding and rectal trauma from bowel care. Specimens obtained from the central portion of stools may be more reliable. In the face of persistent diarrhea without an obvious cause, clostridium difficile toxin, stool culture, and examination for ova and parasites may

be helpful, especially if there is a history of travel or antibiotic use in the recent past (84). Flat and upright radiographs of the abdomen can be useful to assess colon size and rule out impaction (118), obstruction, or rupture of a hollow viscous. Fecal retention and megacolon are increasingly common findings in persons with SCI (85, 104).

Patient and Family Education: Problems Explained and Solutions Demonstrated

There are a few education tools available that explain neurogenic bowel dysfunction and adaptive techniques for compensation. The first step in patient education is a verbal explanation of the problem. Pointing out the lack of sensation and reasons for deficits in sphincter control is a good preface to patient reading. Then, a read of the chapter on neurogenic bowel in a spinal cord patient education book, such as *Yes You Can!*, provides a foundation for further study (119).

Interactive software provides images, animation, and short video clips that bring the subject of neurogenic bowel to life and dramatize the challenges that patients experience. This media allows for patient-driven selection of lecture material, patient-to-patient advice, and creatively depicted animated situations for the learner. These are utilized in *Fantastic Voyage* from Take Control III, a series of interactive software products available on CD ROM (Figure 31.10). *Fantastic Voyage* brings the viewer through the gastrointestinal system from mouth to anus as a virtual passenger in a space ship (120).

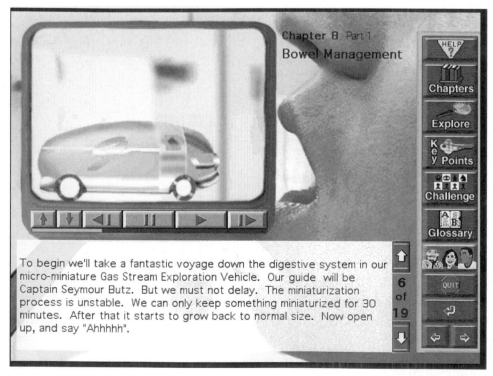

Figure 31.10 *Fantastic Voyage* from Take Control III. Sample frame from the interactive CD-ROM chapter designed to teach about bowel anatomy, function, and adaptation after SCI. The viewer is guided through the gastrointestinal system and learns methods for bowel care thereafter. (Kepplinger F, Stiens SA. *Bowel Management: A Fantastic Voyage.* Take Control III [an education series for persons with SCI and their families]. CD-ROM. VanBiervliet A, PVA-ETF, 1998.)

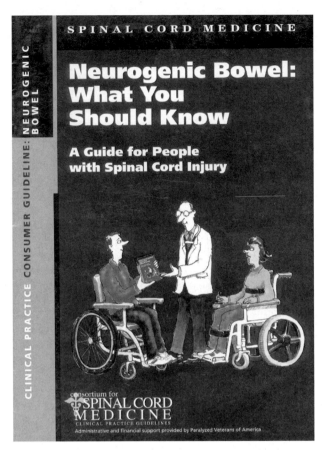

Figure 31.11 Cover of the Consortium for Spinal Cord Medicine guide for neurogenic bowel management after SCI.

Bowel program design and bowel care technique are also outlined in booklet form and illustrated with cartoons (Figure 31.11) (121). This reference breaks bowel care down into simple steps for first time understanding and performance of bowel care (Tables 31.6 and 31.7). Introducing the subject of bowel care assistance to patients with recent SCI, relatives, or new attendants can be challenging. Video-based material can also be used to illustrate the pertinent anatomy, to outline the need for bowel care, and to present the steps performed by an attendant. *Accidents Stink!: Bowel Care 202* reviews the steps with an anatomic model, and then a person with tetraplegia and his attendant demonstrate bowel care (122). Persons with SCI who need to train attendants can utilize these media products to introduce attendants to the topic and train them in the most effective techniques.

Bowel Program: The Comprehensive Personalized Treatment Plan (CPG)

Best results are achieved with intervention strategies that minimize as many of impairments and functional deficits as possible. This comprehensive individualized treatment plan is termed a *bowel program* and is designed to eliminate incontinence, achieve effective and efficient colonic evacuation, and prevent the secondary complications of neurogenic bowel dysfunction (84, 114). Individualization of a bowel program requires prescription of unique diet, physical activity, equipment, oral medications, rectal

medications, and scheduling of bowel care. *Bowel care* is the procedure for scheduled stool elimination. This is an individually developed and prescribed procedure carried out on a regular schedule by the patient or caregiver to evacuate stool from the colon (114).

Bowel programs are designed within the first few weeks after SCI and are modified as needed throughout the patient's life (115). A particular effort is made during acute rehabilitation and early community reentry in the pursuit of a long-term bowel management strategy that can be used to prevent both short- and long-term sequelae of neurogenic bowel dysfunction (85, 114). In an effort to derive a consensus on knowledge related to neurogenic bowel dysfunction and rehabilitative interventions, a panel was

---

Table 31.6   Bowel Care Steps: Areflexic Bowel

1. *Getting ready and washing hands*—empty bladder.
2. *Setting up and positioning*—transfer to a toilet or commode. If you don't sit up, lie on your left side.
3. *Starting and repeating digital rectal simulation*—to keep stool coming, repeat digital rectal stimulation every 5 to 10 minutes as needed, until all stool has passed.
4. *Doing manual evacuation*—use one or two gloved and well-lubricated fingers to break up stool, hook it, and gently pull it out.
5. *Use repeated Valsalva maneuvers*—breathe in and try to push air out, but block the air in your throat to increase the pressure in your abdomen. Try to contract your abdominal muscles as well to help you increase pressure around the colon to push stool out.
6. *Bending and lifting*—to help change the position of the colon and expel stool, lift yourself as if doing a pressure release or do forward and sideways bending with Valsalva maneuvers.
7. *Checking the rectum*—to make sure the rectum is empty, do a final check with a gloved and well-lubricated finger.
8. *Cleaning up*—wash and dry the anal area.

Table 31.7   Bowel Care Procedure: Reflexic Bowel

1. *Getting ready and washing hands*—empty bladder.
2. *Setting up and positioning*—transfer to a toilet or commode. If you don't sit up, lie on your left side.
3. *Checking for stool*—remove any stool that would interfere with inserting a suppository or mini-enema.
4. *Inserting stimulant medication*—using a gloved and lubricated finger or assistive device, place the medication right next to the rectal wall.
5. *Waiting*—wait about 5–15 minutes for the stimulant to work.
6. *Starting and repeating digital rectal stimulation*—to keep stool coming, repeat digital rectal stimulation every 5–10 minutes as needed, until all stool has passed.
7. *Recognizing when bowel care is completed*—you'll know that stool flow has stopped if: (a) no stool has come out after two digital stimulations at least 10 minutes apart, (b) mucus is coming out without stool, or (c) the rectum is completely closed around the stimulating finger.
8. *Cleaning up*—wash and dry the perianal area.

convened by the Consortium for Spinal Cord Medicine to research the literature and write clinical practice guidelines (115). Subsequently, the guidelines were utilized to write a consumer's guide (*Neurogenic Bowel: What You Should Know*) (Figure 31.11) on neurogenic bowel management that presents pathophysiology and patient-centered interventions in clear language, outlined in sequential steps (121). Effective use of a CPG improves the outcome of healthcare and optimizes resource use. Derivation of the CPG should lead to change in clinical practice and physician behavior in managing patients in order to benefit the patients. This does not happen simply by publishing guidelines; rather, there should be wide dissemination and implementation of these guidelines in order to increase provider adherence (123). In a study, physicians managing adult patients with SCI and neurogenic bowel at six different VA Medical Centers were surveyed. The study results showed that provider adherence to a CPG by King et al. did not change after the publication was released in 1998, but increased significantly ($p < 0.0001$) after these guidelines were implemented in 2000–2001 (124).

The bowel program is broken down into essential components for consideration in history-taking and intervention (84). These components consist of diet, exercise, equipment, oral medications, rectal medications, and scheduled bowel care (115).

The diet component of the bowel program is modulated to control stool consistency (Figure 31.12) and to prevent gut irritation. The diet is reviewed to ensure that foods do not trigger incontinence, cause constipation, or contribute to loose stools. Dietary patterns before and after SCI are reviewed for frequency and amount of food in meals and for discussion of the various food groups. Refined carbohydrates and dairy products tend to produce hard, dry stools. Spicy foods, such as certain chili peppers, cayenne pepper, paprika, and excessive garlic, can promote increased transit and excess fluids in stools. These spices can cause diarrhea and bowel accidents. Raw or partially cooked vegetables soften stools and decrease transit time.

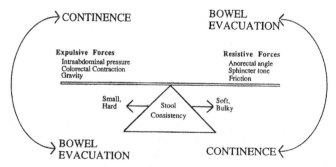

Figure 31.12 Balance of stool consistency. Stool consistency ideally should be titrated to allow for efficient propulsion as well as continence between bowel care procedures. The balance above relates the variables that affect stool consistency and the resulting outcome. Small hard stools move the fulcrum to the left and facilitate continence and, in the extreme, impaction. Soft bulky stools move the fulcrum to the right favoring stool propulsion and bowel evacuation. Expulsive influences and retention mechanisms must be balanced to retain stool yet promote easy complete evacuation at the time of scheduled bowel care. (From Linsenmeyer T, Stone J. Neurogenic bladder and bowel dysfunction. In: DeLisa J, et al., eds. *Rehabilitation Medicine: Principles and Practice.* 3rd ed. Philadelphia: Lippincott-Raven, 1998:1073–1106.)

A review of the type and amount of insoluble fiber is essential for planning a diet. Soluble fiber from fruits and vegetables in combination with adequate water intake contributes to softer, moister stools. Adequate fiber intake in the form of whole grains, fruits, and vegetables allows the stool to form sufficient bulk and to retain water (16). The hydrated fiber maintains a plastic consistency that promotes successful propulsion through the colon (84). Intracolonic material in a viscous fluid phase can be propelled 32 to 100 times faster than a solid (74). Dairy products and high-fat meals tend to work in the opposite way, slowing stool transit (125).

Stool consistency modulation preserves continence by keeping stools formed and eases propulsion and evacuation with moist, soft stools (Figure 31.12). Maintaining a pliable stool with a balance of fiber and adequate fluid facilitates its transit and prevents impaction (118). Fluid intake is therefore an important part of the diet as well. Sufficient fluid intake to produce urinary outputs of 2000–3000 cc's per day is optimal. Caffeinated beverages often produce unpredictable results and may have a laxative as well as a diuretic effect. Fruit juices such as prune juice or apricot nectar provide fluid but also may stimulate stool transit.

Vegetable matter or roughage has varied effects on bowel function. Dietary fiber includes a variety of indigestible plant-derived materials that are primarily composed of nonstarch polysaccharides. A rough separation of these substances based on capacity for suspension in water can be made. They are considered as soluble and insoluble fiber. Soluble fiber consists of multibranched hydrophilic substances such as pectins, guar, and ispaghula, which form viscous gels and colloids that delay gastric emptying and nutrient absorption. They alleviate constipation by keeping stool pliable and propulsive. Two types of insoluble fiber are cellulose and lignin, which markedly accelerate colonic transit time in subjects without spinal cord injury (84). This effect is proportional to dose and increased basal stool weight (126).

Various types of fiber produce different effects depending upon particular segments they traverse along the gastrointestinal tract. These effects depend on fiber volume, the degree of water solubility, and the location within the gastrointestinal tract. Inside the stomach, dietary fiber tends to produce early satiety and to prolong gastric emptying time, whereas in the small intestine, absorption may be delayed while transit time is decreased or increased (127). In the colon, fiber provides bulk to stimulate peristalsis and retain fluid to keep stool pliable. Fiber softens and expands stool and eases the transit through the lower bowel, increasing the frequency of bowel movements and the volume of stools. Coarsely ground fiber tends to be more effective than finely ground fiber (126).

Food sources rich in fiber include whole grain breads and cereals, particularly bran. There are a variety of ways of boosting fiber intake. Common additions to the diet include whole grain breads, cereals, wheat germ, legumes, and salad vegetables. Changing to a breakfast cereal that has more whole grain content is a good first step. To further add fiber to the breakfast, bran muffins and fresh fruit are good choices. Switching to whole grain breads increases fiber intake throughout the day. If flatus is not a problem, then increasing the content of beans and legumes in the diet offers fiber and protein. Dietary supplementation with fiber must be carried out gradually. The expected impact will be a larger volume of softer stools, a requirement for bowel movements with greater frequency, and an improvement in bowel care efficiency. Therefore, changes in the frequency of bowel care will likely be required.

There are a variety of potential complications that could result from fiber additions to the diet. The increase in indigestible material will certainly increase stool bulk. This may induce the need for more frequent bowel movements and lead to more stool output during the bowel care process. Nonetheless, dietary changes are preferable to prescription of laxatives and should be the first step. There is growing evidence that foods high in dietary fiber may also enhance health by lowering blood cholesterol (126, 128), increasing feelings of satiety resulting in weight loss, and promoting transit of stool through the colon (126).

More research needs to be directed toward understanding the effects of dietary fiber in SCI. The findings of studies completed so far suggest there may be differences in the physiologic effect of fiber in gastrointestinal function after SCI. Two significant differences are decreased and varied peristalsis patterns and the problem of the spastic anal sphincter after SCI, which retains stool and suppresses defecation (97). A study of SCI subjects who were supplemented with 40 g of bran per day for a three-week period revealed either no change or prolongation of colonic transit times. The increased fiber, in itself, did not produce changes in evacuation frequency, time required for bowel care, or stool weight per defecation (129). It is clear that the addition of fiber to the diet of a person with SCI makes stools softer by retaining fluid. However, the expected increase in stool bulk may require an increase in the frequency and/or duration of bowel care to fully eliminate the excess stool and prevent colonic overdistension (84, 94, 115).

Exercise is the next component of a complete bowel program. It is well known that mechanical movement of the intestines generates peristalsis. Patients report that range-of-motion exercises before bowel care seem to increase the speed of the fecal elimination and result in larger stool volumes. Regular activity during each day is recommended on a case-by-case basis, depending on independent movement capability. Movement that lifts the perineum up off of the cushion reduces pressure on the anus, and allows flatus to expel, preventing over-distention. At a minimum, regular turns in bed, transfers up to a power wheelchair, and regular tilt or recline pressure releases are expected to provide some gut stimulation.

Appropriate adaptive equipment for bowel care should be prescribed based on the individual's functional needs and discharge environment (115). Seating for upright bowel care utilizes gravity and places the abdominal muscles at maximum mechanical advantage to facilitate the efficient passage of stool (84). Trial and proper identification of the most effective commode chair that provides ease of transfer, stable seating, and skin protection are all important. Nelson and her co-investigators studied patient satisfaction with commode chairs and found that 37% of 147 respondents did not feel safe in their shower commode chairs. Transfers in and out can be problematic. Many commode chairs have fixed, nonremovable armrests, as well as wheel locks that are not effective. Falls were reported during transfers in 35% of respondents, and 23% said their injuries were severe enough to require hospitalization.

Careful measures should be taken to avoid pressure ulcers related to fecal incontinence transfers or to seating during bowel care (115). Pressure ulcer development during commode chair use (130) is a significant risk, especially because the typical bowel care session may last longer than an hour and may be followed by a shower. Regular pressure releases every 15 minutes that allow for a shift of the patient's position on the seat can be helpful. This can be accomplished with a tip back of the commode chair or with assisted leans forward and to the side. The seating of the patient on the commode chair should be reviewed to ensure that excessive pressure and shear does not threaten skin over the sacrum and ischial tuberosities. Focal pressure along the edges of the toilet seat is often a problem. Foot support should be carefully fitted and padding utilized as needed to maintain knee and hip flexion just beyond 90 degrees and to protect skin from focal pressure and shear.

The frequency of bowel care and the time of day are planned based on the patient's life schedule before the SCI. The clinical guidelines for SCI medicine recommend that bowel care be completed no less than three times per week (115). Adhering to a regular schedule of bowel care is essential. Neglected bowel care sessions can contribute to excessive accumulation of stool, which may become increasingly dry, less plastic, and more difficult to eliminate (84). This can stretch the colon, reducing the effectiveness of peristalsis (94) and resulting in extended bowel care with poor results. The establishment of rehabilitation and spinal cord unit–wide standards for bowel management can result in uniformity of procedures, greater patient satisfaction, and improved continence of stool (115, 131).

Bowel Care: The Procedure for Facilitated Defecation

Scheduled bowel care is a subcomponent of the total bowel program. Bowel movements are essential life events that have ramifications for health, personal assistance needs, modesty, self-esteem, and role function of the person with SCI. Normal or effective defecation can be operationally defined as the easy volitional passage of enough soft formed stool on a regular basis to prevent the sensation of incomplete evacuation and overdistention of the colon (84). Achievement of assisted defecation that meets this definition with efficiency, convenience, and privacy is imperative. After SCI, the sensations of need for a bowel movement, control of the anal sphincter, and capability for positioning and clean-up for a bowel movement are often absent. Therefore, a preemptive strategy must be utilized to trigger defecation before reflex-mediated incontinence occurs. As a result, *bowel care* is done as the procedure for initiating and assisting defecation to avoid incontinence and colonic overdistention. The goals of bowel care are to facilitate predictable defecation of the maximal stool volume in the least amount of time, with avoidance of stool incontinence between bowel care sessions (84).

Immediately after SCI, there is a period of spinal shock operationally defined as the period when reflex responses are absent below the level of the injury. Typically, gastric emptying and intestinal peristalsis may slow. Bowel care is done in side-lying, with the left side down. Stool is expelled by hooking it with the gloved finger and pulling it out, a maneuver termed manual evacuation. Excessive, constantly oozing liquid stool can be managed by placement of a rectal tube or an adhesive fecal collection bag. After colonic function stabilizes, one of the two basic bowel care procedures is utilized. These techniques use residual motor function after UMN and LMN injuries in order to meet the goals of bowel care.

Bowel Care with Lower Motor Neuron Bowel: Frequent Manual Evacuation

Patients with lower levels of SCI (T12 spinal cord level and below) typically have cauda equina syndromes, and therefore LMN injuries. Persons with SCI who have LMN injuries often have more difficulty with their bowel care due to the absence of spinal cord–mediated reflex peristalsis, termed *areflexic bowel*. The rectum must be cleared of stool more frequently, usually one or more times per day, to prevent unplanned release of stool that cannot be retained by the patulous external sphincter (84, 92). Bowel care is often timed to follow a meal to take advantage of the gastrocolonic reflex, which may trigger advancement of stool into the rectum. Between bowel care sessions, patients should be taught to avoid Valsalva during transfers in order to avoid increased intra-abdominal pressure and inadvertent expulsion of stool. Some persons with SCI use tight underwear or bicycle pants to retain stool by supporting the pelvic floor and anal sphincter with gluteal adduction (84). When any elastic clothing is used, care should be taken to prevent skin breakdown by checking for skin tolerance along seams (114). An air or gel cushion can be cleaned easily and is also helpful to evenly distribute pressure across the descending perineum. Due to the lack of gluteal muscle mass, SCI patients are at particular risk for shear and pressure ulcers. Padded toilet seats and frequent repositioning can prevent breakdown.

The procedure for bowel care for SCI persons with LMN injuries usually consists of removing stool with the finger (manual evacuation) and may include digital rectal stimulation, which may trigger proximal segmental peristasis to help propel stool out. The procedure has been broken down into steps and published in an illustrated consumer guide (Tables 31.6 and 31.7) (121). Bowel care starts with hand-washing setup and careful transfer and positioning on the commode. *Digital rectal stimulation* is done by sliding the gloved and lubricated finger into the rectum to relax the internal sphincter with circular finger movement and proximal rectal dilatation. Deep inhalation, Valsalva maneuver, abdominal wall contraction, and transabdominal colonic massage in a clockwise manner help to trigger peristalsis and propel the stool. At the rectum, stool is hooked with the finger and guided past the sphincter with the help of gravity. Manual evacuation is repeated alternating with digital stimulation until there is no further palpable stool. The absence of palpable stool, the passage of mucus, and the tightening of the internal anal sphincter are all signals that defecation (bowel care) is complete.

Bowel Care with Upper Motor Neuron Bowel: Reflex Facilitation

Upper motor neuron SCI results from a lesion above the level of the conus medullaris. This produces a variety of impairments that create problems with defecation. There is a limitation in production of effective intra-abdominal pressure in patients with lesions above T12. There is no conscious contraction or relaxation of the external anal sphincter and impairment of discriminate sensation of rectal contents. However, many people with clinically complete SCI have demonstrated the ability to perceive rectal distention (102). The external anal sphincter is typically spastic and retains stool and flatus. The external anal sphincter may persistently constrict, impeding defecation during rectal contraction, termed anorectal dyssynergia (93). Defecation may be spontaneous due to reflex relaxation of the external anal sphincter with poor accommodation of the rectum to stretch (132). Without bowel care, there is a tendency to produce and accumulate stool and overfill the colon. Stool is retained too long and desiccates, resulting in proximal colon impaction with dry, hard stool. The person with SCI experiences significant disability that has a pervasive effect on the defecation process. Recumbency impairs motility, the gastrocolonic reflex is blunted or absent (79), rectal sensation is impaired, and chest and abdominal musculature are paralyzed.

Bowel care procedures for UMN SCI bowel are designed to overcome these impairments. Persons with UMN need to do scheduled bowel care based on time rather than on the urge for defecation. This prevents uncontrollable reflex defecation (132) in response to rectal distention. Filling of the colon can trigger a giant migratory colonic contraction with advancement of stool into the rectum (84). Therefore, elimination of stool before spontaneous reflex defecation extrudes it requires a scheduled trigger to start bowel care and completion of defecation every one to three days (115). The patient or attendant stimulates reflex defecation manually with a finger (or assistive device) inserted in the rectum (digital rectum stimulation) and/or with an appropriate chemical or electrical stimulus. The initiating stimulus should be of the minimal intensity required to start and sustain the defecation process. Typical initiating stimuli in order of intensity include abdominal massage, digital perianal stimulation, digital rectal stimulation, glycerin suppository, Enemeez mini enema, and bisacodyl suppository (7, 94).

The steps for bowel care for persons with reflexic (UMN) bowel have been outlined in a consumer guide (Table 31.7) (121). The chemical trigger stimulus for defecation is typically a suppository, enema, or mini-enema, which provides a mucosal contact stimulus that is transmitted to the conus to trigger reflex mediated peristalsis (84). Ideal placement of the chemical stimulant is directly against the mucosa in the upper rectum. A waiting interval (*time to flatus*) (Figure 31.13) then starts, as the active ingredients dissolve, disperse, and stimulate. The beginning of propulsive peristalsis for defecation is signaled by flatus or *first flatus*. Soon thereafter, *stool flow* begins and is promoted as necessary with manual evacuation and regular digital stimulations (133).

After bowel care has been initiated, and flatus and stool flow have occurred, peristalsis and stool flow can be maintained by repeatedly triggering the rectocolic reflex. *Digital rectal stimulation* is the technique for relaxing anal sphincter tone and inducing a reflex peristaltic wave from the colon to evacuate stool (84). This technique starts with gentle insertion of the entire gloved and lubricated finger into the rectum. Glove choice is a consideration, as latex allergy prevalence is increasing and may develop with repeated exposure (134). Nonlatex gloves are recommended. The finger is first directed toward the sacrum and then turned toward the umbilicus in order to follow the course of the anal canal as it turns. After the stimulation finger is fully inserted, the puborectalis muscle sling is palpated. Gentle sustained pressure toward the sacrum relaxes the puborectalis muscle, making the rectal angle less acute and reducing outflow resistance (7). This opens the external anal sphincter and provides a stretch stimulus that reduces spastic external sphincter tone and rectal outflow

Intervals:

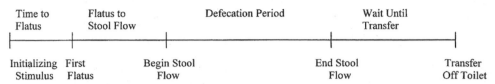

Figure 31.13 Bowel care outcome. Events and intervals of bowel care. Bowel care events separate the bowel care total period into discrete intervals on a timeline. Pharmacologically or mechanically initiated bowel care begins with insertion of rectal medication or with digital rectal stimulation, which acts as an initializing stimulus. First flatus ends the interval time to flatus (initializing stimulus until first gas is passed). Begin stool flow ends the second interval, termed flatus to stool flow, and begins the defecation. The event transfer off toilet ends the wait until transfer period, which represents the time spent to ensure that defecation is complete. The time of transfer off toilet ends the bowel care procedure. (From Stiens SA, Biener Bergman S, Goetz LL. Neurogenic bowel dysfunction after SCI: Clinical evaluation and rehabilitative management (focused review). *Arch Phys Med Rehabil* 1997; 78:S86–S102, with permission.)

resistance. Rectal irritation with rapid movement or force should be avoided as this can precipitate anal sphincter spasm.

Digital rectal stimulation (DRS) is done with a gentle circular movement dilating and relaxing the distal rectum and anal canal. Continual contact with the rectal mucosa and gradual dilatation of the rectum provides the stimulus for peristalsis and opens a space for the stool to descend into and fill. Rotation is continued until relaxation of the bowel wall is felt, flatus passes, stool comes down, or the internal sphincter constricts. Digital rectal stimulation activates the recto-anal inhibitory reflex, producing relaxation of the internal sphincter, and the rectocolic reflex, stimulating pelvic nerve–mediated peristalsis and promoting local enteric-coordinated peristalsis as well (84). In addition to clinical experience, there is some experimental evidence for the practice. In a study on six subjects with SCI, Korsten et al. showed an increase in frequency as well as amplitude of contractions of the left colon in response to DRS (135). These changes were associated with increased peristaltic activity of the left colon as studied by the documentation of the movement of the barium oatmeal paste in the left colon, and finally by expulsion of this oatmeal paste by the fifth DRS in all six of the individuals (135). The mechanism for these changes is believed to be stimulation of the internal sphincter mechanoreceptors in response to DRS. This, in turn, seems to evoke the anorectal excitatory reflex, producing defecation (132, 135). Mechanical stimulation of the rectum has been demonstrated to produce supranormal rectal and sigmoid contractions in UMN chronic SCI (100, 102, 136). Rectal contractions in response to rectal distention are stronger in persons with upper motor neuron spinal cord injury (102). Section of the posterior roots eliminates the rectal contractile response to rectal distention, confirming that this response is spinal reflex mediated (102). Typically, digital stimulation is usually continued for 30 seconds to a minute at a time. Thereafter, the peristaltic activity and stool delivery in response to a digital rectal stimulation occurs within seconds to a few minutes. Digital rectal stimulations are repeated every 3 to 10 minutes as required to sustain the progress of defecation (84).

Without experience with a given patient, it can be difficult to determine when the bowel movement has ended. The completion of defecation is signaled by cessation of flatus and stool flow, expulsion of mucus from the rectum, palpable internal sphincter closure, and the absence of stool results from the last two digital rectal stimulations. Some persons with SCI report a relaxed feeling in the abdomen and rectum that coincides with cessation of active peristalsis and a band of rectal wall construction. This perception could potentially be mediated by visceral afferents transmitted through the vagus from the proximal colon and the sympathetic chain, or could be from partial sacral sparing of anal afferents relayed through the spinal cord (84).

Various practices have been suggested to enhance bowel care effectiveness. Increased activity may help; some do range-of-motion exercises before bowel care. Some people with UMN SCI report triggering and sustaining defecation with cutaneous stimulation of sacral dermatomes. Transabdominal massage starting in the right lower quadrant and following the course of the colon in an aboral direction has been used in an attempt to enhance promulgated peristalsis and bring stool to the rectum. Gentle palmar massage with a lubricant along the course of the colon has been included as a prelude and an adjunct to bowel care for those with SCI by many for years (137). A trial of abdominal wall massage of neurally intact subjects with constipation did not demonstrate effectiveness of the modality (138). The effect of abdominal massage as an adjunct measure to the standard BCP was tested in twenty-four SCI subjects (139). The authors showed improvement in symptoms of abdominal distention and fecal incontinence along with improved colonic transit time, as assessed with the use of radiological markers (139). Abdominal wall compression is not an entirely benign maneuver and should be used gently, taking care to avoid excessive pressure in the colon or the urinary bladder. Antimesenteric perforation of the sigmoid has been reported in association with the use of Crede method by a patient for bladder and bowel evacuation (140). Abdominal wall stimulation using a belt with electrodes (patient blinded) has also shown encouraging results with a decrease in the average time to first stool (50 to 25 minutes, $p < 0.005$) and total bowel care time (115 to 80 minutes, $p < 0.01$) (110).

There are a large variety of other methods for initiating and sustaining defecation of patients with UMN (reflexic) bowels. Various medications utilized to trigger defecation have been compared in clinical trials (Figure 31.14). High-volume tap water enemas were used in the past as a mechanical stimulus to trigger defecation, soften stool, and cleanse the colon after SCI (137, 141). Currently, large-volume enemas are used infrequently in the bowel care of persons with SCI (115), although tap water enemas continue to be used with success by patients who have stool continence problems (142). However, in the care of persons with

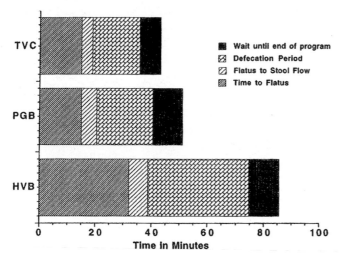

Figure 31.14 Comparison of triggering medications for bowel care. The time intervals of the experimental bowel care sessions were averaged and are presented in minutes for hydrogenated vegetable oil–based (HVB) and polyethylene glycol–based (PGB) bisacodyl suppositories and Theravac® mini-enemas. The time to flatus was comparable for PGB and TVC, although HVB was significantly longer than PGB. Flatus to stool flow was not significantly different between the agents. The HVB defecation period was significantly longer than that for PGB. PGB and TVC defecation periods were comparable. Wait until transfer was significantly longer for PGB compared with TVC, whereas PGB and HVB showed no differences. (From House JG, Stiens SA. Pharmacologically initiated defecation for persons with spinal cord injury: effectiveness of three agents. *Arch Phys Med Rehabil* 1997; 78:1062–1065, with permission.)

spina bifida, enemas are still in common use. The enema continence catheter has been used to help retain fluid during infusion (143, 144). With enemas, bowel care was done once every 1–2 days. The rate of spontaneous bowel incontinence was reduced from 64% of bowel movements to 4%. In a study of forty children with myelomeningocele and neurogenic bowel, use of tap water enema with transrectal irrigation was shown to be effective in 85% cases to relieve constipation and incontinence. However, the major problem was dependence on the caregiver; only one child could do this procedure independently (145). Pulsed irrigation–enhanced evacuation (PIEE) is a hydraulically driven enema delivered in a series of tap water pulses that rehydrate, suspend, and drain away the stool (146). The water is carried through a tube via a rectal speculum that is retained with an inflatable cuff. Effluent with suspended feces from the colon is guided out through the rectal speculum down a drain tube to a stool reservoir. This modality does not require assistance from other caregivers and can be easily used even by those who are immobilized and those who have poor hand function. PIEE has been used successfully to clear impaction (147). Devices that deliver PIEE have also been used for regular bowel care of persons with LMN and UMN bowels. A modification of this technique (Peristeen anal irrigation system) was shown to be superior to standard bowel care in managing adult patients with neurogenic bowel in a prospective randomized multicenter European study (148). The authors showed that transanal irrigation was significantly better in improving patients' symptoms (constipation and fecal incontinence) and provided a better quality of life as compared to standard bowel care (148).

Functional electric stimulation of defecation has been available for the last 25 years but has been only recently aggressively marketed in the United States (149, 150). Urination (150) and defecation have been triggered with electrical stimuli by some investigators with selective nerve root activation in patients with UMN bowels (150–152). Systems are now FDA approved and are being implanted at academic centers in the United States. Implantable stimulators are placed, and selective S2, S3 dorsal root rhizotomies are done to reduce sphincter tone. Electrodefecation with neuroprosthetic stimulation is achieved by radio frequency activation of a surgically implanted subcutaneous receiver that then stimulates the S2, S3, and S4 nerve roots bilaterally (153). Repeated series of electrical stimuli are transmitted at low or high frequency and are sustained for up to 10 seconds. In the colon, complex high-pressure phasic contractions, reminiscent of propulsive peristaltic activity, are induced. Stool is propelled out through the anal sphincter. Experimental use of functional magnetic stimulation has recently demonstrated an increase in rectal pressure upon stimulation and a reduction in colonic transit time with chronic transabdominal stimulation (154). In another recent study, an abdominal belt with implanted electrodes has been employed to stimulate the abdominal muscles to expel stool by increasing intra-abdominal pressure, with encouraging results (108).

Constipation: Difficulty with Evacuation and Colonic Fecal Distention

Constipation has been variously defined and includes prolonged difficult bowel movements, infrequent bowel movements (less than three times per week), and incomplete evacuation. In particular, constipation for the individual is any change in the person's stool elimination pattern that limits defecation frequency or effectiveness. This definition is problematic when applied to the spinal cord injury population because defecation is not frequently willful, and the bowel care procedure varies between patients. Fecal impaction, chronic constipation, and fecal incontinence are common, affecting more than 80% of persons with SCI (6). Unfortunately, colonic function does deteriorate with time after SCI. Constipation-related symptoms are less frequent during the 5-year period immediately after SCI (27, 155). Progressive dysfunction has been attributed to colonic overdistention over time. Symptoms include prolonged and difficult evacuation during bowel care, abdominal distention, and abdominal pain.

A recent radiologic study of the volume of colon contents of persons with SCI admitted for annual evaluations or non–bowel related medical problems sought to quantify the prevalence of radiologic constipation and megacolon (85). Radiologic constipation has been defined as severe-to-moderate stool retention in all segments, and megacolon as colon diameter greater than 6 cm. Abdominal radiographs revealed 74% of subjects as having megacolon, and 55% as having radiologic constipation. Subjects with radiologic constipation frequently complained of constipation, and particularly of abdominal distention. More than a third of the subjects reported spending more than 1 hour on bowel care; stool retention was most common in the right colon. Factors significantly associated with megacolon were older age, longer duration of injury, abdominal distention symptoms, radiologic constipation, urinary outlet surgery, laxative drug use, anticholinergic medication, and use of calcium containing laxatives (85). Hypotheses for this progression of constipation include less frequent or regular bowel care, less effective bowel care, and deficits in colonic peristalsis. Interventions have included use of laxatives and prokinetic agents. Of the various laxatives, oral agents such as docusate and lactulose are commonly used. Administration of laxatives must be based on the knowledge of onset of action of various laxatives (Table 31.8) and time at which bowel movement is desired. Of the prokinetic agents, cisapride showed the most promise (156); however, the drug has been withdrawn from the market in the United States, due to its potential to cause life-threatening cardiac arrhythmias (157). A newer prokinetic agent, neostigmine, has been successfully used in patients with neurogenic bowel after chronic SCI (158). Neostigmine is a competitive inhibitor of the enzyme acetylcholinesterase; hence, it increases the concentration of acetylcholine at the nerve endings. This action at the level of the colon results in an increase in colonic peristalsis. However, this cholinergic action outside the colon has the potential to cause unwanted effects such as bradycardia and bronchospasm. In this respect, the addition of glycopyrrolate (an anticholinergic agent that spares the muscarinic receptors of the colon) to neostigmine is useful (159). Intravenous infusion of neostigmine, as well as neostigmine + glycopyrrolate, was superior for bowel evacuation compared to infusion of normal saline (158). Bowel evacuation was measured by fluoroscopic assessment of the movement of barium oatmeal paste having the consistency of stool (Figure 31.15). The bowel evacuation score was 3 or more in 57% of cases receiving neostigmine infusion and in 64% of cases receiving a combination of neostigmine and glycopyrrolate. In contrast, none of the patients receiving a normal saline infusion received a score of 2 or more. Neostigmine in combination with glycopyrrolate was well tolerated, and there were no adverse effects reported in this study (158). The intravenous route has obvious limitations for chronic

use in patients with SCI and neurogenic bowel. Studies are under progress assessing the intranasal use of neostigmine.

Bowel care can be modified to include upright position, stronger triggering medications, small enemas, more frequent and prolonged digital stimulation, and abdominal massage. Changes in bowel care should be followed with monitoring of bowel care parameters for at least 3 weeks. Should bowel care become prolonged, be associated with frequent autonomic dysreflexia, or produce insufficient results in spite of a period of adaptive modification of the entire bowel program, surgical intervention should be considered.

Diarrhea: Liquid Stool with Risk for Incontinence

The World Health Organization defines diarrhea as stool that takes the shape of the container. Patients with SCI commonly have diarrhea as a result of treatment of urinary tract infections with broad-spectrum antibiotics. This is one of many reasons why treatment of urinary tract infections should include cultures and antibiotics that are targeted specifically at the pathogen. Initial management includes doing bowel care to clear as much of the liquid stool from the colon as possible. Application of an occlusive cream to the perineum after clean-up offers some protection from stool irritation. Patients should remain on regularly scheduled bowel care to prevent spontaneous liquid incontinence episodes (121).

Patient-driven dietary interventions to prevent and manage loose stools are essential. Inclusion of a moderate amount of fiber in the diet such as psyllium regularizes stool consistency by absorbing excess liquid to maintain formed stools. Ongoing patient experience with gut tolerance for various foods, especially spicy or pepper-seasoned dishes, allows for moderation. Preemptive management of gut irritation from such indulgences includes use of calcium antacids for symptoms of heartburn and doing bowel care 6 to 12 hours after such food has been consumed to clear soft stools before a spontaneous defecation occurs. Stool consistency should be modulated by dietary choices based

Table 31.8 **Pharmacological Agents Used in Bowel Care**		
MEDICATION	**DOSE**	**ONSET OF ACTION**
Bulk laxatives		
• Docusate sodium	100–300 mg daily once or in divided doses	12–72 hours
• Psyllium	1 tsp (3.6 g of fiber) 1–2 times a day	12–72 hours
Stimulant laxatives		
• Senna	15–30 mg orally, maximum 60 mg/day	6–12 hours
• Bisacodyl tablet	5–15 mg orally	6–12 hours
• Bisacodyl suppository	10 mg per rectum	0.25–1 hour
• Castor oil	15–60 ml daily	6–8 hours
• Cascara	1–2 tablets daily (325-mg tablet)	6–8 hours
Saline laxatives		
• Magnesium hydroxide	15–30 ml 1–2 times a day	0.5–6 hours
• Sodium phosphate	45–90 ml once a day orally or 45 ml rectal enema	0.5–6 hours
Hyperosmolar laxatives		
• Lactulose	15–60 ml 1–3 times a day	0.5–3 hours
• Sorbitol 70%	15–60 ml 1–3 times a day	0.5–3 hours
• Polyethylene glycol	17 g in 8 oz of water 12 times a day	0.5–3 hours

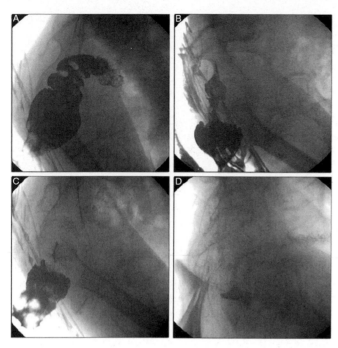

Figure 31.15 Semi-quantitative measure (score 0 to 4) of bowel emptying using barium oatmeal paste. Evacuation score: A = 1, B = 2, C = 3, D = 4.

on regular bowel care results (121). Attendants who do bowel care should report consistency to their clients. Foods that firm the stool are starches and dairy products.

The first step in treatment is to restore the balance in the gut ecology. Lactobacillus is a friendly symbiotic resident that may need to be reintroduced to the gut microbe population with Lactinex capsules and active cultured yogurt in the diet. Should loose stools persist, abdominal and rectal examination should be done to rule out partial obstruction from an inspissated fecal mass causing a "ball valve" effect with intermittent obstruction of liquid fecal flow (160).

Carcinoma of the colon and rectum remains a significant health threat. Reduction in mortality is a consequence of earlier detection and surgical removal of adenomatous polyps (161) and malignant colorectal tumors. The presence of neurogenic bowel can complicate screening and diagnosis. The efficacy and safety of colonoscopy was assessed in subjects with SCI in prospective randomized studies (162, 163). Preparation of the colon (assessed by the Ottawa scale), even with dual preparation for 2 consecutive days, was poorer in SCI subjects. Poor preparation of the colon in subjects with SCI is notorious for missing findings and having a poorer polyp detection rate (164). Colonoscopy was a safe procedure in these patients and none of the subjects developed autonomic dysreflexia (162). In another randomized prospective study on 165 subjects (139 able-bodied and 26 SCI), the use of oral sodium phosphate solution for the bowel preparation was found to be safe, and none of the subjects developed any clinically significant renal failure (165). The myriad of chronic gastrointestinal symptoms after SCI may mask a change in pattern or function that would trigger evaluation. The question of the contribution of SCI to relative risk for colorectal carcinoma is not fully answered. Some have suggested an increased risk (166), whereas others have reported similar incidences in controlled retrospective studies. Screening is problematic. Hemorrhoids are highly prevalent. The process of bowel care with digital stimulation can cause some mucosal irritation and bleeding. Consequently, false positive stool guiac studies are common (167). Yet annual or biannual fecal occult-blood screening reduces the incidence of colorectal cancer (168). Annual digital rectal examination as screening is recommended for patients over 40, and after age 35 in patients with a first-degree relative with a history of colorectal carcinoma or polyps. Endoscopic screening and polypectomy is recommended every 3 to 5 years after age 50 (161). Colonic cleansing in preparation for examination may require assistance at home or hospitalization. Preparations are prolonged and can be incomplete. Future studies of endoscopic screening frequency and methods for efficiency and yield in colon preparation are needed.

Surgical Options: Anatomic Revisions to Enhance Function, Hygiene, and Quality of Life

Appendicocecostomy: A Catheterizable Stoma for Antegrade Enemas to Trigger Bowel Care

An alternative method of enema delivery is through a surgically created continent catheterizable appendicocecostomy stoma (169). This procedure requires a right lower quadrant laparotomy with mobilization of the cecum to bring the appendix through the abdominal wall (Figure 31.16). A stoma is fabricated by amputating the tip to expose the lumen. This opening into the appendix is sewn into a perforation in the abdominal wall, where it is most convenient for independent catheterization by the patient. Functional use of the stoma is best if the location has been identified previously with the help of an occupational therapist and rehabilitation nurse. This technique has been in widespread use for persons with spinal cord dysfunction due to spina bifida (169–171).

Recently, there have been a few case reports of the Malone procedure being used on adults after traumatic SCI (172, 173).

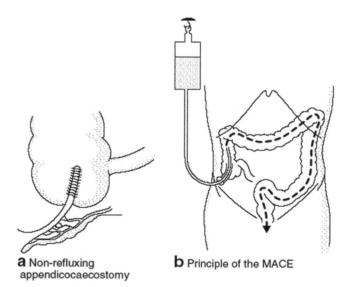

a Non-refluxing appendicocaecostomy   **b** Principle of the MACE

Figure 31.16 Diagram of the Malone antegrade continence enema (MACE) showing (**a**) the nonrefluxing appendicocecostomy and (**b**) the principle of the MACE procedure. (From Malon PS. *Lancet* 1990; 336:1217–1218, with permission.)

In a single-subject design, it was demonstrated that the use of the antegrade continence enema to trigger bowel care can reduce the time required by 50% (2 hours to 1 hour). The bowel care procedure with the antegrade enema requires the infusion of 200 to 500 cc of normal saline into the stoma through a catheter. Peristalsis begins minutes thereafter, and bowel care is then carried out with the steps described for the upper motor neuron bowel (Table 31.7). Once the technique is established, a variety of laxative medications and stimulant medications previously used to trigger bowel care can be removed from the bowel program (172). Long-term results in adults with traumatic SCI after the Malone procedure have not been as favorable as in children with spina bifida. Up to 95% of children continue to use their stoma successfully for bowel care at 6 years, whereas only 77% of adults continue to use the antegrade enema technique after a stoma is fashioned (174). Retrospective review on long-term (4.5-year) results on the use of MACE in six patients showed that the procedure decreased the bowel care time from an average of 190 minutes in the pre-ACE period to 28 minutes after the ACE ($p <$ 0.0001) (175). This was associated with improvement in fecal incontinence and overall quality of life in five of the six (83%) patients. However, one limitation of this procedure over the long term is the need for re-exploration in three of five (60%) cases. Therefore, one should select the cases very carefully. Physicians should involve the patients in the decision-making process and explain to them in detail the benefits and problems related to the procedure. The procedure has the obvious problems of morbidity related to the surgery needed for creating the appendicocecostomy. To overcome this, cecostomy has been created with the use of a colonoscope. This percutaneous endoscopic cecostomy (PEC) is then used for providing the antegrade continence enema (ACE) (176). ACE by this method was successful in decompression of the colon and in providing effective evacuation. However, one problem with long-term use of a catheter for PEC is frequent rupture of the balloon. This problem is tackled by changing the catheter to a Chait Trapdoor Cecostomy catheter (CTCC), which is placed radiologically and is left in the cecum (176).

Colostomy: An Accessible Colonic Stoma with a Collection Bag for Continence

Colostomy is a reasonable management option for persons with neurogenic bowel if a sustained effort has failed to develop a bowel program design that meets the patient's person-centered goals and life demands (115, 177, 178). Failure of bowel care to fully evacuate the colon may call for more attention to stool consistency. A common indication is an extremely long bowel care time with insufficient evacuation (179). Bowel care with tap water irrigation of the colon as an enema three to five times per week has been effective in patients without SCI who have stool continence problems. Many patients receive colostomies as a means to divert the fecal stream away from high-grade buttock pressure ulcers (155). However, pressure ulcers alone may not be the best indication, as these often large wounds have multifocal etiologies and may heal poorly in the chronic state. A single intervention to prevent fecal contamination may not have sufficient impact to promote healing (180). The best candidates for the procedure report significant difficulty or complications with typical bowel care as well as demonstrate the capacity to manage and benefit from a colostomy (178). Colostomy requires major abdominal

surgery and includes complication risks. There are a variety of conditions that can result from surgical stomas: diversion colitis (181), bowel obstruction, stomal ischemia, retraction, prolapse, peristomal hernia fistula, and variceal bleeding (115, 182). Death during the postoperative course after colostomy with concurrent large pressure ulcers has been reported in as much as 15% of patients in a small series (180).

Colostomies in use by people with SCI effectively reduce the burden of care and can contribute to quality of life (178, 183). Total bowel care time is reduced, as are incontinence episodes, as compared with these aspects of bowel program outcomes before colostomy (155, 166, 178, 180). The best outcomes are achieved with careful patient selection and individualization of the procedure to meet person-centered needs and capabilities. Consideration of fecal diversion therefore should include a broad assessment of bowel program, bowel care, personal assistance, body image, and lifestyle issues (7). In a survey on veterans with SCI, patients' satisfaction with their bowel program (BP) and health-related quality of life (HRQOL) were noted for 74 subjects with colostomy and compared with results for 296 subjects who received standard BP (184). Respondents in both the groups claimed to have received adequate training for their BP and to have good HRQOL. One limitation of this study is that the authors did not assess the time taken for the BP or individual gastrointestinal symptoms related to bowel dysfunction. However, more than 40% of patients in each group were dissatisfied with their bowel program (184). This should be taken into consideration before making a decision for surgical diversion of stools or colostomy.

Once the decision for fecal diversion is made, the surgical procedure and the location of the stoma require interdisciplinary assessment including primary rehabilitation nursing and occupational therapy (115). It has been shown that evaluation of the transit time of the colon may be useful to decide the site of colostomy (2, 155). Sigmoid colostomy is suited for those with normal transit time of the colon but with inability to evacuate the rectum, whereas transverse colostomy is useful for patients with delayed transit of the left colon. Patients with dilated and nonfunctional right colon are best candidates for ileostomy (155). When the standard bowel care fails in management of neurogenic bowel after chronic SCI, there are a few options available, such as ACE, sacral root stimulation, and enterostomy. As of today, there are no guidelines available to choose either of these methods, and mostly it depends on the local expertise and availability of the procedure and on patient preference. In a review of published studies to assess the effect of colostomy, ileostomy, sacral root implantation, and Malone ACE in patients with severe chronic SCI, a decision analytic model was created which showed that the MACE provided the best quality adjusted life expectancy. The authors concluded that the MACE procedure is most preferred by the patients and may provide the best outcome in terms of improvement of bowel function and reduction in complication rates, including autonomic dysreflexia (185).

References

1. Stiens SA, O'Young BJ, Young MA. Person-centered rehabilitation: interdisciplinary intervention to enhance patient enablement. In: O'Young B, Young M, Stiens S, eds. *Physical Medicine and Rehabilitation Secrets.* 3rd ed. Philadelphia: Hanley & Belfus, Mosby, 2008:118–125.

2. Singal AK RA, Bauman WA, Korsten MA. Recent concepts in the management of bowel problems after spinal cord injury. *Adv Med Sci* 2006; 51:15–22.

3. Roach MJ, Frost FS, Creasey G. Social and personal consequences of acquired bowel dysfunction for persons with spinal cord injury. *J Spinal Cord Med* 2000; 23:263–269.

4. Hanson R, Franklin M. Sexual loss in relation to other functional losses for spinal cord injured males. *Arch Phys Med Rehabil* 1976; 57:291–293.

5. Stone J, Nino-Murcia M, Wolfe V, Perkash I. Chronic gastrointestinal problems in spinal cord injury patients: a prospective analysis. *Am J Gastroenterol* 1990; 85:1114–1149.

6. Krogh K, Nielsen J, Djurhuus JC, Mosdal C, et al. Colorectal function in patients with spinal cord lesions. *Dis Colon Rectum* 1997; 40:1233–1239.

7. Stiens SA, O'Young BJ, Young MA. Person-centered rehabilitation: interdisciplinary intervention to enhance patient enablement. In: O'Young B, Young M, Stiens S, eds. *Physical Medicine and Rehabilitation Secrets.* 3rd ed. Philadelphia: Hanley & Belfus, Mosby, 2008:118–125.

8. World Health Organization. *International Classification of Functioning Disability and Health.* Geneva: WHO, 2001.

9. Durnan JR, Thaler R. Dental care for the patient with a spinal cord injury. *J Am Dent Assoc* 1973; 86:1318–1321.

10. Schluger S. *Periodontal Diseases: Basic Phenomena, Clinical Management, and Occlusal and Restorative Interrelationships.* 2nd ed. Philadelphia: Lea & Febiger, 1990.

11. Stiefel DJ, Truelove EL, Persson RS, Chin MM, Mandel LS. A comparison of oral health in spinal cord injury and other disability groups. *Spec Care Dentist* 1993; 13:229–235.

12. Gibbons R, Houte J. On the formation of dental plaques. *J Periodontol* 1973; 44:347–360.

13. Almstahl A, Wikstrom M. Oral microflora in subjects with reduced salivary secretion. *J Dent Res* 1999; 78:1410–1416.

14. Taricco M, Adone R, Pagliacci C, Telaro E. Pharmacological interventions for spasticity following spinal cord injury. *Cochrane Database Syst Rev* 2000; (2):CD001131.

15. Nance PW, Bugaresti J, Shellenberger K, Sheremata W, Martinez-Arizala A. Efficacy and safety of tizanidine in the treatment of spasticity in patients with spinal cord injury. North American Tizanidine Study Group. *Neurology* 1994; 44:S44–51; discussion S51–S52.

16. Banwell JG, Creasey GH, Aggarwal AM, Mortimer JT. Management of the neurogenic bowel in patients with spinal cord injury. *Urol Clin North Am* 1993; 20:517–526.

17. Watson AD. Diet and periodontal disease in dogs and cats. *Aust Vet J* 1994; 71:313–318.

18. Stiens S. Reduction in bowel program duration with polyethylene glycol based bisacodyl suppositories. *Arch Phys Med Rehabil* 1995; 76:674–677.

19. Eichel B. Tobacco smoke toxicity: loss of human oral leukocyte function and fluid cell metabolism. *Science* 1969; 166:1424.

20. Blaine HL, Nelson EP. A mouthstick for quadriplegic patients. *J Prosthet Dent* 1973; 29:317–322.

21. Budning BC, Hall M. A practical mouthstick for early intervention with quadriparetic patients. *J Can Dent Assoc* 1990; 56:243–244.

22. Cloran AJ, Lotz JW, Campbell HD, Wiechers DO. Oral telescoping orthosis: an aid to functional rehabilitation of quadriplegic patients. *J Am Dent Assoc* 1980; 100:876–879.

23. Duncan JD, Puckett AD Jr. A one-appointment mouthstick appliance. *J Prosthodont* 1993; 2:196–198.

24. Kozole KP, Gordon RE, Hurst PS. Modular mouthstick system. *J Prosthet Dent* 1985; 53:831–835.

25. Norris M. A mouthstick prosthesis for independence. *Am J Occup Ther* 1968; 22:174–175.

26. Turner C, Bennett CG. A simple mouthstick prosthesis for a quadriplegic patient. *Spec Care Dentist* 1985; 5:178–179.

27. Gore RM, Mintzer RA, Calenoff L. Gastrointestinal complications of spinal cord injury. *Spine* 1981; 6:538–544.

28. Pollock RA, Purvis JM, Apple DF Jr., Murray HH. Esophageal and hypopharyngeal injuries in patients with cervical spine trauma. *Ann Otol Rhinol Laryngol* 1981; 90:323–327.

29. Roffi RP, Waters RL, Adkins RH. Gunshot wounds to the spine associated with a perforated viscus. *Spine* 1989; 14:808–811.

30. Colachis S, Murray K. Esophageal perforation: a delayed complication following traumatic spinal cord injury. Case report. *Paraplegia* 1992; 30:449–453.

31. Weiman DS, Walker WA, Brosnan KM, Pate JW, Fabian TC. Noniatrogenic esophageal trauma. *Ann Thorac Surg* 1995; 59:845–850.

32. Kirshblum S, Johnston MV, Brown J, O'Connor KC, Jarosz P. Predictors of dysphagia after spinal cord injury. *Arch Phys Med Rehabil* 1999; 80:1101–1105.

33. Wolf C, Meiners TH. Dysphagia in patients with acute cervical spinal cord injury. *Spinal Cord* 2003; 41:347–353.

34. Neville AL, Crookes P, Velmahos GC, Vlahos A, et al. Esophageal dysfunction in cervical spinal cord injury: a potentially important mechanism of aspiration. *J Trauma* 2005; 59:905–911.

35. Kewalramani LS. Neurogenic gastroduodenal ulceration and bleeding associated with spinal cord injuries. *J Trauma* 1979; 19:259–265.

36. Singh G, Triadafilopoulos G. Gastroesophageal reflux disease in patients with spinal cord injury. *J Spinal Cord Med* 2000; 23:23–27.

37. Stinneford JG, Keshavarzian A, Nemchausky BA, Doria MI, Durkin M. Esophagitis and esophageal motor abnormalities in patients with chronic spinal cord injuries. *Paraplegia* 1993; 31:384–392.

38. Hinder RA, Libbey JS, Gorecki P, Bammer T. Antireflux surgery: indications, preoperative evaluation, and outcome. *Gastroenterol Clin North Am* 1999; 28:987–1005.

39. Johnson DA. Medical therapy for gastroesophageal reflux disease. *Am J Med* 1992; 92:88S–97S.

40. Richter JE, Long JF. Cisapride for gastroesophageal reflux disease: a placebo-controlled, double-blind study. *Am J Gastroenterol* 1995; 90:423–430.

41. Carone R, Vercelli D, Bertapelle P. Effects of cisapride on anorectal and vesicourethral function in spinal cord injured patients. *Paraplegia* 1993; 31:125–127.

42. Ganzini L, Casey DE, Hoffman WF, McCall AL. The prevalence of metoclopramide-induced tardive dyskinesia and acute extrapyramidal movement disorders. *Arch Intern Med* 1993; 153:1469–1475.

43. Thanik KD, Chey WY, Shah AN, Gutierrez JG. Reflux esophagitis: effect of oral bethanechol on symptoms and endoscopic findings. *Ann Intern Med* 1980; 93:805–808.

44. Katzka DA. Motility abnormalities in gastroesophageal reflux disease. *Gastroenterol Clin North Am* 1999; 28:905–915.

45. Fealy R. Effect of traumatic spinal cord transection on human upper-gastrointestinal motility and gastric emptying. *Gastroenterology* 1984; 89:69–75.

46. MacLellan DG, Shulkes A, Hardy KJ. Profile of gastric stress ulceration following acute cervical cord injury: an animal model. *Aust N Z J Surg* 1986; 56:499–504.

47. MacLellan DG, Shulkes A, Yao CZ, Hardy KJ, Thompson JC. Role of vagal hyperactivity in gastric stress ulceration after acute injury to the cervical cord. *Surg Gynecol Obstet* 1988; 166:441–446.

48. Von Rokitansky C. *Lehrbuch der Pathologisen Anatomk.* 1861.

49. Wilkie D. Chronic duodenal ileus. *Am J Med* 1927; 173:643–649.

50. Roth E, Fenton L, Gaebler-Spira D, Frost F, Yarkony G. Superior mesenteric artery syndrome in acute traumatic quadriplegia: case reports and literature review. *Arch Phys Med Rehabil* 1991; 72:417–420.

51. Wilkinson R, Huang C. Superior mesenteric artery syndrome in traumatic paraplegia: a case report and literature review. *Arch Phys Med Rehabil* 2000; 81:991–994.

52. Vannatta J, Cagas C, Cramer R. SMA (Wilkie's) syndrome: a report of three cases and a review of the literature. *South Med J* 1976; 69:1461–1465.

53. Raissi B, Taylor B, Taves D. Recurrent superior mesenteric artery (Wilkie's) syndrome: a case report. *Can J Surg* 1996; 39:410–416.

54. Carey ME, Nance FC, Kirgis HD, Young HF, et al. Pancreatitis following spinal cord injury. *J Neurosurg* 1977; 47:917–922.

55. Berlly MH, Wilmot CB. Acute abdominal emergencies during the first four weeks after spinal cord injury. *Arch Phys Med Rehabil* 1984; 65:687–690.

56. Apstein MD, Dalecki-Chipperfield K. Spinal cord injury is a risk factor for gallstone disease. *Gastroenterology* 1987; 92:966–968.

57. Moonka R, Stiens S, Resnick W, McDonald J, et al. The prevalence and natural history of gallstones in spinal cord injured patients. *J Am Coll Surg* 1999:274–281.

58. Tola V, Chamberlain S, Kostyk S, Soybel D. Symptomatic gallstones in patients with spinal cord injury. *J Gastrointest Surg* 2000; 4: 642–647.

59. Friedman G, Kannel W. The epidemiology of gallbladder disease: observations in the Framingham study. *J Chronic Dis* 1966; 19:273–292.

60. Ketover SR, Ansel HJ, Goldish G, Roche B, Gebhard RL. Gallstones in chronic spinal cord injury: is impaired gallbladder emptying a risk factor? *Arch Phys Med Rehabil* 1996; 77:1136–1138.

61. Nino-Murcia M, Burton D, Chang P, Stone J, Perkash I. Gallbladder contractility in patients with spinal cord injuries: a sonographic investigation [see comments]. *AJR Am J Roentgenol* 1990; 154:521–524.

62. Tandon RK, Jain RK, Garg PK. Increased incidence of biliary sludge and normal gall bladder contractility in patients with high spinal cord injury. *Gut* 1997; 41:682–687.

63. Xia CS YX, Hong GX. 99 Tcm–DISIDA hepatobiliary imaging in evaluating gall bladder function in patients with spinal cord injury. *Hepatobiliary Pancreatic Dis Int* 2007; 6:204–207.

64. Heruti RJ, Bar-On Z, Gofrit O, Weingarden HP, Ohry A. Acute acalculous cholecystitis as a complication of spinal cord injury. *Arch Phys Med Rehabil* 1994; 75:822–824.

65. Moonka R, Stiens S, Eubank W, Stelzner M. The presentation of gallstones and results of biliary surgery in a spinal cord injured population. *Am J Surg* 1999:246–250.

66. Frost F, ed. *Gastrointestinal Dysfunction in Spinal Cord Injury.* Gaithersburg, MD: Aspen Publishers; 1994.

67. Chen CY, Chuang TY, Tsai YA, Tai HC, et al. Loss of sympathetic coordination appears to delay gastrointestinal transit in patients with spinal cord injury. *Dig Dis Sci* 2004; 49:738–743.

68. Charney K, Juler G, Comarr A. General surgery problems in patients with spinal cord injuries. *Arch Surg* 1975; 110:1083–1088.

69. Rajan RK, Nemchausky BA. Gastrointestinal emergencies in patients with spinal cord injury. In: Eltorai IM, Schmitt IM, eds. *Emergencies in Chronic Spinal Cord Injury Patients.* Jackson Heights, NY: Eastern Paralyzed Veterans Association, 2001:47–65.

70. Sheridan R. Diagnosis of the actue abdomen in the neurologically stable spinal cord–injured patient: a case study. *J Clin Gastroenterol* 1992; 15:825–828.

71. Alobaidi M GR, Jafri SZ, Fink-Bennett DM. Current trends in imaging evaluation of acute cholecystitis. *Emerg Radiol* 2004; 10:256–258.

72. Goyal R, Hirano K. The enteric nervous system. *N Engl J Med* 1996; 334:1106–1115.

73. Horowitz B, Ward SM, Sanders KM. Cellular and molecular basis for electrical rhythmicity in gastrointestinal muscles. *Annu Rev Physiol* 1999; 61:19–43.

74. Christensen J: The motor function of the colon. In: Yamada T, ed. *Gastroenterology.* JB Lippincott, 1991:180–196.

75. Menardo G, Bausano G, Corazziari E, Fazio A, et al. Large-bowel transit in paraplegic patients. *Dis Colon Rectum* 1987; 30:924–928.

76. Connell A, Logan C. The role of gastrin in gastroileocolic responses. *Am J Dig Dis* 1967; 12:277–284.

77. Saltzstein R, Mustin E, Koch T. Gut hormone release in patients after spinal cord injury. *Am J Phys Med Rehabil* 1995; 74:339–344.

78. Aaronson MJ, Freed MM, Burakoff R. Colonic myoelectric activity in persons with spinal cord injury. *Dig Dis Sci* 1985; 30:295–300.

79. Glick M. Colonic dysfunction in patients with thoracic spinal cord injury. *Gastroenterology* 1984; 86:287–295.

80. Schweiger M. Method for determining individual contributions of voluntary and involuntary anal sphincters to resting tone. *Dis Colon Rectum* 1979; 22:415–416.

81. Frenckner B. Function of the anal sphincters in spinal man. *Gut* 1975; 16:638–644.

82. Sapsford R, Hodges P. Contraction of the pelvic floor muscles during abdominal maneuvers. *Arch Phys Med Rehabil* 2001; 82:1081–1088.

83. Rasmussen O. Anorectal function. *Dis Colon Rectum* 1994; 37:386–403.

84. Stiens SA, Bergman SB, Goetz LL. Neurogenic bowel dysfunction after spinal cord injury: clinical evaluation and rehabilitative management. *Arch Phys Med Rehabil* 1997; 78:S86–102.

85. Harari D, Minaker KL. Megacolon in patients with chronic spinal cord injury. *Spinal Cord* 2000; 38:331–339.

86. De Looze DA, De Muynck MC, Van Laere M, De Vos MM, Elewaut AG. Pelvic floor function in patients with clinically complete spinal cord injury and its relation to constipation. *Dis Colon Rectum* 1998; 41:778–786.

87. Richardson SE, Rotman TA, Jay V, Smith CR, et al. Experimental verocytotoxemia in rabbits. *Infect Immun* 1992; 60:4154–4167.

88. Devroede G, Lamarche J. Functional importance of extrinsic parasympathetic innervation to the distal colon and rectum in man. *Gastroenterology* 1974; 66:273–280.

89. Devroede G, Arhan P, Duguay C, Tetreault L, et al. Traumatic constipation. *Gastroenterology* 1979; 77:1258–1267.

90. Stiens S, Goetz LJS: Neurogenic bowel dysfunction: evaluation and adaptive management. In: O'Young B, Young M, Stiens S, eds. *Physical Medicine and Rehabilitation Secrets.* 3rd ed. Philadelphia: Hanley & Belfus, 2008:531–539.

91. Beuret-Blanquart F, Weber J, Gouverneur JP, Demangeon S, Denis P. Colonic transit time and anorectal manometric anomalies in 19 patients with complete transection of the spinal cord. *J Auton Nerv Syst* 1990; 30:199–207.

92. Bartolo D, Read N, Jarratt J, Read M, et al. Differences in anal sphincter function and clinical presentation in patients with pelvic floor descent. *Gastroenterology* 1983; 85:68–75.

93. Linsenmeyer TA, Stone JM, Stiens SA. Neurogenic bladder and bowel management. In: Delisa J, ed. *Rehabilitation Medicine: Principles and Practice.* 3rd ed. Philadelphia: Lippincott, 2005:1619–1644.

94. Badiali D, Bracci F, Castellano V, Corazziari E, et al. Sequential treatment of chronic constipation in paraplegic subjects. *Spinal Cord* 1997; 35:116–120.

95. Kellow J, Gill R, Wingate D. Modulation of human upper gastrointestinal motility by rectal distention. *Gut* 1987; 28:864–868.

96. Rajendran S, Reiser J, Bauman W, Zhang R, et al. Gastrointestinal transit after spinal cord injury. *Am J Gastroenterol* 1992; 87:614–617.

97. Shafik A. Electreorectogram study of the neuropathic rectum. *Paraplegia* 1995; 33:346–349.

98. Tjandra J, Ooi B, Han W. Anorectal physiologic testing for bowel dysfunction in patients with spinal cord lesions. *Dis Colon Rectum* 2000; 43:927–931.

99. Stiens SA, Rodriguez G, King JC. Neurogenic bowel dysfunction: evaluation and rehabilitation. In: Brandom RA, ed. *Physical Medicine and Rehabilitation* (in press).

100. Mc Mahon S, Morrison J, Spillane K. An electrophysiological study of somatic and visceral convergence in the reflex control of the external sphincters. *J Physiol (Lond)* 1982; 328:379–387.

101. White J, Verlot M, Ehrentheil O. Neurogenic disturbances of the colon and their investigation by the colonmetrogram. *Ann Surg* 1949; 112:1042–1057.

102. Sun WM, MacDonagh R, Forster D, Thomas DG, et al. Anorectal function in patients with complete spinal transection before and after sacral posterior rhizotomy. *Gastroenterology* 1995; 108:990–998.

103. Meshkinpour H, Nowroozi F, Glick ME. Colonic compliance in patients with spinal cord injury. *Arch Phys Med Rehabil* 1983; 64:111–112.

104. Nino-Murcia M, Stone JM, Chang PJ, Perkash I. Colonic transit in spinal cord–injured patients. *Invest Radiol* 1990; 25:109–112.

105. MacDonagh R, Sun WM, Thomas DG, Smallwood R, Read NW. Anorectal function in patients with complete supraconal spinal cord lesions. *Gut* 1992; 33:1532–1538.

106. Keshavarzian A, Barnes WE, Bruninga K, Nemchausky B, et al. Delayed colonic transit in spinal cord–injured patients measured by indium-111 Amberlite scintigraphy. *Am J Gastroenterol* 1995; 90: 1295–1300.

107. Wald A. Colonic and anorectal motility testing in clinical practice. *Am J Gastroenterol* 1994; 89:2109–2115.

108. Fajardo N, Hussain K, Korsten M. Prolonged ambulatory colonic manometric studies using endoclips. *Gastrointest Endosc* 2000; 51: 199–201.

109. Fajardo NR PR, Modesta-Duncan R, Creasey G, Bauman WA, Korsten MA. Decreased colonic motility in persons with chronic spinal cord injury. *Am J Gastroenterol* 2003; 98:128–134.

110. Korsten MA FN, Rosman AS, Creasey GH, Spungen AM, Bauman WA. Difficulty with evacuation after spinal cord injury: colonic motility during sleep and effects of abdominal wall stimulation. *J Rehabil Res Dev* 2004; 41:95–100.

111. Krough K, Mosdal C, Laurberg S. Gastrointestinal and segmental colonic transit times in patients with acute and chronic spinal cord lesions. *Spinal Cord* 2000; 38:615–621.

112. Arhan P, Devroede G, Jehannin B, Lanza M, et al. Segmental colonic transit time. *Dis Col* 1981; 24:625–629.

113. Von Der Ohe M, Camilleri M. Subspecialty clinics: gastroenterology. Measurement of small bowel and colonic transit: indications and methods. *Mayo Clin Proc* 1992; 67:1169–1179.

114. Stiens SA, Goetz LL, Strayer J. Neurogenic bowel dysfunction: evaluation and adaptive management. In: O'Young B, Young M, Stiens S, eds. *Physical Medicine and Rehabilitation Secrets.* 3rd ed. Philadelphia: Hanley & Belfus, Mosby, 2008:118–125.

115. King R, Biddle A, Braunschweig C, Cowel F, et al. *Clinical Practice Guidelines: Neurogenic Bowel Management in Adults with Spinal Cord Injury.* Washington, DC: Consortium for Spinal Cord Medicine, Paralyzed Veterans of America, 1998.

116. Blackwell T, Krause J, Winkler T, Stiens S. *A Desk Reference for Life Care Planning for Persons with Spinal Cord Injury.* New York: Demos Medical Publishing, 2001.

117. Correa G, Rotter K. Clinical evaluation and management of neurogenic bowel after spinal cord injury. *Spinal Cord* 2000; 38:301–308.

118. Wrenn K. Fecal impaction. *N Engl J Med* 1989; 321:658–662.

119. Burns S, Hammond M. eds. *Yes, You Can! A Guide to Self-Care for Persons with Spinal Cord Injury.* 4th ed. Washington, DC: Paralyzed Veterans of America, 2009.

120. Kepplinger F, Stiens S. Bowel management: a fantastic voyage. In: *PVA-ETF*, 1998.

121. Stiens S, Cowel J, Dingus M, Montufar M, Matthews-Kirk P. *Clinical Practice Guidelines. Neurogenic Bowel: What You Should Know: A Guide for People with Spinal Cord Injury.* Washington, DC: Consortium for Spinal Cord Injury Medicine, Paralyzed Veterans of America, 1999.

122. Stiens S, Pidde T, Veland B, David M, Chadband C. *Accidents Stink!: Bowel Care 202.* Seattle: Paralyzed Veterans of America, 2002.

123. Davis DA TM, Oxman AD, Rayes RB. Changing physician performance: a systematic review of the effect of changing continuing medical education strategies. *JAMA* 1995; 274:700–705.

124. Goetz LL NA, Guihan M, Bosshart HT, Harrow JJ, Gerhart KD. Provider adherence to implementation of clinical practice guidelines for neurogenic bowel in adults with spinal cord injury. *J Spinal Cord Med* 2005; 28:394–406.

125. Harari D, Quinlan J, Stiens S. *Constipation and Spinal Cord Injury: A Guide to Symptoms and Treatment.* Washington, DC: PVA Spinal Cord Injury Education and Training Foundation, 1996.

126. Spiller RC. Pharmacology of dietary fibre. *Pharmacol Ther* 1994; 62:407–427.

127. Hillemeier C. An overview of the effects of dietary fiber on gastrointestinal transit. [Review]. *Pediatrics* 1995; 96:997–999.

128. Anderson J, Zettwoch N, Feldman T, Tietyan-Clark J, et al. Cholesterol-lowering effects of psyllium hydromucilloid for hypercholesterolemic males. *Arch Int Med* 1988; 148:292–296.

129. Cameron KJ, Nyulasi IB, Collier GR, Brown DJ. Assessment of the effect of increased dietary fibre intake on bowel function in patients with spinal cord injury. *Spinal Cord* 1996; 34:277–283.

130. Nelson A, Malassigne P, Murry J. Comparison of seat pressures on three bowel care/shower chairs in spinal cord injury. *Sci Nurs* 1994; 11:105–107.

131. Davis A, Nagelhout M, Hoban B, Barnard B. Bowel management: a quality of assurance approach to upgrading programs. *J Gerontol Nurs* 1986; 12:13–17.

132. Shafik A, El-Sibai O, Shafik I. Physiologic basis of digital-rectal stimulation for bowel evacuation in patients with spinal cord injury: identification of an anorectal excitatory reflex. *J Spinal Cord Med* 2000; 23:270–275.

133. House J, Stiens S. Pharmacologically initiated defecation for persons with spinal cord injury: effectiveness of three agents. *Arch Phys Med Rehabil* 1997; 78:1062–1065.

134. Shenot P, Rivas D, Kalman D, Staas WJ, Chancellor M. Latex allergy manifested in urological surgery and care of adult spinal cord injured patients. *Arch Phys Med Rehabil* 1994; 75:1263–1265.

135. Korsten MA SA, Monga A, Chaparala G, Khan AM, Palmon R. Anorectal stimulation causes increased colonic motor activity in subjects with spinal cord injury. *J Spinal Cord Med* 2007; 30:31–35.

136. Shafik A. Ano-vesical reflex: role in inducing micturition in paraplegic patients [see comments]. *Paraplegia* 1994; 32:104–107.

137. Comarr A. Bowel regulation for patients with spinal cord injury. *JAMA* 1958; 167:18–20.

138. Klauser A, Flaschentrager J, Gehrke A, Muller-Lissner S. Abdominal wall massage: effect on colonic function in healthy volunteers and in patients with chronic constipation. *Gastroenterology* 1992; 30:247–251.

139. Ayas S LB, Sozay S, Bayramoglu M, Niron EA. The effect of abdominal massage on bowel function in patients with spinal cord injury. *Am J Phys Med Rehabil* 2006; 85:951–955.

140. Rajan R, Juler G, Eltorai I. Sigmoid colon rupture secondary to Crede's method in a patient with spinal cord injury. *J Spinal Cord Med* 2000; 23:90–91.

141. Baird F. Giving enemas to paraplegic patients. *Am J Nurs* 1949:358.

142. Briel J, Schouten W, Vlot E, Smits S. Clinical value of colonic irrigation in patients with continence disturbances. *Dis Colon Rectum* 1997; 40:802–805.

143. Shandling B, Gilmore R. The enema continence catheter in spina bifida: successful bowel management. *J Pediatr Surg* 1987; 22:271–273.

144. Liptak G, Revell G. Management of bowel dysfunction in children with spinal cord disease or injury by means of the enema continence catheter. *J Pediatr* 1992; 120:190–194.

145. Mattsson S GG. Tap water enema for children with myelomeningocele and neurogenic bowel dysfunction. *Acta Pediatr* 2006; 95:369–374.

146. Puet T, Phen L, Hurst D. Pulsed irrigation enhanced evacuation: new method for treating fecal impaction. *Arch Phys Med Rehabil* 1991; 72:935–936.

147. Puet TA, Jackson H, Amy S. Use of pulsed irrigation evacuation in the management of the neuropathic bowel. *Spinal Cord* 1997; 35:694–699.

148. Christensen P BG, Coggrave M, Abel R, Hultling C, et al. A randomized, controlled trial of transanal irrigation versus conservative bowel management in spinal-cord injured patients. *Gastroenterology* 2006; 131:738–747.

149. Katona F, Eckstein H. Treatment of the neuropathic bowel by electrical stimulation of the rectum. *Dev Med Child Neurol* 1974; 16:336–339.

150. Brindley G. *Control of the Bladder and Urethral Sphincters by Surgically Implanted Electrical Stimulators.* London: Heinemann, 1982:464–470.

151. Chia YW, Lee T, Kour N, Tung K, Tan E. Microchip implants on the anterior sacral roots in patients with spinal trauma: does it improve bowel function? *Dis Colon Rectum* 1996; 39:690–694.

152. Frost F, Hartwig D, Jaeger R, Leffler E, Wu Y. Electrical stimulation of the sacral dermatomes in spinal cord injury: effect on rectal manometry and bowel emptying. *Arch Phys Med Rehabil* 1993; 74:696–701.

153. Varma JS. Autonomic influences on colorectal motility and pelvic surgery. *World J Surg* 1992; 16:811–819.

154. Lin V, Nino-Murcia M, Frost F, Wolfe V, et al. Functional magnetic stimulation of the colon in persons with spinal cord injury. *Arch Phys Med Rehabil* 2001; 82:167–173.

155. Stone JM, Wolfe VA, Nino-Murcia M, Perkash I. Colostomy as treatment for complications of spinal cord injury. *Arch Phys Med Rehabil* 1990; 71:514–518.

156. Rajendran SK RJ, Bauman WA, Zhang RL, Gordon SK, Korsten MA. Gastrointestinal transit after spinal cord injury: effect of cisapride. *Am J Gastroenterol* 1992; 87:1614–1617.

157. Wysowski DK BJ. Cisapride and fatal arhythmia. *N Engl J Med* 1996; 335:290–291.

158. Korsten MA RA, Ng A, Cavusoglu E, Spungen AM, et al. Infusion of neostigmine-glycopyrrolate for bowel evacuation in persons with spinal cord injury. *Am J Gastroenterol* 2005; 100:1560–1565.

159. Radulovic M SA, Wecht JM, Korsten MA, Schilero GJ, et al. Effects of neostigmine and glycopyrrolate on pulmonary resistance in spinal cord injury. *J Rehabil Res Dev* 2004; 41:53–58.

160. Suckling P. The ball-valve rectum due to impacted feces. Lancet 1962;2:1147.

161. Winawer S, Fletcher R, Miller L. Colorectal cancer screening: clinical guidelines and rationale. *Gastroenterology* 1997; 112:594–642.

162. Singal AK RA, Shaw S, Galea M, Spungen AM, Bauman WA. Colonoscopy in persons with spinal cord injury: a prospective study of the safety and efficacy of colon preparation [Abstract]. *J Spinal Cord Med* 2007; 30:402.

163. Ancha HR GM, Bauman WA, Jerudi M, Rosman AS, et al. Bowel cleansing prior to screening colonoscopy in persons with spinal cord injury: lack of efficacy using standard regimens [Abstract]. *Gastrointest Endosc* in press.

164. Korsten MA SA. Polyp detection rates are lower in persons with spinal cord injury: a prospective study. Unpublished data, 2007.

165. Singal AK RA, Shaw S, Hunt K, Post JB, Korsten MA. Renal safety of the bowel preparation in subjects with spinal cord injury: a prospective randomized study [Abstract]. *Gastrointest Endosc* in press.

166. Frisbie JH, Chopra S, Foo D, Sarkarati M. Colorectal carcinoma and myelopathy. *J Am Paraplegia Soc* 1984; 7:33–36.

167. McConnaughey D, Stiens S, Moonka R, Dominitz J. Fecal occult blood testing in spinal cord injured patients leads to high positivity rates. *Am College of Gastroenterology* 1999; 94:2678.

168. Mandel J, Church T, Bond J, Ederer F, et al. The effect of fecal occult-blood screening on the incidence of colorectal cancer. *N Engl J Med* 2000; 343:1603–1645.

169. Malone P, Ransley PG, Kiely EM. Preliminary report: the antegrade continence enema. *Lancet* 1990; 336:1217–1218.

170. Koyle M, Kaji D, Duque M, Wild J, Galansky S. The Malone antegrade continence enema for neurogenic and structural fecal incontinence and constipation. *J Urol* 1995; 154:759–761.

171. Geopel M, Sperling H, Stohrer M, Otto T, Rubben H. Management of neurogenic fecal incontinence in myelodysplastic children by a modified continent appendiceal stoma and antegrade colonic enema. *Urology* 1997; 49:758–761.

172. Yang C, Stiens S. Antegrade continence enema for the treatment of neurogenic constipation and fecal incontinence after spinal cord injury. *Arch Phys Med Rehabil* 2000; 81:683–685.

173. Christensen P, Kvitzau B, Krogh K, Buntzen S, Laurberg S. Neurogenic colorectal dysfunction—use of new antegrade and retrograde colonic wash-out methods. *Spinal Cord* 2000; 38:255–261.

174. Gerharz E, Vik V, Webb G, Leaver R, et al. The value of the MACE (Malone Antegrade Colonic Enema) procedure in adult patients. *J Am Coll Surg* 1997; 185:544–547.

175. Teichman JMH ZN, Kraus SR, Harris JM, Barber DB. Long-term results of Malone antegrade continence enema for adults with neurogenic bowel disease. *Urology* 2003; 61:502–506.

176. Uno Y. Introducer method of percutaneous endoscopic cecostomy and antegrade continence enema by use of Chait Trapdoor cecostomy catheter in patients with adult neurogenic bowel. *Gastrointest Endosc* 2006; 63:666–673.

177. Pfeifer J, Agachan F, Wexner S. Surgery for constipation: a review. *Dis Colon Rectum* 1996; 39:444–460.

178. Saltzstein R, Romano J. The efficacy of colostomy as a bowel management alternative in selected spinal cord injured patients. *J Am Paraplegia Soc* 1990; 13:9–13.

179. Borwell B. How acceptable are current methods of bowel management in the person with spinal cord injury? *World Council of Enterostomal Therapists Journal* 1996; 16:6–8.

180. Deshmukh G, Barkel D, Sevo D, Hergenroeder R. Use or misuse of colostomy to heal pressure ulcers. *Dis Colon Rectum* 1996; 39:737–738.

181. Lai JM, Chuang TY, Francisco GE, Strayer JR. Diversion colitis: a cause of abdominal discomfort in spinal cord injury patients with colostomy. *Arch Phys Med Rehabil* 1997; 78:670–671.

182. Arun H, Ledgerwood A, Lucas C. Ostomy prolapse in paraplegic patients: etiology, prevention, and treatment. *J Am Paraplegia Soc* 1990; 13:7–9.

183. Randell N, Lynch A, Anthony A, Dobbs B, et al. Does a colostomy alter quality of life in patients with spinal cord injury? A controlled study. *Spinal Cord* 2001; 39:279–282.

184. Luther SL NA, Harrow JJ, Chen F, Goetz LL. A comparison of patient outcomes and quality of life in persons with neurogenic bowel: standard bowel care program vs colostomy. *J Spinal Cord Med* 2005; 28:387–393.

185. Furlan JC UD, Fehlings MG. Optimal treatment for severe neurogenic bowel dysfunction after chronic spinal cord injury: a decision analysis. *Br J Surg* 2007; 94:1139–1150.

32 Sexual Dysfunction and Infertility in Men with Spinal Cord Injury

Stacy Elliott

The majority of traumatic spinal cord injuries (SCI) happen to men, and often to relatively young men in their reproductive years. For them, the area of sexual and fertility rehabilitation is extremely important. When men and women with SCI were surveyed about what "gain of function" was most important to their quality of life, they put sexuality as a major priority even above the return of sensation, walking, and bladder and bowel function (1). Of 681 participants (approximately 75% male), the majority of individuals with paraplegia felt regaining sexual function was their highest priority, and was the second highest priority for individuals with quadriplegia (preceded only by regaining hand and arm function). In the past, lack of knowledge and general discomfort among both professionals and clients alike resulted in sexual rehabilitation and fertility being underrepresented in many rehabilitation centers. Fortunately, two advances have brought the areas of sexual function and reproduction out in the open: the highly publicized success of the new oral treatments for erection dysfunction (ED), and improvements in assisted reproductive technologies (ART) for male factor infertility. These have reduced the stigmatization concerning sexual function and increased the chance of biologic fatherhood among men with SCI.

This chapter focuses on changes to the sexual functioning of men following SCI, with an emphasis on erectile function, ejaculation, and fertility. However, it should be remembered that issues such as the motor ability to perform sexual acts, bladder and bowel management, and general health (fatigue, skin breakdown, medications, etc.) all have a major impact on sexuality. Aging, disease processes, and other damage sustained from the initial injury also influence sexual functioning, aside from the neurogenic insult.

Men with traumatic SCI are sexual beings like anyone else. Their innate personalities and experiences prior to injury will dictate their readiness to explore and adapt to the sexual changes after their injury. Their interpretation of the sexual experiences they have after their injury will dictate their motivation to pursue assessment and treatment of remaining sexual concerns.

OVERVIEW OF CHANGES TO MALE SEXUAL FUNCTION FOLLOWING SCI

The classic 1960 paper of Bors and Comarr (2) is one of the original studies most often quoted on self-reported sexual function following SCI. Table 32.1 summarizes their findings. Although their results give a general idea of the sexual problems experienced then, it may not be the same today. When this and other older studies were conducted, sexual capacities were done by self-report, and management of issues such as bladder care and spasticity were less than optimal. Additionally, the level and extent of the spinal injuries were not that well defined, and the surgical procedures and medications used for rehabilitation were more likely than today's procedures and medications to interfere with erection and fertility. Most importantly, because the subject of sex was not discussed as openly as it is today in the "post-Viagra" era, many patients may not have been encouraged to be sexually active. Today, with our knowledge of erection and ejaculation physiology and a better appreciation of the softer science of the mind-body interaction involved in sexual arousal and gratification (3), men with SCI can have a full and rewarding sexual life after SCI.

What is the capacity for erection and ejaculation after injury? As Table 32.1 illustrates, without any assisted devices or medications, those men with incomplete injuries and upper motor neuron (UMN) injuries had a better prognosis for erection than men with complete and lower motor neuron (LMN) injuries. However, self-reports do not always accurately reflect the physiologic responsiveness to erotic stimulation. For example, penile tumescence was demonstrated in male SCI patients who believed they could not get erections when they were exposed to erotic stimulation via film, text, and fantasy (4). Furthermore, although erection capacity is vitally important to the majority of men post injury (5), sexuality for men with SCI goes beyond erection. Interpretation of, and acting on, sexual signals post-injury may be different than pre-injury. Some men with SCI have even stated that they feel they would not have appreciated the breadth of their

Table 32.1   Sexual Functioning Self-Reported in Men with Spinal Cord Injuries According to Level and Completeness of Injury

	ERECTION	SUCCESSFUL INTERCOURSE	EJACULATION	CHILDREN SIRED
Complete UMN lesions (n = 287, cervical–sacral)	93%	53%	5%	1%
Complete LMN lesions (n = 109, thoracic 9–sacral only as T5–T6 were totally flaccid)	26%[a]	23%	18%	<6%
Incomplete UMN lesions (n = 123, cervical–sacral)	99%	63%	32%	6%
Incomplete LMN lesions (n = 10, lumbar only)	90%[a]	80%	70%	10%

[a] Psychogenic erections only.
Source: Bors E, Comarr AE. Neurological disturbances of sexual function with special reference to 529 patients with SC spinal cord injury. *Urol Surv* 1960; 10:191–222.

sexual and intimate capacities unless they were injured. Yet others struggle, feeling their sexual lives are relegated to vicarious appreciation of their partner responses.

Because natural ejaculation is generally reported in less than 10% of men with SCI, fertility after SCI is affected. Fortunately, with the advent of vibrostimulation, electroejaculation, and operative sperm retrieval, the potential for biological fatherhood is almost always possible. The main fertility issue, aside from erection and ejaculatory dysfunction, is the poor quality of retrieved semen (normal to high sperm count but more abnormal forms and classically poor motility). Assisted insemination is necessary in most cases.

Before embarking on describing the changes following SCI, it is important to understand what is known to date about sexual functioning in those men without SCI. This knowledge has expanded rapidly in the last decade, allowing for advanced therapeutic modalities to be available.

MALE SEXUAL NEUROPHYSIOLOGY

Numerous components of the central and peripheral nervous system are involved in sexual behaviors and in the highly coordinated mechanisms comprising the mechanics of sexual function. There is moment-to-moment brain assessment during sexual arousal that will alter neurotransmitter levels and neural transmission, which ultimately affects sexual genital capacity (3). To add to the complexity, neurotransmitters relaying sexual signals may be excitatory in the brain but inhibitory in the periphery (noradrenaline, for example), or vice versa. Such complexity helps explain the wide variation of sexual effects of medications and emotions on sexual functioning. In addition, spinal cord injury may have a major effect on the ascending sensory signals coming from physical stimulation (decreasing positive sexual feedback), on muscle tone and spasticity, and in persons with higher and/or complete lesions, the spinal cord injury can exaggerate respiratory and cardiovascular reflexes secondary to the lack of neural control and descending autonomic regulation (autonomic dysreflexia) (6).

Sexual triggers from the brain (auditory, visual, gustatory and olfactory inputs, and imaginative or erotic stimuli), modulated by appropriate hormonal influences, are integrated with sensory afferents from skin and viscera. A generated neuronal signal is coordinated in the midbrain and carried distally through the brainstem and spinal tracts. Although the brain has a regulatory (excitatory and inhibitory) role on the spinal reflexes for sexual function, it is practical to think of supratentorial control as primarily inhibitory. It is the removal of this inhibition that allows for descending signals to be relayed to the various spinal nuclei, and in some cases, release specific spinal reflexes. However, these spinal nuclei can also receive afferent information from the genitalia and can also initiate autonomic and motor output by activating spinal cord systems directly (7). Concomitant brain injury, along with SCI, may alter the degree of cerebral modulation, resulting in sexual dysfunctions additive to the SCI, including sexual disinterest or hypersexuality, and in some cases, inappropriate sexual behavior.

ERECTION

Anatomy

The penis is composed of three tubes of erectile tissue surrounded by a fibroelastic sheath (see Figure 32.1). An erection is primarily a vascular event, with blood entering and expanding the penis from a flaccid state to an elongated, erect state.

In the penis, dorsal bilateral tubes called the corpora cavernosa lie above a third, smaller tube called the corpus spongiosum. The corpus spongiosum dilates at the distal end of the penis to form the penile glans. The urethra passes from the bladder through the corpus spongiosum and exits distally through the glans, terminating as the urethral meatus. Proximally, the two parallel corpora cavernosa enter the body and become the root of the penis, then internally bisect into paired crura that adhere to each ramus of the ischium respectively, ending at the ischial tuberosities. Each crus is surrounded by the ischiocavernosus muscle, which when contracted, is responsible for the increased

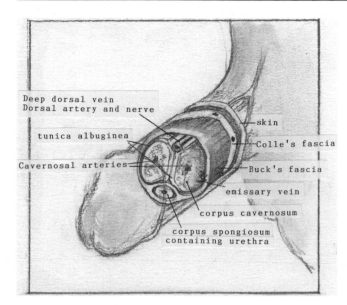

Figure 32.1 Cross-sectional anatomy of the penis.

intracavernosal pressure in a tumescent penis that leads to penile rigidity. Internally, the corpus spongiosum expands into the bulbous penis, which in turn is surrounded by the bulbospongiosus muscle that is responsible for clonic contractions during ejaculation (8).

Each corpus cavernosum is made up of spongy erectile tissue consisting of multiple interconnecting endothelial lined sinusoidal spaces or lacunae capable of filling with blood. The sinusoids are surrounded by a trabecular meshwork of elastin, smooth muscle, fibroblasts, and collagen. Both corpora are encased by a fibroelastic covering called the tunica albuginea forming a perforated septum between them in a figure-eight manner. This allows blood (and medications) to go from one corpus to the other. The corpus spongiosum is also surrounded by a thinner tunica and has a higher ratio of sinusoidal to trabecular components than the corpora cavernosa. Surrounding the three corporal bodies in layers is Buck's fascia (a thick layer of connective tissue), the dartos muscle, and finally skin. The penile arterial is supplied from the internal pudendal artery, which becomes the common penile artery, whose branches give rise to the bulbourethral (supplies the penile bulb and corpus spongiosum), cavernous (courses centrally through each corpora, giving off numerous helicine arteries that can lengthen without blood flow compromise during the expanding erection), and dorsal arteries (penile surface). The venous drainage is from three systems; the superficial, intermediate, and deep. Of primary importance is the venous drainage from the sinusoidal spaces of the corpora cavernosa; these drain into subtunical venules that exit through emissary veins that pierce the tunica. These veins drain primarily into the deep dorsal vein of the intermediate system (8).

Neurophysiology of Arousal

Most studies indicate that two key areas, the hypothalamus and the limbic region, are involved in the supraspinal control of erection function. Various inputs from imagination, emotion and memory, olfactory (rhinencephalon), visual, and somatosensory (thalamus) regions appear to be integrated in the medial pre-optic

and anterior hypothalamic regions (MPOA) and paraventricular nucleus (PVN) of the hypothalamus. The efferent pathways then enter the medial forebrain bundle, pass caudally to the mesencephalon, pons, and medulla, and finally down into the spinal cord (9). The brain stem provides primarily an inhibitory input to the spinal cord circuits regulating sexual reflexes (7). During rapid eye movement (REM) sleep, men will normally have more than three erections per night, each with duration greater than 10 minutes (10). Neurogenic stimuli can therefore bypass cortical inhibitions to cause nocturnal penile tumescence (NPT). Interestingly, NPT is not necessarily related to erotic content (11).

The penis receives innervation from three systems: the sacral parasympathetic (pelvic nerve), thoracolumbar sympathetic (hypogastric nerve and lumbar sympathetic chain), and somatic (pudendal nerve) systems. The three systems appear to reinforce one another. In particular, the sympathetic system has a role in the development of psychogenic erections and detumescence (12), and may contribute to the maintenance of erections after injury to parasympathetic pathways (9).

There are two neurogenic pathways for erections. Psychogenic or mentally induced erections are initiated by various afferent stimuli generated within, or received by, the brain. The brain receives afferent sensory inputs from various erogenous parts of the body, including the genitalia. In the sacral segments, afferent sensory impulses cross over to the lateral spinothalamic tracts (carrying pain-, heat-, and cold-sensory fibers) and other tracts (carrying touch and vibration), and continue up to the brain. Descending pathways from the brain control two outflows, the thoracolumbar (T10–L2) sympathetic and sacral (S2–S4) parasympathetic to the penis, both of which are responsible for psychogenic erections (9).

Reflexogenic erections are mediated by a reflex arc exclusively in the sacral spinal cord. The afferent limb consists of two pathways: touch and rub sensations go through the pudendal nerve that accompanies the motor fibers, and deep pressure and visceroreceptive stimuli likely travel along the pelvic and hypogastric nerves. The efferent limb consists of preganglionic axons that travel via the pelvic nerve to the pelvic plexus, and from there via the cavernous nerve to the penis.

It is probable that both the reflex and psychogenic pathways, along with their neurotransmitters, act synergistically to a final pathway involving the sacral parasympathetics (9).

Erectile Physiology

Erectile response is a dynamic process. Signals from either neurogenic pathway will result in a final vascular event that leads to erection. In the flaccid state, sympathetic tone causes the smooth muscle fibers of the helicine arteries, arterioles, and sinusoids within the cavernosal bodies to be tonically contracted, allowing for minimal or basal blood flow. For an erection to occur, the smooth muscle of the penis relaxes, allowing for a rapid increase in blood flow and volume (up to eight times) (13). The increased blood flow expands the interconnected sinusoidal spaces and enlarges the cavernosal bodies. This elongation and widening of the penis is termed tumescence. As the tunica albuginea stretches to encompass the enlarging corpora, most of the venular plexuses are compressed between the tunica albuginea and the peripheral sinusoids, reducing the venous outflow (see Figure 32.1). When the tunica albuginea is maximally stretched, the emissary veins that pierce the tunica are obliquely compressed, effectively stopping the venous outflow. This venous occlusion leads to an intracavernosal pressure of about 100 mmHg, which results in maximal tumescence. The contraction of the ischiocavernosus muscle causes the intracavernosal pressure to rise to several hundred mmHg, at which point the rigid erection phase is achieved, and blood is virtually trapped within the system. The maintenance of an erection requires a balance between arterial inflow and venous outflow. Detumescence occurs when the arterial inflow no longer meets or exceeds the venous drainage, and a rapid initial fall in intracorporal pressure is followed by a slower decrease in penile circumference.

The dominant autonomic input for tumescence is parasympathetic, and for flaccidity, sympathetic. However, certain parasympathetic and sympathetic pathways to the penis work synergistically and can compensate for one another, presumably through cotransmission between various neurotransmitters (9). Noradrenaline (NE), through predominately alpha-adrenoreceptors, is the major peripheral neurotransmitter controlling flaccidity. Acetylcholine (Ach) is required for ganglionic transmission and vascular smooth muscle relaxation (14). Nitric oxide (NO) is the principle neurotransmitter dictating penile erection. NO increases the activation of guanosine monophosphate (cGMP) in the cavernosal smooth muscle cell, causing a relaxation of the arterial, arteriolar, and sinusoidal smooth muscle. Prostaglandin E1 (PGE1) and vasoactive intestinal peptide (VIP) work primarily by increasing the level of cyclic adenosine monophosphate (cAMP), which also relaxes smooth muscle (Figure 32.2). Gap junctions and intercellular electrical activity allow for a synchronized and coordinated erectile response (14).

Erection is dependent on a balance between agents that cause smooth muscle contraction (NE, endothelin from endothelial damage, angiotensin, and vasopressin) and smooth muscle relaxation (Ach, NO, VIP, PGE1, calcitonin gene-related peptide [CGRP]). Pharmacotherapy for erection dysfunction (ED) utilizes these known modulators by increasing the erectogenic ones and/or inhibiting the erectolytic ones, alone or in combination. For example, PGE1 (alprostadil), delivered via intracavernosal injection or intraurethral micro-pellet, directly relaxes corporal smooth muscle, promoting erection. Phosphodiesterase Type V, a dominant isoenzyme that destroys cGMP, can be inhibited by phosphodiesterase type V inhibitors (PDE5i). By indirectly extending the duration of available cGMP in the penile tissues, PDE5i enhances the erection. However, unlike PGE1, PDE5i's require sexual arousal to liberate neuronal NO from the nerve ending. Disease states and aging generally influence the balance toward flaccidity because of such things as decreased smooth muscle/connective tissue balance from lack of oxygenation secondary to reduced erections, decreased cell-to-cell contacts, sinusoidal endothelial changes (the endothelium is a also source of NO), and degenerative changes in nerve fibers (14). It is understandable how hypertension, hyperlipidemias, smoking, diabetes, and nerve disorders are common risk factors for erection dysfunction (ED).

Androgens are necessary in the development (organization) and maintenance (activation) of sexual function. The precise role of androgen in erection through peripheral (endothelial dependant and independent) and central mechanisms is becoming

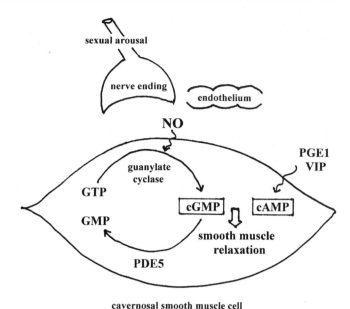

Figure 32.2 Cavernosal smooth muscle relaxation. Nitric oxide (NO) from neuronal and endothelial sources crosses the plasma membrane of the smooth muscle cell, increasing the activity of guanylate cyclase, the enzyme that catalyzes the formation of cGMP. Prostaglandin E1 (PGE1) and vasoactive intestinal peptide (VIP), from autonomic nerves and smooth muscle respectively, stimulate receptors that result in the formation of cAMP. Both cGMP and cAMP coordinate to allow for relaxation of the arterial, arteriolar, and sinusoidal smooth muscle of the corpus cavernosum. Phosphodiesterase V (PDE5) breaks down cyclic cGMP: PDE5 inhibitors allowing cGMP to accumulate, promoting erection. PGE1 can be administered by injection or intraurethral suppository to activate cAMP, promoting erection.

delineated, but has special importance in its role of nitric oxide synthase (NOS), and therefore NO production (15, 16). A minimal amount of androgen is required to maintain erection, with some men (especially younger) able to retain erectile capacity despite low levels of serum testosterone. PDE5i lose efficacy in low-androgen environments, and androgen replacement therapy improves PDE5i efficacy in hypogonadal men (16). Physiologic erections that occur during REM sleep decline rapidly when androgen levels drop, but there is a slower decline in the loss of erotic or daytime erections. The most consistent sexual symptoms of decreasing levels of testosterone are, in order, lack of sexual interest, followed by delayed ejaculation or orgasm, smaller ejaculate volumes, loss of nocturnal erections, and eventually ED in erotic situations. However, endocrinologic ED per se accounts for a minority of all ED. Hypogonadal men, however, require androgen replacement, not just for sexual function, but to reduce other cardiovascular, muscle, fatigue, and osteoporotic risks (17) that are of particular importance in the spinal cord population.

CHANGES TO GENERAL AROUSAL PATTERNS FOLLOWING SCI

How arousal is interpreted after SCI was looked at in a unique survey of 199 men with various levels of SCI (18). After SCI, the predominant sexual stimulation for men that led to best arousal was still genital, but touching of the head/neck area and torso/shoulder/arm area were also arousing. Approximately half the subjects reported difficulty with becoming psychologically aroused, and the vast majority felt it was difficult to become physically aroused. Almost half of the subjects with psychological feelings of arousal felt it translated to their genitals as a physical sensation (this was positively correlated with having genital sensation), whereas about 20% were undecided regarding this phenomenon, and a third of subjects disagreed that psychological arousal translated to feeling anything in the genitals. Many men developed new areas of arousal above the level (42%) or at the level (27.6%) of lesion, especially those who did not have genital sensation and or lower motor function, but men who reported having chronic pain were less likely to develop these new areas of arousal above the level of their lesion. This suggests two phenomena: men with complete injuries affecting their lower body become more psychologically adaptive or open to trying new or nontraditional sexual stimulation, and neuroplasticity can result in formerly nonsexually responsive areas becoming responsive to sexual stimuli with time (18).

CHANGES TO ERECTION FOLLOWING SCI

Because both spinal and supraspinal inputs act synergistically in sexual functioning, it follows that one system can also compensate for the other with variable success, and this is well evidenced in the SCI population (15). Men with complete SCI above the thoracolumbar outflow (T6) who have interrupted psychogenic pathways will have their reflex erections preserved, or even enhanced (no cortical inhibition) (15). Those with sacral damage have abolished reflexogenic response but intact thoracolumbar pathways in which to mediate a psychogenic erection. It appears there are similar neurological pathways for the control of sexual arousal in both men and women after SCI, as psychogenic arousal (as defined in a laboratory-based study as increase in penile circumference with audiovisual stimulation) can be predicted in males by the degree of preservation of the combined ability to perceive surface sensation to pinprick and light touch in the T11–L2 dermatomes (19), similar to the findings seen in women with SCI (20). Men with lesions between the two pathways would seem to be spared both psychogenic and reflex erections; however, the synergism must be lost between the connecting spinal nuclei as erections are not clinically as reliable as one might expect. Those men with conus terminalis lesions may be spared psychogenic erections because of intact thoracolumbar fibers. The lower motor lesions seen in cauda equina injuries result in variable loss of function, from complete (T12–L1 injury results in loss of psychogenic and reflex erections because of inclusive damage below the level of injury) to partial (S4–S5 injury retains psychogenic erection and even partial reflexogenic capacity) (21). Although we can expect men with complete injuries above neurological level T10 to have reflexogenic erections, and those with sacral reflex arc damage to be capable of psychogenic erections, there are clinical exceptions to these predictions. This may be because of inaccurate assessment of the level of injury or unrecognized syringomyelia, inaccurate assessment of completeness of injury, or because of unknown alternate erection pathways that are outside of the spinal cord. Obviously, more study must be done in this area. It is also important to remember that there may be other reasons (depression, use of antispasmodic medications, concomitant diabetes, etc.) for ED in men with SCI in addition to neurological changes.

In clinical practice, many men with SCI who are able to obtain an erection do not have "usable" erections, have difficulty maintaining their erections, do not have as firm an erection as pre-injury, or have difficulty attaining a second erection if the first is lost. Some may have detumescence triggered by movement or pressure, or from unwanted seminal emission triggered neurologically. In a recent survey, without the use of erection enhancement, about 15% of men felt they had an erection that would last, 60% could attain an unreliable erection, and about 25% felt they could only attain a soft erection (18). It is understandable, with this frustrating unpredictability despite erectile potential, that at least two-thirds to three-fourths of men with SCI choose to use erection enhancement (18).

A self-report instrument has been developed to assess the rigidity and usability of erections. The International Index of Erectile Function (IIEF) is a widely used, multi-dimensional instrument for the evaluation of male sexual function, most often used for clinical trials of ED therapies and for diagnostic evaluation of ED severity (22). It has been used in the SCI population to evaluate several therapeutic modalities, and is considered one of the few preferred instruments in the measurement of sexual capacities after SCI (23). Traditional methods of ED investigation may also not be applicable to the SCI population. For example, despite some controversy, in the able bodied, abnormal NPT findings have often been used to differentiate "organic" from "psychologic" causes of ED, assuming the psychologic causes of ED when awake and sexual cause supraspinal inhibition that would be bypassed in sleep, thus resulting in normal NPT tracings. Organic causes (nerve, vascular, receptor, or other end organ issues or medication use) would result in abnormal tracings. However, one author and colleagues (24), using SCI subjects, proposed and confirmed the hypothesis that nocturnal erections were primarily of reflexogenic origin transmitted via the sacral pathway. They showed that positive NPT recordings were primarily among those SCI subjects who maintained reflexogenic erection capacity. Moreover, subjects with impaired reflexogenic erections generally lost nocturnal erections even if they maintained psychogenic-induced erections. Nocturnal erections of normal quality after SCI require preservation of thoracolumbar and sacral neuronal control as well as partially intact connections of the spinal erection centers with brain areas responsible for sexual arousal (24). NPT recordings should, therefore, be used with caution in the SCI population.

EJACULATION AND ORGASM

In neurologically intact men, ejaculation and orgasm usually occur simultaneously, even though they represent different neurophysiologic events. Ejaculation is the process of sperm transference, starting from the testes to the final expulsion of semen from the urethral meatus. Ejaculation is divided into two phases: seminal emission and propulsatile ejaculation, or expulsion. In neurologically intact men, the brain interprets the processing of genital efferent stimuli during ejaculation, such as smooth muscle contraction of the accessory sex organs, the buildup and release of pressure in the posterior urethra, distension of the distal urethra, contractions of the urethral bulb and perineum, and other unidentified components, as generally pleasurable and a component of orgasm. However, orgasm can also be experienced in the absence of sexual organs (penis, prostate, or testicles) and during sleep.

Ejaculation and orgasm are not specifically linked to penile tumescence. Therefore, it is not only possible to have erection, ejaculation, and orgasm as separate events, but also one alone without the others, or two in combination without the third.

Ejaculation

Ejaculation consists of two stages and is mediated through the T10–S4 segments of the spinal cord. While under supraspinal control, it can be triggered through these spinal cord segments alone if supraspinal control is lost. Alternately, supraspinal afferents can stimulate ejaculation by themselves, as evidenced by nocturnal emissions.

Stage 1 or seminal emission begins at high arousal and has a component of voluntary control. Sympathetic outflow from the presacral and hypogastric nerves (T10–L2) causes sperm transport from the storage site in the tail of the epididymis to the more distal genital ducts and initiates smooth muscle peristalsis of the vas deferens and the contraction of the seminal vesicles (storing spermatozoa and seminal fluid) and prostate, forming the seminal bolus. Because this phase is related to subjective arousal, this stage is under some voluntary control in the able-bodied man. The seminal bolus is then deposited into the prostatic urethra via the ejaculatory ducts, and simultaneously, sympathetic input via the hypogastric nerve (L1–L2) causes a functional closure of the bladder neck by stimulation of alpha-adrenergic receptors. This closure prevents the seminal bolus from entering the bladder in a retrograde fashion. In addition, the external sphincter also remains closed during the seminal bolus deposition, increasing the prostatic pressure and instigating a feeling of impending release, called ejaculatory inevitability. Cerebral control of impending ejaculation is minimal at this point (25). Increased prostatic pressure and the general vasocongestion of the pelvic organs correspond with pleasurable feelings of fullness or tension in the genital area.

Stage 2 or propulsatile ejaculation is the process of expulsion of the seminal fluid distally down through the urethra (antegrade ejaculation). A seminal bolus in the posterior urethra does not appear to be necessary to trigger propulsatile ejaculation after seminal emission, as evidenced by post-prostatectomy patients. The pelvic nerve (parasympathetic fibers of S2, S3, S4) is responsible for the spasmodic contractions of the seminal vesicles, prostate, and urethra, which along with intermittent relaxation of the external sphincter and the three to seven rhythmic contractions about 0.8 seconds apart of the bulbospongiosus, ischiocavernosus, levator ani, and related muscles (pudendal nerve carrying somatic signals S2–S4 signals), propel the seminal bolus distally down the urethra to be ejaculated in a propulsatile fashion (25). Orgasmic sensations usually accompany this stage of ejaculation. Stage 2 is under very poor voluntary control, including the contractions of the pelvic floor striated muscle. After men experience ejaculation and orgasm, they undergo a refractory period where a second ejaculation and orgasm is not possible for a variety of reasons (neurotransmitter replenishment, age, etc.) until a finite amount of time passes. The duration of the refractory periods lengthens with age.

Normal antegrade ejaculation requires close coordination of sympathetic, parasympathetic, and somatic components, and the efferent pathways innervating the structures involved drive motor outputs originating from spinal thoracolumbar and lumbosacral nuclei (26). A spinal ejaculation generator, proposed to be in the lumbosacral cord, integrates the sensory inputs necessary to trigger ejaculation and coordinates the emission and expulsion phases (27). A population of spinothalamic neurons in the lumbar spinal cord of male rats (LSt cells), thought to be integral to the spinal ejaculation generator, send projections to the autonomic nuclei and motor neurons involved in the emission and expulsion phase, and are thought to be under the control of both peripheral afferents coming from the genital areas and supraspinal information arising from specific brain regions (28). LSt cells are only activated with ejaculation and not with other components of sexual behavior in male rats, and these spinothalamic neurons are not activated by vaginocervical stimulation in female rats (29). Lesions of LSt cells completely ablate ejaculatory function (27).

Orgasm

During orgasm, the rhythmic pelvic floor contractions, along with smooth muscle contractions and distensions of the internal genitalia, are interpreted by the cerebral cortex as pleasurable, especially in the pelvic area (genital orgasm). However, orgasm can also be experienced as more of a total body or cerebral orgasm that is not necessarily focused in the pelvic area. The definition of orgasm is one area of difficulty when interpreting self-reports or studies looking at orgasm in the neurogenic population. As there is no agreed-upon definitive definition of orgasm, only description can be used. For genital orgasm to occur, it is thought that specific acceptable genital or pelvic stimuli provide afferent signals to the brain via the lateral spinothalamic tracts. Cerebral stimuli (variable in nature and intrinsic to each person in the waking and sleep states) can enhance or inhibit these afferents from the body. The efferent pathway for genital orgasm appears to be the corticospinal tract. Cerebral stimuli can be effective afferents on their own (nongenital orgasm), even if the pathways for genital orgasm are disrupted. Furthermore, it is well known that nocturnal emission and orgasmic release can occur without genital stimulation during sleep, and that some men are capable of orgasmic release through mental Tantric sex practices, nipple stimulation, or other nongenital sources of erotic arousal, resulting in orgasm derived from non-genital sources (even if the orgasmic perception has a pelvic component). For example, the distressing sexual dysfunction of severe premature ejaculation is associated with spontaneous ejaculation through mental arousal alone, but orgasm is felt to occur primarily in the pelvis.

The neurophysiology of orgasm is only partially understood. The main hypothesis of orgasm is that it is a reflex response of the sacral autonomic and somatic nervous system that can be either facilitated or inhibited by cerebral input. There are likely multiple contributory afferent systems—somatic and autonomic inputs from the brain, spinal cord, local spinal reflexes, interpretations of visceral sensations, and possibly even hormonal influences that have not all been identified to explain the variations of genital and nongenital orgasmic experiences.

CHANGES TO EJACULATION AND ORGASM FOLLOWING SCI

In a survey of men with various levels of lesions (54% cervical), 48% had successfully achieved ejaculation post-injury and the most commonly used methods were hand stimulation, sexual intercourse, and vibrostimulation (18): the most commonly cited reasons for trying to ejaculate were for pleasure and for sexual intimacy, the least common reason being fertility.

Because ejaculation is a highly complex process requiring the smooth coordination of the sympathetic, parasympathetic, and somatic nervous systems, ejaculatory dysfunction after SCI is common. Loss of seminal emission occurs if the transmission of the thoracolumbar sympathetic chain is disrupted, retrograde ejaculation occurs if there is inadequate closure of the bladder neck, and failure of propulsatile ejaculation takes place if the parasympathetic or somatic pathways are disrupted. In the latter case, after orgasm, semen may be slowly released with gravity over time or go unnoticed in a urinary collection device. Because the majority of men with SCI do not report seeing antegrade ejaculate, they are usually considered anejaculatory (failure of both phases of ejaculation). However, some of these men with SCI may be having undetected retrograde ejaculation, especially if they experience orgasm.

In those men with UMN lesions above T10 and loss of supraspinal control, the potential for complete ejaculation remains because of the intact T10–S4 cord. Sperm retrieval methods such as vibrostimulation are able to use this potential and are frequently successful at obtaining an ejaculate. However, those men with complete lower injuries involving the sacral cord, although maintaining a higher potential for ejaculation with sexual practices, may also experience unwanted seminal emission and resultant detumescence from stimulation of the thoracolumbar pathways when erotic thoughts are maintaining their psychogenic erections.

Men with incomplete injury have spared descending spinal cord pathways that may maintain some coordination of the various nervous systems involved in ejaculation. Men with incomplete LMN are most likely to ejaculate because their thoracolumbar and/or sacral pathways have been partially spared. Having spasticity during sexual activity, being able to empty the bladder with controlled voiding, and/or having voluntary bowel control are predictive functions of ejaculation capacity (18). However, although those men with complete UMN lesions are the least likely to ejaculate through private sexual practices, they are the most likely to ejaculate with the intense stimulation of the penis by vibrostimulation because their sacral reflex is intact and enhanced by loss of supratentorial control. Those men with high incomplete lesions may be more likely to ejaculate than their complete counterparts in private sexual experiences, but the cerebral interference in a clinical, asexual, and potentially embarrassing situation may inhibit the reflex. Electroejaculation, on the other hand, electrically stimulates only the peripheral nerves eliciting seminal emission, and therefore does not require coordination within the spinal reflex centers.

What is the capacity for men with SCI to experience orgasm? One self-report study of men with SCI stated 42% to 47% of men reported orgasms of a similar, weaker, or different quality from those pre-SCI (30, 31). Another survey reported 41% of men having experienced orgasm post-injury, with the likelihood of experiencing orgasm post-SCI being positively influenced by longer duration of injury, presence of genital sensation, having reliable erections ≥75% of the time, and having the ability to successfully ejaculate (18). Although it is assumed that those men with complete lesions may not experience genitally derived orgasm (because both the upgoing lateral spinothalamic tract and the downgoing corticospinal tract are interrupted), 38% of men with complete SCI reported they retained the ability to achieve orgasm (30). There may be several explanations for this, including a limited assessment of "completeness of injury" via the traditional methods of the American Spinal Injury Association (ASIA) Impairment Scale (AIS), which tests only for sensory and motor scores, negating the effect stimulation may have on autonomic and visceral sensations interpreted as pleasurable. An incomplete spinal injury that spares some or all of the tracts necessary for genital orgasm increases the chance of that person experiencing a familiar pelvic-centered orgasm, even if the required stimulus may have to be strong or for a protracted period of time. It may be that sparing of the reflex sacral arc (i.e., positive bulbocaversnosus reflex) elicits a specific orgasmic pathway. In short, the topic of orgasmic definition, orgasmic potential, and modulating factors requires further study and the neurology is not yet fully defined.

Clinicians working in the area are aware of those men with SCI who are able to experience altered orgasmic sensations, whether the afferent input is from the genitalia, non-genital areas of sensitivity, or the brain itself. It is this author's experience with sperm retrieval methods that about 5% to 10% of men undergoing these procedures for the first time may experience some surprising, pleasurable sensations, even if this was not predicted by traditional neurologic understanding. Some men with disconcerting symptoms of autonomic dysreflexia (AD) with ejaculation have experienced adaption to their symptoms over time such that milder autonomic cardiovascular symptoms of AD turn sexually pleasurable.

A recent controlled, laboratory-based analysis of 45 men with SCIs and 16 able-bodied controls demonstrated that although men with SCIs were less likely than controls to achieve orgasm, characteristics (mean latency to orgasm, blood pressure and heart rates at orgasm) of orgasm were similar (32). Historically, 84.2% of the study subjects with incomplete injury versus 50% of those with complete injuries reported the ability to achieve orgasm in private personal settings, and in the laboratory, 78.9% of the subjects with incomplete injures and 28.0% of those with complete injuries achieved orgasm. Although orgasm and ejaculation were more likely to occur together, a number of men with SCI achieved orgasm without ejaculation. This is also reported in able-bodied men (33). Men with incomplete SCIs were more likely to achieve orgasm than those with complete SCIs, and men with complete lower motor neuron dysfunction affecting their sacral segments were less likely to achieve orgasm than men with any other patterns of SCI (32). Although this is predictive utilizing the local orgasmic reflex theory, there were exceptions. Besides considering the genital versus nongenital orgasmic explanation, it should be remembered that AISA scores do not test for intactness of the autonomic nervous system. Men with complete SCI who are orgasmic may therefore retain the necessary autonomic component of their sacral orgasmic reflex even if the somatic component is affected. Furthermore, AIS scores documenting skin, pinprick, and anal-digital testing to determine SCI completeness do not examine for sensate deeper internal genital structures (i.e., prostate or seminal vesicle sensitivity). Undamaged visceral afferent fibers could therefore remain untested, and account for the ability of men with higher-level complete SCI to feel discomfort from rectal probe electroejaculation, abdominal pain (34), and rectal distention (35). Current work has been done to develop a standard terminology to be able to communicate effectively about the remaining autonomic function, and to document its role in sexual and reproductive function after spinal cord injury (36). Also, the fact that men with complete SCI may experience variants of autonomic dysreflexia that are recognized as pleasurable helps explain the cardiovascular component of the subjective experience of orgasm after SCI (37). Men and women with SCI who are open to experimentation and adaptation may be the ideal model to study the phenomenon of orgasm.

THERAPEUTIC OPTIONS FOR MALE SEXUAL DYSFUNCTIONS

Erection Enhancement for Erectile Dysfunction (ED)

There are four main methods to medically enhance erections:

- Oral phosphodiesterase V inhibitors (PDE5i), including sildenafil (Viagra®), vardenafil (Levitra®), and tadalafil (Cialis®)
- Local penile medicinal therapy (intracavernosal injections, intraurethral micropellets, and topical agents)
- Mechanical, noninvasive therapy (constrictor bands and vacuum devices)
- Surgical therapy (surgical prosthesis and sacral anterior root stimulation)

The effectiveness of these options significantly improve when they are combined with talk-oriented therapy aimed at the integration of their use in the client's life or couple situation. The choice of option depends on the client (knowledge of efficacy and safety, personal preference), whether there is a partner (and if so, whether that person is comfortable with the method of enhancement or even willing to administer the method), the healthcare professional (experience and biases), and availability of the option (price, pharmaceutical limitations, etc.). PDE5i's and penile injections dominate the market, with little need for the irreversible method of penile prosthesis except when reversible methods fail.

Client preference is usually based on simplicity, invasiveness, comfort with the method, and cost. Other determinants include visual acuity, hand function, spasm, and issues of bladder management. In general, a reflex erection that is unreliable may be helped by less-invasive methods: those men who are unable to obtain an erection satisfactory for intercourse at any time will likely require local penile medicinal therapy, because oral medications may not result in the same penile rigidity or reliability, but the latter should still be tried. Any erection enhancement

method should not be used in those men in whom sexual activity itself is deemed unsafe (a caution that applies particularly to cardiovascular patients).

In a systematic review of 49 reports on male sexual dysfunction in men with SCI, several interventions (behavioral therapy, topical agents, intraurethral alprosatadil, intracavernous injections, vacuum tumescence devices, penile implants, sacral stimulators, and oral medication) were evaluated (38). Penile injections resulted in successful erectile function in 90% of men, sildenafil resulted in 79% success, and the difference in efficacy between the two was not statistically significant. Five case-series reports involving 363 participants with penile implants demonstrated a high satisfaction rate, but a 10% complication rate. The authors noted that these interventions positively affected sexual activity in the short term, but that long-term sexual adjustment and holistic approaches beyond erections remained to be studied.

First line treatments in the SCI population are noninvasive oral therapies and mechanical devices, with second choices being the more invasive intracavernosal injections, followed by surgical options (39). One survey of men with SCI demonstrated the diversity of erection enhancement currently used: although 23.1% used nothing, 60% of the men had tried using some type of erection enhancement or drug, including Viagra® (20.6%), penile injections (7.5%), Cialis® (5.5%), penile ring at base (3.5%), vacuum device (3%), Levitra® (2.5%), penile prosthesis (1.5%), or other (1%) (18).

Oral Medications

The PDE5i's currently on the market are orally active, potent, and selective inhibitors of phosphodiesterase type 5 (PDE5) enzyme, an important regulator of cGMP, an essential nucleotide in the sequence of smooth muscle relaxation in the corpus cavernosum via the NO-cGMP pathway (see earlier discussion). They begin to work in the majority of men within 1 hour, but approximately 1/3 of men will notice the therapeutic effects sooner (within 30 minutes), and some younger men with SCI claim the effect happens within 15 minutes. PDE5i's are contraindicated with the use of nitrates. On-demand (prn) Viagra® is available in doses of 25, 50 and 100 mg, and prn Levitra® in doses of 5, 10, and 20 mg. The therapeutic window for Viagra® and Levitra® prn is between 1–4 hours after taking the drug. Many men will state morning erections are also improved if they have taken the drug the night before. A high-fat meal will slow the absorption of both these drugs. On-demand Cialis®, a longer acting PDE5i, should work within 1 hour and last up to 36–48 hours: some men with SCI claim it can last for several days. Prn Cialis® comes in doses of 10 and 20 mg, and is not affected by food intake. For some men with SCI, the longer duration of the drug, although advantageous from a sexual spontaneity point of view, triggers more spontaneous, unwanted erections from movement of their clothes on their genitalia or from pelvic vibration while wheeling. Others do not mind or do not notice this effect. A daily Cialis® 5 mg pill (Cialis® 5 mg OD) has also recently been added to the market. Cialis® 5 mg OD requires approximately 5 days to reach therapeutic blood levels, and has not been evaluated specifically in men with SCI. Daily use of any of the PDE5i in reduced doses (i.e. Cialis® 5 mg OD, the use of Viagra® 25 mg OD, or Levitra® 10 mg OD) can be used as long as there is no clinically relevant symptomatic hypotension: it is this author's clinical experience that men with SCI who have significantly unreliable erectile quality can benefit psychologically and physically from improved morning, spontaneous, and sexual erections without attaching this to prn use. Limitations of PDE5i use is concomitant nitrate use for the duration of prn PDE5i metabolism, and the additional expense and total nitrate contraindication with daily PDE5i.

Because the use of PDE5i in men with SCI requires the release of NO either through mental arousal or penile stimulation, once this stimulation is removed, the erection should dissipate. This makes the potential of priapism with PDE5i remote even in men with SCI, unless other sensory sources (i.e., hot tub) continue to provide excessive stimulation to a reflex erection.

Those men with upper motor neuron lesions will respond better than those with lower motor neuron lesions or cauda equina lesions to PDE5i because peripheral nerve damage diminishes the neuronal source of NO (40). Similarly, those men with endothelial damage from hypertension, smoking, or hyperlipidemias also have a reduced source of endothelial-derived NO, and therefore may not respond as well. PDE5i's are therefore most beneficial to those men with SCI who have retained their reflex erections (generally UMN lesions) and who do not also have other risk factors for ED. One study, utilizing home and clinic-based assessments in 90 men with SCI, found prn PDE5i's to be effective (rigidity enough for penetration) in 85% of the patients on sildenafil, 74% of the patients on vardenafil, and 72% of the patients on tadalafil, with the mean duration of erection being 34, 28, and 26 minutes respectively (40). Another study suggests that men with incomplete lesions do better with sildenafil than those men with complete or higher-level lesions (41). In general, headache (10–15%) and flushing (6–10%) were noted to be the most common side effect for men with SCI using the PDE5i's, followed by dyspepsia, nasal congestion, dizziness, and visual disturbances (mostly under 5%), and a slight decrease in blood pressure. PDE5i's have not been found to add to the risk of cardiovascular events or stroke in able-bodied men who do not take nitrates.

Three studies in men with SCI were published from the approval process of the first PDE5i to market, sildenafil (42–44). In these studies, those men who were able to get a reflex erection in response to vibratory stimulation responded to sildenafil (80% compared to placebo of 10%). Even though men without reflex erections did not fare as well, they still noted an improvement in their erections. The most common side effects (15% and below) were headaches, vasodilatation (flushing and rhinitis), dyspepsia, and blue-tinged vision at higher dosage levels, similar to those seen in able-bodied subjects. Sildenafil dropped the blood pressure (BP) on average by 8.0 mmHg systolic and 5.5 mmHg in the clinical trials in able-bodied men, but this was thought not to be of significance in that population. In the trials of sildenafil and men with SCI, there was also no evidence that the alterations in blood pressure were clinically relevant, but it should be noted that those men with chronic hypotension or with BP < 80/50 mmHg were excluded from the trials (Pfizer data on file). Theoretically, the low blood pressures typically seen in men with injuries above T6 could be exacerbated with the hypotensive effects of any PDE5i, but practically, this is not seen to be a big issue, and is often managed by a reduction in initial dose and accommodation to the effects over time (45). In all studies on sildenafil (45–48) except one (49) it was felt that the decrease in BP had no significant

clinical implications even in those men who were naturally hypotensive (high level lesions). Still, some men with SCI are unable to take PDE5i because of the side effects, including dizziness. Others find the dizziness transient and acceptable. Additionally, if the level of SCI is high, they are also at risk of autonomic dysreflexia. Symptoms of autonomic dysreflexia are similar to the side effects of PDE5i (headache and flushing). Because nitrates, which are contraindicated with concomitant use with PDE5i, are sometimes used to treat autonomic dysreflexia, one must be sure that a person is experiencing true autonomic dysreflexia and not the flushing side effect of a PDE5i. If the person has ingested Viagra® or Levitra® within the past 24 hours, then nitrate administration is contraindicated, because nitrates can potentiate the hypotensive effects of the PDE5i and cause severe hypotension. For Cialis users, this restriction is extended to 48 hours. It follows that men on daily Cialis® 5 mg OD or any daily PDE5i should not use nitrates at all.

Vardenafil was studied in men with SCI in a double-blind, placebo-controlled, parallel group study and was found to be significantly more effective than placebo. Over 12 weeks of treatment, mean per-patient penetration (76% vs. 41%), maintenance (59% vs. 22%), and ejaculation (19% vs. 10%) success rates were reported, and the drug was relatively well tolerated (50). The main side effects were headache, flushing, and nasal congestion. Tadalafil has also been recently studied in men with SCI in a randomized, double-blind, placebo-controlled, flexible dose-titration, parallel group study (51). Again, after treatment, the tadalafil group, compared with the placebo group, was significantly greater in mean per-patient percentage of successful penetration attempts and intercourse attempts, percentage of improved erections, and ejaculatory frequency. The two most common treatment-emergent adverse events were headache and urinary tract infections. In general, studies of men with SCI show that PDE5i's are well tolerated, safe, and effective for men with ED following SCI, regardless of the cause of injury, neurological level, ASIA grade, and time since injury (52).

PDE5i's only influence erectile ability and overall sexual satisfaction, and pharmacologically are not made to increase libido or ejaculatory/orgasmic changes. However, it appears that there may be a mild positive ejaculatory effect in men with SCI, possibly secondary to the improved erection. Data from early clinical trials utilizing sildenafil in men with SCI suggested that some men experienced an improvement in their ejaculation and orgasmic ability although this was not statistically significant (Pfizer data on file). Pooling all papers on PDE5i use in men with SCI, statistical impact on ejaculation success rates was shown in at least one paper for all PDE5i ($p < 0.05$) and very few men with SCI-discontinued use of PDE5i due to drawbacks (52). Unfortunately the statistically significant improvement in ejaculation data from the vardenafil and tadalafil studies do not outline which category of SCI was the most influenced.

The use of other oral medications such as yohimbine and trazadone are basically ineffective in this population, with the exception that trazadone may cause priapism. Other oral therapies including Apomorphine (a dopamine-receptor agonist) and 4–aminopyridine (a channel-blocking agent noted for increasing neurotransmitter release at neuroneuronal sites), have also not proven effective in the SCI population (53, 54). Apomorphine, relatively successful in men without SCI, has a low rate of response in men with SCI and a 40% side effect rate (headache, nausea, tiredness) (53). Testosterone deficiency or hypogonadism should also be looked for when sexual function and libido decline in men with SCI (especially those with concomitant head injury), and testosterone replacement therapy should be considered if found (16, 31).

Local Penile Delivery Systems

PENILE INJECTIONS   Intracavernosal injections have been the gold standard in treating men with SCI because of the reliability and rigidity of the erection produced by the medications injected, and the dose response efficacy.

The use of alprostadil or PGE1 is relatively safe in the correct dose. Alprostadil is commercially available in kits, such as Caverject®. The invasiveness of the technique and the potential for intracavernosal calcium deposition and fibrosis (especially with papaverine) or tunical scarring (penile curvature) from the injection method is a drawback. Penile pain or aching associated with alprostadil is not usually an issue in the SCI population, although other men with neurogenic ED and normal penile sensation are prone to this side effect of alprostadil. Dose titration of alprostadil should be done carefully and slowly, starting with no more than 2 μg (0.1 cc of a 20 μg/ml solution), because of the higher risk of prolonged erection and priapism. The latter is likely caused by denervation hypersensitivity (55). The medication must be accurately delivered to one corpus (it will diffuse unaided to the other corpus) by a short, fine (28–30 gauge) insulin needle. The technique must be carefully shown to the patient and demonstrated by the patient before a prescription is given. Alternatively, the method can be taught to a partner if limited hand function or poor visibility makes this method impractical for the client. The use of autoinjectors can be helpful for those with poor hand function or fear of needles.

Complication rates of injections have been reported in the 15–31% range with the caveat that accumulated experience of clinicians and dosage adjustments reduce this substantially (56). The most common side effects of injections are transient, such as pain and swelling at the injection site. Lower frequency of injections, lower doses of medication, and post-injection pressure on the injection site reduce the risk of intracavernosal or tunical fibrosis. Any erection sustained over 3 hours must be seen by medical personnel: priapism unreactive to oral sympathomimetics must be treated with blood irrigation of the cavernosal bodies, injections of alpha-adrenergic drugs, or potentially surgical intervention to avoid the permanent penile tissue damage from prolonged anoxia from low-flow priapism.

Penile injection is successful in all men with SCI except those with significant penile arterial insufficiency, a large venous leak, or other anatomical abnormalities. Slowly increasing PGE1 doses (up to 20 μg) or the use of combination mixtures (i.e., Trimix, which consists of alprostadil, papaverine, and phentolamine, or Quad mixes that add other alpha-antagonists to the mixtures) may improve the efficacy. It is recommended injections not be done more than once in 24 hours and not more than three times per week to reduce the complication risk. In the pre-PDE5i-era, it was reported that after 2 years of use, approximately 50% of SCI patients would drop out of the injection method (57). It does, however, have a high acceptance rate of 70% in the SCI population (56). This author's informal survey shows a lower drop-out

rate (<20 %) and virtually no cases of priapism: this is likely due to the longer instruction time (including and watching the patient demonstrate the actual injection), utilizing incremental test dosing at home, and active follow-up.

INTRAURETHRAL PELLET OR MUSE®   Alprostadil or PGE1 can also be administered as a tiny pellet into the urethra. The urethra must first be straightened and then lubricated with urine before placement of the pellet, the latter of which may not be easily done by some men with SCI. Absorption of the medication is encouraged by rolling the penis between the hands for at least 1 minute and standing or sitting (not lying down) after insertion. Occasionally, the stimulus of the applicator into the urethra may cause reflex voiding, and the medication will be washed out. In general, this method is easier for most quadriplegics who are able to self-catheterize than the injection method, which requires better hand function. MUSE® can be used up to two times in a 24-hour period. Because of the potential long-term side effects of using an invasive method such as injection, intraurethral alprostadil has a role in men with SCI, but doses are several fold (250, 500, and 1000 μg) that of the injection route. One study (58) noted that the erection quality, especially when compared to intracavernosal injection, was poor and that the highest dose of MUSE® was required to obtain any tumescence. Because this method is reliant on vascular connections between the corpus spongiosum and cavernosal bodies, and the production of a pressure gradient that encourages retrograde venous flow, it is likely that this vascular transference is poor in the spinal cord population, even when aided by an Actis® ring at the base of the penis to discourage venous outflow. Without the ring, men with SCI can experience hypotension from the medication. Furthermore, the urethral mucosa itself may be less likely to absorb the medication when it has been repeatedly catheterized. The addition of other erectogenic drugs such as prazosin to the alprostadil may well improve the efficacy but this has not been evaluated in men with SCI.

Topical Agents

Topical vasodilators such as minoxidil, PGE1, papaverine, and nitroglycerin, although generally safe, are not found to be effective beyond 24–40% in the general population (56), and lack of absorption through the tunica albuginea is the probable reason. The use of topical agents has not been studied in men with SCI, probably due to the efficacy of PDE5i and injection therapy and the reluctance to use topical solutions that may be absorbed intravaginally by the female partner.

Mechanical Methods

Many men with SCI can attain, but not maintain, a firm erection for the act of intercourse. A simple, proper medical constriction band at the base of the penis may assist with erectile maintenance, but should not be left on for more than 30–45 minutes. In men with no genital sensation, leaving the ring on for too long or falling asleep will not result in pain and therefore fail to raise alarm. Although serious corporal damage will likely not be experienced unless the penile tissues are anoxic for several hours, removal of the ring immediately after sexual activity must be emphasized. The removal of the ring is aided by wings or pull-tabs attached to the sides, but still requires some strength and dexterity of the hands.

Vacuum devices (VD) consist of a cylinder that encloses the penis, a pump to create a vacuum, and a constriction ring. VDs are a noninvasive, nonpharmaceutic, and successful method of attaining (via the vacuum) and maintaining (via constriction band) an erection. In one study of 20 couples, 93% of men with SCI and 83% of their female partners reported sufficient penile rigidity for intercourse obtained by the use of a vacuum device after 3 months, but by 6 months less than half the couples were satisfied with the device, although 60% reported improvement of their sexual relationships (59). A fair amount of manual dexterity is required, although there are battery-operated models for those with poor hand function. Because the erection is in the external (visible) corpora only with the internal corporal tissues and associated crura not engorged, the erection tends to swivel at the base. The constriction ring may also cause pain or block ejaculation, but this is not usually a concern in the SCI population. Premature loss of rigidity, petechiae, and penile skin edema can occur, but are usually temporary. Vacuum devices have the advantage of being able to be used more than once in a 24-hour period, and can also be used as a back-up method when other enhancement methods have failed. They can also be used in men with penile implants and in those who have had implants removed.

Penile Prosthesis (Implants)

Penile prosthesis, especially in a population with sensory loss, should only be done in those patients in whom the reversible methods have failed or who require penile straightening procedures or reconstructive genitourinary surgery. Men with SCI experience a much higher infection and erosion rate with these devices when compared to nonneurologic patients (60), although surgical technique and the devices themselves have improved considerably. Because these devices are physically inserted into the corpora cavernosal bodies, the erectile tissue is destroyed, so other erection enhancement methods will no longer be effective, except potentially the vacuum device.

Devices are either malleable, semi-rigid, or multicomponent (two- or three-piece) inflatable prostheses. Although the former is less aesthetically appealing, the latter is more prone to malfunction. The procedures are primarily done as a permanent solution to sexual difficulties, and they have been helpful for bladder management such as condom drainage. Overall, there is a high level of satisfaction amongst men with SCI who opted for this therapy (61).

Surgical Solutions: Penile Prosthesis and Sacral Anterior Root Stimulator Implants (SARSI)

The Brindley Finetech SARSI® is successful for control of micturition with continence in more than 80% of one series of men who have had the device implanted. Because the implantation requires the division of the sacral posterior roots, there is a consequential loss of reflex erections: only 60% of patients were able to use implant-driven erection (62). A similar device, VOCARE Bladder System®, is an FDA-approved system that has a surgically implanted pacemaker-type receiver that stimulates sacral nerves and an external controller that is about the size of a personal CD player. It is used to assist men with SCI to empty their bladder on demand, but a secondary use has been to aid bowel evacuation and promote penile erection. These devices have not been commonly utilized for managing sexual dysfunction.

Future Therapies for ED

The effects of behavioral management for erectile dysfunction should not be forgotten, as maximization of innate potential after SCI should be pursued before or in conjunction with the above current therapeutic modalities. Courtois et al (63) found perineal training combined with biofeedback and home exercises resulted in significant differences in tumescence in 10 men with SCI who retained some voluntary pelvic floor contraction. On the other end of the scale, new knowledge about the underlying mechanisms of erectile dysfunction suggest that penile rehabilitation may include the daily use of PDE5i to improve endothelial function and even reverse the pathology. In the future, biological correction of some facets of the defective erectile mechanism may be possible. Therapeutic prospects on the horizon include novel pharmacotherapies, growth factor therapy, gene therapy, and regenerative medicine (64). Genes that stimulate smooth muscle relaxation, such as neuronal, inducible, and endothelial nitric oxide synthase, or that inhibit smooth muscle cell constriction, can be targeted. Gene therapy studies for ED are currently being evaluated.

Therapies for Orgasmic Improvement

Tepper, after interviewing 12 men and 10 women following SCI, elucidated several conditions that facilitate sexual pleasure and orgasm, including relaxation, meditation, dreams, fantasy, recalling positive experiences, breathing, going with the flow, trust or being with a partner who is trusted, and addition of nongenital touch, plenty of time, and added stimulation of a vibrator (65). Anything that will increase the likelihood of ejaculation will also increase the likelihood of orgasmic feelings, even if learned over time. This means increased intimacy, more and longer stimulation in erotic areas, and even the use of PDE5i may be beneficial. Autonomic dysreflexia can be experienced during sexual activity, and is not limited to the stimulation from the more aggressive sperm-retrieval techniques. In a survey of 199 men with SCI, roughly one third (28.6%) reported experiencing AD symptoms during sexual activity, but only 16.1% indicated that AD interfered with sexual activity and only 6% found AD symptoms during sexual activity to be pleasurable or arousing (18). Of the subjects who did experience AD, the vast majority had injuries at or above T6.

FERTILITY FOLLOWING SPINAL CORD INJURY

It is well recognized that fertility in men is affected following SCI. Ejaculatory disorders and poor semen quality account for the natural lowered fertility, but advances in both sperm-retrieval and reproductive technology can assist with improved outcomes. Ejaculatory disorders after spinal cord injury are primarily neurogenic in etiology. Occasionally, post-injury epididymitis can result in an obstructive cause of infertility. Anejaculation, a term used to describe the inability to ejaculate or produce an antegrade (forward) semen sample, is the most common problem after SCI, because the ejaculation reflex (seminal emission and propulsatile ejaculation) fails to occur. Retrograde ejaculation, caused by either lack of closure of the internal bladder neck (sympathetic) or lack of relaxation of the external sphincter (parasympathetic) can also occur after SCI. As compared to natural rates (see Table 32.1), in a 2005 systematic review of 22 studies utilizing either vibrostimulation or electroejaculation interventions to assist in sperm retrieval, the overall ejaculation response rate was 86%, with a large degree of heterogeneity being observed when the data are pooled (61). However, studies published after 1997 reported response rates of 100% utilizing these two methods (61). Over the last 15 years, both pregnancy and live birth rates have improved considerably, with a respectable pregnancy rate (pooled data) of 51% and a live birth rate of 40% being reported in the partners of men with SCI (61).

Semen quality invariably deteriorates after SCI, likely within the first two weeks after injury, with sperm motility being most affected. Attempts to collect seminal fluid within days or weeks after injury has inherent problems. Because spinal shock eliminates reflex activity and precludes vibrostimulation from working, the clinical stability of the patient must be determined before electroejaculation or aspirative techniques take place (66). However, once this time period has passed, further deterioration in semen quality does not seem to occur (67, 68). Because semen from men with SCI and from controls both lose approximately 65% motility with freezing (69, 70), there does not seem to be much advantage to cryopreserving sperm obtained in the earlier window because the reduction in sperm quality may be equivalent to the improvement in results using current assisted reproductive technology (ART), such as in vitro fertilization (IVF) and intracytoplasmic sperm injection (ICSI). In most cases, men suffering from anejaculation due to SCI are excellent candidates for ejaculation induction procedures and low-level assisted reproductive techniques (71).

The suggested causes of altered sperm quality following SCI include stasis of prostatic fluid, alterations of the seminal fluid composition, higher free radical composition secondary to dead sperm and increased white blood cells, high testicular temperature, recurrent urinary tract infections, exposure of sperm to urine in retrograde ejaculates, abnormal testicular histology, altered antisperm antibodies, disordered storage of spermatozoa in the seminal vesicles, and the long-term use of various medications (67, 72, 73). Evidence is suggesting that hormonal abnormalities, immunologic causes, and scrotal temperature do not seem to explain the poor semen quality in men with SCI (74). Brown-colored semen can also be seen in men with SCI, but does not seem to worsen the quality: this may be related to seminal-vesicle dysfunction (75). Recent studies have pointed to altered seminal components as the main culprit causing the lowered motility: there is higher seminal platelet-activating factor acetyl-hydrolase activity (which results in impairment of motility and sperm capacitation and fertilization) in semen from men with SCI (76), as well as higher levels of cytokines, which when immunoneutralized at the receptor level, appear to improve sperm motility (77). Bladder management also appears important to semen quality. Better semen quality is noted with intermittent self-catheterization than from any other form of bladder management. This may be due to maintenance of lower bladder pressures with less risk of reflux into the ejaculatory ducts and infections (78, 79). It also appears thoracic paraplegics and

those with complete injuries had better overall semen parameters (78). Semen quality is also better when obtained by vibratory stimulation versus electroejaculation, likely because the entire ejaculation reflex is mobilized as compared to seminal emission alone (80, 81). Vibrostimulation usually promotes antegrade ejaculation, but both antegrade and/or retrograde ejaculation can occur (82). Semen parameters have been shown to both improve and stay the same with weekly ejaculations in uncontrolled studies using repeated vibrostimulations for varying times between 3 and 12 months (82–84), but a prospective randomized controlled study suggests some improvement in morphology and forward progression with a trend toward improved motility after weekly vibrostimulation (VS) for three months (85). Asthenospermia of chronic SCI was improved by consecutive day electroejaculation (86), and repeated electroejaculations were shown to have a positive effect on sperm concentration, motility, and ICSI outcome (87). However, other studies suggest repeated electroejaculation has no effect on volume, sperm concentration, motility, or the total motile count (88). Although more research needs to be done to elucidate and possibly prevent the underlying etiology of altered semen parameters and fertility following SCI, biologic fatherhood is possible now due to successful treatments for ejaculatory dysfunction and the use of ART.

Treatment of Ejaculatory Dysfunction

There are two main reasons men with SCI seek assistance with ejaculatory dysfunction: they want to know if there is any method that can be introduced to successfully allow ejaculation for either sexual or reproductive reasons, and/or they wish to know their realistic fertility potential. Knowing their fertility potential removes the question that will undoubtedly need to be answered—will biological fatherhood be possible? An assessment of how semen can be obtained and whether there is live, motile spermatozoa in the ejaculate will lead to an estimation of what would be expected in terms of technical assistance to have a partner conceive. Except for those men who require fertility investigations for medico-legal purposes, most men will pursue sperm retrieval options when they feel ready to seek answers to these questions, or gain access to an appropriate SCI center with experience in fertility. Although it is important to communicate to the man or couple that with today's technology, poor semen quality does not preclude biologic fatherhood, discussions should include up front, realistic discussions on chances of conception depending on semen quality, age of the female partner, financial and emotional cost, philosophies on medical intervention, as well as viable alternatives such as donor insemination and adoption.

The most common methods of obtaining ejaculates from men with SCI make use of the neurophysiology explained earlier. Pharmaceutical methods enhance the ejaculatory reflex at either the efferent or supraspinal level. Methods such as penile vibrostimulation (PVS) utilize heightened afferent stimulation to instigate efferent discharge of the ejaculation reflex via spinal cord intermedularies in those men with intact lumbosacral spinal cord. PVS usually produces an antegrade, propulsatile ejaculation. Electroejaculation (EEJ) "jump starts" the distal efferent fibers of the reflex arc, and stimulates the sympathetic efferent fibers and smooth muscles of the seminal vesicles and terminal vasa (and in some case the obturator nerve resulting in leg movement), resulting in seminal emission that will need to be milked from the urethra (88). However, both PVS and EEJ may produce antegrade, retrograde, propulsatile, and non-pulsatile ejaculations depending on the level of lesion and the stimulus applied. It is accepted practice that, in all men with SCI (especially those whose injury is above neurologic level T12 and in those with incomplete lesions below this level) PVS should be tried first because it is simpler, less invasive, and more easily repeated at lower cost. On the very rare occasion that both PVS and EEJ fail, operative sperm retrieval, which is independent of nerve pathways or intact structures, can be used. Sperm retrieved through operative means commits the couple to the higher technology methods and expense. In contrast, in many men with SCI, PVS can be performed by the patient himself and home insemination performed as a very low cost alternative (71). However, ease of semen retrieval, semen quality, female fertility potential, and type of assisted reproductive measures required (and their affordability) will determine pregnancy rates. If fertility funding is available, as it is in some countries outside North America, then higher technology and operative retrieval may provide the best chance of conception.

Other nerve stimulation techniques (such as transperineal electroejaculation and hypogastric plexus stimulators) and implanted capsules connected to the vas deferens for direct sperm aspiration have not been as successful. For men with SCI, between the techniques of PVS and EEJ, semen collection is virtually assured. To date, unlike PVS, EEJ has not been routinely done at home, nor is it as readily available or affordable as PVS. Operative retrieval requires the use of ART in some form.

Two methods of inducing physiological ejaculation, intrathecal neostigmine (89) and subcutaneous physostigmine (90), have been less popular because of invasiveness and/or the severity of side effects, including a death from cerebral hemorrhage in the former. Some clinics still offer this successfully, however. The reader is referred to a good review of the use of pharmacologic agents that can be used to induce an ejaculation (67).

Risk of Autonomic Dysreflexia

Sperm retrieval methods in those with injuries at or above T6 should only be attempted by a medical team familiar with the management of autonomic dysreflexia (AD). AD is a condition of episodic hypertension triggered by noxious and non-noxious afferent stimuli below the level of lesion of the spinal cord, and is characterized by headache, upper body flushing and sweating, or pallor, nausea, photophobia, bradycardia, and possible cardiac arrhythmias (91). AD may have serious consequences, including intracerebral hemorrhage and death. Common stimuli below the level of the lesion eliciting AD in men with SCI are pain, pressure sores, distension or inflammation of the bladder or gastrointestinal tract, muscle spasm, and sexual activity (92, 93). Pudendal nerve stimulation alone can produce AD (94). AD usually occurs near or at an ejaculation, but can also be heightened with prolonged genital stimulation or the use of any sympathomimetic drugs (such as pseudoephedrine or midodrine, which are often recommended to enhance ejaculation) prior to sperm retrieval. Therefore, with the use of PVS and EEJ, precautionary methods must be practiced. First-time experimental use of PVS at home alone in a man with injury above T6 should be discouraged (91), and patients are advised to do so in a supervised, clinic setting. Pre-procedural antihypertensive medication, such as nifedipine (10 to 20 mg taken 20 minutes prior to the procedure) or prazosin (1 mg taken 12 hours and 1 hour before the procedure, respectively), can be used for prophylaxis. AD is modulated by spinal or general anesthesia by interfering with the uncontrolled sympathetic discharge. During PVS and EEJ procedures, AD should be watched for (and can often be minimized) by continuous blood pressure monitoring and observing, along with listening to the patient and decreasing or stopping either the vibratory stimulus or stimulating current when the man begins to exhibit signs of AD (91, 95). Often with time and experience, symptomatic AD will decrease, but there is no assurance blood pressure elevations are reduced, as silent AD can still be occurring (91, 95). Despite several reports in the literature about modest increases in BP (20–50 mmHg) during ejaculation (32, 37), it should be cautioned that these measurements were not done with beat-to-beat recordings, so peak systolic and diastolic blood pressures at ejaculation may have been missed. It is this author's experience that systolic blood pressure can often approach or exceed 200 mmHg during ejaculation, and that AD can be silent, or even malignant (91, 93, 95). The reality is AD is part of daily life for some men with SCI, but the severity of blood pressure elevation should be respected during elective sperm retrieval, even if AD symptoms are tolerable.

Pharmaceutical Methods

There is little in the way of pharmaceutical treatment to compensate for the neurologic deficits seen with ejaculatory disorders in men with SCI. Sympathomimetic drugs such as pseudoephedrine or midodrine can potentiate seminal emission, or if retrograde ejaculation is occurring because of nerve damage or bladder neck surgery, may encourage antegrade ejaculation. The use of sympathomimetics to promote seminal emission and antegrade ejaculation is fairly successful in the testicular cancer population among those who have undergone retroperitoneal lymph node dissection, disrupting the sympathetic chain. Because of the action of sympathomimetics on the sympathetic nervous system, blood pressure will invariably be increased and could cause urinary retention in some patients (67), so the use of sympathomimetic drugs for enhanced sperm retrieval should be approached with caution in the SCI population with history of AD or hypertension from other causes. In some cases, cautionary use of sympathomimetics can be helpful in combination with other modalities, such as vibrostimulation, that may not induce ejaculation on their own. Midodrine has been studied and found to be a safe and efficient adjunct to PVS for anejaculation in SCI patients who underwent BP monitoring (37). Finally, the rare but distressing problem of severe premature emission after injury at the T12–L1 level is very difficult to treat, but slight improvement has been noted in a few patients with the use of phenoxybenzamine, terazocin, or prazosin (96).

Vibrostimulation

PVS is the first line of treatment for anejaculatory men with SCI. PVS involves the application of a high-speed, high-amplitude vibrator around the glans penis to induce ejaculation via an intact sacral ejaculatory reflex (see Figure 32.3). If recognizable orgasm without antegrade ejaculation can be reached through sexual

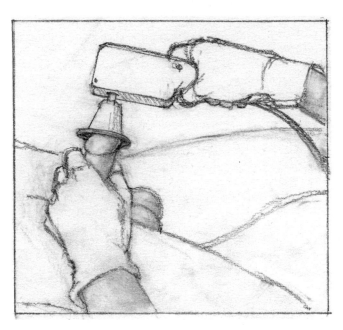

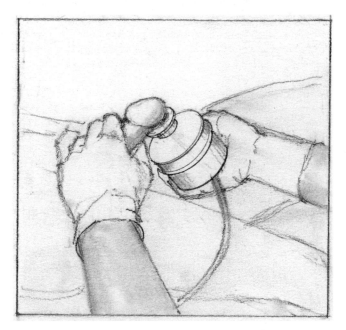

Figure 32.3   The inexpensive, store-purchased WAHL™ vibrator has been rewired to deliver high amplitude. The bell shaped cup distributes the stimulation over most of the glans simultaneously, and does not diminish intensity applied to the penis. (WAHL Model 4196, Div Swenson Canada, Inc., 80 Orfus Road, Toronto, Ontario, M6A 1M1).

Figure 32.4   The FertiCare® Clinic vibrator is commercially available for use in sperm retrieval clinics, and is adjustable in speed and amplitude. The vibrator is applied to the frenulum until ejaculation occurs. (Multicept APS, Rungsted, Denmark). FertiCare® Personal is a smaller model available through the Internet for private purchase.

practices, it can be predicted that PVS will not likely increase the chance of antegrade ejaculation. For men with SCI, ejaculation with PVS may or may not result in orgasm. Although the vibrator usually induces a reflex erection before ejaculation, it is not unusual to lose the erection with the strong stimulus, or to not achieve an erection at all if ejaculation occurs very fast (under 30 seconds). In any event, ejaculation is commonly triggered within one to five minutes of the vibrator being applied or reapplied after a 1- to 2-minute rest interval. Four to six cycles should be tried before abandoning the procedure: however, most positive responders do so within one to two cycles. Because of the risk of AD, it is important to undergo initial trials in a monitored, clinic setting.

Vibrostimulation is both an art and a science. Specific vibrator speeds and amplitudes are more likely to induce the reflex. Sønksen et al. (97) demonstrated that the optimal peak-to-peak amplitude of a vibrator was 2.5 mm at a speed of 100 Hz, and this has been confirmed by several other investigators (98). Inexpensive store-bought vibrators are rarely powerful enough, and most require internal rewiring to deliver higher amplitude (see Figure 32.3). Caution is advised if the casing is not adequate to sustain the increased heat generated by the adaptation. Other more expensive, powerful massagers available commercially may not require rewiring. Sønksen and colleagues were instrumental in the development of a Food and Drug Administration- (FDA) registered PVS device (FertiCare®) that has adjustable speeds and amplitudes. FertiCare® Clinic (Figure 32.4) is a large, durable version used in SCI fertility clinics, but a smaller, rechargeable version (FertiCare® Personal) is available for purchase on-line. The art of PVS consists of effective placement and pressure of the vibrator on the glans, with appropriate rest periods to avoid

exhausting the reflex, and reading the patient for signs of impending ejaculation while monitoring for autonomic dysreflexia. "Trigger spots," or signature areas, can be used to reliably elicit the reflex: these may be at the frenulum, but are often found on the dorsal surface of the glans also. Although single PVS is often effective, some men may require the use of one vibrator on the dorsal and another on the ventral surface of the glans. Positive signs of impending ejaculation include abdominal and leg spasms, hip or knee flexion, abduction or adduction of the thighs, testicular elevation, and generalized piloerection (99, 100). Tonic spasm, periurethral contractions, and an acute distension of the glans (with or without an erection) just prior to ejaculation are premonitory signs of imminent ejaculation (97–99). Sometimes multiple ejaculations can be safely done at one sitting, increasing the total semen volume for insemination purposes. The PVS procedure is more fully explained in other readings (88, 97–99). Vibrostimulation to ejaculation has also been found to relieve leg spasm for up to 3 hours (101), and has been associated with a significant increase in bladder capacity at leak point after 4 weeks of frequent treatment (102).

The efficacy of PVS has been reported in the range of 24% to 96% (98), but higher rates are no doubt related to proper vibrator amplitudes and clinician experience. In men with SCI, especially in those with higher-level lesions, the presence of a bulbocavernosus reflex (BCR) and a hip flexor response is a good predictor of successful PVS, although all patients should be tried initially (100). An anesthetic block of the dorsal nerve will inhibit vibratory-induced ejaculation, erectile response, and signs of autonomic dysreflexia in men with spinal cord injury who would normally exhibit all of the above to PVS (103). In general, it is the author's opinion that clinics using proper PVS techniques should attain at least a 75% success rate for those men with lesions above neurologic level T6, with the higher, complete cervical lesions faring the best. Patient positioning, degree of bladder fullness, and concurrent bedsores or bladder infections may affect the efficacy of PVS. PVS is noninvasive and simple, with the major side effect being AD. Occasionally self-limited minor chafing of the glans or distal penile edema may be experienced with prolonged PVS. Furthermore, the use of two simultaneous vibrators can be tried, as this "sandwich technique" may salvage a single vibrator failure (104). Similarly, case reports of the use of a simple, over-the-counter abdominal muscle stimulator (AES) along with PVS has rescued failures to PVS alone (105, 106). This rescue method is currently undergoing a multicentered trial, and if effective, should be used with PVS before going onto other more invasive and expensive sperm-retrieval techniques.

Semen retrieval with PVS can be done at home using the syringe method during timed ovulation (timed with ovulation predictor kits, for example) if semen quality is adequate and AD is controlled. Because sperm from men with SCI lose motility faster than sperm from uninjured men, samples should be used for insemination as soon as possible, and transported at room versus body temperature (107). If AD is a risk, and/or experienced clinicians and better PVS equipment is required, PVS should be done in a medical clinic setting.

Electroejaculation

PVS failure leads to the need for rectal probe EEJ or operative sperm retrieval. During EEJ, there is likely direct sympathetic stimulation to the prostate gland and seminal vesicles, with indirect sympathetic stimulation to the cauda epididymis (see Figure 32.6). Whereas PVS evokes a true ejaculation (shown by semen markers) (82), EEJ would appear to artificially contract the internal ejaculatory structures and release stored semen in their possession. This may partially explain the recognized better semen quality with PVS than EEJ (80, 82).

A polyvinyl chloride probe with three stainless steel electrodes is inserted into an emptied rectum. The current is administered through the electrodes that are placed firmly against the prostate. AC current generation is controlled by the operator, and probe temperature regulation is done by the electroejaculation equipment (see Figure 32.5). Antegrade flow is encouraged through external milking of the urethral bulb and corpora spongiosum. This emission usually appears within 4 to 15 V of current. Interrupted versus continuous current delivery is preferred because higher volumes and higher mean total motile sperm are found in the antegrade fraction using the interrupted method (108).

The procedure is most commonly done in a left lateral decubitus position but can also be done in lithotomy (Figure 32.6). Short sigmoidoscopy (10–15 cm) before and after the procedure is necessary to rule out any preexisting anorectal conditions or postprocedural thermal injury to the bowel. The bladder is emptied before the procedure by catheter and a phosphate buffer or human tubal fluid solution is instilled to neutralize the urine in case of retrograde semen flow. Some clinicians leave a Foley catheter in the bladder in order to pull it tightly against the bladder neck to reduce the chances of retrograde flow, in which case semen will flow around the outside of the catheter. Regardless of the technique, both antegrade emission and the contents of

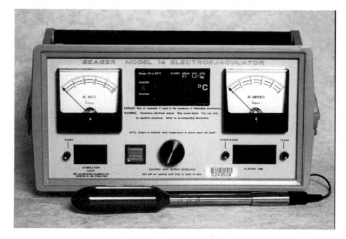

Figure 32.5   The Seager Electroejaculation Stimulation Equipment and Rectal Probes (Distributor: NeuroControl Corporation, 8333 Rockside Road, 1st floor, Valley View, Ohio 44125–6104.)

the bladder (retrograde fraction) are sent for analysis and sperm harvesting at the andrology laboratory.

EEJ can be done as an outpatient clinic procedure in those patients whose injuries have resulted in loss of sensation in the lower pelvis and internal ejaculatory structures. In patients who are partially sensate, some preprocedural sedation or local anesthetic may be adequate for comfort, thus avoiding the more costly operating room time. The current may evoke abdominal pain, tightness, and sometimes chest discomfort, especially if the probe is placed slightly high, near the seminal vesicles, even in those men with "complete" injuries. Some relief can be obtained by moving the probe distally away from this area. Patients who are unable to tolerate the stimulation need either a spinal or general anesthetic.

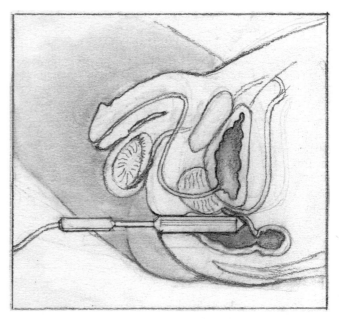

Figure 32.6   The rectal probe for EEJ should be held against the bowel wall, making firm contact with the prostate. Antegrade emission is encouraged by external massage forward from the perineum to the urethra.

During the procedure, adduction of the thighs, testicular retraction, penile erection, and piloerection are usually seen. Autonomic dysreflexia is the major side effect in those patients with injury above T6 (unless under anesthesia). Serious complications with EEJ are very rare. Rectal injury occurs in less than 0.1% of patients, but may require surgical repair (98). The use of spinal or general anesthesia for the EEJ procedure does not seem to alter the success of inducing seminal emission (98). The reader is referred to other readings (73, 109) for procedural information.

Electroejaculation is a highly successful method of sperm retrieval in men with SCI, and has been successfully used to induce ejaculation in men with multiple sclerosis, diabetic neuropathy and surgical injury, and in rare cases, psychogenic anejaculation. However, in the SCI population, PVS should always be tried first because it is very simple to use, is noninvasive, does not require anesthesia, and is preferred by the patients when compared with EEJ (73).

Operative Techniques

Operative sperm retrieval includes the removal of sperm directly from the vas deferens, epididymis, or testes, and is reserved for those cases in men with SCI where sperm retrieval methods fail or there is an obstructive cause of ejaculatory dysfunction. Direct testicular or epididymal sperm removal is popular in able-bodied men who are unable to ejaculate with sexual or gentle vibratory stimulation because the equipment to perform EEJ is not readily available in general infertility clinics.

Because of the lower numbers of sperm and low sperm motility associated with operative retrieval, assisted reproductive technology (ART) is required. In men with SCI, if semen quality is especially poor and higher-level technology, such as in vitro fertilization (IVF) and intracytoplasmic sperm injection (ICSI), is required anyway, there may be a financial benefit to removing sperm operatively rather than use other sperm retrieval techniques, even though much larger numbers of sperm can be obtained using PVS and EEJ. Close coordination is needed with a reproductive team if an operative sperm retrieval method is going to be employed. Aspiration of the vas deferens and implantation of alloplastic spermatoceles, which have a higher risk of scarring, have basically been abandoned, since the improved methods of direct testicular or epididymal sperm removal. The various methods include micro-epididymal sperm aspiration (MESA), percutaneous epididymal sperm aspiration (PESA), or testicular sperm extraction (TESE).

Pregnancy Rates Utilizing Sperm Retrieval Methods

Pregnancy rates are difficult to interpret from the literature because of various patient selection, PVS techniques, and insemination methods. A recent systematic review of the literature (110) looked at 66 reports and found ejaculation interventions in the last decade resulted in response rates of 95% (95% confidence intervals (CI) 91%, 99%), with 100% response rate reported in several recent publications. A total of 13 studies dating from 1993 to 2001 yielded pregnancy rates of 51% (95% CI 42%, 60%) in partners of SCI males. Of these, 11 studies (1993–2003) yielded live birth rates of 41% (95% CI 33%, 49%):

there were no documents relating a superior fertility outcome between PVS and EEJ. Despite higher DNA damage seen in men with SCI compared with controls (111), there is no evidence that men with SCI will father children with a higher incidence of congenital abnormalities than the general population.

Intrauterine insemination (IUI), with or without ovulation induction or other assisted reproductive techniques such as IVF and ICSI, can be employed depending on semen quality and practicalities such as travel and finances. The simplest, most repeatable methods of insemination should be used first as long as the female partner age is under 35. In the author's experience, half the couples where the man was able to safely use PVS at home, had a least one child using intravaginal insemination over time (112, 113), but the literature shows that use of higher ART gives the best chance per cycle of conception, and that to achieve overall pregnancy rates of 50% or greater, ART needs to be used (61). However, ART cost can be prohibitive, and another literature review shows IUI pregnancy rates to be between 9–18% per cycle, and 30–60% per couple, which makes IUI an acceptable alternative (114). Timing of IUI is also important: in a study comparing non-stimulated cycles and cycles stimulated with clomiphene citrate and hCG, it was found that delayed timing of IUI of the stimulated cycles (38–40 hours after the hCG shot) resulted in higher pregnancy rates in the female partners of quadriplegic men (115).

A survey administered to professionals to determine current treatment methods for infertility in couples with SCI male partners found that one-fourth of the infertility clinics did not offer either PVS or EEJ, stating they were untrained or unfamiliar with the sperm retrieval methods and equipment, and about one-third did not offer IUI, but only direct sperm retrieval from the testes or epididymis. This was first-line treatment for anejaculation, committing couples to the more invasive ICSI (114). However, a chart review by the same authors found that semen could be retrieved by PVS or EEJ in 95% of the patients, and that the majority of men with SCI could have semen retrieved with low-cost PVS and have reasonable yields of total motile sperm conducive to trials of IUI. Therefore, centers should consider offering PVS, EEJ, and IUI as a reasonable alternative to ART in couples with SCI male partners.

EVALUATION OF MALE SEXUAL HEALTH AFTER SCI

Doctors and other healthcare professionals must take responsibility for actively addressing sexual concerns in men with SCI. Sexual health should be addressed with the same priority as issues about mobility, bladder management, and bowel control. Although a man with SCI may ask directly about sexual functioning and fertility, he will more often wait for questions to be directed to him. Unspoken or unattended queries about sexual concerns will present themselves in numerous ways in a rehabilitation setting. He may turn to the nurse or occupational therapist for some indirect but encouraging word about sexual attractiveness or functioning. A physiotherapist may face queries about the ability to manage certain positions that simulate sexual acts. Sometimes efforts to have this area addressed may be interpreted as inappropriate, or be rejected or even punished. It is more helpful to determine what provoked the question in the first place, so that respectful information and reassurance can be delivered.

Because sexuality and fertility are legitimate areas of rehabilitation, it is far more effective to have these areas addressed up front. After an assessment of patient readiness and interest, a discussion of various treatments for erectile and ejaculatory dysfunction should occur early on in the rehabilitation process, even if they are not an immediate concern. The knowledge that it is possible to be sexually functional and to potentially father a child will prevent damaging secondary consequences of ignorance and misinformation. More detailed discussions can then be undertaken when appropriate.

A thorough sexual history and a physical examination are essential in the evaluation of sexual and fertility concerns, and can be found in other readings (21, 116, 117). It is critical to assess persons with SCI within the biopsychosocial context of their injury, because that context will affect the rehabilitation of the sexual and fertility concerns (118). Neurophysiologic testing to delineate motor and sensory pathways will be aided in the future by autonomic assessment (36), and this will assist with clinical decision making. Patient education should be part of the agenda; once a patient understands some simplified physiology and why sexual function is altered, he is more likely to creatively access his remaining pathways and persevere in attaining erection, ejaculation or orgasm. Partner participation is always encouraged. If there is an additional factor of brain injury or lack of sexual disinterest based on a reversible cause, this must also be investigated by a medical professional.

The cornerstones to sexual rehabilitation are maximization of existing function, adaptation to limitations, and staying open and positive to new experiences. The principle of maximization can be illustrated by the example of erection dysfunction. The psychogenic component of erectile functioning is important in the rehabilitation of many SCI patients, especially those with lower or incomplete injuries. In the absence of genital or penile sensory afferents from SCI, the brain can still interpret (or learn to interpret) other sensate zones to be erogenous: the thoracolumbar pathway can then convey this maximized supraspinal input and produce an erectile response even when the sacral reflex pathways are unavailable. In men with higher lesions, reflexogenic erections can be maximized by learning which type of penile stimulation or physical pressure facilitates versus diminishes the erection.

The second principle of sexual rehabilitation, adaptation, means integrating the patient's limitations within the context of the whole person. This context includes his:

- Sexual self-view, including body image and ability to attract a partner
- Bladder and bowel issues (which are invariably affected if sexual function is neurologically altered, and have a profound effect on the patient's sense of well being and willingness to be sexual)
- Ability to feel skin sensations in erogenous zones and/or interpret other sensate areas as sexual
- Ability to transfer, turn, or support himself, or to caress, hold, or turn a partner
- Medical concerns (skin problems, pain, spasm, medications, etc.)
- Psychologic status
- Relationships and wish/ability to parent
- Occupational interests and financial stability

The fact that these issues are beyond the scope of this chapter in no way diminishes their extreme importance to overall sexual health and function.

Lastly, staying open to new experiences, including the use of sexual stimuli in areas not appreciated pre-injury, is critical in the development of pleasure and even orgasmic capacity. As time passes and experimentation occurs, greater comfort with the new sexuality is achieved, resulting in improved sexual self-esteem. Neuroplasticity of the brain can occur with dedicated repetition of a new task, and this is what is likely occurring for men and women after SCI who rely on extragenital sensation for arousal and even orgasm. The author and colleagues are currently working on an initial proof of concept study regarding the use of sensory substitution technologies to reestablish sexual sensations in individuals with chronic spinal cord injury (SCI) (119). Neuroplasticity has surely played a role in those men who have learned to maximize their new sexual bodies following SCI and is currently critical in new therapies for all rehabilitation.

CONCLUSION

Men with SCI primarily pursue sexual activity for intimacy need, as well as sexual need and for self-esteem (18). The majority of men with SCI state that their SCI had altered their sexual sense of self and that improving sexual function would improve their quality of life (18). The availability of choices open to men with SCI and their partners in the field of sexual rehabilitation and fertility has improved immensely over the last 15 years and will continue to do so with the exponential growth in knowledge of male sexual physiology and neuroplasticity.

Sexual health care is an integral part of any rehabilitation program, and rehabilitation programs are now accountable to provide assistance with sexual and fertility issues. Healthcare professionals working with men with SCI should be aware of the need to bring up the topic of sexual health, have general knowledge and compassion in the areas of sexual rehabilitation and fertility, and take responsibility to refer to the necessary experts when required. A multidisciplinary team approach to this specialized area is best in order to allow the man with SCI to live his life to the fullest.

ACKNOWLEDGMENTS

The author wishes to acknowledge ICORD (International Collaboration of Repair Discoveries) and RHI (Rick Hansen Institute) for support; Dr. George Szasz, her patients, and her clinical and research colleagues for their teachings; and the artist, Winston Elliott.

References

1. Anderson K. Targeting Recovery: Priorities of the spinal cord injured population. *J Neurotrauma* 2004; 21(10):1371–1383.
2. Bors E, Comarr AE. Neurological disturbances of sexual function with special reference to 529 patients with SC spinal cord injury. *Urol Surv* 1960; 10:191–222.
3. Stevenson RWD, Elliott SL. *Sexuality and Medical Illness in Principles and Practice of Sex Therapy*, 4th ed. New York: Guilford Publications, 2007.
4. Kennedy S, Over R. Psychophysiological assessment of sexual arousal of males with spinal cord injury. *Arch Sex Behav* 1990; 19:15–27.

5. Hultling CP. Partner's perception of the efficacy of sildenafil citrate (Viagra®) in the treatment of erectile dysfunction. *Int J Clin Pract* 1999; (Suppl 102):16–18.

6. Krassioukov AV, Fehlings MG. Effect of graded spinal cord compression on cardiovascular neurons in the rostro-ventro-lateral medulla. *Neuroscience* 1999; 88(3):959–973.

7. Marson L. Central nervous system control. In: Carson C, Kirby R, Goldstein I, eds. *Erectile Dysfunction.* Oxford: ISIS Medical Media, 1999; 73–88.

8. Roberts K, Pryor J. Anatomy and physiology of the male reproductive system. In: Hellstrom W, ed. *Male Infertility and Sexual Dysfunction.* New York: Springer, 1997; 1–21.

9. Chuang AT, Steers WD. Neurophysiology of penile erection. In: Carson C, Kirby R, Goldstein I, eds. *Erectile Dysfunction.* Oxford: ISIS Medical Media, 1999; 59–72.

10. Heaton JPW, Morales A. Facts and controversies on the application of penile tumescence and rigidity: Recording for erectile dysfunction. In: Hellstrom W, ed. *Male Infertility and Sexual Dysfunction.* New York: Springer, 1997; 579–592.

11. Fisher C, Gross J, Zuch A. Cycle of penile erection synchronous with dreaming (REM) sleep. *Arch Gen Psychiatry* 1965; 12:29–45.

12. Beck RO. Physiology of male sexual function and dysfunction in neurogenic disease. In: Fowler C ed., *Neurology of Bladder, Bowel and Sexual Dysfunction.* Boston: Butterworth-Heinemann, 1999; 47–56.

13. Iribarren M, Saenz de Tejada I. Vascular physiology of penile erection. In: Carson C, Kirby R, Goldstein I, eds. *Erectile Dysfunction.* Oxford: ISIS Medical Media, 1999; 51–57.

14. Nitahara NS, Lue TF. Microscopic anatomy of the penis. In: Carson C, Kirby R, Goldstein I, eds. *Erectile Dysfunction.* Oxford: ISIS Medical Media, 1999; 31–41.

15. Giuliano F, Rampin O, McKenna KE. Animal models used in the study of erectile dysfunction. In: Carson C, Kirby R, Goldstein I, eds. *Erectile Dysfunction.* Oxford: ISIS Medical Media, 1999; 43–49.

16. Guay AT. Testosterone and erectile physiology. *Aging Male* 2006; 9:201–206.

17. Laughlin GA, Barrett-Connor E ,Bergstrom J. Low Serum Testosterone and Mortality in Older Men. *J Clin Endocrin Metab* 2008; 93(1):68–75.

18. Anderson KD, Borisoff JF, Johnson RD, et al. Long-term effects of spinal cord injury on sexual function in men: Implications for Neuroplasticity. *Spinal Cord* 2007; 45:338–348.

19. Sipski M, Alexander C, Gómez-Marín O, Spalding J. The effects of spinal cord injury on psychogenic sexual arousal in males. *J Urol* 2007; 177:247–251.

20. Sipski ML, Alexander CJ, Rosen RC. Physiological parameters associated with psychogenic sexual arousal in women with complete spinal cord injuries. *Arch Phys Med Rehab* 1995; 76:811–818.

21. Courtois FJ, Charvier KF, Leriche A et al. Clinical approach to erectile dysfunction in spinal cord injured men: A review of the clinical and experimental data. *Paraplegia* 1995; 33:628–635.

22. Rosen RC, Cappelleri JC, Gendrano N III. The International Index of Erectile Function (IIEF): a state-of-the-science review. Int J Impot Res. 2002 Aug; 14(4):226–244.

23. Alexander M, Brackett N, Bodner D, Elliott S, Jackson A, Sonksen J. National Institute on Disability and Rehabilitation Research. Measurement of sexual functioning after spinal cord injury: preferred instruments. *J Spinal Cord Med* 2009; 32(3):226–236.

24. Schmid DM, Hauri D, Schurch B. Nocturnal penile tumescence and rigidity (NPTR) findings in spinal cord injured men with erectile dysfunction. *Int J Impot Res* 2004;16:433–440.

25. Shaban SF. Treatment of abnormalities of ejaculation. In: Lipshultz L, Howards S eds., *Infertility in the Male.* St. Louis: Mosby Year Book, 1991; 409–427.

26. Giuliano F, Clement P. Neuroanatomy and physiology of ejaculation. *Annu Rev Sex Res* 2005;16:190–216.

27. Allard J, Truitt WA, McKenna KE, Coolen LM. Spinal cord control of ejaculation. *World J Urol* 2005; 23:119–126.

28. Johnson RD. Descending pathways modulating the spinal circuitry for ejaculation: effects of chronic spinal cord injury. *Prog Brain Res.* 2006; 152:415–426.

29. Truitt WA, Shipley MT, Veening JG, Coolen LM. Activation of a subset of lumbar spinothalamic neuron after copulatory behavior in male but not female rats. *J Neurosci* 2003; 23:325–331.

30. Alexander CJ, Sipski ML, Findley TW. Sexual Activities, desire, and satisfaction in males pre- and post-spinal cord injury. *Arch Sex Behav* 1993; 22(3):217–228.

31. Phelps G, Brown M, Chen J et al. Sexual experience and plasma testosterone levels in male veterans after spinal cord injury. *Arch Phys Med Rehabil* 1983; 64:47–52.

32. Sipski M, Alexander CJ, Gomez-Marin O. Effects of level and degree of spinal cord injury on male orgasm. *Spinal Cord* 2006; 44:798–780.

33. Chia M, Arvava DA. *The multiorgasmic man.* New York: HarperCollins Publishers. 1996.

34. Miller LS, Staas WE, Herbison GJ. Abdominal problems in patient with spinal cord lesion. *Arch Phys Med Rehabil* 1975; 56:405–408.

35. Sun W-M, MacDonagh, Forter D, et al. Anorectal function in patients with complete spinal transection before and after sacral posterior rhizotomy. *Gastroenterology* 1994; 108:990–998.

36. Alexander MS, Biering-Sorensen F, Bodner D, Brackett NL, Cardenas D, Charlifue S, Creasey G, Dietz V, Ditunno J, Donovan W, Elliott SL, Estores I, Graves DE, Green B, Gousse A, Jackson AB, Kennelly M, Karlsson AK, Krassioukov A, Krogh K, Linsenmeyer T, Marino R, Mathias CJ, Perkash I, Sheel AW, Shilero G, Schurch B, Sonksen J, Stiens S, Wecht J, Wuermser LA, Wyndaele JJ. International standards to document remaining autonomic function after spinal cord injury. Spinal Cord 2009 Jan; 47(1):36–43.

37. Courtois FJ, Charvier KF, Leriche A, Vezina JG, Cote M, Belanger M. Blood pressure changes during sexual stimulation, ejaculation and midodrine treatment in men with spinal cord injury. *BJU Int* 2008; 101:331–337.

38. DeForge D, Blackmer J, Garritty C, Yazdi F, Cronin V, Barrowman N, Fang M, Mamaladze V, Zhang L, Sampson M, Moher D. Male erectile dysfunction following spinal cord injury: a systematic review. *Spinal Cord* 2006; 44:465–473.

39. Ramos AS, Samso JV. Specific aspects of erectile dysfunction in spinal cord injury. *Int J Impot Res.* 2004; 16(Supp 2):S42–45.

40. Soler JM, Previnaire JG, Denys P, Chartier-Kastier E. Phosphodiesterase inhibitors in the treatment of erectile dysfunction in spinal cord injured men. *Spinal Cord* 2007; 45:169–173.

41. Derry F, Hultling C, Seftel AD, Sipski ML. Efficacy and safety of sildenafil citrate (Viagra) in men with erectile dysfunction and spinal cord injury: a review. *Urology* 2002; 60:49–57.

42. Gardner BP, et al. Sildenafil (Viagra®): A double blind, placebo controlled, single dose, two way cross-over study in men with erectile dysfunction caused by traumatic spinal cord injury. *J Urol* 1997; 702:S157–S181.

43. Derry FA, Dinsmore WW, Fraser M et al. Sildenafil (Viagra®): Efficacy and safety of oral sildenafil (Viagra®) in men with erectile dysfunction caused by SCI. *Neurology* 1998; 51:1–5.

44. Glass C, Derry F, Dinsmore WW, et al. Sildenafil (Viagra TM): An oral treatment for men with erectile dysfunction caused by traumatic spinal cord injury—a double blind, placebo controlled, single dose, two way cross-over study using Rigiscan. *J Spinal Cord Med* 1997; 20(1):145.

45. Sheel W, Krassioukov A, Inglis T, et al. Autonomic dysreflexia during sperm retrieval in spinal cord injury influence of lesion level and sildenafil citrate. *J Applied Physiol* 2005; 99(1):53–58.

46. Del Poplo G, Marzi VL, Mondaini N, Lombardi G. Time/duration effectiveness of sildenafil versus tadalafil in the treatment of erectile dysfunction in male spinal cord-injured patients. *Spinal Cord.* 2004; 42:643–648.

47. Sipski M, Alexander C, Guo X, Gousse A, Zlamal R. Cardiovascular effects of sildenafil in men with SCIs at and above T6. *Top Spinal Cord Inj Rehabil.* 2003; 8(3):26–34.

48. Garcia-Bravo AM, Suarez-Hernandez D, Ruiz-Fernandez MA, Silva Gonzalez O, Barbara-Bataller E, Mendez Suarez JL. Determination of changes in blood pressure during administration of sildenafil (Viagra®) in patients with spinal cord injury and erectile dysfunction. *Spinal Cord.* 2006; 44:301–308.

49. Ethans KD , Casey AR, Schryvers OI, MacNeil BJ. The effects of sildenafil on the cardiovascular response in men with spinal cord injury at or above the sixth thoracic level. *J Spinal Cord Med.* 2003; 26(3):222–226.

50. Giuliano F, Rubio-Aurioles E, Kennelly M, et al. Efficacy and safety of vardenafil in men with erectile dysfunction caused by spinal cord injury. *Neurology* 2006; 66:210–216.

51. Giuliano F, Sanchez-Ramos A, Lochner-Ernst D, et al. Efficacy and safety of tadalafil in men with erectile dysfunction following spinal cord injury. *Arch Neurol* 2007; 64:1584–1592.

52. Lombardi G, Macchiarella A, Cecconi F, Del Popolo G. Ten years of phosphodiesterase type 5 inhibitors in spinal cord injured patients. *J Sex Med* 2009 May; 6(5):1248–1258.

53. Strebel RT, Reitz A, Tenti G, Curt A, Hauri D, Schurch B. Apomorphine sublingual as a primary or secondary treatment for erectile dysfunction in patients with spinal cord injury. *BJU Int.* 2004; 93:100–104.

54. Potter PJ, Hayes KC, Segal JL, et al. Randomized double-blind crossover trial of fampridine-SR (sustained Release 4-aminopyridine) in patients with incomplete spinal cord injury. *J Neurotrauma* 1998;15:837–849.

55. Benard F, Lue TF. The role of the urologist and patient in autoinjection therapy for erectile dysfunction. *Contemporary Urology* 1990; 2:21–26.

56. Elliott S, McBride K, Breen S, Abramson C. Sexual health following spinal cord injury. In: Eng JJ, Teasell RW, Miller WC, Wolfe DL, Townson AF, Aubut J, Abramson C, Hsieh JTC, Connolly S, eds. *Spinal Cord Injury Rehabilitation Evidence (SCIRE)*, Vancouver, 2006; 11.1–11.40.

57. Bodner DR, Leffler E, Frost F. The role of intracavernous injection of vasoactive medications for the restoration of erection in spinal cord injured males: A three year follow-up. *Paraplegia* 1992; 30:118–120.

58. Seftel A, Bodner D, Krueger B. MUSE for erectile dysfunction in spinal cord injured patients. Abstracts of papers presented at AAPS 44th Annual Conference. *J Spinal Cord Med* 1998; 21(4):381.

59. Denil J, Ohl DA, Smythe C. Vacuum erection device in spinal cord injured men: Patient and partner' satisfaction. *Arch Phys Med Rehabil* 1996; 77:750–753.

60. Collins KP, Hackler RH. Complications of penile prosthesis in spinal cord injured patients. *J Urol* 1988; 140:984–985.

61. DeForge D, Blackmer J, Moher D, Garritty C, Cronin V, Yazdi F, Barrowman N, Mamaladze V, Zhang L, Sampson M. Sexuality and reproductive health following spinal cord injury. *Evid Rep Technol Assess (Summ)* 2004; Dec(109):1–8.

62. Brindley GS, Rushton DN. Long term follow-up of patients with sacral anterior root stimulator implants. *Paraplegia* 1990; 28:469–475.

63. Courtois FJ, Mathieu C, Charvier KF, Leduc B, Belanger M. Sexual rehabilitation for men with spinal cord injury : preliminary report on a behavioral strategy. *Sex Disabil* 2001; 19:149–157.

64. Burnett AL. Erectile dysfunction management for the future. *J Androl* 2009; 30(4):391–396.

65. Tepper MS, Whipple B, Richard E, et al. Women with complete spinal cord injury: a phenomenological study of sexual experiences. *J Sex Marital Ther* 2001; 27:615–623.

66. Das S, Soni BM, Sharma SD, et al. A case of rapid deterioration in sperm quality following spinal cord injury. *Spinal Cord* 2006; 44:56–58.

67. Linsenmeyer TA. Management of male infertility. In: Sipski M, Alexander C, eds. *Sexual Function in People with Disability and Chronic Illness*. Gaithersburg, MD: Aspen Publisher, 1997; 487–507.

68. Brackett NL, Ferrell SM, Aballa TC. Quality in spinal cord injured men: Does it progressively decline post injury? *Arch Phys Med Rehabil* 1998; 79:625–628.

69. Pardon OF, Brackett NL, Weizman MS, et al. Semen of spinal cord injured men freezes reliably. *J Androl* 1994; 15:266–269.

70. da silva BF, Borrelli M Jr, Fariello RM, Restelli AE, Del Giudice PT, Spaine DM, Bertolla RP, Cedenho AP. Is sperm cryopreservation an option for fertility preservation in patients with spinal cord injury-induced anejaculation? *Fertile Steril* 2009 May 5 [Epub ahead of print].

71. Ohl DA, Quallich SA, Sonksen J, Brackett NL, Lynne CM. Anejaculation: an electrifying approach. *Semin Reprod Med* 2009 Mar; 27(2): 179–185.

72. Brackett NL, Lynne CM, Weizman MS, et al. Endocrine Profiles and semen quality of spinal cord injured men. *J Urol* 1994; 151:114–119.

73. Sonksen J, Ohl DA. Penile vibratory stimulation and electroejaculation in the treatment of ejaculatory dysfunction. *Int J Androl* 2002; 25:324–332.

74. Sønksen J, Ohl DA, Giwercman A, Biering-Sørensen F, Kristensen JK. Quality of semen obtained by penile vibratory stimulation in men with spinal cord injuries: observations and predictors. *Urology* 1996 Sep; 48(3):453–457

75. Wieder JA, Lynne CM, Ferrell SM, Aballa TC, Brackett NL. Brown-colored semen in men with spinal cord injury. *J Androl* 1999; 20: 594–600.

76. Zhu J, Brackett NL, Aballa TC, et al. High seminal platelet-activating factor acetylhydrolase activity in men with spinal cord injury. *J Androl* 2006; 27:429–433.

77. Brackett NL, Cohen DR, Ibrahim E, Aballa TC, Lynne CM. Neutralization of cytokine activity at the receptor level improves sperm motility in men with spinal cord injuries. *J Androl.* 2007 Sep–Oct; 28(5): 717–721.

78. Ohl DA, Bennett CJ, McCabe M, et al. Predictors of success in electroejaculation of spinal cord injured men. *J Urol* 1989; 142:1483–1486.

79. Rutkowski SB, Meddleton JW, Truman G, et al. The influence of bladder management on fertility in spinal cord injured males. *Paraplegia* 1995; 33:263–266.

80. Brackett NL, Padron OF, Lynne CM. Semen quality of spinal cord injured men is better when obtained by vibratory stimulation verses electroejaculation. *J Urol* 1997; 157:151–157.

81. Lochner-Ernst D, Stohrer M, Kramer G, Ippsich H, Mandalka B, Fiedler K. Long-term results of a fertility program in spinal cord injured males. *J Urol* 1996; 155:366A, abstract 224.

82. Chen D, Hartwig DM, Roth EJ. Comparison of sperm quantity and quality in antegrade V retrograde ejaculates obtained by vibratory penile stimulation in males with spinal cord injury. *Am J Phys Med Rehabil* 1999; 78:46–51.

83. Siosteen A, Forssman L, Steen Y, et al. Quality of semen after repeated ejaculation treatment in spinal cord injured men. *Paraplegia* 1990; 28:96–104.

84. Sonksen J, Ohl DA, Giwercman A, et al. Effect of repeated ejaculation on semen quality in spinal cord injured men. *J Urol* 1999; 161:1163–1165.

85. Hamid R, Patki P, Bywater H, et al. Effects of repeated ejaculation on semen characteristics following spinal cord injury. *Spinal Cord* 2006; 44:369–373.

86. Mallidis C, Lim TC, Hill ST, et al. Necrospermia and chronic spinal cord injury. *Fertil Steril* 2000; 74(2):221–227.

87. Giulini S, Pesce F, Madgar I, et al. Influence of multiple transrectal electroejaculation on semen parameters and intracytoplasmic sperm injection outcome. *Fert Steril* 2004; 82:2000–2004.

88. Oates RD, Kasabian NG. The use of vibratory stimulation for ejaculatory abnormalities. In: Whitehead D, Nagler H, eds. *Management of Impotence and Infertility*. Philadelphia: JB Lippincott, 1994; 314–320.

89. Guttman L, Walsh JJ. Prostigmine assessment test of fertility in spinal man. *Paraplegia* 1971; 9:39–51.

90. Chapelle PA, Blanquart F, Puech AJ, Held JP. Treatment of anejaculation in the total paraplegic by subcutaneous injection of physostigmine. *Paraplegia* 1983; 21:30–36.

91. Claydon VE, Elliott SL, Sheel AW, et al. Cardiovascular responses to vibrostimulation for sperm retrieval in men with spinal cord injury. *J Spinal Cord Med* 2006; 29:207–216.

92. Krassioukov AV, Claydon VE. The clinical problems in cardiovascular control following spinal cord injury: an overview. In: Weaver LC, Polosa C, eds. Prog Brain Res. Amsterdam, NL: Elsevier B.V.: 2006; 152:223–229.

93. Elliott S, Krassioukov A. Malignant autonomic dysreflexia following ejaculation in spinal cord injured men. *Spinal Cord* 2006; 44(6): 386–392.

94. Reitz A, Schmid DM, Curt A, et al. Autonomic dysreflexia in response to pudendal nerve stimulation. *Spinal Cord* 2003; 41:539–542.

95. Sheel W, Krassioukov A, Inglis T, Elliott S. Autonomic dysreflexia during sperm retrieval in spinal cord injury influence of lesion level and sildenafil citrate. *J Applied Physiol.* 2005; 99(1):53–58.

96. Kuhr CS, Heiman J, Cardenas D, Bradley W, Berger RE. Premature emission after spinal cord injury. *J Urol* 1995; 153:429–431.

97. Sonksen J, Biering-Sorenson F. Fertility in men with spinal cord or cauda equina lesions. *Semin Neurol* 1992; 12:98–105.

98. Ohl DA, Sonksen J. Penile vibratory stimulation and electroejaculation. In: Hellstrom W, ed. *Male Infertility and Sexual Dysfunction*. New York: Springer, 1997; 219–229.

99. Szasz G, Carpenter C. Clinical observations in vibratory stimulation of the penis in men with spinal cord injury. *Arch Sex Behav* 1989; 8:461–474.

100. Bird VG, Brackett NL, Lynne CM, Aballa TC, Ferrell SM. Reflexes and somatic responses as predictors of ejaculation by penile vibratory stimulation in men with spinal cord injury. *Spinal Cord* 2001; 39: 514–519.

101. Laessoe L, Nielsen JB, Biering-Sorensen F, Sonksen J. Antispastic effect of penile vibration in men with spinal cord lesion. *Arch Phys Med Rehabil* 2004; 85:919–924.

102. Laessoe L, Sonksen J, Bagi P, Biering-Sorensen F, Ohl DA, McQuire EJ, Kristensen JK. Effects of ejaculation by vibratory stimulation on bladder capacity in men with spinal cord lesions. *J Urol* 2003; 169:2216–2219.

103. Wieder JA, Brackett NL, Lynne CM, Green JT, Aballa TC. Anesthetic block of the dorsal nerve inhibits vibratory-induced ejaculation in men with spinal cord injuries. *Urology* 2000; 55:915–917.

104. Brackett NL, Kafetsoulis A, Ibrahim E, Aballa TC, Lynne CM. Application of 2 vibrators salvages ejaculatory failures to 1 vibrator during penile vibratory stimulation in men with spinal cord injuries. *J Urol* 2007; 177:660–663.

105. Goetz LL, Stiens SA. Abdominal electric stimulation facilitates penile vibratory stimulation for ejaculation after spinal cord injury: a single-subject trial. *Arch Phys Med Rehabil* 2005; 86:1879–1883.

106. Kafetsoulis A, Ibrahim E, Aballa TC, Goetz LL, Lynne CM, Brackett NL. Abdominal electrical stimulation rescues failures to penile vibratory stimulation in men with spinal cord injury: a report of two cases. *Urology* 2006; 68:204.e9–204.e11.

107. Brackett NL, Santa-Cruz C, Lynne CM. Sperm from spinal cord injured men lose motility faster than sperm from normal men: the effect is exacerbated at body compared to room temperature. *J Urol* 1997; 157:2150–2153.

108. Brackett N, Ead D, Aballa S, Ferrell S, Lynne C. Semen retrieval in men with spinal cord injury is improved by interrupting current delivery during electroejaculation. *J Urol* 2002; 167:201–203.

109. Ohl DA. The use of electroejaculation for ejaculatory abnormalities. In: Whitehead D, Nagler H, eds. *Management of Impotence and Infertility.* Philadelphia: JB Lippincott, 1994; 294–313.

110. DeForge D, Blackmer J, Garritty C, Yazdi F, Cronin V, Barrowman N, Fang M, Mamaladze V, Zhang L, Sampson M, Moher D. Fertility following spinal cord injury: a systematic review. *Spinal Cord* 2005; 43:693–703.

111. Brackett NJ, Ibrahim E, Grotas JA, et al. Higher sperm DNA damage is seen from men with spinal cord injuries compared with controls. *J Androl* 2008; 29:93–99.

112. Elliott SL, Fluker MR. Fertility options for men with ejaculatory disorders. *J Soc Obstet Gynecol* Can 2000; Jan:26–32.

113. Elliott S, Nigro M, Ekland M, Griffin S, Allison G. The Vancouver Experience: Sperm Retrieval Program. Abstract in ASIA/ IMSOP Compendium for the International Medicine Society of Paraplegia and American Spinal Injury Association Meeting. May 3–6, 2002; 7.

114. Kafetsoulis A, Brackett NL, Ibrahim E, Attia G, Lynne C. Current trends in the treatment of infertility in men with spinal cord injury. *Fert Steril* 2006; 86:781–789.

115. Pryor JL, Kuneck PH, Blatz SM, et al. Delayed timing of intrauterine insemination results in significantly improved pregnancy rates in female partners of quadriplegic men. *Fertil Steril* 2001; 76:1130–1135.

116. Elliott, S. Sexuality after spinal cord injury. In: Field-Forte E, ed., *Spinal Cord Rehabilitation.* FA Davis (in press 2008).

117. Sipski ML ,Richards JS. Spinal cord injury rehabilitation: state of the science. *Am J Phys Med Rehabil* 2006; 85:310–342.

118. Elliott SL. In: Fehlings MG, Vaccaro A, Boakye M, Rossingnol S, Burns A, DiTunno J, eds. *Sexual Health and SCI in Essentials of Spinal Cord Injury.* New York: Thieme Medical Publishers (in press 2010).

119. Borisoff J, Research Associate, and Gary Birch, PI, Neil Squire Society, Brain Interface Lab, GF Strong Rehabilitation Center, Vancouver, British Columbia, Canada.

33 Sexual Dysfunction in Women with Spinal Cord Injury

Stacy Elliott

Sexuality is an essential component of rehabilitation after spinal cord injury (SCI). When surveyed about what "gain of function" was most important to their quality of life, men and women with SCI put sexuality as a major priority even above the return of sensation, walking, and bladder and bowel function (1). Of 681 participants (approximately 25% female), the majority of individuals with paraplegia felt regaining sexual function was their highest priority, and it was the second highest priority for individuals with quadriplegia (preceded only by regaining hand and arm function) (1). So what progress has been made in investigating and treating female sexual dysfunction following SCI?

On the tail of the explosive knowledge gain and therapeutic breakthroughs for male sexual function over the last decade, the world of female sexual functioning has more recently been inundated with new information. Although male erection and ejaculation therapies have been around for several decades, therapies for women are just starting to be investigated. However, to date more physiological studies have been done on female arousal than male arousal following SCI. This chapter will outline what is known about the sexual neurophysiology and what happens to sexual function and overall sexuality after spinal cord injury. Female sexuality after SCI must be put in the same contextual framework as noted in the sexuality chapter on men (see Chapter 32, Sexual Dysfunction and Infertility in Men with Spinal Cord Injury) and in other readings (2, 3). This chapter will summarize the literature and speculations on genital arousal and orgasm, as well as outline new therapies for female sexual dysfunction on the horizon.

SEXUAL ADJUSTMENT FOR WOMEN AFTER SCI

In general, sexual activity and satisfaction declines after SCI for both sexes (4), although the majority of women remain sexually active after SCI (5, 6). Birth control use in women after SCI is variable. In the United States, two studies reported use in the range of 30–41% (5, 7), whereas use was found to be 48% in Spain (6) and 75% in India (8). The marriage rate for women

with SCI is lower than that for men with SCI or for the general population (9).

In studying sexual concerns after SCI, the Female Sexual Function Index (FSFI) has been found to be one of only a handful of measures that can be considered useful in the measurement of sexual function in women after SCI (10). Developed by a panel, tested and validated with healthy volunteers, the FSFI consists of sex domains of sexual function—desire, arousal, lubrication, orgasm, satisfaction, and pain/discomfort, with a maximum score of 36 achievable (11). One study of 157 Japanese women living with SCI (average age 56 years) found the average FSFI score to be 11.1 and that FSFI scores gradually declined with age (12).

However, after SCI, women do not appear to be all that sexually dissatisfied, despite changes to their sexual abilities, body image, and sexual self-esteem. In the literature, when sexual adjustment for women after SCI is surveyed, the range is wide, with 40–88% of subjects quoted as achieving satisfactory sexual activity (13, 14). Sexual intercourse is often the major sexual activity after SCI, but there is a noticeable decrease in the frequency of intercourse as well as a significant reduction in the capability to reach orgasm compared to pre-injury status (6, 15, 16). In addition, women with cervical injuries have to adjust their sexual practices secondary to reduced hand and arm function, making transfer, balance, self-care, and even masturbation difficult, and leaving them more dependent on others to access social environments and prepare for sexual activities. Yet even women with severe cervical injuries who were found to have lower sexual activity levels had no difference in desire, emotional quality of sexual life, and overall sexual satisfaction than age-economic-educational level and marital status–matched general population controls (17). In contrast, women who are injured before the age of 18 years are at greater risk than other women with SCI of not having an active sexual life in adulthood (6).

Sometimes women who are newly injured feel less sexually attractive, think they were viewed by others as less attractive, and question their ability to perform in a sexually satisfying role (18). However, women become more comfortable with their sexuality and develop improved sexual self–esteem as time passes and as they have experiences with their changed bodies (18, 19). A phenomenological study of sexual experiences in women with complete spinal cord injury that looked beyond the physiological factors described the trajectory of sexuality post-injury (19). Three themes emerged sequentially from the researcher's interviews: cognitive-genital dissociation, sexual disenfranchisement, and sexual rediscovery. The authors encouraged readers to use such findings to provide guidance for educational and therapeutic interventions. Other common themes cited in the literature are the lack of and essential need for education and information from health care professionals to help with sexual adjustment following injury, as well as an overwhelming desire for exchange of information and experience with other women with SCI (6, 12, 14, 18, 20).

Sexual Neurophysiology in Women

Numerous components of the somatic and autonomic nervous system are involved in sexual behaviors and in the highly coordinated mechanisms of sexual arousal and orgasm in women. The reader is referred to the accompanying chapter on male sexuality (see Chapter 32, Sexual Dysfunction and Infertility in Men with Spinal Cord Injury) for a discussion on central arousal mechanisms. Alterations in cardiovascular parameters (increased heart and respiratory rate, sexual flush, and perspiration), increased muscle tone and piloerection, pupil dilatation, and increased sensitivity to "erogenous zones" occur with sexual arousal (21). Women undergo pelvic vasocongestion, lubrication, and swelling of the external genitalia and breasts during sexual arousal. Orgasm is the release of this vasocongestion and neuromuscular tension accompanied by pleasurable sensations, after which the genitalia return to a quiescent state. Women do not have the equivalent of the male refractory period, and are therefore capable of more than one sequential orgasm, or variations of multiple orgasms (21).

With arousal, genital erectile tissue in women becomes engorged with blood, or tumescent. The structures that undergo this engorgement are similar to men's: two dorsal corpora cavernosa form the shaft or body of the corpus clitoris with the ventral corpus spongiosum terminating as the glans clitoris, usually the only structure seen under the hood of the clitoris (an extension of the labia minora). These erectile tissues are composed of small sinusoidal vascular spaces amongst a trabecular extracellular matrix. The sinusoidal spaces are lined by endothelium and surrounded by smooth muscle capable of contraction and relaxation. A thick and relatively effective tunica albuginea, or fibroelastic stocking, surrounds the corpus clitoris. With clitoral engorgement, the tunica is stretched, obliterating venous outflow channels, resulting in blood entrapment (veno-occlusive mechanism) and improved firmness of the clitoris. The deep extensions of the corpora diverge under the pubic arch as long bilateral crura, which are attached to the undersurface of the ischiopubic rami on either side and are covered by the ischicavernosus muscle. The paired bulbs of the clitoris, posteroinferior to the body of the clitoris, lie deep to a thin sheet of bulbospongiosus muscle, fill the space between the crus and the body of the clitoris, and flank the corresponding lateral wall of the urethra and distal vagina to a variable extent (22). The urethral meatus is found separate from and below the glans clitoris, just anterior to the vagina. Periurethral glands and spongy tissues around the urethra, once massaged during a sexual experience through the anterior vaginal wall, can sometimes be felt as a swelling or prominence commonly called the G-spot. Vasocongestion of the pelvis results in a transudate forming through the vaginal epithelium and labia minora (21), resulting in lubrication. With continued arousal the vagina also elongates and the uterus elevates, tenting the distal vagina (21). These physiological changes of clitoral tumescence, vaginal and labial lubrication, and accommodation assist the comfortable entry of a male erection during the act of sexual intercourse. The reproductive role of the tenting seems to be to elevate the cervix so that there is delayed entrance of the pooled ejaculate into the cervix and fallopian tubes, allowing time for sperm capacitation (21). Recent magnetic resonance imaging (MRI) during sexual intercourse has illustrated these mechanics (23).

Relaxation of cavernosal smooth muscle allows for vascular filling of the spongy, erectile tissues, resulting in tumescence. This relaxation is primarily initiated by the nitric oxide (NO) pathway in both men and women, although vasoactive intestinal polypeptide (VIP) and others are also important (24). NO and other neurotransmitters act as modulators for erectile smooth muscle, encouraging contraction or relaxation (flaccidity and erection, respectively). NO is released from nerve endings upon initiation of sexual arousal from the brain, but healthy endothelial tissue is another source of NO (25). Pharmacological methods of increasing NO or its secondary messengers, or inhibiting their breakdown, target this physiology for therapeutic purposes. Damaged endothelium or nerves affect the sources of NO and therefore reduce the efficacy of these drugs.

Three nervous systems, the sacral parasympathetic (pelvic nerve), thoraco-lumbar sympathetic (hypogastric nerve and lumbar sympathetic chain), and somatic (pudendal nerve) are involved in genital arousal. Both mental and physical stimuli contribute to the moment-to-moment, mind-body interaction that will result in either an excitatory or inhibitory descending signal from the brain (3). In general, one autonomic system dominates as sexual arousal progresses, similar to men: the parasympathetic nervous system is predominant during genital arousal, with the sympathetic system activating at higher arousal and orgasm. Besides parasympathetic stimulation, decrease in the sympathetic activity is known to have a positive impact on genital arousal (26). The somatic system is involved in muscular pelvic floor contractions. The afferent pathway involved in sensory innervation of the genitalia includes the hypogastric, pelvic, and vagus nerves, and consists of pressure stimulus (mechanosensitivity), temperature (thermosensitivity), and chemosensitivity (i.e., irritants) (27). The clitoris, the main source of sensory input for eliciting orgasm, sends touch, temperature, and vibration stimulation through the pudendal nerve to the S1–S3 level of the spinal cord. Mechanical and chemical sensations from the vagina travel through the pelvic nerve to S1–S3. The pelvic nerve also sends mechanical and chemical stimulations from the cervix to S1–S3, but afferents from the cervix also travel through the hypogastric nerve (to T12–L1), and also, it appears, through the vagus nerve to the nucleus of the solitary tract (NTS). Mechanical stimulation of the uterus travels through the hypogastric nerve to T12–L1. The efferent pathway also mirrors that seen in men: the parasympathetic pathway is responsible for the clitoral swelling, vaginal congestion, lubrication, and lengthening of the vagina (26). There also appears to be a facilitory effect of sympathetic activation on sexual arousal in women, depending on the timing of the activation (28, 29), before parasympathetic dominance emerges (26). The supporting ligaments of the uterus contain large numbers of autonomic nerves and ganglia as extensions of the inferior pelvic plexus, destined for the clitoris and vulvar structures. More attention has recently been paid to preservation of these autonomic nerves that affect sexual function during hysterectomy and other operative procedures. The striated pelvic-perineal musculature, which plays an additional role in the pleasurable sexual response for women, is innervated by the pudendal nerve (27).

Changes to Genital Arousal after SCI

There are basically two distinct control mechanisms that induce female genital arousal: the psychogenic pathway, located between T11–L2 in the spinal cord, and the reflex pathway located in the sacral cord (S2–S4). In the psychogenic pathway, mental sexual stimuli, along with any sensory inputs from the genitalia and other erogenous zones that ascend spinal pathways, are processed in the higher centers. The resulting signal descending from the brain then activates the parasympathetic neural pathways and probably simultaneously inhibits sympathetic outflow at the genital level (30). The reflex pathway for genital arousal, triggered by genital stimulation, has both an afferent and efferent limb that must be at least partially physiologically intact for activation. In spinal cord lesions above T6, the reflex pathway becomes critical for lubrication. If the pudendal or pelvic nerve is destroyed or the sacral spinal cord injured, reflexogenic ability can be lost (31). Spinal cord injury has a major effect not only on the sensory signals coming from physical stimulation, but on muscle tone and spasticity, as well as exaggerated respiratory and cardiovascular reflexes secondary to the lack of neural control and descending autonomic regulation (32).

The impact of SCI on the psychogenic and reflexogenic pathway will depend on the level and completeness of injury. Most studies have concentrated on the contributions of the psychogenic and reflex pathways generating genital sexual arousal in women with varying levels of SCI: subjective reporting as well as objective measurements of vaginal congestion using vaginal photoplethysmography or vaginal pulse amplitude (VPA) (33), heart rate, respiratory rate, and blood pressure readings (15) are often utilized. Studies have shown the neurological ability to achieve psychogenic arousal after SCI can be predicted in females by the degree of preservation of surface sensation to pinprick and light touch in the T11–L2 dermatomes (15). Women with more feeling in these dermatomes were more likely to demonstrate psychogenic genital vasocongestion than women with lower scores, and this was interpreted by the researchers as evidence for the role of the sympathetic preganglionic neurons (with cell bodies at the T11–L2 level) in the control of psychogenic genital arousal. As evidence of maintenance of reflex genital arousal in women with upper motor neuron (UMN) injuries affecting their sacral spinal segments, women with incomplete SCI who were first subjected to psychogenic, then to manual genital stimulation, showed further increases in their level of objective genital arousal with manual stimulation (regardless of concomitant increase in level of subjective arousal) (34). Women with UMN vs. lower motor neuron (LMN) lesions tended to show a trend to increased

VPA, as would be expected in the presence of reflex genital vasocongestion (15, 34). These findings suggest that the only subset of women who should not have the potential for reflex lubrication should be those women with complete LMN injuries. Women with injuries to their sacral cord or lower are therefore often dependant on intact psychogenic pathways via the hypogastric nerve to elicit genital arousal. Women with complete UMN SCI, when asked to arouse themselves manually, used genital stimulation to achieve reflex lubrication: those with complete LMN injuries at S2–S5 did not choose this method but some (25%) could obtain psychogenic lubrication due to their intact lumbosacral cord (34).

Sexual Activity, Arousal, and Orgasm Experienced after SCI

Sexual Practices

In one large survey by the Kinsey Institute (35), about one-half of the women reported vaginal lubrication and only a third experienced orgasm after injury. Although women do report lubrication difficulties after SCI, a significant percentage of women also report they do not have any knowledge of their ability to lubricate (36). Arousal can be described as that which is felt psychologically (mental arousal) or physically (tension, congestion, or tingling in the pelvis called genital arousal). Women with SCI report difficulty becoming psychologically as well as physically aroused, and this is correlated with the feeling that SCI alters sexual sense of self (5). In both men and women with SCI, especially when genital sensation is altered, extragenital stimulation can be critical for arousal. When sensation and movement originating from the lower cord are lost, there is motivation to try more adaptive, non-genital stimulation, and neuroplasticity likely occurs (37). Pelvic anesthesia and poor hand function dictate different masturbatory approaches, including heightened use of breast and nipple stimulation and vibrators (38). Similarly, kissing, hugging, and touching ranked high amongst most favorite or enjoyable sexual activities post-injury (5, 36).

Compared to pre-injury, the overall frequency of vaginal intercourse post-injury is lower (67%–72%), and duration of injury is a significant predictor for participation in sexual intercourse (7, 35). Major problems associated with sexual intercourse include difficulty with positioning, lack of lubrication, lack of enjoyment, increased spasticity, problems with bladder or bowel incontinence, autonomic dysreflexia, and painful intercourse (7). In a survey of 87 women with chronic SCI (5), the majority (92%) that were having intercourse felt their main difficulties were positioning during foreplay (72.4%) and intercourse (77.0%), vaginal lubrication (65.5%), and spasticity (63.2%), with the least reported difficulty being vaginal pain with intercourse (18.4%). In this survey, one third of women had cervical injuries, and they reported the greatest difficulties. Additionally, 28.7% of women had experienced anal penetration post-injury, an incidence that was unexpectedly high, and possibly adaptive, but still within the normal range of 23–51% of non-disabled women that experience anal intercourse some time in their lives (39, 40). However, anal intercourse is a higher-risk sexual activity, and those more prone to dysreflexia, chronic pain, or spasticity were less likely to participate in this activity (5).

Subjective and Objective Arousal

Because SCI significantly affects the emotional aspects of sexuality and sexual function, women who feel their sexual sense of self is altered have the most difficulty becoming psychologically and physically aroused. In the same survey above (5), where 40% of the women had some remaining genital sensation, physical and mental sources of arousal were defined during sexual activity. The most reported physical cognitions of physical arousal were tingling sensations (41.4%) and spasm (37.9%). The recognition of build-up in the body of sexual tension during sexual stimulation was noted in about two-thirds of the women, and this was positively correlated with the presence of some genital sensation. Autonomic dysreflexia (AD) was also noted with self or partnered sexual activity in just fewer than half the respondents, and one fourth felt AD was significant enough to interfere with sexual activity to some extent. For this latter group, becoming physically aroused was difficult. A small minority of women (7%) had been able to interpret the symptoms of AD during sexual activity as pleasurable or arousing.

What happens to the subjective interpretation of arousal after SCI? Of this same group of women, 64.4% stated they could feel arousal build up in their head: these women were also more likely to experience AD during sexual activity or bladder or bowel care. The majority of women who did not feel a build-up of sexual tension either in their body or their head stated their primary reasons for seeking sexual activity was to keep their partner, versus having a need for intimacy. This subset of women appeared not to be enjoying sex either emotionally or physically, felt their injury had altered their sexual sense of self, but felt improving their sexual function would improve their quality of life (5).

Orgasmic Potential

Across almost all laboratory-based studies or questionnaire surveys of women with various levels or completeness of spinal cord injuries, four findings around orgasmic potential appear constant: it can be expected that about half the women will experience orgasm post injury; the likelihood of experiencing orgasm appears to increase over time; longer and more intense stimulation may be required to reach orgasm; and those with sparing of the sacral reflex arc and/or genital sensation will have more predictive potential. However, many factors, including fear of incontinence, pain, spasm, AD, being self-conscious, or being given inadequate information or misinformation about sexual responses following SCI will also affect orgasmic potential.

The ability for women to achieve orgasm stemming from genital stimulation after SCI has been noted in many studies. In a study of 472 respondents, Jackson and Wadley found that 31.7% of women with cervical, 40.5% with thoracic, and 51.5% with lumbar/sacral injuries reported orgasm. Regardless of level of injury, orgasm is reported more in women with incomplete injuries than complete injuries (7, 38). Sipski and colleagues researched 68 premenopausal women with SCI (along with 21 able-bodied controls) and found that historically less than 50% of them reported the ability to achieve orgasm after injury. They also found the level and type of lesion influenced the ability to reach orgasm: only 17% of women with complete LMN dysfunction affecting the S2–S5 spinal segments were able to achieve orgasm, compared to 59% of women with other levels and degrees of SCIs (16). In the laboratory, latency to orgasm for women with SCI was found to be significantly different than able-bodied controls (mean time 26.37 minutes as compared to 16.33 minutes), along with ability to even achieve orgasm (44% vs. 100%). Subjective descriptions of orgasmic characteristics given both by able-bodied and SCI women were remarkably similar when rated in a blinded fashion by two independent reviewers (16). In the view of the authors, orgasmic potential should remain with all levels and degrees of spinal cord dysfunction except those with LMN dysfunction affecting the S2–S5 spinal cord segments. If there is at least a partially intact sacral reflex arc, it appears there is neurological potential for orgasm generated by manual stimulation.

The Orgasmic Debate: What Is It after SCI?

It should be remembered that American Spinal Injury Association (ASIA) scores used to document motor and sensory preservation do not test for intactness of the autonomic nervous system. Women with complete SCI who are orgasmic may therefore retain the necessary autonomic component of their sacral orgasmic reflex even if the somatic component is affected. Furthermore, ASIA scores documenting touch, pinprick, and anal-digital testing to determine SCI level and completeness do not include examination of deeper vaginal, cervical, or uterine sensibility. Undamaged visceral afferent fibers could therefore remain untested, and account for the ability of women with complete SCI to feel menstrual discomfort (41), abdominal pain (42), labor (14), and rectal distention (43). A standard terminology to be able to communicate effectively about the remaining autonomic function, and to document its role in sexual and reproductive function after spinal cord injury, has recently been developed (44). In addition, the work of Komisaruk and colleagues (45) goes on to propose that the vagus nerve, a functional afferent pathway from the vagina and cervix that completely bypasses the spinal cord and projects directly to the brain, may be a route for women with complete SCI to internally feel vaginocervical stimulation and to perceive orgasm, since their injury is above the level of entry into the spinal cord of all known afferent genitospinal nerves. The vagus nerve projects directly to the nucleus of the solitary tract (NTS) in the medulla oblongata, and the NTS was shown to be activated during functional MRI in four women with complete SCI and one women with incomplete SCI, all above the T10 level, when they stimulated themselves to orgasm using mechanical vaginocervical stimulation (46). The four women were defined as complete SCI by ASIA scoring, demonstrating no sensation or motor movement below the level of lesion and having an absence of feeling with rectal digital stimulation.

The neurology of orgasm is not yet fully understood. A few theories exist, and are not necessarily in conflict with one another. The perception of both orgasm and visceral sensation after complete SCI is likely a multi-facilitated sensation. In humans, there is laboratory evidence that genital arousal and orgasm occur at the spinal cord level in those women with SCI whose sacral reflex arc is intact (15). Similarly, in female rats transected at the T8 level to remove descending inhibition, a spinal sexual reflex called the urethrogenital reflex, consisting of autonomic and somatic nerve activity, has been identified. In this reflex, urethral stimulation results in vaginal, uterine, and anal sphincter contractions, mimicking orgasm (47, 48). Spinal neurons involved in the urethrogenital reflex of the female rat have been identified after stimulation of the pudendal sensory and pelvic nerves (49), and there may be some similarities of these cells to the lumbar spinothalamic cells (LSt) which have been demonstrated in male rats as a spinal ejaculation generator (50). While these LSt cells are not activated during vaginocervical stimulation in female rats, they are activated during the urethrogenital reflex in female rats (51). However, the urethrogenital reflex is not abolished after transection of the vagal nerve (26, 50). Since there is likely an intraspinal organization involved in the coordination between parasympathetic and sympathetic output to the genitalia, then potentially the vagus nerve can represent several things: it may be a supplemental afferent pathway to the spinal system only activated after SCI; it may be involved in the central feeling of orgasm in women with complete SCI; or it may exert a facilitory role in addition to the spinal-to-brain pathway in able-bodied women (27). The researchers of the vagus nerve, who have shown that vaginal-cervical stimulation leads to analgesia in the fingers of women with complete injuries above T10 and in the forepaws of female rats, postulate that this is a similar route for orgasm. In the rat, the analgesia from vaginal-cervical pressure stimulation persists even after bilateral transection of the known genitospinal nerves (pudendal, pelvic, and hypogastric), but is abolished after subsequent bilateral transection of the vagus nerves. The speculation of the role of the human vagal nerve in orgasm after SCI cannot be definitively proven because bilateral transection of the vagal nerves in human females to show loss of orgasmic capacity cannot be done, but evidence for at least supplementary orgasmic sensations and visceral awareness via the vagal nerve in women with SCI is building. Furthermore, despite there being no way to document or prove orgasm in female rats, some of the same brain regions activated in the orgasmic women with SCI have been reported to be activated during mating or vaginocervical stimulation in female rats (46).

It is also well known that for some women, orgasm can be derived from imagery alone (52). Orgasm has been achieved through Tantric sex practices or during sleep, as well as with nongenital (breast, ear, etc.) stimulation. This non-genital orgasmic potential may help explain the preference for arousing non-genital sexual touch for women after SCI with poor or no genital sensation, but may also be the primary source for orgasm for those women with SCI who are unable to attain orgasm by lengthy genital stimulation, or who also lack visceral sensation of their internal pelvic organs. Tepper, after interviewing 12 men and 10 women following SCI, elucidated several conditions that facilitate sexual pleasure and orgasm, including relaxation, meditation, dreams, fantasy, recalling positive experiences, breathing, going with the flow, trust or being with a partner who is trusted, and addition of non-genital touch, plenty of time, and added stimulation of a vibrator (53). Neuroplasticity of the brain can occur with dedicated repetition of a new task, and this is what is likely occurring for men and women who rely on extra-genital sensation for arousal and even orgasm. The author and colleagues are currently working on an initial proof of concept study regarding the use of sensory substitution technologies to reestablish sexual sensations in individuals with chronic spinal cord injury (54).

In summary, the main hypothesis on the neurology of orgasm is that it is a reflex response of the autonomic and somatic nervous systems that can be either facilitated or inhibited by cerebral input, parallel to the presence of the urethrogenital reflex in spinalized female rats. In able-bodied women, the reflex theory is also the most likely explanation for the successful practice of regular manual or vibratory self-stimulation to learn orgasm. In women with and without SCI, practice of this reflex does reinforce the orgasmic potential. However, there are likely multiple contributory afferent systems—brain, spinal cord, local reflex, non-spinal neurological pathways, visceral sensations, and after SCI, variants of autonomic dysreflexia—triggering the recognition of an efferent release called orgasm. Persons with SCI open to experimentation and adaptation may be the ideal model to study this phenomenon of orgasm.

Research around orgasm is difficult because orgasm lacks a clear definition in the research setting. Objective laboratory findings of elevated blood pressure and heart rate in both able–bodied men and women with SCI (or in the latter, bradycardia if the woman is becoming dysreflexic) can objectively assume, but not prove, orgasm has occurred (15). It is often helpful to define orgasm after SCI as genital (triggered by genital stimulation) or non-genital (orgasm arising from sensate nongenital areas or by brain arousal only). To date, only the woman with SCI can define what constitutes an orgasm for her, and that has to be respected during research endeavors. It is clear much more work in the area of well-defined measurement capacities and agreed-upon definitions for orgasm must be done.

Defining Sexual Dysfunction after SCI

The *Diagnostic and Statistical Classification Manual of Mental Disorders*, 4th ed. (DSM-IV) defines a sexual dysfunction as a disturbance in sexual desire and/or in the psychophysiologic changes (including pain) that characterize the sexual response cycle (desire, arousal, and orgasm in women), which causes marked distress and/or interpersonal difficulty. In 2000, a panel at the International Consensus Development Conference on Female Sexual Dysfunction developed specific dysfunction categories dividing arousal, orgasm, and pain disorders into more detailed categories involving differentiation of awareness of genital versus mental arousal, with emphasis on the complaint of personal distress (55). For women with SCI, this can pose a problem, because alterations in their sexual neurophysiology may preclude the mental versus genital arousal differentiation, and the changes may not be distressing to them. Therefore, the prevalence of what may seem to be obvious sexual dysfunction post-injury (as compared to pre-injury) function will be affected. Sipski proposed a more physiologically based Female Spinal Sexual Function Classification system (FSSFC), which defines four categories of sexual function after spinal cord injury and their presence/absence or degree of ability based on a neurological exam: sexual dysfunction (present or absent), psychogenic genital arousal, reflex genital arousal, and orgasm (34, 56). It should be noted in the FSSFC that orgasm is classified as "not possible" if there is no S2–S5 sensation and absent bulbocavernosus and anal wink reflexes, so it is genitally induced orgasm that is being referred to here, because only the somatic pathways are being included in the testing criteria. Based on the performance of the neurological examination and detailed history, the FSSFC should be not only be helpful as a clinical guide to predict sexual response following spinal cord injury in women, but also to document whether the women defines herself as having a sexual dysfunction. At present, international forums are pursuing a unified consensus of definitions of female sexual dysfunctions.

It is important for women with SCI to report sexual dysfunction to their healthcare provider or researchers so that the investigation of dysfunction prevalence and research trials directed at therapeutics for the relief of sexual symptomatology can take place (34).

Treatment of Arousal and Orgasmic Difficulties after SCI

To date there are no approved medications for sexual difficulties in women, let alone women with SCI, although a few for desire are currently being considered. The testosterone patch, developed for the treatment of women with hypoactive sexual desire disorder (HSDD), so far has not been approved by the FDA in North America, citing incomplete safety data, although it has been approved in Europe for surgically menopausal women (57). There is some concern with testosterone use and possible risk of breast cancer and cardiovascular disease (58), but this may potentially be avoided by the use of selective androgen receptor modulators (59). Other products are currently being tested, including a testosterone gel (LibiGel®) (60) and flibanserin, a centrally acting agent that is currently under investigation for HSDD (61, 62). Although exogenous testosterone improves sexual function in postmenopausal women with hypoactive sexual desire with inadequate levels of natural testosterone, replacement of "physiologic levels" in any women is highly controversial because long-term safety has not been assured, and testosterone is rarely the underlying issue perpetuating altered sexual desire levels, especially in premenopausal women (59, 63).

In women, the relationship between desire and androgens is very complicated, and virtually no work has been done around this issue in women with SCI. In able-bodied women, serum levels of androgen show minimal correlation with women's sexual function, and studies have confirmed that women's sexual satisfaction, desire, and function correlate with a woman's mental health, her past experiences, her feeling for her partner generally and during sexual engagement, the duration of the relationship, and partner sexual function (59). Furthermore, androgen metabolites may be more informative than serum testosterone levels (59). Testosterone replacement, along with estrogen replacement, has been used in select women following surgical menopause or in those postmenopausal women who have been found to be especially low in testosterone without any other significant psychosocial or relationship issues. Estrogen improves dyspareunia associated with vulvovaginal atrophy in postmenopausal women (63).

For women with SCI, major contributing factors to altered sexual drive are depression, altered self-image and self-esteem, and concerns about attaining or keeping a relationship. The use of testosterone in women for HSDD following SCI has not been studied, and should be considered in the same light as its use in able-bodied women—that is, only for rare postmenopausal cases that have been thoroughly evaluated in a multidisciplinary fashion. However, hormone replacement per se after SCI is a subject requiring special consideration, as osteoporotic risk is already present with immobility (see Chapter 34, Women's Health Issues).

Arousal and orgasmic difficulties in women are often treated as a continuum. In able-bodied women, those therapies that improve pelvic vasocongestion and genital arousal are also likely to improve the chances of orgasmic attainment. Although the use of phosphodiesterase inhibitors (PDE5i) may improve arousal, genital sensation, orgasm, and sexual function in some able-bodied women with sexual dysfunction (primarily those with normal hormone profiles), there is a substantial placebo effect up to about 40% (63). In healthy, naturally postmenopausal women given the PDE5i sildenafil, clitoral and uterine blood flow improved without erotic stimulus (64). Furthermore, PDE5i can increase physiological sexual arousal (i.e., vaginal photoplethysmography) in women without showing a congruent increase in subjective or mental sexual arousal (65). However, this is not surprising because the effect of PDE5i would be to increase the tumescence of the erectile tissues in the clitoris and the extending erectile tissues located behind the vulva, a subjective experience most women are not particularly aware of. However, because PDE5i can also increase the pelvic vasocongestion, improved lubrication is noticed in some women with lubrication impairment. Potentially, those women with impaired corporal erectile ability and decreased lubrication due to vascular or neurogenic issues, or those who have impaired genital or clitoral sensory sensation (such as with multiple sclerosis or incomplete SCI), may benefit from a PDE5i if clitoral sensitivity and/or pelvic vasocongestion and lubrication increases (63, 66).

In a study of the effect of PDE5i in women with SCI, 14 women with UMN lesions and 5 with LMN affecting their sacral cord were randomly assigned to receive either 50 mg of sildenafil or placebo in a double-blind, crossover design study. Significant increases in subjective arousal were observed with both drug and sexual stimulation conditions, and a borderline significant effect of drug administration on VPA was noted: maximal response occurred when sildenafil was combined with visual and manual stimulation (67). Mild increases in heart rate (±5 bpm) and mild decreases in blood pressure (±4 mmHg) were seen across all stimulation conditions, consistent with the peripheral vasodilatory mechanism of a PDE5i. Nonpharmacologic approaches can also be used. Women with SCI and with impaired, but not absent, ability to achieve psychogenic genital vasocongestion appeared to have some improvement with cognitive-based therapies and the use of sympathetic nervous system manipulation such as anxiety-provoking videos (68, 69). These researchers also regarded their data from the anxiety study as further evidence of the regulatory role of the sympathetic nervous system in psychogenic arousal (69).

EROS-CT® (Clitoral Therapy Device, Urometrics Inc., St. Paul, MN) a small, battery-powered vacuum device designed to enhance clitoral engorgement by increasing blood flow to the clitoris, has been shown to cause significant increases in clitoral and corpus spongiosum diameter and vascular flow (70). It is the only U.S. Food and Drug Administration cleared-to-market device available by prescription to treat female sexual dysfunction (71). EROS-CT® has also alleviated some of the sexual dysfunction seen in irradiated cervical cancer patients by improving blood flow to the area (72). For women with SCI, there may be a training effect from EROS-CT® on the pelvic floor in those women who have retained a bulbocavernosus reflex, which in turn may reinforce remaining sacral reflexes. Studies to date with EROS-CT® are with small numbers of subjects, and there are no published studies on the use of EROS-CT specifically in women with neurological injury and with altered genital sensation to see whether clitoral sensitivity or orgasmic potential is improved. The use of vibratory stimulation to improve pelvic floor tone and/or strength may also contribute to improved psychogenic or reflexogenic arousal. The use of vibrators, usually placed externally around the clitoral area, has been a mainstay for female arousal and orgasmic difficulties. For women with SCI, the use of vibrators has been helpful, and the site of effective stimulation may vary from around the area of injury, to the clitoris, inside the vagina or on the cervix. Based on the theory that orgasm is a spinal cord reflex, studies to test the efficacy of EROS-CT and vibratory stimulation on the stimulation of the reflex response are currently underway (34). Theoretically, by initiating the BCR reflex and encouraging reflex vasocongestion through either method, sensory awareness in those women with some genital or perineal sensory preservation may also improve.

Because the neurological potential to achieve orgasm exists in approximately 50% of women with all levels of SCI, it is important to try and find the intervening variable precluding orgasm (15). Women should be encouraged to learn new body maps of erogenous areas, and to learn and practice mindfulness techniques around sexual inputs. If using genital stimulation, women with SCI need to take longer periods of time and use more intense genital stimulation and/or vibrators in their pursuit of orgasm. Anecdotally, the chance of orgasmic attainment is often improved with a higher degree of comfort, sexual intimacy, and love women feel for their partners. Like the context of Tepper's conditions that facilitate pleasure and orgasm (53), persistence with physical stimulation in the context of security and intimacy can lead to reinforcement of new neural pathways and contribute to neuroplasticity. Neuroplasticity depends on focused repetition to a new task, attention to signals occurring in the moment and being open and positive in their interpretation. Healthcare professionals can assist women with SCI in this process by actively intervening with therapeutic suggestions to reduce medical interferences, such as pain, spasticity, autonomic dysreflexia, and incontinence, allowing the woman more freedom to focus.

CONCLUSION

Sexuality in women with SCI has many biological, psychological, social, and relationship facets. Sexual health must also be reviewed in the context of other medical concerns that can interfere with sexuality. What has been learned in the area of psychogenic and reflexogenic arousal and orgasmic potential in women with SCI has been critical to our understanding of the neurophysiology of human sexual response. Treatment of sexual disorders in women with SCI is most successful when patients and clinicians follow three principles of sexual rehabilitation:

- *Maximize* the remaining capacities of the total body before relying on medications or aids (learning new body maps, breathing, visualization methods, mindfulness exercises, etc.).
- *Adapt* to residual limitations by utilizing specialized therapies (use of vibrators, training aids, PDE5i or EROS-CT®, etc.).
- *Stay open* to rehabilitative efforts and new forms of sexual stimulation, with a positive and optimistic outlook.

Although the nuts and bolts of physiological sexual response appear to be worked out, the many facets involved in

the interpretation of arousal and pleasure are not. After SCI, unlike motor and sensory recovery, sexuality has the potential to keep on evolving long after the physical body has reached its maximum recovery, in what is best described as an extended form of neuroplasticity. Because men and women with SCI provide the best research models to answer our future questions, research efforts around sexual rehabilitation in this population must continue to be supported. Improvement in quality of sexual health will lead to improvement in quality of life (5).

ACKNOWLEDGMENTS

The author wishes to acknowledge her patients who have taught her so much, her clinical and research colleagues, ICORD (International Collaboration of Repair Discoveries), and RHI (Rick Hansen Institute) for support.

References

1. Anderson K. Targeting Recovery: Priorities of the spinal cord injured population. *J Neurotrauma* 2004; 21(10):1371–1383.
2. Elliott S. Sexuality after Spinal Cord Injury. In: Field-Forte E, ed. *Spinal Cord Injury Rehabilitation*. Philadelphia: FA Davis, 2009:513–529.
3. Stevenson RWD, Elliott SL. *Sexuality and Medical Illness In Principles and Practice of Sex Therapy*, 4th ed. New York: Guilford Publications, 2007.
4. Reitz A, Tobe V, Knapp PA, et al. Impact of spinal cord injury on sexual health and quality of life. *In J Impot Res* 2004; 16:167–174.
5. Anderson KD, Borisoff JF, Johnson RD, et al. Spinal cord injury influences psychogenic as well as physical components of female sexual ability. *Spinal Cord* 2007; 45:349–359.
6. Ferrerio-Velasco ME, Barca-Buyo A, Salvador DeLaBarrera S. Sexual issues in a sample of women with spinal cord injury. *Spinal Cord* 2005; 43(1):51–55.
7. Jackson AB, Wadley V. A multicenter study of women's self-reported reproductive health after SCI. *Arch Phys Med Rehabil* 1999; 80:1420–1428.
8. Singh R, Sharma SC. Sexuality and women with spinal cord injury. *Sex Disabil* 2005; 23:21–33.
9. Pentland W, Walker J, Minnes P, et al. Women with spinal cord injury and the impact of aging. *Spinal Cord* 2002; 40:374–387.
10. Alexander M, Brackett N, Bodner D, Elliott S, Jackson A, Sonksen J; National Institute on Disability and Rehabilitation Research. Measurement of sexual capacity after spinal cord injury: preferred instruments. *J Spinal Cord Med* 2009; 32(3):226–236.
11. Rosen R, Brown C, Heiman J, et al. The Female Sexual Function Index (FSFI): A multidimensional self-report instrument for the assessment of female sexual function. *J Sex Marital Ther* 2000; 26:191–208.
12. Kimoto Y, Otani T, Ushiyama T, et al. Sexual dysfunction in female patients with spinal cord injury: Abstract C4.2 ISSIR meeting. *Int J Impot Res* 2002; 14(Supp3):S27.
13. Sipski ML. The impact of spinal cord injury on female sexuality, menstruation and pregnancy: A review of the literature. *J Am Parap Soc* 1991; 14:122–126.
14. Charlifue SW, Gerhart KA, Menter RR, et al. Sexual issues of women with spinal cord injuries. *Paraplegia* 1992; 30:192–199.
15. Sipski ML, Alexander CJ, Rosen R. Sexual arousal and orgasm in women: Effects of spinal cord injury. *Ann Neurol* 2001; 49:35–44.
16. Sipski ML, Alexander CJ, Rosen RC. Orgasm in women with spinal cord injuries: A laboratory-based assessment. *Arch Phys Med Rehabil* 1995; 76:1097–1102.
17. Matzaroglu C, Assimakopoulos K, Panagiotopoulos E, et al. Sexual function in females with severe cervical spinal cord injuries: A controlled study with Female Sexual Function Index. *Int J Rehab Res* 2005; 28:375–377.
18. Ekland M, Lawrie B. How a woman's sexual adjustment after sustaining a spinal cord injury impact sexual health interventions. *SCI Nursing* 2004; 21(1):14–19.
19. Tepper MS, Whipple B, Richard E, et al. Women with complete spinal cord injury: a phenomenological study of sexual experiences. *J Sex Marital Ther* 2001; 27:615–623.

20. Forsythe E, Horsewell JE. Sexual rehabilitation of women with spinal cord injury. *Spinal Cord* 2006; 44:234–241.
21. Levin RJ. Critically revisiting aspects of the human sexual response cycle of Masters and Johnson: Correcting errors and suggesting modifications. *Sex Relationship Ther* 2008; 23:393–9.
22. O'Connell HE, Sanjeevan K. Anatomy of female genitalia. In: Goldstein I, Meston C, Davis S, Traish A, eds. *Women's Sexual Function and Dysfunction*. New York: Taylor & Francis, 2006:105–112.
23. Wallboard Weijmar S, van Andel P, Sabelis I, et al. Magnetic resonance imaging of male and female genitals during coitus and female sexual arousal. *Brit Med J* 1999; 319:1596–1600.
24. Levin RJ. VIP, vagina, clitoral and periurethral glans—an update on female genital arousal. *Exp Clin Endocrinol* 1991; 98:61–69.
25. Chuang AT, Steers WD. Neurophysiology of penile erection. In: Carson C, Kirby R, Goldstein I, eds. *Textbook of Erection Dysfunction*. Oxford, UK: ISIS Medical Media Inc., 1999:59–72.
26. Levin RJ. Sexual arousal—its physiological roles in human reproduction. *Annu Rev Sex Res* 2005; 16:154–89.
27. Giuliano F, Julia-Guilloteau V. Neurophysiology of female genital response. In: Goldstein I, Meston CM, Davis SR, Traish AM, eds. *Women's Sexual Function and Dysfunction*. New York: Taylor & Francis, 2006: 168–173.
28. Meston CM, Gorzalka BB. The effects of immediate, delayed and residual sympathetic activation on sexual arousal in women. *Behav Res Ther* 1996; 34:143–148.
29. Meston CM. Sympathetic nervous system activity and female sexual arousal. *Am J Cardiol* 2000; 86:30F–34F.
30. Giuliano FA, Rampin O, Benoit G, et al. Neural control of penile erection. *Uro Clin North Am* 1995; 22(4):747–766.
31. Wieder JA, Brackett NL, Lynne CM, Green JT, Aballa TC. Anesthetic block of the dorsal nerve inhibits vibratory-induced ejaculation in men with spinal cord injuries. *Urology* 2000; 55:915–917.
32. Krassioukov AV, Fehlings MG. Effect of graded spinal cord compression on cardiovascular neurons in the rostro-ventro-lateral medulla. *Neuroscience* 1999; 88(3):959–73.
33. Rosen RC, Beck JF. Genital blood flow measurement in the female: Psychophysiological techniques. In: Rosen RC, Beck JF, eds. *Patterns of Sexual Arousal*. New York: Guilford Press, 1988:78–107.
34. Sipski ML, Arenas A. Female sexual function after spinal cord injury. In: Weaver LC, Polosa C, eds. *Progress in Brain Research*. Amsterdam: Elsevier B. V., 2006; 152:441–447.
35. White MJ, Rintala DH, Hart KA, et al. Sexual activities, concerns and interests of women with spinal cord injury living in the community. *Am J Phys Med Rehabil* 1993; 72(6):372–378.
36. Sipski ML, Alexander CJ. Sexual activities, response and satisfaction in women pre-and post-spinal cord injury. *Arch Phys Med Rehabil* 1993; 74:1025–1029.
37. Anderson KD, Borisoff JF, Johnson RD, et al. Long-term effects of spinal cord injury on sexual function in men: Implications for neuroplasticity. *Spinal Cord* 2007; 45:338–348.
38. Donohue J, Gebhard P. The Kinsey Institute/Indiana University report on sexuality and spinal cord injury. *Sexuality and Disability* 1995 (Special Issue); 13(1):7–85.
39. Baldwin JI, Baldwin JD. Heterosexual anal intercourse: An understudied, high-risk sexual behavior. *Arch Sex Behav* 2000; 29:357–373.
40. Flannery D, Ellingson L, Votaw KS, et al. Anal intercourse and sexual risk factor among college women, 1993–2000. *Am J Health Behav* 2003; 27:228–234.
41. Axel SJ. Spinal cord injured women's concerns: Menstruation and pregnancy. *Rehab Nurs* 1982; Sept–Oct:10–15.
42. Miller LS, Staas WE, Herbison GJ. Abdominal problems in patient with spinal cord lesion. *Arch Phys Med Rehabil* 1975; 56:405–408.
43. Sun W-M, MacDonagh, Forter D, et al. Anorectal function in patients with complete spinal transection before and after sacral posterior rhizotomy. *Gastroenterology* 1994; 108:990–998.
44. Alexander MS, Biering-Sorensen F, Bodner D, Brackett NL, Cardenas D, Charlifue S, Creasey G, Dietz V, Ditunno J, Donovan W, Elliott SL, Estores I, Graves DE, Green B, Gousse A, Jackson AB, Kennelly M, Karlsson AK, Krassioukov A, Krogh K, Linsenmeyer T, Marino R, Mathias CJ, Perkash I, Sheel AW, Shilero G, Schurch B, Sonksen J, Stiens S, Wecht J, Wuermser LA, Wyndaele JJ. International standards to document remaining autonomic function after spinal cord injury. *Spinal Cord* 2009; 47(1):36–43.
45. Komisaruk B, Sansone G. Neural pathways mediating vagal function: The vagus nerves and spinal cord oxytocin. *Scand J Psychol* 2003; 44:241–250.
46. Komisaruk BR, Whipple B, Crawford A, et al. Brain activation during vaginocervical self-stimulation and orgasm in women with complete spinal cord injury: fMRI evidence of mediation by the vagus nerves. *Brain Res* 2004; 1024:77–88.
47. Giuliano F, Allard J, Compagnie S, et al. Vaginal physiological changes in a model of sexual arousal in anesthetized rats. *Am J Physio Regul Integr Physiol* 2001; 281:R140–149.
48. Chung SK, McVary KT, McKenna KE. Sexual reflexes in male and female rats. *Neurosci Lett* 1988; 94:343–348.
49. Wiedey J, Alexander MS, Marson L. Spinal neurons activated in response to pudendal or pelvic nerve stimulation in female rats. *Brain Res* 2008; 4(1197):106–114.
50. Truitt WA, Shipley MT, Veening JG, et al. Activation of a subset of lumbar spinothalamic neurons after copulatory behavior in male but not female rats. *J Neurosci* 2003; 23:325–31.
51. Marson L, Cai R, Makhanova N. Identification of spinal neurons involved in the urethrogenital reflex in the female rat. *J Comp Neurol* 2003; 462(4):355–370.
52. Whipple B, Ogden G, Komiaruk BR. Relative analgesic effect of imagery compared to genital self-stimulation. *Arch Sex Beh* 1992; 21:121–133.
53. Tepper A, Tepper, M. Pleasure and orgasm in people with SCI. Presented at the 15th World Congress on Sexology Paris, France. June 2001.
54. Borisoff J, Research Associate, and Gary Birch, PI, Neil Squire Society, Brain Interface Lab, GF Strong Rehabilitation Center, Vancouver, British Columbia, Canada.
55. Basson R, Berman J, Burnett, et al. Report on the international consensus development conference on female sexual dysfunctions: Definitions and classifications. *J Urol* 2000; 163:888–893.
56. Sipski ML, Alexander CJ. Documentation of the impact of spinal cord injury on female sexual dysfunction: The female spinal sexual function classification. *Top Spinal Cord Inj Rehabil* 2002; 8:63–73.
57. Wierman ME, Basson R, Davis SR, et al. Androgen therapy in women: An endocrine society clinical practice guideline. *J Clin Endocrinol Metab* 2006; 91:3697–710.
58. Schover LR. Androgen therapy for loss of desire in women: Is the benefit worth the breast cancer risk? *Fertil Steril* 2008 Jul; 90(1):129–40.
59. Basson R. Hormones and sexuality: Current complexities and future directions. *Maturitas* 2007; 57:66–70.
60. Snabes MC, Simes SM, Zborowski JG, et al. A clear pathway to approval for Libigel® treatment of women with hypoactive sexual desire disorder (HSDD): Abstract from International Society for the Study of Women's Sexual Health (ISSWSH) annual meeting, San Diego, California, Feb 21–24, 2008: Poster 24:167.
61. Jolly E, Clayton A, Thorp J, Lewis-D'Agostino D, Wunderlich G, Lesko L. Design of phase III pivotal trials of flibanserin in female hypoactive sexual desire disorder (HSDD). *Sexologies* 2008; 17(Supp 1):S133–S134.
62. Goldfischer E, Cotton D, Miki J, et al. Efficacy of continued flibanserin treatment on sexual functioning in premenopausal women with HSDD: results from the Rose study. Abstract from International Society for the Study of Women's Sexual Health (ISSWSH) annual meeting, San Diego, California, Feb 21–24, 2008; 97.
63. Frank JE, Mistretta P, Will J. Diagnosis and treatment of female sexual dysfunction. *Am Fam Physician* 2008; 77:635–42.
64. Alatas E, Yagci AB. The effect of sildenafil citrate on uterine and clitoral blood flow in postmenopausal women. *Med Gen Med* 2004; 6:51. www.medscape.com
65. Goldstein I, Meston CM, Traish AM, et al. Future directions. In: Goldstein I, Meston CM, Davis SR, Traish AM, eds. *Women's Sexual Function and Dysfunction*. New York: Taylor & Francis, 2006:745–748.
66. Dasgupta R, Wiseman OJ, Kanabar G, et al. Efficacy of sildenafil in the treatment of female sexual dysfunction due to multiple sclerosis. *J Urol* 2004; 171(3):1189–1193.
67. Sipski L, Rosen RC, Alexander CJ, et al. Sildenafil effects on sexual and cardiovascular responses in women with spinal cord injury. *Urology* 2000; 55(6):812–815.
68. Sipski ML, Rosen R, Alexander CJ, et al. A controlled trial of positive feedback to increase sexual arousal in women with spinal cord injuries. *Neuro Rehabil* 2000; 15:145–53.

69. Sipski ML, Rosen RC, Alexander CJ, et al. Sexual responsiveness in women with spinal cord injuries: Differential effects of anxiety—eliciting stimulation. *Arch Sex Behav* 2004; 33:295–302.

70. Munarriz R, Kim SW, Kim NN, Traish A, Goldstein I. A review of the physiology and pharmacology of peripheral (vaginal and clitoral) female genital arousal in the animal model. *J Urol* 2003; 170 (2 pt 2):S40–44.

71. Billups KL. The role of mechanical devices in treating female sexual dysfunction and enhancing the female sexual response. *World J Urol* 2002; 20:137–141.

72. Schroder M, Mell LK, Hurteau JA, et al. Clitoral therapy device for treatment of sexual dysfunction in irradiated cervical cancer patients. *Int J Radiat Oncol Biol Phys* 2005; 61(4):1078–1086.

34 Women's Health Issues

Amie Brown Jackson

WOMEN AND SPINAL CORD INJURY

Never before has there been a more pressing need for understanding the medical management of women with spinal cord injury (SCI). Providing clinical care to women after SCI involves knowledge not only of spinal cord injury medicine, but also the interrelationship and impact of the disability on their health issues. As the number of women with spinal cord injuries has increased over the years, a much-needed focus on the total health care of these women has emerged. The changes that a woman undergoes neurologically may have a dramatic affect on her gynecologic, obstetric, menopausal, and psychosocial health. Furthermore, acute and long-term neural responses to traumatic or acquired central nervous system (CNS) injury are affected by the female reproductive neuro-endocrine system. Medical management of these multifaceted responses requires full understanding of the female reproductive system as well as the adaptations that occur as a consequence of the neural injury.

It is estimated that 40,000 to 45,000 women with spinal cord injury are living in the United States (1). The newest figures from the National Spinal Cord Injury Statistical Center (NSCISC) at the University of Alabama at Birmingham show that 19% of all people enrolled in the National SCI Database (NSCID) are female. Compared to men, each year women are sustaining proportionately more ($p < .0001$) spinal cord injuries (SCI) than in the previous years. Figure 34.1 shows the etiology of injury for women and men for the last three decades. The most common etiology of SCI is motor vehicle crashes (MVC), which is the same for both sexes; however, women have a statistically greater incidence ($p < .001$) of being injured in a MVC than men (55.0% and 39.3%, respectively). Falls are the second most common cause of SCI for women, whereas acts of violence are the second most common cause for men. Interestingly, NSCISC reports the most dramatic etiology trend changes for women since data collection began in the early 1970s (Figure 34.2). Compared to decades ago, a woman sustaining an SCI after 2000 is more likely to experience it by MVC, sports, or "other causes," yet less likely from violence or falls. It is important to keep in mind, however, that these are trends of percentages and not actual numbers. Trends of violence to women—able bodied or disabled—also show annual increases (2).

The average age at injury is increasing each year, which parallels the aging population as a whole in the United States (3). In fact, for all individuals sustaining an SCI since 2000 the average age has climbed to 38.0 years ± 24.5 years (median 34 years). Analysis of the greater than 30,000 people enrolled within 48 hours of injury in the NSCID (since 1973) reveals that women are statistically older than males at the time of injury (33.4 ± 16.8 years and 31.4 ± 14.5 years, respectively; $p < .001$) (4). Furthermore, at the time of injury, women are statistically less likely ($p < .001$) to have a complete injury than men (49.4% of all women; 53.3% of all men, respectively). Trends for neurologic level at injury, however, show no statistical gender differences, although women tend to have paraplegia more than tetraplegia compared to their male counterparts (1).

FEMALE REPRODUCTIVE SYSTEM

The female reproductive system consists of breasts, uterus, cervix, vagina, fallopian tubes, ovaries, and external genitalia or vulva. The autonomic nervous system directs the coordinated function of the internal reproductive organs, and Figure 34.3 illustrates the neuro-control of the female reproductive system (5). The sympathetic chain, with its origins at spinal cord levels T10–L1, is generally responsible for pelvic organ contraction and vasoconstriction. Parasympathetic nerves, via the sacral spinal segments, direct organ relaxation and vasodilatation. These components of the autonomic nervous system form groups of pelvic nerves, or plexi, often in continuous chains composed of ganglia, preganglionic and postganglionic fibers, and afferent (sensory) neurons. For example, the most rostral segments of the aortic and renal plexi contribute to the ovarian plexus, which supplies the ovary and its contiguous segment to the fallopian tube. Its afferent fibers enter the spinal cord through T10. With contributions from spinal levels T11–L1,

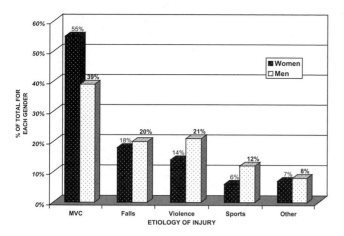

Figure 34.1 Etiology of spinal cord injury since 1973, stratified by gender. (From the University of Alabama at Birmingham, National Spinal Cord Injury Statistical Center, funded by the National Institute on Disability Rehabilitation Research, Grant # H133A060039.)

the aorticorenal plexi caudally join with the inferior mesenteric ganglion/plexus retroperitoneally to create the superior hypogastric plexus. This is the primary conduit for distribution of the autonomic nervous system to the reproductive organ structures. At the level of the common iliac arteries, this system forms the inferior hypogastric plexus (6).

The pelvic plexus consists of extensions from the inferior hypogastric (T10–L1) plexus and parasympathetic fibers (S2–S4). Somatic motor and sensory fibers also contribute to the pelvic plexus via the pelvic nerves. The pelvic plexus further organizes into the uterovaginal and Frankenhauser's plexi to provide afferent and efferent neural control to the latter segment of the fallopian tubes, uterus, and cervix. It also provides small branches to the vagina and urinary bladder. Sensory control is separate for the cervix whereby afferent cell bodies convey pain via S2 through S4 nerve roots.

The external genitalia are primarily innervated by the pudendal nerve, which is a branch of the sacral plexus. Its

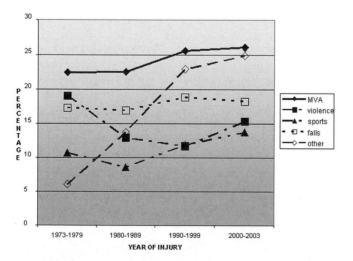

Figure 34.2 Trends for SCI etiologies for women over 30 years.

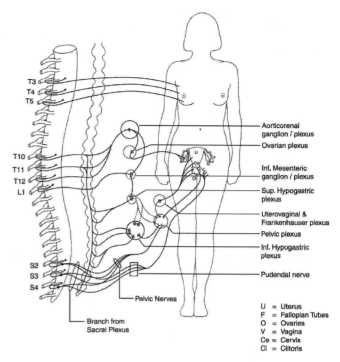

Figure 34.3 Neurology of the female reproductive system.

branches, the deep perineal and superficial perineal nerves, carry motor and sensory fibers to the perineum. Sensory feedback is also provided by the anterior branch of the ilioinguinal (L1) nerve, which supplies the mons pubis and labia majora. The genitofemoral nerve (L1, L2) supplies the rest of the labia majora, and the posterior femoral cutaneous nerve supplies the posterior vulva.

The average 28-day menstrual cycle occurs in a controlled sequence of events to ensure precise hormonal regulation of the hypothalamus, pituitary, and ovary (hypothalamus-pituitary-gonadal axis, or HPG axis) (7). (See Figure 34.4.) Gonadotropin-releasing hormone (GNRH) is secreted from the hypothalamus in a defined pulsating frequency. During the initial "follicular phase" of the cycle, ovarian-produced estrogen levels increase and the resultant acceleration in GNRH pulse frequency exerts positive expression on the pituitary to release the gonadotropins—follicle-simulating hormone (FSH) and luteinizing hormone (LH). These modulators stimulate ovarian follicular growth and steroidogenesis, respectfully. Also during this follicular growth phase, the endometrial wall hypertrophies. GNRH pulse frequency and levels reach an intensity whereby FSH and LH rapidly increase (= LH/FSH surge) and ovulation occurs.

Following ovulation, the luteal phase of the cycle corresponds with deceleration in the GNRH pulse frequency. More recently, specific ovarian peptides such as inhibin and activin have been identified that also regulate selective FSH action. Specific positive and negative feedback mechanisms also direct other end-organ functions such as endometrial lining composition, cervical mucous secretions, and vaginal cell properties; all of which are important for successful fertilization (8). (See Figures 34.3 and 34.5.)

The vertebral thoracic nerves, 3, 4, and 5 supply the breasts. Their stimulation is important for prolactin secretion and breast milk production (Figure 34.5). The neurotransmitter dopamine

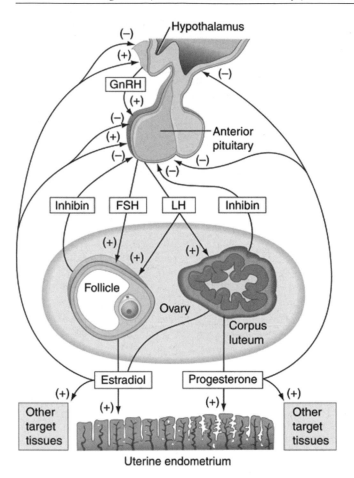

Figure 34.4 Endocrine feedback components of the hypothalamus-pituitary-gonadal axis. (FSH, follicle stimulation hormone; LH, luteinizing hormone; GnRH, gonadotropin releasing hormone.)

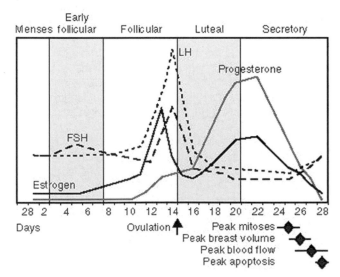

Figure 34.5 Serum reproductive hormone levels during the menstrual cycle. (FSH, follicle stimulation hormone; LH, luteinizing hormone.)

suppresses prolactin secretion and GNRH release (9). When the breasts are stimulated, the resultant afferents of the T3–T5 spinal-intercostal nerves are activated. These impulses provide input to the hypothalamus and pituitary, which in turn create substances that obstruct dopamine biosynthesis and/or its repressive action. This "disinhibition" results in prolactin synthesis and its binding to receptors at the target organ (i.e. breast tissue) to produce milk. Lactation—or release of breast milk—requires oxytocin and continued stimulation. An elevation in prolactin may also occur even in the absence of direct breast stimulation. In fact, any interference of the normal pulsatile or cyclical activity of the HPA that effects GNRH secretion or dopamine production and/or activity may result in hyperprolactinemia with or without galactorrhea.

REPRODUCTIVE ENDOCRINE EFFECTS ON NEUROLOGIC INJURY

The HBG axis is influenced by other substances besides its direct hormonal substrates. Many central nervous system (CNS) neurotransmitters (i.e., dopamine, endogenous opioids, prostaglandins, gamma-aminobutyric acid (GABA), substance P, acetylcholine, serotonin [10, 11, 12, 13]) and CNS injury repair modulators (i.e., nerve growth factor [NGF], and brain-derived neurotrophic factor [BDNF]) have both excitatory and inhibitory effects at target organs, depending on the system's requirements for hormonal homeostasis (14, 15). In addition, in animals the presence of receptors stained for estrogen and progesterone proves the presence and activity of these reproductive hormones in specific regions of the brain (16), the dorsal root ganglia and axon terminals of the spinal cord (17, 18). We know that estrogen and progesterone control many CNS functions via receptor-membrane and receptor-genetic interactions. These actions, in turn, direct neurotransmitter and modulator activity (19, 20).

From these facts we can speculate that the many interactions between the HPG axis and the CNS are, at least in part, responsible for the sexual dimorphism found in the response to neurologic injury (21, 22, 23), the expression of various psychiatric diseases (24), and the emergence of some diseases more common at menopause (25). Observations (26, 27) confirm that in some neurologic disorders (acquired or inherited), estrogen provides neuroprotective properties when the CNS is challenged. More specifically, in female rats, investigators have shown that estrogen will lessen CNS injury by blocking N-methyl-D-aspartate (NMDA) receptor-mediated neuronal death (28). Furthermore, they have demonstrated that estrogen is a powerful antioxidant that retards neuronal apoptosis (29, 30). Estrogen and other sex hormones have also been shown to promote neuronal cell repair by potentiating the effects of NGF (31, 32). NGF produced in peripheral tissues has been shown to travel in a retrograde direction via the sympathetic nervous system to the dorsal root ganglion in the spinal cord where it promotes neuronal survival (33, 34).

Other hormones, with or without estrogen, may influence the neuro-immune response after CNS injury. GNRH (via LH release) (35) has pro-estrogenic effects, but progesterone may exert neuro-immune responses by blocking estrogen's action. We are just beginning to understand how gender plays a part in spinal cord and brain injury.

GYNECOLOGIC ISSUES AFTER SCI

At the time of spinal cord injury, the spinal cord enters a state of spinal shock, which is a state of time-dependent, complete cessation of neural activity and feedback with disruption of neurochemical synaptic interactions (36). It has been hypothesized that the disruption of the internal neurobiologic communication that ensues also has repercussions on the feedback systems of the hypothalamic pituitary axis (37, 38). Thus the neural receptors of the hypothalamus and the pituitary do not receive the neurochemical substances at the bioactive levels and delivery rate required to positively or negatively activate feedback responses. Studies in animals (39–47) support this premise by demonstrating estrogen receptors in many parts of the spinal cord, as well as peripheral sensory ganglion neurons and axons. Thus, injury to the neural components of the spinal cord will influence the normal reproductive cycles, which in turn can alter hormones or neurochemical substances, concentrations, and actions, which can further affect the neural circuitry.

Endocrine Balance

Following a spinal cord injury, the menstrual cycle is usually disrupted and gynecologic dysfunction may occur. Table 34.1 defines several conditions experienced by women with SCI. Secondary amenorrhea, menorrhagia, metrorrhagia (48) and neurogenic prolactinemia with and without galactorrhea (49–51) have been described in the initial post-injury months. Other conditions following a traumatic spinal cord injury, however, may also have an influence on gynecologic endocrine balance. Nutrition, stress, serum mineral and electrolyte disturbances, and medications (especially steroids) (52) have been shown to affect hypothalamic-pituitary communication. In a pilot study of 25 women post-injury (53), almost two-thirds of 25 women studied had mild to greatly elevated prolactin levels at some point after their injury. Of these women, 12% developed

galactorrhea. Other endocrine abnormalities such as hypoestrogenemia were also documented. Interestingly, those women with injuries involving thoracic levels T3–T5 tended to have a greater frequency of prolactinemia with galactorrhea. This has also been shown to occur in chest wall injuries (54). Neurogenic prolactinemia-galactorrhea syndrome mimics lactation, whereby the thoracic nerves are stimulated and initiates disinhibition of dopamine control, thereby producing breast milk.

Endocrine function should be assessed post-injury in all women. Hormone alterations can interfere with bone metabolism, vasomotor regulation, skin integrity, and emotional well-being. If, after six months, menstruation has not returned to pre-injury patterns, checking FSH, LH, estradiol, thyroid stimulating hormone, and prolactin levels will identify the underlying imbalance. Standard interventions (55, 56) include oral contraceptives to regulate menstrual cycling, or bromocryptine to correct prolactinemia or galactorrhea. One must keep in mind, however, that the potential for increasing vascular thrombotic events with these agents in this patient population has not been well studied. Regardless of whether or not a woman resumes menstruation, if she develops abnormal uterine bleeding at a later time, full evaluation for non-SCI-related etiologies is important to differentiate benign from pathologic disorders (60). Abnormal uterine bleeding can be due to reproductive and nonreproductive endocrine dysfunction, malignancies, medications, intra-cranial or brain disorders, and many other organ system problems.

Resumption of Menstruation

With the resumption of regular menstruation (usually 3–6 months after injury), women usually return to pre-injury fertility status. Ovulation, and thus conception, may occur in the absence of menstruation, so birth control counseling is advisable if pregnancy is not sought during this time. The resumption of a regular menstrual cycle may also exacerbate the sequelae of SCI.

Table 34.1   Menstrual Cycle Abnormalities

CONDITION	TYPES	DEFINITION
Abnormal Uterine Bleeding	Dysfunctional uterine bleeding (DUB)	Excessive menstrual blood flow (MBF), usually of endocrine etiology
	Menometrorrhagia	*Prolonged* uterine bleeding at *irregular* intervals
	Menorrhagia	*Prolonged* heavy uterine bleeding at *regular* intervals
	Metrorrhagia	*Frequent irregular* menses
Dysmenorrhea	Primary	Painful abdominal cramping occurring just before or during menstruation, often associated with other somatic symptoms such as nausea vomiting, headache, and diaphoresis AND occurs at the time of menarche but not related to pelvic pathological conditions
	Secondary	Same condition and symptoms as primary BUT occurrence is due to pathological pelvic condition and after menarche has been established
Amenorrhea	Primary	Failure to undergo menarche before 16.5 years of age
	Secondary	Cessation of menstruation for at least 3–12 months after a woman has had a previous pattern of spontaneous menstruation.

In a self-reported multi-center study of 472 women (53) with spinal cord injury, when asked about perimenstrual problems, 25% experienced increased autonomic symptoms (sweating, flushing, headaches, or goose flesh), 18% had more frequent bladder spasms, and 22.5% said they had worsening of muscle spasticity. These symptoms are analogous to the dysmenorrhea or cramping some able-bodied women describe at the time of menstruation (58). Studies of able-bodied women link these premenstrual symptoms to elevated prostaglandin F2 alpha in the endometrium (57, 59). Often anti-inflammatory agents such as naproxen, ibuprofen, or mefenamic acid can alleviate these SCI symptoms.

Return of menstruation and its long-term management is a significant concern for women with SCI. The previously mentioned self-reported study reported no significant changes in menstrual cycle length (25.1 days vs. 27.9 days) or length of menstruation (5.1 days and 5.0 days) in pre- and post-injury experiences, respectively. Problems in menstrual management and bladder continence during menses include tampons and pads creating catheter occlusion or interference with its placement. Labial pressure sores from catheters more commonly occur during this time. Mobility limitations affect menstrual hygiene, which place these women at higher risk for toxic shock syndrome if tampons are not changed frequently or are forgotten from lack of sensation. Higher levels of SCI prevent independent self-care for many women during this time of the month. It is not surprising that some women seek a solution by undergoing a hysterectomy, endometrial ablation procedure, or by taking hormones for suppression of menses.

Candidiasis

Another condition becoming more problematic in women with SCI, especially during menstruation, is significant outbreaks of vaginal and perineal candidiasis. This patient population is prone to this chronic infection due to the persistent moist state of the perineum and the increased utilization of antibiotics for urinary tract infections. Often dismissed as clinically inconsequential, it is very common and can contribute to disruption of dermal integrity and pressure sores. As there is minimal information written on candidiasis and SCI, the more serious sequelae, such as occult systemic infection, is rarely considered as a possible condition that can contribute to illness. Reports concerning the able-body population provide some evidence that chronic "yeast infections" may predispose individuals to systemic yeast infections, which then colonize the woman's body tissues (60). When this occurs in the intestinal tract, the harmless form of the yeast often transforms to the invasive hyphal form that breaks down mucosal integrity allowing leakage of inappropriate substances into the bloodstream. This is called "leaky gut syndrome." Chronic symptoms may be nonspecific, and therefore missed, and can include fatigue, lethargy, headaches, weakness, constipation, food sensitivities, menstrual and premenstrual problems, bladder discomfort, and mental and emotional disturbances (61). Other uncommon consequences of systemic yeast infections include osteomyelitis (vertebral body or other bone structure) (62), uro-vaginal fistula, and fungicemia. There is a lack of sufficient study of these consequences in the SCI literature, but they are described as comorbid manifestations in the immune-compromised

population who also are subject to multiple antibiotic requirements (63). Women with SCI and chronic vaginal or dermatologic yeast infections may be more prone to any of these more invasive infections, including pelvic candidal abscesses. Visual inspection of skin and stain/cultures of vaginal discharge are the only diagnostic tests available for the less severe infections. Unfortunately, blood and cerebral spinal fluid (CSF) cultures may be negative and only helpful in diagnosing the more severe infections involving sepsis and fever. Newer biochemical phenotypic identification methods are being developed that hold more promise (61). Pelvic imaging should be considered for women with a history of chronic UTIs and yeast infections, and additional signs and symptoms of abdominal or pelvic abscess, vaginal fistula, or osteomyelitis. Treatment (61) should be according to cultures and sensitivities, but in absence of these, oral fluconazole, topical anti-candidal agents, and judicious use of antibiotics are appropriate. Prophylactic antifungal therapy effectiveness, especially after a course of antibiotics for another medical condition, is unknown.

Birth Control

Birth control practices are important for those women sexually active and not wanting pregnancy. The multi-center women's health study shows that 70.3% of those women sexually active after spinal cord injury practice birth control. Following spinal cord injury, there was a preference for partners using condoms (38.9%) followed by permanent sterilization (26.1%), and then oral contraceptives (OCPs) (22.1%). Oral contraceptive usage (57.2%) was the birth control of choice before injury.

Some combinations of OCPs with higher estrogen concentrations have risks for deep venous thrombosis (DVT) or myocardial infarction in some able-bodied women, especially if they are greater than 35 years of age and smoke tobacco products (64). Although the immediate immobility in women with spinal cord injury predispose them to DVT (65) acutely post-injury, there are no data to prove that risks are greater with OCPs in women with chronic SCI than in the able-bodied population. OCPs or any form of hormonal manipulation for birth control such as depot-medroxyprogesterone acetate (DPMA) injections, the "mini-pill," or subdermal hormonal implants should be prescribed with caution and avoided in most women within one year of injury who have a positive existing smoking history or migraine, past history of DVT (pre or post-injury), or cardiovascular conditions. If a woman with chronic SCI is to have any surgical procedure and is on OCPs, the risk for DVT and pulmonary thrombo-embolism (PTE) increases and she should be watched closely for any signs or symptoms post-operatively. If not contraindicated, appropriate prophylactic anticoagulation should be considered. Not much is known about SCI and the newer forms of OCPs, which alter menstruation patterns to occur only three to four times a year. The same considerations should be observed as with the monthly or tri-monthly DPMA injections. These alternatives for birth control often produce amenorrhea through mechanism of hypoestrogenemia, which with long term use may lead to worsening immobility-related osteoporosis and cardiovascular disorders (66, 67).

Other birth control options must also be carefully considered before being prescribed. The intrauterine device (IUD) (68) is associated with increased risk of pelvic inflammatory disease in some women whose sexual activity includes multiple partners.

This becomes more important in women with spinal cord injury who have chronic indwelling bladder catheters, bacteriuria, and urinary tract infections. Another complication of the IUD is displacement or perforation of the uterus. As many women with SCI do not perceive pain, the presenting symptoms of pelvic inflammatory disease or uterus perforation may be untimely diagnosed. Before IUD placement in these women, complete sexual and urologic history should be obtained and appropriate counseling given.

Diaphragms, cervical caps, or vaginal sponges are other options. Women with higher levels of injury, however, cannot place them independently. A diaphragm must remain in place at least six hours after intercourse to be effective and prolonged pressure against the vaginal wall may create mucosal breakdown. For those women with latex allergies, latex-free diaphragms must be special ordered.

Sexually Transmitted Diseases

Sexually transmitted diseases (STD) have been reported as being less frequent following injury—in about 2.5% of women who are sexually active (51). More study is needed to explore this health issue in this patient population. Concern exists that STDs may not be recognized and thus under-diagnosed and untreated. In 2006 the first vaccine was FDA approved for prophylaxis against human papilloma virus (HPV) (69, 70). HPV is sexually transmitted, and many strains produce moderate and high-grade cervical neoplasia (71). The American Cancer Society recommends that women between the ages 11 and 26 should receive counseling for HPV vaccination (72). Availability and purpose of vaccination should be discussed with all appropriate-age females who have SCI. This should not, however, substitute for continuing yearly gynecologic examination, especially if the woman is sexually active.

PREGNANCY

Although some data suggest (53) that women with spinal cord injury become pregnant for the first time at an older age than able-bodied women, social issues may play a major role. In a cross-sectional study, 66 (13.9%) out of 472 women with SCI (average age 40) reported having had a total of 101 pregnancies post-injury. The relatively lower pregnancy rate makes prospective studies about obstetrical complications difficult, and no studies have examined female fertility following SCI (73). Unique medical problems, however, appear to occur in these women during pregnancy, labor, and delivery.

Unique Medical Problems

Neurogenic bladder dysfunction and pregnancy increase the incidence of urinary tract infections. Chronic antibiotic suppression may be warranted but must be managed judiciously according to the trimester. The growth of the fetus and abdomen places pressure on the bladder, predisposing to urine leakage either around the catheter or between catheterizations (74). Interference of diaphragm movement will diminish respiratory capacity and increase the risk of pneumonia or respiratory compromise, especially in women with tetraplegia. The growth of the fetus also exerts pressure on the inferior vena cava and common femoral veins, which will worsen edema and possibly further predispose these women to deep venous thrombosis (75–77).

As transfers become difficult and weight alterations change seating contours, pressure ulcers may develop. Furthermore, changing nutritional demands and anemia of pregnancy impairs skin healing once a decubitus ulcer develops. Bowel motility decreases during pregnancy as a result of increased progestin and iron supplementation. Bowel programs must be modified to adjust to this dramatic change. Again, the temporary loss of mobility makes maintaining independence with bowel management difficult.

Other pregnancy difficulties described by women with SCI include frequent autonomic dysreflexia, worsening spasticity, and loss of pre-pregnancy independence (51). As many individuals with SCIs are on multiple medications, each medication should be examined for its appropriate use during each trimester of pregnancy and post-partum if the woman chooses breast feeding (lactation). The U.S. Food and Drug Administration classifies drugs by a use-in-pregnancy rating system (Table 34.2) based on risks and benefits to the fetus and mother. Table 34.3 includes commonly prescribed medicines for spinal cord injury sequelae and potential maternal fetal contraindications. To avoid withdrawal symptoms, careful weaning is advisable.

Labor and Delivery

The level of spinal cord injury will have an effect on the perception of labor. It has been recommended that after 28 weeks of gestation, the woman should be frequently checked for effacement and dilation (76, 78, 79). Tocodynamometry or early hospitalization may be necessary. Labor is mediated by neurohumoral factors (76, 77). The change in estrogen, in part, influences parasympathetic mediated uterine contractions. Progesterone indirectly exerts its effect on sympathetic control to adjust strength of contractions. In able-bodied women, pain during the first stage of labor is primarily from uterine contractions via the T10–L1 spinal cord levels. This is followed by dilation of the cervix and perineal stretching, which produces pain via the pudendal nerve and its branches (S2–S4) during the end of the first stage and throughout the second stage of labor.

Unrecognized conventional labor symptoms and delivery can occur, especially in women whose levels are T10 and above. Often women experience atypical labor symptomatology. Pain above the level of injury, referred pain to the shoulders or upper back, abnormal nonspecific pain, increased spasticity, autonomic dysreflexia, and increased bladder spasms may indicate labor (77). Prenatal education should include explanation of these possible symptoms.

By far the most critical complication of labor and delivery is autonomic dysreflexia. It has been reported that 60–80% (80, 81) of women with SCI with lesions above T6 and a small percentage below T6 (82) will experience autonomic dysreflexia during labor and delivery uterine contractions. Sequelae of fetal distress, maternal intracranial hemorrhage, coma, seizures, and even death have been described (83–85) if this condition goes unrecognized and untreated. Treatment is prompt delivery of the baby and placenta or regional epidural or general anesthesia (86). Occasionally, parental anti-hypertensives (87) are required. It is important to distinguish autonomic dysreflexia from

Table 34.2   Pregnancy Risk Categories

CATEGORY	DESCRIPTION
A	Controlled studies show no risk. Adequate, well-controlled studies in pregnant women have failed to demonstrate a risk to the fetus in any trimester of pregnancy.
B	No evidence of risk in humans. Adequate, well-controlled studies in pregnant women have not shown increased risk of fetal abnormalities despite adverse findings in animals, or, in the absence of adequate human studies, animal studies show no fetal risk. The chance of fetal harm is remote, but remains a possibility.
C	Risk cannot be ruled out. Adequate, well-controlled human studies are lacking, and animal studies have shown a risk to the fetus or are lacking as well. There is a chance of fetal harm if the drug is administered during pregnancy, but the potential benefits may outweigh the potential risk.
D	Positive evidence of risk. Studies in humans, or investigational or post-marketing data, have demonstrated fetal risk. Nevertheless, potential benefits from the use of the drug may outweigh the potential risk. For example, the drug may be acceptable if needed in a life-threatening situation or serious disease for which safer drugs cannot be used or are ineffective.
X	Contraindicated in pregnancy. Studies in animals or humans, or investigational or post-marketing reports have demonstrated positive evidence of fetal abnormalities or risk which clearly outweighs any possible benefit to the patient.

pre-eclampsia (88), which occurs with the same frequency in both able-bodied women and women with disabilities. The cardiovascular symptoms of dysreflexia are hypertension, severe headache, bradycardia, or tachycardia and occurrence of these symptoms during uterine contractions only. The hypertension, tachycardia, and proteinuria of eclampsia occur throughout labor.

Delivery may be further complicated by the musculoskeletal sequelae of spinal cord injury, which may include hip disarticulation, contractures, heterotopic ossification, previous femur fractures, scoliosis, and severe spasticity. Positioning on the delivery table may be problematic. These conditions may contribute to more frequent use of forceps, vacuum, or cesarean section delivery (53, 75).

Pregnancy Outcomes

Early reports (76, 89, 90) of pregnancy outcomes for women with spinal cord injury suggested a higher incident of cesarean section, episiotomy dehiscence, failure to progress in labor, breech presentation, and low birth weight. Other studies, however, support that women with spinal cord injury have similar outcomes to able-bodied women (53, 88). Good prospective studies are needed to confirm the risks of these delivery complications.

SEXUAL FUNCTION

Spinal cord injury has a significant impact on the sexual behavior and function of women (91, 92). Although a more complete discussion of sexual function after SCI can be found in another section of this text, the following is included for completeness of women's health concerns. In reports of women with SCI, the percentage that had sexual intercourse before injury (87%) was comparable to national surveys of able-bodied women (53). This

study showed that participation in sexual intercourse decreased after spinal cord injury and did not reach pre-injury level, although it did increase significantly over time. The physiologic changes following spinal cord injury, as they affect the sexual response cycle (93), are neurologic-level dependent. The excitation phase of lubrication and clitoral enlargement is primarily mediated by the parasympathetics (S2–S4). The components of orgasm, which include the rhythmic contractions of fallopian tubes, uterus, and paraurethral muscles, are predominantly controlled by the sympathetics (T10–L1). The final stage of orgasm (which is analogous to ejaculation in males) is directed by parasympathetic and somatic afferents (94). Studies by Sipski (95, 96) showed that women with complete or incomplete upper motor neuron spinal cord injuries can have reflex lubrication. Although these women were significantly less likely than able-bodied women to achieve orgasm, there was no significant difference among their different levels and completeness of injury to achieve orgasm. Another phenomenon unique to women with spinal cord injury is the ability to experience paraorgasms or intensely pleasurable feelings above the injury level (97). Sensitive areas such as the breasts or neck may become focal erogenous zones for sexual fulfillment (98).

Some women report problems encountered during sexual activity that are SCI dependent. Among these are difficulties with positioning for intercourse, problems with foley catheter, occurrence of bowel and bladder incontinence, and unanticipated muscle spasms and physiologic responses of autonomic dysreflexia. If lubrication does not occur, prescribing commercial lubricant is a simple intervention. Female vibratory aids are available for individuals with upper extremity functional limitations. Prophylactic anti-spasticity or autonomic dysreflexia medications before intercourse may be helpful if not too sedating. Emptying the bowel or bladder and taping or removing the indwelling catheter are helpful hints for unreliable bowel and bladder reflexes

Table 34.3   Drug Use Indications During Pregnancy

Drug Indication or Types	Examples	FDA Use-in-Pregnancy Rating Category	Secreted in Breastmilk	Comments
Antispasticity	Baclofen			
	Oral	C	Unknown	No studies for intrathecal baclofen.
	Intrathecal	Unknown	Unknown	
	Diazepam	D	Yes	As with all benzodiazepams there is increased risk of congenital malformations if taken during first trimester of pregnancy.
	Tizanidine	C	Unknown	Animal studies showed increase in spontaneous abortion and developmental retardation.
	Dantrolene	C	Unknown	Infant risks cannot be ruled out.
Bladder Management	Oxybutinin chloride	B	Unknown	Possibly excreted in breast milk but no known infant effects.
	Tolterodine tartrate	C	Unknown	(a) Secreted in breast milk in animals. (b) Animal studies, using high dosages, showed increase incleft palate, digital abnormalities, and intra-abdominal hemorrhage.
	Pseudoephedrine	C	Yes	American Academy of Pediatric feels it is compatible with lactation although it may cause mild excitation in infant.
	Anticholinergic tricyclic antidepressants (e.g., Amitryptyline, Imipramine)	C	Yes	(a) Possibility of fetal abnormalities or delayed development. (b) Do not take while lactating.
Chronic Pain	Opioids (general) (e.g., hydrocodone, morphine)	C	Yes	For lactation, infant risk is minimal if used in very limited doses.
Non-Steroidal Anti-inflammatory Drugs (NSAIDS)	Naproxen	B (1st and 2nd trimester) D (3rd trimester)	Yes	(a) If taken in 3rd trimester, associated with premature closure of ductus arteriosus and neonatal hypertension. (b) Causes prolongation of labor and delivery.
	Ibuprofen	B (1st and 2nd trimester) D (3rd trimester)	Yes	Same as above.
	Indomethicin	B (1st and 2nd trimester) D (3rd trimester)	Yes	Same as above.
	Celecoxib	C	Yes	No studies have examined effects on ductus arteriosus or labor and delivery.
Steroids	Dexamethasone	C	Yes	(a) Especially harmful during 1st trimester (b) Immunosuppressive effects in newborn. (c) Associated with malformations.
	Methylprednisolone	C	Yes	Same as above.
Common Oral Antibiotics	Sulfamethoxazole trimethoprim	C	Yes	(a) Contraindicated while lactating, as it may cause kernicterus in infant. (b) Caution while pregnant, as it interferes with folic acid metabolism.
	Quinolones (e.g., ciprofloxin, fluoroquinolones)	C	Yes	Therapeutic doses during pregnancy unlikely to pose substantial teratogenic risk.

Table 34.3 *(Continued)*

DRUG INDICATION OR TYPES	EXAMPLES	FDA USE-IN-PREGNANCY RATING CATEGORY	SECRETED IN BREASTMILK	COMMENTS
	Tetracyclines	D	Yes	(a) Detrimental effect on fetal skeletal development. (b) During lactation, can affect dental development in infants.
	Cephalosporins	B	Yes	Use with caution while breast feeding.
	Macrodantin	B (only until 38 weeks' gestation)*	Yes	Avoid in latter weeks of pregnancy (38–42 weeks) due to increased risk of hemolytic anemia in neonates.
Bowel Management	Diphenylmethane (e.g., biscadyl)	Not studied	Unknown	No evidence for contraindication in animal studies.
	Senna compounds	Not studied	Unknown	No evidence for contraindication in animal studies.
	Magnesium Salts			
	Parental	A	Yes	
	Oral	B	Yes	
Antidepressants	Selective serotonin reuptake inhibitors (SSRIs)	C	Yes	(a) Possibility of fetal abnormalities or delayed development. (b) Check with FDA for individual medication. (c) Do not take while lactating.
	Tricyclic antidepressives (general)	C	Yes	Same as above.
Anti-eleptics	Gabapentin	C	Yes	(a) Infant risk cannot be ruled out. (b) Also used for chronic pain.
	Pregabalin	C	Yes	Same as above.
	Carbamazepine	D	Yes	(a) Crosses placenta and has been implicated in increased risk of spina bifida in fetus. (b) 60% of maternal blood concentrations appear in breast milk.
	Phenytoin	Unknown	Probably	Likely produces teratogenic effects in the offspring.
	Valproic acid	D	Yes	Same as above.
Multiple Sclerosis (ref. 213)	Cyclosphosphamide	D	Yes	(a) Severe skeletal and ocular malformations. (b) Fetal growth retardation.
	Azathioprine	D	Yes	(a) Fetal prematurity and distress, chromosomal abnormalities, and growth retardation. (b) Neonatal immunoglobulin deficiency and other permanent immune deficiencies.
	Methotrexate	X	Yes	(a) Probable miscarriage. (b) Severe CNS, craniofacial, and skeletal deformities.
	Interferon β-1b and β-1a	C	Unknown	Increase in spontaneous abortion.
	Glatiramer acetate or copolymer 1	B	Yes	Less information on this drug.

during intercourse. Deflating the intravesicle balloon of the catheter diminishes its physical intrusion and prevents traumatic urethral tearing should catheter expulsion occur. Creative changes in positioning are helpful in addressing musculoskeletal changes. Finally, for sexual well-being, any psychologic factors such as poor body image, fear of pregnancy, being a mother with a disability, and social avoidance should be addressed in an appropriate counseling environment. To aid the woman in dealing with these physiologic changes as they affect her sexual function, practitioners must openly discuss sexual issues with these women. Books such as *Sexuality after Spinal Cord Injury* (99), and internet sites developed by the American College of Obstetrics and Gynecology, and Disability/SCI advocates are helpful consumer references for these women.

UROLOGIC MANAGEMENT

In the past, urologic management has been unimaginative at best for the woman with spinal cord injury. The lack of an external collection device has, for the most part, confined her to indwelling catheters or incontinence unless she has an areflexive bladder and can perform intermittent self-catheterizations or reliable credé maneuvers. Today, however, the knowledge of this aspect of women's health has virtually exploded, giving women with SCI many options (100–102). As spinal cord injury urologic management is addressed in another chapter of this book, details will not be provided here. One must remember, however, that the ultimate goal of satisfactory bladder management is to decrease urologic complications and to preserve renal function long-term (103–105). Bladder management methods are successful only when individualized to a woman's neurologic level, completeness of injury, hand function, caretaker support, employment or social activities, and desire to perform one type over the other.

MENOPAUSE AND AGING ISSUES

It is known that individuals with spinal cord injury experience various pathophysiologic changes as a result of their neurologic deficits. Aging can further add new disability (106) from advancing osteoporosis (107), cardiovascular disorders (108), osteoarthritic conditions (109, 110), spine deformity, joint pain, respiratory decline, obesity (111), and impingement neuropathies (112–114). Individuals who achieve a specific level of function post-injury may find that they are not able to maintain that level and will require wheelchair adaptation, new assistive devices, pain therapy intervention, musculoskeletal corrective surgeries, or even increased or new attendant care.

As women who have had chronic SCI transition through menopause, they undergo the compounded effects of processes involved in normal reproductive aging and aging with SCI. The physiologic effects of decline in estrogen levels potentiate the ongoing post-injury sequela resulting in newer deficits of dermatologic, musculoskeletal, urologic, and cardiovascular conditions (107, 115–118).

As previously mentioned, many female sex hormones such as estrogen exert positive influences on the nervous and immune systems. As a woman ages and estrogen production diminishes, these beneficial properties may weaken (119,120) and instigate (for some women) autoimmune, neuro-degenerative, and cardiovascular disorders. This may especially have an impact for those women who have an SCI at younger ages and prior to menopause.

Osteoporosis

Immobility is a consequence of paralysis, contractures, sensorimotor deficits, or other neurologic disorders. Years of diminished weight-bearing activities predispose women and men with disabilities to disuse osteoporosis (121). For the women, however, the menopausal transition heralds estrogen deficiency that further compounds loss of bone mass. Unfortunately, quantification of bone loss in women with spinal cord injury has not been standardized. No indicators exist for determining typical bone loss from either the disuse or menopausal state. It is unknown what therapies are efficacious or when the appropriate interventions could be initiated to delay the progression of osteoporosis (122, 123).

Concern exists that the osteoporosis that occurs following spinal cord injury may lead to further compression fractures, scoliosis, and kyphosis. Severe spinal curvature changes are associated with predisposing individuals with spinal cord injury to spondylitic, post-traumatic tethering and syringomyelia (124), which can produce new neurologic loss. Curvature and postural changes can lead to pain, radiculopathies (above the injury level [125]), decrease in respiratory function (126) (with predisposition to pneumonia), worsening spasticity, and difficulty with swallowing (127). Finally, as the spine ages, cumulative, abnormal interarticular forces create destructive pressures on the lower lumbar vertebral bodies and discs. The altered tone, muscle strength, and sensation perpetuate this process with resultant formation of charcot joints, often at the L4–L5 or L5–S1 spine levels. This is readily seen by plane x-rays due to the characteristic degenerative changes, bone spurring, and syndesmophyte. Women will present with symptoms of autonomic dysreflexia, sweating, catheter flow interference, bladder spasms, or worsening overall spasms (128–130). These problems are often positional and worsen upon sitting. Nonsteroidal anti-inflammatory drugs may help, and some trials with spinal epidural blocks are encouraging. Interestingly, one study suggests these symptoms can be lessened with caudal or bladder afferent blocks (131).

Lower extremity fractures are a consequence of osteoporosis in able-bodied, post-menopausal women. Recently an analysis of the National Spinal Cord Injury database revealed a trend for women with spinal cord injury to more likely develop lower extremity long bone fracture as time post-injury increased (132). In fact, for women seen 20 years post-injury with an average age of 52 years (average age of menopause for able-bodied is 51) (4), there was a statistically higher reported incidence of lower extremity long bone fractures than for the males during that follow up.

Estrogen Deficiency

Estrogen deficiency has also been postulated to worsen arteriosclerosis and cardiovascular disease (133) by altering lipoprotein metabolism (134). Women with spinal cord injury are also prone to atherosclerosis as they participate less in aerobic activities and have a greater tendency to lead sedentary lifestyles. Premature heart disease, hypertension, or stroke becomes problematic, especially in light of the fact that these women may undergo menopause at an earlier age than able-bodied women (135). Estrogen deficiency also contributes to skin changes such as dermal thinning, loss of elasticity, and diminished subcutaneous blood flow (118). The physically challenged are at higher risk for developing pressure sores, especially if there is a sensorimotor impairment (136). Post-menopausal women with spinal cord injury will have an increased risk of developing pressure sores compared to the pre-menopausal women with disabilities. Furthermore, wound healing may be delayed in comparison to able-bodied women. Related skin changes in the vaginal and urethral mucosa lead to atrophy of the vaginal epithelium. Conditions such as vaginal and urethral drying, vaginitis, and patulous urethra may affect bladder management and continence in those women who have had stable and previously satisfactory neurogenic bladder function.

Vasomotor Instability

Vasomotor instability is another menopausal consequence that may be exaggerated in women with spinal cord injuries. It has been reported that women with spinal cord injury often experience labile vasomotor responses from the primary neurologic disorder (137). These manifest in wide blood pressure swings, bradycardia, tachycardia, flushing, sweating, and chills. The menopausal transition with hormonal alterations can exaggerate these conditions. Furthermore, autonomic dysreflexia, which is a condition that occurs in high paraplegia and tetraplegia, has been a reported symptom of hormonal changes during the menstrual cycle (138). It presents as symptoms of hypertension, headache, flushing, and bradycardia. Although studies are lacking to confirm the prevalence of autonomic dysreflexia in menopausal women with spinal cord injuries, its symptoms and appropriate intervention may not be recognized. On the other hand, symptoms of vasomotor disturbances and hypothalamic thermoregulation are pathognomonic for decreasing estrogens during menopause. "Hot flashes" are, in part, controlled by the central nervous system (139) but have never been studied in women with spinal cord injury and may be confused with symptoms of autonomic dysreflexia.

Hormone Replacement Therapy

Treatment of menopausal symptoms and sequelae has always been controversial, regardless of whether the woman does or does not have SCI. Hormone replacement therapy (HRT), using combinations of estrogen and progesterone, is advocated for amelioration of symptoms such as hot flashes, sleep disturbances, vaginal changes, and mood swings. For able-bodied women, earlier studies advocated HRT for reducing post-menopausal heart disease, osteoporosis, and Alzheimer's (140, 141), although some cautioned there was a risk of increased breast and uterine cancer (142,143). Then in 2002, peri- and postmenopausal medical management changed almost overnight when the results of the Woman's Health Initiative (WHI) were published (144). The report revealed that HRT contributed to an increase in mortality for women who began HRT after menopause compared to those who did not. Unfortunately, these initial publicized results minimized possible confounding influences, such as study participants being able-bodied women with the mean age of 63 ± 7

years. Furthermore, 73.9% of the women had never been on HRT and began HRT (0.625 mg/day conjugated estrogen with or without (=placebo) 2.5 mg/day medroxy progesterone acetate) only after the study began, which was often many years after menopause. Since then, further research has inundated the scientific community with continuous debate on the merits (or failings) of HRT. Consensus at the time of this writing, however, supports that HRT can be beneficial at the time of menopause, for a defined period of time and for an appropriate selection of women (145). Women without potentially negative risk factors (cardiovascular disease or family history of breast cancer) may opt for short-term use of low-dose HRT for alleviation of peri- and postmenopausal symptoms. Women at significant risk for developing morbidity and mortality from osteoporotic fractures (e.g., many women with SCI) may also want to consider HRT for osteoporosis if they do not have a personal or family history of breast or uterine cancer, cannot tolerate other osteoporosis medications, or have other co-morbid contraindications. There are no data, however, to indicate when HRT should be initiated in these women. Regardless, it is important for the health care provider and the woman to understand, communicate, and discuss all ramifications of benefits, risks, and side effects of HRT as it relates to her family and past medical history.

Some women with SCI may have relative contraindications to conventional HRT or may not wish to take it. Other options such as calcitonin (146), selective estrogen receptor modulators (SERMSs) (147, 148), calcium supplements (149), and vitamin D (150) may be explored for specific post-menopausal problems. "Natural" hormone treatments and alternative therapies such as phytoestrogens, polyphenols, and soy products (151, 152) may relieve menopausal symptoms and be safer alternatives, but studies in recent years have yielded equivocal guidance on any actual physiologic benefits. Nutritionally balanced soy products are more convincingly advantageous. The long term post-menopausal benefits of the bisphosphonates (ibandronate, pamidronate, clodrinate, zolidonic acid, allendronate) (153, 154) in preventing and treating postmenopausal osteoporosis are encouraging. Oral administration of these medications, however, specifies protracted upright sitting and significant fluid requirements. As many of these medications now can be taken once a week or even once a month, they are much more tolerable for women whose SCI predisposes them to more frequent gastrointestinal (GI) problems such as esophageal reflux, dysphagia, dysmotility, or decreased GI transit time of neurogenic bowel. There is some rationale for use of these medications in those women (and possibly men) with chronic SCI following a lower extremity fracture with the purpose of maximizing bone healing. Evidence exists that these agents may also have positive cardiovascular health benefits (155). Unfortunately, the discovery that several bisphosphonates may contribute to osteonecrosis of the jaw (ONJ) (but mostly in women who have a history of cancer treatments) (156) may limit widespread use.

Encouraging data are evolving that link the benefits of statin drugs for hypercholesterolemia with improvement in osteoporosis and Alzheimer's disease (157). Further research in the many positive (or potentially negative) health benefits of these medications is imperative for women aging with SCI. This is even more important in light of the significant phenomenon of increased obesity in mobility impaired women (and men).

CONSIDERATION FOR WOMEN WITH SPECIAL SPINAL CORD DISABILITIES

Spina Bifida

Women with a history of meningomyelocele (i.e. spina bifida), with or without hydrocephalus, have special health care concerns similar to women with spinal cord injury due to their unique congenital spinal cord disorder. As the life expectancy of this population is increasing, they are transitioning from adolescence to womanhood and entering their reproductive years often with minimal preparation and a paucity of information. A number of studies (158–165) have demonstrated that sexual maturation and puberty often occurs earlier in girls with spina bifida, with the average age of menarche earlier, compared to able-bodied girls (10.9 to 11.4 years of age and 12.7 years of age [160, 165] respectively.) This makes timing of reproductive health education for these young women even more important.

Latex Allergies

It is well known that individuals with spina bifida have an increased risk of developing latex allergies (166,167). Of all women with spina bifida, 23% have a natural rubber latex allergy that is postulated to correspond to the number of surgical interventions they have undergone. The belief that an inherent state of atopy was the primary etiology has been declared to be only a minor contributing factor (168). It is imperative that questions about latex allergies are included in the medical history so that gynecologic examinations, surgical interventions, and use of reproductive health products, such as condoms and diaphragms, are latex-free.

Gynecologic Issues

Few studies examine specific gynecologic problems or reproductive endocrine dysfunction unique to women with spina bifida. It is known that a few of these women have congenital anomalies of the female reproductive tract such as bicornate uterus (169); however, no detailed studies have actually looked at the extent of these and other possible anatomical changes. Often these women present with a prolapsed uterus due to incomplete innervations of the pelvic floor musculature. Surgical intervention may be ineffective due to the imbalance of pelvic tone. This may also affect the use of a pessary-like device. Latex allergies, commonly acquired by individuals with spina bifida, and vaginal wall pressure points, which predispose to mucosal breakdown, further prevent use of these devices. Mobility limitations and unique body habitus make management of these conditions, as well as menstruation, very difficult.

Orthopedic conditions such as kyphoscoliosis, hip dislocation/subluxation, lower extremity contractures, and pelvic obliquity are other secondary conditions seen in individuals with spina bifida (170, 171). These conditions may physically alter the woman's reproductive anatomy, which may make a gynecologic exam difficult. In addition, positioning on an exam table may require special attention. If a satisfactory exam cannot be performed and the woman presents with specific abnormal symptoms related to her reproductive tract, a pelvic CT or ultrasound should be obtained.

Any intra-peritoneal gynecologic or urologic procedure must be approached cautiously for women with spina bifida and cerebral spinal fluid (CSF) shunts. Hydrocephalus is a common co-morbid condition for individuals with meningomyelocele and is often initially treated at infancy (or later) with ventriculoperitoneal or ventriculoatrial shunting. A previous study (172) reported a 41.4% incidence of shunt and other related complications following these procedures. Although this high incidence was thought to have some association with bowel contamination, these findings have significant ramifications if not recognized.

When treating women with spina bifida, it is imperative that full sexual histories be cautiously elicited due to their possible naiveté and lack of sexual education (173), or in the event of a past history of sexual abuse (which has been reported to be greater in women with disabilities) (174). The need for birth control and what methods are safest for women with spina bifida has not been examined and must be extrapolated from information regarding women with SCI as discussed in a previous section.

Pregnancy and Delivery

As the population and average age of women with spina bifida have increased (175), more have become pregnant. Though large series of surveys and case studies have contributed to the medical management of these women, standards for their obstetrical care still do not exist. Retrospective studies (176–181) have examined pregnancy experiences and the complications arising from co-morbid conditions such as neurogenic bowel/bladder—with or without urinary or gastrointestinal diversion(s), abdominal-pelvic neurologic loss from spinal cord dysfunction, kyphoscoliosis, or other pelvic or lower extremity orthopedic changes, and previous shunting for hydrocephalus. Common problems associated with urinary tract infections were reported, including symptomatic bacteremia and pyelonephritis. Almost 10% of pregnancies exhibited urologic compromise from the growing fetus causing hydronephrosis, intestinal obstruction (177), and renal decline (182). Urinary and bowel incontinence often became problematic (183).

A descriptive case series (184) reported on 17 women with spina bifida who experienced 29 pregnancies. Of these pregnancies, 23 (79%) progressed to live offspring. Although none of the offspring had spina bifida, three (13%) were born with other congenital malformations such as tetralogy of fallot. In one study of 138 pregnancies, the spontaneous abortion rate was relatively high (20%), but 105 live births occurred. In this study, about 11% of the infants had congenital abnormalities, although none with spina bifida.

Pelvic/hip bony abnormalities and lower extremity contractures may interfere with vaginal delivery and necessitate C-sections. During pregnancy, UTIs are even more common for women with spina bifida and can contribute to low birth weight and pre-term infants (185). Another high-risk condition is the possibility of urinary or gastrointestinal stomal or diversion displacement and obstruction (186). It is also possible that obstruction and renal failure (178, 187) may develop, especially if the abdomen is further compromised by exaggerated spine curvature. C-section rates are high and are estimated to be about 42% (193) to 50% (183).

The frequency of seizures may increase in women who have had a history of seizures. Many anticonvulsant medications are contraindicated in pregnancy and their discontinuation further exacerbates this problem.

Liakos (183) retrospectively reported on seven women (out of 70) who had a history of hydrocephalus and pre-pregnancy shunt placement and then had return of hydrocephalus requiring shunt revisions during pregnancy. Other shunt-related problems reported in the literature include increased seizures, headaches, abdominal discomfort, and back pain (188–192). On the other hand, studies have described a high undiagnosed prevalence of increased intracranial pressure (193), arrested hydrocephalus (AH) syndrome, and Chiari/hydro-syringomyelia complex (194) in adults (male and female) with spina bifida who have never been shunted. Obviously these unrecognized conditions could have serious implications in pregnancy management or delivery procedures.

The incidence of spine alignment abnormalities has been reported to be 43% to 50% (175,195) of patients with spina bifida. In addition, lower extremity contractures and pelvic deformities can affect 70% of these individuals. Skeletal abnormalities (187) predispose to maternal respiratory compromise, cardiac failure (188), alterations of center of gravity, and difficulties with labor and delivery progression (189).

Genetic and Environmental Risks

Questions of genetic and environmental risks to the offspring of women with spina bifida are significant considerations. The majority of genetic investigation has examined the role of the inheritance and/or environmental factors that contribute to the risk of able-bodied women having a child with spina bifida. However, 95% of babies with spina bifida and other neural tube defects are born to parents with no family history of these disorders (196). Previous studies (197, 198), however, suggest a recurrence risk for neural tube deficits/spina bifida of 4% to 7% in offspring of women with spina bifida. Historical data provide evidence that although the risk of offspring of women with spina bifida developing congenital or developmental abnormalities is higher than for able-body women, the actual cases of offspring with spina bifida have not been documented. Reasons are multifactorial and possibly related to the higher miscarriage and spontaneous abortion rate, improved genetic counseling, intrapartum amniocentesis evaluation, and understanding of folate supplementation during pregnancy. It is known that nutritional deficits of folic acid during pregnancy increase the risk of having a child with spina bifida (199, 200). Some investigations have focused on a variety of possible mutations involved in fetal folate metabolism, such as reduced folate carrier gene (201) and methionyl tetrahydrofolate reductase (202) gene. It is felt that these genetic contributions, and others currently unrecognized, increase the likelihood of the woman with spina bifida to have offspring with neural tube deficit (203).

All women should have sufficient folate supplementation to lessen the risk of having a newborn with spina bifida. Past literature has recommended an intake of .4 mg of folate per day for pregnant able-body women (204). More recent recommendations (205) have utilized new standards in measuring the amount and forms of folate required for able-body women who become pregnant. These guidelines look at all forms of biologically available folate and recommend 1362 nmol (600 µg) of DFE/d (= Dietary Folate Equivalent per day). This is based on the maintenance of normal red cell folate concentrations required in pregnancy. There are some data, however, to suggest that women with spina

bifida should have even larger doses of folate than their able-body counterparts. Recommendations are that these women should have 4.0 mg of folate every day before and during pregnancy (206). Obviously this question requires urgent investigation.

Multiple Sclerosis

Women with multiple sclerosis (MS) have varying degrees of spinal cord dysfunction. Many of their reproductive health concerns mirror those of women with spinal cord injuries. Neurologically the CNS undergoes autoimmune demyelination that creates paresis, incoordination, paresthesias, visual disturbances, and bowel and bladder dysfunction. Increased tone and spasms are also common. Endocrine imbalances and menstrual irregularities occur as well as sexual dysfunction and pregnancy complications.

It is estimated that the prevalence of MS is 130 per 100,000 women in the United States and 2.6 greater than for men (207). As the onset of MS affects mainly women who are entering their childbearing age (208–210), focus has been on the interrelationship of the course of their disease and pregnancy. The significant numbers of young women who consider pregnancy often seek knowledge concerning the possibilities and extent of disease exacerbations from conception to post-partum. Fetal survival to term and neonate health at delivery become important concerns of the disease effects on pregnancy outcomes.

Pregnancy

Knowledge of pregnancy-related relapse and other problems encountered by women with multiple sclerosis have been expanded by the Pregnancy in Multiple Sclerosis (PRIMS) study (211). This observational, prospective, multicenter study enrolled and followed 254 women with MS during and after 269 pregnancies. This initial report by Confavreaux et al. followed the women throughout their pregnancy, labor and delivery, and 12 months post-partum. Variables studied included relapse rates of MS prior, during, and after pregnancy and delivery, and progressive changes (if any) of function as measured by the Kurtzke Expanded Disability Status Scale (212). Other pregnancy-related outcomes such as epidural anesthesia sequela, fetal-maternal health not related to MS, practices of breast-feeding, and utilization of medications were also studied. Results (Figure 34.6) demonstrated that women with MS exhibited increasingly less episodes of disease relapse (compared to their documented 12-month pre-pregnancy relapse rate) as a function of advancing pregnancy trimester, but experienced significantly greater ($p < .001$) relapse episodes in the 12-month post-partum time frame. Interestingly, only 28% of these women accounted for this significant trend and these women tended to have more severe forms of MS with greater disabling symptoms through all time periods studied (213). A pregnancy with MS did not affect the mean Kurtzke disability scores and the health of the infant (214). Additionally, the underlying disease was not affected by epidural anesthesia, and lactation (215).

This and other studies (216–219) have examined the effects of many medications utilized in the management of MS on pregnancy. Table 34.3 lists several of these medications that may be required by women with MS who are of child bearing age. Regardless of planned or unplanned pregnancy, these women

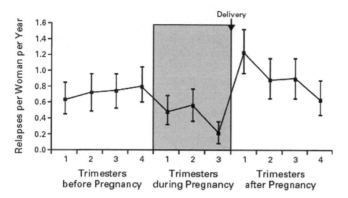

Figure 34.6 Annualized relapse rate in the year before pregnancy, during pregnancy, and in the 2 years after delivery, among 227 women with multiple sclerosis. (From The Pregnancy in Multiple Sclerosis (PRIMS) study. Rate of pregnancy-related relapse in multiple sclerosis. *The New England Journal of Medicine,* 1998; 339(5):285–291, p. 289.)

should receive information from their neurologists, obstetricians, and family practitioners about the effects—either on the fetus or course of disease progression—depending on whether she chooses to discontinue or remain on the medication.

Endocrine Deficiency

As previously mentioned with other types of CNS injury in women, the relationship of reproductive endocrine interactions with neurologic injury and repair in MS has been extensively reviewed. The disorder occurs more commonly in women and is influenced by menstrual cycle and other hormonal fluctuations. Menopause is often a time whereby women with MS enter a stage of many changes. Osteoporosis, advanced heart disease, and conditions similar to SCI are concerns (220–222). Interesting theories of the female-hormonal, neuro-endocrine feedback systems on cell-mediated and humoral immunity (223) give evidence to understanding how these systems interact. Finally, this information can target further investigation strategies for women with MS, depending on their reproductive stages (224).

PSYCHOSOCIAL ISSUES AND WELLNESS

Marital Status

Many important psychosocial issues face women with disabilities. The impact of SCI is just as pronounced on the woman with "standard" as well as nontraditional roles in life. Studies in the past have compared the short-term impact on the marital status of both men and women who have sustained an SCI. DeVivo (225) looked at divorce rates and marriage rates in individuals married at the time of injury and compared them with the general population. Although they were unable to predict which gender would be least likely to marry post-injury, it was interesting to find that for those married at the time of injury, being female, younger age at injury, being African-American, being without children, and higher levels of injury were all associated with the greater likelihood of divorce. Later, a study (226) examining the divorce rate of individuals who married after their injuries showed the opposite effect: males and individuals previously

divorced were 2.2 times more likely to get divorced than females or individuals married for the first time.

Parenting

Parenting issues are paramount for mothers or mothers-to-be with SCI. Ensuring the safety, care, and discipline of their children direct creative support systems and adaptation to manage with their physical challenges (227). Acceptance of extra support can free the mother to focus on those critical parenting skills based on love, bonding, and leadership that define her as "the child's mother" (228).

Abuse

Abuse against women is a significant social problem. Awareness of this problem in women with disabilities has just begun to surface (229). In one study, 40% of 245 women with disabilities reported experiencing abuse by spouses (37%), strangers (28%), parents (15%), service providers (10%) and dates (7%). Of these, 12% were raped. Less than half of these women, however, reported their abuse. As with child protection laws, many states have mandatory reporting for health care clinicians who suspect abuse or neglect to any individual with a disability.

Preventive Health Care

Preventive health care is another social issue often neglected in women with disabilities. A study by Nosek (230) reported that women with disabilities were less likely to receive regular pelvic examinations than women without disabilities. Lack of facility accessibility, trained personnel, and clinician knowledge of a disability set up physical and attitudinal barriers. In addition, the women with a disability may not know what preventive health practices are recommended. Current recommendations by The American College of Obstetrics and Gynecology are for Papicolaou (PAP) tests and other screening procedures to be performed annually, depending on the age of the women (231). PAP smears are to be performed at onset of sexual activity with follow up examinations at least every three years or annually if the woman has multiple or new sexual partners. Mammography for breast cancer detection should be initiated between the ages of 40 and 45, testing every one to two years for women until age 50, and annually after 50. For women with a family history of breast cancer or who have never had a baby, annual screening should begin during the early 40s. Education by the health care practitioner for monthly breast self-examinations should be addressed with all women. Table 34.4 illustrates other recommended preventive health screening for women. HIV testing, TB skin tests, hemoglobin, lipid profiles, stool guiac, colonoscopy, and other tests are appropriate for women with risk factors for co-morbid problems.

Obesity

Obesity is a major problem in the United States today. New statistics from the Center for Disease Control (CDC) (232) report this to be one of the most rapidly growing health concerns today. It is even more concerning for women with physical disabilities who have an even greater incidence of obesity and obesity-related

Table 34.4 Recommended Medical Tests for Women

AGE	PAP	MAMMOGRAPHY	STOOL GUIAC	SIGMOIDOSCOPY	IMMUNIZATION	OTHER
13–18	Baseline and annually if sexually active	—	—	—	Hepatitis B recommended for adolescents and high-risk adults: 3 doses on a 0, 1, 6-month schedule Influenza: given annually Pneumococcal polysaccharide, if at high risk: one-time dose	—
19–39	Annually unless monogamous and has had 3 consecutive normal tests then 1–3 years	—	—	—	Hepatitis B for high risk adults: 3 doses on a 0, 1, 6-month schedule Influenza: given annually Pneumococcal polysaccharide, if at high risk: one-time dose.	Cholesterol every 5 years
40–64	Same as above	Every 1–2 years until age 50, then annually	3 times annually	Every 3–4 years for ages 50–65	Hepatitis B for high-risk adults: 3 doses on a 0, 1, 6-month schedule Influenza: given annually Pneumococcal polysaccharide, if at high risk: one-time dose	Cholesterol every 5 years; consider serum glucose, TSH, colonoscopy
65 and older	Same as above	Annually	Same as above	Every 3–5 years	Hepatitis B for high risk adults: 3 doses on a 0, 1, 6-month schedule Influenza: given annually Pneumococcal polysaccharide: one-time dose	Cholesterol; TSH, and colonoscopy every 3–5 years

problems (233). Preventive health care and heightened vigilance for obesity-related problems such as the metabolic syndrome (= diabetes mellitus, hypercholesterolemia, and hypertension) are paramount for women with SCI.

The medical management of women following an SCI requires a vast knowledge of all aspects of women's health. Unfortunately, our understanding of the full effect of SCI on a woman's body is just beginning. As this population grows, a collaborative approach between physiatry, obstetrics, gynecology, urology, and family practice must evolve to give the comprehensive medical care needed. Finally, women with disabilities must accept the responsibility to demand appropriate and accessible health care.

References

1. Facts & Figures. Available at http://www.spinalcord.uab.edu/show.asp?durki=21446SCISC. Accessed October 15, 2007.
2. McFarlane J, Hughes RB, Noek MA, Groff JY, Swedlen N, Dolan Mullen P. Abuse assessment screen-disability (AAS-D): measuring frequency, type, and perpetrator of abuse toward women with physical disabilities. J Women's Health Gend Based Med 2001; 10(9):861–866.
3. Kung HC, Hoyert DL, Xu J, Murphy SL. Deaths: Preliminary data for 2005. Health E-Stats. National Center for Health Statistics, CDC, Sept 2007. Available at: http://www.cdc.gov/nchs/products/pubs/pubd/hestats/prelimdeaths05/prelimdeaths05.htm Accessed October 17, 2007.
4. Jackson AB, Dijkers M, DeVivo MJ, Poczatek RB. A demographic profile of new traumatic spinal cord injuries: Change and stability over 30 years. Arch Phys Med Rehabil 2004; (85):1740–1748.
5. Mishell DR. Reproductive Endocrinology, in DR Mishell, MA Stenchever, W Droegemuller, AL Herst, eds. Comprehensive Gynecology, 3rd edition, St. Louis, Mosby, 1997; pp 73–128.
6. Aguado LI. Role of the central and peripheral nervous system in the ovarian function. Microscopy Research and Technique 2002; (59):462–473.
7. Backstrom CT, McNeilly AS, Leask RM et al. Pulsatile secretion of LH, FSH, prolactin, estradiol and progesterone during the human menstrual cycle. Clin Endocrinol 1982; 17:29–42.
8. Garcia CR, Mastruianni L, Amelar RD, Dubin L. Current Therapy in Infertility. St. Louis, Mosby-Year Book, 1988.
9. Anderson N, Hagen C, Lange P, et al. Dopaminergic regulation of gonadotropin levels and pulsatility in normal women. Fertil Steril 1987; 47:391–397.
10. Luine VN. Estradiol increases choline acetyltransferase activity in specific basal forebrain nuclei and projection areas of female rats. Exp Neurol. 1985; 89:484–490.

11. Biver F, Lostra F, Monclus M, et al. Sex differences in 5HT2 receptor in the living human brain. Neuroscience 1966; (204):25–28.

12. Wong DF, Broussolle EP, Wand G, et al. In vivo measurements of dopamine receptors in human brain by position emission tomography. Age and sex differences. Ann N Y Acad Sci 1998; (515):205–214.

13. Schomer DL. Ovarian hormones and the nervous system, in Kaplan PW (ed.). Neurologic disease in women, New York, Demos, 1998; pp 45–52.

14. Marchietti B, Guarcello V, Triolo G, et al. Luteinizing hormone-releasing hormone (LHRH) as natural messenger in neuron-immune-endocrine communications, in Hadden JW, Masek K, Nistico G, eds. Interactions among CNS, neuroendocrine and immune systems, Rome: Pythagora Pr, 1989; pp 127–146.

15. Toran-Allerand CD, Miranda RC, Bentham WD, et al. Estrogen receptors colocalize with low-affinity nerve growth factor receptors in cholinergic neurons of the basal forebrain. Proc Natl Acad Sci USA, 1992; 89:4668–4672.

16. Greenspan FS, Stewler GJ, eds. Basic and Clinical Endocrinology. 5th ed. Stamford, Appleton & Lange; 1997.

17. McEwen BS, Wooley CS. Estradiol and progesterone regulate neuronal structure and synaptic connectivity in adult as well as developing brain. Exp Gerontol 1994; 29:431–436.

18. Huang TS, Wang YH, Lai JS, Chang CC, Lien IN. The hypothalamus-pituitary-ovary and hypothalamus-pituitary-thyroid axes in spinal cord-injured women. Metabolism. 1996; 45(6):718–722.

19. Sohrabji F, Miranda RC, Toran-Allerand D. Estrogen differentially regulates estrogen and nerve growth factor receptor mRNAs in adult sensory neurons. J Neurosci 1994; 14:459–471.

20. Mermelstein PG, Becker JB, Surmeier DJ. Estradiol reduces calcium currents in rat neostriatal neurons via a membrane receptor. J Neurosci 1996; 16:595–604.

21. Farace E, Alves WM. Do women fare worse: a metaanalysis of gender differences in traumatic brain injury outcome. J Neurosurg 2000; 93:539–545.

22. Alkayed NJ, Harukuni I, Kimes AS, London ED, Traystam RJ, Hurn PD. Gender-linked brain injury in experimental stroke. Stroke 1998; 29:159–166.

23. Hauben E, Mizrahi T, Agranov E, Schwartz M. Sexual dimorphism in the spontaneous recovery from spinal cord injury: a gender gap in beneficial autoimmunty? Eur J Neurosci 2002; 16:1731–1740.

24. Guarda AS, Swartz KL. Psychiatric disorder in women. In: Kaplan PW, ed. Neurologic disease in women, New York, Demos, 1998. pp 379–403.

25. Garcia-Segura LM, Azcota I, Don Carlos LL. Neuroprotection by estradiol. Prog Neurobiol 2001; 63:79–95.

26. Smith YR, Zebieta JK. Neuroimaging of aging and estrogen effects on central nervous system physiology. Fertil Steril 2001; 76:651–659.

27. Hoffman GE, Le WW, Murphy AZ, Koski CL. Divergent effects of ovarian steroids on neuronal survival during experimental allergic encephalitis in Lewis rats. Exp Neurol 2001; 171:272–284.

28. Weaver Jr CE, Park-Chung M, Gibbs TT, Far DH. 17 beta-estradiol protects against NMDA-induced excitotoxicity by direct inhibition of NMDA receptors. Brain Res 1997; 761:338–341.

29. Mooradian AD. Antioxidant properties of steroids. J Steroid Biochem Mol Biol 1993; 45:59–111.

30. Tan S, Wood M, Maher P. Oxidative stress induces a form of programmed cell death with characteristics of both apoptosis and necrosis in neuronal cells. J Neurochem 1998; 71:95–105.

31. Gibbs RB. Levels of trkA and BDNF mRNA, but not NGF mRNA, fluctuate across the estrous cycle and increase in response to acute hormone replacement. Brain Res 1998; 787:259–68

32. Bjorling DE, Beckman M, Clayton MK, Wang ZY. Modulation of nerve growth factor in peripheral organ by estrogen and progesterone. Neuroscience 2002; 110:155–167.

33. Kaplan DR, Miller FD. Neurotrophin signal transduction in the nervous system. Neurobiology 2000; 10:381–391.

34. Papka RE, Mowa CN. Estrogen receptors in the spinal cord, sensory ganglia, and pelvic autonomic ganglia. Int Rev Cytol 2003; 231:91–127.

35. Marchetti B, Gallo F, Farinella Z, et al. Gender, neuroendocrine-immune interactions and neuron-glial plasticity. Role of luteinizing hormone-releasing hormone (LHRH). Ann NY Acad Sci 2000; 917:678–709.

36. Ahn YH, Lee G, Kang SK. Molecular insights of the injured lesions of rat spinal cords: inflammation, apoptosis, and cell survival. Biochem Biophys Res Commun 2006; 348(2):560–570.

37. Lee K, Jeong J, Tsai MJ, Tsai S, Lydon JP, DeMayo FJ. Molecular mechanisms involved in progesterone receptor regulation of uterine function. J Steroid Biochem Mol Biol 2006; 102(1–5):41–50.

38. Stocco C, Telleria C, Gibori G. The molecular control of corpus luteum formation, function, and regression. Endocr Rev 2007; 28(1):117–149.

39. Papka RE, Srinivasan K., Miller E, Hayashi S. Localization of estrogen receptor protein and estrogen receptor mRNA in peripheral autonomic and sensory neurons. Neuroscience 1997; 79:1153–1163.

40. Papka RE, Storey-Workley M, Shughrue PJ, Merchenthaler , Collins JJ, Usip S, Saunders PTK, Shupnik M. Estrogen receptor-α and–β immunoreactivity and mRNA in neurons of sensory and autonomic ganglia and spinal cord. Cell Tissue Res 2001; 304:193–214.

41. Papka RE, Hafemeister J, Puder BA, Usip S, Storey-Workley M. Estrogen receptor- and neural circuits to the spinal cord during pregnancy. J Neurosci Res 2002; 70:808–816.

42. Papka RE, Traurig HH. Autonomic and visceral sensory innervation of the female reproductive system: special reference to neurochemical markers in nerves and ganglionic connections, in Maggi CA (ed.), 1993. The Autonomic Nervous System, Vol. VI: Nervous Control of the Urogenital System. Harwood Academic Publishers, CHUR, Switzerland, pp 421–464.

43. Papka RE, McCurdy JR, Williams SJ, Mayer B, Marson L, Platt KB. Parasympathetic preganglionic neurons in the spinal cord involved in uterine innervation are cholinergic and nitric oxide-containing. Anta Rec 1995; 241:554–562.

44. Puder BA, Papka RE. Characterization of uterine cervical-related lumbosacral spinal cord neurons. Soc. Neurosci. Abst 2001; 27:840–844.

45. Puder BA, Papka RE. Activation and circuitry of uterine-cervix-related neurons in the lumbosacral dorsal root ganglia and spinal cord at parturition. J Neurosci Res 2005; 82(6):875–889.

46. Amandusson A, Hermanson O, Blomqvist A. Estrogen receptor-like immunoreactivity in the medullary and spinal dorsal horn of the female rat. Neurosci Lett 1995; 196:25–28.

47. Gandelman R. Gonadal hormones and sensory function. Neurosci Biobehav Rev 1983; 7:1–17

48. Terbizan AT, Schneewess WD. The value of gynecological examinations in spinal cord injured women. Paraplegia 1983; 21(4):266–269.

49. Berezin M, Ohry H, Shemesh Y, Zeilig G, Brooks ME. Hyper-prolactinemia, galactorrhea and amenorrhea in women with spinal cord injury. Gynecol Endocrinol. 1989; 3:159–163.

50. Boyd AE, Spare S, Bower B, Reichlins. Neurogenic galactorrhea amenorrhea. J Clin Endocrinol Metab1978; 47:1374–1377.

51 Jackson AB. Hyperprolactinemia following SCI. Eighteenth Annual Scientific Meeting of the American Spinal Cord Injury Association. Abstract Digest. San Diego 1992.

52. Jabbour HN, Kelly RW, Fraser HM, Critchley HO. Endocrine regulation of menstruation. Endocr Rev 2006; 27(1):17–46.

53. Jackson AB, Wadley VA. A multicenter study of women's self-reported reproductive health after spinal cord injury. Arch Phys Med Rehabil 1999; 80:1420–1428.

54. Morley JE, Dawson M, Hodgkinson H, Kalk WJ. Galactorrhea and hyperprolactinemia associated with chest wall injury. J Clin Endocrinol Metab 1997; 45:931–935.

55. Mishell D. Primary and Secondary Amenorrhea. In Mishell DR, Stencheneuer MA, Droegemueller W, Herbst AL, editors. Comprehensive Gynecology, 3rd ed. St. Louis, Mosby, 1997.

56. Hatasaka H. The evaluation of abnormal uterine bleeding. Clin Obstet Gynecol 2005; 48(2):258–273.

57. Bulletti C, Ziegler DE, Setti PL, Cicinelli E, Polli V, Flamigni C. The patterns of uterine contractility in normal menstruating women: from physiology to pathology. Ann N Y Acad Sci 2004; 1034:64–83.

58. French L. Dysmenorrhea. American Family Physician 2005; 71(2):285–291.

59. Speroff L, Ramwell P. Prostaglandins in reproductive physiology. Am J Obstet Gynecol 1970; 107:1111–1130.

60. Pick, M. . Digestive problems—or systemic yeast? / Candida? Available at: http://www.womentowomen.com/digestionandgihealth/candida.asp. Accessed October 29, 2007.

61. Pincus DH, Orenga S, Chatellier S. Yeast identification—past, present, and future methods. Medical Mycology 2007; (45)2:97–121.

62. Eismont FJ, Bohlman HH, Soni PL, Goldberg VM, Freehafer AA. Pyogenic and fungal vertebral osteomyelitis with paralysis. J Bone Joint Surg 1983; 65:19–29.

63. Bohme A, Just-Nubling G, Bergmann L, Shah PM, Stille W, Hoelzer D. Itraconazole for prophylaxis of systemic mycoses in neutropenic patients with haematological malignancies. J Antimicrob Chemother 1996; 38:953–961.

64. Mileikowsky GN, Nadler JL, Huey F et al. Evidence that smoking alters prostocyclin formation and platelet aggregation in women who use oral contraceptives. Am J Obstet Gynecol 1988; 159:1547–1552.

65. Brah BB, Moser KM, Cedar L, Minteer M, Convery R. Venous thrombosis in acute spinal cord paralysis. J. Trauma 1977; 17:289–292.

66. Cundy T, Reid IR. Bone loss and depot medroxy progesterone. Am J Obstet Gynecol 1997; 176(5):1116–1117.

67. Reape KZ. Current contraceptive research and development. Adolesc Med 2005; 16:617–633.

68. Farley TM, Rosenberg MJ, Rowe PJ, Chen JH, Meirik O. Intra-uterine devices and pelvic inflammatory disease: an international perspective. Lancet 1992; 339:785–788.

69. Farrell RM, Rome ES. Adolescents' access and consent to the human papillomavirus vaccine: a critical aspect for immunization success. Pediatrics 2007; 120:434–437.

70. Lowy DR, Schiller JT. Prophylactic human papillomavirus vaccines. J Clin Investigation 2006; 116:1167–1173.

71. Garland SM, Hernandez-Avila M, Wheeler CM, Perez G, Harper DM, Leodolter S, Tang GWK, Ferris DG, Steben M, Bryan J, Taddeo FJ, Railkar R, Esser MT, Sings HL, Nelson M, Boslego J, Sattler C, Barr E, Koutsky LA, the Females United to Unilaterally Reduce Endo/Ectocervical Disease (FUTURE). Quadrivalent vaccine against human papillomavirus to prevent anogenital diseases. N Engl J Med 2007; 356:1928–1943.

72. Saslow D, Castle PE, Cox JT, Davey DD, Einstein MH, Ferris DG, Goldie SJ, Harper DM, Kinney W, Moscicki AB, Noller KL, Wheeler CM, Ades T, Andrews KS, Doroshenk MK, Kahn KG, Schmidt C, Shafey O, Smith RA, Partridge EE (for the Gynecologic Cancer Advisory Group), Garcia F. American Cancer Society Guideline for Human Papillomavirus (HPV) Vaccine Use to Prevent Cervical Cancer and Its Precursors. CA: A Cancer Journal for Clinicians 2007; 57:7–28.

73. DeForge D, et al. Fertility following spinal cord injury: a systematic review. 2005; 43(12):693–703.

74. Nicolle LE. Asymptomatic bacteriuria. Review and discussion of the IDSA guidelines. Int J Antimicrob Agents 2006; 28 (1 suppl):S42–S48.

75. Cross L, Meythaler JM, Tuel SM, Cross AL. Pregnancy following spinal cord injury. In: Rehabilitation Medicine Adding Life to Years. (special issue) West J Med 1991; 157:607–611.

76. Ohry A, Peleg D, Goldman J, David A, Rozin R. Sexual function, pregnancy and delivery in spinal cord injured women. Gynecol Obstet Invest 1978; 9:281–291.

77. Greenspoon JS, Paul RH. Paraplegia and quadriplegia: special considerations during pregnancy, labor and delivery. Am J Obstet Gynecol 1986; 155:738–741.

78. ACOG Committee Opinion: Number 275. Obstetric management of patients with spinal cord injuries. Obstet Gynecol 2002; 100(3):625–627.

79. Kang AH. Traumatic spinal cord injury. Clin Obstet Gynecol. 2005; 48:67–72.

80. Guttman L, Paeslack V. Cardiac irregularities during labor in paraplegic women. Paraplegia 1965; 3:144–147.

81. Wanner MB, Rageth CJ, Zach OA. Pregnancy and autonomic hyperreflexia in patients with spinal cord lesions. Paraplegia 1986; 6:482–490.

82. Gimousky ML, Ojeda A, Ozaki R, Zerne S. Management of autonomic hyperreflexia associated with low spinal cord lesion. Am J Obstet Gynecol 1985; 153(2):223–224.

83. McGregor JA, Meeuwsen J. Autonomic hyperreflexia: mortal danger for spinal cord damaged women in labor. Am J Obst Gynecol 1985; 151(3):330–333.

84. Young BK, Katz M, Klein SA. Pregnancy after spinal cord injury: altered maternal fetal response to labor. Obstet Gynecol 1983; 62(1):59–63.

85. Rossier A, Ruffiex A, Zieglar W. Pregnancy and labor in high traumatic spinal cord lesions. Paraplegia 1969; 7:210–215.

86. Tabsh KMA, Brinkmau CR, Reff RA. Autonomic dysreflexia in pregnancy. Obstet Gynecol 1981; 60:119–121.

87. Schonwald G, Fish KJ, Perkash I. Cardiovascular complications during anesthesia in chronic spinal cord injured patients. Anesthesiology 1981; 55:550–558.

88. Baker ER, Cardena DD, Benedetti TJ. Risks associated with pregnancy in spinal cord injury women. Obstet Gynecol 1992; 80(3):425–428.

89. Goller H, Paeslack V. Our experiences about pregnancy and delivery of the paraplegic woman. Paraplegia 1970; 8:161–166.

90. Goller H, Paeslack V. Pregnancy damage and birth complications in children of paraplegic women. Paraplegia 1972; 10:213–217.

91. Westgren N, Huttling C, Levi R, Serger A, Westgren M. Sexuality in women with traumatic spinal cord injury. Acta Obstet Gynecol Scandinavia 1997; 76:977–983.

92. Elliott SL. Problems of sexual function after spinal cord injury. Prog Brain Res. 2006; 152:387–399.

93. Masters WH, Johnson VE. Human Sexual Response. Boston, MA, Little, Brown, 1966.

94. Sipski ML. Spinal cord injury: what is the effect on sexual response? J Am Paraplegia Soc 1991; 14:40–43.

95. Sipski ML. Sexual response in women with spinal cord injuries: implications for our understanding of the able bodied. J Sex Marital Ther 1999; 25(1):11–22.

96. Sipski ML, Alexander CJ, Rosen RC. Physiologic parameters associated with sexual arousal in women with incomplete spinal cord injuries. Arch Phys Med Rehabil 1997; 78(3):305–313.

97. Berard EJJ. The sexuality of spinal cord injured women: physiology and pathophysiology. A review. Paraplegia 1989; 27:99–112.

98. Thornton CE. Sexual counseling of women with spinal cord injuries. Sex Disability. 1979; 2:267–277.

99. Duchan SH, Gill K. Sexuality after Spinal Cord Injury: Answers to your questions. Baltimore, Paul H Brooks Publishing, 1997.

100. Wein AJ. Pharmacological treatment of lower urinary tract dysfunction in the female patient. Urol Clin North Am 1985; 12:259–269.

101. Jackson AB. Bladder management in women. PM&R Clin North Am 1993; 4(2):321–327.

102. Wan J, McGuire EJ. Augmentation cystoplasty and closure of the urethra for the destroyed lower urinary tract. J Am Paraplegia Soc 1990; 13(3):40–45.

103. Timoney AG, Shaw PJR. Urological outcome in female patients with spinal cord injury: the effectiveness of intermittent catheterization. Paraplegia 1990; 28:556–563.

104. McQuire J, Savastano J. Comparative urological outcome in women with spinal cord injury. J Urol 1986; 135:730–731.

105. Jackson AB, DeVivo M. Urological long-term follow-up in women with spinal cord injury. Arch Phys Med Rehabil 1992; 73:1029–1034.

106. Mentor RR. Aging with a spinal cord injury. Arc Phys Med Rehabil 1998; 36:186–189.

107. Jiang SD, Dai LY, Jiang LS. Osteoporosis after spinal cord injury. Osteoporos Int 2006; 17:180–192.

108. Bauman WA, Spungen AM. Disorders of carbohydrate and lipid metabolism in veterans with paraplegia or quadriplegia. A model of premature aging. Met: Clin Exp 1994; 43:749–756.

109. Avimadje AM, Pellieux S, Goupille P, Zerkak D, Valat JP, Fouquet B. Destructive hip disease complicating traumatic paraplegia. Joint, Bone, Spine: Revue du Rhumatisme 2000; 67(4):334–336.

110. Lal S. Premature degenerative shoulder changes in spinal cord injury patients. Spinal Cord 1998; 36:186–189.

111. Bauman WA, Spungen AM, Wang J, Pierson RN, Jr., Schwartz E. Relationship of fat mass and serum estradiol with lower extremity bone in persons with chronic spinal cord injury. Women to Women 2006; 290:E1098–E1103.

112. Barber DB, Janus RB, Wade WH. Neuroarthropathy: an overuse injury of the shoulder in quadriplegia. J Spinal Cord Med 1996; 19(1):9–11.

113. Sie IH, Waters RL, Adkins RH, Gellman H. Upper extremity pain in the postrehabilitation spinal cord injured patient., Arch Phys Med Rehabil 1992; 73:44–48.

114. Campbell CC, Koris MJ. Etiologies of shoulder pain following cervical spinal cord injury. Clin Ortho Rel Res 1996; 322:140–145.

115. Verdier-Sevrain S, Bonte F, Gilchrest B. Biology of estrogens in skin: implications for skin aging. Exp Dermatol 2006; 15(2):83–94.

116. Sarrel PM. Ovarian hormones and the circulation. Maturitas 1990; 590:287–298.

117. Niskanen L, Laitinen T, Tuppurainen M, Saarikoski S, Kroger H, Alhava E, Hartikainen J. Does postmenopausal hormone replacement therapy affect cardiac autonomic regulation in osteoporotic women? Menopause 2002; 9:52–57.

118. Bolognia JL, Braverman IM, Rousseau ME, Sarrel PM. Skin changes in menopause. Maturitas 1989; 11:295–304.

119. Yin W, Gore AC. Neuroendocrine control of reproductive aging: roles of GnRH neurons. Reproduction 2006; 131(3):403–414.

120. Ottolenghi C, Uda M, Hamatani T, Crisponi L, Garcia JE, Ko M, Pilia G, Sforza C, Schlessinger D, Forabosco A. Aging of oocyte, ovary, and human reproduction, Ann N Y Acad Sci 2004; 1034:117–131.

121. Uebelhart D, Demiaux-Domenec B, Roth M. Chantraine A. Bone metabolism in spinal cord injured individuals and in others who have prolonged immobilization. A review. Paraplegia 1995; 33:669–673.

122. Welner S. Contraception, sexually transmitted diseases and menopause, in Women with Physical Disabilities: Achieving and Maintaining Health and Well-being. Krotoski DM, Nosek MA, Turk MA, eds. Paula H. Brookes Publishing Co., Baltimore, MD, 196, pp 81–90.

123. Management of osteoporosis in postmenopausal women: 2006 position statement of The North American Menopause Society. Menopause. 2006; 13:340–367.

124. Abel R. Gerner HJ, Smit C, Meiners T. Residual deformity of the spinal canal in patients with traumatic paraplegia and secondary changes of the spinal cord. Spinal Cord 1999; 37:14–19.

125. Winter RB, Lonstein JE, Denis F. Pain patterns in adult scoliosis. Ortho Clin No Am 1988; 19:339–345.

126. Nash CL, Kevins K. A literal look at pulmonary function in scoliosis. In Proceedings of the Scoliosis Research Society. J Bone and Joint Surg 1974; 46A:440.

127. Coonrad RW, Feierstein MS. Progression of scoliosis in the adult. J Bone Joint Surg 1976; 58A:156.

128. Klingbeil H, Baer HR, Wilson PE. Aging with a disability. Arch Phys Med Rehabil 2004; 85:68–73.

129. Mohit AA, Mirza S, James J, Goodkin R. Charcot arthropathy in relation to autonomic dysreflexia in spinal cord injury: case report and review of the literature. J Neurosurg Spine 2005; 2(4):476–480.

130. Selmi F, Frankel HL Kumaraguru AP, Apostopouos V. Charcot joint of the spine, a cause of autonomic dysreflexia in spinal cord injured patients. Spinal Cord 2002; 40(9):481–483.

131. Yamauchi Y, Kojh T, Miyazaki H, Kimura S, Arai T. Treatment of hyperhidrosis with caudal epidural alcohol block in a patient with cervical cord injury. Masui. Japanese J of Anesthes 1993; 42(4):606–610.

132. McKinley WO, Jackson AB, Cardenas DD, DeVivo MJ. Long-term medical complications after traumatic spinal cord injury: a regional model systems analysis. Arch Phys Med Rehabil 1999; 80:1402–1410.

133. Matthew KA, Meilahan EN, Kuller LH, et al. Menopause and risk factors for coronary heart disease. N Engl J Med 1989; 321:641–646.

134. Cauley JA, Gutais JP, Kuller LH, Powel JG. The relation of endogenous sex steroid hormone concentrations to serum lipid and lipoprotein levels in the post menopausal women. Am J Epid 1990; 132:884–894.

135. Welner S. Physiologic changes in menopause-effects on women with disabilities. Proceedings of conference on promoting health and wellness of women with disabilities. August 2, 1999, San Antonio, TX.

136. Yarkony GM, Heinemann AW. Pressure ulcers, in Stover SL, DeLisa JA, Whiteneck GG, eds. Spinal Cord Injury: Clinical Outcomes from the Model Systems. Aspen Publishing, Gaithersburg, MD. 1995, pp 199–219.

137. Colachis SC. Autonomichyperflexia with spinal cord injury. J of Am Paraplegia Soc 1990; 15:171–186.

138. Allen JB, Stover SL, Jackson AB, Richards JS. Autonomic dysreflexia and the menstrual cycle in women with spinal cord injury: A case report. NeuroRehabilitation 1991; 1(4):58–62.

139. Erlik Y, Meldrun DR, Judd HL. Estrogen levels in post menopausal women with hot flashes. Obstet Gynecol 1982; 49:403–407.

140. Nosek MA, Gill CJ, National Center for Health Statistics, CDC. Use of cervical and breast cancer screening among women with and without functional limitations, U.S. 1994–95. Morbidity and Mortality Weekly Report. 1998; 47(4):853–856.

141. Grady D, Rubin SM, Petitti DB et al. Hormone therapy to prevent disease and prolong life in postmenopausal women. Ann Int Med 1992; 177:1016.

142. Shairer C, Lubin J, Troisi R, Sturgeon S, Brinton L, Hoover R. Menopausal estrogen and estrogen-progestin replacement therapy and breast cancer risk. JAMA 2000; 283(4):485–491.

143. Krieger N, Lowy I, Aronowitz R, Bigby J, Dickersin K, Garner E, Gaudilliere JP, Hinestrosa C, Hubbard R, Johnson PA, Missmer SA, Norsigian J, Pearson, Rosenberg CE, Rosenberg L, Rosenkrantz BG, Seaman B, Sonnenschein C, Soto AM, Thornton J, Weisz G. Hormone replacement therapy, cancer, controversies, and women's health: historical, epidemiological, biological, clinical, and advocacy perspectives. J Epidemiol Community Health 2005; 59:740–748.

144. Bhavnani B. Women's health initiative study. J Obstet Gynaecol Can 2002; 24:689–690.

145. Johnson SR. Hormone replacement therapy: applying the results of the Women's Health Initiative. Clev Clin J Med 2002; 69:682, 685.

146. Cranney A, Tugwell P, Zytaruk N, Robinson V, Weaver B, Shea B, Wells G, Adachi J, Waldegger L, Guyatt G. Meta-analysis of calcitonin for the treatment of postmenopausal osteoporosis. Endocrine Reviews 2002; 23(4):540–551.

147. Cranney A, Tugwell P, Zytaruk N, Robinsdon V, Weaver B, Adachi J, Wells G, Shea B, Guyatt G. Meta-analysis of raloxifene for the prevention and treatment of postmenopausal osteoporosis. Endocrine Reviews 2002; 23(4):524–528.

148. Fitzpatrick LA. Selective estrogen receptor modulator and phytoestrogens: new therapies for the postmenopausal woman. Mayo Clinic Proc 1999; 74:601–607.

149. Shea B, Wells G, Cranney A, Zytaruk N, Robinson V, Griffith L, Ortiz Z, Peterson J, Adachi J, Tugwell P, Guyatt G. Endocrine Reviews. 2002; 23(4):552–559.

150. Papadimitropoulos E, Wells G, Shea B, Gillespie W, Weaver B, Zytaruk N, Cranney A, Adachi J, Tugwell P, Josse R, Greenwood C, Guyatt G. Meta-analysis of the efficacy of vitamin D treatment in preventing osteoporosis in postmenopausal women. Endocrine Reviews 2002; 23(4):560–569.

151. Kessel B. Alternatives to estrogen for menopausal women. Proceedings of the Society for Experimental Biology and Medicine 1998; 217:38–44.

152. Tham DM, Gardner CD, Haskell WL. Potential health benefits of dietary phytoestrogens: a review of clinical, epidemiological and mechanistic evidence. J Clin Endocrinol Metab 1998; 83:2223–2235.

153. Atmaca A, Gedik O. Effects of alendronate and risedronate on bone mineral density and bone turnover markers in late postmenopausal women with osteoporosis. Adv Ther 2006; 23:842–853.

154. Black DM, Schwartz AV, Ensrud KE, Cauley JA, Levis S, Quandt SA, Satterfield S, Wallace RB, Bauer DC, Palermo L, Wehren LE, Lombardi A, Santora AC, Cummings SR. Effects of continuing or stopping alendronate after 5 years of treatment: the Fracture Intervention Trial Long-Term Extension (FLEX): a randomized trial. JAMA 2006; 296:2927–2938.

155. Price PA, Faus SA, Williamson MK. Bisphosphonates alendronate and ibandronate inhibit artery calcification at doses comparable to those that inhibit bone resorption. 2001. Arterioscler Thromb Vasc Bio 2001; 21(5):817–824.

156. Heras R, Zubillaga R, Castrillo TM, Montalvo Moreno JJ. Osteonecrosis of the jaws and bisphosphonates. Report of fifteen cases. Therapeutic recommendations. Med Oral Pathol Oral Cir Bucal 2007; 12:E267–E271.

157. Mueck AO, Seeger H. Statins and menopausal health. J Br Menopause Soc 2002; 8(4):141–146.

158. Coakly RM, Holmbeck GN, Friedman D, Greenley RN, Thill AW. A longitudinal study of pubertal timing, parent-child conflict and cohesion in females of young adolescents with spina bifida. J Pediatr Psych 2002; 27:471–473.

159. Hochhaus F, Butenandt O, Schwarz HP, Ring-Mrozik E. Auxological and endocrinological evaluation of children with hydrocephalus and/or meningomyelocele. Eur J Pediatr 1997; 156:597–601.

160. Trollmann R, Strehl E, Dorr HG. Precocious puberty in children with myelomeningocele: treatment with gonadotropin-releasing hormone analogues. Develop Med & Child Neurol 1998; 40:38–43.

161. Trollman R, Dorr HG, Strehl E, Katalinic A, Beyer R, Wenzel D. Growth and pubertal development in patients with meningomyelocele: a retrospective analysis. Acta Paediatr 1996; 85:76–80.

162. Meyers, Landau H. Precocious puberty in myelomeningocele patients. J Ped Ortho. 1984; 4:28–31.

163. Greene SA, Frank M, Zachmann M, Prader A. Growth and sexual development in children with meningomyelocoele. Eur J Pediatr 1985; 144:146–148.

164. Elias ER, Sadeghi-Nejad A. Precocious puberty in girls with myelodysplasia. Pediatrics 1994; 3:521–522.

165. Hayden PW, Davenport SLH, Campbelle MM. Adolescents with myelodysplasia: Impact of physical disability on emotional maturation. Pediatrics 1979; 1:53–59.

166. Michael T, Niggeman B, Moers A, et al,. Risk factors for latex allergy in patients with spinal bifida. Clin Exp Allergy 1996; 26:934–939.

167. Nieto A, Estornell F, Mazon A et al. Allergy to latex in spina bifida: A multivariate study of associated factors in 100 consecutive patients. J Allergy Clin Immunol 1996; 98:501–507.

168. DeSwert La, Van Laser KM, Verpoorten CM, et al. Determination of independent risk factors and comparative analysis of diagnostic methods for immediate type latex allergy in spina bifida patients. Clin Exp Allergy 1997; 27:1067–1076.

169. Reitberg CCT, Lindhout D. Adult patients with spina bifida cystica: genetic counseling, pregnancy and delivery. Eur J Obstet Gynecol 1993; 52:63–70.

170. Broughton NS. Medelaus' orthopeaedic management of spina bifida cystica. 3rd ed. Ed. by Broughton NS & Menelaus MB, 1998.

171. McLaurin RL, Oppenheimer S, Dias L, Kaplan WE eds. Spina bifida: a multidisciplinary approach. Praeger Publishers, 1986.

172. Aldana PR, Ragheb J, Sevald J, et al. Cerebrospinal fluid shunt complications after urological procedures in children with myelodysplasia. Neurosurgery 2002; 50(2):313–320.

173. Sipski ML. A Physiatrists view regarding the report of the international consensus conference of female sexual dysfunction: Potential concerns regarding women with disabilities. J Sex Marital Ther 2001; 27:215–216.

174. McRarlane J, Hughes RB, Nosek MA, Groff JY, Swedlend N, Dolan Mullen P. Abuse assessment screen–disability (AAS-D):measuring frequency, type, and perpetrator of abuse toward women with physical disabilities. J Women's Health Gend Based Med. 2001; 10(9):861–866.

175. McDonnell GV, McCann JP. Issues of medical management in adults with spina bifida. Child Nerv Syst 2000; 16(4):222–227.

176. Fujimoto A, Ebbin AJ, Wilson MG, Nakamoto M. Successful pregnancy in women with meningomyelocele. Lancet 1973; 1:104.

177. Powell B, Garvey M. Complications of Maternal spina bifida. Ir J Med Sci 1984; 153(1):20–21.

178. Ellison FE. Term pregnancy in a patient with myelomeningocele, uretero-ileostomy, and partial paraparesis. Am J Obstet Gynecol 1975; 123(1):33–34.

179. Mann WJ, Jones DED. Pregnancy complicated by maternal neural tube defect and an ileal conduit: A case report. J Repro Med 1976; 17(6):339–341.

180. Opitz JM. Pregnancy in women with meningomyelocele. Lancet 1973; 1:368–369.

181. Wynn JS, Mellor S, Morewood GA. Pregnancy in patients with spina bifida cystica. The Practitioner 1979; 222:543–549.

182. Farine D, Jackson U, Portale A, Baxi l, Fox HE. Pregnancy complicated by maternal spina bifida: A report of two cases. J Repro Med 1988; 33(3):323–326.

183. Liakos AM, Bradley NK, Magram G, Muszynski C. Hydrocephalus and reproductive health of women: The medical implications of maternal shunt dependency in 70 women and 138 pregnancies. Neurol Res 2000; 22:69–88.

184. Arata M, Grover S, Dunne K, Bryan D. Pregnancy outcome and complications in women with spina bifida. J Repro Med 2000; 43(9):743–748.

185. Shieve LA, Handler A, Hershow R, Persky V, Davis S. Urinary tract infection during pregnancy: Its association with morbidity perinatal outcome. Am J Public Health 1994; 84:405–410.

186. Hudson CN. Ileostomy in pregnancy. Proc R Soc Med 1972; 65:281–283.

187. To WWK, Wong MWN. Kyphoscoliosis complicating pregnancy. Int J Gynecol Obstet 1996; 55:123–128.

188. Samuel P, Driscoll DA, Landon MB, et al. Cerebrospinal Fluid shunts in pregnancy: Report of two cases and review of the literature. Am J Perinatol 1988; 5(1):22–25.

189. Monfared AH, Koh KS, Apuzzo MLJ, Collea JV. Obstetric management of pregnant women with extracranial shunts. CMA Journal 1979; 120:562–563.

190. Cusimano MD, Meffe FM, Gentili F Sermer M. Ventriculoperitoneal shunt malfunction during pregnancy. Neurosurgery 1990; 27(6):969–971.

191. Kleinman G, Sutherling W, Martinez M, Tabsh K. Malfunction of ventriculoperitoneal shunt during pregnancy. Obstet Gynecol 1983; 61:753–755.

192. Gast MJ, Grubb RL, Strickler RC. Maternal hydrocephalus and pregnancy. Obstet Gynecol 1983; 62:29S–31S.

193. Iborra J, Pages E, Cuxart A, Poca A, Sahuquillo J. Increased intracranial pressure in myelomeningocele (MMC) patients never shunted: Results of a prospective preliminary study. Spinal Cord 2000; 38:495–497.

194. McDonnell GV, McCann JP, Craig JJ, Crone M. Prevalence of the Chiari/Hydrosyringomelia Complex in adults with spina bifida: Preliminary results. Eur J Pediatr Surg 2000; 10(suppl 1):18–19.

195. Bowman RM, McLone DG, Grant JA, Tomita T, Ito JA. Spina bifida outcome: A 25-year prospective. Pediatr Neurosurg 2001; 34:114–120.

196. American College of Obstetricians and Gynecologists (ACOG). Neural Tube Defects. ACOG Practice Bulletin number 44, July 2003.

197. Laurence KM, Beresford A. Continence, friends, marriage and children in 51 adults with spina bifida. Dev Med Child Neurology 1975; 17(supp 35):123–128.

198. Carter CO, Evans K. Children of adult survivors with spina bifida cystica. Lancet 1973; 2:924–926.

199. Czeizel AE, Dudas I. Prevention of the first occurrence of neural tube defects by periconceptional vitamin supplementation. N Engl J Med 1992; 327:1832–1835.

200. Igbal MM. Birth defects: Prevention of Neural tube defects by periconceptional use of folic acid and screening. J Prev Soc Med 1999; 18(1):52–65.

201. Shaw GM, Lammer EJ, Zhu H, et al. Maternal periconceptional vitamin use, genetic variation of infant reduced folate carrier (A80G), and risk of spina bifida. Am J Med Gen 2002; 108:1–6.

202. van der Put NMJ, van den Heuvel LP, Steegers-Theunissen RPM, et al. Decreased methylene tetrahydrofolate reductase activity due to the 677-T mutation in families with spina bifida offspring. J Mol Med 1996; 74:691–694.

203. Neumann PE, Frankel WN, Letts VA, et al. Multifactorial inheritance of neural tube defects: localization of the major gene and recognition of modifiers in ct mutant mice. Nat Genet 1994; 49:143–149.

204. Daly S, Mills JL, Molloy AM, Conley M, Lee YJ, Kirke PN, Weir DG, Scott JM. Minimum effective dose of folic acid for food fortification to prevent neural-tube defects. Lancet 1997; 350:1666–1669.

205. Bailey LB. New standard for dietary folate intake in pregnant women. Am J Clin Nutr 2000; 71(suppl):1304S–1307S.

206. Children's Memorial Hospital. Spina bifida information for teens and young adults. Available at: http://www.childrensmemorial.org/depts/motionanalysis/conditions/tipsforteens.asp. Accessed October 31, 2007.

207. Noonan CW, Kathman SJ, White MC. Prevalence estimates for MS in the United States and evidence of an increasing trend for women. Neurology 2002; 58:136–138.

208. Sadovnick AD, Ebers GC. Epidemiology of multiple sclerosis: a critical overview. Can J Neurol Sci 1993; 20:17–29.

209. Confaverux C, Aimard G, Devic M. Course and prognosis of multiple sclerosis assessed by the computerized data processing of 349 patients. Brain 1980; 103:281–300.

210. Weinshenker BG, Bass B, Rice GPA, et al. The natural history of multiple sclerosis: a geographically based study. I. Clinical course and disability. Brain 1989; 112:133–146.

211. Confavreux C, Hutchinson M, Hours MM, Cortinovis-Tourniaire P, Moreau T, and the Pregnancy in Multiple Sclerosis Group. Rate of pregnancy-related relapse in multiple sclerosis. N Eng J Med 1998; 339(5):285–291.

212. Confavreux C, Compston DAS, Hommes OR, McDonald WI, Thompson AJ. EDMUS, a European database for multiple sclerosis. J Neurol Neurosurg Psychiatry 1992; 55:671–676.

213. Ferrero S, Pretta S, Ragni N. Multiple sclerosis: management issues during pregnancy. Eur J Obstet Gynecol Reproduc Biol 2004; 115:3–9.

214. Vukusic S, Hutchinson M, Hours M, Moreau T, Cortinovis-Tourniaire P, Adeleine P, Confavreux C. Pregnancy and multiple sclerosis (the PRIMS study): clinical predictors of post-partum relapse. The Pregnancy In Multiple Sclerosis Group. Brain 2004; 127(6):1353–1360. Epub 2004 May 6. Erratum in: Brain. 2004; 127(8):1912.

215. Dorotta IR, Schubert A. Multiple sclerosis and aesthetic implications. Curr Opin Anaesthesiol 2002; 15:365–370.

216. Janssen NM, Genta S. The effects of immunosuppressive and anti-inflammatory medications on fertility, pregnancy and lactation. Arch Inter Med 2000; 160:610–619.

217. Committee on Drugs, American Academy of Pediatrics. Transfer of drugs and other chemicals into human milk. Pediatrics 2001; 108:776–779.

218. Sandberg-Wollheim M, Frank D, Goodwin TM, Giesser B, Lopez-Bresnahan M, Stam-Moraga M, Chang P, Francis GS. Pregnancy outcomes during treatment with interferon beta-1a in patients with multiple sclerosis. Neurol 2005; 65:802–806.

219. Vukusic S, Confavreux C. Pregnancy and multiple sclerosis: the children of PRIMS. Clin Neurol Neurosurg 2006; 108:266–270.

220. Lublin FD, Reingold SC. Defining the clinical course of multiple sclerosis: results of an international survey. Neurology 1996; 46:907–911.

221. Sharts-Hopko NC, Sullivan MP. Beliefs, perceptions, and practices related to osteoporosis risk reduction among women with multiple sclerosis. Rehabil Nurs 2002; 27(6):232–236.

222. Sharts-Hopko NC, Smeltzer S. Perceptions of women with multiple sclerosis about osteoporosis follow-up. J Neurosci Nurs 2004; 36(4):189–194, 199.

223. Wegmann TG, Lin H, Guilbert L, Mosmann TR. Bidirectional cytokine interactions in the maternal-fetal relationship: is successful pregnancy a TH2 phenomenon? Immunol Today 1993; 14:353–356.

224. National Multiple Sclerosis Society. The MS information sourcebook. 2001. Available at: http://www.nationalmssociety.org/Sourcebook-Pregnancy.asp. Accessed October 22, 2007.

225. DeVivo MJ, Fine PR. Spinal cord injury: its short term impact on marital status. Arch Phys Med Rehabil 1985; 66:501–504.

226. DeVivo MJ, Jenkins KD, Go BK. Outcomes of post-spinal cord injured marriages. J Am Paraplegia Soc 1990; 13:39–40.

227. Reis JP. Parenting with a disability: how different is it really? Resourceful Woman 1992; 1.

228. American Medical Association. Diagnostic and Treatment Guidelines on Domestic Violence. Chicago, 1992.

229. Doucette J. Violent acts against disabled women. Toronto: Disabled Women's Network, 1986.

230. Nosek MA, Howland CA. Breast and cervical cancer screening among women with physical disabilities. Arch Phys Med Rehabil 1997; 78(suppl 5):39–44.

231. ACOG Task Force in Primary and Preventive Health Care. The Obstetricians and Gynecologists and Primary Preventive Health Care, Washington, D.C., American College of Obstetricians and Gynecologists, 1993.

232. Chevarley FM, Thierry JM, Gill CJ, Ryerson AB, Nosek MA. Health, preventive health care, and health care access among women with disabilities in the 1994–1995 National Health Interview Survey, Supplement on Disability. Women's Health Issues. 2006; 16(6):297–312.

233. Nosek MA, Hughes RB, Robinson-Whelen S, Taylor HB, Howland CA. Physical activity and nutritional behaviors of women with physical disabilities: physical, psychological, social, and environmental influences. Women's Health Issues, 2006; 16:323–333.

V

NEUROLOGIC ASPECTS OF SPINAL CORD CARE

35 Acute Nontraumatic Myelopathies

Florian P. Thomas
Robert M. Woolsey

This chapter and Chapter 36 on acute and chronic nontraumatic myelopathies describe the pathology, clinical features, and treatment of spinal cord disorders not directly caused by trauma. Some formerly important spinal cord diseases such as tabes dorsalis and poliomyelitis for practical purposes no longer exist in the United States or Canada, and will not be discussed.

In this chapter a description of the symptoms and signs of spinal cord injury and dysfunction (SCI) is followed by a review of how clinical features lead to conclusions as to the white and gray matter structures involved in a given patient. Six possible spinal cord, one conus medullaris, and one cauda equina configurations are discussed (Table 35.1).

Under each of these syndromes are listed the acute and chronic spinal cord diseases that might produce it. Finally, each of the listed diseases is described in detail.

To use this chapter and Chapter 36 for clinical management, the reader should (a) make an inventory of the patient's neurologic features and consider if they represent central (CNS) vs. peripheral (PNS) nervous system involvement such as spinal cord vs. spinal nerve root disease; (b) identify the parts of the spinal cord that appear to be involved; (c) match this patient-derived diagram with one of the six syndromes; (d) look at the differential diagnosis of acute and chronic disorders listed as possible causes; (e) review the description of those conditions and order appropriate diagnostic tests; and (f) having established the diagnosis, prescribe the indicated treatment. This syndromic approach has proved useful even though many patients have incomplete lesions that may not fully meet the classical descriptions.

THE NEUROLOGIC MANIFESTATIONS OF SPINAL CORD DISEASE

Motor Abnormalities

Motor abnormalities result from dysfunction of descending upper motor neuron (UMN) pathways that target the anterior horn cells (AHC) and mediate movement. Pathways include the corticospinal, rubrospinal, and reticulospinal tracts. The most important one is the corticospinal tract, but both the reticulospinal and rubrospinal tracts have connections from the cerebral cortex, and movement is possible following destruction of the corticospinal tract (1).

The initial feature of UMN dysfunction is incoordination of movement. Weakness and paralysis occur when 50% and 90%, respectively, of UMNs stop functioning (2). Weakness caused by lower motor neuron (LMN) disease reflects the loss of about 50% of AHC function (3). AHC disease can cause severe muscle atrophy (up to 80% of volume), while paralysis from UMN disease usually causes no more than 20% loss of muscle bulk. AHC dysfunction is frequently accompanied by fasciculations in the muscle that it innervates.

Acute paralysis due to spinal cord disease is accompanied by muscle hypotonia and loss of tendon and cutaneous reflexes, and is also referred to as spinal shock (4). It is caused by the sudden withdrawal of neural activity descending to the AHCs from the cerebral cortex and brain stem. Some of these pathways inhibit AHCs and others facilitate them, but the overall effect is facilitation. Lack of facilitation causes motor neuron hyperpolarization, so that the preserved connections with dorsal root afferents from muscle spindles and cutaneous receptors cannot adequately depolarize membranes and generate action potentials in the AHCs. Over several days to several weeks, muscle tone and reflexes return, probably because of the activation of "silent synapses," i.e. synapses on motor neurons connected to dorsal root afferent fibers that have not been active. Also, dorsal root afferent fibers "sprout" to occupy synaptic sites vacated by the degenerating descending fibers (5). When this occurs, muscle hypertonicity and tendon reflex hyperactivity develop (spasticity). Spastic paralysis is often associated with the presence of an extensor plantar response (Babinski sign).

In more slowly progressive weakness of spinal origin, a gradual replacement of descending facilitatory influences by dorsal root and horn facilitatory influence results in slowly developing spasticity without an intervening phase of hypotonia and hyporeflexia.

Table 35.1 Classification of Spinal Cord and Cauda Equina Syndromes

Syndrome	Affected Pathways	Features	Causes
Total Cord (Bilateral)	All pathways	Complete or near complete loss of strength, sensation, and sphincter control below the level of the lesion	Acute: vascular malformation decompression sickness intramedullary abscess, transverse myelitis, non-organic, cord hemorrhage
Anterior or Ventral Cord (Bilateral)	Anterior 2/3 of cord: Spinothalamic tracts Corticospinal tracts	Loss of pain/temperature sensation Weakness and reflex changes	Acute: cord infarction (anterior spinal artery syndrome), disk herniation Chronic: radiation myelopathy disk herniation
	Descending autonomic tracts to sacral segments:	Incontinence	
Dorsal Cord (Bilateral)	Dorsal columns: Corticospinal tracts:	Gait ataxia/paresthesia Acute: flaccid, hyporeflexia Chronic: hypertonia, hyperreflexia, Babinski sign	Acute: MS Chronic: Friedreich ataxia, B12 deficiency, tumors, HIV, vascular malformation, cervical spondylosis, atlantoaxial subluxation
	Descending autonomic tracts to sacral segments:	Incontinence	
Lateral Cord Brown-Séquard (Unilateral)	Spinothalamic tract:	Contralateral: impaired pain/temperature sensation	Acute: infarction, MS, trauma
	Dorsal columns:	Ipsilateral: paresthesias (often spared)	Chronic: intramedullary or intradural extramedullary tumors
	Corticospinal tract:	Ipsilateral: weakness	
Central Cord (Bilateral)	Disruption of crossing fibers: Spinothalamic tract:	Impaired pain/temperature at the level of the lesion, but normal above/below	Acute: neck hyperextension in presence of spondylosis, hemorrhage
	Dorsal Columns spared: Reflex arch:	Proprioception, vibration intact Reflex loss in the analgesic area	Chronic: syringomyelia, intramedullary tumor
	Large lesions involving anterior horns or corticospinal tracts	Weakness	
Pure Motor Syndrome (Bilateral)	UMN	Incoordination, weakness, hyperreflexia, Babinski signs	HTLV-1 or HIV-1 associated myelopathy, spondylosis, hereditary spastic paraplegia, motor neuron diseases, post-polio syndrome, electric shock
	LMN	Weakness, atrophy, fasciculations	
	UMN and LMN	Combination of both	
Cauda Equina (Unilateral or bilateral)	5 lumbar, 4 sacral pairs of roots supplying the legs & perineum	L5–S1 involvement: lower back pain radiating to posterior thighs and calves, weak foot plantar flexion, loss of ankle jerks, sphincter and sexual dysfunction, fasciculations Lesions at higher levels add higher level motor, sensory, and reflex loss	Acute: disk herniation, trauma Chronic: disk herniation, Paget, spondylosis, arachnoiditis, ankylosing spondylitis, infection, intradural, extramedullary or extradural tumors
Conus Medullaris Syndrome (Usually bilateral)	Distal end of the spinal cord	Back and radicular pain, UMN signs Incontinence and sexual dysfunction Variable leg weakness Perianal sensory loss	Trauma, tumors, inflammation (e.g., ankylosing spondylitis)

Spasms are a phenomenon related to but not identical with spasticity, in which activation of small myelinated and unmyelinated dorsal root afferents excites motor neurons in several adjacent spinal segments to cause contraction of synergistic muscles. The most common types of spasms are flexor, adductor, or extensor spasms in the legs of patients with paraplegia or tetraplegia (6).

Sensory Abnormalities

All sensory information passing from the periphery to the brain, except from the head, passes through the dorsal columns or the spinothalamic tracts of the spinal cord. The dorsal columns convey joint position, vibration, and touch sensation from the ipsilateral body and information about visceral distention. The lateral spinothalamic tract mediates temperature and pain sensation from the opposite side. An anterior spinothalamic tract also carries touch sensation.

Dorsal column dysfunction causes gait ataxia because the brain is deprived of knowledge about leg position. If a lesion affects the cervical cord, there is also arm ataxia. Vision can compensate for impaired proprioception to some degree. Dorsal column disease also causes paresthesias described as crawling, numbness, deadness, or tingling mainly in the distal limbs. Paresthesias probably result from ectopic discharges in damaged dorsal column axons and may be present before abnormalities can be detected on neurologic examination (7). Similar sensations can be evoked by electrical stimulation of the dorsal columns. A special type of paresthesia of dorsal column origin is the Lhermitte, an electric shock sensation over the neck that extends into the back and sometimes the limbs, often provoked by changes in head or neck position. Position sense is lost when ~75% of dorsal column axons have ceased working (2). Dorsal column function is tested by examining the ability to perceive both tuning fork vibration and changes in the position of toes and fingers without visual cues.

Lateral spinothalamic tract dysfunction reduces pain and temperature perception on the contralateral side of the body, one or two dermatomes below the level of the lesion, but rarely causes paresthesias. Patients become aware of their pain and temperature deficit when they experience painless cuts or burns. Bilateral lesions affect erection, ejaculation, and orgasm.

Pain

Spinal cord and nerve root disorders can produce several types of pain (8). Local and radicular pain is nociceptive, is generated from receptors, and is mediated through spinothalamic pathways. Central neuropathic pain, rarely seen as a presenting or early manifestation of spinal cord dysfunction, results from damage to spinal cord pain transmission pathways. A separate chapter deals with pain in greater detail.

Local pain arises from pain receptors in the paravertebral muscles, bones, or ligaments of the spine, although it may originate in the spinal cord itself, probably from blood vessel receptors in the cord. This pain is most intense over its source and can extend laterally to some degree. Vertebral involvement in the cervical and lumbar areas can result in pain in the shoulder and hip or buttock area, respectively, while pain originating in thoracic vertebrae may spread several inches of the midline. Less than 5% of local back or neck pain originates from the spinal cord or cauda equina. About 20% is caused by abnormalities of the spine. In 75% the cause is unknown (9); presumably it originates in the paravertebral structures. When local pain originates in the spinal cord, it often points to a mass lesion (tumor, abscess, hematoma), transverse myelitis, or infarction.

Radicular or nerve root pain is caused by the involvement of or traction on dorsal root ganglia, exemplified by the pain produced by a herniated intervertebral disk. It radiates into the dermatome of the involved root, i.e. arms, trunk, or legs.

Central pain is common in SCI but is, except for intramedullary tumors, multiple sclerosis (MS), and syringomyelia, rare in other spinal cord disorders. Onset is often months or years after injury. Usually described as burning or lancinating, it occurs in an area of impaired or absent sensation. It may occur in the perianal area and buttocks or diffusely below the level of SCI (10).

Neurogenic intermittent claudication, probably a type of peripheral neuropathic pain, occurs with lumbar spinal stenosis and spinal vascular abnormalities. Standing or walking cause dull back and leg pain, sometimes associated with numbness and leg weakness. The neurogenic presentation differs from intermittent peripheral vascular claudication by absence of signs of vascular insufficiency in the legs, although not uncommonly older patients have clinical features of both. Standing without walking causes symptoms in patients with neurogenic claudication, but standing does not produce symptoms in vascular claudication (11).

Sphincter Dysfunction

Bladder dysfunction occurs in practically all acute spinal cord conditions in which the cord is affected bilaterally, with resulting leg weakness. The bladder participates in the syndrome of spinal shock. Like limb muscles, the paralyzed detrusor and bladder sphincter muscles become flaccid and areflexic, which results in inability of the bladder to store urine; continual dribbling incontinence results. The detrusor and sphincter muscles eventually become hypertonic and hyperreflexic, and automatic voiding is provoked by bladder distention. If the condition involves the conus medullaris or cauda equina, detrusor and sphincter muscle flaccidity persists. In either case urinary tract infections are a common consequence.

If the spinal cord condition is of slower onset, there is no stage of flaccidity and areflexia, but rather slow onset spasticity. Due to a small-capacity hyperreflexic bladder, patients experience urinary frequency, urgent micturition, and urge incontinence. If the slowly progressive condition affects the conus medullaris or cauda equina, the bladder and sphincter muscles slowly become atonic and hyporeflexic, producing symptoms of infrequent urination, urinary retention, and overflow incontinence. Bladder symptoms are usually late and frequently inconspicuous in slowly progressive cord conditions (12).

The gastrointestinal system is analogously affected. LMN lesions result in slow stool propulsion and low anal sphincter tone, causing fecal incontinence. With UMN lesions, fecal retention develops due to external anal sphincter contraction. In either case, voluntary control over defecation is lost.

Altitudinal Neurologic Deficit

A "level," below which the patient has sensory, motor, or reflex abnormalities and above which sensory, motor, and reflex function is normal, is the hallmark of spinal cord disease.

SPINAL CORD AND CAUDA EQUINA SYNDROMES

All spinal cord disorders, whether acute or chronic, will present with neurologic signs and symptoms indicating that the spinal cord is involved primarily laterally, centrally, dorsally, ventrally, or totally. A syndrome of pure motor involvement exists. Intraspinal abnormalities can also cause neurologic symptoms by involving the conus medullaris or the cauda equina. Each of these syndromes may be complete, in which there is a total loss of function, or incomplete, in which case function is impaired but not totally lost. The neurologic history and examination provide the data by which these syndromes can be identified, greatly simplifying the differential diagnosis (Table 35.1).

Total Cord Syndrome

The cessation of function in all ascending and descending spinal cord pathways results in the loss of movement and all types of sensation below the level of the lesion, and the loss of bladder and bowel control (Figure 35.1).

The causes of a total cord syndrome include acute myelopathies, such as spinal cord vascular malformation, decompression sickness, epidural or intramedullary abscess, transverse myelitis, spinal cord hemorrhage, and simulated paraplegia.

Ventral Cord Syndrome

Here, tracts in the anterior two-thirds of the spinal cord are involved bilaterally; these encompass the corticospinal and spinothalamic tracts, and the descending autonomic tracts to the sacral centers for bladder control (Figure 35.2). Corticospinal tract involvement produces weakness and reflex changes, as in the dorsal cord syndrome. Spinothalamic tract deficits result in bilateral loss of pain and temperature sensation. Tactile, position, and vibratory sensation are normal. Urinary incontinence is usually present.

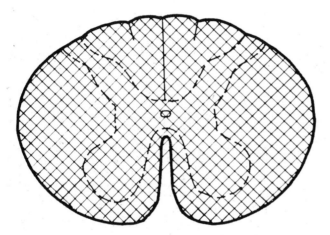

Figure 35.1   Total cord syndrome. Shading indicates a complete transverse spinal cord lesion. (From: Blackwood, W., Dodds, T. C., and Sommerville, J. C. *Atlas of Neuropathology*. Williams & Wilkins, Baltimore, 1964.)

Ventral cord syndrome results from acute myelopathies, such as infarction, disk herniation, and chronic disorders, such as disk herniation or radiation myelopathy.

Dorsal or Posterior Cord Syndrome

These presentations result from bilateral involvement of the corticospinal tracts, the dorsal columns, and the descending central autonomic tracts to bladder control centers in the sacral cord (Figure 35.3). Clinical features include paresthesias and gait ataxia. Corticospinal tract dysfunction produces weakness that if acute is accompanied by muscle flaccidity and hyporeflexia, and, if chronic, by muscle hypertonia and often by hyperreflexia. Extensor plantar responses and urinary incontinence may be present.

Causes include acute conditions such as relapsing-remitting MS, or chronic myelopathies such as Friedreich ataxia, HIV-associated myelopathy, vitamin B12 deficiency (subacute combined degeneration [SCD]), vascular malformations, primary or secondary progressive MS, cervical spondylolytic myelopathy, epidural or intradural extramedullary tumors, and atlanto-axial subluxation.

Lateral Cord Syndrome

Also known as Brown-Séquard syndrome, this unilateral constellation of dorsal column, corticospinal tract, and spinothalamic tract involvement produces paresthesias and weakness on the side of the lesion, and loss of pain and temperature on the opposite side, usually two to three levels below the level of the lesion (Figure 35.4). The dorsal column is at times not involved; then the partial syndrome consists of weakness and reflex changes on the side of the lesion and loss of pain and temperature on the opposite side. Unilateral involvement of descending autonomic fibers does not produce bladder symptoms.

Causes include acute myelopathies such as MS, trauma, or spinal cord infarction, or chronic myelopathies such as intramedullary or intradural extramedullary tumors.

Central Cord Syndrome

Central cord syndrome presents typically with loss of pain and temperature sensation in the distribution of one or many adjacent dermatomes at the site of the spinal cord lesion, caused

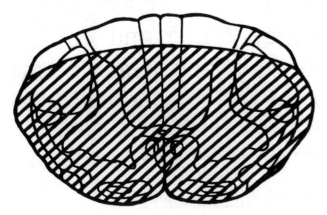

Figure 35.2   Ventral cord syndrome. Shading indicates affected areas. With permission of the American Spinal Injury Association (ASIA).

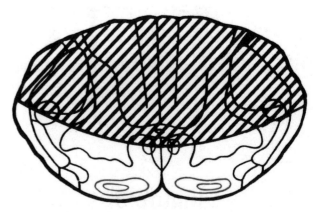

Figure 35.3   Dorsal cord syndrome. Shading indicates affected areas. With permission of ASIA.

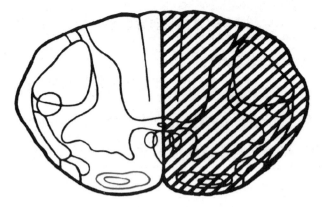

Figure 35.4 Lateral cord syndrome. Shading indicates affected areas. With permission of ASIA.

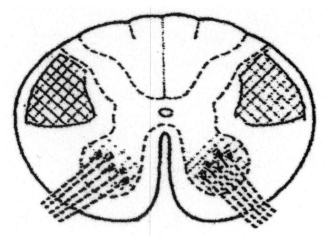

Figure 35.6 Pure motor syndrome. Shading indicates affected areas. (From Blackwood, W., Dodds, T. C., and Sommerville, J. C. *Atlas of Neuropathology.* Williams & Wilkins, Baltimore. 1964.)

by the disruption of crossing spinothalamic fibers. Dermatomes above and below the level of the lesion have normal pain and temperature sensation. Within the involved dermatomes, touch sensation is normal because touch fibers pass into the posterior columns immediately after entering the spinal cord. As a central lesion enlarges, it may encroach on the medial aspect of the corticospinal tracts or on the anterior horn gray matter; in either case, weakness in the analgesic areas may result. Fibers mediating the deep tendon reflexes are interrupted as they pass from the dorsal to the ventral horn, thus causing tendon reflex loss in the analgesic areas. As most lesions occur in the lower cervical region, the arms are predominantly affected. The sphincters and sacral sensation usually remain uninvolved (Figure 35.5).

The causes of a central cord syndrome include acute myelopathies, such as hemorrhage or hyperextension with cervical spondylolysis, or chronic myelopathies such as syringomyelia or intramedullary tumor.

Pure Motor Syndrome

When only UMNs are involved bilaterally, patients develop incoordination and weakness with hyperreflexia and extensor plantar responses. When LMN function is impaired bilaterally,

patients present with weakness, muscle atrophy, and fasciculations. Or, both UMN and LMN dysfunction may develop bilaterally and simultaneously (Figure 35.6).

Classical and West Nile virus poliomyelitis and MS may cause an acute pure motor syndrome. Chronic causes include HTLV-I, hereditary spastic paraplegia, cervical spondylolytic myelopathy, amyotrophic lateral sclerosis (ALS), primary lateral sclerosis, progressive muscular atrophy, post-polio syndrome, and electric shock-induced myelopathy.

Cauda Equina Syndrome and Conus Medullaris Syndrome

A cauda equina syndrome results from the loss of functions of two or more of the 18 nerve roots constituting the cauda equina. Each nerve root has incoming sensory fibers from one of the lower extremity or perineal dermatomes and outgoing motor fibers to a lower extremity myotome. Bilateral involvement of the cauda equina at the L5–S1 vertebral level produces low back and prominent radicular pain, weakness of plantar flexion of the feet, muscle atrophy and fasciculations, loss of ankle jerks, and (later) incontinence. Lesions at higher levels (e.g., L4–L5, L3–L4, L2–L3, or L1–L2) add progressively higher-level sensory, motor, and reflex loss to the syndrome (Figure 35.7).

This is often difficult to differentiate from conus medullaris lesions in which sexual and sphincter dysfunctions present earlier and more severely, and lower limb motor features are more symmetrical, distal, milder, or absent. Typically, sensory features are perianal and radicular pain is minor. UMN features may be present (Figure 35.7).

Both conditions also must be distinguished from lumbosacral plexopathies and mononeuropathy multiplex.

Acute causes include trauma and intervertebral disk herniation. Chronic syndromes may be caused by intervertebral disk herniation, lumbar spondylolysis, arachnoiditis, infections, Paget disease, and epidural or intradural extramedullary tumors.

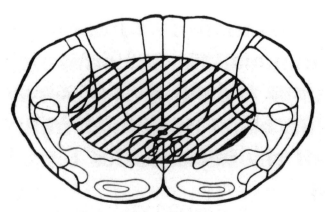

Figure 35.5 Central cord syndrome. Shading indicates affected areas. With permission of ASIA.

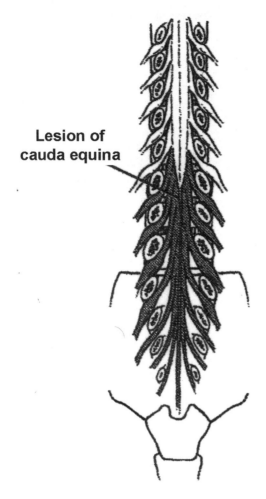

**Lesion of
cauda equina**

Figure 35.7   Cauda equina syndrome and conus medullaris syndrome. Shading indicates affected areas.

DIAGNOSTIC PROCEDURES TO EVALUATE SPINAL CORD DISEASE

Magnetic resonance imaging (MRI) has revolutionized the imaging of spinal cord diseases, and technical and interpretative advances continue to provide additional insights into the nature of spinal disease, rendering MRI the procedure of choice for most diagnostic questions. It can provide images in multiple planes and directly display images of the spinal cord and column, vertebral bone marrow, vessels, exiting nerve roots, and cerebrospinal fluid (CSF). While MRI is very motion sensitive and thus requires extensive patient cooperation, if artifacts are eliminated, gray and white matter can be distinguished. Fluid attenuated inversion recovery (FLAIR), short tau inversion recovery (STIR), and spectroscopy promise to help diagnose acute cord infarct, distinguish spinal cord compression from metastatic versus osteoporotic spine fractures, identify the cell type of tumors, and distinguish radiation myelitis from tumor and infection. Spinal magnetic resonance angiography may provide a noninvasive screen for vascular malformations. For cortical bone and calcified structures and in MR-incompatible patients, computed tomography (CT), without or with intravenous or intrathecal contrast, can often substitute.

Electrophysiologic testing is useful in some spinal cord conditions. Somatosensory-evoked potentials (SSEP) will be abnormal in conditions involving the dorsal columns (13). In cases that show abnormalities of position and vibratory sensation, the procedure is mostly redundant unless spinal cord disease and polyneuropathy coexist. In some conditions, the SSEP become abnormal before clinical symptoms appear, which may afford the opportunity to treat the condition earlier. SSEPs are valuable in the evaluation of simulated paraplegia when they turn out to be normal in the absence of reported sensory perception. Central motor conduction studies can be used in the same manner in patients who consider themselves paralyzed. Nerve conduction studies (NCS) are abnormal in several spinal cord conditions with associated peripheral neuropathy such as B12 deficiency (14) and Friedreich ataxia (15). NCS in patients thought to have ALS occasionally show multifocal motor conduction block neuropathy instead, thus revealing a potentially treatable condition. Needle electromyography (EMG) is useful in confirming muscle denervation in ALS.

Lumbar puncture (LP) is done less frequently than even a decade ago. Although many spinal cord conditions are associated with CSF abnormalities, routine studies, such as increased protein content, are nonspecific. LP should not be done until an MRI has excluded a mass lesion, because up to 10% of patients with mass lesions deteriorate afterwards, presumably due to impaction of the mass against the spinal cord, provoked by the creation of a CSF pressure differential above and below the lesion. In myelopathies thought to be caused by MS, abnormal immunoglobulins and oligoclonal bands specific to the CSF support the diagnosis (16, 17). CSF pleocytosis and the identification of a specific infectious agent by polymerase chain reaction (PCR) are helpful in patients with acute transverse myelitis (18). A very high CSF protein (>100 mg/dl) is rare in patients with spinal cord disease, except in association with neoplasms.

Relapsing-Remitting Spinal Multiple Sclerosis

With a putative prevalence of 1:1000 and some 400,000 people affected in the United States, relapsing-remitting spinal MS (16, 19, 20) is the most common cause of an acute spontaneous spinal cord syndrome in patients age 15 to 50. MS plaques tend to occur dorsally, bilaterally, and symmetrically, and involve the cervical and upper thoracic cord more frequently than the lower thoracic or lumbar areas.

Bilateral plaques in the thoracic dorsal columns produce leg paresthesias and trunk and gait ataxia. If one thoracic dorsal quadrant is involved, unilateral leg weakness and paresthesias result. With bilateral lesions, patients have paraparesis, sphincter and sexual dysfunction, and impaired position and vibration sense in the legs. With cervical lesions, the arms are similarly involved.

MS attacks typically evolve from first symptom to maximal deficit over one day to one week, although onset may be faster or slower. Remission from maximal deficit to maximal improvement usually occurs over one to three months, but may again be slower or faster. Most commonly, patients have an attack about every two years.

Some symptoms and signs of MS are more likely to improve than others: Sensory symptoms remit completely in >75%.

Monoparesis or hemiparesis remit completely in 50%, but fewer than 20% of patients with tetraparesis or paraparesis recover to normality. With sphincter symptoms, only 15% regain complete control.

When spinal cord symptoms occur in a patient with known MS, there is no diagnostic problem. When cord symptoms are the first manifestation of the disease (21, 22), "silent" lesions in the brainstem or optic nerves may be documented using brainstem auditory or visual-evoked potentials. At least half of patients in whom spinal cord symptoms are the first manifestation of MS show typical brain MRI findings. CSF selective oligoclonal banding or gammaglobulin abnormalities are found in some 95% of patients (17).

Subcutaneous or intramuscular interferon beta or subcutaneous glatiramer acetate decrease the frequency of MS attacks, reduce disease activity by MRI, and slow disease progression. In some cases of disabling MS attacks, methylprednisolone given intravenously or by mouth is indicated to hasten recovery. Drugs such as mitoxantrone and natalizimab may be used to "rescue" patients unresponsive to more benign drugs.

Acute Transverse Myelitis

Acute transverse myelitis (ATM) is a clinical syndrome manifested by weakness and sensory loss, generally in a symmetrical pattern, below the affected spinal segment (23). The term transverse myelitis implies that the whole cross-sectional area of the spinal cord is involved. Symptoms evolve over several hours to several weeks.

Initial symptoms are usually paresthesias involving the legs. Pain over the involved cord segments, usually the upper thoracic, affects about one-third of patients. Weakness and incontinence follow. Sensory and motor loss may be total or partial.

In a series of 288 patients with the clinical syndrome of ATM, the etiology was idiopathic in 15.6%, systemic disease (mainly systemic lupus erythematosus and sarcoidosis) in 20.5%, spinal cord infarction in 18.8%, MS in 10.8%, infectious and parainfectious in 17.3%, and neuromyelitis optica in 17% (24).

Rare causes of infection include herpes simplex types 1 or 2, cytomegalovirus, varicella-zoster, or Epstein-Barr virus. Patients are usually immunocompromised. Agents can be identified by serological or PCR CSF studies.

Support for a parainfectious or immune etiology stems from the occasional close temporal association of ATM with vaccinations (rabies, smallpox, tetanus, influenza, polio) or some specific viral disease (measles, mumps, chicken pox). The immunologic hypothesis is further supported by animal models of experimental allergic encephalomyelitis induced via injection of CNS tissue.

CSF may be normal but frequently shows a lymphocytic pleocytosis and protein elevation. Gamma globulin may be selectively elevated.

MRI may be normal but usually shows an intramedullary fusiform cord enlargement over several segments. There is a subtle to obvious hyperintense signal on T2-weighted imaging. Contrast enhancement is variable. In ATM due to sarcoid, a characteristic pattern of intramedullary and leptomeningeal enhancement may be present. Brain MRI is useful because it may point to an alternate diagnosis (e.g., MS), or to associated manifestations of the same etiology (e.g., in lupus or sarcoid).

Pathologically, several or many spinal cord segments are involved. In some cases, the process is primarily one of demyelination; in others, necrosis involves all cord elements.

About one-third of patients with ATM recover completely, about one-third do not improve at all, and about one-third improve with significant residual neurological deficit.

In 5% to 10% of cases, ATM is the presenting feature of MS. These patients are likely to have asymmetric clinical findings, MR lesions extending over fewer than two spinal segments, abnormal visual-evoked responses, and CSF oligoclonal bands (25).

Autoimmune forms of ATM can respond to intravenous steroids, IVIG, plasma exchange, and immunosuppression. Acyclovir may be helpful with viral etiologies (26).

Spinal Cord Infarction

Spinal cord infarction (27) can be caused by insufficient blood flow in the aorta or in segmental arteries, or in arteries of the spinal cord itself. Some causes include dissecting aortic aneurysm and thrombosis, surgical procedures on the aorta, or embolic or atherosclerotic obstruction of segmental or spinal arteries. Infarction is frequently precipitated by severe hypotension.

The two most common pathologic patterns are (1) infarction of all of the gray matter below a certain spinal cord level with relative sparing of the white matter, and (2) infarction of the gray and white matter of the anterior two-thirds of the cord over one or several segments, with sparing of the dorsal column. Interestingly, both patterns produce a similar clinical picture, i.e. the "stroke like" onset of bilateral leg weakness and loss of pain sensation below the level of the lesion and loss of sphincter control. Position and vibratory sensation are intact in the affected areas. Back pain is common. This is called the "anterior spinal artery syndrome," even though occlusion of the anterior spinal artery is rarely the cause. Less commonly, unilateral sensory-motor loss may occur. Most infarcts occur in the thoracic spinal cord.

MRI is usually normal for 24 hours after onset. The first abnormality is usually hyperintensity on T2-weighted images, while on T1-weighted images, the infarct is darker than the spinal cord. On strongly T2-weighted sequences, the bright CSF signal may hinder the detection of the infarct and therefore proton density or FLAIR images are preferred. Swelling of the infarcted spinal cord area may be noted, which might raise concern about a tumor. In the subacute stage, contrast enhancement may occur.

There is no effective treatment for spinal cord infarction. About half of all patients show substantial motor recovery. These are usually younger patients who never had total paralysis during the acute stage of infarction.

Intraspinal Hemorrhage

At the onset, such cases present with back or neck pain localized at the site of bleeding, rapidly followed by weakness and sensory loss below the level of the hematoma. Bladder control is lost. Intraspinal hemorrhage (28) may occur into the epidural space, the subdural space, the subarachnoid space, or the spinal cord itself (hematomyelia). Subarachnoid hemorrhage does not produce cord compression, because blood spreads throughout the CSF.

In about 10% of cases, the cause is trauma; in 5% bleeding from a vascular malformation or tumor; some 25% are anti-coagulated or have a coagulopathy. No cause is found in approximately 60%.

Imaging studies are complex because findings depend on location, age, and state of oxygenation of the blood. CT shows a simpler pattern than does MRI. Imaging patterns permit classifying the hemorrhage as hyperacute (<24 hours), acute (24–72 hours), subacute (>3 days), and chronic (3 weeks–years).

In the hyperacute stage, blood is usually invisible (isodense) on both CT and MRI. In the acute stage, blood is hyperdense (bright) on CT and dark on T2 weighted MRI. In the subacute stage, blood again becomes isodense on CT but appears bright on both T1- and T2-weighted MRI (Figure 35.8). Finally, with the further passage of time, the hematoma resolves. As it does

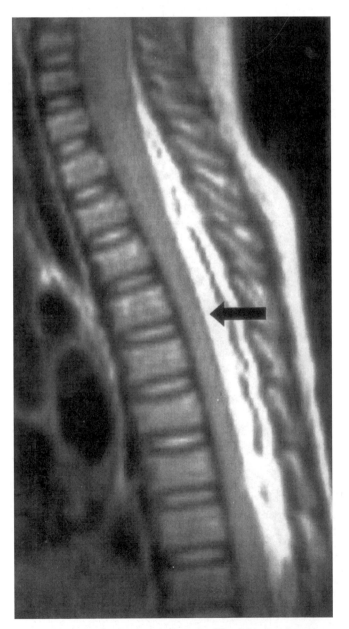

Figure 35.8 Subacute posterior spinal hematoma, compressing the thecal sac and spinal cord and appearing hyperintense on sagittal T1 non-contrast MRI of the thoracic spine.

so, any mass effect resolves and the signal of the hematoma progresses toward the T1 and T2 relaxation time of CSF. At all stages, epidural, subdural, and intraspinal hematomas appear as a mass encroaching upon the subarachnoid space and compressing or expanding the spinal cord.

The treatment of spinal hematomas is emergent surgical removal. About 50% of patients who have total loss of sensory and motor function at the time of operation recover to some degree, and approximately 10% recover completely.

Decompression Sickness

Decompression sickness (29) occurs mainly in recreational divers using SCUBA (self-contained underwater breathing apparatus) equipment. About 250 to 300 cases are reported each year in the United States, likely an underestimation. A few cases result from loss of cabin pressure in aircraft.

The rapid change from a higher to a lower pressure environment causes inert dissolved gases in blood and tissue to form intra- or extravascular bubbles. Within the CNS, extravascular bubbles may compress or tear axons, whereas intravascular bubbles may obstruct arteries or veins and cause infarction. With CNS involvement, the spinal cord is affected in 75% of cases.

Clinical features in the form of paresthesias, weakness, and incontinence occur almost immediately after surfacing from a dive. If the brain is involved, there may be confusion, coma, seizures, vertigo, or amaurosis.

The mainstay of treatment is urgent recompression. This requires the use of a specialized chamber, which is usually available in areas where recreational diving is common. The location of the nearest recompression center can be furnished by the Divers Alert Network (www.DiversAlertNetwork.org) at 919–684–8111 or 919–684–4DAN (collect). Outcome is favorable in 90% of cases, if treatment starts within 30 minutes of surfacing, whereas only 50% avoid sequelae if treatment is delayed over 6 hours. Decompression sickness has a mortality rate of 5–10%.

Intervertebral Disk Herniation

Intervertebral disk herniation usually occurs in a dorsolateral direction into the nerve root canal, producing radiculopathy. This is by far the most common clinically significant event, but because it does not involve the spinal cord, it will not be further discussed. Midline herniation is not common, because the annulus fibrosis is reinforced by the posterior longitudinal ligament. However, sometimes a herniating disk will detach the ligament from the vertebral body and push it into the spinal canal. Even more rarely, will it tear through the ligament (30). In either case, the spinal cord or cauda equina may be compressed (Figure 35.9).

Disk herniation usually occurs in the lower cervical or lower lumbar spine. Less commonly, it may occur in the lower half of the thoracic spine. Herniation may occur suddenly, or the disk may slowly extrude through the annulus. Thus, neurologic deficit may be of sudden onset or slowly progressive (31). Moderate to severe neck or back pain occurs at the site of disk herniation.

Compression of the spinal cord by a disk in the cervical or thoracic area causes an anterior or total cord syndrome. Sometimes, in the cervical area, a lateral cord (Brown-Séquard)

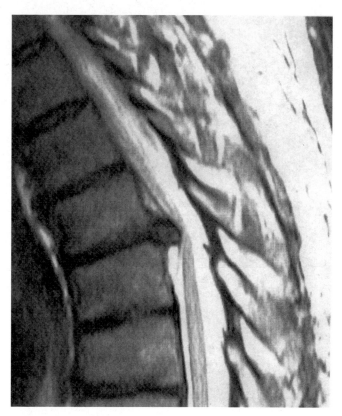

Figure 35.9 Sagittal T2-weighted image of a portion of the thoracic spine demonstrating a large disc protrusion, creating a ventral extradural deformity of the thecal sac and deforming and compressing the spinal cord.

occurs. There is sensory and motor loss below the level of herniation. With bilateral cord compression, bladder symptoms occur (32, 33).

Almost all lumbar disk herniations that produce a cauda equina syndrome occur at the L4–L5 or L5–S1 disk space. Spine pain at the site of herniation and bilateral sciatica are usually present. Herniation at the L5–S1 disk space causes sensory deficit in the distribution of all sacral roots and loss of ankle reflexes bilaterally. There may be weak foot plantar flexion. Urinary retention and overflow incontinence are common.

The MRI appearance of a herniated disk shows a soft tissue mass of disk intensity protruding posteriorly and compressing the spinal cord or cauda equina. However, the signal intensity of discs changes depending on their biochemical state. Desiccated or calcified discs are often dark. Also, other items may mimic discs in signal intensity, particularly scars. Also, discs that have herniated may migrate a considerable distance from their origin, even into the dural sac or posterior to the sac. Lastly, as asymptomatic ruptured disks are found in 15% to 20% of normal individuals, their presence does not predict symptomatology.

In patients with disk herniation causing spinal cord compression or a cauda equina syndrome, the disk should be surgically removed. Following disk removal, only about half of patients with cord compression improve. With lumbar disk removal, almost all patients recover sensory and motor function, but about 30% do not recover normal bladder function (31).

Spinal Epidural Abscess

Spinal epidural abscess (34, 35) is a collection of pus within the spinal canal external to the dura. In about one-third of cases, the abscess forms by extension of a local infection such as vertebral osteomyelitis or discitis; then, the abscess lies anterior to the spinal cord. In another third, hematogenous spread from a distant infection is responsible. This typically occurs in the immunologically suppressed, the intravenous drug user, the patient with bacterial endocarditis, and the occasional patient with genitourinary infection. In at least one-third of patients, no source is identified. In both latter situations, the abscess is lateral or posterior to the dura.

The initial symptom is local pain, usually severe, over the site of the abscess. Fever is present in about two-thirds. Radicular pain and leg weakness, usually bilateral, occur in about 50%. Sensory and bladder symptoms are less common. Symptoms evolve over a few days to weeks and have been present for more than two weeks before diagnosis in more than two-thirds of cases. The evolution of symptoms and signs reflect gradual enlargement of the abscess with progressive root and cord compression.

In some cases, symptoms evolve more slowly with inconspicuous fever and leucocytosis. Such patients may appear to have an epidural tumor until surgical exploration or postmortem examination reveals the true nature of the lesion.

Abscess formation within the spinal cord itself (intramedullary abscess) is rare. Clinical features resemble those of epidural abscess (36).

Laboratory examination shows a leucocytosis. CSF cell count and protein are elevated, but glucose content is normal. However, LP should be avoided because of the danger of increasing spinal cord or cauda equina compression and of introducing infection into the subarachnoid space, thus producing meningitis.

MRI is the optimal diagnostic procedure (Figure 35.10). The abscess is shown as a pocket of T1 and T2 prolongation with ring-like or peripheral contrast enhancement. When the infection is local, there will be signal abnormality and the anatomic deformity within the disc (discitis) or the bone (osteomyelitis). With hematogenous abscesses, the intraspinal ring-enhancing mass with T1 and T2 prolongation is present without signs of adjoining infection.

Treatment consists of surgical drainage and excision of abscess tissue. Broad spectrum intravenous antibiotics should be started immediately (usually including an anti-staphylococcal penicillin, third-generation cephalosporins, and aminoglycosides). When the bacterium has been identified (staphylococcus aureus in over 50% of cases), antibiotic coverage can be narrowed. In selected cases intravenous antibiotics with or without CT-guided percutaneous needle drainage may be as effective as surgery (37).

The relationship between the time of spinal cord decompression and outcome is well known. Patients treated before the development of paralysis usually recover completely, whereas patients paraplegic for more than 36 to 48 hours usually do not.

West Nile Virus Poliomyelitis

Before 1955, poliomyelitis occurred in epidemic form in the USA, with 25,000 to 50,000 cases annually, 90% of patients being children under age 10. Symptoms began as an aseptic meningitis with headache, fever, and nuchal rigidity. After several days, about 75% of patients developed some degree of flaccid paresis of various limb muscles. CSF analysis showed a

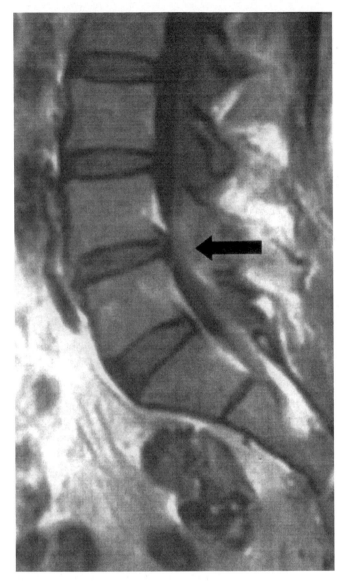

Figure 35.10 Spinal epidural abscess. Sagittal T1-weighted post-contrast image of the lumbar spine showing a soft tissue mass within the spinal canal.

polymorphonuclear or lymphocytic pleocytosis and moderate protein elevation. About 75% of patients recovered completely. The rest were left with persistent muscle weakness and atrophy. With the advent of the polio vaccine, the disease became rare after 1962, with only sporadic cases occurring caused by other enteroviruses or the vaccine itself. Since 1999, there have been no cases of polio in the United States or Canada.

In 1999, the first cases of infection with the West Nile virus were reported in the United States. This is a single-stranded RNA virus, related to those causing Japanese and St. Louis encephalitis and Yellow Fever. Since then, small annual nationwide epidemics have occurred. Patients can present with a neurological disorder that closely resembles the now extinct poliomyelitis except that adults rather than children are involved, i.e. acute, painless, asymmetric weakness, sometimes in a single limb, with CSF pleocytosis, particularly in the setting of an acute febrile illness (38). This form of polio occurs in isolation or is associated with several other CNS and PNS syndromes. While most individuals seropositive for the virus remain asymptomatic; the risk of clinical disease and of death increases dramatically with age. Treatment is symptomatic. Recovery may be limited.

EMG/NCS show evidence of AHC and motor axonal involvement. The condition can be confused with numerous other conditions, including stroke (due to the asymmetric presentation) and Guillain-Barré syndrome (GBS); imaging studies help rule out stroke, and GBS is distinguished by predominance of motor neuronal and axonal involvement, asymmetry, and CSF findings. Autopsy studies reveal an anterior myelitis closely resembling polio.

Simulated Paraplegia

In simulated paraplegia, a patient without dysfunction of the CNS or PNS claims to have sensory loss and weakness of the legs. There are two varieties of simulated paraplegia; hysterical paraplegia and malingered paraplegia. In hysterical paraplegia, patients truly believe they have the symptoms of which they complain (conversion reaction). In malingered paraplegia, the patient is simply lying, usually for financial gain. Simulated tetraplegia is extremely rare, because tetraplegia is too complex and disabling to serve any conscious or unconscious purposes.

The diagnosis of simulated paraplegia requires that (1) there are no signs of nervous system disease that would explain the clinical presentation, and (2) there are positive signs of hysteria (conversion reaction) or malingering. The positive signs of hysterical or malingered paraplegia are muscle weakness without changes in muscle tone or tendon reflexes, and normal plantar responses. Alleged sensory loss does not correspond to that found in lesions of the spinal cord, nerve roots, or peripheral nerves (Figure 35.11). Bowel and bladder functions are almost always preserved.

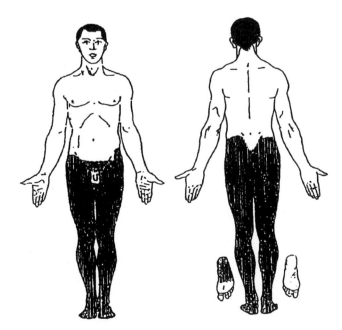

Figure 35.11 Illustration from Charcot's original description of "hysterical paraplegia" (39). Note the pattern of sensory loss. The upper border of the anesthetic area outlines the iliac crest and the inguinal ligament, rather than a dermatome. There is also sensory sparing of the penis and scrotum.

Simulated paraplegia was first described by Charcot more than a century ago (39). The findings that he described have proven to be remarkably consistent in cases described by others since (40).

Somatosensory-evoked potentials and central motor-evoked potentials are especially useful in evaluating patients with simulated paraplegia because they will be normal in patients claiming to have lower extremity paralysis and anesthesia.

References

1. Alexander GE, DeLong MR. Central mechanisms of initiation and control of movement. In: Asbury AK, McKhann GM, McDonald W, eds. *Diseases of the Nervous System*. Philadelphia: WB Saunders, 1992:304.

2. Kakulas BA. A review of the neuropathology of human spinal cord injury with emphasis on special features. *Spinal Cord Med* 1999; 22:119–124.

3. Dalakas MC. The post-polio syndrome as an evolving clinical entity definition and clinical description. *Ann NY Acad Sci* 1995; 753:68–80.

4. Hiersemenzel LP, Curt A, Dietz V. From spinal shock to spasticity, neuronal adaptations to a spinal cord injury. *Neurology* 2000; 54: 1574–1582.

5. Rothwell J. *Control of Human Voluntary Movement*. 2nd ed. London: Chapman & Hall, 1994:199.

6. Young RR. Spastic paresis. In: Young RR, Woolsey RM, eds. *Diagnosis and Management of Disorders of the Spinal Cord*. Philadelphia: WB Saunders, 1995:367.

7. Lindblom U, Ochoa J. Somatosensory function and dysfunction. In: Asbury AK, McKhann GM, McDonald WI, eds. *Diseases of the Nervous System*. 2nd ed. Philadelphia: WB Saunders, 1992:222.

8. Woolsey RM. Chronic pain following spinal cord injury. *J Am Paraplegia Soc* 1986; 9:39–41.

9. Bigos S, Bowyer O, Braen G, et al. *Acute Low Back Problems in Adults*. Clinical Practice Guideline No. 14. AHCPR Publication No 95–0642. Rockville, MD: Agency for Health Care Policy and Research, Public Health Service, U.S. Department of Health and Human Services, 1994:8.

10. Pagni CA. Central pain due to spinal cord and brainstem damage. In: Wall PD, Melzack R, eds. *Textbook of Pain*. 3rd ed. Edinburgh: Churchill Livingstone, 1994.

11. Bryne TN, Benzel EC, Waxman SG. *Diseases of the Spine and Spinal Cord*. New York: Oxford University Press, 2000:143–151.

12. Tanagho EA, Schmidt RA. Neuropathic bladder disorders. In: Tanagho EA, McAnisch W, eds. *Smith's General Urology*. 14th ed. Norwalk, CT: Appleton & Lange, 1995:496–513.

13. Kiers L, Chiappa KH. Motor and somatosensory evoked potentials in spinal cord disorders. In: Young RR, Woolsey RM, eds. *Diagnosis and Management of Disorders of the Spinal Cord*. Philadelphia: WB Saunders, 1995:153–169.

14. Healton EB, Savage DG, Brust JCM, et al. Neurologic aspects of cobalamin deficiency. *Medicine* 1991; 70:229–244.

15. Harding AE. *The Hereditary Ataxias and Related Disorders*. Edinburgh: Churchill Livingstone, 1984:74.

16. Paty DW, Ebers GC. *Multiple Sclerosis*. Philadelphia: FA Davis, 1998:66.

17. Freedman MS, Thompson EJ, Deisenhammer E, Giovannoni G, Grimsley G, Keir G; Öhman S, Racke MK, Sharief M, Sindic DJM, Sellebjerg F, Tourtellotte WW. Recommended standard of cerebrospinal fluid analysis in the diagnosis of multiple sclerosis: a consensus statement. *Arch Neurol* 2005; 62:865–870.

18. Fishman RA. Lumbar puncture and cerebrospinal fluid examination. In: Rowland LP. ed. *Merritt's Textbook of Neurology*. 10th ed. Philadelphia: Lippincott Williams & Wilkins, 2000.

19. Noseworthy JH, Lucchinetti C, Rodriguez M, et al. Multiple sclerosis. *N Eng J Med* 2000; 343:938–952.

20. Compston A, Ebers G, Lassmann H, et al. *McAlpine's Multiple Sclerosis*. 3rd ed. London: Churchill Livingstone, 1998.

21. Shibasaki H, McDonald WI, Kuroiwa Y. Racial modifications of clinical picture of multiple sclerosis: Comparison between British and Japanese patients. *J Neurol Sci* 1981; 49:253–271.

22. Hawkins CP. Spinal features of multiple sclerosis. In: Engler GL, Cole J, Merton WL, eds. *Spinal Cord Diseases*. New York: Marcel Dekker Inc., 1998:401.

23. Ropper AH, Poskanzer DC. The prognosis of acute and subacute transverse myelopathy based on early signs and symptoms. *Ann Neuro* 1978; 451–459.

24. de Seze J, Lanctin C, Lebrun C, et al. Idiopathic acute transverse myelitis: Application of the recent diagnostic criteria. *Neurology* 2005; 65:1950–1953.

25. Scott TF, Bhagavatula K, Snyder PJ, et al. Transverse myelitis—comparison with spinal cord presentations of multiple sclerosis. *Neurology* 1998; 50:429–433.

26. de Silva SM, Mark AS, Gilden DH, et al. Zoster myelitis: Improvement with antiviral therapy in two cases. *Neurology* 1996; 47:929–931.

27. Cheshire WP, Santos CC, Massey EW, et al. Spinal cord infarction: Etiology and outcome. *Neurology* 1996; 47:321–330.

28. Wisoff HS. Spontaneous intraspinal hemorrhage. In: Wilkins RH, Rengachary SS, eds. *Neurosurgery, Vol. II*, 2nd ed. New York: McGraw-Hill, 1996:2559–2565.

29. Pearson RR. Decompression illness and the spinal cord. In: Critchley E, Eisen A, eds. *Spinal Cord Disease. Basic Science, Diagnosis and Management*. London: Springer, 1997:443–460.

30. De Palma AF, Rothman RH. *The Intervertebral Disk*. Philadelphia: WB Saunders, 1970:52.

31. Kostuik JP, Harrington I, Alexander D, et al. Cauda equina syndrome and lumbar disk herniation. *J Bone and Joint Surg* 1986; 68A:386–391.

32. Arce CA, Dohrmann GJ. Herniated thoracic disks. *Neurol Clin* 1985; 3:383–392.

33. Hoh JT, Japadopoulos SM. Cervical disc disease and cervical spondylosis. In: Wilkins RH, Rengachary SS, eds. *Neurosurgery Vol. III*, 2nd ed. New York: McGraw-Hill, 1996:3767.

34. Darouiche RO, Hamill RJ, Greenberg SB, et al. Bacterial spinal epidural abscess: Review of 43 cases and literature survey. *Medicine* 1992; 71:369–385.

35. Mackenzie AR, Laing RBS, Smith CC, et al. Spinal epidural abscess: The importance of early diagnosis and treatment. *J Neurol Neurosurg Psychiatry* 1998; 65:209–212.

36. Menezes AH, VanGilder JC. Spinal cord abscess. In: Wilkins RH, Rengachary SS, eds. *Neurosurgery, Vol. 3*, 2nd ed. New York: McGraw-Hill, 1996; 3323–3326.

37. Siddiq F, Chowfin A, Tight R, et al. Medical vs. surgical management of spinal epidural abscess. *Arch Intern Med* 2004; 164:2409–2412.

38. Flaherty ML, Wijdicks EFM, Stevens JC, et al. Clinical and electrophysiologic patterns of flaccid paralysis due to West Nile virus. *Mayo Clin Proc* 2003; 78:1245–1248.

39. Charcot JM. *Diseases of the Nervous System, Vol. 3* (Savill T, Translator) London: The New Sydenham Society, 1889:374–389.

40. Baker JHE, Silver JR. Hysterical paraplegia. *J Neurol Neurosurg Psychiatry* 1987; 50:375–382.

36 Chronic Nontraumatic Myelopathies

Florian P. Thomas
Robert M. Woolsey

AMYOTROPHIC LATERAL SCLEROSIS

Amyotrophic lateral sclerosis (ALS) (1) is a disorder of unknown cause in which motor neurons of the cerebral cortex, brain stem, and spinal cord atrophy and die (Figure 36.1). It is more common in men than women, 90% of cases begin after age 40, and 5%–10% are familial. Mutations in three genes, superoxide dismutase 1, alsin, and senataxin, and several additional loci have been identified for the hereditary forms.

Because both the upper (UMN) and lower motor neurons (LMN) are involved, the disease can present in a variety of ways. About 15% of cases present with UMN onset—i.e., ataxia, spasticity, and hyperreflexia. When anterior horn cells (AHC) or LMNs are involved first, weakness, muscle atrophy, and fasciculations are evident; this is known as progressive spinal muscular atrophy; some 30% of patients present this way. In over 50% of cases, UMN and LMN features are present at onset, i.e. classical ALS. In 85% of cases, limb muscles are involved first, the arm five times more often than the leg (2). In some 20%, muscles innervating the hypoglossal or vagal nuclei are involved first producing dysarthria and dysphagia, i.e. the syndrome of progressive bulbar or progressive pseudobulbar palsy. A significant number of ALS patients develop dementia, mostly of the frontotemporal type (3). Clinically apparent sensory abnormalities, sphincter dysfunction, and ocular palsy are rare.

Regardless of initial presentation, the disease eventually progresses to widespread muscle weakness and atrophy, with fasciculations, hyperreflexia, dysarthria, and dysphagia, i.e., the syndrome of ALS. Some patients never exhibit extensor plantar responses. Life expectancy is generally 3–5 years after the onset of symptoms, with death from respiratory failure due to loss of neurons of the phrenic nerve.

A definite diagnosis of ALS requires that UMN and LMN signs be present in more than one area of the nervous system such as the oropharynx and the arms, or the arms and the legs, or the like. The "El Escorial Criteria" of the World Federation of Neurology recommend that a diagnosis of "definite ALS" be supported by the presence of UMN and LMN signs in three of four possible areas (brain stem, cervical, thoracic, and lumbar cord). MRI of the spinal cord, along with EMG/NCS (also to support the clinical findings of LMN affection) and numerous laboratory studies tailored to the individual case are indicated to exclude a host of conditions that must be considered in the differential diagnosis (2). Considering the gravity of the diagnosis, the El Escorial Criteria make sense; however, some patients never satisfy all of them even at the time of death.

No treatment reverses or halts disease progression, but early diagnosis and intense ongoing care by a team that focuses on physical and occupational therapy, assistive technology and communication devices, symptomatic, nutritional, and psychological support, and the eventual need for gastrostomy and positive pressure ventilation prolong life and maximize patients' comfort and independence. Riluzol 50 mg twice daily extends life for several months. Some 10% of patients opt for tracheostomy and ventilator support, particularly if respiratory failure occurs early during the course.

OTHER PURE OR PREDOMINANTLY MOTOR SYNDROMES

This group of conditions is very heterogeneous (4). It comprises disorders involving the LMN, including hereditary diseases such as Werdnig-Hoffman and Kugelberg-Welander and the post-infectious post-polio syndrome, as well as disorders involving the UMN such as Hereditary Spastic Paraplegia, retroviral HTLV-I associated myelopathy, sporadic primary lateral sclerosis, and myelopathy induced by electric shock.

The spinal muscular atrophies (SMA) comprise a group of mostly autosomal recessive conditions characterized by AHC degeneration, which leads to generalized muscle weakness. They are classified based on genetics and onset age, maximal muscular activity achieved, and life expectancy (4). A detailed discussion is beyond the scope of this chapter. Severe infantile acute SMA or type I (Werdnig-Hoffman), infantile chronic SMA or type II, juvenile SMA or type III (Kugelberg-Welander), and adult onset SMA or type IV are almost all caused by homozygous deletions in

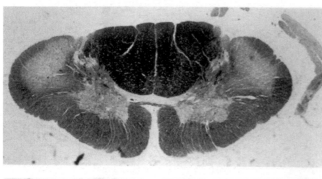
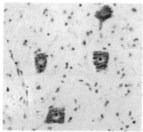
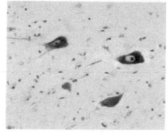

Figure 36.1 Upper figure is a myelin-stained section of the lower cervical spinal cord of an ALS patient illustrating demyelination secondary to corticospinal tract degeneration. The lower figures are H&E stains: the left shows normal AHCs; the right shows degenerative changes in AHCs in ALS.

the SMN1 (survival of motor neuron) gene. An X linked recessive form is Kennedy disease, which results from a triplet repeat expansion in the androgen receptor gene, and is associated with sensory neuropathy, gynecomastia, congenital fractures, and contractures.

Hereditary spastic paraplegia (HSP), also known as familial spastic paraplegia (FSP), is the most common of the "pure" or primarily UMN syndromes (4, 5). HSP is most often autosomal dominantly inherited; autosomal recessive forms are less common, and X linked forms are rare. Over 30 loci and 10 genes have been identified. In "complicated HSP," numerous central nervous system (CNS) features may be associated.

Onset is usually between ages 10 and 30, but can be in childhood or old age. Early on, gait becomes awkward. Examination shows hyperreflexia and extensor plantar responses. In some patients, vibratory sense is mildly impaired at the toes and ankles. Weakness is limited and a late feature. The arms are uninvolved except for hyperreflexia in some patients. Symptoms progress slowly and disability is delayed until late in life, when bladder symptoms can develop as well.

Electrophysiologic tests are normal, except for somatosensory-evoked potentials (SSEPs), which are absent or show low amplitude. Pathologic changes are confined to the spinal cord, in which the longest axons in the corticospinal tracts, those innervating the legs, degenerate, and those supplying the arms are minimally involved or not at all. Most cases show less intense degenerative changes in fasciculus gracilis, which mediates position and tactile sensation from the legs.

The diagnosis is based upon family history and clinical findings. Genetic tests are commercially available for HSP 1 and 2. Treatment with spasticity drugs may be helpful.

Primary lateral sclerosis (PLS) is another condition caused by degeneration of the corticospinal tract, but is not hereditary

(6). Symptoms commence at age 50–55 with progressive leg stiffness. Subsequently, the arms are involved and hand movement becomes awkward. Weakness is minimal. There is hyperreflexia and extensor plantar responses, but no sensory abnormalities. The condition is very slowly progressive and patients continue to be able to walk decades after onset. Bladder symptoms are delayed until late in the course. MRI is normal or shows spinal cord atrophy. Cerebrospinal fluid (CSF) is normal or shows slight protein elevation but no selective gamma globulin elevation or oligoclonal bands. PLS is differentiated from autosomal recessive HSP by a later onset and arm involvement. Treatment with spasticity drugs may be helpful.

Originally described by Raymond and Charcot (7), the term "post-polio syndrome" was coined by patients, who noticed that, after 15–30 years of stable deficit, they developed new muscle weakness and atrophy. Acute poliomyelitis results from infection with the neurotropic polio virus, which destroys AHCs and causes a random pattern of muscle paralysis and atrophy that ranges from mild to severe and persists in 25% of patients as a permanent motor deficit. Currently there are 1–1.5 million polio survivors in the United States.

Diagnosis of this condition can be difficult. It requires (1) an established past diagnosis of polio, (2) a stable neurologic status for at least 15 years, (3) the development of new muscle weakness and/or atrophy, (4) persistence of the condition for at least 1 year, and (5) exclusion of other causes for the symptoms or signs.

The prevalence remains controversial. According to some estimates, about 30% of survivors of paralytic polio develop the syndrome (7). However, a study of polio survivors in Olmsted County, Minnesota, detected no cases of muscle weakness and atrophy that followed the initial infection that could not be explained by other causes (8).

HTLV-I associated myelopathy (HAM) (Tropical Spastic Paraplegia, TSP) (10) is caused by infection with human T-lymphotropic virus type I (HTLV-I) and is a disease mainly found in the Caribbean basin, equatorial Africa, and Japan. The virus is transmitted by sexual intercourse or exposure to contaminated blood and hypodermic needles.

Symptoms usually occur at age 30–40. HAM is twice as common in women as in men. Patients present with leg weakness or gait ataxia caused by spasticity. Some have leg pain or paresthesias and urinary, bowel, and sexual dysfunction. Examination shows leg weakness, hyperreflexia, and extensor plantar responses. Gait impairment usually leads to wheelchair use 5–10 years after onset. Cerebral and cranial nerve deficits are rare.

Pathologically, the spinal cord shows a chronic meningeal and perivascular mononuclear reaction. HTLV-I can be demonstrated in mononuclear cells. There is demyelination of the corticospinal tracts and nerve roots, mainly in the thoracic cord.

Serum HTLV-l antibodies are present. The CSF shows lymphocytic pleocytosis and elevated protein in 50% of patients and is normal in the rest: Oligoclonal bands may be present. SSEPs are usually abnormal, even in the absence of sensory symptoms. MRI of the spinal cord is usually normal, but multifocal high-signal intensity cerebral white matter lesions on T2-weighted images are common. Anti-spasticity drugs may be helpful.

Myelopathy induced by electric shock can occur when high-voltage electrical current or lightning passes through the spinal cord (10). In one series, 37% of patients struck by lightning experienced an immediate paraparesis, or less commonly tetraparesis that resolved within 24 hours. In a few such patients, the symptoms are persistent. Some patients have no neurological symptoms until days or weeks after the electrical event, most commonly 1 week. They then experience a progressive paraparesis or tetraparesis with hyperreflexia and extensor plantar responses, which worsens over several days to two weeks. Some patients develop LMN signs in the spinal segments through which the current passed. Sensory features are minimal and bladder function is usually unaffected. The few autopsy studies have shown extensive demyelination with axonal preservation and little evidence of damage to spinal cord neuronal cell bodies. Very rarely patients develop ALS after a high voltage shock or lightning strike; however, whether there is a causal connection is unknown.

SPONDYLOLYTIC COMPRESSION OF THE SPINAL CORD OR CAUDA EQUINA

Spondylosis is an almost universal correlate of aging; prevalence numbers reflect the imaging technology used and the age range studied (12, 13).

Spondylosis begins with loss of water content in the intervertebral disk, resulting in decreased volume of the disk and laxity of annulus fibrosis, which then bulges outward in all directions. Disk degeneration destabilizes the posterior joints. Bone proliferates at the margins of the disk and the posterior joints, resulting in the formation of osteophytes, which protrude into both the anterior spinal and nerve root canals. Osteophytes, which narrow the nerve root canal, may compress nerve roots, producing radiculopathy, and those that narrow the spinal canal may produce myelopathy or cauda equina compression. Usually, multiple levels are involved. A similar process may affect the articular facets of the vertebrae posteriorly. Because these spondylotic joints are mobile, neural compression is intermittent so that symptoms tend to be episodic and show spontaneous resolution.

Radiculopathy due to spondylosis tends to occur in the lower half of the cervical spine or in the lower lumbar spine. The symptoms and findings produced by nerve root compression by osteophytes resembles those produced by herniated intervertebral disks, i.e. neck or back pain that radiates into the arm or leg associated with loss or depression of appropriate tendon reflexes, and in the case of severe compression, with sensory loss and weakness.

Myelopathy due to spondylosis likewise usually occurs in the lower half of the cervical spinal cord. Most patients have neck pain. Spastic gait, hyperreflexia, and hypertonicity are the most clinical features. Weakness if present is not severe, and sensory abnormalities, if present, usually consist of decreased position and vibratory sense. Urinary frequency and urgency are common, but patients are seldom incontinent. Some patients show a pure motor syndrome with atrophy and weakness of intrinsic hand muscles and lower-extremity ataxia and hyperreflexia, which may raise the issue of ALS. Traumatic neck hyperextension in patients with canal narrowing caused by osteophytes may result in severe, acute compression of the spinal cord and a central cord syndrome in which sensory and (or) motor deficits are greater in the upper than lower limbs, colloquially referred to as "upside-down paraplegia."

Cauda equina compression due to spondylosis usually causes neurogenic intermittent claudication. One or both legs ache and feel numb or weak when the patient stands or walks. By contrast, symptoms with vascular claudication do not occur with standing only, and signs of vascular disease are present in the legs, although it is not uncommon for older patients to have clinical features of both. Because the spinal canal becomes wider with flexion, symptoms of neurogenic claudication disappear quickly when the patient bends forward or sits down. Low back pain is frequently present but is not severe. There are no or only minor abnormalities on neurologic examination.

On MRI, sagittal views often display the loss of height of intervertebral discs. The long TR sequences show the loss of water (disc desiccation) that appears as signal loss. The sagittal views also demonstrate degenerative spondylolisthesis. Coronal views can display scoliosis and resulting disc deformities. Spurs with accompanying annular bulges can be seen as extradural thecal sac deformities on T2-weighted sequences. Axial views demonstrate the remaining width of the spinal canal and show the status of the articular facets and facet joints. Loss of disc height, annular bulging, and facet hypertrophy in combination narrow the central canal, the lateral recesses, the neural foramina, or all of the above. If the patient also has congenitally short pedicles, sagittal-oriented facet joints, or both, the situation is exacerbated. If there is motion at the facet joints, synovial cysts may develop that also encroach on the spinal canal from the posterior lateral direction. If the narrowing occurs in an area of the spine where the cord may be compromised, the thecal sac will be narrowed (particularly visible on long TR axial views) and the cord will appear to take up a larger percentage of the spinal canal (and may superficially appear to be enlarged). Later in the course of the disease, as the spinal cord atrophies, the thecal sac assumes a more "normal" size. The spinal cord signal will not necessarily change during the course of the disease.

Studies of the natural history of spondylosis show a pattern of symptomatic periods alternating with asymptomatic periods, each of which may last for weeks, to months, to years. Much less commonly, the pattern is one of steady deterioration.

Because the natural history is so highly variable, it is difficult to evaluate treatment options (13). In patients with mild symptoms, a cervical collar may be all that is needed. Patients with more severe symptoms or neurologic deficit frequently undergo surgery. Foramenotomy has been recommended for radiculopathy. Cervical myelopathy has been treated with posterior decompression by laminectomy, or anterior decompression by discectomy or vertebrectomy, and cauda equina compression by laminectomy.

Although all of these procedures have been reported to be successful, they may be unnecessary and can have serious complications. About two-thirds of patients improve after surgery. The remainder are unchanged or worse. Patients suffering steady, serious deterioration of neurological function probably have no prospect for stabilization or improvement without surgical intervention.

RHEUMATOID ARTHRITIS OF THE CERVICAL SPINE

When dealing with rheumatoid arthritis it is important to bear in mind the plethora of neurological sequelae and pathogenic processes that may be active: The CNS, PNS, and muscle may be involved in numerous ways and simultaneously in any given patient. As to the spinal cord, the transverse atlantal ligament that holds the odontoid process of C2 (the axis) against the anterior arch of C1 (the atlas) is frequently disrupted in rheumatoid arthritis (14). This allows C1 to move forward and produce atlantoaxial subluxation. Once present, subluxation progresses in 35–85% of patients. About 21% of rheumatoid arthritis patients develop subluxation of vertebrae at other cervical levels. About 50% of patients eventually develop signs of myelopathy, and if untreated, about half will die within six months. Treatment consists of surgical reduction and stabilization of the subluxed vertebrae; this usually arrests progression, and most patients improve.

On MRI the inflammatory change that causes ligamentous laxity shows T1 and T2 prolongation. In flexion, C1–C2 instability shows the spinal cord draped over the odontoid peg. There may be an inflammatory rheumatoid mass called pannus at C1–C2 with an intermediate T1 and T2 signal that may compress the cervical cord regardless of neck position. The sagittal spin-echo sequences are sufficient to display the abnormalities, but obtaining a second plane of view is standard.

SUBACUTE COMBINED DEGENERATION

Subacute combined degeneration (SCD) (15) is a myelopathy caused by vitamin B12 (cobalamin) deficiency. Young individuals can be involved, and the prevalence varies with the group studied (3%–16% in the general population, 11% among HIV seropositive individuals, 21% among the elderly, according to different studies).

As neurologic and psychiatric features resulting from pathology in the brain, spinal cord, peripheral, and optic nerves often coexist, it may be difficult to attribute findings in a given patient to particular anatomic structures. Onset is subacute or chronic, although more acute courses have been described, in particular after N$_2$O exposure, which oxidizes the cobalt core of cobalamin, thus depleting vitamin stores (Figure 36.2B). Early symptoms include hand and foot paresthesias. Untreated patients may develop limb weakness and ataxia. One study found both neuropathy and myelopathy in 41% of patients, neuropathy only in 25%, and myelopathy only in 12%, and a normal exam in 14%. Early on, most patients show impaired vibratory or position sense in the legs. On presentation, 50% have absent ankle reflexes with relative hyperreflexia at the knees. Plantars are initially flexor and later extensor. A Hoffman sign may be found. As the disease progresses, ascending loss of pinprick, light touch, and temperature sensation occurs. Later, depending on the predominance of posterior column vs. cortical spinal tract involvement, ataxia or spastic paraplegia predominates and PNS involvement causes distal limb atrophy. Rare autonomic features include orthostasis, sexual dysfunction, and bowel and bladder incontinence.

The pathogenesis of SCD remains under investigation. Traditional concepts have focused on a role of cobalamin in methylation reactions needed for myelin synthesis and maintenance, and in serotonin, norepinephrine, and dopamine synthesis. However, more recent findings indicate that the clinical and histological changes of SCD may result from up-regulation of neurotoxic cytokines (TNFα) and down-regulation of neurotrophic factors (epidermal growth factor).

Pathologically, cobalamin deficiency causes degenerative changes in the CNS and PNS. The term SCD describes the process

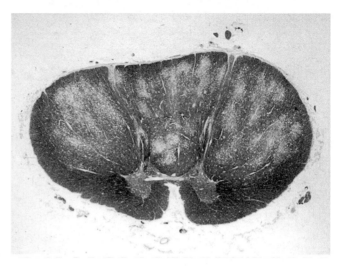

Figure 36.2A A myelin-stained section of upper cervical spinal cord of a patient with subacute combined degeneration caused by vitamin B12 deficiency. Note multifocal vacuolated and demyelinated lesions in the dorsal and lateral funiculi, resulting in a "spongelike" appearance.

of initial demyelination in the center of the posterior columns of the upper thoracic cord, with lesions then spreading laterally and cranially to the lateral corticospinal tracts in the cervical segments and the medulla (Figure 36.2A). Myelin breakdown, foamy macrophages, and occasional lymphocytes are characteristic, predominantly in a perivascular location. As demyelination and vacuolation increase, axons degenerate. Gliosis may be present in older lesions.

The cause of cobalamin deficiency in 75% of patients is pernicious anemia (PA), in which intrinsic factor (IF) antibodies block the formation of the cobalamin-IF complex required from normal absorption. Inactivation of B12 by recreational ("whippets") or iatrogenic N$_2$O use, dietary deficits, achlorhydria, various disorders of the terminal ileum, infections (*H. pylori*, fish tapeworm, blind loop syndrome), and medications (metformin, proton pump inhibitors, colchicin, neomycin, *p*-aminosalicylic acid) must be considered.

The diagnosis is confirmed by showing a below-normal cobalamin (radioassay: 170–900 pg/mL; chemiluminescence assay: 250–1100 pg/mL). However, these normal levels are insensitive, because when homocysteine (HC) and methylmalonic acid (MMA) are measured (whose levels rise when B12 is lacking), 5–10% of patients with true deficiency have B12 levels of 200–300 pg/mL, and 0.1% have levels greater than 300 pg/mL. Thus, MMA and/or HC should be measured as well. Finding IF or parietal cell antibodies (60% and 90% sensitivity, respectively) confirms the diagnosis of PA. If these are absent, a Schilling test is done, in which radioactive cobalamin is given by mouth and urinary cobalamin is assayed. If this is low, a second dose of radioactive cobalamin is given with IF, which in the presence of PA will increase the urinary excretion of radioactive cobalamin. Hematologic abnormalities are often absent at the time of neurologic presentation, especially because numerous food items now contain folate supplements. SSEP may reveal prolongation of the L3–P27 latency, reflecting a defect in conduction in the large-fiber sensory pathway between the cauda equina and the

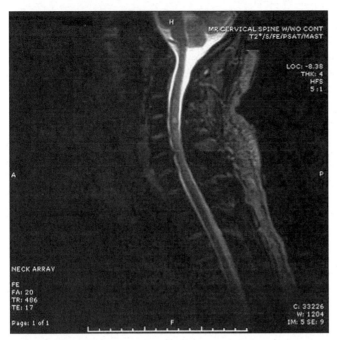

Figure 36.2B   T2-weighted sagittal MRI (TR = 4000; TE = 135). 31-year-old patient with cobalamin deficiency (B12 = 98 pg/ml) due to recreational N_2O use ("whippets"), who presented with mild leg weakness, gait ataxia, paresthesias in the arms and legs, impaired vibration and joint position sense, hyporeflexia, neutral plantar responses, and normal mental status; the clinical features had developed over 3 months (16). CSF including immunoglobulin analysis was normal except for protein elevation to 81 mg/100 ml. Intrinsic factor antibodies were absent. The neurological features resolved with cessation of N_2O use and B12 supplementation. MRI shows an area of hyperintensity posteriorly from the upper cervical to thoracic cord as well as multilevel disk herniation. T1-weighted images with and without gadolinium contrast showed no spinal cord abnormality. Brain MRI was normal. While this patient was treated fairly quickly, in patients with chronic disease, atrophy of the spinal cord is observed.

contralateral sensory cortex. EMG/NCS are abnormal in the majority of patients.

Once the diagnosis is made, oral daily supplements of 1,000 micrograms are given for life. As even in the absence of IF, 1% of oral B12 is absorbed in the gut, this results in uptake of 10 micrograms, or twice the daily requirement of 2–6 micrograms. However, following gastric surgery, e.g. barosurgery, it is preferable to rely on traditional protocols of 500–1,000 micrograms of vitamin B12 daily by injection for 5 days, followed by the same dose given monthly.

Half of treated SCD patients recover when treated. Patients with severe neurologic deficit prior to treatment and patients who have been symptomatic for over 6 months before treatment also improve when treated but are unlikely to recover completely.

FRIEDREICH ATAXIA

Autosomal recessive Friedreich ataxia (17) is the most common form of hereditary ataxia, with multiple other neurological and non-neurological manifestations. It results from a GAA triplet repeat expansion in the frataxin gene on chromosome 9q13–21.1. This reduces the gene product, which is required in mitochondrial metabolism. Pathologically, the spinal cord shows axonal loss and gliosis in the dorsal columns and the corticospinal and dorsal spinocerebellar tracts. Neuronal loss occurs in the dorsal root ganglia and anterior horn, Clarke's column, brainstem, cerebellar dentate nucleus, and cortex.

Patients usually become symptomatic in late childhood or adolescence. A cerebellar and sensory gait ataxia is universal. Neurologic examination shows loss of position and vibratory sense in the legs and areflexia at the knees and ankles. Most patients also show extensor plantar responses, ataxic movements of the arms, emotional lability, dysarthria, pes cavus, and kyphoscoliosis. Hypertrophic cardiomyopathy occurs in nearly all patients; diabetes or glucose intolerance and optic and peripheral neuropathies are rare manifestations. Patients usually become unable to walk 10–15 years after onset and die in early middle age, most commonly of cardiomyopathy. Because the genetic defect was identified in 1996, an adult form has been recognized with onset after age 25, which comprises about 15% of all cases. It may lack some of the typical features, notably scoliosis, pes cavus, and absent tendon reflexes.

The diagnosis is made on the basis of the clinical features and confirmed by demonstrating the size of GAA repeats by commercially available testing, which is especially useful in "form fruste" and adult cases. While antioxidants, chelators, tryptophan, and other agents have been tried, currently treatment remains symptomatic.

VACUOLAR MYELOPATHY

HIV-associated or vacuolar myelopathy (VM) occurs during the late stages of AIDS, when CD4$^+$ lymphocyte counts are very low, often in conjunction with AIDS dementia complex, peripheral neuropathies, and opportunistic CNS and PNS infections or malignancies (e.g., cytomegalovirus [CMV], progressive multifocal leukoencephalopathy, lymphoma) (17). Since the introduction of HAART (highly active antiretroviral therapy), fewer than 10% of patients develop clinical VM, although it remains common at autopsy.

Although relapsing-remitting courses and asymmetric features occur, typically patients have progressive, painless leg weakness, stiffness, sensory loss, imbalance, and sphincter dysfunction, in the absence of a sensory level or prominent back pain. Arm function remains normal until advanced stages. The exam reveals slowly progressive spastic paraparesis, sensory ataxia, hyperreflexia, and extensor plantar responses.

In isolated VM, CSF is usually normal, but associated neuropathies or chronic aseptic meningitides may result in protein elevation; CSF analysis is useful to rule out other viral causes of myelopathy such as CMV, varicella-zoster, herpes simplex, and HTLV. B12, MMA, and HC levels should be assayed. SSEPs are usually abnormal.

MRI may be normal, but is useful because it can reveal unsuspected coexisting conditions such as extramedullary or intramedullary infections and neoplasms, degenerative disk, or joint disease of the spine. However, typical findings include cervical and thoracic cord atrophy, as well as usually symmetric nonenhancing high-signal areas on T2

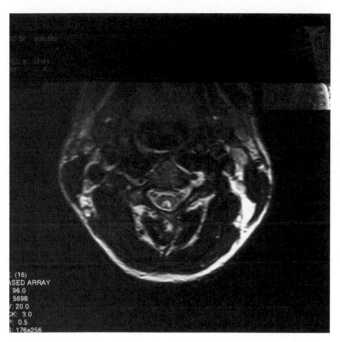

Figure 36.3A T2-weighted axial MRI (TR = 5698; TE = 96) of patient with VM.

images due to extensive vacuolation; this may be confined to the posterior columns, especially the gracile tracts, or may be diffuse (Figure 36.3A, B).

Pathologically, there is intramyelinic or periaxonal vacuolation and myelin pallor involving the dorsal and lateral more than the anterior and anterolateral tracts, and affecting the cervical and thoracic more than the lumbar segments or the

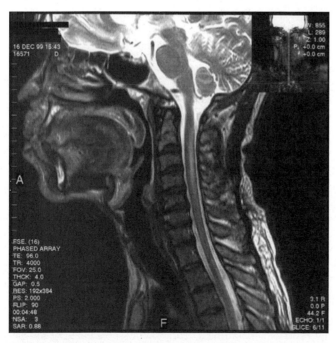

Figure 36.3B T2-weighted sagittal MRI (TR = 4000; TE = 96) of patient with VM.

brainstem, accompanied by astrogliosis. Axons are rarely disrupted. HIV is identified in activated, lipid-laden macrophages and microglia. The changes resemble those of SCD.

Anecdotal reports show improvement and remission with HAART. The prognosis is poor, but is determined by the underlying immune deficiency.

VASCULAR MALFORMATIONS OF THE SPINAL CORD

The nomenclature of vascular malformations has lacked consensus, resulting in many names for the same abnormality (19). Here, they are classified as extramedullary malformations on the surface of the spinal cord and intramedullary malformations within the substance of the spinal cord.

Extramedullary malformations result from the establishment of a fistula between an artery supplying and a vein draining the cord. Direct shunting of high-pressure arterial blood into veins causes them to dilate and elongate; it usually takes place in the nerve root canal or involves the anterior spinal artery on the ventral surface of the cord. These dilated serpentine tangles of vessels most commonly lie on the dorsal surface of the lower thoracic or lumbar cord. Less often, when the anterior spinal artery is involved, they are on the ventral or lateral surface. For the most part, they are considered to be acquired lesions, because they are not seen in children. Spinal cord symptoms are produced by compression by the venous mass or a "steal" phenomenon. This group accounts for about 75% of spinal vascular malformations (20).

Middle-aged and older men make up 80–90% of patients; they develop progressive leg weakness and sensory loss. Back pain, usually not severe, is frequent. Bladder symptoms occur, but are not an early symptom. Neurogenic intermittent claudication, in which symptoms are produced or exaggerated by walking, is frequent. If untreated, significant gait impairment occurs after several years.

Intramedullary vascular malformations usually become symptomatic in childhood or young adult life. They may also cause progressive weakness and sensory loss, but about one-third of patients have a sudden spinal cord event, sometimes of catastrophic proportions, because of hemorrhage into or infarction of the cord, which may occur as the presenting manifestation or be superimposed on a syndrome of progressive deficit.

MRI scan usually shows increased signal within the spinal cord on T2-weighted images. However, this finding is nonspecific. Flow voids from dilated vessels are seen only in about half the cases. MR angiography may provide additional information; definitive diagnosis is by spinal angiography.

Vascular malformations are treated by obliteration of the fistulae by embolization or surgical techniques. Most treated patients cease to deteriorate and about half improve.

PRIMARY PROGRESSIVE SPINAL MULTIPLE SCLEROSIS

Ten to 15% of MS patients have primary progressive MS (PPMS) without exacerbations or remissions, with onset usually after age 40. A female preponderance is less apparent. About half have a progressive myelopathy with occasional plateaus with spastic weakness, gait ataxia, impairment of position and vibratory sense, and sphincter and sexual dysfunction; it culminates in wheelchair dependency after about 20 years (21, 24).

Typical MS lesions seem to be less common and smaller on brain MRI in PPMS; enhancement is rare (22). Spinal MRI shows diffuse T2 lesions that often extend over many segments (23). As in RRMS and SPMS, CSF (oligoclonal banding or elevated gamma globulin) and evoked potential studies are typically abnormal (24).

No medications have received FDA approval, though many practitioners use the same drugs as in RRMS and SPMS. Treatment is otherwise symptomatic.

ARACHNOIDITIS

Arachnoiditis is a condition in which the arachnoidal membrane becomes adherent to the spinal cord and spinal nerve roots, causing partial or total obliteration of the subarachnoid space. The initiating event is thought to be an inflammatory reaction in the arachnoidal membrane. Various provocative events have been reported, including bacterial meningitis, surgical manipulation of the arachnoid membrane, and injection of chemical agents, especially myelographic dye, into the subarachnoid space. As arachnoiditis develops, fibrous tissue contraction progressively strangulates the nerve roots and spinal cord.

Reports before about 1980 emphasize a spinal cord syndrome with progressive paraparesis or tetraparesis and nerve root involvement, usually bilateral, at the upper level of the neurologic deficit, whereas more recent reports describe almost exclusively a progressive cauda equina syndrome or single lumbosacral nerve root involvement (25).

Patients develop back pain and usually bilateral sciatica. About 25% develop urinary incontinence. Neurologic examination shows paraparesis with muscle atrophy and fasciculations, and sensory and reflex loss in the distribution of the involved roots. This clinical picture is similar to that produced by lumbar spinal stenosis or central herniation of a lumbar intervertebral disk.

MRI findings depend on the severity of the inflammation and scarring. One pattern is a central clump of nerve roots within the spinal canal; this may be a single soft tissue mass or multiple cords of adherent roots. Alternatively, roots adhere to the peripheral walls of the thecal sac, producing so-called "empty sac" pattern: the spinal canal appears devoid of nerve roots. The least common pattern is of a single, large, nonspecific soft tissue mass within the spinal canal. Although variable, almost always some enhancement occurs; this may help identify clumped nerve roots or distinguish between tumor and arachnoiditis in that the former is brighter with contrast than the latter. If arachnoiditis leads to calcification or ossification, MR images lose signal where ossification is densest.

Surgical treatment consists of stripping the adhesive arachnoid tissue from nerve roots. This is controversial, but some authors claim it is beneficial in some patients (26).

SYRINGOMYELIA

Syringomyelia (27) is a disorder in which a cavity forms within the spinal cord, thus destroying segmental neurons and long ascending and descending tracts passing through the involved spinal segments. The exact mechanism of cavity formation is uncertain but appears to be in some way related to the obstruction of normal CSF flow by scar tissue or a congenital posterior fossa malformation. Two conditions are notably associated with syringomyelia. Syringomyelia associated with Chiari type I malformation, i.e. herniation of the cerebellar tonsils into the spinal canal, may become symptomatic at any age but most commonly does so in adolescents or young adults. Syringomyelia associated with spinal cord injury (SCI) may develop shortly after the trauma or years later. This is the subject of a separate chapter and will only be briefly dealt with here. Cavity formation also occurs in some intramedullary spinal cord tumors.

Because the syrinx usually begins in the central part of the lower half of the cervical cord (Figure 36.4), the first neural elements are likely to be involved two-fold: Destroyed are the fibers entering the dorsal horns from muscle stretch receptors and passing to AHCs, resulting in a loss of tendon reflexes. Also involved are fibers entering the dorsal horn from pain receptors that, after synapse, cross the cord to enter the spinothalamic tract; this destruction causes a loss of pain perception in the hands and arms. Fibers mediating touch, vibration, and position sense are uninvolved. This has been called dissociated sensory loss. Patients may present with unilateral features.

As the syrinx grows larger, symptoms and signs become bilateral. Invasion of the anterior horn gray matter produces muscle weakness, fasciculations, and atrophy in the arms. Eventually, pressure upon or actual invasion of the white matter pathways produces UMN signs and leg weakness as well as loss of position and vibration sense in the arms and legs. A Horner sign may be present. Bladder symptoms occur late or not at all. Syringomyelia is steadily

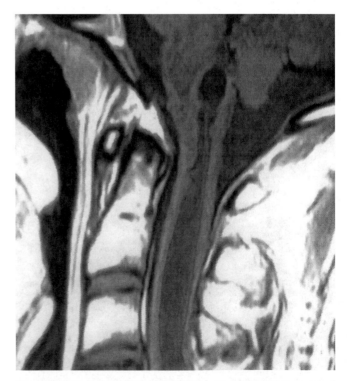

Figure 36.4 Sagittal T1-weighted image of the craniometrical junction demonstrating a central syrinx involving the cervical spinal and medulla.

progressive in about 50% and progressive with periods of stability in 25%. Some patients spontaneously cease to progress.

Pain is a common symptom in syringomyelia. Aching pain occurs over the site of the syrinx and extends upward in the neck and into the occipital area of the head. Many patients experience upper limb central neuropathic pain in the areas of altered sensation. The pain has a burning, shooting, or tingling quality, and may be severe. Patients with a Chiari I malformation frequently have cough-induced headache.

Clinically, it is difficult to distinguish syringomyelia from slow-growing intramedullary spinal cord tumors, so imaging studies can be very helpful. On MRI, syringomyelia is well demonstrated as an area of T1 and T2 prolongation within the spinal cord and is particularly obvious on FLAIR sequences. There is no enhancement. A collapsed syrinx appears similar to spinal cord atrophy with decreased cord diameter.

Surgery is the only effective treatment. With malformations at the craniospinal junction, a suboccipital decompression is done. In purely spinal forms, arachnoidal scarring is resected to reestablish normal CSF flow. If this is not possible, the syrinx cavity is shunted to the subarachnoid, the pleural, or the peritoneal spaces. About 80% of patients improve or cease to progress after surgery, but some 20% become worse (29).

SPINAL TUMORS

Spinal epidural tumors comprise about 55% of all spinal cord tumors (30, 31). Almost all are metastatic lesions of the vertebral column that extend into the epidural space to compress the spinal cord or cauda equina. Only about 5% are direct metastases to the epidural space. Lung, breast, and prostate are the site of the primary lesion in some 60%; a variety of other carcinomas, myelomas, and lymphomas account for the rest. Although some patients with epidural tumors are known to have cancer, spinal metastasis is commonly the first manifestation of malignancy. Rarely, the spinal cord itself is the site of a metastatic tumor, usually from the lung; the clinical features are indistinguishable from metastatic epidural tumor (32).

Local pain is the presenting symptoms in 95% of cases. The pain is moderate to severe and aching. Often it is worse when supine. Only about 50% report tenderness at the site of pain. Radicular pain is common as well, especially in lumbosacral lesions involving the cauda equina.

After a variable interval, patients develop signs of myelopathy with weakness and sensory abnormalities below the level of the lesion, which only then may bring them to medical attention and lead to diagnosis of the local lesion and the primary malignancy. Bladder symptoms are present in over 50% of cases. Reflexes are increased when the spinal cord is involved and decreased with cauda equina involvement. Patients with demonstrable neurologic abnormalities are at risk of developing sudden paralysis, indicating the need to begin treatment as soon as possible.

Lumbar puncture (LP) should not be done because of the risk of provoking clinical deterioration.

Plain spine films miss at least 20% of spinal metastatic tumors and often delay definitive diagnosis. The procedure of choice is MRI. The entire neuraxis should be surveyed to identify clinically silent additional lesions, including in the brain. In general, tumor masses show bone destruction with loss of the normal hypointense margin of cortical bone and bone marrow replacement, T1 and T2 prolongation, and contrast enhancement. The distinction of metastatic marrow replacement from acute osteoporotic compression fractures can be challenging.

The prognosis is poor and is related to that of the primary tumor. Only 50% of patients survive more than 6 months, and only 25% for more than one year. The goals of treatment are to preserve bowel and bladder control and ambulation as long as possible.

Untreated, patients progress to an anesthetic paraplegia or tetraplegia with total loss of bowel and bladder function. When an epidural lesion is the first indication of cancer and no primary tumor site can be identified, CT-guided percutaneous needle biopsy is diagnostic in 95% of cases. For over 50 years, standard of care was decompression by laminectomy followed by radiation therapy. About 25 years ago, a consensus developed that radiation without laminectomy is equally effective. Steroids, given at diagnosis to control vasogenic spinal cord edema, produce a rapid response; this is followed by radiation. Various steroids in various doses have been used. A commonly used protocol is 10 mg dexamethasone IV followed by 4 mg four times daily, tapering over several weeks. Combined steroids and radiation result in better outcome than radiation alone. When longer than usual survival is expected and the general condition permits, circumferential spinal cord decompression with surgical removal of maximal tumor tissue, usually by an anterior approach, is performed, followed typically by a stabilization procedure. Patients then receive radiation therapy (33).

Intradural extramedullary tumors (34) lie in the subarachnoid space. They are benign histologically and grow slowly. Meningiomas arise from arachnoidal cells. Schwannomas or neurofibromas arise from Schwann cells of the spinal roots. Each constitutes about 25% of primary spinal cord tumors. They arise lateral to the spinal cord and may involve any portion of the cord, although meningiomas most commonly occur in the cervical and thoracic areas. Both become symptomatic between ages 30–60. Meningiomas are more common in women.

Both meningiomas and Schwannomas present with local neck or back pain and frequently with radicular pain as well. Because of the slow growth, spinal cord symptoms may not appear until months or even years later. Eventually patients notice weakness and sensory symptoms below the level of the tumor. Bladder symptoms occur late in the course. Despite the lateral location, a lateral cord (Brown-Séquard) syndrome occurs in only about 5% of patients, although motor weakness usually begins on the side of the tumor.

MRI can reveal remodeling of the adjacent bone, but no destruction. The tumors have a characteristic "dumbbell" shape, because they grow through the neural foramen. They show T1 and T2 prolongation and enhance intensely. Dural AVMs, when large, may simulate an extramedullary-intradural mass, but can be identified by focusing on the signal void on T2-weighted sequences and abnormal T2 prolongation within the spinal cord due to ischemia.

The treatment of meningiomas and Schwannomas is surgical removal, which is usually curative.

Intramedullary tumors (35) arising within the spinal cord itself are most commonly ependymomas or astrocytomas, the former being about twice as common as the latter. Ependymomas tend to occur in the lower half of the spinal cord and cauda equina, whereas astrocytomas are mostly in the upper half of the spinal cord. Ependymomas are usually well demarcated and histologically benign. Astrocytomas, conversely, are more infiltrative, and about 25% are histologically malignant. Other histologies, including hemangioblastomas and metastases, are rare.

Ependymomas and benign astrocytomas are slowly growing lesions; patients are frequently symptomatic months or years before the tumor is detected. Local neck or back pain is usually the first symptom, followed by weakness and sensory symptoms below the level of the lesion. A lateral or central cord syndrome is present in some patients. Because about half of all ependymomas arise from the filum terminale, a cauda equina syndrome frequently occurs. Bladder symptoms develop late.

These cord tumors show T1 and T2 prolongation, widen the spinal cord, and enhance variably. They may be associated with syrinxes or may have cystic components (hemangioblastomas).

The optimal treatment of intramedullary spinal cord gliomas is surgical removal. In cases of incomplete removal of benign astrocytomas or with histological signs of malignancy, radiation therapy is given. Treatment is often curative with ependymomas and benign astrocytomas; the 10-year postoperative survival is about 80%. In malignant astrocytomas, however, postoperative 10-year survival is only about 15%.

RADIATION MYELOPATHY

Radiation myelopathy, in the form of a progressive myelopathy, is rare (36, 37). Among 1,048 patients who received radiation treatment for lung cancer, 0.5% developed radiation myelopathy (38). The cause is thought to be a radiation-induced vasculopathy.

The disorder has several curious clinical features, among them the long latency between the completion of radiation and symptom onset. Symptoms almost never appear until 6 months later and most commonly begin after 9 to 15 months. Also unusual is early spinothalamic involvement in the form of an anterior cord or Brown-Séquard syndrome with unilateral or bilateral loss of pain and temperature sensation. However symptoms begin, total transverse cord involvement occurs over about 6 months, producing paralysis and sensory loss below the radiated cord segment. There is no effective treatment.

Pathologically, the white matter of the cord is primarily affected with axonal loss and demyelination in the area exposed to radiation. There is a vasculopathy involving arteries and veins. Although it is assumed that the myelopathy results from the vasculopathy, alternatively the neural and vascular pathology develop independently.

Another radiation-related syndrome called acute transient radiation myelopathy consists of a Lhermitte's phenomenon in patients who have had radiation exposure of the cervical cord. There are no associated abnormal sensory or motor findings. The onset of symptoms usually occurs about 4 months after radiation therapy, and symptoms spontaneously resolve several months later.

References

1. Rowland LP, Schneider NA. Amyotrophic lateral sclerosis. *N Engl J Med* 2001; 344:1688–1700.
2. Parry GJ. Motor neuropathy with multifocal conduction block. In: Dyck PJ, Thomas PK, Griffin JW, et al. eds. *Peripheral Neuropathy.* 3rd ed., Philadelphia: WB Saunders, 1993:1518–1524.
3. Lomen-Hoerth C, Murphy J, Langmore S, et al. Are amyotrophic lateral sclerosis patients cognitively normal? *Neurology* 2003; 60:1094–1097.
4. Rowland LP, Mitsumoto H, De Vivo DC. Hereditary and acquired motor neuron diseases. In: Rowland LP. ed. *Merritt's Textbook of Neurology.* 11th ed. Philadelphia: Lippincott Williams & Wilkins, 2005:861–862.
5. Harding AE. *The Hereditary Ataxias and Related Disorders.* Edinburgh: Churchill Livingstone, 1984:174–190.
6. Pringle CE, Hudson A, Munoz DG, et al. Primary lateral sclerosis: Clinical features, neuropathology and diagnostic criteria. *Brain* 1992; 115:495–520.
7. Raymond F, Charcot M. Note sur deux cas de paralysie essentielle de l'enfance. atrophic musculaire consécutive. *Gaz Med Paris* 1875; 4:225–226.
8. Dalakas MC. The post-polio syndrome as an evolving clinical entity definition and clinical description. *Ann N Y Acad Sci* 1995; 753:68–80.
9. Windebank A, Litchy WJ, Daube JR, et al. Lack of progression of neurologic deficit in survivors of paralytic polio: A 5-year prospective population based study. *Neurology* 1996; 46:80–84.
10. Engstrom JW. HTLV-I infection and the nervous system. In: Aminoff MJ, ed. *Neurology and General Medicine.* 3rd edition, New York. Churchill Livingstone, 2001:777–788.
11. Lammertse DP. Neurorehabilitation of spinal cord injuries following lightning and electrical trauma. *NeuroRehabilitation* 2005; 20:9–14.
12. Byrne TN, Benzel EC, Waxman SG. *Diseases of the Spine and Spinal Cord.* Oxford: Oxford University Press, 2000:124–165.
13. Rowland LP. Surgical treatment of cervical spondylotic myelopathy: time for a controlled trial. *Neurology* 1992; 42:5–13.
14. Dvorak M, McGraw RW. Rheumatoid arthritis of the cervical spine. In: Critchley E, Eisen A, eds. *Spinal Cord Disease.* London: Springer, 1997:297–314.
15. Singh NN, Thomas FP. Vitamin B12 associated neurological diseases. http://emedicine.medscape.com/article/1152670-overview.
16. Diamond AL, Diamond R, Freedman SM, Thomas FP. "Whippets" induced cobalamin deficiency manifesting as cervical myelopathy. *J Neuroimaging* 2004; 14:277–280.
17. Delatycki MB, Williamson R, Forrest SM. Friedreich's ataxia: an overview. *J Med Genet* 2000; 37:1–8.
18. Singh NN, Thomas FP. HIV-1 associated vacuolar myelopathy. http://emedicine.medscape.com/article/1167064-overview.
19. Detwiler PW, Porter RW, Spetzler RF. Spinal arteriovenous malformations. *Neurosurg Clin N Am* 1999; 10:89–100.
20. Watson JC, Oldfield EH. The surgical management of spinal dural vascular malformations. *Neurosurg Clin N Am* 1999; 10:73–87.
21. Andersson PB, Waubant E, Gee L, et al. Multiple sclerosis that is progressive time of onset. *Arch Neurol* 1999; 56:1138–1142.
22. Thompson AJ, Kermode AG, Wicks D, et al. Major differences in the dynamics of primary and secondary progressive multiple sclerosis. *Ann Neurol* 1991; 29:53–62.
23. Nijeholt GJL, Barkhof F, Scheltens P, et al. MR of the spinal cord in multiple sclerosis: Relation to clinical subtype and disability. *Am J Neuroradiol* 1997; 18:1041–1048.
24. Bashir K, Whitaker JN. Clinical and laboratory features of primary progressive and secondary progressive MS. *Neurology* 1999; 53:765–771.
25. Shaw MD, Russell JA, Grossart KW. The changing pattern of spinal arachnoiditis. *J Neurol Neurosurg Psychiatry* 1978; 41:97–107.
26. Dolan RA. Spinal adhesive arachnoiditis. *Surg Neurol* 1993; 39:479–484.
27. Barnett HJM, Foster JB, Hudgson P. *Syringomyelia.* London: WB Saunders, 1973:11–29.

28. Milhorat TH, Capocelli AL, Anzil AP, et al. Pathological basis of spinal cord cavitation in syringomyelia: analysis of 105 autopsy cases. *J Neurosurg* 1995; 82:802–812.

29. Batzdorf U. Primary spinal syringomyelia. Invited submission from the joint section meeting on disorders of the spine and peripheral nerves. *J Neurosurg Spine* 2005; 3:429–435.

30. Byrne TN, Benzel EC, Waxman SG. *Diseases of the Spine and Spinal Cord.* Oxford: Oxford University Press, 2000; 166–205.

31. Siegal T, Seigal T. Spinal metastases. In: Schiff D, O'Neill BP, eds. *Principles of Neuro-Oncology.* New York: McGraw-Hill, 2005:581–598.

32. Schiff D, O'Neill BP. Intramedullary spinal cord metastases: Clinical features and treatment outcome. *Neurology* 1996; 47:906–912.

33. Patchell RA, Tibbs PA, Regine WF, et al. Direct decompressive surgical resection in the treatment of spinal cord compression caused by metastatic cancer: a randomized trial. *Lancet* 2005; 366:643–648

34. Schutta HS. Spinal tumors. In: Joynt RJ, Griggs RC, eds. *Clinical Neurology,* revised edition, Vol 3, Chapter 44. Philadelphia: Lippincott Williams and Wilkins, 1998:26–36.

35. Stieber VW, Tatter SB, Shaffrey ME, Shaw EG. Primary spinal tumors. In: Schiff D, O'Neill BP, eds. *Principles of Neuro-Oncology.* New York: McGraw-Hill, 2005:501–517.

36. Goldwein JW. Radiation myelopathy: A review. *Med Fed Oncol* 1987; 15:89–95.

37. Schultheiss TE, Stephens LC. Invited review: permanent radiation myelopathy. *Brit J Radiol* 1992; 65:737–753.

38. Macbeth FR. Radiation myelopathy: Estimates of risk in 1,048 patients in three randomized trials of palliative radiotherapy for non-small cell lung cancer. The Medical Research Council Lung Cancer Working Party. *Clin Oncol* 1996; 8:176–181.

37 Multiple Sclerosis

Jack Burks
George Kim Bigley
Haydon Harry Hill

Multiple sclerosis (MS) was first described in depth by the famous French neurologist Jean-Martin Charcot in 1868 (1). However, multiple sclerosis had likely been present for the preceding several centuries. In the United States, multiple sclerosis was considered a rare disease until the mid-twentieth century. The current estimates of multiple sclerosis in the United States exceed 400,000 cases. In addition to cerebral and ophthalmic involvement, spinal cord damage is seen in most MS patients. In fact, much of the disability is secondary to spinal cord damage. Many of the challenges facing MS patients are similar to those facing others with spinal cord dysfunction. Weakness, spasticity, pain, decreased mobility, as well as bowel, bladder, and sexual dysfunction, are common occurrences from spinal cord involvement in MS.

As we learn more of the pathogenesis of MS, the definition is evolving from the standard older textbook definition of a relapsing-remitting, inflammatory, demyelinating disorder. In fact, the disease course and pathogenesis are much more complex. Axonal and neuronal damage, along with a degenerative type of pathology, lead to continual damage and repair processes (2). Without treatment, most patients who begin with relapsing-remitting MS (RRMS) will develop a progressive disease after several years.

This chapter provides an overview of the pathogenesis, immunology, demographics, definition, epidemiology, etiologic considerations, diagnosis, disease course, differential diagnosis, clinical manifestations, disease modifying therapies, symptom management, rehabilitation, and emerging therapies for MS.

DEMOGRAPHICS

Multiple sclerosis is one of the leading causes of disability in young adults in the United States. The onset is usually between the ages of 18 and 40, but some children and older adults are also being diagnosed (3). Women are more often affected than men (3:1) with relapsing-remitting MS (RRMS). In primary progressive MS (PPMS), the disease is progressive from the onset, and gender differentiation is not found. In the United States,

Caucasians who live in temperate climates and whose families have emigrated from Northern Europe have the highest risk. Multiple sclerosis was thought to be uncommon or rare in Latin America, Asia, and Middle East. However, the prevalence of MS in these countries has increased (sometimes dramatically) in the last several years. Although African Americans are less likely to get MS than Caucasians, African Americans still have a significant risk. People who live in a high-risk area before adolescence and then move to a low-risk area are less likely to get MS than those who remain in a high-risk area. If one moves from a high-risk area to a low-risk area after adolescence, the risk of MS remains high. Environmental exposure to a virus(es) or toxic influences combined with a genetic susceptibility are the most likely explanation of this high-risk, low-risk phenomenon. Clusters of MS also support the hypothesis of environmental exposure. However, MS is not thought to be a communicable disease. Epidemiology studies continue to evaluate factors associated with the pathogenesis (4).

A genetic link has been demonstrated (5, 6). The risk of MS in close family members of MS patients is increased from the general population risk of 1 per 1,000 (0.1%) to 2%–5%. In monozygotic twins when one twin has MS, the risk of MS is as high as 30% in the other twin.

RISK FACTORS FOR DEVELOPING MULTIPLE SCLEROSIS

Some risk factors implicated in MS include environmental exposure, genetics, gender, age, lack of exposure to sunlight, less exposure to parasites, and other factors not yet identified.

Environmental Exposure

Environmental exposures have led to the postulation that the cause of MS is related to a virus or viral exposure, especially in childhood. In addition, industrial exposures or other toxic influences have often been considered but not proven. No specific toxic exposure has been convincingly incriminated.

A number of infectious agents have been linked to the etiology of MS. Those have included canine distemper, measles, corona virus, HTLV1, HTLV6, chlamydia, and Epstein Barr virus (EBV). Molecular mimicry may play an important role (7). Currently, Herpes virus 6 (8), chlamydia, and Epstein Barr virus are the leading candidates for potential infectious agents. Efforts to incriminate chlamydia and HHV6 have been mixed. However, substantial evidence is accumulating to link the association of MS with Epstein Barr virus (9–11). Epstein Barr virus (EBV) has been previously linked to Burkitt's lymphoma and Hodgkin's lymphoma as well as primary CNS lymphoma, nasopharyngeal carcinoma, posttransplant lymphoproliferative diseases, and gastric cancer. EBV is a neurotrophic virus that has been isolated from the brain and spinal fluid, primarily from B cells. It remains in the body in a latent state and has been identified as the cause of infectious mononucleosis that usually affects adolescents and young adults. Type 1 EBV is the predominate strain in developed countries. Antibodies to EBV virus are more common in MS patients than in the general population, although as many as 90% of members of the general population have EBV antibodies. The EBV antibodies titers are higher during MS relapses, and MS patients are more likely to have had mononucleosis than the general population. EBV antibodies have been identified in oligoclonal bands in the spinal fluid of patients with MS. Children with MS are more likely to be antibody positive for EBV virus. Elevated EBV titers associated with HLA DR15 haplotype increase the risk for MS even more (12, 13).

Another environmental exposure issue is lack of vitamin D and sunlight, which increase the risk of MS (14–17). Vitamin D has immunomodulatory activity, and lower levels of vitamin D in the blood are more likely found in areas of less sunlight exposure. Studies have found that nurses who took more than 400 IU of supplemental vitamin D a day were less likely to get MS. A Defense Department study showed that higher levels of vitamin D in the blood were associated with a lower risk of MS. Therefore, vitamin D and sunlight may have an effect on reducing the risk of developing MS. Nevertheless, these findings have not led to general recommendations of supplementing vitamin D for patients who have already contracted the disease. However, research continues in this area.

The relationship between parasitic diseases and MS is intriguing. Traditionally, underdeveloped countries have had a low risk of MS and a high risk of parasitic diseases. Parasitic diseases have a known immunomodulating effect. MS patients who also have parasitic diseases are likely to have a milder form of the disease (18). An MS treatment trial using parasites is under way (19).

Genetics and Multiple Sclerosis

Although MS is not considered a specific hereditary disease, the risk of MS is higher in close relatives than in controlled populations (20, 21). The risk of MS in the general population in the United States is approximately 0.1 per 1,000. In close family relatives, the risk is 1%–5%; in identical twins, the rate is approximately 30%, compared to like-sex fraternal twins, which is 2%–5%. In a Canadian study, genetic factors were considered the primary association for familial cluster cases, versus environmental factors. MRI studies have shown that 4% of relatives of patients with sporadic MS and 10% of relatives of patients with familial MS have asymptomatic brain lesions resembling MS.

However, these findings do not necessarily indicate clinical MS in these patients. Clustering of autoimmune disease in females with high risk for MS has been described (22).

The strongest genetic influence of MS appears to lie in the HLA-DRB1 gene, located on chromosome 6. The HLA Class II DR2, DR3, and DR4 haplotypes are overrepresented in MS. A polygenetic inheritance in MS with a number of genes contributes to the risk factors in MS. However, only chromosome 6 haplotypes have been consistently linked to MS. Recently, IL2 and IL7R polymorphisms have also been directly linked to MS (23). Therefore, the search for the associated genes in MS is narrowing.

Some evidence also shows that there may be genetic influence in the course of MS and the response to therapy. Some research suggests that the APOE4 gene is associated with a more aggressive MS (24). In addition, some groups, such as African Americans, may not respond as well to current interferon betas compared to other ethnic groups (25).

In summary, there seems to be a clear genetic link to the risk of MS. However, except for identical twins, the risk appears to be less than 5% in relatives of MS patients.

Gender Differences in Multiple Sclerosis

Women are at greater risk for MS than men, and that ratio may be increasing. Women also have an increased risk for other autoimmune diseases such as lupus, rheumatoid arthritis, and Sjögren syndrome. The increased risk may be related to the influence of sex hormones on the immune system. As early as 1969, birth control pills were shown to have an ameliorating effect on experimental autoimmune encephalomyelitis (EAE) in rodents (26). More recently, Estriol, a naturally occurring estrogen, has been shown to have a beneficial effect on MS in pilot studies (27, 28). Pregnancy reduces the exacerbation rate in MS during pregnancy. The risk of MS attacks in the last trimester of pregnancy declines by 70%. However, there was a 70% increase in exacerbation rate during the first 3 months postpartum. These changes are presumably related to the immunomodulating effects of hormones.

Breastfeeding does not appear to increase the risk of postpartum exacerbations. MS does not seem to have an effect on reproductive functions. Some studies have indicated that symptoms of MS and MRI activities are associated with hormonal fluctuations during the menstrual period (29, 30). Hormone replacement therapy and contraceptives have not been proven to reduce MS exacerbations.

The FDA-approved immunomodulating therapies of interferon betas, glatiramer acetate, Mitoxantrone, and Natalizumab are not recommended if pregnancy is contemplated. If an MS patient becomes pregnant while on one of these therapies, it is recommended that she stop the therapy until after the pregnancy is completed. Interferon beta is an abortifacient, but it has not been demonstrated to increase the risk of teratogenesity. Glatiramer acetate has not been associated with either abortions or fetal malformations. Nonetheless, caution is advised for all MS therapies.

PATHOLOGY OF MULTIPLE SCLEROSIS

MS damage is associated with results from immune dysregulation (2). This complex subject is not completely understood. An acute attack of MS is thought to begin with antigen-activated

T cells in the peripheral blood system. These activated T cells cross the blood-brain barrier and initiate a series of immunologic events involving cytokines, monocytes, plasma cells, macrophages, microglia, astrocytes, and chemokines. The activated T cells in the presence of antigen-presenting cells (APC) initiate a series of events where activated macrophages produce myelin toxic substances such as nitric oxide, free radicals, and pro-inflammatory cytokines, such as interferon gamma and TNF alpha. As a result, myelin, axons, and neurons are damaged.

Immunologic events both up-regulate and down-regulate the immune system in a complex series of interactions during an MS relapse. T cells, B cells, T regulatory cells, IL17 cells, and macrophages interact to up- or down-regulate the immune system, and through cytokines (pro- and anti-inflammatory) and chemokines. Based on these complex interrelated processes, current treatment goals include efforts to promote anti-inflammatory cytokines-producing cells, T regulatory cells, and brain-derived neurotrophic factors, while reducing pro-inflammatory cytokines-producing cells, IL 17 cells, and nitric oxide production.

Four specific immunopathologic patterns are described (31, 32). Pattern I involves a T cell and macrophage interaction. Pattern II appears to be related to antibody-mediated lesions associated with deposition of immunoglobulin and complement activation. Both patterns I and II are associated with partial oligodendrocytes survival and remyelination. Pattern III is a diffuse oligodendrogliopathy with apoptosis of oligodendrocytes and a preferential loss of myelin-associated glycoprotein protein (MAG). Type III resembles the diffuse pathology as might be seen in hypoxia or diffuse viral or toxic encephalitis. In pattern IV, the primary event appears to be oligodendrocyte degeneration.

Pattern II pathology was seen in 58% of cases compared to pattern III in 26%, pattern I in 15%, and pattern IV in 1% of cases studied. The patterns were exclusive in any individual patient (i.e., the pattern of pathology was the same in all lesions from any individual patient), indicating that there may be four distinct pathogenic subgroups.

Patterns I and II represent autoimmune demyelination, either T cell/macrophage associated or antibody/complement associated. Patterns III and IV involve oligodendrocyte damage primarily with less of an apparent immunology base. Patterns I and II are associated with remyelination, but not patterns III and IV.

Barnett and Prineas offer an alternative explanation, in that a primary injury to oligodendrocytes may represent the initial lesions in RRMS patients (33). They postulate that MS may not be primarily an autoimmune disease and that inflammation may be secondary to damage of oligodendrocytes. They are not convinced that four separate immunogenic subtypes of MS exist.

Remyelination

Remyelination may be extensive in MS (34). Remyelination can be related to the survival of oligodendrocytes or from stem cell-type differentiation. In addition, T cells can also release anti-inflammatory cytokines such as interleukin 4 and 10, as well as brain-derived neurotropic factor (BNDF), which may promote repair and remyelination.

Axonal Injury

Axonal injury and loss is well documented in MS (35–37). Dark spots or "black holes" in T-1 MRI are indicative of axonal damage or loss. Inflammation is associated with axonal loss as well as myelin damage. Neurotoxic substances such as nitrous oxide can damage both axons and myelin. In pattern II immunopathology, antibodies and compliment also damage axons as well as myelin. However, noninflammatory chronic lesions also show axonal loss, which may indicate that subtle inflammation occurs even in late secondary progressive MS (SPMS) or primary progressive MS (PPMS). Other factors may play a role in MS lesion development and progression.

Late pathology may result from early damage. Earlier demyelination, which is associated with repair, may leave the damaged cells susceptible to eventual programmed death or apoptosis after several years. Axons that are relatively intact, but that have lost their protective myelin cover, may be more susceptible to local environmental influences and further damage. Early transected axons may undergo Wallerian degeneration (antegrade from the site of the initial myelin damage). Damage to the axon can increase intranodal calcium, which leads to impaired axon transport and further disruption of axonal function.

Gray Matter

Gray matter pathology can be present in very early multiple sclerosis (38, 39). Current MRI technology usually does not usually detect gray matter abnormalities. However, utilizing higher MRI magnets, some gray matter lesions are extensive and can involve the entire cortical gray matter thickness. Cortical lesions affect both myelin and neurons. Monocytes are rarely seen in cortical lesions. Cortical lesions are more likely seen in progressive types of MS than in RRMS. Demyelination in the gray matter may be extensive. Cortical lesions may explain some of the cognition dysfunction as well as the poor correlation between the clinical examination and the white matter lesion load on MRI.

Normal-appearing White Matter

Normal-appearing white matter may not be normal in MS (40). By newer imaging techniques, diffuse white matter changes are seen even in areas where the routine MRI is normal. This may be secondary to Wallerian degeneration or other silent mechanisms of damage.

Degenerative Changes

Degenerative changes in the CNS are prominent in later stages of MS. The rate of progression in MS may not be related exclusively to relapses or inflammation as seen by the MRI. Although immunomodulating therapies have a marked effect on inflammation, they have less effect on progressive types of MS. Progressive axonal loss may occur in areas without widespread white matter lesions. Magnetic resonance spectroscopy reveals a decrease in n-acetyl aspartate (NAA) in gray and white matter, which suggests primarily neuronal and axonal degeneration (41, 42).

In summary, at least two mechanisms of damage are noted in the CNS. In addition to the inflammatory lesions, a separate neurodegeneration process exists. Damage in the progressive MS disease types may be related to separate degenerative processes or to an intrinsic CNS inflammatory process without associated blood-brain barrier abnormalities. In other words, instead of the activation of the immune system occurring in the periphery, the destructive process might be compartmentalized to the central nervous system.

CLINICAL SUBTYPES IN MULTIPLE SCLEROSIS

Types of MS include relapsing/remitting MS disease (RRMS), secondary progressive MS (SPMS), primary progressive MS (PPMS), and progressive relapsing MS (PRMS) (43). A newly defined early MS type is called clinically isolated syndrome (CIS). CIS is the earliest clinical manifestation of RRMS, although damage may precede this first event. This diagnosis, along with specific MRI damage, allows for treatments to commence earlier in patients who are destined to get clinically definite RRMS, but have not had a second attack.

Clinically Isolated Syndrome (CIS)

This syndrome is defined as the onset of the first acute clinical demyelinating event with MRI evidence of subclinical demyelination not related to the clinical symptoms (44, 45). These patients are considered to be at very high risk for clinically definite MS and are likely to benefit from treatment before the second clinical episode. Other causes of demyelinating pathologies must be excluded such as those listed in Table 37.1. Patients with clinically isolated syndrome and a T-2 lesion load greater than 1.23 cc have a 90% chance of developing clinically definite MS (CDMS) within 5 years. Of these patients, 52% will have an expanded disability status scale (EDSS) score greater than 3 at

---

Table 37.1 Differential Diagnosis of Multiple Sclerosis

- Acute disseminated myelitis (ADEM)
- Neuromyelitis optica (devic)
- Collagen vascular disease (SLE)
- CADASIL
- Thyroid disease
- Hypoglycemia
- Vitamin deficiencies (B12)
- Sjögren syndrome
- Behçet disease
- Myasthenia gravis
- Spinocerebellar degeneration
- Adrenoleukodystrophies
- Lyme disease
- Syphilis
- TB, other CNS infections
- Sarcoidosis
- CNS malignancy
- CNS embolic disease
- AVM
- AIDS
- PML
- Migraine headache
- Psychosomatic

---

5 years. Patients with normal MRIs with clinically isolated syndrome have less than a 20% chance of developing clinically definite MS. Patients with two or more MRI lesions unrelated to the clinical event have an 85% chance of developing clinically definite MS by 2 years (46).

Relapsing-Remitting MS (RRMS)

This form is the most common type of MS. Relapses are defined as new or recurrent clinical signs or symptoms lasting more than 24 hours. These episodes may take months to resolve. They are followed by either partial or complete remissions. In relapsing-remitting MS, the patient remains stable between attacks. However, relapses may lead to residual deficits over time (47).

Secondary Progressive Disease (SPMS)

This version of MS is defined in patients who initiated their MS symptoms with RRMS but, after a period of time, came to have progression between attacks. Later, they came to have progression without evidence of clinical attacks. Approximately 50% of untreated RRMS patients will develop SPMS within 10 years, and 90% may develop SPMS after 25 years (48, 49). SPMS is described as a slow, insidious, progressive neurologic deterioration with or without relapses, following RRMS.

Primary Progressive MS (PPMS)

This form is found in approximately 10% of MS patients and is characterized as a slowly progressive deterioration without relapsing or remissions from the onset of neurologic symptoms. Patients with PPMS tend to experience onset at an older age and to have prominent spinal cord symptoms leading to progressive weakness, sensory loss, and spasticity, as well as bowel, bladder, and sexual dysfunction over a period of several years.

Progressive Relapsing MS (PRMS)

This form is relatively rare (5%). In PRMS, patients start with progressive MS but will have occasional exacerbations. Patients continue to deteriorate between relapses.

In a cross-sectional analysis of one MS population, 55% of patients had RRMS, 31% SPMS, 9% PPMS, and 5% PRMS.

Benign or Mild MS

The definition of benign MS has been controversial. Some studies have shown that patients with "benign MS" after 10 years will continue to deteriorate (50). In one study, only 20% maintained their true benign status after another 10 years of follow-up. Factors favorable to forecast benign MS include RRMS onset before age 40, fewer areas of CNS involvement on MRI, optic neuritis, sensory and brainstem symptoms, female gender, and infrequent relapses. Unfavorable prognostic factors include onset after age 40; multiple areas of CNS involvement, including motor, cerebellar, and sphincter involvement; male gender; and frequent relapses early in the disease. The percentage of patients that have sustained "benign MS" is debated but is likely around 10%, if patients are untreated.

"Burned Out" MS

The existence of "burned out" MS is a controversial issue. However, some patients with severe disability stabilize, usually after age 50 or 60.

DIAGNOSIS OF MULTIPLE SCLEROSIS

Lesions in Time and Space

The diagnosis of MS is usually determined by a detailed neurologic history and examination, which indicate "multiple lesions in time and space." In other words, multiple areas of the central nervous system are involved, and damage occurs at different times. Lesions can be documented by clinical findings, such as a second confirmed attack, or by MRI findings of subclinical demyelinating lesions. Initially these new subclinical lesions were defined by a second MRI at least 3 months after the clinically isolated syndrome (McDonald criteria) (51). Recently, the McDonald criteria have undergone revision to include new T-2 lesions at 1 month after CIS, to indicate MS if other MS mimickers have been eliminated (52). Also, spinal cord lesions are included in the latest criteria. Even newer criteria are being developed to suggest that treatment immediately following a CIS is reasonable.

Early clinical signs of MS may include visual loss, fatigue, numbness, parasthesias, weakness, visual disturbances such as double vision or an intranuclear opthalmoplegia, trigeminal neuralgia, facial nerve paralysis, cerebral ataxia, neuropathic pain (including L'Hermitte's sign), or even cognitive dysfunction.

Imaging in Multiple Sclerosis

After a thorough history and examination, an MRI may reveal multiple subclinical lesions, which involve the periventricular white matter, subcortical area, brainstem, cerebellum, or spinal cord. Hyperintense lesions on the T-2 MRI are the most common early lesions. In addition, contrast-enhancing (GAD) lesions are often seen early in many MS patients on T-1 MRI images. The enhancement may take several forms, from a mild enhancement to an intense ring enhancement pattern. Higher-dosed contrast material and higher magnet strength may increase the diagnostic accuracy. T-1 hypo-intense lesions, or "black holes," are thought to correlate with axonal loss, but a recent study has shown that "black holes" may not lead to persistent hypo-intensities on a T-1 MRI (53). Increasing T-2 lesion volume loss is correlated with increased risk of SPMS and increased disability over a 20-year period (54).

Cerebral Atrophy

Cerebral atrophy on MRI decreases brain volume and increases the ventricular size. Quantifying atrophy is often one of the MRI criteria in clinical trials. However, in routine clinical practice, cerebral atrophy on MRI may not be obvious.

Spinal Cord MRI Abnormalities

Spinal cord MRI abnormalities are detectable in most patients with MS in clinical research evaluations (55).

New MRI technology has not been incorporated in most clinical settings but is becoming more available. For example,

magnetic resonance spectroscopy (MRS) allows one to measure various tissue metabolites such as n-Acetylaspartate (NAA), a marker for axons and neurons. Flare MRI is incorporated in most MRI centers, which increases the sensitivity for identifying and quantifying MS lesions. Functional MRI relates blood oxygen level–dependent signals to the brain during activation while completing a complex task. Diffusion tensor imaging measures the diffusion of water as an indication of tissue damage. Magnetization transfer imaging is another research tool used to increase sensitivity for detecting brain damage and repair.

Other Tests in Multiple Sclerosis

Cerebral Spinal Fluid

Cerebral spinal fluid (CSF) analysis is a recommended diagnostic test by many neurologists. Before the advent of the MRI, it was a mainstay for ancillary MS testing. CSF protein is usually normal, as is glucose. Cell counts usually do not exceed 10 to 20 white blood cells per cc in MS. In MS the cerebral spinal fluid will often indicate an increased IGG production in the spinal fluid as well as showing oligoclonal bands within the IGG range. Serum values of immunoglobulins need to be obtained at the same time as the CSF. Routine spinal fluid evaluations also are performed to rule out infection, neoplastic disease, or other central nervous system disorders.

Evoked Potentials

Evoked potentials measure the speed of impulse within the central nervous system from the sensory pathways of the extremities, as well as visual and auditory brainstem pathways. Visual evoked potential abnormalities are most consistently seen in MS or optic neuritis.

Cognitive Testing

Cognitive testing is not used routinely in most clinics but is found to be abnormal in many patients, even with clinically isolated syndrome. User-friendly and computer-based cognitive testing systems are being developed (56–58).

Other Tests

Other evaluations done in MS patients involve measuring disability, usually with the EDDS, the MS functional composite scale (MSFCS), or the Scripps scale. These evaluations are usually utilized to measure serial disability scores in clinical trials.

Other tests are usually included to rule out possibilities of other diseases, which may mimic MS, listed in Table 37.1. The most common screening tests include a complete blood count (CBC), thyroid studies, antinuclear antibody testing, syphilis serology, vitamin B-12 levels, folic acid levels, lime titers in high-risk areas, and erythrocyte sedimentation rate. Other special tests for the MS mimics are also available.

Optical Coherence Tomography

Optical coherence tomography (OCT) is an emerging clinical trial evaluation that measures infrared light reflected from the retina (59). OCT measures the thickness and integrity of the retinal nerve fiber layer. Because these nerve cells have no myelin, one can get a direct view of the axon and axonal damage. An abnormal nerve fiber layer indicates loss of axons in MS patients. OCT may become recognized as a test to follow specific damage to axons in the central nervous system. OCT is now being used in several clinical trials to test its validity in measuring progressive damage to axons in MS.

DIFFERENTIAL DIAGNOSES OF MULTIPLE SCLEROSIS

The differential diagnoses of MS are in Table 37.1. They include metabolic, neoplastic, vascular, inflammatory, granulomatous, infectious, and psychosomatic conditions (60–65). Acute disseminated encephalomyelitis (ADEM) and neuromyelitis optica (NMO) are two conditions that can be easily confused with MS.

Acute Disseminated Encephalomyelitis (ADEM)

This disorder can be difficult to distinguish from MS clinically isolated syndrome (66). ADEM may be seen more frequently in children, the elderly, or after an infection or vaccination. However, ADEM can occur without an antecedent event. It is usually monophasic but can be recurrent. Seizures and encephalopathy are more common than in RRMS. Spinal fluid protein and white cells may be elevated, but there is less likelihood of oligoclonal bands in the spinal fluid. ADEM is treated with IV steroids without MS disease–modifying therapies. The long-term prognosis is usually favorable, if recovery occurs.

Neuromyelitis Optica (NMO)

Neuromyelitis optica, also known as Devic's disease, can be confused with MS (67). The gender predilection in NMO is more strongly female-to-male than in MS, with an approximate ratio of 10:1. There is less ethnic predilection compared to MS. In fact, NMO can be seen throughout the world. Distinguishing features of NMO include an optic neuritis and a transverse myelitis occurring together or within a matter of several months. White blood cell counts may exceed 50 per cc in the cerebrospinal fluid (CSF). Polymorphonuclear white cells may also be detected in the CSF. Oligoclonal banding is usually negative in the CSF. The spinal cord MRIs may show longitudinally extensive lesions greater than three spinal segments with central necrotic lesions in the spinal cord. Some cerebral lesions are permitted in the diagnosis. An Aquaporin-4 antibody or NMO antibody is found in approximately 70% of cases, indicating that this may be an antibody-mediated disease.

Optica Spinal MS

In Asia, an optica spinal form of MS is reported. This form has also been reported in Latin America. The female-to-male ratio is approximately 3:1. The brain MRI may be normal or may show typical MS lesions, and spinal cord lesions can be of variable length. Oligoclonal bands are seen in approximately 30% of cases, and NMO antibody is found in over 50% of patients, especially if long cord spinal lesions are present (68). The specific relationship between NMO and optica spinal MS is under investigation.

DISEASE-MODIFYING THERAPIES IN MS

Before the release of Betaseron in 1993, there was no widely accepted or FDA-approved treatment to alter the long-term disease course. Corticosteroids, especially given intravenously at very high doses (1,000 mg per day) for 3 to 10 days, were utilized for patients with moderate-to-severe exacerbations of MS. No evidence showed that this treatment altered the long-term prognosis of the patient.

Five disease-modifying therapies (DMTs) have now been approved by the FDA as first-line therapies in multiple sclerosis. They are Betaseron (interferon B-1b, sc 1993), Avonex (interferon B-1a, I.M., 1996) Copaxone (glatiramer acetate, SC, 1996), Rebif (interferon B-1a, subcutaneous, 2002) and Extavia (interferon B-1b, sc, 2009). In addition, Mitoxantrone (Novantrone, 2000), an immunosuppressant anti-neoplastic agent, is indicated for worsening MS, and Natalizumab (Tysabri, 2004), a monoclonal antibody (anti-VLA-4), is approved for relapsing MS but is currently used primarily as a "rescue therapy," when other drugs have produced suboptimal responses or shown significant toxicity.

Interferon Betas (Betaseron, Extavia, Avonex, Rebif)

Interferon betas have anti-inflammatory effects by suppressing pro-inflammatory T cells and cytokines, such as interferon gamma, as well as reducing blood-brain barrier permeability, which inhibits activated lymphocytes from migrating into the brain.

Interferon B-1b: Betaseron and Extavia

Betaseron was the first interferon beta approved by the FDA after it was shown to reduce exacerbation rates by one-third and MRI lesions by more than 80% in relapsing-remitting MS cases (69). In secondary progressive MS, one study from Europe demonstrated reduced relapses, progression of disability, and MRI lesions (70). Betaseron was approved for the treatment of SPMS in Europe and Canada. A North American trial in SPMS showed some of the same positive effects but did not show an effect on disability (70). In the United States, Betaseron is approved for relapsing forms of MS, which includes patients with secondary progressive disease who are still having relapses.

Extavia, which was FDA approved in 2009, is a bio-identical product to Betaseron.

In a recent CIS trial, Betaseron reduced the risk for clinically definite MS by 55% after 2 years, compared to a placebo treatment. It also decreased the risk of progression of disability by 40% at the end of 3 years in patients who received continuous Betaseron treatments versus those who got delayed Betaseron treatments (46). The delayed group was treated with Betaseron after they had a second episode, or after 2 years, whichever came first.

Interferon Beta 1-a

This drug is available in two preparations—Avonex and Rebif—which are similar but are given at different frequency doses and through different routes of administration. Avonex is given intramuscularly, once weekly at 30 mg and is approved by the FDA for relapsing forms of MS. The pivotal trial showed an effect on the exacerbation rate and disability progression. It is also approved in CIS to reduce the risk of clinically definite MS at 2 years (72). A follow-up study at 5 years showed continued benefit in those taking Avonex for CIS (73).

Rebif is usually given in the United States as a 44-mg dose subcutaneously three times a week. The pivotal trial showed a positive effect on relapses, MRI, and disability (74). An SPMS clinical trial with Rebif showed a positive effect in patients who were still having relapses (75).

Adverse events from interferon beta include flu-like side effects, which can be minimized with dose escalation and prophylactic analgesics such as ibuprofen, acetaminophen, or aspirin. Injection site reactions are another potential problem with subcutaneous interferons. However, auto-injectors and better injection techniques have minimized these problems considerably. Depression may occur and should be evaluated by the treating physician on a regular basis. Increase in liver abnormalities and decrease in white blood cell counts, as well as thyroid abnormalities, are also occasionally seen in interferon therapies. Blood tests are followed over the course of treatment. Injection site pain is another potential problem.

Neutralizing Antibodies

Neutralizing antibodies (NAbs) (76, 77) have been detected in interferon-treated patients. Their significance is debated. The American Academy of Neurology does not recommend routine testing. Antibodies to Betaseron are more frequent, but are usually of lower titer and are more transient. Rebif has less likelihood of antibodies than Betaseron but may be of a higher titer and more persistent. Avonex has the lowest titer of interferon antibodies, with only about 5% of patients having neutralizing antibodies on Avonex. The association of high-titered and persistent NAbs with reduced efficacy is likely (77).

Glatiramer Acetate (Copaxone)

A random sequence of four amino acids within the myelin basic protein structure, glatiramer acetate (GA) is approved for relapsing-remitting MS. It has been shown to positively affect the relapse rate and the MRI. The mechanism of action reveals that it reduces pro-inflammatory T cells and cytokines and converts pro-inflammatory Th1 cells to anti-inflammatory Th2 cells, which can migrate into CNS and produce brain-derived nerve growth factor (BDNF) (78, 79). BDNF may have a neuro-protective affect. Recently, Copaxone has also been shown to act on antigen presenting cells (APC) as well (80).

Given subcutaneously, at 20 mg per day, GA side effects include transient injection site pain, skin redness, and lipoatrophy. An infrequent adverse event is a postinjection systemic reaction, which is manifest by chest tightness, pain, flushing, anxiety, and shortness of breath, usually lasting for only a few seconds to a few minutes, without sequelae. Binding antibodies in glatiramer acetate have been detected, but neutralizing antibodies have not been consistently demonstrated.

Data have shown effectiveness of GA in CIS (81) and now GA has been approved for CIS by the FDA. In a pilot study, doubling the dose of GA to 40 mg per day was more effective than the 20-mg dose in RRMS (82). A larger trial is under way. A study

in PPMS was not successful, although a post hoc analysis indicated a possible effect in males. GA is not FDA approved for PPMS.

Long-Term Data from Immunomodulating Therapies

Encouraging long-term data have been presented. Betaseron, Copaxone, Avonex, and Rebif have all demonstrated that patients who stay on therapy continue to show beneficial effects. The scientific rigor of these data has been challenged because patients who stop therapy may be lost to follow-up. However, all long-term data demonstrate the benefits of staying on therapy continually.

Head-to-Head Class I Trials

The results of four Class 1 head-to-head trials have been published. The INCOMIN trial demonstrated greater efficacy with Betaseron over Avonex in class 1 MRI data at 2 years (83). The second is the EVIDENCE trial, which showed clinical and MRI superiority of Rebif over Avonex at 24 and 48 weeks (84). The REGARD trial showed there was no difference in relapse rate between Copaxone and Rebif (85). The BEYOND trial showed no difference in relapses or disability between Copaxone and Betaseron (86). In the Copaxone vs. interferon trials, some MRI data favored the interferons. The annualized relapse rate for Copaxone, Betaseron, and Rebif were all much better than demonstrated in the pivotal trials. These low relapse rates were likely due to early treatment in these recent trials. The CombiRx trial, which is in progress, compares Copaxone, Avonex, and a combination of the two.

Mitoxantrone (Novantrone)

Mitoxantrone is a chemotherapeutic agent used to treat neoplastic disease. MS clinical trials of Mitoxantrone have lead to the FDA approval of Mitoxantrone for "worsening MS." The recommended dosage is 12 mg per meter square every 3 months, not to exceed 140 mg per meter square total dose. This limitation is to avoid cardiotoxicity, which may be permanent. Amenorrhea and the risk of secondary leukemia with Mitoxantrone are also potential adverse events. Mitoxantrone is usually used as a rescue therapy for patients who have not responded adequately to the immunomodulating therapies discussed earlier.

Natalizumab (Tysabri)

Natalizumab is a monoclonal antibody (anti-VLA-4) that reduces the transmigration of lymphocytes across the blood-brain barrier. In the pivotal trial against placebo, a 68% reduction in relapse rate and an 85% reduction in active MRI lesions, as well as a 42% reduction in disability, were noted (87). After FDA approval, two cases of progressive multifocal leukoencephalopathy (PML) were reported (88, 89). One case was fatal. At that point, the drug was voluntarily withdrawn from the market. A third case of PML, which was also fatal, was found in a non-MS trial. After a thorough safety evaluation, Natalizumab was reapproved with added monitoring. It is mainly used as a rescue therapy for patients who have a suboptimal response to the immunomodulating therapies.

More safety data may modify its utilization. Currently over 60,000 patients have gone through the safety monitoring programs for Natalizumab. To date thirty-one new cases of PML have been detected. It is recommended that Natalizumab only be used as monotherapy for MS. Since the re-release, not enough long-term data are available to determine Natalizumab's ultimate safety profile.

Comprehensive Team Care, Rehabilitation, and Symptom Management

Since the introduction of disease modifying therapies beginning in 1993, the long-term benefits have become obvious to most MS experts. Patients with relapsing forms of MS are being helped substantially by a reduction in attacks and in the progression of disability. However, none of these treatments "cures" the disease. Therefore, the need for aggressive rehabilitation and symptom management care remain high. In recent years, numerous studies have evaluated the effectiveness of MS rehabilitation in both the inpatient and outpatient settings (90–93). The effort to maintain the highest function and quality of life, despite progressive disease, is a major challenge facing MS patients. Also, no FDA-approved treatments are available for primary progressive MS. Therefore, rehabilitation is the mainstay of therapy.

Comprehensive MS Team Care

In addition to disease modifying therapies, comprehensive team care for rehabilitation and symptom management is the "gold standard" for caring for MS patients (Figure 37.1). The MS healthcare team works to maximize quality of life and independence in the community for the patients. The MS "medical model" approach utilizes healthcare professionals to provide direct care to reduce tissue damage and symptoms. This approach is combined with a "functional model" of care, where the healthcare professionals function as educators and coordinators of care and the patient takes a more active role in the decisions that affect his or her well-being (Table 37.2). This care team provides knowledgeable, comprehensive, and timely care, while educating patients, family, and caregivers, and providing information to help patients understand their condition and available community resources. Examples of patients' needs include "best practice" healthcare, emotional support, family support, employment counseling, equipment and aids, modification in the home, work and transportation, insurance guidance, disability guidance, legal guidance, and transportation, among others. Mobility and

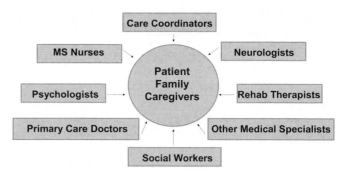

Figure 37.1 Integrated medical and functional model: patient-centered and seamless.

activity levels, as well as supporting family, friends, caregivers, and the patient, are addressed. The teams strive for functional improvement and safety while helping the patients adapt and cope with their MS. The goals of the functional model are to enhance patient function and to improve psychosocial well-being and quality of life.

An integrated comprehensive MS team care model includes neurologists, primary care doctors, MS nurses, other medical specialists, rehabilitation therapists, psychologists, social workers, health educators, care coordinators, the patient's family, and the patient's caregivers (Table 37.3). The aim is a seamless patient-centered combination of a medical and functional model of care (Table 37.2).

Tables 37.3–37.10 are examples of the roles of the various MS specialty team members. As one can see from the variety of interventions from each of the healthcare professionals, an integrated comprehensive approach can cover most of the patient's medical and functional issues.

Integrating Western Medicine with Complementary and Alternative Medicine

Alternative medicine can be a major support to people with MS. However, MS patients can become victimized by some care providers, especially those who promote items that "enhance immune function." MS patients already have an up-regulated immune system. Therefore, products that increase immune system activity may actually be harmful to MS patients. *Dietary Supplements and Multiple Sclerosis: A Health Professional's Guide* and *Complementary and Alternative Medicine and Multiple Sclerosis* are recommended reading (94, 95).

Table 37.2   Integrating Medical and Functional Health Care

	MEDICAL MODEL	FUNCTIONAL MODEL
Goal orientation	Disease state	Quality of life
Healthcare professional's role	Director	Educator, coordinator
Patient's role	More passive	More active
Organization	Fragmented: no integrated team	Interdisciplinary team
Objectives	Reduce tissue damage and symptoms	Enhance function and psychosocial well-being

Table 37.3   Integrated Comprehensive MS Care: The Team (Medical Model)

- Neurologists
- MS nurses
- Primary care doctors
- Other medical specialists
- Rehabilitation therapists
- Psychologists
- Social workers
- Health educators
- Care coordinators/Patient navigators
- The patient/family/caregivers

Table 37.4   The Role of the MS Specialist Team— Physicians

- Diagnosis of MS
- Medical care, including other medical conditions
- Disease-modifying therapies
- Prevent and manage adverse events
- Symptomatic MS treatments
- Clinical trial principal investigator (PI)
- Team leader
- Champion for patients and healthcare professional team

Table 37.5   The Role of the MS Specialist Team—Nurses

- First contact for patient follow-up (often)
- MS education
- Help keep patients on therapy
- Clinical trial coordination
- Self-care skills
- Counseling and support
- Bowel, bladder, and sexuality programs
- Nutrition
- Skin care
- Champion for patients and healthcare professional team

Table 37.6   The Role of the MS Specialist Team— Physical Therapists

- Strength, range of motion
- Tone
- Balance, coordination, and safety
- Ambulation/mobility
- Bed mobility/transfers
- Breathing exercises
- Adaptive equipment
- General conditioning
- Fatigue management

Table 37.7   The Role of the MS Specialist Team— Occupational Therapists

- Strength/range/tone/coordination
- Sensory/perceptual compensation
- Activities of daily living (ADL)
- Fatigue management
- Adaptive equipment
- Home management and modification
- Vocational evaluation
- Driving evaluation
- Wheelchair evaluation

Table 37.8   The Role of the MS Specialist Team— Speech/Language Pathologists

- Dysphagia
- Dysarthria/voice disorders
- Communication pragmatics
- Cognitive impairments: retraining

Table 37.9   The Role of the MS Specialist Team— Psychologists/Psychiatrists/Other Psychotherapists

- Affective (depression)/anxiety/personality changes
- Cognitive impairment: retraining and adaptation
- Psychologic problems (family, work, coping)
- Clinical trials: cognitive evaluations
- Psychiatric medications
- Teach strategies to enhance quality of life
- Family and caregiver support
- Team counseling

Table 37.10   The Role of the MS Specialist Team— Social Workers

- Resource identification
- Counseling and family support
- Disposition planning

Caregiver Support

The importance of caregiver support cannot be underestimated for MS patients. Fifty million family caregivers are in the United States. The risk of anxiety, stress, and depression in caregivers has been called a national crisis, with over 50% of caregivers suffering significantly. In fact, 50% of caregivers feel their own health has deteriorated within the first six months of assuming their role. Caregivers' immunologic dysfunction continues for at least 3 years after their role ends (96). Caregivers need information about MS and available resources as much as patients. Psychosocial and emotional support for caregivers is critical. Respite care, which provides caregivers independent time and space, can be an important break for caregivers. An interdisciplinary approach to the disease provides help for caregivers and family members as well as MS patients.

Coordination of the various aspects of care "through the system" is a major challenge in MS. In cancer, the concept of a patient navigator to provide support and referrals to needed resources is gaining support. Voluntary health organizations for MS such as the National MS Society (NMSS), the MS Association of American (MSAA), the MS Foundation (MSF), and others provide some of these resources. A care coordinator or patient navigator helps to identify financial, home, health, transportation, and other resources. He or she can coordinate clinical trial opportunities and can work with insurance companies and employers to reduce nonreimbursed care. He or she can help patients, families, and caregivers to navigate the healthcare system independently, resulting in less dependency on the caregivers. Patient navigators provide timely and compassionate help at a time of need. Unfortunately, other members of the MS comprehensive healthcare team are often too overcommitted to take on this added responsibility.

In summary, the comprehensive care team integrates the medical and functional healthcare models with professionals who understand that maintaining a high quality of life is a complex challenge necessitating interdisciplinary teamwork.

Disease Management and Rehabilitation

The ideal long-term management of MS patients resides in the interdisciplinary rehabilitation model using a team approach to patients. Most physicians treating MS patients are troubled by a fragmented healthcare system for people with chronic disabilities. This fragmentation, miscommunication, and lack of collaboration are problematic for MS patient care. The management of MS patients involves not only diagnosis and medical management but also preventive maintenance, by addressing family, caregiver, employment, and avocational issues. Education and care coordination are key to successful long-term disease management. Patient self-responsibility and empowerment are integral components of disease management. The systematic use of patient advocacy groups in the community (NMSS, MSAA, MSF, and other organizations) increases quality of life for MS patients (97–99).

The specific components of disease management include prevention, diagnosis, acute medical treatment, treatment of MS exacerbations and combined complications, long-term medical treatment, rehabilitation, psychosocial adaptation, community integration, and end-of-life issues. The "best practice" approach to the MS patient starts with a better doctor-patient communication system and with the integration of healthcare providers and services. As team care concepts increasingly become part of the management strategy of MS patients, the patient's quality of life will benefit greatly.

Basic and clinical trial research results have provided positive disease modifying outcomes. However, rehabilitation to minimize functional loss remains critically important. The concept of "maximum rehabilitation potential" is a perpetual challenge in MS care because the issues for the MS patient continually change and are lifelong.

Should rehabilitation start only when the patient has significant disability? Some doctors believe, erroneously, that MS patients do not benefit from active rehabilitation early, or that those with severe disabilities cannot benefit from rehabilitation. In fact, active rehabilitation interventions must start early—soon after the diagnosis. The issues of adaptation, wellness, exercise, nutrition, energy conservation, psychosocial equilibrium, stress management, and education are part of the postdiagnosis treatment plan. Family involvement cannot be overemphasized: for example, divorce rates decrease in comprehensive care centers that can focus on family issues.

Rehabilitation plays a role to maximize function and to create safe environments, as well as to prevent secondary disabilities and medical complications. This facilitates improved independence and quality of life in the community with decreased cost and burden of care.

The maintenance rehabilitation concept for MS patients was pioneered by Dr. Randall Schapiro, of Minnesota. His active ongoing rehabilitation interventions have successfully increased function and decreased complications over a long period of time.

Symptom Management

Almost any neurologic symptom can be associated with MS, depending on the location and scope of lesions within the central nervous system. The following is a brief description and therapeutic recommendations for the most common of MS symptoms. The textbook *Managing the Symptoms of Multiple Sclerosis* (2007), Demos, is recommended reading.

Fatigue

Fatigue is the most common symptom in MS and requires a combination of rehabilitation and medical management (100). Heat often exacerbates fatigue. However, this may be temporarily relieved by cooling via cooling vests, sucking on ice chips, and taking cool baths (101). Fatigue counseling to maximize the patient's ability to function on a daily basis can be very helpful. For example, most MS patients experience fatigue in the late afternoon. Therefore, important daily activities are often done in the morning, so that the patient can rest in a cooler environment in the late afternoon. Often, a 30-minute rest period can reduce fatigue significantly.

Exercise and conditioning programs, which can reduce fatigue, are important activities for patients with MS. Increased strength and physical fitness improves the MS patient's mobility and function. These programs must be individualized for each patient (102).

Medications play a role in the treatment of MS fatigue as well. Amantadine (Symmetrel®) or selective serotonin reuptake inhibitors (SSRIs) may be given initially. However, modafinil (Provigil®) or armodafinil (Nuvigil®) are frequently the first-line treatments for MS fatigue (103). CNS stimulants such as methylphenidate (Ritalin®) and dexedrine sulfate (Dexedrine®) are usually second-line treatments because of the risk of side effects, habituation, and tolerance.

Spasticity

Spasticity management requires a combination of rehabilitation and medications. Stretching exercises and cooling often relieve mild spasticity. Baclofen (Lioresal®) and tizanidine (Zanaflex®) are usually the initial medications for spasticity. These medications must be initiated with slowly increasing doses because of the tendency to produce drowsiness and fatigue in some patients. Many patients tolerate these medications beyond the common or usual recommended dose. Intrathecal baclofen is underutilized, because it involves an intrathecal pump. However, it can be very helpful in selected patients who do not respond to oral medications (103–104). Diazepam (Valium®), Clonzapan (Klonipin), gabapentine (Neurontin), dopamine agents, and sodium dantrolene (Dantrium®) are also used sometimes by neurologists. Motor point blocks, botulinum toxin (Botox) injections, and ablative procedures are also used in selected circumstances (105).

Weakness and Mobility

Weakness is a difficult problem. Attempts to strengthen the affected muscles sometimes have limited success. However, complementary muscles may be strengthened. Combined with rehabilitation, this increased muscle strength may help overcome the weaker muscles. Difficulty with mobility and ambulation can create additional hardships for MS patients. The approach to the patient with mobility difficulties is similar to other conditions with reduced mobility encountered by the rehabilitation team. Assistive technology such as ankle-foot orthoses (AFOs), canes, scooters, and wheelchairs can reduce fatigue and increase mobility. Many MS patients delay use of these aids. Recent studies with 4-aminopyridine (Ampyra) have shown this drug's effectiveness in helping gait as well as increasing strength and endurance. It has been FDA approved for improving gait.

Vertigo, Dizziness, Cerebellar Incoordination, and Tremor

Vertigo, dizziness, cerebellar incoordination, and tremor are difficult to treat. Balancing exercises and vestibular stimulation therapy may be helpful. Safety issues are a major concern because some MS patients may fall because of imbalance. Medications are usually not very helpful. Vertigo may respond temporarily to transdermal scopolamine, meclizine (Antivert®), diphenhydramine (Benadryl®), and dimenhydrinate (Dramamine®). Cerebellar tremors are also very difficult to treat in MS patients. Clonazepam (Klonopin®), propanolol, Primidione, Busprione, Isoniazod, Ondagatram, and some sedative drugs have been shown to help tremors somewhat. A weighted walker and wrist weights may be helpful. Stereotactic brain stimulation can be considered in selected patients with refractory tremors (106, 107).

Paroxysmal Disorders

Some of the most frequently neglected symptoms in MS are paroxysmal disorders. Paroxysmal muscle spasm, pain, sensory symptoms, ataxia, and dysarthria are often not recognized. If healthcare professionals are aware that up to 10% of MS patients experience paroxysmal disorders, then they can be alerted to treat earlier. Paroxysmal disorders are temporary signs or symptoms that occur suddenly and last from seconds to several minutes. The clinician is urged to identify patients who are having "spells" of neurologic dysfunction. Trigeminal neuralgia, L'Hermittes phenomenon, and tonic spinal cord seizures with tonic spasms are the most easily recognized paroxysmal disorders in MS. Anticonvulsants are the first-line therapies for paroxysmal disorders. Gabapentin (Neurontin®) is the most frequently used treatment. Pregabalin (Lyrcia) is now available with a similar mode of action. Carbamazepine (Tegretol®), phenytoin (Dilantin®), and other anticonvulsants are other potential treatments.

Pain

In the past, pain was thought to be an unusual symptom in MS patients. However, studies have shown pain to be present in as many as 75% of MS patients (108). The pain is usually one of two varieties. The first is central neurogenic pain, which is often described as burning, hot, painful, dysesthesia with numbness and tingling that is deep and "indescribable." Anticonvulsants, such as gabapentin (Neurontin), are first-line therapies (109). Pregabalin (Lyrcia) and Duloxetine (Cymbalta) may also be helpful. The second type is musculoskeletal pain, which occurs frequently in MS because of abnormal postures, muscle spasms, and contractures. These patients are treated like other neuromuscular pain patients in rehabilitation: stretching, range of motion, active exercises, cooling, and removal of pain-precipitating factors are the mainstays of treatment. Headache, including migraine headaches, are often seen in MS. Other treatments for pain, such as biofeedback and acupuncture, can be helpful in some patients.

Depression and Other Affective States

Depression is seen in most MS patients at some time during the course of the illness. Therefore, psychotherapy and counseling to deal with adaptation and coping are important. Early intervention can help prevent later disruptions. Family counseling is also an integral part of better understanding the disease. When depression becomes manifest, psychotherapy and medications are often used concurrently. Tricyclic antidepressants (TCAs) were the mainstay of MS depression treatment for many years. However, their anticholinergic side effects made many MS symptoms worse. Blurred vision, cognitive blunting, dry mouth, constipation, and urinary retention are some of the problems with tricyclic antidepressants. Therefore, SSRIs and non-SSRIs such as Effexor (Venlafaxine), Trazodone (Desyrel), Nefazodone (Serzone®), Bupropion (Wellbutrin®), Duloxetine (Cymbalta) and many other drugs are also used in the medical management of moderate depression. Careful selection and monitoring of antidepressants are important. Depression can be associated with anxiety and/or bipolar states, which require added attention. The drug treatment of depression need not be lifelong, especially if there is adequate psychological support. Bipolar disease and mania are also seen in MS.

Cognitive Dysfunction

Cognition dysfunction previously was not thought to be a major part of MS symptomatology. Now we realize that cognitive dysfunction is frequent (>50%), may occur early, and may be unrecognized for a long period of time. Therefore, cognitive testing might be helpful early in the disease course. Depression, fatigue, and medications for other MS symptoms may worsen cognitive dysfunction. The medical treatment for cognitive dysfunction has not been adequately studied. Anticholinesterase inhibitors and other "Alzheimer drugs" are often tried in MS cognitive dysfunction. The results of small studies have been mixed (57, 58). However, cognitive retraining helps patients adapt and increases quality of life for patients with cognitive problems. Immunomodulating therapy has also been shown to have favorable results to reduce the progression of impaired cognition.

Bladder Dysfunction

Bladder problems are among the most common MS symptoms, causing social isolation and a reduced quality of life (110). The evaluation of bladder dysfunction starts with an assessment of a post-void residual volume and evaluation of bladder emptying by ultrasound, if indicated. More formal bladder dysfunction testing using urodynamics may be performed by urologists. The treatment for bladder dysfunction starts with education and counseling. Volume and timing of fluid intake is extremely important. Drinking more fluid, especially at night, may lead to urine leakage or frank incontinence. However, fluid deprivation can lead to dehydration, bladder infection, stone formation, constipation, and other side effects such as dry mouth, dizziness, and nausea. For Nocturia, evening fluid restriction, anticholinergic agents, and desmopressin given by nasal spray at bedtime can be useful.

Rehabilitation of bladder voiding and incontinence problems begins with timed voiding and ultrasound scans to assess voiding patterns and postvoid residual bladder volume. The goals are continence and avoiding overdistending the bladder beyond 400 cc. Management of the large, hypotonic bladder is challenging. Bethanechol (Urecholine®) is the only agent available to stimulate Detrusor bladder contractions. Results are variable. Intermittent catheterization is often the best treatment for patients who have urinary retention.

A dyssynergic bladder, where both the bladder wall and the urinary sphincter contract at the same time, can cause urinary retention and reflux of urine to the kidneys. Baclofen (Lioresal®) and alpha-blockers may help the dyssynergic bladder. Medication for a small spastic bladder usually begins with Tolterodine tartrate (Detrol®), because it has the least anticholinergic side effects. Oxybutynin (Ditropan XL®) can be given once a day with fewer anticholinergic side effects than regular Oxybutynin. Many other anticholinergic drugs are also available. Alpha-blockers inhibit the urethral internal sphincter contraction with resultant decreased bladder outflow resistance. Available alpha-blockers include Flomax (Tamsulosin Hydrochloride), Terazosin (Hytrin®), and Phenoxybenzamine (Dibenzyline®). Alpha-blockers may cause orthostatic hypotension, and follow-up blood pressure assessments are important.

Bowel Dysfunction

Bowel dysfunction usually means constipation, but diarrhea and incontinence also occur (110). Medications for other MS symptoms, which are complicated by dehydration, can play a significant role in aggravating constipation. The first step in treating bowel dysfunction is an assessment of the patient's bowel habits and time of day including frequency of bowel movements, laxative medication, and episodes of incontinence. Patients are trained to establish a regular pattern of bowel elimination.

A high-fiber diet and hydration are the cornerstones to treatment of most bowel dysfunction. The gastrocolic reflex, especially after breakfast, can be utilized if the patient adequately prepares for a bowel movement at that time. A warm beverage may also help stimulate a bowel movement.

Stool softeners and bulk agents may also be helpful. Chemical stimulant cathartics (laxatives) for bowel movements can lose their effectiveness over time because of habituation. A rectal suppository administered after the preferred meal can be useful. A glycerin suppository, which contains no medication, is preferred over the stimulant suppositories such as Bisacodyl (Ducolax®). Enemas are effective, but should be saved for failures with the preceding treatments. Digital stimulation can also be effective if other treatments fail.

Sexual Dysfunction

Physicians and patients historically seem to be joined in a conspiracy not to discuss or treat most sexual dysfunction (111, 112). Sexual dysfunction is common in both men and women. Sexual dysfunction in women may be as prevalent as in men. However, erectile dysfunction seems to be the center of attention of most treatment efforts. Both men and women may have altered libidos, altered genital sensation, decreased frequency and intensity of orgasms, and/or pain during sexual intercourse. Vaginal dryness and pain are common complaints in women. Sometimes, sexual intercourse may stimulate massive muscle spasms or pain. Adductor muscle spasms may hamper intercourse. Urinary incontinence may accompany intercourse.

The management of sexual dysfunction begins with education and counseling about the specific pathophysiology of sexual dysfunction. If sexual intercourse is extremely problematic, sexual activities can occur in many forms that do not require sexual intercourse. Intimacy is a special connection that is not necessarily tied to intercourse. Communication is often the key to intimacy.

The medical treatments for fatigue, depression, bladder dysfunction, bowel dysfunction, and muscle spasms are important considerations in the treatment of sexual dysfunction. For women, lubrication, estrogen creams, and vibrators may be helpful. Sildenafil citrate (Viagra), Vardenalfil (Levitra), and Tadalafil (Cialis) have been very effective for erectile dysfunction (ED) in some males. One additional problem associated with these medications is that patients may focus on the act of sexual intercourse as the ultimate in sexuality. However, communication and intimacy may actually play a greater role in quality of life in the long run.

Dysphagia

Dysphagia occurs in 20% to 25% of MS patients (112). Patients may have a delay in swallowing, where food enters the pharynx before the pharyngeal motor response has been initiated. This leaves the airway open, which leads to aspiration and possibly pneumonia. The motility of food through the pharynx may also lead to inefficient swallowing and aspiration. Reduced tongue movement, incoordination, and poor lip closure or facial tone may also decrease swallowing. Esophageal peristalsis dysfunction is theoretically possible in MS, although very few studies have been published.

The treatment of dysphagia is difficult, but a speech and language pathologist can provide treatments to improve dysphagia. Surgical procedures to prevent aspiration have not been very successful in MS patients. Dysphagia is also related to fatigue: for example, some MS patients take a long time to finish a meal. Chewing becomes difficult and, by the end of the meal, fatigue may produce coughing, regurgitation of food, and aspiration. Therefore, it is recommended that patients having problems with dysphagia have more frequent but smaller meals to prevent fatigue.

Dysarthria

Dysarthria is very complex in MS and may involve spasticity, weakness, or ataxic incoordination of the muscles of the lip, tongue, mandible, soft palate, vocal cords, and diaphragm. A speech and language pathologist can be helpful in the evaluation and treatment of dysarthria. Dysarthria is thought to occur in between 25% and 50% of MS patients. The medical treatment of dysarthria involves the treatment of fatigue and spasticity as well as attempts to treat ataxia and tremor.

POTENTIAL NEW MULTIPLE SCLEROSIS THERAPIES IN TRIALS

Emerging Oral Therapies in Clinical Trials

There are several oral therapies that are being tested and are yielding encouraging results (113).

Cladribine

This is a small nonpeptide molecule, cytotoxic to lymphocytes and monocytes (114), that is used in leukemia therapy. Phase III clinical trial data have shown substantial efficacy of oral Cladribine vs. placebo (115). In one MS study it was given orally 20 days the first year and 10 days the second year. It is currently being tested versus placebo and as an induction agent before interferon beta therapy. Parenteral Cladribine was used several years ago and was shown to have a positive effect on relapses and MRI but not on progression of disease in patients who had progressive MS. In current trials, it is used orally in relapsing-remitting MS patients.

Fingolimod (FTY720)

This drug is an oral Sphingosine receptor modulator that blocks lymphocytes from leaving the lymph nodes, and therefore prohibits them from entering the central nervous system (116). Fingolimod was shown to be more effective than interferon B-1a intramuscularly. Adverse events included bradycardia, increased blood pressure, airway obstruction, macular edema, and infections. Other positive effects, such as neuroprotection, have been noted in animal models.

Fumaric Acid Ester (Fumarate BG-12)

This is another oral agent with anti-inflammatory and possibly neuroprotective properties (117). It is used in psoriasis. In a phase IIB study in MS patients, BG-12 showed a 69% reduction in the formation of new gadolinium-enhanced lesions and a 32% reduction in relapse rate over a 48-week period. The toxicity profile was favorable.

Laquinimod

This is an immunomodulating agent that converts pro-inflammatory TH-1 cells to anti-inflammatory TH-2 cells (118). A phase II trial in RRMS demonstrated that MRI activity was reduced by 40%, and the annual relapse data were also positive. Laquinimod was derived from Linomide, which was tested in MS previously and found to be effective but with significant adverse events. Laquinimod has an improved safety profile.

Teriflunomide

This is an oral immunomodulator primarily affecting T cell synthesis (119). It is an active metabolite of Leflunomide, which is currently approved for rheumatoid arthritis. The drug inhibits new RNA and DNA synthesis. In a phase II trial, a marked reduction in new MRI activity was noted in 9 months. Treatment was well tolerated. Studies adding Teriflunomide to patients taking interferon and Copaxone are in progress.

Monoclonal Antibodies (120)

Alemtuzumab (Campath)

This is a monoclonal antibody directed against the CD-52 receptor on T cells and monocytes (121). It induces long-term T cell depletion, and it is currently indicated for B cell leukemia. In a study comparing Alemtuzumab to Rebif, a reduction in the Alemtuzumab group was noted for relapses and sustained disability over a 36-month period, even though Alemtuzumab was given only at baseline and year one (5 days and 3 days, respectively). Over 50% of Campath patients improved in this trial, suggesting the possibility of reduced neurodegeneration or increased neuroprotection. In another study, Alemtuzumab produced a dramatic reduction in the annualized relapse rate. Adverse events include idiopathic thrombocytopenia purpura (ITP), which produced one fatality, as well as Graves disease (about 8%), infusion reactions, and infections. Additional trials are under way.

Rituximab (Rituxan)

This is a monoclonal antibody to CD-20, which induces B cell depletion. In a relapsing-remitting MS study, two infusions of Rituximab were given, and the patients were followed for 48 weeks versus placebo. All clinical and MRI outcomes favored Rituximab over placebo (122). Rituximab has been associated with serious adverse events, including progressive multifocal leukoencephalopathy (PML) in non-MS patients. A trial in PPMS failed to show clinical efficacy over placebo. However, PPMS patients under 55 years of age with enhanced MRI lesions showed some benefit in a post-hoc analysis (123).

Rituximab has also been studied in neuromyelitis optica (NMO) (Devic's disease) (124). Ten patients who were doing poorly on current therapy were given Rituximab, and the relapse rate reduced from 3.7 to 0.57 over a 9-month period. Of these patients, 70% were NMO antibody positive.

Daclizumab

This drug is a monoclonal antibody that binds to the receptor of the inflammatory cytokine interleukin 2 (IL2), which results in a decrease in an IL2-mediated stimulation of T cell function. It is used for renal transplants. In interferon beta–treated MS patients who had continual disease activity, two recent studies have shown that daclizumab was effective in reducing MRI lesions and relapses and/or improving EDSS scores. Adverse events were not serious but included decreased platelet counts, infections, and infusion reactions (125).

Other Therapies for Multiple Sclerosis

BHT-3009

This is a plasmid DNA "vaccine," which encodes the entire molecule of myelin basic protein and induces tolerance, which turns off the immune system. In a 13-week study versus placebo, the treated group had decreased MRI lesions, decreased myelin reactive T cells, and decreased myelin antibodies in the spinal fluid. BHT-3009 was well tolerated (126).

Bone Marrow Transplant

This treatment is under evaluation in specialty centers (127). For active relapsing MS, a new study has been encouraging, but adverse events, including death, are still being reported (128). Embryonic stem cells and remyelination research are in early phases of study.

Atorvastatin (Lipitor) and Simvastatin (Zocor)

These are oral statins currently being tested in MS (129). Zocor 80 mg a day was shown to reduce MRI-enhanced lesions in an uncontrolled study (130). A controversy exists regarding whether statins may interfere with the interferon mechanism of action (131). The latest two studies did not show a specific interference (132–134), but the controversy remains. The potential mechanism of statin interference with interferons is not an issue with Copaxone. Other trials with statins are in progress.

Minocycline

This is a tetracycline-type antibiotic, which decreases matrix metalloproteinase and decreases the transmigration of lymphocytes across the blood-brain barrier. It has been shown to be effective in experimental autoimmune encephalitis (EAE) in animals. It also decreases a neurotoxin, nitric oxide, in the CNS. Pilot studies with Minocycline have found an effect on decreasing enhancing lesions and relapse rates (135, 136).

Estriol

This is an oral estrogen that has anti-inflammatory effects and potential neuroprotective properties. Increased Estriol production is thought to be one of the mechanisms by which MS disease activity is reduced during pregnancy. A pilot study showed a reduction in enhancing lesions. A study utilizing Copaxone with and without Estriol in relapsing-remitting MS showed a more robust effect on MRI and a lower relapse rate with the combination therapy versus Copaxone alone (137, 138).

Fluoxetine (Prozac)

This is an SSRI antidepressant that has an immunomodulating effect by decreasing inflammation. It decreases lesions in experimental autoimmune encephalitis. Also, Fluoxetine is a sodium channel blocker and has been shown to increase brain-derived nerve factor (BDNF) in the CNS. In a small trial, it reduced MRI lesions and increased n-Acetylaspartate, an axonal marker, on magnetic resonance spectroscopy. These data are considered preliminary.

NeuroVax

This T cell vaccine is composed of three T cell receptor peptides. NeuroVax induces T suppressor cells, which have been found effective in animal models of EAE. Clinical trials are forthcoming (129).

Erythropoietin

This drug has encouraging preliminary data as a disease-modifying agent (130).

Other Potential Disease-Modifying Therapies in Multiple Sclerosis

Aziathiaprine (Imuran), pulse steroids, cyclophosphamide (Cytoxan), intravenous immunoglobulins (IVIG), methotrexate, plasma exchange (131), and micophenolate (CellCept) are currently in use in MS patients by some neurologists. They are not FDA approved.

Other Potential Disease-Modifying Therapies in Multiple Sclerosis

Aziathiaprine (Imuran), pulse steroids, cyclophosphamide (Cytoxan), intravenous immunoglobulins (IVIG), methotrexate, plasma exchange (140), and micophenolate (CellCept) are currently in use in MS patients by some neurologists. They are not FDA approved.

Potential Symptom Management Treatments in Clinical Trials

Zenvia (Formerly Neurodex)

This drug is being tested to treat pseudobulbar affect, which is characterized by sudden and unpredictable episodes of laughing, crying, and other displays of emotion. It is a combination of dextromethorphan and low-dose quinidine. Preliminary trials are encouraging (141).

Cannabis (Sativer)

Cannabis (142, 143) is used in Canada and the United Kingdom for symptomatic treatment in MS, including pain, bladder symptoms, and spasticity. In addition, cannabis may have immunomodulator and neuroprotective effects, but more data are needed. A recent study showed deleterious effects on cognition in MS with cannabis.

Botulinum Toxin Type A

This has been effective in treating overactive bladder symptoms, as well as muscle spasticity in MS (144).

Low-Dose Naltrexone (LDN)

This opioid receptor blocker is currently being tested in MS patients in trials in the United States and Italy. A higher dose of LDN (50 mg) is currently approved for alcohol and opioid addiction. Results in MS have not been published. One study did not show benefits in MS patients (145).

Vitamin D

This substance is being evaluated for possible effectiveness in MS. Reduced vitamin D and sunlight exposure have been linked to an increased risk of MS (56).

COMPARING MULTIPLE SCLEROSIS AND SPINAL CORD INJURY ISSUES

The most obvious difference between MS and SCI is the natural history of the disorder. MS patients tend to progress over time, whereas SCI patients tend to stabilize or get better. However, other differences are important to recognize. MS patients tend to be older than SCI patients. MS patients tend to come from higher socioeconomic backgrounds and are more likely to be college educated. Childbearing issues and genetics are often more relevant in MS. A major goal in MS is to find treatments to prevent damage over time, whereas SCI damage prevention management is currently confined to the immediate postinjury phase. Because of the location of many MS lesions above the spinal cord level, more problems with cognition, vision and eye movement, speech and swallowing disturbances, paroxysmal symptoms, cerebellar tremors, and incoordination are likely.

Most MS symptoms are treated with rehabilitation techniques, as well as with medication (146–147). Much of the disability in MS is related to spinal cord involvement; therefore, some rehabilitation issues in MS are similar to those in SCI. However, there are many key differences in the treatment of the symptoms of MS versus SCI. Rehabilitation medicine physicians are often the principal physician care providers for SCI, whereas neurologists are more often the principal physician care providers for MS. Their backgrounds and orientation to disease management can be different, although that difference has been narrowing in the last several years.

Reimbursement for rehabilitation in SCI is somewhat less difficult to obtain than long-term rehabilitation for MS. Although it is obvious that SCI patients need rehabilitation, the benefit of rehabilitation in MS is less utilized, in spite of numerous recent articles demonstrating efficacy.

CONCLUSION

This chapter previews some of the complexities in the diagnosis, pathogenesis, disease courses, and treatments of MS symptoms. Disease modifying therapies, especially when initiated early, have favorably altered the short- and long-term prognosis. Emerging therapies may facilitate treatment even more. However, dramatic efficacy results may be tempered by the adverse event profiles. Clinical trials will help establish future approved therapies. The integrated, comprehensive treatment approach among rehabilitation therapists, physicians, and other members of the healthcare team is an impor-

tant aspect to successful long-term management of MS in patients.

The disease management approach in MS provides education, self-management, and empowerment opportunities for the patient. This not only helps the patient but also helps the caregiver and healthcare professionals involved in the treatment. A well-designed system of care accomplishes the ultimate goal of a higher quality of life for MS patients. Symptom management is often underutilized but can increase functioning in most MS patients.

References

1. Murray TJ. *Multiple Sclerosis: The history of a disease.* New York: Demos Medical Publishing, 2005.
2. Dhib-Jalbut S. Pathogenesis of myelin/oligodendrocyte damage in multiple sclerosis. *Neurology* 2007; 68:S13–S21.
3. Bandwell B, Krupp L, Tellier R, et al. Clinical features and viral serologies in children with multiple sclerosis: results of a multinational cohort study. *Lancet Neurol* 2007; 6(9):773–781.
4. Kantarci O, Wingerchuk D. Epidemiology and natural history of multiple sclerosis: new insights. *Curr Opin Neurol* 2006; 19(3):248–254.
5. Oksenberg JR, Hauser SL. Genetics of multiple sclerosis. *Neurol Clin* 2005; 23(1):61–75.
6. International Multiple Sclerosis Genetics Consortium, Hafler DA, Compston A, et al. Risk alleles for multiple sclerosis identified by a genomewide study. *N Engl J Med* 2007; 357(9):851–862.
7. Fujinami RS, von Herrath MG, Christen U, Whitton JL. Molecular mimicry, bystander activation, or viral persistence: infections and autoimmune disease. *Clin Microbiol Rev* 2006; 19(1):80–94.
8. Clark D. Human herpesvirus type 6 and multiple sclerosis. *Herpes* 2004; 11(Suppl 2):112A–119A.
9. Alotaibi S, Kennedy J, Tellier R, et al. Epstein-Barr virus in pediatric multiple sclerosis. *JAMA* 2004; 291(15):1875–1879.
10. Levin LI, Munger KL, Ruberston MV, et al. Multiple sclerosis and Epstein-Barr virus. *JAMA* 2003; 289(12):1533–1536.
11. Levin L, Munger KL, Ruberstone MV, et al. Temporal relationship between elevation of Epstein-Barr virus antibody titers and initial onset of neurological symptoms in multiple sclerosis. *JAMA* 2005; 293(20):2496–2500.
12. Marrie RA. When one and one make three: HLA and EBV infection in MS. *Neurology* 2008; 70(13 Pt 2):1067–1068.
13. De Jager PL, Simon KC, Munger KL, et al. Integrating risk factors: HLA-DRB1*1501 and Epstein-Bar virus in multiple sclerosis. *Neurology* 2008; 70(13 Pt 2):1113–1118.
14. Munger KL, Zhang SM, O'Reilly E, et al. Vitamin D intake and incidence of multiple sclerosis. *Neurology* 2004; 62(1):60–65.
15. Hayes CE, Acheson DE. A unifying multiple sclerosis etiology linking virus infection, sunlight, and vitamin D, through viral interleukin-10. *Med Hypotheses* in press.
16. Munger KL, Levin LI, Hollis BW, et al. Serum 25-hydroxyvitamin D levels and risk of multiple sclerosis. *JAMA* 2006; 296(23):2832–2838.
17. Islam T, Gauderman J. Cozen W, Mack T. Childhood sun exposure influences risk of multiple sclerosis in monozygotic twins. *Neurology* 2007; 69:381–388.
18. Correale J, Farez M. Association between parasite infection and immune responses in multiple sclerosis. *Ann Neurol* 2007; 61(2):97–108.
19. Fleming J. society funds novel clinical trial of harmless worms, based on "hygiene hypothesis." National MS Society, 2008; http://www.nationalmssociety.org/news/news-detail/index.aspx?nid=215.
20. Gregersen JW, Kranc KR, Ke X, et al. Functional epistasis on common MHC haplotype associated with multiple sclerosis. *Nature* 2006; 443(7111):574–577.
21. Oksenberg JR, Barcellos LF. Multiple Sclerosis genetics: leaving no stone unturned. *Genes Immun* 2005; 6(5):375–387.
22. Barcellos LF, Kamdar BB, Ramsay PP, et al. Clustering of autoimmune diseases in families with a high-risk for multiple sclerosis: a descriptive study. *Lancet Neurol* 2006; 5(11):924–931.
23. Komiyama Y, Nakae S, Matsuki T, et al. IL-17 plays an important role in the development of experimental autoimmune encephalomyelitis. *J*

Immunol 2006; 177(1):566–573.

24. Frzekas F, Strasser-Fuchs S, Kollegger H, et al. Apolipoprotein E epsilon 4 is associated with rapid progression of multiple sclerosis. *Neurology* 2001; 57(5):853–857.

25. Cree BA, Khan O, Bourdette D, Goodin DS, et al. Clinical characteristics of African Americans vs. Caucasian Americans with multiple sclerosis. *Neurology* 2004; 63(11):2039–2045.

26. Arnason BG, Richman DP. Effect of oral contraceptives on experimental demyelinating disease. *Arch Neurol* 1969; 21(1):103–108.

27. Sicotte NL, Liva SM, Klutch R, et al. Treatment of multiple sclerosis with the pregnancy hormone Estriol. *Ann Neurol* 2002; 52(4):465–475.

28. Soldan SS, Alvarez Retuerto AI, Sicotte NL, Voskuhl RR. Immune modulation in multiple sclerosis patients treated with the pregnancy hormone Estriol. *J Immunol* 2003; 171(11):6267–6274.

29. Giesser BS, Halper J, Cross AH, et al. Multiple sclerosis symptoms fluctuate during menstrual cycle. *MS Exchange* 1991; 3:5.

30. Pozzilli C, Falaschi P, Mainero C, et al. MRI in multiple sclerosis during the menstrual cycle: relationship with sex hormone patterns. *Neurology* 1999; 53:622–624.

31. Lucchinetti C, Bruck W, Parisi J, et al. Heterogeneity of multiple sclerosis lesions: implications for the pathogenesis of demyelination. *Ann Neurol* 2000; 47(6):707–717.

32. Lucchinetti CF, Bruck W, Lassmann H. Evidence for pathogenic heterogeneity in multiple sclerosis. *Ann Neurol* 2004; 56(2):308.

33. Barnett MH, Prineas JW. Relapsing and remitting multiple sclerosis: pathology of the newly forming lesion. *Ann Neurol* 2004; 55(4):458–468.

34. Patrikios P. Stadelmann C, Kutzenlnigg A, et al. Remyelination is extensive in a subset of multiple sclerosis patients. *Brain* 2006; 129(Pt 12):3165–3172.

35. Trapp BD, Peterson J, Ransoff RM, et al. Axonal transection in the lesions of multiple sclerosis. *N Engl J Med* 1998; 338(5):278–285.

36. DeLuca GC, Ebers GC, Esiri MM. Axonal loss in multiple sclerosis: a pathological survey of the corticospinal and sensory tracts. *Brain* 2004; 127(Pts):1009–1018.

37. Kuhlmann T, Lingfeld G, Bitsch A, et al. Acute axonal damage in multiple sclerosis is most extensive in early disease stages and decreases over time. *Brain* 2002; 125(Pt 10):2202–2212.

38. Bo L, Vedeler CA, Nyland HI, et al. Subpial demyelination in the cerebral cortex of multiple sclerosis patients. *J Neuropathol Exp Neurol* 2003; 62(7):723–732.

39. Kutzelnigg A, Lucchinetti C, Stadelmann C, et al. Cortical demyelination and diffuse white matter injury in multiple sclerosis. *Brain* 2005; 128(Pt 11):2705–2712.

40. Allen IV, McQuaid S, Mirakhur M, Nevin G. Pathological abnormalities in the normal-appearing white matter in multiple sclerosis. *Neurol Sci* 2001; 22(2):141–144.

41. Arnold DL. Magnetic resonance spectroscopy: imaging axonal damage in MS. *J Neuroimmunol* 1999; 98(1):2–6.

42. Khan O, Shen Y, et al. Long-term study of brain (1)H-MRS study in multiple sclerosis: effect of glatiramer acetate therapy on axonal metabolic function and feasibility of long-term (1)H-MRS monitoring in multiple sclerosis *J Neuroimmunol* 2007; 20:1–6.

43. Lublin FD, Reingold SC. Defining the clinical course of multiple sclerosis: results of an international survey. National Multiple Sclerosis Society (USA) Advisory Committee on Clinical Trials of New Agents in Multiple Sclerosis. *Neurology* 1996; 46(4):907–911.

44. Tintore M, Rovira A, Rio J, et al. New diagnostic criteria for multiple sclerosis: application in first demyelinating episode. *Neurology* 2003; 60(1):27–30.

45. Tintore M, Rovira A, Rio J, et al. Baseline MRI predicts future attacks and disability in clinically isolated syndromes. *Neurology* 2006; 67(6):968–972.

46. Kappos L, Freedman MS, Polman CH, et al. Effect of early versus delayed interferon beta-1b treatment on disability after a first clinical event suggestive of multiple sclerosis: a 3-year follow-up analysis of the BENEFIT study. *Lancet* 2007; 370(9585):389–397.

47. Lublin FD, Baier M, Cutter G. Effect of relapses on development of residual deficit in multiple sclerosis. *Neurology* 2003; 61(11):1528–1532.

48. Weinshenker BG, Bass B, Rice GPA, et al. The natural history of multiple sclerosis: a geographically based study. *Brain* 1989; 112:133–146.

49. Weinshenker BG, Bass B, Rice GPA, et al. The natural history of multiple sclerosis: a geographically based study II. Predictive value of the early clinical course. *Brain* 1989; 112:1419–1428.

50. Hawkins SA, McDonnell GV. Benign multiple sclerosis? Clinical course, long-term follow up, and assessment of prognostic factors. *J Neurol Neurosurg Psychiatry* 1999; 67:148–152.

51. McDonald W, Compston A, Edan G, et al. Recommended diagnostic material for multiple sclerosis: guidelines from the International Panel on the Diagnosis of Multiple Sclerosis. *Ann Neurol* 2001; 50:121–127.

52. Polman CH, Reingold SC, Edan G, et al. Diagnostic criteria for multiple sclerosis: 2005 revisions to the "McDonald Criteria." *Ann Neurol* 2005; 58(6):840–846.

53. Wolansky LJ, Haghighi MH, Sevdalis E. et al. Safety of serial monthly administration of triple-dose gadopentetate dimeglumine in multiple sclerosis patients: preliminary results of the BECOME trial. *J Neuroimaging* 2005; 15(3):289–290.

54. Fisniku LK, Brex PA, Altmann, DR, et al. Disability and T2 MRI lesions: a 20-year follow-up of patients with relapse onset of multiple sclerosis. *Brain* 2008; 131(Pt 3):808–817.

55. Neema M, Stankiewicz J, Arora A, Guss ZD, Bakshi R. MRI in multiple sclerosis: what's inside the toolbox? *Neurotherapeutics* 2007; 4(4):602–617.

56. Zarei M, Chandran S, Compston A, Hodges J. Cognitive presentation of multiple sclerosis: evidence for a cortical variant. *J Neurol Neurosurg Psychiatry* 2003; 74(7):872–877.

57. Krupp LB, Christodoulou C, Melville P, et al. Donepezil improved memory in multiple sclerosis in a randomized clinical trial. *Neurology* 2004; 63(9):1579–1585.

58. Carone DA, Benedict RH, Munschauer FE, et al. Interpreting patient/informant discrepancies of reported cognitive symptoms in MS. *J Int Neuropsychol Soc* 2005; 11(5):574–853.

59. Pulicken M, Gordon-Lipkin E, et al. Optical coherence tomography and disease subtype in multiple sclerosis. *Neurology* 2007; 69(22): 2085–2092.

60. Younger DS. Vasculitis of the nervous system. *Curr Opin Neurol* 2004; 17(3):317–336.

61. Zakrzewska JM. Diagnosis and differential diagnosis of trigeminal neuralgia. *Clin J Pain* 2002; 18(1):14–21.

62. McArthur JC, Brew BJ, Nath A. Neurological complications of HIV infection. *Lancet Neurol* 2005; 4(9):543–555.

63. Singhal S, Rich P, Markus HS. The spatial distribution of MR imaging abnormalities in cerebral autosomal dominant arteriopathy with subcortical infarcts and Leukoencephalopathy and their relationship to age and clinical features. *AJNR Am J Neuroradiol* 2005; 26(10):2481–2487.

64. Stern BJ. Neurological complications in rheumatic diseases. *Curr Opin Neurol* 2004; 17(3):311–316.

65. Theodoridou A, Settas L. Demyelination in rheumatic diseases. *J Neurol Neurosurg Psychiatry* 2006; 77(3):290–295.

66. Menge T, Hemmer B, Nessler S, et al. Acute disseminated encephalomyelitis: an update. *Arch Neurol* 2005; 62(11):1673–1680.

67. Wingerchuk DM, Lennon VA, Pittock SJ, et al. Revised diagnostic criteria for neuromyelitis optica. *Neurology* 2006; 66(10):1485–1489.

68. Lennon VA, Kryzer TJ, Pittock SJ, et al. IgG marker of optic-spinal multiple sclerosis binds to Aquaporin-4 water channel. *J Exp Med* 2005; 202(4):473–477.

69. The IFN Multiple Sclerosis Study Group. Interferon beta 1b is effective in relapsing-remitting multiple sclerosis. I. Clinical results of a multicenter, randomized, double-blind, placebo-controlled trial. *Neurology* 1993; 43:655–661.

70. European Study Group on Interferon β-1b in Secondary Progressive MS. Placebo-controlled multicenter randomized trial of interferon β-1b in treatment of secondary progressive multiple sclerosis. *Lancet* 1998; 352:1491.

71. Goodkin DE, North American Study Group on Interferon Beta-1b in Secondary Prevention MS. Interferon beta-1b in secondary progressive MS: clinical and MRI results of a 3-year randomized controlled trial. *Neurology* 2000; 54(Suppl):2352.

72. Jacobs LD, et al. Intramuscular interferon beta-1a therapy initiated during a first demyelinating event in multiple sclerosis. *N Engl J Med* 2000; 343:898.

73. CHAMPIONS Study Group (R. P. Kinkel chair writing committee). IM interferon B-1a delays definite multiple sclerosis 5 years after a first demyelinating event. *Neurology* 2006; 66(5):678–687.

74. Prevention of Relapses and Disability by Interferon B-1a Subcutaneously in Multiple Sclerosis (PRISMS) Study Group. Randomized double-blind placebo-controlled study of interferon B-1a in relapsing/remitting multiple sclerosis. *Lancet* 1998; 352:1498.

75. Kappos L, Traboulsee A, Constantinescu C, et al. Long-term subcutaneous interferon beta-1a therapy in patients with relapsing-remitting MS. *Neurology* 2006; 67(6):944–953.

76. Goodin DS, Frohman EM, Garmany GP Jr. Therapeutics and Technology Assessment Subcommittee of the American Academy of Neurology; MS Council for Clinical Practice Guidelines. Disease modifying therapies in multiple sclerosis: report of the Therapeutics and Technology Assessment Subcommittee of the American Academy of Neurology and the MS Council for Clinical Practice Guidelines. *Neurology* 2002; 58(2):169–178.

77. Goodin DS, Frohman EM, Hurwitz B, et al. Neutralizing antibodies to interferon beta: assessment of their clinical and radiographic impact: an evidence report: Report of the Therapeutics and Technology Assessment Subcommittee of the American Academy of Neurology. *Neurology* 2007; 68:977–984.

78. Agrawal SM, Yong VW. Immunopathogenesis of multiple sclerosis. *Int Rev Neurobiol* 2007; 79:99–126.

79. Yong VW. Prospects for neuroprotection in multiple sclerosis. *Front Biosci* 2004; 9:864–872.

80. Schrempf W, Ziemssen T. Glatiramer acetate: mechanisms of action in multiple sclerosis. *Autoimmun Rev* 2007; 6(7):469–475.

81. Comi G, O'Connor P, Montalban X, et al. Phase II study of oral fingolimod (FTY720) in multiple sclerosis: 3-year results. *Mult Scler* 2009.

82. Cohen JA, Rovaris M, Goodman AD, et al. Randomized, double-blind, dose-comparison study of glatiramer acetate in relapsing-remitting MS. *Neurology* 2007; 68(12):939–944.

83. Durelli L, Verdun E, Barbero P, et al. Independent Comparison of Interferon (INCOMIN) Trial Study Group. Every other day interferon beta-1b versus once weekly interferon beta-1a for multiple sclerosis. *Lancet* 2002; 359:1453–1460.

84. Panitch H, Goodin DS, et al. Randomized comparative studies of interferon B1a treatment regimens in MS: the EVIDENCE Trial. *Neurology* 2002; 59:1496–1506.

85. Mikol DD, Barkhof F, Chang P, et al. Comparison of subcutaneous interferon beta-1a with glatiramer acetate in patients with relapsing multiple sclerosis (the Rebif vs Glatiramer Acetate in Relapsing MS Disease [REGARD] study: a multicentre, randomised, parallel, open-label trial. *Lancet Neurol* 2008; 7(10):903–914.

86. O'Conner P, Filippi M, Arnason B, et al. 250 µg or 500 µg interferon beta-1b versus 20 mg glatiramer acetate in relapsing-remitting multiple sclerosis: a prospective, randomised, multicentre study. *Lancet Neurol* 2009; 8(10):889–897.

87. Miller DH, Soon D, Fernando KT, et al. MRI outcomes in a placebo-controlled trial of Natalizumab in relapsing MS. *Neurology* 2007; 68(17):1390–1401.

88. Stuve O, Marra CM, et al. Potential risk of progressive multifocal leukoencephalopathy with Natalizumab therapy: possible interventions. *Arch Neurol* 2007; 64(2):169–176.

89. Ransohoff RM. Natalizumab and PML. *Nat Neurosci* 2005; 8(10):1275.

90. Thompson AJ. The effectiveness of neurological rehabilitation in multiple sclerosis. *J Rehabil Res Dev* 2000; 37(4):455–461.

91. Freeman JA, Langdon DW, Hobart JC, Thompson AJ. The impact of inpatient rehabilitation on progressive multiple sclerosis. *Ann Neurol* 1997; 42(2):236–244.

92. Kesselring J, Beer S. Symptomatic therapy and neurorehabilitation in multiple sclerosis. *Lancet Neurol* 2005; 4(10):643–652.

93. Khan F, Turner-Stokes L, et al. Multidisciplinary rehabilitation for adults with multiple sclerosis. *Cochrane Database Syst Rev* 2007; (2)DC006036.

94. Bowling A, Stewart T. *Dietary Supplements and multiple sclerosis: A Health Professional's Guide.* New York: Demos Medical Publishing, 2004.

95. Bowling A. *Complementary and Alternative Medicine and Multiple Sclerosis.* New York: Demos Medical Publishing, 2007.

96. Kiecolt-Glaser JK, Preacher KJ, et al. Chronic stress and age-related increases in the proinflammatory cytokine IL-6. *Proc Natl Acad Sci U S A* 2003; 100(15):9090–9095.

97. Britell CW, Burks JS, Schapiro RT. Introduction to symptom and rehabilitative management: disease management model. In: Burks JS, Johnson KP, eds. *Multiple Sclerosis: Diagnosis, Medical Management, and Rehabilitation.* New York: Demos Medical Publishing, 2000.

98. Schapiro RT. *Symptom Management in Multiple Sclerosis.* 3rd ed. New York: Demos Medical Publishing, 1998.

99. Maloney FP, Burks JS, Ringel SP. *Interdisciplinary Rehabilitation of Multiple Sclerosis and Neuromuscular Disorders.* Philadelphia: J.B. Lippincott Company, 1985.

100. Mathiowetz VG, Finlayson ML, Matuska KM, et al. Randomized controlled trial of an energy conservation course for persons with multiple sclerosis. *Mult Scler* 2005; 11(5):852–601.

101. Schwid SR, Petrie MD, Murray R, et al. A randomized controlled study of the acute and chronic effects of cooling therapy for MS. *Neurology* 2003; 60(12):1955–1960.

102. Petajan JH, Gappmaier E, et al. Impact of aerobic training on fitness and quality of life in multiple sclerosis. *Ann Neurol* 1996; 39(4):432–441.

103. Rammohan KW, Rosenberg JH, et al. Efficacy and safety of Modafinil (Provigil) for the treatment of fatigue in multiple sclerosis: a two centre phase 2 study. *J Neurol Neurosurg Psychiatry* 2002; 72(2): 179–183.

104. Zahavi A, Geertzen JH, Middel B, et al. Long-term effect (more than five years) of intrathecal Baclofen on impairment, disability, and quality of life in patients with sever spasticity of spinal origin. *J Neurol Neurosurg Psychiatry* 2004; 75(11):1553–1557.

105. Sheean G. Botulinum toxin treatment of adult spasticity: a benefit-risk assessment. *Drug Saf* 2006; 29(1):31–48.

106. Bittar RG, Hyam J, Nandi D, et al. Thalamotomy versus thalamic stimulation for multiple sclerosis tremor. *J Clin Neurosci* 2005; 12(6):638–642.

107. Yap L, Kouyialis A, Varma TR. Stereotactic neurosurgery for disabling tremor in multiple sclerosis: thalamotomy or deep brain stimulation? *Br J Neurosurg* 2007; 21(4):349–354.

108. Solaro C, Brichetto G, Amato MP, et al. The prevalence of pain in multiple sclerosis: a multicenter cross-sectional study. *Neurology* 2004; 63(5):919–921.

109. Ross EL. The evolving role of antiepileptic drugs in treating neuropathic pain. *Neurology* 2000; 55(5 Suppl 1):41–46.

110. DasGupta R, Fowler CJ. Bladder, bowel, and sexual dysfunction in multiple sclerosis: management strategies. *Drugs* 2003; 63(2):153–166.

111. Zorzon M, Zivadinov R, Bosco A, et al. Sexual dysfunction in multiple sclerosis: a case-controlled study. I. Frequency and comparison of groups. *Mult Scler* 1999; 5(6):418–427.

112. Prosiegel M, Schelling A, Wagner-Sonntag E. Dysphagia and multiple sclerosis. *Int MS J* 2004; 11(1):22–31.

113. Kieseier BC, Wiendl H. Oral disease-modifying treatments for multiple sclerosis: the story so far. *CNS Drugs* 2007; 21(6):483–502.

114. Leist T, Vermersch P. The potential role for Cladribine in the treatment of multiple sclerosis: clinical experience and development of an oral tablet formulation. *Curr Med Res and Opin* 2007; 23(11):2667–2676.

115. Giovannoni G, Comi G, Cook S, et al. A placebo–controlled trial of oral Cladribine for relapsing multiple sclerosis. *N Engl J Med* 2010 [Epub ahead of print].

116. Kappos L, Antel J, Comi G, et al. Oral Fingolimod (FTY720) for relapsing multiple sclerosis. *N Engl J Med* 2006; 355(11):1124–1140.

117. Schimrigk S, Brune N, et al. Oral fumaric acid esters for the treatment of active multiple sclerosis: an open-label, baseline-controlled pilot study. *Eur J Neurol* 2006; 13:604–610.

118. Polman C, Barkhof F, et al. Treatment with Laquinimod reduces development of active MRI lesions in relapsing MS. *Neurology* 2005; 64:987–991.

119. O'Connor P, Freedman M, et al., on behalf of the Teriflunomide Multiple Sclerosis Trial Group and the University of British Columbia MS/MRI Research Group. *Neurology* 2006; 66:894–900.

120. Buttmann M, Rieckmann P. Treating multiple sclerosis with monoclonal antibodies. *Expert Rev Neurother* 2008; 8(3):433–455.

121. Coles AJ, Cox A, Le Page E, et al. The window of therapeutic opportunity in multiple sclerosis: evidence from monoclonal antibody therapy. *J Neurol* 2006; 253(1):98–108.

122. Hauser S, Waubant E, et al. B-cell depletion with Rituximab in relapsing-remitting multiple sclerosis. *N Engl J Med* 2008; 358:676–688.

123. Cree B. Emerging monoclonal antibody therapies for multiple sclerosis. *Neurology* 2006; 12(4):171–179.

124. Hawker K, O'Conner P, Freedman M, et al. Rituximab in patients with primary progressive multiple sclerosis: results of a randomized double-blind placebo-controlled multicenter trial. *Ann Neurol* 2009; 66(4): 460–471.

125. Rose JW, Burns JB, et al. Daclizumab phase II trial in relapsing and remitting multiple sclerosis: MRI and clinical results. *Neurology* 2007; 69(8):785–789.

126. Correale J, Fiol M. BHT-3009, a myelin basic protein-encoding plasmid for the treatment of multiple sclerosis. *Curr Opin Mol Ther* 2009; 11(4):463–470.

127. Bar-Or A, Vollmer T, Antel J. Induction of antigen-specific tolerance in multiple sclerosis after immunization with DNA encoding myelin basic protein in a randomized, placebo-controlled phase 1/2 trial. *Arch Neurol* 2007; 64(10):1407–1415.

128. Freedman MS. Bone marrow transplantation: does it stop MS progression? *J Neurol Sci* 2007; 259(1–2):85–89.

129. Neuhaus O, Hartung HP. Evaluation of Atorvastatin and Simvastatin for treatment of multiple sclerosis. *Expert Rev Neurother* 2007; 7(5): 547–556.

130. Vollmer T, Key L, Durkalski V, et al. Oral simvastatin treatment in relapsing-remitting multiple sclerosis. *Lancet* 2004; 363:1607–1608.

131. Birnbaum G, Cree B, Altafullah I, et al. Combining beta interferon and Atorvastatin may increase disease activity in multiple sclerosis. *Neurology* 2008; 71(18):1390-1395.

132. Sorensen PS, Frederiksen JL, Lycke J, Sellebjerg F. Does simvastatin antagonise the effect of interferon beta? Interim safety analysis of the ongoing SIMCOMBIN study. *Mult Scler* 2007; 13:S25. [Abstract]

133. Rudick R, Pace A, Panzara M, et al. Effects of statins on intramuscular interferon beta-1a for relapsing-remitting multiple sclerosis. *Mult Scler* 2007; 13:S57. [Abstract]

134. Giuliani F, Metz LM, et al. Additive effect of the combination of glatiramer acetate and Minocycline in a model of MS. *J Neuroimmunol* 2005; 158(1–2):213–221.

135. Giuliani F, Fu SA, Metz LM, Yong WV. Effective combination of Minocycline and interferon-beta in a model of multiple sclerosis. *J Neuroimmunol* 2005; 165(1–2):83–91.

136. Sicotte NL, Liva SM, Klutch R, et al. Treatment of multiple sclerosis with the pregnancy hormone Estriol. *Ann Neurol* 2002; 52(4):421–428.

137. Antonio M, Patrizia F, Ilaria I, Paolo F. A rational approach on the use of sex steroids in multiple sclerosis. *Recent Pat CNS Drug Discov* 2008; 3(1):34–39.

138. Gold SM, Voskuhl RR. Estrogen and testosterone therapies in multiple sclerosis. *Prog Brain Res* 2009; 175:239–251.

139. Keegan M, Konig F, McCleeland R, et al. Relation between humoral pathological changes in multiple sclerosis and response to therapeutic plasma exchange. *Lancet* 2005; 366(9485):579–582.

140. Panitch HS, Thisted RA, Smith RA, et al. Randomized, controlled trial of dextromethorphan/quinidine for pseudobulbar affect in multiple sclerosis. *Ann Neurol* 2006; 59(5):780–787.

141. Ghaffar O, Feinstein A. Multiple Sclerosis and cannabis: a cognitive and psychiatric study. *Neurology* in press.

142. Smith PF. Symptomatic treatment of multiple sclerosis using cannabinoids: recent advances. *Expert Rev Neurother* 2007; 7(9): 1157–1163.

143. Gallien P, Reymann JM, Amarenco G, et al. Placebo controlled, randomized, double blind study of the effects of botulinium A toxin on detrusor sphincter dyssynergia in multiple sclerosis patients. *J Neurol Neurosurg Psychiatry* 2005; 76(12):1670–1676.

144. Gironi M, Martinelli-Boneschi F, Sacerdote P, et al. A pilot trial of low-dose naltrexone in primary progressive multiple sclerosis. *Mult Scler.* 2008; 14(8):1076–1083.

145. Halper J, Burks JS. Care patterns in multiple sclerosis: principal care, comprehensive team care, consortium care. *Neuro Rehab* 1994; 4(2):67–75.

146. Burks JS. Multiple sclerosis care: an integrated disease management model. *J Spinal Cord Med* 1998; 21(2):113–116.

147. Burks JS. Is case management the solution to the managed care conundrum? *MS Quarterly* 1998; 17(2):4–7.

38 Pain Management in Persons with Spinal Cord Injury

Thomas N. Bryce

PROBLEM SCOPE

Pain is a common and significant problem for persons with spinal cord injury (SCI). Almost four out of five persons with SCI report chronic pain, and approximately one-third report chronic severe pain that interferes with activity and affects quality of life (1–11). These statistics hold true in different cultures, among persons enrolled in the Model Systems for Spinal Cord Injury, as well as in the American veteran population (8, 11–13).

Studies reported by Siddall and Cardenas are illustrative of the pervasiveness of the problem. In 1999, Siddall reported the results of a survey of 100 persons with new SCI, consecutively admitted to a spinal injury unit. Of these, 91% noted pain at 2 weeks after SCI, whereas 64% noted pain at 6 months. In those who reported pain at 6 months, 21% rated it as severe. Two-thirds of the pain at 2 weeks and 40% of the pain at 6 months was identified by the investigators as musculoskeletal; the remainder was considered neuropathic (see Table 38.1) (10). In 2005, Cardenas reported the results of a survey of 7,379 individuals with traumatic-onset SCI from sixteen Spinal Cord Injury Model Systems. Pain prevalence remained stable over time, ranging from 81% among persons 1 year postinjury to 83% for those at 25 years, while the overall prevalence of pain interfering with work or usual activity decreased over time, ranging from 70% at year 1 to 51% at 25 years (11).

Persons with pain after SCI typically do not have just one pain problem. Moreover, if a person has two or more pain problems, they are usually of different pain types. In a large German survey, Stormer et al. found that 64% of subjects with pain and/or dysesthesia had at least two distinct pains or dysesthesias, and a small percentage had four or five (8). In two small Australian studies, Siddall and his group reported a range of from 0 to 5 pain components, with an average of 2.3 (14, 15).

IDENTIFICATION OF PAIN GENERATORS

There is no universally accepted classification of pain after SCI. There are classification systems based upon location related to injury level (i.e., above-level, at-level, and below-level) (16, 17). There are systems based upon clinical syndromes: nerve root and diffuse pain of central origin (18); local segmental and remote pain (19); visceral, root, and burning—tingling—poorly localized pain (1); musculoskeletal, visceral, root, phantom, psychic, and sympathetic pain (20); visceral, root, and diffuse pain in areas with sensory loss (3); and mechanical, visceral, segmental, spinal cord, and psychogenic pain (21). Recently, hybrid systems based upon both location relative to injury level and clinical syndrome have been proposed (22, 23). For one hybrid system, Siddall included the following categories: musculoskeletal pain, visceral pain, neuropathic pain at the level of the lesion, neuropathic pain below the level of lesion, and other types of pain (22). For another, Ragnarsson included nociceptive pain at the level of the cord lesion, and radicular, segmental, visceral, and deafferentation central pain (23).

In 2000, Bryce and Ragnarsson expanded on the hybrid classifications of Siddall and Ragnarsson to include all the categories of pain more common after SCI (12, 24, 25). For this classification, the Bryce-Ragnarsson SCI Pain Taxonomy (BR-SCI-PT), the neurological level of injury is defined as the most caudal segment of the spinal cord with normal sensory and motor function bilaterally (26). Above-level pain is defined as being localized rostral to the two dermatomes above the neurological level, at-level pain to within the two dermatomes above or below the neurological level, and below-level pain to the dermatomes localized caudally to the two dermatomes below the neurological level. Persistent nociceptive pain is defined as pain that occurs when intact peripheral nociceptors in partially or fully innervated areas of the body are activated by local damage or ongoing irritation to non-neural tissues such as bone, ligaments, muscle, skin, or other organs. Neuropathic pain, in contrast, is defined as pain that occurs as a result of damage to neural tissue either in the peripheral or central nervous system. A simple three-tier decision tree organizes the schema: first, the pain is regionally localized relative to the neurological level of SCI (i.e., either above-level, at-level, or below-level); second, the pain is identified as either nociceptive or neuropathic pain; third, the pain is stratified into subtypes of the regionally localized nociceptive or neuropathic pain types.

Table 38.1   Prevalence of Types and Characteristics of Pain after SCI

	MUSCULOSKELETAL	BELOW-LEVEL NEUROPATHIC	VISCERAL	AT-LEVEL NEUROPATHIC	ALLODYNIA
Barrett et al. (ref. 14) (total $N = 88$)					
Number of cases with pain type	29	16	10	7	5
Percent of cases	44%	24%	15%	11%	6%
Average pain intensity on 0 (no pain) to 10 (worst possible pain) scale	6	6	7	6	5
Siddall et al. (ref. 15) (total $N = 73$)					
Number of cases with pain type	43	25	4	30	10
Percent of cases	59%	34%	5%	41%	14%
Average pain intensity on 0 (no pain) to 10 (worst possible pain) scale	5	6	8	6	Not specified

The same year the International Association for the Study of Pain (IASP), building on the preliminary published classification scheme for SCI pain of one of its members (22), published a similar three-tiered system, albeit with a reversal of the first two tiers. The nociceptive versus neuropathic distinction is made first, and then, within the nociceptive category, a division is made into musculoskeletal and visceral subtypes, whereas within the neuropathic category, there is a division into three subtypes: above-, at-, and below-level pain. Within the third tier of both systems, further subdivisions are made. There are fifteen specific subcategories within the BR-SCI-PT. Within the IASP scheme, there are further subcategories based on specific underlying structural causes of pathology, when identified. Another recently cited classification is the Cardenas scheme (27), which was developed for a funded study, prior to the publication of the IASP and Bryce-Ragnarsson schemes, although those publications were cited by the time the results of the study by Cardenas et al. were published (28). Cardenas proposed two major categories: neurologic and musculoskeletal. For neurologic pain, there are four subcategories: SCI pain, transition zone pain, radicular pain, and visceral pain. For musculoskeletal pain, there are two subcategories: mechanical spine pain and overuse pain.

These three classification systems, upon close examination, seem to include many of the same subtypes of pain, and the use of any one of these will allow one to identify most of the common subtypes of pain found after SCI. Nevertheless, none of the classifications has achieved universal acceptance. Perhaps this is due in part to a lack of demonstrated reliability and validity or perhaps it is due to a number of limitations of the systems, as described below.

Evoked pain is not specifically considered in any classification system. Subtypes of pain are designated as either nociceptive or neuropathic, with no accommodation for mixed neuropathic and nociceptive pain. Measures of the degree of certainty of classification for any subtype of pain are not included (i.e., users of the classification systems are unable to express confidence in their classification of subtype). Pain generators are not always specifically identified, either by anatomic tissue type or specific site. And finally, the systems are all biologically based, without incorporating any of the concepts inherent in a biopsychosocial model of pain.

Evoked pains are not uncommonly seen after SCI (14, 15). Evoked pains are, by definition, only felt when something is done to provoke the pain. Superficial cutaneous evoked pains are commonly elicited by noxious or non-noxious stimulation of the skin. If, during the sensory examination, pain is elicited with a stimulus that does not normally provoke pain, then this evoked pain is often defined as allodynia. The pain threshold is defined as the lowest intensity of a stimulus at which a subject experiences pain. Hypoalgesia is an increased pain threshold, compared to what an average person may experience or compared to noninvolved areas of a person's body. Hyperalgesia is a decreased pain threshold (an exaggerated painful response to a pain-provoking stimulus). Wind-up pain is hyperalgesia resulting from high-frequency (greater than 3 Hz) repetitive noxious stimuli; it is also sometimes referred to as hyperpathia. Allodynia, hyperalgesia, and wind-up pain are findings commonly associated with neuropathic etiologies of pain, although they can be seen with nociceptive and mixed nociceptive-neuropathic etiologies.

In at least one intervention trial, treatment of evoked neuropathic pain after SCI has been more effective than treatment of spontaneous neuropathic pain (29). This differential treatment effect on spontaneous and evoked pain with a single intervention has also been suggested in another study where persons with incomplete injuries with neuropathic pain and persons with complete injuries with neuropathic pain responded differently to medication (30). These findings suggest that different mechanisms are responsible for different components of pain, at least when it comes to spontaneous and evoked pain. Therefore, if a component of pain, such as evoked pain, is not evaluated and measured in a study, then the true effectiveness of the treatment being studied is not being captured.

With few exceptions, pain after SCI that is thought to be neuropathic in origin is rarely just neuropathic in presentation. Significant injury to a nerve root, nerve plexus, or peripheral nerve usually leads to denervation of muscle and secondary pain with all the hallmarks of nociceptive pain. Complex regional pain syndrome (CRPS) type I, which by definition is not triggered by identifiable nerve injury, often acquires the hallmarks of both nociceptive and neuropathic pain. Neuropathic pain resulting from injury to the spinal cord, root, plexus, or peripheral nerve by an unstable local fracture or dislocation often is coexistent with the nociceptive pain attributable to the unstable local fracture or dislocation. When the fracture is stabilized or the dislocation is reduced, both subtypes of pain, neuropathic and nociceptive, may resolve. The one notable exception to the coexistent presentations of nociceptive and neuropathic pain after damage to a single neurologic structure is below-level pain in persons with complete SCI, which is attributed to damage to the spinal cord. Here, there is usually no nociceptive component, as the persons have no retained somatic sensation in the area where the pain is perceived.

A related concept concerns the hypothesis that pain which initially is thought to be nociceptive may evolve over time into a neuropathic type as plastic changes within the pain transmission system occur. The prototypical example of this is pain triggered by herpes zoster infection. The mechanisms underlying the pain of the acute herpes zoster lesion are thought to be nociceptive ones, whereas the mechanisms underlying the pain of postherpetic neuralgia are thought to be neuropathic.

The degree of certainty of a diagnosis is a concept that has been used as part of diagnostic criteria guidelines for many years (31). It also has utility in pain classification systems, as it allows the user of a classification system to express confidence in a particular classification based upon the strength of supporting evidence and the degree to which the clinical presentation is consistent with what is expected for the particular attributed pain generator. One method of expressing certainty includes three levels: "definite," "probable," and "possible." It is suggested that, in classifying pain, three criteria typically must be fulfilled to qualify a diagnosis as definite. First, the pain history must fit what is expected for pain originating from the attributed pain generator. Second, there must be findings on a physical exam that corroborate the pain history. Third, there must be confirmation of appropriate damage to the specific pain generator, which corroborates both the pain history and the physical exam findings. Adequate confirmation might, for example, include identification of a lesion during surgical exploration, findings of appropriate pathology on imaging (magnetic resonance imaging, computed tomography, ultrasound, etc.), or findings on pathologic specimen review. A confirmatory test for a specific nerve root as a source of pain could be an isolated nerve root impingement seen on an MRI, which corroborates the history and physical exam, whereas a confirmatory test for the sacroiliac joint as a source of pain might be temporary relief of the pain after interarticular injection of the joint with a short-acting anesthetic medication. The first two of these criteria, that the pain history must fit what is expected and that there must be findings on the physical exam that corroborate the pain history, must be fulfilled to qualify as probable. To qualify as possible, the clinical presentation may be atypical or there may be a lack of findings on the physical exam that corroborate the pain history. Diagnoses with less than definite certainty encourage further scrutiny.

Finally, it should not be forgotten that specific pain generators are the ultimate targets for treatment, especially if they can be identified and addressed before permanent plastic changes have been made throughout the neuroaxis. For example, although determining that a specific pain is musculoskeletal in nature and above-level in location is useful, it is much more useful for a treating clinician to identify the specific pain generator as the supraspinatus tendon. Only by knowing the specific pain generator during an early critical window can an effective

treatment plan be devised. Therefore, whenever possible, specific pain generators should be specified. Moreover, as alluded to above, injury to a nerve root, nerve plexus, or peripheral nerve usually leads to changes that include pain within affected muscles. In this case the injured nerve root, nerve plexus, or peripheral nerve is defined as the primary pain generator, whereas the muscle, secondarily affected, is defined as the secondary pain generator. Several pain generators, primary and secondary, may be active for any particular pain complaint.

COMMON PAIN GENERATORS

This section reviews many of the common pain generators that may develop after SCI. In addition to a description of the various generators, treatment suggestions are included for many of the musculoskeletal pain conditions. For a more in-depth review of musculoskeletal pain and overuse injuries, including their prevention, see Chapter 46. For those pain generators where treatment is not addressed, a separate section reviewing pharmacologic, psychologic, and nonpharmacologic/nonpsychologic interventions follows.

Shoulder Pain

The prevalence of shoulder pain in persons with chronic paraplegia ranges from 40% to 50% (data taken from questionnaires sent to community resident individuals) (32–34). Bayley, who reported a prevalence of shoulder pain of 30% in hospitalized veterans with paraplegia independent of transferring, noted that 75% of these had chronic impingement syndrome and subacromial bursitis, and 16% had aseptic necrosis of the humeral head (four out of five of this latter group used alcohol at least moderately) (35). Sie, who reported a prevalence of shoulder pain of 36% in outpatients with paraplegia followed in an SCI clinic, noted that of the fifteen persons clinically evaluated, two had pain referred from the cervical spine; eleven had pain that was "orthopedically related," including tendinitis, bursitis, capsulitis, and osteoarthritis; and for two the cause remained undetermined (36). An earlier study of a similar group revealed bicipital tendonitis as the most common cause of shoulder pain (37). When twenty wheelchair athletes with paraplegia, both with and without a rotator cuff impingement syndrome, were compared with regard to shoulder strength, the athletes with rotator cuff impingement exhibited decreased shoulder adduction and external and internal rotation strength and increased abduction-to-adduction and abduction-to-internal rotation strength ratios. These findings led the authors to conclude that shoulder muscle imbalance, with relative weakness of the adductors and external and internal rotators, may be a factor in the development and perpetuation of rotator cuff impingement in wheelchair athletes with paraplegia (38). In another small study of wheelchair propulsion biomechanics in persons with long-standing paraplegia, it was found that those who later developed pain had a smaller push arc, with a more forward initial hand placement and a greater vertical force on the push rim (39).

Specific treatment (and prevention) strategies for shoulder pain originating from the rotator cuff in persons with SCI should include strengthening, stretching, optimizing posture, and avoiding activities that promote impingement (40). Strengthening of the dynamic shoulder stabilizers should occur in a balanced fashion. A program should emphasize strengthening the posterior shoulder musculature, including the external rotators, the posterior scapular muscles (rhomboids and trapezius), and the adductors, as wheelchair use strengthens the antagonists to these muscles (i.e., the anterior shoulder musculature) (38, 40). Stretching of the dynamic shoulder stabilizers, especially the anterior shoulder musculature, which often has become hypertrophied and contracted through constant use during wheelchair propulsion and transfer activities, is also necessary in achieving a strength-balanced shoulder. In one controlled study of wheelchair users, a 6-month exercise protocol that included two exercises for stretching anterior shoulder musculature and three exercises for strengthening posterior shoulder musculature was found to be effective in decreasing the shoulder pain that interfered with functional activities (41). Optimizing sitting posture with a goal of achieving normal alignment of shoulder, head, and spine, both through posture exercises and through provision of proper wheelchair seating systems, can also help decrease impingement during everyday activities (40). Activities that promote impingement—that is, activities in which the arm is abducted or flexed more than 90 degrees—especially when combined with internal rotation, should be identified by a thorough functional evaluation, and alternatives sought and implemented (40). It has been found that, in transferring from a mat to a wheelchair using a popover technique, ground reaction forces beneath the trailing hand are greater than those beneath the leading hand (42). It is suggested that, if there is weakness or pain in one arm, this arm should be selected as the leading arm. If there is pain in neither or both arms, then the direction of transfer should be varied in order to minimize selective arm overuse. For manual wheelchair users, proper positioning and fit in a wheelchair to allow the most efficient and least stressful propulsion pattern is indicated—the provision of the lightest-weight wheelchair that requires the least amount of force to propel and that meets a person's needs is essential.

Adjuncts to the active treatment strategies for shoulder pain originating from the rotator cuff outlined above should also include, as necessary, application of ice; relative rest; anti-inflammatory medications; injections of steroid into appropriate bursae or joints; and direct or indirect suprascapular nerve blocks. Most of these have been shown to be effective in decreasing the pain originating from the rotator cuff, at least in persons without SCI (43–45).

Caution is warranted in deciding on surgical treatment of rotator cuff tendonopathies in persons with SCI, as the outcomes literature is sparse and not particularly favorable. Five persons with paraplegia for a total of six shoulders with rotator cuff tears underwent surgical repair at one institution, but only one repair of a small tear limited to the supraspinatus muscle was deemed successful, as evidenced by decreased pain and increased strength and range of motion (ROM) postoperatively. The other repairs of large tears did not result in an improvement in shoulder function or ROM (40). Another study reported three persons with paraplegia and one with tetraplegia, for a total of six shoulders with rotator cuff tears, who underwent repair with anterior acromioplasty, and when indicated, repair of the supraspinatus tendon. All were noted, at least initially, to have decreased pain and a functional capacity that approached or equaled preoperative levels (46).

There has been little written concerning replacement arthroplasties in the weight-bearing shoulder of persons with paraplegia. One study reported the results of this procedure in five subjects (47). Four had generalized osteonecrosis, and one had avascular necrosis; three of these had associated full-thickness rotator cuff tears. Pain decreased and function improved in four of the five; in the fifth, the glenoid implant migrated at 30 months.

The prevalence of shoulder pain in persons with chronic tetraplegia is similar to that in paraplegia, ranging from 40% to 60% (33, 34). Sie, reporting an overall prevalence of 46% in outpatients with tetraplegia, noted that twenty-seven of sixty-two individuals had shoulder pain that was orthopedically related, twenty had pain referred from the cervical spine, and nine had pain due to a variety of other known and unknown causes, including spasticity, heterotopic ossification, and syringomyelia (36). A convenience sample of eleven veterans with tetraplegia, half of whom had one painful shoulder, the other half two, all painful for less than 6 months, underwent workup for their shoulder pain using a protocol designed to determine the etiology of musculoskeletal shoulder pain using physical exam, plain radiography, and arthrography. Six shoulders were determined to have capsular contracture or capsulitis; four had rotator cuff tears; two had anterior instability; and one shoulder each had rotator cuff impingement, osteoarthritis, and osteonecrosis (48). Using this same protocol in thirteen veterans with a total of fifteen shoulders that had been painful for more than 6 months, five shoulders were determined to have anterior instability; three shoulders had multidirectional instability; three shoulders had capsular contracture or capsulitis; and one shoulder each had Charcot arthropathy, rotator cuff tear, rotator cuff impingement, and scapular pain (48).

In 1991 Silfverskiold observed that, although 78% of persons with tetraplegia noted shoulder pain within the first 6 months of injury, this decreased to 33% 6–18 months later; the persons whose pain persisted all exhibited spasticity (49).

Another type of pain occasionally seen in persons with mid-cervical levels of tetraplegia is a musculoskeletal pain originating in the muscles supporting the shoulder girdle, labeled scapular pain by Silfverskiold. In a convenience sample of forty persons with tetraplegia for less than 6 months who were evaluated for shoulder pain, six were diagnosed with scapular pain. Six to eighteen months later, only three reported persistent pain (49). Scapular pain is centered along the medial-dorsal border of the scapula with associated tenderness to palpation over the rhomboids, levator scapulae, and supraspinatus and infraspinatus muscles. A postulated mechanism for scapular pain is the presence of a relative imbalance in residual innervation to muscles of the shoulder girdle caused by a mid-cervical spinal cord lesion, whereby increased scapular retractor muscle strength compared to scapular protractor muscle strength may lead to abnormal scapulothoracic motion and secondary inflammation and contracture of muscles and joint capsule.

Although the treatment of musculoskeletal shoulder pain in persons with tetraplegia depends upon the exact etiology, a few principles should be emphasized. With regard to positioning, if a person with tetraplegia has weak shoulder stabilizers and shoulder pain that is lessened when the humeral head is manually reduced by an examiner into the glenoid fossa, then emphasis should be placed on proper positioning in the wheelchair with adequate arm support, whether through use of an arm trough or a lap tray, so that the humerus remains within the glenoid fossa. When ROM exercises are performed, the shoulder should not be flexed or abducted beyond 90 degrees unless upward rotation of the scapula and external rotation of the humerus also occurs; this will both minimize stress on the glenoid capsule and minimize impingement of the rotator cuff. If transfers, positioning, and bed mobility are performed with the assistance of another person, the assistant must be trained to assist without putting undue stress on the arms of the assisted. Excess strain on a shoulder with already weak dynamic shoulder stabilizers can lead to a sprain of the static shoulder stabilizers, the ligaments of the capsule, and, in the long term, single or multidirectional instability. If there is some active motor strength in the dynamic shoulder stabilizers, then a balanced strengthening program can theoretically help reduce a functional instability. Finally, performance of a daily stretching program, especially if there is spasticity or a significant muscle imbalance, with the goal of obtaining balanced shoulder muscle strength with full ROM in all directions, is important for the prevention of capsular contracture and capsulitis.

Occasionally, shoulder pain is experienced by persons with tetraplegia with all the signs and symptoms of the primary pain generators being the muscles and tendons of the rotator cuff complex. However, the primary pain generator is actually the spinal cord, affected by either tethering or syringomyelia, causing pain only secondarily to be generated by the muscles and tendons of the rotator cuff complex. Clues that the primary generator is actually the spinal cord may include the presence of allodynia or hyperpathia to repetitive pinprick over the shoulder region and the ineffectiveness of treatment of the musculoskeletal pain generators.

Autonomic Dysreflexia Headache Pain

A severe headache, usually described as "pounding," associated with an elevated blood pressure, and often with diaphoresis, piloerection, and cutaneous vasodilation above the level of injury, bradycardia or tachycardia, nasal stuffiness, conjunctival congestion, and mydriasis in a person with SCI and a neurologic level most commonly above T6, indicates the presence of autonomic dysreflexia (AD) (50–52). The syndrome occurs in response to noxious stimulation below the neurological level and usually responds promptly to the removal of the offending stimulus. The most common cause is a distended bladder, but other causes may include bowel impaction, tight clothing, a localized abscess, a broken bone, or a urinary system calculus.

Compressive Neuropathy Pain

In 1992 Sie reported a total prevalence of 66% for signs and symptoms of carpal tunnel syndrome (CTS) (i.e., numbness or tingling of thumb, index, or middle fingers; abnormal sensation on testing; or numbness or tingling with provocative tests) for a sample of 103 persons with paraplegia undergoing routine annual SCI follow-up. The reported prevalence correlated for the most part with time since injury; it was 42% for the group 0–5 years postinjury, 63% for the group 5–9 years postinjury, 74% for the group 10–14 years postinjury, 92% for the group 15–20 years postinjury, and 86% for the group 20+ years postinjury (36). Previous studies with fewer subjects showed similar trends (53, 54), and studies in which screening for CTS in persons with paraplegia was done using electrodiagnostic techniques found similar overall prevalences (53, 55).

Unlike in persons without SCI who have CTS, resting pressures in the carpal tunnel of persons with paraplegia and CTS often are normal, and the presenting complaints are usually of hyperesthesias of the thumb and index finger and not of night, wrist, and hand pain (56). Sie has suggested the syndrome could be more accurately labeled as repetitive contact neuropathy (36). The pathophysiology of this syndrome is thought to result from a combination of (1) repetitive trauma, as occurs with propulsion of manual wheelchairs, and (2) ischemia from repetitive marked increases in carpal canal pressures, as occurs with push-up ischial pressure reliefs, and transfers from one seating surface to another (54). Persons who use a larger ROM of the wrist while propelling their wheelchairs tend to use less force and fewer strokes to travel at a given speed, indicating that long, smooth strokes may benefit nerve health in manual wheelchair users (57). Furthermore, body mass has been associated both with the peak resultant force applied to the push rim and to median nerve latency and median sensory amplitude (i.e., median nerve health) (58).

The ulnar nerve may be involved in a manner similar to the median nerve; Davidoff found in a convenience sample of thirty-one persons with paraplegia three who had electrodiagnostic evidence of an ulnar mononeuropathy at the wrist (55).

Prevention and treatment of repetitive contact neuropathies at the wrist should begin with the cushioning of the volar aspect of the wrist by use of padded gloves and the avoidance of weight bearing on an extended wrist by substituting a neutral wrist position whenever possible. A side-to-side ischial pressure relief or forward lean ischial pressure relief can often be substituted for the push-up relief as well. In addition, for manual wheelchair users, proper positioning and fit in a wheelchair to allow the most efficient and least stressful propulsion pattern, provision of the lightest-weight wheelchair that requires the least amount of force to propel, and the use of ergonomically designed hand rims all have been postulated to minimize stress upon the nerves and other structures about the wrists.

Surgical carpal tunnel release should only be performed for pain that doesn't respond to conservative measures or when progressive neurological deterioration is observed, as a carpal tunnel release may actually leave a nerve more exposed to the direct trauma that is thought to be a major contributory factor to this condition (59).

The presumed pathophysiology compressive neuropathy pain in persons with tetraplegia is the same as in persons with paraplegia: repetitive trauma combined with ischemia from repetitive marked increases in carpal tunnel canal pressures (54). However, because of the impaired sensation, intrinsic to tetraplegia, in the dermatomes overlying the peripheral nerves usually affected by mononeuropathies at the wrist or elbow, the prevalence of symptomatic compressive neuropathies after tetraplegia is presumably low, occurring only in those persons with relatively preserved sensation of the lower cervical dermatomes. As a result, there have been no studies that have critically evaluated this entity.

Visceral Pain

The nociceptive pain sensation that originates from damage, irritation, or distention of internal organs or their supporting ligamentous structures is often altered by SCI. Causes of visceral pain in persons with SCI that have been reported include fecal impaction, bowel obstruction, bowel infarction, bowel perforation, cholecystitis, choledocholithiasis, pancreatitis, appendicitis, splenic rupture, urinary bladder perforation, pyelonephritis, and the superior mesenteric artery syndrome (60–66).

The sensory innervation to the parietal peritoneum is segmental and correlates roughly with the truncal dermatomes. Therefore, when the parietal peritoneum is irritated at a level with at least some retained sensation, precise localization is usually possible. In contrast, sensation from the internal organs is not segmental. Thus, when the visceral peritoneum or an internal organ is irritated, localization is usually not precise in those without SCI, and even less so in those with SCI.

The anatomical pathways for visceral sensation are less understood than the anatomical pathways for somatic sensation. One putative anatomical pathway for the conduction of visceral sensation is that visceral afferents follow sympathetic pathways. Evidence of this was found by Ray in 1947 in persons without SCI who had undergone sympathectomies for hypertension and underwent gut distention and temperature stimulation via catheter and direct gut stimulation during laparatomy under local anesthesia (67). The visceral afferents are thought to follow postganglionic sympathetic fibers from internal organs in the abdomen and pelvis to the paravertebral sympathetic chains (60, 64, 68). These visceral afferents have wide and overlapping receptive fields from which they originate. They may pass directly into the spinal cord at the level where they reach the paravertebral chain, or they may travel either down or up the chain before entering the spinal cord along pathways paralleling the exiting preganglionic sympathetic fibers from the spinal cord (i.e., at levels anywhere from T1 through L3, the only levels from which preganglionic sympathetic fibers exit the spinal cord) (64). Because visceral afferents may enter the spinal cord at a level more rostral than that at which they joined the paravertebral chain, it is thought that a person with an upper thoracic– (or lower–) level lesion may have at least some preserved visceral sensation through this pathway (64).

In persons with visceral pain and a neurologic level of injury below the mid-thoracic, nociceptive stimuli from the internal abdominal and pelvic organs presumably travel rostrally along visceral afferents following the sympathetic pathways. If these sympathetic pathways are intact and the visceral afferents from an inflamed organ join the spinal cord at a level rostral to the neurologic level, then the visceral sensation from this inflamed organ will presumably be unaltered by SCI. Moreover, depending on the neurologic level below the mid-thoracic, the parietal peritoneum has at least some retained sensation. Therefore, although visceral pain in these individuals may be quite altered, it is of a less vague character and is more often accurately localized than the visceral pain that occurs in individuals with a higher neurological level who lack any sensation originating from the parietal peritoneum (60).

In 1985 Juler reported a case series of various abdominal emergencies in persons with SCI (63). There were two persons with paraplegia, one with a T11 neurological level, the other with a T12 level, who were operated upon for acute appendicitis. Each was able to localize abdominal pain to the right lower quadrant of the abdomen early in the disease course. There were three persons with paraplegia, one with a T11 neurological level, another with a T12 level, and a third with an L4 level, who were operated upon for perforated bowel. Only one developed increased abdominal spasm, but all three were able to localize abdominal pain well. There were ten persons with paraplegia, neurological levels between T6 and L1, who were operated upon for acute bowel obstruction; all but one, a person with a T12–L1 level, experienced crampy abdominal pain, similar to what has been described in persons without a SCI who have experienced this condition (63).

For persons with a neurologic level of injury above the mid-thoracic, depending on the degree of retained sensation below the level of injury, visceral pain can be characteristically vague and poorly localized.

As mentioned previously, visceral afferents are thought to follow postganglionic sympathetic fibers from the abdominal and pelvic organs to the paravertebral sympathetic chains and from there to the spinal cord at segmental levels between T1 and L3. This is thought to be the main pathway by which the brain receives nociceptive input from the viscera. A cervical SCI can disrupt this main pathway, as there is no sympathetic outflow rostral to the T1 level. Nevertheless, because persons with anatomically complete cord transections above this level are often still able to describe visceral pain, other neural pathways, not yet defined in humans, are assumed to exist (66, 69). One such purported pathway is the vagus nerve (60, 69, 70).

In one case series, initially reported by Charney and later by Juler, of eight persons with both neurologically complete and incomplete SCI, at levels ranging from C4 to T6, who were reported to have perforated appendicitis, seven were able to localize pain to the right lower quadrant (RLQ); the other, who had a C5 complete injury, noted only shoulder pain (60, 63). Seven of the eight, not including a person with a C4 incomplete SCI, exhibited an elevated pulse rate, an elevated blood pressure, increased abdominal spasticity, and sweating above the level of the lesion. The majority also exhibited early anorexia and elevated temperature (60, 63). Eight persons with both complete and incomplete SCI, at levels ranging from C3 to T4, who were reported to have other areas of perforated bowel, all had generalized abdominal and shoulder pain, but only one could localize his pain to the upper abdomen (60, 63). In addition, all these individuals with perforated bowel exhibited an elevated pulse rate, blood pressure, and temperature, as well as sweating above the level of the lesion. Increased abdominal spasm was also present in most (60, 63).

These cases illustrate several points that should be remembered in the evaluation of abdominal pain in persons with SCI: (1) localization and intensity of nociceptive visceral abdominal pain is dependent upon the level and completeness of neurologic injury; (2) referred pain to other sensate areas may overshadow the classical patterns of pain typically produced by intra-abdominal pathologies, if those classical patterns of pain are located in insensate areas; (3) for persons with SCI who have a neurologic level above the mid-thoracic level, signs and symptoms of AD may provide more of a clue that there is intra-abdominal pathology than the visceral pain itself; and (4) other associated symptoms may include anorexia, altered bowel patterns, nausea and/or vomiting, and a change in the intensity or pattern of abdominal spasticity.

Radicular Pain

Radicular pain is neuropathic pain arising from nerve root damage. It commonly occurs within the dermatome representing the neurologic level of injury or within three dermatomal levels below the neurologic level of injury. Causes usually relate to impingement or irritation of the nerve roots by bone fragments, disc material, or scar. The character of the pain is often described as "stabbing," "shooting," or "electric shock–like," although it has also been described as "burning" or "aching" (1, 21, 71). It is generally unilateral and paroxysmal in its presence, radiating in a dermatomal pattern. Hyperesthesia or allodynia (i.e., pain evoked by non-noxious stimuli) is common in the dermatomes innervated by the damaged nerve roots, although hypoalgesia or analgesia can be seen, especially if the dorsal root ganglions are affected. It is often difficult and sometimes impossible to distinguish between at-level neuropathic pain due to damage to the nerve roots and pain due to damage to the spinal cord, especially if imaging does not allow clear visualization of the nerve roots. In these cases, diagnostic nerve root blocks performed with fluoroscopic guidance may provide both diagnostic and therapeutic benefit.

Facet Joint Pain

When a zygapophyseal joint is the pain generator, the most intense area of evoked pain is localized to one segment inferior and slightly lateral to the affected joint (72, 73). The medial extent of the pain elicited by any pain-generating zygapophyseal joint approaches midline but does not cross it and can extend laterally to the posterior axillary line, becoming less intense at its lateral extent (72). The pain is typically worsened with extension of the spine and is improved with flexion. The character of the pain often is a deep, dull ache (72). This type of pain often is generated at the vertebral levels, either just above or just below a fusion mass, often several years after the fusion is performed. This is thought to occur as a result of arthritic degeneration of the facet joints due to compensation and overuse of these joints adjacent to the now fused segments.

Treatment of the facet joint pain should include strengthening of the dynamic stabilizers of the spine with a slight flexion bias if possible, and may include fluoroscopically guided facet joint injections or median branch blocks and radiofrequency denervation. The median branches provide sensory innervation to the facet joints. Bracing and possible extension of the fusion to incorporate the degenerated segments are other potential treatment options.

Sacroiliac Joint Pain

When a sacroiliac joint is a pain generator, the distribution of pain is usually localized to a 3-cm by 10-cm vertical column extending from the posterior superior iliac spine caudally (74–76). There is typically tenderness to palpation over this area.

The pain typically worsens with extension of the lower spine and pelvis, and usually is more severe on one side than the other.

Treatments may include core and pelvic stabilization exercises, injections into the joint under fluoroscopic guidance, and most importantly, addressing of underlying biomechanical imbalances, which are likely the precipitating activation of a sacroiliac joint pain generator. Treatments aimed at the biomechanical abnormalities may include spasticity management with oral, intrathecal, or local injections of medication and strengthening of the relevant core and extremity musculature.

Discogenic Pain

When a vertebral disc is a pain generator, the character is often described as burning or aching (77). Pain is worsened with activities that cause compressive forces on the spine; pain while sitting is a hallmark. The pain is often worse while leaning forward without support (78). The pain is primarily in the low back but often radiates to the legs. L3–4 discs often provoke pain in the anterior thigh; L4–5 discs frequently provoke pain in the anterior leg and sometimes in the posterior leg, whereas L5–S1 discs often provoke pain in the posterior thigh (79).

At-Level Spinal Cord Pain

At-level spinal cord pain, also called at-level central pain, is neuropathic pain that is not related to nerve root damage but to actual segmental spinal cord damage that occurs within the dermatome representing the neurologic level of injury and/or within the three dermatomes below this level and not in any lower dermatomes (80). The character is typically one of "tightness," "pressure," or "burning" in thoracic-level injuries and of "numbness," "tingling," "heat," or "cold" in cervical injuries (23). The distribution is typically bilateral, involving single or multiple adjacent dermatomes over the shoulders, arms, or hands for cervical injuries; single or multiple dermatomal bands about the chest for thoracic injuries; and single or multiple adjacent dermatomes to the groin or legs for lumbar injuries. Furthermore, rather than being paroxysmal, SCI at-level spinal cord pain is typically continuous in its presence. Nevertheless, as noted above, it is often difficult to distinguish SCI at-level spinal cord pain from SCI at-level radicular pain, as both may present in the same manner.

Spinal Cord Pain of Syringomyelia

One specific common subtype of spinal cord pain is pain of syringomyelia. A delayed onset of pain after SCI, especially beginning after one year, should raise the suspicion of syringomyelia as the cause of pain (81–85). Nashold found a prevalence of syringomyelia of 65% in persons who had a late onset of spinal cord pain (86). Bulbar signs and symptoms, especially facial pain, associated with at-level pain of late onset, are rare but virtually diagnostic of syrinx (87).

Historically, syringomyelia of clinical significance has been found in approximately 2% to 5% of persons after SCI (83–85, 88, 89). The most common initial symptom is pain, either unilateral or bilateral (83, 84, 90). In one early series of seventeen persons with SCI and syringomyelia, seven presented with pain on coughing, seven presented with spontaneous pain, one each presented with temperature sensation loss and excessive sweating above the injury, and one was asymptomatic (81). The pain of posttraumatic syringomyelia often will begin at the segment marking the neurologic level of injury or in a segment just proximal to this; its presence is often intermittent initially (87). As the syrinx enlarges, the segment may then develop anesthesia to pin and temperature sensation. Subsequently, the pain at the level often will transform into a temporally continuous and characteristically burning type of pain (83, 87). Burning pain and dull, aching pain have been the most commonly reported characters of pain in several large series, although sharp pain, electrical pain, and stabbing pain have been reported as well (83–87, 91). Other presenting symptoms that may reflect the presence of a syrinx, although occurring less frequently than pain, include worsening spasticity and loss of motor strength (84, 90).

Magnetic resonance imaging (MRI) is the diagnostic study of choice in the evaluation of syringomyelia, although a computed tomography (CT) myelogram with up to 24-hour delayed imaging often will show contrast dye within a syrinx cavity in those for whom an MRI is unobtainable.

Treatment of posttraumatic syringomyelia can include (1) untethering if there is an associated tethering of the spinal cord with the syrinx, (2) untethering and placement of a shunt if untethering alone is unsuccessful, or (3) shunting if there is no associated tethering (90, 92). Surgery, in addition to theoretically preventing further neurologic deterioration, often will alleviate pain; in one study, 56% had substantial improvement in neurogenic pain after detethering (92).

Complex Regional Pain Syndrome Pain

Spontaneous or evoked pain, allodynia, or hyperalgesia that fulfills the following three criteria can be classified as complex regional pain syndrome (CRPS) pain: (1) it is not limited to the territory of a single peripheral nerve or root; (2) it is disproportionate in intensity to what is expected; and (3) it is associated with edema, skin blood flow abnormality, or abnormal sudomotor activity (93). In the IASP classification of chronic pain syndromes, the term reflex sympathetic dystrophy has been replaced by CRPS type I, and the term causalgia has been replaced by CRPS type II (93). CRPS type I differs from CRPS type II, in that in the latter, there is an identifiable root or peripheral nerve injury. This syndrome generally encompasses elements of both nociceptive and neuropathic pain. One theory relating to the development of CRPS type I, namely compartmental ischemia (94), would suggest that there is damage to both neural and non-neural tissue, with muscle ischemia leading to inflammatory pain and nerve ischemia leading to neuropathic pain.

There have been a number of small retrospective case reports, as well as case series, which have noted an association between cervical SCI and CRPS (95–101). The diagnostic criteria utilized in these reports vary. One prospective study of sixty persons consecutively admitted to an SCI unit revealed six who complained of diffuse hand pain, swelling, and stiffness and had a pattern of diffuse uptake in the third phase of a triple-phase bone scan (98).

There are no controlled studies of treatment of CRPS after SCI. Of five persons reported by Cremer as having CRPS after SCI, three improved after a short course of oral corticosteroids with or without desensitization and ROM exercises (99). Of the

six persons reported by Gellman, three underwent stellate ganglion blocks with relief of symptoms (98).

It is generally thought that an intensive hand therapy program should underlie the treatment of CRPS, with pharmacologic approaches only being added as adjuncts, although the evidence garnered through controlled studies to support the use of physical modalities is limited, even for persons without SCI who have CRPS (102).

Muscle Pain Due to Spasticity

Pain due to spasticity can usually be classified as muscular pain. Depending on the degree of retained sensation and the pattern of muscles affected, the degree of nociceptive pain associated with spasticity may vary. Painful muscle spasms respond best to stretching and positioning, local nerve or muscle blocks, or anti-spasticity medications. Common antispasticity medications that have been shown to be effective in treating spasticity after SCI include baclofen, a gamma-aminobutyric acid (GABA) B receptor agonist; tizanidine, an α_2 receptor agonist; and diazepam, a benzodiazepine that interacts with the GABA A receptor (103–106). Another medication, gabapentin, which is commonly used in the treatment of neuropathic pain after SCI, has also been shown to have some effect in treating spasticity after SCI and may be a good choice when treating both neuropathic pain and below-level muscular pain secondary to spasticity (107, 108). Opioids have also been shown to have antispasticity effects, especially when administered intrathecally. Both tricyclic antidepressants and SSRIs, drugs that often are prescribed for persons with SCI, may worsen spasticity, however (109, 110).

Below-Level Spinal Cord Pain

Below-level spinal cord pain or central pain is neuropathic pain that is perceived more than three dermatomes below the dermatome representing the neurologic level of injury and may or may not be perceived within the dermatome representing the neurologic level of injury and the three dermatomes below this level. Its distribution is generally not dermatomal but regional, enveloping large areas such as the anal region, the bladder, the genitals, the legs, or commonly the entire body below the neurologic level. The character is often described as "burning" or "aching," although other descriptors have included "pressure," "heaviness," "cold," "numbness," and "pins and needles" (1, 2, 6–8, 71). It is usually continuous in presence, although the intensity of the pain can fluctuate in response to a number of factors including psychologic stress, anxiety, fatigue, smoking, noxious stimuli below the level of injury, and weather changes (1, 2, 4, 5, 9, 111).

PATHOPHYSIOLOGY OF NEUROPATHIC PAIN AFTER SCI

The pathophysiology of pain thought to be due to damage to the spinal cord itself or to the nerve roots has not been well defined, although there has been significant progress recently in elucidating some of the underlying processes occurring at the spinal cord and root levels as well as the brain.

By definition, at-level and below-level spinal cord pain arises from injury to the spinal cord. In persons with SCI and pain presumed to be the result of damage to the spinal cord, abnormal spontaneous and evoked electrical activity has been recorded in both the superficial dorsal horn of the spinal cord and the somatosensory thalamus (112–114). This spontaneous activity differs in location and characteristics between persons with SCI with pain and without pain (115). For persons with SCI whose typical pain is experienced in a deafferented region (i.e., an area with altered or absent sensation), this same pain can be provoked by electrical stimulation of the ventrocaudal thalamic nucleus or rostral medial midbrain (116, 117).

Neuronal reorganization in the thalamus of persons with SCI and pain has been shown to occur with an increased somatotopic representation of the body regions at the level of injury or border zone areas (114). Multiple thalamic subregions have been demonstrated in animals to undergo change after SCI. In one study in animals, hypersensitivity of somato-visceral convergent neurons within the thalamus was demonstrated (118). This provides a potential mechanism where pain, which may be referred to at-level or above-level regions, can be triggered by noxious stimuli of pelvic and visceral origin, analogous to the situation in persons with SCI in whom pain is exacerbated by the presence of a distended bladder or an impacted rectum.

Action potential generation and propagation is dependent on voltage-gated sodium channels. Multiple isoforms of these channels have been isolated. One particular isoform, the $Na_V1.3$ sodium channel, is up-regulated in neurons after nerve injury. It has been shown that after SCI in animals, there are changes in sodium channel expression both within the dorsal horn of the spinal cord and within the thalamus (119, 120).

Other changes seen within the spinal cord of animals after SCI that are thought to contribute to neuronal hyperexcitability are changes in the expression of glutamate and s-hydroxytryptamine receptors (121, 122). A greater reduction of GABAergic inhibition within the spinal cord of animals after SCI with at-level evoked pain (allodynia) as compared to animals with SCI but without at-level evoked pain has been noted. Endogenous opioids also likely play a role in the development of evoked pain. When spinal opioid receptor antagonists are administered to spinally injured animals, evoked pain is generated in those animals that do not develop such behavior spontaneously (123).

Dysrhythmia, defined as a spontaneous firing of neurons in an oscillatory mode, has been demonstrated within the thalamus in animals with SCI both with and without evoked pain (124). However, in comparing animals with SCI alone with animals with SCI and evoked pain, those with evoked pain exhibit more frequent afterdischarges and evoked responses within both the spinal cord and thalamus. One theory explaining why some animals, and by extension some people, develop evoked pain (allodynia) and others do not is that, in those with evoked pain, there is exaggerated spinal input being processed by a dysrhythmic thalamus. In other words, there must be both abnormal discharges originating from the spinal cord in the case of spinal cord pain or from the periphery in the case of radicular pain, as well as a dysrhythmic thalamus that processes these ectoptic discharges. The initial effectiveness of a cordotomy or a spinal anesthetic block performed above a lesion may be attributed to blocking the peripheral or spinal ectoptic discharges, originating in the injured nerve roots or injured spinal cord caudal to the block or cordotomy, from reaching the thalamus. The lack of effect in some could relate to the establishment of abnormal

bursting within the thalamus, now independent of the peripheral or spinally originating ectoptic discharges.

In possible contrast to the mechanisms responsible for allodynia associated with spinal cord damage, sprouting may explain the allodynia that is common in the dermatomes innervated by the damaged roots. Normally, primary afferent Aβ (non-pain) fibers terminate in Rexed's lamina III and above and not in Rexed's laminas I and II of the dorsal horn, where primary afferent C fibers terminate. However, after peripheral nerve injury, primary afferent Aβ (non-pain) fibers may sprout to terminate in laminas I and II (125, 126). A second long-term adaptive mechanism which may be important in radicular pain occurring after prolonged noxious stimulation is phenotypic switching with regard to the synthesis of modulating neuropeptides by primary afferents. Primary afferent Aβ (non-pain) fibers have been shown to begin synthesizing substance P after receiving noxious stimulation for longer than 48 hours, thus functionally resembling primary afferent C fibers (127).

TREATMENT

Chronic pain is often defined as pain that persists beyond 6 months, an interval which surpasses the expected healing time for injuries in which healing is expected to occur. Chronic pain has been described as a disease entity in and of itself with different levels of pathology (128). In a model proposed by Siddall, three levels or components of pathology are described. The first is the damaged tissue that generates pain. The second is those pathophysiologic consequences induced in areas distant from the primary pathology by the persistent noxious stimuli. The third is those environmental factors, both internal such as depression or anxiety and external such as family-induced stress, which contribute to the presence of chronic pain. All of these components must be addressed in order to successfully treat chronic pain.

As is typical of any problem in medicine without an identified single effective treatment, there is a plethora of treatments that persons with pain after SCI utilize. In addition, because pain is a significant problem affecting all aspects of life, most individuals may be using a variety of treatments at the same time, or in succession, trying to find that combination of medications and other interventions that will reduce their pain. There are a few survey studies in the literature that document the percentage of subjects who are using or have used particular treatments, and their perceived benefit. These studies are summarized in Tables 38.2 and 38.3. It should be noted that all of these data come from questionnaires and that the types of pain being treated are not specified.

Pharmacologic Interventions

The available analgesics used to treat pain for which the primary pain generator is within the musculoskeletal system include primarily nonsteroidal anti-inflammatory drugs (NSAIDs) and opioids. The available analgesics used to treat pain for which the primary pain generator is the spinal cord or nerve roots specifically (i.e., neuropathic pain) include antidepressants, anticonvulsants, and opioids, among others (see Table 38.4). The published randomized controlled trials of the pharmacological treatment of neuropathic pain after SCI can be summarized as

Table 38.2 Pharmacologic Treatments of Chronic Pain after SCI: A Summary of Surveys

Lead Author	Warms Survey 1 (Ref. 178)		Warms Survey 2 (Ref. 178)		Widerstrom-Noga (Ref. 179)		Budh (Refs. 180–181)		Cardenas (Ref. 182)	
Total # of Subjects in Sample (all with SCI and pain of unspecified type)	308		163		120		90		117	
	% using	Mean "helpfulness" rating[c]	% using	Mean "helpfulness" rating[a]	% using	% "Considerably better" or "Pain-free"	% using	% reporting "rather good," "good"/"very good" effect	% using	Average relief[b]
Acetaminophen	58	2	53	2	18	18			70	4
Amitriptyline	26	2	21	2						
Anticonvulsants (unspecified)					18	24	12	NR		
Antidepressants (unspecified)					13	13	11	NR	41	3
Anti-spasticity meds					17	15				
Aspirin					9	9				
Baclofen	44	2	42	3					50	3
Carbamazepine	12	2	10	2					14	2
Clomipranine										
Diazepam	41	3	31	3						
Dilantin									13	3
Gabapentin	5	3	26	3						
Intrathecal infusion pump	3	4	5	4					38	3
Mexiletine	2	2	2	3					3	6
NSAIDS	66	2	55	2	20	21	16	NR		
NSAIDS/aspirin									71	4
Opioids	52	3	60	3	23	33	34	NR	58	6
Sedatives					15	22			39	5

NR = not reported
[c]Scale of 1–5 where 1 = "not at all helpful" and 5 = "extremely helpful."
[b]Scale of 0 (no relief) to 10 (complete relief)
Source: Compiled by Jeane Zanca, PhD, MPT.

Table 38.3 Nonpharmacologic Pain Treatments of Chronic Pain after SCI: A Summary of Surveys

Lead Author	Warms Survey 1 (Ref. 178)		Warms Survey 2 (Ref. 178)		Widerstrom-Noga (Ref. 179)		Budh (Refs. 180–181)		Cardenas (Ref. 182)	
Total # of subjects in sample (all with SCI and pain of unspecified type)	308		163		120		90		117	
	% using	Mean "helpfulness" rating[a]	% using	Mean "helpfulness" rating[a]	% using	% "Considerably better" or "Pain-free"	% using	% reporting "rather good," "good"/"very good" effect	% using	Average relief[b]
Acupressure	0 (n=1)	5	7	3						
Acupuncture	4	3	14	3			36	28	28	3
Biofeedback/relaxation	22	2	18	2					23	4
Chiropractic	1	4	2	4					27	5
Cold/Ice					13	NR	10	NR	43	3
Counseling/psychotherapy/ mental training	21	2	23	2	11	15	6	NR	21	3
Exercise/physical activity/ physical training (type unspecified)	2	4	3	5			4	100		
Exercise-range of motion									54	4
Exercise-strengthening									68	4
Heat					17	NR	24	77	57	4
Hypnosis	6	2	6	2					9	3
Magnets									17	2
Massage	6	4	38	3	27	NR	34	87	55	6
Nerve blocks	17	2	14	2					18	4
Physical therapy	67	3	68	3	33	50			64	4
TENS	3	3	23	2			32	28	35	3
Spinal cord stimulator	12	2	6	2						

NR = not reported.

[a]Scale of 1–5 where 1 = "not at all helpful" and 5 = "extremely helpful."

[b]Scale of 0 (no relief) to 10 (complete relief).

Source: Compiled by Jeane Zanca, PhD, MPT.

Table 38.4 Common Oral Medications Used to Treat Neuropathic Pain after SCI

Drug Class	Drug	Mechanism of Action	Type of Pain Typically Treated	Associated Symptoms That May Suggest Use	Drug Interactions	Adverse Effects[a]	Starting Dose	Comments
Local anesthetic	topical lidocaine 5% patch or other delivery vehicle	Blocks sodium channels	Evoked neuropathic and nociceptive pain	Dislikes or unable to tolerate oral medication	Possible systemic absorption and interaction with class 1 antiarrhythmics	Skin erythema, rash	1–3 patches for 12 out of 24 hours	Topical application to painful areas.
Tricyclic antidepressants	amitriptyline, nortriptyline, imipramine	Releases NE onto α₂ receptors in the dorsal horn. (123) Binds the NMDA-receptor complex[184]	Spontaneous neuropathic	Depressed mood, difficulty sleeping	Metabolized by CYP450 2D6	Cardiac conduction block, orthostatic hypotension, confusion, dry mouth, urinary retention, constipation	Start 25 mg before sleep	Use of secondary amine compound (e.g., desipramine and nortriptyline) in lieu of a more AC tertiary amine compound (e.g., amitriptyline, imipramine, and doxepine) may also improve tolerability. Contraindicated in persons who have significant cardiac conduction abnormalities.
Selective serotonin and norepinephrine reuptake inhibitor (SSNRI)	duloxetine	Potent inhibitor of neuronal serotonin and norepinephrine reuptake and a less potent inhibitor of dopamine reuptake	Spontaneous neuropathic	Depressed mood	Metabolized by CYP450 2D6 and 1A2	Nausea, dizziness, somnolence, fatigue, constipation, dry mouth, anorexia	30 mg daily for one week then increase to 60 mg	
SSNRI	venlafaxine	Potent inhibitor of neuronal serotonin and norepinephrine reuptake and weak inhibitor of dopamine reuptake	Spontaneous neuropathic	Depressed mood	Metabolized by CYP450 2D6 and 3A4	Hypertension, ataxia, insomnia, anxiety, anorexia, nausea	37.5 mg daily	
Anticonvulsant	topirimate	Blocks voltage-dependent sodium channels, augments the activity of GABA at some subtypes of the GABA-A receptor, antagonizes the AMPA/kainate subtype of the glutamate receptor, and inhibits the carbonic anhydrase enzyme, particularly isozymes II and IV	Spontaneous and evoked neuropathic	Seizures	Not extensively metabolized	Paresthesia, weight loss, somnolence, anorexia, dizziness, difficulty with memory, depression, insomnia, psychomotor slowing, dizziness, nausea, metabolic acidosis	25 mg twice per day	

continued on next page

Table 38.4 *(Continued)*

Drug Class	Drug	Mechanism of Action	Type of Pain Typically Treated	Associated Symptoms That May Suggest Use	Drug Interactions	Adverse Effects[a]	Starting Dose	Comments
Anticonvulsant	lamotrigine	Inhibits voltage-sensitive sodium channels	Spontaneous and evoked neuropathic	Seizures	Metabolized by glucuronic acid conjugation.	Stevens-Johnson syndrome, toxic epidermal necrolysis, angioedema	25 mg once daily	Discontinue at first sign of rash. Very slow titration.
Anticonvulsant	carbamazepine	Blocks sodium channels	Historically has been used for treatment of lancinating or shooting neuropathic pain (185–190)	Seizures	Metabolized by CYP450 3A4	Sedation, ataxia, rash, vertigo, blurred vision, nausea, vomiting, hepatic toxicity, aplastic anemia, agranulocytosis, Stevens-Johnson syndrome	100 mg twice a day	Monitor complete blood count and serum chemistry tests.
Anticonvulsant	oxcarbazepine	Blocks voltage-sensitive sodium channels; increases potassium conductance and modulates high voltage activated calcium channels	Similar to carbamazepine	Seizures	Can inhibit CYP450 2C19 and 3A4/5	Dizziness, diploplia, nausea, vomiting, somnolence, fatigue, hyponatremia, Stevens-Johnson syndrome, toxic epidermal necrolysis	150 mg twice per day	
Anticonvulsant	gabapentin	Limits high-frequency repetitive firing of sodium-dependent action potentials (191, 192); binds alpha-2-delta subunit of voltage-sensitive calcium channels (193, 194); decreases glutamate levels in brain (195); increases free plasma serotonin (196); and decreases release of serotonin, dopamine, and norepinephrine (191)	Continuous and paroxysmal spontaneous, as well as dynamic mechanical and cold allodynia evoked neuropathic pain (197)	Anxiety, seizures, difficulty sleeping	Negligible metabolic interactions; taking with protein may increase absorption of drug	Dizziness, sedation	100 mg 3–4 times per day	
Anticonvulsant	pregabalin	Binds to alpha-2-delta subunit of voltage-gated Ca channels and modulates influx of Ca ions into hyperexcited neurons, reducing release of neurotransmitters such as glutamate and substance P137	Spontaneous and evoked neuropathic	Anxiety, seizures, difficulty sleeping	Negligible metabolic interactions.	Somnolence, dizziness, edema, asthenia, dry mouth, constipation	50 mg twice a day	

Class	Drug	Mechanism	Indication	Metabolism	Adverse effects	Dosage	Comments
Opioid	methadone	μ receptor agonist (see morphine), N-methyl-D-aspartate (NMDA) receptor channel blocker (198)	Spontaneous and evoked neuropathic	Metabolized by CYP450 3A4 and 2B6; avoid prescribing with other drugs known to prolong the QT interval as has rarely been associated with torsade de pointes; grapefruit juice may increase levels; contraindicated with MAO inhibitors	Sedation,[b] constipation,[c] respiratory depression, nausea, confusion, cardiac conduction abnormalities	2.5–5 mg 3–4 times per day to start; may decrease dosing frequency over time	Equianalgesic oral dose 10 mg. Addiction risk.[d]
Opioid	fentanyl	(See morphine)	All	Metabolized by CYP450 3A4	Sedation,[b] constipation,[c] respiratory depression, nausea, confusion	25 mcg/hr; change patch every 2–3 days depending on response	Addiction risk.[d]
Opioid	tramadol	Binds μ-opioid receptors and weakly inhibits reuptake of norepinephrine and serotonin	All	Metabolized by CYP450 2D4; risk of serotonin syndrome with co-administration of SSRIs	Dizziness, sedation, constipation, nausea, headache, seizures	50 mg 3–4 times per day for short-acting formulation	Less physical dependence and abuse potential than other opioids in table. Caution should be observed if co-administered with selective serotonin reuptake inhibitors or tricyclic antidepressants.
Opioid	morphine	Binds μ-opioid receptors and thus inhibits primary afferent neurotransmitter release by suppression of voltage-sensitive calcium currents, and direct inhibition of dorsal horn neurons (199)	All	Metabolized by glucuronidation not P450 enzymes; UGT 2B7 and UGT 1A3 are the major enzymes involved	Sedation,[b] constipation,[c] respiratory depression, nausea, confusion	15 mg 3–4 times per day for short acting formulation; change to long-acting formulation if effective; Available for intrathecal use[e]	Equianalgesic oral dose 30 mg. Addiction risk.[d]
Opioid	oxycodone	(see morphine)	All	Metabolized by CYP450 2D6	Sedation,[b] constipation,[c] respiratory depression, nausea, confusion	10 mg 3–4 times per day for short-acting formulation; change to long-acting formulation if effective	Equianalgesic oral dose 20 mg. Addiction risk.[d]

Abbreviations used: NE = norepinephrine, AC = anticholinergic.

[a] With the exception of topical lidocaine, all drugs in this table can cause central nervous system (CNS) adverse effects. These adverse effects can be minimized by slow dose escalation.

[b] The addition of a stimulant medication, e.g., methylphenidate, as an adjunct is often helpful to maintain alertness.

[c] The addition of stimulant laxatives, bulking agents, and/or stool softeners is often necessary along with close monitoring for ileus in persons with SCI who may lack, depending on the completeness and the neurologic level of injury, the warning sensation of discomfort that accompanies constipation, normal bowel transit times, and voluntary bowel control.

[d] Due to addiction risk, opioids should be used in accordance with guidelines that have been developed for their use in persons with nonmalignant pain (see Table 38.5) (200, 201).

[e] If systemically administered opioids are not tolerated because of side effects, intrathecally administered opioids should be considered. Long-term intrathecal infusion of morphine administered by implanted drug pumps has been found to be safe; although granuloma formation at the catheter tip, which may progress to cause neural impingement, has been reported especially when higher concentrations of drug are used (202).

follows: Amitriptyline, a tricyclic antidepressant and norepinephrine reuptake inhibitor, has shown mixed efficacy in treating pain after SCI (110, 203). Trazodone, a selective serotonin reuptake inhibitor, has not been shown to be effective (129). The opioid alfentanil, given intravenously, has been found to be effective in one small study (130), and in another investigation, morphine given intravenously has been found to be effective in attenuating brushed evoked allodynia, but not spontaneous pain (29). In a study that evaluated the effect of intrathecal morphine, clonidine, and their combination on below-level and at-level neuropathic pain after SCI, only the combination was found to be effective (131). Intravenous lidocaine, a sodium channel blocker, has been found to be effective in treating at-level and below-level pain, irrespective of the presence or absence of evoked pain, and intrathecal lidocaine has also been shown to be effective (132, 133). However, the oral analogue to lidocaine, mexilitine, has not been shown to be effective (134). The atypical anticonvulsants topirimate and lamotrigine have not been found to be effective, whereas pregabalin and gabapentin have been found to be more effective than placebo in treating pain after SCI (30, 135–137). Although controlled studies seem to support the use of at least pregabalin and gabapentin, pharmacologic or other therapy remains unsatisfactory for many or most persons with pain after SCI. Intravenous administration is, of course, not an option for treatment of persons with SCI residing in the community who experience neuropathic pain, however severe. In clinical practice, because many of these medications are not efficacious in and of themselves, they are often used in combination. The combinations are chosen to target different mechanisms thought to be active in the transmission of the pain signals throughout the neuroaxis up to the cortex, where the pain is perceived. An algorithm for the pharmacologic treatment of at-level and below-level neuropathic pain related to SCI based upon differing mechanisms of action and the limited published evidence of drug efficacy is shown in Table 38.6.

During the treatment of the pain, the treating clinician should ensure that potentially correctable causes of the pain are not missed (e.g., ongoing nerve root compression due to bony fragments at the level of injury).

Nonpharmacologic/Nonpsychologic Interventions

Spinal stabilization with instrumentation and fusion is indicated for an unstable spine causing SCI at-level mechanical pain. Surgical decompression and stabilization is also indicated to relieve compression on nerve roots causing at-level radicular pain. Pain originating from a syrinx often will disappear with drainage of the syrinx, and SCI at-level nociceptive pain caused by spinal instrumentation often will be relieved by the removal of the offending instrumentation. There are few other instances where nonpharmacologic and nonpsychologic interventions are of proven benefit for chronic pain after SCI, except possibly the dorsal root entry zone (DREZ) procedure and cranial electrical stimulation, which are reviewed below. One reason for this lack of proven benefit may be the paucity of studies that have been performed; another may be the presence of multiple pain generators, which have arisen all along the neuroaxis, as described in the neurobiology section; with multiorigin pain, one single modality acting at a single locale is unlikely to be efficacious.

Table 38.5 Proposed Guidelines for the Management of Opioid Therapy in Persons with Intractable Spinal Cord Pain

1. Long-term opioid therapy should be considered only after reasonable analgesic modalities have failed.
2. Opioids should be viewed as a complementary therapy that might be combined with other analgesic and rehabilitative approaches.
3. A single practitioner should take responsibility for administration and monitoring of therapy.
4. A prior history of substance abuse, severe character pathology, or a chaotic social situation should be viewed as a relative contraindication to therapy.
5. Informed consent should be documented in the medical record. The consent discussion should include information about side effects (including the risk of additive side effects from other centrally acting drugs and the need to avoid driving and other potentially dangerous activities if cognitive impairment should occur), the small risk of addiction, and the need for clearly defined parameters for dosing.
6. "Around the clock" dosing with long-acting medication is preferred for the management of chronic pain, but "as needed" dosing may be considered in some patients with widely fluctuating pain.
7. Opioid dosing should be titrated until either satisfactory pain relief or undesirable opioid-induced side effects occur. Side effects should be managed and a trial with alternative opioids should be considered if dose-limiting side effects are a major problem in establishing a favorable treatment. If a dose cannot be stabilized at a level associated with benefits that clearly exceed disadvantages, therapy should be discontinued.
8. Following dose titration, the dose should be stabilized and not changed by the patient without prior consent of the physician. A monthly quantity of drug should be established. Some patients should be offered a defined smaller quantity to be used for transient exacerbation of the pain (so-called rescue doses).
9. Initially, patients should be evaluated at least monthly. Once dosing is stable, visits may be less frequent.
10. At each visit, the physician should assess the patient for (1) the degree of analgesia, (2) the occurrence of side effects, (3) functional status (physical and psychosocial), and (4) any evidence of aberrant drug-related behavior. This assessment should be clearly documented in the medical record.
11. Evidence of aberrant drug-related behavior, such as drug hoarding or uncontrolled dose escalation, should be carefully evaluated. The clinical response developed from the assessment should stop the behavior and appropriately manage the underlying cause. In rare cases, this may involve referral for formal treatment of an addiction disorder; more often, therapy must be adjusted and strict controls reestablished. Repeated episodes of aberrant drug-related behavior necessitate tapering and discontinuation of treatment.

Source: Slightly modified from Hegarty and Portenoy (1994) (201).

Table 38.6 An Algorithm for the Pharmacologic Treatment of At-Level and Below-Level Neuropathic Pain Related to SCI Based on Differing Mechanisms of Action and the Limited Published Evidence of Drug Efficacy

Correctable causes for each pain should be sought and addressed concurrently. Nonpharmacologic treatments should be used concurrently and environmental factors addressed as appropriate.

STEP NUMBER	SIMPLIFIED PRIMARY MECHANISM OF ACTION (PRESUMED ANATOMIC SITE OF ANALGESIC EFFECT)	SUGGESTED DRUGS OR DRUG CLASSES (SEE TABLE 38.4 FOR ADDITIONAL DRUG DETAILS)	COMMENTS
1 (Skip this step if pain is not of a superficial cutaneous evoked type).	Sodium channel blockade (root/peripheral nerve)	lidocaine patch	Apply to area of problematic evoked pain.
2	Voltage-gated Ca channel blockade (brain/spinal cord)	gabapentin pregabalin	
3 (Skip this step if pain is not paroxysmal and lancinating),	Sodium channel blockade (brain/spinal cord/root/ peripheral nerve)	carbazamepine oxcarbazepine	
4	Norepinephrine release for TCA (brain/spinal cord) Serotonin and norepinephrine reuptake inhibition for SSNRI (brain/spinal cord)	TCA SSNRI (see Table 38.5 for examples from each class)	If sedation is preferable, choose TCA; if sedation is to be avoided, choose SSNRI.
5	Opiate receptor agonist (brain/spinal cord)	Opioid (see Table 38.5 for examples)	Methadone is preferred due to additional mechanism of NMDA receptor blockade.

```
                          ┌──────────────┐
                          │  Start at    │
                          │  Step 1      │
                          └──────┬───────┘
                                 │
                                 ▼
             ┌─────────────▶ ╔══════════════╗ ◀─────────────┐
             │               ║ Titrate drug ║               │
             │               ║  to effect   ║               │
             │               ╚══════════════╝               │
  ┌──────────┴──────┐              │              ┌──────────┴──────┐
  │ Continue last   │              │              │ Stop last drug  │
  │ drug and add    │              │              │ added and       │
  │ drug from       │              │              │ add drug*       │
  │ the next step   │              ▼              │ from the same   │
  └──────────┬──────┘      ◇─────────────◇        │ or next step    │
             │             ╱  Level of   ╲        └──────────┬──────┘
             │            ╱  pain relief  ╲                  │
             └───────────◇    at 4-6       ◇─────────────────┘
  Partial but           ╲   weeks?**      ╱         None or
  not                    ╲               ╱          intolerable
  adequate                ◇─────────────◇           adverse
                                 │                  effects
                                 │ Adequate
                                 ▼
                          ┌──────────────┐
                          │  Stop at     │
                          │  this step   │
                          └──────────────┘
```

* If during any step, one of the available drugs is not effective or causes intolerable adverse effects, consider switching to another drug within the same step before continuing to the next step.
** The speed of adding medication with a different mechanism of action can be quicker than the algorithm suggests, i.e., adding a drug every 4–6 weeks, for pain which has not been long established, that is, pain that has not induced significant plastic changes within the nervous system, and for severe pain. A slower than indicated titration within a step may allow improved tolerability if this becomes an issue.

continued on next page

TABLE 38.6   *(Continued)*

Step Number	Simplified Primary Mechanism of Action (presumed anatomic site of analgesic effect)	Suggested Drugs or Drug Classes (see Table 38.4 for additional drug details)	Comments
6	NMDA receptor–mediated Ca channel blockade (brain/spinal cord)	dextromethorphan memantine methadone	
7	Sodium channel blockade (brain/spinal cord/root/ peripheral nerve)	TCA carbazamepine oxcarbazepine topiramate lamotrigine gabapentin lidocaine	If this step is reached and pain relief is not adequate and another drug in this step is considered, choose a drug with an additional different mechanism of action.

TCA = tricyclic antidepressant; SSNRI = selective serotonin and norepinephrine reuptake inhibitor.

Spinal Cord Stimulation

Spinal cord stimulation involves the percutaneous implantation and electrical activation of single or multiple channel electrodes within the epidural space over the dorsum of the spinal cord. It has not been found to be effective in treating spinal cord pain after SCI (138–143).

DREZ Ablation Procedures

The dorsal root entry zone (DREZ) has been defined as the proximal portion of a dorsal nerve root and its adjacent superficial layers of dorsal horn. Destruction of this area with either radiofrequency or laser coagulation, as first described by Nashold, has been shown to be somewhat effective in reducing SCI at-level radicular and spinal cord pain, but not SCI below-level spinal cord pain (112, 144–148). As conventionally performed, the coagulation is performed two levels above and one or two levels below the level of injury, causing an ascent of the sensory neurologic level by two segments. In a large series with persons with SCI at-level radicular or SCI at-level spinal cord pain treated with conventional DREZ lesioning, Friedman reported that twenty-three of thirty-one persons undergoing the procedure had good relief (defined as lack of pain or pain that did not require analgesics or interfere with daily activities). In a second large series, Rath reported that twelve of seventeen had fair or good relief (146, 148).

In 1993, Edgar reported a method of recording abnormal signals in the DREZ before selectively lesioning the areas with abnormal signals. He noted that forty-two of forty-six persons with spinal cord pain in his series, predominantly with SCI below-level spinal cord–type pain, treated with selective lesioning, had at least 50% relief (112). Falci reported in 1999 that nine of eleven persons with SCI below-level spinal cord pain treated with DREZ guided only by spontaneous intramedullary electrical recordings had at least 50% relief, whereas twenty-one of twenty-five persons with SCI below-level spinal cord pain treated with DREZ guided by intramedullary electrical recordings of both spontaneous and C fiber–evoked signals had 100% relief at 3 months to 5 years (149). These results contrast starkly with

what had been previously reported by other investigators using the conventional approach.

The DREZ procedure may have limited use in the treatment of intractable SCI at-level radicular or spinal cord pain as it has been conventionally performed and in the treatment of SCI below-level spinal cord pain if guided by intramedullary recordings, but it is not recommended currently, as it has been conventionally performed for the treatment SCI below-level spinal cord pain.

Motor Cortex and Deep Brain Stimulation

Motor cortex stimulation involves placement and electrical activation of an implanted subdural electrode grid over the motor cortex. It has been described for the treatment of various types of neuropathic pain in a limited number of uncontrolled studies (150–152). Only a few persons with pain after SCI have been treated with this technique, and the results have been mixed (150).

Deep brain stimulation involves placement and electrical activation of implantable electrodes within the somatosensory thalamus, which includes the ventroposterior lateral and ventroposterior medial nuclei; the caudal medial thalamic areas around the third ventricle including the periventricular gray matter (PVG) and adjacent nuclei, centralis medialis, and parafascicularis; and near the junction of the third ventricle and the sylvian aqueduct, the rostral ventral periaqueductal gray matter and caudal ventral PVG. This intervention has not been found to be effective for pain after SCI (153, 154).

Acupuncture

Acupuncture is a neurostimulatory technique in which small solid needles are inserted into the skin at varying depths, typically penetrating the underlying musculature (155). Meta-analyses evaluating its efficacy in multiple types of chronic pain have been inconclusive (156–159). In 2001 Dyson-Hudson reported the results of a prospective trial of the efficacy of ten sessions over 5 weeks of either acupuncture or Trager manual therapy in eighteen persons with SCI who used manual wheelchairs as their primary means of mobility. Subjects served as their own controls. Both groups had significant decreases in pain scores (160). In another prospective study of twenty-two persons with chronic pain after SCI, in which subjects served as their own controls, 46% of those treated had a significant improvement in pain, but 26% actually had worsened 3 months posttreatment (161). Acupuncture may be a useful adjunct for the treatment of certain types of pain after SCI.

Transcutaneous Electrical Stimulation

In 1975 Davis reported the results of the use of transcutaneous electrical stimulation (TENS) on thirty-one persons with various types of pain after SCI, including radicular, spinal cord, and pain "at the site of injury." Effectiveness, defined as a reduction in pain medication or continued use of the device, was noted only in those who had a component of the pain "at the site of injury," and not in those with radicular or spinal cord pain (162). Hachen reported the use of TENS in thirty-nine persons with a similar array of pain types, finding at 3 months slight or moderate pain relief for most of the persons with pain "at the site of vertebral trauma," almost complete relief for one-half of the persons who had radicular pain, and no effect for most of the persons with spinal cord pain (163). Thus, TENS may be a useful adjunct for persons with SCI at-level mechanical/musculoskeletal pain or radicular pain.

Cranial Electrical Stimulation

In 2006 Tan reported the results of a double-blinded placebo-controlled study where, for 21 days for 1 hour each day, a microcurrent was delivered via ear clip electrodes or not (sham) to the brain of thirty-eight individuals with SCI and chronic pain. The group that received the active treatment reported decreased pain and pain interference (164). In 2007 Fregni reported the results of a double-blinded placebo-controlled parallel group trial of five daily sessions of transcranial direct current stimulation for seventeen persons with spinal cord pain (central pain). A constant current of 2 mA was delivered to the scalp (C3 or C4 on the electroencephalogram 10/20 system) for 20 minutes on 5 consecutive days. There was a significant decrease in pain measured at the four last sessions and a trend toward a significant effect 16 days after the final session. Cognition and mood were not affected (165). Cranial electrical stimulation may be a useful adjunct for the treatment of pain after SCI.

Psychologic Interventions

The goal of cognitive-behavioral, relaxation, and hypnotic techniques for treating chronic pain after SCI is to teach the person with the pain to perform the techniques himself in order to manage his pain over the long term and minimize the impact of the pain on his life. These techniques are not brief interventions that will abolish pain. However, they are commonly thought to be integral to the effective management of chronic pain.

Clinical trials of psychologic interventions for pain after SCI are sparse in the literature. In 2006, Budh reported the results of a prospective parallel group trial in Sweden for persons with SCI and neuropathic pain, for which the intervention was education, behavioral therapy, relaxation, stretching, light exercise, and body awareness training. The interventions occurred during twenty sessions over 10 weeks. At 12 months, levels of anxiety and depression in the treatment group were decreased compared with baseline values; however, pain intensity, health-related quality of life, and life satisfaction did not change significantly (166).

Commonly employed psychologic interventions that have shown promise in other chronic pain conditions and are often used in clinical practice to treat pain after SCI are described below.

Education

Education of the person with pain about pain after SCI by addressing the purported cause of the pain and its meaning can and should be addressed by all treating clinicians. This is an important first step in treatment, which may have a significant effect on reducing pain-associated anxiety, selective attention to pain, and misattribution of the sources of pain (167).

Cognitive-Behavioral Therapy

Cognitive-behavioral therapy (CBT) promotes the self-management of pain. CBT aims to alter negative thoughts, attitudes, and emotions through education, skills acquisition, cognitive and behavioral rehearsals, and generalization (168). CBT emphasizes learning of self-regulation and control skills as well as learning how to take personal responsibility for lifestyle changes, especially as related to maladaptive beliefs about pain. Training in cognitive strategies is performed with a goal of replacing abnormal coping strategies such as catastrophizing and ruminating (169). For chronic pain of multiple etiologies, not necessarily related to SCI, CBT has been shown in a meta-analysis to be effective in changing pain experience, mood/affect, cognitive coping and appraisal (reduction of negative coping and increase in positive coping), and pain behavior and activity level when compared to waiting list control conditions (170). Other meta-analyses that evaluated CBT for chronic back pain also showed effectiveness in decreasing pain, changing mood, and changing behavior (171–173).

Relaxation

Relaxation techniques aim for nondirected relaxation, often achieved by repetitive focusing on a word, sound, prayer, phrase, sensation, or muscle activity to the exclusion of intruding thoughts (168). There are several different relaxation techniques, including: autogenic training, where a peaceful environment and comforting body sensations are imagined; meditation; progressive muscle relaxation; paced respiration, where persons are taught to maintain slow breathing during stressful periods; and deep breathing. There is strong evidence that relaxation techniques are able to reduce chronic pain from a variety of conditions (168). There have been uncontrolled studies showing their efficacy for pain after SCI (174, 175).

Hypnosis

Hypnotic techniques aim to induce states of selective attentional focusing or diffusion through three phases: a presuggestion phase, a suggestion phase, and a postsuggestion phase (168). In the presuggestion phase, subjects attentionally focus through imagery, distraction, or relaxation. In the suggestion phase, a specific strategy or suggestion is introduced to modify the pain experience; this may include time reorientation to a time when pain was of minor consideration; pain displacement from one area of the body to another less threatening area; replacement of painful sensations with more tolerable sensations; or a direct or indirect suggestion that the pain will no longer be experienced (176). The postsuggestion phase involves continuation of the new behavior following termination of hypnosis (168). There is strong evidence that hypnosis is effective in cancer pain and some evidence that it is effective for other chronic pain types as well (168, 176, 177).

CONCLUSIONS

The vast majority of pain after SCI generally falls into two categories: neuropathic pain due to spinal cord damage and nociceptive pain due to overuse.

Identification and treatment of the primary pain generators are the first steps toward eliminating these pains. The next steps are to identify and address those environmental factors, both internal and external, which contribute to the presence of the pain or may have even caused the pain to occur in the first place. Next, if addressing the primary pain generators and environmental factors is not completely successful, then it is important to address those pathophysiologic consequences induced in areas distant to the primary pathology due to the plasticity of the nervous system in the presence of persistent noxious stimuli.

Finally, use of a combination of pharmacologic interventions, perhaps using multiple drugs, each with different mechanisms of actions; nonpharmacologic and nonpsychologic interventions; and psychologic interventions is likely to be the most efficacious approach to the treatment of chronic pain after SCI, although this has yet to be proven.

References

1. Davis L, Martin J. Studies upon spinal cord injuries. II. The nature and treatment of pain. *J Neurosurg* 1947; 4:483–491.
2. Botterell EH, Callaghan JC, Jousse AT. Pain in paraplegia; clinical management and surgical treatment. *Proc R Soc Med* 1954; 47:281–288.
3. Burke DC. Pain in paraplegia. *Paraplegia* 1973; 10:297–313.
4. Nepomuceno C, Fine PR, Richards JS, et al. Pain in patients with spinal cord injury. *Arch Phys Med Rehabil* 1979; 60:605–609.
5. Richards JS, Meredith RL, Nepomuceno C, Fine PR, Bennett G. Psychosocial aspects of chronic pain in spinal cord injury. *Pain* 1980; 8:355–366.
6. Davidoff G, Roth E, Guarracini M, Sliwa J, Yarkony G. Function-limiting dysesthetic pain syndrome among traumatic spinal cord injury patients: a cross-sectional study. *Pain* 1987; 29:39–48.
7. Cairns DM, Adkins RH, Scott MD. Pain and depression in acute traumatic spinal cord injury: origins of chronic problematic pain? *Arch Phys Med Rehabil* 1996; 77:329–335.
8. Stormer S, Gerner HJ, Gruninger W, et al. Chronic pain/dysaesthesiae in spinal cord injury patients: results of a multicentre study. *Spinal Cord* 1997; 35:446–455.
9. Rintala DH, Loubser PG, Castro J, Hart KA, Fuhrer MJ. Chronic pain in a community-based sample of men with spinal cord injury: prevalence, severity, and relationship with impairment, disability, handicap, and subjective well-being. *Arch Phys Med Rehabil* 1998; 79:604–614.
10. Siddall PJ, Taylor DA, McClelland JM, Rutkowski SB, Cousins MJ. Pain report and the relationship of pain to physical factors in the first 6 months following spinal cord injury. *Pain* 1999; 81:187–197.
11. Cardenas DD, Bryce TN, Shem K, Richards JS, Elhefni H. Gender and minority differences in the pain experience of people with spinal cord injury. *Arch Phys Med Rehabil* 2004; 85:1774–1781.
12. Bryce TN, Ragnarsson KT. Epidemiology and classification of pain after spinal cord injury. *Top Spinal Cord Inj Rehabil* 2001; 7:1–17.
13. Rintala DH, Holmes SA, Fiess RN, Courtade D, Loubser PG. Prevalence and characteristics of chronic pain in veterans with spinal cord injury. *J Rehabil Res Dev* 2005; 42:573–584.
14. Barrett H, McClelland JM, Rutkowski SB, Siddall PJ. Pain characteristics in patients admitted to hospital with complications after spinal cord injury. *Arch Phys Med Rehabil* 2003; 84:789–795.
15. Siddall PJ, McClelland JM, Rutkowski SB, Cousins MJ. A longitudinal study of the prevalence and characteristics of pain in the first 5 years following spinal cord injury. *Pain* 2003; 103:249–257.
16. Michaelis LS. The problem of pain in paraplegia and tetraplegia. *Bull N Y Acad Med* 1970; 46:88–96.
17. Maury M. About pain and its treatment in paraplegics. *Paraplegia* 1978; 15:349–352.
18. Holmes G. Pain of central origin. *Contributions to Medical and Biological Research.* 1919; 1:235–246.
19. Riddoch G. The clinical features of central pain. *Lancet* 1938; 234:1150–1156.
20. Kaplan LI, Grynbaum BB, Lloyd KE, Rusk HA. Pain and spasticity in patients with spinal cord dysfunction: results of a follow-up study. *JAMA* 1962; 182:918–925.
21. Donovan WH, Dimitrijevic MR, Dahm L, Dimitrijevic M. Neurophysiological approaches to chronic pain following spinal cord injury. *Paraplegia* 1982; 20:135–146.
22. Siddall PJ, Taylor DA, Cousins MJ. Classification of pain following spinal cord injury. *Spinal Cord* 1997; 35:69–75.
23. Ragnarsson KT. Management of pain in persons with spinal cord injury. *J Spinal Cord Med* 1997; 20:186–199.
24. Bryce TN, Ragnarsson KT. Pain after spinal cord injury. *Phys Med Rehabil Clin N Am* 2000; 11:157–168.
25. Bryce TN, Dijkers MP, Ragnarsson KT, Stein AB, Chen B. Reliability of the Bryce/Ragnarsson spinal cord injury pain taxonomy. *J Spinal Cord Med* 2006; 29:118–132.
26. Marino RJ, Ditunno JF, Donovan WH, et al., eds. *International Standards for Neurological and Functional Classification of Spinal Cord Injury.* Chicago: American Spinal Injury Association, 2000.
27. Cardenas D. Current concepts of rehabilitation of spinal cord injury patients. *Spine State Art Rev* 1999; 13:575–585.
28. Cardenas DD, Turner JA, Warms CA, Marshall HM. Classification of chronic pain associated with spinal cord injuries. *Arch Phys Med Rehabil* 2002; 83:1708–1714.
29. Attal N, Guirimand F, Brasseur L, Gaude V, et al. Effects of IV morphine in central pain: a randomized placebo-controlled study. *Neurology* 2002; 58:554–563.
30. Finnerup NB, Sindrup SH, Bach FW, Johannesen IL, Jensen TS. Lamotrigine in spinal cord injury pain: a randomized controlled trial. *Pain* 2002; 96:375–383.
31. Poser CM, Paty DW, Scheinberg L, et al. New diagnostic criteria for multiple sclerosis: guidelines for research protocols. *Ann Neurol* 1983; 13:227–231.
32. Nichols PJ, Norman PA, Ennis JR. Wheelchair user's shoulder? Shoulder pain in patients with spinal cord lesions. *Scand J Rehabil Med* 1979; 11:29–32.
33. Dalyan M, Cardenas DD, Gerard B. Upper extremity pain after spinal cord injury. *Spinal Cord* 1999; 37:191–195.
34. Curtis KA, Drysdale GA, Lanza RD, Kolber M, et al. Shoulder pain in wheelchair users with tetraplegia and paraplegia. *Arch Phys Med Rehabil* 1999; 80:453–457.
35. Bayley JC, Cochran TP, Sledge CB. The weight-bearing shoulder: the impingement syndrome in paraplegics. *J Bone Joint Surg Am* 1987; 69:676–678.
36. Sie IH, Waters RL, Adkins RH, Gellman H. Upper extremity pain in the postrehabilitation spinal cord injured patient. *Arch Phys Med Rehabil* 1992; 73:44–48.
37. Gellman H, Sie I, Waters RL. Late complications of the weight-bearing upper extremity in the paraplegic patient. *Clin Orthop Relat Res* 1988; 233:132–135.
38. Burnham RS, May L, Nelson E, Steadward R, Reid DC. Shoulder pain in wheelchair athletes: the role of muscle imbalance. *Am J Sports Med* 1993; 21:238–242.
39. Mulroy S, Newsam C, Gronley J, Bontrager E. Impact of wheelchair propulsion biomechanics on development of shoulder pain in individuals with spinal cord injury. *Gait Posture* 2006; 24:S37–S38.
40. Goldstein B, Young J, Escobedo EM. Rotator cuff repairs in individuals with paraplegia. *Am J Phys Med Rehabil* 1997; 76:316–322.
41. Curtis KA, Tyner TM, Zachary L, et al. Effect of a standard exercise protocol on shoulder pain in long-term wheelchair users. *Spinal Cord* 1999; 37:421–429.

42. Forslund EB, Granstrom A, Levi R, Westgren N, Hirschfeld H. Transfer from table to wheelchair in men and women with spinal cord injury: coordination of body movement and arm forces. *Spinal Cord* 2007; 45:41–48.

43. van der Windt DA, van der Heijden GJ, Scholten RJ, Koes BW, Bouter LM. The efficacy of non-steroidal anti-inflammatory drugs (NSAIDS) for shoulder complaints: a systematic review. *J Clin Epidemiol* 1995; 48:691–704.

44. Goupille P, Sibilia J. Local corticosteroid injections in the treatment of rotator cuff tendinitis (except for frozen shoulder and calcific tendinitis). Groupe Rhumatologique Francais de l'Epaule (G.R.E.P.). *Clin Exp Rheumatol* 1996; 14:561–566.

45. Blair B, Rokito AS, Cuomo F, Jarolem K, Zuckerman JD. Efficacy of injections of corticosteroids for subacromial impingement syndrome. *J Bone Joint Surg Am* 1996; 78:1685–1689.

46. Robinson MD, Hussey RW, Ha CY. Surgical decompression of impingement in the weightbearing shoulder. *Arch Phys Med Rehabil* 1993; 74:324–327.

47. Garreau De Loubresse C, Norton MR, Piriou P, Walch G. Replacement arthroplasty in the weight-bearing shoulder of paraplegic patients. *J Shoulder Elbow Surg* 2004; 13:369–372.

48. Campbell CC, Koris MJ. Etiologies of shoulder pain in cervical spinal cord injury. *Clin Orthop Relat Res* 1996; 322:140–145.

49. Silfverskiold J, Waters RL. Shoulder pain and functional disability in spinal cord injury patients. *Clin Orthop Relat Res* 1991; 272:141–145.

50. Kewalramani LS. Autonomic dysreflexia in traumatic myelopathy. *Am J Phys Med* 1980; 59:1–21.

51. Pryor J. Autonomic hyper-reflexion. *N Engl J Med* 1971; 285:860.

52. Wayne EM, Vukov JG. Eye findings in autonomic hyperreflexia. *Ann Ophthalmol* 1977; 9:41–42.

53. Aljure J, Eltorai I, Bradley WE, Lin JE, Johnson B. Carpal tunnel syndrome in paraplegic patients. *Paraplegia* 1985; 23:182–186.

54. Gellman H, Chandler DR, Petrasek J, Sie I, et al. Carpal tunnel syndrome in paraplegic patients. *J Bone Joint Surg Am* 1988; 70:517–519.

55. Davidoff G, Werner R, Waring W. Compressive mononeuropathies of the upper extremity in chronic paraplegia. *Paraplegia* 1991; 29:17–24.

56. Gelberman RH, Hergenroeder PT, Hargens AR, Lundborg GN, Akeson WH. The carpal tunnel syndrome: a study of carpal canal pressures. *J Bone Joint Surg Am* 1981; 63:380–383.

57. Boninger ML, Impink BG, Cooper RA, Koontz AM. Relation between median and ulnar nerve function and wrist kinematics during wheelchair propulsion. *Arch Phys Med Rehabil* 2004; 85:1141–1145.

58. Boninger ML, Cooper RA, Baldwin MA, Shimada SD, Koontz A. Wheelchair pushrim kinetics: body weight and median nerve function. *Arch Phys Med Rehabil* 1999; 80:910–915.

59. Sie I, Waters R, Adkins R. Upper extremity disability due to lower extremity paralysis in paraplegia. *Current Orthopedics* 1991; 5:88–91.

60. Charney KJ, Juler GL, Comarr AE. General surgery problems in patients with spinal cord injuries. *Arch Surg* 1975; 110:1083–1088.

61. Miller LS, Staas WE, Herbison GJ. Abdominal problems in patients with spinal cord lesions. *Arch Phys Med Rehabil* 1975; 56:405–408.

62. Gore RM, Mintzer RA, Calenoff L. Gastrointestinal complications of spinal cord injury. *Spine* 1981; 6:538–544.

63. Juler GL, Eltorai IM. The acute abdomen in spinal cord injury patients. *Paraplegia* 1985; 23:118–123.

64. Sheridan R. Diagnosis of the acute abdomen in the neurologically stable spinal cord-injured patient: a case study. *J Clin Gastroenterol* 1992; 15:325–328.

65. Roth E. Pain in spinal cord injury. In: Yarkony G, ed. *Spinal Cord Injury: Medical Management and Rehabilitation*. Gaithersburg, MD: Aspen, 1994:141–158.

66. Moonka R, Stiens SA, Eubank WB, Stelzner M. The presentation of gallstones and results of biliary surgery in a spinal cord injured population. *Am J Surg* 1999; 178:246–250.

67. Ray B, Neill C. Abdominal visceral sensation in man. *Ann Surg* 1947; 126:709–724.

68. Tunks E. Pain in spinal cord injured patients. In: Bloch RF, Basbaum M, eds. *Management of Spinal Cord Injuries*. Baltimore: Williams and Wilkins, 1986:180–211.

69. Ingberg HO, Prust FW. The diagnosis of abdominal emergencies in patients with spinal cord lesions. *Arch Phys Med Rehabil* 1968; 49:343–348.

70. Hoen T, Cooper I. Acute abdominal emergencies in paraplegics. *Am J Surg* 1948; 75:19–24.

71. Burke D, Woodward J. Pain and phantom sensation in spinal paralysis. In: Vinken P, Bruyn G, eds. *Handbook of Clinical Neurology*. Amsterdam: North Holland, 1976:489–499.

72. Dreyfuss P, Tibiletti C, Dreyer SJ. Thoracic zygapophyseal joint pain patterns: a study in normal volunteers. *Spine* 1994; 19:807–811.

73. McCall IW, Park WM, O'Brien JP. Induced pain referral from posterior lumbar elements in normal subjects. *Spine* 1979; 4:441–446.

74. Fortin JD, Dwyer AP, West S, Pier J. Sacroiliac joint: pain referral maps upon applying a new injection/arthrography technique. Part I: asymptomatic volunteers. *Spine* 1994; 19:1475–1482.

75. Fortin JD, Aprill CN, Ponthieux B, Pier J. Sacroiliac joint: pain referral maps upon applying a new injection/arthrography technique. Part II: clinical evaluation. *Spine* 1994; 19:1483–1489.

76. van der Wurff P, Buijs EJ, Groen GJ. Intensity mapping of pain referral areas in sacroiliac joint pain patients. *J Manipulative Physiol Ther* 2006; 29:190–195.

77. Ohnmeiss DD, Vanharanta H, Ekholm J. Degree of disc disruption and lower extremity pain. *Spine* 1997; 22:1600–1605.

78. Zhou Y, Abdi S. Diagnosis and minimally invasive treatment of lumbar discogenic pain—a review of the literature. *Clin J Pain* 2006; 22:468–481.

79. Ohnmeiss DD, Vanharanta H, Ekholm J. Relation between pain location and disc pathology: a study of pain drawings and CT/discography. *Clin J Pain* 1999; 15:210–217.

80. Bryce TN, Dijkers M. Anatomic localization of 'at level' central pain after complete spinal cord injury. *J Spinal Cord Med* 2004; 27:190.

81. Barnett H, Jousse A. Syringomyelia as late sequel to traumatic paraplegia and quadriplegia: clinical features. In: Barnett H, ed. *Syringomyelia*. Philadelphia: Saunders, 1973:129–152.

82. Williams B, Terry AF, Jones F, McSweeney T. Syringomyelia as a sequel to traumatic paraplegia. *Paraplegia* 1981; 19:67–80.

83. Alcazaren E. Post-traumatic cystic myelopathy: a late neurologic complication of spinal cord injury. *Curr Concepts Rehabil Med* 1984; 1:15–24.

84. Rossier AB, Foo D, Shillito J, Dyro FM. Posttraumatic cervical syringomyelia: incidence, clinical presentation, electrophysiological studies, syrinx protein and results of conservative and operative treatment. *Brain* 1985; 108(Pt 2):439–461.

85. Schurch B, Wichmann W, Rossier AB. Post-traumatic syringomyelia (cystic myelopathy): a prospective study of 449 patients with spinal cord injury. *J Neurol Neurosurg Psychiatry* 1996; 60:61–67.

86. Nashold B. Paraplegia and pain. In: Ovelmen-Levitt J, ed. *Deafferentation Pain Syndromes: Pathophysiology and Treatment*. New York: Raven, 1991:301–319.

87. Tasker R, De Carvalho G. Central pain of spinal cord origin. In: North R, Levy R, eds. *Neurosurgical Management of Pain*. New York: Springer-Verlag, 1997:110–116.

88. Griffiths ER, McCormick CC. Post-traumatic syringomyelia (cystic myelopathy). *Paraplegia* 1981; 19:81–88.

89. el Masry WS, Biyani A. Incidence, management, and outcome of post-traumatic syringomyelia. In memory of Mr. Bernard Williams. *J Neurol Neurosurg Psychiatry* 1996; 60:141–146.

90. Lee TT, Alameda GJ, Gromelski EB, Green BA. Outcome after surgical treatment of progressive posttraumatic cystic myelopathy. *J Neurosurg* 2000; 92:149–154.

91. Frisbie JH, Aguilera EJ. Chronic pain after spinal cord injury: an expedient diagnostic approach. *Paraplegia* 1990; 28:460–465.

92. Falci SP, Lammertse DP, Best L, et al. Surgical treatment of posttraumatic cystic and tethered spinal cords. *J Spinal Cord Med* 1999; 22:173–181.

93. Stanton-Hicks M, Janig W, Hassenbusch S, Haddox JD, et al. Reflex sympathetic dystrophy: changing concepts and taxonomy. *Pain* 1995; 63:127–133.

94. Coderre TJ, Xanthos DN, Francis L, Bennett GJ. Chronic post-ischemia pain (CPIP): a novel animal model of complex regional pain syndrome-type I (CRPS-I; reflex sympathetic dystrophy) produced by prolonged hindpaw ischemia and reperfusion in the rat. *Pain* 2004; 112:94–105.

95. Ohry A, Brooks ME, Steinbach TV, Rozin R. Shoulder complications as a cause of delay in rehabilitation of spinal cord injured patients (case reports and review of the literature). *Paraplegia* 1978; 16:310–316.

96. Wainapel SF, Freed MM. Reflex sympathetic dystrophy in quadriplegia: case report. *Arch Phys Med Rehabil* 1984; 65:35–36.

97. Wainapel SF. Reflex sympathetic dystrophy following traumatic myelopathy. *Pain* 1984; 18:345–349.

98. Gellman H, Eckert RR, Botte MJ, Sakimura I, Waters RL. Reflex sympathetic dystrophy in cervical spinal cord injury patients. *Clin Orthop Relat Res* 1988; 233:126–131.

99. Cremer SA, Maynard F, Davidoff G. The reflex sympathetic dystrophy syndrome associated with traumatic myelopathy: report of 5 cases. *Pain* 1989; 37:187–192.

100. Philip PA, Philip M, Monga TN. Reflex sympathetic dystrophy in central cord syndrome: case report and review of the literature. *Paraplegia* 1990; 28:48–54.

101. Aisen PS, Aisen ML. Shoulder-hand syndrome in cervical spinal cord injury. *Paraplegia* 1994; 32:588–592.

102. Bengtson K. Physical modalities for complex regional pain syndrome. *Hand Clin* 1997; 13:443–454.

103. Duncan GW, Shahani BT, Young RR. An evaluation of baclofen treatment for certain symptoms in patients with spinal cord lesions: a double-blind, cross-over study. *Neurology* 1976; 26:441–446.

104. Roussan M, Terrence C, Fromm G. Baclofen versus diazepam for the treatment of spasticity and long-term follow-up of baclofen therapy. *Pharmatherapeutica* 1985; 4:278–284.

105. Neill RW. Diazepam in the relief of muscle spasm resulting from spinal-cord lesions. *Ann Phys Med* 1964; Suppl:33–38.

106. Nance PW, Bugaresti J, Shellenberger K, Sheremata W, Martinez-Arizala A. Efficacy and safety of tizanidine in the treatment of spasticity in patients with spinal cord injury. North American Tizanidine Study Group. *Neurology* 1994; 44:S44–51.

107. Gruenthal M, Mueller M, Olson WL, Priebe MM, et al. Gabapentin for the treatment of spasticity in patients with spinal cord injury. *Spinal Cord* 1997; 35:686–689.

108. Priebe MM, Sherwood AM, Graves DE, Mueller M, Olson WH. Effectiveness of gabapentin in controlling spasticity: a quantitative study. *Spinal Cord* 1997; 35:171–175.

109. Stolp-Smith KA, Wainberg MC. Antidepressant exacerbation of spasticity. *Arch Phys Med Rehabil* 1999; 80:339–342.

110. Cardenas DD, Warms CA, Turner JA, Marshall H, et al. Efficacy of amitriptyline for relief of pain in spinal cord injury: results of a randomized controlled trial. *Pain* 2002; 96:365–373.

111. Summers JD, Rapoff MA, Varghese G, Porter K, Palmer RE. Psychosocial factors in chronic spinal cord injury pain. *Pain* 1991; 47:183–189.

112. Edgar RE, Best LG, Quail PA, Obert AD. Computer-assisted DREZ microcoagulation: posttraumatic spinal deafferentation pain. *J Spinal Disord* 1993; 6:48–56.

113. Lenz FA, Tasker RR, Dostrovsky JO, et al. Abnormal single-unit activity recorded in the somatosensory thalamus of a quadriplegic patient with central pain. *Pain* 1987; 31:225–236.

114. Lenz FA, Kwan HC, Martin R, Tasker R, et al. Characteristics of somatotopic organization and spontaneous neuronal activity in the region of the thalamic principal sensory nucleus in patients with spinal cord transection. *J Neurophysiol* 1994; 72:1570–1587.

115. Hirayama T, Dostrovsky JO, Gorecki J, Tasker RR, Lenz FA. Recordings of abnormal activity in patients with deafferentation and central pain. *Stereotact Funct Neurosurg* 1989; 52:120–126.

116. Tasker RR, Gorecki J, Lenz FA, Hirayama T, Dostrovsky JO. Thalamic microelectrode recording and microstimulation in central and deafferentation pain. *Appl Neurophysiol* 1987; 50:414–417.

117. Lenz FA, Gracely RH, Baker FH, Richardson RT, Dougherty PM. Reorganization of sensory modalities evoked by microstimulation in region of the thalamic principal sensory nucleus in patients with pain due to nervous system injury. *J Comp Neurol* 1998; 399:125–138.

118. Hubscher CH, Johnson RD. Chronic spinal cord injury induced changes in the responses of thalamic neurons. *Exp Neurol* 2006; 197:177–188.

119. Hains BC, Saab CY, Waxman SG. Changes in electrophysiological properties and sodium channel Nav1.3 expression in thalamic neurons after spinal cord injury. *Brain* 2005; 128:2359–2371.

120. Waxman SG. Neurobiology: a channel sets the gain on pain. *Nature* 2006; 444:831–832.

121. Mills CD, Hulsebosch CE. Increased expression of metabotropic glutamate receptor subtype 1 on spinothalamic tract neurons following spinal cord injury in the rat. *Neurosci Lett* 2002; 319:59–62.

122. Hains BC, Willis WD, Hulsebosch CE. Serotonin receptors 5-HT1A and 5-HT3 reduce hyperexcitability of dorsal horn neurons after chronic spinal cord hemisection injury in rat. *Exp Brain Res* 2003; 149:174–186.

123. Hao JX, Yu W, Xu XJ. Evidence that spinal endogenous opioidergic systems control the expression of chronic pain-related behaviors in spinally injured rats. *Exp Brain Res* 1998; 118:259–268.

124. Gerke MB, Duggan AW, Xu L, Siddall PJ. Thalamic neuronal activity in rats with mechanical allodynia following contusive spinal cord injury. *Neuroscience* 2003; 117:715–722.

125. Woolf CJ, Shortland P, Coggeshall RE. Peripheral nerve injury triggers central sprouting of myelinated afferents. *Nature* 1992; 355:75–78.

126. Lekan HA, Carlton SM, Coggeshall RE. Sprouting of A beta fibers into lamina II of the rat dorsal horn in peripheral neuropathy. *Neurosci Lett* 1996; 208:147–150.

127. Neumann S, Doubell TP, Leslie T, Woolf CJ. Inflammatory pain hypersensitivity mediated by phenotypic switch in myelinated primary sensory neurons. *Nature* 1996; 384:360–364.

128. Siddall PJ, Cousins MJ. Persistent pain as a disease entity: implications for clinical management. *Anesth Analg* 2004; 99:510–20.

129. Davidoff G, Guarracini M, Roth E, Sliwa J, Yarkony G. Trazodone hydrochloride in the treatment of dysesthetic pain in traumatic myelopathy: a randomized, double-blind, placebo-controlled study. *Pain* 1987; 29:151–161.

130. Eide PK, Stubhaug A, Stenehjem AE. Central dysesthesia pain after traumatic spinal cord injury is dependent on N-methyl-D-aspartate receptor activation. *Neurosurgery* 1995; 37:1080–1087.

131. Siddall PJ, Molloy AR, Walker S, Mather LE, et al. The efficacy of intrathecal morphine and clonidine in the treatment of pain after spinal cord injury. *Anesth Analg* 2000; 91:1493–1498.

132. Finnerup NB, Biering-Sorensen F, Johannesen IL, et al. Intravenous lidocaine relieves spinal cord injury pain: a randomized controlled trial. *Anesthesiology* 2005; 102:1023–1030.

133. Loubser PG, Donovan WH. Diagnostic spinal anaesthesia in chronic spinal cord injury pain. *Paraplegia* 1991; 29:25–36.

134. Chiou-Tan FY, Tuel SM, Johnson JC, Priebe MM, et al. Effect of mexiletine on spinal cord injury dysesthetic pain. *Am J Phys Med Rehabil* 1996; 75:84–87.

135. Harden RN, Brenman E, Saltz S, Houle TT. Topiramate in the management of spinal cord injury pain: a double-blind, randomized, placebo-controlled pilot study. In: Yezierski RP, Burchiel KJ, eds. *Spinal Cord Injury Pain: Assessment, Mechanisms, Management. Progress in Pain Research and Management, Vol. 23.* Seattle: IASP Press, 2002:393–407.

136. Levendoglu F, Ogun CO, Ozerbil O, Ogun TC, Ugurlu H. Gabapentin is a first line drug for the treatment of neuropathic pain in spinal cord injury. *Spine* 2004; 29:743–751.

137. Siddall PJ, Cousins MJ, Otte A, Griesing T, et al. Pregabalin in central neuropathic pain associated with spinal cord injury: a placebo-controlled trial. *Neurology* 2006; 67:1792–1800.

138. Richardson RR, Meyer PR, Cerullo LJ. Neurostimulation in the modulation of intractable paraplegic and traumatic neuroma pains. *Pain* 1980; 8:75–84.

139. North RB, Ewend MG, Lawton MT, Piantadosi S. Spinal cord stimulation for chronic, intractable pain: superiority of "multi-channel" devices. *Pain* 1991; 44:119–130.

140. Cole J, Illis L, Sedgwick E. Intractable pain in spinal cord injury is not relieved by spinal cord stimulation. *Paraplegia* 1991; 29:167–172.

141. Kumar K, Nath R, Wyant GM. Treatment of chronic pain by epidural spinal cord stimulation: a 10-year experience. *J Neurosurg* 1991; 75:402–407.

142. Cioni B, Meglio M, Pentimalli L, Visocchi M. Spinal cord stimulation in the treatment of paraplegic pain. *J Neurosurg* 1995; 82:35–39.

143. ten Vaarwerk IA, Staal MJ. Spinal cord stimulation in chronic pain syndromes. *Spinal Cord* 1998; 36:671–682.

144. Nashold BS, Ostdahl RH. Dorsal root entry zone lesions for pain relief. *J Neurosurg* 1979; 51:59–69.

145. Nashold BS, Bullitt E. Dorsal root entry zone lesions to control central pain in paraplegics. *J Neurosurg* 1981; 55:414–419.

146. Friedman AH, Nashold BS. DREZ lesions for relief of pain related to spinal cord injury. *J Neurosurg* 1986; 65:465–469.

147. Young RF. Clinical experience with radiofrequency and laser DREZ lesions. *J Neurosurg* 1990; 72:715–720.

148. Rath SA, Seitz K, Soliman N, Kahamba JF, et al. DREZ coagulations for deafferentation pain related to spinal and peripheral nerve lesions: indication and results of 79 consecutive procedures. *Stereotact Funct Neurosurg* 1997; 68:161–167.

149. Falci S, Best L, Lammertse D, Starnes C. Surgical treatment of spinal cord injury (SCI) pain using a new technique of intramedullary electrical analysis. *J Spinal Cord Med* 1999; 22.

150. Nguyen JP, Lefaucheur JP, Decq P, et al. Chronic motor cortex stimulation in the treatment of central and neuropathic pain: correlations between clinical, electrophysiological and anatomical data. *Pain* 1999; 82:245–251.

151. Carroll D, Joint C, Maartens N, Shlugman D, et al. Motor cortex stimulation for chronic neuropathic pain: a preliminary study of 10 cases. *Pain* 2000; 84:431–437.

152. Saitoh Y, Shibata M, Hirano S, Hirata M, et al. Motor cortex stimulation for central and peripheral deafferentation pain: report of eight cases. *J Neurosurg* 2000; 92:150–155.

153. Levy RM, Lamb S, Adams JE. Treatment of chronic pain by deep brain stimulation: long term follow-up and review of the literature. *Neurosurgery* 1987; 21:885–893.

154. Duncan GH, Bushnell MC, Marchand S. Deep brain stimulation: a review of basic research and clinical studies. *Pain* 1991; 45:49–59.

155. Jacox A, Carr D, Payne R. *Management of Cancer Pain: Clinical Practice Guideline No. 9*. Rockville, MD: Agency for Health Care Policy and Research, U.S. Department of Health and Human Services, Public Health Service, 1994.

156. Patel M, Gutzwiller F, Paccaud F, Marazzi A. A meta-analysis of acupuncture for chronic pain. *Int J Epidemiol* 1989; 18:900–906.

157. ter Riet G, Kleijnen J, Knipschild P. Acupuncture and chronic pain: a criteria-based meta-analysis. *J Clin Epidemiol* 1990; 43:1191–1199.

158. Ernst E, White AR. Acupuncture for back pain: a meta-analysis of randomized controlled trials. *Arch Intern Med* 1998; 158:2235–2241.

159. van Tulder MW, Cherkin DC, Berman B, Lao L, Koes BW. The effectiveness of acupuncture in the management of acute and chronic low back pain: a systematic review within the framework of the Cochrane Collaboration Back Review Group. *Spine* 1999; 24:1113–1123.

160. Dyson-Hudson TA, Shiflett SC, Kirshblum SC, Bowen JE, Druin EL. Acupuncture and Trager psychophysical integration in the treatment of wheelchair user's shoulder pain in individuals with spinal cord injury. *Arch Phys Med Rehabil* 2001; 82:1038–1046.

161. Nayak S, Shiflett SC, Schoenberger NE, et al. Is acupuncture effective in treating chronic pain after spinal cord injury? *Arch Phys Med Rehabil* 2001; 82:1578–1586.

162. Davis R, Lentini R. Transcutaneous nerve stimulation for treatment of pain in patients with spinal cord injury. *Surg Neurol* 1975; 4:100–101.

163. Hachen HJ. Psychological, neurophysiological and therapeutic aspects of chronic pain: preliminary results with transcutaneous electrical stimulation. *Paraplegia* 1978; 15:353–367.

164. Tan G, Rintala DH, Thornby JI, Yang J, et al. Using cranial electrotherapy stimulation to treat pain associated with spinal cord injury. *J Rehabil Res Dev* 2006; 43:461–474.

165. Fregni F, Boggio PS, Lima MC, et al. A sham-controlled, phase II trial of transcranial direct current stimulation for the treatment of central pain in traumatic spinal cord injury. *Pain* 2006; 122:197–209.

166. Norrbrink Budh C, Kowalski J, Lundeberg T. A comprehensive pain management programme comprising educational, cognitive and behavioural interventions for neuropathic pain following spinal cord injury. *J Rehabil Med* 2006; 38:172–180.

167. Mittenberg W, Tremont G, Zielinski RE, Fichera S, Rayls KR. Cognitive-behavioral prevention of postconcussion syndrome. *Arch Clin Neuropsychol* 1996; 11:139–145.

168. Integration of behavioral and relaxation approaches into the treatment of chronic pain and insomnia. NIH technology assessment panel on integration of behavioral and relaxation approaches into the treatment of chronic pain and insomnia. *JAMA* 1996; 276:313–318.

169. Turk DC. Understanding pain sufferers: the role of cognitive processes. *Spine J* 2004; 4:1–7.

170. Morley S, Eccleston C, Williams A. Systematic review and meta-analysis of randomized controlled trials of cognitive behaviour therapy and behaviour therapy for chronic pain in adults, excluding headache. *Pain* 1999; 80:1–13.

171. Flor H, Fydrich T, Turk DC. Efficacy of multidisciplinary pain treatment centers: a meta-analytic review. *Pain* 1992; 49:221–230.

172. Turner JA. Educational and behavioral interventions for back pain in primary care. *Spine* 1996; 21:2851–2857.

173. McCracken LM, Turk DC. Behavioral and cognitive-behavioral treatment for chronic pain: outcome, predictors of outcome, and treatment process. *Spine* 2002; 27:2564–2573.

174. Grzesiak RC. Relaxation techniques in treatment of chronic pain. *Arch Phys Med Rehabil* 1977; 58:270–272.

175. Mariauzouls C, Michel D, Schiftan Y. Vibrationsgestützte musiktherapie reduziert schmerz und fördert entspannung bei para- und tetraplegikern. eine pilotstudie zur psychischen und vegetativen wirkung von simultaner akustischer und somatosensorischer musik-stimulation als schmerztherapie [Vibration-assisted music therapy reduces pain and promotes relaxation of para- and tetraplegic patients: a pilot study of psychiatric and physical effects of simultaneous acoustic and somatosensory music stimulation as pain management]. *Rehabilitation (Stuttg)* 1999; 38:245–248.

176. Gaupp L, Flinn D, Weddige R. Adjunctive treatment techniques. In: Tollison C, Satterthwaite J, Tollison J, eds. *Handbook of Pain Management*. Baltimore, MD: Williams and Wilkins, 1994:108–135.

177. Montgomery GH, DuHamel KN, Redd WH. A meta-analysis of hypnotically induced analgesia: how effective is hypnosis? *Int J Clin Exp Hypn* 2000; 48:138–153.

178. Warms CA, Turner JA, Marshall HM, Cardenas DD. Treatments for chronic pain associated with spinal cord injuries: many are tried, few are helpful. *Clin J Pain* 2002; 18:154–163.

179. Widerstrom-Noga EG, Turk DC. Types and effectiveness of treatments used by people with chronic pain associated with spinal cord injuries: influence of pain and psychosocial characteristics. *Spinal Cord* 2003; 41:600–609.

180. Norrbrink Budh C, Lundeberg T. Use of analgesic drugs in individuals with spinal cord injury. *J Rehabil Med* 2005; 37:87–94.

181. Norrbrink Budh C, Lundeberg T. Non-pharmacological pain-relieving therapies in individuals with spinal cord injury: a patient perspective. *Complement Ther Med* 2004; 12:189–197.

182. Cardenas DD, Jensen MP. Treatments for chronic pain in persons with spinal cord injury: a survey study. *J Spinal Cord Med* 2006; 29:109–117.

183. Millan M. The role of descending noradrenergic and serotoninergic pathways in the modulation of nociception: focus on receptor multiplicity. In: Dickerson A, Besson J, eds. *Pharmacology of Pain. (Handbook of Experimental Pharmacology: Vol 130)*. Germany: Springer-Verlag, 1997:385–446.

184. Boireau A, Bordier F, Durand G, Doble A. The antidepressant metapramine is a low-affinity antagonist at N-methyl-D-aspartic acid receptors. *Neuropharmacology* 1996; 35:1703–1707.

185. Campbell FG, Graham JG, Zilkha KJ. Clinical trial of carbazepine (tegretol) in trigeminal neuralgia. *J Neurol Neurosurg Psychiatry* 1966; 29:265–267.

186. Rockliff BW, Davis EH. Controlled sequential trials of carbamazepine in trigeminal neuralgia. *Arch Neurol* 1966; 15:129–136.

187. Killian JM, Fromm GH. Carbamazepine in the treatment of neuralgia: use of side effects. *Arch Neurol* 1968; 19:129–136.

188. Nicol CF. A four year double-blind study of tegretol in facial pain. *Headache* 1969; 9:54–57.

189. Swerdlow M, Cundill JG. Anticonvulsant drugs used in the treatment of lancinating pain: a comparison. *Anaesthesia* 1981; 36:1129–1132.

190. McQuay H, Carroll D, Jadad AR, Wiffen P, Moore A. Anticonvulsant drugs for management of pain: a systematic review. *BMJ* 1995; 311:1047–1052.

191. McLean MJ. Gabapentin in the management of convulsive disorders. *Epilepsia* 1999; 40(Suppl 6):S39–S50.

192. Wamil AW, McLean MJ. Limitation by gabapentin of high frequency action potential firing by mouse central neurons in cell culture. *Epilepsy Res* 1994; 17:1–11.

193. Suman-Chauhan N, Webdale L, Hill DR, Woodruff GN. Characterisation of [3H]gabapentin binding to a novel site in rat brain: homogenate binding studies. *Eur J Pharmacol* 1993; 244:293–301.

194. Gee NS, Brown JP, Dissanayake VU, Offord J, et al. The novel anticonvulsant drug, gabapentin (neurontin), binds to the alpha2delta subunit of a calcium channel. *J Biol Chem* 1996; 271:5768–5776.

195. Stewart BH, Kugler AR, Thompson PR, Bockbrader HN. A saturable transport mechanism in the intestinal absorption of gabapentin is the underlying cause of the lack of proportionality between increasing dose and drug levels in plasma. *Pharm Res* 1993; 10:276–281.

196. Rao ML, Clarenbach P, Vahlensieck M, Kratzschmar S. Gabapentin augments whole blood serotonin in healthy young men. *J Neural Transm* 1988; 73:129–134.

197. Attal N, Brasseur L, Parker F, Chauvin M, Bouhassira D. Effects of gabapentin on the different components of peripheral and central neuropathic pain syndromes: a pilot study. *Eur Neurol* 1998; 40:191–200.

198. Gorman AL, Elliott KJ, Inturrisi CE. The d- and l-isomers of methadone bind to the non-competitive site on the N-methyl-D-aspartate (NMDA) receptor in rat forebrain and spinal cord. *Neurosci Lett* 1997; 223:5–8.

199. Dougherty PM, Staats PS. Intrathecal drug therapy for chronic pain: from basic science to clinical practice. *Anesthesiology* 1999; 91:1891–1918.

200. Portenoy RK, Sciberras A, Eliot L, Loewen G, et al. Steady-state pharmacokinetic comparison of a new, extended-release, once-daily morphine formulation, avinza, and a twice-daily controlled-release morphine formulation in patients with chronic moderate-to-severe pain. *J Pain Symptom Manage* 2002; 23:292–300.

201. Hegarty A, Portenoy RK. Pharmacotherapy of neuropathic pain. *Semin Neurol* 1994; 14:213–224.

202. Hassenbusch SJ, Portenoy RK, Cousins M, et al. Polyanalgesic consensus conference 2003: an update on the management of pain by intraspinal drug delivery—report of an expert panel. *J Pain Symptom Manage* 2004; 27:540–563.

203. Rintala DH, Holmes SA, Courtade D, et al. Comparison of the effectiveness of amitriptyline and gabapentin on chronic neuropathic pain in persons with spinal cord injury. *Arch Phys Med Rehabil* 2007; 88:1547–1560.

39 New Advances in the Surgical Treatment of Nontraumatic Myelopathies

Stacey Quintero-Wolfe
Michael Y. Wang
Glen Manzano
Barth A. Green

Although trauma is a dramatic and devastating cause of spinal cord injury (SCI), nontraumatic myelopathies remain an important cause of spinal cord disease and dysfunction. Although the incidence of nontraumatic myelopathy has not been well studied, Mckinley et al. reported 39% of all spinal cord injuries admitted to a regional SCI inpatient rehabilitation center to be nontraumatic in nature (Figure 39.1) (1).

There are numerous causes of nontraumatic myelopathy, the most common of which is degenerative spondylosis with canal stenosis. However, neoplastic lesions, vascular anomalies, inflammatory arthropathies, infectious processes, and congenital disorders may all cause spinal cord injury and be amenable to surgical treatment.

The basic tenets of surgical management for treating these patients include (1) spinal cord decompression and vertebral column stabilization, (2) maintenance of normal vascular perfusion of the neural tissues, and (3) safe removal of offending or compressive intradural pathologies.

Over the last two decades, significant technological advances have occurred that have altered the surgical management of these pathologies. These advances have improved the safety and efficacy of neurosurgical endeavors to prevent or treat paralysis in the operating theatre.

ADVANCES IN THE NEUROSURGICAL OPERATING ROOM

Neuromonitoring

Intraoperative electromyography (EMG), somatosensory evoked potentials (SSEP), and motor-evoked potentials (MEP) are of integral importance in the surgical management of myelopathy. Evoked potentials record the electrical signals produced after stimulation of specific neural tracts, thereby demonstrating the integrity of those pathways. SSEP measures the time in milliseconds for a distal stimulation (median, ulnar, common peroneal, and posterior tibial nerves) to reach the contralateral parietal sensory cortex through the dorsal columns. MEP measures the time from stimulation of the motor cortex to peripheral muscles through the corticospinal tract, and may be an earlier predictor of impending spinal cord damage than SSEP (2). A prolonged latency or decreased amplitude of the SSEP or MEP thus suggests impairment of the dorsal column or corticospinal tracts. EMG allows for motor monitoring of individual nerve roots, which can be useful when treating lumbar disorders at the cauda equina level.

For the neurological surgeon, neuromonitoring provides intraoperative feedback regarding the integrity of the spinal cord tracts. Should there be dampening of the amplitude or prolongation of latency, the surgeon can reevaluate the clinical situation. For example, this feedback can alert the surgeon that the degree of spinal cord manipulation has been excessive or that the blood pressure is inadequate. Neuromonitoring also allows the surgeon to monitor the brachial and lumbosacral plexus and adjust patient positioning to prevent compressive neuropathies, identify inadvertent hypotension, and evaluate the depth of anesthesia (as the anesthetic lightens, spontaneous movement is usually noted in the hand intrinsics). The continuous evaluation of neural functioning in the asleep patient thus enhances patient safety and assists in intraoperative decision making.

Contemporary Neuroanesthesia

The goals of anesthesia for myelopathy surgery should include maintenance of cord perfusion and oxygenation, and balanced anesthesia that allows for neuromonitoring and maintenance of normoglycemia. Maintenance of perfusion and oxygenation is of utmost importance when operating for myelopathy, as the neural tissues are already in a state of compromise. Adequate cardiac output and a mean arterial blood pressure of 70 mmHg or greater

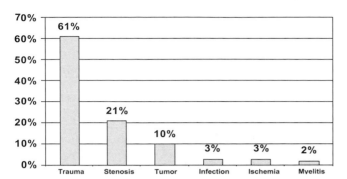

Figure 39.1 Etiology of spinal cord injury. (Adapted from Mckinley et al., *Arch Phys Med Rehabil,* 1999 [1].)

has been shown to prevent secondary injury to the spinal cord (3). Fluid administration to maintain adequate intravascular volume, reduction of anesthetic depth, and discontinuation of all myocardial depressant anesthetic agents should be augmented with administration of inotropic agents with beta-agonist activity, such as dopamine and dobutamine (2). Alpha-adrenergic agents, such as phenylephrine, increase systemic vascular resistance and blood pressure at the expense of increased afterload and reduced cardiac output (2). Spinal shock is uncommon in nontraumatic myelopathy but must always be entertained and urgently treated in the setting of cervical surgery and a sudden decrease in blood pressure.

Anesthesia should be given with consideration to neuromonitoring. Inhalational halogenated agents (desflurane, enflurane, halothane, isoflurane, sevoflurane) produce a dose-related decrease in evoked potentials when greater than 0.5 minimum in alveolar concentration (MAC) (4), so a balanced mix of nitrous oxide, narcotics, and propofol should be used. SSEPs may also be affected by hypotension and hypothermia. Should paralytics be needed at surgery onset, only short-acting nondepolarizing agents should be employed, and succinylcholine should generally be avoided in severe, cervical myelopathy, as there exists a risk of hyperkalemia related to the proliferation of extrajunctional myoneural receptors and abnormal muscle cell membrane responses (5).

Intraoperative glucose control is also important, as raised plasma glucose levels can adversely affect neurologic outcomes (6). This is most likely due to anaerobic glucose metabolism that occurs in ischemic neuronal tissue with resultant acidosis, again stressing the importance of cord perfusion and oxygenation.

Finally, in patients with severe cervical stenosis, compression, and/or instability, great care must be taken during intubation. For such patients, we use fiberoptic intubation with in-line traction held by the surgeon to prevent neurologic deterioration. Likewise, care must be taken when positioning these patients in the prone position. We place them in skeletal fixation with a head clamp, which is controlled at all times by the surgeon as positioning occurs.

Pharmacologic Agents

There is much controversy over the use of steroids for spinal cord injury following the National Acute Spinal Cord Injury Studies (NASCIS). Although NASCIS I (7) showed no benefit to the use of steroids, the dose was felt to be inadequate, and in the

follow-up studies, NASCIS II (8) and III (9) demonstrated mild neurologic improvement with methylprednisolone. These analyses, however, were made using subgroups of the study populations; functional recovery was not clinically significant (10). Additionally, high-dose methylprednisolone administration was associated with significantly more infectious complications (8). Consequently, many centers have abandoned the routine use of high-dose steroids for traumatic SCI.

However, the situation may be different for steroids given *prior* to an insult to the spinal cord, as is the case with an intraoperative injury. In addition, corticosteroids have clearly been shown to be of benefit in neoplastic disease (11–13). Steroids are believed to decrease vasogenic edema, stabilize membranes, inhibit lipid peroxidation, and enhance Na/K ATPase ionic pump function (9, 11). Thus, steroids given prophylactically may confer an element of neuroprotection, which has been demonstrated in several animal studies (14, 15). At the University of Miami, patients undergoing surgery for primary or metastatic neoplastic disease, vascular malformation, syringomyelia and untethering, or any planned violation of the spinal cord pia that places them at risk for spinal cord injury are given a loading dose of methylprednisolone (30 mg/kg) over 1 hour before surgery and continue bolus doses for 24 hours postoperatively (250 mg/kg every 8 hours).

Hypothermia

Hypothermia has been used since the 1960s for spinal cord cooling with mixed results (16). The benefits of hypothermia include decreased cellular metabolism, reduced inflammation, edema, excitotoxicity, free radical production, oxidative stress, and apoptosis (17). In experimental animal studies, the histologic volume of injury has also been found to be smaller following traumatic SCI with hypothermia, probably due to decreased cascades secondary injury (17). Although studies for reactive hypothermia, occurring after the insult, have shown equivocal effectiveness (18), preventative hypothermia, induced before the injury, has resulted in good functional recovery in animal studies (19).

Hypothermia may be induced either locally or systemically. Local cooling of the spinal cord minimizes the potential for systemic complications but is invasive, cannot be instituted without violation or exposure of the spinal canal, and may have poor control to a target temperature. Systemic cooling is less invasive and may be performed by surface methods or intravascularly. Using either methodology, the profound systemic changes may increase the risk of complications such as infection (sepsis, pneumonia, wound infections), coagulopathy, hypotension, electrolyte disturbances, cardiac arrhythmias, and myocardial dysfunction. Additionally, patients may experience significant discomfort, resulting in the need for sedation or intubation to prevent shaking chills, which may counteract the hypothermic effects.

The degree of cooling necessary for adequate neuroprotection remains a topic of debate. Mild hypothermia (34–36°C), moderate hypothermia (30–33°C), and severe hypothermia (less than 30°C), have all been utilized in animal and clinical studies with varying degrees of success. At the University of Miami, patients undergoing intradural tumor removal, treatment of spinal vascular malformations, or spinal cord untethering for syringomyelia are placed into a state of moderate hypothermia following the induction of general anesthesia. A femoral, subclavian, or jugular intravenous cooling catheter is placed percutaneously, and the patient cooled to between 33ºC (91.4ºF) and 34ºC (93.2ºF). We use the Alsius cooling catheter (Alsius Co., Irvine, CA), which consists of a triple lumen catheter with a saline-filled polyethylene balloon at its tip. This catheter has the advantage of combining cooling capabilities with central venous access. Following surgery, the patient is awakened, and his/her neurologic status is assessed. If no new deficits are seen, then the patient is warmed at 1 degree per hour, and the catheter is subsequently removed. If, during surgery, there was significant cord manipulation, neuromonitoring showed decreased signal potentials, or the patient demonstrated a worsened neurologic state, then moderate hypothermia is maintained postoperatively for 48–72 hours. Rewarming then begins at 1°C every 8 hours, as rapid rewarming may lead to rebound phenomena and enhance deleterious neurologic effects (23).

Microsurgical Technique and Operative Adjuncts

Many advances have been made in intraoperative visualization. From the onset of the operating microscope in neurosurgery, beginning in the late 1950s, microneurosurgery has become increasingly safe (24). Improved lighting, superior magnification, and a rotational field of view allow for less tissue manipulation and for precision in manipulating vital structures and delicate tissues. With contemporary microscopy, it is even possible to see the dorsal median sulcus, which has improved the accuracy of placing a midline myelotomy for the resection of intramedullary tumors, potentially reducing the incidence of postoperative dorsal dysfunction.

Improvements in tissue disruption technology have provided the surgeon with a new generation of ultrasonic aspirators. The CUSA Ultrasonic Surgical System (Integra Radionics, Burlington, MA) is a tissue aspirating system that allows for the simultaneous ultrasonic emulsification and aspiration of neoplastic tissue in small areas. Likewise, the Orion-1 EMF System (Traatek, Ft. Lauderdale, FL) is a tissue vaporizer that removes tumor and scar with extremely high radio frequency and low power output to achieve instantaneous pinpoint vaporization with minimal heat spread to surrounding tissue. The operative laser (Nd:YAG) allows us to burn or disrupt structures without mechanical or electrical damage to the surrounding tissue and is particularly useful for treating intradural lipomas.

Intraoperative imaging has also advanced. Ultrasound is very useful in localizing intradural lesions. It provides immediate feedback as to the craniocaudal extent of the lesions, which allows us to limit the length of laminectomy. In addition, it is invaluable in our treatment of CSF disruptions, allowing localization of spinal cord scarring and syringomyelia. This helps us to plan both our dural and pial incisions to best maintain cord integrity. Intraoperative computed tomography (CT) has also become available and can be helpful in assessing placement of instrumentation or assessment of the adequacy of spinal canal decompression for stenosis.

Endovascular advancements have been essential in the safe treatment of both neoplastic and vascular disease. Through endovascular access, one is able to embolize intra- and extradural spinal cord tumors, in order to reduce vascularity that would otherwise preclude surgical excision due to blood loss. This is especially helpful in hemangioblastomas, in which devascularization makes for a significantly shorter and safer surgery (25). Vascular metastases, such as renal cell carcinoma or melanoma, are also easily seen on angiography and embolized to reduce their blood flow, making resection more feasible (26). Endovascular treatment for vascular lesions has in some cases obviated the need for open surgical treatment, such as in certain intramedullary arteriovenous malformations (AVM) and dural arteriovenous fistulae (DAVF).

Finally, the Cyberknife (Accuray Inc., Sunnyvale, CA) is an image-guided, frameless stereotactic radiosurgery system. The system utilizes the coupling of an orthogonal pair of X-ray cameras to a dynamically manipulated robot-mounted lightweight linear accelerator in order to target lesions to within 1 mm of spatial accuracy. This form of radiosurgery has been adapted to use for the spinal cord and vertebral column. Ongoing investigations are examining its use for spinal cord neoplasms (27) and metastases (28) and for AVMs (29), with promising results.

ADVANCES IN THE SURGICAL MANAGEMENT OF NONTRAUMATIC MYELOPATHIES

Any surgical intervention to treat nontraumatic myelopathy requires a sober evaluation of the pathology, natural history, and prognosis by both the surgeon and the patient. Many nonstructural causes of myelopathy remain nonoperative, including multiple sclerosis, transverse myelitis, radiation-induced myelopathy, paraneoplastic myelitis, motor neuron diseases, nutritional diseases, and herpes, syphilis, AIDS, and other infectious diseases. Potentially operative etiologies may be subacute in onset with a progressive disease course, may have underlying systemic pathologies, and may require additional adjuvant therapy. Realistic informed consent must take into account the expectations of possible increased deficits with the potential for short- and long-term improvement or deterioration.

Degenerative Spondylosis

Myelopathy secondary to degenerative disease of the cervical spinal column, commonly referred to as cervical spondylotic myelopathy, is the most common cause of spinal cord dysfunction in middle-aged and elderly patients. Static and dynamic factors are postulated to play a role in the pathophysiology of spondylotic myelopathy (30). The static factors can include stenosis from congenital canal narrowing, disc herniations, bony osteophytes, and ossification and hypertrophy of the posterior longitudinal ligament (PLL) and ligamentum flavum. In concert, these may result in circumferential compression of the spinal cord. The dynamic aspect involves abnormal forces experienced by the spinal column and spinal cord during normal physiologic loads, resulting in the progression of degenerative changes and in repeated microtrauma to the spinal cord as it is contused and/or infarcted by the surrounding herniated discs, osteophytes, and hypertrophied ligaments (Figure 39.2).

Although conservative therapy is an option for patients with mild, nonprogressive symptoms (31), patients with progressive or debilitating myelopathy should be managed surgically. It has been shown that the majority of patients with symptomatic myelopathy will experience pervasive symptoms, and that as many as 50% will continue to deteriorate neurologically (32–34).

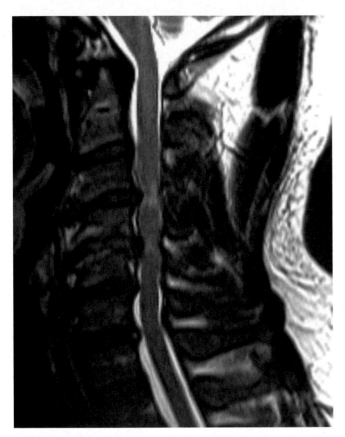

Figure 39.2 A T2-weighted sagittal MRI showing circumferential, multifactorial, multi-segmental spinal cord compression resulting in cervical myelopathy.

The goal of surgery is to halt the progression of myelopathy by adequately decompressing the spinal cord.

Achieving the extensive decompression necessary to surgically treat cervical spondylotic myelopathy, while at the same time preserving cervical spine lordosis, range of motion, and stability, has challenged spine surgeons for many years. Controversy still exists regarding which surgical approach, anterior versus posterior, and which surgical procedure best accomplishes these goals. Laminectomy was originally the procedure of choice in treating myelopathy from multilevel cervical spondylosis. In the 1950s and 1960s, the anterior approach to the cervical spine was introduced and popularized (35, 36). Subsequently, in Japan, the laminoplasty technique was developed in the 1970s as another treatment option (37, 38). Each procedure has associated risks and benefits, and there is a lack of strong evidence in the literature to support one over the other. There is agreement, however, among most surgeons that the configuration of the cervical spine (i.e., lordotic or kyphotic) should help dictate which approach is used. Posterior approaches rely somewhat on dorsal migration of the spinal cord away from ventral disc herniations, osteophytes, or calcified PLL, and this occurs preferentially with a lordotic configuration. Thus, patients with a significant kyphosis are often best managed with an anterior approach. Exceptions do exist, however, as some degrees of kyphosis can be corrected with posterior supplemental instrumentation.

Multilevel anterior discectomies, without or with partial corpectomies to remove osteophytes, and fusion with interbody grafts and plating can be used to treat cervical spondylotic myelopathy. The advantages of this approach include direct decompression of the spinal cord and anterior spinal artery via removal of the compressive pathology, including herniated discs, osteophytes, and calcified PLL. Anterior plating allows for correction of kyphosis and immediate stability until fusion occurs. Disadvantages with this procedure include increasing rates of pseudoarthrosis reported when these anterior constructs span multiple levels, as is frequently the case in decompression for spondylotic myelopathy (39, 40), as well as the approach-related morbidity associated with anterior neck dissections (recurrent laryngeal nerve injury and postoperative dysphagia) (42–44). Anterior fusions are also known to carry a well-documented risk of symptomatic degeneration in adjacent spinal segments (41).

Posterior approaches for cervical spondylotic myelopathy are based on the premise that a wide decompression will allow the cord to migrate dorsally away from ventral compression, so long as spinal lordosis is maintained. However, extensive bone, ligament, and muscular disruption are associated with a risk of postoperative delayed spinal instability. Thus, laminectomy without instrumentation and fusion has gradually fallen out of favor with contemporary spine surgeons, as this has been postulated to be the cause of postlaminectomy failures and kyphosis reported in some adult series (45, 46). This has made laminectomy with instrumented fusion increasingly popular among spine surgeons. The instrumentation usually consists of lateral mass screws coupled with plates or rods (Figure 39.3). Proponents of this technique claim that the benefit of adding instrumentation lies not only in providing immediate stability and decreasing the risk of postlaminectomy kyphosis, but also in addressing the dynamic factors associated with spondylotic myelopathy most effectively. The disadvantages of this technique include the increased potential morbidity associated with spinal instrumentation, including spinal cord, nerve root, or vascular injury; the increased associated costs; and the long-term consequences of rigidly fusing the cervical spine, especially in young patients.

A multitude of variations in laminoplasty have been described, including the open door laminoplasty (37), which we use preferentially at the University of Miami (Figure 39.4). Other popular variants include the "Z-plasty" (38), and the French-door laminoplasty (47), and a minimally invasive laminoplasty technique has also been described (48, 49). These are all variations that involve opening the lamina with a high-speed drill and keeping them elevated as a construct with suture, strut grafts, or mini-plates. The premise behind cervical laminoplasty is that a thorough decompression is performed while preserving as much of the dorsal bony arch and posterior tension band as possible, thereby decreasing the risk of postoperative kyphosis without subjecting patients to the risks of spinal instrumentation. In addition, the dorsal arch keeps the spinal musculature from contacting and adhering to the dura, which can result in progressive neurologic deterioration from this "pseudomembrane" formation. Another inherent advantage to laminoplasty is that, by using a drill to elevate the laminae en bloc, the risk of spinal cord injury from introducing instruments into a narrow spinal canal is minimized. One criticism of laminoplasty has been that it does not afford immediate stability and that, until the spine heals and "stiffens," patients are still at risk for postoperative kyphosis. In addition, some also have reported that the "stiffening" effect

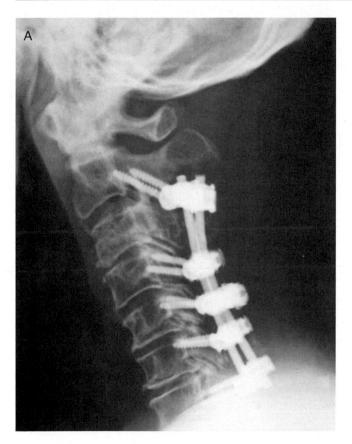

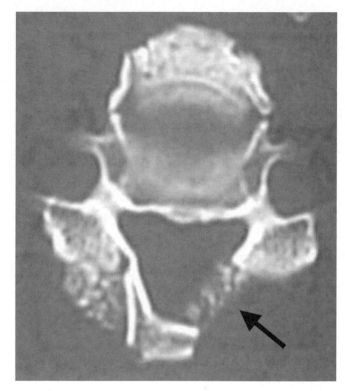

Figure 39.4   An axial CT showing expansion of the vertebral canal by a left open-door laminoplasty and rib allograft (**arrow**).

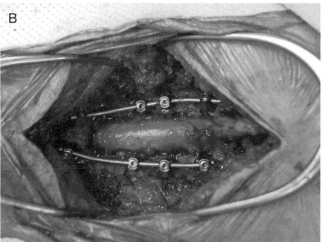

Figure 39.3   A lateral radiograph (**A**) and an intraoperative photo (**B**) showing a laminectomy and segmental instrumentation for decompression of cervical myelopathy and instability.

that laminoplasty has on the spine eventually leads to a loss of cervical range of motion comparable to that seen with cervical instrumented fusion (50, 51). Other potential problems with laminoplasty include the potential for neurologic injury from collapse of the construct and a high incidence of C5 root palsy associated with dorsal cord migration and traction on this root (52, 53).

There is a paucity of literature directly comparing outcomes after each of these procedures for cervical spondylotic myelopathy. Herkowitz published a retrospective review comparing clinical and radiographic outcomes in patients undergoing laminectomy ($n = 12$), anterior fusion ($n = 18$), and laminoplasty ($n = 15$) for patients with radiculopathy and myelopathy (54). He found better clinical results with laminoplasty. However, he also found that cervical range of motion was most limited in laminoplasty patients. Heller et al. retrospectively reviewed matched cohorts of thirteen patients undergoing laminoplasty and thirteen undergoing laminectomy with fusion for cervical myelopathy (55). Their major findings included greater symptomatic improvement in the laminoplasty cohort and a greater incidence of complications in the laminectomy and fusion group. These papers are limited by the fact that they are retrospective reviews and that they analyze a relatively small number of patients, making the results somewhat less significant. However, the use of these surgical techniques varies greatly between institutions and surgeons.

Compression of the spinal cord in the thoracic segments can lead to lower extremity myelopathy. Although this may be caused by congenital stenosis, ligamentum flavum hypertrophy, abnormalities of ossification, or spinal column deformities, by far the most common cause of thoracic myelopathy is a thoracic herniated disc. The preferred approach for these lesions is anteriorly through a transthoracic or thoracoabdominal approach, if they are centrally located or severely calcified. Posterolateral lesions may be accessed through a transpedicular, costotransversectomy, or lateral extracavitary approach. Additionally, minimally invasive thoracoscopic approaches can also be used to treat these lesions.

Inflammatory Disease

Rheumatoid arthritis can manifest as inflammation and instability of the occipitocervical spine, which may result in severe cervical myelopathy. Basilar impression and atlantoaxial subluxation are the most common mechanisms causing significant neurologic disability, the result of erosive synovitis causing destruction of the joints, ligaments, and bone of the atlantooccipital and atlantoaxial joints. Subaxial disease may be as a result of either instability or ankylosis, and superimposed deformities may be either fixed or mobile. Aggressive management should be established early, as patients who progress to a Ranawat III-B status (objective weakness with long tract signs, and who have become nonambulatory) have a much higher morbidity and mortality rate associated with surgical intervention than do patients who ambulate (56).

Surgical management of atlantoaxial instability in patients with rheumatoid arthritis is complex and must be individualized for each patient, but always requires arthrodesis. This is usually is performed posteriorly and may require preoperative cervical traction to restore proper alignment and correct basilar impression. The cause of myelopathy is most often an inflammatory, retroodontoid pannus causing spinal cord compression. Transoral odontoidectomy and resection may be required (56), but the inflammatory mass often regresses with posterior fusion alone (57). Despite the fact that these patients are severely disabled, osteoporotic, and treated chronically with anti-inflammatory medications, fusion rates can be quite acceptable, with high solid arthrodesis rates (88%) and good clinical outcomes (66% improved, 38% stabilized) (57).

Calcium pyrophosphate dehydrate deposition, or pseudogout, is a rare cause of retroodontoid mass lesions in elderly individuals, which presents with neck pain, myelopathy, and, not infrequently, lower cranial nerve deficits. Calcification of the mass or transverse ligament is common, necessitating transoral odontoidectomy and mass resection, unlike the rheumatoid pannus (58). Dorsal fusion is not always mandatory, as concomitant ligamentous calcification and atlantoaxial joint ankylosis may provide added stability (58).

Infection

Discitis and osteomyelitis usually occur due to hematogenous spread from skin and soft tissue infections or IVDA but can also occur due to direct inoculation, from surgery, from epidural injections, or from lumbar punctures. These vertebral infections can result in epidural extension with potentially devastating neurologic sequelae and are the most common cause of epidural abscess, although spontaneous epidural abscess occur rarely. The incidence seems to be increasing over the past decade, possibly due to an increase in intravenous drug abuse (IVDA) and instrumentation (59), with the predominant organism being the staphlyococcus species. Over 70% of epidural abscesses present with neurologic deficits (59).

In the acute infection, liquid pus is present, but most epidural abscesses present after several weeks, when there is a combination of pus and granulation tissue. This precludes a small laminotomy to wash out the infection and usually mandates a multilevel laminectomy with evacuation of abscess and granulation tissue. Despite care to preserve facets for stabilization,

should the laminectomy be greater than 2–3 levels or the epidural abscess be associated with osteomyelitis or discitis, we perform a posterolateral fusion with autologous iliac crest bone graft. Significant kyphosis or instability may require anterior and/or posterior decompression with instrumented fusion. Despite the difficulties in treating infection in the face of a foreign body, debridement and instrumentation as a single-stage procedure for spinal infection is becoming more prevalent, with good results. In one series, there was no recurrence of the initial infection during an 18-month follow-up, and there was a fusion rate of 90.5% (60).

Antibiotics should be started immediately after obtaining surgical cultures (90% yield from abscess, 60%–70% CT guided biopsy, 60% yield from blood) (61), with 67% of gram positive cultures caused by staphylococcus aureus (59). Antibiotics should be continued for 4–6 weeks for epidural abscess alone and 6–8 weeks for concomitant osteomyelitis/discitis (61). Medical management is reserved for those without neurologic deficit or poor surgical candidates, but without surgical evacuation, there may be a 37% incidence of paralysis and death (62). With surgery, 78% of patients have either a full recovery or mild residual weakness, although those with complete paralysis for over 36 hours or complete paralysis within the first 12 hours of presentation carry a more dismal prognosis (63).

Tuberculous osteomyelitis is now much less common than bacterial osteomyelitis but can still cause compressive myelopathy. Surgical treatment of thoracic and lumbar tuberculous spondylitis has classically aimed at debriding the infected bone and restoring correction of kyphosis from an anterior approach, but posterior debridement and instrumentation also appears efficacious (64).

Neoplastic Disease

Historically, it was thought that, as the majority of tumors within the substance of the cord are infiltrating in character, they were therefore not removable (65), and a conservative approach consisting of biopsy and adjuvant radiotherapy was adopted. Recently, however, a more aggressive surgical approach has been advocated, with good results after aggressive resection of intramedullary tumors in both pediatric and adult patients (66–68). Although treatment of these tumors may alleviate progressive neurologic deterioration and pain, the potential complications are formidable. CSF leak and pseudomeningocele, wound infection and/or dehiscence, worsened neurological deficits, intractable pain, and spinal cord scarring, or tethering, must be discussed with the patient prior to surgery, and caution should be exercised at all times by the surgeon. As mentioned above, we use both prophylactic steroids and moderate hypothermia, if any spinal cord manipulation is expected. All cases are monitored with evoked potentials (MEP and SSEP).

Intradural tumors can be subcategorized into intramedullary and extramedullary, as the ramifications of surgery for each are different. Intramedullary tumors, such as astrocytomas, ependymomas, and hemangioblastomas, carry a risk of neurologic deterioration after resection as the integrity of the spinal cord must be violated in order to access the tumor. After an adequate laminectomy is performed to allow for possible duraplasty, intraoperative ultrasound is used to locate the lesion. After opening the dura well above and below the tumor, we tack the dura to the paraspinal

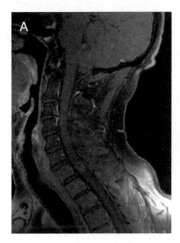
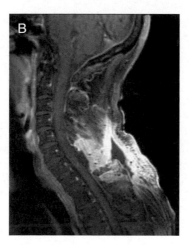
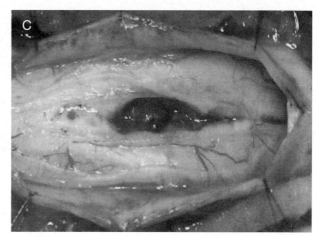

Figure 39.5 Pre- (**A**) and postoperative (**B**) sagittal T1-weighted MRI with gadolinium showing an intramedullary ependymoma. Intraoperative resection showing establishment of a plane between the tumor and gliotic spinal cord (**C**).

muscles with nonabsorbable sutures, to help prevent the spinal cord from scarring postoperatively. We place a small piece of Gelfoam (Pfizer, New York, NY) at the cranial and caudal ends of the durotomy to prevent blood from entering the subarachnoid space and causing arachnoiditis. At this point, the operating microscope is used to identify the dorsal median sulcus, located by following the course of penetrating vessels arising from the midline dorsal medullary vein, and this plane is opened until the tumor is encountered. In cases where the lesion is laterally situated in the cord, an approach via the dorsal root entry zone is employed. Should the tumor have an associated cyst, this is aspirated with a 25-gauge needle to reduce pressure on the spinal cord substance, which may worsen with the manipulation of surgery.

Using microsurgical dissecting tools, we gently develop a plane circumferentially around the lesion (Figure 39.5). As described earlier, the Orion or CUSA ultrasonic aspirator is used to debulk the lesion in order to minimize traction on the spinal cord, lessening the trauma to the cord parenchyma. With the onset of any change in the MEP or SSEP, our policy is to stop the resection, remove all cord retraction, and allow the cord to "rest" for several minutes. After ensuring that the signals are not being affected by hypotension, depth of anesthesia, or temperature, we reassess the evoked potentials and continue only if these have returned to baseline. If the plane between tumor and spinal cord is ill defined, then it is incumbent on the surgeon to cease tumor removal before any destruction of the spinal cord tracts may occur, keeping in mind the ultimate goal of preserving neurologic function. In a recent review of our series of intramedullary tumors at the University of Miami (sixty-four patients, 50% ependymomas), patients did not manifest significant motor weakness postoperatively, but 43.6% exhibited dorsal column dysfunction. With the possible exception of hemangioblastomas, which can be cured and are usually well defined, caution should be exercised above all else. Hemangioblastomas should be embolized preoperatively but usually have an excellent plane, allowing for complete tumor removal. These tumors should not be entered and debulked, due to vascularity, but should be bipolared over the surface of the capsule and removed in total (69).

Extramedullary tumors, such as schwannomas, neurofibromas, and meningiomas, cause myelopathy due to compression and can be cured with complete resection. In order to protect the spinal cord, the first goal of surgery for intradural, extramedullary tumors is adequate bone removal in order to remove the tumor without untoward manipulation of the spinal cord. Often, the pedicle and facet of the involved side must be removed, and instrumentation used, if multiple levels are involved. Ultrasound is then used to locate the cranial and caudal limits of the tumor. After opening the dura, all work is performed with the use of the operating microscope, for enhanced lighting and visualization. The tumor should be internally debulked as much as possible to prevent tumor manipulation from being transferred to the spinal cord. Intradural tumors are rarely adherent to the spinal cord, but if one can not easily separate the tumor from the cord, it is better to leave a small amount of residual tumor. As most intradural, extramedullar tumors are slow-growing and benign, they can be followed or treated with Cyberknife.

Prior to dural closure, we find it useful to repeat the ultrasound and ensure that there is no blood clot, unsuspected residual tumor, or cord compression. If there is any doubt regarding adequate space in the intradural compartment, or if residual tumor with the propensity to grow was left, we perform a duraplasty with cadaveric dura. We use a lumbar drain if the duraplasty is larger or if there is any doubt regarding a watertight closure. If, during surgery, there was significant cord manipulation, neuromonitoring showed decreased signals, or the patient demonstrated a worsened neurologic exam, we maintain hypothermia for 48–72 hours. Postoperatively, the patients are positioned laterally or semiprone and are moved frequently to avoid spinal cord tethering.

Metastatic spinal cord compression is a devastating complication of cancer. Its natural history is one of progressive pain, paralysis, sensory loss, and sphincter dysfunction, and those with paralysis, either at presentation or following treatment, have a much shorter life expectancy (70). Historically, simple decompressive laminectomy was performed for myelopathy for metastatic spinal cord compression. Due to segmental instability and poor functional outcomes, Posner recommended radiation treatment only (71). Harrington, Siegal and Siegal, and Sunderesan ushered in the new era of circumferential decompression of spinal cord with instrumented stabilization followed by radiation, with much better functional outcomes (70, 72, 73). This has been established as the standard of care by a multicenter prospective randomized trial, which showed the posttreatment rate of ambulation to be 84% following surgery and radiation, but only 57% following radiation alone (74). Better functional outcomes with surgery followed by radiation are seen because surgical decompression is immediate, and decompression occurs prior to secondary vascular injury and spinal cord infarction.

Similar to Patchell's inclusion criteria (74), we consider for surgical decompression those with greater than 3 months' survival, no major medical contraindications to surgery, and a focal area of neural compression. We consider surgery for both neurologic deterioration and intractable pain, unless the tumor is very radiosensitive, such as myeloma or lymphoma. As patients with metastatic disease may have limited longevity, we should do everything possible to optimize their quality of life during that time.

Vascular Lesions

Spinal arteriovenous malformations can be classified into four types, each with different pathophysiology and clinical presentation (75, 76). Type I lesions are dural arteriovenous fistula (DAVF), which present with progressive myelopathy due to venous congestion of the spinal cord (Figure 39.6). DAVFs are usually located between T6 and L5 in the root sleeve, with the feeding arteries often being at a different level than the fistulous point. The surgical treatment consists of intradural interruption of the draining vein with coagulation or excision of the dural fistula. Endovascular embolization may now be used to treat DAVF, but it is crucial that the embolic material reach and occlude the draining vein for persistent and successful obliteration (77). Obliteration rates for endovascular occlusion of DAVF range from 25% to 50% (77, 78). As open surgical obliteration is

minimally invasive, quick, and durable, with occlusion rates near 100%, this is still our first line of treatment.

Type II and III lesions are intramedullary AVMs, with Type III being the juvenile variant, which is both intra- and extramedullary. These high-flow and high-pressure malformations usually present with hemorrhage, although they can also present with progressive myelopathy from cord congestion. These are difficult lesions to treat surgically, as the feeders usually arise from both anterior and posterior, and the nidus lies within the substance of the spinal cord. A small subset of high, posterior AVMs are amenable to surgical resection, as all arterial feeders come from the posterior. Endovascular therapy has provided an alternative for treatment of these lesions, which is often palliative, with complete obliteration achieved in only 37.5% of cases. Despite this, a good clinical outcome was realized in over 80% of cases (79). It is important to remember, however, that the potential for devastating complications is always present when treating intramedullary AVMs.

Type IV lesions, or perimedullary fistulae, are intradural, extramedullary direct arteriovenous fistulas, involving the intrinsic arterial supply of the spinal cord, which present with venous hypertension. These can best be treated by surgical ligation of the fistula through an anterior or posterior approach, as needed (76).

Cavernomas can present either with hemorrhage and acute neurological decline or with chronic progressive myelopathy, occurring due to microhemorrhages and resultant gliosis. Surgery and complete removal of the lesion tends to halt the progression of symptoms (80). If a cavernoma has bled and abuts the surface of the spinal cord, then we have an excellent chance of success in removing these lesions, again using the operative adjuncts of steroids, moderate hypothermia, intraoperative monitoring, and meticulous operative techniques.

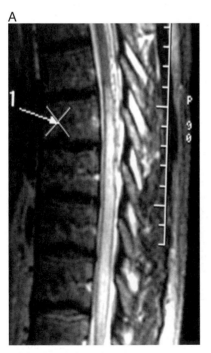
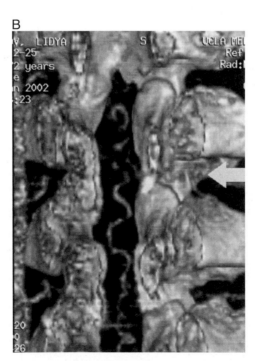
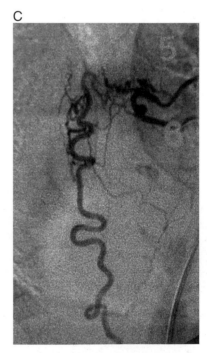

Figure 39.6   Thoracic (T7) dural AV fistula shown on T2-weighted MRI (**A**), CT angiography (**B**), and digital subtraction angiography (**C**) before endovascular embolization.

CSF Flow Alterations

Cerebrospinal fluid dynamics may be altered by congenital malformations, Chiari malformations, infections, spinal cord tumors, posttraumatic scarring, and iatrogenic injury, such as postsurgical scarring or epidural injections, among many other causes.

Almost all cases involve a blockage of normal CSF flow, for which treatment includes reestablishment of normal or adequate CSF flow. Cine MRI has become very helpful for evaluating the presence or absence of CSF flow, although quantification of flow remains elusive.

Syringomyelia was historically treated by diverting CSF from the cyst within the spinal cord to the subarachnoid space, the peritoneum, or the pleural space. These methods may still be used today, but in combination with treatment for the cause of the syrinx, whenever possible. Reestablishment of normal CSF flow dynamics nearly always results in regression, and most often collapse, of the syrinx. Should the syringomyelia be secondary to an arachnoid cyst or tumor, resection will result in spontaneous resolution over time. When the syrinx is due to Chiari malformation, the posterior fossa should be enlarged with bony and dural decompression. Ultrasound can be used following duraplasty to view tonsillar and spinal cord pulsations, and cine MRI can be used pre- and postoperatively to view CSF flow.

Progressive posttraumatic myelomalacic myelopathy presents with sensorimotor function deterioration, local and/or radicular pain, increased spasticity, increased autonomic dysreflexia, and sphincter dysfunction (81). This may be as a result of adhesion of the spinal cord to the dura, or tethering (Figure 39.7). This can result in devastating progressive myelopathy and is most often a delayed result of trauma or intradural surgery. Tethering blocks the flow of CSF and is often associated with syringomyelia, due to a confluence of microcystic changes. Deterioration of motor function was the most frequent manifestation in our series, present in thirty-one of forty patients (81). Following untethering combined with expansive duraplasty to reestablish CSF flow, there were significant improvements in motor function (79%), autonomic dysreflexia (75%), pain (62%), sphincter dysfunction (50%), and sensory function (43%) of the patients

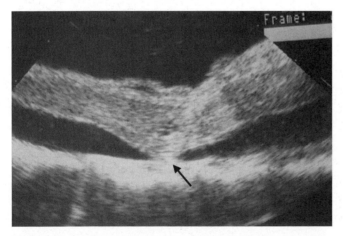

Figure 39.7 Intraoperative ultrasound showing dorsal tethering of the spinal cord to the dura (**arrow**).

(81). Two patients experienced retethering of the spinal cord, and one underwent a second operation (81).

In order to untether the spinal cord, a wide laminectomy is required in order to expose the area of dural adhesion and allow for an adequate expansile duraplasty. All arachnoidal bands are cut, and, if present, the syrinx is fenestrated or shunted to the subarachnoid, pleural, or peritoneal spaces. In the case of kyphotic deformity, consideration is given to corrective reconstruction and stabilization to prevent further cord damage and scarring. If the expansile duraplasty with cadaveric dura is not watertight with a valsalva, then a small muscle graft is placed, and lumbar drainage is used for 5 to 7 days. We position these patients prone or semiprone for 6 weeks postoperatively to prevent cord adhesion to the point of duraplasty.

Despite relative advances in the treatment of CSF flow disorders, much additional information, tools, and research are needed. The development of better imaging software for CSF flow dynamics would increase our understanding and help us develop better preventative and treatment strategies. Improved tissue adhesives and synthetic dural grafting materials to seal dural holes and materials to prevent soft tissue scarring are needed. Finally, a national database and multicenter long-term follow-up studies of surgical and nonsurgical patients for natural history and treatment outcome analysis are paramount to the definitive treatment of this group of disorders.

Areas of ongoing research include the use of cellular therapy to treat neuropathic pain caused by syringomyelia. The transplant of a human neuronal cell line to act as cellular "minipumps" has been extremely successful in animal models (82, 83). Subarachnoid transplantation of the hNT2.17 cell line secretes inhibitory neurotransmitters; this process is hypothesized to reestablish the chemical balance of the sensory interneurons in the dorsal horn. Transplantation of donor adrenal chromaffin cells has also proven advantageous (84).

CONCLUSIONS

Many advances have been made in the surgical treatment of nontraumatic myelopathy. Neuroprotection with the use of monitoring, hypothermia, perioperative steroids, and better operating and imaging technology is paramount to our treatment of spinal cord injury and to creating improved patient outcomes. The long-term treatment of traumatic and nontraumatic myelopathies is comparable, and patients with each have been shown to achieve similar functional outcomes with rehabilitation (1). Nevertheless, the myriad underlying pathophysiologies of nontraumatic myelopathy and the tendency toward older age presents us with a different set of challenges, which underscores the need for continually improving acute treatments. Further development and investigation of minimally invasive approaches, imaging and image guidance, robotics, motion preservation, biomaterials, and genetic engineering remains an exciting endeavor for those treating myelopathy.

References

1. Mckinley WO, Seel RT, Hardman JT. Nontraumatic spinal cord injury: incidence, epidemiology, and functional outcome. *Arch Phys Med Rehabil* 1999; 80:619–623.
2. Cottrell J, Smith D. *Anesthesia and Neurosurgery.* 4th ed. Mosby Yearbook, 2001.

3. Levi L, Wolf A, Belzberg H. Hemodynamic parameters in patients with acute cervical cord trauma: description, intervention, and prediction of outcome. *Neurosurgery* 1993; 33:1007–1016.

4. Porkkala T, Jantti V, Kaukinen S. Somatosensory evoked potentials during isoflurane anesthesia. *Acta Anaesthesiol Scand* 1994; 38:206–210.

5. Gronert G, Theye R. Pathophysiology of hyperkalemia induced by succinylcholine. *Anesthesiology* 1975; 43:89–99.

6. Nagamizo D, Tsuruta S, Matsumoto M, Matayoshi H, et al. Tight glycemic control by insulin, started in the preischemic, but not postischemic, period, protects against ischemic spinal cord injury in rabbits. *Anesth Analg* 2007; 105:1397–1403.

7. Bracken M, Shepard M, Hellenbrand K, Collins W, et al. Methylprednisolone and neurological function 1 year after spinal cord injury: results of the national acute spinal cord injury study. *J Neurosurg* 1985; 63:704–713.

8. Bracken M, Shepard M, Collins W, Holford T, et al. A randomized, controlled trial of methylprednisolone or naloxone in the treatment of acute spinal-cord injury: results of the second national acute spinal cord injury study. *N Eng J Med* 1990; 322:1405–1411.

9. Bracken M, Shepard M, Holford T, Leo-Summers L, et al. Administration of methylprednisolone for 24 or 48 hours or tirilizad mesylate for 48 hours in the treatment of acute spinal cord injury: results of the third national acute spinal cord injury randomized controlled trial. National acute spinal cord injury study. *JAMA* 1997; 277:1597–1604.

10. Sayer F, Kronvall E, Nilsson O. Methylprednisolone treatment in acute spinal cord injury: the myth challenged through a structured analysis of published literature. *Spine* 2006; 6:335–343.

11. Ushio Y PR, Posner JB, Shapiro WR. Experimental spinal cord compression by epidural neoplasm. *Neurology* 1977; 27:422–429.

12. Delattre J, Arbit E, Thaler H, Rosenblum M, Posner J. A dose-response study of dexamethasone in a model of spinal cord compression caused by epidural tumor. *J Neurosurg* 1989; 70:920–925.

13. Sorensen S, Helweg-Larsen S, Mouridsen H. Effect of high-dose dexamethasone in carcinomatous metastatic spinal cord compression treated with radiotherapy: a randomised trial. *Eur J Cancer* 1994; 1:22–27.

14. Fu E, Saporta S. Methylprednisolone inhibits production of interleukin-1beta and interleukin-6 in the spinal cord following compression injury in rats. *J Neurosurg Anesthesiol* 2005; 17:82–85.

15. Harms C, Albrecht K, Harms U, Seidel K, et al. Phosphatidylinositol 3-akt-kinase-dependent phosphorylation of p21(waf1/cip1) as a novel mechanism of neuroprotection by glucocorticoids. *J Neurosci* 2007; 27:4562–4571.

16. Albin M, White R, Donald D, Maccarty C, Faulconer A. Hypothermia of the spinal cord by perfusion cooling of the subarachnoid space. *Surg Forum* 1961; 12.

17. Inamasu J, Nakamura Y, Ichikizaki K. Induced hypothermia in experimental traumatic spinal cord injury: an update. *J Neurol Sci* 2003; 209:55–60.

18. Clifton G, Miller E, Choi S, Levin H, et al. Lack of effect of induction of hypothermia after acute brain injury. *N Eng J Med* 2001: 556–563.

19. Jou I. Effects of core body temperature on changes in spinal somatosensory-evoked potential in acute spinal cord compression injury: an experimental study in the rat *Spine* 2000; 25:1878–1885.

20. Busto R, Globus M-T, Dietrich W, Martinez E, et al. Effect of mild hypothermia on ischemia-induced release of neurotransmitters and free fatty acids in rat brain. *Stroke* 1989; 20:904–910.

21. Toyoda T, Suzuki S, Kassell N, Lee K. Intraischemic hypothermia attenuates neurotrophil infiltration in the rat neocortex after focal ischemia-reperfusion injury. *Neurosurgery* 1996; 39:1200–1205.

22. Dietrich W, Busto R, Halley M. The importance of brain temperature in alternations of the blood-brain barrier following cerebral ischemia. *J Neuropathol Exp Neurol* 1990; 49:486–497.

23. Steiner T, Friede T, Aschoff A, Schellinger P, et al. Effect and feasibility of controlled rewarming after moderate hypothermia in stroke patients with malignant infarction of the middle cerebral artery. *Stroke* 2001; 32:2833–2835.

24. Kriss T, Kriss V. History of the operating microscope: from magnifying glass to microneurosurgery. *Neurosurgery* 1998; 42:899–907.

25. Eskridge J, McAuliffe W, Harris B, Kim D, et al. Preoperative endovascular embolization of craniospinal hemangioblastomas. *AJNR* 1996; 17:525–531.

26. Shi H, Suh D, Lee H, Lim S, et al. Preoperative transarterial embolization of spinal tumor: embolization techniques and results. *AJNR* 1999; 20:2009–2015.

27. Dodd R, Ryu M, Kamnerdsupaphon P, Gibbs I, et al. Cyberknife radiosurgery for benign intradural extramedullary spinal tumors. *Neurosurgery* 2006; 58:674–685.

28. Gerszten P, Welch W. Cyberknife radiosurgery for metastatic spine tumors. *Neurosurg Clin N Am* 2004; 15:492–501.

29. Sinclair J, Chang S, Gibbs I, Adler J. Multisession cyberknife radiosurgery for intramedullary spinal cord arteriovenous malformations. *Neurosurgery* 2006; 58:1081–1089.

30. White A, Panjabi M. Biomechanical considerations in the surgical management of cervical spondylotic myelopathy. *Spine* 1988; 13:856–860.

31. Kadanka Z, Mares M, Bednanik J, Smrcka V. Approaches to spondylotic cervical myelopathy: conservative versus surgical results in a 3-year follow-up study. *Spine* 2002; 27:2205–2210.

32. Epstein J, Epstein N. The surgical management of cervical spinal stenosis, spondylosis, and myeloradiculopathy by means of the posterior approach. In: Sherk HH, Dunn EJ, Eismont FJ, et al., eds. *The Cervical Spine*. 2nd ed. Philadelphia: J.B. Lippincott Co., 1989:625–643.

33. Syman L, Lavender P. The surgical treatment of cervical spondylotic myelopathy. *Neurology* 1967; 17:117–126.

34. Roberts A. Myelopathy due to cervical spondylosis treated by collar immobilization. *Neurology* 1966; 16:951–954.

35. Bailey R, Badgley C. Stabilization for the cervical spine by anterior fusion. *J Bone Joint Surg Am* 1960; 42:565–594.

36. Smith G, Robinson R. The treatment of certain cervical spine disorders by anterior removal of the intervertebral disc and interbody fusion. *J Bone Joint Surg Am* 1958; 40:607–623.

37. Hirabayashi K. Expansive open-door laminoplasty for cervical spondylotic myelopathy. *Jpn J Surg* 1978; 32:1159–1163.

38. Oyama M, Hattori S, Moriwaki N. A new method of posterior decompression. *Chubuseisaisi* 1973; 16:792.

39. Paramore C, Dickman C, Sonntag V. Radiographic and clinical follow-up review of caspar plates in 49 patients. *J Neurosurg* 1996; 84:957–961.

40. Vaccaro A, Falatyn S, Scuderi G, Eismont F, et al. Early failure of long segment anterior cervical plate fixation. *J Spinal Disord* 1998; 11:410–415.

41. Hilibrand A, Carlson G, Palumbo M, Jones P, Bohlman H. Radiculopathy and myelopathy at segments adjacent to the site of a previous anterior cervical arthrodesis. *J Bone Joint Surg Am* 1999; 81A:519–528.

42. Morpeth J, Williams M. Vocal fold paralysis after anterior cervical diskectomy and fusion. *Laryngoscope* 2000; 110:43–46.

43. Riley L, Skolasky R, Albert T, Vaccaro A, Heller J. Dysphagia after anterior cervical decompression and fusion: prevalence and risk factors from a longitudinal cohort study. *Spine* 2005; 30:2564–2569.

44. Wang M, Green B. Open-door cervical expansile laminoplasty. *Neurosurgery* 2004; 54:119–123.

45. Kato Y, Iwasaki M, Fuji T, Yonenobu K, Ochi T. Long-term follow-up results of laminectomy for cervical myelopathy caused by ossification of the posterior longitudinal ligament. *J Neurosurg* 1998; 89: 217–223.

46. Kaptain G, Simmons N, Replogle R, Pobereskin L. Incidence and outcome of kyphotic deformity following laminectomy for cervical spondylotic myelopathy. *J Neurosurg* 2000; 93:199–204.

47. Kurokawa T, Tsuyama N, Tanaka H. Enlargement of spinal canal by sagittal splitting of the spinous process. *Bessatsu Seikei Geka* 1982; 2: 234–240.

48. Santiago P, Fessler R. Minimally invasive surgery for the management of cervical spondylosis. *Neurosurgery* 2007; 60:S160–165.

49. Wang M, Green B, Coscarella E, Baskaya M, et al. Minimally invasive cervical expansile laminoplasty: an initial cadaveric study. *Neurosurgery* 2003; 52:370–373.

50. Houten J, Cooper P. Laminectomy and posterior cervical plating for multilevel cervical spondylotic myelopathy and ossification of the posterior longitudinal ligament: effects on cervical alignment, spinal cord compression, and neurological outcome. *Neurosurgery* 2003; 52:1081–1087.

51. Ratliff J, Cooper P. Cervical laminoplasty: a critical review. *J Neurosurg* 2003; 98:230–238.

52. Satomi K, Nishu Y, Kohno T, Hirabayashi K. Long-term follow-up studies of open-door expansive laminoplasty for cervical stenotic myelopathy. *Spine* 1994; 19:507–510.

53. Tsuzuki N, Abe R, Saiki K, Zhongshi L. Extradural tethering effect as one mechanism of radiculopathy complicating posterior decompression of the cervical cord. *Spine* 1996; 21:203–211.

54. Herkowitz HN. A comparison of anterior cervical fusion, cervical laminectomy, and cervical laminoplasty for the surgical management of multiple level spondolytic radiculopathy. *Spine* 1988; 13:774–780.

55. Heller J, Edwards C, Murakami H, Rodts G. Laminoplasty versus laminectomy and fusion for multilevel cervical myelopathy: an independent matched cohort analysis. *Spine* 2001; 26:1330–1336.
56. Casey A, Crockard H, Pringle J, O'Brien M, Stevens J. Rheumatoid arthritis of the cervical spine: current techniques for management. *Orthop Clin North Am* 2002; 33:291–309.
57. Clark C, Goetz D, Menezes A. Arthrodesis of the cervical spine in rheumatoid arthritis. *J Bone Joint Surg Am* 1989; 71:381–392.
58. Fenoy A, Menezes A, Donovan K, Kralik S. Calcium pyrophosphate dihydrate crystal deposition in the craniovertebral junction. *J Neurosurg Spine* 2008; 8:22–29.
59. Rigamonti D, Liem L, Sampath P, Knoller N, et al. Spinal epidural abscess: contemporary trends in etiology, evaluation and management. *Surg Neurol* 1999; 52:189–197.
60. Suess O, Weise L, Brock M, Kombos T. Debridement and spinal instrumentation as a single-stage procedure in bacterial spondylitis/spondylodiscitis. *Zentralbl Neurochir* 2007; 68:123–132.
61. Currier B, Eismont F. Chapter 39: infections of the spine. In: Herkowitz HN, ed. *The Spine.* Philadelphia: WB Saunders, 1999.
62. Wheeler D, Kisser P, Rigamonte D. Medical management of spinal epidural abscesses: case report and review. *Clin Infect Dis* 1992; 15:22–27.
63. Tang H, Lin H, Liu Y, Li C. Spinal epidural abscess: experience with 46 patients and evaluation of prognostic factors. *J Infect* 2002; 45:76–81.
64. Güzey F, Emel E, Bas N, Hacisalihoglu S, et al. Thoracic and lumbar tuberculous spondylitis treated by posterior debridement, graft placement, and instrumentation: a retrospective analysis in 19 cases. *J Neurosurg Spine* 2005; 3:450–458.
65. Elsberg C. *Tumors of the Spinal Cord and the Symptoms of Irritation and Compression of the Spinal Cord and Nerve Roots: Pathology, Symptomatology, Diagnosis and Treatment.* New York: Hoeber, 1925.
66. Raco A, Esposito V, Lenzi J, Piccirilli M, et al. Long-term follow-up of intramedullary spinal cord tumors: a series of 202 cases. *Neurosurgery* 2005; 56:972–981.
67. Constantini S, Miller D, Allen J, Rorke L, et al. Radical excision of intramedullary spinal cord tumors: surgical morbidity and long-term follow-up evaluation in 164 children and young adults. *J Neurosurg* 2000; 93:183–193.
68. Shrivastava R, Epstein F, Perin N, Post K, Gallo G. Intramedullary spinal cord tumors in patients older than 50 years of age: management and outcome analysis. *J Neurosurg Spine* 2005; 2:249–255.
69. Lonser RR OE. Microsurgical resection of spinal cord hemangioblastomas. *Neurosurgery* 2005; 57:372–376.
70. Sundaresan N, Galicich J, Lane J. Treatment of neoplastic epidural cord compression by vertebral body resection and stabilization. *J Neurosurg* 1985; 63:676–684.
71. Posner J. Management of central nervous system metastases. *Semin Oncol* 1977; 4:81–91.
72. Harrington K. Anterior cord decompression and spinal stabilization for patients with metastatic lesions of the spine. *J Neurosurg* 1984; 61:107–117.
73. Siegal T, Siegal T. Surgical decompression of anterior and posterior malignant epidural tumors compressing the spinal cord: a prospective study. *Neurosurgery* 1985; 17:424–432.
74. Patchell R, Tibbs P, Regine W, Payne R, et al. Direct decompressive surgical resection in the treatment of spinal cord compression caused by metastatic cancer: a randomised trial. *Lancet* 2005; 366:643–648.
75. Rosenblum B, Oldfield E, Doppman J, Di Chiro G. Spinal arteriovenous malformations: a comparison of dural arteriovenous fistulas and intradural AVM's in 81 patients. *J Neurosurg* 1987; 67:795–802.
76. Heros R, Debrun G, Ojemann R, Lasjaunias P, Naessens P. Direct spinal arteriovenous fistula: a new type of spinal AVM. Case report. *J Neurosurg* 1986; 64:134–139.
77. Jellema K, Sluzewski M, van Rooij W, Tijssen C, Beute G. Embolization of spinal dural arteriovenous fistulas: importance of occlusion of the draining vein. *J Neurosurg Spine* 2005; 2:580–583.
78. Van Dijk J, TerBrugge K, Willinsky R, Farb R, Wallace M. Multidisciplinary management of spinal dural arteriovenous fistulas: clinical presentation and long-term follow-up in 49 patients. *Stroke* 2002; 33: 1578–1583.
79. Corkill R, Mitsos A, Molyneux A. Embolization of spinal intramedullary arteriovenous malformations using the liquid embolic agent, onyx: a single-center experience in a series of 17 patients. *J Neurosurg Spine* 2007; 7:478–485.
80. Jallo G, Freed D, Zareck M, Epstein F, Kothbauer K. Clinical presentation and optimal management for intramedullary cavernous malformations. *Neurosurg Focus* 2006; 21.
81. Lee T, Arias J, Andrus H, Quencer R, et al. Progressive posttraumatic myelomalacic myelopathy: treatment with untethering and expansive duraplasty. *J Neurosurg* 1997; 86:624–628.
82. Wolfe S, Garg M, Cumberbatch N, Furst C, et al. Optimizing the transplant dose of a human neuronal cell line graft to treat SCI pain in the rat. *Neurosci Lett* 2007; 414:121–125.
83. Eaton M, Wolfe S, Martinez M, Hernandez M, et al. Subarachnoid transplant of a human neuronal cell line attenuates chronic allodynia and hyperalgesia after excitotoxic spinal cord injury in the rat. *J Pain* 2007; 8:33–50.
84. Guenot M, Lee J, Nasirinezhad F, Sagen J. Deafferentation pain resulting from cervical posterior rhizotomy is alleviated by chromaffin cell transplants into the rat spinal subarachnoid space. *Neurosurgery* 2007; 60:919–925.

40 Spasticity: Pathophysiology, Assessment, and Management

Melanie Adams
Audrey L. Hicks

Unequivocally, "spasticity" is understood to be among the symptoms resulting from injury to the upper motor neurons within the central nervous system (CNS) and is a common, but not an inevitable, sequelae of spinal cord injury (SCI) (1–3). Although much of what is known concerning the clinical features and management of spasticity of spinal cord origin has been derived from the study of individuals with spinal cord injury, many of the same principles apply to spasticity associated with the various nontraumatic spinal cord disorders. A commonly cited definition for spasticity was published by Lance in 1980 (4): "Spasticity is a motor disorder characterized by a velocity-dependent increase in tonic stretch-reflexes (muscle tone) with exaggerated tendon jerks, resulting from hyperexcitability of the stretch reflex, as one component of the upper motoneuron syndrome." There remains, however, discrepancy in the literature about the definition of spasticity; whereas some authors include symptoms such as clonus, hyperactive tendon reflexes, and spasms within the umbrella term "spasticity" (1, 5–8), others discuss these same symptoms as related to, but separate from, spasticity, which is defined by these authors as increased muscle tone (3, 9–12). Decq (2) recently has suggested the use of a modified definition, whereby spasticity, in general, is defined as a symptom of the upper motor neuron syndrome characterized by an exaggeration of the stretch reflex secondary to hyperexcitability of spinal reflexes. He follows by separating the various components of spasticity into sub-definitions: (1) *intrinsic tonic spasticity:* exaggeration of the tonic component of the stretch reflex (manifesting as increased tone), (2) *intrinsic phasic spasticity:* exaggeration of the phasic component of the stretch reflex (manifesting as tendon hyperreflexia and clonus), and (3) *extrinsic spasticity:* exaggeration of extrinsic flexion or extension spinal reflexes. Throughout the discussion to follow, the modified definition of spasticity suggested by Decq (2) will be utilized in order to clearly differentiate between the various spasticity-related symptoms that are experienced by individuals with SCI.

The literature has shown that 65%–78% of sample populations of individuals with chronic SCI ($\geq$1 year postinjury) have symptoms of spasticity (6, 13). Although unclear, it has been suggested that the American Spinal Injury Association (ASIA) classification of SCI (severity) and level of injury may predict the likelihood of developing spasticity; for example, in individuals with a cervical SCI, 93% of those diagnosed as ASIA A and 78% of those diagnosed as ASIA B–D reported having symptoms of spasticity, whereas in individuals with thoracic SCI, 72% of those diagnosed as ASIA A and 73% of those diagnosed as ASIA B–D reported symptoms of spasticity (6). The greater incidence of lower motor neuron injury associated with lower-level injuries results in a reduced tendency for spasticity development in these individuals (6, 13). Whereas the resolution of spinal shock may coincide with an increase in spasticity symptoms (13), there is no clear relationship between the presence of spasticity symptoms and time since injury beyond the spinal shock period (6).

Spasticity has the potential to negatively influence quality of life (QOL) through restricting activities of daily living (ADL); inhibiting effective walking and self-care; causing pain and fatigue; disturbing sleep; compromising safety; contributing to the development of contractures, pressure ulcers, infections, and a negative self-image; complicating the role of the caretaker; and impeding rehabilitation efforts (3, 6, 7, 14–18). Reports of problematic spasticity 1, 3, and 5 years following SCI occurred in 35%, approximately 31%, and approximately 27% of a sample of a population-based cohort of SCI survivors reported to the Colorado Spinal Cord Injury Early Notification System (19). Similarly, of those individuals reporting spasticity in the Stockholm Spinal Cord Injury Study, 40% reported their spasticity to be problematic, in that ADL were restricted and/or the spasticity caused pain (20). In a study by Sköld and colleagues (6), 20% and 4% of their total sample perceived their spasticity to restrict ADL and cause pain, respectively. Although Krawetz and Nance (21) have identified that severity of spasticity is among the factors that can reduce the degree to which walking is effective in functional ambulators after SCI, Norman and colleagues (22) have emphasized that, despite the common association between spasticity and clinical signs of abnormal gait, the nature of this relationship remains unclear. Furthermore, it must be noted that, although spasticity can have a negative impact on QOL, it has been suggested that symptoms of spasticity may increase stability in sitting and standing, facilitate the performance of some ADL and transfers, increase muscle bulk and strength of spastic muscles (thereby helping prevent osteopenia), and increase venous return (possibly diminishing the incidence of deep vein thrombosis) (11, 15–17). This potential for a beneficial effect of spasticity on QOL has a large impact upon decisions regarding its management (7, 17).

PATHOPHYSIOLOGY OF SPASTICITY AFTER SCI

In general, spasticity is classified as a symptom of the upper motor neuron syndrome, characterized by an exaggeration of the stretch reflex secondary to hyperexcitability of spinal reflexes (2). Upper motor neurons originate in the brain and brainstem and project to lower motor neurons within the brainstem and spinal cord (12). The lower motor neurons are of two types, both of which originate in the ventral horn of the spinal cord: (1) alpha motor neurons project to extrafusal skeletal fibers, and (2) gamma motor neurons project to intrafusal muscle fibers within the muscle spindle (12). With a lesion of the CNS comes interruption of the signals sent via the upper motor neurons to the lower motor neurons or related interneurons. Immediately following SCI, a period exists whereby the individual presents with flaccid muscle paralysis and loss of tendon reflexes below the level of the lesion (5). This period was first described in 1750, with the term "spinal shock" being introduced by Marshall Hall in 1850 (23). Spinal shock has been reported to end from 1–3 days (24) to a few weeks postinjury, with the gradual development of exaggerated tendon reflexes, increased muscle tone, and involuntary muscle spasms (5): the symptoms of spasticity. Recent animal research has suggested that a recovery of relatively normal motor neuron excitability and plateau potential behavior (sustained depolarizations), in the absence of normal inhibitory control to turn off plateaus and associated sustained firing, may be implicated in the recovery of spinal shock following SCI (25).

Intrinsic Tonic Spasticity

Decq (2) has differentiated intrinsic *tonic* spasticity (increased muscle tone) as that component of spasticity resulting from an exaggeration of the *tonic* component of the stretch reflex. Briefly, the stretch reflex is a monosynaptic reflex pathway that originates in the muscle spindles embedded parallel to the muscle fibers and travels via a Ia afferent to the spinal cord, where it synapses either first with interneurons, or directly with an alpha motor neuron innervating the muscle from which the stimulus originated (12). The tonic component of the stretch reflex associated with increased muscle tone results from a maintained stretch of the central region of the muscle fibers and the reflex is polysynaptic (12). Upon a sustained stretch, both type Ia and type II afferents (from secondary spindle endings) synapse with interneurons within the ventral horn of the spinal cord. Synapses of the interneurons with alpha motor neurons facilitate contraction in the muscle being stretched (12).

It is the hyperexcitability of this tonic stretch reflex that is commonly thought to result in increased muscle tone in response to passive stretch following SCI (3). This hypertonia is velocity dependent, with faster stretching velocities being associated with greater amounts of reflex activity (3). The development of tonic stretch

reflex hyperexcitability could be due to a lower threshold, an increased gain of the stretch reflex, or a combination of the two (26). The resultant increase in muscle tone is thought to be due to a combination of increased denervation hypersensitivity (2, 3, 5, 10, 27) and changed muscle properties (12, 14, 26, 28, 29). Denervation leads to an initial down-regulation of neuronal membrane receptors, followed by an up-regulation, with enhanced sensitivity to neurotransmitters (2). Gradual changes in muscle properties also occur following SCI, such as fibrosis, atrophy of muscle fibers, decrease in the elastic properties, decrease in the number of sarcomeres, accumulation of connective tissue, and alteration of contractile properties toward tonic muscle characteristics, which likely contribute to the increased passive tension (12, 14, 26, 28–30).

Intrinsic Phasic Spasticity

Intrinsic phasic spasticity encapsulates symptoms such as tendon hyperreflexia and clonus, and is due to exaggeration of the *phasic* component of the stretch reflex (2). Tendon hyperreflexia is identified as an exaggerated muscle response to an externally applied tap of deep tendons (7). Reduced presynaptic Ia inhibition is thought to play an important role in this hyperreflexia, as the occurrence of reduced presynaptic inhibition of group Ia fibers appears to correlate with the excitability of tendon reflexes (30).

Clonus has been defined as "involuntary rhythmic muscle contraction that can result in distal joint oscillation" (31) and most often occurs at the ankle (2, 7, 10). Clonus is elicited by a sudden rapid stretch of a muscle (32). The prevailing theory explaining the underlying mechanism responsible for clonus is that of recurrent activation of stretch reflexes (12, 31, 32). According to this theory, dorsiflexing the ankle causes activation of the Ia muscle spindle afferents and induces a reflex of the triceps surae, resulting in plantar flexion of the ankle (12, 31, 32). This reflex contraction is brief and essentially phasic, and it ceases rapidly (2). The muscle then relaxes, causing the ankle to be dorsiflexed once again, due either to gravity or to the sustaining of the stretch by an examiner (2). The result is a new stretch reflex, and so forth (2, 31). Ultimately, it is the disinhibition of the stretch reflex due to interruption of descending influences with SCI that is thought to cause exaggeration of the phasic stretch reflex pathway and, hence, clonus (3).

The second theory is that clonus is the result of activity of a central oscillator or generator within the spinal cord that rhythmically activates alpha motor neurons in response to peripheral events (31, 32). Beres-Jones and colleagues (31) have outlined observations that they feel support such a hypothesis: (1) reports of similar frequencies of clonus among ankle, knee, and wrist muscles, (2) observations that the clonus frequency is not entrained by the input frequency, which suggests that clonus cannot be solely stretch-mediated, (3) the finding that stimuli other than stretch evoke clonus, and (4) the observation of a refractory period following the clonic EMG burst, where tendon tap, H-reflex stimulation, and vibration fail to elicit an efferent response. Therefore, whereas reduced presynaptic inhibition of group Ia fibers appears to be among the contributing factors to tendon hyperreflexia, the underlying mechanism of clonus has not been clearly elucidated.

Extrinsic Spasticity

In addition to the various intrinsic factors that contribute to symptoms of spasticity, involuntary muscle spasms can also occur in response to a perceived noxious stimulus originating extrinsic to the muscle: *extrinsic spasticity* (2, 3, 7). Flexion spasms are the most common form of extrinsic spasticity and are triggered by afferent input from skin, muscle, subcutaneous tissues, and joints (collectively referred to as "flexor reflex afferents"). These flexor reflex afferents mediate the polysynaptic reflexes involved in the flexion withdrawal reflex (3, 29, 33). SCI can interrupt the inhibition of these reflexes by supraspinal pathways, making them hyperexcitable (2, 3, 34). In other words, whereas flexor withdrawal reflexes occur normally in individuals without SCI, upon disruption of normal descending influences, the threshold for the flexor withdrawal reflex may become lowered, the gain of the system may become raised, or both may occur together (3). A recent study has provided evidence to implicate plateau potentials in the spinal interneuronal and motoneuronal circuitry in the hyperexcitability of flexion withdrawal reflexes in individuals with chronic SCI (35). Intrasegmental polysynaptic connections cause the flexor reflex initiated by a localized stimulus to generate a widespread flexor spasm, which can appear as a coordinated flexion of all joints of the leg (29, 33).

ASSESSMENT OF SPASTICITY AFTER SCI

In order to make well-informed decisions about spasticity management and to evaluate the effects of treatment in people with SCI, it is necessary to apply measurement instruments shown to be valid and reliable in this population. It is important to note that, generally, there are poor correlations among different measures of spasticity and furthermore, that reductions in spasticity are not necessarily correlated with improvements in function (36–38). Therefore, it is now commonly suggested that a variety of different evaluation approaches be combined to obtain a representative assessment of spasticity (8, 36–40). The assessment of the symptoms of spasticity can be achieved using various methods performed by the examiner, including clinical, biomechanical, and electrophysiological techniques (26, 41–44). In addition, self-reporting of spasticity by the *individual* (41, 45) is also being recognized as an important adjunct, as examiner-based physical examination does not necessarily elicit spasticity in individuals who report the symptom (6), and individuals with SCI may experience spasticity in body segments that are not tested by an examiner (46).

Examiner-Administered Clinical Scales

Examiner-administered clinical scales of spasticity are often applied because of their simplicity and low financial cost. Widely used, the Ashworth Scale (47) (or Modified Ashworth Scale [48]) allows an examiner to numerically rate muscle hypertonicity in response to passive movement (Table 40.1). Recently, a clinical scale for the numerical rating of spasms and

Table 40.1   Clinical Scales of Spasticity

Scale/Scale Component	Grade	Description
Ashworth Scale	1	No increased tone.
Resistance to passive movement	2	Slight increase in tone, giving a "catch" when the affected part is moved in flexion or extension.
	3	More marked increase in tone but affected part is easily flexed.
	4	Considerable increase in tone, passive movement is difficult.
	5	Affected part is rigid in extension.
Modified Ashworth Scale	0	No increase in muscle tone.
Resistance to passive movement	1	Slight increase in muscle tone, manifested by a catch and release, or by minimal resistance at end ROM when affected part is moved in flexion or extension.
	1+	Slight increase in muscle tone, manifested by a catch, followed by minimal resistance throughout the remainder (>50%) of ROM.
	2	More marked increase in muscle tone through most of ROM but affected part is easily moved.
	3	Considerable increase in muscle tone, passive movement difficult.
	4	Affected part is rigid in flexion or extension.
SCATS—Clonus	0	No reaction.
Imposed dorsiflexion of plantarflexors	1	Mild: clonus < 3 sec.
	2	Moderate: clonus 3–10 sec.
	3	Severe: clonus > 10 sec.
SCATS—Flexor Spasms	0	No reaction.
Pinprick perturbation to bottom of foot	1	Mild: <10° flexion at knee and hip / extension of great toe.
	2	Moderate: 10° to 30° of flexion at knee and hip.
	3	Severe: >30° flexion at knee and hip.
SCATS—Extensor Spasms	0	No reaction.
Imposed extension of hip and knee	1	Mild: extensor spasm (displacement of patella) <3 sec.
	2	Moderate: extensor spasm (displacement of patella) 3–10 sec.
	3	Severe: extensor spasm (displacement of patella) >10 sec.

ROM = range of motion.

clonus has also become available (the Spinal Cord Assessment Tool for Spinal reflexes—SCATS); examiners rate each spasticity symptom in response to a standard perturbation (Table 40.1) (49). Evaluation of functional ability has also been employed, as the motor impairment resulting from spasticity may translate to impairment in the performance of daily tasks; although not direct assessments of spasticity, assessment of mobility, performance of ADL, and ease of caregiving may provide insight to the effects that spasticity can have during daily life (44, 50).

There are potential limitations of clinical assessment of spasticity related, in part, to the inherent subjectivity of these methods. There has been some question about the reliability and validity of the Ashworth and Modified Ashworth scales, depending on the assessment protocol and the population and limb(s) of interest (51, 52). Furthermore, when assessing functional tasks performed by individuals with spasticity and SCI, it can be difficult to determine whether an observed impairment is related to the presence of spasticity or to another motor complication. The assumed relationship between spasticity and activity limitation remains unproven, a challenge that is compounded and complicated by limited evidence for the impact of spasticity treatment on activity, participation, and independence (53).

Biomechanical Techniques

Pendulum testing with goniometry, isokinetic dynamometry, and biomechanical gait analysis have been used to quantify and characterize limb movement in individuals with spasticity (36, 41). During pendulum testing, the leg (that is hanging over the edge of a testing surface) of the individual with spasticity is extended and subsequently released, allowing it to swing freely. Identification of reduced swing by goniometry is considered to be reflective of the presence of spasticity (52). Only motion about the knee joint can be assessed with this test, however, and the ability of the individual to relax can influence the outcome. Isokinetic dynamometry allows for standardization during application of applied stretch and, therefore, allows for examination of the effects of velocity and amplitude on muscle hypertonicity in response to stretch (52). Analysis of gait using biomechanical techniques, although not an assessment of spasticity alone, has been performed in order to evaluate an important functional task that can be influenced by the presence of spasticity (21).

Electrophysiological Techniques

Electrophysiological assessment of affected skeletal muscle can help to identify underlying neurophysiologic abnormalities in spasticity. For example, the H-reflex is believed to represent the excitation of motor neurons via antidromic stimulation of Ia fibers (26, 54). For the H-reflex to be compared from session to session or between individuals, it is important to express the outcomes relative to the evoked response to the supramaximal stimulation of all motor neurons supplying the muscle of interest (M-wave) (54). It is also important to control for possible confounding factors, such as position of the assessed joint and of the head (54). The H/M ratio provides an indication of the excitability of the motor neuron pool (55, 56) and, therefore, tends to be increased in individuals with spasticity

(57). Electrophysiological assessment is only useful for the assessment of certain muscle groups (56), and there is some question as to the relevance of such measures to the clinical symptoms of spasticity and their impact on daily life (36, 41). Therefore, such techniques tend to be limited to research settings for the purpose of acquiring an understanding of the pathophysiology of spasticity symptoms.

Self-Ratings of Spasticity

Routine clinical work often includes self-evaluation or self-descriptions of the extent and impact of spasticity (46). Although limited, there are also examples of research studies that have begun to include self-ratings among the outcome measures of spasticity in the SCI population. Examples of these self-ratings include measures of both (1) spasticity severity, such as the visual analogue scale (58), the Penn Spasm Frequency Scale (59), single-item self-ratings of spasticity (60), and change in spasticity after treatment (61), and (2) spasticity impact, such as the relation of spasticity with function and pain (38) and single items to assess the helpful and problematic effects of spasticity on daily life (46). In general, assessment of the reliability and/or validity of these self-report measures is lacking. Recently developed, the Spinal Cord Injury Spasticity Evaluation Tool (SCI-SET) is a reliable and valid self-report measure of the impact of spasticity on daily life in people with SCI, taking into account both the problematic and potentially useful effects of spasticity (45). Because not all individuals with SCI who report *having* spasticity indicate that spasticity has an *impact* on their daily life (46), inclusion of various self-report tools may be the best approach.

MANAGEMENT OF SPASTICITY AFTER SCI

In contrast to the general lack of agreement within the literature about the definition and evaluation of spasticity, there appears to be widespread agreement that decisions regarding the management of spasticity must be based on the goal of achieving balance between the useful and detrimental effects of spasticity on an individual's QOL (2, 11, 17, 28). The management of spasticity may be desired for the reduction of "passive problems," such as preventing contracture, reducing pain, facilitating splint wearing, easing positioning and hygiene, and preventing contractures, or of "functional problems," including the individual's reduced ability to perform useful work with the motor system (10).

In general, no one treatment option will successfully manage spasticity in all individuals; the most conservative tactics are utilized first, with a progression from physical rehabilitation modalities to pharmacologic interventions, injection techniques, intrathecal baclofen, and lastly, surgery (16). In general, local treatments are used primarily by individuals with spasticity predominating in only certain muscle groups, such as occurs mainly in individuals with stroke or traumatic brain injury (28). In the case of SCI, the distribution of spasticity tends to be more diffuse, making regional or systemic treatment preferable (28). The decision of whether or not to treat spasticity and, if so, in what manner, is summarized nicely in a flow chart by Parziale and colleagues (Figure 40.1 [17]).

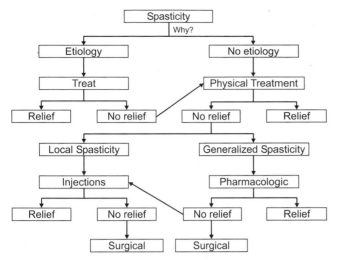

Figure 40.1 Spasticity management (adapted from Parziale and colleagues [17]).

Conservative/Physical Rehabilitation Management

It is generally agreed that physical therapy/rehabilitation is an essential component in the management of spasticity as a first line of defense, as well as in a long-term regimen during and after the implementation of pharmacological or surgical strategies (11, 18, 30). The goal of physical therapy is to diminish spasticity in order to allow expression of voluntary mobility and movements and/or to improve the comfort and independence in tasks related to QOL, such as transfers, dressing, and using the washroom (62). The literature on the conservative/physical treatment of spasticity is sparse and some have questioned the effectiveness of these management strategies (30). Table 40.2 summarizes the most common physical therapy approaches to spasticity management.

Pharmacologic Management

Systemic pharmacological treatments of spasticity symptoms are often prescribed in the SCI population (28). Most antispasticity medications can be grouped roughly into three functional categories: (1) "GABAergic"—drugs that act at interneurons that use the neurotransmitter gamma-aminobutyric acid (GABA) in the CNS (e.g., baclofen and diazepam), (2) alpha-2-adrenergic—those that act at alpha-2 receptors in the CNS (e.g., tizanidine and clonidine), and (3) peripheral acting—those that act at the neuromuscular level (e.g., dantrolene) (63). Numerous factors are taken into consideration when the physician and patient are deciding upon the role of pharmacologic management, including time since injury, onset of spasticity, severity, prognosis, available support system, cognitive status, concurrent medical problems, geographic location, symptom location, and financial issues (10). Each type of medication has potentially serious side effects and no single medication has a beneficial effect in all individuals (16, 28). Table 40.3 summarizes the most common pharmacologic agents, recommended dosages, and side effects.

Diazepam

GABA is an inhibitory neurotransmitter typically found in short interneurons (64). There are two types of GABA receptors, with diazepam acting at the $GABA_A$ receptor, the more prominent of the two (28). When GABA is released from a presynaptic membrane and binds to $GABA_A$ receptors on the postsynaptic membrane, chloride channels are opened, allowing chloride ions to flow into the postsynaptic membrane, hyperpolarizing the membrane (28). As a result, GABA inhibits action potential transmission. Presynaptic inhibition occurs when a GABAergic interneuron connects with the terminal of a Ia afferent and, therefore, decreases the excitability of the Ia afferent terminal and causes a decrease in the transmitter released from the Ia afferent to, ultimately, the motor neuron (28).

Diazepam is the most commonly used agent among the benzodiazepines to treat spasticity. Benzodiazepines, as a group, act by enhancing the efficiency of GABAergic transmission (10, 11, 14, 63). Diazepam does not directly mimic GABA (16, 28). Rather, it binds postsynaptically near $GABA_A$ receptors, facilitates GABA-mediated chloride conductance and, therefore, hyperpolarizes the membrane (10, 11, 16, 63). The result of diazepam administration is an increase in presynaptic inhibition of afferent neuronal terminals and, thus, a reduction of monosynaptic and polysynaptic reflexes (10, 14, 28). Diazepam is often mentioned as being most effective in the treatment of hyperactive reflexes and painful spasms in individuals with SCI (compared to individuals with stroke or multiple sclerosis) (10, 11, 14, 16). Functional measures, however, have been shown not to improve with diazepam treatment (10). Doses of diazepam typically begin at 2 mg twice daily, with a recommended maximum of 60 mg per day in divided doses (11, 16, 17, 41).

Negative side effects of diazepam include sedation, cognitive impairment, reduction of motor coordination, depression, impaired memory and attention, weakness, ataxia, and possible addiction (10, 11, 16). Anxiety; agitation; restlessness; irritability; tremor; muscle fasciculation and twitching; nausea; hypersensitivity to touch, taste, smell, light, and sound; insomnia; nightmares; and seizures have all been associated with abrupt cessation of diazepam (11, 28). Clonazepam (Klonopin®, Rivotril®), another benzodiazepine, causes less sedation than diazepam and has a slightly lower risk for dependence; it is typically used for the reduction of nighttime spasms (16, 28).

Baclofen

Unlike diazepam, baclofen is a structural analogue of GABA and an agonist of $GABA_B$ receptors (10, 11, 14, 16, 63). When baclofen binds to $GABA_B$ receptors both presynaptically and postsynaptically, monosynaptic and polysynaptic spinal reflexes are inhibited (10, 11, 14, 16, 63). Upon binding of baclofen presynaptically, influx of calcium into the presynaptic terminal is restricted, and neurotransmitter release in excitatory spinal pathways is decreased, leading to a decrease in alpha motor neuron activity (10, 11, 16, 28, 64). When baclofen binds to $GABA_B$ receptors on the postsynaptic membrane of a Ia afferent, potassium channels allow the flow of potassium out of the Ia afferent terminal, resulting in membrane hyperpolarization and, hence, interruption of action potential transmission (10, 11, 28).

Table 40.2   Physical Techniques in the Management of Spasticity

PHYSICAL THERAPY TECHNIQUE DESCRIPTION AND COMMENT ON EFFECTIVENESS	PURPOSE/SUGGESTED MECHANISMS
Positioning (16, 62) • In bed and during sitting. • Reports of clinical effectiveness; impact remains to be proven scientifically (15).	• Important to the maintenance of muscle length (16, 62).
Range of motion/stretching • Includes passive stretch and passive lengthening (15, 62). • Benefits may carry over for several hours (16, 17). • Effects remain to be quantified and the efficacy remains to be determined despite the clinical evidence for the benefits (15).	• Prevents contractures (28, 62). • Causes temporary reduction in intensity of muscle contraction in reaction to muscle stretch (62). • May cause plastic changes within the central nervous system and/or mechanical changes at the muscle, tendon, and soft-tissue level (15).
Weight-bearing • Using a tilt table or standing frame. • Benefits are greater than stretching alone and may persist into next day (9). • Effectiveness has been questioned (15).	• Prolonged stretch of ankle plantar flexor muscles (9, 15, 16). • Mechanism remains uncertain; suggested to include a modulating influence from cutaneous and joint receptor input to the spinal motor neurons, resulting in decreased excitability (9).
Muscle strengthening • Progressive addition of resistance to muscles with voluntary control (17, 62).	• Emphasis of balance of agonist and antagonist groups of muscles with voluntary control (17, 62).
Electrical stimulation • Various methods: stimulation to the antagonist muscle, application of tetanic contraction to the spastic muscle, functional electrical stimulation (FES), and transcutaneous electrical nerve stimulation (TENS) (15–17, 62). • Reports of beneficial effects between only 10 minutes and 3 hours[15,16,62]	• Stimulation of the antagonist muscle: augmentation of reciprocal inhibition of the spastic muscle (15). • Repetitive tetanic stimulation of spastic muscle: fatigue of the muscle due to repetitive tetanic stimulation (15). • FES: change the mechanical properties of a spastic joint by strengthening the antagonists of the spastic muscle or might decrease the hyperactivity of spastic muscles through reciprocal inhibition (74). • TENS: may involve the stimulation of large-diameter afferent fibers that travel from mechanoreceptors to the spinal cord (15).
Epidural spinal cord stimulation • For mild spasticity and incomplete lesions: stimulation below the level of the lesion found effective (spasms) (75). • For severe spasticity: stimulation of dorsal roots of the upper lumbar cord segment found effective (hypertonus and spasms) (76). • Shown to lack long-term effectiveness (77).	• May involve the activation of inhibitory networks within the spinal cord (76). • More strongly affected patients require stronger stimuli and/or higher frequencies (76).
Cold/heat application • Application of a cold pack or of a vapocoolant spray, or of superficial heat. • Following cold application: tendon reflex excitability and clonus may be reduced for a short period of time (e.g., <1 hr), allowing for intermittent improved motor function (16, 17). • Following heat application: subsequent passive stretch is facilitated (17).	• Cold: may cause slowing of nerve conduction, decrease in sensitivity of cutaneous receptors, and alteration of CNS excitability (15–17). • Heat: facilitation of uptake of released neurotransmitters and return of calcium to the sarcoplasmic reticulum (17).
Splinting/orthoses • Helpful in the continuous application of muscle stretch. • Use of splints is questioned (15).	• Enables long-term stretch (28, 62). • Joint can be maintained in a position that does not elicit a spasm (16).

Baclofen is a commonly used drug for spasticity in the SCI population (22). It has been reported to be particularly effective for reducing flexor spasms (10, 11, 28). The literature also suggests, however, that baclofen may have no positive effect on walking ability or the performance of ADL (10, 22, 28, 63). Similar to other muscle relaxants, baclofen may impair the ability of the patient to walk or stand (14, 16). Baclofen has been shown to be safe and effective for long-term use, with no evidence for tolerance (16). The initiating dose of baclofen is 5 mg twice or three times per day (11, 16, 17, 41). The maximum recommended dose of baclofen is 80 mg per day in divided doses (11, 16, 17, 41), although good effects have also been reported with much higher doses (200 to 300 mg per day) (16, 41).

Table 40.3 Commonly Used Pharmacologic Agents to Treat Spasticity

Agent	Starting Dosage	Maximum Recommended Dosage	Effects Adverse	Monitoring	Attention Special
Diazepam	2 mg/day or 5 mg at bedtime	40–60 mg/day in divided doses	Sedation, cognitive impairment, depression	Dependence potential	Withdrawal syndrome
Baclofen	5 mg/day increasing to 15 mg/day in 3 divided doses	80 mg/day in divided doses	Muscle weakness, sedation, fatigue, dizziness, nausea	Periodic liver function tests	Abrupt associated with seizures
Clonidine	0.1 mg/day	Not approved for spasticity; in patients with hypertension, doses as high as 2.4 mg in divided doses have been studied but rarely employed Usual dose in hypertension, 0.2–0.6 mg/day	Bradycardia, hypotension, dry mouth, drowsiness, constipation, dizziness, depression		Add-on agent Hypotension may result Not to be used with tizanidine
Tizanidine	2–4 mg/day	36 mg/day in divided doses	Drowsiness, dry mouth, dizziness, reversible dose-related elevated liver transaminases	Periodic liver function tests	Not to be used with antihypertensives or clonidine
Dantrolene	25 mg/day	400 mg/day in divided doses	Hepatotoxicity (potentially irreversible), weakness, sedation, diarrhea	Periodic liver function tests	Hepatotoxicity
Cyproheptadine	4 mg	36 mg/day in divided doses	Sedation, dry mouth		

Source: Adapted from Kita M, Goodkin DE. Drugs used to treat spasticity. *Drugs* 2000; 59:487–495.

Reported side effects of baclofen are related to CNS depression and include sedation, drowsiness, insomnia, fatigue, muscle weakness, ataxia, hypotonia, paresthesia, nausea, mental confusion, interference with attention and memory, hallucinations, and dizziness (10, 11, 14, 16, 28). Abrupt cessation of baclofen following chronic administration treatment has been associated with withdrawal symptoms such as auditory and visual hallucinations, anxiety, tachycardia, markedly increased or rebound spasticity, confusion, and seizures (11, 14, 17, 28).

Clonidine

Clonidine is a centrally acting alpha-2 adrenergic agonist commonly used to treat hypertension (10, 28). Alpha-2 receptors are located, among other regions, on presynaptic nerve terminals in the CNS and are termed adrenergic because they are involved in release of norepinephrine and acetylcholine (64). Generally speaking, an alpha-2-adrenergic agonist can bind to alpha-2 receptors, thereby preventing the normal action of norepinephrine to act as a neurotransmitter (64). Therefore, clonidine can act spinally

to reduce spasticity by enhancing alpha-2-mediated presynaptic inhibition of sensory afferents, thereby suppressing spinal polysynaptic reflexes (10, 16). Clonidine has been found to be associated with improved walking ability in individuals with incomplete SCI (e.g., longer cycles, increased treadmill speed, and more upright posture) (22, 65). Doses starting at 0.1 mg per day and increasing up to 0.2–0.6 mg per day have been suggested for the treatment of spasticity (11, 16, 41). Adverse effects include bradycardia, hypotension, dry mouth, drowsiness, constipation, dizziness, depression, orthostasis, lethargy, and syncope (10, 11, 14, 16).

Tizanidine

Tizanidine is an imidazole derivative and, like clonidine, is a centrally acting (spinally and supraspinally) alpha-2-adrenergic agonist (10, 11, 14, 28, 63). Therefore, it acts by inhibiting the release of excitatory amino acids from the presynaptic terminals of excitatory spinal neurons (10, 11). It may also facilitate the inhibitory neurotransmitter glycine (10, 11, 14). Tizanidine has been shown to reduce muscle tone and frequency of muscle spasms in individuals with SCI, but no increase in functional measures has been noted (10, 11, 14, 16, 28). Manual muscle testing while being treated with tizanidine has indicated that strength is not decreased (11, 16), although weakness has been reported (28). Doses of tizanidine have been suggested to begin at 2 mg per day (usually at night), with a gradual increase to a maximum of 36 mg per day in divided doses (11, 16, 17, 41). Adverse effects include dry mouth, sedation, drowsiness, dizziness, weakness, hypotension, nausea, and vomiting (10, 11, 14, 28). There is no evidence of dependency, withdrawal, or tolerance effects (16).

Dantrolene Sodium

Dantrolene sodium is the only oral medication that acts peripherally at the muscle tissue, rather than at the spinal cord level, to weaken muscles that are overexcited (10, 16, 28). It is a hydantoin derivative that inhibits muscle action potential–induced release of calcium from the sarcoplasmic reticulum to the active myosin fibers during muscle contraction by increasing the binding of calcium to the sarcoplasmic reticulum (10, 11, 14, 16, 28, 63). The result is interference with excitation-contraction coupling that is necessary to produce muscle contraction (11, 63). It has also been suggested that dantrolene may alter muscle spindle sensitivity by acting on the gamma motor neurons (10, 28). Dantrolene appears to have a greater effect on phasic than on tonic stretch reflexes and on fast twitch rather than slow twitch muscle fibers, with the clinical significance of these discrepancies remaining unclear (10, 11, 16, 28). There is evidence that individuals with SCI respond well to dantrolene sodium, with possible reductions in muscle tone, tendon reflexes, and clonus, and increases in range of motion (10, 28). Improvement in performance of ADL is less evident (28). Individuals with SCI are rarely treated with dantrolene, likely because its peripheral site of action results in its most common adverse effect: muscle weakness (10, 11, 14). Initiating doses of dantrolene are 25 mg per day with a gradual increase to the maximum recommended dose of 400 mg per day (11, 16, 17, 41). Other negative side effects of dantrolene include paresthesias, nausea, diarrhea, drowsiness, malaise, vomiting, and dizziness (10, 11, 16, 28). Liver toxicity, sometimes irreversible, is the most concerning possible adverse reaction with dantrolene, occurring in 1% to 2% of cases (10, 11, 14, 16, 28).

Cyproheptadine

Although less commonly reported among the drugs used to treat spasticity, cyproheptadine has been associated with an improvement in walking pattern in individuals with SCI (e.g., reduced need for manual assistance, increased treadmill speed, and reduced ankle clonus) (22, 66, 67). Cyproheptadine is a histamine and a serotonin antagonist, which is proposed to reduce spasticity via inhibition of motor neurons by "neutralizing the spinal and supraspinal serotoninergic excitatory inputs" (28). It is recommended that cyprohepatadine be initiated at 4 mg at bedtime, with a maximum recommended dose of 36 mg per day (16). Side effects may include sedation and dry mouth (28).

Cannabis

Tetrahydrocannabinol (THC), available in the drug dronabinol, is the main active ingredient in cannabis (16). Cannabinoids have been shown to have efficacy in treating spasticity and are currently being studied (10). Anecdotal reports by individuals with SCI have also revealed a beneficial effect of marijuana on the management of spasticity (28). Some literature supports the hypothesis that the relaxing effect of marijuana on muscles in patients with SCI-related spasticity is due to an antispastic effect, perhaps inhibition of polysynaptic reflexes, rather than to simply a general relaxation response (28, 63). A study investigating the effects of oral THC on spasticity in individuals with SCI used an initiating dose of 10 mg, with maximum daily doses ranging from 15 to 60 mg based on tolerance and achievement of treatment aim (68).

Intrathecal Administration of Baclofen

Intrathecal administration of baclofen combines the pharmacologic administration of baclofen with a surgical technique (16). In individuals who do not respond to oral administration of medications or to other techniques or who have had intolerable side effects from medications, intrathecal baclofen may be indicated and should be considered prior to surgical intervention (11, 16, 28). Briefly, a pump with reservoir (~4 inches in diameter) is surgically implanted in the subcutaneous tissue of the abdominal wall, allowing the direct delivery of the drug to the cerebrospinal fluid (11, 16, 28). A percutaneous puncture into the access port allows access to the pump reservoir (16). The dose and flow rate of baclofen are individualized through external computer communication with a computer chip within the pump (16).

Bypassing the blood–brain barrier allows as much as four times the concentration of baclofen to be delivered to the spinal cord with only 1% of the oral dose (11, 16). One of the main advantages is the reduction in negative systemic side effects compared to oral administration (16). The effectiveness of intrathecal baclofen as an anti-spasticity management therapy has been shown in individuals with SCI, with little data on functional improvements or QOL being reported (18, 28, 63, 69). Recent reviews have described the effects of intrathecal baclofen on reducing hypertonus, spasm frequency, reflex intensity, and/or spasticity-related discomfort, as well as improving QOL through allowing the individual to eat, feel, and look better and facilitating transfers, nursing care, sleep, and, in some, walking ability (18, 70).

The long-term effects of treatment with intrathecal baclofen are not yet known (18). Possible complications as a result of the surgical implantation of the pump include dislodgement, disconnection, migration, catheter kinking, blockage, pump failure, battery depletion, infection, and accidental overdose (11, 16). As with oral baclofen, drowsiness, dizziness, nausea, hypotension, headache, weakness, and withdrawal syndrome are possible side effects (16).

INJECTION TECHNIQUES— CHEMODENERVATION AGENTS

Injection for the purpose of local chemodenervation is one of the four possible routes of administration of a pharmacologic agent (with enteral, transdermal, and intrathecal administration being the other three) (10). The technique actually treats the upper motor neuron syndrome by simulating a lower motor neuron lesion (10). Injection techniques are preferred for treatment of focal spasticity and when agonist muscles have the functional strength once freed from antagonist spasticity (10, 16). One of the benefits of injection is the minimization of systemic side effects (10, 16). The injections can be applied as nerve blocks or motor point blocks, which are temporary, or as chemical neurolysis, which permanently destroys a portion of the nerve; whether an injection results in temporary or permanent chemodenervation depends on the concentration of the agent administered (28). The chemodenervation agents used include phenol, ethanol, and, more recently, botulinum toxin (10).

Phenol and Ethanol Injections

Local injections of phenol or ethanol are utilized less commonly in individuals with SCI; for a detailed review, see Gracies and colleagues (28). Briefly, administration of phenol or ethanol to a nerve trunk causes short-term effects similar to a local anesthetic: blocking of sodium channels reduces nerve depolarization (17). The mechanism of the longer-term nerve block involves denaturing of protein and fibrosis of neural tissue, causing disruption of nerve conduction and interruption of the reflex arc and, hence, muscle relaxation (15–17, 28). Recovery is variable between individuals, from a few days to months, as axons regenerate and reach motor end plates (Wallerian degeneration and regeneration) (15, 17, 28). A number of factors may influence the duration of the effects, including the concentration and volume used for injection, the site of the block, vascular complications, cutaneous side-effects, excessive motor weakness, sensory loss, wound infection, treatment variables after the block, and systemic side effects (28). A progressive reduction in motor unit activity tends to occur with repeated injections, however, as there is some permanent denervation with every injection (18).

There have been fewer reports of adverse effects of ethanol injection compared to phenol (28). Among the complications of these are injection site pain (particularly when intramuscular), vascular complications (phlebitis), permanent nerve damage, skin irritation, acute systemic effects (tremor, convulsions, central nervous system depression, and cardiovascular collapse), chronic dysesthesia, tissue necrosis, sensory dysesthesia, postblock pain due to an incomplete block, and muscular weakness (15–18, 28). Most individuals who undergo a phenol or an ethanol injection have preservation of motor strength (28).

Botulinum Toxin

Botulinum toxin is the most potent neurotoxin known to humans and is a product of the anaerobic bacteria *clostridium botulinum* (11, 16, 71). It was initially developed for clinical use in 1980 by an ophthalmologist to treat involuntary contractions and spasms of the eyelid muscles and "crossed eyes," and first was examined formally for the treatment of spasticity in 1989 (16, 71). Seven immunologically distinct toxins have been identified (type A through G) (11, 16), with types A and B being currently available for treatment (10). Compared with ethanol and phenol, the actions of which are mediated by their ability to denature protein at the nerve, the botulinum toxins manifest their effects at the neuromuscular junction, where they inhibit the release of acetylcholine from presynaptic motor axons (10, 11, 15, 16).

More specifically, botulinum toxin is injected into a muscle at its end plate region and spreads throughout the muscle and fascia approximately 30 mm (11, 14). The mechanism of action of botulinum toxin then occurs in three stages, through coordinated action of the heavy and light chain components of the toxin: (1) *binding:* botulinum toxin binds to the presynpatic neuron at the neuromuscular junction via the heavy chain (11, 14, 15), (2) *internalization:* the toxin is internalized into the cell by endocytosis, where the heavy chain forms a channel to allow the light chain to enter the cytosol, and (3) *inhibition of acetylcholine release:* the release of acetylcholine from presynaptic vesicles is inhibited (16). In step 3, the system involved in ACh exocytosis (the soluble N-ethlylmaleimide-sensitive fusion protein attachment protein receptor [SNARE] complex) is proteolytically cleaved in different critical sections by the different toxin types (10, 16, 71). Type A has been described as activating zinc-dependant proteolysis of SNAP-25 (a synaptosome-associated protein), whereas toxin B is active on synaptobrevin-2, a protein attached to the acetylcholine vesicle (involved in docking and fusion of the synaptic vesicle to the presynaptic membrane) (10, 15, 16, 71). With a disrupted SNARE complex, acetylcholine cannot be released from the presynaptic terminal, and muscle contraction is inhibited. Therefore, without affecting the synthesis of acetylcholine, botulinum toxin causes reversible chemical denervation atrophy, thereby weakening muscle (11, 14, 16).

Because of the complex mechanism of action, chemical denervation subject to botulinum toxin injection develops slowly over the course of 24 to 72 hours, peaking at 2 to 6 weeks (11, 14, 16). Collateral sprouting and slow reinnervation of chemically denervated nerve terminals allows for a gradual reversal of the clinical response (15, 16, 71). The duration of the botulinum toxin response can depend on a number of factors, including muscle size, the dose of the toxin administered, activity of the muscle, and perhaps factors including physiotherapy and bracing (15). In general, the duration has been reported to be between 2 and 6 months, with approximately 3 months being common (11, 14–16, 71).

Botulinum toxin has recently been touted "the pharmacological treatment of first choice for focal spasticity" (18) because of the evidence for its effectiveness in reducing pain and tone, and improving range of motion, function, brace tolerance, and walking ability (15, 18). Although botulinum toxin is not as commonly used in individuals with generalized spasticity (such as in SCI), improvements in pain, nursing care, hygiene, comfort, and functional activities can be induced by botulinum toxin injections into isolated muscle groups (16). Botulinum toxin therapy can also be combined with other treatments to enhance rehabilitation and function (16). In general, the literature indicates that botulinum toxin injections potentially can be useful in the treatment of spasticity secondary to SCI (16, 71, 72).

There have been very few reports of severe adverse reactions due to the injection of botulinum toxin (16). Any possible complications of botulinum toxin are often related to the blocking of acetylcholine release from parts of the autonomic nervous system by the toxin (dry mouth, reduced sweating), or to the spreading of the toxin beyond the desired area, resulting in excessive weakness (which is ultimately reversible) (11, 14–16, 71).

Surgical Management

As most surgeries performed on patients with spasticity take place at the muscle or the tendon, they are useful for treatment of focal spasticity with a purpose of improving function, correcting a deformity, or for cosmetic reasons (15, 73). Although there are and have been several possible surgical techniques to treat spasticity (for a review, see Chambers [73]), only those currently relevant to individuals with SCI will be discussed here. For example, selective rhizotomy (cutting of posterior roots to interrupt the peripheral reflex arc), although shown to be encouraging for children with cerebral palsy, is not frequently used in individuals with SCI (14, 16, 73). Intrathecal baclofen administration, often discussed under the topic of surgical management of spasticity (14, 16), has been discussed above; currently, it is considered to be the most commonly used and successful of the surgical treatments for spasticity in individuals with SCI (14).

Orthopedic surgical techniques (as opposed to neurosurgical) are reserved for only selected cases (15). A tenotomy, the release of a tendon from a severely spastic muscle, might be performed in individuals with severe spasticity and without voluntary movement (15). Tendon lengthening serves to reduce the pull on spastic muscles, thereby positioning the joints at a more natural and useful angle (15). A tendon transfer, moving the tendon attachment to bone closer to the muscle, is performed in muscles that have at least partial voluntary function, with the goal of allowing these muscles to produce useful movements (15). The mechanism of action of tendon lengthening and tendon transfers in terms of spasticity reduction is via alteration of the tension in the intrafusal muscle spindle, resulting in a decreased stimulus for further contraction and, hence, in theory, reduced spasticity (73). It has been reported, however, that the effects of tendon lengthening and tendon transfer on spasticity are variable and unpredictable (73).

CONCLUSION

Symptoms of spasticity are experienced by the majority of individuals with SCI and are a possible contributor to reduced QOL (3, 6, 7, 14–18). The emerging understanding of the different pathophysiologies of the various presentations of spasticity symptoms has led to a recent suggestion that distinct terminology be used for these symptoms (2). By considering intrinsic tonic spasticity, intrinsic phasic spasticity, and extrinsic spasticity as having distinct etiologies, the identification and classification of troubling symptoms becomes more specific, thereby allowing for more effective application of management strategies. Our growing understanding of spasticity in the SCI population is serving to further enhance the QOL of those who find their spasticity symptoms to be problematic.

*R*eferences

1. NINDS Spinal Cord Injury Information Page. http://www.ninds.nih.gov/health_and_medical/disorders/sci.htm, 2001.
2. Decq P. Pathophysiology of spasticity. *Neurochirurgie* 2003; 49:163–184.
3. Sheean G. The pathophysiology of spasticity. *Eur J Neurol* 2002; 9(Suppl 1):3–9.
4. Lance JW. The control of muscle tone, reflexes, and movement. Robert Wartenberg Lecture. *Neurology* 1980; 30:1303–1313.
5. Dietz V. Spastic movement disorder. *Spinal Cord* 2000; 38:389–393.
6. Sköld C, Levi R, Seiger A. Spasticity after traumatic spinal cord injury: nature, severity, and location. *Arch Phys Med Rehabil* 1999; 80:1548–1557.
7. St George CL. Spasticity: mechanisms and nursing care. *Nurs Clin North Am* 1993; 28:819–827.
8. Burridge JH, et al. Theoretical and methodological considerations in the measurement of spasticity. *Disabil Rehabil* 2005; 27:69–80.
9. Bohannon RW. Tilt table standing for reducing spasticity after spinal cord injury. *Arch Phys Med Rehabil* 1993; 74:1121–1122.
10. Elovic E. Principles of pharmacological management of spastic hypertonia. *Phys Med Rehabil Clin N Am* 2001; 12:793–816.
11. Kita M, Goodkin DE. Drugs used to treat spasticity. *Drugs* 2000; 59:487–495.
12. Lundy-Ekman L. *Neuroscience: Fundamentals for Rehabilitation.* Toronto: W.B. Saunders Company, 1998.
13. Maynard FM, Karunas RS, Waring WP III. Epidemiology of spasticity following traumatic spinal cord injury. *Arch Phys Med Rehabil* 1990; 71:566–569.
14. Burchiel KJ, Hsu FP. Pain and spasticity after spinal cord injury: mechanisms and treatment. *Spine* 2001; 26:S146–S160.
15. Jozefczyk PB. The management of focal spasticity. *Clin Neuropharmacol* 2002; 25:158–173.
16. Kirshblum S. Treatment alternatives for spinal cord injury related spasticity. *J Spinal Cord Med* 1999; 22:199–217.
17. Parziale JR, Akelman E, Herz DA. Spasticity: pathophysiology and management. *Orthopedics* 1993; 16:801–811.
18. Ward AB. Long-term modification of spasticity. *J Rehabil Med* 2003:60–65.
19. Johnson RL, Gerhart KA, McCray J, Menconi JC, Whiteneck GG. Secondary conditions following spinal cord injury in a population-based sample. *Spinal Cord* 1998; 36:45–50.
20. Levi R, Hultling C, Seiger A. The Stockholm Spinal Cord Injury Study: 2. Associations between clinical patient characteristics and post-acute medical problems. *Paraplegia* 1995; 33:585–594.
21. Krawetz P, Nance P. Gait analysis of spinal cord injured subjects: effects of injury level and spasticity. *Arch Phys Med Rehabil* 1996; 77:635–638.
22. Norman KE, Pepin A, Barbeau H. Effects of drugs on walking after spinal cord injury. *Spinal Cord* 1998; 36:699–715.
23. Bastian HC. On the symptomatology of total transverse lesions of the spinal cord, with special reference to the condition of the various reflexes. *Med Chir Trans (Lond)* 1890; 73:151–217.
24. Ditunno JF, Little JW, Tessler A, Burns AS. Spinal shock revisited: a four-phase model. *Spinal Cord* 2004; 42:383–395.
25. Bennett DJ, Li Y, Siu M. Plateau potentials in sacrocaudal motoneurons of chronic spinal rats, recorded in vitro. *J Neurophysiol* 2001; 86:1955–1971.
26. Sehgal N, McGuire JR. Beyond Ashworth: electrophysiologic quantification of spasticity. *Phys Med Rehabil Clin N Am* 1998; 9:949–979.
27. Noth J. Trends in the pathophysiology and pharmacotherapy of spasticity. *J Neurol* 1991; 238:131–139.
28. Gracies JM, Nance P, Elovic E, McGuire J, Simpson DM. Traditional pharmacological treatments for spasticity. Part II: general and regional treatments. *Muscle Nerve Suppl* 1997; 6:S92–S120.
29. Mayer NH. Clinicophysiologic concepts of spasticity and motor dysfunction in adults with an upper motoneuron lesion. *Muscle Nerve Suppl* 1997; 6:S1–S13.
30. Dietz V. Spinal cord lesion: effects of and perspectives for treatment. *Neural Plast* 2001; 8:83–90.
31. Beres-Jones JA, Johnson TD, Harkema SJ. Clonus after human spinal cord injury cannot be attributed solely to recurrent muscle-tendon stretch. *Exp Brain Res* 2003; 149:222–236.
32. Rossi A, Mazzocchio R, Scarpini C. Clonus in man: a rhythmic oscillation maintained by a reflex mechanism. *Electroencephalogr Clin Neurophysiol* 1990; 75:56–63.
33. Schmit BD, Benz EN, Rymer WZ. Reflex mechanisms for motor impairment in spinal cord injury. *Adv Exp Med Biol* 2002; 508:315–323.
34. Schmit BD, McKenna-Cole A, Rymer WZ. Flexor reflexes in chronic spinal cord injury triggered by imposed ankle rotation. *Muscle Nerve* 2000; 23:793–803.
35. Hornby TG, Rymer WZ, Benz EN, Schmit BD. Windup of flexion reflexes in chronic human spinal cord injury: a marker for neuronal plateau potentials? *J Neurophysiol* 2003; 89:416–426.
36. Pierson SH. Outcome measures in spasticity management. *Muscle Nerve Suppl* 1997; 6:S36–S60.
37. Sherwood AM, Graves DE, Priebe MM. Altered motor control and spasticity after spinal cord injury: subjective and objective assessment. *J Rehabil Res Dev* 2000; 37:41–52.
38. Priebe MM, Sherwood AM, Thornby JI, Kharas NF, Markowski J. Clinical assessment of spasticity in spinal cord injury: a multidimensional problem. *Arch Phys Med Rehabil* 1996; 77:713–716.
39. Robinson CJ, Kett NA, Bolam JM. Spasticity in spinal cord injured patients: 2. Initial measures and long-term effects of surface electrical stimulation. *Arch Phys Med Rehabil* 1988; 69:862–868.
40. Hsieh JTC, Wolfe DL, Connolly S, Townson AF, Curt A, Blackmer J, Sequeira K, Aubut J. Spasticity following spinal cord injury. In: Eng JJ,

Teasell RW, Miller WC, Wolfe DL, Townson AF, Aubut J, Abramson C, Hsieh JTC, Connolly S, eds. *Spinal Cord Injury Rehabilitation Evidence.* Vancouver, 2006; 21.1–21.56.

41. Elovic EP, Simone LK, Zafonte R. Outcome assessment for spasticity management in the patient with traumatic brain injury: the state of the art. *J Head Trauma Rehabil* 2004; 19:155–177.

42. Damiano DL, et al. What does the Ashworth Scale really measure and are instrumented measures more valid and precise? *Dev Med Child Neurol* 2002; 44:112–118.

43. Haas BM, Crow JL. Towards a clinical measurement of spasticity? *Physiotherapy* 1995; 81:474–479.

44. Hinderer SR, Gupta S. Functional outcome measures to assess interventions for spasticity. *Arch Phys Med Rehabil* 1996; 77:1083–1089.

45. Adams MM, Martin Ginis KA, Hicks AL. Spinal Cord Injury Spasticity Evaluation Tool (SCI-SET): development and evaluation. *Arch Phys Med Rehabil* 2007; 88:1185–1192.

46. Lechner HE, Frotzler A, Eser P. Relationship between self- and clinically rated spasticity in spinal cord injury. *Arch Phys Med Rehabil* 2006; 87:15–19.

47. Ashworth B. Preliminary trial of carisoprodol in multiple sclerosis. *Practitioner* 1964; 192:540–542.

48. Bohannon RW, Smith MB. Interrater reliability of a modified Ashworth scale of muscle spasticity. *Phys Ther* 1987; 67:206–207.

49. Benz EN, Hornby TG, Bode RK, Scheidt RA, Schmit BD. A physiologically based clinical measure for spastic reflexes in spinal cord injury. *Arch Phys Med Rehabil* 2005; 86:52–59.

50. Platz T, Eickhof C, Nuyens G, Vuadens P. Clinical scales for the assessment of spasticity, associated phenomena, and function: a systematic review of the literature. *Disabil Rehabil* 2005; 27:7–18.

51. Haas BM, Bergstrom E, Jamous A, Bennie A. The inter rater reliability of the original and of the modified Ashworth scale for the assessment of spasticity in patients with spinal cord injury. *Spinal Cord* 1996; 34:560–564.

52. Biering-Sorensen F, Nielsen JB, Klinge K. Spasticity-assessment: a review. *Spinal Cord* 2006; 44:708–722.

53. Pandyan AD, et al. Spasticity: clinical perceptions, neurological realities and meaningful measurement. *Disabil Rehabil* 2005; 27:2–6.

54. Voerman GE, Gregoric M, and Hermens HJ. Neurophysiological methods for the assessment of spasticity: the Hoffmann reflex, the tendon reflex, and the stretch reflex. *Disabil Rehabil* 2005; 27:33–68.

55. Barboi AC, Barkhaus PE. Electrodiagnostic testing in neuromuscular disorders. *Neurol Clin* 2004; 22:619–641.

56. Fisher MA. H reflexes and F waves: fundamentals, normal and abnormal patterns. *Neurol Clin* 2002; 20:339–360.

57. Bischoff C. Neurography: late responses. *Muscle Nerve* 2002; Suppl 11:S59–S65.

58. Skold C. Spasticity in spinal cord injury: self- and clinically rated intrinsic fluctuations and intervention-induced changes. *Arch Phys Med Rehabil* 2000; 81:144–149.

59. Penn RD. Intrathecal baclofen for severe spasticity. *Ann N Y Acad Sci* 1988; 531:157–166.

60. Hagenbach U, et al. The treatment of spasticity with Delta(9)-tetrahydrocannabinol in persons with spinal cord injury. *Spinal Cord* 2007; 45:551–562.

61. Seib TP, Price R, Reyes MR, Lehmann JF. The quantitative measurement of spasticity: effect of cutaneous electrical stimulation. *Arch Phys Med Rehabil* 1994; 75:746–750.

62. Albert T, Yelnik A. Physiotherapy for spasticity. *Neurochirurgie* 2003; 49:239–246.

63. Rode G, Maupas E, Luaute J, Courtois-Jacquin S, Boisson D. Medical treatment of spasticity. *Neurochirurgie* 2003; 49:247–255.

64. Rang HP, Dale MM, Ritter JM, Gardner P. *Pharmacology.* New York: Churchill Livingstone, 1995.

65. Stewart JE, Barbeau H, Gauthier S. Modulation of locomotor patterns and spasticity with clonidine in spinal cord injured patients. *Can J Neurol Sci* 1991; 18:321–332.

66. Fung J, Stewart JE, Barbeau H. The combined effects of clonidine and cyproheptadine with interactive training on the modulation of locomotion in spinal cord injured subjects. *J Neurol Sci* 1990; 100:85–93.

67. Wainberg M, Barbeau H, Gauthier S. The effects of cyproheptadine on locomotion and on spasticity in patients with spinal cord injuries. *J Neurol Neurosurg Psychiatry* 1990; 53:754–763.

68. Hagenbach U, et al. The treatment of spasticity with Delta9-tetrahydrocannabinol in persons with spinal cord injury. *Spinal Cord* 2007; 45:551–562.

69. Korenkov AI, Niendorf WR, Darwish N, Glaeser E, Gaab MR. Continuous intrathecal infusion of baclofen in patients with spasticity caused by spinal cord injuries. *Neurosurg Rev* 2002; 25:228–230.

70. Emery E. Intrathecal baclofen. Literature review of the results and complications. *Neurochirurgie* 2003; 49:276–288.

71. Barnes M. Botulinum toxin—mechanisms of action and clinical use in spasticity. *J Rehabil Med* 2003: 56–59.

72. Al Khodairy AT, Gobelet C, Rossier AB. Has botulinum toxin type A a place in the treatment of spasticity in spinal cord injury patients? *Spinal Cord* 1998; 36:854–858.

73. Chambers HG. The surgical treatment of spasticity. *Muscle Nerve Suppl* 1997; 6:S121–S128.

74. Mirbagheri MM, Ladouceur M, Barbeau H, Kearney RE. The effects of long-term FES-assisted walking on intrinsic and reflex dynamic stiffness in spastic spinal-cord-injured subjects. *IEEE Trans Neural Syst Rehabil Eng* 2002; 10:280–289.

75. Barolat G, et al. Epidural spinal cord stimulation in the management of spasms in spinal cord injury: a prospective study. *Stereotact Funct Neurosurg* 1995; 64:153–164.

76. Pinter MM, Gerstenbrand F, Dimitrijevic MR. Epidural electrical stimulation of posterior structures of the human lumbosacral cord: 3. Control of spasticity. *Spinal Cord* 2000; 38:524–531.

77. Midha M, Schmitt JK. Epidural spinal cord stimulation for the control of spasticity in spinal cord injury patients lacks long-term efficacy and is not cost-effective. *Spinal Cord* 1998; 36:190–192.

41 Autonomic Dysfunction in Spinal Cord Disease

Brenda Mallory

Autonomic dysfunction is a universal problem clinicians will encounter in caring for persons with spinal cord disease. The autonomic nervous system (ANS) regulates visceral function and maintains internal homeostasis through its innervation of smooth muscle, cardiac muscle, and glandular tissue (1). The ANS is deranged by spinal cord injury (SCI). The derangement of ANS function in SCI results not only from the loss of normal supraspinal control of the ANS, but also from changes caused by the synaptic reorganization and neuronal plasticity of the damaged spinal cord. An understanding of the three components of the ANS (sympathetic, parasympathetic, and enteric), their function, and their supraspinal, spinal, and peripheral organization is essential for appreciating autonomic dysfunction in persons with SCI.

ANATOMY OF THE AUTONOMIC NERVOUS SYSTEM

The parasympathetic and sympathetic nerves comprise an efferent pathway consisting of preganglionic and postganglionic neurons. Preganglionic neurons (PGNs) are located in either the brainstem or the spinal cord. Postganglionic neurons are located in a number of ganglia and plexuses outside of the central nervous system (CNS). The second-order postganglionic neurons synapse upon smooth and cardiac muscle and also control glandular secretion. In addition to preganglionic and postganglionic neurons, the control systems of the ANS also involve (1) supraspinal controlling and integrative neuronal centers, (2) supraspinal, spinal, ganglionic, and peripheral interneurons, and (3) afferent neurons. Afferent neurons have cell bodies in the dorsal root ganglia or cranial nerve somatic sensory ganglia (1). Afferent axons travel in somatic peripheral nerves or along with autonomic efferent nerves.

The parasympathetic preganglionic component of the ANS has a supraspinal and spinal portion. Parasympathetic nerves have also been referred to as craniosacral nerves and cholinergic nerves. Parasympathetic PGNs are found in four parasympathetic brainstem nuclei: the nucleus Edinger-Westphal, the superior salivatory nucleus, the inferior salivatory nucleus, and the dorsal vagal complex of the medulla. Their axons exit via cranial nerves 3 (oculomotor), 7 (facial nerve), 9 (glossopharyngeal nerve), and 10 (vagus nerve), respectively.

Preganglionic parasympathetic efferent axons in the oculomotor nerve synapse in the ciliary ganglion and postganglionic axons travel in the short ciliary nerve and innervate the pupiloconstrictor fibers of the iris and the ciliary muscle. Preganglionic parasympathetic efferent axons exit in the facial nerve to the level of the geniculate ganglion (sensory ganglion of the facial nerve), and then branch to form the greater superficial petrosal nerve and synapse in the pterygopalatine ganglion. Postganglionic axons from the pterygopalatine ganglion join the maxillary nerve and innervate the lacrimal glands and the blood vessels of the palate, nasopharynx, and sinuses. Other preganglionic axons in the facial nerve travel in the chorda tympani and join the lingual nerve to synapse in the submandibular ganglion and innervate the submandibular and sublingual glands. Preganglionic axons in the glossopharyngeal nerve branch at the level of the jugular foramen and course to the lesser superficial petrosal nerve, which exits the foramen ovale with the third division of the trigeminal nerve to synapse on postganglionic neurons in the otic ganglia. Postganglionic axons from the otic ganglia form the auriculotemporal nerve and innervate the parotid gland. The dorsal vagal complex consists of the nucleus ambiguus and the dorsal motor nucleus. Preganglionic parasympathetic efferent axons in the vagus nerve synapse with postganglionic parasympathetic neurons in ganglia on or near the organs they innervate (heart, bronchi, esophagus, stomach, pancreas, kidney, and intestine to the splenic flexure of the colon) (Figure 41.1).

Parasympathetic PGNs are also found in the intermediolateral cell column (IML) of the sacral spinal cord in segments S2–S4 and exit the CNS via the sacral ventral roots and the spinal nerves and then continue to the pelvic viscera as the pelvic nerve. The sacral preganglionic parasympathetic efferent axons of the pelvic nerve synapse with postganglionic parasympathetic neurons in the ganglia of the pelvic plexus. Postganglionic

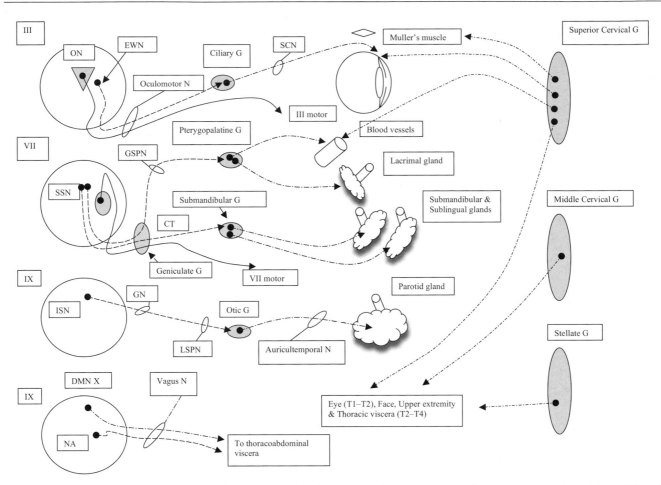

Figure 41.1   Autonomic nervous system of the head and neck. ON = oculomotor nerve nucleus; EWN = nucleus Edinger-Westphal; SSN = superior salivatory nucleus; GSPN = greater superficial petrosal nerve; SCN = short ciliary nerve; CT = chorda tympani; G = Ganglion; GN = glossopharyngeal nerve; ISN =inferior salivatory nucleus and dorsal vagal complex of the medulla; DMN = dorsal motor nucleus of the vagus nerve; T = thoracic; NA = nucleus ambiguus; III = oculomotor nerve; VII = facial nerve; IX = glossopharyngeal nerve; X = vagus nerve.

axons innervate the descending colon, rectum, urinary bladder, and sexual organs (1).

The sympathetic preganglionic component of the ANS is purely spinal. Sympathetic preganglionic neurons (SPNs) are found in the IML of the thoracic and lumbar spinal cord in segments T1–L2 (1) and exit the CNS via the thoracolumbar ventral roots. The sympathetic segmental outflow can vary if the brachial plexus is prefixed or postfixed, so that the outflow can start as high as C8 or as low as T2 and end at L1 or L3 (1). The thinly myelinated preganglionic fibers exit via the ventral roots as the white rami communicantes. Many sympathetic preganglionic fibers will synapse in the paravertebral ganglia, which are paired, and lie next to the spine from the cervical to the sacral segments. There are three cervical paravertebral ganglia, the superior cervical ganglion, the middle cervical ganglion, and the stellate ganglion. There are usually eleven thoracic ganglia, four lumbar ganglia, and four or five sacral ganglia (1). At the level of the coccyx, the two sympathetic ganglia chains join in the single ganglion impar (1). Sympathetic preganglionic axons can synapse in paravertebral ganglia at the segment of their exit or can pass

up or down several segments of the sympathetic chain before synapsing. One sympathetic preganglionic axon will synapse with several postganglionic neurons. Postganglionic axons are unmyelinated, leave the paravertebral ganglia via the gray rami communicantes, and exit via the segmental spinal nerves.

Some sympathetic preganglionic axons pass through the paravertebral ganglia without synapsing and constitute the splanchnic nerves that innervate three prevertebral ganglia: (1) the celiac ganglion, (2) the superior mesenteric ganglion, and (3) the inferior mesenteric ganglion, as well as the adrenal medulla. Sympathetic nervous system (SNS) stimulation of the adrenal medulla results in the release of norepinephrine (NE) and epinephrine (E). NE excites α-receptors with only slight excitation to beta-receptors. E excites both alpha- and beta-receptors (1). Postsynaptic axons from the prevertebral ganglia course to the abdominal and pelvic viscera as the hypogastric, splanchnic, and mesenteric plexuses.

Sweat glands, piloerector muscles, and most small blood vessels receive only sympathetic innervation. Diffuse SNS discharge results in pupillary dilatation, increased heart rate, and contractility, bronchodilation, vasoconstriction of the mesenteric circulation, and vasodilation of skeletal muscle arterioles. This is the "fight or flight" defense reaction.

There is evidence that the supraspinal inputs to SPNs come from five main brain regions and include the rostral ventrolateral medulla, the rostral ventromedial medulla, the caudal raphe nuclei, the A5 region, and the paraventricular nucleus of the hypothalamus (2). Although the SNS is capable of producing highly selective responses, the specific supraspinal neurons that are responsible for a given response are not well understood (2).

SPINAL CORD REFLEX ORGANIZATION OF THE AUTONOMIC NERVOUS SYSTEM

The SNS and the parasympathetic nervous system (PNS) regulate visceral function largely by autonomic reflexes (1). Experimentally, a variety of distinct autonomic reflex pathways can be elicited by electrical stimulation of afferent nerves. These reflexes are characterized by their afferent spinal input and by the autonomic efferent pathway function. Some of these reflexes are relayed at the level of the spinal cord, whereas others require a relay in supraspinal structures. The relay in the CNS can be modulated by a wide range of afferent inputs as well as by descending inputs such as those from the hypothalamus. The details of the integration of autonomic spinal reflex pathways with descending supraspinal systems are largely unknown (3). The control circuits in the spinal cord consist of PGNs; spinal interneurons, both segmental and propriospinal (project over many spinal segments); and their synaptic connections (3). The various autonomic control circuits in the spinal cord interact with afferent spinal input from the periphery and descending spinal pathways. In a recent review, Schramm presents evidence that spinal sympathetic interneurons have a limited role in sympathetic regulation when the spinal cord is intact (4). However, following SCI, spinal sympathetic interneurons become important in generating ongoing activity in sympathetic nerves and in mediating segmental and intersegmental sympathetic reflexes (4).

Central regulation of autonomic function occurs chiefly in the hypothalamus, brainstem, and spinal cord. Unlike the relay of the central message to the target organ in the somatic motor system, the autonomic target can be innervated by more than one final common autonomic pathway. In addition, the central autonomic message may be changed quantitatively in the autonomic ganglia or at the neuroeffector junction by neural, hormonal, or other processes (3). Following interruption of the spinal cord, there is residual autonomic function of the isolated spinal cord associated with thermoregulation, evacuation of the urinary bladder and colon, regulation of sexual function, regulation of blood pressure, and other reflexes.

AUTONOMIC PHARMACOLOGY

Glutamate, gamma-aminobutyric acid (GABA), and glycine are the amino acid neurotransmitters that are present in the axons of the supraspinal neurons and spinal neurons that synapse on SPNs (5). Catecholamines (E and NE), as well as serotonin (5-hydroxytryptamine [5-HT]), derived from supraspinal neurons, also have inputs on the SPNs. Axons containing a number of neuropeptides also form synapses either in the IML or on identified SPNs (5).

Acetylcholine (Ach) is the neurotransmitter for all preganglionic axons, both parasympathetic and sympathetic. Ach is also the neurotransmitter for all postganglionic parasympathetic axons. NE is the neurotransmitter released by most sympathetic postganglionic axons, with some exceptions such as those that innervate sweat glands and release Ach.

Ach receptors are of two types: muscarinic and nicotinic. Preganglionic axons synapse upon nicotinic receptors, and postganglionic axons synapse upon muscarinic receptors. There are five identified subtypes of muscarinic receptors, M1–M5. Muscarinic receptors are involved in peripheral and central cholinergic responses. Information on the subtype selectivity of muscarinic agonists and antagonists, as well the pattern of expression of muscarinic subtypes in the many tissues of the body, continues to grow.

The M3 receptor has been shown to mediate the direct contractile response in human detrusor muscle tissue taken from individuals with neurogenic and idiopathic detrusor overactivity and those with normal bladder function. The M2 receptor also appears to mediate detrusor contraction by an indirect and/or possibly a minor direct effect (6). Compared to tolterodine and oxybutynin, new muscarinic receptor antagonists, darifenacin, solifenacin, and trospium, have a lower incidence of adverse events and comparable efficacy rates in the treatment of the overactive bladder (7). See Table 41.1.

Although salivation is primarily mediated by M3 receptors, M1 receptors are required for maximum salivation. The low drop-out rates due to dry mouth (<3%) during darifenacin treatment suggest that sparing the M1 receptors in the salivary glands may be enough to limit the severity of dry mouth. M2 and M3 receptors are thought to be the most functionally important muscarinic receptors in the human gut (6). The M3 receptor is the most prevalent (60%–75%) in the human eye, which contains all five muscarinic receptor subtypes. In animal studies, the M3 and M5 receptors control iris sphincter contraction (6). The predominant muscarinic receptor within the mammalian heart is the M2 subtype, which modulates pacemaker activity and atrioventricular conduction (8).

NE receptors are divided into alpha (α) and beta (β) adrenoceptors (AR). Although there are many exceptions, α-AR are excitatory, and β-AR are inhibitory. α-AR are divided into α1-AR and α2-AR based on the relative potency of certain alpha agonists and antagonists (9). α-AR are further divided into α1A-, α1B-, and α1D-AR. α2-AR are further divided into α2A-, α2B-, and α2C-AR. α1-AR are coupled to a G protein to stimulate phospholipase C, which promotes the hydrolysis of phosphatidylinositol bisphosphate, producing inositol triphosphate

Table 41.1   Muscarinic Receptor Antagonists

MUSCARINIC ANTAGONIST	SELECTIVITY	TISSUE
Tolterodine (Detrol)	Nonselective	Bladder
Oxybutynin (Ditropan)	Nonselective	Bladder
Darifenacin (Enablex)	M3-selective	Bladder
Solifenacin (Vesicare)	M3-selective	Bladder
Trospium (Sanctura)	Nonselective	Bladder
Tiotropium (Spiriva)	Nonselective	Lung

and diacyldlycerol, which are second messengers that mediate intracellular Ca2+ release and smooth muscle contraction (9). α1-AR are mostly postsynaptic and excitatory, and α2-AR are usually presynaptic and inhibitory. Presynaptic α2-AR inhibit the release of NE from sympathetic axons and result in sympathetic inhibition.

β-AR are divided into β1-, β2 -, and β3-AR. β2-AR that do not respond to NE can be considered as hormone receptors for circulating E from the adrenal medulla and are not functionally innervated by sympathetic nerves (9). Smooth muscles from different tissues have specific patterns of β-AR subtypes, and multiple subtypes of β-adrenoceptor are often coexpressed in smooth muscle. Airway smooth muscle expresses predominantly β2-adrenoceptors. β3-AR are important in gastrointestinal tract smooth muscle, except for the esophageal smooth muscle, which expresses β1-AR. The urinary bladder has large quantities of the β3-AR (10).

Peptides coexist in individual neurons with the classical Ach and NE transmitters. Dozens of neuropeptides have been identified, and one of their functions is to augment the action of the classical transmitter.

CARDIOVASCULAR DYSFUNCTION

In high SCI, the SNS is decentralized, and the isolated spinal cord is no longer under control from supraspinal structures. The cardiovascular results of SNS decentralization range from the potentially life-threatening autonomic dysreflexia (AD), reflex bradycardia, and cardiac arrest to a low resting blood pressure, orthostatic hypotension, limited cardiovascular responses to exercise, and changes in the skin microcirculation (11). See Table 41.2.

Table 41.2 **Cardiovascular Effects of Quadriplegia**

	ACUTE QUADRIPLEGIA	CHRONIC QUADRIPLEGIA
MAP	↓	↓
Cardiac output	↓	↓
Total peripheral vascular resistance	↓	Normal or ↑
Resting heart rate	↓	↓
Peak exercise heart rate		↓
Orthostatic hypotension	+	+/−
Orthostatic tachycardia	+	+/−
Resting plasma catecholamines		↓
Resting plasma renin		↑
Resting plasma aldosterone		↑
Nocturnal plasma aldosterone		No ↑
Autonomic dysreflexia	+/−	+/−
Sympathetic nerve activity (in animal model)	↓	
Nocturnal urine output		↑
Urinary sodium excretion		↓
Extracellular fluid compartment		↑

Arterial pressure is regulated by a rapid neuronal mechanism, as well as by slower hormonal and renal control systems (12). Supraspinal vasomotor centers generate the resting tone of sympathetic nerve discharges, whereas reflex activity, central respiratory modulation, and brainstem and spinal neural circuits all may generate the periodic discharges of sympathetic nerves (12). The descending input to SPNs involved in regulating resistance vessels is predominantly sympathoexcitatory from the glutamatergic neurons of the rostroventrolateral medulla (RVLM). There are also sympathoinhibitory descending inputs from GABAergic, glycinergic, and adrenergic neurons onto SPNs, although it is thought that inhibiting excitatory inputs, such as those from the RVLM, largely produce SPN inhibition (12). In humans, the pathways from the lower brainstem to the SPNs run in the dorsal aspect of the lateral funiculus of the white matter (13).

SPNs that project to the heart are located in spinal cord segments T1 to T4, whereas the SPNs for the peripheral vasculature are found mainly in spinal cord segments T1 to L2 (14). A small proportion of the neurons in the IML are interneurons. The cholinergic SPNs innervate the adrenal medulla as well as noradrenergic neurons in sympathetic ganglia, which in turn innervate blood vessels and the heart. The heart is also innervated by three branches of the vagus nerve (superior cervical cardiac, inferior cervical cardiac, thoracic cardiac). Preganglionic efferent parasympathetic axons in these branches form synapses with neurons in the ganglia of the cardiac plexus.

The adrenoceptors that are innervated by the SNS and contribute to basal vascular tone are α1-AR in arteries, α1- and β1-AR in the heart, and α2- and β2-AR in the veins (9). α1-AR are the most important in the maintenance of vascular tone by the SNS. Although the α1-AR subtype mediating vasoconstriction in humans is unclear, in rats, α1A-AR are prominent, and α1B-AR and α1D-AR are involved in the responses to exogenous agonists (9).

Afferent fibers from the heart project via either the sympathetic cardiac nerves or the vagus nerve (15). Parasympathetic afferent fibers from sensory receptors in the heart are conveyed via the cardiac branches of the parasympathetic vagus nerve, have cell bodies in the jugular and nodose ganglia, and project centrally to the nucleus tractus solitarius (NTS). There is also evidence in animals that a portion of vagal afferent neurons in the nodose ganglion project to the upper cervical spinal cord via a supraspinal pathway not involving dorsal root ganglia (16) The sympathetic afferents course in the inferior cervical and thoracic sympathetic cardiac nerves, then via white rami communicantes to cell bodies in the dorsal root ganglia (T1 to T5).

The traditional view is that afferent sympathetic cardiac fibers mediate cardiac nociception, and afferent vagal cardiac fibers mediate cardiovascular reflexes (15). However, vagal afferent fibers may have some role in the mediation of cardiac nociception, such as pain referred to the head and neck (perhaps via afferent projections to the cervical spinal cord), and afferent sympathetic fibers may also transmit some cardiovascular reflexes.

The arterial baroreflex is the most important mechanism for the CNS regulation of arterial pressure (12). The arterial or high-threshold baroreceptors are located in carotid sinus and walls of the aortic arch. The cardiac or low-threshold baroreceptors are located in the atria and ventricles. A decrease in arterial blood pressure inhibits firing, and a rise in blood pressure increases firing in afferent arterial baroreceptor fibers that project through the vagus and glossopharyngeal nerves, with cell bodies in the petrosal and nodose ganglia, to terminate in the NTS of the medulla (12). A fall in arterial blood pressure activates three limbs of the baroreceptor response: (1) a reduction of excitatory drive from the NTS to the nucleus ambiguus, which increases heart rate by slowing vagal firing, (2) a reduction of excitation on inhibitory interneurons in the caudal ventrolateral medulla that project to neurons in the RVLM, which in turn excite vasoconstrictor SPNs in the IML of the thoracic and lumbar spinal cord segments T1–T2 (1), and (3) the activation of vasopressin-synthesizing neurons in the hypothalamus (17). There is also evidence that baroreceptor inhibition of sympathetic activity can be exerted at the spinal cord level, suggesting that some fibers conveying baroceptor afferent information course directly to the spinal cord (18).

Peripheral chemoreceptors that sense a fall in oxygen or a rise in carbon dioxide are located in the carotid bodies and the aorta and have afferent fibers in the glossopharyngeal and vagus nerves. The brain also has chemoreceptors that sense carbon dioxide. Peripheral chemoafferents terminate in the NTS and relay sympathoexcitatory responses via the RVLM to spinal vasomotor neurons. In spinal animals, the chemoreflex may also stimulate the release of arginine vasopressin (AVP) (also known as antidiuretic hormone) (19).

In response to systemic hypoxia, perfusion of vital organs needs to be maintained. Hypoxia results in activation of peripheral chemoreceptors, and hypercapnia results principally in activation of central chemoreceptors (20). Chemoreceptor reflexes result in vasoconstriction principally in skeletal muscle vascular beds via activation of the SNS (21). Research on the cardiovascular responses to hypercapnia in quadriplegic subjects is inconclusive. In one study of mechanically ventilated quadriplegic subjects, no change in heart rate was detected in response to elevation of carbon dioxide (22). Another study of six quadriplegic subjects with complete lesions above the sympathetic outflow responded to breathing carbon dioxide by increased blood pressure, both in the horizontal and the tilted positions, which suggests either a peripheral or spinal cord effect of hypercapnia (23). As chemoreceptor stimulation in spinal animals has been shown to produce a pressor response that seems to be mediated via excitatory amino acids in the RVLM and increases in AVP release (19), it is interesting to speculate that the increased blood pressure response to hypercapnia in quadriplegic subjects may have resulted from AVP release.

Hypotension

After a high spinal cord transection, systemic arterial pressure drops (24), owing to a drop in cardiac output and in total peripheral resistance. Resistances of the muscle and visceral vascular beds are decreased equally (25). Mathias et al. found the average resting blood pressure in recently injured quadriplegic individuals to be 130/57 (mean 82) mmHg, in chronic quadriplegic individuals to be 107/82 (mean 73) mmHg, and in control individuals to be 122/82 (mean 95) mmHg (26). A strong treatment option included in the "Guidelines for the Management of Acute Cervical Spine and Spinal Cord Injuries" is to maintain the MAP at 85–90 mmHg for 7 days following acute

cervical spinal cord injury with the use of crystalloid, colloid, dopamine, and phenylephrine, as this may improve neurologic outcomes (27).

Animal studies have found a reduction in sympathetic nerve activity following acute SCI, with the exception of the mesenteric and splenic nerves (28–33). However, the firing pattern of sympathetic nerves following acute SCI in animals changed from a rhythmic synchronized discharge to a less synchronized one (31, 34, 35). It has been postulated that the less synchronized firing pattern of sympathetic nerve activity that remains following SCI in experimental animals may not support vascular tone adequately, regardless of the magnitude of SPN discharge (31, 32, 34, 35).

With no connection between the medullary baroreceptor systems and the spinal cord, sympathetic activity cannot be increased to compensate for postural changes. In humans, orthostatic hypotension, defined as a decrease in systolic blood pressure (SBP) of more than 20 mmHg or a fall in diastolic blood pressure of more than 10 mmHg, within 3 minutes of standing or during head-up tilt to 60 degrees (36), occurs after acute SCI (37). Orthostatic tachycardia also occurs with head-up tilt in acute SCI and is thought to be due to baroreceptor withdrawal of vagal tone. The heart rate rise is usually less than 100 beats per minute, which is less than the tachycardia associated with hypotensive shock in non-SCI individuals (38). Mathias, in a recent review, provides a list of nonpharmacologic strategies for the management of orthostatic hypotension, which includes things to avoid (sudden head-up postural change, prolonged recumbency, straining during bowel and bladder elimination, high ambient temperatures, and vasodepressor drugs), things to do (elevate the head of bed, encourage high salt intake, and adopt different body positions), and things to consider (elastic stockings, thigh cuffs, abdominal binders, and water ingestion) (38). Most of the time, drug treatment is not necessary; however, when symptoms are not relieved with first-line strategies, there are several drugs with at least some evidence of efficacy, and they have recently been reviewed by Krassioukov et al. They conclude that midodrine should be included in the management protocol for orthostatic hypotension in individuals following SCI (39). In one double-blind, placebo-controlled, randomized trial, Nieshoff found that midodrine also improved exercise performance in three of four individuals with complete C6–C8 SCI (40).

After a time, the ability to maintain blood pressure in a sitting position improves (41). Improvement may be due to the development of spinal reflex control of blood pressure, long-term regulation by renal fluid control, increased vascular resistance, spasticity, increased α-AR responsiveness, or dominant autoregulatory controllers of blood flow (11). Alternatively, Bravo and coworkers suggest that the decrement in arterial pressure and heart rate immediately after SCI may result from Ach release from parasympathetic fibers and from the cholinergic stimulation of nitric oxide (NO) release from endothelium (42).

Several studies have shown that vascular resistance in the lower limbs of chronic SCI subjects is higher than in control subjects (43, 44). This may be due to structural changes resulting from venous atrophy and stiffness, which would limit venous dispensability, and thereby maintain central volume and prevent orthostasis (45). Furthermore, the development of spasticity may contribute to the recovery of arterial pressure, owing to increased central venous volume resulting from enhanced venous return and to physical compression on the arterial side of the skeletal muscle beds, which would increase vascular resistance (46).

In contrast to intact subjects, quadriplegic subjects have a lower resting concentration of catecholamines (47–50), and there is no significant increase in either NE or E when quadriplegic subjects change from a lying to a sitting position (47). This appears to be due to a reduction in NE release and not to a decrease in NE clearance (51). Resting skin blood flow is greater in quadriplegic than in control subjects (47, 52). This is in keeping with observations of diminished resting vasoconstrictor tone and much lower plasma NE levels. Submaximal and maximal exercise results in increases in plasma NE in controls and paraplegic subjects, but not in quadriplegic subjects (48).

Animal studies have been unable to attribute the normalization of arterial pressure following spinal cord transection to either (1) increased vascular sensitivity to a constantly low level of sympathetic activity or (2) a steadily increasing level of sympathetic nerve discharge (46). The enhanced pressor response to NE in humans with cervical SCI reported by Mathias and colleagues (53) may not have been due to denervation sensitivity, as suggested, but may have resulted from the absence of baroreceptor-mediated sympathoinhibition (46). Arnold and coworkers found a left shift of the dose-response curve for local infusions of NE to reduce dorsal foot vein diameter, suggesting that α-AR responsiveness is increased in quadriplegic persons (54). Kooijman et al. found that α-AR-mediated vascular tone in the lower limbs of subjects with T4–T12 complete chronic SCI was preserved and postulated that this was related to a spinal sympathetic reflex, a local venoarteriolar reflex, or an α-AR hypersensitivity to circulating catecholamines (43).

Normalization of blood pressure following SCI may occur because autoregulatory controllers of blood flow completely dominate within 24 hours following spinal cord transection, with the result being that any remaining sympathetic vasoconstrictor activity is without effect. Hypotension following spinal cord transection may therefore be principally the result of a decrease in sympathetic activity to vascular beds with relatively weak autoregulatory properties, such as skin and skeletal muscle (46).

Renin-Angiotensin System and AVP

Animal studies have indicated that, after lesions of RVLM, arterial pressure is maintained by the renin-angiotensin system and by AVP secretion (55). Animal studies have also shown that arterial pressure following spinal cord transection is related to the level of salt and water intake (56) and is in part dependent on angiotensin II vasoconstrictor activity (46).

The secretion of AVP by the posterior pituitary gland is predominantly controlled by (1) changes in plasma osmolality, which are sensed by osmoreceptors in the hypothalamus, and (2) changes in blood volume and blood pressure relayed from cardiovascular receptors in the carotid sinus and thorax via the glossopharyngeal and vagal cranial nerves to the NTS, and thence to the paraventricular and supraoptic nuclei of the hypothalamus (57).

Renin release is controlled by neural and nonneural stimuli. An increase in efferent renal nerve activity causes renin release via stimulation of postjunctional β-AR on the renin-containing juxtaglomerular granular cells (58). Nonneural stimuli that control renin release are (1) NaCl sensed at the macula densa, (2) humoral factors with angiotensin II, vasopressin, endothelin, and adenosine triphosphate (ATP) inhibiting renin release, and (3) the renal vascular baroreceptor mechanism, with increases in renal perfusion pressure decreasing renin secretion and with decreases in renal perfusion pressure resulting in increased prostacyclin synthesis and increased renin secretion (59).

The vasoconstrictor activity of the renin-angiotensin system and AVP, as well as renal sympathetic nerve activity, all may enhance renal retention of sodium and water, which would influence arterial pressure in the long term. Persons with chronic quadriplegia exhibit decreased urinary sodium excretion and expansion of the extracellular fluid compartment (60). Research findings show that quadriplegic persons have increased plasma renin levels and high normal aldosterone (a mineralocorticoid produced in the adrenal cortex, which increases renal sodium and water reabsorbtion) levels (37, 61), probably owing to renin release by the juxtaglomerular cells in response to the decreased renal perfusion that accompanies low arterial pressures (62). Renin acts on angiotensinogen in the plasma, forming angiotensin, which is converted to angiotensin II, a major vasoconstricting hormone. Increased release of aldosterone is probably a direct effect of the increased serum renin level (41).

In one study by Kilinc and coworkers, control subjects without SCI had a nocturnal increase in AVP level, whereas quadriplegic or paraplegic individuals did not (63). Quadriplegic or paraplegic individuals had an increased urine volume at night relative to controls. Kilinc hypothesized that daytime pooling of blood in paralyzed legs with associated reduction of central venous pressure was followed by a redistribution of volume during recumbency, resulting in increased blood pressure, which prevented nocturnal increases in AVP, resulting in nocturnal polyuria. It has been suggested that SCI individuals with severe nocturnal polyuria should have AVP levels checked and, if necessary, be treated with DDVAP at bedtime (64).

Infusion of hypertonic saline causes plasma AVP to rise in both control and quadriplegic subjects; however, at any given level of plasma osmolality, plasma AVP tended to be higher in the quadriplegic subjects than in the control subjects (61). Unlike control subjects, quadriplegic subjects demonstrated an increase in MAP without an increase in heart rate as a result of hypertonic saline infusion. In quadriplegic subjects, water loading resulted in normal suppression of urine osmolality, but in subnormal free water clearance during maximal water diuresis, despite appropriately suppressed levels of plasma AVP (61). Plasma AVP increased following head-up tilt in both control and quadriplegic subjects, but the increase was significantly greater in the quadriplegic group (57). These studies indicate that quadriplegic persons have appropriate cardiovascular and osmotic control of AVP secretion, but increased sensitivity to the pressor effect of AVP. The increase in postural release of AVP may be responsible for the oliguria seen in persons with SCI after prolonged sitting (57).

Infusion of AVP did not change MAP or heart rate in control subjects but did result in a marked rise in MAP and bradycardia in quadriplegic subjects. The bradycardic effect of AVP in quadriplegic subjects was probably the result of baroreflex activation of the intact vagal efferents secondary to the rise in MAP. The reason for the pressor response is not clear; it may have been due to increased sensitivity to peripheral or spinal-mediated pressor vascular effects of AVP or because baroreflex-mediated inhibition of sympathetic tone was interrupted by the spinal cord lesion (57, 65).

In control subjects and in persons with SCI below the L1 level, blood pressure rises with sitting and falls with recumbency. In quadriplegic subjects, blood pressure is lower when sitting than when lying down (61). This rise in blood pressure during recumbency has been attributed to fluid shifts into the central compartment and subsequent increased venous return and stroke volume. This expansion of central blood volume after recumbency, and the accompanying elevation in blood pressure inhibiting the release of AVP, may explain the diuresis associated with recumbency in quadriplegic persons (66).

Autonomic Dysreflexia (AD)

AD is manifested by hypertension, sweating, headache, and bradycardia (67–70) and is most often associated with SCI at or above the T6 level. The SBP will increase 20 mmHg or more during a dysreflexic episode. This disorder is reported to affect 30% to 90% of quadriplegic and high paraplegic persons with chronic SCI (71) and 6% of individuals in the acute phase (within 1 month) after SCI (72). In individuals with SCI, common sources of afferent stimulation that result in AD include bladder distension, pressure sores, childbirth, and rectal distension (73).

Somatic and visceral afferent input enters the spinal cord below the level of the spinal cord lesion and projects to the IML via propriospinal pathways. Spinal sympathetic pathways linking the supraspinal cardiovascular centers with the peripheral sympathetic outflow are interrupted at the level of the injury, but the parasympathetic efferent pathways through the vagus nerve, as well as the afferent arc of the baroreceptor reflex through the glossopharyngeal and vagus nerves, are intact after SCI. Bradycardia results from activation of efferents in the vagus nerve coursing to the sinoatrial node. Descending sympathoinhibitory projections through the spinal cord that would normally result in vasodilatation are disrupted by SCI, and the bradycardia alone is not adequate to reduce blood pressure. Treatment requires that the eliciting cause be eliminated or that pharmacologic treatment be instituted. For reviews, see Lee et al. (74), Naftchi et al. (75), Comarr and Eltorai (76), Amzallag (77), and Blackmar (78).

Several pathophysiologic mechanisms responsible for AD have been postulated and include (1) disinhibition of sensory pathways, (2) disinhibition of the sympathetic systems, (3) altered reflex responses in SPNs, (4) reinnervation of SPNs by spinal interneurons, and (5) denervation hypersensitivity.

In intact animals, noxious cutaneous mechanical stimulation elicited increases in heart rate, blood pressure, efferent renal sympathetic nerve activity, and cardiac sympathetic efferent nerve activity, whereas the same stimulus in acutely spinalized animals elicited even larger increases in cardiovascular responses (79). In animals, spinal cord transection was shown to convert a previously sympathoinhibitory response to a nonnoxious stimulus into a sympathoexcitatory one. Chemo- and mechanoreceptors in the small intestine, peripheral vasculature, or urinary bladder of spinal cord intact rats, activated by capsaicin, result in depression of cardiovascular SPNs (80). However, bladder distension or intravesical capsaicin (which activates afferent C fibers [81]) in spinal cord–transected rats activated a reflex excitatory response conveyed by pelvic nerve afferents that probably involved activation of SPNs via propriospinal pathways (80). In a rat model of SCI, visceral or cutaneous stimuli that were noxious or nonnoxious both resulted in pressor responses, with the noxious stimuli eliciting the greater increases in MAP (82). A larger percentage of sympathetically correlated spinal interneurons are excited by noxious and innocuous cutaneous stimulation in rats with chronic SCI compared to those with acute SCI (83). In the rat, spinal cord transection can convert a previously sympathoinhibitory response to a nonnoxious stimulus into a sympathoexcitatory response (80).

The afferent pathway that mediates the AD in response to bladder distension in humans is not clear. Complete sacral dorsal rhizotomy reduced but did not eliminate AD in response to intradural sacral ventral root stimulation for bladder emptying (84). However, dorsal rhizotomy alone may not eliminate all bladder afferents, as the existence of ventral root afferents has been well established (85, 86). It is also possible that the afferent pathway was via thoracic and lumbar dorsal roots via afferent fibers in the hypogastric nerve.

Krassioukov and Weaver identified morphological changes in SPNs following spinal cord transection in rats (87). SPNs caudal to the spinal transection demonstrated dendritic degeneration and a decrease in soma size within 1 week after transection, which was reversed by 1 month posttransection. They also found that the timeframe of degeneration and recovery of the dendritic arbor of SPNs correlated to the timeframe for first reduced and then enhanced vasomotor reflexes in the rat (88). However, the return to a normal preganglionic neuronal soma size and dendritic tree did not reverse the loss of 50%–70% of the synaptic input attributed to bulbospinal input, indicating that lost bulbospinal synaptic inputs to thoracic SPNs were not replaced by intraspinal inputs (89). Weaver suggests that the dense networks of fibers that appear following spinal transection are new inputs on neurons antecedent to the preganglionics (82).

In a mouse model of SCI, Jacob and coworkers described the development of AD in association with sprouting of calcitonin gene–related peptide (CGRP) fibers in the primary afferent arbor below the level of injury (90). Krentz and coworkers found that blocking nerve growth factor (NGF) prevented primary afferent sprouting in spinal cord–transected rats and decreased the hypertension induced by colon stimulation (91). Weaver reviews evidence that afferent sprouting in the spinal cord dorsal horn occurs in the same timeframe as the development of hypertensive responses to sensory stimulation, characteristic of AD, and that the sprouting is caused by an intraspinal action of NGF (82). Treatment of acute SCI in rats with a monoclonal antibody (mAb) against the CD11d subunit of the leukocyte integrin CD11d/CD18 (known to decrease intraspinal inflammation and oxidative damage) improved dysreflexia evoked by colon distension via a mechanism that appeared to be related to preservation or sprouting of spared descending pathways (82).

Treatment of Autonomic Dysreflexia

The Consortium for Spinal Cord Medicine has established a protocol for the management of AD (70). Treatment requires that the eliciting cause be eliminated or that pharmacologic treatment be instituted (74–78, 92, 93). Pharmacologic treatment is aimed primarily at producing direct vasodilatation (calcium-channel blockers, nitrates, hydralazine, diazoxide), central (spinal) (α2-adrenoceptor agonist activity (clonidine) (94), or ganglionic blockade (mecamylamine). Esmail and coworkers suggest that 25 mg of captopril be administered sublingually as a first-line treatment, if SBP is at or greater than 150 mmHg (95). The Joint National Committee on Detection, Evaluation and Treatment of High Blood Pressure has discouraged use of immediate release nifedipine (96).

α1-adrenoceptor blocking agents have been used in the prophylactic management of AD. Prazosin, 3 mg *bid,* was effective in reducing the number of severe episodes of AD and in reducing the average rise in systolic and diastolic blood pressure during an episode (97). Recurrent symptoms of AD such as headache, sweating, and flushing of the face together with an increase in blood pressure have been successfully treated with the once-a-day selective α1-adrenergic blocking drug terazosin (1–10 mg in adults and 1–2 mg in children) (98). In one randomized, controlled trial, tamsulosin (an α1a-adrenergic-blocking drug) treatment in individuals with neurogenic bladder secondary to suprasacral SCI was able to improve bladder storage and emptying, and decrease symptoms of AD (99).

Phenoxybenzamine is a long-acting α-adrenergic blocker that has been used to prevent AD; however, there are conflicting reports as to its effectiveness in preventing AD (69). The long-term use of phenoxybenzamine should be avoided, as it is a known carcinogen in rodents and may also be carcinogenic in humans (100).

DISORDERS OF MICTURITION

The lower urinary tract functions are to store and periodically release urine. These functions are performed by the smooth muscle of the urinary bladder (detrusor) and urethra and by the striated muscle of the external urethra sphincter. Micturition requires the coordinated activation of these muscles, which is controlled by supraspinal structures controlling autonomic and somatic nerves.

Complete SCI proximal to the sacral spinal cord results in an upper motor neuron lesion characterized by a hyperreflexic detrusor, whereas injuries involving the sacral cord or cauda equina result in a lower motor neuron lesion characterized by an areflexic detrusor (101). Reflex detrusor activity is abolished in spinal shock but returns in most cases in 2–12 weeks (102). About 15% of individuals classified as having a complete SCI will have some sensation in response to bladder filling or electric stimulation (103). In a study of 489 persons with spinal cord lesions due to a variety of causes, all those who had suprasacral spinal cord lesions without evidence of additional sacral spinal cord or cauda equina involvement had either detrusor hyperreflexia (defined as involuntary bladder contractions with increased detrusor pressure of at least 60 cm H2O) or detrusor-external urethral sphincter dyssynergia (DESD) (101). DESD has been defined as the presence of involuntary contractions of the external urethral sphincter during involuntary detrusor contractions (104). DESD has been reported to occur during bladder contractions that are evoked either during urodynamic studies or by suprapubic tapping in as many as 86% of persons with SCI (105). For a review of the urodynamics of SCI, see Watanabe (106).

Bladder mechanoreceptors are activated by bladder distension, mucosal deformation, and a shift in bladder position (107). Fluid-induced bladder distension results in the activation of mechanoreceptors, which provide the sensory input needed to facilitate the activation of both supraspinal- and spinal-mediated micturition reflexes (108).

Sensory inputs from the bladder to the human lumbar spinal cord arise from T11 to L1, and perhaps as far proximal as T9; sensory inputs from the bladder to the human sacral spinal cord arise from S2 to S4 (109). Afferent fibers in the pelvic nerve projecting to the sacral spinal cord are responsible for the initiation of micturition. In cats, Aδ-fiber bladder afferents respond to bladder distension, whereas C fiber bladder afferents respond primarily to noxious stimulation (110). In the rat, A fiber and C fiber bladder afferents are both mechano- and chemosensitive (102). Aδ-fiber bladder afferents initiate the supraspinal micturition reflex, whereas C fiber bladder afferents are thought to contribute to bladder hyperactivity following SCI in humans. Most C fiber bladder afferents are conveyed in the hypogastric nerve (111). Mitsui et al. proposed that the hypogastric afferents are linked to the development of urinary frequency caused by chemical bladder irritation (111).

Neuropeptides may be important transmitters in the afferent pathways from the urinary bladder. Many bladder afferent neurons contain CGRP, vasoactive intestinal polypeptide (VIP), pituitary-adenyl cyclase–activating polypeptide (PACAP), tachykinins, galanin, and opioid peptides (102). Most bladder C fibers are sensitive to capsaicin, a neurotoxin that can release peptides from afferent terminals. When the urinary bladder is exposed to capsaicin, it produces an inflammatory response including plasma extravasation and vasodilatation (102). Capsaicin activates the vanilloid receptor subtype 1 (VR1), now called transient receptor potential (TRP)V1, on sensory neurons (110). Intravesical capsaicin or resiniferatoxin (a potent analog of capsaicin) can reduce both bladder hyperactivity and AD induced by bladder distention (112). NGF can induce hyperexcitability of C fiber bladder afferent pathways after spinal cord transection in rats that is reversed by intrathecal NGF antibodies (113). DESD in chronic spinalized rats is associated with an increase in NGF levels in the spinal cord that can be neutralized by subcutaneous capsaicin, which desensitizes C fiber afferents or the application of intrathecal NGF-Ab (113). NGF and its receptors in the bladder and/or spinal cord are potential targets for new therapies for DESD (102).

The urothelium has been shown to have both sensory and signaling properties, in that it can express molecules that respond to thermal, mechanical, and chemical stimuli and can release factors/transmitters (114). ATP is one transmitter that is released from the urothelial cells in response to bladder distension and activates $P2X_3$ and/or $P2X_{2/3}$ receptors on bladder submucosal primary afferents (115). Chronic spinal cord–injured cats have an augmented stretch-evoked ATP release from urothelial cells, which Birder suggests may contribute to bladder hyperreflexia (114). In spinal cord–injured rats, Khera et al. demonstrated that urothelial ATP release is exocytotic (secreted to the extracellular environment) and inhibited by botulinum toxin A (BTX-A) (116).

Preganglionic parasympathetic neurons in the IML of the sacral cord segments S2 to S4 project preganglionic fibers in the pelvic nerve to the pelvic plexus (107). In the human bladder, some pelvic plexus neurons are in the bladder wall (107). Parasympathetic postganglionic nerves excite detrusor smooth muscle via release of Ach acting on muscarinic receptors in the bladder muscle or by the release of ATP acting on purinergic receptors in the bladder muscle (110). The M3 muscarinic receptor subtype mediates bladder contractions (110). ATP excites detrusor smooth muscle via $P2X_1$ purinergic receptors (102), and although purinergic excitatory transmission may not be important in normal human detrusor functioning, it is involved in the bladders of individuals with conditions such as bladder outlet obstruction (117). The parasympathetic input to the urethral smooth muscle is inhibitory and is mediated by NO (118). See Table 41.3.

SPNs that project to the lower urinary tract are found in spinal cord segments T10 to L2 in humans (107). Most preganglionic sympathetic fibers project through the lumbar splanchnic nerves to the IMG, and a smaller number of preganglionic sympathetic fibers project via the sacral paravertebral chain ganglia into the pelvic nerve to the pelvic plexus (119). The hypogastric nerve (also known as the presacral nerve) is composed of both preganglionic and postganglionic sympathetic fibers that pass from the IMG to the pelvic plexus (120). Most preganglionic sympathetic fibers innervating the pelvic viscera form synapses in the IMG or the pelvic plexus (107, 120).

The sympathetic postganglionic nerves release NE, which (1) inhibits detrusor smooth muscle via β2- or β3-AR, (2) contracts the smooth muscle of the bladder trigon and urethra via α1-AR, and (3) inhibits (via α2-AR) or facilitates (via α1-AR) parasympathetic ganglionic transmission (121). The α1A-adrenoceptor is the major subtype in the prostate and urethra (110). The α1-AR blockers doxazosin and terazosin, used in the treatment of bladder outlet obstruction, are not selective enough on the urethra to eliminate cardiovascular side effects. The selective α1A-adrenoceptor antagonist tamsulosin has fewer cardiovascular side effects (9) and has been shown to be safe and effective in individuals with suprasacral SCI (99). Alfuzosin (a selective α1A-adrenoceptor antagonist) was shown to significantly decrease urethral pressure in twenty of twenty-one individuals with SCI (122).

The urethral sphincter mechanism has two parts: the internal and external urethral sphincter (EUS) (123). The internal sphincter is the smooth muscle of the urethra that extends from the bladder outlet through the pelvic floor (123). The striated muscle of the EUS also has two components: (1) the intrinsic EUS, which lies completely within the urethral wall, and (2) the extrinsic EUS, which is formed by the skeletal muscle fibers of the pelvic floor and urogenital diaphragm (124). The EUS is innervated by the somatic pudendal nerve (125). The EUS is the most important active mechanism for maintenance of urinary continence (123).

Activation of the parasympathetic pathways to the detrusor muscle and inhibition of somatic input to the intrinsic EUS are the essential neuronal events that initiate release of urine. Reflex contractions of the urinary bladder and release of urine that occurs in response to bladder distension are mediated via a parasympathetic reflex pathway consisting of an Aδ-fiber afferent limb and a preganglionic parasympathetic efferent limb in the pelvic nerve (126, 127). Spinal afferent pathways ascend in the lateral funiculus or the dorsal funiculus of the spinal cord and terminate in the nucleus gracilis and periaqueductal gray (PAG). It is thought that neurons in the PAG relay information to the pontine micturition center (PMC) to initiate micturition (121). The descending pathway of the micturition reflex is also in the dorsolateral funiculus (128). The PMC coordinates the reciprocal activation of the detrusor muscle and inhibition of the EUS. Voiding dysfunction caused by lesions above the PMC is not associated with DESD, whereas lesions affecting the PMC or the afferent/efferent pathways of the spinobulbospinal micturition reflex result in prominent DESD. The spinobulbospinal micturition reflex can be modulated at the spinal level by a variety of afferent inputs from the colon, vagina, penis, or perineum, and the modulation can occur at different sites, including primary afferent terminals, interneurons, or bladder PGNs (129).

The PAG also has connections to suprapontine centers such as the thalamus, insula, cingulate, and prefrontal cortices that could influence the appropriate timing for micturition (130). The PMC is under inhibition until the appropriate desire and circumstance to void occurs. In intact individuals, the *first sensation to void* occurs around 40% bladder capacity, the *first desire to void* occurs around 60% bladder capacity, and a *strong desire to void* occurs at about 90% bladder capacity (130). Positron emission tomography (PET) studies in humans have shown that the anterior cingulate gyrus, the insula, and the prefrontal cortex are involved in the central control of micturition (130). Damage to these areas of the cortex results in a loss of their inhibition of the anterior hypothalamic area that normally provides an excitatory input to micturition centers in the brainstem (102).

Table 41.3 Autonomic Innervation of the Urinary Tract

ANS	NEUROTRANSMITTER	RECEPTOR	TISSUE	EFFECT
Parasympathetic	Ach	Muscarinic	Detrusor smooth muscle	Contraction
Parasympathetic	ATP	Purinergic	Detrusor smooth muscle	Contraction
Parasympathetic	NO	Nitrergic	Urethral smooth muscle	Inhibition
Sympathetic	NE	β2- or β3-AR	Detrusor smooth muscle	Inhibition
Sympathetic	NE	α1-AR	Trigone	Contraction
Sympathetic	NE	α1A-AR	Urethral smooth muscle	Contraction

Abbreviations: Ach = acetylcholine; ANS = autonomic nervous system; AR = adrenoreceptor; NE = norepinephrine; NO = nitrous oxide; ATP = adenosine triphosphate.

The major excitatory neurotransmitter in the CNS control of micturition is glutamic acid (110). Both N-methyl-D-aspartate (NMDA) and α-amino-3-hydroxy-5-methyl-4-isoxazolepropionic acid (AMPA) receptors are involved. Glutamate receptors at the level of the lumbosacral spinal cord in the rat are involved in processing the afferent input from the urinary bladder, and they mediate segmental interneuronal excitation of parasympathetic PGNs (110). The PMC elicits voiding in response to glutamate injection in the cat (131).

The PMC is under tonic GABAergic inhibition (131). At the spinal cord level, GABA agonists inhibit sacral parasympathetic PGNs (110). Baclofen, a GABAB agonist, decreases bladder hyperactivity in individuals with spinal cord pathology (132). Glycine, an inhibitory amino acid, contributes to the inhibition of EUS motor neurons during micturition (133).

During continence, a spinal vesicosympathetic reflex pathway allows the urinary bladder to accommodate larger volumes by increasing the tone of the bladder neck, by depressing impulse transmission from the sacral spinal cord in pelvic vesical ganglia, and by directly inhibiting the detrusor muscle (134). An intersegmental spinal pathway elicits vesicosympathetic reflexes with afferents in the pelvic nerve and efferents in the hypogastric nerve (121). The vesicosympathetic reflex pathway is inhibited via a supraspinal mechanism when bladder pressure reaches the threshold for producing micturition (102).

In addition to the spinobulbospinal pathway, which is thought to mediate normal micturition, a spinal micturition reflex pathway has been identified (135). Research by deGroat and Ryall found that the spinal micturition reflex was present in some intact cats and in all cats with chronic spinal cord transection (127). It is thought that this spinal pathway, which has a C fiber afferent limb and parasympathetic postganglionic efferent limb in the pelvic nerve, mediates automatic micturition following chronic spinal cord transection (126). C fiber afferents, which usually do not respond to bladder distention, may become mechanosensitive after SCI and may elicit the spinal micturition pathway as well as bladder hyperreflexia following SCI.

Cutaneovesical reflexes have also been described. In rats, cutaneous stimulation resulted in a reflex bladder contraction both before and after spinal cord transection (136). Neonatal cats exhibit a perineal bladder reflex mediated in the spinal cord that disappears in adult life, and this reflex reappears after spinal cord transection in adult cats (137). Activation of spinal cutaneous somatovesical reflexes may be responsible for voiding elicited by suprapubic tapping or pulling pubic hair in persons with SCI above the sacral outflow.

MALE SEXUAL DYSFUNCTION

Most cases (82%) of SCI occur in males in their reproductive years (mean age, 26 years) (138). The male genital response includes erection and ejaculation. Ejaculation consists of emission and expulsion (139). Male sexual dysfunction following SCI can be classified as an upper motor neuron lesion or lower motor neuron lesion. An upper motor neuron lesion occurs when the SCI is above the sacral (S2–S4) level, so that sacral reflex arcs are intact. Lower motor neuron lesions occur when there is direct injury to the conus medullaris or cauda equina.

The penis receives innervation from both somatic (motor/sensory) and autonomic (sympathetic/parasympathetic)

pathways. Somatic afferent innervation to penile skin is carried in a terminal branch of the pudendal nerve, called the dorsal nerve of the penis (DNP), which projects to the sacral spinal cord via the S2–S4 dorsal root ganglia (140). Physiologic activation of afferent pathways in the DNP elicits multiple sexual responses, including penile erection, seminal emission, and ejaculation (141, 142). Afferent pathways to the medullary reticular formation (MRF) from the dorsal nerve of the penis are conveyed in the dorsal portion of the lateral funiculus (143).

Somatic efferent innervation to the ischiocavernosis and bulbospongiosus striated muscles arise in Onuf's nucleus in sacral segments S2–S4 and are conveyed in the pudendal nerve. The contraction of the perineal striated muscles enhances an erection that is already present (144).

Sympathetic preganglionic fibers from T11 to L2 and parasympathetic preganglionic fibers from S2 to S4 are involved in erection and ejaculation (145). Parasympathetic preganglionic fibers from the sacral spinal cord project in the pelvic nerve to the pelvic plexus (140). One pathway for sympathetic preganglionic fibers to the penis is from the thoracolumbar spinal cord through the paravertebral chain ganglia to project via (1) the pelvic nerve and plexus into the penile nerve (also known as the cavernous nerve) or (2) the pudendal nerve to the penis. The other pathway for sympathetic preganglionic fibers is through the lumbar splanchnic nerves to the IMG. Sympathetic postganglionic fibers from neurons in the IMG as well as preganglionic fibers project through the hypogastric nerves to the pelvic plexus. Sympathetic and parasympathetic postganglionic efferent fibers project from the pelvic plexus to the penis via the penile nerves (146).

In female rats, afferent nerves from the reproductive organs conveyed in the hypogastric nerve respond to noxious stimuli; however, it is unknown if hypogastric afferents also play a role in nociception in the male (147). The role of pelvic nerve afferents from the male reproductive organs is unknown (147). There are many spinal afferent pathways that convey sensory information from the internal reproductive organs and external genitalia, including dorsal column, postsynaptic dorsal column, spinoreticular, spinothalamic, spinosolitary, spinoparabrachial, spinohypothalamic, spinoamygdalar, spinomesencephalic, and spinocerebellar pathways (147). The areas of the brain that receive convergent somatic and pelvic visceral sensory inputs include the nucleus reticularis gigantocellularis and surrounding nuclei within the medullary reticular formation, the nucleus gracilis and solitarius, and various subregions of the thalamus (147).

Erectile Dysfunction

Erections occur in most individuals with UMN lesions (94%) and are usually *reflex erections* obtained by tactile stimulation of the penis (148). However, these erections often lack the desired penile rigidity and/or duration needed for successful intercourse (149). In individuals with an LMN lesion, erections occur less often (26%) and are usually *psychogenic* in origin, obtained by visual or imaginative stimuli (148). Erection is primarily a spinal reflex modulated by supraspinal influences and results from the relaxation of smooth muscle in the penis (150). See Table 41.4.

The SNS is responsible for detumescence. Penile flaccidity is maintained by sympathetic efferents and α-AR (151). Both α1- and α2-AR have been found in human corpus cavernosum (152).

Table 41.4 Male Sexual Reflexes

	AFFERENT	EFFERENT	SPINAL	SUPRASPINAL	NEUROTRANSMITTER
Reflex erection	Pudendal nerve	Pelvic to penile nerve	S2–S4		NO VIP
Psychogenic erection	CNS	Hypogastric to penile nerve		+	NO VIP
Detumescence		SNS	T11–L2		α1-AR
Secretion		Pelvic to penile nerve	S2–S4		?Ach ?NPY
Secretion		Hypogastric to penile nerve	T11–L2		?Ach ?VIP
Emission		SNS	T11–L2		α1-AR
Ejaculation		Pudendal nerve	S2–S4		Ach

The predominant subtype is the α1-adrenoceptor, although stimulation of prejunctional α2-AR may inhibit the release of the nonadrenergic noncholinergic (NANC) mediator of penile erection thought to be NO (153).

Reflex erections are mediated via the sacral parasympathetics with afferent input from the pudendal nerve and efferent output via the pelvic, then penile (cavernous), nerves. Reflex erections are organized in the sacral spinal cord (145). The phenomenon of *psychogenic erections* in paraplegic men with complete sacral lower motor neuron lesions and abolished reflexogenic erections indicates that a pathway for erection from the sympathetic outflow exists (145). The sympathetic proerectile outflow may be via the hypogastric to the penile (cavernous) nerves (144). Spinal reflex erections are under tonic inhibition from the ventral medial reticular formation (154).

Vasodilatation of the arterioles that supply the erectile tissue of the corpora cavernosa causes the erectile tissue to fill with blood and occlude the venous outflow, resulting in penile erection (149). Erection involves parasympathetic cholinergic and NANC mechanisms (144, 155). The NANC neurotransmitter primarily thought to mediate erection is NO, a smooth muscle relaxant and vasodilator (138). It is unlikely that Ach causes erection by a direct action on smooth muscle fiber postjunctional muscarinic receptors because isolated human corpus cavernosum smooth muscle cells contract in response to cholinergic stimulation (138). Ach may contribute to erection by inhibiting the release of NE via stimulation of muscarinic receptors on adrenergic nerve terminals (156) or by modulating NO release by endothelial cells and/or nerves in the penis (152). Toda et al. reviewed the evidence that supports the widely accepted theory that NO synthesized from L-argenine via neuronal NO synthase (nNOS) acts as a neurotransmitter of NANC inhibition of the smooth muscle of the penile corpus cavernosum and is essential for the initiation and maintenance of penile erection (157). Furthermore, the release of NO from the endothelial cells lining the sinuses of the corpus callosum in response to neurogenic Ach also participates in the erection (157).

NO and VIP are colocalized in cholinergic nerves in the human penis (152). VIP has also been implicated as a mediator of the NANC mechanism of erection (153, 155) and is known to relax smooth muscle from the human penis (153, 158). VIP stimulates VIP receptors in the penis, which leads to an increase in cAMP, which in turn activates a cAMP-dependent protein kinase (152).

NO relaxation of vascular smooth muscle is mediated through activation of guanylate cyclase to produce cyclic guanosine monophosphate (cGMP) (138). Activation of a cGMP-dependent protein kinase (cGK I) leads to penile erection (152). Neurons and endothelial cells in the corpus cavernosum synthesize and release NO. Phosphodiesterases (PDEs) catalyze the hydrolysis of cAMP and cGMP (152). Sildenafil increases cGMP by inhibition of cGMP-specific phosphodiesterase V and results in penile erection (138). Phosphodiesterase Type 5 Inhibitors (sildenafil, tadalafil, vardenafil) have been found to be safe and effective for erectile dysfunction caused by SCI (159–162).

Intracavernosal drug injection is the most effective nonsurgical treatment of erectile dysfunction; however, it is invasive (160). Penile injectable medications useful for erectile dysfunction after SCI include papaverine, phentolamine, and prostaglandin E1 (PGE1) (alprostadil). The main action of PGE1 is probably to increase the intracellular concentration of cAMP in corpus cavernosum smooth muscle cells. The main action of papaverine is nonselective PDE inhibition. Phentolamine is a competitive antagonist of α1- and α2-AR.

Ejaculatory Dysfunction

The secretion of seminal fluid is under parasympathetic control, whereas the closure of the bladder neck and contraction of the ductus deferens, which move the seminal fluids into the proximal urethra, are under sympathetic control (163). Emission is followed by contraction of the bulbourethral striated muscles (primarily the bulbocavernosus muscle), the latter being mediated by pudendal somatic efferents (145). Some 5% to 10% of men with complete SCI experience ejaculation or seminal emission (145, 164, 165).

For purposes of obtaining semen for artificial insemination, an ejaculation reflex can be obtained by vibratory stimulation of the frenulum and lower surface of the glans penis (166). The afferent pathway of this ejaculation reflex likely involves the pudendal nerves (DNP) and ascending tracts from the sacral spinal cord to the thoracolumbar T12 to L1 preganglionic sympathetic nerves (164, 167). Penile vibratory stimulation (PVS) is more successful in lesions above T10 (81%) than T10 or below (12%) and is more successful if hip flexion and bulbocavernosus reflexes are present (77%) than absent (14%) (168).

Electroejaculation is the electrical stimulation of efferent sympathetic nerves via a rectal probe. Biering-Sorensen and Sonksen recommend PVS as the first treatment choice for management of ejaculatory dysfunction in men with SCI, followed by electroejaculation if PVS fails (169).

FEMALE SEXUAL DYSFUNCTION

A woman's libido and reproductive capability remain intact following SCI (170); however, sexual dysfunction is common (171, 172). There is transient anovulation in about 50% of women with SCI, but the preinjury menstrual pattern is reestablished in 3 to 6 months (170, 171, 173). Anovulation is thought to be a result of the stress of the trauma and is not related to the level of injury or its degree of completeness. Mean menstrual cycle length and the duration of menses have been shown to fall within the normal range for fertile, able-bodied women, regardless of level or completeness of injury (173). Menarche is not delayed if the SCI is preadolescent. The fertility rate and miscarriage rate are the same for women with SCI as for the general population of sexually active women (170).

Three pathways are thought to convey sensory information from the uterus, cervix, and vagina to the CNS. These pathways are (1) via the hypogastric nerves to the thoracolumbar spinal cord (T10–L1), (2) via the pelvic nerve to the sacral spinal cord (S2–S4), and (3) via the vagal nerve to the nodose ganglia and NTS (174). In the rat, the pelvic nerve primarily conveys afferent genitosensory input from vaginal cervical stimulation to the CNS (175).

The four components of the sexual response cycle—excitement, plateau, orgasm, and resolution—are all present but may vary in degree in women with SCI (171, 172). The normal female sexual excitation phase consists of vaginal lubrication, swelling of the clitoral gland, and congestion of the labia (171). A psychogenic pathway and a reflex pathway control female sexual arousal (176). With complete SCI, there is absence of lubrication (reflex or psychogenic) when the injury is situated between T10 and T12, indicating that SPNs at this level of the spinal cord constitute the final efferent pathway for both reflex and centrally mediated lubrication (171). Reflex lubrication does occur with lesions above T9, and psychogenic lubrication is present with injuries below T12 (171). Sipski and coworkers found that preservation of T11–L2 sensory function was associated with psychogenic genital vasocongestion (177).

About 50% of women of women with SCI report the ability to achieve orgasm (176). Sipski found that 17% of women with complete lower motor neuron dysfunction involving S2–S5 spinal segments were able to achieve orgasm, whereas 59% of women with other levels and degrees of SCI were able to achieve orgasm; however, time to orgasm was increased in women with SCI compared to non-SCI controls (26 minutes vs. 16 minutes) (177). The quality of orgasm appeared to be similar for SCI and non-SCI women (177).

Whipple and Komisaruk hypothesize that the orgasms obtained in women with complete SCI in response to genital stimulation are mediated by sensory fibers in the vagus nerve (178). Komisaruk et al. 2004 demonstrated that three of five women studied with complete T10 or above SCI were able to experience orgasm with vaginal-cervical self-stimulation (CSS), and during orgasm, there was activation in the hypothalamic paraventricular nucleus; medial amygdale; anterior cingulated; frontal, parietal, and insular cortices; and cerebellum, as visualized by functional magnetic resonance imaging (fMRI). In these women, as well as those SCI females who did not experience orgasm, there was activation of the inferior region of the NTS during CSS, leading to the conclusion that the vagus nerve conveys sensory information from the genital area in females and that this afferent input is sufficient to stimulate orgasm in some women (179).

Sildenafil may partially reverse the sexual dysfunction commonly associated with SCI in women (180). Sildenafil has been shown to result in significant increases in subjective arousal in women with SCI, with maximal responses occurring when sildenafil was combined with visual and manual sexual stimulation. Sildenafil was found to be well tolerated with no evidence of significant adverse events (180).

Pain in the first stage of labor is due to uterine contraction and cervical dilatation (170). Because the afferent innervation of the uterus arises from T10 to LI, labor is painless for women with an SCI above T10. In the second stage, labor pain is from the perineum, innervated by the pudendal nerve and spinal cord segments S2 to S4. About 25% of pregnant spinal cord–injured women are unable to detect the onset of labor (170).

Efferent uterine innervation arises from T10 to T12 (171). In women with SCI above the T10 level, uterine contractions are effective, and labor progresses normally (171). The intensity of uterine contractions is not reduced, and labor is of short duration, often with spasm of the abdominal muscles (181). Most women with an SCI level above T6 will develop AD with uterine contractions (101, 182). A significant increase in the incidence of premature delivery has not been documented (170). Women with SCI may be expected to have a reasonably normal pregnancy outcome, provided that specific complications, particularly AD, are anticipated and managed properly (181, 183).

GASTROINTESTINAL DYSFUNCTION

The function of the gastrointestinal (GI) tract is to retain nutrients and eliminate waste. The motility, secretion, and absorption processes of the GI tract are regulated via exocrine, endocrine, and neural mechanisms (184). Paracrine regulation occurs when a sensing cell releases a mediating chemical, which influences the function of nearby cells. Endocrine regulation occurs when a sensing cell releases a hormone into the circulation to effect the function of a distant target cell. Neural mechanisms involve sensory receptors that reflexively alter the secretory or motor activity of the gut. GI reflex pathways may be located entirely within the gut or may involve the brain and/or spinal cord. SCI results in abnormalities of the motor function of the gut rather than in absorptive or secretory dysfunction.

Enteric Nervous System

The stomach and intestinal wall contain intrinsic neurons that are part of the enteric nervous system, a system that has been referred to as the third division of the ANS. It is noteworthy that there are as many neurons in the enteric nervous system (108) as there are in the spinal cord (184). Neurons of the enteric nervous system are not postganglionic parasympathetic neurons, and the majority of enteric neurons do not have direct contact with parasympathetic preganglionic axons. The enteric nervous system has two ganglionated divisions that are connected by nerve processes: (1) the submucosal plexus (Meissner's plexus), which innervates the mucosa and regulates secretion, and (2) the myenteric plexus (Auerbach's plexus), which innervates the circular and longitudinal smooth muscle layers and regulates motility. In addition, there are several aganglionated plexuses that supply all layers of the gut (185).

The enteric nervous system has three types of nerve cells: (1) motor neurons that innervate smooth muscle cells, (2) interneurons that connect different neurons, and (3) intrinsic primary afferent neurons (IPANs). The neurotransmitters of excitatory motor neurons to the circular smooth muscle of the small intestine of the guinea pig are accounted for by Ach and tachykinins (TK) (186). Inhibitory neurons use multiple neurotransmitters, which vary with species and location in the digestive tract and include ATP, NO, VIP, and pituitary adenylyl cyclase–activating peptide (PACAP) (186). In human isolated colon circular muscle, 5-hydroxytryptamine-4 (5-HT$_4$) receptor agonists facilitate both inhibitory neurons which release NO and excitatory neurons which release Ach (187, 188).

Enteric motor neurons are categorized as muscle motor neurons, secretomotor neurons, enteric vasodilator neurons, and motor neurons to enteric endocrine cells and can be excitatory or inhibitory. Secretomotor neurons result in water and electrolyte secretion in the small and large intestine, bicarbonate secretion in the duodenum, and gastric acid secretion in the stomach (189).

In the guinea-pig, IPANs have been identified with cell bodies in the wall of the small intestine (190, 191). Three classes of IPANs have been identified: tension sensitive neurons, mucosal mechanosensitive neurons, and chemosensitive neurons (189). The intrinsic primary afferents are thought to be indirectly excited by an intermediate substance. Submucosal IPANs can initiate peristaltic and secretory reflexes when stimulated by 5-HT released into the lamina propria by enteric endocrine cells, which have microvilli projecting into the lumen of the GI tract and stores of 5-HT in secretion granules at their bases (192).

Enteric interneurons are involved in motor reflexes and send axons orally or anally, and so are called ascending or descending and form multisynaptic pathways the length of the gut.

Extrinsic Innervation of the Gastrointestinal Tract

Extrinsic primary afferent neurons have cell bodies in the nodose ganglia with axons in the vagus nerve or cell bodies in the dorsal root ganglia with axons in the pelvic nerve and sympathetic nerves. They convey sensations of satiety, nausea, and pain to the CNS (189). Vagal and spinal afferents innervate the entire gastrointestinal tract; however, there are more vagal afferents proximally and more pelvic afferents distally (193). In general, physiologic stimuli are conveyed in the vagus, and pelvic nerve afferents and noxious stimuli are conveyed in the splanchnic nerves (193). Extrinsic primary afferent neurons are described as mucosal receptors, muscle receptors, and serosa receptors.

Mucosal receptors respond to mechanical stimuli such as gentle stroking of the epithelium, lumenal chemicals, cold, or lumenal osmolarity (194). Cholecystokinin (CCK) and 5-HT released from enteroendocrine cells in the mucosa area are likely involved in the activation of vagal mucosal afferents (193). *Muscle receptors* in the gastric, duodenal, and jejunal smooth muscle respond to distension and contraction of the viscus and have afferent fibers in the vagus nerve (195). *Serosal receptors* are activated by mechanical stimuli. The splanchnic nerves, which convey afferents from the gut to the spinal cord, are thought to mediate painful sensations, although vagus nerve afferents may also be involved in gut nociception (196). The sensation of hunger is reduced in vagotomized individuals, but it is not eliminated, perhaps because the hypothalamus monitors the levels of circulating nutrients (195, 197).

Extrinsic efferent innervation of the GI tract occurs through the parasympathetic and sympathetic divisions of the ANS. The GI tract from the esophagus to the distal colon is innervated by vagal nerve efferents with preganglionic neurons in the dorsal motor nucleus of the vagus nerve (DMV). There is more proximal and lesser distal vagal innervation of the GI tract. Preganglionic parasympathetic neurons project from the sacral segments S2 to S5 through the pelvic nerves and pass to the left colon and anorectum via the pelvic plexus (120). It is unclear exactly where in the colon the vagal nerve innervation stops and the pelvic nerve innervation starts. The vagal nerve has been described as stopping at the splenic flexure or innervating the entire colon to the rectum, whereas the pelvic nerve may also provide innervation of the entire colon (198).

Mechano- and chemotransmission from the GI tract elicit a number of different vago-vagal reflexes, which consist basically of sensory vagal afferents, second-order integrative neurons of the NTS, and efferent vagal neurons of the DMV. One vagal efferent pathway from the DMV is cholinergic-muscarinic and induces an increase of GI functions such as motility and acid output, and the second is NANC and causes a decrease in gastric motility when activated, mainly via release of NO onto gastric smooth muscle (199).

SPNs in the IML of the spinal cord send efferent fibers through the splanchnic nerves to the celiac and superior mesenteric prevertebral ganglia (plexuses). The stomach receives sympathetic postganglionic fibers principally from the celiac plexus but also from the left phrenic plexus, the bilateral gastric and hepatic plexuses, and the sympathetic trunk. Postganglionic sympathetic efferent nerves emerge from the celiac and SMG to run along mesenteric blood vessels and innervate the small intestine. The sympathetic supply to the right colon arises from T6 to T12, and that to the left colon and upper rectum arises from L1 to L3 (200). SPNs to the colon and pelvic viscera project to the superior mesenteric ganglion (SMG) and IMG via the lumbar splanchnic nerves. Postganglionic fibers from the SMG innervate the colon from the cecum to the distal transverse colon. Postganglionic fibers from the IMG project via lumbar colonic nerves that run along the inferior mesenteric artery to innervate the left side of the colon. Postganglionic fibers from the IMG also project via the hypogastric nerves and join the pelvic plexus (also known as the inferior hypogastric plexus) to innervate the distal colon (120). Other sympathetic preganglionic axons enter paravertebral chain ganglia and form synapses with postganglionic neurons there (119).

Sympathetic ganglia receive synaptic input from (1) PGNs with cell bodies in the spinal cord, (2) primary sensory neurons with cell bodies in the dorsal root ganglia, and (3) neurons arising in visceral intramural ganglia (enteric nervous system). The apparent convergence of multiple synaptic inputs onto individual principal ganglionic neurons suggests that the outflow from these neurons is the result of integration of synaptic information from several sources (201). The peripheral ANS may therefore mediate complex reflex functions of the gastrointestinal system without the involvement of either supraspinal or spinal cord influences.

Some sympathetic postganglionic neurons are visceral vasoconstrictor neurons and innervate vascular smooth muscle, whereas others are motility-regulating (MR) neurons that innervate visceral smooth muscle (200). Whereas some sympathetic postganglionic neurons control the effector organs directly, other sympathetic postganglionic neurons control the effector organs indirectly by influencing other peripheral neurons such as those in the submucosal ganglia (Meissner's plexus) or myenteric ganglia (Auerbach's plexus) of the enteric nervous system or in the prevertebral ganglia, via pre- or postsynaptic mechanisms (181).

The lumbar sympathetic outflow exerts a tonic inhibitory influence on the motility of the colon. Studies in rats show that there is differential sympathetic inhibition of the proximal, transverse, and distal colon (202). The distal colon receives a tonic inhibitory influence with a supraspinal organization, the transverse colon receives a tonic inhibitory influence with a spinal organization, and the proximal colon appears to be influenced by neither spinal nor supraspinal tonic inhibition.

Electrical stimulation of the sympathetic supply to the colon results in contraction of the internal anal sphincter and relaxation of the colon and rectum (120). Studies in the rat have shown that the sympathetic inhibition is mediated by postjunctional β-AR on colon smooth muscle, whereas sympathetic induced contractions, which are most prominent in the distal colon although also present in the proximal colon, are mediated by postjunctional smooth muscle α-AR (203).

The majority of lumbar sympathetic postganglionic neurons are noradrenergic, but many contain a peptide as well (201, 204). In the guinea pig ileum, activation of α_2-AR on interneurons in the myenteric plexus and intrinsic sensory neurons is needed for sympathetic inhibition of intestinal motility (205).

Upper Gastrointestinal Dysfunction

Upper GI tract dysfunction following SCI includes impairment of gastric motility, gastric emptying, and intestinal motility. One third of persons with complete quadriplegia for more than 1 year have been found to have mild GI symptoms such as nausea, diarrhea, constipation, and fecal incontinence (206).

In the abdomen, the parasympathetic preganglionic efferent fibers to the stomach are conveyed in the vagus nerve, which in turn gives rise to gastric branches that form synapses with neurons in the myenteric and the submucosal plexuses of the stomach. The actions of the stomach in response to a meal are storage, secretion, mixing, and emptying. The fundus of the stomach acts as a reservoir to accommodate the meal, whereas the antrum is both a pump and a grinder. The vagus nerve is important for the motor activity of the stomach. Vagal stimulation induces relaxation of the fundus and contraction of the antrum (194).

Mesenteric sympathetic nerve stimulation inhibits contraction in the small intestine (194).

In the normal interdigestive state of the gastrointestinal tract of humans, a cyclic wave begins in the stomach and duodenum and migrates to the terminal ileum. This activity, characterized by recurring periods of intense regular motor activity, is known as phase III of the interdigestive motor complex (IDMC) and is also referred to as the migrating myoelectric complex (MMC) (207). The IDMC usually begins in the antrum and migrates to the proximal duodenum in a coordinated manner that is interrupted by feeding. Phase III activity is followed by a period of less intense activity (phase IV), then by quiescence (Phase I), and then by irregular contractions (phase II) (208). The phases of the interdigestive state disappear after a meal and are replaced by the ongoing phasic contractile activity of the fed pattern (208). The phases of the IDMC and the fed pattern of gastrointestinal contractile activity occur independent of nerves extrinsic to the enteric nervous system (208). It is thought that in humans, the hormone motilin acts on enteric nervous system neurons in the gastric antrum to control gastric emptying and trigger the MMC (209). Erythromycin has motilin agonist properties, and its administration can induce an MMC (209). One case report describes the successful resolution of refractory SCI–induced gastroparesis with erythromycin lactobionate (210).

In humans, gastric distension and ileus occur immediately after traumatic spinal cord transection, suggesting abnormal gastrointestinal motility. In long-term quadriplegic persons, an intact supraspinal sympathetic pathway is not an absolute requirement for initiation and propagation of antral phase III motor activity, as there are no significant differences in the duration of phases of the IDMC, the cycle length of the duodenal IDMC, or the propagation velocity of phase III of the IDMC from the duodenum to the jejunum between subjects with quadriplegia (neurologic level above T1), low paraplegia (neurologic level below T10), or an intact spinal cord (211). In normal subjects, 90% of phase IIIs originated in the antrum and migrated to the duodenum and jejunum, whereas in subjects with high SCI, fewer than 40% of phase IIIs originated in the antrum. Some 80% of quadriplegic subjects had dissociation between antral and duodenal phase III motility, manifested primarily as a pattern of persistent antral activity. In one subject with prominent recurrent AD, there was marked antral hypomotility. Antral quiescence was associated with the degree of reflex vascular hypertension resulting from spontaneous and suprapubic pressure-induced AD, whereas duodenal motility was unaffected (211). This suggests that motility in the antrum is modified by central sympathetic input and that excessive splanchnic sympathetic outflow may delay gastric emptying by inhibiting antral motility (211). Fealey and coworkers suggested that sympathetic activity may influence gastric motility via a direct neural pathway to the gut wall or via indirect pathways that modulate the release of polypeptide gastrointestinal hormones (211).

Gastric emptying has been reported as delayed in chronic quadriplegic subjects when data on gastric emptying is studied for at least 2 hours (211, 212). Segal and coworkers identified a biphasic pattern of gastric emptying, where the initial (20–30 minutes of) gastric emptying (which resembled the patterns seen in control and paraplegic subjects) was followed by a delayed second phase (212). Lu and coworkers demonstrated a normal cutaneous electrogastrogram (EGG) in twelve patients with complete cervical SCI (206). Abnormalities in the EGG have been associated with gastric motor dysfunction, but if there is antral-duodenal motor incoordination after SCI, as described by Fealey (211) and coworkers, then abnormal gastric myoelectrical activity may correlate poorly with gastric emptying (206). Paraplegic persons have been reported to have delayed gastric emptying, but this appears to be a nonspecific finding related to prolonged immobilization (213). Metoclopramide, a dopamine receptor antagonist known to interact with serotonergic receptors (moderate 5-HT$_4$ receptor agonist and weak 5-HT$_3$ antagonist), has been shown to improve delayed gastric emptying in quadriplegics and paraplegics (214, 215).

Lower Gastrointestinal Dysfunction

The most obvious lower gastrointestinal dysfunction associated with SCI is the loss of voluntary control of the initiation of defecation. The most common problems complicating the neurogenic bowel are poorly localized abdominal pain (in 14% of cases studies by Stone's group), difficulty with bowel evacuation (20%), hemorrhoids (74%), abdominal distension (43%), and AD arising from the gastrointestinal tract (43%) (216). As many as 27% of persons with SCI have significant chronic gastrointestinal problems, and those with more complete injuries are more likely to have symptoms (33%) than those with incomplete injuries (6%) (216). In one survey of individuals with SCI, 30% regarded colorectal dysfunction as worse than both bladder and sexual dysfunction (217).

When food is ingested into the stomach, there is an increase in colonic motor activity that is called the gastrocolic reflex (218). The afferent limb of this reflex can be blocked by intragastic lidocaine, and the increase in distal colonic spike activity can be blocked by anticholinergics or naloxone, indicating participation of cholinergic and opiate receptors. Colonic cyclical organization in the rat, including enhancement of distal colonic cyclical activity as a secondary response to feeding (gastrocolic reflex), persists after ablation or section of the spinal cord (202). This demonstrates that—at least for the distal colon—colonic cyclical organization is not initiated by lumbar spinal or supraspinal influences. The local enteric nervous system or the prevertebral ganglionic system, or both, are probably responsible for the cyclical organization of distal colonic motility in rats. The gastrocolic reflex in the transverse colon also persists in rats after spinal cord transection but is abolished by spinal cord ablation, suggesting that it is organized in the spinal cord (202).

Analysis of colonic myoelectric spike activity of the rectal mucosa 6 to 15 cm from the anus revealed that, in the fasting state, persons with SCI above T10 who were also more than 3 months postinjury had significantly greater basal colonic myoelectric spike activity than control subjects (219). Meal stimulation increased basal spike activity (gastrocolic reflex) in the control group compared to the fasting state. In the spinal cord–injured group, there was no significant increase in myoelectric spike activity after the meal, compared to the fasting state. Because feeding did not significantly increase the already high basal spike activity of persons with SCI, the gastrocolic reflex could not be demonstrated. The loss of a tonic inhibitory supraspinal influence may cause the increase in basal colonic spike activity following SCI (219). The absence of a gastrocolic reflex in this study is consistent with studies by Glick and colleagues (220), who

recorded at 12 to 18 cm from the anus, but the findings differ from those of the study of Connell and associates (221), who recorded intact gastrocolic reflexes at 15, 20, and 25 cm from the anus (181).

Fecal material entering the rectum results in relaxation of the internal anal sphincter (IAS) (rectoanal inhibitory reflex) but contraction of the external anal sphincter (EAS) to prevent incontinence (holding reflex) (216, 222). This allows defecation to be delayed to an appropriate time. Stool elimination results from voluntary relaxation of the EAS and the puborectalis muscle (223). Sacral parasympathetic spinal reflex activity independent of supraspinal pathways and having afferent and efferent limbs in the pelvic nerve is needed for the initiation of propulsive activity during defecation (224). Complete sacral posterior rhizotomy did not eliminate the IAS relaxation induced by rectal distention. The recto-ano inhibitory reflex (RAIR) is an entero-enteric reflex dependent on the myenteric nervous system (225). However, reflex contraction of the EAS in response to either rectal distention or increased intra-abdominal pressure was eliminated by sacral posterior rhizotomy, indicating that these contractions are mediated by a spinal reflex (223). Distension-mediated relaxation of the IAS is inhibited by sympathetic outflow through the lumbar colonic nerves (226).

Individuals with complete SCI have been variously reported to have decreased, normal, or increased basal IAS pressure and to have absent or present rectoanal reflexes to rectal distension (225). Valles et al. found three patterns of colorectal dysfunction in individuals classified as complete using the International Standards for Neurological and Functional classification of SCI and the ASIA impairment scale. The three patterns were based on neurologic level above or below T7 and the presence or absence of sacral reflexes. Individuals with SCI above T7 with sacral reflexes were most likely to be constipated (86%), whereas those with SCI below T7 without sacral reflexes were most likely to suffer more severe fecal incontinence, and those with SCI below T7 with sacral reflexes were less likely to suffer from either constipation (50%) or fecal incontinence.

In persons with complete SCI above T12, transit of contents is slowed throughout the large bowel, regardless of the level of the spinal cord lesion (227). Studies have identified (1) prolonged rectosigmoid transit times (227), (2) transit delays more marked in the descending colon, sigmoid, and rectum than in the cecum, ascending colon, and transverse colon (228, 229), and (3) transit delays involving the entire colon (230). Krough and coworkers found that persons with supraconal SCI had generalized colonic dysfunction, whereas persons with conal or cauda equina lesions had severe rectosigmoid dysfunction (151). Increases in colonic transit time (CTT) are present in about half of individuals with SCI, and besides an association between shorter CTT and successful rectal emptying, Leduc et al. found little relationship between CTTs and chronic intestinal symptoms (231).

The obvious clinical implication of prolonged transit time throughout the left and right colon is that treatment of colorectal dysfunction in individuals with SCI should include not only rectal agents but also prokinetic agents to reduce transit time in the entire colon (230). Cisapride (a nonselective 5-HT$_4$ receptor agonist) has been shown to improve chronic constipation and colonic transit times in persons with quadriplegia or paraplegia (232–234). Cisapride has been withdrawn from the United States market, although it will continue to be available under a limited-access program for individuals for whom other drug treatments fail (235). Prucalopride (a highly selective 5-HT$_4$ receptor agonist), in a double-blind, placebo-controlled phase II study, reduced colonic transit time in individuals with constipation due to SCI (236); however, clinical trials have been discontinued because of carcinogenicity in animals (215). Nizatidine, an H2-receptor inhibitor, appears to exert a prokinetic action in the human colon, but studies in individuals with SCI are lacking (237).

PULMONARY DYSFUNCTION

Although pulmonary problems are common following SCI, they are usually secondary to impairments in inspiratory and expiratory function, with associated abnormalities in gas exchange that are largely the result of ineffective cough mechanisms and not autonomic dysfunction. However, changes in breathing patterns, airway hyperresponsiveness, ventilatory drive, and control of ventilatory responses have been identified.

The PNS via the vagus nerve is the dominant pathway in the control of bronchial smooth muscle tone (238). Stimulation of parasympathetic nerves results in bronchoconstriction, mucus secretion, and bronchial vasodilation mediated by muscarinic M$_3$ receptors (238, 239). Chemical and physical stimuli arising from receptors in the lungs, heart, arterial baroreceptors and chemoreceptors, and mucosa of the upper airways and esophagus mediate reflex cholinergic contractions of airway smooth muscle (240). There is also an inhibitory nonadrenergic noncholinergic (i-NANC) parasympathetic pathway that mediates bronchodilitation (238). The neurotransmitters of the i-NANC pathway are colocalized with ACH in the parasympathetic nerves. The main neurotransmitter of the i-NANC system in human airways appears to be NO that may be coreleased with ACH and VIP (238). Both NO and VIP have potent smooth muscle relaxing properties. The i-NANC airway parasympathetic nerves are activated in response to noxious chemical and mechanical stimulation of bronchopulmonary C fibers and rapidly adapting receptors and are thought to restore airway patency following defensive reflexes such as coughing or reflex bronchospasm (240). Although β2-adrenergic receptors are expressed on human bronchial smooth muscle, no innervation from the SNS has been shown (238). These β2-adrenoceptors are activated by circulating NE or E released from the adrenal medulla (223).

The bronchial circulation is controlled by sympathetic vasoconstrictor and parasympathetic vasodilator nerves (241). It is thought that the bronchial vasculature is under tonic sympathetic influence, resulting in vasoconstriction mediated by α-AR (241). Pulmonary vascular tone is also regulated by NANC neural mechanisms and humoral mechanisms.

Pulmonary receptors convey afferent information via the vagus nerve (242). Slowly adapting receptors (SAR) and rapidly adapting receptors (RAR) detect lung volume and changes in lung volume (243). Afferents fibers from these receptors terminate in the NTS in the medulla and can reflexively inhibit or excite inspiration (243). The RAR in the large bronchi and carina appear to be the most important receptors for the initiation of cough (244). There is also sensory C fiber nociceptor innervation of the airways. C fiber axon stimulation causes bronchial vasodilatation via a peripheral vagal axon reflex mechanism dependent on the release of vasodilator neuropeptides from axon terminals (245).

An axon reflex occurs when the impulse propagated centrally by the stimulation of one branch of the peripheral end of an afferent axon invades a second peripheral branch of the same axon, resulting in the release of neuropeptides from the peripheral end of the second afferent axon branch. Activation of C fiber afferents in the lungs and airways also causes reflex bronchial vasodilation with afferent and parasympathetic efferent pathways in the vagus nerve (245). Respiration is also controlled by chemosensors that detect hypoxia and hypercapnia. Peripheral chemoreceptors are located in the carotid and aortic bodies and also project to the NTS (243). Medullary neurons are also chemosensitive to CO$_2$ (246).

Loveridge and coworkers identified impaired ventilatory lung function in sitting following complete C5–C8 SCI at 3 months postinjury with improvement between 3 and 6 months. They also found that the sigh reflex is retained in quadriplegic subjects, although they take more big breaths in supine than in sitting positions (247).

Otherwise healthy subjects with quadriplegia have been shown to have airway hyperresponsiveness to aerosolized methacholine, histamine, and ultrasonically nebulized distilled water (248–251). Aerosol treatment with the Ach receptor antagonist ipratropium bromide blocked airway hyperreactivity associated with aerosolized methacholine and ultrasonically nebulized distilled water but did not inhibit airway hyperreactivity associated with histamine inhalation (249). Nebulized β-agonist metaproterenol sulfate blocked both histamine- and methacholine-associated airway hyperreactivity (249). In one report, subjects with high paraplegia (T1–T6) who demonstrated airway hyperresponsiveness to methacholine had significantly lower FEV1.0 than subjects who did not demonstrate hyperreactivity (251). Singas and coworkers hypothesized that loss of the ability to stretch airways by deep breathing may cause airway hyperresponsiveness in quadriplegic subjects (251).

Several studies have evaluated cholinergic bronchomotor tone in individuals with cervical SCI using plethysmography to assess airway conductance and have found that quadriplegic individuals have reduced baseline conductance compared to controls without SCI. Furthermore, the reduced conductance improved 134%–235% after inhalation of an anticholinergic drug (252). As sympathetic innervation of bronchial smooth muscle in humans is sparse or absent (240), the increase in bronchomotor tone in quadriplegic individuals may be due to denervation of the adrenal medulla (252). Schmid et al. previously had found that quadriplegics had low levels of circulating E and NE, whereas T1–T4 paraplegics had normal levels of NE and low levels of E, which were attributed to denervation of the adrenal medulla (48).

There are conflicting reports on the response of quadriplegics to hypercapnia. Normally, ventilatory drive is increased by hypercapnia (primarily via central chemoreceptor stimulation) and hypoxia (primarily via peripheral chemoreceptor stimulation) (20). Several studies have found a blunted ventilatory drive in response to hypercapnia (253–255), whereas another reports normal ventilatory chemosensory responses to hypercapnia and hypoxia (256). The latter results may have been due to the inclusion of quadriplegic subjects with incomplete spinal lesions. Manning (254) and coworkers could not contribute the blunted respiratory drive found in quadriplegic subjects to expiratory muscle weakness nor to altered chest wall mechanics. They hypothesized that the blunted ventilatory drive in response to hypercapnia may be due to loss of supraspinal control of the SNS, as similar blunted responses have been reported previously in individuals with autonomic dysfunction. Unlike Manning and colleagues, Lin (255) and coworkers found that the reduction of minute ventilation (VE) per increase in PCO2 was normalized by maximal voluntary ventilation (MVV) (i.e., ΔVE /ΔPCO2/ΔMVV), suggesting that muscle weakness was the primary factor contributing to the diminished ventilatory response.

The control of a range of ventilatory responses—tidal volume, respiratory frequency, inspiratory and expiratory durations, and mean inspiratory airflow—does not appear to require afferent pathways from the rib cage and intercostal muscles (257, 258). A group of ventilated quadriplegic subjects detected changes in tidal volume of as little as 100 ml just as well as did a group of ventilated control subjects (259). The sensory information that allowed the quadriplegic group to detect changes in lung volume could arise from visceral lung afferents that project to the CNS in the vagus nerve. Mechanical ventilation is known to inhibit inspiratory muscle activity in humans (260). In control and C2 quadriplegic subjects with intact sternocleidomastoid (SCM) efferents and afferents, inspiratory effort as evidenced by EMG activity in the SCM muscle was elicited by increasing end-tidal PCO_2. In both these groups, onset of inspiratory muscle activity occurred at a higher end-tidal PCO_2, when inspiratory activity was elicited by increasing the inspired fraction of CO_2 ($FICO_2$), than when it was elicited by decreasing the tidal volume or frequency during mechanical ventilation. In C1 quadriplegic subjects with efferent innervation of the SCM muscle via the accessory nerve, but lacking afferent innervation of the SCM, the onset of inspiratory muscle activity occurred at the same level of end-tidal PCO_2, independent of whether end-tidal PCO_2 was increased by increasing $FICO_2$ or by decreasing tidal volume or frequency. Simon (260) and coworkers concluded that afferent feedback from some part of the chest wall was needed to produce a volume- and frequency-dependent inhibition of inspiratory muscle activity during mechanical ventilation.

Sensation of the need to cough and of congestion has been reported to remain after high cervical spinal cord lesions (259). It has also been shown that ventilated quadriplegic subjects can reliably perceive an increase in PCO_2 in the physiologic range as an uncomfortable sense of "air hunger" (22). Ventilated quadriplegic subjects maintained at a constant but elevated level of end-tidal PCO_2 experienced a similar sensation of "air hunger" when tidal volume was decreased (254). The sensation of dyspnea in response to increases in end-tidal PCO_2 is preserved in SCI intact humans, paralyzed with total neuromuscular blockade, suggesting that chemoreceptor activity can lead to discomfort in the absence of any respiratory muscle contraction (261).

THERMOREGULATORY DYSFUNCTION

Impairment of temperature regulation is a recognized hazard for persons with SC1 (262). Body temperature control in homeotherms is regulated by behavioral and autonomic mechanisms. Behavioral mechanisms include changing the thermal environment, changing posture, and changing the amount of insulating clothing. Physiological mechanisms include vasomotor adjustment, sweating, shivering and nonshivering thermogenesis, piloerection, and panting, of which only the first three are of importance in humans.

Thermoregulatory dysfunction is most severe for persons with a complete cervical SCI because *shivering* can only occur above the level of the injury and hypothalamic control of sympathetically mediated *vasomotor control* and *sweating* is lost below the level of the lesion. Some degree of thermoregulation via activation of local or spinal vasomotor and sudomotor reflexes has been identified in individuals with spinal cord injuries. Behavioral modification remains an important mechanism for thermoregulation in persons with complete high-level spinal cord injuries (263). See Table 41.5.

Most central thermosensory neurons are warm sensitive, and the most important ones for temperature regulation are located in the preoptic anterior hypothalamus (POA) (264). However, there is evidence of mesencephalic, medullary, and spinal temperature sensors (265). Peripheral thermomosensors are superficial in the skin or deep in the esophagus, stomach, large intra-abdominal veins, and other organs (264). Most superficial thermoreceptors are cold sensitive and are located in the epidermis, and they convey their signals by Aδ fibers. The less common warm sensitive superficial thermoreceptors convey their signals by C fibers (264). Afferent fibers from peripheral warm and cold receptors with cell bodies in the dorsal root ganglia enter the spinal cord, synapse on lamina I neurons that in turn ascend contralaterally in the lateral funiculus, and project to the insular cortex with a relay in the thalamus (264). This spino-thalmo-cortical pathway is thought to be involved in the behavioral decisions that determine one's interaction with the environment (264). Lamina I neurons also project to the brainstem reticular

Table 41.5 Thermoregulatory Reflexes

REFLEX	AFFERENT	EFFERENT	SPINAL	SUPRASPINAL
Shivering	Superficial cold thermoreceptors	Skeletal muscle motor neurons and nerves	−	+
Vasodilatation	Superficial warm thermoreceptors	Axon reflex	−	−
Vasodilatation	Superficial warm thermoreceptors	Sympathetic cholinergic system	+ (late)	+ (early)
Vasodilatation	Deep warm thermoreceptors	Sympathetic cholinergic system	+ (attenuated)	
Vasoconstriction	Deep cold thermoreceptors	Sympathetic cholinergic system	−	+
Sweating	Deep warm thermoreceptors	Sympathetic cholinergic and adrenergic system	+ (attenuated)	

formation neurons, which project to the POA (264). Efferents from the hypothalamus control thermoregulatory vasomotor and sudomotor tone as well as nonshivering and shivering thermogenesis via descending noradrenergic and cholinergic fibers that exit the spinal cord below C7 (266). Vagal afferents, conveying metabolic information from the periphery to the brain, are important for thermoregulation during fever and may also play a role in body temperature regulation (267).

Cooling the skin—regardless of whether central body temperature changes—causes increased heat production via shivering (268). In paraplegic subjects, deep or central temperature receptors sensitive to cold are also able to initiate shivering above the level of the SCI, and these receptors can act independently of the temperature of the skin above the SCI (268). Researchers have postulated that, in normal humans, these central cold receptors may be a backup mechanism that comes into play if there is a loss or diminution of skin cold receptor reflex activity (268). In humans, shivering does not occur below the level of a complete SCI, and therefore shivering is thought not to be a spinal reflex (268).

Cooling of peripheral or central areas results in a reduction of skin blood flow and a simultaneous increase in flow to central vascular regions (266). In control subjects, cooling or warming of one hand elicits a cutaneous vasomotor response of the contralateral hand and both legs (269). Several investigations (269–271) have failed to observe a similar cutaneous vasomotor response below the level of SCI; others have observed vasomotor responses below the level of SCI in both primates and humans (272–275). Tsai and coworkers reported that all vasomotor responses to cooling or warming in the paraplegic lower extremities of men were absent following acute SCI (T5 to T11), but by 4 months after injury, the ipsilateral local vasomotor responses to warming and cooling in the paraplegic lower extremities returned to normal, and by 18 months after injury, the crossed vasomotor reflex to cooling and warming recovered to normal (272).

Skin is known to be innervated by a sympathetic adrenergic vasoconstrictor system and a cholinergic vasodilator system (276). Cutaneous vasoconstriction is tonically active in thermoneutral environments, and hyperthermia triggers active cutaneous vasodilation, which dissipates heat (277). The sympathetic cholinergic system is the principal mediator of thermoregulatory vasodilatation; however, local heating of skin mediates vasodilation via a local axon reflex and also by the local production of nitrous oxide (276).

Paraplegic men have been shown to have significant differences in skin blood flow response to hyperthermia when compared to intact control subjects (278). When only insensate skin was heated (to 40°C) in paraplegic subjects, little or no increases in forearm blood flow (FBF) occurred, even with an elevation of oral temperature of 1° to 1.5°C over 59 to 71 minutes, though the subjects exhibited mild sweating on the upper body. In contrast, a normal subject exhibited vigorous vaso- and sudomotor responses to the same pattern of heating that was given to the paraplegic subject. With whole-body heating of paraplegic subjects, all but one exhibited sweating above the level of the spinal cord lesion, and FBF increased in all subjects. However, the increase in FBF in the paraplegic subjects was less than that reported for hyperthermic spinal cord–intact men. Nicotra et al. found that local cutaneous heating above and below the level of

SCI resulted in increases in skin vasodilation similar to that in control subjects, thus demonstrating that axon reflex vasodilatation is preserved below the level of lesion in chronic complete SCI (273).

Tam and colleagues (279) reported that a person with T6 paraplegia had to achieve a higher core temperature threshold (37.2° to 37.9°C) to generate sweating and related vasodilatation responses, compared to the core temperature threshold (36.2° to 37.1°C) of a normal control subject. It can be concluded that paraplegic persons appear to exhibit markedly attenuated skin blood flow in response to hyperthermia and thus are limited in their ability to dissipate excess heat (278).

The primary and principal stimulus that elicits the thermoregulatory sweating response is a change in core temperature (280). Sweat glands receive dual innervation by both cholinergic and adrenergic fibers and are stimulated by cholinergic, α-adrenergic, and β-adrenergic agonists; however, cholinergic stimulation provokes the largest response (281). Spinal segments T2 to T4 supply sweat glands on the head and neck, T2 to T8 to glands of the upper limbs, T6 to T10 to the trunk, and T11 to L2 to the lower extremities (281). Normell (282) provides an outline of the segmental arrangement of the thermoregulatory vasomotor innervation of the skin of the trunk and lower extremities. Autonomic dermatomes overlap several segments above and below the somatic level. In several reports, spinal lesions are associated with anhidrosis below the level of the lesion (281, 282). Normal evaporative cooling is maintained in persons with spinal injury by increased compensatory sweating from sentient skin (280, 281).

Reflex sweating occurs below the level of lesion in SCI during AD. There is also evidence for thermal reflex sweating below the level of SCI in humans. A 1961 study by Seckendorf and Randall demonstrated low-intensity sweating in five individuals with anatomically complete lesions of the spinal cord (T3–T8) (283). In 1991 Silver, Randall, and Guttmann recorded sweat responses of nine individuals with physiologically complete lesions of the spinal cord, including six with cervical lesions (284). Although sweating (up to 30% of what would be expected in controls) occurred on the entire cutaneous surface below the level of SCI in every individual in response to environmental heating, the sweating was not sufficient to prevent an elevation in body temperature in individuals with cervical SCI.

In quadriplegic subjects, sympathetic skin nerve recordings of vasoconstrictor and sudomotor impulses from below the level of SCI, made while ambient temperature was varied, demonstrated no changes in sympathetic outflow despite cooling that reduced tympanic temperature 2°C (285). During this study, abdominal pressure over the bladder, as well as mechanical and electrical skin stimulation applied distal to the level of SCI, induced bursts of neural impulses recorded in the sympathetic skin nerve fascicles also below the level of SCI, indicating the presence of spinal vesicosympathetic and somatosympathetic reflexes. It has long been noted that increases in urinary bladder pressure elicit an increase in arterial blood pressure in quadriplegic persons (286). Of note is that reflex vasoconstriction (below the level of SCI) induced by suprapubic pressure is prolonged during body cooling. The finding of increased vasoconstriction during cooling in persons with SCI may therefore not be a thermoregulatory response but simply an artifact induced by facilitation of vesicosympathetic reflexes (285). This argues against the presence of physiologically significant spinal sympathetic thermoregulatory reflexes.

Conscious control of behavior depends on sensory appreciation of temperature. In one study, paraplegic subjects did feel hot as their oral temperature was raised 1° to 1.5°C by heating insensate skin (278). However, in the case of one T8 paraplegic individual, researchers reported that a fall in central temperature to 36.2°C was not associated with a conscious appreciation of cold (287). The perception of warm and cold after SCI appears to depend on the temperature of the sentient skin.

Animal studies have shown an inferior locomotor and histopathologic outcome following acute SCI, in which the core temperature was increased to 39.5°C and maintained for a 4-hour period, compared to normothermic (37°C) animals (288). Temperatures over 99.9°F are common following acute SCI, with an incidence of 60.4% in acute care and 50% in rehabilitation (289). Treatment and prevention of elevated temperature in the immediate postinjury period may prevent the secondary excitotoxic, apoptotic, and inflammatory cascades that result in irreversible cell injury and neurologic deficits (288).

References

1. Shields RW Jr. Functional anatomy of the autonomic nervous system. *J Clin Neurophysiol* 1993; 10:2–13.
2. Sved AF, Cano G, Card JP. Neuroanatomical specificity of the circuits controlling sympathetic outflow to different targets. *Clin Exp Pharmacol Physiol* 2001; 28:115–119.
3. Janig W. Spinal cord reflex organization of sympathetic systems. *Prog Brain Res* 1996; 107:43–77.
4. Schramm LP. Spinal sympathetic interneurons: their identification and roles after spinal cord injury. *Prog Brain Res* 2006; 152:27–37.
5. Llewellyn-Smith IJ, Weaver LC, Keast JR. Effects of spinal cord injury on synaptic inputs to sympathetic preganglionic neurons. *Prog Brain Res* 2006; 152:11–26.
6. Abrams P, Andersson KE, Buccafusco JJ, et al. Muscarinic receptors: their distribution and function in body systems, and the implications for treating overactive bladder. *Br J Pharmacol* 2006; 148:565–578.
7. Hesch K. Agents for treatment of overactive bladder: a therapeutic class review. *Proc (Bayl Univ Med Cent)* 2007; 20:307–314.
8. Dhein S, van Koppen CJ, Brodde OE. Muscarinic receptors in the mammalian heart. *Pharmacol Res* 2001; 44:161–182.
9. Guimaraes S, Moura D. Vascular adrenoceptors: an update. *Pharmacol Rev* 2001; 53:319–356.
10. Tanaka Y, Horinouchi T, Koike K. New insights into beta-adrenoceptors in smooth muscle: distribution of receptor subtypes and molecular mechanisms triggering muscle relaxation. *Clin Exp Pharmacol Physiol* 2005; 32:503–514.
11. Teasell RW, Arnold JM, Krassioukov A, Delaney GA. Cardiovascular consequences of loss of supraspinal control of the sympathetic nervous system after spinal cord injury. *Arch Phys Med Rehabil* 2000; 81:506–516.
12. Sun MK. Central neural organization and control of sympathetic nervous system in mammals. *Prog Neurobiol* 1995; 47:157–233.
13. Krassioukov A. Which pathways must be spared in the injured human spinal cord to retain cardiovascular control? *Prog Brain Res* 2006; 152:39–47.
14. Schwaber JS. Neuroanatomical substrates of cardiovascular and emotional-autonomic regulation. In: Magro AM, North Atlantic Treaty Organization, Scientific Affairs Division, eds. *Central and Peripheral Mechanisms of Cardiovascular Regulation.* 109th ed. New York: Plenum Press, 1986:353–384.
15. Malliani A, Lombardi F, Pagani M. Sensory innervation of the heart. *Prog Brain Res* 1986; 67:39–48.
16. McNeill DL, Chandler MJ, Fu QG, Foreman RD. Projection of nodose ganglion cells to the upper cervical spinal cord in the rat. *Brain Res Bull* 1991; 27:151–155.
17. Saper CB. The central autonomic nervous system: conscious visceral perception and autonomic pattern generation. *Annu Rev Neurosci* 2002; 25:433–469.
18. Coote JH, Lewis DI. The spinal organisation of the baroreceptor reflex. *Clin Exp Hypertens* 1995; 17:295–311.
19. Amano M, Asari T, Kubo T. Excitatory amino acid receptors in the rostral ventrolateral medulla mediate hypertension induced by carotid body chemoreceptor stimulation. *Naunyn Schmiedebergs Arch Pharmacol* 1994; 349:549–554.
20. Somers VK, Mark AL, Zavala DC, Abboud FM. Contrasting effects of hypoxia and hypercapnia on ventilation and sympathetic activity in humans. *J Appl Physiol* 1989; 67:2101–2106.
21. Somers VK, Mark AL, Zavala DC, Abboud FM. Influence of ventilation and hypocapnia on sympathetic nerve responses to hypoxia in normal humans. *J Appl Physiol* 1989; 67:2095–2100.
22. Banzett RB, Lansing RW, Reid MB, Adams L, Brown R. 'Air hunger' arising from increased PCO2 in mechanically ventilated quadriplegics. *Respir Physiol* 1989; 76:53–67.
23. Downey JA, Chiodi HP, Miller JM III. The effect of inhalation of 5 per cent carbon dioxide in air on postural hypotension in quadriplegia. *Arch Phys Med Rehabil* 1966; 47:422–426.
24. Hilton S. The central nervous contribution to vasomotor tone. In: Magro A, North Atlantic Treaty Organization, Scientific Affairs Division, eds. *Central and Peripheral Mechanisms of Cardiovascular Regulation.* New York: Plenum Press, 1986:465–486.
25. Yardley CP, Fitzsimons CL, Weaver LC. Cardiac and peripheral vascular contributions to hypotension in spinal cats. *Am J Physiol* 1989; 257:H1347–H1353.
26. Freeman R. Treatment of orthostatic hypotension. *Semin Neurol* 2003; 23:435–442.
27. Hadley MN, Walters BC, Grabb PA, et al. Guidelines for the management of acute cervical spine and spinal cord injuries. *Clin Neurosurg* 2002; 49:407–498.
28. Gootman PM, Cohen MI. Sympathetic rhythms in spinal cats. *J Auton Nerv Syst* 1981; 3:379–387.
29. Mannard A, Polosa C. Analysis of background firing of single sympathetic preganglionic neurons of cat cervical nerve. *J Neurophysiol* 1973; 36:398–408.
30. Meckler RL, Weaver LC. Splenic, renal, and cardiac nerves have unequal dependence upon tonic supraspinal inputs. *Brain Res* 1985; 338:123–135.
31. Qu L, Sherebrin R, Weaver LC. Blockade of spinal pathways decreases pre- and postganglionic discharge differentially. *Am J Physiol* 1988; 255:R946–R951.
32. Stein RD, Weaver LC. Multi- and single-fibre mesenteric and renal sympathetic responses to chemical stimulation of intestinal receptors in cats. *J Physiol* 1988; 396:155–172.
33. Meckler RL, Weaver LC. Characteristics of ongoing and reflex discharge of single splenic and renal sympathetic postganglionic fibres in cats. *J Physiol* 1988; 396:139–153.
34. McCall RB, Gebber GL. Brain stem and spinal synchronization of sympathetic nervous discharge. *Brain Res* 1975; 89:139–143.
35. Stein RD, Weaver LC, Yardley CP. Ventrolateral medullary neurones: effects on magnitude and rhythm of discharge of mesenteric and renal nerves in cats. *J Physiol* 1989; 408:571–586.
36. Schatz IJ, Bannister R, Freeman RL, et al. Consensus statement on the definition of orthostatic hypotension, pure autonomic failure and multiple system atrophy. *Clin Auton Res* 1996; 6:125–126.
37. Johnson RH, Park DM. Effect of change of posture on blood pressure and plasma renin concentration in men with spinal transections. *Clin Sci* 1973; 44:539–546.
38. Mathias CJ. Orthostatic hypotension and paroxysmal hypertension in humans with high spinal cord injury. *Prog Brain Res* 2006; 152:231–243.
39. Krassioukov A, Warburton DER, Teasell RW, Espey MJ. Orthostatic hypotension following spinal cord injury. In: Eng J et al., eds. *Spinal Cord Injury Rehabilitation Evidence: Systematic Reviews.* Version1.0. Canada: Kristin Konnyu, 2006.
40. Nieshoff EC, Birk TJ, Birk CA, Hinderer SR, Yavuzer G. Double-blinded, placebo-controlled trial of midodrine for exercise performance enhancement in tetraplegia: a pilot study. *J Spinal Cord Med* 2004; 27:219–225.
41. Groomes TE, Huang CT. Orthostatic hypotension after spinal cord injury: treatment with fludrocortisone and ergotamine. *Arch Phys Med Rehabil* 1991; 72:56–58.

42. Bravo G, Rojas-Martinez R, Larios F, et al. Mechanisms involved in the cardiovascular alterations immediately after spinal cord injury. *Life Sci* 2001; 68:1527–1534.

43. Kooijman M, Rongen GA, Smits P, Hopman MT. Preserved alpha-adrenergic tone in the leg vascular bed of spinal cord-injured individuals. *Circulation* 2003; 108:2361–2367.

44. Hopman MT, Groothuis JT, Flendrie M, Gerrits KH, Houtman S. Increased vascular resistance in paralyzed legs after spinal cord injury is reversible by training. *J Appl Physiol* 2002; 93:1966–1972.

45. Wecht JM, De Meersman RE, Weir JP, Spungen AM, Bauman WA. Cardiac homeostasis is independent of calf venous compliance in subjects with paraplegia. *Am J Physiol Heart Circ Physiol* 2003; 284:H2393–H2399.

46. Osborn JW, Taylor RF, Schramm LP. Determinants of arterial pressure after chronic spinal transection in rats. *Am J Physiol* 1989; 256:R666–R673.

47. Mathias CJ, Christensen NJ, Corbett JL, Frankel HL, et al. Plasma catecholamines, plasma renin activity and plasma aldosterone in tetraplegic man, horizontal and tilted. *Clin Sci Mol Med* 1975; 49:291–299.

48. Schmid A, Huonker M, Barturen JM, et al. Catecholamines, heart rate, and oxygen uptake during exercise in persons with spinal cord injury. *J Appl Physiol* 1998; 85:635–641.

49. Dela F, Stallknecht B, Biering-Sorensen F. An intact central nervous system is not necessary for insulin-mediated increases in leg blood flow in humans. *Pflugers Arch* 2000; 441:241–250.

50. Schmid A, Halle M, Stutzle C, et al. Lipoproteins and free plasma catecholamines in spinal cord injured men with different injury levels. *Clin Physiol* 2000; 20:304–310.

51. Krum H, Brown DJ, Rowe PR, Louis WJ, Howes LG. Steady state plasma [3H]-noradrenaline kinetics in quadriplegic chronic spinal cord injury patients. *J Auton Pharmacol* 1990; 10:221–226.

52. Kooner JS, Birch R, Frankel HL, Peart WS, Mathias CJ. Hemodynamic and neurohormonal effects of clonidine in patients with preganglionic and postganglionic sympathetic lesions: evidence for a central sympatholytic action. *Circulation* 1991; 84:75–83.

53. Mathias CJ, Frankel HL, Christensen NJ, Spalding JM. Enhanced pressor response to noradrenaline in patients with cervical spinal cord transection. *Brain* 1976; 99:757–770.

54. Arnold JM, Feng QP, Delaney GA, Teasell RW. Autonomic dysreflexia in tetraplegic patients: evidence for alpha-adrenoceptor hyperresponsiveness. *Clin Auton Res* 1995; 5:267–270.

55. Cochrane KL, Nathan MA. Pressor systems involved in the maintenance of arterial pressure after lesions of the rostral ventrolateral medulla. *J Auton Nerv Syst* 1994; 46:9–18.

56. Mikami H, Bumpus FM, Ferrario CM. Hierarchy of blood pressure control mechanisms after spinal sympathectomy. *J Hypertens Suppl* 1983; 1:62–65.

57. Poole CJ, Williams TD, Lightman SL, Frankel HL. Neuroendocrine control of vasopressin secretion and its effect on blood pressure in subjects with spinal cord transection. *Brain* 1987; 110(Pt 3):727–735.

58. DiBona GF, Kopp UC. Neural control of renal function. *Physiol Rev* 1997; 77:75–197.

59. Burns KD, Homma T, Harris RC. The intrarenal renin-angiotensin system. *Semin Nephrol* 1993; 13:13–30.

60. Cardus D, McTaggart WG. Total body water and its distribution in men with spinal cord injury. *Arch Phys Med Rehabil* 1984; 65:509–512.

61. Kooner JS, Frankel HL, Mirando N, Peart WS, Mathias CJ. Haemodynamic, hormonal and urinary responses to postural change in tetraplegic and paraplegic man. *Paraplegia* 1988; 26:233–237.

62. Mathias CJ, Christensen NJ, Frankel HL, Peart WS. Renin release during head-up tilt occurs independently of sympathetic nervous activity in tetraplegic man. *Clin Sci (Lond)* 1980; 59:251–256.

63. Kilinc S, Akman MN, Levendoglu F, Ozker R. Diurnal variation of antidiuretic hormone and urinary output in spinal cord injury. *Spinal Cord* 1999; 37:332–335.

64. Szollar S, North J, Chung J. Antidiuretic hormone levels and polyuria in spinal cord injury: a preliminary report. *Paraplegia* 1995; 33:94–97.

65. Riphagen CL, Pittman QJ. Vasopressin influences renal function via a spinal action. *Brain Res* 1985; 336:346–349.

66. Kooner JS, da Costa DF, Frankel HL. Recumbency induces hypertension, diuresis and natriuresis in autonomic failure, but diuresis alone in tetraplegia. *J Hypertens Suppl* 1987; 5:S327–S329.

67. Cole JD. The pathophysiology of the autonomic nervous system in spinal cord injury. In: Illis LS, ed. *Spinal Cord Dysfunction Assessment.* Oxford: Oxford Medical Publications, 1988:201–235.

68. Kewalramani LS. Autonomic dysreflexia in traumatic myelopathy. *Am J Phys Med* 1980; 59:1–21.

69. Braddom RL, Rocco JF. Autonomic dysreflexia: a survey of current treatment. *Am J Phys Med Rehabil* 1991; 70:234–241.

70. Consortium for Spinal Cord Medicine. Acute management of autonomic dysreflexia: adults with spinal cord injury presenting to health-care facilities. *J Spinal Cord Med* 1997; 20:284–308.

71. Lindan R, Joiner E, Freehafer AA, Hazel C. Incidence and clinical features of autonomic dysreflexia in patients with spinal cord injury. *Paraplegia* 1980; 18:285–292.

72. Krassioukov AV, Furlan JC, Fehlings MG. Autonomic dysreflexia in acute spinal cord injury: an under-recognized clinical entity. *J Neurotrauma* 2003; 20:707–716.

73. Giannantoni A, Di Stasi SM, Scivoletto G, et al. Autonomic dysreflexia during urodynamics. *Spinal Cord* 1998; 36:756–760.

74. Lee BY, Karmakar MG, Herz BL, Sturgill RA. Autonomic dysreflexia revisited. *J Spinal Cord Med* 1995; 18:75–87.

75. Naftchi NE, Richardson JS. Autonomic dysreflexia: pharmacological management of hypertensive crises in spinal cord injured patients. *J Spinal Cord Med* 1997; 20:355–360.

76. Comarr AE, Eltorai I. Autonomic dysreflexia/hyperreflexia. *J Spinal Cord Med* 1997; 20:345–354.

77. Amzallag M. Autonomic hyperreflexia. *Int Anesthesiol Clin* 1993; 31:87–102.

78. Blackmer J. Rehabilitation medicine. 1. Autonomic dysreflexia. *CMAJ* 2003; 169:931–935.

79. Kimura A, Ohsawa H, Sato A, Sato Y. Somatocardiovascular reflexes in anesthetized rats with the central nervous system intact or acutely spinalized at the cervical level. *Neurosci Res* 1995; 22:297–305.

80. Giuliani S, Maggi CA, Meli A. Capsaicin-sensitive afferents in the rat urinary bladder activate a spinal sympathetic cardiovascular reflex. *Naunyn Schmiedebergs Arch Pharmacol* 1988; 338:411–416.

81. Holzer P. Local effector functions of capsaicin-sensitive sensory nerve endings: involvement of tachykinins, calcitonin gene-related peptide and other neuropeptides. *Neuroscience* 1988; 24:739–768.

82. Weaver LC, Marsh DR, Gris D, Brown A, Dekaban GA. Autonomic dysreflexia after spinal cord injury: central mechanisms and strategies for prevention. *Prog Brain Res* 2006; 152:245–263.

83. Krassioukov AV, Johns DG, Schramm LP. Sensitivity of sympathetically correlated spinal interneurons, renal sympathetic nerve activity, and arterial pressure to somatic and visceral stimuli after chronic spinal injury. *J Neurotrauma* 2002; 19:1521–1529.

84. Schurch B, Knapp PA, Jeanmonod D, Rodic B, Rossier AB. Does sacral posterior rhizotomy suppress autonomic hyper-reflexia in patients with spinal cord injury? *Br J Urol* 1998; 81:73–82.

85. Coggeshall RE. Law of separation of function of the spinal roots. *Physiol Rev* 1980; 60:716–755.

86. Schenker M, Birch R. Intact myelinated fibres in biopsies of ventral spinal roots after preganglionic traction injury to the brachial plexus: a proof that Sherrington's 'wrong way afferents' exist in man? *J Anat* 2000; 197(Pt 3):383–391.

87. Krassioukov AV, Weaver LC. Morphological changes in sympathetic preganglionic neurons after spinal cord injury in rats. *Neuroscience* 1996; 70:211–225.

88. Krenz NR, Weaver LC. Changes in the morphology of sympathetic preganglionic neurons parallel the development of autonomic dysreflexia after spinal cord injury in rats. *Neurosci Lett* 1998; 243:61–64.

89. Llewellyn-Smith IJ, Weaver LC. Changes in synaptic inputs to sympathetic preganglionic neurons after spinal cord injury. *J Comp Neurol* 2001; 435:226–240.

90. Jacob JE, Pniak A, Weaver LC, Brown A. Autonomic dysreflexia in a mouse model of spinal cord injury. *Neuroscience* 2001; 108:687–693.

91. Krenz NR, Meakin SO, Krassioukov AV, Weaver LC. Neutralizing intraspinal nerve growth factor blocks autonomic dysreflexia caused by spinal cord injury. *J Neurosci* 1999; 19:7405–7414.

92. Karlsson AK. Autonomic dysreflexia. *Spinal Cord* 1999; 37:383–391.

93. Krassioukov A, Warbuton DER, Teasell RW, Eng J. Autonomic dysreflexia following spinal cord injury. In: Eng J et al., eds. *Spinal Cord Injury Rehabilitation Evidence.* Version 1. Canada: Kristin Konnyu, 2006.

94. Lindan R, Leffler EJ, Kedia KR. A comparison of the efficacy of an alpha-1-adrenergic blocker in the slow calcium channel blocker in the control of autonomic dysreflexia. *Paraplegia* 1985; 23:34–38.

95. Esmail Z, Shalansky KF, Sunderji R, Anton H, et al. Evaluation of captopril for the management of hypertension in autonomic dysreflexia: a pilot study. *Arch Phys Med Rehabil* 2002; 83:604–608.

96. Anton HA, Townson A. Drug therapy for autonomic dysreflexia. *CMAJ* 2004; 170:1210.

97. Krum H, Louis WJ, Brown DJ, Howes LG. A study of the alpha-1 adrenoceptor blocker prazosin in the prophylactic management of autonomic dysreflexia in high spinal cord injury patients. *Clin Auton Res* 1992; 2:83–88.

98. Vaidyanathan S, Soni BM, Sett P, Watt JW, et al. Pathophysiology of autonomic dysreflexia: long-term treatment with terazosin in adult and paediatric spinal cord injury patients manifesting recurrent dysreflexic episodes. *Spinal Cord* 1998; 36:761–770.

99. Abrams P, Amarenco G, Bakke A, et al. Tamsulosin: efficacy and safety in patients with neurogenic lower urinary tract dysfunction due to suprasacral spinal cord injury. *J Urol* 2003; 170:1242–1251.

100. Vaidyanathan S, Mansour P, Soni BM, Hughes PL, Singh G. Chronic lymphocytic leukaemia, synchronous small cell carcinoma and squamous neoplasia of the urinary bladder in a paraplegic man following long-term phenoxybenzamine therapy. *Spinal Cord* 2006; 44:188–191.

101. Kaplan SA, Chancellor MB, Blaivas JG. Bladder and sphincter behavior in patients with spinal cord lesions. *J Urol* 1991; 146:113–117.

102. De Groat WC, Yoshimura N. Mechanisms underlying the recovery of lower urinary tract function following spinal cord injury. *Prog Brain Res* 2006; 152:59–84.

103. Wrathall JR, Emch GS. Effect of injury severity on lower urinary tract function after experimental spinal cord injury. *Prog Brain Res* 2006; 152:117–134.

104. Blaivas JG, Sinha HP, Zayed AA, Labib KB. Detrusor-external sphincter dyssynergia. *J Urol* 1981; 125:542–544.

105. Wyndaele JJ. Urethral sphincter dyssynergia in spinal cord injury patients. *Paraplegia* 1987; 25:10–15.

106. Watanabe T, Rivas DA, Chancellor MB. Urodynamics of spinal cord injury. *Urol Clin North Am* 1996; 23:459–473.

107. Andersson KE, Sjogren C. Aspects on the physiology and pharmacology of the bladder and urethra. *Prog Neurobiol* 1982; 19:71–89.

108. Maggi CA, Barbanti G, Santicioli P, et al. Cystometric evidence that capsaicin-sensitive nerves modulate the afferent branch of micturition reflex in humans. *J Urol* 1989; 142:150–154.

109. Janig W, McLachlan EM. Identification of distinct topographical distributions of lumbar sympathetic and sensory neurons projecting to end organs with different functions in the cat. *J Comp Neurol* 1986; 246:104–112.

110. De Groat WC, Yoshimura N. Pharmacology of the lower urinary tract. *Annu Rev Pharmacol Toxicol* 2001; 41:691–721.

111. Mitsui T, Kakizaki H, Matsuura S, Ameda K, et al. Afferent fibers of the hypogastric nerves are involved in the facilitating effects of chemical bladder irritation in rats. *J Neurophysiol* 2001; 86:2276–2284.

112. Chancellor MB, De Groat WC. Intravesical capsaicin and resiniferatoxin therapy: spicing up the ways to treat the overactive bladder. *J Urol* 1999; 162:3–11.

113. Seki S, Sasaki K, Igawa Y, et al. Suppression of detrusor-sphincter dyssynergia by immunoneutralization of nerve growth factor in lumbosacral spinal cord in spinal cord injured rats. *J Urol* 2004; 171:478–482.

114. Birder LA. Role of the urothelium in urinary bladder dysfunction following spinal cord injury. *Prog Brain Res* 2006; 152:135–146.

115. Ford AP, Gever JR, Nunn PA, et al. Purinoceptors as therapeutic targets for lower urinary tract dysfunction. *Br J Pharmacol* 2006; 147(Suppl 2):S132–S143.

116. Khera M, Somogyi GT, Kiss S, Boone TB, Smith CP. Botulinum toxin A inhibits ATP release from bladder urothelium after chronic spinal cord injury. *Neurochem Int* 2004; 45:987–993.

117. Burnstock G. Physiology and pathophysiology of purinergic neurotransmission. *Physiol Rev* 2007; 87:659–797.

118. Yoshimura N. Bladder afferent pathway and spinal cord injury: possible mechanisms inducing hyperreflexia of the urinary bladder. *Prog Neurobiol* 1999; 57:583–606.

119. Kuo DC, Hisamitsu T, De Groat WC. A sympathetic projection from sacral paravertebral ganglia to the pelvic nerve and to postganglionic nerves on the surface of the urinary bladder and large intestine of the cat. *J Comp Neurol* 1984; 226:76–86.

120. Janig W, McLachlan EM. Organization of lumbar spinal outflow to distal colon and pelvic organs. *Physiol Rev* 1987; 67:1332–1404.

121. De Groat WC. A neurologic basis for the overactive bladder. *Urology* 1997; 50:36–52.

122. Cramer P, Neveux E, Regnier F, Depassio J, Berard E. Bladder-neck opening test in spinal cord injury patients using a new i.v. alpha-blocking agent, alfuzosin. *Paraplegia* 1989; 27:119–124.

123. McGuire EJ. The innervation and function of the lower urinary tract. *J Neurosurg* 1986; 65:278–285.

124. Elbadawi A. Functional anatomy of the organs of micturition. *Urol Clin North Am* 1996; 23:177–210.

125. Elbadawi A. Ultrastructure of vesicourethral innervation. II. Postganglionic axoaxonal synapses in intrinsic innervation of the vesicourethral lissosphincter: a new structural and functional concept in micturition. *J Urol* 1984; 131:781–790.

126. Mallory B, Steers WD, De Groat WC. Electrophysiological study of micturition reflexes in rats. *Am J Physiol* 1989; 257:R410–R421.

127. De Groat WC, Ryall RW. Reflexes to sacral parasympathetic neurones concerned with micturition in the cat. *J Physiol* 1969; 200:87–108.

128. Sakakibara R, Hattori T, Tojo M, Yamanishi T, et al. The location of the paths subserving micturition: studies in patients with cervical myelopathy. *J Auton Nerv Syst* 1995; 55:165–168.

129. Shefchyk SJ. Spinal mechanisms contributing to urethral striated sphincter control during continence and micturition: "how good things might go bad". *Prog Brain Res* 2006; 152:85–95.

130. Fowler CJ. Integrated control of lower urinary tract—clinical perspective. *Br J Pharmacol* 2006; 147(Suppl 2):S14–S24.

131. Mallory BS, Roppolo JR, De Groat WC. Pharmacological modulation of the pontine micturition center. *Brain Res* 1991; 546:310–320.

132. Steers WD, Meythaler JM, Haworth C, Herrell D, Park TS. Effects of acute bolus and chronic continuous intrathecal baclofen on genitourinary dysfunction due to spinal cord pathology. *J Urol* 1992; 148:1849–1855.

133. Shefchyk SJ, Espey MJ, Carr P, Nance D, et al. Evidence for a strychnine-sensitive mechanism and glycine receptors involved in the control of urethral sphincter activity during micturition in the cat. *Exp Brain Res* 1998; 119:297–306.

134. De Groat WC. Nervous control of the urinary bladder of the cat. *Brain Res* 1975; 87:201–211.

135. De Groat WC, Nadelhaft I, Milne RJ, Booth AM, et al. Organization of the sacral parasympathetic reflex pathways to the urinary bladder and large intestine. *J Auton Nerv Syst* 1981; 3:135–160.

136. Sato A, Sato Y, Shimada F, Torigata Y. Changes in vesical function produced by cutaneous stimulation in rats. *Brain Res* 1975; 94:465–474.

137. Thor KB, Blais DP, De Groat WC. Behavioral analysis of the postnatal development of micturition in kittens. *Brain Res Dev Brain Res* 1989; 46:137–144.

138. Monga M, Bernie J, Rajasekaran M. Male infertility and erectile dysfunction in spinal cord injury: a review. *Arch Phys Med Rehabil* 1999; 80:1331–1339.

139. Motofei IG, Rowland DL. Neurophysiology of the ejaculatory process: developing perspectives. *BJU Int* 2005; 96:1333–1338.

140. Steers WD, Mallory B, De Groat WC. Electrophysiological study of neural activity in penile nerve of the rat. *Am J Physiol* 1988; 254:R989–R1000.

141. Rampin O, Giuliano F, Dompeyre P, Rousseau JP. Physiological evidence of neural pathways involved in reflexogenic penile erection in the rat. *Neurosci Lett* 1994; 180:138–142.

142. Rampin O, Bernabe J, Giuliano F. Spinal control of penile erection. *World J Urol* 1997; 15:2–13.

143. Hubscher CH, Johnson RD. Effects of chronic dorsal column lesions on pelvic viscerosomatic convergent medullary reticular formation neurons. *J Neurophysiol* 2004; 92:3596–3600.

144. Giuliano F, Rampin O. Central neural regulation of penile erection. *Neurosci Biobehav Rev* 2000; 24:517–533.

145. Yarkony GM. Enhancement of sexual function and fertility in spinal cord–injured males. *Am J Phys Med Rehabil* 1990; 69:81–87.

146. Steers WD. Neural pathways and central sites involved in penile erection: neuroanatomy and clinical implications. *Neurosci Biobehav Rev* 2000; 24:507–516.

147. Hubscher CH, Kaddumi EG, Johnson RD. Brain stem convergence of pelvic viscerosomatic inputs via spinal and vagal afferents. *Neuroreport* 2004; 15:1299–1302.

148. Comarr AE. Sexual function among patients with spinal cord injury. *Urol Int* 1970; 25:134–168.

149. Brown DJ, Hill ST, Baker HW. Male fertility and sexual function after spinal cord injury. *Prog Brain Res* 2006; 152:427–439.

150. Andersson KE. Neurophysiology/pharmacology of erection. *Int J Impot Res* 2001; 13(Suppl 3):S8–S17.

151. Krogh K, Mosdal C, Laurberg S. Gastrointestinal and segmental colonic transit times in patients with acute and chronic spinal cord lesions. *Spinal Cord* 2000; 38:615–621.

152. Andersson KE. Pharmacology of penile erection. *Pharmacol Rev* 2001; 53:417–450.

153. Simonsen U, Prieto D, Hernandez M, Saenz de Tejada I, Garcia-Sacristan A. Prejunctional alpha 2-adrenoceptors inhibit nitrergic neurotransmission in horse penile resistance arteries. *J Urol* 1997; 157:2356–2360.

154. Marson L, McKenna KE. The identification of a brainstem site controlling spinal sexual reflexes in male rats. *Brain Res* 1990; 515:303–308.

155. Gu J, Polak JM, Probert L, et al. Peptidergic innervation of the human male genital tract. *J Urol* 1983; 130:386–391.

156. Hedlund H, Andersson KE, Mattiasson A. Pre- and postjunctional adreno- and muscarinic receptor functions in the isolated human corpus spongiosum urethrae. *J Auton Pharmacol* 1984; 4:241–249.

157. Toda N, Ayajiki K, Okamura T. Nitric oxide and penile erectile function. *Pharmacol Ther* 2005; 106:233–266.

158. Dail WG, Minorsky N, Moll MA, Manzanares K. The hypogastric nerve pathway to penile erectile tissue: histochemical evidence supporting a vasodilator role. *J Auton Nerv Syst* 1986; 15:341–349.

159. Derry FA, Dinsmore WW, Fraser M, et al. Efficacy and safety of oral sildenafil (Viagra) in men with erectile dysfunction caused by spinal cord injury. *Neurology* 1998; 51:1629–1633.

160. Montague DK, Jarow JP, Broderick GA, et al. Chapter 1: the management of erectile dysfunction: an AUA update. *J Urol* 2005; 174:230–239.

161. Maytom MC, Derry FA, Dinsmore WW, et al. A two-part pilot study of sildenafil (VIAGRA) in men with erectile dysfunction caused by spinal cord injury. *Spinal Cord* 1999; 37:110–116.

162. Gans WH, Zaslau S, Wheeler S, Galea G, Vapnek JM. Efficacy and safety of oral sildenafil in men with erectile dysfunction and spinal cord injury. *J Spinal Cord Med* 2001; 24:35–40.

163. Coolen LM, Allard J, Truitt WA, McKenna KE. Central regulation of ejaculation. *Physiol Behav* 2004; 83:203–215.

164. Sarkarati M, Rossier AB, Fam BA. Experience in vibratory and electro-ejaculation techniques in spinal cord injury patients: a preliminary report. *J Urol* 1987; 138:59–62.

165. Brindley GS. The fertility of men with spinal injuries. *Paraplegia* 1984; 22:337–348.

166. Brindley GS. Reflex ejaculation under vibratory stimulation in paraplegic men. *Paraplegia* 1981; 19:299–302.

167. Chapelle PA, Roby-Brami A, Yakovleff A, Bussel B. Neurological correlations of ejaculation and testicular size in men with a complete spinal cord section. *J Neurol Neurosurg Psychiatry* 1988; 51:197–202.

168. Ohl DA, Menge AC, Sonksen J. Penile vibratory stimulation in spinal cord injured men: optimized vibration parameters and prognostic factors. *Arch Phys Med Rehabil* 1996; 77:903–905.

169. Biering-Sorensen F, Sonksen J. Sexual function in spinal cord lesioned men. *Spinal Cord* 2001; 39:455–470.

170. Nygaard I, Bartscht KD, Cole S. Sexuality and reproduction in spinal cord injured women. *Obstet Gynecol Surv* 1990; 45:727–732.

171. Berard EJ. The sexuality of spinal cord injured women: physiology and pathophysiology. A review. *Paraplegia* 1989; 27:99–112.

172. Westgren N, Hultling C, Levi R, Seiger A, Westgren M. Sexuality in women with traumatic spinal cord injury. *Acta Obstet Gynecol Scand* 1997; 76:977–983.

173. Reame NE. A prospective study of the menstrual cycle and spinal cord injury. *Am J Phys Med Rehabil* 1992; 71:15–21.

174. Collins JJ, Lin CE, Berthoud HR, Papka RE. Vagal afferents from the uterus and cervix provide direct connections to the brainstem. *Cell Tissue Res* 1999; 295:43–54.

175. Pfaus JG, Manitt C, Coopersmith CB. Effects of pelvic, pudendal, or hypogastric nerve cuts on Fos induction in the rat brain following vaginocervical stimulation. *Physiol Behav* 2006; 89:627–636.

176. Sipski ML, Arenas A. Female sexual function after spinal cord injury. *Prog Brain Res* 2006; 152:441–447.

177. Sipski ML, Alexander CJ, Rosen R. Sexual arousal and orgasm in women: effects of spinal cord injury. *Ann Neurol* 2001; 49:35–44.

178. Whipple B, Komisaruk BR. Sexuality and women with complete spinal cord injury. *Spinal Cord* 1997; 35:136–138.

179. Komisaruk BR, Whipple B, Crawford A, Liu WC, et al. Brain activation during vaginocervical self-stimulation and orgasm in women with complete spinal cord injury: fMRI evidence of mediation by the vagus nerves. *Brain Res* 2004; 1024:77–88.

180. Sipski ML, Rosen RC, Alexander CJ, Hamer RM. Sildenafil effects on sexual and cardiovascular responses in women with spinal cord injury. *Urology* 2000; 55:812–815.

181. Young BK, Katz M, Klein SA. Pregnancy after spinal cord injury: altered maternal and fetal response to labor. *Obstet Gynecol* 1983; 62:59–63.

182. McGregor JA, Meeuwsen J. Autonomic hyperreflexia: a mortal danger for spinal cord-damaged women in labor. *Am J Obstet Gynecol* 1985; 151:330–333.

183. Baker ER, Cardenas DD. Pregnancy in spinal cord injured women. *Arch Phys Med Rehabil* 1996; 77:501–507.

184. Furness JB, Costa M. Types of nerves in the enteric nervous system. *Neuroscience* 1980; 5:1–20.

185. Hansen MB. The enteric nervous system I: organisation and classification. *Pharmacol Toxicol* 2003; 92:105–113.

186. Bornstein JC, Costa M, Grider JR. Enteric motor and interneuronal circuits controlling motility. *Neurogastroenterol Motil* 2004; 16(Suppl 1):34–38.

187. Cellek S, John AK, Thangiah R, et al. 5-HT4 receptor agonists enhance both cholinergic and nitrergic activities in human isolated colon circular muscle. *Neurogastroenterol Motil* 2006; 18:853–861.

188. Goyal RK, Hirano I. The enteric nervous system. *N Engl J Med* 1996; 334:1106–1115.

189. Furness JD, Bornstein JD, Kunze WA, Clerc N. The enteric nervous system and its extrinsic connections. In: Yamada T, Alpers D H, eds. *Textbook of Gastroenterology*. 3rd ed. Philadelphia: Lippincott Williams & Wilkins, 1999.

190. Furness JB. Types of neurons in the enteric nervous system. *J Auton Nerv Syst* 2000; 81:87–96.

191. Furness JB, Kunze WA, Bertrand PP, Clerc N, Bornstein JC. Intrinsic primary afferent neurons of the intestine. *Prog Neurobiol* 1998; 54:1–18.

192. Gershon MD. Review article: serotonin receptors and transporters—roles in normal and abnormal gastrointestinal motility. *Aliment Pharmacol Ther* 2004; 20(Suppl 7):3–14.

193. Grundy D. Sensory signals from the gastrointestinal tract. *J Pediatr Gastroenterol Nutr* 2005; 41(Suppl 1):S7–S9.

194. Read NW, Houghton LA. Physiology of gastric emptying and pathophysiology of gastroparesis. *Gastroenterol Clin North Am* 1989; 18:359–373.

195. Andrews PL. Vagal afferent innervation of the gastrointestinal tract. *Prog Brain Res* 1986; 67:65–86.

196. Berthoud HR, Neuhuber WL. Functional and chemical anatomy of the afferent vagal system. *Auton Neurosci* 2000; 85:1–17.

197. Kral JG. Behavioral effects of vagotomy in humans. *J Auton Nerv Syst* 1983; 9:273–281.

198. Chung EA, Emmanuel AV. Gastrointestinal symptoms related to autonomic dysfunction following spinal cord injury. *Prog Brain Res* 2006; 152:317–333.

199. Travagli RA, Hermann GE, Browning KN, Rogers RC. Musings on the wanderer: what's new in our understanding of vago-vagal reflexes? III. Activity-dependent plasticity in vago-vagal reflexes controlling the stomach. *Am J Physiol Gastrointest Liver Physiol* 2003; 284:G180–G187.

200. Longo WE, Ballantyne GH, Modlin IM. The colon, anorectum, and spinal cord patient: a review of the functional alterations of the denervated hindgut. *Dis Colon Rectum* 1989; 32:261–267.

201. Keef KD, Kreulen DL. Comparison of central versus peripheral nerve pathways to the guinea pig inferior mesenteric ganglion determined electrophysiologically after chronic nerve section. *J Auton Nerv Syst* 1990; 29:95–112.

202. Du C, Ferre JP, Ruckebusch Y. Spinal cord influences on the colonic myoelectrical activity of fed and fasted rats. *J Physiol* 1987; 383:395–404.

203. Luckensmeyer GB, Keast JR. Activation of alpha- and beta-adrenoceptors by sympathetic nerve stimulation in the large intestine of the rat. *J Physiol* 1998; 510(Pt 2):549–561.

204. Lundberg JM, Hokfelt T, Anggard A, et al. Organizational principles in the peripheral sympathetic nervous system: subdivision by coexisting peptides (somatostatin-, avian pancreatic polypeptide-, and vasoactive

intestinal polypeptide-like immunoreactive materials). *Proc Natl Acad Sci U S A* 1982; 79:1303–1307.

205. Stebbing M, Johnson P, Vremec M, Bornstein J. Role of alpha(2)-adrenoceptors in the sympathetic inhibition of motility reflexes of guinea-pig ileum. *J Physiol* 2001; 534:465–478.

206. Lu CL, Montgomery P, Zou X, Orr WC, Chen JD. Gastric myoelectrical activity in patients with cervical spinal cord injury. *Am J Gastroenterol* 1998; 93:2391–2396.

207. Rees WD, Malagelada JR, Miller LJ, Go VL. Human interdigestive and postprandial gastrointestinal motor and gastrointestinal hormone patterns. *Dig Dis Sci* 1982; 27:321–329.

208. Kunze WA, Furness JB. The enteric nervous system and regulation of intestinal motility. *Annu Rev Physiol* 1999; 61:117–142.

209. Tack J. Georges Brohee Prize 1994. Motilin and the enteric nervous system in the control of interdigestive and postprandial gastric motility. *Acta Gastroenterol Belg* 1995; 58:21–30.

210. Clanton LJ Jr., Bender J. Refractory spinal cord injury induced gastroparesis: resolution with erythromycin lactobionate, a case report. *J Spinal Cord Med* 1999; 22:236–238.

211. Fealey RD, Szurszewski JH, Merritt JL, DiMagno EP. Effect of traumatic spinal cord transection on human upper gastrointestinal motility and gastric emptying. *Gastroenterology* 1984; 87:69–75.

212. Segal JL, Milne N, Brunnemann SR. Gastric emptying is impaired in patients with spinal cord injury. *Am J Gastroenterol* 1995; 90:466–470.

213. Rock E, Malmud L, Fisher RS. Motor disorders of the stomach. *Med Clin North Am* 1981; 65:1269–1289.

214. Segal JL, Milne N, Brunnemann SR, Lyons KP. Metoclopramide-induced normalization of impaired gastric emptying in spinal cord injury. *Am J Gastroenterol* 1987; 82:1143–1148.

215. Karamanolis G, Tack J. Promotility medications—now and in the future. *Dig Dis* 2006; 24:297–307.

216. Stone JM, Nino-Murcia M, Wolfe VA, Perkash I. Chronic gastrointestinal problems in spinal cord injury patients: a prospective analysis. *Am J Gastroenterol* 1990; 85:1114–1119.

217. Krogh K, Nielsen J, Djurhuus JC, Mosdal C, et al. Colorectal function in patients with spinal cord lesions. *Dis Colon Rectum* 1997; 40:1233–1239.

218. Hertz A, Newton A. The normal movement of the colon in man. *J Physiol (Lond)* 1913; 47:57–65.

219. Aaronson MJ, Freed MM, Burakoff R. Colonic myoelectric activity in persons with spinal cord injury. *Dig Dis Sci* 1985; 30:295–300.

220. Glick ME, Meshkinpour H, Haldeman S, Hoehler F, et al. Colonic dysfunction in patients with thoracic spinal cord injury. *Gastroenterology* 1984; 86:287–294.

221. Connell AM, Frankel H, Guttmann L. The motility of the pelvic colon following complete lesions of the spinal cord. *Paraplegia* 1963; 1:98–110.

222. Banwell JG, Creasey GH, Aggarwal AM, Mortimer JT. Management of the neurogenic bowel in patients with spinal cord injury. *Urol Clin North Am* 1993; 20:517–526.

223. Sun WM, MacDonagh R, Forster D, Thomas DG, et al. Anorectal function in patients with complete spinal transection before and after sacral posterior rhizotomy. *Gastroenterology* 1995; 108:990–998.

224. De Groat WC, Krier J. The sacral parasympathetic reflex pathway regulating colonic motility and defaecation in the cat. *J Physiol* 1978; 276:481–500.

225. Valles M, Vidal J, Clave P, Mearin F. Bowel dysfunction in patients with motor complete spinal cord injury: clinical, neurological, and pathophysiological associations. *Am J Gastroenterol* 2006; 101:2290–2299.

226. Yamanouchi M, Shimatani H, Kadowaki M, et al. Integrative control of rectoanal reflex in guinea pigs through lumbar colonic nerves. *Am J Physiol Gastrointest Liver Physiol* 2002; 283:G148–G156.

227. Beuret-Blanquart F, Weber J, Gouverneur JP, Demangeon S, Denis P. Colonic transit time and anorectal manometric anomalies in 19 patients with complete transection of the spinal cord. *J Auton Nerv Syst* 1990; 30:199–207.

228. Menardo G, Bausano G, Corazziari E, et al. Large-bowel transit in paraplegic patients. *Dis Colon Rectum* 1987; 30:924–928.

229. Leduc BE, Giasson M, Favreau-Ethier M, Lepage Y. Colonic transit time after spinal cord injury. *J Spinal Cord Med* 1997; 20:416–421.

230. Keshavarzian A, Barnes WE, Bruninga K, Nemchausky B, et al. Delayed colonic transit in spinal cord-injured patients measured by indium-111 Amberlite scintigraphy. *Am J Gastroenterol* 1995; 90:1295–1300.

231. Leduc BE, Spacek E, Lepage Y. Colonic transit time after spinal cord injury: any clinical significance? *J Spinal Cord Med* 2002; 25:161–166.

232. Binnie NR, Creasey GH, Edmond P, Smith AN. The action of cisapride on the chronic constipation of paraplegia. *Paraplegia* 1988; 26:151–158.

233. Geders JM, Gaing A, Bauman WA, Korsten MA. The effect of cisapride on segmental colonic transit time in patients with spinal cord injury. *Am J Gastroenterol* 1995; 90:285–289.

234. Rajendran SK, Reiser JR, Bauman W, Zhang RL, et al. Gastrointestinal transit after spinal cord injury: effect of cisapride. *Am J Gastroenterol* 1992; 87:1614–1617.

235. Richter JE. Cisapride: limited access and alternatives. *Cleve Clin J Med* 2000; 67:471–472.

236. Krogh K, Jensen MB, Gandrup P, et al. Efficacy and tolerability of prucalopride in patients with constipation due to spinal cord injury. *Scand J Gastroenterol* 2002; 37:431–436.

237. Sun WM, Hasler WL, Lien HC, Montague J, Owyang C. Nizatidine enhances the gastrocolonic response and the colonic peristaltic reflex in humans. *J Pharmacol Exp Ther* 2001; 299:159–163.

238. Van der Velden VHJ, Hulsmann AR. Autonomic innervation of human airways: structure, function, and pathophysiology in asthma. *Neuroimmunomodulation* 1999; 6:145–159.

239. Belvisi MG. Overview of the innervation of the lung. *Curr Opin Pharmacol* 2002; 2:211–215.

240. Canning BJ. Reflex regulation of airway smooth muscle tone. *J Appl Physiol* 2006; 101:971–985.

241. Coleridge HM, Coleridge JC. Neural regulation of bronchial blood flow. *Respir Physiol* 1994; 98:1–13.

242. Canning BJ, Fischer A. Neural regulation of airway smooth muscle tone. *Respir Physiol* 2001; 125:113–127.

243. Bianchi AL, Denavit-Saubie M, Champagnat J. Central control of breathing in mammals: neuronal circuitry, membrane properties, and neurotransmitters. *Physiol Rev* 1995; 75:1–45.

244. Yu J, Zhang JF, Roberts AM, Collins LC, Fletcher EC. Pulmonary rapidly adapting receptor stimulation does not increase airway resistance in anesthetized rabbits. *Am J Respir Crit Care Med* 1999; 160:906–912.

245. Coleridge HM, Coleridge JC. Pulmonary reflexes: neural mechanisms of pulmonary defense. *Annu Rev Physiol* 1994; 56:91.

246. Neubauer JA, Gonsalves SF, Chou W, Geller HM, Edelman NH. Chemosensitivity of medullary neurons in explant tissue cultures. *Neuroscience* 1991; 45:701–708.

247. Loveridge B, Sanii R, Dubo HI. Breathing pattern adjustments during the first year following cervical spinal cord injury. *Paraplegia* 1992; 30:479–488.

248. Almenoff PL, Alexander LR, Spungen AM, Lesser MD, Bauman WA. Bronchodilatory effects of ipratropium bromide in patients with tetraplegia. *Paraplegia* 1995; 33:274–277.

249. DeLuca RV, Grimm DR, Lesser M, Bauman WA, Almenoff PL. Effects of a beta2-agonist on airway hyperreactivity in subjects with cervical spinal cord injury. *Chest* 1999; 115:1533–1538.

250. Grimm DR, Arias E, Lesser M, Bauman WA, Almenoff PL. Airway hyperresponsiveness to ultrasonically nebulized distilled water in subjects with tetraplegia. *J Appl Physiol* 1999; 86:1165–1169.

251. Singas E LM, Spungen A, Bauman WA, Almenoff PL. Airway hyperresponsiveness to methacholine in subjects with spinal cord injury. *Chest* 1996; 110:911–915.

252. Mateus SR, Beraldo PS, Horan TA. Cholinergic bronchomotor tone and airway caliber in tetraplegic patients. *Spinal Cord* 2006; 44:269–274.

253. Kelling JS, DiMarco AF, Gottfried SB, Altose MD. Respiratory responses to ventilatory loading following low cervical spinal cord injury. *J Appl Physiol* 1985; 59:1752–1756.

254. Manning HL, Shea SA, Schwartzstein RM, Lansing RW, et al. Reduced tidal volume increases 'air hunger' at fixed PCO2 in ventilated quadriplegics. *Respir Physiol* 1992; 90:19–30.

255. Lin KH, Wu HD, Chang CW, Wang TG, Wang YH. Ventilatory and mouth occlusion pressure responses to hypercapnia in chronic tetraplegia. *Arch Phys Med Rehabil* 1998; 79:795–799.

256. Pokorski M, Morikawa T, Takaishi S, Masuda A, et al. Ventilatory responses to chemosensory stimuli in quadriplegic subjects. *Eur Respir J* 1990; 3:891–900.

257. Axen K. Ventilatory responses to mechanical loads in cervical cord–injured humans. *J Appl Physiol* 1982; 52:748–756.

258. O'Donnell DE, Sanii R, Dubo H, Loveridge B, Younes M. Steady-state ventilatory responses to expiratory resistive loading in quadriplegics. *Am Rev Respir Dis* 1993; 147:54–59.

259. Banzett RB, Lansing RW, Brown R. High-level quadriplegics perceive lung volume change. *J Appl Physiol* 1987; 62:567–573.

260. Simon PM, Leevers AM, Murty JL, Skatrud JB, Dempsey JA. Neuromechanical regulation of respiratory motor output in ventilator-dependent C1–C3 quadriplegics. *J Appl Physiol* 1995; 79:312–323.

261. Gandevia SC, Killian K, McKenzie DK, et al. Respiratory sensations, cardiovascular control, kinaesthesia and transcranial stimulation during paralysis in humans. *J Physiol* 1993; 470:85–107.

262. Schmidt KD, Chan CW. Thermoregulation and fever in normal persons and in those with spinal cord injuries. *Mayo Clin Proc* 1992; 67:469–475.

263. Downey JA, Chiodi HP, Darling RC. Central temperature regulation in the spinal man. *J Appl Physiol* 1967; 22:91–94.

264. Romanovsky AA. Thermoregulation: some concepts have changed. Functional architecture of the thermoregulatory system. *Am J Physiol Regul Integr Comp Physiol* 2007; 292:R37–R46.

265. Simon E. Temperature regulation: the spinal cord as a site of extrahypothalamic thermoregulatory functions. *Rev Physiol Biochem Pharmacol* 1974; 1–76.

266. Downey RJ, Downey JA, Newhouse E, Weissman C. Fatal hyperthermia in a quadriplegic man: possible evidence for a peripheral action of haloperidol in neuroleptic malignant syndrome. *Chest* 1992; 101:1728–1730.

267. Nagashima K, Nakai S, Tanaka M, Kanosue K. Neuronal circuitries involved in thermoregulation. *Auton Neurosci* 2000; 85:18–25.

268. Lemons DE, Riedel G, Downey JA. Thermoregulation and the effects of thermomodalities. In: Gonzalez EG, Myers SJ, Lieberman JS, Downey JA, eds. *Physiological Basis of Rehabilitation Medicine.* 3rd ed. Boston: Butterworth Heinemann, 2001:507–520.

269. Cooper KE, Ferres HM, Guttmann L. Vasomotor responses in the foot to raising body temperature in the paraplegic patient. *J Physiol (Lond)* 1957; 136:547–555.

270. Appenzeller O, Schnieden H. Neurogenic pathways concerned in reflex vasodilatation in the hand with especial reference to stimuli affecting the afferent pathway. *Clin Sci* 1963; 25:413–421.

271. Benzinger TH. Heat regulation: homeostasis of central temperature in man. *Physiol Rev* 1969; 49:671–759.

272. Tsai SH, Shih CJ, Shyy TT, Liu JC. Recovery of vasomotor response in human spinal cord transection. *J Neurosurg* 1980; 52:808–811.

273. Nicotra A, Asahina M, Young TM, Mathias CJ. Heat-provoked skin vasodilatation in innervated and denervated trunk dermatomes in human spinal cord injury. *Spinal Cord* 2006; 44:222–226.

274. Corbett JL, Frankel HL, Harris PJ. Cardiovascular reflex responses to cutaneous and visceral stimuli in spinal man. *J Physiol* 1971; 215:395–409.

275. Sahs AL, Fulton JR. Somatic and automatic reflexes in spinal monkeys. *J Neurophysiol* 1940; 3:258–268.

276. Minson CT, Berry LT, Joyner MJ. Nitric oxide and neurally mediated regulation of skin blood flow during local heating. *J Appl Physiol* 2001; 91:1619–1626.

277. Charkoudian N. Skin blood flow in adult human thermoregulation: how it works, when it does not, and why. *Mayo Clin Proc* 2003; 78:603–612.

278. Freund PR, Brengelmann GL, Rowell LB, Halar E. Attenuated skin blood flow response to hyperthermia in paraplegic men. *J Appl Physiol* 1984; 56:1104–1109.

279. Tam HS, Darling RC, Cheh HY, Downey JA. The dead zone of thermoregulation in normal and paraplegic man. *Can J Physiol Pharmacol* 1978; 56:976–983.

280. Downey JA, Huckaba CE, Kelley PS, Tam HS, et al. Sweating responses to central and peripheral heating in spinal man. *J Appl Physiol* 1976; 40:701–706.

281. Quinton PM. Sweating and its disorders. *Annu Rev Med* 1983; 34:429–452.

282. Normell LA. Distribution of impaired cutaneous vasomotor and sudomotor function in paraplegic man. *Scand J Clin Lab Invest* 1974; 138:25–41.

283. Seckendorf R, Randall WC. Thermal reflex sweating in normal and paraplegic man. *J Appl Physiol* 1961; 16:796–800.

284. Silver JR, Randall WC, Guttmann L. Spinal mediation of thermally induced sweating. *J Neurol Neurosurg Psychiatry* 1991; 54:297–304.

285. Wallin BG, Stjernberg L. Sympathetic activity in man after spinal cord injury: outflow to skin below the lesion. *Brain* 1984; 107(Pt 1):183–198.

286. Guttmann L, Whitteridge D. Effects of bladder distension on autonomic mechanisms after spinal cord injuries. *Brain* 1947; 70:366–404.

287. Johnson RH. Neurological studies in temperature regulation. *Ann R Coll Surg Engl* 1965; 36:339–352.

288. Dietrich WD, Bramlett HM. Hyperthermia and central nervous system injury. *Prog Brain Res* 2007; 162:201–217.

289. McKinley W, McNamee S, Meade M, Kandra K, Abdul N. Incidence, etiology, and risk factors for fever following acute spinal cord injury. *J Spinal Cord Med* 2006; 29:501–506.

42 Syringomyelia

Jelena N. Svircev
James W. Little

Syringomyelia is a clinical syndrome that results from an enlarging syrinx; that is, an enlarging fluid-filled cyst within the gray matter of the spinal cord. The word syrinx is derived from the Greek word for pipe and myelos meaning marrow; a syrinx cavity is often like an elongated fluid-filled tube or pipe within the spinal cord.

Two types of syringomyelia are often distinguished: communicating and noncommunicating (1, 2, 3). Communicating syringomyelia (also called hydromyelia) is caused by an enlargement of the central canal within the spinal cord. The more common noncommunicating syringomyelia is caused by syrinx developing within the gray matter of the spinal cord. Communicating and noncommunicating syringomyelia have also been called cannilicular and extracannilicular syringomyelia, respectively. Because the type of syrinx is unclear in some cases, and because the two types may be associated, the terms syringohydromyelia and hydrosyringomyelia have been used. Two common types of syringomyelia are reviewed here: posttraumatic following spinal cord injury and congenital due to Chiari malformation.

POSTTRAUMATIC SYRINGOMYELIA

A posttraumatic syrinx originates at the site of spinal cord injury (SCI) and extends rostrally or caudally. This type of syrinx is most often noncommunicating. Such a posttraumatic syrinx develops in 0.2% to 8% of SCI patients as neurologic decline (4–8), in 12% to 28% by magnetic resonance imaging (MRI) (8–13), and in 17% to 20% at autopsy (14, 15). The clinical syndrome, manifest as neurologic and functional decline, is known as posttraumatic syringomyelia (PTS); it is also called ascending cystic degeneration or progressive posttraumatic cystic myelopathy. Small intramedullary cysts that do not extend longitudinally over time and that do not cause neurologic decline are seen in 39–59 percent of SCI patients (13, 16, 17); these are often referred to as posttraumatic cysts or cystic myelomalacia.

PTS can develop in 2 months to 30 years post-SCI. The incidence of PTS is similar following paraplegia and tetraplegia (11).

It is one of the most common causes of worsening myelopathy after SCI (18). It can be psychologically devastating, because it can cause worsening disability after an SCI individual has completed initial rehabilitation (19).

The pathogenesis of posttraumatic syrinxes is not known. The cavity originates in the gray matter at the site of cord injury (20). Initiating factors are likely cord hematoma, edema, inflammation (21), and enzymatic lysis contributing to formation of an intramedullary posttraumatic cyst (22, 23). Other factors may be arachnoidal scarring, residual spinal canal stenosis, and residual spinal kyphotic deformity; such deformities may cause cord tethering with resulting increased cord tension on spine flexion and impaired cerebrospinal fluid (CSF) flow in the subarachnoid space (14, 24, 25, 26, 27). SCI patients with more than 15 degrees residual kyphosis and more than 25% canal stenosis are twice as likely to develop a posttraumatic syrinx (12). Cord tension may pull open cystic cavities and cause traction to cord vessels, leading to gray matter ischemia; recurrent gray matter infarction may coalesce into a syrinx (11, 12, 24, 28). PTS extends rostrally in 81%, caudally in 4%, and in both directions in 15% of patients (5). Non-traumatic spinal cord pathology (e.g., spinal cord tumors, spinal stenosis, infectious meningitis, disc protrusion, spinal cord arteriovenous malformation, spinal cord infarction, and transverse myelitis) (21) can predispose to syringomyelia, perhaps also by tethering the spinal cord, causing spinal cord ischemia, and impairing CSF flow in the subarachnoid space. Uncommon traumatic cyst-to-subarachnoid fistulas may allow the more direct transmission of subarachnoid pressure surges to the cyst and lead to more rapid syrinx development (2, 5, 29).

A variety of factors may contribute to syrinx enlargement. PTS, as a type of noncommunicating syrinx, does not communicate with the fourth ventricle or with the central canal (30–32); rather, it likely arises from posttraumatic cysts at the zone of cord injury that take on fluid from the subarachnoid space, increase in pressure, and extend rostrally and/or caudally by dissecting through the intermediate zone of the gray matter—often unilaterally (33). The longitudinal fluid dissection may result from pulsatile increases in subarachnoid fluid pressure caused by cough, sneeze, straining or Valsalva, Credé pressure over abdomen, weight lifting, forward-lean pressure release, and manual assisted (quad) coughing (19, 34–38). These intraabdominal or intrathoracic pressure surges are transmitted via the valveless inferior vena cava and azygous veins to the epidural venous plexus; increased subarachnoid pressure either surges pump fluid into the syrinx cavity via perivascular spaces (Virchow–Robin spaces; 32, 34, 39) or causes fluid in the syrinx to "slosh" rostrally (30, 40). In an ovoid syrinx, pressure is greatest where the curvature is greatest—thus, syrinxes extend at the poles and become long, tubular structures (41). The perivascular spaces of Virchow–Robin may act as one-way valves, allowing fluid from subarachnoid space into the syrinx but limiting egress; this may explain the high intrasyrinx pressures and protein concentrations in some syrinxes (4, 42). The dilated spinal cord may also be compressed against spondylotic spurs, thus leading to additional neurologic decline (43). New theories are being developed to describe the pathophysiology of PTS, and principles of fluid dynamics and dynamic imaging are being applied to support the theories (27).

The symptoms and signs of early PTS are often nonspecific. The symptoms and signs, such as ascending reflex and sensory loss, are often unilateral early in PTS (4, 7, 44), consistent with a unilateral syrinx on MRI; the syrinx may become bilateral later. Pain is a common presenting symptom and is seen in 36% to 80% of PTS patients (4–6, 44, 45). The pain is often localized to the site of the original injury or may radiate to the neck or upper limbs. The pain is often aching or burning and is aggravated by coughing, sneezing, straining, postural change, body vibration, or active limb movement. Functional MRI (fMRI) studies suggest that the spontaneous neuropathic pain and the allodynic neuropathic pain of syringomyelia may be due to different pathophysiologic mechanisms (45). Ascending loss of deep tendon reflexes and ascending loss of pain and temperature sensation are common early signs (4–6, 46). Loss of pain and temperature sensation with preserved touch, position, and vibration sense is referred to as dissociated sensory loss (4–6, 46), which is caused by a disruption of crossing spinothalamic fibers by the syrinx but sparing of posterior column fibers. Worsening weakness is also common in PTS (4–6, 46, 47) but typically develops after ascending sensory loss (7, 20).

Less-common findings are increased or decreased spasms, muscle fasciculations, muscle atrophy, hyperhidrosis, loss of reflex bladder emptying, worsening orthostatic hypotension, scoliosis, central and/or obstructive sleep apnea, new Horner's syndrome, reduced respiratory drive, impaired vagal cardiovascular reflexes, and sudden death (4, 48). With high cervical and brainstem involvement by the syrinx, diaphragm paralysis, sensory loss in the trigeminal nerve distribution, dysphagia, dysphonia, and nystagmus may be seen. Neurogenic arthropathy (Charcot joint), pressure sores, and burns can develop due to loss of protective pain and temperature sensation.

Syringomyelia is variable in its presentation and in its natural history. Long, dilating, sudden-onset syrinxes often worsen most rapidly. These manifest as weakness and loss of function, but some long and dilated syrinxes manifest minimal symptoms (Figure 42.1). Syrinx size on MRI does not correlate directly with symptoms or degree of disability. Short syrinxes may manifest as weakness and loss of function, particularly in lower limbs of patients with incomplete SCI. Short or long, dilated or

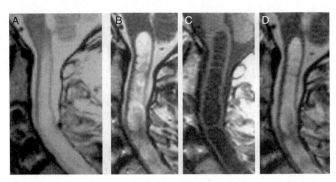

Figure 42.1 MRI of posttraumatic syrinx. Serial magnetic resonance images are shown of a posttraumatic syrinx in a 57-year-old male with T3 traumatic paraplegia, who developed L hand weakness and pain at 8 months post-SCI; examination revealed loss of tendon reflexes and loss of pinprick sensation in the L upper limb. The initial MRI (**A**) showed a large dilating syrinx ascending rostrally from the thoracic level of SCI through the cervical spinal cord to the medulla. He underwent arachnoid dissection/duraplasty at 12 months post-SCI with gradual resolution of his L hand weakness and partial resolution of pain. Despite sustained recovery of L hand strength and improvement in pain symptoms, follow-up MRIs at 21 months (**B, C**) and 30 months (**D**) post-SCI showed a persisting, dilating syrinx extending rostrally to the medulla. MRI images A, B, and D are T2-weighted; image C is T1-weighted.

nondilated syrinxes can cause neuropathic pain. Regarding natural history, syrinx manifestations can spontaneously resolve, worsen then plateau, worsen intermittently, or worsen continuously. Syrinxes with an early onset post-SCI often cause the most rapid neurologic decline.

MRI is usually definitive for diagnosing PTS. An intramedullary cyst with well-defined margins that is eccentric, extends beyond the limits of the original cord injury, does not communicate with the central canal or the fourth ventricle, and is isodense with CSF (i.e., low-density T1-weighted image, high-density T2-weighted image) is characteristic. Syrinx MRI features that are associated with neurologic decline include long and wide dimensions (7, 12, 49), CSF flow from cardiac-gated images (50), poorly demarcated T2-weighted signal hyperintensity at the rostral extent (51), flow void sign on T2-weighted images suggesting high pressure (25), and association with spinal stenosis (12). MRI may be limited by metal that may distort cord images (e.g., rods, wires, plates, screws, bullet fragments, etc.). Rarely, false-positive and false-negative MRIs can occur. False-positive MRI diagnosis may be caused by myelomalacia (i.e., ischemic cord damage/gliosis and microcystic degeneration), cord hemorrhage, or tumor (34, 52, 53). False-negative MRIs for PTS can occur when the signal density of the proteinaceous syrinx fluid is similar to neural tissue (53). Gadolinium, as an intravenous contrast agent, can improve the distinction between PTS and intra- or extramedullary tumors, arteriovenous malformation, and multiple sclerosis plaques. MRI can provide information on CSF flow velocity using images gated to the cardiac cycle and can aid in distinguishing syrinxes from cystic myelomalacia and arachnoid cysts (54).

Other imaging studies may be useful for evaluating PTS and for distinguishing it from other progressive myelopathies. Conventional spine radiography with flexion and extension views may help diagnose spinal instability, disc space infection, and spinal stenosis. Metrizamide myelogram with immediate and delayed computed tomography (CT) scans can aid diagnosis of PTS, arachnoiditis, and disc herniation, particularly in those in whom MRI can not be performed (55).

Electrodiagnostic findings in PTS include features of mixed upper and lower motoneuron involvement (4, 56, 57, 58, 59). Early findings are (a) prolonged segmental conduction on F-wave studies, and (b) prolonged descending motor conduction on motor-evoked potential (MEP) testing. Later electrodiagnostic findings include (a) reduced compound muscle action potential (CMAP) amplitude; (b) enlarged motor-unit action potential (MUAP) amplitude consistent with motoneuron loss and compensatory motor axon sprouting by spared motoneurons; and (c) reduced maximal firing rate of motor units during maximal voluntary effort, consistent with reduced upper motoneuron input to motoneurons. Sensory nerve action potentials (SNAP) are preserved except when there is associated peripheral nerve entrapment, which is common (58). Muscle membrane instability is a late finding, likely because lower motoneuron loss is gradual and there is ongoing compensatory sprouting to minimize persisting denervation in a muscle.

Neurologic monitoring guides treatment. Large syrinxes on MRI may be minimally symptomatic. Some argue to surgically decompress a syrinx only when the patient becomes symptomatic. Others warn that early treatment is needed or neuronal loss may advance silently and become irreversible. If nonoperative treatment is chosen, then close neurologic monitoring is needed to assure that the patient is neurologically stable. The clinical neurologic examination, including sensory pinprick exam and manual strength testing, may not be sufficiently sensitive to detect neurologic decline before irreversible damage has occurred. Additional monitoring with serial quantitative strength testing (60), such as handheld myometry or measurements of grips and pinches, electrodiagnostic studies (F-waves, MEP, electromyography), or serial MRI may be considered. Neurologic monitoring is also needed postoperatively to assure persisting benefit from the syrinx surgical decompression.

PTS can lead to a neurologic decline of sufficient degree to cause functional loss. In severe cases, a fully independent person with paraplegia may decline to tetraplegia with total dependence for transfers and self-care (3, 61). Another scenario for functional loss in PTS is in a patient with incomplete SCI; such persons regain walking and bowel/bladder control early after injury and then lose walking and bowel/bladder control years later due to PTS. In addition to disability from either ascending cord involvement or long-tract cord involvement in those with incomplete SCI, other factors can contribute to functional loss in PTS. These include severe neuropathic pain, extensor spasms, and neuropathic joints. Noncystic myelopathy, such as myelomalacia and cord tethering, may also cause pain, sensory loss, and weakness, but the degree to which they cause functional decline is less clearly described.

Conservative treatments have been advocated for PTS (6, 7, 62, 63); however, they are not well studied. Nonoperative treatment is favored by some if there is no apparent or minimal neurologic decline (6, 7, 62, 63), although in most studies, followup was for less than 10 years. Rossier and colleagues (4) stated that "a patient, if followed long enough, will eventually show some signs of progression." Syrinx patients who are managed conservatively must be monitored closely; if they show significant decline, then prompt surgical treatment may be needed.

Conservative treatment is often clinical observation without any specific intervention, but may also include activity precautions aimed at altering spinal fluid dynamics by reducing CSF production and by lowering venous pressures, percutaneous drainage of the syrinx, assuring no secondary causes of myelopathy, and providing ongoing rehabilitation. Activity precautions include avoiding maneuvers that transmit venous pressures to the subarachnoid space, such as high-force exercise, Valsalva and Credé, manual assisted (quad) coughing with direct compression over the inferior vena cava, and forward-lean (chest-on-thigh) pressure releases. Attempts to alter spinal fluid dynamics may include agents to reduce CSF production, head-of-bed elevation to 20 degrees at night to lessen rostral "slosh" of fluid in the syrinx, agents to promote venous dilation and lower venous pressures, and agents (venous compression stockings, the alpha-adrenergic vasoconstrictor midodrine, etc.) to lessen daytime fluid accumulation caused by orthostatic hypotension. Other treatable causes of myelopathy should be addressed, including B12 deficiency and spinal stenosis. Percutaneous drainage of the syrinx under CT guidance can provide benefit (64), but often fluid reaccumulates rapidly (65). Perhaps a combination of conservative measures can prevent neurologic decline without surgery, but this has not been examined in rigorous clinical studies.

Surgical treatment is usually indicated if there is ongoing or rapid neurologic decline. Surgery should not be delayed until there is severe weakness. It should be considered at the first sign of weakness, because deficits can become irreversible if surgery is delayed (5, 21, 35, 66). Surgical options include (a) syringostomy to drain the syrinx (67); (b) shunting (syringo-subarachnoid, syringo-pleural, or syringo-peritoneal; 35, 66–71); (c) dissection of arachnoidal scar and duraplasty to reconstruct the subarachnoid space (72–74); and (d) cordectomy (39, 42, 66, 75, 76).

Surgery yields improved strength and improved pain control in some but not all patients, whereas sensation does not usually recover (66, 77). Reduced syrinx size on postoperative MRI (78) and restored intrasyrinx fluid motion during the cardiac cycle (79) predict a good surgical result, but complete syrinx resolution is not essential for a good clinical outcome. With either shunting or arachnoid dissection/duraplasty, there is recurrence of neurologic decline by five years in as many as 50% of patients (66, 74). In some, the failure is caused by a recurrence of fluid within the syrinx; shunts can occlude because of syrinx cavity collapse around the catheter tip and glial ingrowth into the shunt openings (73). Shunts or duraplasty may fail even though the syrinx remains decompressed on MRI; cord tethering by the shunt or recurrent arachnoidal scarring may contribute to recurrent symptoms. Patients with SCI who ambulate (i.e., ASIA D or E) are at risk for new neurologic decline after shunting (78, 80); the shunt tube may compromise descending motor axons adjacent to the syrinx. These particular patients may benefit most from conservative treatment or arachnoid dissection with duraplasty. Persons with complete SCI (ASIA A) may benefit from syringo-pleural or syringo-peritoneal shunting. Cordectomy or complete surgical transection of the cord, a procedure regarded as "radical" by some and infrequently performed, has been shown to yield long-term benefit in most cases reported in the literature (39, 66, 75, 76). Whether a conservative or surgical approach is used to manage PTS, rehabilitation therapies should play an integral role in management. As patients experience functional decline, their mobility, ability to perform activities of daily living, and method of bowel/bladder management may change as well. Patients' functional abilities and equipment needs should be assessed regularly by physical and occupational therapy. Individuals with PTS should be educated on syringomyelia and the physical and functional implications. Care needs should be reviewed, as patients who were once independent in all activities may now require assistance. Consultation by a social worker or case manager may guide the patient in seeking home support services in the community.

CHIARI MALFORMATION CAUSING SYRINGOMYELIA

Syrinxes that are associated with congenital foramen magnum encroachment (e.g., Chiari I or Chiari II malformation) may result from either central canal dilation (i.e., communicating syringomyelia or hydromyelia) or from an eccentric syrinx cavity in the gray matter of the cord (noncommunicating syringomyelia) (1, 81–86). Because the two types of syrinxes are often indistinguishable by imaging studies, particularly later in the disease, they may be referred to as syringohydromyelia or hydrosyringomyelia.

Chiari I malformation is a congenital downward displacement of the cerebellar tonsils through the foramen magnum, into the cervical subarachnoid space. The more severe Chiari II malformation is downward displacement of the cerebellar vermis, pons, and medulla into the foramen magnum and elongation of the fourth ventricle. Chiari I malformation typically presents clinically in young adults, whereas Chiari II malformation presents in infants and is usually associated with myelomeningocele and hydrocephalus. More recently, Chiari 0 (syringohydromyelia without cerebellar tonsillar herniation) and Chiari 1.5 (tonsillar herniation with brain stem herniation) malformations have been described, but management principals are based on the guidelines developed for the treatment of more common Chiari I and II malformations (86).

Chiari I malformation is the most common cause of syringomyelia; syringohydromyelia and scoliosis are present in 10–20% of patients who have Chiari I malformation (86). Although it usually presents clinically in young adult years, it may present early in an infant or later in a middle-aged or elderly adult (1, 87, 88). The duration from onset of symptoms to diagnosis is typically 3 to 7 years (1). The earliest symptom is often headache, neck, or arm pain aggravated by straining or cough; neck pain may be accompanied by torticollis. Neurologic findings depend on the structures involved. It is sometimes difficult to distinguish direct foramen magnum compression from cervical syrinx compromise. The syrinx is often noted at the C4–C6 bony levels but may extend rostrally or caudally the full length of the cord. Dissociated sensory loss in a capelike distribution over the neck and arms is characteristic (i.e., loss of pain and temperature sense with sparing of touch, vibration, and position sense); dissociated sensory loss results because crossing spinothalamic tract fibers carrying pain and temperature sensation are most affected, whereas posterior column sensory fibers are spared. Hand and arm weakness develop as lower motoneurons

of the cervical cord are affected. Long-tract myelopathic symptoms develop in the lower limbs with further expansion of the cervical syrinx. Worsening scoliosis is common, particularly in childhood-onset syringomyelia of Chiari I malformation. Other associated craniocervical abnormalities of Chiari I malformation may include basilar impression, Klippel–Feil anomaly (congenital fusion of cervical vertebrae), and atlanto-occipital assimilation. Syrinx extension into the brainstem can lead to sleep apnea, eye movement abnormalities (e.g., nystagmus, oscillopsia), dysphagia, aspiration, vertigo, truncal ataxia, and poor balance.

Chiari II malformation often presents in infancy as stridor, weak cry, nystagmus, and apnea, or in childhood as gait abnormality, spasms, worsening incoordination, and nystagmus. Later it may lead to loss of head control, arm weakness, spasms, and tetraparesis. Deficits associated with Chiari II malformation are often related to a larger extent to the myelomeningocele and hydrocephalus rather than the syringomyelia itself.

MRI confirms the diagnosis, but asymptomatic cerebellar tonsilar herniation is common. Because cerebellar tonsils retract upward with age, MRI interpretation depends on age-appropriate controls. Tonsilar herniations greater than 6 mm are significant up to age 10, greater than 5 mm for ages 10 to 30, and greater than 4 mm for ages over 30. However, 30% of persons with cerebellar herniations of 5 to 10 mm are asymptomatic.

Differential diagnosis for syringomyelia of Chiari I malformation includes multiple sclerosis, spinal muscular atrophy, amyotrophic lateral sclerosis, spinocerebellar ataxias, cervical disc and posttraumatic syringomyelia from trauma, arteriovenous malformation, arachnoiditis or meningitis, neurofibromatosis, and from spinal cord or brainstem tumors (e.g., ependymoma, astrocytoma, hemangioblastoma).

Syringohydromyelia may arise from abnormal fluctuations in subarachnoid fluid pressures and abnormal CSF flow at the foramen magnum (89, 90). The causes of these alterations in CSF pressure include bony narrowing of the foramen magnum, as in achondroplasia or basilar invagination, Chiari I and II malformations, intramedullary and extramedullary tumors, and subarachnoid scarring secondary to trauma, hemorrhage, or infection. In patients with Chiari II malformations, hydrocephalus may contribute to syrinx formation. Rostral or caudal extension of the syrinx may result from rapid changes in intraspinal pressure, such as those caused by coughing, straining, or sneezing.

Treatment of Chiari I malformation involves posterior fossa decompression with a suboccipital craniectomy, with or without dural patch grafting, and cervical laminectomy with fenestration or shunting of the syrinx cavity is performed to restore the normal physiologic CSF flow at the cranio-cervical junction (86). In patients with mild symptoms, 70% to 90% report improvement (91–95). Self-reported quality of life also improved in 84% after surgical decompression (96). Some suggest that direct surgery of the syrinx should be undertaken only after craniocervical decompression has failed (1, 91, 92). MRI CSF flow studies may be helpful in deciding the type of surgery to be performed (97). A "top-down" approach has been suggested for surgical treatment of Chiari II malformation: closure of the myelomeningocele within 72 hours of birth (86), shunt for hydrocephalus, then posterior fossa decompression for Chiari malformation, then syringo-pleural shunt for syringomyelia if needed. Surgical decompression of the posterior fossa typically involves occipital craniectomy, laminectomies of C1 and C2, lysis of arachnoidal adhesions, and generous fascia lata dural grafting to attempt to restore CSF flow across the foramen magnum (1). Surgery for syringohydromyelia is similar to that described for PTS: shunting or dural graft. After posterior fossa decompression, with or without syrinx shunting, 50% or more patients improve. In those with syrinxes, about one third improve, one third stabilize, and one third deteriorate further after surgery (1). Postoperative neurologic decline can result from recurrent syringomyelia, occipital C1–C2 instability, pseudomeningocele, tethering of the spinal cord, meningitis, and extradural abscess (1, 91–93). Spinal deformity (scoliosis, kyphosis) can develop in association with syringomyelia from any cause, particularly in those patients with prior complete laminectomies (98). Hemilaminectomy or instrumented spinal fusion can be considered to minimize disruption of soft tissue, which may weaken axial musculature and contribute to spinal deformity. The optimal management for recurrent syringohydromyelia is controversial.

Chiari II malformation that becomes symptomatic in infancy is the leading cause of death in children with myelomeningocele (1, 99, 100). Respiratory compromise and recurrent aspiration are particularly worrisome. Less-severe symptoms may stabilize by 1 year of age. Older children with Chiari II malformation do better with cervical spinal cord decompression; improvement is reported in 60% to 80% of patients.

CONCLUSIONS

Syringomyelia, whether caused by a congenital Chiari malformation or a spinal cord injury, can be severely disabling and even fatal, yet some patients are stable for decades. Syrinxes should be diagnosed early by identifying the characteristic dissociated sensory loss and tendon reflex loss, and by obtaining an MRI. If little or no ongoing neurologic decline is evident, then conservative treatment can be advocated, but close monitoring is needed. If neurologic decline is noted, either by functional decline, strength decline on quantitative testing, or electrodiagnostic changes, then surgical decompression of the syrinx should be considered. Resection of arachnoid scar and duraplasty may be most appropriate in those with some lower limb function preserved. Shunting or cordectomy may be most appropriate in those with no lower limb function. Ongoing monitoring is needed after surgery, because syrinxes can recur. Continuing rehabilitation is often needed to adjust to functional changes.

References

1. Hurlbert RJ, Fehlings MG. The Chiari malformations. In: Engler GL, Cole J, Merton WL, eds. Spinal Cord Diseases: Diagnosis and Treatment. New York: Marcel Dekker, 1998; 65–100.
2. Milhorat TH, Capocelli AL Jr, Anzil AP, Kotzen RM, Milhorat RH. Pathological basis of spinal cord cavitation in syringomyelia: Analysis of 105 autopsy cases. J Neurosurg 1995; 82:802–812.
3. Barnett HJM, Jouse AT. Post-traumatic syringomyelia (cystic myelopathy). In: Vinken, Bruyn, eds. Handbook of Clinical Neurology, Vol. 26. North Holland Publishing Company 1976; 113–157.
4. Rossier AB, Foo D, Shillito J, Dyro FM. Post-traumatic syringomyelia: Incidence, clinical presentation, electrophysiological studies, syrinx protein and results of conservative and operative treatment. Brain 1985; 108:439–461.
5. Edgar R, Quail P. Progressive post-traumatic cystic and non-cystic myelopathy. Br J Neurosurg 1994; 8:7–22.
6. El Masry W, Biyani A. Incidence, management, and outcome of post-traumatic syringomyelia. J Neurol Neurosurg Psychiat 1996; 60:141–146.
7. Schurch B, Wichmann W, Rossier AB. Post-traumatic syringomyelia (cystic myelopathy): A prospective study of 449 patients with spinal cord injury. J Neurol Neurosurg Psychiatry 1996; 60:61–67.
8. Carroll AM, Brackenridge P. Post-traumatic syringomyelia: a review of the cases presenting in a regional spinal injuries unit in the north east of England over a 5-year period. Spine 2005; 30:1206–1210.
9. Frisbie JH, Aquilera EJ. Chronic pain after spinal cord injury: An expedient diagnostic approach. Paraplegia 1990; 28:460–465.
10. Isu T, Iwasaki Y, Nunomura M, et al. Magnetic resonance imaging of post-traumatic syringomyelia and its surgical treatment. No Shinkei Geka 1991; 19:41–46.
11. Abel R, Gerner HJ, Smit C, et al. Residual deformity of the spinal canal in patients with traumatic paraplegia and secondary changes of the spinal cord. Spinal Cord 1999; 37:14–19.
12. Perrouin-Verbe B, Lenne-Aurier K, Robert R, Auffray-Calvier E, Richard I, Mauduyt de la Grieve, et al. Post-traumatic syringomyelia and post-traumatic spinal canal stenosis: A direct relationship: review of 75 patients with a spinal cord injury. Spinal Cord 1998; 36:137–143.i
13. Sett P, Crockard H. The value of magnetic resonance imaging (MRI) in the follow-up management of spinal injury. Paraplegia 1991; 29:396–410.
14. Wozniewicz B, Filipowicz K, Swiderska S, Deraka K. Pathophysiological mechanism of traumatic cavitation of the spinal cord. Paraplegia 1983; 21:312–317.
15. Squier MV, Lehr RP. Post-traumatic syringomyelia. J Neurol Neurosurg Psychiatry 1994; 57:1095–8 99.
16. Backe HA, Betz RR, Mesgarzadeh M, Beck T, Clancy M. Post-traumatic spinal cord cysts evaluated by magnetic resonance imaging. Paraplegia 1991; 29:607–612.
17. Silberstein M, Hennessy O. Cystic cord lesions and neurological deterioration in spinal cord injury. Paraplegia 1992; 30:661–668.
18. Bursell J, Little JW, Stiens SA. Electrodiagnosis in spinal cord injured patients with new weakness or sensory loss. Arch Phys Med Rehabil 1999; 80:904–909.
19. Hilton EL, Henderson LJ. The nature, meanings, and dynamics of lived experiences of a person with syringomyelia: a phenomenological study. SCI Nurs 2003; 20:10–17.
20. Biyani A, Masri WS. Post traumatic syringomyelia: A review of literature. Paraplegia 1994; 32:723–731.
21. Broadbent AR, Stoodley MA. Post-traumatic syringomyelia: a review. J Clin Neurosci 2003; 10:401–408.
22. Williams B. Pathogenesis of post-traumatic syringomyelia [editorial]. Br J Neurosurg 1992; 6:517–520.
23. Silberstein M, Hennessy O. Implications of focal spinal cord lesions following trauma: Evaluation with magnetic resonance imaging. Paraplegia 1993; 31:160–167.
24. Caplan LR, Norohna AB, Amico LL. Syringomyelia and arachnoiditis. J Neurol Neurosurg Psychiatry 1990; 53:106–113.
25. Asano M, Fujiwara K, Yonenobu K, Hiroshima K. Posttraumatic syringomyelia. Spine 1996; 21:1446–1453.
26. Carpenter PW, Berkouk K, Lucey AD. Pressure wave propagation in fluid-filled co-axial elastic tubes. Part 2: Mechanisms for the pathogenesis of syringomyelia. J Biomech Eng. 2003 Dec; 125(6):857–63.
27. Greitz D. Unraveling the riddle of syringomyelia. Neurosurg Rev. 2006; 29:251–263.
28. Bertram CD, Bilston LE, Stoodley MA. Tensile radial stress in the spinal cord related to arachnoiditis or tethering: a numerical model. Med Biol Eng Comput 2008; 46:701–707.
29. Van den Bergh R. Pathogenesis and treatment of delayed post-traumatic syringomyelia. Acta Neurochir (Wien) 1991; 110:82–86.
30. Jensen F, Reske-Nielsen E. Post-traumatic syringomyelia. Scand J Rehabil Med 1977; 9:35–43.
31. Anton HA, Schweigel JF. Posttraumatic syringomyelia: The British Columbia experience. Spine 1986; 11:865–868.
32. Ball MJ, Dayan AD. Pathogenesis of syringomyelia. Lancet 1972; 2:799–801.
33. Hida K, Iwasaki Y, Imamura H, Abe H. Posttraumatic syringomyelia: Its characteristic magnetic resonance imaging findings and surgical management. Neurosurg 1994; 35:886–891.

34. Bertrand G. Dynamic factors of syringomyelia and syringobulbia. Clin Neurosurg 1972; 20:322–333.

35. Tator CH, Briceno C. Treatment of syringomyelia with syringosubarachnoid shunt. Canad J Neurol Sci 1988; 15:48–57.

36. Williams B, Terry AF, Jones F, McSweeney T. Syringomyelia as a sequel to traumatic paraplegia. Paraplegia 1981; 19:67–80.

37. Vernon JD, Silver JR, Symon L. Post-traumatic syringomyelia: The results of surgery. Paraplegia 1983; 21:37–46.

38. Balmaseda MT, Wunder JA, Gordon C, Cannell CD. Posttraumatic syringomyelia associated with heavy weightlifting exercises: Case report. Arch Phys Med Rehabil 1988; 69:970–972.

39. Durward QJ, Rice GP, Ball MJ, Gilbert JJ, Kaufmann JCE. Selective spinal cordectomy: clinicopathological correlation. J Neurosurg 1982; 56:359–367.

40. Kruse A, Rasmussen G, Borgesen SE. CSF dynamics in syringomyelia: Intracranial pressure and resistance to outflow. Br J Neurosurg 1987; 1:477–484.

41. Martins G. Syringomyelia, an hypothesis and proposed method of treatment. J Neurol Neurosurg Psychiatry 1983; 46:365 (letter).

42. Shannon N, Symon L, Logue V, Cull D, Kang J, Kendall BE. Clinical features, investigation and treatment of post-traumatic syringomyelia. J Neurol Neurosurg Psychiatry 1981; 44:35–42.

43. Shoukimas GM. Thoracic spine. In: Stark DD, Bradley WG Jr., eds. Magnetic Resonance Imaging, 2nd ed. New York: Mosby Year Book, 1992; 1302–1338.

44. Kramer KM, Levine AM. Post-traumatic syringomyelia: A review of 21 cases. Clin Ortho Rel Res 1997; 334:190–199.

45. Ducreux D, Attal N, Parker F, Bouhassira D. Mechanisms of central neuropathic pain: a combined psychophysical and fMRI study in syringomyelia. Brain 2006; 129(Pt 4):963–976.

46. Lyons BM, Brown DJ, Calvert JM, Woodward JM, Wriedt CHR. The diagnosis and management of post traumatic syringomyelia. Paraplegia 1987; 25:345–350.

47. Tobimatsu H, Nihei R, Kimura T, et al. Magnetic resonance imaging of spinal cord injury in chronic stage. Rinsho Seikei Geka (Clin Ortho Surg) 1991; 26:1173–1182.

48. Nogues MA, Gene R, Encabo H. Risk of sudden death during sleep in syringomyelia and syringobulbia. J Neurol Neurosurg Psychiatry 1992; 55:585–589.

49. Wang D, Bodley R, Sett P, Gardner B, Frankel H. A clinical magnetic resonance imaging study of the traumatised spinal cord more than 20 years following injury. Paraplegia 1996; 34:65–81.

50. Quencer RM, Post MJD, Hinks RS. Cine MR in the evaluation of normal and abnormal CSF flow: Intracranial and intraspinal studies. Neuroradiology 1990; 32:371.

51. Jinkins JR, Reddy S, Leite CC, Bazan C 3rd, Xiong L. MR of parenchymal spinal cord signal change as a sign of active advancement in clinically progressive posttraumatic syringomyelia. AJNR (Am J Neuroradiol) 1998; 19:177–182.

52. Lee TT, Arias JM, Andrus HL, Quencer RM, Falcone SF, Green BA. Progressive posttraumatic myelomalacic myelopathy: Treatment with untethering and expansive duraplasty. J Neurosurg 1997; 86:624–628.

53. Pojunas K, Williams A, Daniels D, Haughton VM. Syringomyelia and hydromyelia: Magnetic resonance evaluation. Radiology 1984; 153:679–683.

54. Baledent O, Gondry-Jouet C, Stoquart-Elsankari S, Bouzerar R, Le Gars D, Meyer ME. Value of phase contrast magnetic resonance imaging for investigation of cerebral hydrodynamics. J Neuroradiol 2006 Dec; 33(5):292–303.

55. Quencer RM, Green BA, Eismont FJ. Post traumatic spinal cord cysts; clinical features and characterization with metrizamide computed tomography. Radiology 1983; 146:415–423.

56. Little JW, Robinson LR, Goldstein B, Stewart D, Micklesen P. Electrophysiologic findings in post-traumatic syringomyelia: Implications for clinical management. J Am Para Soc 1992; 15:44–52.

57. Nogues MA, Stalberg E. Electrodiagnostic findings in syringomyelia. Muscle Nerve 1999; 22:1653–1659.

58. Rittenberg JD, Burns SP, Little JW. Worsening myelopathy masked by peripheral nerve disorders. J Spinal Cord Med 2004; 27:72–77.

59. Roser F, Ebner FH, Liebsch M, Dietz K, Tatagiba M. A new concept in the electrophysiological evaluation of syringomyelia. J Neurosurg Spine 2008; 8:517–23.

60. Jacquemin G, Little JW, Burns SP. Measuring hand intrinsic muscle strength: normal values and interrater reliability. J Spinal Cord Med 2004; 27:460–467

61. Dworkin GE, Staas WE. Posttraumatic syringomyelia. Arch Phys Med Rehabil 1985; 66:329–331.

62. Watson N. Ascending cystic degeneration of the cord after spinal cord injury. Paraplegia 1981; 19:89–95.

63. Ronen J, Catz A, Spasser R, Gepstein R. The treatment dilemma in posttraumatic syringomyelia. Disability and Rehab 1999; 21:455–457.

64. Schlesinger EB, Antunes JL, Michelsen J, Louis KM. Hydromyelia: Clinical presentation and comparison of modalities of treatment. Neurosurgery 1981; 9:356–365.

65. Peerless SJ, Durward QJ. Management of syringomyelia: A pathophysiological approach. Clin Neurosurg 1983; 30:531–576.

66. Sgouros S, Williams B. Management and outcome of posttraumatic syringomyelia. J Neurosurg 1996; 85:197–205.

67. Adelstein LJ. The surgical treatment of syringomyelia. Am J Surg 1938; 40:384–395.

68. Suzuki M, Davis C, Symon L, Gentili F. Syringoperitoneal shunt for treatment of cord cavitation. J Neurol Neurosurg Psychiatr 1985; 48:620–627.

69. Barbaro NM, Wilson CB, Gutin PH, Edwards MSB. Surgical treatment of syringomyelia: Favorable results with syringoperitoneal shunting. J Neurosurg 1984; 61:531–538.

70. Dautheribes LW, Pointillart V, Gaujard E, Petit H, Barat M. Mean term follow-up of a series of post traumatic syringomyelia patients after syringo-peritoneal shunting. Paraplegia 1995; 33:241–245.

71. Perin NI. Posttraumatic syrinx: Diagnosis and treatment. In: Engler GL, Cole J, Merton WL, eds. Spinal Cord Diseases: Diagnosis and Treatment. New York: Marcel Dekker, 1998; 65–100.

72. Levi ADO, Sonntag VKH. Management of posttraumatic syringomyelia using expansile duraplasty. Spine 1998; 23:128–132.

73. Batzdorf U, Klekamp J, Johnson JP. A critical appraisal of syrinx cavity shunting procedures. J Neurosurg 1998; 89:382–388.

74. Klekamp J, Batzdorf U, Samil M, Bothe HW. Treatment of syringomyelia with subarachnoid scarring caused by arachnoiditis or trauma. J Neurosurg 1997; 86:233.

75. Laxton AW, Perrin RG. Cordectomy for the treatment of posttraumatic syringomyelia. Report of four cases and review of the literature. J Neurosurg Spine 2006; 4:174–8.

76. Kasai Y, Kawakita E, Morishita K, Uchida A. Cordectomy for posttraumatic syringomyelia. Acta Neurochir (Wien) 2008; 150:83–86.

77. Cao F, Yang X, Liu W, Li G, Zheng, Z, Wen L. Surgery for posttraumatic syringomyelia: a retrospective study of seven patients. Chinese Journal of Traumatology 2007; 10(6):366–370.

78. Wiart L, Dautheribes M, Pointillart V, Gaujard E, Petit H, Barat M. Mean term follow-up of a series of post-traumatic syringomyelia patients after syringo-peritoneal shunting. Paraplegia 1995; 33:241–245.

79. Park CH, Chung TS, Kim DJ, Suh SH, Chung WS, Cho YE. Evaluation of intrasyrinx fluid motion by spatial modulation of magnetization-magnetic resonance imaging in syringomyelia with long-term follow-up: a predictor of postoperative prognosis? J Comput Assist Tomogr 2008; 32:135–140.

80. Wester K, Pedersen PH, Krakenes J. Spinal cord damage caused by rotation of a T-drain in a patient with syringoperitoneal shunt. Surg Neurol 1989; 31:224–227.

81. Klekamp J, Raimondi AJ, Samii M. Occult dysraphism in adulthood: Clinical course and management. Childs Nerv Syst 1994; 10:312.

82. Menezes AH. Primary craniovertebral anomalies and the hindbrain herniation syndrome. Pediatr Neurosurg 1995; 23:260.

83. Milhorat TH, Johnson RW, Milhorat RH, et al. Clinicopathological correlations in syringomyelia using axial magnetic resonance imaging. Neurosurgery 1995; 37:206.

84. Bindal AK, Dunsker SB, Tew JM. Chiari I malformation: Classification and management. Neurosurgery 1995; 37:1069–1074.

85. Paul KS, Lye RH, Strang FA, Dutton J. Arnold-Chiari malformation: Review of 71 cases. J Neurosurg 1983; 58:183–187.

86. Hankinson TC, Klimo P Jr, Feldstein NA, Anderson RC, Brockmeyer D. Chiari malformations, syringohydromyelia and scoliosis. Neurosurg Clin N Am 2007; 18:549–68.

87. Wu YW, Chin CT, Chan KM, Barkovich AJ, Ferriero DM. Pediatric Chiari I malformations: Do clinical and radiologic features correlate? Neurology 1999; 53:1271.

88. Geroldi C, Frisoni GB, Bianchetti A, Trabucchi M, Bricolo A. Arnold-Chiari malformation with syringomyelia in an elderly woman. Age Ageing 1999; 28:399–400.

89. Heiss JD, Patronas N, DeVroom HL, Shawker T, Ennis R, Kammerer W, Eidsath A, Talbot T, Morris J, Eskioglu E, Oldfield EH. Elucidating the pathophysiology of syringomyelia. J Neurosurg 1999; 91:553–562.

90. Ellenbogen RG, Armonda RA, Shaw DW, Winn HR. Toward a rational treatment of Chiari I malformation and syringomyelia. Neurosurg Focus 2000; 8:E6.

91. Klekamp J. The surgical treatment of Chiari I malformation. Acta Neurochir (Wien) 1996; 138:788–801.

92. Hida K, Iwasaki Y, Koyanagi I, Abe H. Pediatric syringomyelia with Chiari malformation: Its clinical characteristics and surgical outcomes. Surg Neurol 1999; 51:383–390.

93. Depreitere B, Van Calenbergh F, van Loon J, Goffin J, Plets C. Posterior decompression in syringomyelia associated with Chiari malformation: A retrospective analysis of 22 patients. Clin Neurol Neurosurg 2000; 102:91–96.

94. Tubbs RS, McGirt MJ, Oakes WJ. Surgical experience in 130 pediatric patients with Chiari I malformations. J Neurosurg 2003; 99:291–296.

95. Wetjen NM, Heiss JD, Oldfield EH. Time course of syringomyelia resolution following decompression of Chiari malformation Type I. J Neurosurg Pediatrics 2008; 1:118–123.

96. Mueller D, Oro' JJ. Prospective analysis of self-perceived quality of life before and after posterior fossa decompression in 112 patients with Chiari malformation with or without syringomyelia. Neurosurg Focus 2005; 18:ECP2.

97. Panigrahi M, Praveen Reddy B, Reddy AK, Reddy JJM. CSF flow study in Chiari I malformation. Childs Nerv Syst 2004; 20:336–340.

98. Batzdorf U, Khoo LT, McArthur DL. Observations on spine deformity and syringomyelia. Neurosurgery 2007; 61:370–377.

99. Stevenson KL. Chiari Type II malformation: past, present, and future. Neurosurg Focus 2004; 16:E5.

100. Tubbs RS, Oakes WJ. Treatment and management of the Chiari II malformation: an evidence-based review of the literature. Childs Nerv Syst 2004; 20:375–81.

43 Surgical Treatment of Posttraumatic Tethered and Cystic Spinal Cords

Scott P. Falci
Charlotte Indeck
Daniel P. Lammertse

It is well known that spinal cord-injured patients suffer many sequelae of spinal cord injury (SCI), including sensory, motor, and functional loss, pain, and spasticity. This chapter discusses the relationship of posttraumatic spinal cord tethering, myelomalacia, and cyst development (syringomyelia) to the progression of these sequelae, as well as surgical treatment and outcomes.

HISTORY

Progressive posttraumatic cystic myelopathy (PPCM) as a cause of progressive neurological deterioration has been well described (1–5). One hallmark is cyst (syrinx) development and progression within the spinal cord, along with progression or new development of myelopathic symptoms. Because the cyst itself had historically been treated as the pathologic entity causing the progressive myelopathy, standard treatment evolved into simple drainage or shunting the syrinx to the subarachnoid space, pleural space, or peritoneal space. These techniques met with limited long-term success, even with persistent collapse and successful shunting of the syrinx. A search for the pathophysiologic mechanism of PPCM ensued, as well as improved surgical techniques.

POSTTRAUMATIC SPINAL CORD TETHERING

Edgar and Quail (1) reported cases of patients continuing to experience symptoms of a progressive myelopathy in the face of successfully shunted posttraumatic cysts by radiographic evaluation. Surgically releasing the spinal cord of its "tether" of arachnoidal scar to the surrounding dura resulted in arrest of the progressive myelopathy, and the term progressive posttraumatic noncystic myelopathy (PPNM) given.

Edgar and Quail additionally recognized that a posttraumatically tethered spinal cord without radiographic evidence of significant myelomalacia or cyst formation could lead to the identical progression of symptoms seen in PPCM, and that surgical detethering could arrest the progressive myelopathy. Others subsequently recognized the same (1–6). A new understanding of the progressive posttraumatic myelopathies evolved, suggesting that posttraumatic tethering of the spinal cord is a necessary precursor to the progressive myelopathy, with progressive myelomalacia and cyst development and progression being an endpoint of the process.

SYMPTOMS

Clinically evident neurologic loss from PPNM or PPCM can occur within a few months of, or more than 40 years subsequent to a spinal cord injury. Symptoms correlated with these entities include progressive loss of sensation, strength, muscular fatigue with repetitive motion, loss of bowel, bladder, or sexual function, neuropathic pain, spasticity, hyperhidrosis, autonomic dysreflexia, Horner's syndrome, headache, cognitive impairment, blurred vision, hypothermia, extremity edema, piloerection, and patchy erethemic blushing of the skin (Table 43.1).

DIAGNOSIS

Patient history and physical examination findings are critically important in determining the relevance of imaging findings consistent with posttraumatic tethered and cystic spinal cords to a progressive myelopathy. The progression of the symptoms previously described must be correlated to objective clinical findings and other potential contributing factors such as spinal instability and anatomic compression of the spinal cord. Primary neurodegenerative processes such as multiple sclerosis and ALS should be ruled out. Additionally, one must evaluate common sequelae of SCI with the understanding of their ability to mimic symptoms of a progressive myelopathy. It is not unusual for spinal cord-injured patients to experience significant comorbidities such as urinary tract infections, urinary tract stones, gall stones, heterotopic ossification, and skin sores, all of which can exacerbate symptoms of neuropathic pain, spasticity, autonomic dysreflexia, and hyperhidrosis. These may in turn manifest as functional loss, which is sometimes interpreted by the patient as motor deterioration. These comorbidities, however, never mimic

Table 43.1   Most Common Presenting Symptoms in Descending Order of Frequency

Motor loss (including bowel, bladder, sexual function)
Sensory loss (including bowel, bladder, sexual function)
Spasticity
Neuropathic pain
Autonomic dysreflexia
Hyperhidrosis
Horner's syndrome
Extremity edema/dermatologic changes
Headache/blurred vision/cognitive impairment
Hypothermia

IMAGING STUDIES

Magnetic resonance imaging (MRI) is the best modality for assessing regions of spinal cord tethering, myelomalacia, and cystic cavitation. Spinal cord tethering is recognized as an absence of subarachnoid space or abnormal position of the spinal cord within the canal. Myelomalacia is recognized as a widened spinal cord with low signal on T1-weighted images, signal hyperintense to cerebrospinal fluid (CSF) in proton density (PD) images, or increased signal in T2-weighted images. Cystic cavitation is recognized as signal isointense with CSF on T1-, PD-, and T2-weighted images. (Figures 43.1 and 43.2). If metal artifact from instrumentation does not allow a quality MR image, then delayed CT myelography can be helpful. With CT myelography, cord tethering is recognized as an absence of subarachnoid space or abnormal positioning of the spinal cord within the spinal canal, and cystic cavitation as evidence of myelographic dye within the spinal cord. CINE MRI CSF flow studies can show regions of impaired or absent CSF flow around the spinal cord, implying cord tethering from arachnoidal scar. However, such studies can miss small, localized regions of tethering, and quality studies can be hard to obtain in patients with any degree of spasticity.

progressive sensory loss. Pulmonary issues and pregnancy are noteworthy of discussion. Any pulmonary process (e.g. atelectasis, pulmonary embolus, pneumonia) can initiate a progressive myelopathy in patients with tethered and cystic spinal cords who were otherwise neurologically stable. Resolution of the pulmonary process often results in arrest of the progressive myelopathy. The same can occur in SCI patients who become pregnant. Pregnancy can initiate a progressive myelopathy, and childbirth can result in subsequent arrest and even reversal of the process. We believe both conditions result in temporary increases in intraspinal pressures poorly tolerated by the tethered and cystic spinal cord.

SURGICAL METHODS

Surgical technique for treatment of posttraumatic tethered and cystic spinal cords has evolved substantially over the last 15 years. Presently, surgical objectives include (1) minimizing traction of the spinal cord and rootlets, (2) improving spinal cord and rootlet

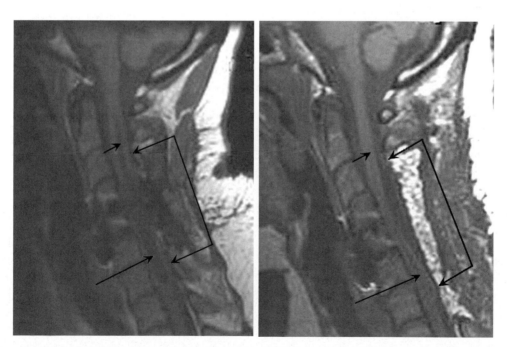

Figure 43.1   The panel on the left shows a preoperative T1-weighted MR image of the spinal cord of a patient with a traumatic quadriplegia and suffering a progressive myelopathy. Note the region of cord tethering (double arrow), regions of myelomalacia (short arrow), and region of descending cystic cavitation (long arrow).

The panel on the right shows a postoperative T1-weighted MR image after spinal cord detethering, expansion duraplasty, and placement of a descending cyst-subarachnoid shunt. Note the region of detethering, duraplasty placement, and reconstitution of posterior subarachnoid space (double arrow), decrease in ascending cord myelomalacia (short arrow), and collapse of descending cyst cavity (long arrow).

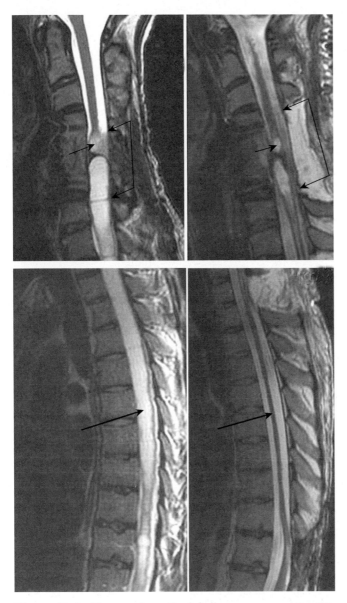

Figure 43.2 The panels on the left show a preoperative T2-weighted MR image of the spinal cord of a patient with a traumatic quadriplegia and suffering a progressive myelopathy. Note the region of cord tethering (double arrow), region of myelomalacia (short arrow, above), and large descending cyst cavity (long arrow, below).

The panels on the right show a postoperative T2-weighted MR image after spinal cord detethering, expansion duraplasty, and placement of a descending cyst-peritoneal shunt. Note the region of detethering, duraplasty placement, and reconstitution of posterior subarachnoid space (double arrow), decrease in cord myelomalacia (short arrow, above), and marked collapse of the descending cyst cavity (long arrow, below).

mobility demonstrated by increased motion with CSF pulsation, (3) improving CSF flow, and (4) facilitating the egress of cyst fluid. Laminectomies are performed to expose dura in regions of tethering, determined by preoperative imaging studies. Intraoperative ultrasonography is then used to assess regions of myelomalacia and cystic cavitation within the spinal cord, as well as

regions of scar tethering the spinal cord to the surrounding dura. Spinal cord and rootlet detethering is then performed with use of the intraoperative microscope, with attention given to reestablishment of cord and rootlet motion with CSF pulsation and release of tension off these elements. Anterior detethering is performed to the limits of a posterior exposure. If a spinal cord cyst does not collapse subsequent to the detethering process, as determined by intraoperative ultrasonography, or if the cyst expands with Valsalva, then a myelotomy is performed in the midline, at the most caudal end of the cyst, for placement of a shunt tube. In general, a shunt tube the caliber of a lumbar drain is used for shunting, but tubes even less than 1 mm in diameter are used for small cysts. We choose to thread the shunt tubes the entire length of the cysts, those tubes having perforations along their lengths. The distal end of the shunt tubes are placed in normal subarachnoid space caudal to regions of tethering, or in the peritoneal space for larger cysts when it is believed that the craniospinal axis will be unable to reabsorb the large amount of cyst fluid. An expansion duraplasty is subsequently placed to minimize the chance of retethering.

CSF Shunting

A small percentage of patients (less than 5% in our experience) will additionally benefit from permanently shunting spinal fluid from the subarachnoid space to the peritoneum. We employ this technique in patients in whom successful detethering and cyst shunting by imaging criteria fail to arrest a progressive myelopathy. We believe that decreasing the intraspinal pressures in these patients improves spinal cord perfusion and cord function.

Cyst Shunting

In our experience, approximately 20% of patients require shunting of the syrinx, in addition to spinal cord detethering.

RESULTS

Long-term outcome from spinal cord detethering and cyst shunting using both rigorous objective evaluation measures such as American Spinal Injury Association (ASIA) sensory and motor scoring, and subjective patient self-assessment measures is sparse, if nonexistent in the literature, although reports using various outcome measures can be found (1–6).

We recently published a long-term study using both objective and subjective patient outcome measures of more than 400 patients who had previously sustained traumatic spinal cord injuries and underwent surgery for progressive myelopathies attributed to tethering of the spinal cord to the surrounding spinal canal, with or without myelomalacia and cyst formation (7). Our findings show that spinal cord detethering and cyst shunting is a successful treatment for a progressive posttraumatic myelopathy related to posttraumatic tethered and cystic spinal cords in the long term. Treatment is best for functional sensory and motor loss, less so for neuropathic pain.

DISCUSSION

Spinal cord injury from any cause can result in tethering of the cord to the surrounding dura with delayed neurologic deterioration occurring from months to more than 40 years subsequently. Varying degrees of myelomalacia and cystic cavitation can be sequelae to tethering. In our experience, tethering occurs in all cases of spinal cord injury from skeletal trauma. It may occur in cases of nonskeletal trauma, such as from hemorrhage, infection, previous surgery to the spinal cord, and prolonged compression from stenosis.

Of imaging modalities, MRI is most diagnostic of spinal cord tethering, myelomalacia, and cystic cavitation, although CT myelography can be helpful if a metal artifact makes MR imaging nondiagnostic. History is critical in determining the relevance of a posttraumatic tethered spinal cord to a progressive myelopathy. A progression of symptoms previously described, unrelated to anatomic compression of the spinal cord, spinal instability, and primary neurodegenerative processes such as MS and ALS, is highly correlative. Nevertheless, one must always evaluate common comorbidities of spinal cord injury and their ability to mimic symptoms consistent with a progressive myelopathy. As previously discussed, the comorbidities of urinary tract infections, bladder stones, kidney stones, gallstones, heterotopic ossification, and skin sores can all exacerbate symptoms of central pain, spasticity, autonomic dysreflexia, hyperhidrosis, and indirectly exacerbate motor and functional loss from muscular disuse while recovering from these sequelae. Never, however, have the above mimicked progressive sensory loss. It should always be kept in mind that pulmonary issues and pregnancy can cause a self-limited exacerbation of symptoms.

Once the diagnosis of a progressive myelopathy has been made, one must help the patient assess the need to undergo surgical treatment. Spasticity, neuropathic pain, autonomic dysreflexia, and hyperhidrosis can often be treated pharmacologically. Functional change can often be improved with adaptive equipment. In some patients, poor baseline health makes surgical risk unacceptable. However, for the symptoms described refractory to pharmacological management, and progressive functional loss unacceptable to the patient, surgery can be an excellent option.

References

1. Edgar R, Quail P. Progressive post-traumatic cystic and non-cystic myelopathy. *Br J Neurosurg* 1994; 8:7–22.
2. Small JA, Sheridan PH. Research priorities for syringomyelia: a national institute of neurological disorders and stroke workshop summary. *Neurology* 1996; 46:577–582.
3. Klekamp J, Batzdorf U, Samii M, Bothe HW. Treatment of syringomyelia associated with arachnoid scarring caused by arachnoiditis or trauma. *J Neurosurg* 1997; 86:233–240.
4. Falci SP, Lammertse DP, Best L, et al. Surgical treatment of posttraumatic cystic and tethered cords. *J Spinal Cord Med* 1999; 22:173–181.
5. Falci SP. Surgical treatment of posttraumatic tethered, myelomalacic and cystic spinal cords. *Semin Spine Surg* 2005; 17:40–45.
6. Lee TT, Arias JM, Andrus HL, et al. Progressive posttraumatic myelomalacic myelopathy: treatment with untethering and expansive duraplasty. *J Neurosurg* 1997; 86:624–628.
7. Falci SP, Indeck C, Lammertse DP. Posttraumatic spinal cord tethering and syringomyelia: surgical treatment and long-term outcome. *J Neurosurg Spine* 2009; 11:445–460.

44 Dual Diagnosis: Spinal Cord Injury and Brain Injury

Ziyad Ayyoub
Dixie Lynne Reiko Aragaki

Rehabilitation after spinal cord injury (SCI) involves an intensive program of learning new information and skills, and adapting to a new lifestyle (1). Patients with SCI need to learn radically new methods for mobility, self-care, and integration into the community. This process requires the ability to attend to, concentrate on, understand, process, retain, retrieve, integrate, and utilize information. The number of tasks and skills that the patient is required to learn can be daunting. Thorough and meticulous evaluation of relative cognitive strengths and weaknesses provides information that can be helpful in developing a focused rehabilitation treatment plan. Achievement of the goals of rehabilitation, which include maximal independence in self-care and mobility skill performance, prevention of medical complications, optimal emotional adjustment to the disability, and complete reintegration into the community after hospitalization, may be adversely affected by inability to learn or effectively apply the knowledge and skills taught during inpatient rehabilitation.

Rehabilitation specialists are becoming increasingly aware of the impact of occult closed head injury (CHI) on functional outcome after SCI. Recognition of the presence and nature of these deficits during this initial phase of the post-injury course of recovery is important because this is the period during which maximal rehabilitation takes place (2). It would seem prudent to identify CHI patients as early as possible during acute care and rehabilitation. These patients may benefit from a motor-free neurocognitive screen to evaluate deficits in problem-solving and executive-level functioning. The identification of deficits would allow for appropriate modification of the rehabilitation program to take advantage of the remaining intellectual strengths of the patient (3). It is reasonable to expect that an impact that is severe enough to injure the spinal cord may also cause varying degrees of traumatic brain injury (TBI). All SCI patients, regardless of level, deserve a systematic evaluation of occult CHI during their acute care evaluation.

Several considerations are necessary to perform a proper and thorough assessment of neuropsychologic functioning in SCI patients. Factors such as reduced or absent upper-extremity function, poor endurance, and limited sitting tolerance require that appropriate modifications be made in the design and administration of a comprehensive test battery.

Occult head injury is often not diagnosed until the patient is in the rehabilitation setting. The head injury may first be apparent when the patient demonstrates an inability to learn adaptive skills because of cognitive deficits such as impaired new learning, decreased short-term memory, and the inability to organize information. In addition, there are indications that the SCI population as a whole tends to function intellectually in the low average range, even when there is no evidence of cognitive impairment (3, 4).

Some patients with traumatic SCI also have a history of TBI before the onset of SCI. In addition, the long-term cognitive effects of alcohol and substance abuse, which have been found to approach a prevalence of 50% in this population, may contribute to cognitive or behavioral disorders (5). Medications commonly used in the acute care setting by SCI patients may interfere with cognitive functioning. These include antidepressants, anticonvulsants, antispasticity agents, sedative-hypnotics, and analgesics. Further, premorbid learning disabilities and limited pre-injury education, along with motivational problems, severe depression, pain, fatigue, and preoccupation with adjustment may impair neuropsychologic test performance (5–8). The results of neurologic evaluation for TBI may be normal in SCI patients, however, neuropsychologic examination may reveal cognitive deficits. These tests are sensitive to problems of attention, concentration, memory, and judgment in these patients.

The reported prevalence figures for cognitive deficits in patients with SCI vary, depending on which definition of cognitive deficits is used and on the specific procedures that are used for assessment and measurement in a particular study. According to a number of studies (2–17), 40% to 60% of acute SCI patients demonstrate cognitive dysfunction. These cognitive deficits result from various forms of cerebral damage, including concurrent or premorbid traumatic brain injury (TBI), chronic alcohol or substance abuse, premorbid learning disability, the use of psychoactive medication, or motivational or other problems. Other studies have demonstrated similar findings that associate the rate of TBI in SCI populations, when SCI is the primary injury (18–26).

When TBI is the primary diagnosis, the incidence of SCI is much lower than the incidence of TBI when the primary diagnosis is SCI. Data from the Spinal Cord Model Systems report that 28.2% of SCI patients have at least a minor brain injury with loss of consciousness, whereas 11.5% have a TBI severe enough to demonstrate cognitive or behavioral changes (25).

Several investigators have reported the magnitude and nature of neuropsychologic test abnormalities among SCI patients using a broad range of assessments of cognitive function. Unfortunately, applicability of the findings from many of these studies has been limited. The distinction between the diagnosis of a "concomitant TBI," which is a specific diagnosis, and "cognitive deficits," which are a more general problem with many potential contributing factors, is often ignored. It is important to separate these two issues, because they have different definitions, frequencies, and implications (22).

Roth (2) and associates administered a comprehensive motor-free neuropsychologic test battery to 81 acute SCI patients and 61 controls matched on age, gender, level of education, and geographic location. Patients were tested a mean of 72 days post-injury. The results of this study suggested that patients had generalized cognitive deficits. Although attention, concentration, and initial learning were often impaired, long-term memory for well-established verbal material was relatively preserved. Abilities to acquire new knowledge, adapt to new situations, and shift to new mental sets also were relatively impaired, as was word retrieval and syntax use.

Davidoff and associates (7), in one of the first studies of the prevalence of cognitive deficits in SCI patients, found that, based on the clinical histories of impaired consciousness and posttraumatic amnesia at the time of injury, 12 (40%) of the 30 patients had sustained mild TBI concurrently with SCI. Six of the remaining 18, or 20% of the entire sample, had a premorbid history of TBI. Only 12 patients (40%) had no history of TBI at any time, as defined by loss of consciousness, posttraumatic amnesia, or both, before or at the time of SCI. Wilmot and associates (8) studied 67 SCI patients who were considered at high risk for what they called "occult head trauma." "High risk patients" were defined as those who met one or more of the four selection criteria, which were tetraplegia from deceleration trauma, history of loss of consciousness, presence of neurologic indicators, and the need for ventilatory support. Of these "high-risk" SCI subjects, 64% were rated as mildly impaired or worse. The patients who had pre-SCI learning disabilities (one-third of the sample) had scores reflecting the greatest impairment. The group with cognitive deficits but no preinjury learning disabilities was found to be the most likely to have sustained TBI at the time of SCI.

To identify the incidence of cognitive deficits in SCI patients with no obvious TBI, Kreutzer and associates (11) conducted neuropsychologic testing of 62 consecutive SCI patients. Their testing revealed a variety of deficits when compared with the normal ranges reported in the neuropsychologic testing literature. Impairments were found to be most prevalent in visual learning, verbal learning, visual organization, and attention.

To determine the relative contribution that concomitant TBI and alcohol or substance abuse may have on cognitive performance, Davidoff and associates (10) administered a comprehensive, motor-free neuropsychologic test battery to 116 patients with acute SCI and 69 control subjects. The SCI patients were divided into three groups: SCI only, SCI-TBI, and SCI-abuse (alcohol or drug abuse history with no concomitant TBI). Statistically significant differences were found between all patient and control mean scores for all but three of the eighteen tests used. Impairments were present in the SCI-abuse group, suggesting chronic deficits in this group of patients.

It has been asserted that mood can affect attention, concentration, memory, and other cognitive functions. This is a particularly relevant factor in SCI patients, who have a depression rate estimated about one third (27–29). Richards and associates (30), in their study of 31 SCI inpatients, noted that deficits in arousal and performance did not show up strongly in an unnatural and deprived environment. However, they believed that depression or anxiety might be major contributing factors in performance and arousal deficits in recently injured patients. Davidoff and associates (31) found a minimal relationship between neuropsychologic performance and depression. Their findings suggest that the magnitude and nature of cognitive deficits are unrelated to the presence or severity of depression in SCI patients, and that these two psychologic issues should be treated as separate problems.

In summary, the presence of a head injury in combination with spinal cord injury dramatically impacts the rehabilitation process. Cognitive deficits will impair the patient's ability to adapt to physical limitations, learn compensatory skills, and achieve a higher level of independence, as compared to those with SCI alone. Behavioral dysregulation is a common sequela of head injury. The resultant emotional lability, poor impulse control, treatment nonadherence, and decreased insight could impair the patient's ability to fully comprehend and adjust to a state of disability. The patient with a dual diagnosis of head injury and SCI usually has a longer length of stay. Once discharged from the rehabilitation setting, these individuals are at greater risk for hospital readmission, urinary tract infections, bowel impaction, skin breakdown, substance abuse, noncompliance with care, depression, and delayed adjustment to injury (32–35). To avoid complications, treatment guidelines must be customized, with great attention paid to the individual's specific cognitive limitations. A comprehensive, multidisciplinary approach is crucial to form a successful, long-term plan of care that addresses the complex needs of this population.

RISK FACTORS FOR CONCOMITANT SPINAL CORD INJURY AND BRAIN INJURY

As in SCI, TBI has a peak incidence in males between the ages 15 and 35 years and has a second peak in the elderly greater than 65 years of age. Alcohol and/or drug use combined with impulsive risk-taking behaviors are common factors found to be associated with the majority of these injuries in the young, but falls cause more cases in the elderly. Alcohol intoxication is also a frequent factor at the onset of injury (32). The mechanism of injury varies and is regional. In urban areas, motor vehicle accidents (MVAs), acts of violence, and falls predominate, whereas farming injuries and falls are seen more in rural areas. Beach communities and summer months have a large number of surfing, skiing, and recreation-related injuries. Ethnic breakdown varies and is regional (32–34).

Numerous studies have examined the association between traumatic cervical spine and head injuries. Alker (36) found a 16% incidence (10/61) of concurrent cerebral and cervical injury in a 1975 review of 146 patients who died at the scene or in the emergency room shortly after arrival. Shrago (20) reviewed the records of 50 survivors of highway accidents with injury to the cervical spine and reported a 53% incidence of concurrent head trauma when the upper cervical spine was injured, and a 9% rate when the damage occurred at lower levels. Head trauma was not well defined in this paper and included "contusions, abrasions, lacerations, or skull fractures."

Bivins (37) reported a series of 17 victims of cardiorespiratory arrest seen in the emergency department following blunt trauma and found a 24% incidence of injury to the cervical spine. It is possible that the more serious head injuries do not survive the dangerous aggravation of depressed respiration following the head injury by decreased ventilation resulting from the paralysis of respiratory muscles by the spinal injury.

Bucholz (38) reported a postmortem series of 100 consecutive patients dying in motor vehicle accidents. He found twenty-four cervical injuries (24%), twenty of which were located between the occiput and the axis. There was no statistically significant difference in associated injuries, including cerebral damage, between patients with cervical injury and those without such injury. Porter (39) found that in 62 (29%) of 216 nonacute SCI mortalities there was evidence of significant associated injury to the brain or skull on pathologic examination. Davis (40) and associates reported that 46% of autopsied spinal cord injuries had demonstrated pathology of the brain. Most cases were upper as compared to lower cervical lesions. Young (41) recorded major head injuries coincident with paraplegia at 16% and with tetraplegia, 7%. Wagner and associates (42) found that of those with head injuries, complete tetraplegic individuals had severe head injuries, as clinically assessed at 24 hours, whereas complete paraplegic individuals had mild injuries. Patients with incomplete lesions also sustained head injuries, but these more often were mild in both paraplegic and tetraplegic individuals. Numerous authors have stressed that the cervical spine injuries seen in association with head injury primarily involve the atlanto-occipital junction, C1, or C2. Damage to the cervical spinal cord at this level is generally fatal and may account for the greater rate of combined injury seen in autopsy reviews.

Traumatic brain injury is also becoming labeled a signature injury of modern military conflicts as a higher proportion of returning combat soldiers are surviving serious head and neck injuries due to more effective body armor and helmets (43). Although this protective gear may shield soldiers from bullets and shrapnel, thus lowering penetrating head injuries, it cannot completely prevent blast injuries caused by concussive forces. The exact proportion of troops who have traumatic brain injury is not known, but estimates range from 6–20% (43–44) and are potentially underestimating the occult mild brain injuries that can go undiagnosed despite increasing efforts for appropriate screening of returning veterans.

DEGREES OF BRAIN INJURY

The severity of a TBI is often assessed according to Glasgow Coma Scale (GCS) score, duration of loss of consciousness (LOC), and post-traumatic amnesia (PTA). A Mild TBI is usually not associated with visible brain imaging abnormalities and is the most common type of brain injury. A mildly brain-injured individual will have a GCS score of 13–15 and less than an hour LOC or PTA. Moderate TBI, which corresponds to a lower GCS score of 9–12, can produce LOC or PTA for up to 24 hours. Injuries resulting in loss of consciousness or amnesia beyond 24 hours are considered Severe TBI and correspond to the lowest GCS score range of 3–8. The moderate and severe injuries may cause punctate hemorrhages in the corpus callosum or other signs of bleeding or swelling in regions to become visible on brain magnetic resonance imaging.

BIOMECHANICS OF DUAL INJURY

The forces associated with traumatic SCI are contact/impact with axial loading (subsequent crushed vertebrae) and noncontact/indirect with sudden deceleration/acceleration (subsequent torn ligaments). Most SCIs are secondary to indirect forces transmitted to the spine through the head (45). Direct forces are penetrating, such as bullets or stab wounds. Contact/impact forces may be associated with local brain damage. The brain injury occurs at the site of impact on the skull. The damage ranges from mild (contusion) to severe (hematoma/edema). Polar brain damage is associated with acceleration/deceleration forces. The sudden stop in motion causes the brain to move within the skull and dura. This causes brain injury at two opposing sites of the brain. Again, injury may be mild (contusion) or severe (hematoma/edema) (46). Diffuse axonal injury (DAI) is diffuse brain injury secondary to the shearing of axons within the myelin sheath (47). This type of injury (DAI) can be associated with contact/impact, rotational/shear, or acceleration/deceleration movements. TBI is a general category that includes closed brain injury, open head injury, and penetrating brain injury. A closed brain injury denotes that the dura remained intact; and open head injury indicates that the dura was opened. Both closed and penetrating brain injuries may result in both localized and diffuse brain damage. The term "penetrating" brain damage denotes that a foreign object penetrated the dura and entered the brain; stab wounds and missile wounds are included as subcategories.

The location of SCI will also be associated with specific types of trauma. Upper cervical injuries are associated with high-energy trauma, and these forces have a high likelihood of causing a concurrent brain injury. Lower cervical injuries can be associated with vertical compression (axial compression), compressive flexion ("tear drop" fracture), distractive flexion (hyperflexion, bilateral facet dislocation), compressive extension (hyperextension), distractive extension (whiplash), and lateral flexion (includes lateral mass fracture and unilateral facet dislocation) (48).

PATHOPHYSIOLOGY

The pathophysiology of both SCI and brain injury is generally classified as primary injury or secondary injury. Primary injury consists of initial neurochemical damage, which occurs at initial contact. This phase can only be modified by injury prevention. Secondary injury is the progressive, degradative cellular damage that is set at the time of primary insult (49). The phases of injury may be classified as acute (hours to days), recovery (hours to months), chronic/plateau (months to years). In this schema, primary injury occurs in the acute phase, and the secondary injury occurs in the acute and recovery phase (50). The pathophysiology of injury has critical implications for acute recovery and regenerative neuroprotective interventions. Secondary systemic insults include cerebral ischemia, decreased perfusion pressure, arterial hypoxemia, arterial hypotension, hypercapnea, anemia, pyrexia, hyponatremia, hypoglycemia, and vasospasm. Secondary

Table 44.1   Secondary Insults

SYSTEMIC	INTRACRANIAL
Arterial hypoxemia	Hematoma—extradural, subdural, intracerebral
Arterial hypotension	Raised pressure—swelling, edema, hydrocephalus
Hypercapnia	Infection—meningitis, abscess
Anemia	Seizures
Pyrexia	Vasospasm

intracranial insults (Table 44.1) are hematoma (extradural, subdural, intracerebral), raised intracranial pressure (brain swelling or edema, acute hydrocephalus), infection (meningitis, abscess), seizures, and cerebral vasospasm.

Hypoxia, which results from ischemia, disrupts aerobic oxidative respiration. The following mechanisms have been proposed as disruptive to cell membranes: progressive loss of phospholipids, cytoskeletal abnormalities, reactive oxygen species, lipid breakdown products, and loss of intracellular amino acids. Prolonged ischemia contributes to permanent damage of the cell membrane, irreversible injury, and cell death. Key events in any ischemic lesions include energy depletion and activation of anaerobic glucolysis. Cytoskeletal integrity and homeostatic mechanisms are disrupted and contribute to the cellular death because of the presence of excess calcium, sodium, and chloride (50–52). Hypoxia and perfusion status play a significant role in the secondary injury process in TBI and SCI. After an ischemic insult, the complex buildup of metabolic products such as free radicals, dysregulation of calcium, and excitatory neurotransmitters contribute to the disruption of neuronal cellular integrity. The death of cells is the final and ultimate result of cellular injury and occurs by two distinct processes: necrosis and apoptosis. In necrosis there is a rapid decline in the ability of the cell to maintain homeostasis, and it quickly becomes swollen and disintegrates, releasing its content. Apoptosis occurs as a normal process during which abnormal and defective cells are removed. Apoptosis occurs in more orderly fashion because it is a gene-regulated mechanism. Adequate perfusion to the penumbra region can potentially preserve neuronal cell function after a CNS insult. The penumbra contains cells that are at risk unless reperfusion is reestablished within a certain window.

Treatment programs based on the maintenance of cerebral perfusion and the control of intracranial pressure have proven to be of critical importance to the functional outcome of TBI survivors. The correction of systemic parameters such as hypoxia, hypotension, and hyperglycemia is critical to the current concept of limiting secondary injury. Novel pharmacologic therapies are currently being developed, all geared at inhibiting and limiting the extent of secondary injury.

ACUTE INTERVENTION GUIDELINES

The combination of a head injury with SCI poses special problems of management. A severe head injury may initially mask the diagnosis of a spinal injury, because the inability to move the limbs may be attributed to the head injury, and the lack of cooperation may make it difficult to assess sensory function. The main objectives in the treatment of the severely head-injured patient are to treat the complications of TBI (e.g., increased intracranial pressure) and to limit secondary brain damage. Ischemia is probably the greatest factor contributing to secondary damage in TBI.

The 3rd edition of the Brain Trauma Foundation's (BTF) *Guidelines for the Management of Severe Traumatic Brain Injury* was last updated in 2007 (53). The clinical guidelines were originally developed in 1995 and remain a joint initiative of the Brain Trauma Foundation, the American Association of Neurological Surgeons, the Congress of Neurological Surgeons, and the Joint Section on Neurotrauma and Critical Care. An independent analysis of their effect on TBI outcome and cost savings by the Centers for Disease Control and Prevention (CDC) found that more routine use of the BTF guidelines would reduce deaths, improve quality of life, and save $288 million per year in medical and rehabilitation costs (54). These guidelines will be summarized.

Blood Pressure and Oxygenation

Post-injury hypotension or hypoxia increases morbidity and mortality. In a helicopter transport study, in patients with an oxygen saturation <60%, the mortality rate was 50% and all of the survivors were severely disabled (55). The guidelines define hypotension as systolic blood pressure (SBP) <90 mmHg, and hypoxia as apnea, cyanosis, oxygen saturation <90%, or PaO_2 <60 mmHg. Treatment recommendations are to monitor blood pressure and oxygenation, and to avoid or rapidly correct hypotension and hypoxia to improve outcomes. Exact target values and treatment thresholds are key issues for future investigation.

Hyperosmolar Therapy

Mannitol and hypertonic saline (HS) are hyperosmolar agents currently in clinical use for treatment of raised intracranial pressure (ICP) in traumatic brain injury. The BTF guidelines report mannitol is effective in the management of traumatic intracranial hypertension, but the current evidence is not strong enough to make recommendations regarding hypertonic saline.

Mannitol is thought to have two effects. First, it has an immediate plasma-expanding effect that reduces the relative concentration of hematocrit, thereby decreasing blood viscosity, and increases both cerebral blood flow and cerebral oxygen delivery (56–57). The second osmotic effect of mannitol is delayed for 15 to 30 minutes until plasma and cell gradients are established. This effect can last 1.5 hours to 6 or more hours. Because mannitol is excreted entirely in the urine, a risk of renal failure exists when serum osmolarity exceeds 320 mOsm. Indications for mannitol prior to ICP monitoring should be restricted to patients with signs of transtentorial herniation or progressive neurologic decline not due to extracranial causes. Limited data suggest that intermittent bolus therapy may be more effective than continuous infusion, but most recent analysis revealed insufficient data to support one form of infusion over the other. The effective dose range is 0.25–1 g/kg body weight.

Hypertonic saline (HS) is theorized to reduce cerebral water content by osmotic mobilization across the intact blood-brain barrier. It may also enhance microcirculation because it dehydrates endothelial cells and erythrocytes, thus increasing the diameter of the blood vessels and deformability of the blood cells to expand plasma volume and improve blood flow. Because of the risk of central pontine myelinolysis if HS is given to patients with chronic hyponatremia, hyponatremia should be excluded prior to HS administration. Current studies suggest that HS may be an effective adjuvant or alternative to mannitol infusion for intracranial hypertension treatment, but there is insufficient evidence to make recommendations for specific use, concentration, or method of administration.

Prophylactic Hypothermia

There is insufficient evidence to clearly demonstrate consistent and statistically significant benefits of hypothermia on mortality in traumatic brain injury. However, patients who were treated with hypothermia were more likely to have favorable neurological outcomes. Also, preliminary findings suggest that there is a higher chance of reducing mortality if cooling is maintained for greater than 48 hours. Serious quality flaws were noted in the majority of reviewed studies, which limited these BTF recommendations to level III. This remains an intriguing area of future research.

Infection Prophylaxis

The incidence of infection is increased with mechanical ventilation and invasive monitoring techniques commonly employed in the care of patients with severe TBI. BTF guidelines recommend that ventriculostomies and ICP monitors be placed under sterile conditions to closed drainage systems with minimal manipulation for flushing or catheter exchanges. There is support for a short course of antibiotics at the time of intubation to reduce pneumonia incidence, but no data suggesting need for longer-term antibiotics during intubation. Early tracheostomy may reduce the duration of mechanical ventilation but did not appear to improve pneumonia or nosocomial infection rates.

DVT Prophylaxis

Patients with both traumatic brain injury and spinal cord injury are at increased risk for deep vein thrombosis (DVT) and venous thromboembolic events (VTE). A clear incidence is difficult to determine due to the varying methods of screening and detection in symptomatic and asymptomatic patients. Pulmonary emboli (PE) are more likely to occur in the setting of proximal DVTs and are associated with high mortality and morbidity. There are mechanical and pharmacological prevention strategies, and both have their advantages and disadvantages. The BTF recommendations are limited to level III because of the limited quality of available studies. Graduated compression or intermittent pneumatic compression stockings are recommended for DVT prophylaxis in all severe TBI patients unless lower extremity injuries prohibit their use. Low-dose heparin and low-molecular weight heparin is also supported for DVT prophylaxis, but there is a trend toward higher rate of major bleeding complications and insufficient data to provide specific guidance on the optimal timing or dosing regimen.

Intracranial Pressure Monitoring

The aggressive treatment of elevated intracranial pressure (ICP) has become critical to acute brain injury management. Normal ICP is 0 to 10 mmHg. Most use 20 to 25 mmHg as the arbitrary upper limit, but it may vary among medical centers. Effective management of elevated ICP (defined as >20–25 torr) has been shown to have significant impact on outcome (52, 58–60). ICP monitoring is not without risks and is generally not recommended in mild or moderate head injuries, although it may be used in a conscious patient with traumatic mass lesion. Intracranial pressure (ICP) monitoring is recommended for patients with severe head injury (Glasgow Coma Scale of 3 to 8 after cardiopulmonary resuscitation) and abnormal CT (hematoma, contusion, or compressed basal cistern). ICP monitoring is recommended in those with a normal CT if two or more of the following are present: age >40 years, unilateral or bilateral motor posturing, and systolic BP <90 mmHg.

The goal of ICP monitoring is to maintain adequate cerebral perfusion and oxygenation. Continuous monitoring of ICP and blood pressure is the only reliable measurement of cerebral perfusion pressure (CPP). The CPP is the mean arterial blood pressure minus the ICP. Low CPP can be deleterious to vulnerable or ischemic parts of the brain. Conversely, increasing CPP can increase cerebral perfusion. The recommendation is to maintain a CPP at minimum of 70 mmHg. A hypotensive patient can sustain harmful sequelae from only marginal elevations of the ICP. In contrast, an elevated blood pressure could be protective in a patient with high ICP. In persons with brain injury, the Monro–Kellie doctrine establishes that within the confines of the cranium, ICP is governed by three factors: brain parenchymal volume, volume of cerebrospinal fluid (CSF), and cerebral blood volume (CBV). Cerebral parenchymal volume (CPV) increases after head injury because of the cerebral edema, which results in increased ICP. To compensate, CSF is initially displaced from the cranium, and subsequently changes in CBV occur. The arterial system, with one third of the total CBV, is responsible for autoregulation. Autoregulation allows the blood vessels to change in diameter in response to metabolic effect. Because autoregulation is compromised in moderate and severe ischemia, CBF varies passively with perfusion pressure. Ventricular drainage is an important management technique for the treatment of elevated ICP. The ventricular catheter allows the physician not only to monitor ICP but to treat it effectively by draining CSF either continuously or intermittently.

Anesthetics, Analgesics, and Sedatives

Barbiturates are not recommended for prevention of intracranial hypertension, but high doses may be useful to control high ICP that is refractory to all other management. The most commonly used barbiturate in clinical situations is pentobarbital. The reported effect is through alterations in vascular tone, decreased metabolism (with subsequent decreased blood flow needs), and the inhibition of free radical mediated lipid peroxidation. Hemodynamic stability should be monitored and maintained before and during barbiturate administration. Clinical use is normally limited to the critical care setting.

Propofol is a sedative-hypnotic anesthetic agent with a rapid onset and short duration of action. It may also have a neuroprotective effect through its ability to depress cerebral metabolism and oxygen consumption. Propofol is listed in the new recommendations for controlling ICP, but high doses can cause significant morbidity and it was not shown to improve mortality or 6-month outcome.

Other commonly used analgesics and sedatives were mentioned and included in a table, but there were insufficient data to form an evidence base for recommendations (morphine sulfate, midazolam, fentanyl, sufentanyl, and propofol).

Nutrition

Traumatic brain injury can cause hypermetabolism and nitrogen wasting, which could result in up to 15% weight loss per week in starved TBI patients. Full nutritional caloric replacement is recommended by day 7 post-injury. Gastric, jejunal, and parenteral options for early feeding methods were reviewed, but there is insufficient evidence to clearly state which method is superior in terms of nitrogen retention, complications, or outcomes. More investigation is needed to determine the best timing and method for delivering nutrients.

Antiseizure Prophylaxis

Posttraumatic seizures (PTS) are classified as immediate (occurring within 24 hours of brain injury), early (within first 7 days of brain injury), or late (beyond the first week). Certain factors associated with higher risk of developing PTS include Glasgow Coma Scale (GCS) score <10, cortical contusion, depressed skull fracture, subdural hematoma, epidural hematoma, intracerebral hematoma, penetrating head wound, or a seizure with 24 hours of injury. Phenytoin is recommended to reduce the incidence of early PTS. Valproic acid can also reduce risk of early PTS, but has been associated with higher mortality. The current available evidence does not indicate that prevention of PTS leads to better outcomes. Phenytoin and valproic acid have not been shown to be effective in preventing late posttraumatic seizures (PTS). In addition, potential adverse effects of anticonvulsant use include neurobehavioral side effects, ataxia, hematolic abnormalities, and Stevens-Johnson syndrome. Therefore, routine seizure prophylaxis is not recommended later than 1 week following traumatic brain injury.

Hyperventilation

Hyperventilation remains a highly effective, acute treatment for increased ICP via changes in cerebral blood volume (CBV) (61). However, studies have demonstrated that prophylactic treatment with hyperventilation is not beneficial. In some cases, the vasoconstriction obtained with hyperventilation causes the cerebral blood flow (CBF) to drop below ischemic levels. Thus, hyperventilation should not be used for an extended period of time, and PCO_2 should not be reduced below 25 mmHg. In the absence of increased ICP after head injury, it is recommended to avoid chronic, prolonged hyperventilation therapy. Brief periods of hyperventilation may be warranted in the setting of acute neurologic deterioration. Longer periods of hyperventilation may be necessary if intracranial hypertension was unresponsive to sedation, paralysis, CSF drainage, and osmotic diuretics.

This guideline recommends avoiding prophylactic hyperventilation ($PaCO_2$ of 25 mmHg or less) during the first 24 hours after severe head injury. It can decrease cerebral perfusion (by causing cerebral vasoconstriction) during the time that cerebral blood flow is reduced.

Steroids

Glucocorticoids have been shown to be deleterious in patients with traumatic brain injury and are not recommended for improving outcomes or reducing ICP in patients with severe head injury. In one study, 161 patients were randomized to placebo or high-dose dexamethasone (100 mg/day), followed by a tapering dose. There was no difference in one-month survival or six-month outcome. High dose methylprednisolone is associated with higher mortality in patients with moderate or severe TBI. This information is in contrast to the proven benefits of the methylprednisolone protocols used in acute SCI management and should be heavily weighed when managing the SCI patient with concomitant moderate to severe TBI.

REHABILITATION OF THE PATIENT WITH DUAL TBI AND SCI

The combination of a transverse lesion of the spinal cord with an associated cerebral lesion requires different rehabilitation principles. Because of high incidence of this compound injury, centers that are primarily set up for spinal paralyzed patients must ensure an adequate program for this patient group. The rehabilitation of these patients is made more difficult because of the psychologic effects of cerebral lesions, such as disorders in performance and personality. The rehabilitation should ideally begin while the patient is still in acute care. At this stage, the psychiatrist can intervene to prevent complications that could compound the patient's disability later in recovery. Transfer to the acute rehabilitation unit should be done when the patient is medically stable.

Rehabilitation of the Unconscious Patient

The goals of rehabilitation in the unconscious TBI patient are three-fold: (a) to remove obstacles to recovery to allow patients who have the potential to regain consciousness to do so; (b) to treat medical complications that can increase disability in those patients who do recover; and (c) to provide education, counseling, and support to family members. During this phase, reversible medical factors must be ruled out as a possible cause of coma. Sedating drugs, systemic illness, malnourishment, and other medical problems that can be corrected can impair arousal and responsiveness. Several rating scales have been developed to assess the responsiveness of unconscious or low-level patients. These scales include the Coma/Near-Coma Scale, the Coma Recovery Scale, the Western Neuro Sensory Stimulation Profile, and the Sensory Stimulation Assessment Measure.

Various terms have been used to describe programs aimed at treating unconscious patients, including "coma arousal therapy," "multisensory therapy," and "coma stimulation." This sensory stimulation provides an organized presentation of direct stimulation in multiple modalities with the hope of advancing patients from an unconscious state. There is insufficient data to support that a specific therapy will accelerate emergence from coma, but an organized treatment approach permits routine assessment and more opportunity to recognize any changes or recovery. Common treatment strategies include visual, auditory, olfactory, cutaneous, kinesthetic, and oral stimulation. Pharmacologic treatment is an intervention often used to directly increase arousal and facilitate recovery of consciousness of these patients. Medications include stimulants (e.g., methylphenidate, dextroamphetamine) and antiparkinsonian medications (bromocriptine and amantadine).

The unconscious patient should undergo range-of-motion (ROM) exercise in order to prevent contractures and other joint abnormality. The patient should be positioned to prevent pressure ulcers, edema, and contractures. Intervention for spasticity, nutrition, and bowel or bladder incontinence should be provided.

Rehabilitation during Posttraumatic Amnesia (PTA) and Agitated States

A patient's ability to learn new information is minimal or nonexistent during this period. After emerging from PTA, patients usually also have a memory gap for events that occurred during the short period leading up to the moment of injury. A standard technique for assessing PTA is the Galveston Orientation and Amnesia Test (GOAT).

During PTA, many patients exhibit agitation, which includes cognitive confusion, extreme emotional lability, motor overactivity, and physical or verbal aggression. The agitated patient is typically unable to sustain attention and effort long enough to perform simple tasks, and can overreact to frustration by crying or shouting. The patient can be easily frustrated and irritated, and show grossly inappropriate behavior toward staff or family members. During the agitation stage it is important to rule out medical reasons as a possible cause for agitation, such as electrolyte imbalance, seizure activity, and sleep disturbances. Agitation can be a reaction to discomfort or musculoskeletal injury, and can be caused by medications.

The goals of therapy during this stage are to decrease the intensity, duration, and frequency of agitation, and to increase attention to environment. Structure is the foundation of treatment at this level. Because patients at this level have a decreased ability to process environmental stimuli, it is imperative that the surroundings remain constant and nonthreatening. Environmental management is the first line of intervention, with the major goals to lower the level of stimulation and cognitive complexity in the

Table 44.2 Agents that Influence Neurotransmitters

NEUROCHEMICAL	AFFECT
Cholinergic	Memory, concentration, attention
Dopaminergic	Movement, arousal
Noradrenergic	Arousal, sleep/wake, memory, learning
Serotonergic	Sleep, mood, arousal

patient's immediate surroundings, and protect the patient from harming himself and others.

Psychotropic medications are often needed, but should be used sparingly.

Cognitive Enhancement

Neuropharmacologic agents are used in TBI to enhance cognitive functions, treat emotional disorders, and minimize behavioral dysfunction. Few controlled studies have evaluated the enhancement of cognitive functions after TBI using neuropharmacologic agents. These agents usually influence neurotransmitters (Table 44.2) that are widely spread throughout the brain. Some of the medications used as neurostimulants in the management of TBI are listed in Table 44.3.

COGNITIVE SYMPTOMS AND BEHAVIORAL PROBLEMS OF BRAIN INJURY AND INTERVENTIONS

An individual who sustains a head injury is left with cognitive impairments, behavioral problems, emotional disturbances, and personality changes that he cannot completely control. Cognitive deficits include shortened attention span, memory problems, impaired judgment, safety awareness, problem solving, and slowed processing. Cognitive impairments can sabotage or

Table 44.3 Some of the Medications used as Neurostimulants

MEDICATION	MECHANISM OF ACTION	SIDE EFFECTS
Methylphenidate (Ritalin®)	Increases dopamine and norepinephrine activity	Increases BP, agitation, insomnia, headache, dysphoria
Pemoline (Cylert®)	Similar to Ritalin®	Reported fewer sympathomimetic side effects
Amantadine (Symmetrel®)	Presynaptic and postsynaptic dopamine receptor	Lowered seizure threshold; increases BP, arrhythmias, headache, nausea
Bromocriptine (Parlodel®) L-Dopa + Carbidopa (Sinemet®)	Dopamine agonist	Same as above
Modafinal (Provigil®)	Exact mechanism unknown	Headache, nausea, nervousness, insomnia
Naltrexone (Revia®)	Opioid antagonist	Nausea

complicate a patient's rehabilitation by negatively affecting his ability to learn his care. A patient with any degree of head injury may exhibit emotional lability, impaired impulse control, and a complete host of other behavioral impairments. Behavioral impairments and acting out can leave him socially isolated, without any support network. A detailed assessment of the individual by the neuropsychologist is of key importance. The neuropsychologist performs a detailed assessment that identifies cognitive impairments and target behaviors. From this follows the development of a comprehensive plan of care, which includes a behavioral management plan. Cognitive impairments and behavioral issues manifest themselves differently from person to person and must be handled on an individual basis. Evaluations, plans, and goals must be established to address whatever impairments are found, especially those that have the greatest impact on functioning. A patient with impaired attention and concentration, and decreased ability to screen out irrelevant information is easily distracted and finds it difficult to follow long discussions. He usually does better in settings that are structured and short in duration. This patient learns new information more effectively in an environment that is distraction-free (no TV, radio). Information can be given in written form for purposes of reinforcement.

Some patients may have an impaired ability to read and write. Packaging directions on medical equipment, prescription information, and medical information may get left at the wayside if they cannot be read and understood. Patient teaching will have to be done by explanation and demonstration. Having the patient provide a return explanation or demonstration is one way of assessing what he has learned.

Impaired new learning and decreased short-term memory is another problem. The individual cannot learn catheterization programs or other aspects of care as quickly as others. In this situation, written materials (when appropriate), repetition, and family and caregiver training are necessary.

Other cognitive consequences of TBI include a decreased ability to solve problems, organize information, and correctly sequence complex actions. Patients cannot problem-solve their way through small or big problems that arise in their daily activities; for example, what to do if they drop a catheter on the floor. They may fail to anticipate when medications and supplies run out and plan ahead to reorder. Managing their money and keeping an accurate checkbook may be impossible without help. Bills may not get paid in a timely manner because they cannot prioritize which should be paid first. Patients will have difficulty following a recipe, or planning or making a dinner start to finish.

Patients with decreased processing skills and an inability to divide attention have difficulty understanding and integrating information. It takes them longer to read instructions, follow a recipe, and perform most functional tasks. They cannot do two things at once. Do not expect them to be able to watch the kids and make dinner at the same time and not get frustrated or make a mistake.

Behavioral problems are common following head injury. Impulsivity may be caused by poor insight and judgment when a patient has impaired self-regulation of desires. He decides on an action and does not think it through first or consider the consequences of the action. Personal safety can often be compromised.

A patient will perform unsafe transfers and then fall. He may overeat, drink, or smoke. He may be careless with power tools or driving. He demonstrates apathy, poor initiation, poor motivation, and the inability to follow through. The patient may desire to take action, but cannot motivate himself to initiate the action. He appears to be "lazy" and uninvolved with his care. Bowel and bladder routines, pressure releases, and medications will be missed. He demonstrates emotional instability, lower frustration tolerance, resulting in overstimulation characterized by agitation, angry outbursts, crying, and lability. This patient appears to be easily irritated by minor things. He may want to quit a task after one try. He has great difficulty in tolerating (normal) daily stressors without breaking down.

Because of shortened temper and poor frustration tolerance, issues of safe and effective parenting may arise. Attention should be paid to his environment to keep it structured, simple, and free of elements that trigger agitation. Periods of activity must be balanced with periods of rest. Disinhibition may be demonstrated by inappropriate comments or sexual behaviors. Behavioral management plans that target specific behaviors are successful in extinguishing these annoying events. Anxiety requires psychologic intervention. Medication management is required when it is acute enough to prevent a patient from participating in therapy or learning self-care. A patient may have extreme fears of falling that prevent him from fully participating in gait training, transfers, and fall recovery. Noncompliance, denial, and refusal to participate may be demonstrated by a patient listing numerous reasons why he is not going to therapy. In these situations a behavioral contract with mutually agreed-on goals, rewards, and consequences is valuable in increasing compliance.

Extinguishing problem behaviors successfully requires a customized behavioral management plan. The neuropsychologist is responsible for performing a detailed assessment to identify specific target behaviors and designing the behavioral plan. The team is responsible for carrying it out. A successful behavior management plan includes structure, consistency, repetition, and practicality. Structure the plan to be well constructed and sound; otherwise it will fail. The brain-injured patient cannot deal with generalized, unstructured environments. Lack of structure often results in overstimulation, acting out, and a sense of failure. Consistency requires that the patient adhere to the same tasks with the same people at the same time. Unpredictability leads to confusion. Repetition is the primary means by which learning can be accomplished.

Practicality involves choosing a target behavior that, when eliminated, results in increased functioning in the home, community, or self-care. Goals must be directed at increasing basic functioning and addressing long-term goals. Specific consequences must be established for targeted behaviors. A patient with brain injury cannot generalize information; he needs to focus on specific goals or consequences and meaningful rewards. The goals that are selected must be viewed as valuable and desirable to the patient and family.

MEDICAL COMPLICATIONS

Medical issues arise in both brain injury and SCI, although the etiologies of these issues are often different. An overview of medical complications related to SCI is provided in another chapter.

Neurologic Complications

Posttraumatic Epilepsy (PTE)

It is estimated that approximately 5% of all persons with TBI who are hospitalized will develop posttraumatic epilepsy. Patients are at increased risk of developing PTE after certain injuries, acute intracranial hemorrhage requiring surgical evacuation within two weeks of injury, early epilepsy, and depressed skull fracture. Other factors, such as dural tearing, focal signs, posttraumatic amnesia >24 hours, and the presence of foreign bodies are also considered as increased risks. Seventy five to 80% of TBI patients develop PTE within 2 years; the rate is no different from the general population after 5 years (62). Most PTE, 50% to 80%, is thought to be of the partial variety, either simple partial or complex partial; 20% to 50% of PTE is of generalized type. Recent studies have shown that using phenytoin (Dilantin®) beyond the first week following a brain injury does not prevent the development of late PTE.

Posttraumatic Hydrocephalus

True posttraumatic hydrocephalus (PTH) is relatively uncommon. One study estimated the incidence to be in the range of 1% to 8% (63). The Model System National Database showed that PTH, defined as an enlargement of the ventricles that requires the placement of a shunt or drain, was detected in only 5% of patients (64). PTH should be suspect when a patient is not progressing as expected or is deteriorating. The symptoms of PTH may range from coma to arrest of progress in rehabilitation. An atypical presentation such as seizures and emotional problems is possible. Generally, shunting is successful if the pressure is elevated >180 mmH₂O or if the ventricles progressively increase in size.

Respiratory Complications

Early in SCI, respiratory complications are the primary cause of death. In fact, respiratory system complications, most commonly pneumonia, are the most common cause of mortality in SCI patients at any time. Pulmonary complications are common in higher-level injuries, especially at the C1 to C4 levels. Complications include acute respiratory distress syndrome (ARDS); aspiration, atelectasis, bronchitis, bronchospasm, lung abscess, pleural effusion, pneumonia, pneumo/hemothorax, pulmonary edema, pulmonary thromboembolism, tracheitis, upper respiratory infection, and ventilatory failure.

Persons with injury below T12 essentially have no impairment of respiratory function. Injuries between T1 and T12 result in some impairment of the abdominal muscles, which reduces forceful expiration and cough. With higher thoracic level injuries there is also impairment of intercostal muscles, which reduce inspiratory and expiratory function. With injuries above C8, loss of all abdominal and intercostal muscles occurs with further impairment of inspiration and expiration. C4 is generally the highest level of injury at which spontaneous ventilation can be sustained. Injury above this level generally requires mechanical ventilation.

Respiratory failure is one of the most common complications seen in severely brain-injured patients, necessitating the use of artificial respiration. A multicenter study revealed that 39% of all severe TBI patients are affected. Patients with combined SCI and TBI are at very high risk for respiratory complications. Laryngeal and tracheal disorders are not uncommon in this patient population.

Deep Venous Thrombosis (DVT)

Incidence of DVT in SCI is very high in the first 12 weeks, with the first 2 weeks having the highest rate following acute injury. The venous stasis that results from muscle paralysis, and hypercoagulability as a result of the stimulation of thrombogenic factors following injury are the two major factors contributing to the development of DVT in the SCI population. Damage to the vessel wall can occur in SCI patients as a direct result of trauma from the original injury or indirectly from external pressure on the paralyzed leg. The incidence of DVT in the TBI population is lower than in SCI population. In some instances, prophylaxis and treatment of DVT in SCI patients with concomitant TBI requires the use of mechanical devices for prophylaxis and inferior vena cava (IVC) filter placement when anticoagulation is contraindicated.

Gastrointestinal Complications

Gastric emptying and gastric acid secretion may be altered in SCI patients. The SCI patient is at high risk to develop gastric atony and ileus. As with most polytrauma patients, the patient with SCI and TBI has an increased risk of stress ulceration during the acute phase. The risk is greater in patients with complete injuries above the T5 level; bleeding is unusual in patients with lesions below the T5 level.

A large number of patients have impaired liver function, which in most cases is drug induced, mostly from phenytoin and phenobarbital; the remainder of cases are caused by acute viral hepatitis. Diarrhea in patients with SCI and TBI may be caused by osmotic overload from tube feeding or due to *Clostridium difficile* colitis.

Swallowing Disorders

Dysphagia is a common problem in both SCI and brain injury. The SCI patient with a concomitant head injury is at a greater risk for a swallowing disorder. Dysphagia can be difficult to detect in the head-injured patient. Often, these patients are unable to communicate effectively, have difficulty swallowing, or can be silent aspirators. Dysphagia as a result of a head injury may be attributed to a variety of causes. TBI patients usually have one or more of the following findings on a videofluoroscopy:

- A delay or absence of swallowing responses
- Reduced tongue control
- Reduced pharyngeal transit
- Reduced laryngeal closure, elevation, or spasms

Most patients have two functional problems in their swallowing, such as impaired tongue control and a delayed triggering mechanism. Left unchecked, swallowing difficulties can result in aspiration pneumonia, death, or malnutrition. Head-injured patients can exhibit a wide range of behaviors that vary in severity. Impulsivity and poor self-regulation combined with any degree of dysphagia can lead to aspiration. Swallowing is also unsafe when patients are disoriented, confused, agitated, or exhibit fluctuating levels of alertness. The successful management of these patients requires an integrated interdisciplinary approach that includes extensive family involvement and training. These individuals require the expertise of the speech therapist, the dietitian, and the neuropsychologist to ensure that they eat safely and adequately. In addition, swallowing disorders in some patients with dual SCI and TBI may be caused by anterior cervical reconstruction surgeries. Intraoperative damage or postoperative swelling can result in impairments to the recurrent laryngeal nerve or the vagus nerve. Both of these nerves are essential for effective swallowing. Swallowing difficulties may also occur when patients are immobilized in Gardener–Wells traction, halo devices, and rigid collars, where the patient's neck tends to be in extension, thus resulting in decreased laryngeal elevation and closure (65). This places the patient at risk for aspiration caused by an open airway during swallowing. High cervical injuries that require tracheotomies and are ventilator-dependent are obviously at high risk to develop dysphagia or aspiration. Endotracheal intubation can cause peripheral nerve damage (recurrent laryngeal nerve) from prolonged mechanical compression and also result in dysphagia.

It is necessary to ensure adequate and safe oral intake. Feeding tubes are used when the swallowing disorder and/or behaviors are severe enough that adequate nutrition cannot be maintained. The role of the dietitian cannot be stressed enough during these situations to assist in calorie counts, menu selection, and prescribing dietary supplements or enteral nutrition.

Endocrine Complications

Endocrine complications include syndromes of inappropriate antidiuretic hormone secretion, diabetes insipidus, thyroid dysfunction, and anterior hypopituitarism. Anterior pituitary insufficiency should be suspected in patients who have anorexia, low temperature, malaise, hypoglycemia, hyponatremia, bradycardia, and hypotension.

Metabolic Changes

Changes in metabolism include hypercalcemia, hyperphosphatemia, and hypermagnesuria, and osteoporosis may be seen in SCI patients with concomitant TBI.

Musculoskeletal Complications

Musculoskeletal complications are found in SCI patients and in TBI patients. It is not unusual for patients with both SCI and TBI to sustain concomitant extremity injuries. Some of these injuries go undiagnosed in the acute setting.

Spasticity

Spasticity in SCI manifests itself once spinal shock has resolved at or below the level of injury. Incomplete SCI tends to have severe spasticity. Spasticity as seen in the brain-injured population presents itself differently when compared to spasticity seen in the SCI population. The severity and types of complications resulting from spasticity can vary. There can be minor twitching, which has no impact on function, to severe spasticity, which does have an impact on function. Severe spasticity can override functional activities and

create increased dependence in activities of daily living. Contractures and frozen joints are the result of a decreased range of motion. Skin breakdown can occur when spasticity interferes with proper positioning. Frequent episodes of uncontrolled spasticity can interrupt sleep and result in falls from wheelchairs. It can cause severe pain and fatigue. Depression can develop when spasticity dramatically impacts activities of daily living by decreasing a person's level of independence. It can increase when issues of infection, pressure sores, or heterotopic ossification are present. Patients with dual diagnosis are at greater risk to develop these complications because of cognitive impairments. To avoid complications, treatment guidelines must be customized, with great attention paid to the patient's specific cognitive limitations. Lack of insight can result in the inability of the individual to recognize causative factors that increase spasticity. In these situations, the physician must be proactive in anticipating and identifying causative agents. Short-term memory loss can result in the patient's forgetting therapy regimens, pressure releases, follow-up doctor appointments, and medication schedules. When appropriate, memory devices may be employed or developed to assist the individual in areas of self-reliance and independence. If a memory device is not helpful, the caretaker or family member must be familiarized and made responsible for the execution of therapeutic regimens.

Treatment can be pharmacologic and nonpharmacologic. Performing regular range-of-motion exercises is standard procedure. The use of diazepam (Valium®) should be avoided in the head-injured patient, because it can further impair cognition and cause sedation. Baclofen, dantrolene (Dantrium®), and tizanidine hydrochloride (Zanaflex®) are commonly used oral agents. In severe cases, intrathecal baclofen pumps are another treatment option. Botulinum toxin and phenol injections can be useful in selected patients.

Heterotopic Ossification (HO)

Heterotopic ossification (HO) is the formation of new bone in periarticular soft tissues. The methods of diagnosis and treatment for HO are the same for brain-injured patients as they are for SCI patients. As HO develops in joints, it manifests itself as a loss of range of motion, edema, and heat. It is a major complication common to both brain injury and SCI. The incidence of HO in SCI alone is 16% to 53%. In SCI, HO usually does not occur above the level of the injury. There is an increased incidence of HO in SCI individuals with complete lesions. In the head-injured population, HO occurs at a rate of 11% to 75%, depending on the center and method of study (66). The incidence of HO in TBI patients is most likely 10% to 20%. A clinically significant HO is associated with pain or decreased range of motion. HO usually presents one to three months after injury. It can mimic thrombophlebitis. Shoulder HO consistently forms inferomedially to the joint. HO at the elbow originates anterior to the elbow if flexor spasticity is present and posterior to the elbow if extensor tone is initially present. Although posterior HO forms in small amounts, the elbow is the most likely joint to ankylose. The hip has three major sites of involvement. HO inferomedial to the hip joint is associated with adductor spasticity and is the most frequent. The anterior HO forms between the anterosuperior iliac spine of the pelvis and the proximolateral femur. The final site of hip HO is situated posterior, 70% of which is seen in the affected part of the body. HO is seen most commonly with brain injured individuals who have experienced prolonged comatose and vegetative states and hypoxic episodes. Spasticity, venous stasis, and immobility are risk factors for HO that are common to both brain injured and SCI individuals. Therefore the person with the dual diagnosis of SCI and brain injury is probably at greater risk to develop HO.

Treatment options for HO are both pharmacologic and non-pharmacologic. They usually consist of aggressive range of motion, IV and oral dosing of didronel, use of anti-inflammatory drugs (Indocin®), and in some cases, radical surgical resection. Patients receiving treatment require frequent, thorough physician monitoring and follow-up. The successful treatment of HO is dependent on compliance with medication and therapeutic regimens. Cognitively impaired individuals are limited in their ability to adhere to this type of regimen. In some cases, surgical resection is indicated. Because most neurologic recovery occurs by 1.5 years, resection should be considered at this time. The classification of patients according to neurologic status was proposed by Garland (66) as the best predictor for functional improvement and rate of HO recurrence after resection:

- Class I, near-normal neurologic recovery
- Class II, mild to moderate motor and mild cognitive dysfunction
- Class III, significant motor impairment with minimal cognitive dysfunction
- Class IV, moderate cognitive impairment with minimal motor involvement
- Class V, severe cognitive and physical impairment

Class I patients have zero or minimal recurrence and best functional improvement. Class V patients have minimal or no gain in motion, and HO recurs in each instance. Good outcome and low recurrence are anticipated in Class I or II patients regardless of location or site of HO.

Autonomic Dysregulation

Autonomic dysregulation may be found in patients with dual SCI and TBI, which includes hypertension, orthostatic hypotension, and temperature instability (central fever, hypothermia). Hypertension must be controlled to avoid added neurologic insult. Patients may have diaphoresis, which requires close monitoring for possible dehydration. It is important to monitor for skin breakdown, because the patient's skin will be intermittently soaked. Autonomic dysregulation can take two forms in the SCI patient. The first form is orthostatic hypotension, which is commonly seen in the early phases of recovery. The second form is autonomic dysreflexia (67). Both situations require prompt medical intervention. Autonomic dysreflexia is always considered a medical emergency and should be treated as such. Both these conditions can sometimes be prevented when the patient is well educated and vigilant in his or her care. Learning the difference between the two is often difficult for the cognitively impaired patient, so family members and caregivers must also be educated. The patient should always carry a medical alert card that can instruct anyone in the steps necessary to stop dysreflexia. The SCI patient who has a concomitant head injury is more likely to experience orthostatic hypotension and dysreflexia. Because of cognitive deficits and behavior issues, these patients often fail to take the actions necessary to prevent these conditions. These patients often require more

family, caretaker, and physician involvement to ensure that their day-to-day care is of a standard that will prevent these situations.

Hyperthermic states often result from a defect in the central thermoregulatory system (68). It is not uncommon to see a rapid rise in temperature. Left untreated, a hyperthermic state will result in further brain damage. Assessing and diagnosing the situation correctly is crucial in developing the correct treatment. A diagnostic work-up must take place to rule out the possibility of drug fever, DVT, pulmonary embolism, infection, HO, and others. After all these and other causes have been ruled out, then the physician can consider the possibility that a "central" fever is present. If hyperthermia is a regularly occurring event for the patient, he will then need frequent monitoring of his temperature. A cooling blanket that employs a rectal temperature probe is helpful. Other useful interventions include cool showers, fans, and not overdressing the patient. Autonomic dysfunction may resolve over time. However, if a patient is discharged from the hospital still exhibiting symptoms, patient, family, and caregiver education regarding the monitoring and management of this situation is critical in avoiding harmful sequelae.

Skin Breakdown

Skin breakdown is a multifactoral complication of both brain injury and SCI. There are similarities and differences regarding the risk factors of skin breakdown for both of these populations. Therefore, when these risk factors are combined, as seen in someone with the dual diagnosis of brain injury and SCI, it should be understood that the risk for skin breakdown is very great. Appropriate interventions in the areas of behavioral management, treatment of depression, and identification of cognitive deficits are beneficial in the prevention of skin breakdown. The SCI individual is at risk for skin breakdown primarily because of issues of immobility, pressure relief, impaired sensation, and spasticity. Secondary issues tend to be those of a psychologic nature, such as noncompliance, depression, anger, adjustment to disability, denial, and loss. Other causes of skin breakdown are indirect, such as substance abuse, smoking, and impaired cognition. Immobility combined with a decreased level of consciousness places the individual at particular risk for skin breakdown. The involvement of nursing, enterostomal therapy, and dietary professionals in the planning and implementation of aggressive turn schedules, frequent skin checks, and adequate nutrition are crucial interventions in prevention of breakdown. Cognitive deficits often limit the patient's ability to adhere to a turning schedule, perform adequate pressure releases, or perform dressing changes. In these situations, frequent reinforcement, use of memory devices, and family training and education are important factors for home care.

Bowel and Bladder Management

Managing the bowel and bladder for the SCI patient who also has a significant head injury can be difficult because of both physical and cognitive impairment. In addition, some patients may have behavioral problems as a result of TBI. Decreased new learning and impaired executive functioning results in an inability to make practical, simple adjustments to the program. Impaired memory results in missed catheterizations or improper bowel care technique. Patients may forget key steps that are critical to complete evacuation in their bowel program. The end result is often bowel impaction or chronic UTI. The treating team involved in the care of a patient with dual SCI and TBI must be very proactive, aware of the exact nature of the patient's cognitive deficits, and develop a plan that includes compensatory strategies. Extra time is always necessary to provide the extra reinforcement of the teaching. Often, in the course of teaching, patients become overwhelmed by the volume of information being presented to them. They then confuse facts later on and make errors when carrying out their programs. Printed information (memory books) is often necessary to clarify critical aspects of care. Memory devices and family involvement are key in preventing complications and setting the patient up for success. The presence of SCI in the TBI patient further complicates the bladder function. Urodynamic studies are usually helpful to accurately determine the bladder dysfunction if the patient is cooperative. Bowel incontinence and constipation may be found in patients with SCI and TBI. If the level of injury is C5 or higher, or the head injury is severe, a caretaker must become responsible for the bowel and bladder program. If the patient is cognitively capable, he should be well versed in directing another in his care. A daily or every other day Dulcolax® suppository followed by digital stimulation is a good start. Bowel care should be done at the same time of day and in an upright sitting position. The dietitian can review the current diet of enteral feeding to ensure that the patient is receiving a balanced, high-fiber diet. If constipation or impaction becomes a chronic problem, consider prescribing laxatives or stimulants on a daily basis.

Miscellaneous Disorders

Regulatory disturbances including fatigue, changes in sleep patterns, dizziness, and headaches are not uncommon problems in TBI patients.

Perceptual deficits such as possible changes in hearing, vision, taste, smell, and touch are found in some patients.

PHARMACOLOGIC CONSIDERATIONS

Multiple and varied medications are used acutely and long term in the trauma patient. In the SCI patient with mild to moderate brain injury, the physician may choose medications that, although appropriate to spinal cord medicine, may be undesirable to use in patients with a brain injury. Specific pharmacologic points and recommendations are made in the previous sections, but general concepts include the following:

- Avoid sedating medications
- Normalize sleep/wake patterns
- Maximize medical condition
- Treat adjustment issues, mood, and anxiety

Potentially sedating medications that are often given to patients with dual SCI and TBI include anticonvulsants such as phenytoin and phenobarbital. Phenytoin decreases attention, concentration, mental processing, and motor speed. As much as possible, the use of sedating anticonvulsants should be avoided in SCI patients with TBI. Antispasticity (baclofen, diazepam) medications have varying degrees of sedation. Dantrolene sodium is preferred to other agents when treating spasticity in persons with TBI (69). Benzodiazepines should be avoided in the brain injured (except when necessary for severe agitation or behavioral issues). Long-elimination half-life benzodiazepines may be more sedating (70). Benzodiazepines should not be used as first-choice anxiolytics. Buspirone hydrochloride can be used instead as an antianxiety drug (71).

Antihypertensive (propranolol, metoprolol, methyldopa) and psychoactive agents (neuroleptics, amitriptyline, doxepin, imipramine, trazadone) should be avoided in patients with TBI because of their sedating effect. Gastrointestinal medications (histamine H2 receptor antagonists) may cause cognitive and behavioral disturbances in TBI patients. These agents should be withdrawn as soon as possible once the risk of stress ulceration has passed. Metoclopramide hydrochloride (Reglan®) and antiemetics may cause sedation, dystonia, restlessness, and tardive dyskinesia. All narcotics must be used sparingly because of their sedating effect. Tramadol hydrochloride (Ultram®) is reported to be less sedating (72), but can lower the seizure threshold, and should be used with caution.

OUTCOMES

The assessment of physical and mental status is done using a variety of clinical scales. Some of these scales commonly used are the Glasgow Coma Scale (GCS); Glasgow Outcome Scale (GOS); Rappaport Disability Rating Scale (DRS); Galveston Orientation and Amnesia Test (GOAT); Functional Independence Measure (FIM); Rancho Level of Cognitive Functioning Scale (RLCF) (73–76); Disability Rating Scale (DRS); Community Integration Questionnaire (CIQ); Repeatable Battery for the Assessment of Neuropsychological Status (RBANS); and the Neurobehavioral Functioning Inventory (NFI). RLCF and DRS measure recovery; GCS and GOAT scales are used to measure injury severity. GOS, FIM, CIQ, and NFI measure outcome, and RBANS measures neuropsychologic function.

The GOS classifies outcomes in five categories: Death, Persistent Vegetative State, Severely Disabled, Moderately Disabled, and Good Recovery. The severely disabled population includes those who are partially or totally dependent in performing activities of daily living (ADL) tasks. Moderately disabled are essentially independent and resume almost all ADLs, but are not at their prior level of function. This includes limitations in social and vocational activities. To be classified as achieving good recovery, the patient has returned to prior level of function, including social, recreational, and vocational activities. An advantage of the GOS is that it is easy to assign a category and it correlates strongly with the Glasgow Coma Scale. A disadvantage is that it is simplistic, with limited sensitivity. For example, the Severely Disabled category is broad and encompasses a wide range of disability.

The Rappaport Disability Rating Scale is the sum of a variety of disabilities and impairments, ranging from coma to community reintegration. The scale ranges from 0 (no level of disability) to 30 (death). Categories included in this scale are eye opening, communication ability, motor response, cognitive disability, and employability. Many studies have reported good reliability and validity coefficients for the DRS, although the GCS and DRS consist largely of items that tend to lose their predictive value after the acute period (74).

The Rancho Los Amigos Scale (Table 44.4) was designed to measure recovery; it is widely used to describe neurobehavioral function. The scale ranges from 1 (no response) to 8 (purposeful and appropriate). This scale can be used to guide the rehabilitation team in a treatment plan (75).

Table 44.4   Rancho Los Amigos Scale

I. NO RESPONSE	Unresponsive to any stimulus
II. GENERALIZED RESPONSE	Limited, inconsistent, nonpurposeful, often only to pain
III. LOCALIZED RESPONSE	Purposeful, may follow simple commands, may focus on object
IV. CONFUSED, AGITATED	Heightened state of activity, confused, disoriented, aggressive behavior, agitation appears to relate to internal confusion, unable to do self-care, unaware of present events
V. CONFUSED, INAPPROPRIATE	Not agitated, appears alert, responds to commands, distractible, unable to concentrate on tasks, agitation to external stimuli, verbally inappropriate, does not learn new information
VI. CONFUSED, APPROPRIATE	Good directed behavior, needs cueing, can relearn old skills, memory problems, some awareness of self and others
VII. AUTOMATIC, APPROPRIATE	Appears appropriate, oriented, robotlike in daily routine, minimal or absent confusion, increased awareness of self, lacks insight into disability; decreased judgment and problem solving; interacts in environment
VIII. PURPOSEFUL, APPROPRIATE	Alert, oriented, recalls and integrates new activities, independent in home and living, capable of driving; deficits in stress tolerance/judgment/abstract reasoning; may function at reduced levels in society

The Functional Independence Measure (FIM) is widely used in the general rehabilitation population. The assessment incorporates 18 items, including bowel, bladder, self-care, and mobility. The Functional Assessment Measure (FAM) with the FIM (FIM-FAM) adds 12 items to FIM to improve sensitivity in assessing the brain injured (76–77).

The physician must remember to factor the brain injury component into the outcome of the dual diagnosis patient. In general, a better outcome is more challenging for patient and treating team in the dual diagnosis. Recovery in the TBI patient is most rapid after the injury and slows down with the passage of time. Many people with severe head injuries end up with almost no noticeable problems, but others require constant care for the rest of their lives. In general terms, the longer a person remains in coma, the less likely he or she will recover completely. The full extent of a brain injury may be unknown for months or even years. A significant relationship exists between the impairments in memory, concentration, and learning skills demonstrated during initial inpatient rehabilitation, and the rate of rehospitalization for SCI patients. The prevention of medical morbidity and enhancement of function are two of the major goals of SCI rehabilitation. Awareness of the potentially adverse effects of cognitive deficits on hospitalization, medical care use, and functional abilities may help to reduce their impact on the post-SCI course.

CONCLUSION

When an SCI patient sustains a concomitant head injury, his care becomes complex and challenging. Brain injury results in a variety of cognitive impairments. Some of these impairments, such as limited insight, reduced short-term memory, decreased attention, and impaired new learning can profoundly affect the successful rehabilitation of these individuals. Patients suffering concomitant head injuries have poorer recoveries than do non–head-injured SCI patients. These patients require comprehensive rehabilitation services. To optimize outcomes and avoid complications, treatment guidelines must be customized with great attention to the patient's specific cognitive limitations and needs.

References

1. Bleiberg J, Merbitz C. Learning goals during initial rehabilitation hospitalization. *Arch Phys Med Rehabil* 1983; 64:448–450.
2. Roth E, Davidoff G, Thomas P, et al. A controlled study of neuropsychological deficits in acute spinal cord injury patients. *Paraplegia* 1989; 27:480–489.
3. Davidoff G, Roth EJ, Richards S. Cognitive deficits in spinal cord injury: Epidemiology and outcome. *Arch Phys Med Rehabil* 1992; 73:275–284.
4. Fine PR, Kuhlemeier KV, De Vivo MJ, Stover SL. Spinal cord injury: An epidemiologic perspective. *Paraplegia* 1979; 17:237–250.
5. Grant I, Adams KM, Reed R. Aging, abstinence, and medical risk factors in the prediction of neuropsychologic deficits among long-term alcoholics. *Arch Gen Psychiatry* 1984; 4:710–718.
6. Hillbom M, Holm L. Contribution of traumatic head injury to neuropsychologic deficits alcoholics. *J Neurosurg Psychiatry* 1986; 49:1348–1353.
7. Davidoff G, Morris J, Roth E, Bleiberg J. Cognitive dysfunction and mild closed head injury in traumatic spinal cord injury. *Arch Phys Med Rehabil* 1985; 66:489–491.
8. Wilmot CB, Cope DN, Hall KM, Acker M. Occult head injury: Its incidence in spinal cord injury. *Arch Phys Med Rehabil* 1985; 66:227–231.
9. Richards JS, Brown L, Hagglund K, Bua G, Reeder K. Spinal cord injury and concomitant traumatic brain injury: Results of a longitudinal investigation. *Am J Phys Med Rehabil* 1988; 67:211–216.
10. Davidoff GN, Roth E, Thomas P, et al. Three-center study of risk factors for cognitive impairment in acute spinal cord injury patients (abstract). *Arch Phys Med Rehabil* 1987; 68:673–674.
11. Kreutzer JS, Barth J, Ellwood MS, et al. Occult neuropsychological impairments in spinal cord injured patients (abstract). *Arch Phys Med Rehabil* 1988; 69:764.
12. Silver JR, Morris WR, Otfinowski JS. Associated injuries in patients with spinal injury. *Injury* 1980; 12:219–224.
13. Schueneman AL, Morris J. Neuropsychologic deficits associated with spinal cord injury. *SCI Digest* 1982; 4:35–36,64.

14. Wagner KA, Kopaniky DR, Esposito L. Head and spinal cord injury patients: Impact of combined sequelae (abstract). *Arch Phys Med Rehabil* 1983; 64:519.

15. Dubo H, Delaney G. 101 spinal cord injuries due to motor vehicle accidents. *Proceedings of the Tenth Annual Meeting of the American Spinal Injury Association,* March 1984; 35–38.

16. Davidoff G, Morris J, Roth E, Bleiberg J. Closed head injury in spinal cord injured patients: Retrospective study of loss of consciousness and post-traumatic amnesia. *Arch Phys Med Rehabil* 1985; 66:41–43.

17. Davidoff G, Thomas P, Johnson M, et al. Closed head injury in acute traumatic spinal cord injury: Incidence and risk factors. *Arch Phys Med Rehabil* 1988; 69:869–872.

18. Meinecke FW. Frequency and distribution of associated injuries in traumatic paraplegia and tetraplegia. *Paraplegia* 1968; 5:196–211.

19. Harris P. Associated injuries in traumatic paraplegia and tetraplegia. *Paraplegia* 1968; 5:215–220.

20. Shrago GG. Cervical spine injuries: Association with head trauma a review of 50 patients. *Am J Roent* 1973; July:670–673.

21. Steudel WI, Rosenthal D, Lorenz R, Merdes W. Prognosis and treatment of cervical spine injuries with associated head trauma. *Acta Neurochir Suppl* 1988; 43:85–90.

22. Davidoff G, Thomas P, Berent S, Dijkers M, Dolijanac R. Closed head injury in acute spinal cord injury: Incidence and risk factors. *Arch Phys Med Rehabil* 1988; 69:869–872.

23. Michael DB, Guyot DR, Darmody WR. Coincidence of head and spinal injury. *J Neurotrauma* 1989; 6:177–189.

24. Saboe LA, Reid DC, Davis LA, Warren SA, Grace MG. Spine trauma and associated injuries. *J Trauma* 1991; 31:43–48.

25. Go BK, De Vivo MJ, Richards JS. The epidemiology of spinal cord injury. In: Stover SL, Delisa JA, Whiteneck GG, eds. *Spinal Cord Injury; Clinical Outcomes from the Model Systems.* Gaithersburg, MD: Aspen, 1995; 21–51.

26. Lida H, Tachibana S, Kitahara T, Horiike S, Ohwada T, Fujii K. Association of head trauma with cervical spine injury, spinal cord injury, or both. *J Trauma* 1999; 46:450–452.

27. Frank RG, Kashani JH, Wonderlich SA, et al. Depression and adrenal function in spinal cord injury. *Am J Psychiatry* 1985; 142:252–253.

28. Fullerton DT, Harvey RF, Klein MH, Howell T. Psychiatric disorders with spinal cord injuries. *Arch Gen Psychiatry* 1981; 38:1369–1371.

29. Davidoff G, Roth E, Thomas P, et al. Depression among acute spinal cord injury patients: A study utilizing the Zung Self-Rating Depression Scale. *Rehabil Psychol* 1990; 35:171–180.

30. Richards JS, Hirt M, Melamed L. Spinal cord injury: A sensory restriction perspective. *Arch Phys Med Rehabil* 1982; 63:195–199.

31. Davidoff G, Roth E, Thomas P, et al. Depression and neuropsychological test performance in acute spinal cord injury patients: Lack of correlation. *Arch Clin Neuropsychol* 1990; 5:77–88.

32. Watanabe T, Ross Z, Lairson E. Traumatic brain injury associated with acute spinal cord injury: Risk factors, evaluations, and outcomes. *Topics Spinal Cord Injury Rehab* 1999; 5(2):83–90.

33. Heinemann AW, Doll M, Scholl S. Treatment of alcohol abuse in persons with recent spinal cord injuries. *Alcohol, Health, and Research World* 13; 110–117.

34. National Spinal Cord Injury Statistical Center. *Annual Report.* Birmingham, Alabama: University of Alabama, 1995.

35. Hawkins D, Heinemenn A. Substance abuse and medical complications following spinal cord Injury. *Rehabilitation Psychology* 1998; 43(3): 219–231.

36. Alker GJ, Oh YS, Leslie EV, et al. Postmortem radiology of head and neck injuries in fatal traffic accidents. *Radiology* 1975; 114:611–617.

37. Bivins HG, Ford S, Beznalinovic Z, et. al. The effect of axial traction during orotracheal intubation of the trauma victim with an unstable cervical spine. *Ann Emerg Med* 1988; 17:25–29.

38. Bucholz RW, Burkhead WZ, Graham W, et al. Occult cervical spine injuries in fatal traffic accidents. *J Trauma* 1979; 19:768–771.

39. Porter RW. Some problems in management of spinal cord injured patients with associated head or facial trauma. *Proceedings of 19th Veterans Administration Spinal Cord injury Conference* 1973, Feb 1977; 188–196.

40. Davis D, Bohlman H, Walker AE, Fisher R, Robinson R. Pathological findings in fatal craniospinal injuries. *J Neurosurg* 1971; 34:603–613.

41. Young JS. Hospital Study Report. Model systems. *SCI Digest* 1979; 1:11–32.

42. Wagner KA, Kopaniky DR, Esposito L. Head and spinal cord injured patients: Impact of combined sequelae (abstract). *Arch Phys Med Rehabil* 1983; 64:519.

43. Okie S. Traumatic brain injury in the war zone. *N Engl J Med* 2005; 352:2043–2047.

44. Hoge CW, McGurk D, Thomas JL, et al. Mild traumatic brain injury in U.S. soldiers returning from Iraq. *N Engl J Med* 2008; 358:453–463.

45. Mahmoud A, Rengachary S, Zafonte D. Biomechanics of Associated Spine Injuries in Head Injured Patients. *Topics in Spinal Cord Injury Rehabilitation* 1999; 5(2):42–43.

46. Rosenthal M, Griffith E, Bond M, Miller JD. *Rehabilitation of the Adult and Child with Traumatic Brain Injury,* 2nd ed., Philadelphia: FA Davis, 1990; 22.

47. Narayan RK, Wilberger JE, Povlishock JT. *Neurotrauma.* New York: McGraw-Hill 1996; 23.

48. Narayan RK, Wilberger JE, Povlishock JT. *Neurotrauma.* New York: McGraw-Hill 1996; 1102–1106.

49. Zafonte R, Giap B, Coplin W, Pangilian P. Traumatic brain injury and spinal cord injury: Pathophysiology and acute therapeutic strategies. *Topics in Spinal Cord Injury Rehabilitation* 1999; 5(2):21–22.

50. Narayan RK, Wilberger JE, Povlishock JT. *Neurotrauma.* New York: McGraw-Hill 1996; 1078.

51. Siesjo B. Pathophysiology and treatment of focal cerebral ischemia: Part 1. *J Neurosurg* 1992; 77:169–184.

52. Zafonte RD, Giap BT, Coplin WM, Pangilian P. Traumatic brain injury and spinal cord injury: Pathophysiology and acute therapeutic strategies. *Top Spinal Cord Inj Rehabil* 1999; 5(2):21–40.

53. Brain Trauma Foundation, The American Association of Neurologic Surgeons, Congress of Neurological Surgeons, The Joint Section on Neurotrauma and Critical Care, *Guidelines for the Management of Severe Traumatic Brain Injury,* 3rd ed. *J Neurotrauma* 2007; 24 (Supplement 1).

54. Faul M, Wald MM, Rutland-Brown W, et al. Using a Cost-Benefit Analysis to Estimate Outcomes of a Clinical Treatment Guideline: Testing the Brain Trauma Foundation Guidelines for the Treatment of Severe Traumatic Brain Injury, *J Trauma: Injury, Infection, and Critical Care* 2007; 63(6):1271–1278.

55. Stochetti N, Furlan A, Volta F. Hypoxemia and arterial hypotension at the accident scene in head injury. *J Trauma* 1996; 40:764–767.

56. Muizelaar J, Wei E, Kontos H, Becker D. Mannitol causes compensatory vasoconstriction and vasodilation in response to blood viscosity changes. *J Neurosurg* 1984; 59:822–828.

57. Muizelaar J, Lutz H, Becker D. Effect of mannitol on ICP and CBF and correlation with pressure autoregulation in severely head injured patients. *J Neurosurg* 1984; 61:700–706.

58. Marshal L, Smith R, Shapiro H. The outcome with aggressive treatment in severe head injuries: The significance of intracranial pressure monitoring. *J Neurosurg* 1979; 50:20–25.

59. Becker D, Miller J, Ward J. The outcome from severe head injury with early diagnosis and intensive management. *J Neurosurg* 1977; 47:491–502.

60. Marshal L, Gautille T, Klauber M, et al. The outcome of severe head injury. *J Neurosurg* 1992; 77:901–907.

61. Havill J. Prolonged effect of hyperventilation and intracranial pressure. *Crit Care Med* 1984; 12:72–74.

62. Yablon SA. Posttraumatic seizures. *Arch Phys Med Rehabil* 1993; 74:983–1001.

63. Gudeman SK, Kishore PRS, Becker DP, et al. Computed tomography in the evaluation of incidence and significance of post-traumatic hydrocephalus. *Neuroradiology* 1981; 141:397.

64. Bonke CF, Lehmkuhl DL, Englander JS, et al. Medical complications and associated injuries of persons treated in Traumatic Brain Injury Model Systems Programs. *J Head Trauma Rehabil* 1993; 8:34.

65. Black K, DeSantis N. Medical complications common to spinal cord injured patients. *Topics in Spinal Cord Injury Rehabilitation* 1999; 5(2):47–75.

66. Garland D. Clinical observations on fractures and heterotopic ossification in spinal cord and traumatic brain injured populations. *Clinical Orthop Related Res* 1988; 233:86–101.

67. Kavchak M. Autonomic hyperreflexia. *Rehabilitation Nursing* 2000; 25(1):31–35.

68. Childer E, et al. Post Traumatic hyperthermia in acute brain injury rehabilitation. *Brain Injury* 1994; 8(4):335–343.

69. Katz R. Pharmacologic management of spasticity. *State of the Art Reviews-Spasticity* 1994; 8(3):474–476.

70. Greenblatt DJ. Pharmacology of benzodiazepine hypnotics. *Clinical Psychiatry* 1992; 53:7–12.

71. *Physician's Desk Reference,* 54th ed. New Jersey: Medical Economics Company, 2000; 820.

72. *Physician's Desk Reference,* 54th ed. New Jersey: Medical Economics Company, 2000; 2218.

73. Jennet B, Teasdale G, Braakman R, et al. Prediction of outcome in individual patients after severe head injury. *Lancet* 1976; 1:1031–1035.

74. Horn L, Zasler N. *Medical Rehabilitation of Traumatic Brain Injury.* Philadelphia: Hanley & Belfus, 1996; 203.

75. Woo B, Nesathurai S. *The Rehabilitation of People With Traumatic Brain Injury.* Boston: Boston Medical Center, 2000; 7–11.

76. Rosenthal M, Griffith E, Bond M, Miller JD. *Rehabilitation of the Adult and Child with Traumatic Brain Injury,* 2nd ed. Philadelphia: FA Davis Company, 1990; 265.

77. Horn L, Zasler N. *Medical Rehabilitation of Traumatic Brain Injury.* Philadelphia: Hanley & Belfus, 1996; 204–205.

45 Spinal Cord Disorders in Children and Adolescents

Lawrence Cabell Vogel
Randal R. Betz
Mary Jane Mulcahey

This chapter reviews spinal cord injuries (SCI) in children and adolescents, and myelomeningocele, the two most common pediatric spinal cord disorders. Children and adolescents with SCI and myelomeningocele share many of the same clinical characteristics related to spinal cord dysfunction, including paralysis, sensory loss, and bladder, bowel, and sexual dysfunction. Both disorders also exhibit similar complications, such as scoliosis and hip dysplasia, which result from the young age at onset of spinal cord dysfunction. However, because of associated brain abnormalities and onset in utero, children with myelomeningocele demonstrate many distinctive features, including cognitive and behavioral abnormalities and congenital malformations, such as clubfeet.

The general principles of managing children and adolescents with spinal cord disorders are significantly different when compared to adults with similar impairments. Pediatric care must be family centered because of the central role of parents and family in a child or adolescent's life, and it must be developmentally based and responsive to the dynamic changes that occur as a consequence of growth and development (1). The care of children with spinal cord disorders must be developmentally appropriate, with compatible physical and philosophic characteristics, including child-life and recreation therapy. In contrast, adolescents require a unique adolescent-based approach rather than a more traditional pediatric or adult setting.

Children or adolescents with spinal cord disorders and their families must be provided anticipatory guidance in a developmentally based fashion, which is critical to prepare them for potential complications and transitions, such as sexual development and functioning, and transition into adulthood.

Transition into adulthood is a major aspect of caring for children and adolescents with spinal cord disorders (2, 3). Transition planning should be initiated during childhood and increase in intensity as children become adolescents and approach adulthood. Transition planning incorporates many spheres of functioning, including independent living, employment, securing financial resources, socialization, and health care (3–6). From the time of onset of spinal cord dysfunction, even

if present at birth, parents must be reassured that their child has the potential to be an independently functioning adult. In order for these expectations to become ingrained in the child and adolescent, thus assuring a successful transition into adulthood, parents, healthcare providers, and other adults involved with the child must similarly foster these expectations.

An example of the importance that transition planning should begin during early childhood is the central role that employment plays in adult life, including life satisfaction. Adults with childhood-onset SCI or those with myelomeningocele are employed less frequently than the general population (7, 8). This is particularly important, because employment is significantly associated with life satisfaction. Compared to able-bodied peers, children and adolescents with SCI participate in significantly fewer prevocational activities (9). Children with spinal cord disorders should be expected to have age-appropriate chores, and as they grow up, they must be involved in developmentally appropriate prevocational and vocational activities that will adequately prepare them for adult employment (9–11).

Comprehensive primary care for children and adolescents with spinal cord disorders is frequently neglected and overshadowed by tertiary care needs (12–14). In addition to standard childhood immunizations, children and adolescents with spinal cord disorders should be immunized with the pneumococcal vaccine when they are 2 years of age or older, and yearly influenza vaccination should begin at 6 months of age (15). Children who are 12 years of age and younger should receive two doses of the split virus preparation of the influenza vaccine one month apart the first time they are immunized against influenza (15).

SPINAL CORD INJURIES

The distinctive anatomic and physiologic features of children and adolescents, along with growth and development, are responsible for the unique manifestations and complications of SCI in the pediatric population (16–20). SCI without radiologic abnormalities (SCIWORA), lap-belt injuries, birth injuries, upper cervical injuries, and the delayed onset of neurologic deficits are relatively unique to pediatric SCI and are a result of sustaining a SCI at a young age. As a result of growth, children who sustain their SCI before 8 to 10 years experience a higher incidence of scoliosis and hip dislocation. Patient compliance varies with development and is responsible for the untrainable toddler becoming a model patient during the early years of school and then a noncompliant adolescent. In children injured prior to puberty, SCI can affect growth, an example being the failure of paralyzed limbs to grow normally. Impaired mobility associated with an SCI limits the ability of children and adolescents to explore their environment in a developmentally appropriate fashion, thus impairing psychosocial, educational, and vocational development.

Epidemiology

Approximately 3% to 5% of the SCIs that occur each year in the United States occur in individuals younger than 15 years of age, and about 20% occur in those younger than 20 years of age (21–27). Utilizing the Kids' Inpatient Database and the National Trauma Data Bank, the incidence of SCI in individuals 18 years and younger from 1997 to 2000 was 1.99 cases per 100,000 children and adolescents (28). As in adults with SCI, males are more commonly affected than females during adolescence. However, as the age that children sustain an SCI decreases, the preponderance of males becomes less marked, and by 3 years of age the number of females with SCI equals that of males (24, 25, 29–31). The life expectancy of children and adolescents with SCI varies with the neurologic level and the degree of completeness of the SCI (29, 32, 33). The less severe the neurologic deficit with respect to both level of injury and category, the longer the expected survival.

The neurologic level and degree of completeness varies with age, with younger children more likely to be paraplegic and have complete lesions (29, 30, 32). However, in children under 8 years the reliability of neurological classification is significantly limited (34, 35). Among children who sustain their SCI when they are 12 years old or younger, approximately two-thirds are paraplegic and approximately two-thirds have complete lesions. In contrast, approximately 50% of adolescents are paraplegic, and approximately 55–56% have complete lesions. Younger children are more likely to have upper cervical injuries and less likely to have C4–C6 injuries, which is the more common level for tetraplegia in older children and adolescents (24, 29, 30, 32). Evaluation of cervical spine injuries in younger children must take into account the anatomical and biomechanical differences between the pediatric and adult cervical spine (36). Infants and young children are more susceptible to upper cervical injuries because of their disproportionately larger heads and underdeveloped neck musculature.

The most common cause of SCI in children and adolescents is motor vehicle crashes, with violence and sports being the next most common etiologies (29, 30, 32, 37). Violence causes SCI in children of all ages, but is an especially common cause in adolescents, particularly among Hispanics and African-Americans (29, 30, 32). Although violence remains a major cause of SCI in the pediatric population, there has recently been a decrease in the percentage of SCIs attributed to violence done to children and adolescents, as also has been observed in adults (23, 30, 38). All-terrain vehicles (ATVs) are a significant cause of serious injuries, including SCI, in children and adolescents, emphasizing the need for greater legislation and preventive efforts (39).

Those etiologies of SCI that are unique to the pediatric population include lap-belt injuries, child abuse (40) and birth injuries. Spinal cord injuries related to nontraumatic causes include tumors (41, 42) and transverse myelitis (43). There are a variety of causes of nontraumatic upper cervical spine instability related to syndromes such as Down syndrome or skeletal dysplasias, infections (tonsillopharyngitis) (44), and inflammatory conditions (juvenile rheumatoid arthritis) (45).

Lap-belt injuries most commonly affect children weighing between 40 and 60 pounds, because the lap belt rises above the pelvic brim and acts as an anterior fulcrum, resulting in flexion/distraction forces in the mid-lumbar spine (46, 47). The three major components of lap-belt injuries are abdominal wall bruising, intra-abdominal injuries, and spinal cord damage. The abdominal wall bruising is caused by trauma from the lap belt and ranges from abrasions to full-thickness skin loss. The most frequent abdominal injuries are perforations or tears of the small or large intestines, with injuries occurring less frequently to the kidneys, liver, spleen, pancreas, bladder, or uterus. Although the injury forces of a lap-belt injury are concentrated at the mid-lumbar spine, the neurologic level varies from mid-thoracic to the conus or cauda equina. The most common location for vertebral damage is between L2 and L4 (Figure 45.1); however, 23% to 30% of children with lap-belt injuries have SCIWORA. In order to decrease the risk of lap-belt injuries in children who weigh more than 40 pounds and who are 4 to 8 years of age, approved belt-positioning booster seats should be utilized (48, 49).

Neonatal SCIs occur in approximately one per 60,000 births, and most commonly result in upper cervical lesions related to torsional forces during delivery (50–61). In contrast, SCIs associated with breech deliveries are related to traction forces and most commonly involve the lower cervical or upper thoracic spine. The least-common types of neonatal SCIs are thoracic or lumbar lesions, which result from vascular occlusion associated with umbilical artery catheters or paradoxical air embolism through transitional cardiovascular shunts. Associated findings include hypoxic encephalopathy and brachial plexus or phrenic nerve injuries. Affected neonates generally present with a flaccid type of paralysis; the differential diagnosis includes spinal muscular atrophy, congenital myotonic dystrophy, amyotonia congenita, and neural tube defects.

Approximately 15% to 20% of individuals with Down syndrome demonstrate atlantoaxial instability, which is related to ligamentous laxity (62–66). An atlanto–dens interval (ADI) greater than 4.5 mm is considered abnormal. The majority of children with atlantoaxial instability are asymptomatic. In general, only symptomatic patients require surgical intervention with a C1–C2 fusion. However, one study found a similar incidence of neurological symptoms in those with subluxation and those without necessitating thorough roentgenographic examination with MRI or CT prior to surgical correction (66). Restricting high-risk activities in asymptomatic patients with an increased ADI is controversial. Additionally, children with Down syndrome commonly demonstrate occipitalatlanto instability, which must be carefully assessed (63).

Children and adolescents with polyarticular juvenile rheumatoid arthritis (JRA) may experience fusion of the cervical

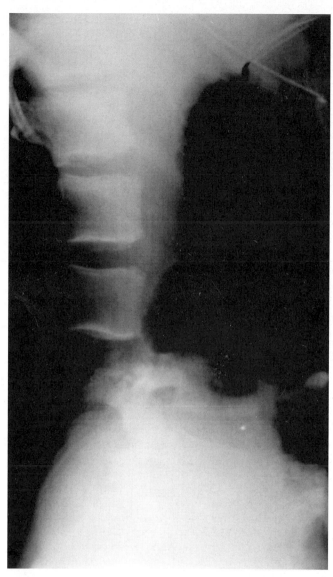

Figure 45.1 Spine radiographs of a 16-year-old male who sustained a complete T7 spinal cord injury as a result of a lap-belt injury. The radiographs demonstrate L3–L4 fracture-dislocation.

vertebra, particularly C2–C3. This may progress to fusion of a significant portion of the cervical spine, placing the patient at risk for a cervical fracture and possible tetraplegic SCI (67). In addition, individuals with JRA may develop instability at C1–C2 because of synovitis of the facet and synovial joints surrounding the odontoid process or from destruction of the odontoid process as a result of the inflammatory process (68).

Skeletal dysplasias, such as achondroplasia, spondyloepiphyseal dysplasia congenita, metatropic dysplasia, brachytelephalangic chondrodysplasia punctata, and Morquio syndrome, may be associated with a cervical myelopathy (45, 69–74). Infants with achondroplasia may have a small foramen magnum, resulting in compression of the upper cervical cord and the caudal medulla (70). Individuals with achondroplasia, primarily males, are also at risk of developing spastic paraplegia because of spinal stenosis (69). Children with dwarfing syndromes with odontoid dysplasia, such as Morquio's mucopolysaccharidosis IV,

may develop atlantoaxial instability. Myelopathy may develop in more than 50% of those with instability (69, 71).

Pathophysiology

Anatomic and physiologic characteristics unique to prepubertal children 10 years of age and younger are responsible for SCIWORA and the delayed onset of neurologic findings. Among children 10 years of age or younger when sustaining an SCI, approximately 60% have SCIWORA; in contrast, SCIWORA is found in approximately 20% of older children (72, 73). Despite the benign radiologic picture of SCIWORA, affected children are more likely to have complete neurologic lesions (31, 75).

The unique anatomic and biomechanical characteristics of the youthful spine are responsible for the higher incidence of SCIWORA in younger children with SCI (75, 76). These include increased elasticity of the spine with a less-flexible spinal cord, shallow and horizontally oriented facet joints, anterior wedging of the vertebral bodies, vulnerability of the growth zone of vertebral end plates, and poorly developed uncinate processes.

Despite normal plain radiographs, tomography, computerized tomography (CT), myelography, and dynamic flexion/extension studies, magnetic resonance imaging (MRI) abnormalities are commonly seen in patients with SCIWORA (Figure 45.2) (75, 77–78). Both extraneural and spinal cord abnormalities may be identified. The primary extraneural MRI findings include rupture of the anterior or posterior longitudinal ligaments, end plate fractures, and intradisk abnormalities. Abnormalities of the spinal cord include disruption, hemorrhage, and edema. The MRI abnormalities correlate with the severity of the neurologic deficit and the prognosis for recovery (77). Complete SCIs are generally associated with cord disruption and extensive cord hemorrhage; incomplete lesions are more likely associated with minor cord hemorrhage or edema, and mild partial cord syndromes correlate with no cord abnormalities on MRI. The use of diffusion-weighted MRI may identify abnormalities in some patients with SCIWORA and a normal conventional MRI (79).

Approximately 25% to 50% of children who sustain an SCI experience a delay in onset of neurologic abnormalities that ranges from 30 minutes to 4 days (25, 76, 80–82). Children with a delayed onset of neurologic findings frequently experience transient and subtle neurologic symptoms, such as paresthesias or subjective weakness. Mechanisms that may be responsible for delayed onset include posttraumatic occlusion of radicular arteries, natural expansion of the cord injury by inflammation, and repeated trauma to the spinal cord as a result of occult spinal instability.

Medical Issues

Deep Venous Thrombosis

The development of deep venous thrombosis (DVT) is relatively rare in children who sustain an SCI (16, 83). In one series no DVT were identified in children 5 years of age and younger and in only 1.9% of those 6 to 12 years of age in comparison to a 7.9% to 9.1% incidence in adolescents (16). In a population-based study, the incidence of DVT was 1.1% in children aged 8 to 13 years old, 4.8% in adolescents, and 4.2% to 7.4% in adults (84). Among

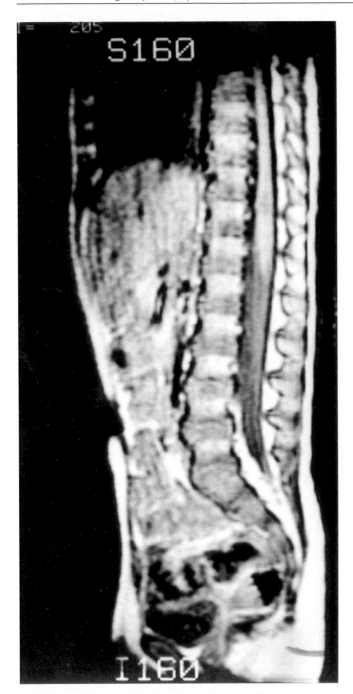

Figure 45.2   Magnetic resonance imaging study of a 2½-year-old male who sustained a complete L2 spinal cord injury as a result of a lap-belt injury, demonstrating a lucent area in the lumbar spinal cord. There were no abnormalities on the plain radiographs, so the patient has a spinal cord injury without radiologic abnormalities (SCIWORA).

children and adolescents with SCI who develop DVT, approximately 25% develop postphlebitic syndrome and 2.3% experience pulmonary emboli (83, 85).

Treatment and prophylaxis for DVT in children and adolescents with SCI is similar to that for adults (86, 87). Individuals who develop a DVT are anticoagulated with intra-

venous heparin. Heparin is initiated as a bolus of 75 units/kg over 10 minutes (5,000 to 10,000 units in adults), followed by continuous infusion of 28 units/kg/hour for infants or 20 units/kg/hour for children over 1 year (20,000 to 40,000 units/day in adults) (88, 89). The dose of heparin is adjusted to maintain the activated partial thromboplastin time between 60 and 85 seconds. Oral anticoagulation with warfarin sodium, 0.2 mg/kg, is started concurrently with heparinization. Dosage adjustments are made to maintain a prothrombin time of 2 to 3 international normalized ratio (INR). An alternative approach to managing DVT is low molecular weight heparin (1 mg/kg q12 hours subcutaneously), monitored with anti-factor Xa levels.

DVT prophylaxis includes anticoagulation and graduated elastic stockings for older children and adolescents. For younger children who cannot wear commercially available graduated elastic stockings, custom-made lower extremity garments, such as Jobst stockings, may be a consideration. Elastic wraps to wrap the legs should not be used because the unevenness of wrapping may result in constrictions with venous obstruction, thus increasing the risk of DVT. In addition, some elastic wraps contain latex, which is contraindicated because of the risk of latex allergy in the SCI population. Alternatives for prophylactic anticoagulation are the same as for adults, with utilization of low molecular weight heparin because of the ease of administration and the fact that laboratory monitoring is not needed. The dosage of low molecular heparin is 0.5 mg/kg administered subcutaneously every 12 hours (0.75 mg/kg for infants younger than 2 months) (90, 91). Because of the low incidence of DVT in children 12 years of age and younger, use of prophylactic anticoagulation in this age group should be limited to those who may be at greater risk, such as those with concomitant pelvic or lower extremity fractures.

Hypercalcemia

Hypercalcemia most commonly involves adolescent and young adult males, usually during the first 3 months after injury (92–95). Hypercalcemia affects 10% to 23% of individuals with SCI. Hypercalcemia presumably occurs as a result of increased bone resorption as a consequence of the immobilization associated with SCI. The increased incidence of hypercalcemia in the pediatric SCI population is caused by the increased bone turnover in growing children and adolescents, and their large and active bone mass, particularly in adolescent males. Because hypercalcemia depresses renal function, the excessive calcium load is not adequately excreted by the kidneys, resulting in decreased calcium excretion and an impairment of renal concentrating ability.

Patients with hypercalcemia typically present with the insidious onset of abdominal pain, nausea, vomiting, malaise, lethargy, polyuria, polydipsia, and dehydration. Patients may also exhibit behavioral changes or an acute psychosis. In a series of 87 individuals younger than 16 years, 18 (24%) experienced hypercalcemia (94). In this series, five of the patients with hypercalcemia had a clinical presentation consistent with an acute abdomen, and two of them underwent exploratory laparotomies. Patients with hypercalcemia may also be asymptomatic.

Serum calcium is elevated above the normal age-adjusted range, which is 10.8 mg/dl in children and 10.2 mg/dl in adolescents. In addition, ionized calcium is elevated above its upper limit of 1.23 mmol/L. Serum phosphorus is normal, and alkaline phosphatase is either normal or slightly elevated above age-appropriate norms. Parathyroid hormone is usually depressed because of the hypercalcemia.

The management of hypercalcemia includes hydration, which may require intravenous normal saline, and furosemide (Lasix® 0.5–2 mg/kg/day Q6–12H) to facilitate renal excretion of calcium (96). Pamidronate is efficacious in managing hypercalcemia (18, 97–100). It is administered intravenously at a dose of 1 mg/kg (usual adult dose of 60 mg) administered over 4 hours. A single dose of pamidronate is usually effective in resolving the hypercalcemia.

The complications of hypercalcemia include nephrocalcinosis, urolithiasis, and renal failure. In the series reported by Tori and Hill, 10 of their 18 (55%) pediatric patients with hypercalcemia experienced urinary stones, compared to an 18% incidence of stones in patients without hypercalcemia (94). Additionally, 2 of their 18 patients developed renal failure and nephrocalcinosis.

Autonomic Dysreflexia

The pathophysiology, clinical manifestations, and management of autonomic dysreflexia in children and adolescents with SCI is comparable to the adult SCI population (101, 102). Differences between the pediatric and adult SCI population include developmental variations of blood pressure in children and adolescents, different blood pressure cuff sizes for children, and the ability of children to communicate (103, 104).

For children and adolescents, blood pressure varies with age and body size. Normal blood pressure increases as children grow older, with older adolescents reaching adult norms. For children and adolescents without SCI, median systolic blood pressure can be estimated by the formula 90 mmHg + (2 × age in years) (105). Similar to adults with SCI, children and adolescents with cervical and upper thoracic SCI have lower baseline blood pressures compared to individuals without SCI. In view of the lower blood pressures in children and adolescents with SCI, as a consequence of both age and neurologic level, it is important that baseline blood pressures be determined. Blood pressure elevations of 20 to 40 mmHg above baseline should be considered a sign of autonomic dysreflexia.

Blood pressure measurement in the pediatric population is complicated by the need to use appropriately sized blood pressure cuffs and the anxiety that children experience with healthcare professionals. Anxiety associated with obtaining blood pressures may make it difficult to obtain accurate measurements during baseline determinations, as well as during an episode of autonomic dysreflexia. A calm and reassuring environment for the child or the adolescent and the presence of parents may be helpful.

In view of the varying cognitive and verbal communication abilities of children as they progress from infancy through adolescence, the symptoms of autonomic dysreflexia may not be expressed at all or may be communicated less clearly compared to adults (103, 104). As an example, in preschool-aged children, even though they are verbal, autonomic dysreflexia may present with vague symptoms rather than expressed complaints of a pounding headache. Medical alert identification should be utilized, and appropriate education must be provided for those adults who are significantly involved in the lives of children with SCI, such as teachers, school nurses, coaches, and community-based healthcare providers. Education about autonomic dysreflexia should include symptom recognition as well as emergency management.

Children and adolescents must take increasing responsibility for the prevention, diagnosis, and treatment of autonomic dysreflexia. This should include the consistent wearing of medical alert identification, maintaining of an information sheet or card about autonomic dysreflexia, and taking responsibility for educating healthcare providers or other significant adults about its diagnosis and management.

The management of autonomic dysreflexia in children and adolescents should be conducted efficiently in a calm and reassuring atmosphere. Symptomatic measures are generally successful in managing the majority of episodes of autonomic dysreflexia. For those not responsive to conservative measures, nifedipine (Procardia®, Adalat®, 0.25 mg/kg or 10 mg in adolescents weighing 40 or more kg) should be administered by chew and swallow for those who can follow directions or sublingually for younger children and infants. Patients with recurrent autonomic dysreflexia may be managed with prazosin (Minipress® 25–150 mcg/kg/24 hours ÷ every 6 hours) or terazosin (Hytrin® 1–5 mg daily).

Hyperhidrosis

Hyperhidrosis is seen primarily in individuals with tetraplegia or upper thoracic paraplegia (106–109). In a series of 154 individuals with SCI, 27% experienced hyperhidrosis (109). The pathogenesis of hyperhidrosis probably involves sympathetic overactivity of the cephalad portion of the spinal cord immediately below the zone of injury (109). Similar to autonomic dysreflexia, increased sympathetic output is a response to noxious stimuli below the zone of the SCI. Stimuli that may incite hyperhidrosis include UTI, urolithiasis (107), post-injury myelopathic changes, including posttraumatic syringomyelia (110–113), tethering of the spinal cord at the injury site (114), or it may be unexplained.

The sympathetics that innervate the sweat glands of the face and neck originate from T1 to T7, those for the trunk from T4 to T12, and those for the legs from T9 to L2 (108). This pattern of sympathetic innervation of the sweat glands is responsible for excessive sweating in the face and neck, which are above the zone of injury, as a result of noxious stimuli occurring below the zone of injury.

The treatment of hyperhidrosis should be initiated if it is embarrassing, impairs function, or increases the risk of developing pressure ulcers. The management of hyperhidrosis should begin with avoidance and alleviation of precipitating factors. Medications that may be beneficial are those that inhibit sympathetic overactivity, such as propantheline (115) or transdermal scopolamine (108).

Temperature Regulation

The severity of defects in temperature regulation is related to the level and completeness of the SCI (101, 106, 116). Lesions at T6 or above produce a poikilothermic state because the SCI interferes with central control of the major splanchnic sympathetics and voluntary muscles of the lower body. The patient is unable to decrease core body temperature by vasodilatation and sweating below the zone of injury. Similarly, the patient is unable to increase core temperature by vasoconstriction and shivering below the zone of the SCI. Therefore, this group of patients is at risk of hypothermia or hyperthermia as a result of environmental temperatures or endogenous factors, such as exercise (117). Infants and young children are especially vulnerable to environmental temperature extremes because of their relatively large surface area and their variable communication, cognitive, and problem-solving abilities. In contrast, adolescents with SCI may be susceptible to hypothermia or hyperthermia because of their erratic judgment and behavior.

Rarely, children with SCI are seen who cannot engage in summertime outdoor activities because their inability to sweat causes heat exhaustion. Functional cooling suits are commercially available for children with this problem (1).

Fever

Fever is a common occurrence during the first few months after an SCI and may pose a diagnostic challenge because of multiple etiologies and loss of sensation (101, 118, 119). Although fever in the acute SCI period is not unique to children with SCI when compared to adults with SCI, children are more prone to becoming febrile and experiencing higher temperature elevations. The most common cause of fever is a UTI. Other common causes include DVT, heterotopic ossification, pathologic fractures, pressure ulcers, surgical site infections, pulmonary disorders, and epididymitis. Patients with intra-abdominal disorders frequently present with subtle signs and symptoms that demand a high index of suspicion when a patient presents with fever, anorexia, nausea, vomiting, and abdominal distension (120). Multiple sources of fever are seen in approximately 15% of febrile individuals, whereas no etiology is found for 8% to 11% of febrile episodes and may reflect thermoregulatory abnormalities (118, 119).

The evaluation of a febrile child with an SCI should begin with a thorough history and physical examination. Appropriate laboratory and imaging studies should be guided by the clinical evaluation. The physical examination must encompass a general evaluation to identify problems such as otitis media, sinusitis, or pneumonia. The evaluation must also be tailored to SCI-specific problems, such as the identification of a swollen scrotum caused by epididymitis or a swollen extremity with limited range, consistent with heterotopic ossification or a pathologic fracture.

Laboratory and imaging studies should be guided by clinical findings, but generally include a urine analysis and culture, a complete blood count with differential, erythrocyte sedimentation rate, and C-reactive protein. Liver function tests, serum amylase and lipase, plain abdominal radiographs, abdominal and pelvic ultrasound, gallium scan, and CT may be helpful in evaluating the patient for potential abdominal disorders.

Pain

Chronic pain is a significant problem among children and adolescents with SCI (121, 122). Pain may be very disabling and negatively affect school, work, and social interactions. Pain may be radicular and originate from the area of trauma because of compression of a nerve root at the level of injury. Pain may also result from mechanical instability of an unhealed fracture or may represent central pain or dysesthesia (122–125). The evaluation of

pain in infants and younger children is complicated by their variable communication abilities.

Self-abusive behavior or self-mutilation is occasionally seen in individuals of all ages with SCI and may be a manifestation of dysesthesia (126–128). The most common presentation of self-abusive behavior is bitten fingertips, which can result in finger amputations. One of the authors has cared for a young boy with C8 tetraplegia who presented with chronic trauma and destruction of his nipples, resulting from constant picking.

The management of dysesthesia should incorporate physical modalities, psychologic interventions, and medications (129, 130). Physical modalities may include physical therapy, hydrotherapy, and transcutaneous electrical neural stimulation (TENS). Children and parents should be reassured that dysesthesia generally resolves within 3 to 6 months. Medications primarily used in the pediatric SCI population for dysesthesia include amitriptyline (Elavil® 0.1 mg/kg/dose at night), carbamazepine (Tegretol® 10–20 mg/kg/day ÷ BID or TID, QID if suspension is used), and gabapentin (Neurontin®), which can be used in children older than 12 years of age (900–1,800 mg/day ÷ TID) (125, 131, 132). Other medications that may be beneficial include clonidine (Catapres® 5–7 mcg/kg/day ÷ Q 6–12 hours) and phenytoin (Dilantin® 3–5 mg/day ÷ QD or BID).

Latex Allergy

Immediate-type allergic reactions to latex have been identified with increasing frequency over the past decade (133, 134). Those populations at greatest risk of latex allergy include children with myelomeningocele, SCI, and congenital genitourinary anomalies, and healthcare workers (101, 135, 136). Approximately 6% to 18% of children and adolescents with SCI are allergic to latex (136). In one report of adults with SCI who had chronic indwelling catheters, 7 of 15 (47%) had evidence of latex allergy (137).

Latex allergy probably results from frequent and extensive contact with latex-containing products, especially medical supplies and equipment. Additional risk factors include young age at initial exposure and longer duration of exposure to latex-containing products. Allergic reactions may be elicited by direct contact with latex via cutaneous, mucosal, serosal, or intravenous routes or by airborne dissemination of latex antigens that adhere to glove powder.

Latex allergic reactions may manifest as localized or generalized urticaria, wheezing, angioedema, or anaphylaxis. Allergic reactions to latex that occur intraoperatively may be life threatening and may be difficult to diagnose because of surgical drapes covering the patient's skin, which may mask the presence of urticaria.

The diagnosis of latex allergy is made by a history consistent with an immediate-type allergic reaction or with in vitro assays or skin tests. Children are considered to be allergic to latex if they have a history of reacting to latex or a positive laboratory or skin test. Clinical manifestations are frequently subtle, such as the child who develops a blotchy rash on his face when he blows up a balloon. Latex allergy should be suspected in individuals who have unexplained intraoperative allergic reactions, or in individuals allergic to kiwi, bananas, avocados, or chestnuts (138). Although skin tests are probably the most sensitive method of identifying latex allergy, the routine use of skin tests is limited by the lack of availability of standardized preparations and the potential for initiating a severe allergic reaction (134).

In view of the potential severity of latex allergy, individuals at risk, such as those with SCI or myelomeningocele, should be cared for in a latex-free environment. This should minimize the risk of sensitizing patients, in addition to preventing allergic reactions both in patients with known, as well as in those with undiagnosed, latex allergies. Patients, their families, and caregivers should be educated about the potential for latex allergy and the necessity to avoid all latex-containing products. Individuals allergic to latex should wear a medical alert identification and carry autoinjectable epinephrine.

Cardiovascular Fitness and Nutrition

Cardiovascular disorders, including hypertension and coronary artery and cerebrovascular diseases, are major causes of morbidity and mortality in adults with SCI (139). The increased risk of cardiovascular disease in individuals with SCI may be a result of their sedentary lifestyles, which is related to volitional motor impairments (140) and an increased incidence of metabolic syndrome (141). Children with SCI have lower resting metabolic rates and decreased total lean tissue mass, predisposing them to obesity (142). The evaluation and management of fitness is complicated in children with SCI for several reasons. Because the traditional measure of obesity, body mass index (BMI), underestimates body fat in children with SCI, the use of dual energy X-ray absorptiometry is needed to accurately assess total body fat and total lean body mass (142, 143). Nutritional interventions need to take into account the fact that resting energy expenditure in children is significantly lower compared to the general population (144, 145). Individuals with SCI should be encouraged to adopt a lifestyle and pursue preventive measures that promote fitness and improve nutrition, thereby reducing their risk of cardiovascular complications. Because of their relatively long life span, it becomes particularly important for children and adolescents with SCI to make adaptations to normally practiced preventive measures, such as exercise, diet, stress reduction, and avoidance of tobacco.

Exercise is a major element in preventing cardiovascular complications. A regular exercise program becomes a significant challenge in children and adolescents with SCI because of their motor limitations, compounded by varying preferences and compliance, which may be limited by their developmental stage. Because of motivation and size, younger children with paraplegia may be physically active by crawling and ambulating with a variety of orthotics. With this exception, the pediatric SCI population shares significant limitations of exercise options with the adult SCI population. Children and adolescents with SCI, especially those with cervical and upper thoracic lesions, may exhibit decreased cardiovascular adaptions to exercise, which may be manifested by decreased cardiac output, reduced aerobic capacity, exertional hypotension, and hyperthermia (117, 146–149). In additional, children and adolescents must take special precautions when exercising; one of the author's patients with a T1-level injury died of a crush injury and suffocation at home during unsupervised weight lifting.

Various exercise programs are available for children and adolescents with SCI, such as adapted physical education and therapeutic recreational activities (150–153). Cardiovascular fitness and increased aerobic capacity, muscle strength, and endurance should be key objectives of an exercise program (154). Exercise programs should be developmentally based, compatible with age-appropriate and contemporary activities, consistent with pre-injury interests, and incorporated into family and community activities (151, 152). Exercise programs should promote independence, be integrated into the child's or adolescent's lifestyle and routine, and most important, be fun.

Children and adolescents with SCI should be assessed for their risk of cardiovascular disorders, which includes factors such as obesity, smoking, sedentary lifestyle, hyperlipidemia, hypertension, and family history. Screening for hyperlipidemia after 2 years of age should be pursued in children with a high-risk family history.

Pulmonary

Pulmonary complications are important problems during both the acute and chronic phase of SCI for children with SCI (18, 139, 155–158). Children with high cervical injuries generally require lifelong ventilatory support or phrenic nerve or diaphragm pacing (159–161). Children who are candidates for phrenic nerve pacing are those with C3 or higher lesions (162). Bilateral phrenic nerve stimulation is usually performed in children to avoid excessive mediastinal shifts. In addition, tracheostomies are needed because of the upper airway obstructions that occur in young children during phrenic nerve pacing. Children may experience failure to thrive if they are entirely dependent on phrenic nerve pacing, so that supplemental nighttime ventilation via a tracheostomy may be required (162). Noninvasive ventilation using systems such as biphasic positive airway pressure (BiPAP) and airway secretion management may be applicable in the pediatric SCI population (163). Although children with high tetraplegia experience significant morbidity and mortality, they generally enjoy a satisfying and relatively independent life (164, 165).

Infants and young children with tetraplegic SCI may be at risk of incipient respiratory failure, which may be manifested by a sleep-disordered breathing disturbance with sleep apnea, snoring, restless sleep, morning confusion, daytime sleeping, headache, and mental dullness (157, 166, 167). A high index of suspicion must be maintained in these young children with tetraplegia, and sleep studies should be ordered if the child demonstrates any symptoms of a sleep-disordered breathing disturbance. Risk factors for sleep-induced respiratory failure include diaphragmatic and intercostal muscle paralysis, obesity, and use of medications such as baclofen or diazepam (166).

Urology

Intermittent catheterization is the standard management of the neurogenic bladder in children and adolescents with SCI (12, 168–174). Clean intermittent catheterization is initiated when the child is approximately 3 years old, or earlier if the child is experiencing recurrent UTIs or exhibiting renal impairment. Self-catheterization is initiated in children with adequate hand function when they are developmentally 5 to 7 years old (172).

The utilization of prophylactic antibiotics and the treatment of asymptomatic bacteriuria in the pediatric SCI population are similar to that of adults with SCI (175). Prophylactic antibiotics should not be routinely used. They should be limited to patients who experience recurrent and severe UTIs and in those with obstructive uropathy or compromised renal function, including hydronephrosis and vesicoureteral reflux. Asymptomatic bacteriuria is generally not treated unless the patient has compromised renal function. Treatment should be limited to those with symptomatic UTIs, as manifested by systemic toxicity (fever, chills, dysreflexia, or exacerbation of spasticity), incontinence, or cloudy and foul-smelling urine. Usage of fluoroquinolones should be limited in children younger than 18 years of age because of the potential of cartilage damage (176). However, fluoroquinolones may be used in children and young adolescents with SCI if alternative safe and effective antimicrobials are not available (176).

Continence and independence are crucial aspects of bladder management of children and adolescents with SCI. The management of incontinence may include anticholinergics, modification of fluid intake and catheterization schedule, Botox (177), and treatment of urologic complications such as UTIs and urolithiasis. Urodynamics should be performed in patients with persistent incontinence. Children and adolescents with limited bladder capacity unresponsive to anticholinergics may be candidates for a bladder augmentation (173, 178, 179).

Continent catheterizable conduits are an alternative for individuals who are not independent in performing intermittent catheterization (173, 180, 181). A continent catheterizable conduit, known as the Mitrofanoff procedure, consists of creating a catheterizable conduit using the appendix or a segment of small bowel, which is used to connect the bladder to a stoma, either on the lower abdominal wall or in the umbilicus (182, 183). Continent catheterizable conduits allow individuals with limited upper extremity function, such as those with C6 or C7 injuries, to catheterize themselves (184–187). Additionally, continent catheterizable conduits may promote independence in bladder management for individuals who have difficulty accessing their urethra, such as females who have difficulty transferring to a commode or toilet or those who cannot actively abduct their legs.

Bowel Management

The crucial issues for bowel management in children and adolescents with SCI include complete and regular emptying, continence, short duration of the bowel program, aesthetics, and prevention of complications (169, 174, 188–193). The necessity for regularity in performing bowel programs often conflicts with the lack of conformity of children and adolescents. However, the anxiety associated with the potential for fecal incontinence is a strong incentive for compliance with bowel program scheduling. Bowel programs are begun when children are 2 to 4 years of age, which is a developmentally appropriate age, or earlier if they are experiencing diarrhea or constipation (194).

The fundamental components of a bowel program include independence, privacy, and regularity with respect to frequency and time of day. The bowel program should take place on a toilet or a commode. A sitting position facilitates defecation, and if neurologically capable, the child should be taught and encouraged to increase intra-abdominal pressure. It is important that these key principles be instituted when a bowel program is initiated, irrespective of the age of the child or adolescent.

For children and adolescents who do not respond to standard bowel program interventions, options include the antegrade continence enema (ACE procedure), enema continence catheters, and pulsed irrigation enemas (195). With the antegrade continence enema procedure, antegrade evacuation of the bowel is accomplished by administering an enema directly into the cecum (196, 197). This is delivered into the cecum via the appendix, which is accessible through an abdominal wall stoma. The ACE procedure has been reported to be useful in improving continence and decreasing constipation (198).

Spasticity

Children with SCI are less likely to demonstrate spasticity compared to the adult SCI population. This may be a reflection of the higher incidence of paraplegia in children with SCI compared to adults (199). Nevertheless, spasticity is an important problem for a significant number of children with SCI (200–202). General management principles of spasticity in children with SCI are no different from those in the adult SCI population (199). Evaluation should include a thorough history and physical examination with attention directed to potential inciting factors. Factors that perpetuate or exacerbate spasticity include noxious stimuli below the zone of injury, which are frequently clinically inapparent. Hence, a high index of suspicion and a thorough evaluation are necessary, particularly in view of the age-dependent variability in the ability to communicate. Hip subluxation or dislocation is an example of a noxious stimulus that may exacerbate spasticity and that is more common in the pediatric SCI population.

The goals of spasticity management are to improve function, prevent complications, and alleviate pain and embarrassment (199, 203). Both the advantages and disadvantages of spasticity must be considered when treating spasticity. The major aspects of spasticity management include prevention, nonpharmacologic interventions, medications, and invasive procedures. Prevention is the foundation of any therapeutic program for spasticity and comprises the avoidance of precipitating factors and the establishment of good bladder, bowel, and skin programs. Nonpharmacologic interventions include relief of inciting factors and a program of stretching and range-of-motion exercises and positioning.

Medications should be considered in patients with spasticity that affects the child's functioning and that is unresponsive to conservative treatment. Baclofen administered orally is the initial medication of choice and is initiated at 0.125 mg/kg/dose BID to TID (5 mg BID to TID in children 12 years and older) (204). Doses are then increased every 3 to 5 days by increments of 0.125 mg/kg/dose (5 mg/dose in children 12 years and older). The usual maximum daily dose is 1 to 2 mg/kg/day administered QID (80 mg/day in children 12 years and older). Although baclofen remains the drug of choice for managing spasticity in adolescents, the potential for illicit drug experimentation must also be considered (205).

Other medications that may be beneficial in the management of spasticity include diazepam, clonidine, dantrolene, gabapentin, and tizanidine. Diazepam (Valium® 0.1 mg/kg/dose QHS to QID) may be used in combination with baclofen or as a single drug for patients who do not tolerate baclofen. Clonidine (5–7 mcg/kg/day 4 Q 6–12 hours) may be effective as a single agent or in combination with other drugs (206). Transdermal administration of clonidine (0.1–0.3 mg patch weekly) may be used in older children or adolescents (207, 208). Dantrolene (Dantrium®) is generally not used to manage spasticity in children and adolescents with SCI. Although not approved for use for spasticity, gabapentin (Neurontin® 900–1,800 mg/day 4 TID for children older than 12 years of age) may assist in controlling spasticity. Although tizanidine (Zanaflex®) is not approved for use in pediatrics, it is used by some clinicians and demonstrates efficacy similar to that in adults with SCI (209). Because of the potential for hepatotoxicity, liver function studies should be performed, especially during the first 6 months of therapy.

For spasticity that does not respond to standard management, options include intrathecal baclofen, selective dorsal root rhizotomies, epidural spinal cord stimulation, and localized injection of botulinum toxin (210–215). Baclofen can be administered intrathecally by an implanted pump and has been utilized increasingly in children and adolescents with SCI, with encouraging results (216). Experience with intrathecal baclofen in the pediatric population also includes children and adolescents with cerebral palsy (217). Disadvantages of intrathecal baclofen are cost—for both the initial implantation and pump refills—and the rare occurrence of serious adverse reactions (218, 219).

Surgical

Halo Fixators

Proper halo ring application on children is crucial in preventing pin loosening and pin tract infections. For infants, multiple pins (10 in comparison to four in adults) with low torque (2 inch-pounds) have been shown to be safe (220). Torque should range from 4 to 6 inch-pounds for children between 2 and 12 years of age and to 8 inch-pounds for children older than 12 years of age. CT scanning of the skull is recommended for pin placement for children under 6 years of age, because of the variability in skull thickness (221, 222). If halo fixation fails, a Minerva-type cervicothoracolumbosacral orthosis is an alternative. Because use of Crutchfield tongs in patients younger than 12 years old may result in skull penetration and dural fluid leaks, halo traction is the preferred method for this age group.

Spine Boards

Because the head is proportionately larger than the rest of the body in children younger than 8 to 10 years of age, their necks will be inadvertently flexed if they are immobilized on a standard spine board (Figure 45.3A, B). Therefore, when spinal stabilization is needed, younger children should be immobilized on child-specific spine boards (Figure 45.3C) (221, 223). However, if a standard spine board must be used for a younger child, excessive cervical flexion can be avoided by raising the torso 2 to 4 cm, leaving the head at the board level (Figure 45.3D).

Spine Deformities

Spine deformities are an extremely common problem in pediatric SCI, especially if the injury is sustained prior to skeletal maturity (224, 227). (See Figure 45.4.) For children injured prior

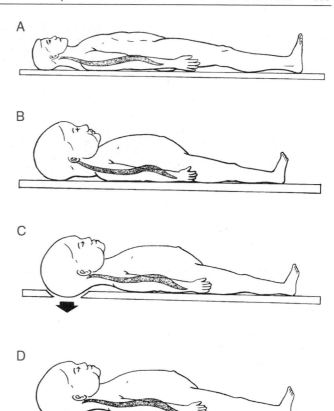

Figure 45.3 **A** depicts an adult immobilized on a standard backboard. **B** shows a young child on a standard backboard; the relatively large head results in a kyphotic position of the neck. In **C**, the child is on a modified backboard with a cut-out to recess the occiput, which provides for safe cervical positioning. In **D** a double mattress pad raises the chest, providing safe cervical positioning. (Source: Herzenberg JE, Hensinger RN, Dedrick DK, et al. Emergency transport and positioning of young children who have an injury of the cervical spine. The standard backboard may be hazardous. *J Bone Joint Surg* 1989; 71A:15–22.)

to skeletal maturity, 98% will develop scoliosis, with 67% requiring surgery (226). In contrast, for children and adolescents whose injuries occurred after skeletal maturity, the risk of scoliosis is reduced to 20%, with approximately 5% requiring surgical correction. The spine deformities may be a result of muscle weakness or imbalance, residual deformity, or may be iatrogenic, as a result of a laminectomy, for example (228). The complications of these spine deformities include pelvic obliquity, pressure ulcers, impaired use of the upper extremities secondary to poor sitting balance, pain, poor fitting of lower extremity orthotics, and gastrointestinal and cardiopulmonary problems. Because of the high incidence of scoliosis, radiographs of the thoracic, lumbar, and sacral spine should be obtained every 6 months prior to puberty and every 12 months thereafter.

Use of prophylactic bracing with thoracolumbosacral orthoses (TLSO) may be effective in delaying the need for spine surgery. In a study of 123 children with SCI, in those who were braced prophylactically when their curve was 20 degrees or less, the time to surgical correction was significantly delayed

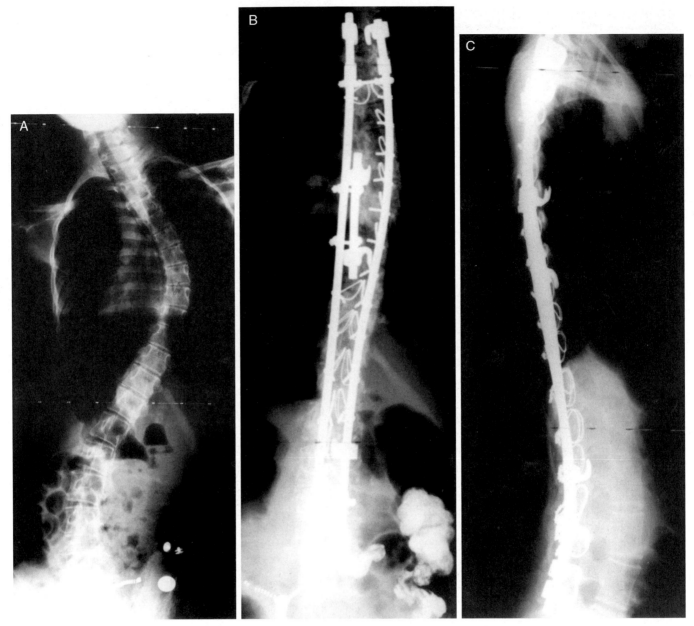

Figure 45.4   Spine radiographs of a 13-year-old female who sustained an incomplete C4 spinal cord injury (ASIA Impairment Scale score of C) when she was 8 years old. **A** demonstrates a 65-degree thoracolumbar curve. **B** and **C** are radiographs obtained after she underwent a posterior spine fusion with instrumentation.

compared to those who were not braced (229). In contrast there was no significant difference in those who were braced compared to those who were not braced when the initial curve at presentation was greater than 20 degrees. The major disadvantages of routine bracing include the interference with mobility and independent functioning, such as self-catheterization (230, 231). Irrespective of the degree of scoliosis, bracing with a TLSO may benefit patients with poor trunk support, which facilitates upper extremity functioning and sitting.

Surgical correction is indicated when the curve progresses beyond 40 degrees in children older than 10 years old (1). For younger children, curves up to 80 degrees are tolerated if they are

flexible and decrease while in a TLSO; otherwise, surgery is indicated regardless of age.

Hip Deformities

Hip subluxation, dislocation, and contractures are frequent complications in children with SCI, especially if they were injured at younger ages (Figure 45.5) (1, 228, 232–234). In one series, hip instability was observed in 100% of children who were injured when they were less than 5 years of age and in 93% of those injured when they were younger than 10 years of age (1, 234). In another report, hip instability was found in 60% of children

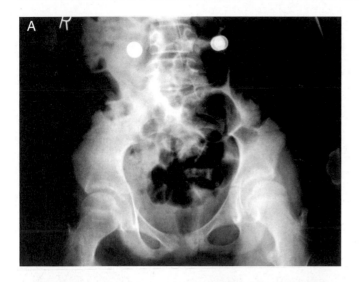

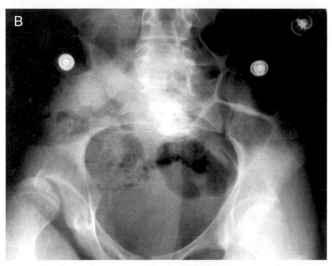

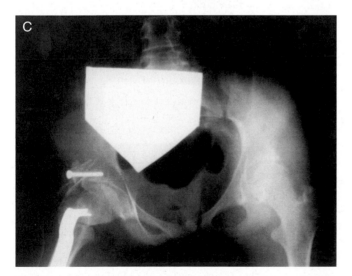

Figure 45.5   Pelvic radiographs of a female with incomplete C4 tetraplegia. Radiographs obtained at 10 years of age (**A**) demonstrate both hips to be located, with subluxation of the right hip when she was 11 years of age (**B**). **C** is a radiograph obtained after surgical correction of the hip dislocation.

injured when they were 8 years of age or younger (235). Hip instability occurs in patients regardless of their neurologic level, presence or absence of spasticity, or their gender (236).

The indications for surgical management of hip instability are not clear-cut. An aggressive approach to managing hip instability should be entertained in view of the future applications of the FES systems for upright mobility and the future possibility for spinal cord regeneration (1, 232, 237). The management of hip instability may include the surgical release of hip contractures, a capsulorrhaphy, varus osteotomies, and anterior or posterior acetabular augmentations (238, 232, 238).

Because of the high incidence of hip instability and contractures in children injured when they are 10 years or younger, an aggressive prevention approach is indicated. This would include active soft tissue stretching, control of spasticity, and prophylactic abduction bracing (232).

Heterotopic Ossification

An accurate incidence of heterotopic ossification (HO) in pediatric SCI is not known but may be approximately 3%, in contrast to a 20% incidence in adults with SCI (228, 239). The hip is most commonly involved in children and adolescents with SCI. In pediatric SCI, HO begins on average 14 months after injury, in contrast to adult onset within 1 to 4 months (240). Etidronate disodium (Didronel®) to prevent HO is not routinely used in the pediatric SCI population because of the relatively low risk of HO (241). In addition, the use of etidronate disodium should be limited in children prior to puberty because of the possible development of a rachitic-like syndrome (242–244). Surgery is indicated if there are significant functional deficits. Resection of HO should be undertaken 1–1.5 years after its onset to avoid the possible progression of femoral neck osteoporosis and intraarticular fibrosis if surgery is postponed until the bone scan and alkaline phosphatase are normal (239, 245). The postoperative use of radiation therapy may be contraindicated in younger children because of the long-term consequences of radiation. However, indomethacin (Indocin® 1–3 mg/kg/day 4TID or QID, maximum dose of 200 mg/day) is used in the postoperative period (246).

Osteopenia and Pathologic Fractures

The onset of osteopenia begins soon after sustaining an SCI and reaches a plateau 6 to 12 months after sustaining an SCI. Children and adolescents with SCI have bone densities that are 60% of normal age- and sex-matched controls (247, 248). A combination of standing, stepping, and FES may increase bone mineral density by approximately 25%.

Pathologic long bone fractures, as a consequence of loss of bone mineral density, occur in approximately 14% of children and adolescents with SCI (1, 228). Gait training, range-of-motion exercises, and minor trauma are responsible for approximately 40% of the pathologic fractures, with the etiology of the remaining fractures not being identified. Children and adolescents with SCI who develop a pathologic fracture may present with fever and a swollen extremity. The supracondylar region of the femur and the proximal tibia are the most common sites of a pathologic fracture. Radiographic abnormalities may initially be subtle, and the diagnosis of a pathologic fracture in growing children requires a high index of suspicion (228, 232).

The treatment of pathologic fractures in children with SCI should consist of removable splints (1, 228, 232, 249). If casts are necessary, they must be well padded over all bony prominences and bivalved to enable inspection to prevent pressure ulcers. Because of osteoporosis, internal or external fixation generally may not hold very well. Fortunately, exuberant callus usually develops within 3 to 4 weeks, at which time splinting or casting can be discontinued with resumption of range-of-motion exercises. However, ambulation should be postponed for 6 to 8 weeks after sustaining a fracture.

Prevention is critical, but is especially challenging in the pediatric SCI population because of the risk-taking behaviors characteristic of children and adolescents. Prevention must focus on safety in risky activities. In addition, bone mineral loss should be minimized by encouraging weight bearing with orthotics or FES. Good nutrition and adequate sunlight are also essential. Appropriate training and adequate equipment for transfers are essential components of pediatric SCI rehabilitation. In the future, bisphosphonates such as alendronate may have a role in preventing pathologic fractures.

Pressure Ulcers

Pressure ulcers are one of the most common complications for children and adolescents with SCI (250, 251). The incidence of pressure ulcers in the pediatric SCI populations is not known. In a retrospective study of people who sustained their SCI when they were less than 13 years of age, 55% developed at least one pressure ulcer during a mean follow-up period of 10.3 years (250). The peak age for pressure ulcer development was 8 years of age. Issues unique to the pediatric population include variable compliance in both preventive and therapeutic endeavors because of the different developmental stages of children and adolescents (250, 252). Toddlers and younger children may be at risk of developing pressure ulcers because of inadvertent trauma from the careless activities and play typical in these age groups. Younger children have limited cognitive abilities to comply with the usual preventive measures that older individuals follow, such as pressure relieves. Preventive measures may include wristwatches with automatic resetting timers to remind children to perform pressure relief. Additionally, preventive interventions should be developmentally based, with responsibility gradually shifted from the parents to the children as they grow up. As children grow up and become physically larger, new equipment must be matched to their size. Properly fitting wheelchairs and adequate cushions must be prescribed, and pressure mapping should be performed to reduce the risk of pressure ulcers.

Rehabilitation

Pediatric SCI rehabilitation must be developmentally based, and goals must be responsive to the dynamic changes that occur as children and adolescents grow up (1, 253–260). The objectives of rehabilitation are to maintain health and restore productivity, with the ultimate goal that the patient experiences a satisfying life. A major challenge in providing care for children and adolescents with SCI is to address the changing needs at each developmental stage, with the ultimate goal being that the patient becomes an adult with a high quality of life (261).

Standard interventions should encompass mobility, activities of daily living, bowel, bladder, and skin programs, recreation, social services, and psychologic and vocational counseling. Conventional rehabilitation must be broadened to incorporate effective mobility and access in the community, and educational, vocational, and recreational interventions that promote a productive and satisfying life. As children and adolescents grow up, they need new equipment because of increasing size and changing needs. Using mobility as an example, infants and young toddlers may crawl, stand, and ambulate in parapodia, and use strollers for wheeled mobility. Although young school-aged children may crawl at home, they use a variety of orthotics for ambulation or standing in school, and they should become independent users of their wheelchairs (262). Older children and adolescents primarily utilize wheelchairs for community mobility, with older adolescents needing access to motor vehicles for community mobility.

Upper Extremity Function

Although hand function in children with tetraplegia may be improved with a variety of static and dynamic orthotics, they generally stop using these braces because of cosmesis, the added stigma, and the burden of carrying additional equipment (263, 264). In contrast, surgical reconstruction, including tendon transfers of the upper extremities to restore hand function, is beneficial for children and adolescents with SCI (265, 266). The usual objectives of surgical reconstruction of the upper extremities are to restore elbow extension, wrist extension, finger extension and flexion, and thumb pinch.

Implantable FES systems have been successfully utilized to restore grasp and release in adolescents with C5 or weak C6 tetraplegia, who would otherwise not be candidates for reconstructive surgeries (267, 268). Similar to adults with SCI, the Freehand System® in adolescents results in increased independence and improved satisfaction (264, 269). Findings in animal studies, and now FDA clinical trials in humans, indicate that children as young as 6 years of age may benefit from this technology (270).

Ambulation

The ability to ambulate depends on a variety of factors, including age, body size, neurologic level and degree of completeness, compliance, and preferences. Children who are most likely to be community ambulators are those who are young, have L3 or lower lesions, or have an American Spinal Injury Association (ASIA) impairment scale score of D (271–273). Compared to adolescents and adults, children tend to be more active ambulators because of their size, increased energy level, and reduced concern for cosmesis (272–277).

Parapodia permit children with SCI to stand without the need for upper extremity weight bearing and allow them to perform activities with both hands (272, 278). Children are also able to ambulate with parapodia. The basic requirements to utilize parapodia include head control and the absence of significant contractures of the lower extremities. In general, patients who utilize parapodia are either therapeutic or household ambulators. However, parapodia provide children with some independence

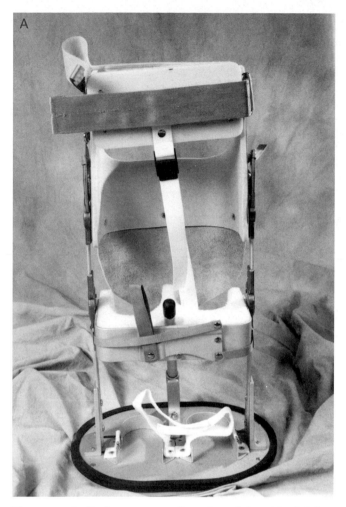

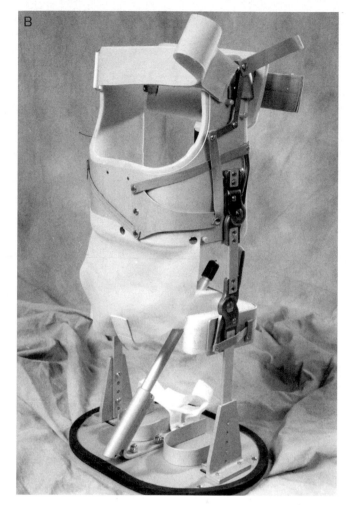

Figure 45.6   Rochester parapodium: front (**A**) and back (**B**) views.

in mobility and an opportunity to be upright and face their peers at eye level.

Children can begin using parapodia as young as 9 to 12 months of age, which is a developmentally appropriate time to start standing and walking. Parapodia may also be helpful in giving the young child an opportunity to be upright prior to initiating other orthotics. Another advantage of parapodia is that they do not require intensive therapy. Parapodia are generally well accepted by preschoolers and early school-aged children, but children tend to stop using parapodia by the time they are 7 to 10 years of age.

Rochester parapodia are the more commonly used parapodia. Rochester parapodia have hip and knee joints that facilitate donning and doffing, allow the patient to sit while wearing the brace, and may facilitate transferring from the floor or chair to standing (Figure 45.6) (278, 279). Children can ambulate with the Rochester parapodia by swiveling, produced by twisting their upper trunks and swinging their arms. They may also choose to perform a swing-to or a swing-through gait utilizing an assistive device, such as a walker or forearm crutches.

A third orthosis is the reciprocating gait orthosis (RGO) frequently used in children or adolescents with upper lumbar

or thoracic paraplegia SCI (Figure 45.7) (272, 277, 278). In comparison to hip–knee–ankle–foot orthoses (HKAFO) or knee–ankle–foot orthoses (KAFO), which may also be utilized in this group of patients, RGOs provide a reciprocating gait and are more energy efficient (280). Children as young as 15 to 18 months old can begin to use RGOs. Children with active hip flexors, or who are young and motivated, are most likely to be community ambulators, although the majority of RGO users will primarily be therapeutic or household ambulators (277, 278).

Standing may have extensive functional and psychologic benefits for children with SCI (277, 281). In addition to parapodia there are a number of static and mobile standing devices that are suitable for children, including standing wheelchairs, standing frames, and mobile standing devices (277). Because of their size, standing wheelchairs are only appropriate for older children and adolescents. The standing Danny (Figure 45.8) and the Rifton standing walker (Figure 45.9) are two examples of mobile standing devices. Mobile standing devices are most appropriate for preschool-aged to pre-adolescent children, and they are primarily used for household or school activities. There are a variety of standers that permit the child or adolescent with an SCI to go

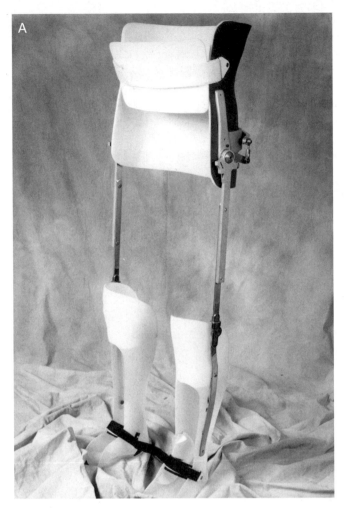
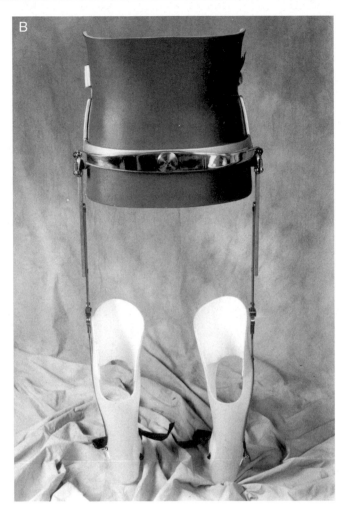

Figure 45.7   Reciprocating gait orthosis (RGO): front (**A**) and back (**B**) views.

from sitting to standing, with some standers allowing the individual to be mobile using arm cranks.

FES systems are another option for upright mobility in children, and these have been demonstrated to be feasible and practical (1, 282). Using an implanted FES system, adolescents were able to stand at home two to four times a week (283). They were able to perform common activities while standing, which included reaching high places and exercising. In another clinical trial, an implanted FES system was compared to KAFOs (284). Compared to KAFOs, the FES system was equal or better in promoting independence and was preferred for the majority of activities. Hip dislocation, lower extremity contractures, severe scoliosis, and myocutaneous flaps that have been performed for pressure ulcers are contraindications to FES for upright mobility. It is therefore critical to prevent these complications in children and adolescents with SCI, who may benefit one day from innovative treatments such as FES.

Psychosocial Issues and Sexuality

Sexuality is an often-overlooked aspect of caring for children with special needs. This is particularly critical because children and

adolescents with disabilities tend to be "infantalized" or treated as asexual beings. Several dimensions of sexuality must be addressed with children and adolescents with SCI and their families. These aspects of sexuality include the general sexuality issues common to all children and adolescents, sexuality issues common to children with special needs, and the SCI-specific sexuality issues (285–288). From the onset of the SCI, patients and parents must be educated in a prospective and optimistic manner about future sexuality issues, including fertility. As children and adolescents grow, sexuality education and counseling must be provided in a developmentally based fashion. Additionally, sexuality counseling must be progressively addressed directly to older children and adolescents without parents being present. Females who have sustained SCI and their parents should be reassured that the SCI will result in minor or no abnormalities, and no delays in onset or resumption of menstruation (289).

Education

As with all children with special needs, federal laws protect the educational rights of children and adolescents with SCI (290). The public laws, the Education for All Handicapped Children Act

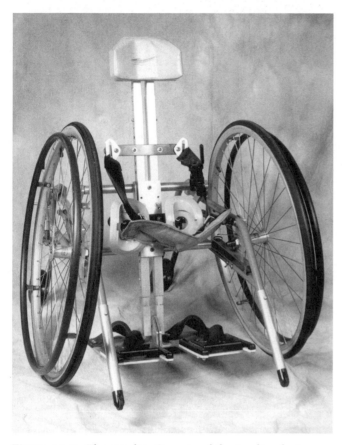

Figure 45.8   The standing Danny mobile standing device.

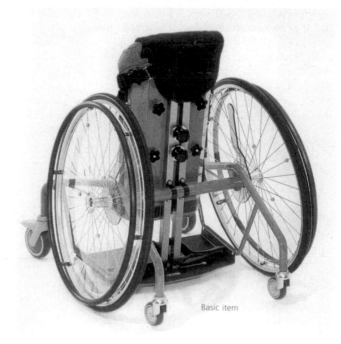

Basic item

Figure 45.9   The Rifton standing walker.

(EAHCA, 1975), and the Individuals with Disabilities Education Act (IDEA, 1990) require that children and adolescents with special needs be educated in the least-restrictive environment (291). In a variety of ways, education is an important part of the lives of children and adolescents with SCI (10, 261, 285, 286). In addition to play, education is the main occupation of children and adolescents. It is critical that they return to school as soon as possible after injury, and ideally they should return to the school that they had previously attended prior to their injury. Returning to school allows the child or adolescent with SCI to reestablish friendships and peer interactions. Additionally, education is a major determinant of adult employment, which in turn is a crucial predictor of life satisfaction for adults with SCI. Returning to school can be a traumatic event for the patient, fellow students, and the teachers. Transition back into school can be significantly improved by having the patient visit his school prior to discharge from inpatient rehabilitation. From the teachers' and fellow students' perspectives, this experience may also be beneficial. If that is not possible, the teachers and students may benefit from viewing a video of the patient in addition to reviewing educational materials about SCI. A teaching manual about SCI designed for school teachers and school nurses may also be helpful (285, 286).

Psychologic Counseling

Children and adolescents who sustain an SCI may experience myriad psychosocial consequences, and these issues will vary as children age. This poses unique challenges during adolescence because of the concurrent psychosocial and physical processes inherent in adolescence (292). Although SCI have a significant impact on psychological well-being, the occurrence of the injury during childhood does not worsen long-term psychologic adjustment compared to those injured as adults (293). Children and adolescents with SCI should receive psychologic evaluation and counseling in an ongoing manner, appropriate for their developmental stage (294). Because of the significant impact that families have on their children or adolescents with SCI, counseling and support must also be provided for parents, siblings, and other significant family members (285, 286). Support and peer groups are also beneficial for patients, parents, and other family members (292).

Attendant Care

Although family members may be available to provide daily care, attendant care should be given consideration for children with tetraplegia. Attendant care assists parents in maintaining their parental role, which includes limit-setting and support and guidance for their children. To perform the roles of both parent and caregiver is a major challenge for most parents. To avoid burning out parents, respite care is essential, particularly if their children have high tetraplegia with complicated and intense needs.

Recreation

Play and recreation should be an integral aspect of the rehabilitation program for children and adolescents with SCI (151–153, 296, 297). The pre-injury interests and experiences of the child or adolescent should provide direction to play and recreation-based therapy. Play is essential for young children during rehabilitation because play is their primary activity of daily living. Play techniques must be incorporated into the rehabilitation program. Recreation and play afford older children and adolescents the necessary break from more traditional rehabilitation. Older children and adolescents must be provided appropriate outlets and access to typical age-appropriate activities, such as sports, television, movies, music, and talk. Similarly, they need knowledge and exposure to community activities and wheelchair sports.

Substance Abuse

As with the adult SCI population, substance abuse and psychologic issues are major problems for children and adolescents with SCI (298). Adolescents with SCI may be at greater risk of suicide because of the tremendous impact of an SCI, superimposed on the usual turbulence of adolescence.

NEURAL TUBE DEFECTS

The two most common forms of neural tube defects, also known as spinal dysraphism, are spina bifida and anencephaly (299–301). Spina bifida lesions are classified depending on whether or not neural tissue is exposed (300). A myelomeningocele is an open spina bifida lesion in which there is either no skin covering, or neural tissue is covered only by a thin membrane. Occult spinal dysraphism refers to a spina bifida lesion with intact skin covering and includes lipomeningocele, meningocele, myelocystocele, dermal sinus, tight filum terminale, and diastematomyelia. Spina bifida occulta is a benign and common abnormality in which there is a failure of fusion of the spinous processes of the lower lumbar or sacral spine. Individuals with spina bifida occulta are asymptomatic, with the diagnosis made as an incidental finding on plain radiographs.

The most common form of nonfatal neural-tube defects are myelomeningoceles, which are characterized by serious brain and spinal cord defects. This section reviews the epidemiology, etiology, pathogenesis, clinical manifestations, management, and prevention of myelomeningoceles.

Epidemiology

The incidence of myelomeningocele in the United States is approximately 3–4 per 10,000 live births (302, 303). The incidence of myelomeningocele has varied as a function of time, geography, race, and ethnicity. Trends in the incidence of myelomeningocele are probably related to a number of factors, including nutritional issues, folic acid usage in the periconceptual period, availability of prenatal diagnosis, and elective pregnancy termination (304, 305). In the United States, the incidence of myelomeningocele has decreased from 4.1 cases per 10,000 births in 1995–1996 to 3.0 cases per 10,000 births in 1999–2000 (306). During this time, the rates of myelomeningocele varied among racial and ethnic groups in the United States with the lowest incidence in Asians/Pacific Islanders (2.3/10,000) and the highest rates for Hispanics (6.0/10,000) (302). However, by 1990 the rates for myelomeningocele were nearly identical for blacks, Hispanics, and whites. A higher incidence of neural-tube defects appears in lower socioeconomic populations (307).

The mortality for individuals with myelomeningocele is highest during infancy, resulting from CNS infection, hydrocephalus, and hindbrain dysfunction (308). Since the introduction of folic acid fortification in the United States in 1998, there has been an improvement in the survival of infants born with spina bifida, suggesting that folic acid may play a role in reducing the severity of neural tube defects in addition to preventing their occurrence (309). During the past half-century, survival has varied dramatically as a result of different treatment approaches utilized. Over the past several decades, a more aggressive approach to treatment has been the norm, so that individuals who would have died as neonates or infants are now surviving. In one report, 56% of patients survived to their 20th birthday (310). In another report, 85% of individuals with spina bifida born after 1975 survived to 16 years of age irrespective of their shunt status (311). Furthermore, of those who survived to 16 years of age, a decreased survival rate past 34 years of age of 75% was found in those with shunted hydrocephalus, compared to 94% survival rate for those without a shunt.

Etiology

The exact etiology of myelomeningocele is not known, and probably includes both genetic and environmental factors (312). Myelomeningocele has been associated with maternal diabetes mellitus (313), obesity (314, 315), fever (316), hyperthermia (317), and maternal use of valproic acid (318) and carbamazepine (319). The increased incidence of neural-tube defects observed in lower socioeconomic groups suggests that nutritional deficiencies, particularly lack of folic acid, may play a significant role in the etiology of neural tube defects (307).

Genetic factors play an important role in the etiology of neural tube defects, as reflected by the increased risk for individuals who have previously had an affected baby, affected first-degree relatives, and individuals who have neural tube defects themselves (300). The recurrence risk ranges from 1% to 5% in a family with one affected child and as high as 10% in families with two affected children (301, 320–322).

Pathophysiology

Neural-tube defects are caused by failure of the neural tube to close between the third and fourth week of gestation, resulting in abnormalities of the brain and spinal cord (323). The main abnormalities of the brain include hydrocephalus in 80% to 90% of children with myelomeningoceles and the Chiari II malformation, which is present in almost all affected individuals (324). The main findings in Chiari II malformations are a small posterior fossa, caudal displacement of the cerebellar vermis and brain stem into the cervical spinal canal, kinking of the cervicomedullary junction, and beaking of the tectum. Hydrocephalus results from obstruction of cerebrospinal fluid movement as a result of the Chiari II malformation.

The defect of the vertebral column and the spinal cord may occur anywhere from the thoracic to the sacral segments. The most common site of the defect is the lumbosacral spine, which is involved in approximately 66% to 75% of the cases (325). At the site of the lesion, the spinal canal is open posteriorly, with defects of the dorsal elements of several contiguous vertebrae (326). At the site of the myelomeningocele lesion, the spinal cord exhibits varying degrees of dysplasia. The spinal cord is present as a flat neural plate and is covered by a thin membrane. Spinal cord damage, with resulting neurologic deficits, results from several factors, including spinal cord dysplasia, tethering of the spinal cord at the myelomeningocele defect, damage to the neural plate during its surgical repair, toxicity of amniotic fluid, and mechanical trauma from the uterine wall during gestation, labor, and delivery (327, 328).

Clinical Manifestations and Management

Surgical repair of the myelomeningocele should be undertaken shortly after birth to reduce the risk of infection and ventriculitis (329). Closure should be undertaken within the first 24 hours of life if the myelomeningocele sac is leaking; otherwise, the closure can be performed within the first 2 to 3 days of life (326, 329, 330). Goals of the initial closure are to cover the defect with skin, untether the spinal cord, and reconstruct the neural tube and dura. Because of the potential development of hydrocephalus, patients need close monitoring after closure of the myelomeningocele defect. Hydrocephalus develops in approximately 80% to 90% of cases and requires ventriculoperitoneal shunting (331, 332).

The primary manifestations of myelomeningocele are a consequence of the brain and spinal cord abnormalities. Individuals with myelomeningocele demonstrate a variety of cognitive defects (333–335). Children who have experienced meningitis or ventriculitis are more likely to have cognitive abnormalities (336). Approximately 30% of children with myelomeningocele have subnormal intelligence, primarily perceptual motor abnormalities, with normal verbal skills. Individuals with myelomeningocele frequently exhibit disorders of visual–spatial organization and may have learning disabilities, hearing and visual impairments, and seizures (337). Children with myelomeningocele commonly demonstrate defects in coordination and dexterity of hand function (338). Children with myelomeningocele may manifest "cocktail chatter," characterized by excessive talking and superficiality of content (339). Lastly, youth with spina bifida frequently exhibit attention-deficit/hyperactivity disorder, with 31% involved in one series (340).

Because most individuals with myelomeningocele have hydrocephalus and require ventriculoperitoneal shunts, they are at risk for shunt infections and shunt malfunction. Shunt malfunction in younger children is manifested by signs and symptoms of increased intracranial pressure, including nausea, vomiting, and severe headache. In contrast, symptoms of shunt malfunction in adolescents and young adults may be more subtle. They may manifest indolent symptoms of shortened attention span, poor school performance, irritability, intermittent headaches, weakness, or worsening scoliosis.

In infants and younger children, symptoms of hindbrain dysfunction resulting from the Chiari II malformation may include feeding and swallowing abnormalities, stridor, vocal cord paralysis, weak cry, apnea, sleep-disordered breathing (341–343), nystagmus, opisthotonus, and weakness and spasticity of the upper extremities (324). Older children and adolescents more commonly present with decreased upper extremity function, progressive scoliosis, neck pain, and depressed respiratory function. Shunting of the hydrocephalus usually results in the resolution of the symptoms related to a Chiari II malformation; however, some patients may require a posterior fossa decompression (324, 344).

Hydrosyringomyelia in association with the Chiari II malformation is a relatively common occurrence in individuals with myelomeningocele (324, 344). The clinical manifestations are similar to those of development hydrosyringomyelia.

Motor paralysis, sensory loss, spasticity, and bladder, bowel, and sexual dysfunction are the major manifestations of spinal cord dysfunction. The extent of the neurologic deficit is determined by the location of the myelomeningocele. In contrast to spinal cord injuries, in which the degree of motor deficits either approximate or exceed the sensory deficits, children with myelomeningocele generally have sensory deficits that are more severe than the motor deficits. In myelomeningocele, the spinal cord deficits are more severe on the dorsal aspect of the cord, including the posterior spinal nerve roots, with relative sparing of the anterior spinal nerve roots. In the absence of normal sensation, the function of muscles under voluntary control is limited. Most patients with myelomeningocele have a flaccid type of paralysis, with approximately 10% to 30% of individuals exhibiting spasticity (345, 346).

Various classification systems are used to categorize spinal cord dysfunction in children with myelomeningocele, and they are generally used to predict ambulation (345, 347, 348). It is imperative that accurate serial documentation be performed of motor and sensory levels and the presence and degree of spasticity. This is particularly important for early recognition of complications such as hydrocephalus, hydrosyringomyelia, and retethering of the spinal cord.

Tethering of the spinal cord at the site of the defect is a major component of the myelomeningocele abnormality at birth. One of the primary goals of the initial surgical correction in the newborn is to untether the spinal cord. However, there is a tendency for retethering, in which the spinal cord becomes adherent to the myelomeningocele repair site (326). The majority of individuals with myelomeningocele demonstrate retethering of the spinal cord with a low-lying spinal cord (349). With growth, the retethered spinal cord cannot migrate cephalad as it normally should. Patients with a retethered spinal cord may experience impairment of the remaining spinal cord function, which may be manifested by the onset or worsening of weakness, spasticity, sensory loss, pain, progressive scoliosis, orthopedic deformities in the lower extremities, or changes in bowel or bladder function. Because the majority of patients with low-lying spinal cords are asymptomatic, the decision to surgically repair the retethered spinal cord must be based on well-documented clinical changes.

Clinical manifestations and management of the neurogenic bladder and bowel in children with myelomeningocele is not significantly different from children and adolescents with SCI. However, individuals with myelomeningocele may have congenital anomalies of the genitourinary system that require additional monitoring or treatment (350). Males with myelomeningocele are at increased risk of cryptorchidism (351, 352).

Once the infant has been stabilized after the myelomeningocele defect has been repaired, urodynamic testing should be performed during the neonatal period (353–357). Neonates with high bladder pressures (leak point pressure >40 cmH$_2$O) or detrusor–sphincter dyssynergia are at risk of developing urinary tract deterioration, and they should be managed with intermittent catheterization and anticholinergics. In contrast to individuals with SCI, those with myelomeningocele have a neurogenic bladder from conception. This may significantly retard bladder growth, particularly in children with high-pressure, low-volume bladders. Bladder augmentation may be indicated in individuals with myelomeningocele who have inadequate bladder capacity despite anticholinergic therapy (357). The standard bladder management of individuals with myelomeningocele is intermittent catheterization (168, 169, 172, 354, 357, 358). The ability to perform self-catheterization may be limited by the visual–motor defects that are frequently present in patients with myelomeningocele and developmental delays that may also be present (172, 359).

Bowel incontinence is a major problem for children with myelomeningocele, especially those without bulbocavernosus or anocutaneous reflexes (360). Education and regular, consistently timed reflex-triggered bowel evacuations are essential elements of a bowel program (360). For children with myelomeningocele with bowel program complications unresponsive to more conservative measures, antegrade continence enemas (196, 197), pulsed irrigation enemas (195), enema continence catheters (198, 361), or biofeedback (362–364) are potential alternatives.

Secondary manifestations or complications may be apparent at birth and would be considered congenital defects, or they may be acquired postnatally. Examples of congenital defects include clubfeet, dislocated hips, or extension knee contractures; these are secondary complications of the primary spinal cord deficit, with resulting in-utero paralysis. Postnatally acquired secondary complications result in significant morbidity and occasionally mortality. The prevention and early management of secondary complications are an integral aspect of the overall management of children and adolescents with myelomeningocele. Meningitis, ventriculitis, tethered cord, and shunt malfunction have already been discussed.

Orthopedic Issues

Individuals with myelomeningocele experience a variety of orthopedic complications, especially disorders of the lower extremities and spine (325, 365). Orthopedic deformities may be a consequence of several factors, including muscle paralysis, unopposed muscle function, spasticity, and congenital malformations (365). Orthopedic deformities may be present at birth and be a consequence of paralysis present in utero, affecting the position of the fetus. Examples of this include clubfeet, dislocated hips, or extension contractures of the knees (325). Other skeletal deformities, such as congenital vertebral and rib anomalies, present in as many as 15% of patients are primary defects associated with myelomeningocele. Postnatally acquired orthopedic complications, such as dislocated hips, hip and knee contractures, and pathologic fractures are a consequence of the neuromuscular defects associated with myelomeningocele. Spine deformities such as scoliosis, kyphosis, and lordosis may be a result of both congenital vertebral anomalies and neuromuscular defects (366, 367). In general, the management of these orthopedic complications is complicated and should be provided by clinicians experienced in caring for individuals with myelomeningocele. Depending on the neurologic level, many children and adolescents with myelomeningocele will ambulate to varying degrees; hence, management of lower extremity deformities should take this into account.

Hip contractures and dislocation are very common in children with myelomeningocele, especially those with thoracic and upper- to mid-lumbar lesions, where up to 90% of patients may be affected (368). In those with thoracic lesions, hip dislocation occurs because all of the hip musculature is denervated (365). In contrast, hip dysplasia in individuals with lumbar-level lesions results from muscle imbalance, with active hip flexors and adductors unopposed by hip extensors and abductors. The treatment of hip dysplasia in the myelomeningocele population is somewhat controversial, particularly because hip dysplasia is usually not painful and may not significantly affect the ability to ambulate (369). For patients with thoracic and upper- to mid-lumbar level lesions, treatment of the hip dysplasia is usually limited to those with pelvic obliquity, placing them at a higher risk of developing pressure ulcers. Children with lower lumbar lesions have good ambulation potential. Their dislocated hips should be surgically corrected by 4 years of age, including both skeletal corrections and muscle transfers to prevent recurrent dislocation.

Hip contractures are common complications in children and adolescents with myelomeningocele. Hip contractures exceeding 30 to 40 degrees can hinder ambulation. Treatment of hip contractures must be individualized and based on the neurologic level, ambulation status, and presence of hip dysplasia. For individuals with thoracic and upper lumbar levels, hip contractures are generally managed by surgical releases and aggressive bracing and physical therapy, postoperatively. For those with mid- to lower-lumbar lesions, a combination of surgical releases and appropriate tendon transfers is performed. Unfortunately, surgical releases are frequently complicated by recurrences of the hip contractures.

Extension and flexion contractures and valgus rotation deformities are the major abnormalities of the knee in children with myelomeningocele (365). Extension contractures of the knee are relatively uncommon and generally are the result of breech deliveries, or are seen in patients with mid-lumbar level lesions who have strong quadriceps without strong knee flexors. Physical therapy and splinting are usually successful in managing knee extension contractures; however, for those that are resistant to conservative management, a modified V-Y quadricepsplasty should be performed.

Knee flexion contractures greater than 20 degrees may limit ambulation. Children under 2 years of age having flexion contractures of their knees may be successfully managed with physical therapy and splinting; otherwise surgical correction is indicated. Valgus rotation deformities of the knee are a result of iliotibial band tightness and the forces of ambulation. Management includes muscle transfers, distal iliotibial band sectioning, and knee–ankle–foot orthoses (KAFOs). Distal femoral osteotomies may be necessary if the deformity becomes fixed.

Ankle and foot deformities are common in children and adolescents with myelomeningocele, and they are frequently resistant to conservative measures and usually require surgical correction (365). Approximately 50% of patients with myelomeningocele have clubfeet, as a result of muscle paralysis and in utero positioning. These clubfoot deformities tend to be rigid, are resistant to casting, and usually require surgical repair (365). Calcaneovalgus deformities result from unopposed contraction of the anterior tibial muscle, peroneal muscles, or the toe extensors and are most commonly seen in patients with low lumbar lesions. The deformity is usually progressive, resulting in a crouch gait, and predisposing to pressure ulcers from shoe or brace wear. Surgical correction consists of an anterior tibial tendon transfer to the calcaneus (365). Individuals with sacral-level lesions may present with cavus deformities of the foot, which are frequently accompanied by claw toe deformities, predisposing to pressure ulcers under the toes or metatarsal heads.

Pathologic fractures most commonly involve children 3 to 7 years of age, and they usually occur after cast immobilization or during skeletal traction. These pathologic fractures generally are in an epiphyseal or metaphyseal location, and they may exhibit exuberant callus formation, raising concerns of a tumor. Fractures usually present with a warm, swollen, and erythematous extremity in a febrile child. The fractures should be managed with splinting, and weight bearing can be initiated within 2 to 3 weeks to prevent further osteoporosis and reduce the risk of further fractures (365).

Scoliosis affects the majority of patients with myelomeningocele and results from a variety of factors, including congenital vertebral anomalies, neuromuscular weakness, pelvic obliquity, and hip contractures (332, 366, 367). Scoliosis affects almost all patients with thoracic-level lesions, with a decreased incidence of scoliosis in patients with lower neurologic levels (366, 370). Progressive scoliosis may be a manifestation of decompensated hydrocephalus, retethered spinal cord, or hydrosyringomyelia (371, 372). The correction of hydrocephalus, a retethered spinal cord, or hydrosyringomyelia may slow or halt progression of scoliosis in patients with spinal curvatures less than 40 degrees, but generally does not change the course of more severe curves (371–373).

The management of scoliosis must include accurate monitoring of the motor and sensory examination, deep tendon reflexes of both the upper and lower extremities, and degree of spasticity. Radiographs of the spine are performed at least annually. Imaging studies to exclude hydrocephalus, retethered cord, and hydrosyringomyelia should be performed on patients who are experiencing progressive scoliosis, particularly if accompanied by progressive weakness or spasticity. Individuals with curves that are greater than 25 degrees or those with unbalanced curves should wear bivalved molded body jackets. Particular care must be taken to prevent the development of pressure ulcers under the body jacket. The timing of the surgical repair and the extent and type of spinal surgery depends on the child's age (preferably after age 10), neurologic level, ambulation status, and location and flexibility of the curve. For children who are ambulators, the lumbosacral joint generally should not be fused. In addition, hip contractures should be corrected prior to spine fusions to avoid excessive torque to the postoperative spine fusion.

Between 8% and 15% of patients with myelomeningocele develop kyphosis, particularly those patients with thoracic lesions (325, 326) (Figure 45.10). Kyphosis can interfere with sitting or wearing orthotics and may cause a pressure ulcer over the kyphos. Progression of the kyphotic deformity can compromise ventilation because abdominal contents are pushed up into the thorax. Surgical correction of kyphosis is complex and technically demanding and may be associated with significant morbidity and mortality (326, 367). Preoperative evaluation of ventriculoperitoneal shunt functioning is critical.

Medical Issues

Children and adolescents with myelomeningocele frequently experience short stature as a result of several factors (374, 375). These factors include spine deformities, decreased growth in paralyzed extremities, nutritional deficiencies, precocious puberty, and growth hormone deficiency. Precocious puberty affects 10% to 20% of individuals with myelomeningocele and is presumably

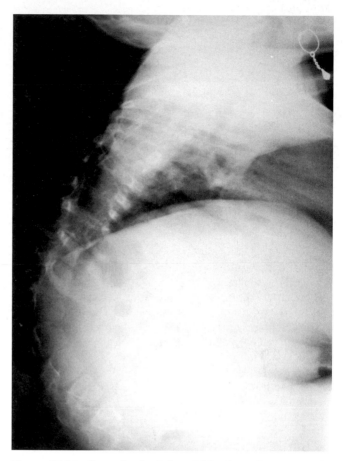

Figure 45.10   Severe kyphosis in a child with myelomeningocele.

caused by brain abnormalities (376–378). Precocious puberty more commonly affects females and those with hydrocephalus. Obesity is also a common problem for children with myelomeningocele, especially as they become adolescents (346, 376, 379–383).

Children and adolescents with myelomeningocele are at a high risk for latex allergy, with 18% to 64.5% of patients affected (384–386). One explanation for the high incidence of latex allergy in the myelomeningocele population may be the multiple surgeries that they undergo beginning at a young age (387–389). The risk of latex sensitization may be decreased in the myelomeningocele population by minimizing exposure to latex (390–393).

Similar to individuals with SCI, children and adolescents with myelomeningocele are at risk for developing pressure ulcers (394, 395). However, the prevention and management of pressure ulcers may be complicated by the associated cognitive and behavioral disturbances frequently exhibited by patients with myelomeningocele.

Psychosocial Issues and Sexuality

Individuals with myelomeningocele face both psychosocial and sexuality issues that are common for all children and adolescents, as well as the additional burdens caused by the physical, psychologic, and cognitive deficits associated with myelomeningocele (381, 396, 397). Psychosocial development and sexual development for individuals with myelomeningocele are complicated by the onset of their disability at birth and the varying expectations that parents have for their child's future (398). Sexuality and reproductive health issues should be addressed in a developmentally appropriate fashion for children and adolescents, as well as for their parents (399, 400). This should include sexual functioning, fertility, and sexual abuse and exploitation.

The majority of children with myelomeningocele should be educated in a regular school setting. However, several factors may significantly affect education, including psychosocial development, cognitive defects, learning disabilities, visuomotor disturbances, and frequent school absences because of healthcare needs (332). The transition into adulthood, including employment and independence, must be an integral component of the comprehensive care for the myelomeningocele population (401, 402).

Prevention

Folic acid taken in the periconceptual period has been shown to be effective in preventing neural tube defects (403–407). Periconceptual use of folic acid may decrease the risk of neural tube defects by 50% in the general population and 72% in individuals who have previously had an affected pregnancy (403). Therefore, the United States Public Health Service recommendations are that all women of childbearing age consume 0.4 mg of folic acid daily, with the total daily intake of folic acid being less than 1 mg (404). For high-risk women who have previously had a neural tube defect–affected pregnancy, 4.0 mg of folic acid should be taken daily from at least 1 month before conception through the first 3 months of the pregnancy (403, 404).

Prenatal Diagnosis and Management

Prenatal screening for neural tube defects is accomplished by maternal serum alpha-fetoprotein testing between the 16th and 18th week of gestation (408–409). Diagnosis is confirmed with high-resolution ultrasound or elevated levels of alpha-fetoprotein or acetylcholinesterase in the amniotic fluid (410). Prenatal diagnosis allows the parents the opportunity to terminate the pregnancy. Alternatively, prenatal diagnosis assists parents and healthcare providers in planning the appropriate prenatal and postnatal care, such as in utero surgery, elective cesarean section, and delivery in a medical center that is experienced in caring for newborns with myelomeningoceles (409).

The neurologic deficits associated with myelomeningocele may in part be caused by prolonged exposure of the dysplastic spinal cord to the intrauterine environment, as a result of physical trauma or toxicity of the amniotic fluid (327, 328, 411). In utero surgical repair of the myelomeningocele sac has been conducted on fetuses of 22 to 28 weeks of gestation, with preliminary reports demonstrating decreased shunt-dependent hydrocephalus, reversal of the Chiari II malformation, and possibly improved leg function. (412–416). However, fetal surgery in this population may result in significant adverse events, namely premature labor and birth. In order to compare the safety and efficacy of intrauterine repair with standard postnatal repair, the "Management of Myelomeningocele Study" (MOMS), a study funded by the National Institute of Child Health and Human Development (NICHD), was initiated in 2003 (415, 416).

To prevent further damage to the dysplastic spinal cord as a result of uterine contractions and passage through the birth canal, elective pre-labor cesarean section has been advocated (301, 417).

Fetuses with lower extremity movement noted on ultrasound, minimal to no hydrocephalus, and neural elements that protrude dorsally may be the most appropriate circumstances for elective pre-labor cesarean section (301). However, there is insufficient evidence to support prophylactic cesarean delivery of infants with myelomeningocele (418).

LIPOMYELOMENINGOCELE

Lipomyelomeningoceles are a form of occult spinal dysraphism in which there is intact skin covering the defect (300, 419, 420). The spinal cord remains within the spinal canal, with the junction between the spinal cord and the lipoma also residing within the canal. (See Figure 45.11.) In general, individuals with lipomyelomeningoceles are normal at birth. Neurologic findings are first noted during the second year of life, with most patients exhibiting some neurologic deficits by early childhood. The most common presentation is a subcutaneous fat collection in the

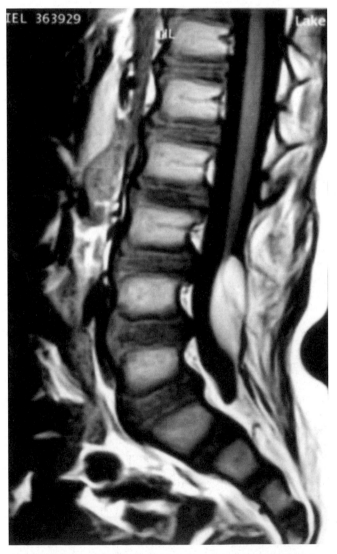

Figure 45.11 Magnetic resonance image of a child with a lipomeningocele, demonstrating tethering of the spinal cord and an intraspinal lipoma.

lower back and upper buttocks. Approximately 50% of affected individuals have cutaneous markings, such as a hairy patch, a midline dimple, or a hemangiomatous nevus. The primary goal of surgery is to untether the spinal cord. Removal of the entire lipoma is usually not performed, because the neural tissue extends into the lipoma and aggressive surgical excision of the lipoma may cause significantly more neurologic damage. Approximately 13% of affected children will have an associated type I Chiari malformation (421)

SACRAL AGENESIS

Sacral agenesis is a relatively uncommon congenital anomaly causing varying degrees of deficiencies of the sacrum and associated neurologic abnormalities (422–426) (Figure 45.12). Sacral agenesis is associated with maternal diabetes mellitus,

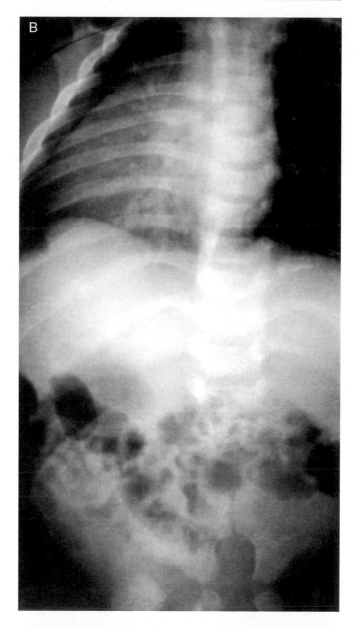

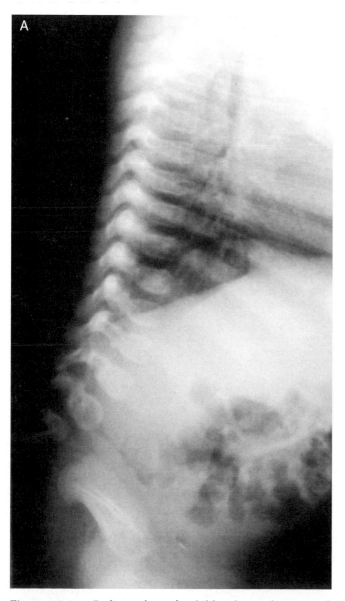

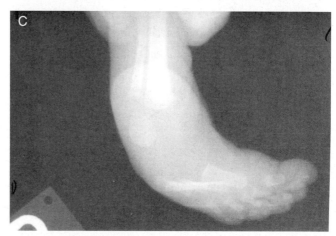

Figure 45.12 Radiographics of a child with sacral agenesis demonstrating abrupt loss of the vertebral column at T12–L1 (**A** and **B**) and foot deformities (**C**).

with 1% of infants born to diabetic mothers having sacral agenesis, and approximately 12% to 16% of infants with sacral agenesis being born to mothers with diabetes mellitus. In general, patients present either during infancy or between 4 and 5 years of age with persistent urinary incontinence and chronic constipation. The majority of affected children have neurologic deficits of their lower extremities, 40% have weakness, and 86% have altered deep tendon reflexes. Interestingly, sensation is usually intact caudally for several segments below the motor level for most individuals with sacral agenesis (422, 423). Severe orthopedic deformities of their lower extremities are present in about two-thirds of affected patients, including clubfeet and webbed knees.

References

1. Betz RR, Mulcahey MJ. Spinal cord injury rehabilitation. In: Weinstein SL, ed. *The Pediatric Spine: Principles and Practice.* New York: Raven Press, 1994; 781–810.
2. Anderson CJ, Johnson KA, Klaas SJ, et al. Pediatric spinal cord injury: Transition to adulthood. *J Voc Rehabil* 1998; 10:103–113.
3. Smith QW, Frieden L, Nelson MR, et al. Transition to adulthood for young people with spinal cord injury. In: Betz RR, Mulcahey MJ, eds. *The Child with a Spinal Cord Injury.* Rosemont, IL: American Academy of Orthopaedic Surgeons, 1996; 601–612.
4. Vogel LC, Klaas SJ, Lubicky, JP, et al. Long-term outcomes and life satisfaction of adults with pediatric spinal cord injuries. *Arch Phys Med Rehabil* 1998; 79:1496–1503.
5. Johnson CP. Transition into adulthood. *Pediatr Ann* 1995; 24:268–273.
6. American Academy of Pediatrics, Committee on Children With Disabilities and Committee on Adolescence. Transition of care provided for adolescents with special health care needs. *Pediatrics* 1996; 98:1203–1206.
7. Anderson, CJ, Vogel, LC. Employment outcomes of adults who sustained spinal cord injuries as children or adolescents. *Arch Phys Med Rehabil* 2002; 83:791–801.
8. Anderson, CJ, Vogel, LC, Betz, RR, Willis, KM. Overview of adult outcomes in pediatric-onset spinal cord injuries: implications for transition to adulthood. *J Spinal Cord Med* 2004; 27:S98–S106.
9. Anderson CJ, Vogel LC. Work experience in adolescents with spinal cord injuries. *Dev Med Child Neurol* 2000; 42:515–517.
10. Massagli, TL, Dudgeon, BJ, Ross, BW. Educational performance and vocational participation after spinal cord injury in childhood. *Arch Phys Med Rehabil* 1996; 77:995–999.
11. White PH. Resilience in children with disability—transition to adulthood. *J Rheumatology* 1996; 23:960–962.
12. Vogel LC. Long-term prophylactic medical care. In: Betz RR, Mulcahey MJ, eds. *The Child with a Spinal Cord Injury.* Rosemont, IL: American Academy of Orthopaedic Surgeons, 1996; 679–688.
13. Tepperman PS. Primary care after spinal cord injury: What every physician should know. *Postgrad Med* 1989; 86:211–218.
14. Bernardez SJ, Brown LT, Nora J, et al. Primary care for the spinal cord injured patient. *J Am Acad Phys Assist* 1994; 8:526–531.
15. American Academy of Pediatrics Committee on Infectious Diseases: Active Immunization. In: Pickering LK, Baker CJ, Long SS, McMillan JA, eds. *Red Book: 2006 Report of the Committee on Infectious Diseases,* 27th ed. Elk Grove Village, IL: American Academy of Pediatrics, 2006.
16. Vogel, LC, Anderson, CJ. Spinal cord injuries in children and adolescents: A review. *J Spinal Cord Med,* 2003; 26:193–203.
17. Betz RR, Mulcahey MJ, eds. *The Child with a Spinal Cord Injury.* Rosemont, IL: American Academy of Orthopaedic Surgeons, 1996.
18. Massagli TL. Medical and rehabilitation issues in the care of children with spinal cord injury. *Phys Med Rehabil Clin N Am* 2000; 11:169–182.
19. Vogel LC, Betz RR, Mulcahey MJ. The child with a spinal cord injury. *Dev Med Child Neurol* 1997; 39:202–207.
20. Vogel LC, ed. Pediatric Issues. *Top Spinal Cord Inj Rehabil* 1997; 3(2).
21. Colorado Department of Public Health and Environment. *1995 Annual Report of the Spinal Cord Injury Early Notification System.* Denver: Colorado Department of Transportation Printing Office, 1996.
22. Bracken MB, Freeman DH, Hellenbrand K. Incidence of acute traumatic hospitalized spinal cord injury in the United States, 1970–1977. *Am J Epidemiol* 1981; 113: 615–622.
23. Nobunaga AI, Go BK, Karunas RB. Recent demographic and injury trends in people served by the Model Spinal Cord Injury Care Systems. *Arch Phys Med Rehabil* 1999; 80:1372–1382.
24. Hadley MN, Zabramski JM, Browner CM, et al. Pediatric spinal trauma. Review of 122 cases of spinal cord and vertebral column injuries. *J Neurosurg* 1988; 68:18–24.
25. Hamilton MG, Myles ST. Pediatric spinal injury: Review of 174 hospital admissions. *J Neurosurg* 1992; 77:700–704.
26. Kewalramani LS, Kraus JF, Sterling HM. Acute spinal-cord lesions in a pediatric population: Epidemiological and clinical features. *Paraplegia* 1980; 18:206–219.
27. Osenbach RK, Menezes AH. Pediatric spinal cord and vertebral column injury. *Neurosurgery* 1992; 30:385–390.
28. Vitale MG, Goss JM, Matsumoto H, Roye DP. Epidemiology of pediatric spinal cord injury in the United States years 1997 and 2000. *J Pediatr Orthop* 2006; 26:745–749.
29. Vogel LC, DeVivo MJ. Etiology and demographics. In: Betz RR, Mulcahey MJ, eds. *The Child with a Spinal Cord Injury.* Rosemont, IL: American Academy of Orthopaedic Surgeons, 1996; 3–12.
30. DeVivo, M.J., Vogel, L.C. Epidemiology of spinal cord injuries in children and adolescents. *J Spinal Cord Med* 2004; 27:S4–S10.
31. Ruge JR, Sinson GP, McLone DG, et al. Pediatric spinal injury: The very young. *J Neurosurg* 1988; 68:25–30.
32. Vogel LC, DeVivo MJ. Pediatric spinal cord injury issues: Etiology, demographics, and pathophysiology. *Top Spinal Cord Inj Rehabil* 1997; 3:1–8.
33. Shavelle RM, DeVivo MJ, Vogel LC, Strauss DJ, Paculdo DR. Long-term survival after childhood spinal cord injury. *J Spinal Cord Med* 2007; 30:S48–S54.
34. Mulcahey MJ, Gaughan J, Betz RR, Johansen KJ. The international standards for neurological classification of spinal cord injury: Reliability of data when applied to children and youth. *Spinal Cord* 2007; 45:452–459.
35. Mulcahey MJ, Gaughan J, Betz RR, Vogel LC. Rater reliability on the ISCSCI motor and sensory scores obtained before and after formal training in testing technique. *J Spinal Cord Med* 2007; 30:S146–S149.
36. Khanna G, El-Khoury GY. Imaging of cervical spine injuries of childhood. *Skeletal Radiol* 2007; 36:477–494.
37. Haffner DL, Hoffer MM, Wiedbusch R. Etiology of children's spinal injuries at Rancho Los Amigos. *Spine* 1993; 18:679–684.
38. Rovinsky D, Haskell A, Huffman GR, et al. Firearm related spinal cord injuries in children and adolescents: A fifteen year experience. *Top Spinal Cord Inj Rehabil* 2000; 6(Suppl):1–6.
39. Mangano FT, Menendez JA, Smyth MD, Leonard JR, Narayan P, Park TS. Pediatric neurosurgical injuries associated with all-terrain vehicle accidents: A 10-year experience at St. Louis Children's Hospital. *J Neurosurg (1 Suppl Pediatrics)* 2006; 105:2–5
40. Gabos PG, Tuten HR, Leet A, et al. Fracture-dislocation of the lumbar spine in an abused child. *Pediatrics* 1998; 101:473–477.
41. Pollono D, Drut R, Ibanez O, Ferreyra M, Cedola J. Spinal cord compression: A review of 70 pediatric patients. *Pediatr Hematology and Oncology* 2003; 20:457–466.
42. Wilson PE, Oleszek JL, Clayton GH. Pediatric spinal cord tumors and masses. *J Spinal Cord Med* 2007; 30:S15–S20.
43. Knebusch M, Strassburg HM, Reiners K. Acute transverse myelitis in childhood: Nine cases and review of the literature. *Dev Med Child Neurol* 1998; 40:631–639.
44. Wilberger JE Jr. Clinical aspects of specific spinal injuries. In: Wilberger JE Jr, ed. *Spinal Cord Injuries in Children.* Mount Kisco, NY: Futura Publishers, 1986; 69–95.
45. Wills BPD, Dormans JP. Nontraumatic upper cervical spine instability in children. *J Am Acad Orthop Surg* 2006; 14:233–245.
46. Apple DF, Murray HH. Lap belt injuries in children. In: Betz RR, Mulcahey MJ, eds. *The Child with a Spinal Cord Injury.* Rosemont, IL: American Academy of Orthopaedic Surgeons, 1996; 169–177.
47. Achildi O, Betz RR, Grewal H. Lapbelt injuries and the seatbelt syndrome in pediatric spinal cord injury. *J Spinal Cord Med* 2007: 30:S21–S24.
48. Centers for Disease Control. Motor-vehicle occupant fatalities and restraint use among children aged 4–8 years—United States, 1994–1998. *MMWR* 2000; 49:135–137.

49. Winston FK, Durbin DR, Kallan MJ, et al. The danger of premature graduation to seat belts for young children. *Pediatrics* 2000; 105: 1179–1183.

50. Bresnan MJ, Abroms IF. Neonatal spinal cord transection secondary to intrauterine hyperextension of the neck in breech presentation. *J Pediatrics* 1974; 84:734–737.

51. Ruggieri M, Smarason AK, Pike M. Spinal cord insults in the prenatal, perinatal, and neonatal periods. *Dev Med Child Neurol* 1999; 41:311–317.

52. Lanska MJ, Roessmann U, Wiznitzer M. Magnetic resonance imaging in cervical cord birth injury. *Pediatrics* 1990; 85:760–764.

53. Vialle R, Pietin-Vialle C, Ilharreborde B, Dauger S, Vinchon M, Glorion C. Spinal cord injuries at birth: a multicenter review of nine cases. *J Maternal-Fetal and Neonatal Medicine* 2007; 20:435–440.

54. Rossitch E, Oakes WJ. Perinatal spinal cord injury: Clinical, radiographic and pathologic features. *Pediatr Neurosurg* 1992; 18:149–152.

55. MacKinnon JA, Perlman M, Kirpalani, et al. Spinal cord injury at birth: Diagnostic and prognostic data in twenty-two patients. *J Pediatrics* 1993; 122:431–437.

56. Rehan VK, Seshia MMK. Spinal cord birth injury—diagnostic difficulties. *Arch Dis Child* 1993; 69:92–94.

57. Brand MC. Part 1: Recognizing neonatal spinal cord injury. *Adv Neonatal Care* 2006; 6:15–24.

58. Menticoglou SM, Perlman M, Manning FA. High cervical spinal cord injury in neonates delivered with forceps: Report of 15 cases. *Obstet Gynecol* 1995; 86:589–594.

59. Perlman M. Neonatal spinal cord injury in the infant: Etiology, diagnosis, treatment and outcome. In: Betz RR, Mulcahey MJ, eds. *The Child with a Spinal Cord Injury.* Rosemont, IL: American Academy of Orthopaedic Surgeons, 1996; 161–167.

60. Medlock MD, Hanigan WC. Neurologic birth trauma. Intracranial, spinal cord, and brachial plexus injury. *Clin Perinatol* 1997; 24:845–857.

61. Hankins GDV. Lower thoracic spinal cord injury—A severe complication of shoulder dystocia. *Am J Perinatol* 1998; 15:443–444.

62. American Academy of Pediatrics, Committee on Sports Medicine. Atlantoaxial instability in Down syndrome. *Pediatrics* 1984; 74:152–154.

63. Tredwell SJ, Newman DE, Lockith G. Instability of the upper cervical spine in Down syndrome. *J Pediatr Orthop* 1990; 10:602–606.

64. Loder RT, Hensinger RN. Developmental abnormalities of the cervical spine. In: Weinstein SL, ed. *The Pediatric Spine: Principles and Practice.* New York: Raven Press, 1994; 397–420.

65. Ward WT. Atlanto-axial instability in children with Down syndrome. In: Betz RR, Mulcahey MJ, eds. *The Child with a Spinal Cord Injury.* Rosemont, IL: American Academy of Orthopaedic Surgeons, 1996; 89–96.

66. Ferguson RL, Putney ME, Allen BL. Comparison of neurologic deficits with atlanto-dens intervals in patients with Down syndrome. *J Spinal Disorders* 1997; 10:246–252.

67. Vogel LC, Lubicky JP. Cervical spine fusion not protective of cervical spine injury and tetraplegia. *Am J Orthopaedics* 1997; 26:636–640.

68. Nathan FF, Bickel WH. Spontaneous axial subluxation in a child as the first sign of juvenile rheumatoid arthritis. *J Bone Joint Surg* 1968; 50A:1675–1678.

69. Goldberg MJ. Orthopedic aspects of bone dysplasias. *Orthop Clin of N Am* 1976; 7:445–455.

70. Yang SS, Corbett DP, Brough AJ, et al. Upper cervical myelopathy in achondroplasia. *Am J Clin Path* 1977; 68:68–72.

71. Gulati MS, Agin MA. Morquio Syndrome: A rehabilitative perspective. *J Spinal Cord Med* 1996; 19:12–16.

72. Miyoshi K, Nakamura K, Haga N, Mikami Y. Surgical treatment for atlantoaxial subluxation with myelopathy in spondyloepiphyseal dysplasia congenita. *Spine* 2004; 29; E488–E491.

73. Leet AI, Sampath JS, Scott CI, MacKenzie WG. Cervical spinal stenosis in metatropic dysplasia. *J Pediatr Orthop* 2006; 26:347–352.

74. Herman TE, Lee BCP, McAlister WH. Brachytelephalangic chondrodysplasia punctata with marked cervical stenosis and cord compression: report of two cases. *Pediatr Radiol* 2002; 32:452–456.

75. Pang D. Spinal cord injury without radiographic abnormality (SCIWORA) in children. In: Betz RR, Mulcahey MJ, eds. *The Child with a Spinal Cord Injury.* Rosemont, IL: American Academy of Orthopaedic Surgeons, 1996; 139–160.

76. Osenbach RK, Menezes AH. Spinal cord injury without radiographic abnormality in children. *Pediatr Neurosci* 1989; 15:168–175.

77. Grabb PA, Pang D. Magnetic resonance imaging in the evaluation of spinal cord injury without radiographic abnormality in children. *Neurosurgery* 1994; 35:406–413.

78. Felsberg GJ, Tien RD, Osumi AK, et al. Utility of MR imaging in pediatric spinal cord injury. *Pediatr Radiol* 1995; 25:131–135.

79. Shen H, Tang Y, Huang L, Yang R, Wu Y, Wang P, Shi, Y, He X, Liu H, Ye J. Applications of diffusion-weighted MRI in thoracic spinal cord injury without radiographic abnormality. *International Orthopaedics* 2007; 31:375–383.

80. Choi JU, Hoffman HJ, Hendrick EB, et al. Traumatic infarction of the spinal cord in children. *J Neurosurg* 1986; 65:608–610.

81. Hamilton MG, Myles ST. Pediatric spinal injury: Review of 174 hospital admissions. *J Neurosurg* 1992; 77: 700–704.

82. Schwartz GR, Wright SW, Fein JA, et al. Pediatric cervical spine injury sustained in falls from low heights. *Ann Emerg Med* 1997; 30:249–252.

83. Radecki RT, Gaebler-Spira D. Deep vein thrombosis in the disabled pediatric population. *Arch Phys Med Rehabil* 1994; 75:248–250.

84. WaJones T, Ugalde V, Franks P, Zhou H, White RH. Venous thromboembolism after spinal cord injury: Incidence, time course, and associated risk factors in 16,240 adults and children. *Arch Phys Med Rehabil* 2005; 86:2240–2247.

85. David M, Andrew M. Venous thromboembolic complications in children. *J Pediatr* 1993; 123:337–346.

86. Consortium for Spinal Cord Medicine. Prevention of thromboembolism in spinal cord injury. *J Spinal Cord Med* 1997; 20:259–283.

87. Ginsberg JS. Management of venous thromboembolism. *N Engl J Med* 1996; 335:1816–1828.

88. Michelson AD, Bovill E, Andrew M. Antithrombotic therapy in children. *Chest* 1995; 108:506S–522S.

89. Andrew M, Michelson AD, Bovill E, et al. Guidelines for antithrombotic therapy in pediatric patients. *J Pediatr* 1998; 132:575–588.

90. Massicotte P, Adams M, Marzinotto V, et al. Low-molecular-weight heparin in pediatric patients with thrombotic disease: A dose finding study. *J Pediatr* 1996; 128:313–318.

91. Dix D, Andrew M, Marzinotto V, et al. The use of low molecular weight heparin in pediatric patients: A prospective cohort study. *J Pediatr* 2000; 136:439–445.

92. Nand S, Goldschmidt JW. Hypercalcemia and hyperuricemia in young patients with spinal cord injury. *Arch Phys Med Rehabil* 1976; 57:553.

93. Steinberg FU, Birge SJ, Cooke NE. Hypercalcemia in adolescent tetraplegia patients: Case report and review. *Paraplegia* 1978; 16:60–67.

94. Tori JA, Hill LL. Hypercalcemia in children with spinal cord injury. *Arch Phys Med Rehabil* 1978; 59:443–447.

95. Maynard FM. Immobilization hypercalcemia following spinal cord injury. *Arch Phys Med Rehabil* 1986; 67:41–44.

96. Bilezikian JP. Management of acute hypercalcemia. *N Engl J Med* 1992; 326:1196–1203.

97. Gallacher SJ, Ralston SH, Dryburgh FJ, et al. Immobilization-related hypercalcaemia—a possible novel mechanism and response to pamidronate. *Postgrad Med J* 1990; 66:918–922.

98. Tamion F, Bonmarchand F, Girault C, et al. Intravenous pamidronate sodium therapy in immobilization-related hypercalcemia. *Clin Nephrol* 1995; 43:138–139.

99. Lteif AN, Zimmerman D. Bisphosphonates for treatment of childhood hypercalcemia. *Pediatrics* 1998; 102:990–993.

100. Kedlaya D, Branstater ME, Lee JK. Immobilization hypercalcemia in incomplete paraplegia: Successful treatment with pamidronate. *Arch Phys Med Rehabil* 1998; 79:222–225.

101. Vogel LC. Management of Medical Issues. In: Betz RR, Mulcahey MJ, eds. *The Child with a Spinal Cord Injury.* Rosemont, IL: American Academy of Orthopaedic Surgeons, 1996; 189–212.

102. Consortium for Spinal Cord Medicine. Acute management of autonomic dysreflexia: Adults with spinal cord injury presenting to health-care facilities. *J Spinal Cord Med* 1997; 20:284–309.

103. Hickey, KJ, Vogel, LC, Willis, KM, Anderson, CJ. Prevalence and etiology of autonomic dysreflexia in children with spinal cord injuries. *J Spinal Cord Med* 2004; 27:S54–S60.

104. McGinnis, KB, Vogel, LC, McDonald, CM, Porth, S, Hickey, KJ, Davis, M, Bush, P, Jenkins, D. Recognition and management of autonomic dysreflexia in pediatric spinal cord injury. *J Spinal Cord Med* 2004; 27:S61–S74.

105. Chameides L, Hazinski MF, eds. *Pediatric Advanced Life Support.* Dallas: American Heart Association, 1997; 2–5.

106. Guttmann L, ed. *Spinal Cord Injuries: Comprehensive Management and Research,* 2nd ed. Oxford: Blackwell Scientific, 1976; 295–330.

107. Fast A. Reflex sweating in patients with spinal cord injury: A review. *Arch Phys Med Rehabil* 1977; 58:435–437.

108. Staas WE, Nemunaitis G. Management of reflex sweating in spinal cord injured patients. *Arch Phys Med Rehabil* 1989; 70:544–546.

109. Anderson LS, Biering-Sorensen F, Muller PG, et al. The prevalence of hyperhidrosis in patients with spinal cord injuries and an evaluation of the effect of dextropropoxyphene hydrochloride in therapy. *Paraplegia* 1992; 30:184–191.

110. Ottomo M, Heimburger RF. Alternating Horner's syndrome and hyperhidrosis due to dural adhesions following cervical spinal cord injury. *J Neurosurgery* 1980; 53:97–100.

111. Stanworth PA. The significance of hyperhidrosis in patients with post-traumatic syringomyelia. *Paraplegia* 1982; 20:282–287.

112. Rossier AB, Foo D, Shillito J, et al. Posttraumatic cervical syringomyelia. Incidence, clinical presentation, electrophysiological studies, syrinx protein and results of conservative and operative treatment. *Brain* 1985; 108:439–461.

113. Glasauer FE, Czyrny JJ. Hyperhidrosis as the presenting symptom in post-traumatic syringomyelia. *Paraplegia* 1994; 32:423–429.

114. Falci SP, Lammertse DP, Best L, et al. Surgical treatment of posttraumatic cystic and tethered spinal cords. *J Spinal Cord Med* 1999; 22:173–181.

115. Canaday BR, Stanford RH. Propantheline bromide in the management of hyperhidrosis association with spinal cord injury. *Ann Pharmcother* 1995; 29:489–492.

116. Formal C. Metabolic and neurologic changes after spinal cord injury. *Phys Med Rehabil Clin N Am* 1992; 3:783–796.

117. Petrofsky JS. Thermoregulatory stress during rest and exercise in heat in patients with a spinal cord injury. *Eur J Appl Physiol* 1992; 64:503–507.

118. Sugarman B, Brown D, Musher D. Fever and infection in spinal cord injury patients. *JAMA* 1982; 248:66–70.

119. Beraldo PSS, Neves EGC, Alves CMF, et al. Pyrexia in hospitalized spinal cord injury patients. *Paraplegia* 1993; 31:186–191.

120. Sheridan R. Diagnosis of the acute abdomen in the neurologically stable spinal cord-injured patient: A case study. *J Clin Gastroenterol* 1992; 15:325–328.

121. Jan FK, Wilson PE. A survey of chronic pain in the pediatric spinal cord injury population. *J Spinal Cord Med* 2004; 27:S50–S53.

122. Lau C, McCormack G. Chronic pain management in pediatric spinal cord injury. In: Betz RR, Mulcahey MJ, eds. *The Child with a Spinal Cord Injury.* Rosemont, IL: American Academy of Orthopaedic Surgeons, 1996; 653–670.

123. Richards JS. Chronic pain and spinal cord injury: Review and comment. *Clin J Pain* 1992; 8:119–122.

124. Siddall PJ, Taylor DA, Cousins MJ. Classification of pain following spinal cord injury. *Spinal Cord* 1997; 35:69–75.

125. Bryce TN, Ragnarsson KT. Pain after spinal cord injury. *Phys Med Rehabil Clin N Am* 2000; 11:157–168.

126. Dahlin, PA, Van Buskirk NE, Novotny RW, et al. Self-biting with multiple finger amputations following spinal cord injury. *Paraplegia* 1985; 23:306–318.

127. Marmolya G, Yagan R, Freehafer A. Acro-osteolysis of the fingers in a spinal cord injury patient. *Spine* 1989; 14:137–139.

128. Vogel, L.C., Anderson, C.J. Self-injurious behavior in children and adolescents with spinal cord injuries. *Spinal Cord* 2002; 40:666–668.

129. Balazy TE. Clinical management of chronic pain in spinal cord injury. *Clin J Pain* 1992; 8:102–110.

130. Umlauf RL. Psychological interventions for chronic pain following spinal cord injury. *Clin J Pain* 1992; 8:111–118.

131. Bowsher D. Central pain following spinal and supraspinal lesions. *Spinal Cord* 1999; 37:235–238.

132. Sandford PR, Lindblom LB, Haddox JD. Amitriptyline and carbamazepine in the treatment of dysesthetic pain in spinal cord injury. *Arch Phys Med Rehabil* 1992; 73:300–301.

133. Kwittken PL, Sweinberg SK, Campbell DE, et al. Latex hypersensitivity in children: Clinical presentation and detection of latex-specific immunoglobulin E. *Pediatrics* 1995; 95:693–699.

134. Landwehr LP, Boguniewicz M. Current perspectives on latex allergy. *J Pediatr* 1996; 128:305–312.

135. Rendeli C, Nucera E, Ausili E, Tabacco F, Roncallo C, Pollastrini E, Scorzoni M, Schiavino D, Caldarelli M, Pietrini D, Patriarca G. Latex sensitization and allergy in children with myelomeningocele. *Childs Nerv Syst* 2006; 22:28–32.

136. Vogel LC, Schrader T, Lubicky JP. Latex allergy in children and adolescents with spinal cord injuries. *J Pediatr Orthop* 1995; 15:517–520.

137. Monasterio EA, Barber DB, Rogers SJ, et al. Latex allergy in adults with spinal cord injury: A pilot investigation. *J Spinal Cord Med* 2000; 23:6–9.

138. Fisher AA. Association of latex and food allergy. *Cutis* 1993; 52:70–71.

139. DeVivo MJ, Krause JS, Lammertse DP. Recent trends in mortality and causes of death among persons with spinal cord injury. *Arch Phys Med Rehabil* 1999; 80:1411–1419.

140. Yekutiel M, Brooks ME, Ohry A, et al. The prevalence of hypertension, ischaemic heart disease and diabetes in traumatic spinal cord injured patients and amputees. *Paraplegia* 1989; 27:58–62.

141. Nelson MD, Widman LM, Abresch RT, Stanhope K, Havel PJ, Styne DM, McDonald CM. Metabolic syndrome in adolescents with spinal cord dysfunction. *J Spinal Cord Med* 2007; 30:S127–S139.

142. Liusuwan A, Wiman L, Abresch RT, McDonald CM. Altered body composition affects resting energy expenditure and interpretation of body mass index in children with spinal cord injury. *J Spinal Cord Med* 2004; 27:S24–S28.

143. McDonald CM, Abresch-Meyer AL, Nelson MD, Widman LM. Body mass index and body composition measures by dual X-ray absorptiometry in patients aged 10 to 21 years with spinal cord injury. *J Spinal Cord Med* 2007; 30:S97–S104.

144. Patt PL, Agena SM, Vogel LC, Foley S, Anderson CJ. Estimation of resting energy expenditure in children with spinal cord injuries. *J Spinal Cord Med* 2007; 30:S83–S87.

145. Liusuwan RA, Widman LM, Abresch RT, Styne DM, McDonald CM. Body composition and resting energy expenditure in patients aged 11 to 21 years with spinal dysfunction compared to controls: Comparisons and relationships among the groups. *J Spinal Cord Med* 2007; 30:S105–S111.

146. Sawka MN, Latzka WA, Pandolf KB. Temperature regulation during upper body exercise: Able-bodied and spinal cord injured. *Med Sci Sports Exerc* 1989; 21:S132–140.

147. Widman LM, Abresch RT, Styne DM, McDonald CM. Aerobic fitness and upper extremity strength in patients aged 11 to 21 years with spinal cord dysfunction as compared to ideal weight and overweight controls. *J Spinal Cord Med* 2007; 30:S88–S96.

148. King ML, Freeman DM, Pellicone JT, et al. Exertional hypotension in thoracic spinal cord injury: Case report. *Paraplegia* 1992; 30:261–266.

149. Hopman MT, Oeseburg B, Binkhorst RA. Cardiovascular responses in persons with paraplegia to prolonged arm exercise and thermal stress. *Med Sci Sports Exerc* 1993; 25:577–583.

150. Liusuwan RA, Widman LM, Abresch RT, Johnson AJ, McDonald CM. Behavioral intervention, Exercise, and Nutrition Education to improve health and Fitness (BENEfit) in adolescents with mobility impairment due to spinal dysfunction. *J Spinal Cord Med* 2007; 30:S119–S126.

151. Johnson KA, Klaas SJ. Recreation therapy. In: Betz RR, Mulcahey, MJ, eds. *The Child with a Spinal Cord Injury.* Rosemont, IL: American Academy of Orthopaedic Surgeons, 1996; 619–624.

152. Johnson KA, Klaas SJ. Recreation issues and trends in pediatric spinal cord injury. *Top Spinal Cord Inj Rehabil* 1997; 3(2)79–84.

153. Johnson KA, Klaas SJ. Recreation involvement and play in pediatric spinal cord injury. *Top Spinal Cord Inj Rehabil* 2000; 6(Suppl):105–109.

154. Cowell LL, Squires WG, Raven PB. Benefits of aerobic exercise for the paraplegic: A brief review. *Med Sci Sports Exerc* 1986; 18:501–508.

155. Porth SC. Recognition and management off respiratory dysfunction in children with tetraplegia. *J Spinal Cord Med* 2004; 27:S75–S79.

156. McKinley WO, Jackson AB, Cardena D, et al. Long-term medical complications after traumatic spinal cord injury: A regional model systems analysis. *Arch Phys Med Rehabil* 1999; 80:1402–1410.

157. Lanig IS, Peterson WP. The respiratory system in spinal cord injury. *Phys Med Rehabil Clin N Am* 2000; 11:29–43.

158. Padman R, Alexander M, Thorogood C, Porth S. Respiratory management of pediatric patients with spinal cord injuries: retrospective review of the duPont experience. *Neurorehabil Neural Repair* 2003; 17:32–36.

159. Frates RC, Splaingard ML, Smith EO, et al. Outcome of home mechanical ventilation in children. *J Pediatr* 1985; 106:850–856.

160. Onders RP, Elmo MJ, Ignagni AR. Diaphragm pacing stimulation system for tetraplegia in individuals injured during childhood or adolescence. *J Spinal Cord Med* 2007; 30:S25–S29.

161. Nelson VS, Lewis CC. Ventilatory support: Preparing for discharge. *Top Spinal Cord Inj Rehabil* 2000; 6(Suppl):16–24.

162. Weese-Mayer DE, Hunt CE, Brouillette RT, et al. Diaphragm pacing in infants and children. *J Pediatr* 1992; 120:1–8.

163. Nelson VS. Non-invasive mechanical ventilation for children and adolescents with spinal cord injuries. *Top Spinal Cord Inj Rehabil* 2000; 6(Suppl):12–15.

164. Nelson VS, Dixon PJ, Warschausky SA. Long-term outcome of children with high tetraplegia and ventilator dependence. *J Spinal Cord Med* 2007; 30:S93–S97.

165. Gilgoff RL, Gilgoff IS. Long-term follow-up of home mechanical ventilation in young children with spinal cord injury and neuromuscular conditions. *J Pediatr* 2003; 142:476–480.

166. Bonekat HW, Andersen G, Squires J. Obstructive disordered breathing during sleep in patients with spinal cord injury. *Paraplegia* 1990; 28:392–398.

167. Flavell H, Marshall R, Thornton AT, et al. Hypoxia episodes during sleep in high tetraplegia. *Arch Phys Med Rehabil* 1992; 73:623–627.

168. Lapides J, Diokno AC, Silber SJ, et al. Clean intermittent self-catheterization in the treatment of urinary tract disease. *J Urol* 1972; 107:458–461.

169. Merenda L, Brown JP. Bladder and bowel management for the child with spinal cord dysfunction. *J Spinal Cord Med* 2007; 27:S16–S23.

170. Patki P, Hamid R, Somayaji S, Bycroft J, Shah PJR, Craggs M. Long-term urological outcomes in paediatric spinal cord injury. *Spinal Cord* 2006; 44:729–733.

171. Fernandes ET, Reinberg Y, Vernier R, et al. Neurogenic bladder dysfunction in children: Review of pathophysiology and current management. *J Pediatr* 1994; 124:1–7.

172. McLaughlin JF, Murray M, Van Zandt K, et al. Clean intermittent catheterization. *Dev Med Child Neurol* 1996; 38:446–454.

173. Pontari MA, Bauer SB. Urologic issues in spinal cord injury: Assessment, management, outcome, and research needs. In: Betz RR, Mulcahey MJ, eds. *The Child with a Spinal Cord Injury*. Rosemont, IL: American Academy of Orthopaedic Surgeons, 1996; 213–231.

174. Vogel LC, Pontari M. Pediatric spinal cord injury issues: Medical issues. *Top Spinal Cord Inj Rehabil* 1997; 3:20–30.

175. National Institute on Disability and Rehabilitation Research Consensus Statement. The prevention and management of urinary tract infections among people with spinal cord injuries. *J Am Paraplegia Soc* 1992; 15:194–204.

176. Schaad UB. Pediatric use of quinolones. *Pediatr Infect Dis J* 1999; 18:469–470.

177. Akbar M, Abelt R, Seyler TM, Gerner HJ, Mohring K. Repeated botulinum-A toxin injections in the treatment of myelodysplastic children and patients with spinal cord injuries with neurogenic bladder dysfunction. *BJU Int* 2007; 100(3):639–645. Epub 2007 May 26.

178. Kass EJ, Koff SA. Bladder augmentation in the pediatric neuropathic bladder. *J Urol* 1983; 129:552–555.

179. Sidi AA, Aliabadi H, Gonzalez R. Enterocystoplasty in the management and reconstruction of the pediatric neurogenic bladder. *J Pediatr Surg* 1987; 22:153–157.

180. Mitrofanoff P. Trans-appendicular continent cystotomy in the management of the neurogenic bladder. *Chir Pediatr* 1980; 21:297–305.

181. Vogel LC. Unique management needs of pediatric spinal cord injury patients. *J Spinal Cord Med* 1997; 20:17–20.

182. Merenda LA, Duffy T, Betz RR, Mulcahey MJ, Dean G, Pontari M. Outcomes of urinary diversion in children with spinal cord injuries. *J Spinal Cord Med* 2007; 30:S41–S47.

183. Chulamorkodt NN, Estrada CR, Chaviano AH. Continent urinary diversion: 10-year experience of Shriners Hospitals for Children in Chicago. *J Spinal Cord Med* 2004; 27:S84–S87.

184. Vogel LC, Anderson CJ, Chaviano AC, et al. Bladder management in pediatric SCI: Continent diversions and upper extremity reconstruction. *J Spinal Cord Med* 1998; 21:382.

185. Vogel LC, Anderson CJ, Chaviano AC, et al. Continent catheterizable conduits improve independence and quality of life for adolescents with spinal cord injuries. *J Spinal Cord Med* 1998; 21:156.

186. Chaviano AC, Anderson CJ, Matkov TG, et al. Mitrofanoff continent catheterizable stoma for pediatric patients. *Top Spinal Cord Inj Rehabil* 2000; 6(Suppl):30–35.

187. Pontari MA, Weibel B, Morales V, et al. Improved quality of life after continent urinary diversion in pediatric patients with quadriplegia after spinal cord injury. *Top Spinal Cord Inj Rehabil* 2000; 6(Suppl): 25–29.

188. Branwell JG, Creasey GH, Aggarwal AM, et al. Management of the neurogenic bowel in patients with spinal cord injury. *Urol Clin N Am* 1993; 20:517–526.

189. Stiens SA, Bergman SB, Goetz LL. Neurogenic bowel dysfunction after spinal cord injury: Clinical evaluation and rehabilitative management. *Arch Phys Med Rehabil* 1997; 78:S86–S102.

190. Kirshblum SC, Gulati M, O'Connor KC, et al. Bowel care practices in chronic spinal cord injury patients. *Arch Phys Med Rehabil* 1998; 79:20–23.

191. Goetz LL, Hurvitz EA, Nelson VS, et al. Bowel management in children and adolescents with spinal cord injury. *J Spinal Cord Med* 1998; 21: 335–341.

192. Consortium for Spinal Cord Medicine. *Neurogenic Bowel Management in Adults with Spinal Cord Injury*. Washington, DC: Paralyzed Veterans of America, 1998.

193. Chen D, Nussbaum SB. The gastrointestinal system and bowel management following spinal cord injury. *Phys Med Rehabil Clin N Am* 2000; 11:45–56.

194. Gleeson RM. Bowel continence for the child with a neurogenic bowel. *Rehabil Nurs* 1990; 15:319–321.

195. Puet TA, Jackson H, Amy S. Use of pulsed irrigation evacuation in the management of the neuropathic bowel. *Spinal Cord* 1997; 35: 694–699.

196. Kim J, Beasley SW, Maoate K. Appendicostomy stomas and antegrade colonic irrigation after laparoscopic antegrade continence enema. *J Laparoendoscopic AdvSurg Techniques* 2006;16:400–403.

197. Herndon CDA, Rink RC, Cain MP, Lerner M, Kaefer M, Yerkes E, Casale AJ. In situ Malone antegrade continence enema in 127 patients: A 6-year experience. *J Urol* 2004; 172:1689–1691.

198. Liptak GS, Revell GM. Management of bowel dysfunction in children with spinal cord disease or injury by means of the enema continence catheter. *J Pediatr* 1992; 120:190–194.

199. Vogel LC. Spasticity: Diagnostic workup and medical management. In: Betz RR, Mulcahey MJ, eds. *The Child with a Spinal Cord Injury*. Rosemont, IL: American Academy of Orthopaedic Surgeons, 1996; 261–268.

200. Little JW, Micklesen P, Umlauf R, et al. Lower extremity manifestations of spasticity in chronic spinal cord injury. *Am J Phys Med Rehabil* 1989; 68:32–36.

201. Hurvitz EA, Nelson VS. Functional evaluation of spasticity and its effect on rehabilitation. In: Betz RR, Mulcahey MJ, eds. *The Child with a Spinal Cord Injury*. Rosemont, IL: American Academy of Orthopaedic Surgeons, 1996; 255–260.

202. Alpiner NM. Spasticity: Pathophysiology and objective assessments. In: Betz RR, Mulcahey MJ, eds. *The Child with a Spinal Cord Injury*. Rosemont, IL: American Academy of Orthopaedic Surgeons, 1996; 233–253.

203. Barnes MP. Local treatment of spasticity. *Clin Neurol* 1993; 2:55–71.

204. Rice GPA. Pharmacotherapy of spasticity: Some theoretical and practical considerations. *Can J Neurol Sci* 1987; 14:510–512.

205. Perry HE, Wright RO, Shannon MW, et al. Baclofen overdose: Drug experimentation in a group of adolescents. *Pediatrics* 1998; 101:1045–1048.

206. Donovan WH, Carter RE, Rossi CD, et al. Clonidine effect on spasticity: A clinical trial. *Arch Phys Med Rehabil* 1988; 69:193–194.

207. Weingarden SI, Belen JG. Clonidine transdermal system for treatment of spasticity in spinal cord injury. *Arch Phys Med Rehabil* 1992; 73:876–877.

208. Yablon SA, Sipski ML. Effect of transdermal clonidine on spinal spasticity. *Am J Phys Med Rehabil* 1993; 72:154–157.

209. Mathias CJ, Luckitt J, Desai P, et al. Pharmacodynamics and pharmacokinetics of the oral antispastic agent tizanidine in patients with spinal cord injury. *J Rehabil Res Dev* 1989; 26:9–16.

210. Apple DF, Murray HH. Spasticity: Surgical management. In: Betz RR, Mulcahey MJ, eds. *The Child with a Spinal Cord Injury*. Rosemont, IL: American Academy of Orthopaedic Surgeons, 1996; 269–283.

211. Hambleton P. Therapeutic application of botulinum toxin. *J Med Microbiol* 1993; 39:243–245.

212. Jankovic J, Brin MF. Therapeutic uses of botulinum toxin. *N Engl J Med* 1991; 324:1186–1194.

213. Ochs GA. Intrathecal baclofen. *Bailliere's Clin Neurol* 1993; 2:73–86.

214. Penn RD, Savoy SM, Corcos D, et al. Intrathecal baclofen for severe spinal spasticity. *N Engl J Med* 1989; 320:1517–1521.

215. Snow BJ, Tsui JKC, Bhatt MH, et al. Treatment of spasticity with botulinum toxin: A double-blind study. *Ann Neurol* 1990; 28:512–515.

216. Armstrong RW, Steinbok P, Farrell K, et al. Continuous intrathecal baclofen treatment of severe spasms in two children with spinal cord injury. *Dev Med Child Neurol* 1992; 34:731–738.

217. Albright AL, Barron WB, Fasick MP, et al. Continuous intrathecal baclofen infusion for spasticity of cerebral origin. *JAMA* 1993; 270:2475–2477.

218. Delhaas EM, Brouwers JRBJ. Intrathecal baclofen overdose: Report of 7 events in 5 patients and review of the literature. *Int J Clin Pharmacol* 1991; 29:274–280.

219. Teddy P, Jamous A, Gardner B, et al. Complications of intrathecal baclofen delivery. *Br J Neurosurg* 1992; 6:115–118.

220. Mubarak SJ, Camp JF, Vuletich W, et al. Halo application in the infant. *J Pediatr Orthop* 1989; 9:612–614.

221. Betz RR, Mulcahey MJ, D'Andrea LP, Clements DH. Acute evaluation and management of pediatric spinal cord injury. *J Spinal Cord Med* 2004; 27:S11–S15.

222. Letts M, Kaylor D, Gouw G. A biomechanical analysis of halo fixation in children. *J Bone Joint Surg* 1988; 70B:277–279.

223. Herzenberg JK, Hensinger RN, Dedrick DK, et al. Emergency transport and positioning of young children who have an injury of the cervical spine. The standard backboard may be hazardous. *J Bone Joint Surg* 1989; 71A:15–22.

224. Mayfield JK, Erkkila JC, Winter RB. Spine deformity subsequent to acquired childhood spinal cord injury. *J Bone Joint Surg* 1981; 63A:1401–1411.

225. Lancourt JE, Dickson JH, Carter RE. Paralytic spinal deformity following traumatic spinal-cord injury in children and adolescents. *J Bone Joint Surg* 1981; 63A:47–53.

226. Dearolf WW III, Betz RR, Vogel LC, et al. Scoliosis in pediatric spinal cord–injured patients. *J Pediatr Orthop* 1990; 10:214–218.

227. Bergstrom EMK, Short DJ, Frankel HL, et al. The effect of childhood spinal cord injury on skeletal development: A retrospective study. *Spinal Cord* 1999; 37:838–846.

228. Betz RR, Orthopaedic problems in the child with spinal cord injury. *Top Spinal Cord Inj Rehabil* 1997; 3:9–19.

229. Mehta S, Betz RR, Mulcahey MJ, McDonald C, Vogel LC. Effect of bracing on paralytic scoliosis secondary to spinal cord injury. *J Spinal Cord Med* 2004; 27:S88–S92.

230. Sison-Williamson MM, Bagley A, Hongo A, Vogel LC, Mulcahey, MJ, Betz RR, McDonald CM. Effect of thoracolumbosacral orthoses on reachable workspace volumes in children with spinal cord injury. *J Spinal Cord Med* 2007; 30:S184–S191.

231. Chavetz RS, Mulcahey MJ, Betz RR, Anderson C, Vogel LC, Gaughan J, O'Del MA, Flanagan A, McDonald CM. Impact of prophylactic thoracolumbosacral orthosis bracing on functional activities and activities of daily living in the pediatric spinal cord injury population. *J Spinal Cord Med* 2007; 30:S178–S183.

232. McCarthy JJ, Betz RR. Hip disorders in children who have spinal cord injury. *Orthop Clin N Am* 2006; 37:197–202.

233. McCarthy JJ, Chavetz RS, Betz RR, Gaughan J. Incidence and degree of hip subluxation/dislocation in children with spinal cord injury. *J Spinal Cord Med* 2004; 27:S80–S83.

234. Miller F, Betz RR. Hip joint instability. In: Betz RR, Mulcahey MJ, eds. *The Child with a Spinal Cord Injury.* Rosemont, IL: American Academy of Orthopaedic Surgeons, 1996; 353–361.

235. Vogel LC, Gogia RS, Lubicky JP. Hip abnormalities in children with spinal cord injuries. *J Spinal Cord Med* 1995; 18:172.

236. Rink P, Miller F. Hip instability in spinal cord injury patients. *J Pediatr Orthop* 1990; 10:583–587.

237. Betz RR, Mulcahey MJ, Smith BT, et al. Implications of hip subluxation for FES-assisted mobility in patients with spinal cord injury. *Orthopedics* 2001; 24:181–184

238. McCarthy JJ, Weibel B, Betz RR. Results of pelvic osteotomies for hip subluxation or dislocation in children with spinal cord injury. *Top Spinal Cord Inj Rehabil* 2000; 6(Suppl):48–53.

239. Garland DE. A clinical perspective on common forms of acquired heterotopic ossification. *Clin Orthop* 1991; 263:13–29.

240. Garland DE, Shimoya ST, Lugo C, et al. Spinal cord insults and heterotopic ossification in the pediatric population. *Clin Orthop* 1989; 245:303–310.

241. Banovac K, Gonzalez F, Renfree KJ. Treatment of heterotopic ossification after spinal cord injury. *J Spinal Cord Med* 1997; 20:60–65.

242. Bellah RD, Zawodniak L, Librizzi RJ, et al. Idiopathic arterial calcification of infancy: Prenatal and postnatal effects of therapy in an infant. *J Pediatr* 1992; 121:930–933.

243. Pazzaglia UE, Beluff G, Ravelli A, et al. Chronic intoxication by ethane-1-hydroxy-1,1-diphosphonate (EHDP) in a child with myositis ossificans progressiva. *Pediatr Radiol* 1993; 23:459–462.

244. Silverman SL, Hurvitz EA, Nelson VS, et al. Rachitic syndrome after disodium etidronate therapy in an adolescent. *Arch Phys Med Rehabil* 1994; 75:118–120.

245. Freebourn TM, Barber DB, Able AC. The treatment of immature heterotopic ossification in spinal cord injuries with combination surgery, radiation therapy and NSAID. *Spinal Cord* 1999; 37:50–53.

246. Wick M, Muller EJ, Hahn MP, Muhn G. Surgical excision of heterotopic bone after hip surgery followed by oral indomethacin application: Is there a clinical benefit for the patient? *Arch Orthop Trauma Surg* 1999; 119:151–155.

247. Betz RR, Triolo RJ, Hermida VM, et al. The effects of functional neuromuscular stimulation on the bone mineral content in the lower limbs of spinal cord injured children. *J Am Paraplegia Soc* 1991; 14:65–66.

248. Lauer R, Johnston TE, Smith BT, Mulcahey MJ, Betz RR, Maurer AH. Bone mineral density of the hip and knee in children with spinal cord injury. *J Spinal Cord Med* 2007; 30:S10–S14.

249. Miller F. Pathologic long-bone fractures: Diagnosis, etiology, management, and prevention. In: Betz RR, Mulcahey MJ, eds. *The Child with a Spinal Cord Injury.* Rosemont, IL: American Academy of Orthopaedic Surgeons, 1996; 331–338.

250. Hickey KJ, Anderson CJ, Vogel LC. Pressure ulcers in pediatric spinal cord injury. *Top Spinal Cord Inj Rehabil* 2000; 6(Suppl):85–90.

251. Yarkony GM, Heinemann AW. Pressure ulcers. In: Stover SL, DeLisa JA, Whiteneck GG, eds. *Spinal Cord Injury: Systems.* Gaithersburg MD: Aspen Publications, 1995; 100–119.

252. Bonner L. Pressure ulcer prevention. In: Betz RR, Mulcahey MJ, eds. *The Child with a Spinal Cord Injury.* Rosemont, IL: American Academy of Orthopaedic Surgeons, 1996; 285–292.

253. Zager RP, Marquette CH. Developmental considerations in children and early adolescents with spinal cord injury. *Arch Phys Med Rehabil* 1981; 62:427–431.

254. Zidek K, Srinivasan R. Rehabilitation of a child with a spinal cord injury. *Seminars Pediatr Neurol* 2003; 10:140–150.

255. Webster G, Kennedy P. Addressing children's needs and evaluating rehabilitation outcome after spinal cord injury: The Child Needs Assessment Checklist and Goal-Planning Program. *J Spinal Cord Med* 2007; 30:S140–S145.

256. Spoltore TA, O'Brien AM. Rehabilitation of the spinal cord injured patient. *Orthop Nurs* 1995; 14:7–14.

257. Nelson MR, Tilbor, AG, Frieden L, et al. Introduction to pediatric rehabilitation. In: Betz RR, Mulcahey MJ, eds. *The Child with a Spinal Cord Injury.* Rosemont, IL: American Academy of Orthopaedic Surgeons, 1996; 461–470.

258. Mulcahey MJ, Betz RR. Considerations in the rehabilitation of children with spinal cord injuries. *Top Spinal Cord Inj Rehabil* 1997; 3:31–36.

259. Mulcahey MJ. Unique management needs of pediatric spinal cord injury patients: Rehabilitation. *J Spinal Cord Med* 1997; 20:25–30.

260. Jarosz DA. Pediatric spinal cord injuries: A case presentation. *Crit Care Nurs Q* 1999; 22(2):8–13.

261. Jaffe KM, McDonald CM. Rehabilitation following childhood injury. *Pediatr Ann* 1992; 21:438–447.

262. Krey CH, Calhoun CL. Utilizing research in wheelchair and seating selection and configuration for children with injury/dysfunction of the spinal cord. *J Spinal Cord Med* 2004; 27:S29–S37.

263. Krajnik S, Bridle M. Hand splinting in tetraplegia: Current practice. *Am J Occup Ther* 1992; 46:149–156.

264. Mulcahey MJ. Upper extremity orthoses and splints. In: Betz RR, Mulcahey MJ, eds. *The Child with a Spinal Cord Injury.* Rosemont, IL: American Academy of Orthopaedic Surgeons, 1996; 375–392.

265. Mulcahey MJ. Rehabilitation and outcomes of upper extremity tendon transfer surgery, In: Betz RR, Mulcahey MJ, eds. *The Child with a Spinal Cord Injury.* Rosemont, IL: American Academy of Orthopaedic Surgeons, 1996; 419–448.

266. Mulcahey MJ, Betz RR, Smith BT, Weiss AA. A prospective evaluation of upper extremity tendon transfers in children with cervical spinal cord injury. *J Pediatr Orthop* 1999; 19:319–328.

267. Mulcahey MJ, Betz RR, Smith BT, et al. Implanted FES hand system in adolescents with SCI: An evaluation. *Arch Phys Med Rehabil* 1997; 78:597–607.

268. Peckham PH, Marsolais EB, Mortimer JT. Restoration of key grip and release in the C6 tetraplegic patient through functional neuromuscular stimulation. *J Hand Surg* 1980; 5:462–469.

269. Kilgore KL, Peckham PH, Keith MW, et al. An implanted upper-extremity neuroprosthesis. Follow-up of five patients. *J Bone Joint Surg* 1997; 79A:533–541.

270. Akers JM, Smith BT, Betz RR. Implantable electrode lead in a growing limb. *IEEE Trans Rehabil Eng* 1999; 7:35–45.

271. Hussey RW, Stauffer ES. Spinal cord injury: Requirements for ambulation. *Arch Phys Med Rehabil* 1973; 54:544–547.

272. Vogel LC, Lubicky JP. Ambulation in children and adolescents with spinal cord injuries. *J Pediatr Orthop* 1995; 15:510–516.

273. Vogel LC, MD; Mendoza MM, Schottler JC, Chlan KM, Anderson CJ. Ambulation in children and youth with spinal cord injuries. *J Spinal Cord Med* 2007; 30:S158–S164.

274. Kelly MA, Stokes KS. Standing and ambulation for the child with paraplegia or tetraplegia. In: Betz RR, Mulcahey MJ, eds. *The Child with a Spinal Cord Injury.* Rosemont, IL: American Academy of Orthopaedic Surgeons, 1996; 519–532.

275. Moynahan M, Hunt M, Halden E. Evaluation of Standing and Ambulation: Needs and Outcomes. In: Betz RR, Mulcahey MJ, eds. *The Child with a Spinal Cord Injury.* Rosemont, IL: American Academy of Orthopaedic Surgeons, 1996; 503–517.

276. Creitz L, Nelson VS, Haubenstricker L, et al. Orthotic Prescriptions. In: Betz RR, Mulcahey MJ, eds. *The Child with a Spinal Cord Injury.* Rosemont, IL: American Academy of Orthopaedic Surgeons, 1996; 537–553.

277. Vogel LC, Lubicky JP. Pediatric spinal cord injury issues: Ambulation. *Top Spinal Cord Inj Rehabil* 1997; 3:37–47.

278. Vogel LC, Lubicky JP. Ambulation with parapodia and reciprocating gait orthoses in pediatric spinal cord injury. *Dev Med Child Neurol* 1995; 37:957–964.

279. Kinnen E, Gram M, Jackman KV, et al. Rochester parapodium. *Clin Prosthet Orthot* 1987; 8:24–25.

280. Katz DE, Haideri N, Song K, et al. Comparative study of conventional hip-knee-ankle-foot orthoses versus reciprocating-gait orthoses for children with high-level paraparesis. *J Pediatr Orthop* 1997; 17:377–386.

281. Fitzsimmons AS. The physiologic benefits of standing. In: Betz RR, Mulcahey MJ, eds. *The Child with a Spinal Cord Injury.* Rosemont, IL: American Academy of Orthopaedic Surgeons, 1996; 533–535.

282. Johnston TE, Betz RR, Smith BT, Mulcahey MJ. Implanted functional electrical stimulation: An alternative for standing and walking in pediatric spinal cord injury. *Spinal Cord* 2003; 41:144–152.

283. Moynahan MA, Mullin C, Cohn J, et al. Home uses of a FES system for standing and mobility in adolescents with spinal cord injury. *Arch Phys Med Rehabil* 1996; 77:1005–1013.

284. Bonaroti D, Akers J, Smith BT, et al. Comparison of functional electrical stimulation to long leg braces for upright mobility in children with complete thoracic level spinal injuries. *Arch Phys Med Rehabil* 1999; 80:1047–1053.

285. Anderson CJ. Psychosocial and sexuality issues in pediatric spinal cord injury. *Top Spinal Cord Inj Rehabil* 1997; 3:70–78.

286. Anderson CJ. Unique management needs of pediatric spinal cord injury patients: Psychological issues. *J Spinal Cord Med* 1997; 20:21–24.

287. Yarkony GM, Anderson CJ. Sexuality. In: Betz RR, Mulcahey MJ, eds. *The Child with a Spinal Cord Injury.* Rosemont, IL: American Academy of Orthopaedic Surgeons, 1996; 625–637.

288. Sipski Alexander M, Alexander CJ. Recommendations for discussing sexuality after spinal cord injury/dysfunction in children, adolescents, and adults. *J Spinal Cord Med* 2007; 30:S65–S70.

289. Anderson CJ, Mulcahey MJ, Vogel LC. Menstruation and pediatric spinal cord injury. *J Spinal Cord Med* 1997; 20:56–59.

290. American Academy of Pediatrics, Committee on Children With Disabilities. Provision of educationally-related services for children and adolescents with chronic diseases and disabling conditions. *Pediatrics* 2000; 105:448–451.

291. The Individuals with Disabilities Education Act (IDEA). 20 USC B 1400 et seq, June 4, 1997.

292. Augutis M, Levi R, Asplund K, Berg-Kelly K. Psychosocial aspects of traumatic spinal cord injury with onset during adolescence: A qualitative study. *J Spinal Cord Med* 2007; 30:S55-S64.

293. Kennedy P, Gorsuch N, Marsh N. Childhood onset of spinal cord injury: Self-esteem and self-perception. *Br J Clin Psychol* 1995; 34:581–588.

294. Sammallahti P, Kannisto M, Aalberg V. Psychological defenses and psychiatric symptoms in adults with pediatric spinal cord injuries. *Spinal Cord* 1996; 34:669–672.

295. Gorman C, Kennedy P, Hamilton LR. Alterations in self-perceptions following childhood onset of spinal cord injury. *Spinal Cord* 1998; 36:181–185.

296. Johnson KA, Klaas SJ, Vogel LC, McDonald C. Leisure characteristics of the pediatric spinal cord injury population. *J Spinal Cord Med* 2004; 27:S107–S109.

297. Johnson KA, Klaas SJ. The changing nature of play: Implications for pediatric spinal cord injury. *J Spinal Cord Med* 2007; 30:S71–S75.

298. Callen L. Substance use and abuse. In: Betz RR, Mulcahey MJ, eds. *The Child with a Spinal Cord Injury.* Rosemont, IL: American Academy of Orthopaedic Surgeons, 1996; 671–677.

299. Sarwark, JF, Lubicky JP, eds. *Caring for the Child with Spina Bifida.* Rosemont, IL: American Academy of Orthopaedic Surgeons, 2002.

300. Northrup H, Volcik KA. Spina bifida and other neural tube defects. *Curr Probl Pediatr* November/December 2000; 317–332.

301. Shurtleff DB, Lemire RJ. Epidemiology, etiologic factors, and prenatal diagnosis of open spinal dysraphism. *Neurosurg Clin N Am* 1995; 6:183–193.

302. CDC. Spina bifida incidence at birth—United States, 1983–1990. *MMWR* 1992; 497–500.

303. Williams LJ, Rasmussen SA, Flores A, Kirby RS, Edmonds LD. Decline in the prevalence of spinal bifida and anencephaly by race/ethnicity: 1995–2002. *Pediatrics* 2005; 116:580–586.

304. Yen IH, Khoury MJ, Erickson JD, et al. The changing epidemiology of neural tube defects, United States 1968–1989. *Am J Dis Child* 1992; 146:857–861.

305. Shurtleff DB, Luthy DA, Nyberg DA, et al. Meningomyelocele: Management in utero and post natum. *Ciba Found Symp* 1994; 181: 270–286.

306. CDC. Spina bifida and anencephaly before and after folic acid mandate-United States, 1995–1996 and 1999–2000. *MMWR* 2004; 362–365.

307. Wasserman CR, Shaw GM, Selvin S, et al. Socioeconomic status, neighborhood social conditions, and neural tube defects. *Am J Public Health* 1998; 88:1674–1680.

308. McLone DG. Continuing concepts in the management of spina bifida. *Pediatr Neurosurg* 1992; 18:254–256.

309. Bol KA, Collins JS, Kirby RS. Survival of infants with neural tube defects in the presence of folic acid fortification. *Pediatrics* 2006; 117:803–813.

310. Hunt GM. The median survival time in open spina bifida. *Dev Med Child Neurol* 1997; 39:568.

311. Davis BE, Daley CM, Shurtleff DB, Duguay S, Seidel K, Loeser JD, Ellenbogen RG. Long-term survival of individuals with myelomeningocele. *Pediatr Neurosurg* 2005; 41:186–191.

312. Mitchell LE. Epidemiology of neural tube defects. *Am J Med Genetics Part C (Semin Med Genet)* 2005; 135C:88–94.

313. Becerra JE, Khoury MJ, Cordero JF, et al. Diabetes mellitus during pregnancy and the risks for specific birth defects: A population based case-control study. *Pediatrics* 1990; 85:1–9.

314. Shaw GM, Velie EM, Schaffer D. Risk of neural tube defect—affected pregnancies among obese women. *JAMA* 1996; 275:1093–1096.

315. Watkins ML, Scanlon KS, Mulinare J, et al. Is maternal obesity a risk factor for anencephaly and spina bifida? *Epidemiology* 1996; 7: 507–512.

316. Graham JM, Edwards MJ, Edwards MJ. Teratogen update: Gestational effects of maternal hyperthermia due to febrile illnesses and resultant patterns of defects in humans. *Teratology* 1998; 58:209–221.

317. Edwards MJ, Shiota K, Smith MSR, et al. Hyperthermia and birth defects. *Reprod Toxicol* 1995; 9:411–425.

318. Lammer EJ, Sever LE, Oakley GP. Teratogen update: Valproic acid. *Teratology* 1987; 35:465–473.

319. Rosa FW. Spina bifida in infants of women treated with carbamazepine during pregnancy. *N Engl J Med* 1991; 324: 674–677.

320. McBride ML. Sib risks of anencephaly and spina bifida in British Columbia. *Am J Med Genet* 1979; 3:377–387.

321. Myers GJ. Myelomeningocele: The medical aspects. *Pediatr Clin N Amer* 1984; 31:165–175.

322. Toriello HV, Higgins JV. Occurrence of neural tube defects among first-, second-, and third-degree relatives of probands: Results of a United States study. *Am J Med Genet* 1983; 15:601–606.

323. Urui S, Oi S. Experimental study of the embryogenesis of open spinal dysraphism. *Neurosurg Clin N Am* 1995; 6:195–202.

324. Rauzzino M, Oakes WJ. Chiari II malformation and syringomyelia. *Neurosurg Clin N Am* 1995; 6:293–309.

325. Swank M, Dias L. Myelomeningocele: A review of the orthopaedic aspects of 206 patients treated from birth with no selection criteria. *Dev Med Child Neurol* 1992; 34:1047–1052.

326. Pang D. Surgical complications of open dysraphism. *Neurosurg Clin N Am* 1995; 6:243–257.

327. Drewek MJ, Bruner JP, Whetsell WO, et al. Quantitative analysis of the toxicity of human amniotic fluid to cultured rat spinal cord. *Pediatr Neurosurg* 1997; 27:190–193.

328. Heffez DS, Aryanpur J, Hutchins GM, et al. The paralysis associated with myelomeningocele: Clinical and experimental data implicating a preventable spinal cord injury. *Neurosurgery* 1990; 26:987–992.

329. Hahn YS. Open myelomeningocele. *Neurosurg Clin N Am* 1995; 6:231–241.

330. Charney EB, Weller SC, Sutton LN, et al. Management of the newborn with myelomeningocele: Time for a decision-making process. *Pediatrics* 1985; 75:58–64.

331. Stein SC, Schut L. Hydrocephalus in myelomeningocele. *Child's Brain* 1979; 5:413–419.

332. Steinbok P, Irvine B, Cochrane DD, et al. Long-term outcome and complications of children born with meningomyelocele. *Childs Nerv Syst* 1992; 8:92–96.

333. Hunt GM, Poulton A. Open spina bifida: A complete cohort reviewed 25 years after closure. *Dev Med Child Neurol* 1995; 37:19–29.

334. Roebroeck ME, Hempenius L, Van Baalen B, Hendriksen JGM, Van Den Berg-Emons HJG, Stam HJ. Cognitive functioning of adolescents and young adults with meningomyelocele and level of everyday physical activity. *Disability Rehabil* 2006; 28:1237–1242.

335. Rose BM, Holmbeck GN. Attention and executive functions in adolescents with spina bifida. *J Pediatr Psychol* 2007; 32:983–994.

336. McLone DG, Czyzewski D, Raimondi AJ, et al. Central nervous system infections as a limiting factor in the intelligence of children with myelomeningocele. *Pediatrics* 1982; 70:338–342.

337. Cull C, Wyke MA. Memory functions of children with spina bifida and shunted hydrocephalus. *Dev Med Child Neurol* 1984; 26:177–183.

338. Jansen J, Taudorf K, Pedersen H, et al. Upper extremity function in spina bifida. *Childs Nerv Syst* 1991; 7:67–71.

339. Swisher LP, Pinsker EJ. The language characteristics of hyperverbal, hydrocephalic children. *Dev Med Child Neurol* 1971; 13:746–755.

340. Burmeister R, Hannay HJ, Copeland K, Fletcher JM, Boudousquie A, Dennis M. Attention problems and executive functions in children with spina bifida and hydrocephalus. *Child Neuropsychology* 2005; 11:265–283.

341. Kirk VG, Morielli A, Brouillette RT. Sleep-disordered breathing in patients with myelomeningocele: The missed diagnosis. *Dev Med Child Neurol* 1999; 41:40–43.

342. Petersen MC, Wolraich M, Sherbondy A, et al. Abnormalities in control of ventilation in newborn infants with myelomeningocele. *J Pediatr* 1995; 126:1011–1015.

343. Waters K, Forbes P, Morielli A, et al. Sleep-disordered breathing in children with myelomeningocele. *J Pediatr* 1998; 132:672–681.

344. Park TS, Cail WS, Maggio WM, et al. Progressive spasticity and scoliosis in children with myelomeningocele. *J Neurosurg* 1985; 62:367–374.

345. Bartonek A, Saraste H, Knutson LM. Comparison of different systems to classify the neurological level of lesion in patients with myelomeningocele. *Dev Med Child Neurol* 1999; 41:796–805.

346. Curtis BH, Brightman, E. Spina bifida: A follow-up of ninety cases. *Conn Med* 1961; 26:145–150.

347. McDonald CM, Jaffe KM, Shurtleff DB, et al. Modifications to the traditional description of neurosegmental innervation in myelomeningocele. *Dev Med Child Neurol* 1991; 33:473–481.

348. McDonald CM. Rehabilitation of children with spinal dysraphism. *Neurosurg Clin N Am* 1995; 6:393–412.

349. Shurtleff DB, Duguay S, Duguay G, et al. Epidemiology of tethered cord with meningomyelocele. *Eur J Pediatr Surg* 1997; 7(Suppl 1):7–11.

350. Shurtleff DB. Selection process for the care of congenitally malformed infants. In: Shurtleff DB, ed. *Myelodysplasias and Exstrophies: Significance, Prevention and Treatment.* Orlando, FL: Grune and Stratton, 1986; 89–115.

351. Jutson JM, Beasley SW, Bryan AD. Cryptorchidism in spina bifida and spinal cord transection: A clue to the mechanism of transinguinal descent of the testis. *J Pediatr Surg* 1988; 23:275–277.

352. Kropp KA, Voeller KKS. Cryptorchidism in meningomyelocele. *J Pediatr* 1981; 99:110–113.

353. Sidi AA, Dykstra DD, Gonzalez R. The value of urodynamic testing in the management of neonates with myelodysplasia: A prospective study. *J Urol* 1986; 135:90–93.

354. Joseph DB, Bauer SB, Colodny AH, et al. Clean, intermittent catheterization of infants with neurogenic bladder. *Pediatrics* 1989; 84:78–82.

355. Kasabian NG, Bauer SB, Dyro FM, et al. The prophylactic value of clean intermittent catheterization and anticholinergic medication in newborns and infants with myelodysplasia at risk of developing urinary tract deterioration. *Am J Dis Child* 1992; 146:840–843.

356. Roach MB, Switters DM, Stone AR. The changing urodynamic pattern in infants with myelomeningocele. *J Urol* 1993; 150:944–947.

357. Stone AR. Neurologic evaluation and urologic management of spinal dysraphism. *Neurosurg Clin N Am* 1995; 6:269–277.

358. Uehling DT, Smith J, Meyer J, et al. Impact of an intermittent catheterization program on children with myelomeningocele. *Pediatrics* 1985; 76:892–895.

359. Hannigan KF. Teaching intermittent self-catheterization to young children with myelodysplasia. *Dev Med Child Neurol* 1979; 21:365–368.

360. King JC, Currie DM, Wright E. Bowel training in spina bifida: Importance of education, patient compliance, age, and anal reflexes. *Arch Phys Med Rehabil* 1994; 75:243–247.

361. Shandling B, Gilmour RF. The enema continence catheter in spina bifida: Successful bowel management. *J Pediatr Surg* 1987; 22:271–273.

362. Wald A. Use of Biofeedback in treatment of fecal incontinence in patients with meningomyelocele. *Pediatrics* 1981; 68:45–49.

363. Whitehead WE, Parker L, Bosmajian L, et al. Treatment of fecal incontinence in children with spina bifida: Comparison of biofeedback and behavior modification. *Arch Phys Med Rehabil* 1986; 67:218–224.

364. Loening-Baucke V, Desch L, Wolraich M. Biofeedback training for patients with myelomeningocele and fecal incontinence. *Dev Med Child Neurol* 1988; 30:781–790.

365. Karol LA. Orthopedic management in myelomeningocele. *Neurosurg Clin N Am* 1995; 6:259–268.

366. Piggott H. The natural history of scoliosis in myelodysplasia. *J Bone Joint Surg* 1980; 62B:54–58.

367. Guille JT, Sarwark JF, Sherk HH, Kumar SJ. Congenital and developmental deformities of the spine in children with myelomeningocele. *J Am Acad Orthop Surg* 2006; 14:294–302.

368. Shurtleff DB. Mobility. In: Shurtleff DB, ed. *Myelodysplasias and Exstrophies: Significance, Prevention and Treatment.* Orlando, FL: Grune and Stratton, 1986; 313–356.

369. Feiwell E, Downey DS, Blatt T. The effect of hip reduction on function in patients with myelomeningocele. *J Bone Joint Surg* 1978; 60A:169–173.

370. Mackel JL, Lindseth RE. Scoliosis in myelodysplasia. *J Bone Joint Surg* 1975; 57A:1031.

371. Hall PV, Lindseth RE, Campbell RL, et al. Myelodysplasia and developmental scoliosis. *Spine* 1976; 1:48–56.

372. Tomlinson RJ, Wolfe MW, Nadall JM, et al. Syringomyelia and developmental scoliosis. *J Pediatr Orthop* 1994; 14:580–585.

373. Hall P, Lindseth R, Campbell R, et al. Scoliosis and hydrocephalus in myelocele patients. *J Neurosurg* 1979; 50:174–178.

374. Rosenblum MF, Rinegold DN, Charney EB. Assessment of stature of children with myelomeningocele, and usefulness of arm-span measurement. *Dev Med Child Neurol* 1983; 25:338–342.

375. Rotenstein D, Reigel DH. Growth hormone treatment of children with neural tube defects: Results from 6 months to 6 years. *J Pediatr* 1996; 128:184–189.

376. Hunt GM. Open Spina bifida: Outcome for a complete cohort treated unselectively and followed into adulthood. *Dev Med Child Neurol* 1990; 32:108–118.

377. Elias ER, Sadeghi-Nead A. Precocious puberty in girl with myelodysplasia. *Pediatrics* 1994; 93:521–522.

378. Trollman R, Strehl E, Dorr HG. Precocious puberty in children with myelomeningocele: Treatment with gonadotropin-releasing hormone analogues. *Dev Med Child Neurol* 1998; 40:38–43.

379. Hayes-Allen MC. Obesity and short stature in children with myelomeningocele. *Dev Med Child Neurol* 1972; 4(Suppl 27):59–64.

380. Hunt GM. Spina bifida: Implications for 100 children at school. *Dev Med Child Neurol* 1981; 23:160–172.

381. Hayden PW. Adolescents with meningomyelocele. *Pediatr Rev* 1985; 6:245–252.

382. Shurtleff DB. Dietary management. In Shurtleff DB ed., *Myelodysplasia and Extrophies: Significance, Prevention and Treatment.* Orlando, FL: Grune and Stratton, 1986; 285–298.

383. Roberts D, Shepherd RW, Shepherd K. Anthropometry and obesity in myelomeningocele. *J Paediatr Child Health* 1991; 27:83–90.

384. Meeropol E, Kelleher R, Bell S, et al. Allergic reactions to rubber in patients with myelodysplasia. *N Engl J Med* 1990; 323:1072.

385. Yassin MS, Sanyurah S, Lierl MB, et al. Evaluation of latex allergy in patients with meningomyelocele. *Ann Allergy* 1992; 69:207–211.

386. Kelly KJ, Pearson ML, Kurup VP, et al. A cluster of anaphylactic reactions in children with spina bifida during general anesthesia: Epidemiologic features, risk factors, and latex hypersensitivity. *J Allergy Clin Immunol* 1994; 53–61.

387. Michael T, Niggemann, B, Moers A, et al. Risk factors for latex allergy in patients with spina bifida. *Clin Exp Allergy* 1996; 26:934–939.

388. Mazon A, Nieto A, Estornell F, et al. Factors that influence the presence of symptoms caused by latex allergy in children with spina bifida. *J Allergy Clin Immunol* 1997; 99:600–604.

389. Niggemann B, Kulig M, Bergmann R, et al. Development of latex allergy in children up to 5 years of age—a retrospective analysis of risk factors. *Pediatr Allergy Immunol* 1998; 9:36–39.

390. De Swert LFA, Van Laer KMIA, Verpoorten CMA et al. Determination of independent risk factors and comparative analysis of diagnostic methods for immediate type latex allergy in spina bifida patients. *Clin Exp Allergy* 1997; 27:1067–1076.

391. Cremer R, Hoppe A, Kleine-Diepenbruck U, et al. Longitudinal study on latex sensitization in children with spina bifida. *Pediatr Allergy Immunol* 1998; 9:40–43.

392. Cremer R, Kleine-Diepenbruck U, Hoppe A, et al. Latex allergy in spina bifida patients—prevention by primary prophylaxis. *Allergy* 1998; 53:709–711.

393. Szepfatusi Z, Seidl R, Bernert G, et al. Latex sensitization in spina bifida appears disease-associated. *J Pediatr* 1999; 134:344–348.

394. Okamoto GA, Lamers JV, Shurtleff DB. Skin breakdown in patients with myelomeningocele. *Arch Phys Med Rehabil* 1983; 64:20–23.

395. Harris MB, Banta JV. Cost of skin care in the myelomeningocele population. *J Pediatr Ortho* 1990; 10:355–361.

396. Hayden PW, Davenport SLH, Campbell MM. Adolescents with myelodysplasia: Impact of physical disability on emotional maturation. *Pediatrics* 1979; 64:53–59.

397. Zurmohle UM, Homann T, Schroeter C, et al. Psychosocial adjustment of children with spina bifida. *J Child Neurol* 1998; 13:64–70.

398. Loomis JW, Javornisky JG, Monahan JJ et al. Relations between family environment and adjustment outcomes in young adults with spina bifida. *Dev Med Child Neurol* 1997; 39:620–627.

399. Joyner BD, McLorie GA, Khoury AE. Sexuality and reproductive issues in children with myelomeningocele. *Eur J Pediatr Surg* 1998; 8:29–34.

400. Sawyer SM, Roberts KV. Sexual and reproductive health in young people with spina bifida. *Dev Med Child Neurol* 1999; 41:671–675.

401. Bodzioch J, Roach JW, Schkade J. Promoting independence in adolescent paraplegics: A 2-week "camping" experience. *J Pediatr Orthop* 1986; 6:198–201.

402. Nehring WM, Faux SA. Transitional and health issues of adults with neural tube defects. *J Nursing Scholarship* 2006; 38:63–70.

403. MRC Vitamin Study Research Group. Prevention of neural tube defects: Results of the Medical Research Council vitamin study. *Lancet* 1991; 338:131–137.

404. Centers for Disease Control. Recommendations for the use of folic acid to reduce the number of cases of spina bifida and other neural tube defects. *MMWR* 1992; 41(No. RR–14):1–7.

405. American Academy of Pediatrics. Committee on Genetics. Folic acid for the prevention of neural tube defects. *Pediatrics* 1999; 104: 325–327.

406. Bell KN, Oakley GP. Tracking the prevention of folic acid-preventable spina bifida and anencephaly. *Birth Defects Research (Part A)* 2006; 76:654–657.

407. De Wals P, Tairou F, Van Allen MI, Uh S-H, Lowry RB, et al. Reduction in neural-tube defects after folic acid fortification in Canada. *N Engl J Med* 2007; 357:135–142.

408. American Academy of Pediatrics. Committee on Genetics. Maternal serum α-fetoprotein screening. *Pediatrics* 1991; 88:1282–1283.

409. Hobbins JC. Diagnosis and management of neural-tube defects. *N Eng J Med* 1991; 324:690–691.

410. Babcook CJ. Ultrasound evaluation of prenatal and neonatal spina bifida. *Neurosurg Clin N Am* 1995; 6:203–218.

411. Meuli M, Meuli-Simmen C, Hutchins GM, et al. The spinal cord lesion in human fetuses with myelomeningocele: Implications for fetal surgery. *J Pediatr Surg* 1997; 32:448–452.

412. Tulipan N, Bruner JP. Myelomeningocele repair in utero: A report of three cases. *Pediatr Neurosurg* 1998; 28:177–180.

413. Johnson MP, Gerdes M, Rintoul N, Pasquariello P, Melchionni J, Sutton LN, Adzick NS. Maternal-fetal surgery for myelomeningocele: Neurodevelopmental outcomes at 2 years of age. *Am J Obstet Gynecol* 2006; 194:1145–1152.

414. Zambelli H, Carelli E, Honorato D, et al. Assessment of neurosurgical outcome in children prenatally diagnosed with myelomeningocele and development of a protocol for fetal surgery to prevent hydrocephalus. *Childs Nerv Syst* 2007; 23:421–425.

415. Bruner JP. Intrauterine surgery in myelomeningocele. *Semin Fetal Neonatal Med* 2007; 12:471–476.

416. Sutton LN. Fetal surgery for neural tube defects. *Best Practice & Research Clinical Obstetrics and Gynaecology* 2008; 22(1):175–188.

417. Luthy DA, Wardinsky T, Shurtleff DB, et al. Cesarean section before the onset of labor and subsequent motor function in infants with meningomyelocele diagnosed antenatally. *N Eng J Med* 1991; 324: 662–666.

418. Owen J. Prophylactic Cesarean for prenatally diagnosed malformations. *Clin Obstet Gynecol* 1998; 41:393–404.

419. Sutton LN. Lipomyelomeningocele. *Neurosurg Clin N Am* 1995; 6:325–338.

420. Forrester MB, Merz RD. Descriptive epidemiology of lipomyelomeningocele, Hawaii, 1986–2001. *Birth Defects Research (Part A)* 2004; 70:953–956.

421. Tubbs RS, Bui CJ, Rice WC et al. Critical analysis of the Chiari malformation type I found in children with lipomyelomeningocele. *J Neurosurg* 2007; 106:196–200.

422. Renshaw TS. Sacral agenesis. *J Bone Joint Surg* 1978; 60-A:373–383.

423. Estin D, Cohen AR. Caudal agenesis and associated caudal spinal cord malformations. *Neurosurg Clin N Am* 1995; 6:377–391.

424. Wilmshurst JM, Kelly R, Borzyskowski M. Presentation and outcome of sacral agenesis: 20 years' experience. *Dev Med Child Neurol* 1999; 41:806–812.

425. Guzman L, Bauer SB, Hallett M, et al. Evaluation and management of children with sacral agenesis. *Urology* 1983; 22:506–510.

426. Caird MS, Hall JM, Bloom DA, Park JM, Farley FA. Outcome study of children, adolescents, and adults with sacral agenesis. *J Pediatr Orthop* 2007; 27:682–685.

VI

MUSCULOSKELETAL CARE

46 Musculoskeletal Pain and Overuse Injuries

Michael L. Boninger
Jennifer L. Collinger
Rory A. Cooper
Alicia M. Koontz

Individuals with spinal cord injury (SCI) have a high incidence of musculoskeletal pain and overuse injuries. Survey studies find the absolute incidence of musculoskeletal pain to be between 50% and 81% (1–4). Because the majority of individuals with SCI rely on their upper extremities for all activities of daily living (ADLs) and for mobility, this pain can have a tremendous impact on their quality of life. All the subjects in one study reported a change or increase in their dependence on personal care assistants with fluctuations in upper extremity pain (5). Even when self-care is not impacted, upper extremity pain can limit an individual's mobility and endurance (6). In one study, pain was the only factor found to be correlated with lower quality-of-life scores (7). Another study found that pain was inversely related to muscle strength and functional outcomes (8). The largest survey study, completed by Sie et al. defined significant pain as pain requiring analgesic medication, pain associated with two or more ADLs, or pain severe enough to result in cessation of activity (1). Using this definition, significant pain was present in 59% of individuals with tetraplegia and 41% of individuals with paraplegia. Unfortunately, clinicians are not effective at treating these complaints. Subbarao et al. found that 51.5% of 451 individuals with SCI had reported upper extremity pain to their doctors, but the majority had not found relief with the offered treatments (5).

ALTERNATIVE DIAGNOSES

Is the individual's pain related to a musculoskeletal problem? Probably, but not definitely. Anyone who treats or works with individuals with SCI needs to have an expanded differential diagnosis. A common diagnosis in individuals with SCI is neuropathic pain. Historical factors that can help differentiate neuropathic pain from musculoskeletal pain are:

- Type of pain
  Neuropathic—can be burning or stabbing and sometimes aching

  Musculoskeletal—usually dull

- Location of pain
  Neuropathic—can occur anywhere, often at the level of injury or below

  Musculoskeletal—usually above the level of injury, often associated with specific joints or trigger points

- Exacerbating factors
  Neuropathic—uncertain; pain can be present constantly

  Musculoskeletal—usually worse with movement and activity involving affected joint or region

The above list is not complete, and differentiating neuropathic from musculoskeletal pain is not an easy task. In addition to the historical factors, musculoskeletal pain can commonly be reproduced on physical examination. This is usually not the case for neuropathic pain.

Syringomyelia is another diagnosis unique to SCI (9). In this condition, fluid collects in the spinal cord itself and eventually compresses the cord in the rigid spinal canal. This condition usually has associated numbness and pain; weakness can also be a presenting symptom. This condition is potentially life threatening and needs to be ruled out if there is clinical suspicion or if a patient with pain does not respond to treatment as expected. Syrinx frequently requires surgical treatment and is diagnosed using magnetic resonance imaging (MRI). Many other, non-musculoskeletal conditions such as radiculopathy can cause upper extremity pain and numbness. A broad differential diagnosis is needed when diagnosing and treating pain in people with SCI.

SHOULDER INJURIES

The shoulder is the most common source of musculoskeletal pain in SCI (10). This finding is not surprising, as the shoulder is built for maximum flexibility and motion—not for weight bearing. The prevalence of pain by survey methods varies from 30% to

100% (1, 11–14). This range in prevalence is due to many differences between the studies, including subject characteristics such as gender, injury level, and years since injury. One study found that 30% of 89 men with traumatic SCI experienced shoulder pain (14), but another found that 73% of 11 women with traumatic paraplegia experienced shoulder pain, compared to only 27% of age, size, and activity-level matched able-bodied women (12). This study raises awareness to the fact that women may be more at risk for developing secondary upper extremity injuries.

Many studies attribute the high prevalence of shoulder pain to "overuse syndrome" (1, 4, 5, 13, 15). Of 239 individuals with less than five years post-SCI, 53% of individuals with tetraplegia and 16% of individuals with paraplegia reported shoulder pain (1). The difference between the groups is likely caused by neuropathic pain at the shoulder in tetraplegia. By 20 years post-injury, over 70% of individuals with paraplegia had pain, a higher percentage than those with tetraplegia. This increase in paraplegic shoulder pain likely represents repetitive strain injuries from years of transfers and manual wheelchair use. Similarly, another study reported 35% of individuals with paraplegia at least one year out from injury experience shoulder pain, and that percentage jumps to 100% for individuals more than 25 years post-injury (13).

To get a better idea of the cause of pain, many studies have incorporated physical examination and imaging studies (15–18). The majority of these studies involve individuals with paraplegia, and found that people with shoulder pain often showed signs of pathology determined by physical exam (15, 16) or X-ray (15). However, one study found that although 38 out of 50 subjects showed degenerative changes on X-ray, only six complained of shoulder pain (17). Older subjects and women were more susceptible to developing degenerative changes at the shoulder.

Two studies to date have looked at MRI abnormalities in individuals with SCI (19, 20). Escobedo et al. found that 57% of veterans with paraplegia had rotator cuff tears, with severity of tears related to age and duration of spinal cord injury. In contrast, Boninger et al. found a relative absence of rotator cuff tears. In the 28 subjects tested (55 shoulders), only a single rotator cuff tear was seen. The most likely cause for the difference between the studies is disparity in populations. The average age of the subjects in Escobedo's study was 59 years, and the average number of years post-injury was 26, which was in contrast to Boninger's study where the average age was 35 years and years post-injury was 11.5. If these subjects were followed for an additional 15 years, the prevalence of rotator cuff tears and pain would likely increase. Boninger recruited from wheelchair vendors and discharge records after acute SCI rehabilitation, thus including individuals not seen by a physician. Individuals who have pain may be more likely to see a physician in regular follow-up. Thus, previous studies may have overestimated the prevalence of rotator cuff tears. Most of the subjects in the study by Boninger used ultralight weight wheelchairs, which, as will be discussed later in this chapter, could lower the incidence of injury.

Another imaging abnormality noted in individuals with paralysis is osteolysis of the distal clavicle, characterized by progressive resorption of the lateral end of the clavicle (Figure 46.1). This finding represents advanced bone degeneration (21). Two separate studies found a prevalence of osteolysis of the distal clavicle of approximately 13% (20, 22). Osteolysis of the distal

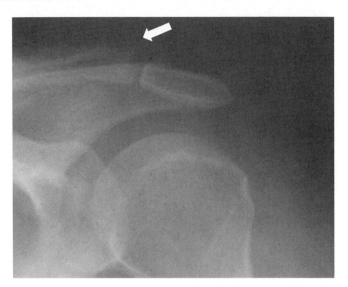

Figure 46.1   Osteolysis of the distal clavicle.

clavicle should be added to the differential diagnosis of shoulder abnormalities in individuals with paraplegia. As stated by Roach, the most likely cause of this finding is repetitive upper limb trauma caused by transfers and wheelchair propulsion (23).

Few direct studies examine the pathophysiology of shoulder pain and injury in SCI. In Bayley's study of shoulder pain, he found that interarticular pressure was over two times arterial pressure when performing a transfer (15). He believed that this increased pressure stressed the vasculature of the rotator cuff tendon leading to injury. Wylie et al. reported that 18% of active wheelchair users had joint space narrowing in the shoulder, which he felt led to impingement of the rotator cuff (18). Muscle imbalance, caused by overuse, is thought to lead to abnormal biomechanics and thus injury. Muscle imbalance has been demonstrated among manual wheelchair users with paraplegia (24) and correlated to shoulder pain in a group of wheelchair athletes (25). Boninger et al. observed a relationship between the number of imaging abnormalities and an individual's weight (20). This relationship was thought to be due to the excess work and strain required to perform transfers and wheelchair propulsion for people with increased body weight.

Recent evidence has linked shoulder pathology determined by MRI and physical exam to propulsion biomechanics (26). Mercer et al. found that subjects who experienced higher directional joint loading were more likely to exhibit CA ligament edema or CA ligament thickening, which has been associated with surgically confirmed rotator cuff tears (27). Subjects who experienced higher superior forces and internal rotation moments showed signs of shoulder pathology during the physical exam.

Researchers have begun using ultrasound to identify acute changes in the biceps tendon resulting from strenuous wheelchair propulsion. An increase in fluid content of the biceps tendon was observed after a wheelchair sporting event (28). Individuals who had more playing time showed a larger increase in biceps tendon diameter, demonstrating a link between activity level and acute tendon changes. Using ultrasound to examine acute changes to musculoskeletal structures may provide a convenient way to evaluate the immediate impact of an intervention designed to reduce the risk of injury.

ELBOW INJURIES

Musculoskeletal problems at the elbow tend to be the result of strained muscles and tendons, or nerve impingement. The prevalence of elbow pain in individuals with SCI is approximately 6–15% (1, 8). Studies of wheelchair athletes found that 12–14% of musculoskeletal injuries occurred at the elbow (29, 30). The propulsive stroke of everyday and athletic users involves pronation of the forearm and extension of the elbow, coupled with extension of the wrist and gripping of the hand at the start of the propulsive stroke (31). This position of the elbow and hand may place an individual with SCI at higher risk for lateral epicondylitis.

Entrapment of the ulnar nerve at the elbow can occur at the cubital tunnel during full flexion of the elbow. Direct trauma can also occur because only a ligament sheath covers the outer surface. Two studies found slower motor conduction velocity of the ulnar nerve across the elbow in wheelchair users compared to a control group (32, 33). These studies show that elbow discomfort and pain are commonly caused by both musculoskeletal and peripheral nerve reasons. No specific study has investigated the etiology of elbow injuries in individuals with SCI.

WRIST INJURIES

As at the elbow, wrist pain can be caused by both musculoskeletal injury and nerve injury. Although the majority of studies in this area have focused on Carpal Tunnel Syndrome (CTS), Sie attempted to separate symptoms of CTS and other causes of wrist pain in a group of individuals with paraplegia (1). Wrist and hand pain not associated with CTS was seen 13% and 11% of the time, respectively, and historical or physical examination evidence of CTS was found in 66% of subjects (1). Gellman et al. found that 49% of 77 individuals with paraplegia had signs and symptoms of CTS (34). Both of these large clinical series found the incidence of CTS increased with a longer duration of paralysis.

To add objective criteria to the diagnosis of CTS, a number of investigators have performed nerve conduction studies on this population (35–38). These investigators observed electrodiagnostic evidence of CTS in 50–80% of individuals with paraplegia, and clinical evidence of CTS was identified in approximately 30–75% of the subjects. Persons with longer duration of injury, greater weight, and body mass index (BMI) were more likely to exhibit symptoms of CTS upon physical exam (38). From these studies it is apparent that CTS is a common problem in individuals with SCI. Most of the studies found a greater prevalence of abnormalities on nerve conduction studies than actual clinical symptoms. This may signify that subclinical nerve damage exists in a number of these individuals. Whether this subclinical damage goes on to become clinically important has not yet been determined.

CTS is generally thought to be caused by compression of the median nerve within the carpal tunnel. Ultrasound has been used to study acute changes of the median nerve resulting from intense wheelchair propulsion (39, 40). The high impact task of wheelchair propulsion causes a compression of the median nerve immediately following the task, resulting in lower fluid content

and smaller size. Extremes of wrist flexion and extension have been shown to greatly increase the pressure within the carpal tunnel, more so in patients with CTS. Gellman et al. studied patients with SCI and found that pressures in the carpal tunnel were higher in wrist flexion compared to a group of controls (34). In a study of 34 individuals with paraplegia, Boninger et al. found that increased weight was related to median nerve slowing and amplitude loss (41). Controlled for weight, those individuals who hit the pushrim more frequently and with greater force also had greater evidence of median nerve damage. This article was the first to find a direct link between daily activities and the incidence of repetitive strain injury in a population of individuals with SCI. Boninger et al. also found that individuals who had a larger range of motion at the wrist during propulsion used less force and fewer strokes to propel their wheelchair and exhibited better nerve function than subjects who had a smaller range of motion (42).

MUSCULOSKELETAL BACK AND NECK PROBLEMS

Surprisingly little is written about back pain in individuals with SCI. As in much of the literature on pain in SCI, when a study reports the prevalence of back pain it likely contains some individuals with neuropathic pain. Nepomuceno performed a mail survey returned by 200 individuals with SCI (2). Neck pain was seen in up to 16% of respondents depending on injury level, with individuals with tetraplegia having the greatest incidence. Back or trunk pain had an incidence as high as 83%, with thoracic level spinal cord injury being most associated with this type of pain. The discussion of this article focused on neuropathic causes for pain, including radiculopathy associated with the initial injury. It is likely, however, that at least some of these pain complaints were related to musculoskeletal causes. Turner et al. surveyed 384 individuals with spinal cord injuries and reported that 61% experienced back pain (3). In a study of 71 participants of the National Veterans Wheelchair Games, 66% reported neck pain since becoming a wheelchair user, and 60% reported pain in the last month (43). Of those individuals reporting pain, 60% visited the doctor about the pain, and 40% limited their activities due to the pain. Using trigger point palpation, this same study reported physical examination findings consistent with myofascial pain in 54% respondents who experienced pain in the last month (43). Clinicians should consider the origin of neck pain during treatment as mechanical neck pain that may be treated more effectively than neck pain that is neuropathic in nature. In addition, patients should be questioned related to sleep disturbance that commonly accompanies myofascial pain. Although the underlying pathology behind myofascial pain may be benign, symptoms related to this disorder can be quite disabling.

It has generally been thought that increased kyphosis and scoliosis lead to neck and back pain, but there has been little research to support this contention. One study of patients with thoracic and lumbar spinal fractures found a positive relationship between kyphosis and pain, although this was not statistically significant (44). Whiteneck et al. reported a 14% incidence of kyphosis and scoliosis in persons more than 20 years post-SCI (45). Boninger et al. found no difference in measures of scoliosis and kyphosis when comparing individuals less than two years post-SCI and a group greater than 10 years post-SCI

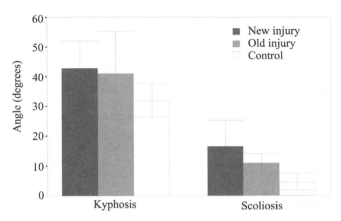

Figure 46.2 Kyphosis and scoliosis by group. (Reprint from *Archives of Physical Medicine and Rehabilitation*, Vol. 79, Boninger ML, Sauer T, Trefler E, Hobson D, Burde HR, Cooper RA, Postural changes with aging in tetraplegia, pp. 910–915, 1998.)

indicating that the increase in spinal curvature occurs early (46) (Figure 46.2). No relationship was seen between the degree of scoliosis or kyphosis and measures of pain. Not surprisingly, this paper recommended early intervention. No formal research has investigated the effect of overhead activities on neck and back pain in wheelchair users. However, due to their seated posture, wheelchair users may frequently need to work with their arms above shoulder height, which may also contribute to the prevalence of neck and back pain observed in this population (43). One study found that sustained neck extension and rotation increased the neck discomfort of wheelchair users (47). Unfortunately, this position is often assumed due to the nature of the environment. Minimizing extreme neck postures should be considered as part of wheelchair, home, and environmental design (48).

For most individuals with SCI, a majority of their day is spent in a wheelchair, where they encounter impact vibrations while traversing curbs, bumps, and other obstacles, and cyclic vibrations while traversing over uneven or rough terrains. These vibrations are a potential cause of back pain. Research has shown that impact vibrations reside in a range of frequencies sensitive to humans (4–12.5 Hz), and that individuals with SCI may experience higher peak frequencies compared to unimpaired persons (49, 50). This higher frequency may be a function of the seating position (e.g., a kyphotic posture) inherent to wheelchair propulsion, or may be related to the amount of active muscle control. Vibrations experienced in a manual wheelchair during usual activities may exceed standards set for industrial occupations, such as truckers, heavy equipment operators, and aircraft crews. DiGiovine et al. found that riders were significantly more comfortable in ultralightweight wheelchairs, defined as having a high degree of adjustability, than in lightweight chairs (51). Although this article does not provide a direct link between back pain and type of wheelchair, it does suggest that such a link may be present. More recently, another research group investigated vibration transmission and comfort in manual wheelchairs by simulating real world vibration conditions using a vertical electro-dynamic vibrator system (52). Discomfort of the neck and lower back was reported by 56% and 28% of the participants respectively during simulated vibrations. This study suggests designing wheelchairs and seat cushions to reduce vibration transmissions around 8 Hz, while also accounting for the variable response of different regions of the body when designing the wheel-

chair damping and stiffness characteristics. Further research into this and other causes of secondary spine injury and pain is needed.

PREVENTION AND TREATMENT OF MUSCULOSKELETAL INJURIES IN SCI

Prevention

As with most conditions, prevention is infinitely preferable to treatment. Recently, Clinical Practice Guidelines were published by the Paralyzed Veterans of America Consortium for Spinal Cord Medicine related to the preservation of upper limb function following spinal cord injury (48). The Clinical Practice Guidelines were established as a reference for health care professionals involved in the care of spinal cord-injured individuals. The first recommendation is that clinicians as well as patients need to be informed about the prevalence and impact of upper limb pain and injury so that appropriate prevention techniques can be implemented.

The guideline goes on to recommend that individuals with SCI seek routine health reviews as part of a risk assessment and upper limb prevention plan. This exam should include an evaluation of transfer and wheelchair propulsion techniques, wheelchair and transfer equipment, and current health status (48). In addition, clinicians should ask patients about pain. A patient may be reluctant to come forth with this information; however, early treatment of pain could result in fewer symptoms in the future, and identification of the problem can serve as a catalyst to healthy lifestyle changes. Additional recommendations are detailed below and fall into the following categories:

1. Ergonomics
2. Equipment Selection, Training, and Environmental Adaptations
3. Exercise

Ergonomics

Repetitive tasks have been linked to upper limb injuries by three major evidence-based reviews (53–55). Task performance modification based on ergonomic analysis has proven effective in reducing risk factors for pain and upper extremity pathology in various work settings (56, 57). Therefore, it seems reasonable to take a similar approach toward the task of manual wheelchair propulsion (58). Ergonomics literature finds that limiting the frequency of repetitive tasks could reduce the risk of injury, specifically to the wrist (59, 60) and shoulder (61, 62). One study found that increased push frequency during wheelchair propulsion was associated with higher oxygen cost and decreased mechanical efficiency and push angle (63).

Peak forces during propulsion should be minimized, as high forces during tasks have been related to joint pain or injury. Maintaining an ideal body weight is another way to reduce peak forces during propulsion and transfers. Manual wheelchair users should be educated about proper propulsion techniques as part of a musculoskeletal injury prevention program (Figure 46.3).

Extreme wrist postures, particularly wrist extension, have been implicated as a risk factor for developing CTS (59). Extreme wrist extension combined with weight bearing, as in a transfer,

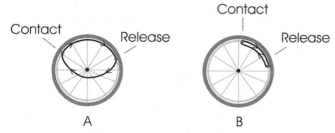

Figure 46.3 The recommended propulsion pattern is shown in **A**. An example of a poor propulsion pattern is shown in **B** (arc pattern). The thick black line on the wheel is the path followed by the hand. (Reprinted with permission from the *Paralyzed Veterans of America (PVA) Preservation of Upper Limb Function Following Spinal Cord Injury: A Clinical Practice Guideline for Health-Care Professionals*. Washington, DC: © Paralyzed Veterans of America, 2005.)

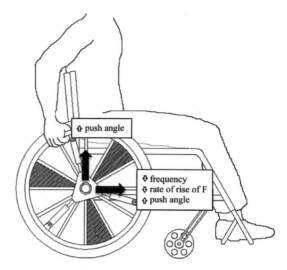

Figure 46.4 The effect of axle position on biomechanics.

should be avoided. A classic position for impingement of the supraspinatus tendon is internal rotation of the humerus combined with abduction or forward flexion (64). Shoulder positioning needs to be considered when training weight-bearing tasks such as transfers. Alternative transfer techniques and home modifications are presented below.

Equipment Selection, Training, and Environmental Adaptations

Providing individuals with the lightest-weight adjustable wheelchairs possible affords many benefits. Ultralight wheelchairs reduce rolling resistance, which in turn lessens the amount of force required to propel the wheelchair. Lighter-weight wheelchairs are adjustable or selectable to better fit the user. Adjusting the axle to a more forward position decreases rolling resistance, improves efficiency, lessens muscle activity in prime movers, and reduces superior force at the shoulder (65–68). Axle position should be adjusted as far forward as is functional while maintaining the level of stability desired by the manual wheelchair user. Figure 46.4 shows biomechanical changes associated with movement of the axle (F = resultant force). The large, black arrows indicate the direction of movement of the axle relative to the shoulder, and the information in the box indicates how this affects propulsion biomechanics. Seat height should be adjusted so that the elbow is flexed between 100 and 120 degrees when the hand is resting on the top dead center of the pushrim. This seat position can reduce stroke frequency and increase push angle mechanical efficiency (69, 70).

Many handrim designs exist that may reduce the risk for overuse injuries during wheelchair propulsion, particularly at the wrist. At the time of writing this chapter, the benefits of one commercially available handrim designed to improve contact with the hand and relieve stress and pressure on the carpal tunnel have been investigated. Research has shown that this handrim can reduce the severity of symptoms such as hand or wrist pain and improve functional outcomes (71).

A wheelchair should provide appropriate seating and stabilization for the pelvis and trunk. Upper limbs may be forced to do more work to compensate for instability if this is not addressed with appropriate seating. Specific recommendations

for seating and positioning can be found in the Clinical Practice Guidelines (48).

Educating patients to use proper propulsion techniques may further reduce their risk of developing upper limb injury. Manual wheelchair users should use a long, smooth, propulsive stroke to distribute force over a longer period of time, reducing stroke frequency, peak forces, and rate of loading. The hand should be allowed to drift naturally below the pushrim during recovery, following an elliptical pattern that eliminates abrupt changes in direction and extra hand movement, and has been shown to result in a lower stroke frequency (48, 72) (Figure 46.3).

Home modifications, both small and large, can help preserve upper limb integrity as well as improve independence with activities of daily living. Home, work, and transportation environments should be addressed. The guiding principle is to limit the stress on joints in positions where they are most vulnerable to injury. Understanding wrist, shoulder, and back biomechanics as well as ADLs is essential to appropriate modification of activities as well as the environment. For example, lowering the height of key kitchen utensils and frequently used cabinets may help reduce the risk of injury.

Transferring to a higher surface (uphill) increases forces on the upper limb (73) and should be avoided if possible. Modifications such as adjustable height surfaces and roll-in shower chairs should be made so that transfers are level. Although transfers and other weight-relief tasks may occur less frequently than propulsion, the shoulder joint forces are much higher (74). It is likely that both transfers and wheelchair propulsion contribute to overuse injuries, and therefore both should be included in an injury-prevention program. Many individuals transfer with a maximally extended wrist, a position implicated in CTS (59). Strategies to avoid loading in extreme joint positions should be explored (48). It is good practice to vary the leading arm during transfers because the trailing arm often experiences increased joint loading (75). The same holds true for pressure relief activities, which can be performed with a variety of techniques including forward leaning, side-to-side shifting, and depression-style maneuvers (48). Maintaining an ideal body weight can reduce the demand placed on joints during transfers.

Assistive devices for transfers are available that may reduce the forces experienced in the upper limb during transfers. One research group found that sliding boards reduce the amount of force needed for lateral movement (76). Reducing stress on the upper extremity should reduce the risk of injury or exacerbation of pain (48). Many types of patient lifts are also available for individuals who are unable to perform a transfer safely, although they are more cumbersome and less convenient.

Old dogma dictated that if you could push a wheelchair you should. This is being rethought as issues of secondary disabilities come to light. For some high-risk individuals, alternative forms of mobility should be considered to preserve upper limb integrity. High risk patients include, but are not limited to, those who have prior upper limb injury, are obese, are elderly, or live in a challenging environment with hills or rough terrain (48). Powered mobility will reduce propulsion-related repetitive strain, and can reduce fatigue because less energy is required for mobility, among other advantages. However, powered mobility is more difficult to transport, costs more, and may potentially lead to weight gain or decreased fitness. Another technology option, pushrim activated power assist wheels (PAPAWs), offers a blend between a power and manual wheelchair (77). PAPAWs have motors in the hub of the wheel that provide extra power when the user applies a force to the pushrim. PAPAWs can often be retrofitted to a current wheelchair and therefore can offload the upper extremity without causing some of the difficulties associated with switching to a power chair. PAPAWs have been found to reduce energy demands for individuals with paraplegia and tetraplegia (78, 79). Because of the hub motors, PAPAWs weigh more than a wheelchair with standard wheels and should not be recommended for someone who is frequently lifting their chair, as in a vehicle transfer.

Exercise

Exercise is an important part of preventing musculoskeletal injury. A stretching routine should be designed to maintain normal glenohumeral motion and pectoral muscle mobility (48). Limited range of motion has been associated with pain, reduced activity, and/or injury (14, 80). A tight capsule can alter biomechanics in such a way as to increase the chances of impingement. As with the general population, cardiovascular fitness needs to be maintained. Patients should be directed to strive for accumulating 30 minutes of moderate exercise most days of the week (81). Although propelling a manual wheelchair is one type of physical activity, it is not necessarily the best choice. For individuals with paraplegia, an upper extremity ergometer or swimming can provide a low-impact form of exercise. For individuals with tetraplegia, more expensive equipment that incorporates electrical stimulation into exercise may be needed to stress the cardiovascular system.

An individualized, progressive, resistance training program may be able to reduce muscle imbalance and selective muscle weakness that have been observed in individuals with SCI (25, 48). The external rotators may be weak compared to the internal rotators (24). The same muscles that provide external rotation also help to depress the shoulder, thus preventing impingement. Additionally, shoulder flexors tend to be stronger than shoulder extensors because of the pushing nature of wheelchair propulsion. Exercises targeting shoulder extensors should be incorporated in a strengthening program. Resistance training has been shown to decrease shoulder pain in men with paraplegia (82). Finally, it is important to keep most exercises below shoulder height as to avoid positions of impingement.

Treatment

Treating individuals with SCI and musculoskeletal injuries requires insight into the special needs of this population. The single most unique factor is related to their use of extremities. For the vast majority of individuals with SCI it is nearly impossible to rest an extremity. For an individual with paraplegia, to rest their arm may mean going from complete independence to complete dependence. In some cases where home care is not an option, it may be necessary to admit a patient to a skilled facility just to assure adequate rest. For this reason, prevention of injuries and early treatment is essential. It is important to remember early treatment of pain can prevent the development of chronic pain and injury (83). Specific treatments for the injuries are numerous and beyond the scope of this text. Instead, a brief summary is provided. Areas where treatment may need to be approached differently for individuals with SCI are highlighted.

Treatment for most musculoskeletal conditions can be summarized in the following categories:

- Exercise
- Modalities
- Modification of activity
- Bracing
- Medications
- Injections
- Diet

Some of these categories, such as exercise and modification of activity, are also part of a prevention plan. If the individual is not following an appropriate prevention plan, these interventions should be addressed immediately as part of treatment.

Exercise is usually the mainstay of treatment. Depending on the condition, focused stretching followed by strengthening can usually help. Cardiovascular fitness should be an important part of a healthy lifestyle.

Modalities are best used initially to help control pain, and in the long term to help with stretching. For the most part, modalities should be a small part of a treatment program.

Modification of activity is a mainstay of treatment. Any modifications that were not part of a prevention plan should be considered at this point. If the feeling is that wheelchair propulsion is, at least in part, related to the injury, it may be warranted to consider switching to a power wheelchair. It is important for clinicians to realize that the choice of switching to a power wheelchair is a significant one. The patient will likely feel a profound sense of loss over this perceived setback. For this reason the discussion of changing wheelchairs must be dealt with in a thoughtful, caring manner, and if possible, peer counseling should be involved.

Bracing can be an effective form of treatment for CTS and should be considered. Another form of bracing that should be considered for shoulder and back pain is related to seating. Appropriate seating can improve posture, and at least theoretically reduce complaints related to back, neck, and shoulder pain. Special care should be taken to reduce the natural kyphotic posture assumed when sitting in a wheelchair. This can be accomplished through tilt of the seat, avoiding sling upholstery, and using specialized cushions and back supports.

Medications such as nonsteroidal anti-inflammatories (NSAIDs) are a mainstay of treatment to reduce inflammation. As with all patients, gastrointestinal and other potential side effects must be explained to the patients. For pain as a result of fibromyalgia or chronic pain not associated with inflammation, NSAIDs may not have a role. In these cases it may be worthwhile to consider a medication with a better side effect profile, such as acetaminophen. Although narcotic analgesics have a potential for addiction, their use should not be ruled out in individuals with chronic pain.

Injections can be helpful in a number of conditions affecting the upper extremities. Although they can relieve symptoms in CTS, symptoms frequently recur (84). Injection of steroids and an anesthetic can also be effective in lateral epicondylitis. Unfortunately, steroid injections can weaken ligamentous tissues for prolonged periods of time (85). This is an important consideration when treating rotator cuff tears. In general, the individual should not use the arm in any lifting activity for three to four days. Because rest of the arm is difficult and the risk of tendon rupture is increased in the presence of a tear, this treatment should be used with caution in individuals with SCI. Injections may also play a role in treatment of trigger points.

Diet, although not traditionally thought of as a treatment for pain, may be an essential component of a comprehensive treatment plan that should not be ignored. A link has been established between weight and both shoulder injuries and CTS (20, 41). This link is not surprising, because heavier patients have to do more work during transfers and wheelchair propulsion, placing more strain on joints. At the same time, the ability to perform cardiovascular fitness exercises is diminished. As in the general population, the mainstay of a weight loss prescription is diet.

Surgery is usually thought of when alternative treatments have not successfully relieved the symptoms. Surgical treatment of CTS and most shoulder injuries requires absolute rest of the arm for extended periods of time. Once again, to assure proper rest, an individual with SCI may need to be admitted to a skilled facility during the recovery period to assure that rest is achieved without compromising the skin. It should also be noted that for rotator cuff injuries there is a greater risk of reinjury when returning to the same activity level. In one study, for example, individuals who had work-related rotator cuff injuries and returned to the same job were at greatly increased risk for reinjury (86). There is also literature showing that individuals with CTS related to repetitive tasks may be at greater risk of a worse outcome from release surgery (87, 88). Evidence regarding the success of rotator cuff repair surgery is inconclusive, and therefore more conservative therapies should be exhausted prior to surgery (89–91).

It may be useful to apply a stepwise approach to the treatment of upper extremity pain in individuals with SCI. Once pain is appropriately diagnosed, initial treatment should consist of

- Exercise, modalities, medications, modification of activity, patient education, and bracing. Consider dietary counseling if the patient is overweight. At this point, continued use of a manual wheelchair is acceptable

⇓

if pain persists

⇓

- Continue treatment outlined above, plus begin exclusive use of a power wheelchair or power assist wheelchair, and offer peer counseling

⇓

if pain persists

⇓

- Surgery as a last resort; power wheelchair use exclusively after surgery to prevent reinjury

As in all types of medical care, the patient should help to guide treatment. Because changes in wheelchairs and ADLs impact the patient's lifestyle to a great extent, it is important for the clinician to understand the patient from a broad perspective, including vocational and avocational activities. These types of discussions help the patient understand the treatment approach and assure greater compliance.

References

1. Sie IH, Waters RL, Adkins RH, Gellman H. Upper extremity pain in the postrehabilitation spinal cord injured patient. *Arch Phys Med Rehabil* 1992; 73:44–48.
2. Nepomuceno C, Fine PR, Richards JS, Gowens H, Stover SL, Rantanuabol U, Houston R. Pain in patients with spinal cord injury. *Arch Phys Med Rehabil* 1979; 60:605–609.
3. Turner JA, Cardenas DD, Warms CA, McClellan CB. Chronic pain associated with spinal cord injuries: a community survey. *Arch Phys Med Rehabil* 2001; 82(4):501–509.
4. Gironda RJ, Clark ME, Neugaard B, Nelson A. Upper limb pain in a national sample of veterans with paraplegia. *J Spinal Cord Med* 2004; 27(2):120–127.
5. Subbarao JV, Klopfstein J, Turpin R. Prevalence and impact of wrist and shoulder pain in patients with spinal cord injury. *J Spinal Cord Med* 1994; 18(1):9–13.
6. Curtis KA, Roach KE, Applegate EB, Amar T, Benbow CS, Genecco TD, Gualano J. Development of the Wheelchair User's Shoulder Pain Index (WUSPI). *Paraplegia* 1995; 33(5):290–293.
7. Lundqvist C, Siösteen A, Blomstrand C, Lind B, Sullivan M. Spinal cord injuries. Clinical, functional, and emotional status. *Spine* 1991; 16(1): 78–83.
8. van Drongelen S, de Groot S, Veeger HE, Angenot EL, Dallmeijer AJ, Post MW, van der Woude LH. Upper extremity musculoskeletal pain during and after rehabilitation in wheelchair-using persons with a spinal cord injury. *Spinal Cord* 2006; 44(3):152–159.
9. Rossier AB, Foo D, Shillito J, Dyro FM. Posttraumatic cervical syringomyelia. Incidence, clinical presentation, electrophysiological studies, syrinx protein and results of conservative and operative treatment. *Brain* 1985; 108:439–461.
10. Dalyan M, Cardenas DD, Gerard B. Upper extremity pain after spinal cord injury. *Spinal Cord* 1999; 37(3):191–195.
11. Nichols PJ, Norman PA, Ennis JR. Wheelchair user's shoulder? Shoulder pain in patients with spinal cord lesions. *Scand J Rehabil Med* 1979; 11(1):29–32.

12. Pentland WE, Twomey LT. The weight-bearing upper extremity in women with long term paraplegia. *Paraplegia* 1991; 29(8):521–530.
13. Gellman H, Sie I, Waters RL. Late complications of the weight-bearing upper extremity in the paraplegic patient. *Clin Orthop & Related Res* 1988; 233:132–135.
14. Ballinger DA, Rintala DH, Hart KA. The relation of shoulder pain and range-of-motion problems to functional limitations, disability, and perceived health of men with spinal cord injury: a multifaceted longitudinal study. *Arch Phys Med Rehabil* 2000; 81(12):1575–1581.
15. Bayley JC, Cochran TP, Sledge CB. The weight-bearing shoulder. The impingement syndrome in paraplegics. *J Bone Joint Surg Am* 1987; 69(5):676–678.
16. Samuelsson K, Tropp H, Gerdle B. Shoulder pain and its consequence in paraplegic spinal cord-injured, wheelchair users. *Spinal Cord* 2004; 42:41–46.
17. Lal S. Premature degenerative shoulder changes in spinal cord injury patients. *Spinal Cord* 1998; 36(3):186–189.
18. Wylie EJ, Chakera TM. Degenerative joint abnormalities in patients with paraplegia of duration greater than 20 years. *Paraplegia* 1988; 26(2):101–106.
19. Escobedo EM, Hunter JC, Hollister MC, Patten RM, Goldstein B. MR imaging of rotator cuff tears in individuals with paraplegia. *Am J Roentgenol* 1997; 168(4):919–923.
20. Boninger ML, Towers JD, Cooper R.A., Dicianno BE, Munin MC. Shoulder imaging abnormalities in individuals with paraplegia. *J Rehabil Res Dev* 2001; 38(4):401–408.
21. Yu YS, Dardani M, Fischer RA. MR observations of posttraumatic osteolysis of the distal clavicle after traumatic separation of the acromioclavicular joint. *J Comput Assist Tomogr* 2000; 24(1):159–164.
22. Roach NA, Schweitzer ME. Does osteolysis of the distal clavicle occur following spinal cord injury? *Skeletal Radiol* 1997; 26(1):16–19.
23. Scavenius M, Iversen BF. Nontraumatic clavicular osteolysis in weight lifters. *Am J Sports Med* 1992; 20(4):463–467.
24. Ambrosio F, Boninger ML, Souza AL, Fitzgerald SG, Koontz AM, Cooper RA. Biomechanics and strength of manual wheelchair users. *J Spinal Cord Med* 2005; 28(5):407–414.
25. Burnham RS, May L, Nelson E, Steadward R, Reid DC. Shoulder pain in wheelchair athletes. The role of muscle imbalance. *Am J Sports Med* 1993; 21(2):238–242.
26. Mercer JL, Boninger ML, Koontz, Ren D, Dyson-Hudson T, Cooper R.A. Shoulder joint pathology and kinetics in manual wheelchair users. *Clin Biomech* 2006; 21(8):781–789.
27. Farley TF, Neumann CH, Steinbach LS, Petersen SA. The coracoacromial arch: MR evaluation and correlation with rotator cuff pathology. *Skeletal Radiol* 1994; 23(8):641–645.
28. van Drongelen S, Boninger ML, Impink BG, Khalaf T. Ultrasound imaging of acute bicep tendon changes after wheelchair sports. *Arch Phys Med Rehabil* 2007; 88(3):381–385.
29. Ferrara MS, Davis RW. Injuries to elite wheelchair athletes. *Paraplegia* 1990; 28(5):335–341.
30. Nyland J, Robinson K, Caborn D, Knapp E, Brosky T. Shoulder rotator torque and wheelchair dependence differences of National Wheelchair Basketball Association players. *Arch Phys Med Rehabil* 1997; 78(4):358–363.
31. Boninger ML, Cooper RA, Shimada SD, Rudy TE. Shoulder and elbow motion during two speeds of wheelchair propulsion: a description using a local coordinate system. *Spinal Cord* 1998; 36(6):418–426.
32. Crane CR, Raptou AD. The effect of exercise training on pulmonary function in persons with quadriplegia. *Paraplegia* 1994; 32(7):435–441.
33. Stefaniwsky L, Bilowit DS, Prasad SS. Reduced motor conduction velocity of the ulnar nerve in spinal cord injured patients. *Paraplegia* 1980; 18:21–24.
34. Gellman H, Chandler DR, Petrasek J, Sie I, Adkins R, Waters RL. Carpal tunnel syndrome in paraplegic patients. *J Bone Joint Surg Am* 1988; 70(4):517–519.
35. Aljure J, Eltorai I, Bradley WE, Lin JE, Johnson B. Carpal tunnel syndrome in paraplegic patients. *Paraplegia* 1985; 23(3):182–186.
36. Tun CG, Upton J. The paraplegic hand: electrodiagnostic studies and clinical findings. *J Hand Surg Am* 1988; 13:716–719.
37. Davidoff G, Werner R, Waring W. Compressive mononeuropathies of the upper extremity in chronic paraplegia. *Paraplegia* 1991; 29(1):17–24.
38. Yang J, Boninger ML, Leath J, Fitzgerald SG, Dyson-Hudson TA, Chang M. Carpal tunnel syndrome in manual wheelchair users with spinal cord injury: A cross-sectional multi-center study. *Am J Phys Med Rehabil* 2009; 88(12):1007–1016.
39. Walker H, Boninger ML, Impink BG, Malkiewicz AJ, Cooper RA. Ultrasound Evaluation of the median nerve before and after intense wheelchair activity. 51st Annual Meeting of the Association of Academic Physiatrists; Tucson, AZ: 2005.
40. Walker H, Boninger ML, Impink BG, Malkiewicz AJ, Cooper RA. Correlation between ultrasonographic median nerve characteristics and clinical symptoms in wheelchair users. 52nd Annual Meeting of the Association of Academic Physiatrists; Daytona Beach, FL: 2006.
41. Boninger ML, Cooper RA, Baldwin MA, Shimada SD, Koontz A. Wheelchair pushrim kinetics: body weight and median nerve function. *Arch Phys Med Rehabil* 1999; 80(8):910–915.
42. Boninger ML, Impink BG, Cooper RA, Koontz AM. Relation between median and ulnar nerve function and wrist kinematics during wheelchair propulsion. *Arch Phys Med Rehabil* 2004; 85(7):1141–1145.
43. Boninger ML, Cooper RA, Fitzgerald SG, Lin J, Cooper R, Dicianno B, Liu B. Investigating neck pain in wheelchair users. *Am J Phys Med Rehabil* 2003; 82(3):197–202.
44. Gertzbein SD. Scoliosis Research Society. Multicenter spine fracture study. *Spine* 1992 May; 17(5):528–540.
45. Whiteneck GG, Charlifue SW, Frankel HL, Fraser MH, Gardner BP, Gerhart KA, Krishnan KR, Menter RR, Nuseibeh I, Short DJ, et al. Mortality, morbidity, and psychosocial outcomes of persons spinal cord injured more than 20 years ago. *Paraplegia* 1992; 30(9):617–630.
46. Boninger ML, Saur T, Trefler E, Hobson DA, Burdett R, Cooper RA. Postural changes with aging in tetraplegia: effects on life satisfaction and pain. *Arch Phys Med Rehabil* 1998; 79(12):1571–1581.
47. Kirby RL, Fahie CL, Smith C, Chester EL, Macleod DA. Neck discomfort of wheelchair users: effect of neck position. *Disabil Rehabil* 2004; 26(1):9–15.
48. Preserving Upper Limb Function in Spinal Cord Injury: A Clinical Practice Guideline for Health-Care Professionals. 4-1-2005. Washington DC, Consortium for Spinal Cord Medicine. Spinal Cord Medicine, Clinical Practice Guideline.
49. DiGiovine CP, Cooper RA, Wolf E, Fitzgerald SG, Boninger ML. Analysis of whole-body vibration during manual wheelchair propulsion: a comparison of seat cushions and back supports for individuals without a disability. *Assist Technol* 2003; 15(2):129–144.
50. VanSickle DP, Cooper RA, Boninger ML, DiGiovine CP. Analysis of vibrations induced during wheelchair propulsion. *J Rehabil Res Dev* 2001; 38(4):409–421.
51. DiGiovine MM, Cooper RA, Boninger ML, Lawrence B, VanSickle DP, Rentschler AJ. User assessment of manual wheelchair ride comfort and ergonomics. *Arch Phys Med Rehabil* 2000; 81(4):490.
52. Maeda S, Futatsuka M, Yonesake J, Ikeda M. Relationship between Questionnaire Survey Results of Vibration Complaints of Wheelchair Users and Vibration Transmissibility of Manual Wheelchair. *Environ Health and Preventive Med* 2003; 8:82–89.
53. Musculoskeletal Disorders and Workplace Factors: A critical review of epidemiology for work related musculoskeletal disorders of the neck, upper extremity, and low back. Cincinnati, OH: National Institute for Occupational Safety and Health, Publications Dissemination, 1997.
54. Work-related musculoskeletal disorders: a review of the evidence. Washington, DC: National Academy Press, 1999.
55. Musculoskeletal Disorders and the Workplace: Low Back and Upper Extremities. Washington, DC: National Academy Press, 2001.
56. Chatterjee DS. Workplace upper limb disorders: a prospective study with intervention. *Occup Med (Lond)* 1992; 42(3):129–136.
57. Carson R. Reducing cumulative trauma disorders: use of proper workplace design. *AAOHN J* 1994; 42(6):270–276.
58. Boninger ML, Koontz AM, Sisto SA, Dyson-Hudson TA, Chang M, Price R, Cooper RA. Pushrim biomechanics and injury prevention in spinal cord injury: recommendations based on CULP-SCI investigations. *J Rehabil Res Dev* 2005; 42(3, Supp. 1):9–19.
59. Loslever P, Ranaivosoa A. Biomechanical and epidemiological investigation of carpal tunnel syndrome at workplaces with high risk factors. *Ergonomics* 1993; 36(5):537–555.
60. Werner RA, Franzblau A, Albers JW, Armstrong TJ. Median mononeuropathy among active workers- are there differences between symptomatic and asymptomatic workers. *Am J Ind Med* 1998; 33(4):374–378.
61. Cohen RB, Williams GR. Impingement syndrome and rotator cuff disease as repetitive motion disorders. *Clin Orthop Relat Res* 1998; (351):95–101.

62. Fredriksson K, Alfredsson L, Thorbjörnsson CB, Punnett L, Toomingas A, Torgén M, Kilbom A. Risk factors for neck and shoulder disorders: a nested case-control study covering a 24-year period. *Am J Ind Med* 2000; 38(5):516–528.

63. Goosey-Tolfrey VL, Lenton JP. A comparison between intermittent and constant wheelchair propulsion strategies. *Ergonomics* 2006; 15:49(11):1111–1120.

64. Neer CS. Impingement lesions. *Clin Orthop Relat Res* 1983; (173):70–77.

65. Brubaker CE, Ross S, McLaurin, CA. *Effect of seat position on handrim force.* Houston, TX, 1982.

66. Hughes CJ, Weimar WH, Sheth PN, Brubaker CE. Biomechanics of wheelchair propulsion as a function of seat position and user-to-chair interface. *Arch Phys Med Rehabil* 1992; 73:263–269.

67. Mulroy S, Newsam CJ, Gutierrez DD, Requejo P, Gronley JK, Haubert LL, Perry J. Effect of fore-aft seat position on shoulder demands during wheelchair propulsion: part 1. A Kinetic Analysis. *J Spinal Cord Med* 2005; 28(3):214–221.

68. Gutierrez DD, Mulroy SJ, Newsam CJ, Gronley JK, Perry J. Effect of fore-aft seat position on shoulder demands during wheelchair propulsion: part 2. An electromyographic analysis. *J Spinal Cord Med* 2005; 28(3):222–229.

69. Boninger ML, Baldwin MA, Cooper RA, Koontz AM, Chan L. Manual wheelchair pushrim biomechanics and axle position. *Arch Phys Med Rehabil* 2000; 81(5):608–613.

70. van der Woude LH, Veeger DJ, Rozendal RH, Sargeant TJ. Seat height in handrim wheelchair propulsion. *J Rehabil Res Dev* 1989; 26(4):31–50.

71. Koontz AM, Yang Y, Boninger DS, Kanaly J, Cooper RA, Boninger ML, Dieruf K, Ewer L. Investigation of the performance of an ergonomic handrim as a pain-relieving intervention for manual wheelchair users. *Assist Technol* 2006; 18(2):123–143.

72. Boninger ML, Souza AL, Cooper RA, Fitzgerald SG, Koontz AM, Fay BT. Propulsion patterns and pushrim biomechanics in manual wheelchair propulsion. *Arch Phys Med Rehabil* 2002; 83(5):718–723.

73. Wang YT, Kim CK, Ford HT, Ford HT. Reaction force and EMG analyses of wheelchair transfers. *Percept Mot Skills* 1994; 79(2):763–766.

74. van Drongelen S, van der Woude LH, Janssen TW, Angenot EL, Chadwick EK, Veeger DH. Glenohumeral contact forces and muscle forces evaluated in wheelchair-related activities of daily living in able-bodied subjects versus subjects with paraplegia and tetraplegia. *Arch Phys Med Rehabil* 2005; 86(7):1434–1440.

75. Perry J, Gronley JK, Newsam CJ, Reyes ML, Mulroy SJ. Electromyographic analysis of the shoulder muscles during depression transfers in subjects with low-level paraplegia. *Arch Phys Med Rehabil* 1996; 77(4): 350–355.

76. Grevelding P, Bohannon RW. Reduced push forces accompany device use during sliding transfers of seated subjects. *J Rehabil Res Dev* 2001; 38(1):135–139.

77. Cooper RA, Fitzgerald SG, Boninger ML, Prins K, Rentschler AJ, Arva J, O'Connor TJ. Evaluation of a pushrim-activated, power-assisted wheelchair. *Arch Phys Med Rehabil* 2001; 82(5):702–708.

78. Algood SD, Cooper RA, Fitzgerald SG, Cooper R, Boninger ML. Effect of a pushrim-activated power-assist wheelchair on the functional capabilities of persons with tetraplegia. *Arch Phys Med Rehabil* 2005; 86(3):380–386.

79. Arva J, Fitzgerald SG, Cooper RA, Boninger ML. Mechanical efficiency and user power requirement with a pushrim activated power assisted wheelchair. *Med Eng Phys* 2001; 23(10):699–705.

80. Waring WP, Maynard FM. Shoulder pain in acute traumatic quadriplegia. *Paraplegia* 1991; 29(1):37–42.

81. Pate RR, Pratt M, Blair SN, Haskell WL, Macera CA, Bouchard C, Buchner D, Ettinger W, Heath GW, King AC, et al. Physical activity and public health. A recommendation from the Centers for Disease Control and Prevention and the American College of Sports Medicine. *JAMA* 1995; 273(5):402–407.

82. Nash MS, van deVen I, van Elk N, Johnson BM. Effects of circuit resistance training on fitness attributes and upper-extremity pain in middle-aged men with paraplegia. *Arch Phys Med Rehabil* 2007; 88(1):70–75.

83. Arnstein PM. The neuroplastic phenomenon: a physiologic link between chronic pain and learning. J Neurosci Nurs 1997; 29(3):179–186.

84. D'Arcy CA, McGee S. The rational clinical examination does this patient have carpal tunnel syndrome? *JAMA* 2000; 283(23):3110–3117.

85. Wiggins ME, Fadale PD, Barrach H, Ehrlich MG, Walsh WR. Healing characteristics of a type I collagenous structure treated with corticosteroids. *Am J Sports Med* 1994; 22(2):279–288.

86. Gazielly DF, Gleyze P, Montagnon C. Functional and anatomical results after rotator cuff repair. *Clin Orthop Relat Res* 1994; (304):43–53.

87. Botte MJ, von Schroeder HP, Abrams RA, Gellman H. Recurrent carpal tunnel syndrome. *Hand Clin* 1996; 12(4):731–743.

88. Nancollas MP, Peimer CA, Wheeler DR, Sherwin FS. Long-term results of carpal tunnel release. *J Hand Surg [Br]* 1995; 20(4):470–474.

89. Robinson MD, Hussey RW, Ha CY. Surgical decompression of impingement in the weightbearing shoulder. *Arch Phys Med Rehabil* 1993; 74(3):324–327.

90. Goldstein B, Young J, Escobedo EM. Rotator cuff repairs in individuals with paraplegia. *Am J Phys Med Rehabil* 1997; 76(4):316–322.

91. Popowitz R, Zvijac J, Uribe J, Hechtman K, Schurhoff M, Green J. Rotator cuff repair in spinal cord injury patients. *J Shoulder Elbow Surg* 2003; 12(4):327–332.

47 Extremity Fractures in Spinal Cord Injury

Douglas E. Garland
Dudley Fukunaga

Extremity fracture management in spinal cord injury (SCI) is summarized by the following principles. Upper extremity (UE) fracture care should follow standard orthopedic principles with a tendency toward surgical fixation in both acute and chronic SCI. Most lower extremity (LE) fractures in acute SCI, including the hip, should undergo open reduction and internal fixation (ORIF). In chronic SCI individuals, femoral neck fractures require an endoprosthesis. Chronic SCI individuals with displaced intertrochanteric (IT) fractures require intramedullary hip fixation. Likewise, femoral shaft and displaced tibia shaft fractures in chronic SCI require intramedullary locked nails. Conversely, nondisplaced IT, distal femur/proximal tibia, tibia shaft, foot, and ankle fractures in chronic SCI may be managed by nonoperative splinting.

The approach to the treatment of fractures in individuals with SCI has evolved over the last century due to the advances in knowledge, newer surgical principles, and improved technologies. The incidence of SCI is approximately 35 people per one million annually. The occurrence of concomitant extremity fractures in acute SCI is 28% (1–4). Motor vehicle accidents remain the most common cause of SCI, as well as associated extremity fractures (5). Gunshot wounds (GSW) are a common etiology of SCI but have few associated fractures and are clustered in urban areas where much of the SCI research is conducted. Few centers develop expertise in SCI, especially in the treatment of concomitant injuries, which leads to a paucity of literature addressing the management of acute extremity fractures with acute SCI. Most studies make only a minor reference to acute fractures or combine them with pathologic fractures in the chronic SCI patient. Furthermore, there has been an unwarranted tendency to apply treatment principles of pathologic fractures to that of the acute situation.

GENERAL

Modern principles of general fracture management were outlined by Comarr in 1962 and have influenced treatment through the last half of the twentieth century (6). Treatment principles were based on the final neurologic outcome, namely completeness. Long bone fractures were divided into four classes: I—fractured UE concomitant with cord injury; II—fractured LE concomitant with cord injury; III—fractured UE after cord injury; and IV—fractured LE after cord injury.

Fractures above the neurologic insult or in individuals with incomplete injuries and functioning extremities were treated according to standard orthopedic principles. Nonoperative treatment with pillow splints was advocated for long bone fractures below the level of a complete neurologic injury.

Alignment and shortening were deemphasized in the nonambulatory patient. Circular casts were discouraged secondary to complications such as limited range of motion and skin breakdown. Open reduction and internal fixation (ORIF) often resulted in complications, sometimes disastrous. Of the 81 LE fractures in Comarr's report, five were nonunions (12.5%) (6).

Multiple authors after Comarr's landmark report have addressed the dilemmas encountered with treatment of pathologic fractures in chronic SCI with ORIF. They usually excluded acute fracture management concomitant with SCI, although some combined them. Their documented complication rate after ORIF (mostly from pathologic fracture experience) reinforced Comarr's conclusions (7–22).

Two later studies emerged however, reporting that ORIF could be predictably and safely performed in the acute setting. Tricot and Hallot reported on 192 paraplegics with 39 concomitant acute fractures from 1963 to 1967 and found no contraindication to surgical osteosynthesis while recommending its use in most instances once spinal shock was resolved. All fractures treated with osteosynthesis achieved union with no complication (7). In 1967, Meinecke, Rehn, and Leitz reported on 128 acute SCI extremity fractures. Fifty-three patients had 64 fractures below the level of SCI. They concluded and recommended ORIF of long bone fractures based on their fracture outcome, as well as the facilitation of rehabilitation (8).

A study by McMaster and Stauffer in 1975 updated Comarr's classification: I—acute fracture suffered in the same accident that rendered the SCI; II—pathologic fracture in an osteoporotic extremity in chronic SCI; and III—traumatic fracture in a chronic SCI-injured patient who is involved in another high-energy accident (16).

Twenty-five participants in Class I had 27 acute fractures. They noted two complications in the ORIF group; one delayed union and one wound infection in 19 surgical procedures, for a complication rate of 11%. The complication rate was higher in the nonoperative group. In that group, 15 of 24 (62%) had complications including 5 delayed unions, 2 nonunions, 4 malunions, and 4 skin pressure sores.

McMaster and Stauffer observed that nonoperative treatment had a prolonged course of healing and a high insufficient union rate despite the concept of exuberant callous in SCI patients (16). Based on these key findings, ORIF was recommended for the class I group with grossly unstable fractures or for those requiring casting for stability. Pillow splints were recommended for fractures when open techniques were contraindicated (16). The Comarr and McMaster studies set the initial standard for acute fracture care in SCI in the United States while the Europeans were drifting toward a more aggressive surgical approach.

FRACTURE IN ACUTE SCI

Fracture in the acute SCI patient is an injury complex that is deserving of special, specific guidelines. The goals of acute fracture care in the acute SCI patient should produce a high rate of union, maintain length, prevent angular deformities, and maximize functional return. Furthermore, fracture management should facilitate medical, nursing, and rehabilitation issues without compounding the patient's disability (6).

During the last century, neurologic dysfunction often dictated treatment principles of fracture management. As a result, treatment principles have often been based on the premise that the complete SCI individual will not ambulate in his or her lifetime. But the new millennium shows promise in improved neurologic function and the possibility of gait. This necessitates a reevaluation of fracture care, both acute and pathologic.

The most common acute long bone injury is the femur, followed by tibia, humerus, radius, and ulna fractures. Recent data have shown improved outcome with operative stabilization regardless of the neurological status.

Femoral Shaft Fractures

The records of individuals with acute SCI and femoral shaft fractures admitted to the SCI service at Rancho Los Amigos National Rehabilitation Center (RLANRC) from 1969 to 1982 were reviewed to compare operative versus nonoperative fracture treatment (17). The femoral shaft was defined as the region from 1 cm inferior to the less trochanter to the supracondylar area. The records identified 23 patients with 27 femoral shaft fractures. Nineteen of these fractures were classified as transverse, 8 were comminuted, and only 1 was open. Eleven of these fractures were treated with nonoperative methods, and 8 fractures were treated with ORIF. Due to angular deformity or lack of callous formation, 8 fractures in the nonoperative group were eventually treated with ORIF after 6 weeks. The average time to union was 14 weeks in the nonoperative group. However, all patients who underwent ORIF developed bridging callous within 12 weeks of

surgery. There was an impending nonunion rate in 6 of 16 patients (31%) who received closed treatment. Eight fractures (73%) developed malunion in the nonoperative group. In contrast, only two patients developed malunion in the operative group. Two complications (12.5%) were related to surgery, which include a painful prominent rod that had to be removed at 6 months, and osteomyelitis that occurred in a diabetic patient after ORIF with plate fixation.

Medical complications were higher in the nonoperative group versus the operative group. There were six decubitus ulcers in the nonoperative group consistent with prolonged bed rest necessary for healing, including four that required surgery. Two patients in the operative group developed deep vein thrombosis (DVT) after ORIF with plates.

Nonoperative treatment was not associated with exuberant callus but displayed a higher rate of nonunion and medical complications (17). Nearly one-third of the femurs failed to demonstrate callus or were impending nonunions. The best results were achieved by early stabilization of femoral shaft fractures with locked intramedullary rods, regardless of neurologic improvement. Surgical fixation facilitates rehabilitation activities and decreases orthopedic and medical complications.

Tibia Fractures

The records of all patients with tibia fractures and acute SCI at RLANRC between January 1968 and December 1982 were reviewed (18). The records identified 28 individuals with 34 tibia fractures. These patients were classified into three groups: nonoperative, operative, and fractures with Type III open injuries. Fractures with joint extension were excluded.

The nonoperative group consisted of 17 fractures; 10 were closed and 7 were open fractures. Six fractures (35%) had delayed union or nonunion, and three fractures (18%) were labeled as radiographic malunions. The average time to union was 6.5 months. Again, the medical complications were significant in the nonoperative group, occurring in 7 of 17 patients (36%). These complications included two pulmonary emboli (PE) and 5 sacral pressures sores that required surgery.

In the operative group, 11 tibia fractures underwent ORIF. Five fractures were closed and six were open. The average time to surgery was 12 days, and the average time to union was 12 weeks, compared to 6.5 months in the nonoperative group. There were only two (18%) surgical complications. One distal fracture developed delayed union that united at 7 months. A superficial wound infection healed uneventfully. The only medical complication was a DVT.

The third group consisted of six tibia fractures with significant Type III fractures with soft tissue injuries. All six patients underwent initial debridement. Three patients underwent ORIF, and the other three were treated with orthotic methods after initial external fixation. All six Type III fractures had delayed or nonunions. Two of the three patients who did not undergo ORIF developed angular deformities of 13 and 17 degrees of varus. Two patients had chronic osteomyelitis. Medical complications occurred in three of the six (50%) patients; two patients developed sacral pressure sores that required surgery and one developed a PE.

Due to a combination of factors including the severity of the injury, poor function, and a mean bone loss of 20% during the

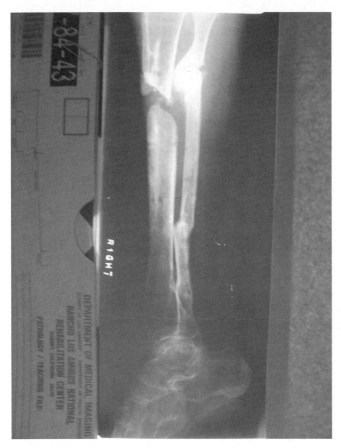

Figure 47.1 A good example of an open acute fracture that barely unites.

Table 47.1 UE Fracture Distribution in Acute SCI			
INJURY	NONOPERATIVE	OPERATIVE	TOTAL
Humerus	12	8	20
Radius	14	5	19
Ulna	0	8	8
Radius and ulna	3	3	6
Total	29	24	53

All eight ulna fractures were managed operatively and achieved union and acceptable ROM and rehabilitation times similar to other groups. There were two minor pin complications that required removal after union was achieved.

Six participants were identified with combined radius and ulna fractures. Two of the three fractures that were managed nonoperatively eventually required surgery for malunion and nonunion. Two open fractures treated operatively developed synostosis.

Upper extremity fractures should be managed according to standard orthopedic rules with a tendency toward ORIF to facilitate predictable fracture outcome and rehabilitation.

Conclusion

Past treatment principles for extremity fractures in the acute SCI individual were based on the premise that the complete SCI individual would never ambulate in their lifetime and therefore standard orthopedic fracture management was not necessary. This often led to nonoperative treatment and subsequent poor fracture outcome.

The trend toward operative fixation of long bone fractures in acute SCI has been evolving over decades. Most fractures were initially treated nonoperatively. Later, nonoperative treatment was reserved for complete injuries with functionless extremities. Recent studies have emerged demonstrating that nonoperative treatment prolongs healing and leads to limb shortening and angular deformities.

The previous misconception that LE fractures heal rapidly due to exuberant callus and that operative fixation often failed served to reinforce nonoperative treatment. Our studies have demonstrated that there are fewer medical complications and more rapid union with intramedullary nailing of femur and tibia fractures. Therefore, acute LE fractures associated with acute SCI should undergo operative fixation whether the patient is neurologically complete or incomplete. Only nondisplaced, low-energy fractures that can be easily and effectively treated with orthoses should be managed nonoperatively.

Upper extremity function is of vital importance to the SCI patient for wheelchair propulsion, transfers, and assisted ambulation. Rehabilitation programs stress the need for early functional skills to maximize the patient's adaptive potential (4). Similar functional results were demonstrated in humerus fractures for the operative versus nonoperative groups. However, operative management may be more desirable for humerus fractures because it can facilitate rehabilitation. Surgical fixation is the accepted management for radius and ulna fractures in the general population, and this may apply to acute SCI patients with

first year of SCI, diaphyseal tibia fractures in SCI do not heal more rapidly than the general population (Figure 47.1). Furthermore, nonoperative treatment of tibia fractures had a higher rate of medical complications and nonunion than the operative group. Therefore, ORIF with an intramedullary nail is recommended for tibia fractures regardless of neurologic lesion. An extremity free of splints and external devices facilitates transfer training, ROM exercises, and activities of daily living (18).

Upper Extremity Fractures

The records of individuals with acute SCI and upper extremity (UE) fractures from 1970 to 1986 were reviewed (23). Fifty-two patients with 59 fractures were identified to compare operative versus nonoperative treatment. Twenty-four patients received operative treatment, and the remaining 29 patients utilized nonoperative treatment (Table 47.1). Treatment outcome was evaluated by comparing time to union, range of motion (ROM), total rehabilitation time, and complications (23).

Humerus fractures comprised 20 of the 53 UE fractures. No difference was seen between the operative and nonoperative groups with respect to time to union, ROM, or rehabilitation time.

Of the 19 radius fractures identified, 5 were managed operatively, and 14 were nonoperative cases. Like the humerus fracture group, there was no significant difference in terms of time to union, ROM, or rehabilitation time.

forearm fractures. UE fracture care should follow general orthopedic principles with a tendency toward surgical fixation.

FRACTURE IN CHRONIC SCI (PATHOLOGICAL FRACTURES)

The overall incidence of pathologic fractures in chronic SCI patients has been reported as high as 40%. These pathologic fractures are caused by relatively minor trauma such as transferring, falls from a wheelchair, or may occur without known injury. However, the incidence may be even higher because many patients with "trivial," painless fractures may never seek medical attention or may be treated at non-SCI centers. Paraplegics have a higher incidence of pathologic fractures than tetraplegics due to the greater degree of function, mobility, and participation in various physical activities (4). Furthermore, the fracture rate is 10 times greater in individuals with complete lesions compared to those with incomplete lesions. Pathologic fractures in chronic SCI often present with soft tissue swelling, increase in limb girth, warmth, spasticity, deformity, or symptoms of autonomic dysreflexia (1, 2, 4, 22).

Chronic SCI patients have numerous altered physiologic factors that affect the management of long bone fractures. These patients have negative nitrogen and calcium balance as well as impaired skin sensitivity, resulting in a propensity to develop decubitus ulcers, along with poor wound and fracture healing.

Fracture site correlates with the specific bone mineral density (BMD) level in chronic SCI patients. Males with complete chronic SCI lose 33% of the bone mineral density at the knee within 1.5–2 years after injury. Females with complete SCI lose 40% to 45% of their BMD at the knee within 1.5–2 years (24). Patients with known LE fractures have 50% or greater bone loss of BMD at their knee. This 50% reduction of BMD at the knee is the fracture breakpoint for this population (25). Females with SCI are at fracture risk at the knee soon after SCI and should be counseled regarding osteoporosis and potential for fracture.

General

Records were reviewed of chronic SCI patients who presented with pathologic extremity fractures to the primary care and orthopedic SCI clinics from January 1991 to December 1995. Seventy-three patients with 99 pathologic fractures were identified. Ninety-three fractures occurred in the LE, and seven occurred in the UE. Thirty-four (35%) of the fractures were about the knee (Table 47.2).

The average time of pathologic fracture from initial SCI was 6.5 years (range, 8 months to 20 years). The majority of the patients were treated as outpatients with nonoperative methods, such as braces, splints, casts, and pillow splints. Circumferential casts were not used, and if used, were bivalved (6, 9, 16, 21). Some patients were admitted for observation of soft tissue swelling, blood loss, possible autonomic dysreflexia, or for surgery.

The most commonly encountered pathologic fractures were supracondylar fractures of the femur, followed by proximal tibia and tibial shaft fractures. Fractures that occurred above the knee frequently required acute hospitalization and have made up the majority of reports from SCI centers. Conversely, fractures below the knee often did not require aggressive treatment (1, 2).

Femoral Neck Fractures

Displaced femoral neck fractures are not commonly encountered but pose a management dilemma. If untreated, the femur may migrate proximally, unbalancing the pelvis and causing pressure sores (22). In the past, displaced femoral neck fractures were often treated nonoperatively, leading to secondary complications such as pelvic obliquity and leg shortening. When reduced and pinned, the result was fixation failure and nonunion. Endoprosthetic replacement is associated with early and late subluxation. Dislocation should be anticipated due to adductor spasticity, and the rate of infection may be higher due to recurrent urinary tract infections.

The fracture complication rate for a displaced femoral neck fracture is much higher in the SCI population than in the general population. Predictors of potential complications include lower extremity spasticity, existing subluxation, displaced fractures, and significant osteoporosis.

Nondisplaced femoral neck fractures also pose management dilemmas. Two of four (50%) nondisplaced femoral neck fractures were treated nonoperatively and had significant complications, including nonunions with subluxation of the distal femoral fragment proximally. Operative treatment with cannulated screw fixation does not ensure stability or union.

Because there is lack of a consensus in the literature to support a clear treatment recommendation, the decision of operative versus nonoperative management is based on the individual situation depending on the patient's age, activity level, general health, and potential complications. Endoprosthetic replacement appears to provide the more predictable outcome.

Table 47.2   Fracture Distribution in Chronic SCI

				NONUNION		COMPLICATION	
FRACTURE TYPE	NUMBER	NONOPERATIVE	OPERATIVE	NONOPERATIVE	OPERATIVE	NONOPERATIVE	OPERATIVE
Femoral neck	20	12	8	3 (25%)	2 (25%)	2 (17%)	2 (25%)
IT	11	7	4	0	0	7 (0%)	2 (50%)
Subtrochanteric	9	7	2	0	0	1 (11%)	
Femoral shaft	31	29	2	2 (6%)	0	9 (31%)	1 (50%)
Supracondylar	34	34	0	0	0	4 (12%)	
Tibia shaft	20	19	0	0	0	1 (5%)	
Tibia metaphysis	17	16	1	0	0	3 (16%)	

Intertrochanteric Fractures

Nonoperative treatment of intertrochanteric fractures is often associated with varus deformity of the hip. This may lead to a pelvic tilt or a prominent trochanter and cause pressure sores. Operative treatment with a side plate and screws may lead to fixation failure due to osteoporosis. The preferred operative management is a locked intramedullary hip fixation that facilitates near-anatomic alignment and union without clinical complications.

Femoral Shaft Fractures

Nonoperative management of femoral shaft fractures is cumbersome, especially in spastic patients. Casts and splints are inadequate for union. Displaced femoral shaft fractures often lead to nonunion. Individuals may require prolonged bed rest, possibly leading to pressure sores.

External fixation may be effective but has its own set of complications, including fixation failure from pin loosening through osteoporotic bone and possible stress fracture through the pin site at a later date. Furthermore, immobilization by external fixation may interfere with patient positioning.

Operative treatment has proven to facilitate union without a significant increase in complications. Therefore, the preferred method of treatment for displaced or nondisplaced femoral shaft fractures is intramedullary rodding with interlocking screws.

Locking screws are necessary for rotational stability due to the large intramedullary canals seen in osteoporosis.

Distal Femur/Proximal Tibia Fractures

Minimally or nondisplaced distal femur or proximal tibial fractures are the most prevalent fractures encountered in the chronic SCI population (Figure 47.2). The treatment of choice is nonoperative management with well-padded splints or knee immobilizers (9). These orthoses provide adequate immobilization and provide access for frequent skin inspection to lower the risk of skin breakdown. Pillow splints have been widely used in the past, but are bulky and make mobilization difficult. Displaced distal femur fractures may require surgery in which retrograde intramedullary nails through the knee are advantageous.

Tibial Shaft Fractures

Tibia shaft fractures heal predictably if minimally or nondisplaced, and can be treated nonoperatively with well-padded splints (Figure 47.3). Displaced tibia shaft fractures or fractures wherein splint treatment is not feasible due to skin breakdown require interlocking intramedullary fixation.

Ankle Fractures

Ankle fractures are usually low-energy fracture patterns that unite uneventfully with nonoperative treatment in a well-padded

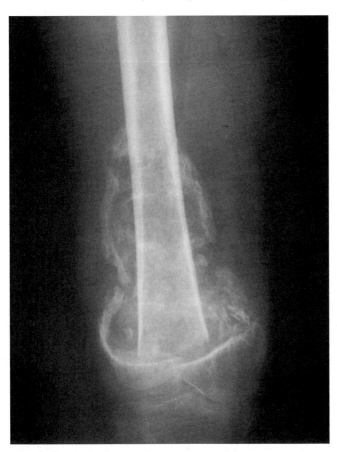

Figure 47.2 This type of supracondylar femur fracture responds well to nonoperative methods. Note the so-called exuberant callus that took many months to evolve, and union was slow.

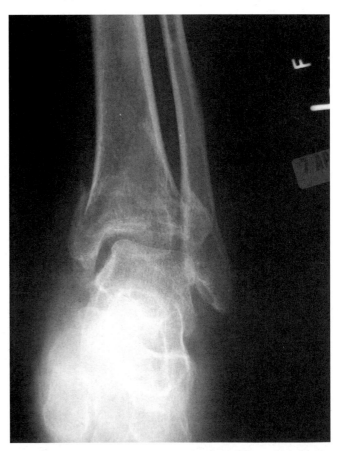

Figure 47.3 A typical low-energy fracture of the distal tibia and fibula. These fractures unite with nonoperative methods.

posterior splint or cam walker. Healing may be either bony or fibrous union without complications. However, alignment is essential. Varus-valgus angular deformities leads to malleolar pressure sores and fixed equinus. Therefore, the ankle should always be maintained in neutral position in the anterior-posterior or lateral planes to avoid skin breakdown from bony prominences and equinus deformities.

Foot Fractures

Foot fractures are usually non-displaced and commonly occur at the metatarsal base or toes. These fractures unite with a soft splint without consequence. The foot should be maintained at a neutral position so that a plantigrade foot can be maintained.

Upper Extremity Fractures

Although fractures in the UE in individuals with SCI are uncommon, preservation of upper extremity function is essential for activities such as wheelchair propulsion and transferring. Management of pathologic fractures that occur in the aged SCI population and in occasional patients with incomplete tetraplegia should follow general orthopedic principles, with an emphasis on preserving function. Nondisplaced, low-energy fractures respond to splinting.

Conclusion

In individuals with chronic SCI and a swollen extremity, a high index of suspicion of an extremity fracture must be made. A careful history of trauma, however minor, should be carefully sought in individuals with SCI, as well as any increase in spasticity or sweating, which should alert the clinician of the possibility of an occult fracture. The only sign on examination may be a late-onset of swelling.

Management of the extremity fracture varies regarding operative versus nonoperative treatment depending on the location of the pathological fracture. Femoral neck fractures continue to pose a difficult management dilemma due to the poor fixation in osteoporotic bone. Endoprosthetic replacement is preferred. Some intertrochanteric and femoral shaft fractures should be managed operatively with interlocking, intramedullary fixation. Conversely, distal femur and proximal tibia fractures may be managed nonoperatively with well-padded splints and knee immobilizers that allow frequent skin inspections. However, displaced tibia shaft fractures should be treated with an interlocking, intramedullary fixation. Fractures in distal tibia, ankle, and foot all respond with splinting, although alignment is essential. Management of UE fractures, although uncommon, should follow general orthopedic principles.

Previous treatment guidelines for SCI LE fractures were based on the premise that the complete SCI individual will not ambulate and does not require near normal fracture outcomes. However, the future for nerve regeneration holds promise, and restoration of some function will eventually become a reality. The new millennium offers the potential of standing and even ambulation in some modified form. Furthermore, new treatment of osteoporosis will assist in future prevention and possibly strengthen bone for improved fixation. Fracture care should begin to mimic that of the able-bodied individual.

References

1. Kraus JF. Epidemiologic aspects of acute spinal cord injury: a review of incidence, prevalence, causes and outcome. In: Becker DP, Povlishock JT, eds. *Central Nervous System Trauma Status Report, 1985*. Washington, DC: National Institutes of Health, 1988; 312–322.
2. Go BK, DeVivo MJ, Richards JS. The epidemiology of spinal cord injury. In: Stover SL, Delisa JA, Whiteneck GG, eds. *Spinal Cord Injury: Clinical Outcomes from the Model Systems*. Gaithersburg, MD: Aspen, 1995; 21–55.
3. Burke DA, Linden RD, Zhang YP, et al. Incidence rates and populations at risk for spinal cord injury: a regional study. *Spinal Cord* 2001; 39:274–278.
4. Wang CM, Chen Y, DeVivo MJ, Huang CT. Epidemiology of extraspinal fractures associated with acute spinal cord injury. *Spinal Cord* 2001; 39(11):589–594.
5. Saboe LA, Reid DC, Davis LA, et al. Spine trauma and associated injuries. *J Trauma* 1991; 31:43–48.
6. Comarr AE, Hutchinson RH, Bors E. Extremity fracture of patients with spinal cord injuries. *Am J Surg* 1962; 103:732–739.
7. Tricot, A, Hallot R. Traumatic paraplegia and associated fractures. *Paraplegia* 1968; (5):211–215.
8. Meinecke FW, Rehn J, Leitz G. Conservative and operative treatment of fractures of the limbs in paraplegia. In: *Proceedings of the Annual Clinical Spinal Cord Injury Conference* 1967; 17:77.
9. El Ghatit AS, Lamid S, Flatley TJ. Posterior splint for leg fractures in the spinal cord injured patients. *Am J Phys Med* 1981; 60:239.
10. Levine AM, Krebs M, Santos-Mendoza N. External fixation in quadriplegia. *Clin Orthop* 1984; 184:169–172.
11. Sobel M, Lyden JP. Long bone fracture in a spinal-cord injured patient: complication of treatment—a case report and review of literature. *J Trauma* 1991; 31(10):1440–1444.
12. Baird RA, Kreitenberg A, Eltorai I. External fixation of femoral shaft fractures in spinal cord injury patients. *Paraplegia* 1986; 24:183–190.
13. Baird RA, Kreitenberg A. Treatment of femoral shaft fractures in the spinal cord injury patient using the Wagner leg lengthening device. *Paraplegia* 1984; 22:366–372.
14. Staub PL. Orthopaedic surgery on paraplegic patients. *Am J Surg* 1950; 79:717.
15. Azaria M, Anner A, Ohry A. Long bone fractures in spinal cord injured patients pose orthopaedic and rehabilitation problems. *Orthop Rev* 1983; 12:69.
16. McMaster WC, Stauffer ES. The management of long bone fracture in the spinal cord injured patient. *Clin Orthop* 1975; 112:44–52.
17. Garland DE, Reiser TV, Singer DI. Treatment of femoral shaft fractures associated with acute spinal cord injuries. *Clin Orthop* 1985; 197:191–195.
18. Garland DE, Saucedo T, Reiser TV. The management of tibial fractures in acute spinal cord injury patients. *Clin Orthop* 1988; 213:237–240.
19. Ragnarsson KT, Sell GH. Lower extremity fractures after spinal cord injury: a retrospective study. *Arch Phys Med Rehabil* 1981; 62:418–423.
20. Eichenholtz SN. Management of long-bone fracture in paraplegic patients. *J Bone Joint Surg* 1963; 45A:299–310.
21. Freehafer AA, Mast WA. Lower extremity fractures in patients with spinal cord injury. *J Bone Joint Surg* 1965; 47A:683.
22. Garland D. Clinical observations on fractures and heterotopic ossification in the spinal cord and traumatic brain injured population. *Clin Orthop* 1988; 233:286.
23. Garland DE, Jones RC, Kunkle RW. Upper extremity fractures in the acute spinal cord injured patient. *Clin Orthop* 1988; 233:110–115.
24. Garland DE, Adkins RH, Stewart CA, Ashford R, Vigil D. Regional osteoporosis in women who have a complete spinal cord injury. *J Bone Joint Surg* 2001; 83A:1195–1200.
25. Garland DE, Adkins RH, Stewart CA, Ashford R. Fracture threshold and risk for osteoporosis and pathologic fractures in individuals with spinal cord injury. *Top Spinal Cord Inj Rehab* 2005; 11:61–69.

48 Functional Restoration of the Upper Extremity in Tetraplegia

Vincent R. Hentz
Catherine M. Curtin
Caroline Leclercq

With continued improvements in the emergency resuscitation of cervical spinal cord injuries, greater numbers of patients with higher levels of injuries are surviving. These patients reach rehabilitation facilities with heightened expectations regarding recovery and with significant rehabilitative demands.

In addition, because of the increasing acceptance that surgery can play an important role in restoring function to the paralyzed upper extremity, greater numbers of tetraplegic patients are knowledgeable about upper extremity surgery and inquire regarding the appropriateness of surgery for their hands and arms. People with tetraplegia express a greater desire to have function restored to their hands than to have, for example, sexual function restored.

HISTORICAL PERSPECTIVE

In the minds of both physiatrists and surgeons, the appropriateness of surgical reconstruction for the tetraplegic's upper extremity has waxed and waned in acceptance since the initial reports of Bunnell (1) in the l940s. The many factors that are responsible for the varying attitudes toward surgery are discussed here.

In l949, Bunnell (1) described his results with procedures designed to provide an automatic finger grasp and release and tip-to-tip, or so-called opposition pinch, for tetraplegic patients possessing active wrist extension. This was accomplished by multiple tenodeses (implanting a tendon into bone) so that the fingers would automatically flex with wrist extension and would automatically open with wrist flexion. Additionally, with wrist extension, the thumb and the index and middle fingertips were brought together in so-called opposition, or three-jawed chuck pinch. Muscle transfers were used occasionally instead of tenodeses, but Bunnell's goal for the thumb remained focused on achieving tip-to-tip pinch because this was felt to represent refined function. In general, Bunnell's patients would be classified at C6 and C7 functional levels according to current standards.

Some years later, at Rancho Los Amigos Hospital, Nickel and his colleagues (2) attempted to extend hand surgery to tetraplegics with less residual upper extremity function. They devised a complex operation involving multiple joint arthrodeses to pre-position the fingers and thumb and multiple tenodeses to achieve an automatic opposition-type or tip-to-tip pinch between thumb, index, and middle fingers. In actuality, it was difficult to achieve the precise digital posture needed for accurate thumb opposition. Some patients were unhappy with the stiff fingers, a consequence of the fusions. Although this surgical procedure fell into disfavor, its external corollary, a mechanical device or orthosis that holds the fingers and thumbs in the necessary position, became the standard orthosis. The Rancho design of the wrist-driven flexor hand splint and various modifications of this splint still remain the standard functional orthosis for the tetraplegic's hand, even today (Figure 48.1.)

During the l960s and early l970s, several pioneer reconstructive extremity surgeons, including Lamb and Landry (3) in Scotland and Zancolli (4) in Argentina, were reporting good results using active muscle-tendon transfers to substitute for missing function. However, during the decade of the 1950s and 1960s, surgery was not held in high regard because of the more than occasional poor result. The results of muscle-tendon transfers were sometimes unpredictable because frequently the transferred muscle was spastic. Patients did not appreciate stiff contracted fingers that could result from transfer of such spastic muscles. Guttmann (5), in his textbook on spinal cord management, stated in l976 that fewer than 5% of tetraplegic patients were candidates for hand surgery.

In l975 a Swedish hand surgeon, Erik Moberg (6), published his philosophy regarding the role of hand surgery in tetraplegia and described his results in reconstructing two important functions missing in the majority of tetraplegic patients (Figure 48.2). Moberg held four strong opinions:

l. Aside from the brain, the hand of the tetraplegic represents his most important residual resource. However the tetraplegic uses his hands differently from any other patient in that he must walk on his hands. Failure to recognize the functional demands of the tetraplegic's hands led to poorly designed arthrodeses and tenodeses that broke down in response to these demands.

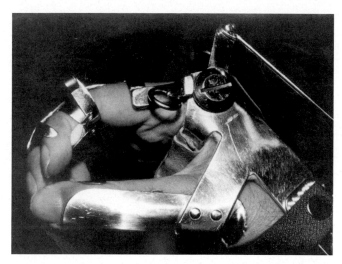

Figure 48.1   The wrist-driven flexor hinge splint was designed by engineers from the Rancho Los amigos Hospital and is referred to as the "Rancho" splint. It is designed to stabilize all joints except the wrist and the metacarpophalangeal joints of the index and middle finger. The thumb is held in a position of opposition as a fixed post. Flexion of the wrist results in extension of the index and middle fingers at their metacarpophalangeal joints. This opens the hand. Wrist extension brings the tips of the index and middle fingers against the rigidly stabilized thumb tip.

2. As the most important residual resource, the hand has three primary roles: gripping, feeling, and human contact. Moberg believed that supple hands are preferred for human contact and that the stiff clawed hands of previous years were unacceptable.
3. When limited functional resources remain after injury, surgery should represent essentially no risk to these residual resources. Therefore, especially for patients whose cervical cord injuries are more proximal, surgery should be reversible.
4. Moberg believed that the key grip, or lateral pinch, between the broad pulp of the thumb and the side of the index finger was far more useful for the tetraplegic patient than the opposition-type pinch favored by almost all his predecessors. Moberg believed that for the so-called C5–C6 patient, the largest single group of tetraplegic patients, the goal of surgery should be reconstruction of active elbow extension and a key grip for at least one extremity.

Moberg remained a champion of the role of surgery for tetraplegic patients until his death in the spring of l993. His philosophy has personally guided the development of our program in surgical reconstruction for tetraplegic patients at the Palo Alto VAMC Spinal Cord Injury Center over the past 25 years. We (7–10) have enlarged upon Moberg's philosophy as we have gained experience. Tetraplegics with greater numbers of residual motor resources are candidates for the reconstruction of more functional hands than can be achieved by the creation of only a key or lateral pinch. Some minimal risk for these patients is acceptable. Even after 20 years, we still follow Moberg's dictums, especially for patients who present with little remaining function in the upper limb. Stimulated by Moberg and recognizing that

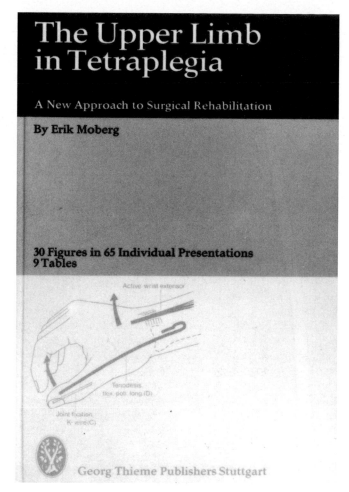

Figure 48.2   The cover of Erik Moberg's monograph *The Upper Limb in Tetraplegia: A New Approach to Surgical Reconstruction* (14).

Moberg's 1978 publication had become somewhat outdated, we combined our experiences from two spinal injury centers and published a more current monograph in 2002 (10).

THE SHOULDER IN THE TETRAPLEGIC PATIENT

Shoulder pain is a common sequela of spinal cord injury (11). Silfverskiold (12) studied a population of spinal cord–injured patients and determined that 78% of tetraplegics experienced some shoulder symptoms during the first 6 months following injury. By 18 months, the percentage had decreased, but there were still patients with significant shoulder pain, which interfered with function. Symptoms of chronic shoulder pathology include pain, stiffness, and weakness. The management of chronic shoulder pathology requires, above all, a correct diagnosis.

The pathophysiology of shoulder dysfunction in the tetraplegic patient depends upon the level of the spinal cord injury and which shoulder muscles are weakened or absent. Muscles that remain well innervated can respond to increased functional demands by hypertrophy. However, the tetraplegic patient's shoulder is at risk to both acute and chronic shoulder pathology by virtue of the lack of full motor power about the shoulder. Moreover, these patients often lack the necessary muscle resources for the familiar muscle-tendon transfers. Because they are dependent on upper limb function for every aspect of their lives, especially movement, operating on them for shoulder pathology is complicated by formidable functional, social, and psychologic risks.

The genesis of shoulder pathology is clear. It begins from the moment of injury. Eliminating all discussion of concomitant or preexisting shoulder injury, let us focus on the etiology of acute shoulder problem. First, the tetraplegic patient lies for long hours in bed recovering from the injury, or surgery for spinal stabilization. In bed, the scapulae are pushed forward into medial rotation (Figure 48.3). The arm frequently rests for long periods in internal rotation at the glenohumeral joint. Without great diligence on the part of the acute care team, capsular tightness rapidly develops. Once even minimally established, attempts at therapy typically trigger a second pathologic feature, spasticity of parascapular and other upper motor neuron–injured muscles. Campbell (11) found the following shoulder pathologies in twenty-four tetraplegic patients during the acute period of rehabilitation: capsular contracture/capsulitis, rotator cuff tears, anterior instability, and osteonecrosis/osteoarthritis. In the end, shoulder pain is a formidable deterrent to rehabilitation goals.

The treatment for the acutely painful shoulder is, of course, prevention and rapid aggressive response to the earliest signs of difficulty. This includes pain control modalities, anti-inflammatory treatments, antispastic and antiadrenergic pharmacology, and gentle but persistent therapy. This can be a big challenge for the patient and rehabilitation team.

Without a full complement of stabilizing muscles, the patient experiences instability, with the principal direction of instability depending on which muscles remain well innervated. Anterior instability predominates, followed by what is termed multidirectional instability. Tears of the rotator cuff, perhaps antecedent to spinal cord injury, complicate the picture. Even-

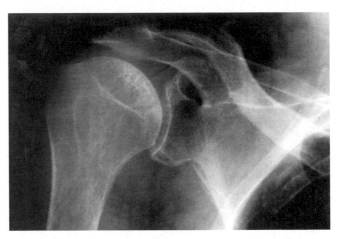

Figure 48.4 Over time, the shoulder of the tetraplegic patient may develop multidirectional instability. The humeral head begins to shift superiorly, impinging on the rotator cuff. The acromion is now acting as an acetabulum, and degenerative arthritis soon develops.

tually, the acromion comes to function as the acetabulum of the hip, with the development of rotator cuff attrition, and arthritis (Figure 48.4).

Conservative treatment includes anti-inflammatory medication, evaluation of ADL activities, modifications in activities, change from manual to motorized wheelchair, and strengthening exercises. Shoulder surgery for the tetraplegic patient is typically a last resort because of the potential long period of extreme dependency the patient may need to accept to rehabilitate the shoulder. Arthroscopic decompression for impingement can be successful but must include some more-or-less permanent modification in activity. Surgery for more significant pathology includes arthroplasty, either complete or hemiarthroplasty and shoulder arthrodesis. The spinal cord literature is generally discouraging of arthroplasty because of the many difficulties already mentioned. The surgeon has difficulty correcting the principal pathology, absent muscle function. The risk of component instability is high. We have performed shoulder arthroplasty in only three shoulders in two tetraplegic patients during the last 7 years. The indications were pain that precluded sleep and unresponsiveness to conservative therapy. Both patients had some elbow problems that mandated trying to maintain good glenohumeral motion. There were no complications, but rehabilitation was prolonged. Arthrodesis is a good operation for the very unstable or arthritic shoulder. We have employed a preliminarily placed external fixator to assist in determining the best position for arthrodesis.

CLASSIFICATION OF THE TETRAPLEGIC UPPER EXTREMITY

An injury to the cervical spinal cord has been classified in many ways, including by the skeletal level of injury or according to the most distal remaining functioning cervical root. However, no two patients even with injuries at the same skeletal level are exactly alike, and the same is frequently true of the right and left extremity in the same patient. There may be discrepancies in the motor

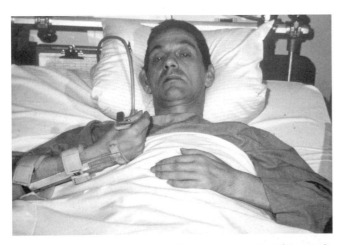

Figure 48.3 The newly injured tetraplegic patient frequently spends long hours supine in bed. In this position, the shoulders are held internally rotated and protracted across the chest. The onset of stiffness and pain can be rapid.

and sensory distribution of an individual patient's injury. In order to develop useful recommendations for treatment, it was necessary to develop a more precise method for classifying the upper limb in the tetraplegic patient (Table 48.1). From these needs arose the international classification used today, based not on the spinal level of injury, but on the limb's remaining useful motor and sensory resources. Muscle strength is assessed using the standard 0–5 scale, and the limb is classified according to the number of grade 4 or 5 muscles still functioning distal to the elbow. The grade 4 level was chosen because one can transfer a grade 4 muscle and expect it to perform useful work. A grade 3 muscle looses so much of its power in transfer that it cannot be reliably expected to do useful work after transfer.

Moberg (13, 14) encouraged us also to consider remaining sensory resources as well. If sufficient proprioception remains in any part of the hand (typically the thumb and index finger), then the patient can control his hand without having to keep it in view. If the hand lacks proprioception, then the patient can instead use his eyes for afferent control. However, lack of proprioception limits the patient in performing bi-manual activities. Today we equate static two-point discrimination of less than l2–l5 mm as indicating the presence of proprioception. The classification was extended somewhat to include a determination of the presence or absence of active elbow extension. This system was adopted by the International Federation of Hand Surgery

Societies, and it is used by essentially all surgeons involved in the care of the upper extremities of these patients.

FORMING A TEAM

Moberg also stressed the need to develop a critical mass of like-minded professionals into a team, which should include physiatrists and rehabilitation medicine specialists involved in the rehabilitation and long-term care of tetraplegic patients. Critical to the concept of a team are well-trained therapists, either physical therapists or occupational therapists (preferably both). The hand and upper extremity surgeon whose primary background may be either orthopedics or plastic and reconstructive surgery constitutes the remaining professional resource. Others, including social workers and psychologists, may play unique roles. However, the most important part of the team, once identified, is the patient; equally important is the patient's support group, including family, attendants, and so forth. The roles of the professionals on this team seem relatively clear cut. The physiatrist or rehabilitation medicine specialist should assist in determining the appropriateness of the patient for surgery as well as the appropriate timing of surgery relative to overall rehabilitation goals and schedules. The therapist frequently serves as the patient's advocate. He or she knows the patient better than anyone else and, in particular, knows the patient's motivation, intelligence, and (most importantly) expectations (voiced or not).

For the tetraplegic patient, upper extremity surgery has perhaps greater emotional impact than for most other patients. The tetraplegic patient is aware of the somewhat precarious nature of his life. Although the goal of surgical reconstruction for the upper extremity is greater independence, this can only be achieved at the expense of an occasionally prolonged period of greater dependence. For family and attendants this greater period of dependence translates into more inconvenience and effort. All the team members must play a role in the decision-making process and must share in the frustrations as well as the rewards.

PALO ALTO EXPERIENCE

In 1977, a multidisciplinary upper extremity clinic was established as part of the Spinal Cord Injury Center at the PAVAHCS. This clinic was staffed by rehabilitation physiatrists, therapists, psychologists, orthotists, and surgeons. During the past 30 years, over 500 tetraplegic Veteran patients were examined. Of this group, 175 patients elected to undergo some type of functionally oriented upper extremity surgery. The primary functional goals depended on those muscle and sensory resources remaining under voluntary control following neurologic stabilization.

PATIENT EVALUATION AND SELECTION

It is our strong belief that the hand and upper extremity team should become part of the routine evaluation of even newly injured patients. The cervical cord–injured patient arrives at a rehabilitation facility or spinal cord injury unit usually with fairly supple upper limbs, although with no or only minimal volitional movement. Fortunately, today's well-educated therapists become involved with patients in the early days or weeks postinjury and are aware of the need for protective splinting to avoid the

---

Table 48.1   International Classification for Surgery of the Hand in Tetraplegia (Edinburgh 1978, Modified—Giens, 1984ª)

SENSIBILITY MOTOR DESCRIPTION

O OR CU GROUP CHARACTERISTICS FUNCTIONª

0	No muscles below elbow suitable for transfer Flexion/supination of elbow
1	Br
2	+ ECRL Extension of wrist (weak or strong)
3ᵇ	+ ECRB Extension of wrist
4	+ PT Extension of wrist and pronation of forearm
5	+FCR Flexion of wrist
6	+Finger extensors Extrinsic extension of fingers, partial or complete
7	+Thumb extension Extrinsic extension of the thumb
8	+Partial digital flexors Extrinsic flexion of the fingers, weak
9	Lacks only intrinsics Extrinsic flexion of the fingers
X	Exceptions

Abbreviations: Br = brachioradialis; ECRL = extensor carpi radialis longus, ECRB = extensor carpi radialis brevis; PT = pronator teres; FCR = flexor carpi radialis.
ªAdvises indicating presence or absence of triceps function.
ᵇCaution, it is not possible to determine ECRB strength without surgical exposure.

insidious development of pathological contractures of the shoulders, elbows, wrists, and digits.

Once the patient's vertebral injury has become stabilized and the patient can begin sitting in a wheelchair, an assessment by the upper extremity team takes on new meaning. By the third or fourth month following injury, the eventual functional level is usually clearly established for the majority of patients. At this time, and based on the patient's ability to adapt to adaptive devices for feeding and hygiene, an early determination regarding the applicability of more complex functional orthoses can be made (15–17). For some patients, early measurement, fabrication, and fitting of a functional orthosis such as a wrist-driven flexor hinge splint (Figure 48.1) will advance the rate of rehabilitation. For patients with early but weak recovery of wrist extension, the wrist-driven flexor hinge splint represents an excellent exercise therapy directed toward strengthening wrist extensors so that they may eventually actuate a surgically reconstructed pinch or grip.

Hand or upper extremity surgery is rarely indicated during the initial months of rehabilitation following injury. The patient needs time to experience neurologic and psychologic stability. From a practical standpoint, there are simply too many more important rehabilitation activities going on. On the other hand, a dogmatic philosophy embracing tired dicta such as "never operate on a patient before 12 months" has no basis in science. Some patients are clearly candidates for surgery prior to this calendar date. For example, early surgical intervention to relieve the pathologic effects of a fixed elbow flexion contracture may allow a patient to participate more vigorously in necessary rehabilitation activities (18). There exists a good rationale for surgically paralyzing for some months a spastic and shortened biceps muscle by an open crush of the musculocutaneous nerve. A good argument can be made for early release of a fixed elbow flexion contracture with simultaneous transfer of the contracted biceps muscle to the triceps. This removes a pathologic or deforming force and reinforces or restores some power to the antagonist.

Once the patient seems to have achieved neurologic and psychologic stability, a formal evaluation to establish the appropriateness of upper extremity surgery can be accomplished by the team. The evaluation should focus on both tangible evidence of recovery, by assessing remaining motor and sensory resources, and the important intangibles, such as motivation and intelligence. In addition, the assessment should include an evaluation of the means by which the patient now accomplishes the tasks of daily living, with particular attention to how he or she performs transfers and pushes a wheelchair (Figure 48.5A, B.)

The motor examination includes an assay of residual motor groups as well as the identification of pathologic conditions such as contracted, painful, or unstable joints. The sensory evaluation includes measuring two-point discrimination in the digits to assess proprioception and the identification of pathologic conditions such as painful hypersensitivity. The currently used grip patterns are assessed (Figure 48.6). Any residual grip or pinch power is measured using standard dynamometers or pinch gauges. It may be necessary to construct a more useful measuring tool for these patients such as a squeeze ball attached to a mercury manometer.

The patient's current functional status is assessed. Is he dependent or independent in bed mobility? How are transfers performed? Does he use a manual or electric wheelchair? What

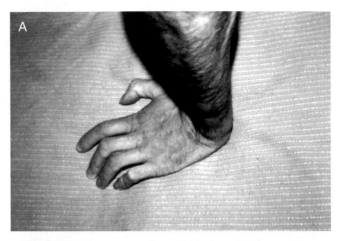

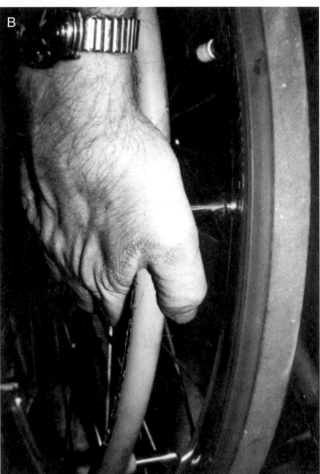

Figure 48.5 Assessment of the upper extremity must include an evaluation of how the patient currently uses his or her upper limbs, including their habitual method of transfers and weight shifts (**A**) and how they use their hands in propelling a manual wheelchair (**B**).

The postures depicted in **A** and **B** should be discouraged because they will lead to breakdown of collateral ligaments at many joints. These postures are incompatible with a long-lasting good outcome following essentially all hand surgery procedures proposed for the tetraplegic patient.

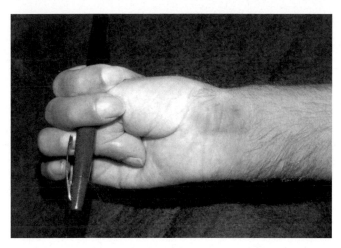

Figure 48.6 This patient found this interlocking grip to be useful. It may be better to concentrate on improving what has been a useful grip pattern rather than simply considering reconstructing only more standard patterns of grip or pinch. This is particularly true for the weak patient now years from the time of injury.

adaptive devices are used for dressing, grooming, and feeding? If surgery is to be performed, is there sufficient support to get the patient through a period of greater functional dependence, or will the extra burden of care result in the patient's attendant quitting. For many patients, upper extremity surgery means restriction to an electric-driven chair. Can this be made available? Does the home situation permit the use of an electric wheelchair? Are the controls of the chair mounted on the non-operated side? We have come to rely on our therapists for the necessary attention to these details in determining these issues.

Often some aspect of the examination will identify features that indicate that surgery at this time is inadvisable. Perhaps a motor group can be made significantly stronger by a period of directed exercise. Frequently this may mean the difference between a mediocre and a truly beneficial result. Occasionally we can assess the level of patient motivation by his or her response to a course of functional therapy. Does the patient respond favorably? Does he or she demonstrate the commitment to achieve a goal? The input and ideas of all team members are sought in the decision-making process. Although the surgeon must accept the ultimate responsibility for the decision, the decision is a team effort, and the fact that decisions are made as a team is made abundantly clear to our patients, again permitting all to share in the rewards of a good result and help bear the frustrations when things don't go as intended.

GENERAL GUIDELINES FOR RECONSTRUCTION

The surgical procedures applicable for improving upper limb function in tetraplegia include surgically immobilizing a joint (arthrodesis, also termed fusion); anchoring tendons to bone (tenodesis), so that another movement will result in the passive tightening of the anchored tendon; and, with this tightening, moving a more distally located joint and transferring the power of an expendable muscle-tendon unit under good volitional

control to compensate for the absence or ineffectiveness of function of another muscle-tendon unit (tendon transfer). These are all well-established surgical techniques, many dating from the era of polio reconstruction. A fourth reconstruction technique has been recently introduced. Termed functional neuromuscular stimulation, or FNS, this technique utilizes the residual contractile properties of upper motor neuron–paralyzed muscles when stimulated by an extra neural source. The remainder of this chapter is devoted to a discussion of the role of surgery in improving function at the elbow, wrist, and fingers. The objective is not to teach surgical techniques. These are referenced if more information is required; rather, it is our goal to discuss what procedures are available to patients at the various international classification levels, and the expected outcomes of surgical reconstruction. Admittedly, it is difficult to present this in a fashion that does not bring to mind a cookbook of recipes; however, nothing could be more divorced from fact. Each patient, and indeed each upper extremity, must be evaluated, and a treatment plan individualized. This cannot be stressed enough.

For cervical spinal cord injuries at the most proximal anatomic level, no expendable, and thus transferable, muscles exist. For patients injured at the more distal anatomic extreme, however, many potentially expendable, and thus transferable, muscles of grade 4 or 5 power exist. Thus reconstructive possibilities range from procedures to merely simplify the mechanics of the hand, such as arthrodesing a wrist joint so that this joint no longer requires external stabilizing by an orthosis, to complex multistaged procedurals involving many muscle-tendon transfers. The choice of procedure depends primarily on the residual resources and, secondly, on the many intangibles such as motivation and support. Although the surgical techniques are exactly those used to overcome the functional loss for patients with peripheral nerve injuries, matching the patient and procedure requires an understanding of the real difference between the tetraplegic patient and someone with, for example, a brachial plexus injury or a combined high median and ulnar nerve palsy. A cautious approach while one gains experience pays great dividends in terms of obtaining the acceptance of team members and patients that surgery can promote greater independence for these patients. A poor outcome early in the team's experience creates a tremendous hurdle.

ORTHOSES

For the patient with no muscles functioning at the grade 4 or greater level distal to the elbow, few reconstructive possibilities exist. For the majority of these patients, some type of functional orthosis must suffice (16, 17). Rarely for this O or OCu-0 patient, fusion of the wrist might permit the patient to employ a less cumbersome functional orthosis, for example a self-donned universal cuff rather than a long opponens splint for which the patient needs assistance donning and doffing (Figure 48.7).

Surgery may also be useful in repositioning a badly positioned part. For example, for the patient whose forearm is fixed in a supinated position, osteotomy of the radius may be useful in placing the hand in a more favorable pronated position. This might permit easier manipulation of the joystick control for an electric wheelchair than can be accomplished by a hand that is perpetually supinated.

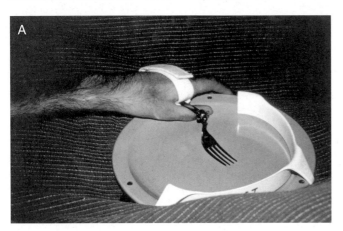

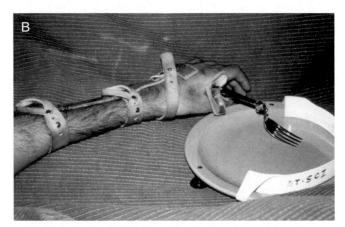

Figure 48.7   This tetraplegic patient, of ICO-0, preferred to have his wrist arthrodesed so that he could use a much more convenient orthosis, such as a "U-cuff (**A**)," rather than his previous, more complex orthosis (**B**). He was able to self-don the simpler orthosis, whereas donning and doffing the more complex brace required the aid of an assistant.

SURGICAL RECONSTRUCTION

Elbow Extension

Erik Moberg brought to our attention the importance of active elbow extension for the spinal cord–injured patient. The wheelchair-bound individual depends upon good shoulder and elbow power and stabilization to push a wheelchair, transfer from bed to chair, and perform pressure releases to prevent pressure sores. For the tetraplegic patient, lack of a functional elbow extension results in a much-reduced functional environment (18). The world of the tetraplegic patient is determined by the range of motion of his or her upper extremity. Without the ability to extend the elbow, the patient's "sphere of influence" is much reduced. The ability to extend the hand in space by an additional 12 inches results in an additional 800% of space that the hand can reach.

There are other reasons why reconstruction of active elbow extension is tremendously useful. Without active elbow extension, the tetraplegic's hands frequently fall into his face when lying supine. One cannot push a manual wheelchair up any incline without triceps function. Even as simple a task as turning on a room light switch may be impossible without active elbow extension.

Deltoid-to-Triceps Transfer

There are two surgical procedures advocated for restoring active elbow extension. In the United States, transfer of the power of the posterior half of the deltoid to the triceps tendon, as described by Moberg (13), is preferred. We prefer this procedure when the posterior deltoid is strong and the elbow has near normal passive extension. The procedure, performed under general anesthesia, involves detaching the insertion of about one-half of the deltoid (usually the posterior half) from the humerus and connecting this portion of the muscle via the triceps tendon insertion into the olecranon process of the ulna (Figure 48.8). Several technical modifications have been described, but the goals are similar. After surgery, the elbow is immobilized in full or near full extension for several weeks, and then the elbow is exercised for several additional weeks by allowing progressively greater elbow flexion in a

specially designed flexion-stop brace (Figure 48.9). Some months of cautious use are necessary to prevent overstretching of the transfer, and many months pass before maximal strength is obtained.

The results have been reasonably consistent in our experience. The great majority of patients can achieve full or near full

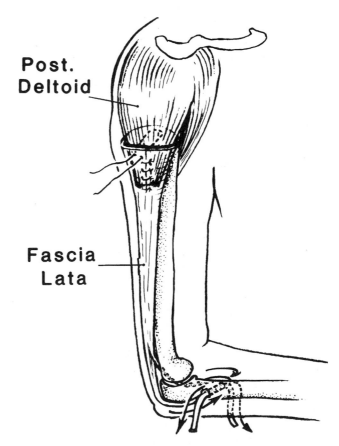

Figure 48.8   The operative steps for the deltoid-to-triceps transfer are illustrated.

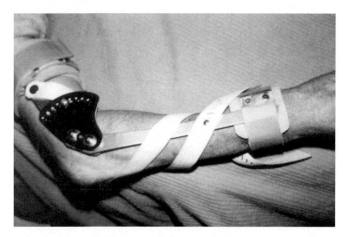

Figure 48.9 Following either procedure for restoring elbow extension, the patient uses a flexion-stop brace for several weeks as he or she is allowed to slowly and progressively regain elbow flexion.

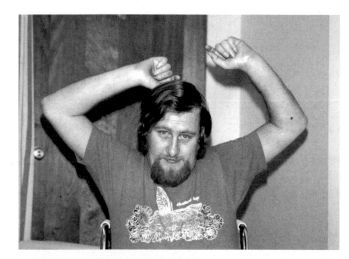

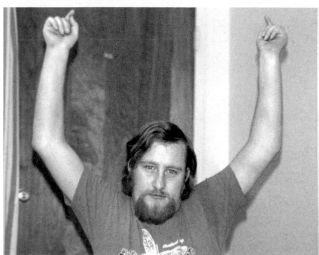

extension against gravity (Figure 48.10). This allows them to more accurately position an arm in space and control its movements. Rarely a patient achieves sufficient power to permit independent transfer in all circumstances, but this is not a realistic goal for most patients. The majority of patients find that they achieve more efficient transfers, pressure releases, and wheelchair mobility.

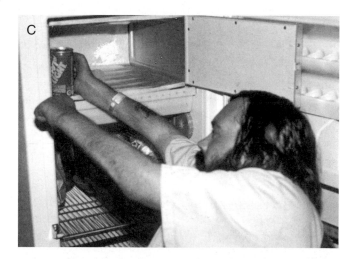

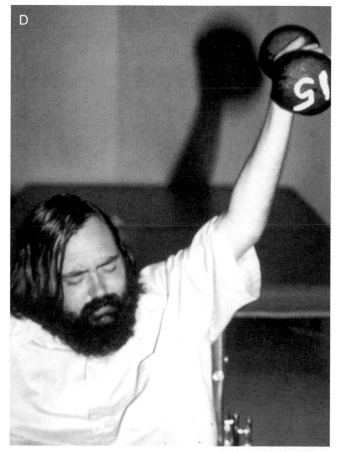

Figure 48.10 Following bilateral deltoid to triceps transfer, the patient (**A** and **B**) could reach overhead and could perform transfers in a much easier fashion. Another patient (**C**), following deltoid to triceps transfer. His ability to position his arm more accurately in space improved his ability to acquire objects from overhead storage. This patient regained sufficient power to lift 15 pounds directly overhead (**D**).

Complications are rare, provided that the patient follows the exercise protocol and does not overstretch the transfer by too rapidly performing full elbow flexion. In two patients, we have transferred the entire deltoid muscle without measurably changing shoulder function. This makes sense because surgery has merely altered the point of attachment of the muscle more distally on the limb.

Biceps-to-Triceps Transfer

A second procedure has been advocated to improve elbow extension. The biceps tendon can be detached from its insertion on the greater tuberosity of the radius and the muscle-tendon unit routed either medially or laterally, and the tendon attached to the triceps aponeurosis (19, 20). We have performed this transfer when there is a preexisting flexion contracture of the elbow greater than 30 degrees. In this case, the biceps is usually a deforming force, and this deforming force must be treated either by tendon lengthening or tenotomy. Rather than lengthen the biceps tendon, we prefer to transfer it. One might anticipate the transfer of an antagonist causing problems in rehabilitating the transfer. However, we have learned that by teaching the patient to conjointly supinate the forearm and extend the elbow, we can take advantage of the supinator function of the biceps in re-education. Our results of biceps-to-triceps transfer are not as impressive as deltoid-to-triceps transfer. Typically the patient cannot actively extend through a large range against the force of gravity. However, the patient does appreciate a gain in the ability to position the arm more accurately in space, and removing a deforming force and strengthening the antagonist decreases the chances for recurrence of the elbow contracture. Biceps-to-triceps transfers performed in younger patients without preexisting elbow flexion contractures have yielded excellent results, and some surgeons now prefer this procedure over deltoid-to-triceps transfer (21).

Reconstruction of elbow extension has been the single most satisfying reconstruction for our patients. Even though the overall time for rehabilitation can be relatively lengthy, the functional gain is substantial, predictable, and easily appreciated by the patient. Furthermore, the risks to residual preoperative function are practically nil. It represents an important addition to our reconstructive surgical armamentarium.

Improving Wrist Extension: The O or OCu-1 Patient

In the class O or OCu-1 patient, the brachioradialis is typically the only muscle with grade 4 function distal to the elbow. However, grade 2+ to grade 3+ radial wrist extensor function is typically present as well. The patient may be able to extend the wrist against gravity but cannot exert any force between digits and thumb through any existing natural tenodesis effect of the paralyzed finger and thumb flexors or cannot utilize a wrist-driven flexor hand splint unless it is equipped with a ratchet mechanism lock and release. For this patient, wrist extensor strength can be augmented by transferring the power of the brachioradialis into the more central of the radial wrist extensors, the extensor carpi radialis brevis (ECRB) tendon that attaches to the base of the third metacarpal (22). From several biomechanical studies, it has been determined that the

brachioradialis becomes a more effective wrist extensor following transfer if the patient can stabilize the elbow in space. If no active elbow extension is present, the brachioradialis, because it crosses the elbow joint, may waste some of its excursion and power in flexing the elbow rather than in extending the wrist. For this reason, we prefer first to reconstruct active elbow extension and occasionally will combine deltoid-to-triceps and brachioradialis-to-ECRB transfers. Following surgery and over time, we have observed impressive gains in wrist extensor strength. The patient can then better utilize a wrist-driven flexor hand splint or, in optimal cases, may become a candidate for surgical reconstruction of key pinch. The brachioradialis is truly a useful spare part.

Key Pinch Procedure

Patients functioning at the O or OCu-2 level can actively extend the wrist against gravity and against some resistance. This is a presenting feature for a large number of our patients. This correlates to the C5–C6 functional classification. They may still have relatively weak wrist extension or very strong wrist extension because grade 4 is such a subjective parameter.

Patients in the O or OCu-2 category are potential candidates for creation of a lateral or key pinch as described by Moberg (6). Conceptually, this is a very simple operative procedure, and, importantly, it is essentially totally reversible should the patient decide he was more functional before surgery. This is a consideration for a patient with weak wrist extension who is many years from his injury. The key pinch procedure may be combined with brachioradialis-to-ECRB transfer if greater wrist extensor power is deemed advantageous. It represents an automatic pinch, in that the tendon of the thumb flexor, the flexor pollicis longus (FPL), is anchored to the palmar surface of the radius under such tension that, with wrist extension, the thumb tip is pulled against the side of the index finger (Figure 48.11). The other fingers are usually left supple, and the patient frequently must learn to roll these

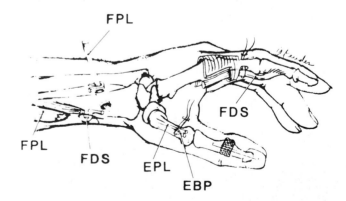

Figure 48.11 The operative design of the Moberg key pinch operation is illustrated. The interphalangeal joint of the thumb is stabilized. The radial wrist extensors are reinforced, if necessary, by brachioradialis-to-extensor carpi radialis brevis transfer. The tendon of the flexor pollicis longus is anchored to the volar surface of the radius. The index and middle finger flexors are adjusted so that these fingers become better platforms for the thumb to work against during key pinch.

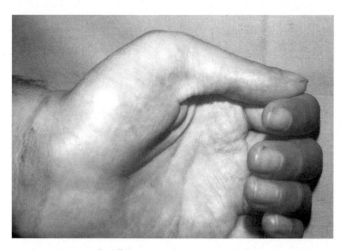

Figure 48.12 The illustration demonstrates the proper position for stable key pinch between the pulp of the thumb and the radial side of the index finger. Note the "bow-stringing" of the tendon of the flexor pollicis longus as forceful pinch is achieved.

digits into some flexion in order to provide a platform against which the thumb can act (Figure 48.12). Gravity is needed to flex the wrist, releasing tension on the tenodesed FPL and allowing opening of the grip. This implies that, preoperatively, the wrist must have a good passive range of motion and that the patient can be sitting much of the time so that gravity can affect opening of the grip.

Several technical modifications have been described to accommodate individual anatomic variations (23, 24). Typically, the hand and wrist are immobilized for 4 to 5 weeks, and cautious use is required for an additional 1 to 2 months to allow firm adherence of the tenodesis. We have performed this procedure on more than fifty hands, and the results have been very satisfying (Figure 48.13). We can measure the gain in pinch strength, and it is typically proportional to the strength of the wrist extensor power but somewhat depends on the stability of the thumb and finger joints. Pinch strengths between 1 and 5 kg have been

uniformly achieved. We have not had any patient ask to have his operative procedure reversed.

Active Key Pinch

After gaining experience with the key pinch procedure, described by Moberg, we have chosen to modify the key pinch operation for the patient with very strong wrist extension, meaning a strong O or OCu-2 or OCu-3 patient. These patients do not require augmentation of wrist extension by, for example, brachioradialis transfer. Instead of tenodesing the FPL to the radius as described above, in a single stage procedure, the following steps are accomplished (Figure 48.14):

1. The carpometacarpal (CMC) is arthrodesed to pre-position the thumb tip to contact the index finger middle phalanx.
2. The extensor pollicis longus (EPL) tendon is anchored to the extensor retinaculum on the dorsum of the wrist.
3. The brachioradialis muscle tendon unit is transferred to the tendon of the flexor pollicis longus.
4. One-half of the flexor pollicis longus is detached from the distal phalanx and routed dorsally to be attached to the tendon of the extensor pollicis longus to prevent the thumb from flexing excessively at the interphalangeal joint during pinch.

With this procedure, the patient depends upon gravity to flex the wrist and tighten the extensor pollicis longus tenodesis, thus opening the grip. Then, by actively contracting the brachioradialis, the thumb flexes against the side of the index finger irrespective of wrist position. Further wrist extension augments the power of the brachioradialis transfer (Figure 48.15). We and other colleagues have enjoyed good results and have worked with very satisfied patients (25). In several instances, we have performed bilateral hand surgery in OCu-2 or OCu-3 patients and have chosen to provide a traditional key pinch via FPL tenodesis on one side and active key pinch via brachioradialis muscle transfer to the flexor pollicis longus tendon on the opposite side. The patients have enjoyed the different functional attributes of each method and find that certain functions are easier with one

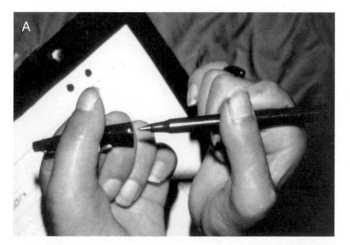

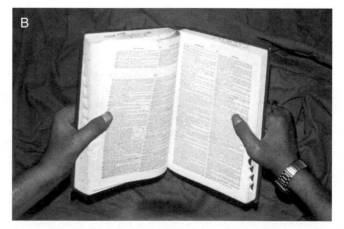

Figure 48.13 This ICOCu-2 patient has undergone bilateral Moberg key pinch procedures as described above (**A** and **B**). He achieved 4 pounds of pinch force. He was able to discard all his orthoses.

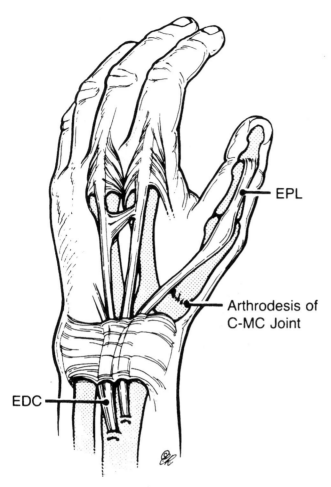

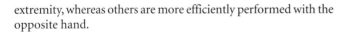

Figure 48.14   The operative steps to achieve active key pinch are illustrated. Power for pinch comes from transferring the brachioradialis into the tendon of the flexor pollicis longus.

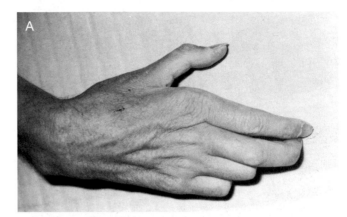

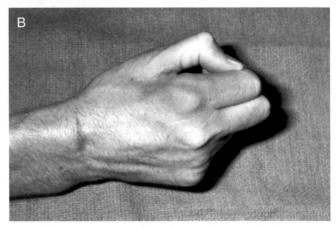

Figure 48.15   Following surgery, the patient is able to open the grip (**A**) by allowing gravity to flex the wrist. This causes the thumb to fully extend. By contracting the brachioradialis, the patient can achieve strong key pinch, irrespective of wrist position (**B**).

extremity, whereas others are more efficiently performed with the opposite hand.

Grasp-and-Release Procedures

For our tetraplegic patients who possess additional motor resources distal to the elbow, more complicated reconstructions are possible but not always indicated. These patients are, of course, also candidates for either procedure described above, if reversibility seems an important consideration. In the early years of our experience, we frequently offered only key pinch reconstruction for OCu-4 and even OCu-5 patients. As we have gained experience, so we have gained confidence in the team's decisions. As we have gained confidence in being able to achieve a reliable outcome, we have extended the risk-benefit equation to include more complex procedures.

The OCu-4 patient has four strong muscles functioning distal to the elbow, usually the brachioradialis, the two radial wrist extensors, the extensor carpi radialis longus, and the extensor carpi radialis brevis, and also the pronator teres muscle. In addition, the majority of OCu-4 patients have some function, albeit minimal, in the flexor carpi radialis. They can flex

the wrist with some force when the forearm is pronated, with gravity assisting the weak flexor carpi radialis. For these patients, we have devised a two-stage procedure that takes advantage of the presence of two expendable muscles for transfer, the extensor carpi radialis longus and the brachioradialis, and occasionally the pronator teres. Prerequisites for surgery include near normal passive wrist movement and reasonably flexible fingers. At the initial procedure, we test the power of the extensor carpi radialis brevis under local anesthesia to be certain that this muscle is sufficiently strong to extend the wrist. If this is the case, we proceed to arthrodese the carpometacarpal joint of the thumb to pre-position the thumb ray for pinch and, at the same time, attach the tendons of the extensor digitorum communis and extensor pollicis longus to the dorsum of the radius. This is referred to as the release phase. We also perform the FPL-to-EPL tenodesis to control the interphalangeal joint of the thumb. After a period of healing, with wrist flexion, the fingers and thumb extend. This is a very natural and synergistic motion and is easily learned.

Some weeks to months later, the flexor phase is performed. Two active muscle-tendon transfers are performed, including transfer of the extensor carpi radialis to the combined tendons of the flexor digitorum profundus so that this muscle smoothly flexes all of the fingers, and transfer the brachioradialis to the tendon to the flexor pollicis longus. These transfers permit the patient to actively close the fingers around an object and flex the fingers to provide a platform against which the thumb can actively pinch through the power of the brachioradialis transfer. The hand and wrist are immobilized for about four weeks, and then exercises are performed under the supervision of our therapist. Because they are synergistic transfers, re-education is relatively easy and quick. Many months are necessary before full strength is achieved. Also, because the patient lacks active finger extension, daily digital extension exercises are necessary to avoid the development of finger flexion contractures. A static night splint that maintains the proximal interphalangeal joints in near full extension should be worn essentially indefinitely.

Strong Grasp and Release

Patients in the international classification OCu-5 category usually have a functioning triceps. They are also functioning at some reasonable level of efficiency because they frequently have some residual effective natural flexor tenodesis in their paralyzed fingers and thumb. Decisions regarding the appropriateness of surgery for this category need careful consideration (26, 27). On the other hand, these patients have the most to gain from carefully planned and executed surgery.

We have performed several variations of a two-stage grasp-and-release procedure described for the OCu-4 group above, except that an additional muscle is available for transfer. Typically, we have tried to avoid arthrodesis of any joints. Extension of the fingers or the release phase is obtained either via extensor tenodesis, as described above, or occasionally by active muscle transfer to the combined tendons of the thumb and finger extensors, using either the pronator teres or the brachioradialis as the source of power. The flexor phase includes several procedures to maximize the versatility of thumb pinch and provide powerful finger flexion. This includes provision for some ability to abduct the thumb away from the palm. The goal of pinch is still directed toward more of a lateral or side or key pinch, but frequently the patient can also pinch closer to the index fingertip and can manipulate smaller objects, such as a coin into a telephone coin receptacle, with some efficiency.

These patients have truly gained the most from their surgery, particularly in terms of efficiency of movement and function. Instead of requiring 1 hour to dress themselves in the morning, they accomplish the same tasks in 10 to 15 minutes. Few do many more tasks postoperatively, but all perform these tasks with much greater efficiency and less expenditure of energy (Figure 48.16).

OCu-6-, OCu-7-, and OCu-8-Level Patients

Patients classified at the OCu-6 level possess active digital extension but lack thumb extension. These patients have the most to gain from surgery because their active digital extensors, in the absence of any finger flexors, frequently prevent them from achieving a tenodesis-type grip. They can achieve truly spectacular results by all parameters, including pinch strengths equal to 5 kg and grasp strengths between l0 and l5 kg. The results of surgery can be a nearly normal hand, except that ulnar intrinsic

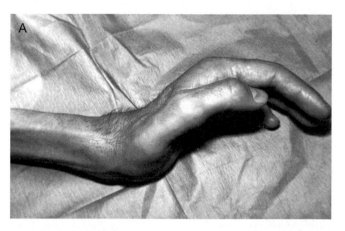

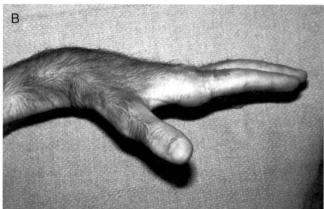

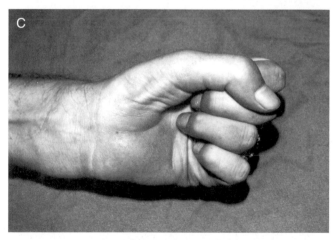

Figure 48.16 The steps of the two-stage grasp-and-release procedure are shown in the accompanying illustrations. The patient is ICOCu-5. Prior to the initial operative procedure (**A**), the release phase, the patient had to fully flex his wrist to allow his fingers to partly open. Following the release phase (**B**), the patient could flex his wrist only to a small degree to open the hand. Following the grasp or flexor phase (**C**), the patient could grasp objects using his reconstructed finger flexors and pinch with his thumb.

function is not reestablished. They require only adding an extensor force for the thumb and, at the same operation, multiple tendon transfer to achieve balanced thumb pinch and strong finger grasp. Therefore, only one procedure is necessary, and their period of dependence is minimal.

Patients with an even greater number of remaining resources can be approached somewhat like patients with lower peripheral nerve injuries. The surgical procedures performed for these patients are more directed at reconstructing some aspects of hand intrinsic muscle function and balance. There are relatively few tetraplegic patients in this category compared to the OCu-2 or OCu-5 categories, and we have operated on insufficient numbers to draw useful conclusions.

Other Presentations

Some injury patterns do not fit easily into the international classification. Patients with so-called central cord injuries have hands that defy classification. These patients require prolonged studies and frequent reexamination before formulating a surgical plan. Temporary nerve blocks have been particularly helpful in determining the procedure of choice.

FUNCTIONAL NEUROMUSCULAR STIMULATION

We have had experience implanting a system of electronics, including a programmable stimulator controlling an array of eight epimyseal electrochannels. This system (Figure 48.17), developed by surgeons and engineers from the Case Western Reserve University and the Cleveland Veterans Administration Medical Center, has the capability of allowing a patient with a very high spinal injury to activate and control a preprogram sequence of muscle contractions and thus achieve a useful grasp for one hand (28–31). The control mechanism is mounted

Components of the NeuroControl Freehand System

Transmitting Coil

Sensory Electrode

Shoulder-Mounted Joystick

Implanted Stimulator

External Control Unit

Electrodes

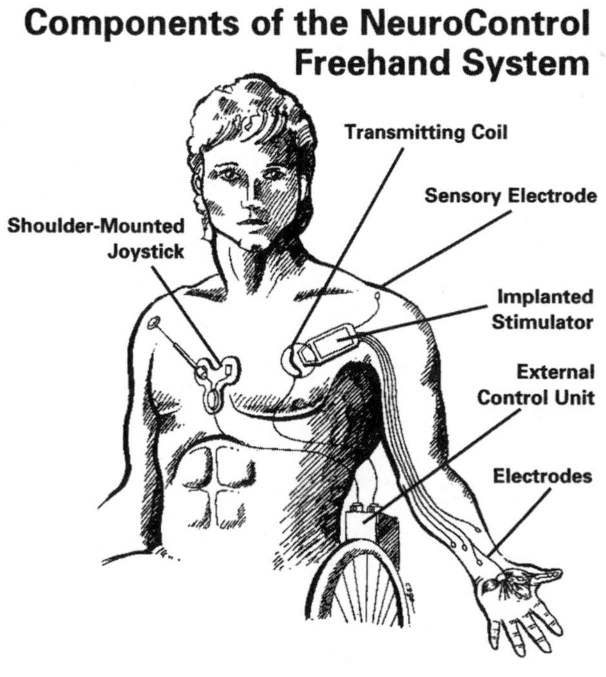

Figure 48.17 The design of the so-called freehand upper extremity functional neuromuscular stimulation system is illustrated. A small computer is attached to the patient's wheelchair. See text for details.

externally about the opposite shoulder, allowing active and volitional shoulder movement to open and close the grip and modulate the force. Some additional movements can lock the grip in a closed position at the desired force of closure. Two different grip-and-release patterns can be programmed, and the patient can switch between the two patterns. These include a lateral or key pinch pattern useful for grasping smaller objects in a secure grip (Figure 48.18) and a tip-to-tip pinch or opposition pinch useful for acquiring and holding larger objects (Figure 48.19). This system of electrodes placed on predetermined upper motor neuron–paralyzed muscles has the potential to restore useful function in limbs heretofore deemed useless and unreconstructable by standard surgical techniques. This device underwent transition from the laboratory to commercialization, and over 250 devices were implanted worldwide, with notable gains in function in the majority of implanted patients. Unfortunately, at the time this chapter is being written, because of business and economic decisions on the part of the industry source, the device is no longer commercially available.

POSTOPERATIVE CARE

The operative procedure is only the prelude to a series of important, if not critical, steps in the rehabilitation of upper limb function (32). All of our patients have benefited from the skills of our therapy team members. Much of their therapy takes place at home, although some occurs in our unit, with the patients being seen on an outpatient basis. Frequently the patient is discharged from the hospital 2 to 3 days following surgery, once the therapists have determined it is safe to discharge the patient. Safety means having a suitable electric wheelchair with an overhead support to assist in elevation of the operated hand and an adequately instructed attendant or family. The patient is readmitted at the proper time to remove his cast or splint, and several days are spent in instructing the patient in the exercise protocols and, importantly, in those activities that must be avoided or modified, particularly transfers and wheelchair mobility. Removable protective splints are fashioned at this time. Depending on circumstances, the patient may be discharged to continue exercising at home. Frequent follow-up is not particularly necessary for the majority of patients once transfers or tenodeses have achieved stable repair through healing. However, long-term follow-up is absolutely essential because the tetraplegic hand is a dynamic structure, and changes do occur over time. Surgical revisions may be necessary if tenodeses stretch out or joints become malpositioned secondary to contractures.

RESULTS

Recent reports show encouraging results for tendon transfers in the tetraplegic upper extremity (32–36). With continued experience, we have found it necessary to modify surgical indications and procedures more or less continually. We recommend videotaping the hand performing several standard functions such as opening a package or holding a pen, both pre- and postoperatively. We recommend formalizing the record-keeping process and the team dynamics and decision-making processes.

Because of the significant functional demands placed by tetraplegic patients on their upper limbs, especially the need to bear weight on their hands, the durability of operative procedures

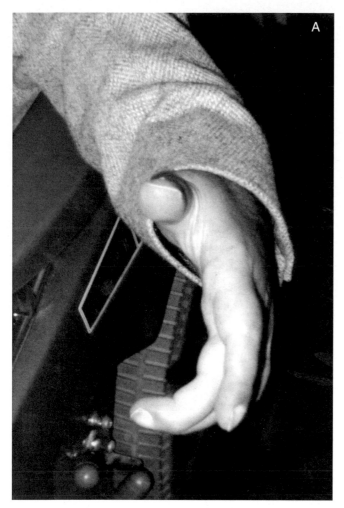 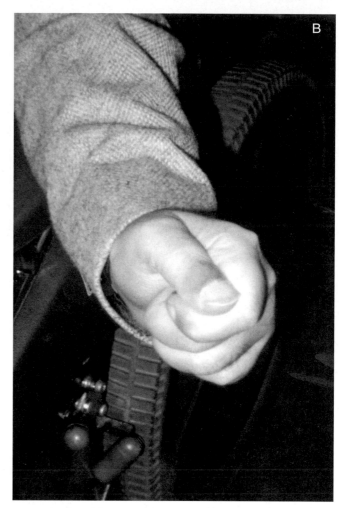

Figure 48.18 The lateral or key pinch grasp pattern is demonstrated. This is useful for acquiring smaller objects. Grasp open (**A**). Grasp closed (**B**).

performed to enhance upper limb function in tetraplegic patients has been questioned. Perceptions about the durability of some of the earlier surgical recommendations, such as the surgically created wrist-driven flexor hinge hand, still influence the referral patterns to surgeons of modern-day physiatrists and spinal cord rehabilitation specialists. To provide some current perspective on this issue, we were able to locate and personally examine forty-five patients who had been operated on at least 10 years prior to evaluation. We analyzed these patients according to the proposed major preoperative goals.

The first goal was restoration of elbow extensor stabilization and active elbow extension. Two surgical procedures were employed, with relatively specific indications for each. Most commonly, transfer of posterior deltoid to triceps, as popularized by Moberg, was performed. It was performed exclusively until 1985. Beginning in 1985, for patients presenting with a preoperative elbow contracture greater than 30 degrees, contracture release was combined with medial routing of biceps to triceps, as popularized by Zancolli.

We examined twenty-one patients who had undergone elbow extensor reconstruction more than 10 years prior. In the

fifteen patients who had had posterior deltoid-to-triceps transfer, ten had had bilateral transfers. All fifteen had required a motorized wheelchair as their primary means of movement before surgery. Ten years following surgery, nine now used a push chair as their standard chair, and four others used a push chair at least some of the time. There were three patients who had undergone bilateral posterior deltoid-to-triceps transfer, who were able to self-transfer in the early postoperative period. All three continued to be able to perform this task—monumental for a tetraplegic. In the posterior deltoid-to-triceps group, four patients had required a preliminary release of elbow flexion contracture. One of the four examined 10 years postsurgery had developed a recurrence of contracture greater than 30 degrees. In the six patients having biceps-to-triceps transfer (all needing contracture release), two could use a push chair, but not exclusively so. None had developed a recurrence of elbow contracture.

The second goal was the restoration of pinch for the weaker patients and pinch and grasp, as well as the ability to open the hand, for the stronger patients. International classification OCu-2 patients typically had key grip fashioned by tenodesis of the flexor pollicis longus to the radius. Seven were evaluated after

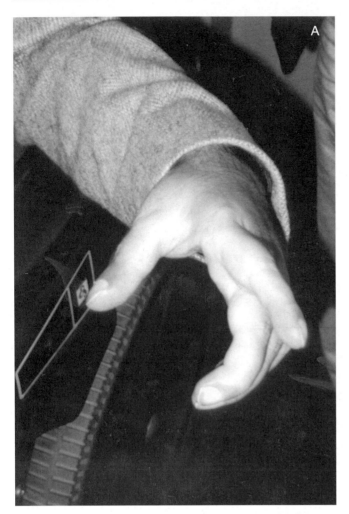

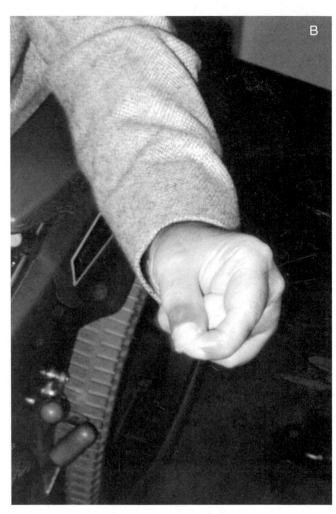

Figure 48.19   The tip-to-tip or opposition pattern is illustrated. This is useful for grasping larger objects. Grasp open (**A**). Grasp closed (**B**).

more than 10 years. Five had maintained pinch strength essentially equivalent to that demonstrated 6–12 months following surgery. Overall pinch strength in this group was 25 newtons.

One patient lost to follow-up for many years was an O2 patient. He presented with hands typical of Hansen's disease, with dissolution of thumb phalanges, presumably the result of forceful thumb use in an insensate and less than fully self-aware patient. This unique finding does point to the potential for harm when strong grasp is restored in a totally insensate limb that is then subjected to weight-bearing.

International classification OCu-3 patients typically had transfer of brachioradialis to flexor pollicis longus to restore dynamic voluntary key pinch. Six were evaluated, and all six had maintained useful power, which averaged 20 newtons. Thumb interphalangeal joint instability seemed to play a strong role in the diminished power seen in several of the BR-FPL patients. We now routinely employ the split FPL attachment described by Mohammed and Rothwell (37) to provide thumb interphalangeal stabilization but to avoid fusion.

Of the OCu-4 and -5 patients, the strong patients, eighteen were reexamined. Almost all had undergone two-stage procedures, and half had elected to have bilateral reconstruction. Flexor

power was by active transfer of extensor carpi radialis longus, brachioradialis or pronator teres, or accessory wrist extensor, always in some combination to the thumb and digital flexors. Six had undergone some type of additional surgery in the period between their initial surgery and the date of long-term evaluation, typically adjustment of the flexor to one or another finger (usually the index) or release of a contracted proximal interphalangeal joint (usually the ring or little). Grip power had not deteriorated in these patients compared to values measured at the 6–12-month evaluation after their initial surgery. Pinch force averaged 34 newtons. Typically, two muscles were devoted to thumb function in these patients. We found, as did House (26), that those patients who had had some type of intrinsic stabilization, either by Zancolli (27) lasso or by House's (26) intrinsic reconstruction procedure, had, on average, more powerful grasp. This may be a product of preselection, however, with the stronger patients having selectively been chosen for intrinsic substitution.

We conclude from this long-term analysis that carefully chosen upper limb reconstructive procedures in properly educated patients are both effective and durable. Systematic postoperative reevaluation of their upper limbs should become a standard part of the more typical interval examinations of more generally studied systems such as renal and bladder function, blood pressure, and pulmonary status. Aside from their brains, tetraplegic patients' upper limbs remain their most important residual resource. Frequent reevaluation of their upper limbs makes ultimate good sense.

As mentioned earlier, few of our patients perform many new activities. Typically, a good or excellent result means that the patient performs many of the same functions but with much greater efficiency. The rewards for surgeons, rehabilitation medicine specialists, and therapists are best expressed by one of our patients who replied to a question requesting his feelings on his outcome: "It is not as much as I hoped for, but it is much more than I ever had."

THE CURRENT STATE OF UPPER LIMB SURGERY FOR TETRAPLEGIA

Reconstructive upper limb surgery for tetraplegia has been well described for many years. The literature has also shown that improvement of upper limb function is a high priority for patients. This is demonstrated by the following quote from a person with tetraplegia: "I've often thought how much easier things would be, even if I were a para. Even if I had use of my hands . . . How useful they are, they're great, everyone should have working hands" (38). Despite these surgeries' long history and seeming congruence with patient desires, upper limb surgery has been slow to diffuse into general spinal cord injury rehabilitation. A survey of national United States databases showed that few of these procedures are performed: less than 10% of people with new cervical spine injuries receive upper extremity reconstruction (39). At Palo Alto, we have found that 35% of patients who were evaluated benefited from some type of upper limb surgery. Although there is debate on exactly how many people are appropriate candidates for these procedures, the current U.S. utilization of these procedures is extremely low.

The cause of the underutilization of upper extremity reconstruction is multifactorial, but some contributory factors have been identified. A primary barrier to the delivery of these surgeries is a disconnect between the physiatrists, who direct the rehabilitation, and hand surgeons, who are willing to perform these procedures. The absence of these interdisciplinary networks leads to inefficiency in referrals. In addition, lack of exposure to these procedures can result in the referring physicians having reservations about the efficacy of these procedures (40). We believe these findings highlight the importance of a multidisciplinary team to provide effective care of the upper limbs in tetraplegia. These teams allow for timely referrals and cross-communication between very different specialties.

Patients also contribute to the underutilization of upper limb surgery. Many people with tetraplegia do not know that these procedures exist or have negative perceptions about the efficacy of these procedures (41). In addition, people with tetraplegia have a variety of rehabilitation goals and may not be willing to make the large time investment for improved but not cured upper extremity function (42). This was demonstrated by Gorman, who found that only 12% of patients screened were eligible and elected to undergo reconstruction with functional electric stimulation (43).

Given that one barrier to care is that both patients and providers have concerns about the efficacy of these procedures, we wanted to better quantify the risk-benefit ratio. Therefore, we performed a systematic review of the current literature. We reviewed 165 limbs that had undergone posterior deltoid-to-triceps transfer, and the average postoperative elbow extension was an MRC grade of 3.3 with a complication rate of 28%. Of these complications, 45% related to loosening or stretching of the repair. More serious complications included functional loss in two patients secondary to unrecognized syrinx and spinal instability. For pinch reconstruction, we found that the postoperative pinch for 377 limbs was 1.8 kg with a complication rate of 47%. The most common complications were difficulties with the stabilization of the thumb IP joint with K wires, loosening/-rupture of repair, and malpositioning of the thumb. Five serious complications were found: two unrecognized syrinxes, one postoperative pneumonia, and two cases of autonomic dysreflexia. These data show that these surgeries give satisfactory functional gains and that complications are common but generally minor. This information should help the patients and the providers in making decisions regarding upper extremity surgery. Ultimately, we hope it will assist with the referral of appropriate patients to a hand surgeon.

*R*eferences

1. Bunnell S. Tendon transfer in the hand and forearm. *American Academy of Orthropaedic Surgeons Instructional Course Lectures* 1949; 6:106–112.
2. Nickel VL, Perry J, Garrett AL. Development of useful function in the severely paralyzed hand. *J Bone Joint Surg Am* 1963; 45:933.
3. Lamb DW, Landry R. The hand in quadriplegia. *Hand* 1971; 3:31–37.
4. Zancolli E. Surgery for the quadriplegic hand with active, strong wrist extension preserved. *Clin Orthop Relat Res* 1975; 112:101–113.
5. Guttmann L. *Spinal Cord Injuries: Comprehensive Management and Research.* 2nd ed. Oxford: Blackwell Scientific Publications, 1976.
6. Moberg E. Surgical treatment for absent single-hand grip and elbow extension in quadriplegia: principles and preliminary treatment. *J Bone Joint Surg Am* 1975; 57(2):196–206.
7. Hentz VR, Hamlin C, Keoshian LA. Surgical reconstruction in quadriplegia. *Hand Clin* 1988; 4(4):601–607.
8. Hentz VR, Brown M, Keoshian LA. Upper limb reconstruction in quadriplegia: functional assessment and proposed treatment modifications. *J Hand Surg Am* 1983; 8(2):119–131.
9. Hentz VR. Historical background and changing perspectives in surgical reconstruction of the upper limb in quadriplegia. *J Am Paraplegia Soc* 1984; 7:36–38.
10. Hentz V, Leclercq C. *Surgical Rehabilitation of the Upper Limb in Tetraplegia.* London: WB Saunders, 2002.
11. Campbell C, Koris M. Etiologies of shoulder pain in cervical spinal cord injury. *Clin Orthop* 1996; 320:140–145.
12. Silverskiold J, Waters R. Shoulder pain and functional disability in spinal cord injury patients. *Clin Orthop Relat Res* 1991; 272:141–145.
13. Moberg E. Reconstructive hand surgery in tetraplegia, stroke, and cerebral palsy: some basic concepts in physiology and neurology. *J Hand Surg Am* 1975; 1:29–34.
14. Moberg E. *The Upper Limb in Tetraplegia: A New Approach to Surgical Rehabilitation.* Stuttgart: Thieme, 1978.
15. Curtin M. Development of a tetraplegia hand assessment and splinting protocol. *Paraplegia* 1994:159–169.
16. DiPasquale-Lehnerz P. Orthotic intervention for development of hand function with C6 quadriplegia. *Am J Occup Ther* 1994; 48:138–144.
17. Krajnik SR, Bridle MJ. Hand splinting in quadriplegia: current practice. *Am J Occup Ther* 1992; 46:149–156.
18. Grover J, Gellman H, Waters RL. The effect of a flexion contracture of the elbow on the ability to transfer in patients who have quadriplegia at the sixth cervical level. *J Bone Joint Surgery Am* 1996; 78(9):1397–1400.
19. Revol M. Biceps-to-triceps transfer in tetraplegia: the medial route. *J Hand Surg Br* 1999; 24(2):235–237.
20. Kuz J, Van Heest AE, House JH. Biceps-to-triceps transfer in tetraplegic patients: report of the medial routing technique and follow-up of three cases. *J Hand Surg Am* 1999; 24(1): 161–172.

21. Mulcahey MJ, Lutz C, Kozin SH, Betz RR Prospective evaluation of biceps to triceps and deltoid to triceps for elbow extension in tetraplegia. *J Hand Surg Am* 2003; 28(6):964–971.

22. Johnson DL, Gellman H, Waters R, Tognella M. Brachioradialis transfer for wrist extension in tetraplegic patients who have fifth-cervical-level neurological function. *J Bone Joint Surg Am* 1996; 78:1063–1067.

23. Bryan RS. The Moberg deltoid-triceps replacement and key-pinch operations in quadriplegia: preliminary experiences. *Hand* 1977; 9(3): 207–214.

24. Newman JH. The use of the key grip procedure for improving hand function in quadriplegia. *Hand* 1977; 9(3):215–220.

25. Paul SD, Gellman H, Waters R, Willstein G, Tognella M. Single-stage reconstruction of key pinch and extension of the elbow in tetraplegic patients. *J Bone Joint Surg Am* 1994; 76(10):1451–1456.

26. House JH, Gwathmey FW, Lundsgaard DK. Restoration of strong grasp and lateral pinch in tetraplegia due to cervical spinal cord injury. *J Hand Surg* 1976; 1(2):152–159.

27. Zancolli E. *Structural and Dynamic Bases of Hand Surgery.* 2nd ed. Philadelphia: JB Lippincott, 1979.

28. Mulcahey MJ, Smith BT, Betz RR, Triolo RJ, Peckham H. Functional neuromuscular stimulation: outcome in young people with tetraplegia. *J Am Paraplegia Soc* 1994; 17:20–35.

29. Smith B, Mulcahey MJ, Betz RR. Quantitative comparison of grasp and release abilities with and without functional neuromuscular stimulation in adolescents with tetraplegia. *Paraplegia* 1996; 34(1):16–23.

30. Triolo RJ, Bets RR, Mulcahey MJ, Gardner ER. Application of functional neuromuscular stimulation to children with spinal cord injuries: candidate selection for upper and lower extremity research. *Paraplegia* 1994; 32:824–843.

31. Wuolle KS, Van Doren CL, Thrope G, Keith M, Peckham P. Development of a quantitative hand grasp and release test for patients with tetraplegia using a hand neuroprosthesis. *J Hand Surg Am* 1994; 19(2): 209–218.

32. Leclercq C. Surgical rehabilitation of the upper limbs in tetraplegic patients. *Chirurgie* 1996; 121:492–495.

33. Freehafer AA. Gaining independence in tetraplegia: Cleveland technique. *Clin Orthop* 1998; 355:282–289.

34. Lo IK. The outcome of tendon transfers for C6-spared quadriparetics. *J Hand Surg Br* 1998; 23(2):156–161.

35. Goloborod'ko SA. A method of restoration of the abduction of the thumb in traumatic tetraplegic patients. *J Hand Surg Am* 1999; 24(2):320–322.

36. Gellman H, Kan D, Waters R, Nicosa A. Rerouting of the biceps brachii for paralytic supination contracture of the forearm in tetraplegia due to trauma. *J Bone Joint Surg Am* 1994; 76(3):398–402.

37. Mohammed KD, Rothwell AG, Sinclair SW, Willems SM, Bean AR. Upper limb surgery for tetraplegia: a 10-year re-review of hand function *J Hand Surg Am* 2003; 28(3):489–497.

38. Manns PJ, Chad KE. Components of quality of life for persons with a quadriplegic and paraplegic spinal cord injury. *Qual Health Res* 2001; 11(6):795–811.

39. Curtin CM, Gater DR, Chung KC. Upper extremity reconstruction in the tetraplegic population: a national epidemiologic study. *J Hand Surg Am* 2005; 30(1):94–99.

40. Curtin CM, Hayward RA, Kim HM, Gater DR, Chung KC. Physician perceptions of upper extremity reconstruction for the person with tetraplegia. *J Hand Surg Am* 2005; 30(1):87–93.

41. Wagner J, Curtin CM, Gater DR, Chung KC. Individuals with tetraplegia: perceptions on upper extremity reconstructive surgery. *J Hand Surg Am* 2007; 32(4):483–490.

42. Snoek GJ, Ijzerman MJ, Post MW, Stiggelbout AM, et al. Choice-based evaluation for the improvement of upper-extremity function compared with other impairments in tetraplegia. *Arch Phys Med Rehabil* 2005; 86(8):1623–1630.

43. Gorman PH, Wuolle KS, Peckham PH, and Heydrick D. Patient selection for an upper extremity neuroprosthesis in tetraplegic individuals. *Spinal Cord* 1997; 35:569–573.

49 Medical Management of Pressure Ulcers

Michael Priebe
Lisa-Ann Wuermser
Heather E. McCormack

Although thought to be completely preventable, pressure ulcers continue to present a leading health problem for people with spinal cord injury (SCI). More attention has been given to pressure ulcers than to any other secondary condition following SCI, but many questions remain unanswered concerning prevention and management. Much of what we know about the etiology, prevention, and treatment of pressure ulcers has been derived from studies of elderly nursing home patients, who are presumably quite different from persons with SCI. Although it is known that many physiologic processes are altered during the acute phase of SCI, very little is known about the long-term effect of SCI on complications such as pressure ulcers. Although much attention is being directed at cure research in SCI, eliminating pressure ulcers as a complication of SCI remains a high priority. The Institute of Medicine report *Spinal Cord Injury: Progress, Promise, and Priorities* (1) states,

> Spinal cord injury research should focus on preventing the loss of function and on restoring lost functions—including sensory, motor, bowel, bladder, autonomic and sexual functions—with the elimination of complications, particularly pain, spasticity, pressure sores (decubitus ulcers), and depression, with the ultimate goal of fully restoring to the individual the levels of activity and function that he or she had before injury.

This chapter will discuss the factors that are involved in pressure ulcer development and healing and provide information about the current state of knowledge regarding the medical management of pressure ulcers for persons with SCI.

INCIDENCE, PREVALENCE, AND COST

Pressure ulcers complicate the care and management of acute SCI, prolong length of stay in acute care and rehabilitation, and increase costs of initial care and rehabilitation for people with SCI.

Acute Hospitalization

The true incidence and prevalence of pressure ulcers are difficult to determine because of varying populations, settings, methodology, and definitions used in research studies. The incidence is reported to range from 0.4% to 38% for hospitalized patients, 2.2% to 23.9% for those in long-term care, and 17% for those in home care (2). The 2006 National Spinal Cord Injury Statistical Center Annual Statistical Report (3) reported that pressure ulcers occur in 33.5% of persons during the acute phase of SCI. In nontraumatic SCI, prevalence at admission to rehabilitation was similar at 31.3% (4).

Long-Term Follow-Up

Chen et al. (5) found the incidence of stage 2 or greater pressure ulcers to be 11.5% in the first year following SCI. This incidence rate increased to 21% by 15 years postinjury. Garber et al. (6), in a prospective study of community-dwelling persons with SCI, found that 32% of their sample had a stage 2 or greater pressure ulcer at the time of evaluation. The strongest risk factors for predicting the occurrence of a pressure ulcer were the presence of a previous pressure ulcer, prior pressure ulcer surgery, and self-reported susceptibility to pressure ulcers.

There is a distinct population of persons with SCI who have recurrent pressure ulcers. Krause and Broderick (7) reported that whereas 70% of persons with traumatic SCI either only had a pressure ulcer in the immediate period following SCI or never had a pressure ulcer, 13% had a clear pattern of recurring pressure ulcers (one or more per year). What sets these patients apart from the rest of the SCI population is fertile ground for research.

Cost

Epidemiologic data not only substantiate that pressure ulcers are a lifelong threat to persons with SCI, but studies have provided insight into the costs to both the individual and healthcare services when pressure ulcers occur. Pressure ulcers account for approximately 25% of the overall cost of treating people with SCI, with an estimated annual cost of $1.2 billion in the United States (8).

Pressure ulcers are one of the most common causes for rehospitalization in people with SCI. Cardenas et al. (9) found diseases of the skin, including pressure ulcers, to be the second most common cause of rehospitalization in their sample, with disease of the genitourinary system being most common. Persons with ASIA grades A, B, and C paraplegia had the highest rate of rehospitalization for pressure ulcers. In a retrospective study of one VA SCI center, 39% of veterans with SCI were seen in clinic or received home care for management of pressure ulcers over a 3-year period. Over half of those with pressure ulcers were hospitalized at least once during the study period. Thirty percent of the hospitalized patients were admitted three or more times. The average length of stay was 150 days (10).

The human and societal costs of pressure ulcers are immeasurable, including human suffering, pain, disfigurement, and body image change (11). The loss of productivity, the effect of prolonged bed rest on health and wellness, and the effect of pressure ulcers on family dynamics, the development or worsening of depression, and community reintegration—although difficult to measure—are significant.

RISK FACTORS AND PRESSURE ULCER DEVELOPMENT

The National Pressure Ulcer Advisory Panel (12) has defined a pressure ulcer as "localized injury to the skin and/or underlying tissue usually over a bony prominence, as a result of pressure, or pressure in combination with shear and/or friction." A pressure ulcer is a soft tissue infarction. As such, the process starts with an ischemic event—usually caused by unrelieved pressure or shear—and has an opportunity for reperfusion with partial or complete recovery if the pressure is adequately relieved and circulation restored within a critical time period. This is a localized event; however, the general health of the individual contributes significantly to the likelihood of developing a pressure ulcer and to the ability to heal it.

To better understand the development and healing of pressure ulcers and to assist with their assessment and management, it is helpful to differentiate between extrinsic and intrinsic risk factors that contribute to pressure ulcer development and delayed healing in the SCI population. Extrinsic risk factors are those factors external to an individual that subject a person to increased risk of developing a pressure ulcer (i.e., pressure, shear, and moisture). Intrinsic risk factors are those physiologic factors that contribute to pressure ulcer development. These may be subdivided into two main groups—those factors that are present as a direct result of the SCI, and those factors that are common in people with SCI, often as a result of concomitant disease or aging (Table 49.1).

Extrinsic Risk Factors

Pressure

Although many factors contribute to the development of a pressure ulcer, pressure is the most important. The age-old saying, "where there is no pressure there is no pressure ulcer," remains true today. Kosiak (13, 14), in his classic animal experiments, found that deep tissue necrosis develops during prolonged episodes of low pressure, recurrent episodes of pressure without adequate relief, or short episodes of high pressure. He reported a positive relationship between tissue damage and duration of

Table 49.1   Risk Factors for Development and Delayed Healing of Pressure Ulcers after Spinal Cord Injury

EXTRINSIC RISK FACTORS	INTRINSIC RISK FACTORS: CONSEQUENCE OF SCI	INTRINSIC RISK FACTORS: CONSEQUENCE OF CHRONIC DISEASE OR AGING
Pressure*	Impaired mobility	Anemia*
Shear*	Impaired sensation	Malnutrition*
Moisture*	Altered Posture* due to spasticity or contractures	Diabetes*
	Impaired vascular responses	Peripheral vascular disease*
	Altered collagen metabolism	Hypogonadism*
	Altered temperature regulation	Thinning skin, muscle atrophy, obesity*
	Impaired immune function	

*Modifiable risk factor.

pressure. He also found that tissue damage could be prevented with frequent episodes of pressure relief, even in the face of high pressures.

Tissues vary in their sensitivity to pressure-induced ischemia. Muscle is most sensitive because of its high metabolic activity and ease of blood vessel compression, whereas skin is most resistive because of its lower metabolic activity and the orientation of capillary loops in the dermis (15). The time between the onset of pressure and occurrence of tissue damage varies from person to person but may require as little as 2 to 6 hours of constant low pressure. Even when initial signs of pressure damage are recognized early and relief measures initiated, necrosis to deep muscle and fat may have already occurred (16).

Shear

Shear forces also contribute to the development of pressure ulcers. Dinsdale et al. (17) demonstrated that the pressure level capable of disrupting blood flow in the skin is reduced by half in the presence of significant shear forces. Because capillary loops in the skin are oriented vertically, they are more resistant to direct, vertically oriented pressure. However, if lateral forces (shear) are exerted on them, they are readily kinked, resulting in dermal ischemia and necrosis. Therefore, any force that exerts both pressure and shear is more likely to result in dermal tissue injury.

Moisture

Excessive moisture and maceration decreases the skin's tolerance to mechanical stress, making dermal injury more likely to occur during an episode of shearing and pressure. Urine, feces, and sweat are potential irritants to tissue and serve to break down the body's normal barrier against damage and infection.

Conversely, skin permitted to become excessively dry because of dehydration, lack of environmental humidity, or extended periods of cold is also susceptible to damage (18).

Intrinsic Factors: Consequence of Spinal Cord Injury

Mobility Impairment

Decreased mobility and the inability to reposition independently are important risk factors for pressure ulcer development. Data on pressure ulcers during acute care and rehabilitation indicate that those with complete tetraplegia have the highest risk (53.4%) of developing a pressure ulcer during this time period, followed by those with complete paraplegia (39.0%), incomplete tetraplegia (28.7%), and incomplete paraplegia (18.3%) (3). These data are similar to data reported by Young (19) over 25 years ago. Fuhrer et al. (20) reported that the presence of a pressure ulcer in community-dwelling individuals was more likely in persons with a lower ASIA motor score and greater disability as measured by the Functional Independence Measure.

Sensory Impairment

The loss of protective sensation results in a decreased awareness of tissue injury and impending ischemia. In the fully sensate person, tissue ischemia is painful and results in a conscious or unconscious shift of the body. However, in a person with decreased or absent sensation, the usual signals of impending tissue damage are not present and no behavioral changes result. Early symptoms allow early interventions. Because of the loss of sensory feedback, persons with SCI are not able to take appropriate action (immediately get off the area of ischemia), and ischemia proceeds to infarction.

Persons with SCI are taught to reposition themselves frequently during the day, independent of sensation, and to inspect their skin at least twice each day (18). However, Krause and Broderick (7) reported that following usual preventive measures, including weight shifts and skin inspection, did not correlate with risk of recurrent pressure ulcers in their study population. This finding raises important questions regarding the efficacy of the usual pressure ulcer prevention techniques used for people with SCI.

Positioning

The presence of limb contractures, scoliosis, pelvic obliquity, or severe spasticity will aggravate positioning problems. These abnormalities in positioning in turn contribute to problems of pressure and shear. Abnormal positioning increases pressures over specific bony prominences and creates a higher risk for pressure ulcer development because of higher pressures and shear forces. The Consortium for SCI Medicine Clinical Practice Guideline on Pressure Ulcer Prevention and Treatment recommends that persons at bed rest be repositioned every 2 hours and notes that most therapists recommend that persons in wheelchairs practice pressure relief maneuvers every 15 to 30 minutes (18). However, studies on healthy individuals and elderly nursing home residents have demonstrated that skin temperature, redness, and pressure at the sacrum, ischium, and trochanter significantly increase and show signs of early tissue destruction

after as little as 1 to 1.5 hours of a static position (21). Pressure over bony prominences of persons with SCI during wheelchair sitting has been demonstrated to increase following as little as 10 to 15 minutes (22, 23). Makhsous et al. found that the transcutaneous oxygen tension ($tcPO_2$) dropped to less than 10 mmHg within 200 seconds of sitting (24). It remains unclear how long a person may remain in one position without pressure injury. The answer will likely depend on the tissue tolerance to pressure and will vary from person to person.

Vascular Responses

Altered circulation is frequently seen after SCI. Decreased venous return because of impaired muscle pump in the legs and loss of normal vasoconstriction during alterations of blood pressure and posture are especially common. Venous and lymphatic congestion may contribute to pressure ulcers in the pelvic region in the same way that venous congestion contributes to venous stasis ulcers in the lower extremities. The alterations in vasoconstriction may result in transient hypotension, which may be clinically important if other factors contribute to put a person at risk for pressure ulcer development.

Reactive hyperemia, the normal physiologic response to pressure, signals an increased vascular perfusion to the upper dermis and corrects the local metabolic debt accumulated during ischemia. However, prolonged pressure may lead to a toxic buildup of metabolites in tissue and ultimately to an inflammatory response. Impaired reactive hyperemia, examined by microcirculation studies, has been demonstrated to occur in persons with SCI (25–28). Researchers have noted normal blood flow and reactive hyperemia, but greatly diminished vascular reactivity to pressure events, in persons with SCI under resting conditions. Vascular capacity for dilation, abnormal vascular tone, and increased venous pressures have also been shown to contribute to a significantly decreased blood content in tissue following reactive hyperemia (26).

Collagen Metabolism

Collagen metabolism appears to be altered below the level of injury in SCI (18). Studies have shown that there is a decrease in numerous components of denervated skin, including in the amino acid content, the activity of enzymes of collagen synthesis, the proportion of type 1 to type 3 collagen fibers, and the density of adrenergic receptors below the level of injury. There is also a large increase in excretion of collagen metabolites in the urine after SCI. These changes may lead to diminished tensile strength of the skin, resulting in an increased risk of mechanical injury, and to impaired healing of pressure ulcers for this population.

Temperature Regulation

Increased tissue temperature leads to higher metabolic demands in deep tissues. This increases the likelihood that a relatively brief episode of pressure will lead to deep tissue damage. Many patients report that their pressure ulcer developed during an illness with accompanying fever (16). Polliack et al. (29) reported that any event accounting for increased body temperature leads to at least a 28% increase in the levels of metabolites, especially lactate and urea, in the sweat. Mahanty et al. (30) noted a significant rise in skin temperature within 2 to 5 minutes about the ischium and sacrum of SCI patients sitting in wheelchairs. The peak temperatures were proportionally related to the magnitude and duration of applied pressures. Vistnes (31) demonstrated that elevated skin temperature is greatest over areas subjected to repeated pressure stress even when pressure relief activities are performed. Finestone et al. (32) determined that a correlation exists between erythema size and skin temperature following prolonged pressure on tissue over bony prominences.

Immune Function

The natural and adaptive immune responses have been noted to be strikingly altered immediately following SCI. Multiple communicating pathways exist between the nervous, endocrine, and immune systems and are associated with blood vessel function and lymphocyte processes. Adhesion molecules, necessary for wound healing and adaptation to inflammation, have been noted to be reduced in immobile persons with SCI, but they return to normal levels when activity is increased. The intricate relationship between nutritional status, functional lifestyle, neuromuscular impairment, and immune function is often disrupted in persons with SCI and is considered by some scientists to prompt the development of pressure ulcers and to affect the rate of healing from pressure ulcers (33).

Intrinsic Factors: Consequence of Concomitant Disease or Aging

Anemia

Many persons with SCI and pressure ulcers have evidence of anemia, often with a hematologic picture of an anemia of chronic disease (18). This is likely due to a combination of decreased nutritional intake, loss of serum protein and electrolytes from the ulcer, secondary infection, and a general debilitated status. Persons with a hemoglobin level of less that 10 mg/dl have delayed wound healing. Tissue metabolism may be impaired because of decreased oxygen carrying capacity, thus resulting in increased risk for pressure ulcer development and poor wound healing. Perkash et al. (34) studied sixty-five males with SCI treated at a Veterans Affairs medical center between 6 months and 32 years following injury and reported that 52.3% experienced anemia without clinical and hematologic evidence of hemolysis or hemorrhage. Approximately half of the subjects with anemia demonstrated decreased serum iron and decreased serum iron binding capacity but no other abnormalities in nutritional status. All subjects studied who had large deep pressure ulcers were anemic, and 83.3% of the persons who were anemic had pressure ulcers. Keast et al. (35) demonstrated that persons with SCI, anemia of chronic disease, and pressure ulcers receiving recombinant human erythropoetin had an improvement in hemoglobin levels and a reduction in ulcer size after 6 weeks of treatment.

Malnutrition

Nutritional problems lead to both increased likelihood of pressure ulcer development and decreased ability of the body to heal. Serum albumin has been found to correlate positively with pressure ulcer stage and to negatively correlate with pressure ulcer risk. It has also been shown that pressure ulcers improve with nutritional support (18). Because of the long half-life of serum albumin, other tests, including pre-albumin and transferrin, may be more sensitive measures of change in nutritional status.

Deficiency of micronutrients, including vitamins A, C, and E, has been demonstrated in persons with SCI living in the community (36). Vitamin C is necessary for the hydroxylation of proline to hydroxyproline, which is critical for normal collagen formation. Deficiencies of vitamins A and E also may contribute to poor wound healing; however, supplementation has not been proven to benefit wound healing. Retinoids antagonize many of the detrimental effects of corticosteroids on collagen metabolism. In patients taking corticosteroids, supplementation with vitamin A may be beneficial, although there is contradictory evidence regarding this (37). Zinc is necessary for collagen synthesis. However, studies of zinc levels do not correlate with pressure ulcer presence, and zinc supplementation has not been demonstrated to increase wound healing (18).

Peripheral Vascular Disease and Smoking

Adequate blood flow is necessary for wound healing. Peripheral vascular disease decreases arterial blood flow to tissues, resulting in a decreased ability to heal. In addition to the vasomotor changes that occur after SCI, smoking, diabetes, and other risk factors for peripheral vascular disease can increase the risk for pressure ulcer development. Age over 60 years, diabetes, SCI, and renal insufficiency were found to be independent risk factors for developing pressure ulcers in a surgical intensive care unit (38). Smoking also decreases arterial oxygen tension and causes an immediate effect on tissue oxygenation. Therefore, smoking has both an acute and a long-term effect on the healing of pressure ulcers.

Hypogonadism

Conditions such as SCI, trauma, major surgery, liver failure, myocardial infarction, burns, alcoholism, and malnutrition have been found to be associated with the suppression of gonadotropin secretion and secondary hypogonadism. Wang (39) reported that 12.7% of sixty-three otherwise healthy men with SCI for an average of 6 years exhibited low serum testosterone levels. Approximately one-third of the subjects had low serum thyroxine, thyrotropin, cortisol, growth hormone, and plasma adrenocorticotropic hormone accompanying the diminished serum testosterone levels. Testosterone, an essential element for collagen integrity and health, influences tissue responsiveness to both pressure ulcer formation and healing. Although there are few studies testing the relationship between hypogonadism and the formation of pressure ulcers in persons with SCI, men who are hypogonadal following SCI may be more likely to develop a pressure ulcer and to experience delayed wound healing.

Thinning Skin, Muscle Atrophy, and Obesity

Thinning skin, which has less tolerance to trauma and shear forces, commonly occurs with advancing age unrelated to SCI. Changes in muscular strength and activity level caused by immobilization, advancing age, or chronic illness may put an individual at higher risk for pressure ulcers. This may be especially true for a person with SCI during prolonged immobilization for medical complications including treatment for another pressure ulcer.

People with cachexia have higher interface pressures compared to people with normal build, increasing their risk for pressure ulcers (40). Atrophy of muscle below the level of injury results in a decreased surface area to distribute pressure during sitting or lying and theoretically provides less "padding" of bony prominences. It is unclear whether "padding" per se is protective, or whether factors, such as malnutrition and anemia, which are frequently associated with cachexia and muscle atrophy, increase the risks of pressure ulcers. Clearly persons with excess adipose tissue can develop pressure ulcers, as can people with severe muscle atrophy. Further research in this area is necessary to understand these factors.

NORMAL WOUND HEALING

In brief, normal wound healing has three phases. The *inflammatory phase,* which begins within 4 hours of injury, usually lasts from 4 to 6 days. Neutrophils arrive first to kill bacteria and prevent colonization of the wound. Macrophages, which arrive later, kill bacteria, clean up the cellular debris, and recruit the fibroblasts needed for tissue repair by secreting soluble cytokines. The balance between collagen synthesis and collagen breakdown is thought to be moderated by activated macrophages (41). The *proliferative phase* occurs between days 2 and 24, when granulation tissue is generated. Fibroblasts stimulate the ongoing production of collagen, which is responsible for the tensile strength and structure of the healed wound. Wound margins contract, granulation tissue fills the defect, and epithelial cells migrate from the wound margins to close the wound. This phase is anabolic, whereas the inflammatory and maturation phases are catabolic. The *maturation phase* occurs from day 21 to 2 years. Collagen fibers reorganize, remodel, and mature, gaining tensile strength. This process continues until the scar has regained 70% to 85% of the tissue's original strength (42).

Superficial partial thickness ulcers will heal without scarring through regeneration of epithelium. This takes only 1 to 2 weeks because the epithelial cells migrate from dermal appendages— hair follicles and sweat glands. Full-thickness superficial wounds heal by epithelial migration from the wound margins. The ulcer size will determine the speed of healing. Deep pressure ulcers require much longer to heal, depending on the size of the wound. These wounds heal by a combination of wound contraction, granulation, and epithelialization.

Pathology of Nonhealing Wounds

Pressure ulcers may stall in any of the phases of healing— somehow losing the ability to move from one phase to another. Pressure ulcers may stall in the inflammatory phase if the onset of this phase is delayed or blocked as is seen with the use of glucocorticoids. Prolonged or heightened intensity of acute inflammation may also retard wound healing. Ongoing acute inflammation is commonly seen in chronic nonhealing wounds. Histologic findings of ongoing acute inflammation include perivascular infiltrates of neutrophils, degraded extracellular matrix and abnormal fibroblasts, and a high content of neutrophil-specific enzymes and proteinases in chronic wound fluid.

Pressure ulcers that stall in the proliferative or tissue-formation phase may do so because of failure to form granulation tissue because of the persistence of causative factors (pressure, ischemia, infection), inadequate components required for healing (protein, vitamins/minerals, growth factors), or a prolonged inflammatory phase. The effectiveness of topical proliferative agents, such as growth factors, is often diminished because the proteins are degraded by inflammatory proteinases in chronic wounds.

The maturation or remodeling phase may be halted by failure to adequately epithelialize because of an inhospitable environment (bacterial colonization, dry wound bed, pressure, or shear) or by excess wound contracture. Scar contracture may result in restricted movement across joints, and reinjury caused by inadequate scar strength during stretching or range of motion exercises may result.

Increased bacterial load is a common complication that causes wounds to stagnate in the healing process (43). The characteristics of unhealthy granulation tissue include superficial bridging, friability, and delay of expected healing rate. Bacterial load may lead to local or systemic infection. Fever, leukocytosis, erythema, edema, induration, odor, and increased drainage are standard signs of infection. Occult infection is thought to be the primary culprit when wounds do not progress in healing. Chronic wounds with bacterial counts of more than 100,000 organisms per gram of tissue or growth of any beta-hemolytic *Streptococcus* from tissue biopsy do not heal. Therefore, any wound that is not healing should undergo wound biopsy for aerobic and anaerobic cultures. Use of topical antimicrobial agents to decrease the bacterial count is recommended. Likewise, unless there is evidence of systemic infection, use of systemic antibiotics is not recommended for pressure ulcers (44).

PRINCIPLES OF PRESSURE ULCER MANAGEMENT

The management of pressure ulcer requires a comprehensive team approach. This approach must focus not only on the wound, but also on the individual's biologic, psychologic, and social systems. The team's primary goals in the medical management of pressure ulcers are to optimize the conditions for healing and to minimize the complications of immobilization created by the treatment approach. These goals can be best achieved by basing clinical decisions on principles of management and on evidence-based approaches, rather than relying on anecdotal experience or use of the newest product on the market. The essential principles for pressure ulcer management include prevention, correction of the underlying causative factors, adequate debridement, and moist wound healing (Figure 49.2).

Principle #1: Prevention

Prevention is a deliberate action taken to minimize the occurrence or impact of those extrinsic and intrinsic factors that place the person at risk for the development of a pressure ulcer. Bergstrom and Braden (1) identify two factors as key in the development of pressure ulcers—the amount and duration of pressure, and the body's ability to tolerate the pressure. Much of our effort to prevent pressure ulcers is focused on three main objectives: (1) prevent pressure-induced ischemia by minimizing or attenuating the degree of tissue compression (e.g., special mattresses, beds, cushions, routine pressure relief maneuvers,

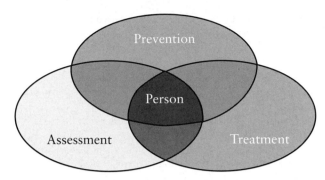

Figure 49.1   Person-oriented philosophy for managing pressure ulcers.

turning regimens); (2) identify early signs of pressure-induced ischemia (e.g., routine skin checks); and (3) minimize the degree of pressure-induced ischemia by taking immediate action (e.g., avoid sitting or lying on an area that looks injured or vulnerable). Unfortunately, only the first objective is proactive. The others are reactive and are likely to be less effective. An important objective not readily accomplished is early detection of impending pressure-induced ischemia so that interventions to maximize reperfusion and limit the degree of ischemia can be initiated before tissue necrosis occurs.

No amount of effort on the part of the healthcare worker to institute measures for preventing pressure ulcers will be effective if the person with SCI fails to accept his or her role in prevention. However, the prevention strategy must incorporate the individual's physical abilities, healthcare beliefs and attitudes, social system, and economic reality. A prevention strategy that fails has likely overlooked one or more of the important factors in a person's life, making compliance with the strategy difficult or impossible. A prevention strategy that identifies the individual at risk, performs regular risk assessment, provides prevention education during every patient interaction, and modifies the prevention strategy throughout a person's life is most likely to be successful. Table 49.2 summarizes prevention strategies for modifiable risk factors. All of these strategies should be reevaluated and continued when a person develops a pressure ulcer, as these factors also contribute to delayed wound healing.

Risk Assessment

Assessment is a process of ongoing observation and decision making about the factors that put a person at risk for the development of a pressure ulcer. The process must become second nature to the person with SCI and to all SCI care providers. Rehabilitation of the person with SCI should emphasize understanding the risk factors that contribute to pressure ulcers, working with the healthcare team for pressure ulcer management, and assuming personal accountability for health maintenance. Medical management of pressure ulcers requires a recurring cycle of prevention, assessment, and treatment with the person as the focal point for all activities (figure 49.1). The degree of healthcare intervention required is directly proportional to the person's ability to independently satisfy the requirements of a prevention strategy.

The Norton scale and the Braden scale are two of the most common tools used by clinicians to assess a patient's risk for pressure ulcer development. The Norton scale has been tested

Table 49.2   Managing Modifiable Risk Factors

Assessment	Prevention Strategies
Extrinsic Factors	
Pressure	Pressure relief every 15–30 minutes during wheelchair sitting. Turning every 2 hours when in bed. Use wheelchair cushions and mattresses that distribute pressure.
Shear	Keep clothing and linen wrinkle-free. Reduce sliding in bed and friction during transfers. Use draw sheet when repositioning in bed.
Moisture	Maintain clean, dry skin
Intrinsic Factors	
Positioning	Correct flexible deformities. Accommodate inflexible deformities.
Anemia	Eat a well-balanced diet with appropriate level of iron supplementation. Maintain hemoglobin above 10 mg/dl. Consider use of erythropoeitin for anemia of chronic disease.
Malnutrition	Maintain healthy body weight and nutritional levels by eating a well-balanced diet. Monitor serum albumin and pre-albumin levels to ensure adequate nutrition.
Diabetes	Monitor and control blood glucose level closely.
Peripheral vascular disease	Smoking results in both short-term and long-term complications for wound healing. Encourage smoking cessation.
Hypogonadism	Evaluate for hypogonadism. Provide replacement therapy if abnormal.
Obesity	Maximize protein in the diet, but avoid excess caloric intake during pressure ulcer healing.

extensively (45). Physical condition, mental state, activity, mobility, and incontinence are each assigned a numeric value from 1 to 4. Scores may range from 5 to 20, with lower scores being indicative of higher risk. The "onset of risk" begins with a score of 14, and a person is at high risk with a score of 12 or less. One study reported low reliability among registered nurses who used the Norton scale and disagreement among experts as to its face validity (46).

The Braden scale, however, has been shown to be highly reliable when used by registered nurses (47). It allows the assessor to assign a numeric value to six different indicators with potential scores from 4 to 23. Sensory perception, skin moisture, physical activity, nutritional intake, friction and shear, and the ability to change body position are each given a numeric value; these values are totaled to indicate a patient's potential for developing pressure ulcers. A patient with a Braden scale score of 16 or less is considered to be at risk. The exception is the geriatric patient, who may be at risk even with a score as high as 18. It is also interesting to note that, in SCI, values for sensory perception, activity, mobility, and friction/shear are all affected. Thus, a person with tetraplegia can achieve a maximum possible score of only 15, putting him at high risk for pressure ulcer development even when not compromised. Risk assessment scales specific to SCI have been proposed (48) but have had limited testing for validity or reliability.

Many intrinsic and extrinsic factors can place a person at risk for the development of pressure ulcers or delayed healing from pressure ulcers. Table 49.2 has been constructed as a general guideline to be used by all individuals on the healthcare team, including the person with SCI.

Education of the staff, patient, and caregivers is also an important component of prevention because these people are the first-line defenders against pressure injury (49). Prevention of pressure ulcers is a multidisciplinary concern requiring full participation by everyone involved, including the person with SCI.

Principle #2: Correct the Underlying Contributing Factors

Once an ulcer develops, a complete assessment should be done to determine the cause of the pressure ulcer, identify underlying contributing factors, document the severity of the wound, and determine an appropriate management strategy. Clark et al. (16) reported that pressure ulcers were most likely to develop when a person who is at a relatively high risk for pressure ulcers experiences an equilibrium-disrupting change. This may be a urinary tract infection, a change in equipment, or the change of a caregiver. Identifying the equilibrium-disrupting change is critical to understanding the cause of the pressure ulcer and the starting place to correct the factors that contributed to the ulcer. One can also learn from the cascade of events that resulted in a pressure ulcer to begin planning to prevent future pressure ulcers. Often the patient knows or has an idea of what caused the pressure ulcer. Many attribute it to a missed transfer, a slip in the bathtub, a cushion failure, or a fall. Sometimes the attributed cause is correct, other times patients attribute the cause to an unlikely source, and other times they do not know. If the patient believes he knows how it happened, one should look carefully at that event, even if is seems trivial.

A comprehensive evaluation of the medical, psychologic, and social factors that may have contributed to the development of the pressure ulcer must be performed before a pressure ulcer can be effectively treated. Each person with a pressure ulcer will have a combination of modifiable and nonmodifiable underlying contributing factors identified. Utilizing a preventive health perspective, one can begin to accommodate those factors that are not modifiable and correct those that are modifiable. The saying, "One can put anything on a pressure ulcer except the patient and it will heal," is only partially true. A more appropriate statement may be, "Correct the underlying factors that contributed to the pressure ulcer, and it will heal, no matter what else you do." Also, its converse is true: "Fail to correct these factors, and the ulcer will not heal, no matter what else you do."

Pressure Shear and Positioning

Some of the most important underlying factors to address are pressure, shear, and positioning. The location of an ulcer provides clues to the cause of the wound. The location of a wound is classically described by the underlying bony prominence (e.g., ischium, sacrum, etc). It is beneficial to be able to determine whether the pressure ulcer was caused by unrelieved pressure and/or poor positioning while lying down or while sitting up. Pressure ulcers involving the occiput, scapulae, sacrum, lateral aspect of the greater trochanter, fibular head, lateral malleoli, and heels are typically developed while lying down either supine or, in the case of the lateral aspect of the greater trochanter, in a lateral decubitus position. Conversely, pressure ulcers over the ischium coccyx and posterior aspect of the greater trochanter are developed while sitting. While most pressure ulcers in people with acute SCI occur at the sacrum and heels, pressure ulcers in persons with SCI who are active in the community occur more commonly over the ischial tuberosities, coccyx, and lateral aspect of the greater trochanter (18).

The location of a pressure ulcer can help determine its underlying cause. A person who sits with scoliosis and a pelvic obliquity is likely to develop a pressure ulcer over the ischium and posterior aspect of the greater trochanter on the low side of the obliquity, whereas a person with tight hamstrings and a posterior pelvic tilt will develop a pressure ulcer over the coccyx. A person who is ill and spends more time in bed without turning will likely develop a pressure ulcer over the sacrum.

Knowing the relationship between location and etiology is critical to healing a current ulcer and preventing a new pressure injury. Modifications of posture and seating systems are frequently necessary in the presence of a "sitting" wound. However, a "lying down" pressure ulcer will require increased nursing care to turn the patient more frequently or the utilization of a specialty bed to minimize pressure during bed rest. Many patients with "lying down" pressure ulcers can sit in their wheelchairs without slowing the healing rate because sitting was not a contributing factor in the development of the pressure ulcer.

Evaluating the wheelchair and cushion of the person with a "sitting" pressure ulcer is essential to understanding the cause of the ulcer and correcting the cause—poor positioning—of the pressure ulcer. Observing the individual sitting in the wheelchair will reveal positioning problems, including scoliosis, pelvic obliquity, or sacral sitting. It will also identify problems of inadequate back support, incorrect footplate height, or other evidence of poor fitting or adjustment of the chair. Looking at the wheelchair cushion itself is also essential. Some key questions to ask include the following: If it is an air cushion, is it overinflated or underinflated? If a gel cushion, is there evidence of too little gel, or is the cushion placed incorrectly in the chair so that the person is not sitting on the gel pads? If the cushion is made of foam, how old is it?

Review of the method and frequency of pressure-relieving weight shifts is also important. Coggrave and Rose (50) studied the effectiveness of typical pressure relief techniques in people with acute and chronic SCI using transcutaneous oxygen measurements at the ischial tuberosity. Tissue oxygen measurements were made during sitting and during pressure relief maneuvers. They found that the mean duration of pressure relief necessary to return tissue oxygen levels to baseline levels following sitting was 111 seconds (range 42 seconds to 210 seconds). Makhsous et al. (24) measured transcutaneous pressure of oxygen (TcPO2) and carbon dioxide (TcCO2) during changes in interface pressure using a dynamic seating system. They found that TcPO2 recovered to baseline levels in an average of 208 to 214 seconds, whereas TcCO2 required 252 to 255 seconds to recover during off-loading. Maximal wheelchair pushups averaged 49 seconds, significantly shorter than necessary for tissue reperfusion. These studies point out that standard wheelchair pushups are inadequate to restore tissue perfusion, and thus recommend alternate methods for pressure relief during sitting (e.g., forward and side leaning or use of a dynamic seating system) to allow time for adequate tissue reperfusion. These findings may shed light on the report by Krause and Broderick (6) that compliance with recommendations for routine pressure relief and skin inspections did not correlate with pressure ulcer recurrence risk. If one of the standard techniques recommended for pressure relief is ineffective in restoring tissue perfusion, it is not surprising that the prevalence of pressure ulcers is not decreasing.

Interface Pressure Measurements

Interface pressure evaluation can be helpful in identifying contributing positional and equipment factors. The goal of interface pressure assessment is to identify areas of high pressure and to adjust the person's sitting posture, wheelchair, or cushion to evenly distribute pressure across the entire seating surface. This method adds important information for tissue pressure management. However, it should not be the only method used to evaluate a cushion or seating system. Hands-on and "hands-under" evaluation of the individual's seating surface is essential. It is not wise to rely on a predetermined target pressure. Interface pressure measurement only measures the interaction occurring at the interface of the support surface and the subject, not pressure or its effects on deeper tissues. These pressure measurements do not tell us how much pressure is too much in the deep tissues, where pressure ulcers begin to develop. Measurement of tissue oxygenation and blood flow, as part of a pressure management strategy, are likely to become more clinically applicable as the devices used become smaller and more readily available.

Nutrition

A careful evaluation of the individual's nutritional state is essential. Pressure ulcers compete with the body for energy stores, amino acids, and micronutrients, usually doubling the body's demand for the specific nutritional intake of protein, calories, vitamin C, and zinc. Most research has focused on the enhanced intake of protein and calories as adjunctive to pressure ulcer healing. Persons with low albumin levels (<3.5 gm/dl) have a higher likelihood of developing and recovering more slowly from pressure ulcers than do persons with normal serum albumin. Persons with chronic pressure ulcers often show signs of malnutrition and require aggressive nutritional management. Dietary supplementation with an average of 1.5 to 2 grams of protein per kilogram of body weight per day and between 3,000 and 3,500 calories per day is generally required for proper wound healing (18, 51). However, care must be taken to avoid replacing lost lean body mass with fat gain. Table 49.3 illustrates the nutritional requirements for SCI patients who have a pressure ulcer.

In a randomized controlled study, Lee et al. (52) demonstrated that the rate of pressure ulcer healing doubled in patients receiving standard care plus a concentrated, fortified collagen protein hydrolysate supplement compared to those receiving

Table 49.3   Twenty-Four-Hour Nutritional Requirements for Persons with SCI

Caloric intake (kcal)	Males = 66 + (13.7 × current weight in kilograms) + (5 × height in centimeters) − (6.8 × age in years)	
	Females = 655 + (9.6 × current weight in kilograms) + (1.7 × height in centimeters) − (4.7 × age in years)	
	WITHOUT A PRESSURE ULCER	**WITH A PRESSURE ULCER**
Harris-Benedict equation (BEE)		Multiply BEE by stress factor: 1.2 for Stage 2; 1.5 for Stages 3 and 4
Protein intake	1.0–1.25 grams/ kilogram of body weight	1.25–2 grams/ kilogram of body weight
Vitamin C	10–20 milligrams	60 milligrams

Source: *Pressure Ulcer Prevention and Treatment Following Spinal Cord Injury: A Clinical Practice Guideline for Health-Care Professionals* (18).

standard care alone. Periodic monitoring of serum albumin, prealbumin, and transferrin, and 24-hour urine analysis for nitrogen balance, are recommended in the management of nutrition for persons with pressure ulcers. Evaluation of the hemoglobin, hematocrit, and lymphocyte count has also been found to provide indicators for nutritional status and should be utilized for persons with pressure ulcers.

Trauma, infection, and chronic illness initiate a physiologic stress response by the body that increases the energy demands and results in a catabolic state of protein breakdown and hypermetabolism. Circulating hormones, prompted by the stress response, result in an increase in cortisol and catecholamines but a decrease in the anabolic steroids, growth hormone, and testosterone. Although catabolism can rapidly appear within weeks following injury, restoration of a steady anabolic state may take months of medical management. Many patients with pressure ulcers are in a severe catabolic state, which must be taken into account when planning treatment. The correction of this catabolic state and restoring sufficient nutrient intake to meet the increased protein and energy needs is necessary before a pressure ulcer will heal. Anabolic steroids, testosterone, and human growth hormone are agents that may increase protein synthesis and restore the body weight necessary for effective wound healing. Clinical trials using oxandrolone, an oral anabolic steroid, have demonstrated an increased rate in wound healing for refractory pressure ulcers (53), and additional studies in SCI are under way (54).

Careful assessment and correction of other factors that can cause and inhibit wound healing, including anemia, smoking, and endocrinologic factors, should be performed. Severe spasticity and muscle contractures will affect sitting and lying posture and positioning. Correction of these is necessary for long-term maintenance and future prevention after the wound is healed. Excess moisture must be managed as well. Psychologic and educational factors must be assessed and corrected where possible.

Limited social support and other environmental complications must also be addressed while the healing process continues so that the person is able to return to an environment in which he can be successful and remain healthy and pressure ulcer free.

Wound Assessment

The purpose of ongoing wound assessment is to document healing (or failure to heal) and to modify the management plan accordingly. By consistently using the same techniques to monitor wound presentation and healing, the clinician will be able to identify the causative factors of the ulcer and direct medical management. By using objective data points to support progress within a treatment plan, the clinician is able to provide justifiable, expeditious care to patients with even the most complex wounds. Frequent assessment of the pressure ulcer location, size, staging, wound bed, exudate, wound margins, and periulcer skin should be performed and recorded. Because variability exists between the assessment skills and approaches for each practitioner, it is advisable to standardize the format for daily recording of pressure ulcer characteristics and assign the task of assessment to a limited number of observers.

Assessing Wound Stage

Staging is often considered the cornerstone of wound assessment. When staging pressure ulcers, two key concepts must be recognized. First, a wound cannot be accurately staged if there is necrotic tissue in the base. Secondly, there is no reverse staging. Wounds do not heal by restoring normal tissue planes, but by scar formation. Therefore, for example, the rule is once a stage 4, always a stage 4, until it is completely healed. Table 49.4 provides the revised NPUAP staging classification system based on the depth of tissue involvement (12).

Assessing Wound Size

Wound size is used to monitor a wound's progress toward closure and provides information to determine the appropriate wound care product to use. Attention must be paid to define how the measurements were taken. Even among skilled clinicians, objective measurement is difficult and may be unreliable. Numerous techniques have been developed to objectively determine wound size. Three-dimensional linear measurement is the most frequently used technique among wound care professionals. The length, width, and depth of the cavity are measured and stated in centimeters. A long-handled cotton-tipped applicator and a disposable ruler are standard tools for measurement. Linear measurements have been thought to be unreliable because of a lack of standardization for which dimensions constitute the length or width. In addition, there is error of up to 0.5 cm with each measurement using this system. It is good practice for the whole team to measure the dimensions using the same technique. One technique is to define length as the wound measurement along the body's head to toe, or longitudinal, axis. Width is the distance from epithelial edges across the hip to hip, or transverse, axis. Depth is measured from the wound base to the surface of the skin at the deepest point, measuring perpendicular to the skin surface.

Undermining and tracking in the wound bed are also measured and recorded. Undermining is defined as an extension

---

Table 49.4 National Pressure Ulcer Advisory Panel Updated Pressure Ulcer Staging System (2007) (12)

Deep Tissue Injury (Suspected): Purple or maroon localized area of discolored intact skin or blood-filled blister due to damage of underlying soft tissue from pressure and/or shear. The area may be preceded by tissue that is painful, firm, mushy, boggy, warmer, or cooler as compared to adjacent tissue.

Stage 1: Intact skin with non-blanchable redness of a localized area usually over a bony prominence. Darkly pigmented skin may not have visible blanching; its color may differ from that of the surrounding area.

Stage 2: Partial-thickness skin loss of dermis presenting as a shallow open ulcer with a red pink wound bed, without slough. May also present as an intact or open/ruptured serum-filled blister.

Stage 3: Full-thickness tissue loss. Subcutaneous fat may be visible, but bone, tendon, or muscle is not exposed. Slough may be present but does not obscure the depth of tissue loss. May include undermining and tunneling.

Stage 4: Full-thickness tissue loss with exposed bone tendon or muscle. Slough or eschar may be present on some parts of the wound bed. Often includes undermining and tunneling.

Unstageable: Full thickness tissue loss in which the base of the ulcer is covered by slough (yellow, tan, gray, green, or brown) and/or eschar (tan, brown, or black) in the wound bed.

---

of the wound under the surface of the skin that is parallel to the surface of the skin. This would be indicative of a combination shear and pressure injury. Tracking or tunneling is defined as a tract heading away from the wound base in any direction. These variables are most effectively documented as components on a clock face (e.g., 2 cm tract at 12 o'clock, undermining from 2 to 5 o'clock position). This provides consistency and allows for reasonably reliable location of the area by other clinicians. The PUSH® tool developed by the NPUAP is a wound assessment tool designed to standardize wound measurements that incorporates these recommendations (55).

Wound tracings are an easily obtained measurement that is both inexpensive and that produces minimal discomfort for the patient. Tracings only provide an assessment of wound area. Pressure ulcers with significant wound depth are not well represented by wound tracings. Tracings also require both consistent patient positioning and agreement by clinicians as to what is the exact edge of the wound. Some clinicians trace the extent of undermining on the surface of the skin and trace or measure the entire wound area, not just the wound opening. Improvements in tracing size are a good indicator of wound contraction, but not of volume changes.

Wound photography is a commonly used method to document wound healing. With the advent of the digital camera and increased use of the Internet, wound photography is being used more widely. Telemedicine, using static digital images (store-and-forward technology) or real-time video, has been used to monitor pressure ulcers in the home setting (56). Digital images may be entered into the computer and retrieved by an off-site assessor for patients in remote locations. Photo images may be displayed in the patient's medical record to document progress toward healing. The saying "a picture is worth a thousand words" is true when attempting to describe a wound, whether to another clinician or to a jury in the courtroom. However, photos are two-dimensional images that do not accurately capture wound depth, undermining, tracking, odor, or exudate. Color may also be distorted because of lighting. Photo images, however, provide visual context to linear measurement.

Assessing Wound Base

A wound base may be described as clean, sloughy, or necrotic. A healthy wound base will be filled with red granulation tissue. Chronic pressure ulcers are often pale pink with a smooth, rather than granulating, base. Slough is identified as soft, yellow, brown, or gray material and is characterized by its stringy, adherent quality. A necrotic ulcer can be covered with a hard, dry eschar, or filled with soft, nonviable tissue at the base. Both sloughy and necrotic wounds require debridement. The amount of slough and necrotic tissue should be documented as an estimated percentage of coverage in the wound base. Underlying support structures, such as bone, tendon, or joint capsule, may also be visible or palpable in the wound.

Assessing Wound Exudate

Wound exudate characteristics include amount, color, and quality. Increased exudate is a frequent indicator of bacterial colonization and is a major determinant in the choice of dressing material used. Drainage may be serous, serosanguinous, sanguinous, or purulent. Pressure ulcers with drainage that is other than serosanguinous are not healthy and require additional evaluation to determine what may be interfering with normal wound healing.

Assessing Wound Edge

Assessment and documentation of the condition of the wound edges can give many clues about the wound. Ideally, at the wound edge, advancing epithelium would be seen migrating across a healthy bed of granulation tissue. This is often not the case in the care of chronic wounds. The assessor should note maceration or desiccation of the margins or whether the edge is mounded, indicating the chronic nature of an injury or continued pressure. Epithelium advancing down the side of a deep wound suggests that the wound is not granulating well, and is healing only through contraction and epithelialization.

Assessing Peri-Wound Skin

The skin surrounding the pressure ulcer may be macerated or desiccated. Damage to tissues by maceration may be evidenced by a white, moist appearance with the skin peeling in layers. Epidermal stripping, associated with tape injuries, bleeds readily and may be full thickness. Another cause of damage of the peri-wound skin may be a fungal infection. Cellulitis or induration may be a sign of infection or evidence of continued pressure-induced injury.

Principle #3: Perform Adequate Debridement

If necrotic tissue is present, it must be removed before healing can occur. Necrotic tissue prevents wound healing, harbors bacteria, and obscures the deep regions of the pressure ulcer. An eschar, the dry leathery covering over a pressure ulcer, should not be considered a biologic dressing. It is necrotic skin and subcutaneous tissue and must be debrided. A scab, on the other hand, is dried serum and may be left on a superficial wound as a biologic covering if there is no evidence of infection. Four methods of debridement are sharp or surgical, mechanical, enzymatic, and autolytic. Each has indications and contraindications for use, and each differs in the degree of selectivity and the speed of debridement. Table 49.5 describes the various methods of debridement.

Sharp

Sharp or surgical debridement is the most aggressive form of debridement. Usually performed with a scalpel or scissors, this is often performed at the bedside but may require the operating room if pain and bleeding may be difficult to manage. In addition

Table 49.5 Approaches for Debridement of Pressure Ulcers: Advantages and Disadvantages

	EXAMPLES	ADVANTAGES	DISADVANTAGES
Sharp/Surgical	Scalpel or scissors used to remove necrotic tissue	Fast, effective, and necessary in presence of infection or large amount of necrotic tissue; converts chronic wound bed to acute wound bed	Nonselective—removes healthy as well as necrotic tissue; risk for excess bleeding, pain, or autonomic dysreflexia
Mechanical	Saline and gauze dressings removed dry (wet-to-dry); hydrotherapy	Relatively fast and effective	Nonselective; may be painful to remove dry dressing if adherent to wound bed; labor intensive
Enzymatic	Use of various commercially available enzymatic debridement products	Selective—removes only nonviable tissue	Slow; patients may complain of burning or stinging sensation; often ineffective with hard, dry eschar
Autolytic	Create moist wound environment with occlusive dressing changed every 1–3 days	Selective; excellent adjunct to prepare wound for sharp debridement	Slow; contraindicated in infected wounds; wound exudate may have odor

to ridding the wound of necrotic and infected tissue, sharp debridement also converts a chronic wound into an acute wound. Although this method is fast and effective, it is nonselective and painful for sensate patients. Nonselective techniques are often necessary for the expedient assessment of infected wounds or those with eschar and may be used alone or in combination with other techniques.

Mechanical

Mechanical debridement involves the use of rough gauze or a soft brush to gently scrub the wound bed and loosen or remove any necrotic tissue. This is not as aggressive as sharp debridement. This also includes application of wet-to-dry dressings. Wet-to-dry dressings use open-mesh gauze that is moistened with normal saline and applied to the wound surface. The gauze is left in place and allowed to dry prior to its removal. When removed, the now dry dressing will pull out any necrotic tissue that is attached. This is usually repeated three times each day in dirty wounds. Wet-to-dry dressings are especially helpful when used in conjunction with sharp debridement and are the dressings of choice for infected wounds. Mechanical debridement is relatively fast and effective, but does have several disadvantages. Most important, removal of the dry dressing is painful for the patient who has sensation. Mechanical debridement is also nonselective, so it may damage new granulation tissue and cause bleeding in the wound bed. It is also labor intensive for the nursing staff.

Wet-to-dry dressings are often used with antimicrobial solutions. Acetic acid, hydrogen peroxide, dilute bleach solutions, and povidone iodine have a limited role in modern wound care. These products may be useful for a short period of time to control bacterial load in conjunction with appropriate debridement. Each of these solutions is, however, toxic to fibroblasts and granulation tissue. However, it may be necessary to first control infection in order for healing to occur. The use of silver sulfadiazine cream has been shown to control bacterial load better than povidone iodine without causing damage to fibroblasts (57).

Hydrotherapy is usually considered a component of mechanical debridement. The gentle movement of the water over the necrotic tissue can help to remove it with less pain or discomfort. In a controlled trial of twenty-three people with stage 3 or 4 pressure ulcers, Burke et al. found that "daily whirlpool significantly enhanced wound healing" (58). The disadvantage of immersion hydrotherapy is that it is costly and requires significant time on the part of a specially trained person to coordinate the setup, use, cleaning, and maintenance of the equipment. Pulsed lavage has been used as an effective alternative to immersion hydrotherapy. This powered irrigation device directs irrigation fluid selectively and can be used to cleanse heavily draining or necrotic ulcers (59). Low-frequency, noncontact ultrasound therapy (MIST ultrasound therapy) is another option for debridement and cleansing of wounds without use of immersion hydrotherapy. The ultrasound energy atomizes sterile saline that is directed at the wound bed (60).

Enzymatic

Chemical agents, also known as enzymatic debridement agents, are used to break down necrotic tissue. This method is slower than sharp or mechanical debridement, but it is selective.

Enzymatic agents are most effective in wounds with a relatively small burden of slough or necrotic tissue. They are virtually ineffective against hard, dry eschars.

Autolytic

Autolytic debridement involves the use of an occlusive dressing over a wound to allow the body's own enzymes to break down necrotic tissue. The viable tissue is separated from the nonviable by the body's own enzymes and white blood cells, and the liquefied necrotic tissue is cleaned away with each dressing change. Selecting the best type of occlusive dressing depends on the wound assessment. Thin film dressings are frequently used for dry eschar because they are not absorptive and the wound bed can be easily visualized. Hydrocolloid dressings are frequently used if the wound has some drainage. This product is effective because it maintains a fluid environment while absorbing excess exudate. In both cases, dressings should be changed every 1 to 3 days, and the wounds must be carefully evaluated for infection. Autolytic debridement is advantageous to the patient because it causes very little discomfort and is highly selective. The disadvantages are that this technique is slow and that an odor is often produced with the liquefaction of the necrotic tissue. The patient or caregivers must be vigilant to identify infection when using this technique. Autolytic debridement is contraindicated when there is evidence of active infection in the wound.

Principle #4: Moist Wound Healing

Once the pressure ulcer is clean, the clinician may proceed with moist wound healing. The choice for the type of dressing will depend on one's knowledge of the properties of the wound care products and a good wound assessment. Although many new products become available every year, there is no conclusive evidence that one dressing is better than another. In fact, studies done typically compare the new dressing with saline and gauze dressings as the current standard of care. The great benefit of many new dressings is their ability to decrease the frequency of dressing changes. This offsets the increased cost of the dressing itself with the decreased cost of nursing or caregiver time.

The depth of the wound and the amount of exudate will frequently determine the type and frequency of dressing change. The ultimate goal is to keep the wound environment moist to allow contraction, granulation, and epithelialization while protecting the surrounding skin, with the least amount of dressing and personnel time.

Dressings can be categorized by how much moisture the dressing can absorb and by whether the dressing is designed for superficial use (wafers and sheets) or for deep wounds, which are packed into the wound and require a secondary dressing to hold it in place. The frequency of dressing changes is determined by the amount of wound drainage and the dressing's ability to manage the drainage. Dressings that can be changed once a day or less provide a significant benefit in time.

Wounds should be regularly monitored for healing. Wounds that do not show improvement within 2 weeks should be reevaluated for underlying factors that are interfering with wound healing (18). The problem is most likely not the dressing, but

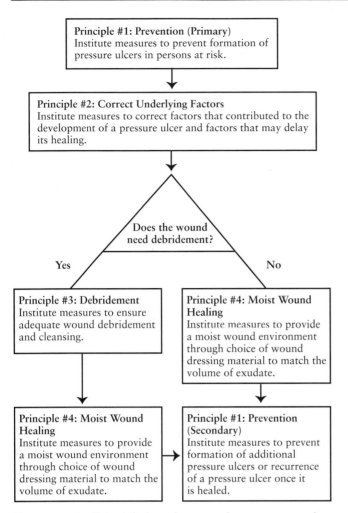

Principle #1: Prevention (Primary)
Institute measures to prevent formation of pressure ulcers in persons at risk.

Principle #2: Correct Underlying Factors
Institute measures to correct factors that contributed to the development of a pressure ulcer and factors that may delay its healing.

Does the wound need debridement?

Yes

No

Principle #3: Debridement
Institute measures to ensure adequate wound debridement and cleansing.

Principle #4: Moist Wound Healing
Institute measures to provide a moist wound environment through choice of wound dressing material to match the volume of exudate.

Principle #4: Moist Wound Healing
Institute measures to provide a moist wound environment through choice of wound dressing material to match the volume of exudate.

Principle #1: Prevention (Secondary)
Institute measures to prevent formation of additional pressure ulcers or recurrence of a pressure ulcer once it is healed.

Figure 49.2 Principle-based approach to pressure ulcer management.

rather an uncorrected intrinsic or extrinsic factor that needs to be addressed.

ADJUNCTIVE TREATMENT FOR PRESSURE ULCERS

Negative Pressure Wound Therapy

Negative pressure wound therapy (NPWT) is widely used to medically manage deep and highly exudative wounds. This therapy involves the use of a foam sponge that is placed into the wound, covered by an occlusive dressing to create an air-tight seal, and connected to a pump that applies negative pressure to the wound bed. Continuous negative pressure is used to remove any excess edema in the peri-wound skin and has been shown to decrease bacterial load in contaminated wounds (61). The removal of excess fluid in the wound bed promotes moist wound healing and evacuates the chronic wound fluid that is thought to retard granulation tissue formation. Negative pressure further assists the body by encouraging angiogenesis. These new blood vessels will carry oxygen and nutrients to the wound bed (62).

There are several advantages of NPWT in relation to patient tolerance and nursing time. The frequency of the dressing change

is most often three times each week, thereby decreasing nursing time. Although nursing duties are increased on dressing change days, nursing activity drops overall when compared to wet-to-dry dressings changed three times each day. Patients also have less pain during their dressing changes.

ELECTRICAL STIMULATION

Electrical stimulation (ES) has been shown to be effective in increasing the healing rate of chronic pressure ulcers. In one study, ES was shown to increase the rate of healing of pressure ulcers compared to placebo at 5, 15, and 20 days using high-voltage pulsed current (HVPC) (63). Stage 2 wounds healed completely in both the ES and placebo groups. All stage 3 and 4 ulcers ($n = 6$) in the ES group, but only three of seven stage 3 and 4 ulcers in the placebo group showed consistent reduction in size compared to baseline. In another study, low-frequency pulsed currents (LFPC) (i.e., alternating current) were compared to direct current and control groups (64). Researchers found that healing is faster when pressure ulcers are treated with ES compared to controls. They found that pressure ulcers treated with LFPC healed twice as fast as those treated with standard care (control). A third survey of SCI-specific pressure ulcers found that electrically balanced asymmetric biphasic waveforms showed the highest rate of complete healing (65). The mechanism of enhanced wound healing using ES is not fully understood. Baker et al. (65) states that the most likely explanation is neural changes caused by the ES, which increases blood flow to the tissue.

Electrical stimulation has not had wide usage throughout the United States. The reasons for this are many; however, this form of treatment should not be overlooked for persons with SCI and difficult-to-heal pressure ulcers.

Growth Factors

Studies of fluids from chronic pressure ulcers have demonstrated a significant degradation of growth factor activity from that found in acute wounds (66, 67). The use of topically applied gels containing platelet-derived growth factor can improve fibroblast activity and shorten healing time for chronic wounds (66). One study (67) showed that once-daily application of becaplermin gel increased the incidence of complete healing (23% versus 0%) and greater-than-90% healing (58% versus 29%) compared to placebo.

Hyperbaric Oxygen

Hyperbaric oxygen (HBO) is a controversial therapy for pressure ulcers. Originally created as a treatment for decompression sickness, HBO involves the administration of 100% oxygen at a pressure of 2 to 3 atmospheres for 1 to 2 hours each day.

HBO is used for treatment of necrotizing fasciitis, refractory osteomyelitis, gas gangrene, and compromised myocutaneous flaps. These uses are directly related to the systemic effects of hyperoxygenation. The reduction of edema in compromised flaps, burns, and crush injuries is a result of the vasoconstrictive effects of HBO. Finally, fibroblast activity and antimicrobial activity are increased with improved oxygenation and the stimulation of the phagocytic activity of the white blood cells (68). Theoretically, pressure ulcers with poor circulation, as demonstrated by decreased TcPO2 in the peri-wound skin, would be candidates for HBO. Further research in this area, however, is needed.

CONCLUSIONS

The medical management of pressure ulcers in persons with SCI requires a comprehensive team approach. Understanding the factors that contribute to the development of pressure ulcers in persons with SCI is essential for all SCI clinicians. Identifying those factors that prevent a pressure ulcer from healing is also essential. Understanding these factors enables the clinician to identify persons at high risk for developing pressure ulcers and allows early intervention. Medical management of pressure ulcers can be accomplished for most patients if the underlying contributing factors can be corrected and the body is given the opportunity to heal. The least important part of medical management of pressure ulcers is the choice of wound dressing, yet this is where most attention is often focused. The skilled clinician will chose a wound dressing that manages the exudate and protects the wound bed while searching out and correcting the factors that contributed to the development of the pressure ulcer and those factors that are preventing the wound from healing.

*R*eferences

1. Liverman CT, Altevogt BM, Joy JE, Johnson RT, eds. *Spinal Cord Injury: Progress, Promise and Priorities/Committee on Spinal Cord Injury, Board on Neuroscience and Behavioral Health.* Washington, DC: The National Academies Press, 2005.
2. Bergstom N. Patients at risk for pressure ulcers and evidence-based care for pressure ulcer prevention. In: Bader D, Bouten C, Colin D, Oomens C, eds. *Pressure Ulcer Research: Current and Future Perspectives.* Berlin: Springer, 2005: 35–50.
3. National Spinal Cord Injury Statistical Center. *Annual Report for the Model Spinal Cord Injury Care Systems.* Birmingham: University of Alabama, 2006.
4. New PW, Rawicki HB, Bailey MJ. Nontraumatic spinal cord injury rehabilitation: pressure ulcer patterns, prediction, and impact. *Arch Phys Med Rehabil* 2004; 85:87–93.
5. Chen Y, DeVivo MJ, Jackson AB. Pressure ulcer prevalence in people with spinal cord injury: age-period-duration effects. *Arch Phys Med Rehabil* 2005; 86:1208–1213.
6. Garber SL, Rintala RH, Hart KA, Fuhrer MJ. Pressure ulcer risk in spinal cord injury: predictors of ulcer status over 3 years. *Arch Phys Med Rehabil* 2000; 81:465–471.
7. Krause JS, Broderick L. Patterns of recurrent pressure ulcers after spinal cord injury: identification of risk and protective factors 5 or more years after onset. *Arch Phys Med Rehabil* 2004; 84:1257–1264.
8. Krause JS, Vines CL, Farley TL, Sniezek J, Coker J. An exploratory study of pressure ulcers after spinal cord injury: relationship to protective behaviors and risk factors. *Arch Phys Med Rehabil* 2001; 82(1):107–113.
9. Cardenas DD, Hoffman JM, Kirshblum S, McKinley W. Etiology and incidence of rehospitalization after traumatic spinal cord injury: a multicenter analysis. *Arch Phys Med Rehabil* 2004; 85:1757–1763.
10. Garber SL, Rintala DH. Pressure ulcers in veterans with spinal cord injury: a retrospective study. *J Rehabil Res Dev* 2003; 40(5):433–442.
11. Langemo DK, Melland H, Hanson D, Olson B, Hunter S. The lived experience of having a pressure ulcer: a qualitative analysis. *Adv Skin Wound Care* 2000; 135:225–235.
12. Black J, Baharestani MM, Cuddigan J, Dorner B, et al. National Pressure Ulcer Advisory Panel's Updated Pressure Ulcer Staging System. *Adv Skin Wound Care* 2007; 20(5): 269–274.
13. Kosiak M. Etiology and pathology of ischemic ulcers. *Arch Phys Med Rehabil* 1959; 40:62–68.
14. Kosiak M. Etiology of decubitus ulcers. *Arch Phys Med Rehabil* 1961; 42:19–29.
15. Linder RM, Morris D. The surgical management of pressure ulcers: a systematic approach based on staging. *Decubitus* 1990; 32:32–38.
16. Clark FA, Jackson JM, Scott MD, Carlson ME, et al. Data-based models of how pressure ulcers develop in daily living contexts of adults with spinal cord injury. *Arch Phys Med Rehabil* 2006; 87:1516–1525.
17. Dinsdale SM. Decubitus ulcers: role of pressure and friction in causation. *Arch Phys Med Rehabil* 1974; 55:147–152.
18. *Pressure Ulcer Prevention and Treatment Following Spinal Cord Injury: A Clinical Practice Guideline for Health-Care Professionals.* Consortium for Spinal Cord Injury Medicine Clinical Practice Guidelines. Paralyzed Veterans of America, 2000.
19. Young JS, Burns PE. Pressure sores and the spinal cord–injured. *SCI Digest* 1981; 3:11–48.
20. Fuhrer MJ, Garber SL, Rintala DH, Clearman R, Hart KA. Pressure ulcers in community-resident persons with spinal cord injury: prevalence and risk factors. *Arch Phys Med Rehabil* 1993; 74(11):1172–1177.
21. Knox DM, Anderson TM, Anderson PS. Effects of different turn intervals on skin of healthy older adults. *Adv Wound Care* 1994; 7:48–56.
22. Seymour RJ, Lacefield WE. Wheelchair cushion effect on pressure and skin temperature. *Arch Phys Med Rehabil* 1985; 66(2):103–108.
23. Fisher SV, Szymke TE, Apte SY, Kosiak M. Wheelchair cushion effect on skin temperature. *Arch Phys Med Rehabil* 1978; 59(2):68–72.
24. Makhsous M, Priebe M, Bankard J, Rowles D, et al. Measuring tissue perfusion during pressure relief maneuvers: insights into preventing pressure ulcers. *J Spinal Cord Med* 2007; 30:497–507.
25. Thorfinn J, Sjoberg F, Sjostrand L, Lidman D. Perfusion of the skin of the buttocks in paraplegic and tetraplegic patients, and in healthy subjects after a short and long period. *Scand J Plast Reconstr Surg Hand Surg* 2006; 40:153–160.
26. Hagisawa S, Ferguson-Pell M, Cardi M, Miller SD. Assessment of skin blood content and oxygenation in spinal cord injured subjects during reactive hyperemia. *J Rehabil Res Dev* 1994; 31:1–14.
27. Schubert V, Schubert PA, Briet G, Intaglietta M. Analysis of arterial flow-motion in spinal cord injured and elderly subjects in an area at risk for the development of pressure sores. *Paraplegia* 1995; 33:387–397.
28. Colin D, Abraham P, Preault L, Bregeon C, Saumet JL. Comparison of 90 degrees and 30 degrees laterally inclined positions in the prevention of pressure ulcers using transcutaneous oxygen and carbon dioxide pressures. *Adv Wound Care* 1996; 93:35–38.
29. Polliack A, Tablor R, Bader C. Sweat analysis following pressure ischaemia in a group of debilitated subjects. *J Rehabil Res Dev* 1997; 34:303–308.
30. Mahanty SD, Roemer RB, Meisel H. Thermal response of paraplegic skin to the application of local pressure. *Arch Phys Med Rehabil* 1981; 62(12):608–611.
31. Vistnes LM. Pressure sores: etiology and prevention. *Bull Prosthet Res* 1980; 17:123–125.
32. Finestone HM, Levine SP, Carlson GA, Chizinsky KA, Kett RL. Erythema and skin temperature following continuous sitting in spinal cord injured individuals. *J Rehabil Res Dev* 1991; 28:27–32.
33. Cruse JM, Lewis RE, Dilioglou S, Roe DL, et al. Review of immune function, healing of pressure ulcers, and nutritional status in patients with spinal cord injury. *J Spinal Cord Med* 2000; 232:129–135.
34. Perkash A, Brown M. Anemia in patients with traumatic spinal cord injury. *J Am Paraplegia Soc* 1986; 91(2):10–15.
35. Keast DH, Fraser D. Treatment of chronic skin ulcers in individuals with anemia of chronic disease using recombinant human erythropoietin (EPO). *Ostomy Wound Manage* 2004; 50(10):64–70.
36. Moussavi RM, Garza HN, Eisele SG, Rodriguez G, Rintala DH. Serum levels of vitamin A, C, and E in persons with chronic spinal cord injury living in the community. *Arch Phys Med Rehabil* 2003; 84:1061–1067.
37. Anstead GM. Steroids, retinoids, and wound healing. *Adv Wound Care* 1998; 11:277–285.
38. Frankel H, Sperry J, Kaplan L. Risk factors for pressure ulcer development in a best practice surgical intensive care unit. *Am Surg* 2007; 73:1215–1217.
39. Wang YH, Huang TS, Lien IN. Hormone changes in men with spinal cord injuries. *Am J Phys Med Rehabil* 1992; 71(6):328–332.
40. Defloor T. The effect of position and mattress on interface pressure. *Appl Nurs Res* 2000; 13(1):2–11.
41. Riches D. The multiple roles of macrophages in wound healing. In: Clark R, Henson P, eds. *The Molecular and Cellular Biology of Wound Repair.* New York: Plenum Press, 1988.
42. Ehrlich HP. The physiology of wound healing: a summary of normal and abnormal wound healing processes. *Adv Wound Care* 1998; 117:326–328.

43. Romanelli M, Mastronicola D. The role of wound-bed preparation in managing chronic pressure ulcers. *J Wound Car* 2002;11(8): 305–310.

44. Whitney J, Phillips L, Aslam R, Barbul A, et al. Guidelines for the treatment of pressure ulcers. *Wound Repair Regen* 1996; 14:663–679.

45. Goldstone LA, Goldstone J. The Norton score: an early warning of pressure sores? *J Adv Nurs* 1982:419.

46. Lincoln R, Roberts R, Maddox A. Use of the Norton pressure sore risk assessment scoring system with elderly patients in acute care. *J Enterostomal Ther* 1986; 13:17.

47. Bergstrom N, Demuth PJ, Braden B. A clinical trial of the Braden scale for predicting pressure sore risk. *Nurs Clin North Am* 1987; 22:417.

48. Salzberg CA, Byrne DW, Cayten CG, Kabir R, et al. Predicting and preventing pressure ulcers in adults with paralysis. *Adv Wound Care* 1998;11(5):237–246.

49. Garber SL, Rintala DH, Holmes SA, Rodriguez GP, Friedman J. A structured educational model to improve pressure ulcer prevention knowledge in veterans with spinal cord dysfunction. *J Rehabil Res Dev* 2002; 39(5):575–588. Erratum in: *J Rehabil Res Dev* 2002; 39(6):711.

50. Coggrave MJ, Rose LS. A specialist seating assessment clinic: changing pressure relief practice. *Spinal Cord* 2003; 41:692–695.

51. Collins N. The right mix: using nutritional interventions and an anabolic agent to manage a stage IV ulcer. *Adv Skin Wound Care* 2004; 17:36–39.

52. Lee SK, Posthauer ME, Dorner B, Redovian V, Maloney MJ. Pressure ulcer healing with a concentrated, fortified, collagen protein hydrolysate supplement: a randomized controlled trial. *Adv Skin Wound Care* 2006; 19:92–96.

53. Spungen AM, Koehler KM, Modeste-Duncan R, Rasul M, et al. 9 clinical cases of nonhealing pressure ulcers in patients with spinal cord injury treated with an anabolic agent: a therapeutic trial. *Adv Skin Wound Care.* 2001; 14(3):139–144.

54. Salcido R. Anabolic steroids for pressure ulcers revisited. *Adv Skin Wound Care* 2005; 18(7):344–346.

55. Gardner SE, Frantz RA, Bergquist S, Shin CD. A prospective study of the pressure ulcer scale for healing (PUSH). *J Gerontol A Biol Sci Med Sci* 2005; 60(1):93–97.

56. Ho CH, Bogie K. The prevention and treatment of pressure ulcers. *Phys Med Rehabil Clin N Am* 2007; 18:235–253.

57. Kucan JO, Robson MC, Heggers JP, Ko F. Comparison of silver sulfadiazine, povidone-iodine and physiologic saline in the treatment of chronic pressure ulcers. *J Am Geriatr Soc* 1981; 295:232–235.

58. Burke DT, Ho CH, Saucier MA, Stewart G. Effects of hydrotherapy on pressure ulcer healing. *Am J Phys Med Rehabil* 1998; 77(5):394–398.

59. Svoboda SJ, Bice TG, Gooden HA, Brooks DE, et al. Comparison of bulb syringe and pulsed lavage irrigation with use of a bioluminescent musculoskeletal wound model. *J Bone Joint Surg* 2006; 88-A(10): 2167–2174.

60. Ennis WJ, Valdes W, Gainer M, Meneses P. Evaluation of clinical effectiveness of MIST ultrasound therapy for the healing of chronic wounds. *Adv Skin Wound Care* 2006; 19:437–446.

61. Argenta L, Morykwas M. Vacuum-assisted closure: a new method for wound control and treatment—clinical experience. *Ann Plast Surg* 1997; 38:563–576.

62. Mendez-Eastman S. Negative pressure wound therapy. *Plast Surg Nurs* 1998; 18:33–37.

63. Griffin JW, Tooms RE, Mendius RA, Clifft JK, et al. Efficacy of high voltage pulsed current for healing of pressure ulcers in patients with spinal cord injury. *Phys Ther* 1991; 716:433–442.

64. Stefanovska A, Vodovnik L, Benko H, Turk R. Treatment of chronic wounds by means of electric and electromagnetic fields. Part 2. Value of FES parameters for pressure sore treatment. *Med Biol Eng Comput* 1993; 313:213–220.

65. Baker L, Rubayi S, Villar F. Effect of electrical stimulation waveform on healing of ulcers in human beings with spinal cord injury. *Wound Repair Regen* 1996; 4:21–28.

66. Mast BA, Schultz G. Interactions of cytokines, growth factors, and proteases in acute and chronic wounds. *Wound Repair Regen* 1996; October–December:411–420.

67. Rees RS, Robson MC, Smiell JM, Perry BH. Becaplermin gel in the treatment of pressure ulcers: a phase II randomized, double-blind, placebo-controlled study. *Wound Repair Regen* 1999; 73:141–147.

68. Thackham JA, McElwain DL, Long RJ. The use of hyperbaric oxygen therapy to treat chronic wounds: a review. *Wound Repair Regen* 2008; 16:321–330.

50 The Surgical Management of Pressure Ulcers

Robert E. Montroy
Ibrahim M. Eltorai
Susan V. Garstang

And a certain poor man named Lazarus was . . .
covered with sores . . . even the dogs were coming
and licking his sores.

—*Luke 16:20–21*

The care of the patient with spinal cord dysfunction, whether caused by trauma or disease, is multifaceted and requires an interdisciplinary team approach. The surgeon is a necessary member of the team and must be knowledgeable about the broad spectrum of spinal cord medicine. Although primarily concerned with the surgical management of the pressure ulcer, the reconstructive surgeon must be familiar with the frequent concomitant lifetime medical and socioeconomic problems encountered in this special patient population. In the same manner, other members of this team should be familiar with the special surgical aspects of the patient's care. With this in view, the focus of this chapter is not so much on the technological aspects of flap surgery but rather on the basic concepts of the role of surgery in the repair of pressure ulcers, and the contributions of the surgeon as a team member in the surgical management of these wounds in this challenging group of patients.

THE PRESSURE ULCER DILEMMA

Until a half-century ago, few surgeons were involved in pressure ulcer treatment, because these wounds were considered indicators of a terminal illness. Even today, the general perception is that they occur in the infirm and aged or in people bedridden with incurable diseases—hence the persistence of the term "bed sores." As a result, the care of these wounds in the past was often neglected and attention was diverted to the other seemingly more pressing medical problems that are common in these patients.

For the individual with a debilitating illness, the infirmities of the aging process, or the sequelae of neurologic dysfunction from any cause, the specter of failed skin integrity is forever present. Although pain may not be a factor in many of these wounds, foul odor, the ritual of numerous dressing changes, the need for modification or cessation of activities, and the need for frequent medical attention at a clinic or even hospitalization can be a heavy burden for patients with these wounds.

For the patient undergoing a rehabilitation program, the development of a pressure ulcer and subsequent obligatory bed rest can severely curtail and prolong the rehabilitation process. Prolonged bed rest in the newly spinal cord–injured patient contributes to the atrophy of muscle (1, 2), to urinary tract infections and stone formation (3), to venous thrombosis, to persistent orthostasis, and to mental depression, as these patients are trying to adjust to their injuries.

Not only are these wounds disruptive of an individual's daily activities, but their treatment is also costly, having an estimated range of between $15,000 and $40,000 to treat a single pressure ulcer (4). The total national cost of the medical treatment of these wounds exceeds $1.335 billion a year (5). Based on the premise that an "ounce of prevention is worth a pound of cure," approximately $500 million is spent each year on the seemingly unlimited number of preventative pressure relief products that are available on the market. An estimate of the cost of the "pound of cure" when prevention fails is in the range of an additional $200 million just for drug therapy alone (4). Hirshberg et al. reported that the cost of hospitalization, durable medical equipment, home nursing care, physician management, and transportation supports a $20-billion-a-year industry (6).

In addition, there are numerous "nonmedical" factors, both social and economic, that have compounded these obvious medical treatment costs at a significantly higher annual multibillion dollar amount. It is clear that the theoretically preventable pressure ulcer is a major player in the competition for society's available healthcare resources and that prevention must be a major goal in the care of the at-risk patient population. To add impetus to the need for prevention, starting in 2009, Medicare will withhold additional payments to hospitals if patients develop stage 3 or 4 pressure ulcers while in the hospital, as these are considered potentially preventable adverse events (7).

FACTORS IN COST ESCALATION

The exponential growth of the chronic wound care marketplace is in part caused by the increased incidence of pressure ulcers during the latter half of the twentieth century. Discounting warfare (euphemistically called "the extension of diplomacy by other means") (8), which was a major impetus to the modern development of the specialty of spinal cord injury (SCI) medicine, such factors as the increased life expectancy of the population, the omnipresent internal combustion engine, internecine urban warfare, and the population explosion have made their contributions to this modern epidemic of pressure ulcers. The main causative factors for this increase in incidence, however, are inherent in medicine itself.

With advances in medical and trauma care, including Dr. Fleming's serendipitous discovery of penicillin in 1928 and the dawning of the antibiotic era in the 1930s and 1940s, many patients have been enabled to weather the storm of serious disease or trauma to live relatively normal life spans. In this past half-century, patients with neurologic impairments have begun to survive in a kind of symbiotic relationship with their formally fatal complications, which often include pressure ulcers.

Prior to these advances, pressure ulcers did not command very much interest. Standard textbooks of surgery only briefly (if at all) referred to the sores of the bedridden; the only surgical treatment mentioned was skin grafting or simple suturing of small ulcers. Fomon, in his 1400-page surgical tome written in the late 1930s, granted only one page to discuss the surgical treatment of these wounds (9).

The reason for the surgeon's neglect of pressure ulcers prior to World War II is that patients with "bed sores" had a short life expectancy. Any significant trauma to the spinal cord was considered a mortal injury, and the development of bed sores was an ominous sign. Of the American combat troops in World War I who sustained injuries to the central nervous system, only 20% survived long enough to be brought home. Of these survivors, half were dead within a year, usually from infection and sepsis originating in the genitourinary tract or in their numerous necrotic pressure ulcers (10).

Because this mortality rate was considered the normal outcome of a central nervous system injury from time immemorial, there was little interest in the "untreatable" ulcer that was considered an integral part of "the neurological syndrome" (11). It was taught that any surgical approach was doomed to failure because of infection and the pathophysiology of SCI. In 1940, Donald Monro, the father of modern SCI treatment in the United States, taught that even the simple lancing of an abscessed wound was contraindicated in SCI patients. Such abscesses should be treated by needle aspiration to avoid spreading the infection by cutting tissue and causing fatal "blood poisoning" (12).

Also in the early 1940s, Guttmann's teachings promoted a new philosophy toward the care of persons with spinal cord injury, including an aggressive approach to rehabilitation and the engagement of these patients in an active lifestyle. This not only decreased the mortality rate of patients with spinal cord injury, but also shifted the patterns of ulceration from sacral (from being bedridden) to ischial (from sitting and wheelchair use) (13).

TO DO OR NOT TO DO

That is the question. Although attitudes are not as dogmatic as Dr. Monro's dictum, the surgical treatment of pressure ulcers in SCI patients still has its detractors. They point out that the high recurrence rate among patients with spinal cord injuries is evidence of the futility of the surgical approach. Although not condemning surgical closure of pressure ulcers, Evans et al. (14) reviewed the problem of recurrence and recidivism and asked the question, Is soft tissue closure "curative" for SCI patients with pressure ulcers? This and other studies (15) raise the question of the management of SCI pressure ulcers by surgical closure. Are these ulcers an inevitable and natural consequence of the injury, and thus part of the SCI syndrome, as taught by Charcot (11) in 1879, or are they just a complication of the syndrome that can be prevented by good nursing care?

In the Evans study, seventy-nine operations were performed in thirty patients. This cohort included both traumatic and nontraumatic SCI patients, as well as debilitated and infirm non-SCI patients. Of the twenty-two SCI patients, 82% had a recurrent ulcer at the surgical site within 1 to 78 months following the surgical repair, with an average time to recurrence of 18.2 months. Fourteen patients developed pressure ulcers at a site remote from the surgical repair in the average time of 20.2 months, with a range between 1 and 72 months. Overall, twenty of the twenty-two paraplegic patients (91%) had developed an ulcer at either the surgical site or at a new site within an average time of 19.2 months. In comparison to these patients, there were no recurrences following surgical closure in four of the nonparaplegic patients, either at the surgical site or at a remote site. The remaining nonparalyzed patients did not undergo surgery because of their unstable medical or geriatric condition.

Schryvers et al. looked at 431 surgically treated pressure ulcers in persons with neurologic impairments; 380 ulcers were treated with 421 surgical procedures (253 fasciocutaneous or cutaneous flaps, 93 muscle or musculocutaneous flaps, 75 primary closures). In this series, there was suture line dehiscence in 31% of cases. Eleven percent of cases required reoperation, 11% healed secondarily, and 2% healed after split-thickness skin grafts. Nine percent of patients had not healed at the time of discharge. Fifty-four percent of patients required readmission for recurrence of ulcers; of these, 31% were at the same site, and 21% were at different sites. Osteomyelitis was diagnosed in 16% of cases (13).

Experiences such as those mentioned above have reinforced the opinion of some physicians that, because of the failure of operative intervention to cure the disease, conservative (nonsurgical) methods of wound care are the treatments of choice for pressure ulcers in SCI patients. It is granted that not all patients should be considered candidates for the surgical closure of their wounds. The elderly, the infirm, or those suffering from terminal disease should be humanely cared for by nonsurgical means in a hospice or nursing home setting. However, with the appreciation of potential complications such as sepsis, osteomyelitis, or even malignant transformation (16, 17) in the chronic pressure ulcer, as well as the cost of care and the effects on the quality of life associated with prolonged bed rest, conservative wound care in the rehabilitative patient is not the answer either. The pre–World War II philosophy of institutional care for these patients is not appropriate today.

The problem remains that when pressure ulcers in the SCI patient are successfully healed by either the conservative "secondary intention" route or by invasive surgery, there is a significant recurrence rate of from 5% to 91% (18). The culprit is not the ulcer and its particular mode of treatment per se but the underlying pathologic condition combined with psychosocial issues that may perpetuate this disease or syndrome.

It is obvious that neither surgery nor nonsurgical treatment of pressure ulcers in SCI patients is curative. The selection of the surgical procedure or the level of the surgical skill employed has not been the issue in recurrence in most studies (14, 18). It is "the ounce of prevention" and not the "pound of cure" that must be addressed to improve the quality of life in these individuals. The education of the SCI patient and caregiver, appropriate rehabilitation, social and economic issues, and psychologic factors such as depression and patient compliance are all elements in the pressure ulcer equation—components as equally important as the SCI pathologic syndrome itself. A lifelong holistic treatment plan must be pursued.

THE PRESSURE ULCER AS A WOUND

A wound is an injury that disrupts the integrity of tissue and normally results in an acute inflammatory response (cause and effect) that is intended to limit further injury and that initiates an incredibly complex wound healing process. This wound healing process is a dynamic interactive process involving hematogenous and tissue cells along with humoral components of the activated clotting and complement pathways. The inflammatory process releases numerous cytokines and other growth factors, eventually leading to the production of extracellular matrix components, proteases, and various cytokine growth factors and inhibitors that interact to result in a healed wound. Wound-healing research into this process has led to the development of recombinant exogenous growth factors that have been applied to wounds in order to promote wound healing (19, 20). A recent study suggests that the preoperative application of these recombinant growth factors may contribute to the successful surgical closure of chronic pressure ulcers (21).

This classic wound healing process has three overlapping phases, distinguished by the prevailing dominant biologic process present during a particular sequential time frame. They are the *inflammation phase,* the *tissue-formation phase,* and the *tissue-remodeling phase.* Numerous reviews are available detailing this incredible and fascinating process (22–24) for those interested; these will not be discussed here.

The different gradations of wounds depend on the extent of the injury. A wound may be relatively trivial, such as a contusion or an abrasion. Here, the wound healing inflammatory cascade normally leads to the restoration of tissue integrity within 1 or 2 weeks by the regeneration of cloned epithelial and/or endothelial cells, so that the healed wound is fully restored to its functional and aesthetic preinjury state. The remodeling phase is minimal to nonexistent, because there is usually no scar tissue formation.

In a laceration, this same wound healing process of inflammation and cellular proliferation leads to the restoration of tissue integrity in a week or two (healing by primary intention). In a cutaneous laceration extending completely through the dermis, there is a combination of the processes of epithelial regeneration and scar tissue formation that results in the formation of a new type of tissue called *scar-epithelium*—an inferior although satisfactory substitute for the destroyed dermis that, unlike epithelium, does not regenerate. The final remodeling or maturation phase of this scar tissue may take 6 months or longer.

In a wound with loss of tissue, as in an ulcer, the healing process is more challenging than in the primary intention healing of a laceration. With time and a prolonged inflammatory process, the tissue deficit, if limited, eventually heals by (1) contraction of scar tissue and (2) epithelialization. This process is known as healing by *secondary intention.* Although restoring the integrity of the protective mechanical barrier of skin, such healed wounds are devoid of skin's normal physiologic functions. Scar epithelium lacks nerve endings, pilosebaceous and sweat glands, and hair follicles, and is relatively ischemic compared to the adjacent normal skin.

The seriousness of the injury and the ability of the wound to heal itself normally correlate with the degree of tissue injured. With significant tissue destruction, the capability of the organism to heal and restore tissue continuity in a reasonable time frame is severely strained, if not arrested (wound healing exhaustion). Wounds that fail to heal become chronic and debilitating to the patient because of the prolonged and enhanced inflammatory process. The systemic catabolic effects of the extended period of inflammation may be seen in the malnutrition and anemia that one frequently sees in patients with chronic pressure sores.

It is now recognized that there is more to the development of wound chronicity than the failure of a wound to heal within a certain time frame. Studies of the molecular environment of acute and chronic wounds indicate a difference in the microenvironment of acute and chronic wounds. Tarnuzzer and Schultz demonstrated that fluid specimens collected from chronic wounds were not mitogenic and blocked the DNA synthesis normally stimulated by acute wound fluid (25).

It has been noted by others that fluid from chronic wounds inhibits the proliferation of keratinocytes, fibroblasts, and vascular endothelial cells, elements necessary for the healing of wounds (26, 27). Bucalo et al. also observed that cell adhesion was inhibited by chronic wound fluid (28). It would appear that the reduced level of growth factors in chronic wounds, along with the presence of cytokine inhibitors and proteases normally involved in the remodeling phase of wound healing, inhibit the reparative processes initiated in an acute wound.

CLASSIFICATION OF PRESSURE SORE SEVERITY

A system of classifying the degree of severity of the wound is helpful in planning the type of treatment needed to heal these wounds. In the case of an acute thermal injury, the tissue destruction is usually relatively superficial but can be serious when it involves a large portion of the body surface area, thus evoking not just a localized inflammatory response, but a severe systemic inflammatory reaction (29). Such an enhanced systemic response is injurious to the entire organism and can be brought under control only by closing the wound with skin grafts.

Table 50.1   Stages of Severity of Pressure Ulcers

Stage 1	Nonblanchable erythema of intact skin.
Stage 2	Partial-thickness skin loss with preservation of deep dermis and adnexal skin glands. May involve entire dermis but not subcutaneous fat (abrasion, blister, contusion, shallow ulcers).
Stage 3	Full-thickness skin loss, with damaged or destroyed subcutaneous fat down to deep fascia. Tendency to undermining and sinus formation.
Stage 4	Full-thickness loss to muscle, bone, joint, and the supporting structures (ligaments, tendons, joint capsule). Undermining, bursa, and sinus tracks not uncommon.

Adapted from Treatment of Pressure Ulcers. In: *Clinical Practice Guidelines*, Number 15. Rockville MD: U.S. Department Health and Human Services, 1994.

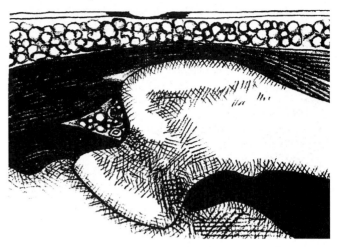

Figure 50.1B   Stage 2 pressure ulcer is a wound with a partial loss of skin that may only involve the epidermis (abrasion, blister) but can include a limited loss of the dermis preserving the deep dermal elements without the involvement of subcutaneous fat.

Like the major and minor burn wounds, the seriousness of a pressure ulcer is determined by the extent of the tissue destruction and the magnitude of the inflammatory response. In thermal injury, the terms "partial-thickness burn" and "full-thickness burn" have replaced the old terminology of first-, second-, and third-degree burns as a measure of wound depth. In the case of the pressure ulcer, where the vertical dimension of depth is the major prognosticator of tissue repair, the term *stage* is used and is analogous to the old burn wound terminology of *degree*. As in burns, this clinical staging of pressure ulcers is useful in assessing the extent of the injury and is used in the development of a surgical or a nonsurgical treatment plan (see Table 50.1). The present consensus grading classification is derived from the original numeric system proposed by Shae in 1975 (30).

In the stage 1 injury, similar to a first-degree burn such as sunburn, the erythema of the invoked localized inflammatory response is the harbinger that tissue injury has occurred (Figure 50.1A). The observable cutaneous vasodilatation is in response to the release of chemotactic cytokines and vasoactive mediators by the injured or activated inflammatory cells. Because there is no tissue loss other than superficial desquamation, this inflammatory phase resolves without calling forth the classic fibroplasia of the proliferative phase of wound repair. Its persistence distinguishes it from the short-lived reactive hyperemia of reperfusion that follows a transitory disruption of capillary flow that may be occasioned by a brief period of external pressure. A stage 1 pressure injury must be heeded as a warning sign that death of tissue is about to take place. Treatment must be instituted in the form of immediate and complete pressure relief until the affected tissue recovers.

The presence of a blister, an abrasion, or the bluish discoloration of a contusion portends a more significant injury than in a stage 1 lesion. This stage 2 injury (Figure 50.1B) results in actual cell death and tissue loss, but any ulceration is limited to the skin and does not clinically involve the subcutaneous fat.

The superficial type of stage 2 injury involving the epidermis or superficial dermis (abrasion) will heal by epithelial regeneration, the result of the replication (mitosis) and migration of surviving epithelial cells across the denuded dermis under the impetus of the released inflammatory cytokines. This regeneration takes place from the viable epithelial cells at the edges of the wound and from the epidermal skin adnexal cells (hair follicles, sweat glands, pilosebaceous glands) residing in the intact dermis.

In deeper stage 2 ulcers involving partial loss of the dermis, the destruction involves cells that do not regenerate and will require replacement by fibrotic scar tissue that is primarily made up of collagen fibers. Residual keratinocytes may be present in the depth of a deep stage 2 ulcer, residing in the surviving skin adnexal cells that often extend into the upper subcutaneous fat layer and are available to contribute to the peripheral epithelial regeneration. These supplementing keratinocyte colonies are visible in the depths of the healing stage 2 wound as tiny white islands or pearls that gradually coalesce to form a new epidermal layer. This same process of scar-epithelium formation is also seen in the healing of deep partial-thickness (second-degree) thermal burns.

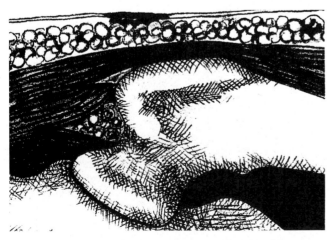

Figure 50.1A   Stage 1 pressure ulcer with injured but intact skin. In patients with darker pigmentation, the erythematous inflammatory reaction to the injury may not be noticed by the casual observer. The underlying bony prominence is a causative factor involved in the formation of pressure ulcers.

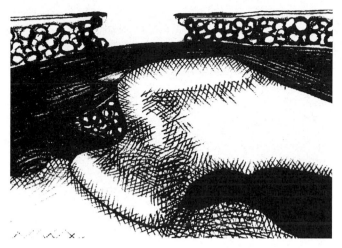

Figure 50.1C Stage 3 pressure ulcer with full-thickness loss of skin. The subcutaneous fat may suffer a partial or full-thickness loss extending to the deep fascia overlying an intact muscle layer.

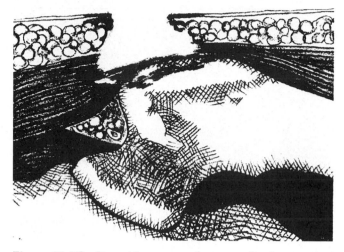

Figure 50.1E Stage 4A pressure ulcer extending into or completely through the underlying muscle layer. A reactive periostitis may be present, but cortical bone is not eroded in a stage 4A ulcer.

The stage 3 injury involves the subcutaneous fat and may extend to the level of the deep fascia overlying the muscle compartment (Figure 50.1C). Because of the superior blood supply of the dermis compared to adipose tissue, there may be a greater loss of the relatively ischemic subcutaneous fat compared to the overlying skin, resulting in an undermining of the ulcerated skin margins. Thus, there may be a more significant tissue loss than is apparent from a casual inspection of the skin defect itself (Figure 50.1D).

The skin over the pocket of devitalized subcutaneous fat may even be intact because of this superior circulation. Such an injury usually manifests itself following bacterial invasion of the liquefying dead or hypoxic fat tissue by an abscess that either spontaneously ruptures through the skin or is drained by scalpel intervention. If small and shallow, stage 3 ulcers may heal in a reasonable time frame by secondary intention through the process of contraction and epithelialization.

Like dermis, muscle tissue is more vascular than subcutaneous fat and more resistant to pressure-induced ischemia. However, if the injury is severe enough, it too will necrose and result in a stage 4 wound (Figures 50.1E and F). Undermining and sinus tract formation is common and difficult to heal without surgical intervention. A more extensive stage 4 pressure ulcer may extend to bone and joint, thus resulting in periostitis, osteomyelitis, or even pyoarthritis. This type of wound involving bone or joint is classified as a stage 4B ulcer by Eltorai (31) because of the more serious nature of the injury and its more complex treatment. Such an ulcer is obviously a more serious wound and is not normally amenable to treatment without surgical intervention (Figure 50.1G).

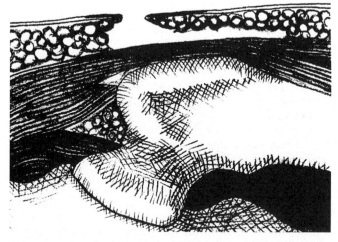

Figure 50.1D Stage 3 pressure ulcer with lateral destruction of the relatively ischemic subcutaneous fat with undermining of the more vascularized skin.

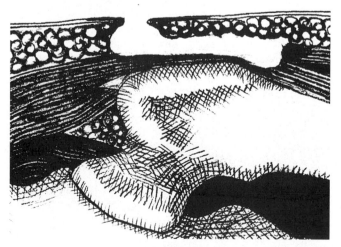

Figure 50.1F A presumed stage 3 ulcer with undermining or sinus formation may actually be a stage 4A ulcer because of unsuspected involvement of muscle tissue remote from the cutaneous wound.

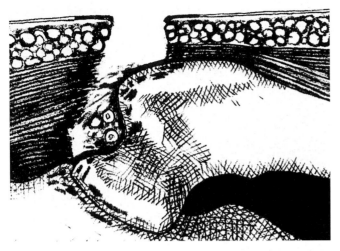

Figure 50.1G Stage 4B ulcer with involvement of muscle with extension through the joint capsule into the joint space. In some systems of pressure ulcer classification, involvement of muscle and joint is considered a single stage 4 wound.

COMPLICATIONS OF PRESSURE SORES

The early and late complications of pressure ulcers must be addressed. The goal of all treatment (surgical and nonsurgical) is healing of the wound, and this requires the prevention of complications that disrupt the normal wound healing process and that can lead to a chronic nonhealing ulcer. The prevention of complications in the acutely injured tissue begins with the recognition of the injury and the removal of the causative agent; treatment begins with pressure relief. Without pressure relief and the control of infection, a superficial stage 1 or 2 ulcer will progress into the deeper tissues and become a more serious stage 3 or stage 4 ulcer.

Bed Rest

Pressure relief in the wheelchair-ambulant patient who develops a pressure ulcer usually entails bed rest that has its own subset of complications. Attempting to avoid further tissue damage and seeking to heal the ulcer requires the removal of the main causative agent of the wound—unremitting pressure. The immobility and reduced physical activity accompanying enforced bed rest, however, increase the loss of bone and muscle mass (1, 2) and encourage the development of joint contractures, particularly in patients with spasticity. Loss of upper body strength in paraplegics confined to bed will require subsequent physical therapy focused on the recovery of muscle strength before they can safely do transfers and operate their manual wheelchairs. Bed rest also places the patient at risk for developing additional pressure ulcers. Consequently, avoidance of this cascade of complications by healing the wound and returning the patient to the ambulant state should be accomplished as early as feasible.

Infection

The invasion of bacteria following the loss of the integrity of the protective skin barrier results in a local invasive wound infection that is nourished by the dead and dying tissue of the pressure ulcer. The establishment of this local infection is a major contributor to the tissue destruction that ensues. It is generally accepted that infection is present when a quantitative assay of the cultured organism(s) exceeds 10^5 organisms per gram of tissue. A bacterial burden that is less than that figure is not considered an infection, but the wound is said to be *colonized*. In the afebrile patient with a normal white blood cell count and a chronic or healing subacute ulcer, wound cultures will reveal a variety of organisms, but only as colonizers, and infection is usually not present. The use of systemic or topical antibiotics is not warranted in colonized ulcers and is, in fact, contraindicated because the end result will be the loss of control of the bacterial invaders and the proliferation of resistant organisms.

An acute infectious process, accompanied by chills, fever, and an elevated white blood cell count, indicates the bacteremia of systemic sepsis. Empirical systemic intravenous antibiotic therapy based on clinical judgment must be initiated and adjusted as soon as sensitivity studies are available. In addition to antibiotics, debridement of the devitalized tissue and drainage of all abscess pockets must be carried out. Appropriate studies should be undertaken if osteomyelitis is suspected.

Sepsis and Septic Shock

In the acute pressure sore setting, the bacterial invasion (infection) of body tissues will initiate a local inflammatory response that seeks to eradicate the undesired invaders. It is frequently accompanied by fever and elevation of the white blood cell count. If uncontrolled, the local infection will lead to further tissue destruction, converting a stage 2 ulcer to a stage 3 or 4 ulcer. Should bacteremia develop, there is the potential for generalized sepsis having a marked systemic inflammatory response that may adversely produce dysfunction in one or more organ systems. Furthermore, this ensuing systemic inflammatory response syndrome (SIRS) can precipitate a potentially lethal septic shock phase, with subsequent multiorgan failure (29, 32).

Periostitis/Osteomyelitis

The stage 4 ulcer may involve bone by direct extension of the infected pressure ulcer and, if inadequately treated, will doom any wound healing treatment plan. The inflammatory involvement of the periosteum (periostitis) is frequently involved in stage 4 ulcers that extend to bone surfaces without involving the bone itself and should not be confused with osteomyelitis. The clinician must know if there is indeed a focus of osteomyelitis underlying the surface periostitis, because one reason for an early recurrence following apparently successful pressure sore surgery is the presence of an unrecognized nidus of chronic bone infection. In such a situation, the chronic infection may manifest itself by the development of a draining sinus tract or an abscess rather than as a typical pressure ulcer.

Preoperative diagnostic efforts involving various radiographic studies and swab cultures are frequently resorted to in an attempt to rule out the presence of infected bone. Such studies not only can be costly but also may be misleading. A preoperative swab culture of the wound with suspected osteomyelitis has poor correlation with the organisms actually infecting the bone and should not be relied on for the selection of antibiotic therapy (33). Other nonbone specimens such as aspirates of pus from soft tissues or swabs of sinus tracts also do not produce reliable concordance with bone culture results (34).

Standard X-rays are the most cost effective imaging studies but may give false-negative or false-positive results for osteomyelitis in 50% of cases (35). The inflammation associated with an adjacent pressure ulcer, pressure-related bone changes, severe osteoporosis, heterotopic bone formation, osteosclerosis, synovitis, and degenerative joint disease (DJD), as well as previous surgeries with partial ostectomies, may confuse the interpretation of these studies (36). However, plain radiographs should be done in the evaluation of osteomyelitis to demonstrate the bony anatomy of the area and delineate preexisting conditions that may influence the selection and interpretation of subsequent procedures (37).

Radionuclide bone scanning can be helpful when using a multiphase flow study protocol but may have a limited degree of sensitivity and specificity depending on the underlying bone condition. Technetium 99m methylene diphosphonate (Tc^{99m}) is still the radiopharmaceutical of choice, as it binds to sites of increased bone metabolic activity and is highly sensitive for the early detection of acute osteomyelitis (38) However, Three-phase bone scans are accurate in settings of normal bone, but the specificity decreases when there are underling osseous abnormalities.

Gallium improves the specificity of the bone scan, as it helps in detection of accompanying soft tissue infection and may also be more sensitive than a Tc^{99m} bone scan in elderly patients (39). The best radionuclide results require the concomitant comparison of the Tc^{99m} bone scan with a gallium^{67} radionuclide scan. Of the five patterns of activity associated with combining a gallium^{67} study with a technetium^{99m} study, when the gallium^{67} scan shows a larger area of relatively more intense uptake than the technetium^{99m} scan, the probability of osteomyelitis approaches 100% (40). A bone scan, as with other diagnostic tests, should be correlated with other laboratory studies and a careful clinical evaluation of the patient.

Other tests to aid in the diagnosis of osteomyelitis include computed tomography (CT) scan and magnetic resonance imaging (MRI). CT is more expensive than plain films and entails a higher radiation dose, but it can be completed quickly and is useful in demonstrating fluid collections, bony erosion, and joint involvement. MRI takes longer to obtain but does not use ionizing radiation and provides excellent anatomic detail. It can also show bone marrow edema before bony involvement is seen on other types of imaging (37). Both CT and MRI have excellent resolution and can reveal destruction of medulla, as well as any periosteal reaction, cortical destruction, articular damage, and soft tissue involvement, even when plain films are still normal. A diagnosis of osteomyelitis by MRI may sometimes precede a positive result on scintigraphy because of the earlier detection of bone marrow involvement with MRI. The addition of gadolinium as a contrast agent can be useful in defining abscesses (37).

Lewis et al. compared plain X-rays, Tc^{99m} bone scans, CT scans, white blood cell counts (WBC), erythrocyte sedimentation rates (ESR), and preoperative needle biopsies done in the operating room prior to debridement (singularly or in various combinations) with the definitively diagnostic postoperative resected bone specimen. His group concluded that the combination of an ESR greater than 120, a WBC greater than 15,000, and a plain pelvic X-ray was as useful as the more costly Tc^{99m} scan alone.

This combination of studies gave a sensitivity of 73% and a specificity of 96%. Their conclusion was that radionuclide scanning was not necessary, if the other criteria were present (41).

The preoperative diagnosis often is simply made the old-fashioned way by exploring the base of the ulcer with a gloved finger and palpating the exposed and eroded bone or bony spicules that confirm bone destruction. Even probing a sinus tract with a cotton-tipped applicator can transmit to the clinician the sensation of roughened and eroded bone.

If a course of preoperative antibiotics is planned for presumed osteomyelitis, then laboratory confirmation of the offending organisms and their antibiotic sensitivities is essential. Histopathology of preoperative bone biopsy specimens is the gold standard for the diagnosis of osteomyelitis (38). The histologic examination of the specimen is done to verify that there is indeed bone involvement. Acute and chronic inflammatory cell infiltration, marrow fibrosis, and microabscesses are the microscopic criteria used to confirm the diagnosis of osteomyelitis. If there is no inflammation, then the bone changes are most likely related to pressure effects. Thus, bone cultures must be correlated with the bone histology, because contamination from the colonized soft tissue wound can occur. In addition, correlation of the histopathology and cultures of the surgically resected osseous specimen should be made in planning postoperative antibiotic therapy.

Adequate ablative surgery of stage 4 ulcers entails the resection of the bone forming the base of the ulcer. Postoperative specimens of resected bone should be sent for gram staining and culture and sensitivity studies *before* placing the surgical specimen in formalin or other fixatives. In addition, a biopsy specimen from bone remaining in the wound bed following a partial ostectomy should be submitted for these same studies, because the results will aid in the decision of whether to embark on a 6-week postoperative course of IV antibiotics. Often the "disease" is cured by the partial ostectomy, and such a prolonged and expensive treatment is not warranted even if the resected bone has changes compatible with osteomyelitis. Again, the definitive diagnosis depends on the results of the culture *and* the histologic examination of the presumed involved bone.

Spasticity and Contractures

Increased spasticity may be considered a complication of unhealed pressure ulcers, because its presence can inhibit or disrupt the healing process whether by surgical or nonsurgical means. The open wound below the level of injury is perceived as a noxious stimulus and may trigger spasms that are a manifestation of hyperactive withdrawal reflexes. A new onset infected pressure ulcer or abscess qualifies as a noxious stimulus, and increased spasticity may be the first clue that an infection is present. Conversely, one of the adverse effects of spasticity is the causation of pressure ulcers secondary to the shear-generated erosions of skin associated with repeated episodic muscle spasms. It therefore goes without saying that control of spasticity is essential in both the prevention and treatment of pressure ulcers. A special section on the medical management of spasticity, a major consequence of SCI, is included in this textbook (see Chapter 40).

In the patient with SCI, contractures are a complication linked with spasticity and aggravated muscle imbalance and are associated with pressure ulcers. Untreated spasticity leads to a myriad of other SCI complications, such as spontaneous fractures of long bones, dislocations, pain, and deformities that prevent proper seating in a wheelchair. Spasticity and associated contractures, being causative agents in pressure ulcers, must be treated both for the maintenance of skin integrity (prevention) and in the treatment of established pressure sores. If these are not addressed, then the most promising surgical closure of a pressure ulcer will fail, either from wound dehiscence in the postoperative period or because of a recurrence following successful wound closure. Medication, splints and positioning, and rigorous stretching are the first treatment modalities to be tried, but they may fail to alleviate the problem. When these conservative measures fail to correct the problem, more invasive treatments such as intrathecal medications, neurolysis, or surgery may be indicated.

In the treatment of pressure ulcers associated with spasticity and contractures, muscle release by peripheral neurectomies, myotomies, and tenotomies has been found to be beneficial in ameliorating the problem by reducing the stretch reflex and correcting joint deformities sufficiently to permit successful healing of the pressure ulcer (42). Patients formerly confined to bed because of contracted lower extremities can be ambulated in their wheelchairs and returned to an active lifestyle in the community (Figure 50.2).

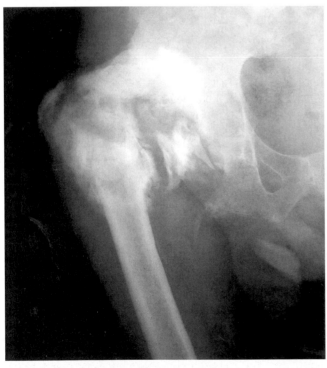

Figure 50.2 Bedridden tetraplegic patient with a nonhealing stage 3 pressure ulcer of the right trochanteric area and marked contractures secondary to severe spasticity that was resistant to conservative methods of therapy. The contractures were treated by iliopsoas and adductor myotomies and tenotomies of the hamstring and achilles tendons. A tensor fascia lata myocutaneous V-Y advancement flap was used to close the pressure ulcer. Following postoperative physical therapy, the patient was discharged ambulant in his wheelchair.

Malignant Transformation

Long-standing indolent wounds of many years duration have demonstrated the potential to develop malignant tumors. There are a number of reports in the literature of squamous cell carcinoma developing in burn scars, the sinus tracts of chronic osteomyelitis, stasis ulcers, unstable scars, and other nonhealing wounds. First described by Dupuytren in 1834 (16), the lesion has been given the eponym of *Marjolin's ulcer,* after Marjolin's earlier description in 1820 of "cancroidal" chronic ulcers (43).

In 1986, Mustoe and coworkers reviewed fourteen cases of malignant degeneration in chronic pressure ulcers that had been previously reported and added four more cases of their own. They noted that, compared to other chronic wound carcinomas, cancers arising in pressure ulcers are highly aggressive and usually follow an unremitting and fatal course. In all cases, the malignancy occurred in chronic ulcers of long-standing duration, averaging 20 years before the malignant transformation to invasive cancer occurred (17).

The patient often seeks a surgical solution to the problem sore because of a change in the character of the ulcer—putrid odor, increased drainage, or even frank bleeding. Frequently, the diagnosis is unsuspected, and the diagnosis is made by the pathologist on histologic examination of the surgical specimen removed at the time of a flap closure. In such a scenario, because most flap repairs of pressure ulcers involve extensive dissection of adjacent tissues in developing the flap, cancer cells are disseminated throughout the various tissue planes and contribute to the high failure rate for disease eradication. When the practitioner has a high clinical index of suspicion based on the chronicity of the wound and its recent change in character, a preoperative tissue biopsy should be done to confirm the diagnosis and further workup done in order to plan for the most appropriate treatment.

The surgical procedure should adhere to basic cancer ablation techniques, using wide en bloc resection, intraoperative frozen sections as needed, and avoidance of tumor cell dissemination. Because of the poor prognosis, delaying the flap repair and packing the resultant open wound until definitive histologic studies of the surgical margins can be obtained is a rational option if complete tumor eradication is in doubt. Oncologic assistance is essential in the total management of these patients.

The authors have treated six cases in the past 30 years. The most recent case was a carcinoma in a paraplegic arising in a chronic sacral ulcer of 25 years' duration. The patient came to the clinic because of recent episodes of bleeding from the ulcer. Malignant degeneration was suspected because of the long history and the change in the characteristics of the sore; a pre-excision frozen section revealed the nature of the disease. Wide local resection was therefore carried out, and the defect was packed open with gauze dressings. Review of the permanent sections revealed a tumor at the deep margin of the resection and invasion of the sacrum. A subsequent wide resection included a subtotal sacrectomy and abdominoperineal resection with an end colostomy and repair using a rectus abdominis myocutaneous flap (Figure 50.3). As with most of these malignancies, local recurrence and distant metastases subsequently developed, and the patient died of his disease.

Recurrence

Following healing of a pressure ulcer, breakdown of the healed wound can be considered a complication of treatment. Once

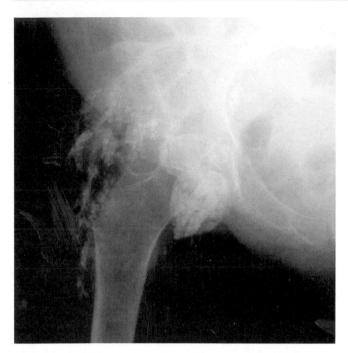

Figure 50.3 Paraplegic patient with rectus abdominis myocutaneous island flap repair of a large sacral defect following abdominal perineal resection and partial sacrectomy for squamous cell carcinoma developing in a chronic pressure ulcer of 25 years' duration.

tissue integrity is destroyed and replaced by scar tissue, the healed wound site will always be at risk for further complications, and this fact should be considered in developing a treatment plan of care. Scar tissue, being an ersatz replacement of the original, is characteristically inferior to normal skin—in tensile strength (80% of normal), blood supply, resiliency, and ability to withstand trauma—because of the reduced protective mechanical barrier afforded by the dense keratin layer of normal skin and the loss of the physiologic protective barrier provided by sebaceous and sweat glands, melanocytes with their protective melanin, and the immunologically important Langerhans's dendritic cells (44). Thus, it is more easily subjected to the complication of recurrent ulceration and the resultant accumulation of avascular scar tissue. There are a number of other factors, such as socioeconomic problems, in the equation of recurrence that make this complication one of the most common problems in the treatment of pressure ulcers in SCI patients.

Other problems associated with the presence of acute and chronic pressure ulcers include increased episodes of autonomic dysreflexia, reduction in serum albumin, amyloidosis, and the anemia of chronic disease.

INDICATIONS FOR INTERVENTION

The surgical closure of pressure ulcers is normally not considered until the wound is "surgically clean," as evidenced by the presence of healthy granulation tissue that is free from devitalized tissue, adjacent cellulites, and purulent drainage. A more exacting surgically clean wound is defined on a quantitative bacterial count of 10^5 gram or less derived from a biopsy tissue specimen, because such wounds are not considered infected but colonized. However, such exactitude is rarely necessary.

As discussed earlier, the presence of necrotic tissue in an unstable pressure ulcer is a source of local infection that can lead to a progression of the ulcerative process and to extension of tissue destruction. It also places the patient at risk for bacteremia and sepsis that can culminate in septic shock syndrome, multiorgan failure, and death.

This devitalized and infected tissue must be eliminated; this is essential to any treatment plan, surgical or nonsurgical. This removal is accomplished by the process called *wound debridement*. Debridement methodologies include mechanical, chemical, and sharp debridement. One should not rely exclusively on any single method, and interventions should be adjusted depending on clinical observations and repeated assessments of the efficacy of the selected treatment plan.

Eradication of necrotic tissue is essential to the well-being of living organisms. Consequently, the body has its own chemical and mechanical self-debridement mechanisms for the elimination of dead tissue. The body's chemical debridement is called *autolysis*—the dissolution of the devitalized tissue, which depends on the release from leukocytes of a number of proteolytic enzymes such as endogenous collagenase, elastase, and other peptases. The presence of these enzymes in the wound is the basis for utilization of occlusive and semiocclusive dressings used in the medical treatment of pressure ulcers (see Chapter 49).

To expedite the autolytic process, a number of commercially available recombinant enzymes may be applied topically to the devitalized tissue. Such agents have been available for decades, but the debridement process is slow, and supplementary sharp debridement is often required to expedite the process. It is unclear whether these preparations are any more effective than properly performed wet-to-dry saline dressings combined with sharp debridement, and poor cost effectiveness diminishes the value of these agents.

Of late, there has been a revival of an exogenous debriding agent that was known to the ancients. Maggot therapy involves the application of larvae of the blowfly. These larvae are nurtured under sterile conditions in the laboratory, placed in the necrotic wound, and sealed off from the surrounding external environment (45). The larvae liquefy and ingest only the devitalized tissue; they debride a wound more rapidly than the topical proteinases available in a tube dispensed by the pharmacist. Some sensate patients, however, may prefer topical ointments and gels to the irritating sensation of the "creepy crawlers."

Mechanical debridement using wet-to-dry saline dressing, when properly performed, is an effective debriding technique. However, the dressings should not be allowed to become too dry if the goal is healing by secondary intention. Wound desiccation can be a problem, particularly for patients in an air-fluidized bed. As they dry, in theory, saline dressings tend to become hypertonic and to absorb fluid from the wound to maintain a physiologic balance, thus helping to reduce wound edema. Wound debris tends to adhere to the gauze, and frequent changing of the dressing mechanically removes the necrotic material. Whirlpool hydrotherapy is a form of mechanical debridement, which is further discussed in Chapter 49.

When confronted with a granulating wound that is obviously not "surgically clean," as manifested by a persistent purulent drainage, the use of a broad spectrum topical antibiotic such as silver sulfadiazine cream 1% might be considered. Topical antiseptic solutions such as providone iodine, hydrogen peroxide, or Dakins's solution and other chemicals utilized to "clean up the wound" are to be used with caution, because they are toxic to keratinocytes and fibroblasts in vitro (46, 47). Clinically, their use for a brief period prior to surgical closure appears to have no observable adverse effect on subsequent wound healing. Nevertheless, use of cytotoxic antiseptic agents and prolonged use of topical silver sulfadiazine are not recommended in a wound healing by secondary intention. Topical agents must never be substituted for good, diligent wound care.

Sharp debridement at the bedside involves resection of the diseased tissue down to viable tissue but has the disadvantage of inducing bleeding and being less selective than enzymatic debridement and maggot therapy. In the toxic and septic patient, surgical debridement is best accomplished in the operating room accompanied by the administration of IV antibiotics.

The surgeon has a variety of tools available for the debridement of abscessed necrotic tissue. The scalpel and scissors have given way to other safer modalities that reduce the likelihood of bacteremia and dissemination of the infection as blood and lymphatic vessels are disrupted. Electrocautery, normally an operating room procedure, is less sanguineous and reduces the dissemination of bacteria, but it can also injure viable tissues and cause coagulation necrosis and tissue desiccation.

The CO_2 laser, although slower than other surgical extirpative methods, is more selective in limiting tissue damage and is usually bloodless. The monochromatic, collimated (laminar) light energy is absorbed by water and is transformed into thermal energy, boiling the cellular water and rapidly vaporizing the purulent debris. Surface tissue injury is limited because the penetration of the destructive beam is confined to only a few hundredths of a millimeter (0.23 mm at 40 watts of power). Because capillaries are sealed (tissue welding) by the thermal energy of the monochromatic light, absorption of debris and bacteria does not readily occur. This markedly reduces the postoperative chills and fever of the bacteremia that often accompany sharp debridement. In addition, swab cultures following laser debridement are uniformly sterile, and the closure of debrided wounds often can be accomplished at the time of debridement (48–52).

An additional pearl concerning wound debridement: the dry, hard eschar, without evidence of putrefaction or surrounding cutaneous inflammation, that is frequently found over the posterior calcaneous usually does not require debridement and is better left intact. Contraction and epithelialization under the periphery of the eschar will take place similar to the mummification and autoamputation that is observed in the dry gangrenous toe. However, should evidence of necrosis under the eschar be noted, as indicated by softening of the eschar and/or the presence of peri-eschar inflammation or frank pus, the eschar should be removed because incipient or frank infection is present (53).

INDICATIONS FOR SURGICAL INTERVENTION

Not all pressure ulcers require surgical closure, particularly if the wound in question is expected to heal in a few weeks or months by an alternative noninvasive method. Neither should a patient

---

Table 50.2   Indications for Surgical Interventions

Necrotic/infected tissue requiring surgical debridement
Stage 3 and 4 ulcers with or without bone/joint involvement
Nonhealing sinus or fistulous tracts
Significant undermining of adjacent tissue
Chronic, nonhealing ulcers
Chronic ulcers with scarred, fibrotic bed and/or keratinized peripheral rim
Heterotopic (ectopic) bone formation
Wound complications not responding to local wound care

---

at the end of life be subjected to a major reconstructive procedure. In general, however, stage 3 and 4 ulcers do not meet the promise of expedient healing and are candidates for a surgical procedure, particularly where bone or joint is involved (see Table 50.2).

Ulcers with sinus tracts usually fail to heal by conservative means and require some surgical intervention, if only to unroof the chronic tract. Sinus tracts leading to bone should suggest the presence of osteomyelitis, and penetration through a joint capsule is indicative of pyarthrosis. With joint involvement, the infectious process usually erodes the joint cartilage and bone, and debridement of the infected tissue followed by wound closure is indicated. The sinogram is a useful tool in determining the course of a sinus tract, particularly where joint involvement is suspected.

Surgery is also indicated where there is significant undermining in the subcutaneous tissue plane (Figures 50.1D and F). Healing of these wounds by secondary intention is significantly delayed or even arrested, thus leading to a chronic nonhealing wound. Any ulcer that becomes chronic and no longer responds to nonsurgical measures should be considered a candidate for surgical closure. Stage 3 or 4 chronic ulcers are often accompanied at the skin level by a hard encircling ischemic fibrous ring (annulus fibrosis) that prevents the process of wound contraction. This situation is often seen when there is a significant ulcer crater. Because epithelial migration requires a skin-level granulating surface, any significant depth to a wound will inhibit epithelial migration. Epithelium does not like to grow "downhill"; this results in the accumulation of new cells at the lip of the ulcer, which, with time, become hyperkeritinized.

In a chronic wound with arrested healing, the deeper tissues may be covered by a dull layer of pale granulation tissue, which indicates the presence of significant chronic fibrous scar tissue having diminished circulation and reduced resiliency. Hypertrophic granulation tissue ("proud flesh") may also be seen in chronic wounds and sometimes is accompanied by polypoid masses of granulation tissue. Such tissue lacks fibrotic scar cells and is spongy to the touch. Granulation tissue of this type is not conducive to epithelial migration and should be removed by the application of silver nitrate or by scraping the wound bed with a tongue blade.

Pressure ulcers complicated by the presence of ectopic bone are a special problem and are discussed more fully in Chapter 51. Surgical repair may fail unless the problem of the associated underlying heterotopic ossification (HO) is addressed also. The pressure effects over the unyielding bone mass can also be a causative factor in the initial development of the ulcer and should be addressed like any osseous pressure point to diminish the probability of recurrence. In addition, osteomyelitis involving this extraskeletal bone, secondary to direct involvement by the ulcer, may be present, as suggested by a chronic sinus tract.

It is important to appreciate that this bone is highly vascular, and care must be taken during excision to avoid excessive blood loss. One strategy suggested by Applet et al. is to perform selective embolization of the feeding vessels to the heterotopic bone prior to definitive resection (54). In addition, this bone may encase neurovascular bundles; thus, removal of the bone requires extra caution to prevent damage to these structures.

BASIC SURGICAL PRINCIPLES

The operative treatment of pressure ulcers in persons with SCI involves not just a surgeon and an agreeable patient. Vital to the program is a multidisciplinary team of operating room personnel, staff nurses, dieticians, the primary care physician, physiatrists and various therapists, infectious disease specialists, medical social workers, case managers, mental health personnel, and chaplains, among others. The definitive goal of pressure ulcer wound care, like all rehabilitation endeavors, is to return the patient to a safe community environment after attaining the maximum restoration of function and the prevention of ulcer recurrence. This is best accomplished by "closing the wound" with the minimal amount of functional disability and including the entire treatment team in the postoperative recovery process.

To accomplish appropriate wound closure by surgical means, there are certain historically proven basic principles and rules of surgery that every well-trained surgeon must know and abide by to achieve these goals while avoiding complications and disastrous outcomes (see Table 50.3). As an obvious example, purulent abscesses should be drained.

The removal (debridement) of all devitalized or necrotic tissue is a basic concept in the surgical treatment of wounds. Exposed tendons, with loss of their nourishing tendon sheath, must be included in the debridement both proximally and distally under the adjacent intact soft tissue because these denuded tendons will not survive. Effective wound debridement is essential in controlling infection prior to any wound closure. During the subsequent surgical closure of pressure ulcers, the excisional debridement of the entire colonized granulating pyogenic membrane lining the ulcer and any involved bone is required. Adjacent ischemic scar tissue secondary to a previously healed ulcer should also be excised, leaving only healthy, well-vascularized tissue.

Other principles include eliminating any "dead space" in the surgically closed wound, ensuring wound hemostasis and control of hemorrhage, promoting postoperative wound drainage by a closed wound evacuation system to avoid potential collections of blood or serum exuding from the raw wound surface, and restoring normal tissue planes by the tension-free and accurate coaptation of anatomic layers.

In restoring the normal tissue planes of muscle-to-muscle, fascia-to-fascia, and skin-to-skin, it is recommended that running sutures be avoided and that only interrupted-type sutures be employed. The reason for mentioning this seemingly insignificant "pearl" is that, should a small wound abscess develop in the sutured wound early in the postoperative period, the simple expedient of removing a few sutures may be adequate to gain drainage of the infected material and promote subsequent healing by secondary intention. If a single continuous suture is used, then the removal of that suture to gain drainage of the localized abscess results in the entire wound being opened and could require a subsequent secondary closure in the operating room.

THE EVOLUTION OF PRESSURE ULCER SURGICAL PRINCIPLES

In the mid-1940s, when surgeons began to close pressure ulcers, caution was the byword because of the tradition and dictates of previous generations of surgeons. Simple primary closure of small granulating and colonized ulcers initially was attempted under the protective cover of penicillin (55). With this success, the use of local random flaps of skin and subcutaneous fat was tried, as encouraged by Davis in 1938, when he replaced the thin unstable scar of a healed pressure ulcer with the more resilient flap of adjacent skin and subcutaneous fat (56).

Subsequent surgeons, using a two-stage approach, applied split-thickness skin grafts to the contaminated granulating ulcers in lieu of Davis's healed scar epithelium to obtain a "sterile field" before attempting the more formidable second-stage flap procedure. With better technology and newer techniques based on a better understanding of wound physiology and the anatomy of the all-important blood supply of soft tissue, some procedures were discarded and new ones developed to give improved results in the repair of these difficult wounds. But it was from the experiences of these pioneering pressure ulcer surgeons that the basic surgical principles evolved that are applied in pressure ulcer surgery (57–59) (see Table 50.4).

Such preliminary wound "sterilization" by skin grafts is not practiced today. Most pressure ulcers are normally closed when infection is controlled and the wound clinically appears "surgically clean," as evidenced clinically by the presence of an ulcer base of bright red granulation tissue that is free from debris and purulent drainage.

The use of large flaps in the repair of pressure ulcers became doctrine early in the beginnings of pressure ulcer surgery. As

---

Table 50.3   Basic Principles of Wound Surgery

Adequate wound debridement	Preservation of blood supply
Obliteration of dead space	Control of infection
Accurate hemostasis	Postoperative wound drainage
Restoration of tissue planes	Adequate nutrition
Tension-free wound closure	Avoidance of secondary injury

Table 50.4   Basic Principles of Pressure Ulcer Surgery

Drain purulent collections	Large, reusable flaps
Debride devitalized tissue	Excision of all scar tissue
Obliteration of dead space	Placement of surgical scar
Accurate wound hemostasis	Removal of osseous pressure points
Tension-free wound closure	Closed wound drainage system

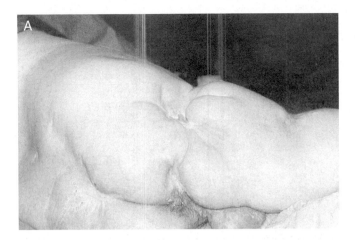

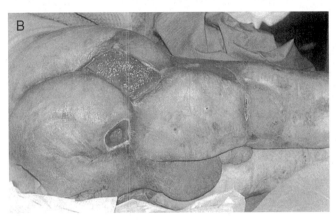

Figure 50.4 (A) Paraplegic patient with marked scarring of the hip and ischial areas following multiple surgical repairs and episodes of wound healing by secondary intention. (B) A tetraplegic patient with a history of multiple surgical procedures utilizing small local random flaps presents the surgeon with the dilemma of exhausted potential flap donor sites.

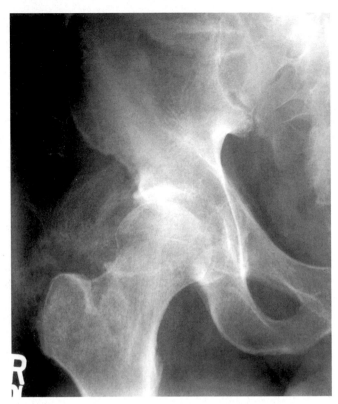

Figure 50.5 Healed large ischial pressure ulcer in a tetraplegic patient requiring the use of a combination gluteal rotation flap and biceps femoris myocutaneous advancement thigh flap. The distal posterior thigh flap donor site was allowed to heal by secondary intention as it was in a nonpressure area. Either flap is reusable should there be a recurrence.

discussed earlier, there is a high recurrence rate of pressure ulcers in the SCI patient population. With this reality in mind, it behooves the surgeon to plan the initial surgical repair knowing that there is a high probability that additional flap repairs will be needed in the future. Small local rotation flaps in patients with SCI, although less traumatic, are unwise because they will interrupt the adjacent blood supply and produce scarring in the area. As a result, when a recurrence does occur, it may be difficult to find adequate unscarred healthy tissue available for a subsequent repair (Figures 50.4A and B). The initial flap, therefore, should be large enough so that it can be used again if needed (Figure 50.5).

In principle, the placement of the surgical scar is best located away from the pressure point of the underlying bone, as long as there is no needless sacrifice of healthy local tissue or it results in a tight closure. A primary closure for a small ulcer, in lieu of a flap, if easily accomplished without tension or a dead space, may serve the patient better by preserving local circulation and adjacent tissue that may be needed for a flap at a later date. The principle is "don't burn your bridges: you will probably need them later."

The reduction of osseous pressure points is another cardinal principle in pressure ulcer surgery. Because most pressure

ulcers develop over bony prominences, the surgical procedure should include the reduction of the underlying osseous protrusion, as recommended by Kostrubala and Greeley in 1947 (57), and thus ameliorate the offending pressure point. Subsequent surgeons, in the case of the ischial pressure ulcer, went a step further and advocated not only the reduction of the ischial tuberosity but also the total extirpation of the offending ischial ramus (60). A subsequent retraction of that recommendation was published a few years later when it was realized that the radical removal of this bony element of the pelvic floor led to urethral trauma in the wheelchair-dependent patient and to the subsequent development of urethral diverticulae or perineal extravasation of urine, with accompanying periurethral abscesses and fistulae (61, 62). Care and conservatism should also be practiced in the reduction of the prominent greater trochanter in osteopenic patients to avoid iatrogenic postoperative fractures of the femur.

Rather than the radical extirpation of the underlying bone, the procedure of choice is a reduction of the osseous prominence by a partial ostectomy. This is accompanied by the addition of soft tissue padding by advancing soft tissue (usually muscle) over the reduced pressure point. In addition to the interposition of healthy padding between the skin and the underlying modified bony pressure point, well-vascularized muscle tissue significantly improved the delivery of antibiotics (63) as well as growth factors and other cytokines released by the wound healing cascades in response to the acute surgical insult. This sacrifice of muscle tissue below the level of injury is normally not a significant functional consideration in nonambulant SCI patients.

In the SCI patient, the use of a nonfunctioning muscle from below the injury level to close a stage 4 ischial pressure ulcer and thus restore the patient's ability to sit in a wheelchair is perfectly proper. However, to utilize a shoulder muscle such as the latissimus dorsi as a free flap to accomplish the same end for a paraplegic in a manual wheelchair is poor judgment. When a free flap repair is the only alternative, a more appropriate muscle selection would be a rectus abdominis myocutaneous free flap—one that would not add an additional disability by weakening the all-important shoulder girdle. The dictum of "do no harm" must prevail.

The goal of rehabilitation medicine is to preserve and strengthen what remains. In some cases, however, the consideration of "function" in planning a pressure ulcer repair must be taken into account just as it would be in non-SCI patients. Case in point: the function of sitting in a wheelchair. Wilms, in 1916, described bilateral thigh amputation for paraplegic patients and noted that without the weight of the lower extremities, patients could turn in bed without assistance (64). Such a plan is partially derived from the perception that because a patient is unable to walk, "functionless" lower extremities are not needed: that the patient is better off without the encumbrance of the useless limbs that are subject to potentially new ulcers and infection. Such a perception is erroneous.

Georgiade et al., in 1956 (65), discussed the amputation or filet procedure in order to harvest a sufficiently large muscle flap for the repair of major wounds in the pelvic region. A second paper by the Georgiade group in 1969 reviewed their series of forty-one total thigh flap repairs of extensive pressure ulcers and emphasized that the procedure was reserved only for extensive ulcers not treatable by alternative means (66).

Other authors in the pioneer days of pressure ulcer surgery advocated amputation of limbs in the treatment of trochanteric ulcers with involvement of the hip joint, osteomyelitis of the proximal femur, ankylosis secondary to heterotopic bone formation, and flexion contractures (67–69). As discussed earlier, there are both nonsurgical and surgical alternative procedures other than amputation that are available to control the lower extremity contractures associated with pressure ulcers.

There are indeed situations where an amputation is necessary, particularly in an ischemic and gangrenous limb or in a case of uncontrolled infection in the distal extremity. Amputation, however, must be weighed against the loss of support granted by the lower limbs and subsequent body imbalance in the wheelchair-confined patient—a problem that can lead to recurrent ulcerations of the buttock and ischial areas. In addition, there are psychologic aspects for the patient who has lost so much and now experiences the addition visible loss of a portion of his body. Serious considerations of alternative methods of wound closure must be pursued and amputation only considered as a last resort. If lower leg amputation is necessary, the ideal level is below the knee or a knee disarticulation to preserve the entire thigh for weight distribution, rather than pursuing amputation above the knee.

Concerning stage 4 ulcers that involve a joint such as the hip, if uncontrolled, the infection not only destroys the joint capsule, synovial lining, and articular cartilage, but also can erode into the adjacent bone and establish frank osteomyelitis (Figure 50.6).

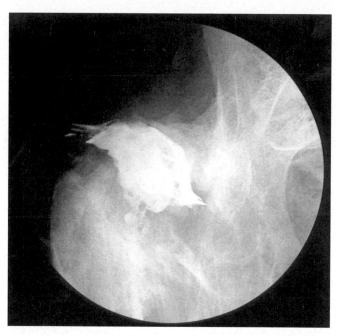

Figure 50.6   Patient with a stage 4B pressure ulcer involving the hip joint with destruction of the joint capsule resulting in dislocation of the femoral head. An upper femorectomy and repair with a vastus lateralis muscle flap and split-thickness skin graft successfully closed the defect with preservation of the limb.

Ulcers involving the interphalangeal joints of the toes are best treated by amputation, because there is minimal morbidity. But amputation for involvement of major joints such as the knee or hip is a significant additional handicap in the patient with SCI. Disarticulation of the extremity in such situations is not always inevitable, and preservation of the limb by a Girdlestone arthroplasty (upper femorectomy) is the preferred treatment.

Garthorne R. Girdlestone originally described his operation in 1943 (70, 71), having developed the procedure earlier in India for the surgical treatment for tuberculosis of the hip. The procedure involves resection of the infected femoral head and any involved proximal femur as well as all involved soft tissue, including the joint capsule. The acetabulum is thoroughly debrided of involved cartilage and synovia with a curette. Repair usually utilizes a local muscle, such as the vastus lateralis or biceps femoris, for obliteration of the resulting dead space (Figure 50.7). The transposed muscle can be covered by a split-thickness skin graft, but usually the wound can be closed primarily or, where there is a large soft tissue deficit, by a more substantial local flap such as the tensor fascia lata flap.

In cases where the infection is not under control, reconstruction following femoral head resection is usually delayed until the wound is clinically free from purulent drainage or other signs of infection. The wound is packed open, with frequent dressing changes as needed, until an elective delayed secondary closure of the wound can be safely accomplished. Careful attention to any nutritional deficit should be corrected during this often protracted time of wound preparation.

Postoperatively, the involved extremity is immobilized by splinting it to the opposite limb, utilizing an abduction pillow

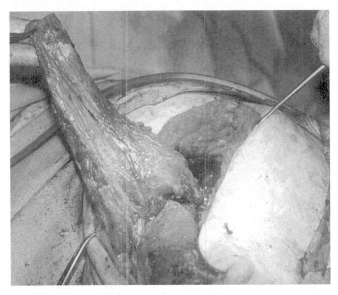

Figure 50.7 Vastus lateralis muscle flap being elevated in preparation for rotation into the acetabulum following resection of the upper femur and femoral head (Girdlestone procedure) for a stage 4B pressure ulcer involving the hip joint.

and a well-padded "mummy wrap" of resilient material and Kerlex® and/or Ace® wrap (72). Some authors have recommended an orthopedic external fixator device with pins in the iliac crest and the posterior femoral shaft (73), but such a device is awkward and presents a difficult nursing problem, as well as requiring a continuous proning position on the part of the patient. Quadriplegics are not able to prone because of the interference with diaphragmatic breathing, and aspiration from eating in the prone position is a real risk. In an osteopenic patient, the use of an external fixator has its own problems, because pins may loosen and become infected.

Successful closures of ulcers involving the hip joint by upper femorectomy have been reported recently in the range of 90% to 100% (74, 75), and the procedure is considered the definitive treatment of hip pyarthrosis associated with stage 4 pressure sores. The only other surgical option, as mentioned previously, is total hip disarticulation.

Other more radical approaches to major pressure ulcers of the pelvic region include the hemipelvectomy and the hemicorporectomy, both of which are accompanied by a high morbidity and a dismal survival rate (76, 77). Although such procedures have been considered in patients with massive pressure ulcers, such procedures are best reserved for the occasional patient with advanced malignancy that requires palliation.

WHEN A GAP, SWING A FLAP

The development and evolution of soft tissue flap surgery has been the basic instrument in the surgeon's weapons system for the closure of chronic pressure ulcers. It is not the intent of this treatise to discuss the technical creation of the variety of such flaps, because there is an abundant literature available on this subject for interested clinicians (78, 79). The intent is to familiarize those caring for SCI patients with the concepts behind the principles of flap reconstruction in the surgery of pressure ulcers.

From the beginnings of pressure ulcer surgery in the late 1940s and early 1950s, the primary workhorse has been advancement or rotational skin and subcutaneous flaps (80, 81). Such transfers of large tissue mass required an intact blood supply, as distinguished from free skin grafts. When planning a procedure, a general principle of reconstructive surgery is to select the least complicated operation that will accomplish the goal of the intended surgery without undue morbidity, because the more complicated the procedure, the greater the risk of complications.

Flap surgery is not always mandated. In the case of a small nonhealing stage 3 ulcer that has failed to heal after a trial of bed rest and appropriate local wound care, it would be unwise to mobilize a large adjacent flap when a simple primary closure would do the job. Careful attention to hemostasis following complete debridement of scar tissue and the contaminated (colonized) pyogenic ulcer bed, along with a tension-free primary closure, should be adequate to close these wounds.

When the above conditions for primary repair are absent, then flap reconstruction is required. Although a split-thickness skin graft is less complicated than a flap in cases with tissue loss, the use of skin grafts is usually not adequate or appropriate in the case of pressure ulcers, particularly over a bony prominence. Skin grafts are easily traumatized over pressure points, and their donor sites add an additional stage 2 wound that frequently is difficult to heal in SCI patients.

Skin grafts can be used in conjunction with flap surgery where there is a distal donor defect, usually in a non-weight-bearing area, following the rotation or advancement of a flap to cover an ulcer site. In such cases, we prefer to obtain the graft from an area where the skin is abundant, such as the anterior abdominal wall. Such donor sites are usually small and can be primarily sutured following excision of the raw dermal bed. This technique avoids the wound healing problems of the classic skin graft donor site (a stage 2 wound left to heal by secondary intention) located on the insensate thigh; these sites are easily traumatized during the required frequent repositioning of the paralyzed patient confined to bed.

The contemporary utilization of muscle in pressure ulcer surgery is partially for the bulk it supplies in the necessary obliteration of any "dead space" following ulcer excision and partially for the theoretical padding over the underlying bony prominence. This initial muscle bulk, however, diminishes in time as the muscle atrophies, losing of 30% to 50% of its mass within a year following surgery. This loss of bulk is probably related to the direct pressure effects in the sitting patient and to the associated periods of pressure-associated ischemia; muscle tissue is less resistant to ischemia than skin.

The main reason to use a muscle flap, however, is because of its superior blood supply. There is an abundant axial (longitudinal) circulation within muscle bellies. Their derivative perforators lead to the overlying subcutaneous fat and skin and are the principal source of blood supply for skin. This axial pattern of blood supply permits the transfer of larger flaps than could be accomplished with the random skin flaps used by earlier surgeons, where the circulation depended on the internal labyrinth of subdermal capillaries. The flap's dominant circulation of low-pressure, subdermal capillaries limits the size of a random flap (Figure 50.8), and its length-to-width dimension can not exceed a 2.5:1 ratio without resorting to a multistaged (delayed) flap. It is now appreciated that the main blood supply to the skin is derived from the perforator vessels

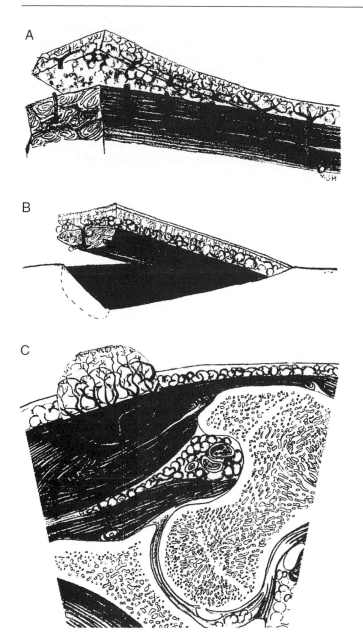

The development of muscular and myocutaneous flaps evolved in the 1960s and 1970s from modern microsurgical and free-flap technology and the subsequent appreciation of the axial pattern of the blood supply of muscles (82). This new fundamental concept enabled the development of the safer transfer of larger pedicle flaps than the classic random lipocutaneous flaps, which frequently required multistaged "delay" procedures designed to encourage the development of an axial pattern of dermal capillary circulation (83). The elucidation of the axial vascular supply of muscle has led to the classification of pedicle flaps by Nakajima and coworkers as: *cutaneous, fasciocutaneous, adipofascial, septocutaneous,* and *musculocutaneous* (84). Although random cutaneous flaps are still useful, the workhorse of pressure sore surgery today is the axial myocutaneous flap. Free flaps, requiring microsurgical techniques, in general are not practical and are rarely used in pressure sore surgery (85, 86). When choosing the surgical approach to a pressure ulcer, consideration should be given to potential recurrence, and to the development of pressure sores in other nearby sites (87). In addition, the vascular supply of the muscles and their arc of rotation must be considered. The vascular supply of muscles is not uniform, and they can be classified into five groups or types having varying degrees of reliability (82). The most dependable are types I, III, and V. The type I muscle has a single, proximal vascular pedicle that will support the entire muscle and its overlying subcutaneous fat and skin over a generous arc of rotation. The tensor fascia lata myocutaneous flap, supplied by the lateral circumflex branch of the femoral artery, is an example (Figure 50.9). The type III muscle has two dominant vascular pedicles from two separate vascular trunks, either of which can carry the entire flap because of the excellent anastomosing intramuscular circulation. An example of a type III muscle is the rectus abdominis muscle or the gluteus maximus. Type V muscles have one dominant vascular pedicle and additional secondary segmental vessels; the latissimus dorsi is an example.

Less dependable and limited in their arc of rotation are the type II and IV muscles. Type II muscles, such as the gracilis, have a dominant proximal vascular supply but require circulatory

Figure 50.8 **(A)** Illustration of the reduced circulation of the subdermal vasculature of a random lipo-cutaneous flap limited by the interruption of multiple perforating vessels originating in the deeper fascial and muscular axial circulation. **(B)** Illustration of the superior blood supply of an axial myocutaneous flap with multiple perforating vessels nourishing a healthy and viable rotation, advancement, or island regional flap. **(C)** Illustration of circulation of the skin with the major source of the fat and dermal blood supply reaching the dermal arterioles and capillaries by way of perforating branches originating from the generous blood supply of the subjacent superficial muscle bellies.

arising from the axial circulation of the underlying superficial muscles that traverse the subcutaneous fat to terminate in the arborescen circulation of the dermal capillaries (Figure 50.8C). An additional type of axial circulation with perforating vessels to the skin from the deep fascia is the basis for the successful use of fasciocutaneous flaps.

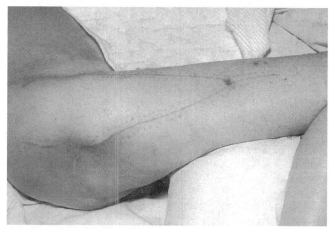

Figure 50.9 C5–C6 tetraplegic patient postrepair of a retrotrochanteric pressure ulcer utilizing a V-to-Y tensor fascia lata (TFL) myocutaneous flap. A small area of the tip of the flap was lost and had to be healed by secondary intention.

supplementation by additional perforating segmental vessels that nourish the distal portion of the muscle. Because of the lack of sufficient anastomosing intramuscular vessels, the division of this supplemental circulation during the elevation of the flap can result in the loss of the distal flap. The type IV muscle is similar in its dependence on multiple segmental perforating vessels but, unlike

the type II muscle, is lacking a dominant proximal arterial or venous supply. An example of a type IV muscle is the sartorius muscle of the thigh. These muscles are not very useful in pressure sore surgery, because they do not support a very large skin paddle.

The inclusion of vascularized muscle in the flap repair of pressure ulcers has allowed the utilization of more remote pedicle tissue that was not available to the pioneer surgeons following World War II. An example is the utilization of anterior abdominal wall tissue via the transverse rectus abdominis myocutaneous (TRAM) flap. The TRAM flap has become the flap of choice for the reconstruction of the female breast following ablative cancer surgery (88, 89). Because this flap is a type III flap with a separate inferior (deep inferior epigastric artery/vein branch of the common femoral artery) and superior blood supply (superior epigastric A/V—the continuation of the internal mammary vascular trunk), it can be rotated either superiorly to cover defects of the anterior chest wall or inferiorly to supply tissue to repair wounds of the sacral, hip, perineum, and ischial areas (90–92). Multiple perforating branches supply the overlying skin and allow the transfer of a large island of skin and subcutaneous fat. Figure 50.3 illustrates the use of a transverse rectus abdominis myocutaneous island flap to repair a large sacral defect following the resection of a squamous cell carcinoma that arose in a chronic pressure sore of 25 years' duration. Figure 50.10 illustrates the vertical rectus abdominis myocutaneous island flap used in the repair of a recurrent ischial pressure ulcer complicated by a large perineal/pelvic floor cavity subsequent to an abscess following a traumatized urethra.

POSTOPERATIVE COMPLICATIONS

Like any invasive procedure, surgery has its complications, such as wound dehiscence, wound infection, bleeding, and hematoma formation. However, in the patient with SCI, complications are more frequent because of the nature of the problems encountered in this special patient population. The loss of pain sensation in SCI patients may appear to be a benefit postoperatively, but actually it is a detriment, because its protective mechanism is absent during the healing process. Thus, tension placed on the wound by the patient inadvertently lying on the surgical site or the necessary act of the frequent turning of the paralyzed patient by the nursing staff can disrupt the sutures and lead to wound dehiscence. In addition, patients with injuries above T6 will be prone to autonomic dysreflexia from the surgical site pain. Another source of stress on the healing suture line that may cause wound dehiscence is the problem of uncontrolled spasticity that may increase following surgery because of the noxious stimuli from the surgical site. Every effort should be made to control any spasticity prior to surgery, but when severe spasticity fails to respond to treatment, the patient probably should not be considered a candidate for flap surgery.

The problem of spasticity in wound healing has its converse side in patients with flaccid paralysis. Over the years, these patients gradually lose their inactive muscular tissue, having it replaced by poorly vascularized adipose tissue that is more easily injured by pressure. Consequently, these "muscles" have a reduced capacity to support any substantial flap that may be needed in the repair of a pressure ulcer.

In addition to disuse atrophy of muscle mass and bone (osteopenia), the vascular tree also atrophies below the level of

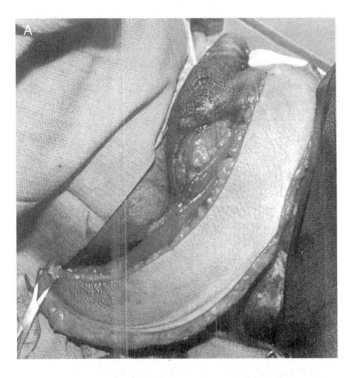

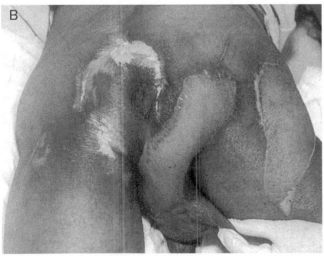

Figure 50.10 (A) Paraplegic patient with a chronic right ischial pressure ulcer and a large pelvic floor abscess cavity following traumatic disruption of the urethra with extravasation of urine requiring closure of the bladder neck and suprapubic catheter placement. A single-stage rectus abdominis myocutaneous island flap was tunneled into the perineum for closure of both the perineal and ischial defects. Note the length-to-width dimensions of the axial flap, which would not be possible with a random flap. (B) Post-op view of healed wound of patient illustrated in (A). The patient has remained healed to date.

injury, as blood is shunted to areas where the metabolic needs are greater. In addition, because persons with SCI have impaired vasoconstrictive responses due to dysregulation of the sympathetic innervation to the vasculature, bleeding and hematoma formation postoperatively can occur.

Combined with the generalized atherosclerosis of aging, there is a relative or absolute ischemia of the affected tissues in long-term SCI patients. Even with the use of a well-vascularized muscle flap in the repair of pressure ulcers, flap circulation can be a problem and lead to flap failure and the loss of essential tissue (the part needed to cover the defect). Smoking is a major contributor to this problem of flap failure. Regarding this well-documented risk factor, some surgeons consider smoking an absolute contraindication to surgical repair. In addition, nicotine replacement via transdermal patch is also contraindicated, due to its vasoconstrictive properties. Circulation difficulties in a flap may either be caused by ischemia (inflow failure) or be secondary to venous congestion (outflow failure), as evident by a dusky cyanotic appearance and a prolonged capillary refill time of greater than 2 to 3 seconds. Hyperbaric oxygen treatments have been useful in the salvage of these vascular-compromised flaps (93).

Because pressure ulcers are colonized under the best of circumstances, the relatively hypoxic and edematous tissue struggling to recover from the surgical insult is an excellent environment for the multiplication of residual pathogenic organisms that may lead to a subsequent wound infection. Most surgeons, therefore, provide intravenous prophylactic antibiosis in the early postoperative period, and it is prudent to extend the perioperative prophylaxis for 72 hours following surgery, rather than the normal single intraoperative dosing recommended for "clean" surgical cases. Antibiotic treatment can then be extended, based on the most recent (collected in the OR) sensitivity studies, if the clinical condition warrants it.

Even with the use of postoperative closed-wound drainage and the careful attention to the obliteration of "dead space" during the surgical repair, collections of blood and serum are not infrequent. Such collections make excellent culture media for bacteria and contribute to the not uncommon wound infection problem. Any significant hematoma will require a return to the operating room for evacuation of the clot and resuturing of the wound. Seromas may persist during the postoperative period and require multiple aspirations. If they do not respond to repeated aspirations, then it is useful to replace the aspirated serum with a sclerosing solution such as sodium morrhuate or tetracycline (94).

It is said that postoperative complications are best treated preoperatively. This maxim is clearly applicable to SCI patients. Comorbid medical conditions should be optimized, not neglecting the problem of malnutrition that is fairly common even in obese patients. Spasticity must be addressed and attention given to clearing the urinary tract of stones and bacteria and attaining a "surgically clean" granulating wound that is free from purulence and necrotic tissue.

POSTOPERATIVE CARE AND MOBILIZATION

Following flap surgery, consideration of the duration of bed confinement and the need for a special pressure relief or pressure reduction bed should be a part of the postoperative care plan. In patients unable to assume a prone position, the use of an air-fluidized (A-F) bed for 2 to 4 weeks postoperatively has been found to be a cost-effective aid in successful surgical outcomes, particularly in the presence of additional pressure ulcers. Patients with sacral flaps are able to tolerate a supine position without compromising the flap repair. The average pressure over the sacrum in an A-F bed is 37.1 mmHg, compared to 52.4 mmHg for a standard hospital bed (95). In fact, the uniformly distributed pressure on the flap in the high-air-loss air-fluidized bed seems to promote the adherence of the flap to the underlying raw wound surface, thus reducing the incidence of seroma and bursa formation under the healed flap.

As soon as the clinical situation is deemed safe, the patient is transferred to a low-air-loss bed and allowed to be on a prone gurney, if that is tolerated. Should the patient be a smoker, the use of the prone gurney is delayed until it is felt that the wound is healed sufficiently to tolerate an expected return to that habit by the patient. A self-contained closed drainage system, such as the Jackson-Pratt device, is a usual accompaniment of pressure ulcer flap surgery. It is usually needed for about 10 to 14 days and its removal is guided by the reduction of the wound drainage to about 5 to 10 cc per 8-hour shift, at which time the drainage in a healthy wound is mostly serous rather than sanguineous. These devices do obstruct by clot formation, so diligence must be maintained.

Staples or sutures are not normally removed before 2 weeks. If sutures are used, it is recommended that running sutures be avoided so that alternate sutures can be removed should there be any concern about the tensile strength of the healing wound, which is only about 20% of normal tissue strength at this time. Also, should a localized superficial "stitch abscess" develop, then evacuation of the pus pocket can be accomplished by the removal of a few select sutures without compromising the entire wound.

There is little literature on the timing of range of motion and progression to sitting postoperatively, with protocols varying from 3 to 8 weeks. Most surgeons prefer at least 2 weeks of complete rest, with no range of motion, sitting, or even head elevation. Some protocols then allow gentle bedside passive range-of-motion exercise of the involved lower extremity, with the goal of getting the hip and knee to 90 degrees of flexion to simulate the tension needed for sitting. The head of the bed may be elevated at this time, as well. Some prefer to wait until 4 to 5 weeks of uncomplicated wound healing have passed before the patients are allowed to elevate the head of the bed to a 30-degree angle for meals (15 to 20 minutes). If there are no untoward events and the extremity can tolerate the sitting position, then brief periods of time up in the wheelchair may be initiated. Some centers start with 15 minutes twice a day, whereas others wait longer to start sitting, then begin with 1 hour twice a day. The surgical site is evaluated by the staff following the return to bed for signs of sitting intolerance such as persistent redness or evidence of bruising. The time is adjusted upward progressively, based on the appearance of the flap. The only study in the literature that defines the postoperative timing for mobilization showed that discontinuation of immobilization at 2 weeks or 3 weeks does not change the rate of complications, nor does it shorten the length of hospitalization (96).

The therapist evaluates the patient's cushion requirements at this time, and adjustments are made to the wheelchair, if needed, to correct any imbalance in seating. The wheelchair time is gradually increased after a few days by additional hourly increments until goals are reached. A reasonable goal is a minimum of 4 hours of wheelchair sitting for at least 3 days before discharge. If travel distance is significant, then this goal is extended. With the patient back in the wheelchair, muscle strength and transfer abilities are evaluated and therapy instituted as needed prior to discharge.

CONCLUSIONS

Although it has been said (mainly by attorneys) that pressure ulcers should never occur given good medical care, they remain a fact of life. Their causes and consequences are numerous and complex and involve much more than the failure of a caregiver to turn the patient every 2 hours. The surgical closure of these wounds is historically a relatively recent option, and even with careful patient selection, the results of the therapeutic effort are notably marred by a high rate of complications, the most common of which is recurrence. Beyond the obvious tissue deficit, there are many sequelae of pressure ulcers that make this wound a challenging task for the surgeon. Nevertheless, the care provider must not lose sight of the goal of rehabilitation, which is to do what it takes to return the victim of this catastrophic event to the best available environment and lifestyle. As stated at the beginning of this chapter, that goal takes a dedicated and compassionate community of people. "It takes a village . . ."

*R*eferences

1. Elias AN, Gwinup G. Immobilization osteoporosis in paraplegia. *J Am Paraplegia Soc* 1992; 15(3):163–170.
2. Krolner B, Toft B. Vertebral bone loss: an unheeded side effect of therapeutic bed rest. *Clin Sci* 1983; 64:537–540.
3. Leadbetter WF, Engster HC. The problem of renal lithiasis in convalescent patients. *J Urol* 1945; 53:269–281.
4. Rodehheaver G, Baharestani MM, Brabec ME, Byrd HJ, et al. Wound healing and wound management: focus on debridement—an interdisciplinary round table, September 18, 1992, Jackson Hole, WY. *Adv Wound Care* 1944; 7(1):22–36.
5. Miller H, Delozier J. Cost implications of the pressure ulcer treatment guideline. Contract No. 282–91–0070. Sponsored by the Agency for Healthcare Policy and Research. Columbia, MD: Center for Health Policy Studies, 1994:17.
6. Hirshberg J, Rees RS, Marchant B, Dean S. Osteomyelitis related to pressure ulcers: the cost of neglect. *Adv Skin Wound Care* 2000; 13(1):25–29.
7. Wachter RM, Foster NE, Dudley RA. Medicare's decision to withhold payment for hospital errors: the devil is in the details. *J Comm J Qual Patient Saf* 2008; 34(2):116–123.
8. Von Clausewitz C. *Vom Kriege [On War]*. New York: Penguin Putman Inc., 1832.
9. Fomon S. *The Surgery of Injury and Plastic Repair.* Baltimore, MD: Williams & Wilkins, 1939.
10. Rao DB, Shane PG, Georgiev EL. Collagenase in the treatment of dermal and decubitus ulcers. *J Am Geriatr Soc* 1975; 23:22–30.
11. Charcot JN. *Lectures on the Diseases of the Nervous System.* Delivered at La-Saltpetrière. 2nd ed. Translation, Sigerson G. Philadelphia: Henry C. Lea, 1879.
12. Monro, D. Care of the back following spinal cord injuries. *N Engl J Med* 1940; 223:391–398.
13. Schryvers OI, Stranc MF, Nance PW. Surgical treatment of pressure ulcers: 20-year experience. *Arch Phys Med Rehabil* 2000; 81:1556–1562.
14. Evans GRD, Dufresne CR, and Manson PN. Surgical correction of pressure ulcers in an urban center: is it effective? *Adv Wound Care* 1994; 7(1):40–46.
15. Disa JJ, Carlton JM, Goldberg NH. Efficacy of operative cure in pressure sore patients. *J Plast Reconstr Surg* 1992; 89(2):272–278.
16. Dupuytren G. *Legons orales de clinique chirurgicale.* 2nd ed., 1834.
17. Mustoe T, Upton J, Marcellino V, Tun CJ, et al. Carcinoma in chronic pressure sores: a fulminant disease process. *J Plast Reconstr Surg* 1986; 77:116–121.
18. Niazi ZB, Salzberg CA, Byrne DW, Viehbeck M. Recurrence of initial pressure ulcer in persons with spinal cord injuries. *Adv Wound Care* 1997; 10(3):38–42.
19. Knighton DR, Ciresi KF, Fiegel VD, Schumerths, et al. Stimulation of repair in chronic non-healing cutaneous ulcers using platelet-derived wound healing formula. *Surg Gynecol Obstet* 1990; 170:56–60.
20. Rees RS, Robson MC, Smiel JM, et al. Becaplermin gel in the treatment of pressure ulcers: a phase II randomized double-blind, placebo-controlled study. *Wound Repair Regen* 1999; 7:141.
21. Kallianinen LK, Hirshberg J, Marchant B, Rees RS. Role of platelet-derived growth factor as an adjunct to surgery in the management of pressure ulcers. *Plast Reconstr Surg* 2000; 106(6):1243–1248.
22. Singer AJ, Clark RAF. Mechanisms of disease: cutaneous wound healing. *N Engl J Med* 1999; 341(10):738–746.
23. Wittee MB, Barbul A. General principles of wound healing. *Surg Clin North Am* 1997; 77:509–528.
24. Clark RAF, ed. *The Molecular and Cellular Biology of Wound Repair.* 2nd ed. New York: Plenum Press, 1996.
25. Tarnuzzer RW, Schultz GS. Biochemical analysis of acute and chronic wound environments. *Wound Repair Regen* 1996; 4:321–325.
26. Bucalo B, Eaglstein WH, Falanga V. The effects of chronic wound fluid on cell proliferation in vitro. *J Invest Dermatol* 1989; 92:408.
27. Bucalo B, Eaglstein WH, Falanga V. Inhibition of cell proliferation by chronic wound fluid. *Wound Repair Regen* 1993; 1:181–186.
28. Bucalo B, Eaglstein WH, Falanga V. The effect of chronic wound fluid on cell proliferation in vitro. *J Invest Dermatol* 1989; 92:408.
29. Bone RC. Systemic inflammatory response syndrome: a unifying concept of systemic inflammation. In: Fein AM, Abraham EM, Balk RA, Bernard GR, et al, eds. *Sepsis and Multiorgan Failure.* Baltimore, MD: Williams & Wilkins, 1997: 3–10.
30. Shae JD. Pressure sores: classification and management. *Clin Orthop* 1975; 112:89–100.
31. Eltorai I, Chung B. The management of pressure sores. *J Dermatol Surg Oncol* 1977; 3:507–510.
32. Wheeler AP, Bernard GR. Current concepts: treating patients with severe sepsis. *N Engl J Med* 1999; 340:207–214.
33. Rousseau P. Pressure ulcers in an aging society. *Wounds* 1989; 1(2):135–141.
34. Zuluaga AF, Galvis W, Saldarriaga JG, et al. Etiologic diagnosis of osteomyelitis. *Arch Intern Med* 2006; 166:95–100.
35. Sugarman B, Hawes S, Musher DM, et al. Osteomyelitis beneath pressure sores. *Arch Intern Med* 1983; 143:683–688.
36. Deloach ED, Check WE, Long R. Diagnosing osteomyelitis underlying pressure sores. *Contemp Orthop* 1993; 27(3):240–246.
37. Palestro CJ, Love C, Miller TT. Infection and musculoskeletal conditions: imaging of musculoskeletal infections. *Best Pract Res Clin Rheumatol* 2006; 20(6):1197–1218.
38. Lew DP, Waldvogel FA. Osteomyelitis. *N Engl J Med* 1997; 336(14): 999–1007.
39. Palestro CJ, Love C. Radionuclide imaging of musculoskeletal infection: conventional agents. *Semin Musculoskelet Radiol* 2007; 11(4):335–352.
40. Tumeh SS, Aliabadi P, Weissman BN, McNeil BJ. Chronic osteomyelitis: bone and gallium scan patterns associated with active disease. *Radiology* 1986; 158:685–688.
41. Lewis VL, Bailey MH, Pulawski G, Kind G, et al. The diagnosis of osteomyelitis in patients with pressure sores. *Plast Reconstr Surg* 1988; 81(2):229–232.
42. Eltorai I, Montroy RE. Muscle release in the management of spasticity in spinal cord injury. *Paraplegia* 1990; 28:433–440.
43. Marjolin JN. Ulcere. In: *Dictionnaire de Medecine,* 1820.
44. Bell D, Young JW, Banchereau J. Dendritic cells. *Adv Immunol* 1999; 72:255–324.
45. Sherman RA, Wyle F, Vulpe M. Maggot therapy for treating pressure ulcers in spinal cord injury patients. *J Spinal Cord Med* 1995; 18(2):71–74.
46. Johnson AR, White AC, McAnalley B. Comparison of common topical agents for wound treatment: cytotoxicity for human fibroblasts in culture. *Wounds* 1989; 1(3):186–192.
47. Teepe RGC, Koebrugge EL, Lowik CWGM, Petit PLC, et al. Cytotoxic effects of topical antimicrobial and antiseptic agents on human keratinocytes in vitro. *Trauma* 1993; 35(1):8–19.

48. Stellar S, Meijer R, Walia S, Mamoun S. Carbon dioxide laser debridement of decubitus ulcers: followed by immediate rotation flap or skin graft closure. *Ann Surg* 1974; 179:230–237.

49. Eltorai I, Glantz G, Montroy RE. The use of the carbon dioxide laser beam in the surgery of pressure sores. *Internat Surg* 1988; 73(1):54–56.

50. Montroy RE. Pressure ulcers. In: Achauer BM, Vander Kam VM, Berns MW, eds. *Lasers in Plastic Surgery and Dermatology*. New York: Thieme Medical Publishers, 1992:164–175.

51. Lutchman GD, Staffenberg DA, Herz BL. The carbon dioxide laser: decubitus debridement and sterilization. In: Lee BY, Herz BL, eds. *Surgical Management of Cutaneous Ulcers and Pressure Sores*. New York: Chapman and Hall, 1998:141–154.

52. Hinshaw JR, Herrea HR, Lanzzafame RJ, Pennino RP. The use of carbon dioxide laser permits primary closure of contaminated and purulent lesions and wounds. *Lasers Surg Med* 1987; 6(6):581–583.

53. *The Treatment of Pressure Ulcers*. Clinical Practice Guideline Number 15. Rockville, MD: The U.S. Department of Health and Human Services, 1994.

54. Applet EA, Kenkel JM, Ballard JR, et al. Preoperative embolization of heterotopic ossification for the treatment of a recalcitrant pressure sore. *Plast Reconstr Surg* 2005; 116(4):50e–53e.

55. Lamon JD Jr, Alexander E Jr. Secondary closure of decubitus ulcers with aid of penicillin. *JAMA* 1945; 127:396.

56. Davis, JS. The operative treatment of scars following bedsores. *Surgery* 1938; 2:1.

57. Kostrubala JC, Greeley PW. The problem of decubitus ulcers in paraplegics. *Plast Reconstr Surg* 1947; 2:403–412.

58. White JC, Hudson HW, Kennard HE. The treatment of bed sores by total excision with plastic closure. *US Nav Bull* 1945; 45:445.

59. Conway H, Kraissl CJ, Clifford RH, Gelb J, et al. The plastic surgical closure of decubitus ulcers in patients with paraplegia. *Surg Gynecol Obstet* 1947; 85:321.

60. Comarr AE, Bors E. Radical ischialectomy in decubitus ischial ulcers complicating paraplegia: report of 100 cases. *Ann West Med Surg* 1951; 5:210–213.

61. Comarr AE, Bors E. Perineal urethral diverticulum—complication of removal of ischium. *JAMA* 1958; 168:2000–2003.

62. Eltorai I, Khonsari F, Montroy RE, Comarr AE. Urinary fistulae after radical ischiectomies in surgery of ischial pressure sores. *Paraplegia* 1985; 23:379–385.

63. Chang N, Mathes SJ. Comparison of the effects of bacterial inoculation in musculocutaneous and random-pattern flaps. *Plast Reconstr Surg* 1982; 70:1.

64. Wilms. Behandlung der ruckenmarkschusse mit totaler Lahmung. *Medizinische Klinik* 1916; 12:435.

65. Georgiade N, Pickrell K, Maguire C. Total thigh flaps for extensive decubitus ulcers. *Plast Reconstr Surg* 1956; 17:220.

66. Royer J, Pickrell K, Georgiade N, Mladick R, Thorne F. Total thigh flaps for extensive decubitus ulcers. *Plast Reconstr Surg* 1969; 44(2):109–118.

67. Van Enst W. Hip disarticulation in patients with paraplegia and a survey of the treatment of pressure sores and its complications *Arch Chir Neerl* 1963; 15:249.

68. Cannon B, O'Leary JJ, O'Neil JW, Steinsieck R. An approach to treatment of pressure sores. *Ann Surg* 1950; 132:760.

69. Garland DE, Dubayi SS, Harway EC, Pompan DC. Proximal femoral resection and vastus lateralis flap in the treatment of heterotopic ossification in patients with spinal cord injury. *Contemp Orthop* 1995; 31(6):341–347.

70. Girdlestone GR. Acute pyogenic arthritis of the hip: an operation giving free access and effective drainage. *Lancet* 1943; 1:419.

71. Girdlestone GR, Somerville EW. *Tuberculosis of Bone and Joint*. Oxford: Oxford University Press, 1952.

72. Eltorai I. The Girdlestone procedure in spinal cord injured patients: a ten year experience. *J Am Paraplegia Soc* 1983; 6(4):85–86.

73. Klein NE, Luster S, Green S, Moore T, Capen D. Closure of defects from sores requiring proximal femoral resection. *Ann Plast Surg* 1988; 21:246–250.

74. Rubayi S, Pompan D, Garland D. Proximal femoral resection and myocutaneous flap for treatment of pressure ulcers in SCI. *Ann Plast Surg* 1991; 27(2):132–138.

75. Evans GRD, Lewis VL Jr, Manson PN, Loomis M, Vander Kolk CA. Hip joint communication with pressure sore: the refractory wound and the role of Girdlestone arthroplasty. *Plast Reconstr Surg* 1993; 91(2):288–294.

76. Pearlman NW, McShane RH, Jochimsen PR, Shirazi SS. Hemicorporectomy for intractable decubitus ulcers. *Arch Surg* 1976; 111(10):1139–1143.

77. Aust JB, Absolon KB. A successful lumbosacral amputation, hemicorporectomy. *Surgery* 1962; 52:756.

78. Mathes JM, Nahai F. *Reconstructive Surgery, Principles, Anatomy, and Technique*. Edinburgh: Churchill Livingstone, 1997.

79. McGraw JB, Arnold PG. *McCraw and Arnold's Atlas of Muscle and Musculocutaneous Flaps*. Norfolk, VA: Hampton Press Publishing Company, 1986.

80. Conway H, Griffith BH. Plastic surgical closure of decubitus ulcers in patients with paraplegia. *Am J Surg* 1956; 91:946.

81. Campbell RM. The surgical management of pressure sores. *Surg Clin N Am* 1959; 39:509.

82. Mathes SJ, Nahai F. Classification of the vascular anatomy of muscles: experimental and clinical correlation. *Plast Reconstr Surg* 1981; 67(2):177–187.

83. Ortichocea M. The musculocutaneous flap method: an immediate and heroic substitute for the method of delay. *Br J Plast Surg* 1972; 25:106.

84. Nakajima H, Fujino T, Adachi S. A new concept of vascular supply to the skin and classification of skin flaps according to their vascularization. *Ann Plast Surg* 1986; 16:1.

85. Yamamoto Y, Nohira K, Shintomi Y, Igawa H, and Ohura I. Reconstruction of recurrent pressure sores using free flaps. *J Reconstr Microsurg* 1992; 8:433.

86. Park S, Koh KS. Superior gluteal vessel as recipient for free flap reconstruction of lumbosacral defect. *Plast Reconstr Surg* 1998; 101:1842.

87. Bauer J, Phillips LG. MOC-PSSM CME article: pressure sores. *Plast Reconstr Surg* 2008; 121:1–10.

88. Hartrampf CR Jr, Scheflan M, Black PW. Breast reconstruction with a transverse abdominal island flap. *Plast Reconstr Surg* 1982; 69(2):216.

89. Drever JM. The lower abdominal transverse rectus abdominis myocutaneous flap for breast reconstruction. *Ann Plast Surg* 1983; 10(3):179.

90. Mixter RC, Wood WA, Dibbell DG. Retroperitoneal transplantation of rectus abdominis myocutaneous flap to the perineum and back. *Plast Reconstr Surg* 1990; 81:437.

91. Kroll SS, Pollock R, Jessup JM, Ota D. Transpelvic rectus abdominis flap reconstruction of defects following abdomininal-perineral resection. *Am Surg* 1989; 55:632.

92. Tobin GR, Day TG. Vaginal and pelvic reconstruction with distally based rectus abdominis myocutaneous flap. *Plast Reconstr Surg* 1988; 81:62.

93. Nemiroff PM. Enhanced healing of compromised skin flaps and skin grafts. In: Camporesi EM, Barker AC, eds. *Hyperbaric Oxygen Therapy*. Bethesda, MD: Undersea and Hyperbaric Medical Society, 1991: 149–157.

94. Baeke JL. Treating seromas (letter). *Plast Reconstr Surg* 2000; 106(5):1224.

95. Sachse RE, Fink SA, Klitzman B. Multimodality evaluation of pressure relief surfaces. *Plast Reconstr Surg* 1998; 102(7):2381–2387.

96. Isik FF, Engray LH, Rand RP, et al. Reducing the period of immobilization following pressure sore surgery: a prospective, randomized trial. *Plast Reconstr Surg* 1997; 100(2):350–354.

51 Heterotopic Ossification

Susan V. Garstang
Robert E. Montroy

Ectopic bone formation had been occasionally described before the early twentieth century but was limited to a few rare medical conditions, usually of a hereditary nature, as first described by Guy Patin in 1692 (1). The discovery of the X-ray by Roentgen in 1895, for which he won the first Nobel Prize granted in physics, and the subsequent development of the X-ray machine based on the Cooledge tube in 1913 enabled a French husband-and-wife team of neurologists to uncover the poorly understood process of the nonhereditary ectopic bone formation in a special patient population, the neuro-injured survivors of the blood-soaked battlefields in northern France of the Great World War of 1914–1918.

Aided by the newly discovered radiograph in a systematic clinical study of seventy-eight paraplegic soldiers, in 1918 Dejerine and Ceillier published their seminal paper describing a new syndrome that they called *paraosteoarthropathy* (POA) (2). The French authors consistently noted the presence of neo-osseous formations near major joints and long bones—real bone that did not involve the integrity of the normal skeletal bone but was separate and lodged in the adjacent soft tissues. In all of their thirty-eight cases of POA, this ectopic bone was consistently located in the region between the pelvis and the knees. The medial knee was the most common site followed by the hip or pelvis and along the femoral diaphysis. From a clinical aspect, the authors felt that the thirty-eight cases (48.7%) revealed by the X-ray did not represent the true incidence of POA, because more than half their patients had convincing clinical evidence of soft tissue ossification.

This condition has now become well recognized as a discrete pathologic process of true bone formation around joints in patients with neurological injury and is called *heterotopic ossification* (HO). With the evolving science of trauma care and spinal cord medicine, following the next world war, that led to the unprecedented survival and successful rehabilitation of an ever-increasing paralyzed patient population, the clinical awareness of the problem of HO began to draw the interest of researchers and clinicians around the world. Nevertheless, many questions remain today: why does bone develop where it shouldn't be? Why does it form in the muscles around major joints such as the hip? How can it be treated? Better yet, can it be prevented?

BACKGROUND

Heterotopic ossification (HO) is a pathologic condition that may be either hereditary or acquired. Acquired HO can be further divided into the categories of posttraumatic HO and neurogenic HO. Posttraumatic HO includes ossification after trauma or procedures such as total hip arthroplasty, and the closely related syndrome of myositis ossificans, which is soft tissue calcification at sites of trauma near long bones (3). The clinical consequences are similar in all types of HO; the outcome is true lamellar bone formation that is indistinguishable from normal skeletal bone, having cortex, marrow, and a Haversian canal system.

The hereditary autosomal dominant type of heterotopic ossification fortunately is quite rare. It is found in at least three distinct genetic disorders: Albright hereditary osteodystrophy; progressive osseous heteroplasia; and fibrodysplasia ossificans progressiva. Each is a unique syndrome in that the genesis and development patterns of disease progression, the distribution of the HO formations, and the histopathologic features are all different. In common, these hereditary disorders are all limited to a few families worldwide, and none has an effective treatment. A recent excellent review by Shore and coworkers is suggested for the interested reader (4).

The acquired type of HO is associated with trauma, and, although not common, its incidence far exceeds the hereditary variety. Traumatic heterotopic ossification has been described following thermal injury (5, 6), poliomyelitis, tetanus, and toxic epidermal necrolysis (7, 8), as well as following major trauma to the central nervous system with resultant spinal cord injury or brain injury (9–11). HO does occur in persons with nontraumatic myelopathy, with an incidence in one study of 6% (12, 13). It is also an unwanted consequence of local hip trauma, such as fractures of the proximal femur or acetabulum and prosthetic hip surgery (14).

The incidence of acquired HO depends on the clinical population. Patients with traumatic spinal cord injury (SCI) have an incidence from 10% to 53%, depending on the study design, detection method, and criteria for diagnosis (13). HO usually occurs near to the time of acute injury, with the peak incidence between 4 to 12 weeks following the SCI (15). HO becomes clinically significant in 20%–30% of cases, and leads to ankylosis in 3%–8% of patients (13).

After total hip arthroplasty (THA), patients have an overall incidence of HO in the range of 15% to 90% (16, 17). The occurrence of clinically significant HO in this group with limited joint mobility and pain is fortuitously less: in the range of 1% to 27%. However, in 1% to 18% of these significant cases, there is complete joint ankylosis caused by osseous bridge fusing the femur to the pelvis (Figure 51.1) (12). Much of the literature that forms the base for our understanding of the prevention and treatment of HO in the SCI-injured population comes from studying the orthopedic literature regarding HO after THA.

Ayers and coworkers identified a group of patients undergoing THA that was at high risk to develop HO postoperatively (18). These included those with a history of posttraumatic arthritis and extensive osteophyte formation, ankylosing spondylitis, or hypertrophic osteoarthrosis. Particularly vulnerable were

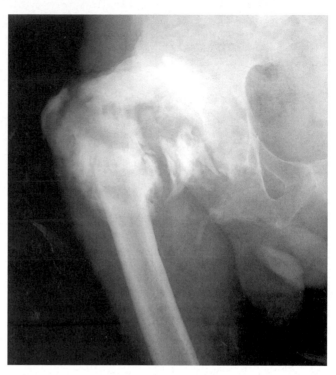

Figure 51.2 A 50-year-old C5 tetraplegic patient with Brooker's class III heterotopic ossification of the right hip. Despite destruction of the femoral head and proximal displacement of the femur, the patient was able to maintain wheelchair mobility.

patients with a prior history of ipsilateral or contralateral HO formation: 80% of these patients undergoing hip surgery suffer a local recurrence or new onset HO at a different site. These risk factors are common in the older patient with advanced degenerative joint disease, and thus may not represent things that increase the risk of HO in the younger SCI population.

Riedel first drew attention to the relationship between ectopic bone formation and traumatic neurologic disorders in 1883 (19). In addition to developing after SCI, neurogenic heterotopic ossification is seen following traumatic brain injuries (TBI), where the severity of the injury (Glasgow coma scale) correlates with the extent of the ossification measured in square centimeters (20). As in the cases reported by Dejerine and Ceillier, it is most commonly associated with spasticity and is always below the level of injury (after SCI) or in neurologically involved extremities (i.e., the affected side after CVA or TBI). Neurogenic HO seemingly differs from that seen following direct muscle trauma, such as in myositis ossificans and invasive hip/pelvis surgery, in that the site of the neurotrauma (brain, spinal cord) is anatomically remote from the affected site.

There are also reports of HO occurring in children with cerebral palsy following iliopsoas and other muscle release procedures and also following rhizotomy with femoral osteotomy, in which local muscle, tendon, and bone trauma occurs in the treatment of a spastic central nervous system disorder (21, 22, 23). The overall risk for HO in pediatric patients with SCI has been reported at 10%, primarily in the acute period (17, 24).

The cause of ectopic bone formation is unknown. In cases such as THA and myositis ossificans, it is reasonable to make an association with the direct muscle injury and the evoked

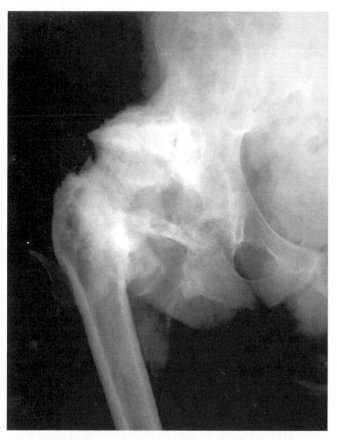

Figure 51.1 A 51-year-old tetraplegic patient with Brooker's class IV ankylosis of the right hip. Anterior bridging between the pelvis and the femur and superior dislocation and partial destruction of the femoral head is present. The femoral dislocation and bone mass created a pressure area resulting in a stage 4 pressure ulcer requiring surgery.

inflammatory response of repair. But the HO following CNS trauma, with no apparent direct relationship to the locus of HO formation, resurrects the ideas of Charcot, who in 1879 put forth a theory, in the case of pressure ulcers, of the traumatic release of a neurogenic "trophic factor" (25). Interestingly, in support of this idea, Kurer et al. took sera from four spinal cord–injured patients with HO and four without HO, and incubated the serum with human osteoblasts in tissue culture (26). The sera from those with HO had much greater levels of osteoblast-stimulating factors than those without HO.

A more contemporary hypothesis, however, concerns the general inflammatory response that follows noninfectious and infectious acute injury and involves cellular, circulating, and locally active mediators and effectors; this is known as the systemic inflammatory response syndrome (SIRS) (27). Such a response can affect the pluripotential mesenchymal stem cells known to be resident in soft tissues and would explain the association of SCI and TBI with HO in the early weeks following the acute injury.

THE PATHOGENESIS OF HETEROTOPIC BONE FORMATION

Heterotopic ossification undergoes the same three main stages of osteogenesis as does skeletal bone: (1) The formation of an extracellular matrix (osteoid); (2) the mineralization of this newly formed osteoid to form bone; and (3) bone remodeling and maturation. The process involves osteogenic cells derived from pluripotential mesenchyme cells of the bone marrow stroma: the osteoblasts, osteocytes, and osteoclasts. Intervention for the prevention or treatment of HO addresses these sequential stages of new bone formation.

The osteoblasts synthesize and lay down the precursors of collagen I that make up 90% to 95% of the extracellular matrix or osteoid tissue. They also produce other noncollagenous proteins of osteoid tissue, such as the proteoglycans of the ground substance, and are rich in alkaline phosphatase. The osteocyte is derived from osteoblasts that are no longer synthesizing collagen and, when exposed to parathyroid hormone, secrete enzymes that begin to dissolve osteoid as part of the third or remodeling phase. The primary cell involved with bone resorption, however, is the osteoclast, which is rich in the enzyme acid phosphatase and secretes collagenase and other enzymes that are involved in the hydrolysis of collagen and demineralization of osteoid. This balanced active metabolic process maintains the equilibrium of the mature bony skeleton throughout life.

The mineralization of the osteoid matrix in the second phase involves the deposition of crystalline hydroxyapatite $[Ca_{10}(PO_4)(6(OH)_2)]$, which is then followed by the last step in osteogenesis—the remodeling phase involving the coupled actions of resorptive osteoclasts and bone-reforming osteoblasts. This synergistic, ongoing process is under the control of various hormones such as estrogens, testosterone, parathormone, and calcitonin, as well as vitamin D metabolites and prostaglandins. In addition, numerous cytokine growth factor superfamilies, such as skeletal growth factor, insulinlike growth factor, transforming growth factor, tumor necrosis factor, acidic/basic fibroblast growth factor, and platelet-derived growth factor are involved (27, 28). The activity of this cascade of inflammatory factors in bone formation suggests the possible mechanism and the

rationale for the use of anti-inflammatory drugs, such as indomethacin, in the prevention of HO in at-risk patients.

The exact cause of the eccentric formation of ossification in the soft tissue of trauma (localized or remote) patients remains unknown, but most investigators believe HO arises as the result of unknown "triggers" (possible inflammatory cytokines) that induce the differentiation of pluripotential mesenchymal stem cells resident in soft tissues into osteoprogenitor cell lines that then differentiate into osteoblasts and the other cell lines involved in bone formation. Such mesenchymal stem cells, common in the bone marrow, are now known to be present in a wide variety of tissues such as adipose tissue and in the connective tissue septa in muscle (26–28). Bosch et al. studied different subpopulations of mouse skeletal muscle and their response to the induction of alkaline phosphatase after exposure to bone morphogenetic protein-2 (BMP-2). An isolated subpopulation of adult muscle cells with an adenovirus construct encoding BMP-2 was injected into the hind limb of immune-compromised mice. These cells appeared to actively participate in the formation of ectopic bone. The authors felt that their data supported their hypothesis that osteoprogenitor cells reside within skeletal muscle and were induced to differentiate into osteoprogenitor cell lines (7).

Bone morphogenetic protein (BMP), first described by Urist, is a bone matrix protein (29). It has been found to have at least fifteen family members, most of which belong to the transforming growth factor beta (TGF-b) superfamily that plays an essential role in the formation and regeneration of the bony skeleton (30). Katagiri and his group demonstrated in vitro that BMP-2 converts the differentiation pathway of myoblasts into that of the osteoblast cell (31). Overexpression of BMP-4 has been shown to occur in genetic forms of HO (32). It has been hypothesized that BMP is released from normal bone in response to inflammation or venous stasis (33). Other possible contributing factors include hypercalcemia, tissue hypoxia, and changes in SNS activity.

Recent studies have shown increased chondroblastic and osteoblastic activity, and an increase in serus osteoblast mitogenic activity, thought to be a consequence of tissue hypoxia after SCI (34). Lotta et al. found subcutaneous microvascular changes in patients with HO, but it is unclear if these are a result of HO or part of the cause (35).

Elevations in prostaglandin E_2 have also been implicated in the formation of HO, as PGE_2 induces a dose-dependant increase in subperiosteal lamellar bone formation, and patients who are developing HO may demonstrate an elevation in urinary prostaglandins (36). However, it is not clear if the PGE_2 elevation is an etiological factor in the development of HO, or merely a marker on the ongoing process.

Much remains to be understood about the molecular events that result in the ectopic bone being formed in para-articular tissues, but with better understanding will come effective prevention and treatment.

THE CLINICAL PATHOLOGIC PROCESS

Regardless of the type of trauma, acquired HO usually becomes clinically apparent in the first 3–4 weeks following the injury, with the peak incidence at 2 months (10). Clinically, the most common early clinical sign is a loss of range of motion of the involved joint that may be confused with the onset of spasticity following recovery from spinal shock. The usual accompanying classical

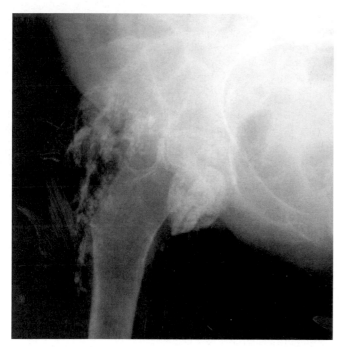

Figure 51.3 A 71-year-old paraplegic patient developed an abscess of the right trochanteric area of the hip 36 years after his SCI injury in 1963. I&D revealed a large collection of infected caseous debris having the appearance and consistency of cottage cheese. Smears and cultures for acid-fast organisms were negative. Postoperative X-rays demonstrated early HO formation with the fluffy flocculation of calcifying osteoid tissue.

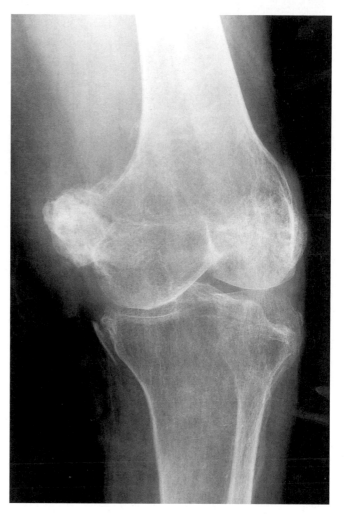

Figure 51.4 A 54-year-old tetraplegic patient with HO of both knees. X-ray showed "diffuse osteoporosis and moderate calcification of the medial collateral ligament." ⁹⁹mTc bone scan indicated "significant osteoblastic activity" of both knees, especially the medial left knee.

signs of acute inflammation are present: swelling, redness, and warmth, (tumor, rubor, and calor), along with pain in those patients whose injury is incomplete. Often there will be a joint effusion, and sometimes even a low-grade fever, causing it to be confused with deep vein thrombosis (DVT), cellulitis, osteomyelitis, or a septic joint.

As observed by Dejerine and Ceillier in their neurogenic POA cases, the process does not involve the normal skeleton and always develops below the cord's level of injury (2). HO does not involve the joint capsule or periosteum; rather, the bone appears to form in the connective tissue between muscle planes (37). Risk factors for the development of HO include spasticity, associated trauma, pressure sores, DVT, age, and the severity and completeness of injury (more common in complete injuries) (15). Although the vast majority of cases of HO occur within 3 months of the acute injury, there are cases of late onset HO years following the original trauma (Figure 51.3).

The location if HO in SCI patients involves tissues around the proximal joints of the extremity, usually involving the hip (60%), and to a lesser degree the more distal medial knee (30%) (Figure 51.4). This reported incidence differs from the findings of Dejerine and Ceillier, wherein the medial knee was most commonly involved (thirty-three of their thirty-eight cases) (2). In tetraplegics, the upper extremities may rarely be involved (10%), with the more proximal shoulder joint affected more often than the elbow. For some unknown reason, not all joints are involved; HO may be unilateral or bilateral and is rarely seen below the elbow or knee.

In SCI HO of the hip, the ossification has a propensity to be located anteromedial to the hip joint, extending between the anterior superior iliac spine (ASIS) and the lesser trochanter. This predilection is interestingly different from TBI's favored anterolateral site between the ASIS and the greater trochanter or posteriorly immediately behind the femoral head and neck (10). When a pressure ulcer is present over the greater trochanter, HO can also be located at that site. A CT scan will help visualize the anatomic location and may be needed where involvement of the femoral vessels is suspected clinically—a useful bit of information should surgery be contemplated.

The classification system used for HO was first described by Brooker in 1973, pertaining to ectopic bone formation that was becoming recognized after total hip replacement (14). The Brooker classification goes from class I, islands of bone within the soft tissue about the hip, to apparent bony ankylosis of the hip—Brooker's class IV (see Table 51.1 and Figures 51.1 and 51.2) (9, 14). Others have modified Brooker's classification by adding the letters A, B, and C to represent the amount of HO expressed as a percentage of the

Table 51.1   Brooker's Classification of Heterotopic Ossification

Class I	Islands of bone within the soft tissues about the hip
Class II	Bone spurs from the pelvis or proximal end of the femur, leaving at least 1 cm between opposing bone surfaces.
Class III	Bone spurs for the pelvis or proximal end of the femur, reducing the space between opposing bone surfaces to <1 cm between opposing ossifying centers
Class IV	Apparent bone ankylosis of hip

Source: Reference 14.

total area on the radiograph. The area is defined at that between a line from the anterior superior iliac spine to the greater trochanter, and the ischium to the lesser trochanter; A is 0%–33%, B is 34%–66%, and C is 67%–100% (18, 22). Schmidt and Hackenbroch developed an alternative classification for HO in 1996, which considers ossifications within the region of the surgical approach (again, primarily used for HO after THA) (see Table 51.2) (38).

Heterotopic ossification in most patients with SCI typically becomes mature by 6 months. However, Garland notes that in 10%–20% of cases the ossification progresses aggressively for much longer and often results in joint ankylosis with increased activity on bone scan and an elevated serum alkaline phosphatase for more than a year (10). He refers to the former patients as type I, and those with the more aggressive course as type II. Often those with type II HO develop huge deposits of bone, which adversely affects sitting balance, contributes to the development

Table 51.2   Classification of Schmidt and Hackenbroch

Region	
I	Heterotopic ossifications strictly below the tip of the greater trochanter
II	Heterotopic ossifications below and above the tip of the greater trochanter
III	Heterotopic ossifications strictly above the tip of the greater trochanter
Grade	
A	Single or multiple heterotopic ossifications smaller than 10 mm maximal extent without contact to pelvis or femur
B	Heterotopic ossifications larger than 10 mm without contact to the pelvis but possibly to the femur; no bridging from caudal to proximal from the greater trochanter
C	Heterotopic ossifications with bridging from the femur to the proximal part of the greater trochanter with no evidence of ankylosis
D	Ankylosis by means of firm bridging from the femur to the pelvis

Source: Reference 38.

of pelvic pressure sores, and aggravates existing spasticity (15, 39). In some cases, wheelchair ambulation is impossible, and the patient is limited to a prone gurney as the sole means of mobility, or may be confined to bed.

METHODS OF EARLY DIAGNOSIS

Routine prophylaxis is not recommended for all patients with acute SCI, as relatively few patients with SCI go on to develop functionally limiting HO, and currently available prophylactic regimens may be poorly tolerated and are not particularly effective. Thus, tests to screen for developing HO are necessary, as are ways to confirm the diagnosis of suspected early HO. Proper identification of HO and elimination of other conditions in the differential diagnosis relies on a combination of laboratory data and imaging studies.

Laboratory Data

Both creatine phosphokinase (CPK) and alkaline phosphate (ALP) have been used as screening tests for developing HO (36, 40–42). ALP is a marker for osteoblast activity, because the cytoplasm and nucleus of these osteoid forming osteoblasts are rich in ALP. ALP is one of the earliest and most convenient markers of developing HO, as it is elevated in a majority of patients who develop clinically significant HO (27). ALP levels become abnormal 2 weeks after injury, and in patients with HO, these levels typically reach a peak of 3.5 times normal by about 10 weeks after the inciting trauma, followed by a return to baseline in 18–20 weeks (43). Nicholas found that a rising ALP consistently appeared before early radiographic changes were noted (44). Of note, the decline in ALP is not useful to predict the maturity of HO, as it may remain elevated for years (8). In addition, serum levels of ALP have not been found in all studies to be a sensitive indicator for early HO (42).

Serum CPK can also be used to predict the development of HO (42). CPK levels may increase after direct muscle injury and can be utilized in screening for skeletal muscle diseases such as polymyositis. Singh et al. found that CPK levels taken at 3 weeks postinjury were higher in patients who went on to develop HO and were correlated with severity of HO (42). In this study, whereas CPK levels were correlated with the formation of HO, elevated serum ALP levels at 3 weeks did not predict the future development of HO (perhaps due to the time after injury it was measured, as other studies above note that ALP peaks at 10 weeks postinjury). Sherman at al. also confirmed the relationship between a more elevated CPK level and more aggressive HO (36).

An elevated C-reactive protein (CRP) level has also been found to be present during the development of HO. Sell and Schleh found a significantly higher CRP level 5 to 7 days following THA in patients who eventually developed HO and consider it a marker that would allow the timely initiation of prophylactic measures (45). Estrores et al. looked at elevations in ESR and CRP in patients with HO confirmed by bone scintigraphy (46). They found that both ESR and CRP are elevated in the acute stage of HO, but CRP returns to normal during treatment with Etidronate as the clinical signs and symptoms of inflammation decrease, whereas ESR remains elevated. Other studies have also shown that elevated ESR and ALP are sensitive indicators of HO, but that they are not specific (36).

Riklin et al. studied the occurrence of DVT and HO in persons with SCI and found that the development of HO was often associated with an increased CRP and a positive D-Dimer, even in patients who did not have evidence of DVT (47). In addition to these markers, a different study showed that an increase in 24-hour urine prostaglandin E_2 was found in patients with immature HO, and that it decreased with the administration of indomethacin (48).

Imaging Studies

Commonly used radiologic studies for the diagnosis of HO include conventional radiographs, bone scintigraphy, ultrasound, and MRI. Plain radiography is not useful early in the development of HO, as the immature bone must ossify before being seen on X-ray. However, plain films will show the appearance of fluffy soft tissue flocculations about 2–4 weeks into the process (Figures 51.3 and 51.5). X-rays are a convenient and inexpensive imaging modality and may be worth using if the diagnosis is being sought further in time from the acute injury, when the HO is more likely to be established.

Early confirmation of suspected HO is best made by seeing the ossification precursors of hyperemia and blood pooling on the first two phases of the three-phase technetium bone scan (49). These first two phases are (1) the dynamic blood phase and (2) the static phase immediately following injection of the

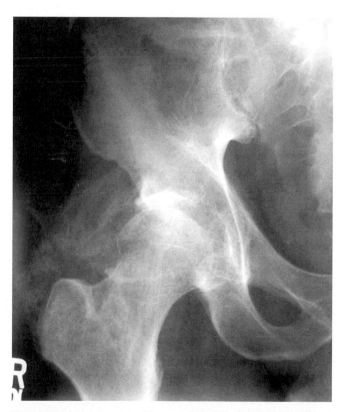

Figure 51.5 A 47-year-old T5 paraplegic patient was admitted for rehabilitation following a motor vehicle accident. An alert therapist noted unilateral reduction in the ROM of the right hip 2 months after admission. An X-ray demonstrated the early development of HO.

isotope; these may be positive as early as 2 to 3 weeks after SCI and 2 to 4 weeks prior to a positive uptake in (3) the third ossification phase of the three-phase bone scan (39). Serial quantitative bone scans can be used to monitor the activity of HO. The only drawback to bone scintigraphy is that, although these scans are very sensitive, they are not specific. If osteomyelitis is in the differential, a ^{67}Gallium bone scan can be compared to a technetium ^{99m}Tc bone scan; ^{67}Ga uptake is proportional to ^{99m}Tc uptake in HO, but in osteomyelitis, there is relatively greater ^{67}Ga uptake (8). Radionuclide scanning, along with the elevated ALP and plain X-ray findings, is also useful in monitoring treatment and the status of the ossification activity. In 80% of cases, the ossification activity has subsided, and the HO matured, within 6 months, as evidenced by the return of the ALP to baseline, inactivity on bone scan, and stable bone formation on the plain X-ray. In the remaining 10% to 20% of patients, these markers have prognostic significance, as the process continues to show activity for many months, resulting in HO progression that is clinically apparent in a reduced range of motion of the limb and even frank ankylosis (10, 15).

Ultrasonography has also been used for the diagnosis of HO. Maier found that 12% of patients showed characteristic findings of HO on sonography, whereas regular X-rays were unremarkable (50). Other studies have also confirmed the utility of ultrasonography in the demonstration of focal soft tissue abnormalities around joints and in muscles in patients with early HO (51). Sonographic findings of HO include a "zone phenomena" around the area of developing HO thought to correspond to tissue inflammation and edema (52).

MRI imaging in patients with early HO demonstrates hyperintense signal on T2-weighted images, with contrast enhancement and muscle swelling in several muscle groups; most patients with acute HO had edema and enhancement of the subcutaneous tissues as well (53). Most patients had concomitant joint effusions. There were consistently found areas with a focal lack of contrast enhancement, which were hyperintense on T2-weighted images. CT correlation with these areas at a later date showed that HO occurred in these formerly nonenhancing regions, primarily at the periphery. Ledermann et al. looked at the imaging characteristics of HO over time and showed that the T2 signal intensity and contrast enhancement decrease, whereas the cortical bone-equivalent signal intensity increases (54). The addition of gadolinium showed an initial ring enhancement, which decreased as the HO matured. One other additional finding in this study was that HO formed in bursa, most commonly the iliopsoas and trochanteric bursae; this finding has been anecdotally confirmed by observations during HO resection.

PREVENTION AND TREATMENT

To prevent the onset of neurogenic HO or to attempt to arrest the progression of ectopic bone formation in the high-risk patient, a number of treatment modalities have been used. Many of the strategies for the primary prevention of neurogenic HO come from the orthopedic literature on the prevention of HO after THA. In cases of surgical resection of established HO, where the rate of recurrence is high, the use of prophylactic measures is indicated and well documented in the literature.

Selection of the most effective interventions currently endorsed depends on the phase of the ossification process—the formation of extracellular matrix (osteoid), the mineralization phase, and the mature bone remodeling phase. Specific selection of nonsurgical treatment is useful only in the early development of HO (immature HO), but it is often marginally successful because of the insidious nature of the ossification process and the dynamics of osteogenesis. In addition, each of the variety of treatment modalities has its own drawbacks and potential complications. In established mature HO, surgical resection is the only treatment available.

Prevention, as in any disease, is preferable to treatment. Patients surviving the effects of severe neurotrauma are at risk for additional disability by developing clinically significant HO, but the risk is sufficiently low so that routine prophylaxis is not warranted in every newly injured patient. Utilizing screening lab tests during the initial rehabilitation of the person with SCI, such as serial determinations of the ALP, CPK, or CRP levels, is an inexpensive way to alert the clinician that the patient is developing HO. Because these tests may not be specific, a confirming triple-phase bone scan is justifiable before starting treatment.

The pharmaceutic interventions most commonly used in the early stages following neurotrauma or orthopedic surgery of the pelvic girdle include anti-inflammatory agents such as nonsteroidal anti-inflammatory drugs (NSAIDs), useful in the preliminary osteoid stage, and the diphosphonate ethane-1-hydroxy-1,1-diphosphonic acid (Etidronate or EHDP), which exerts its effect later in the subsequent mineralization stage.

NSAIDs

Indomethacin is the most commonly used NSAID for the prevention of HO, although ibuprofen, aspirin, and rofecoxib have been reported to be effective. As an inhibitor of cyclooxygenase, NSAIDs hinder the action of prostaglandins in the inflammatory response that probably triggered the induction of HO in the soft tissues (55, 56). NSAIDs also inhibit the differentiation of mesenchymal cells into osteogenic cells (57, 58). The NSAIDs have effects on bone formation, as one might expect from what is known about the osteogenic process in the development of bone involving multiple cytokines and other growth factor superfamilies including the prostaglandins and other mediators of inflammation (56, 57).

Kjaersgaard-Andersen and Schmidt reported that 25 mg of indomethacin three times a day for 6 weeks immediately after hip surgery was effective in preventing clinically significant HO following THA (57, 59). They also noted that it seemed effective if only given for 3 weeks, the period of the dominant inflammatory cellular proliferation phase of wound healing. A recent Cochrane review of studies encompassing 4,587 patients who received NSAIDs after THA showed a 59% reduction in HO formation in patients assigned to active treatment (60).

Banovac et al. used indomethacin SR 75 mg daily for 3 weeks, starting about 3 weeks after SCI (±14 days), and found a significantly lower incidence of both early HO and late HO (61). In another study, Banovac et al. showed a 2.5 times lower relative risk of developing HO in patients on rofecoxib 25 mg daily for 4 weeks (started 3 weeks after SCI) (11). In the newly injured SCI patient on prophylactic DVT anticoagulation therapy, adjustments in dosing should be considered to prevent bleeding secondary to the effect of NSAIDs on platelets. NSAIDs may exacerbate stress-induced peptic ulcer disease with associated upper gastrointestinal tract bleeding, which may follow neurotrauma; thus, GI prophylaxis should be considered.

Etidronate

There has been extensive experience in the use of the diphosphonate etidronate in the prevention and treatment of HO, in both the orthopedic and the neurotrauma populations. Etidronate has no effect on osteoid development but does prevent the conversion of amorphous calcium phosphate compounds into hydroxyapatite crystals, a critical step in the mineralization of the osteoid matrix (10, 62). In 1976, Stover introduced etidronate for the treatment of HO after SCI (63). Several studies have been done since his original work, and they clarify the dose and duration needed for optimal results. Despite some evidence of reduction in HO with etidronate used both prophylactically and for treatment, often the results of etidronate administration are disappointing, and the patient continues to form HO.

Stover et al. prophylactically treated eighty-two patients with disodium etidronate (20 mg/kg/day for 2 weeks and then 10 mg/kg/day for an additional 10 weeks) and compared this group with eighty-four patients in a placebo group (63). There was no difference in the incidence of HO in the two groups, but the treated group had considerably less HO and less functional disability than the control group. Treatment, however, was started relatively late in the natural history of neurogenic HO, ranging from 20 to 121 days after the injury, and treatment was only for 3 months rather than for the 6 months now recommended. Only 35 of the 166 patients in the study had radiographically proven HO; thus, this trial was actually a mixture of prevention and treatment.

Finerman and Stover used the same treatment protocol as the original Stover study but showed a significantly lower incidence of HO after 12 weeks of therapy (64). Repeat radiographic evaluation after 9 months demonstrated a marked increase in HO formation in the group that had received etidronate, raising the concern of a "rebound" phenomena. Garland and colleagues increased the duration of etidronate to 14 months at doses of 10mg/kg/day, followed by an increase in the dose to 20mg/kg/day for 6 months, which resulted in reduced progression of HO from 86% to 47% (30, 65).

Ono, in 1988, treated persons with SCI who had clinical, laboratory, or radiographic evidence of acute HO with etidronate 1,000 mg per day for 12 weeks (66). This study showed that there was a significantly greater likelihood of preventing the progression of HO by treatment with etidronate, as well as an improvement in the clinical and radiographic grade of HO. This and Stover were the two studies reviewed in a 2004 Cochrane review on the pharmacologic treatments for acute HO; this review excluded fifty-four studies in the literature because subjects did not have acute HO at baseline (63, 67). Thus, the body of literature on the treatment of acute HO is lacking, and often studies have a mixture of diagnoses (i.e., SCI and THA) or document both prevention and treatment (due to lack of uniformity of diagnostic criteria).

Banovac et al., in 1996, published the first use of IV etidronate in HO and showed that an initial dose of 300mg/day IV for 3 days followed by oral therapy for 6 months (20mg/kg/day) resulted in less progression of HO (68). The authors did note that those patients with positive radiographic evidence of HO on entry into the study had a poorer response to therapy, with some patients showing continued growth of HO despite treatment. The IV route markedly increases the bioavailability of etidronate and reduces GI intolerance. Unfortunately, since this study has been published, IV etidronate has been taken off the market.

Because etidronate only affects the mineralization of osteoid, theoretically it should be continued indefinitely, and recurrence of varying amounts of HO have been reported following the discontinuance of the drug (10). Although there have been reports of good results with minimal recurrence following treatment for a year or longer, concerns remain for aggravating the sometimes severe osteoporosis found in SCI patients, or impeding the healing of bony fusions from spinal surgeries or fractures related to the acute SCI. Because of this combined detrimental effect of skeletal osteoporosis and reduced osteoid mineralization, a potential complication of prolonged use of diphosphonates is a pathologic (spontaneous) fracture of a long bone; this has been observed in animal experiments (69). This limited window of etidronate treatment of 6 months may permit the process of calcification of nascent osteoid matrix to proceed following discontinuance, because the ossification process was not arrested but only delayed.

Because of the lack of specific data showing effectiveness and the potential negative effects of the prolonged use of etidronate, routine medical prophylaxis of HO in newly injured patients with SCI remains a treatment option rather than being routine clinical practice.

Other Pharmacologic Agents

There are a few other medications that have been used to prevent HO, which are intriguing and will hopefully lead to more research in this area. Colchicine has been shown to strongly inhibit osteoblast cell proliferation and tissue mineralization (70). Dudkiewicz utilized colchicine in a rabbit model to prevent HO (which was induced by injection of bone marrow aspirate into the thigh) (71). The group that received colchicine starting 1 week before the HO induction showed almost complete prevention of HO; the group that received colchicine starting the day of induction had a marked decrease in HO formation, and the control group formed large amounts of new bone at the injection site.

Warfarin is another medication that may contribute to a reduction in the formation of HO. This effect is theorized based on the fact that osteocalcin, one of the proteins that makes up the osteoid matrix, is produced by vitamin K–dependent carboxylation. Buschbacher et al. reviewed patients who were on warfarin for treatment of DVT and showed that none of the patients who had received warfarin went on to develop HO (72). Despite the fact that other studies of patients with DVT on warfarin do show some patients developing HO, the timing of the events and screening protocols have not been fully tested in a prospective study, leaving this treatment as one that should be further evaluated.

Range of Motion

Adjunctive treatment to maintain the mobility of major joints is a basic tenet of rehabilitation medicine. Maintenance of the mobility of the major joints of immobile patients is essential to avoid contractures and fibrous ankylosis of joints from disuse. This goal is usually accomplished by passive range-of-motion (ROM) exercises by trained therapists. The majority of SCI patients in a rehabilitation program do not develop clinically significant HO, and when nascent HO is in the preclinical phase, the first clue to its possible presence may be the recognition by the therapist of diminishing ROM during therapy. However, once HO is diagnosed, the question is invariably raised, "Is it safe to do ROM, and how much should we do?"

Some workers have avoided such manipulation of major joints, believing that such activity may increase the inflammatory response or result in trauma with bleeding and hematoma formation and contribute to the onset of HO or adversely affect the volume of ectopic bone being formed. The basis of these concerns is experiments in rabbits in the early 1980s in which forceful and traumatic manipulation of the limbs caused direct trauma to muscle tissue with hematoma formation that precipitated the development of centers of ossification in the injured muscle tissue (73). Such a setting is more in keeping with myositis ossificans than the HO of neurogenic origin, in which there is no recognized local injury. However, Izumi also showed a relationship between the formation of HO in the paraplegic rabbit and a period of immobilization followed by passive movement (74). Silver has postulated that the timing of initiation of passive movement may play a vital role in the development of HO; if there is a period of immobilization followed by the commencement of ROM, then the HO that develops may be more severe (75). He observed that the longer the period of rest, the more HO forms after the initiation of movement; conversely, patients who receive ROM immediately after injury without a period of immobility seem to be less likely to form aggressive HO. Daud confirmed that clinically apparent HO occurred only in patients in whom the start of passive ROM was delayed by 7 or more days after SCI (76).

Crawford et al. showed that in a population of patients with HO after burn, active ROM in a pain-free range led to improved motion and function, whereas passive ROM past a pain-free range led to worsening of HO and bony ankylosis (77). Thus, there is a consensus that forceful exercises should not be initiated until the inflammatory signs heralding the acute onset of HO, if present, have subsided. More studies need to be conducted to see if immediate ROM would completely eliminate the development of HO.

Radiation

It is theorized that the ionizing radiation alters the nuclear deoxyribonucleic acid (DNA) of rapidly dividing cells and blocks the differentiation of the mesenchymal stem cells into the osteoblastic stem cells that give rise to the osteoblasts, osteoclasts, and osteocytes needed for osteogenesis (78). Radiotherapy has been used for the primary prevention of HO after THA, as well as for secondary prevention of HO after surgical resection (in both the SCI and THA populations). Interestingly, there is little data of primary prevention of HO after SCI, most likely due to concerns over radiation exposure, which may increase risks of malignancy, as well as impair skin integrity and wound healing. In addition, as discussed above, the incidence of clinically significant HO after SCI is not high enough to justify routine prophylaxis with a modality that may have more side effects than benefits for those who do not go on to develop HO.

There is a large body of literature looking at the use of low-dose perioperative radiation for the prevention of HO in patients deemed to be at high risk for developing HO following THA. In addition, low dose radiation has been advocated in the immediate postoperative period for patients undergoing resection of HO and may be combined with an NSAID as an additional prophylactic measure (79). Because of the theoretical danger of inducing malignant change, the use of low-dose radiation therapy is reserved for only those deemed at high risk for developing recurrence of their HO; this includes patients who had an aggressive course in the development of HO and those patients with marked spasticity, who have been shown to have a higher rate of recurrence (10).

Protocols differ as to single-dose or fractionated therapy delivered over a course of several days. Advocates of fractionated protocols feel that 1,000 centigrays (cGy) delivered at 200 cGy per day over 5 days is an effective and safe inhibitor of bone growth. This dose was believed to be equally as effective as a 2,000-cGy fractionated protocol (80). Ayers and his group reported on a number of studies using both single-dose and fractionated radiation protocols that supported the effectiveness of low-dose radiation therapy following THA surgery (78). When therapy was delayed more than 4 to 5 days, however, successful outcomes were reduced in both protocols compared to treatment initiated in the first 24 to 48 hours, even with half the radiation used in delayed protocols. The Ayers group reported that single-dose radiation had greater tissue effects than fractionated radiation of equal or greater total cGy, and they concluded that a single treatment in the immediate postoperative period was superior to delayed or fractionated therapy (78). A number of other authors report equal success with single-dose radiation therapy of between 600 to 700 cGy, given in the immediate postoperative period (81). Therapy should be initiated early in the postoperative recovery phase during the early inductive phase of the pluripotential mesenchymal stem cells' transformation into osteoprogenitor cell lines. In a recent review of prophylaxis and treatment of HO following lower limb arthroplasty, the recommended dose was 7 Gy to 8 Gy given as a single dose either less than 4 hours preoperatively or less than 72 hours postoperatively (32).

Kienapfel et al. (82) compared radiation with the NSAID indomethacin, using a single dose of 600 cGy between the second and fourth postoperative day in one group, and in a comparable second group, 50 mg *bid* of indomethacin for 6 weeks, again starting on the first day following surgery. They found that each method had comparable results in its effectiveness in the prevention of postoperative HO and that both modalities were significantly more helpful than the lack of treatment in a third control group that received no prophylactic postoperative treatment. In a recent meta-analysis of the prevention of HO after major hip procedures, Pakos and Ioannidis found that radiotherapy is more effective than NSAIDS at preventing Brooker class 3 and 4 HO (83).

There are few studies on the primary treatment of HO with radiotherapy, despite its proven efficacy for primary and secondary prevention. Sautter-Bihl and colleagues used low-dose radiotherapy (total dose 7.5–20 Gy) in patients with early HO to prevent progression; thirty of thirty-three irradiated patients showed no progression, and in fact sixteen had no evidence of HO on follow-up plain radiograph (84). In another study by the same group, fifty-eight joints were irradiated as primary

treatment for the inflammatory phase of HO, with doses ranging from 8 Gy in a single dose to 20 Gy in multiple fractions (85). 71% of the irradiated joints did not show progression.

Surgical Treatment

The surgical treatment of established HO should have limited objectives. In the majority of patients who do not have clinically significant HO, surgery is usually not indicated. Where the need to close a pressure ulcer is the goal, however, the underlying ectopic bone mass should be removed to the degree that the "pressure point" is eliminated and flap tissue can be mobilized sufficiently to permit closure of the defect. Because recrudescent HO is common, limiting the surgical trauma is the most acceptable approach, and postoperative HO prophylaxis is indicated (62, 69, 73, 78, 81, 82, 86).

Where there is a need to restore joint mobility in Brooker's class IV fused joints, surgery is the only option (10, 87). In the case of a fused hip joint, the goal should be limited to gaining the degree of mobility that is consistent with sitting in a wheelchair. It should not be the complete ablation of the pathology, because the surgery of extensive HO is difficult and there is a high rate of complications. Limiting the procedure to a simple wedge resection (osteotomy) of a long bone distal to an ankylosed joint, creating a pseudoarthrosis that permits sitting in a wheelchair, is a safer plan than total extirpation of the entire mass of bone. In other cases where HO is associated with osteomyelitis and persistent drainage from a deep sinus tract, a sinogram is indicated to ascertain whether the joint space is involved, because a more major procedure, such as a Girdlestone resection, may be needed (Figure 51.6) (87, 88). Becker et al. described the use of

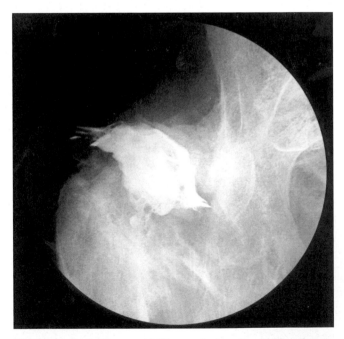

Figure 51.6 A 57-year-old C5 tetraplegic patient with a chronic draining sinus of the hip associated with massive HO formation of many years duration. Sinogram showed a "deep sinus tract but without extravasation into the anatomical acetabulum from which the femoral head has been displaced."

endoprostheses after HO resection to maintain the biomechanics of the hip; the purpose was to maintain appropriate sitting posture and reduce subsequent pressure sore formation (89).

Garland states that resection of HO should not be undertaken during the 6-month period following onset (10). Not only may the process of HO formation be self-limiting and not clinically important, but the majority of workers in the field feel that surgical trauma should be withheld during the inflammatory phase of active ossification if exacerbation of the process is to be limited. Maturation of the process, as evidenced by a return of the ALP to baseline, decreasing activity on ^{99m}Tc bone scan and the radiograph, indicating that only mature bone are criteria assisting the clinician in surgical decision making. Such a situation should exist in the majority of cases within 6 months to a year following the onset of HO. In a limited number of patients, where there is X-ray evidence of continued progression beyond 6 months, the presence of significant amounts of HO, persistent elevation of the ALP, continued radionuclide uptake, and a poor response to prophylactic medications, surgery should be delayed for 18 to 24 months (10). Delaying the needed surgery beyond that time frame, however, increases the risk of intraoperative and postoperative long bone fractures caused by the presence of markedly osteoporotic bone.

Surgical complications include excessive bleeding, a high rate of wound infection including osteomyelitis, delayed wound healing, long bone fractures during and after surgery, and recurrence of HO by the traumatic reactivation of the osteogenic process (78, 81, 90). Blood loss in the operating room routinely requires replacement of from 5 to 10 units of packed red blood cells, because the tissue is highly vascular. Preoperative embolization of the HO mass prior to resection can be utilized to reduce exsanguination (91).

Following surgery, HO prophylaxis is essential and is best initiated on the first postoperative day. Garland recommends a 3- to 6-month course of etidronate accompanied by a consistent program of physical therapy to maintain joint mobility (10). More recently, Schuetz et al. showed that the use of pamidronate infusion starting in the first 12 hours postoperatively and continuing for 10 to 14 days eliminated the recurrence of HO formation (92). This study was limited by a small sample size ($n = 5$). A combination of indomethacin and radiation may be indicated following surgery in high-risk patients (79). This approach in patients after THA using a radiotherapy dose of 7 Gy postoperatively in combination with indomethacin 75 mg for 15 days resulted in only 1 of 54 patients developing clinically significant HO (93). However, overutilization of prophylactic measures must be balanced by the risk of side effects to underlying osteoporotic bone. In a study by van Kuijk and colleagues, the combination of surgery, irradiation, and an NSAID resulted in osteonecrosis of the femoral head (94).

Concerning physical therapy, postoperative fractures of the adjacent osteopenic skeletal bone during the ROM manipulation of limbs are a real danger, particularly following the release of ankylosed joints, in which the long bone atrophy of prolonged disuse may be significant. DEXA assessment of bone density prior to HO resection may not accurately reflect the true underlying bone density (95). Gentle passive range-of-motion therapy and stretching of the involved joint is beneficial but should not be done during the acute inflammatory phase of the immediate postoperative period.

CONCLUSION

The development of soft tissue ectopic bone formation is a common, although rarely disabling, complication of neurotrauma. Its cause is not well understood, but it seems to be the result of postinjury humoral induction of pluripotent mesenchymal stem cells that are resident in soft tissues adjacent to major joints. These mesenchymal stem cells change into osteoprogenitor cell lines that differentiate into osteoblasts and the other cells involved in bone formation. HO is usually self-limiting over a period of 6 months; most patients do not require prophylaxis and respond well to available pharmacologic treatments. However, those patients who develop aggressive HO may progress to bony joint ankylosis; often surgery is the sole option available for treatment to return them to a fully functional state and may be technically difficult. Because recurrence is the most common surgical complication, prophylaxis with NSAIDs, Etidronate, and low-dose radiation, either singularly or in combination early in the postoperative period, is indicated. It is expected that the present line of research into the molecular and cellular causes of this potentially debilitating process will eventually lead to interventions that will prevent this unusual complication of SCI.

References

1. Elsberg CA. The Edwin Smith surgical papyrus and the diagnosis and treatment of injuries to the skull and spine 5000 years ago. *Ann Med Hist* 1931; 3:271–279.
2. Dejerine A, Ceillier A. Para-osteo-arthropathies des paraplégiques par lésion medullaire: etude clinique et radiographique. *Ann Med Hist* 1918; 5:497.
3. Beiner JM, Jokl P. Muscle contusion injury and myositis ossificans traumatica. *Clin Orthop Relat Res* 2002; 403:S110–S119.
4. Shore EM, Glaser DL, Gannon FH. Osteogenic induction in hereditary disorders of heterotopic ossification. *Clin Orthop Relat Res* 2000; 374:303–316.
5. Evans EB. Heterotopic bone formation in thermal burns. *Clin Orthop Relat Res* 1991; 263:94–101.
6. Elledge ES, Smith AA, McManus WF, Pruitt BA Jr. Heterotopic bone formation in burned patients. *J Trauma* 1988; 28(5):684–687.
7. Bosch P, Musgrave DS, Lee JY, et al. Osteoprogenitor cells within skeletal muscle. *J Orthop Res* 2000; 18(6):933–944.
8. Shehab D, Elgazzar AH, Collier BD. Heterotopic ossification. *J Nucl Med* 2002; 43(3):346–353.
9. Singer BR. Heterotopic ossification. *Br J Hosp Med* 1993; 49:247–255.
10. Garland DE. A clinical perspective on common forms of acquired heterotopic ossification. *Clin Orthop Relat Res* 1991; 263(2):13–29.
11. Banovac K, Williams JM, Patrick LD, Levi A. Prevention of heterotopic ossification after spinal cord injury with COX-2 selective inhibitor (rofecoxib). *Spinal Cord* 2004; 42:707–710.
12. Ahrengart L. Periarticular heterotopic ossification after total hip arthroplasty. *Clin Orthop Relat Res* 1991; 263(2):49–58.
13. van Kuijk AA, Geurts ACH, van Kuppevelt HJM. Neurogenic heterotopic ossification in spinal cord injury. *Spinal Cord* 2002; 40:313–326.
14. Brooker AF, Bowerman JW, Robinson RA, Riley L Jr. Ectopic ossification following total hip replacement: incidence and a method of classification. *J Bone Joint Surg* 1973; 55(8):1629.
15. Subbarao JV, Garrison SJ. Heterotopic ossification: diagnosis and management, current concepts and controversies. *J Spinal Cord Med* 1999; 22(4):273–283.
16. Delee J, Ferrari A, Charnley J. Ectopic bone formation following low friction arthroplasty of the hip. *Clin Orthop Relat Res* 1976; 121:53.
17. Rosendahl S, Krogh CJ, Norgaard M. Para-articular ossification following hip replacement. *Acta Orthop Scand* 1977; 48:400.
18. Ayers DC, Evarts CM, Parkinson JR. The prevention of heterotopic ossification in high-risk patients by low-dose radiation therapy after total hip arthroplasty. *J Bone Joint Surg* 1986; 68A:1423.
19. Riedel B. Demonstration line durch ach Hagiges Umhergehen total destruirten kniegelnkes von einem pantienten mit stichverletzing des ruckans. *Vehr Dtsch Gesellschaft Chirurg* 1883; 12:93.

20. Ebinger T, Roesch M, Kiefer H, Kinzl L, Schulte M. Influence of etiology in heterotopic bone formation of the hip. *The Journal of Trauma: Injury, Infection, and Critical Care* 2000; 48(6):1058.

21. Reed MH, McGinn G, Black CB, Larson AG. Heterotopic ossification in children after iliopsoas release. *Can Assoc Radiol J* 1992; 439(3): 195–198.

22. Lee M, Alexander MA, Miller F. Postoperative Heterotopic ossification in the child with cerebral palsy: three case reports. *Arch Phys Med Rehabil* 1992; 73(3):289–292.

23. Payne LZ, DeLuca PA. Heterotopic ossification after rhizotomy and femoral osteotomy. *J Pediatr Orthop* 1993; 13(6):733–738.

24. Jamil F, Subbarao JV, Banaovac K, El Masry WS, Bergman SB. Management of immature heterotopic ossification (HO) of the hip. *Spinal Cord* 2002; 40:388–395.

25. Charcot JM. *Lectures on the Diseases of the Nervous System. Delivered at "La-Saltpetriere."* 2nd ed. Philadelphia: Henry C. Lea, 1879.

26. Kurer MH, Khoker MA, Dandona P. Human osteoblast stimulation by sera from paraplegic patients with heterotopic ossification. *Paraplegia* 1992; 30(3):165–168.

27. Bone RC. Systemic inflammatory response syndrome: a unifying concept of systemic inflammation. In: Fein AM, Abraham EM, Balk RA, et al., eds. *Sepsis and Multiorgan Failure.* Baltimore, MD: Williams & Wilkins. 1997:3–10.

28. Subburaman M, Baylink DJ. Bone growth factors. *Clin Orthop Relat Res* 1991; 263:30–48.

29. Urist MR. Bone formation by autoinduction. *Science* 1965; 150: 893–899.

30. Wozney JM, Rosen V, Celeste AJ. Novel regulators of bone formation: molecular clones and activities. *Science* 1988; 242:1528–1534.

31. Katagiri T, Yamaguchi A, Komaki M. Bone morpho-genetic protein-2 converts the differentiation pathway of 2C12C myoblasts into the osteoblast lineage. *J Cell Biol* 1995; 127:1755–1766.

32. Board TN, Karva A, Board RE, Gambhir AK, Porter ML. The prophylaxis and treatment of heterotopic ossification following lower limb arthroplasty. *J Bone Joint Surg Br* 2007; 89(4):434.

33. Urist MR, Nakagawa M, Nakata N, Nogami H. Experimental myositis ossificans: cartilage and bone formation in muscle in response to a diffusible bone matrix-derived morphogen. *Arch Pathol Lab Med* 1978; 102(6):312–316.

34. Renfree KJ, Banovac K, Hornicek FJ, Lebwohl NH, et al. Evaluation of serum osteoblast mitogenic activity in spinal cord and head injury patients with acute heterotopic ossification. *Spine* 1994; 19(7):740.

35. Lotta S, Scelsi L, Scelsi R. Microvascular changes in the lower extremities of paraplegics with heterotopic ossification. *Spinal Cord* 2001; 39(11):595–598.

36. Sherman AL, Williams J, Patrick L, Banovac K. The value of serum creatine kinase in early diagnosis of heterotopic ossification. *J Spinal Cord Med* 2003; 26(3):227–230.

37. Jensen LL, Halar E, Little JW, Brooke MM. Neurogenic heterotopic ossification. *Am J Phys Med* 1987; 66(6):351–363.

38. Schmidt J, Hackenbroch MH. A new classification for heterotopic ossifications in total hip arthroplasty considering the surgical approach. *Arch Orthop Trauma Surg* 1996; 115(6):339–343.

39. Bravo-Payno P, Esclarin A, Arzoz T, Arroyo O, Labarta C. Incidence and risk factors in the appearance of heterotopic ossification in spinal cord injury. *Paraplegia* 1992; 30:740–745.

40. Furman R, Nicholas JJ, Jivoff L. Elevation of the serum alkaline phosphatase coincident with ectopic bone formation in paraplegic patients *J Bone Joint Surg* 1970; 52A:1131.

41. Garland DE. Clinical observations on fractures and heterotopic ossification in the spinal cord and traumatic brain injured populations. *Clin Orthop* 1988; 233:86.

42. Singh RS, Craig MC, Katholi CR, Jackson AB, Mountz JM. The predictive value of creatine phosphokinase and alkaline phosphatase in identification of heterotopic ossification in patients after spinal cord injury. *Arch Phys Med Rehabil* 2003; 84(11):1584–1588.

43. Orzel JA. Heterotopic bone formation: clinical, laboratory, and imaging correlation. *Soc Nuclear Med* 1985; 26(2):125–132.

44. Nicholas JJ. Ectopic bone formation in patients with spinal cord injury. *Arch Phys Med Rehabil* 1973; 54:354–359.

45. Sell S, Schleh T. C-reactive protein as an early indicator of the formation of heterotopic ossification after total hip replacement. *Arch Orthop Trauma Surg* 1999; 119(3–4):205–207.

46. Estrores IM, Harrington A, Banovac K. C-reactive protein and erythrocyte sedimentation rate in patients with heterotopic ossification after spinal cord injury. *J Spinal Cord Med* 2004; 27(5):434–437.

47. Riklin C, Baumberger M, Wick L, Michel D, et al. Deep vein thrombosis and heterotopic ossification in spinal cord injury: a 3 year experience at the Swiss Paraplegic Centre Nottwil. *Spinal Cord* 2003; 41:192–198.

48. Schurch B, Capaul M, Vallotton MB, Rossier AB. Prostaglandin E2 measurements: their value in the early diagnosis of heterotopic ossification in spinal cord injury patients. *Arch Phys Med Rehabil* 1997; 78(7): 687–691.

49. Freed JH, Hahn H, Menter MD, Dillion T. The use of the three-phase bone scan in the early diagnosis of heterotopic ossification (HO) and in the evaluation of didronel therapy. *Paraplegia* 1982; 20:208.

50. Maier D. Heterotopic ossification spinal cord injury: management through early diagnosis and therapy. *Orthopade* 2005; 34(2):120–122.

51. Bodley R, Jamous A, Short D. Ultrasound in the early diagnosis of heterotopic ossification in patients with spinal injuries. *Paraplegia* 1993; 31(8):500–506.

52. Cassar-Pullicino VN, McClelland M, Badwan DA, McCall IW, et al. Sonographic diagnosis of heterotopic bone formation in spinal injury patients. *Paraplegia* 1993; 31(1):40–50.

53. Wick L, Berger M, Knecht H, Glücker T, Ledermann HP. Magnetic resonance signal alterations in the acute onset of heterotopic ossification in patients with spinal cord injury. *European Radiology* 2005; 15(9):1867–1875.

54. Ledermann HP, Schweitzer ME, Morrison WB. Pelvic heterotopic ossification: MR imaging characteristics. *Radiology* 2001:222101055.

55. Vane JR. Inhibition of prostaglandin synthesis as a mechanism for aspirin-like drugs. *Nature* 1971; 231:232.

56. Ro J, Sudmann E, Marton PF. Effects of indomethacin on fracture healing in rats. *Acta Orthop Scand* 1976; 47:588.

57. Sudmann E, Bang G. Indomethacin-induced inhibition of Haversian remodeling in rabbits. *Acta Orthop Scand* 1979; 50:621.

58. Tornkvist H, Bauer FCH, Nilsson OS. Influence of indomethacin on experimental bone metabolism in rats. *Clin Orthop* 1985; 193:264.

59. Kjaersgaard-Andersen P, Schmidt SA. Indomethacin for prevention of ectopic ossification after hip arthroplasty. *Acta Orthop Scand* 1986; 57:12.

60. Fransen M, Neal B. Non-steroidal anti-inflammatory drugs for preventing heterotopic bone formation after hip arthroplasty. *Cochrane Database Syst Rev* 2004(3):CD001160. DOI: 001110.001002/14651858 .CD14001160.pub14651852.

61. Banovac K, Williams JM, Patrick LD, Haniff YM. Prevention of heterotopic ossification after spinal cord injury with indomethacin. *Spinal Cord* 2001; 39(7):370–374.

62. Fleisch H. Diphosphonates: history and mechanisms of action. *Bone* 1981; 3:279.

63. Stover SL, Hahn HR, Miller JMI. Disodium etidronate in the prevention of heterotopic ossification following spinal cord injury. *Paraplegia* 1976; 14:146.

64. Finerman GA, Stover SL. Heterotopic ossification following hip replacement or spinal cord injury: two clinical studies with EHDP. *Metab Bone Dis Relat Res* 1981; 3(4–5):337–342.

65. Garland DE. Diphosphonate treatment for heterotopic ossification in spinal cord injury patients. *Clin Orthop Relat Res* 1983; 176:197.

66. Ono K, Takaoka K, Kaneda K, Takahashi H, et al. [A double-blind study of EHDP on heterotopic ossification after spinal cord injury using placebo]. *Rinsho Hyoka [Clinical Evaluation]*. 1988; 16(4):581–615.

67. Haran M, Bhuta T, Lee B. Pharmacological interventions for treating acute heterotopic ossification. *Cochrane Database Syst Rev* 2004; 4:CD003321. DOI:003310.001002/14651858.CD14003321.pub14651853.

68. Banovac K. The effect of etidronate on late development of heterotopic ossification after spinal cord injury. *J Spinal Cord Med* 2000; 23(1):40–44.

69. Flora L, Hassing GS, Cloyd GG, Parfitt AM, Villanueva AR. The long-term skeletal effects of EHDP in dogs. *Bone* 1981; 3:279.

70. Salai M, Segal E, Cohen I, et al. The inhibitory effects of colchicine on cell proliferation and mineralisation in culture. *J Bone Joint Surg Br* 2001; 83(6):912–915.

71. Dudkiewicz I, Cohen I, Horowitz S, et al. Colchicine inhibits heterotopic ossification: experimental study in rabbits. *Isr Med Assoc J* 2005; 7(1):31–34.

72. Buschbacher R, McKinley W, Buschbacher L, Devaney CW, Coplin B. Warfarin in prevention of heterotopic ossification. *Am J Phys Med Rehabil* 1992; 71(2):86–91.

73. Michelsson JE, Rauschning W. Pathogenesis of experimental heterotopic bone formation following temporary forcible exercising of immobilized limbs. *Clin Orthop* 1983; 176:265–272.

74. Izumi K. Study of ectopic bone formation in experimental spinal cord injured rabbits. *Paraplegia* 1983; 21(6):351–363.

75. Silver J. Letter to the editor. *Spinal Cord* 2003; 41:421–422.

76. Daud O, Sett P, Burr RG, Silver JR. The relationship of heterotopic ossification to passive movements in paraplegic patients. *Disabil Rehabil* 1993; 15(3):114–118.

77. Crawford CM, Varghese G, Mani MM, Neff JR. Heterotopic ossification: are range of motion exercises contraindicated? *J Burn Care Rehabil* 1986; 7:323–327.

78. Ayers DC, Pellegrini VD, McCollister EC. Prevention of heterotopic ossification in high-risk patients by radiation therapy. *Clin Orthop Relat Res* 1991; 263:87–93.

79. Freebourn TM, Barber DB, Able AC. The treatment of immature heterotopic ossification in spinal cord injury with combination surgery, radiation therapy and NSAID. *Spinal Cord* 1999; 37:50–53.

80. Ayers DC, Evarts CM, Parkinson JR. The prevention of heterotopic ossification in high-risk patients by low-dose radiation therapy after total hip arthroplasty *J Bone Joint Surg* 1986; 68A:1423.

81. Healy WL, Lo TC, DeSimone AA, Rask B, Pfeifer BA. Single-dose irradiation for the prevention of heterotopic ossification after total hip arthroplasty: a comparison of doses of 550 and 700 centigray. *J Bone Joint Surg Am* 1995; 77(4):590–595.

82. Kienapfel H, Koller M, Wust A, et al. Prevention of heterotopic bone formation after total hip arthroplasty: a prospective randomized study comparing postoperative radiation therapy with indomethacin medication. *Arch Orthop Trauma Surg* 1999; 119(5–6):296–302.

83. Pakos EE, Ioannidis JP. Radiotherapy vs. nonsteroidal anti-inflammatory drugs for the prevention of heterotopic ossification after major hip procedures: a meta-analysis of randomized trials. *Int J Radiat Oncol Biol Phys* 2004; 60(3):888–895.

84. Sautter-Bihl ML, Liebermeister E, Nanassy A. Radiotherapy as a local treatment option for heterotopic ossifications in patients with spinal cord injury. *Spinal Cord* 2000; 38(1):33–36.

85. Sautter-Bihl ML, Hültenschmidt B, Liebermeister E, Nanassy A. Fractionated and single-dose radiotherapy for heterotopic bone formation in patients with spinal cord injury. *Strahlentherapie und Onkologie* 2001; 177(4):200–205.

86. Fingeroth RJ AA. Single dose 6 cGy prophylaxis for heterotopic ossification after total hip arthroplasty. *Clin Orthop* 1995; 317: 131–140.

87. Stover SL, Niemann KMW, Tullross JR. Experience with surgical resection of heterotopic bone in spinal cord injury patients. *Clin Orthop Relat Res* 1991; 263(2):71–77.

88. Garland DE, Rubayi SS, Harway EC, Pompan DC. Proximal femoral resection and vastus lateralis flap in the treatment of heterotopic ossification in patients with spinal cord injury. *Contemp Orthop* 1995; 31(6):341–347.

89. Becker SWJ, Röhl K, Weidt F. Endoprosthesis in paraplegics with periarticular ossification of the hip. *Spinal Cord* 2003; 41:29–33.

90. Garland DE, Orwin JF. Resection of heterotopic ossification in patients with spinal cord injuries. *Clin Orthop* 1998; 242:169–176.

91. Appelt EA, Kenkel JM, Ballard JR, Lopez JA, et al. Preoperative embolization of heterotopic ossification for the treatment of a recalcitrant pressure sore. *Plast Reconstr Surg* 2005; 116(4):50e.

92. Schuetz P, Mueller B, Christ-Crain M, Dick W, Haas H. Aminobisphosphonates in heterotopic ossification: first experience in five consecutive cases. *Spinal Cord* 2005; 43:604–610.

93. Pakos EE, Pitouli EJ, Tsekeris PG, Papathanasopoulou V, et al. Prevention of heterotopic ossification in high-risk patients with total hip arthroplasty: the experience of a combined therapeutic protocol. *Int Orthop* 2006; 30(2):79–83.

94. van Kuijk AA, van Kuppevelt HJM, van der Schaaf DB. Osteonecrosis after treatment for heterotopic ossification in spinal cord injury with the combination of surgery, irradiation, and an NSAID. *Spinal Cord* 2000; 38(5):319–324.

95. Jaovisidha S, Sartoris DJ, Martin EME, Foldes K, et al. Influence of heterotopic ossification of the hip on bone densitometry: a study in spinal cord injured patients. *Spinal Cord* 1998; 36(9):647–653.

52

Scoliosis and Spinal Deformities: Avoiding and Managing Neurologic Deficits

Timothy R. Kuklo

Over the past several decades, there have been numerous iterations and technical advancements in spinal instrumentation systems. Consequently, the postoperative correction and surgical outcomes following spinal instrumentation and fusion have continued to improve in both adolescent idiopathic scoliosis (AIS) and adult spinal deformity. Initially, instrumentation systems provided limited correction with long fusion constructs. These were designed to "maintain" the curve. More recently, advanced segmental instrumentation systems have permitted improved curve correction, shorter constructs, and better sagittal contour (21, 27, 28, 31, 49, 53). Additionally, segmental pedicle screw instrumentation has been proven to save fusion levels in AIS (36, 48, 61).

These improvements have also led to more aggressive operative management of adult spinal deformity. Nonetheless, there are only a handful of studies that outline the evaluation and planning of adult spinal deformity, as most of the literature includes retrospective reviews. More importantly, application of these technologic advances requires a thorough understanding of spinal deformity and correction principles aimed at improving outcomes and quality of life, while understanding and managing neurologic risk and/or deficit. This chapter will review the evaluation and management of scoliosis and spinal deformities, the avoidance and surgical management of neurologic deficits in these patients, and the evaluation and management of spinal deformity in spinal cord–injured patients.

EVALUATION OF SCOLIOSIS AND SPINAL DEFORMITIES

Clinical Evaluation

Patients with scoliosis and/or spinal deformity may present on routine referral or with increasing pain or disability. For younger patients, pain is probably more common than originally thought; however, it is generally limited to the thoracic or lumbar region. Pain in association with spinal deformity is much more common in adult patients and will often also be experienced secondary to

degenerative changes of the spine, in the lower extremities as a lumbar radiculopathy, or in a generalized pain pattern consistent with spinal stenosis. A different subset of patients may even be posttraumatic kyphosis patients, who generally present with a history of spinal injury and generalized thoracic and lumbar back pain. In adults, either of these conditions may also present with low endurance and difficulty standing erect. Neurologic progression, although possible, is infrequent.

In addition to a thorough history and neurologic evaluation, examination should include assessment of the overall sagittal and coronal balance. This is done with the patient standing and the knees extended. In adults with thoracolumbar kyphosis or degenerative loss of lordosis, presentation occurs when the patient's lumbar "reserve" is maximized, and further compensation is impossible. Thus, the typical standing posture may include forward tilting of the trunk, which leads to hip and knee flexion and cervical hyperextension in addition to hyperextension of any remaining nonpainful, mobile vertebral segments in the thoracic and lumbar spine. Muscular pain usually follows and is generally associated with fatigue. Furthermore, biomechanical studies have shown increased paraspinal muscular forces required to maintain an erect posture, which may contribute to the fatigue-related etiology of symptoms—much like the fixed sagittal imbalance patient (64, 68).

Additionally, hip flexion contractures can be present in longstanding disease, and the pelvic tilt may be abnormal (29). Patients with severe progression of thoracolumbar kyphosis following lumbar fusion (especially with distraction) may manifest cardiopulmonary or digestive symptoms as well (56). Tension signs are usually not present, although they are possible from associated adjacent segment degeneration with stenosis, especially below a fusion (6, 44).

Radiographic Evaluation

Inherent in the complete evaluation of patients with spinal deformity is a comprehensive radiographic evaluation, in addition to other necessary radiographic studies such as magnetic resonance imaging (MRI), computed tomography (CT), and/or CT myelography. As such, these more advanced imaging techniques are unable to properly capture coronal and sagittal balance, regional spinal deformities, and overall patient "posture"—especially standing. This radiographic evaluation includes process measures (radiographic measurements), which are determined from standing full length (36") anteroposterior (AP) or posteroanterior (PA), and from lateral radiographs (Figure 52.1A and B), also known as "scoliosis" radiographs. In addition to these films, supine side-bending radiographs are frequently included to evaluate regional coronal curves for structural characteristics, instability, and balance, especially when operative intervention is contemplated (Figure 52.1C and D). These give a radiographic view of the clinical picture (Figure 52.1E and H). A 36"–supine lateral or hyperextension lateral radiograph over a bolster may also be indicated and is particularly helpful in evaluating the patient with kyphosis. On occasion, a spot lateral radiograph of the lumbosacral junction, or a Ferguson view of this region, is also necessary.

Reproducible, high-quality scoliosis radiographs are sometimes difficult to achieve, especially with variably skilled radiologic technicians and machines. The onset of digital radiographs has further brought this matter to the forefront, as most institutions are unable to capture single-shot long cassette digital films. More commonly, two 14" × 17" radiographs are obtained and then "stitched" together to reproduce a digital scoliosis radiograph. This can introduce human error in matching, as well as image distortion. Consequently, physicians should carefully monitor these techniques when evaluating scoliosis radiographs.

Obtaining Reproducible Radiographs

A high-quality diagnostic film necessarily includes the cervicothoracic junction proximally and the pelvis distally. This permits a complete spine evaluation, while also identifying pelvic parameters and spinal balance. It should be taken 72" from the patient, and it must include a compensating filter to assure that proper bony density is maintained to view various aspects of the spine. However, numerous generations and models of grid ratios, film and screen combinations, and X-ray machine generators,

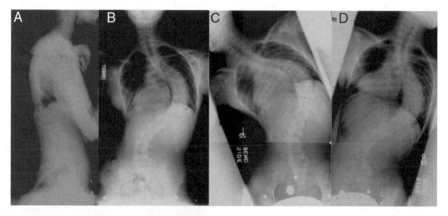

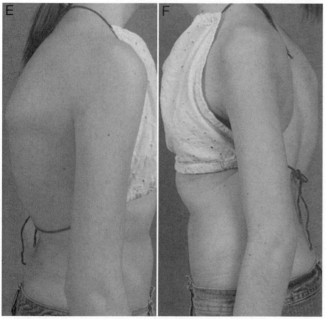

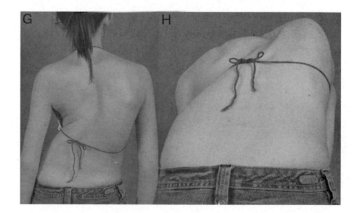

Figure 52.1 AP and lateral standing radiographs of a 13- and 7-year-old female with progressive adolescent idiopathic scoliosis (**A**, **B**), and side-bending supine radiographs (**C**, **D**), with corresponding clinical photographs (**E**, **F**, **G**, **H**).

as well as patient size and shape, preclude recommending standardized film exposure techniques or settings.

As noted earlier, the AP (or PA) and lateral films should be taken in the upright position with the knees extended and the feet shoulder width apart, looking straight ahead, with elbows bent and knuckles in the supraclavicular fossa bilaterally (32). This places the arms at about a 30- to 45-degree angle and helps to keep the humeri forward, thus facilitating visualization of the upper thoracic region on lateral radiographs. Additionally, this does not unnaturally lean the patient backwards. If a limb length discrepancy of over 2 cm is present, then a heel lift or block should be placed under the short extremity to level the pelvis for the AP view (53). Supine side-bending (left and right) radiographs are also obtained when coronal deformity is present and are used to evaluate the flexibility of the various curves. These are generally used only for preoperative planning and are not routinely obtained. For adult scoliosis, this technique may assist in evaluating the ability to posturally correct a degenerative lumbar scoliosis. For younger patients, proximal and distal fusion levels are identified or confirmed from these views.

Classification/Analysis

A well-established or reliable classification of adult scoliosis is not currently available. Nonetheless, various authors have proposed classification schemes (58–59). To date, it is the author's preference to use the Lenke classification as established for adolescent idiopathic scoliosis as a *starting point* in the evaluation of adult scoliosis (46). This provides a comprehensive, systematic evaluation of regional curves. Nonetheless, this should not be misconstrued as definitive for adult deformity.

Using the Lenke classification for adolescent idiopathic scoliosis (AIS), a structural curve is defined by a Cobb angle of greater than or equal to 25 degrees on side-bending radiographs (46). Just as importantly, the overall flexibility is important to note, as this will give an indication of the expected curve correction without utilizing advanced surgical techniques such as osteotomies. In addition to the structural characteristics of the various curves, the radiographs should be evaluated for overall coronal and sagittal balance, with particular attention to the center sacral vertical line (CSVL) and C7 plumbline (C7PL), shoulder height, apical vertebral translation of the thoracic and lumbar curves, curve flexibility, and relative curve magnitudes (52). Unlike AIS, evaluation of the adult deformity patient should also include a critical analysis of degenerative changes and rotatory and/or lateral listhesis, which inherently makes selection of fusion levels more difficult. In addition, clinical assessments of sagittal and coronal balance, curve flexibility, and location of pain (if present) are important and should be analyzed with consideration of degenerative levels (23). In the adult population, foraminal and central stenosis are quite common and are important considerations in the surgical plan. MRI and/or CT myelography are used to evaluate these conditions. When choosing fusion levels, one should avoid ending a fusion adjacent to a severely degenerated disc, especially if there is a fixed tilt or subluxation present on the standing radiographs (48).

Shoulder balance is best determined with close clinical observation; however, the clavicle angle is a useful adjunct that has been shown to correlate with clinical and radiographic evaluations (42). This is particularly useful, as the traditional teaching of evaluating the T1 tilt for proximal thoracic curve characteristics and shoulder balance has not been shown to be reliable (47).

Analysis of the end, neutral, and stable vertebrae is also of critical importance when selecting distal fusion levels in adolescent idiopathic scoliosis (Figure 52.2A and B). This has clinical significance for adult deformity as well. For instance, the stable vertebra should ideally be selected as the lowest instrumented vertebra for most adult deformity, as compensation of the spine post-instrumentation is minimal. This is frequently L5, but it can be L4 as well. A more common scenario in the aging population, however, remains choosing between L5 and S1/ilium. When not accomplished, "adding on" or "falling off" is frequently encountered, and a revision procedure is generally required. The reliability of selecting these levels is variable, with intraobserver reliability determined to be good to excellent for end vertebra (EV) selection, good for neutral vertebra (NV) selection, and good to excellent for stable vertebra (SV) selection (57). Additionally, a trend toward greater intraobserver reliability was noted with increasing levels of observer experience. Interobserver reliability, however, was poor, with complete interobserver agreement between three observers being only 48.7% for EV selection, 41.7% for NV selection, and 51.0% for SV selection (57).

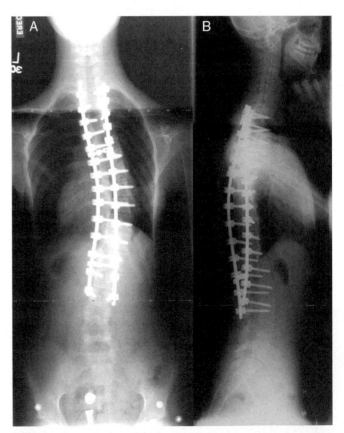

Figure 52.2 Postoperative AP (**A**) and lateral (**B**) radiographs of the 13- and 7-year-old patient in Figure 52.1 after posterior spinal fusion from T2–L3. Note distal fusion level within stable zone with good shoulder balance.

Clinical Decision Making

Proper management of the patient with spinal deformity requires a thorough understanding of coronal and sagittal balance and curve evaluation. The decision of when to operate, however, is more complex. As previously noted, comprehensive physical and medical assessment of the patient is imperative, as is an understanding of patient complaints and expectations. Adult patients with spine deformity generally present with back and/or leg pain, curve progression, and general deconditioning. Cosmesis can also be a presenting concern in some adults. Pain and other dysfunctions are more commonly seen in lumbar or thoracolumbar-lumbar curves than in thoracic curves (23). Curve progression can be severe enough to result in settling of the rib cage within the pelvis, resulting in persistent pain and associated gastrointestinal complaints (Figure 52.3A and B). In most instances, pain is thought to result from a combination of disc degeneration, facet arthrosis, osteopenia, and muscle spasm. Slow curve progression is thought to be fairly common, with severe vertebral tilt and rotatory subluxation being risk factors for rapid progression (commonly seen in elderly women). Clinically, the overall sagittal and coronal balance with the patient standing should be noted, with particular attention to knee and hip flexion and to possible contractures. Due to the three-dimensional nature of scoliosis and associated disc degeneration in adults, lumbar scoliosis frequently results in a significant loss of lumbar lordosis or actual kyphosis, thus driving the patient to a positive sagittal balance position. Loss of lumbar lordosis and increased obliquity of the lumbar end plates are associated with increased pain in adults (59). A supine physical evaluation is also helpful to determine curve flexibility.

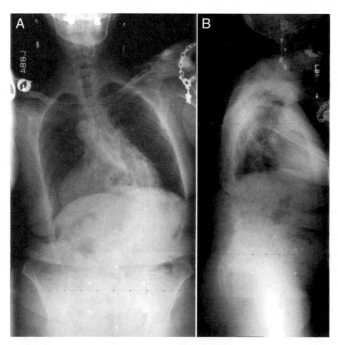

Figure 52.3 AP (**A**) and lateral (**B**) standing radiographs of a 63-year-old female with progressive lumbar scoliosis and coronal imbalance. Note ribs in pelvis on left.

Lumbar Curves

One of the most common presentations in the adult is lumbar scoliosis. However, it is frequently difficult to determine if a particular patient has adult progression of adolescent idiopathic scoliosis or *de novo* degenerative scoliosis. For AIS, typical indications for operative intervention include a Cobb angle of greater than or equal to 40 degrees, usually with significant coronal imbalance and/or trunk shift. Neurologic symptoms, as well as significant pain, are usually not present as they are in the adult. With this scenario and a flexible compensatory curve, an anterior operative approach is often preferred for the adolescent, and fusion levels generally include the Cobb angle, with the lowest instrumented vertebra (LIV) coinciding with the end vertebra (EV). This is not the case with adult lumbar scoliosis.

Typically, the adult patient presents with lumbar back pain, with or without leg pain, and L3–L4 rotatory subluxation, L4–L5 tilt, and L5–S1 disc degeneration on radiographic evaluation. An appreciation of the anatomic changes, especially associated with the lateral/rotatory spondylolisthesis, is helpful (63). Plain radiographs should again be analyzed with particular attention to sagittal balance and loss of lumbar lordosis or possible lumbar kyphosis. In addition, MRI of the lumbar spine is helpful to evaluate for central and/or foraminal stenosis and disc degeneration. Grading schemes have been developed to grade disc degeneration and to correlate operative strategies with postoperative outcomes, yet this has limited application.

Generally, operative levels include fusion of the Cobb angle, extending to L5. The biggest operative decision for the surgeon is to determine the proximal and distal extent of the instrumentation and fusion. Interestingly, Edwards et al. had difficulty recommending fusion to L5 or S1 in a 3–5 year follow-up of a matched cohort of patients following a long fusion, as they reviewed the pros and cons of the differing distal fusion levels (17). Specifically, fusions to the sacral required more additional surgery and had a higher complication rate compared to fusions to L5; however, adjacent segment degenerative changes were frequently noted, in addition to a positive sagittal shift. In one series, this developed in 61% of patients with a long fusion to L5 (18) and was also associated with a forward shift in sagittal balance. As recommended by Bridwell, absolute indications for fusion to the sacrum in adults include (1) L5–S1 spondylolisthesis, (2) previous L5–S1 laminectomy, (3) central or foraminal stenosis at L5–S1, (4) oblique takeoff of L5, and (5) "severe" degenerative changes (5) (Table 52.1). Of note, however, is that if there is significant degeneration of L5–S1 with disc calcification, then this level is likely inherently stable and may not need to be fused. Furthermore, if extension to S1 is undertaken, then iliac fixation should strongly be considered with long fusions (greater than

Table 52.1 Indications for Fusion to the Sacrum in Adults

1. L5–S1 spondylolisthesis
2. Previous L5–S1 laminectomy
3. Central or foraminal stenosis at L5–S1
4. Oblique takeoff of L5
5. Severe degenerative changes

three levels), in addition to an L5–S1 and possibly an L4–L5 interbody fusion (40). Interbody support at L5–S1 should also be considered, as this increases biomechanical stability, restores junctional lordosis, improves the lumbosacral fusion rate, and increases disc and foraminal height, thus reducing foraminal stenosis (8, 55).

The proximal extent of the fusion is often difficult to determine. The proximal instrumented level should at least end at a stable vertebra; this is usually a neutral and nearly horizontal vertebra. If the shoulders are leveled and the main thoracic curve is minimal and well balanced, then the stable end vertebra is an appropriate level to end the fusion. Many degenerative lumbar curves, however, include a Cobb angle from L1–L5, with both the L1 and L5 vertebral bodies being nearly bisected by the CSVL (Figure 52.4). In such instances, one should strongly consider crossing the thoracolumbar junction. As a general rule, it is best to cross the thoracolumbar junction transitional zone to reduce adjacent segment stresses and junctional kyphosis above the instrumented fusion. However, even with this approach, proximal construct pullout or junctional kyphosis can still occur, ultimately requiring extension of the fusion proximally (Figures 52.5A and B). Postoperative physical therapy training with particular attention to body mechanics, posture, and conditioning, and possibly with a thoracolumbar spinal orthosis to assist in reducing proximal junctional issues, is indicated.

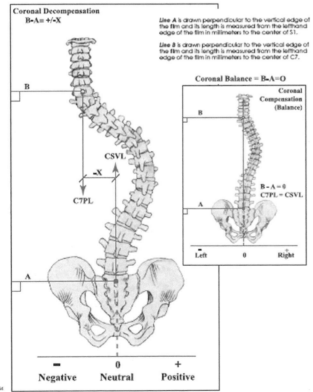

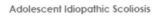

Figure 52.4   Schematic of coronal balance with depiction of the center sacral vertical line (CSVL).

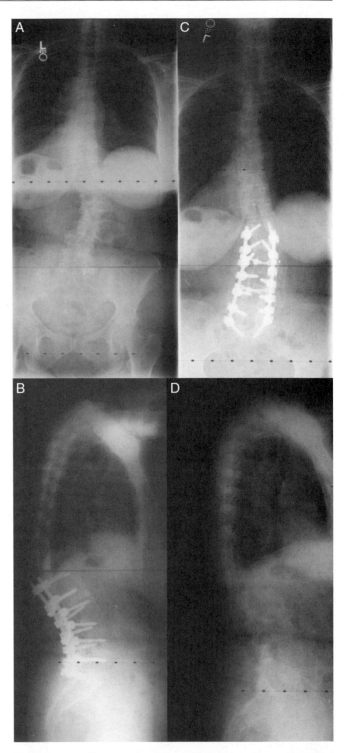

Figure 52.5   Preoperative AP and lateral standing radiographs of a 66-year-old female (**A**, **B**) and after 1 year follow-up for posterior spinal fusion with instrumentation from T12–S1 with decompression for severe stenosis with degenerative scoliosis (**C**, **D**). Note the proximal junctional kyphosis above T12.

Restoration of sagittal balance has been reported as the primary parameter associated with outcome (24); overall sagittal balance should, therefore, be closely evaluated as previously noted. In a retrospective series, Glassman et al. found positive sagittal balance to be the most reliable predictor of clinical symptoms. Because degenerative lumbar curves often present with loss of lordosis, this should be specifically addressed by the surgical plan. Possible surgical approaches include (1) anterior-posterior spinal fusion with multilevel discectomy and interbody spacers, (2) posterior spinal fusion with single- or multilevel posterior lumbar interbody fusion (PLIF) or transforaminal lumbar interbody fusion (TLIF), (3) posterior spinal fusion with wide facetectomies and/or Smith-Petersen osteotomies, and (4) pedicle subtraction osteotomy. Because of frequent association with foraminal stenosis, a TLIF with nerve root decompression, restoration of foraminal height and junctional lordosis, and multiple wide facetectomies can be considered as a suitable option. The inferior aspect of the superior articulating degenerative facet should be the resected portion, as this often limits restoration of lordosis at that level. Whatever the technique, the instrumented proximal level should be bisected by the center sacral line (CSL) on a lateral radiograph and should not be stopped adjacent to the thoracolumbar or thoracic apex.

Double Major Curves

Similar to the presentation of the adolescent, radiographic assessment is critical in the evaluation of the adult with a double major curve. The side-bending views should be evaluated to determine the flexibility of the main thoracic and thoracolumbar-lumbar curves to distinguish between a false double major curve and a true double major curve (5). Major points to consider are (1) the relative apical deviation, (2) the relative rotational comparison, (3) the relative Cobb angles, (4) the clinical status of the patient, and (5) the lifestyle of the patient (5). *If the main thoracic Cobb angle is substantially larger than the lumbar Cobb angle, then the apical vertebral translation is greater, and the rotation of the lumbar spine is minimal. This implies the presence of a false double major curve, in which case a selective thoracic fusion is possible in the adult, as in the adolescent.* This is generally seen in the younger adult patient who presents with progression of adolescent idiopathic scoliosis.

For true double major curves in AIS, the extent of the distal fusion level is frequently L3 or L4, depending on the stable and neutral vertebra and on the amount of tilt at the lowest instrumented vertebra (LIV). However, this is rarely the case in the presentation of double major curves in the adult, as there is frequently associated L4–L5 and/or L5–S1 degeneration. The side-bending radiographs will assist in distinguishing this by identifying the L4–L5 tilt on standing radiographs and curve flexibility on side-bending radiographs. If there is a fixed tilt or subluxation at L4–L5, then L5 should be included in the distal fusion. Otherwise, it is safe to end the fusion at L4. Once again, the major operative decision is whether to stop the fusion at L5 or extend to the sacrum or pelvis, which is associated with an increased incidence of pseudarthrosis and reoperation. If a central or foraminal decompression at L5–S1 is needed, however, then it is mandatory to extend the fusion to the sacrum (4). Additionally, an oblique take-off of L5–S1 should also be extended to the sacrum. A frequent area of debate is the case of a "deep-seated" L5. Various authorities have advocated that, if the L5 pedicles are located below the intercrestal line on a standing radiograph and the transverse processes are fairly large, then the L5–S1 disc is relatively protected from advanced degeneration, and therefore may not need to be included in the fusion. This, however, has not proven to be the case, as this scenario does not appear to afford any protection of

the disc (16, 18). Furthermore, degenerative spondylolisthesis may develop at L5–S1 after stopping at L5 with a long fusion. Therefore, the most common scenario is to extend the fusion to the sacrum and/or the ilium. As with lumbar scoliosis, extension to the ilium is helpful to "protect" the L5 and S1 screws. With time, there appears to be a small halo that appears around the iliac screws as they cross the sacro-iliac joint but do not fuse the joint (40). This is expected and does not appear to lead to problems in the adult, as evidenced by the low incidence of adult patients requiring later removal of the iliac screw. Nonetheless, extension to the ilium does appear to slightly alter the patient's gait. Further research and large multicenter studies are needed to better define the indications for extending the distal fusion to the sacrum and/or ilium, as opposed to stopping at L5.

Ideally, the fusion should include the main thoracic curve and end at a "stable" vertebra proximally. Because adult curves are less flexible than those of adolescents, spontaneous correction of the proximal thoracic curve and shoulder balance should not be expected as in the adolescent (41, 42). More importantly, the proximal extension of the fusion should not stop distal to a structural proximal thoracic curve, and the addition of a crosslink to the construct should also be considered primarily to improve overall construct torsional stiffness (10, 51). This should not be placed at the thoracolumbar junction, which is the main location for pseudarthrosis in adult scoliosis (35).

Complications from adult scoliosis surgery include pseudarthrosis, implant failure such as crosslink breakage, hook or screw pullout, and rod breakage (16, 35). Other surgical complications include wound infection, neurologic deficit, and chronic pain. Medical complications (in the early immediate postoperative period) are especially common in the older adult and include urinary tract infections, pulmonary complications, deep venous thrombosis and pulmonary emboli, and various gastrointestinal problems. Nonetheless, fusion has been shown to provide good to excellent pain relief in 69%–87% of adult scoliosis patients (38, 62). In a comparative study of a group of adult scoliosis patients, a significant decrease in pain and fatigue was also found in surgically treated versus untreated adult scoliosis patients (12).

In general, the surgical management of adult scoliosis is more difficult than AIS due to the associated degenerative changes, back and leg pain, relative inflexibility, and medical comorbidities. This is further complicated by the lack of a comprehensive classification scheme with surgical guidelines. Regardless, there are several biomechanical and surgical principles that should be strictly followed in order to maximize surgical and clinical outcomes following operative intervention. Strict attention to the resultant coronal and especially the sagittal balance are imperative and much more important than saving fusion levels in the adult patient. A comprehensive preoperative assessment of medical and social problems and a close cooperation with the anesthesia team are essential to achieve maximal patient satisfaction and good clinical outcomes.

SURGICAL MANAGEMENT
Approaches and Avoiding Complications

The goal of corrective surgery is to restore spinal alignment to normal or neutral alignment. After evaluation of the location and "flexibility" of the spine, preoperative planning includes selection of operative approach, an estimate of the projected correction from intraoperative positioning, selection of operative levels, and projected bone cuts or osteotomies. The preferred operative approach is primarily posterior, although an anterior or a combined approach is sometimes utilized. Additionally, the use of pedicle screw instrumentation has permitted greater curve correction, maintenance of corrections, and improved biomechanics.

Posterior Approach and Osteotomies

As mentioned above, the posterior approach is the preferred surgical approach in the management of scoliosis. It allows most deformities to be corrected with posterior-based osteotomies, is even suited for rigid kyphosis, and is generally performed at the site of maximal deformity. For patients with preexisting rigid kyphosis of the thoracolumbar spine or those with decompensation of adjacent cephalad segments, osteotomies may be required at cephalad levels. If the deformity is flexible, then correction is generally at or caudal to the apex.

Because extensive forces are applied to the tension side of the spine with these procedures, segmental instrumentation is mandatory. This will maximize construct stability, assist with bilateral compression, and aid bone healing across the osteotomy site(s). At a minimum, a two-level bilateral segmental fixation (four pedicle screws) is necessary cephalad and caudad to a pedicle subtraction osteotomy, and preferably, three levels (six pedicle screws) should be used. Pedicle screws are best, as they provide a rigid, three-column fixation and may also minimize loss of correction. Claw constructs, however, are acceptable, as they provide excellent compression.

Extension Osteotomy (Smith-Petersen)

Smith-Petersen was the first to describe and perform a posterior spinal osteotomy (60). With resection of the posterior elements (facets and undercutting of the spinous process) at the level of correction, sagittal correction is achieved with posterior compression; particular attention should be paid to removing the caudal aspect of the inferior articulating facet. The pivot point is the posterior aspect of the vertebral body, with concomitant distraction at the anterior disc space. By lengthening the anterior column, there is potential destabilization of the spine. Consequently, some authors have recommended anterior release or discectomy, anterior bone grafting, or anterior osteotomy to achieve better correction and anterior stability (7, 19, 20, 30, 39, 43). Distraction of the great vessels anterior to the spine, including superior mesenteric artery syndrome, has also been described following the procedure.

Expected sagittal correction is approximately 1 degree for each millimeter of bone resection, or approximately 5–10 degrees per level. On average, this is about 5 degrees in the thoracic spine and as much as 5–10 degrees per level in the lumbar spine when only a posterior approach is performed. Correction from a Smith-Petersen osteotomy can be quite significant; Chang et al. reported a 37.8-degree average correction in seventeen patients with posttraumatic thoracolumbar kyphosis treated with anterior discectomy and posterior osteotomy (7). Of note, however, in that group, was that multiple osteotomies were performed in twelve of the seventeen patients, and these were significantly enhanced

with the anterior discectomies (7). Similar results have been reported by other authors (6, 60).

Smith-Petersen osteotomies can also be performed asymmetrically. With this approach, coronal correction can be achieved when present. With modern day instrumentation and the use of segmental pedicle screw fixation, significant sagittal correction can be achieved and maintained. A key to correction is repeated compression maneuvers (cantilever bending) directed caudally to the fixed lowest instrumented vertebra in long fusions, or centripetally to the apex of the kyphosis in short constructs.

Pedicle Subtraction Osteotomy

The pedicle subtraction osteotomy (PSO) is a three-column closing wedge osteotomy hinging on the anterior cortex, thus shortening the anterior and middle columns. This is in contrast to the Smith-Petersen osteotomy, which lengthens the anterior column by pivoting on the middle column. Consequently, it is most frequently performed in the lumbar spine, particularly at L2 and L3, but it can be performed at any level. Various modifications of the pedicle subtraction osteotomy have been described, with the primary procedure being a transcortical pedicle decancellation. Expected correction from the posterior only PSO approach is approximately 30–40 degrees per level (6).

It is generally recommended that three levels of bilateral pedicle screws be placed cephalad and caudad to the apex of the deformity. The posterior area of resection is then precisely marked, and all of the posterior elements are resected, including the superior and inferior articulating facets as well as the pedicles. A posterior wedge (apex anterior) is then removed from the vertebral body, including the entire posterior and lateral walls of the body, in order to permit compression across the resected area. Compression is then applied to close the osteotomy. Close observation and palpation can ensure that the exiting nerve roots are not compressed during the procedure. Like the Smith-Petersen osteotomy, asymmetric resection can also help correct coronal deformity.

A PSO is a technically demanding procedure which can result in significant blood loss from the extensive epidural venous plexus, as well as the vascular cancellous bone. This can be minimized with meticulous attention during dissection, with the help of an experienced operative assistant, and with the liberal use of powdered thrombin. Neurologic complication rates vary but are generally considered to be approximately 5% (56). Contraindications to PSO include anterior instrumentation or pseudarthrosis.

Because significant stress is placed on the instrumentation with this procedure, it is best to use larger rod systems, as smaller rods have a tendency to fail with time. Stainless steel instrumentation is sometimes recommended over titanium due to improved rod fatigue strength.

Anterior Approach

The anterior approach can be utilized as a primary procedure or as an adjuvant to a posterior approach. When used as an adjuvant procedure, then resection of the anterior longitudinal ligament, as well as a single or multiple discectomies with or without anterior interbody bone grafting, can be performed. Some authorities prefer the anterior approach, as this permits superior neurologic decompression, potentially greater sagittal alignment, and improved fusion rates.

Management of Intraoperative Neurologic Deficit

Given the potential for severe and long-lasting neurologic injury, avoiding complications from spine surgery is paramount. This begins with meticulous preoperative planning and concludes with appropriate postoperative follow-up. Nonetheless, neurologic deficits will occasionally occur.

The treatment algorithm and rationale to address abnormal neuromonitoring changes have been adapted from research into the pathophysiology and management of acute spinal cord trauma. Other than relieving any elements of the potentially ongoing primary injury within the surgeon's control (e.g., removing misdirected implants, relieving deformity correction, etc.), little can be done about mechanical trauma after it has occurred; our focus will therefore be on methods of reducing secondary injury.

Maintaining spinal cord perfusion and cellular oxygenation is paramount following neurologic injury. Animal studies, as well as clinical series, have shown that removing compression from the anterior spinal circulation as soon as possible helps to improve neurologic recovery. Because only 5%–10% of the nerve fibers in a spinal long tract need to be preserved in order to maintain useful function, literally every neuron counts (50). At the first sign of altered neuromonitoring signals, the anesthesia team should be instructed to increase the patient's mean arterial pressure (MAP) to 85–90 mmHg. This value has been supported by animal studies, as well as retrospective clinical reports (15, 47, 50, 66). Furthermore, the MAP should remain elevated for 5–7 days in cases of acute SCI; this therefore requires recovery in an ICU or step-down unit. Strict MAP control in a monitored unit has been demonstrated to improve neurologic recovery and decrease mortality (1, 54). In addition to increasing blood pressure, the patient should immediately receive supplemental oxygen sufficient to maintain 100% saturations. Although overoxygenation can theoretically lead to increased formation of oxygen free radicals, reasonable increases in FiO2 sufficient to maximize hemoglobin saturation are recommended (26).

Concomitantly, the entire operative team should explore potential causes of false-positive neuromonitoring signals. All monitoring leads should be checked, the neuromonitoring technician or physician should perform a complete systems check and obtain a second set of data for confirmation, and the patient's body temperature should be evaluated and elevated if necessary. Animal studies have shown that even moderate hypothermia (4°C below normal body temperature) can cause a drop in somatosensory evoked potentials (SSEP) amplitude and an increase in latency that may mimic SCI (33). If true neurologic injury is confirmed, the therapeutic response to hypothermia is a matter of controversy. Some authors advocate warming the patient to normal body temperature, whereas others note that hypothermia is neuroprotective in both drowning and certain high-risk neurosurgical procedures (26, 33, 50). The most common culprit in false-positive neuromonitoring is changes in anesthetic medications. Inhaled anesthetics have significant effects on SSEPs and, to a lesser extent, motor evoked potentials (MEPs). Although the effect is dose dependant, usual doses used for all halogenated anesthetics and nitrous oxide can have significant

effect on SSEPs (34). The effect of inhaled anesthetics is diminished if spinal cord electrodes, rather than peripheral (i.e., scalp) electrodes, are used to record potentials (34). Because there are no population-based norms in neuromonitoring, changes from baseline are the standard means of predicting neural tissue injury. Therefore, the baseline data acquisition referenced during the surgical portion of the case should be obtained after the patient is adequately anesthetized and positioned. The anesthesiologist should then attempt to maintain the inhaled anesthetic concentration at a steady state throughout the case.

The subsequent steps in the rapid response to acute neuromonitoring changes or obvious intraoperative traumatic neural tissue injury involve a series of checks, re-checks, and incremental progression of the surgery, as outlined in Table 52.2. If neuromonitoring signals respond to the aforementioned interventions, the case can then proceed as before with only strict maintenance of MAPs greater than 85 mmHg and 100% oxygen saturation. If signals continue to be significantly abnormal, then alternate interventions can be attempted, including testing the true neurologic status of the patient with a wake-up test (67). Although neuromonitoring is highly accurate, the Stagnara wake-up test is still considered the gold standard for perioperative assessment of neurologic function. The literature contains several examples of false-negative neuromonitoring in which no signal changes were noted, yet the patient awoke from anesthesia with a new neurologic deficit.

Although pharmacotherapeutics other than steroids have not gained widespread clinical acceptance to date, they have been the focus of a great deal of research in recent years. Steroids are thought to reduce secondary neurologic injury by reducing edema, stabilizing cell membranes, scavenging free radicals, and decreasing lipid peroxidation. Due largely to the results of the National Acute Spinal Cord Injury Study (NASCIS), steroids, specifically methylprednisolone, have been recommended in patients suffering acute SCI. Acceptance of the NASCIS results was originally robust (unquestioned). More recently, however, the methods and data analysis used in this study have come under (extensive) scrutiny, although some authorities still use the NASCIS III steroid protocol in response to acute intraoperative SCI.

Four emerging agents with limited clinical acceptance, but optimistic animal and early human results, are gangliosides (GM-1), tirilazad (21-aminosteroids), local anesthetics/sodium channel-blockers (lidocaine), and opioid receptor antagonists (naloxone). Gangliosides are complex acidic glycolipids that form a major component of neuronal cell membranes. Parenterally administered, gangliosides stimulate neurite growth and regeneration (22, 50). Monosiaotetrahexosylganglioside (GM-1) is the only ganglioside that has been clinically tested. A randomized, placebo-controlled trial in 1991 demonstrated significant improvement in neurologic recovery when GM-1 (100 mg/day) was started within 72 hours of SCI (22). Tirilazad targets the glucocorticoid receptor that mediates inhibition of lipid peroxidation, sharing the neuroprotective effect of steroids, without the associated side effects. Tirilazad mesylate demonstrated efficacy in cats and was included in the NASCIS III trial; it was found to be no more effective than methylprednisolone (3, 13). Lidocaine possesses two beneficial traits in regard to SCI. First, it is a potent local vasodilator. Second, sodium channel blockade appears to be protective to injured neural tissue (13).

Table 52.2   Intraoperative Interventions for Acute Neuromonitoring Changes

1. Alert entire OR team.
2. Raise MAP to 85–90 mmHg.
   a. Start with fluids—aim for mild hypervolemia.
      i. Don't overload—SCI patients are susceptible to pulmonary edema.
   b. Pressor support—phenylephrine; atropine may be used to increase heart rate to counter unopposed vagal tone.
3. Oxygenate patient to maintain 100% saturation.
4. Check for reasons for false data:
   a. Are neuromonitoring leads intact? (Run a systems check.)
   b. Has an anesthetic agent been changed?
   c. Is the patient hypothermic? (lowers amplitudes and increases latencies) (SSEP > MEP)
5. Reevaluate—obtain a new set of data, and initiate Stagnara wake-up test if neuromonitoring changes do not reverse.
6. Incrementally reverse surgical steps—use intraoperative fluoroscopy or radiography to evaluate instrumentation positioning.
   a. Release correction?
   b. Remove instrumentation?
      i. May be role for screw stimulation to limit amount of instrumentation removed.
7. Reevaluate—obtain a new set of data.
8. If no response—consider NASCIS III methylprednisolone protocol for SCI if abnormal Stagnara wake-up test.
   a. 30 mg/kg bolus; 5.4 mg/kg continuous × 23 hr
   b. Additional pharmacological agents to consider:
      i. GM-1 Ganglioside
      ii. Tirilazad
      iii. Naloxone
      iv. Lidocaine—intravenous or topical to the cord
9. If signals normalize with these interventions—incrementally continue the case:
   a. Re-direct errant instrumentation or omit if the screw is not biomechanically essential.
   b. Correct deformity slowly and possibly accept less correction if signals start to diminish.
10. Consider monitored ICU recovery.

Klemme et al. reported the use of systemically administered lidocaine to partially reverse SCI that occurred during scoliosis surgery (37). In contrast to the other agents, naloxone has demonstrated limited to no beneficial effects on neurologic recovery. However, other more specific opioid-receptor antagonists (Kappa-receptor) may prove to be more efficacious (2, 14). Other than our case report on lidocaine, we have no experience with these agents but continue to be optimistic that, someday, more effective pharmacotherapy will be available to reduce the effects of secondary neurologic injury.

MANAGEMENT OF SPINAL DEFORMITY IN SPINAL CORD–INJURED PATIENTS

Considerations for Surgical and Nonsurgical Management

Following spinal cord injury, various secondary musculoskeletal complications can occur. Specific to the spine, these primarily include progressive deformity and/or scoliosis, osteoporotic fractures, and Charcot changes. Typically, acute spinal cord injury occurs following some type of trauma, and frequently, acute surgical management of any instability is required. Subsequently, adjacent segment problems may arise that must be addressed. Although this more frequently occurs at anatomic transition zones, such as the cervico-thoracic or thoracic-lumbar junction, it can occur anywhere. The result may be further bony and ligamentous destruction and progressive instability known as neuropathic spinal arthropathy or Charcot spine (25, 65, 69)

(Figure 56.6A and B). This often presents as increasing pain, loss of sitting balance, and/or skin problems.

Scoliosis is another frequently recognized spinal deformity, which has been reported to occur in 67% to approximately 100% of pediatric SCI patients (9). Secondary curves, such as

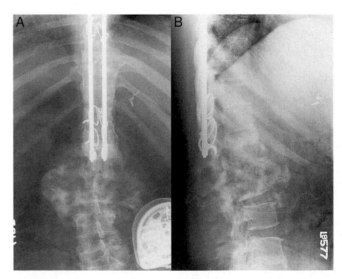

Figure 52.6   AP (**A**) and lateral (**B**) radiographs of a 53-year-old male 15 years after posterior spinal fusion with instrumentation for a fracture dislocation of T10 with resultant paraplegia. Note the Charcot spine inferior to the instrumentation.

hyperlordosis or hyperkyphosis, can also occur. When required, the typical surgical management is a posterior spinal fusion with instrumentation to maintain an upright posture, sitting balance, and pulmonary function. Even after surgery, patient transfers and improper sitting balance can continue to stress the instrumentation. Without a solid fusion, eventual implant failure will occur, thus requiring revision spinal surgery. Every attempt, therefore, should be made by the surgeon to select a strong instrumentation system while ensuring meticulous bone grafting.

Posterior instrumentation of scoliosis involves a long fusion, most often to the sacrum and/or ilium, with the goal of achieving good sitting balance. Due to the high biomechanical forces at the lumbo-sacral junction, every effort should be made to obtain a solid fusion at this level, including consideration of interbody support at L5–S1. Otherwise, all other surgical principles and considerations apply in obtaining a balanced spine centered over the pelvis.

References

1. Anonymous. Management of acute spinal cord injuries in an intensive care unit or other monitored setting. *Neurosurgery* 2002; 50(3 Suppl): S51–7.
2. Bracken MB, et al. A randomized, controlled trial of methylprednisolone or naloxone in the treatment of acute spinal-cord injury. Results of the Second National Acute Spinal Cord Injury Study. *N Engl J Med* 1990; 322(20):1405–1411.
3. Bracken MB et al. Administration of methylprednisolone for 24 or 48 hours or tirilazad mesylate for 48 hours in the treatment of acute spinal cord injury. Results of the Third National Acute Spinal Cord Injury Randomized Controlled Trial. National Acute Spinal Cord Injury Study. *JAMA* 1997; 277(20):1597–1604.
4. Bridwell K, Edwards CC II, Lenke LG. The pros and cons to saving the L5–S1 motion segment in a long scoliosis fusion construct. *Spine* 2003; 28(Suppl 20):S232–S242.
5. Bridwell KH. Selection of instrumentation and fusion levels for scoliosis: where to start and where to stop. Invited submission from the Joint Section Meeting on Disorders of the Spine and Peripheral Nerves, March 2004. *J Neurosurg Spine* 2004; 1(1):1–8.
6. Bridwell KH, Lenke LG, Lewis SJ. Treatment of spinal stenosis and fixed sagittal imbalance. *Clin Orthop Relat Res* 2001; (384):35–44.
7. Chang KW. Oligosegmental correction of post-traumatic thoracolumbar angular kyphosis. *Spine* 1993; 18(13):1909–1915.
8. Cunningham BW, Lewis SJ, Long J, et al. Biomechanical evaluation of lumbosacral reconstruction techniques for spondylolisthesis: an in vitro porcine model. *Spine* 2002; 27(21):2321–2327.
9. Dearwolf WW III, Betz RR, Vogel LC, et al. Scoliosis in pediatric spinal cord–injured patients. *J Pediatr Orthop* 1990; 10:214–218.
10. Dick JC, Zdeblick TA, Bartel B, et al. Mechanical evaluation of cross-link designs in rigid pedicle screw systems. *Spine* 1997; 22(4):370–375.
11. Dickson JH. An eleven-year clinical investigation of Harrington instrumentation: a preliminary report on 578 cases. *Clin Orthop Relat Res* 1973; 93:113–130.
12. Dickson JH, Mirkovic S, Noble PC, et al. Results of operative treatment of idiopathic scoliosis in adults. *J Bone Joint Surg Am* 1995; 77: 513–523.
13. Dumont RJ, Okonkwo DO, Verma S, Hurlbert RJ, et al. Acute spinal cord injury. Part I: contemporary pharmacotherapy. *Clinical Neuropharmacology* 2001; 24(5):254–264.
14. Dumont RJ, Verma S, Okonkwo DO, Hurlbert RJ, et al. Acute spinal cord injury. Part II: contemporary pharmacotherapy. *Clinical Neuropharmacology* 2001; 24(5):265–279.
15. Dutton RP. Anesthetic management of spinal cord injury: clinical practice and future initiatives. *Int Anesthesiol Clin* 2002; 40:103–120.
16. Eck KR, Bridwell K, Patel A, et al. Complications and results of long adult deformity fusions down to L4, L5 and the sacrum. *Spine* 2001; 26(9): E182–92.
17. Edwards CC II, Bridwell KH, Patel A, et al. Long adult deformity fusions to L5 and the sacrum: a matched cohort analysis. *Spine* 2004; 29(18): 1996–2005.
18. Edwards CC III, Bridwell KH, Patel A, Rinella AS, et al. Thoracolumbar deformity arthrodesis to L5 in adults: the fate of the L5–S1 disc. *Spine* 2003; 28(18):2122–2131.
19. Farcy JP, Schwab F. Posterior osteotomies with pedicle subtraction for flat back and associated syndromes: technique and results of a prospective study. *Bull Hosp Jt Dis* 2000; 59(1):11–16.
20. Farcy JP, Schwab FJ. Management of flatback and related kyphotic decompensation syndromes. *Spine* 1997; 22(20):2452–2457.
21. Fitch RD, Turi M, Bowman BE, Hardaker WT. Comparison of Cotrel-Dubousset and Harrington rod instrumentations in idiopathic scoliosis. *J Pediatr Orthop* 1990; 10(1): 44–47.
22. Giesler FH, Dorsey FC, Coleman WP. Recovery of motor function after spinal cord injury—a randomized, placebo-controlled trial with GM-1 ganglioside. *N Engl J Med* 1991; 324(26):1829–1838.
23. Glassman SD, Berven S, Bridwell K, Horton W, Dimar JR. Correlation of radiographic parameters and clinical symptoms in adult scoliosis. *Spine* 2005; 30(6):682–688.
24. Glassman SD, Bridwell K, Dimar JR, Horton W, et al. The impact of positive sagittal balance in adult spinal deformity. *Spine* 2005; 30(18): 2024–2029.
25. Goldman AB, Freiberger RH. Localized infectious and neuropathic diseases. *Semin Roentgenol* 1979; 14:19.
26. Gunnarsson T, Fehlings MG: Acute neurosurgical management of traumatic brain and spinal cord injury. *Curr Opin Neurology* 2003; 16(6): 717–723.
27. Harrington P. Surgical instrumentation for management of scoliosis. *J Bone Joint Surg Am* 1960; 42:1448.
28. Harrington PR. Treatment of scoliosis: correction and internal fixation by spine instrumentation. *J Bone Joint Surg Am* 1962; 44A: 591–610.
29. Hasday CA, Passoff TL, Perry J. Gait abnormalities arising from iatrogenic loss of lumbar lordosis secondary to Harrington instrumentation in lumbar fractures. *Spine* 1983; 8(5):501–511.
30. Herbert J. Vertebral osteotomy. *J Bone Joint Surg Am* 1948; 30:680–689.
31. Horlyck E, Thomasen E. Operative treatment of scoliosis with Harrington instrumentation technique. *Acta Orthop Scand* 1978; 49:350–353.
32. Horton WC, Brown CW, Bridwell KH, Glassman SD, et al Is there an optimal patient stance for obtaining a lateral 36" radiograph? A critical comparison of three techniques. *Spine* 2005; 30(4):427–433.
33. Jou IM. Effects of core body temperature on changes in spinal somatosensory-evoked potential in acute spinal cord compression injury: an experimental study in the rat. *Spine* 2000; 25(15):1878–1885.
34. Jou IM, Chern TC, Chen TY, and Tsai YC. Effects of desflurane on spinal somatosensory-evoked potentials and conductive spinal cord evoked potential. *Spine* 2003; 28(16):1845–1850.
35. Kim YJ, Bridwell KH, Lenke LG, Rinella AS, Edwards C II. Pseudarthrosis in primary fusions for adult idiopathic scoliosis: incidence, risk factors, and outcome analysis. *Spine* 2005; 30(4):468–474.
36. Kim YJ, Lenke LG, Cho SK, Bridwell KH, et al. Comparative analysis of pedicle screw versus hook instrumentation in posterior spinal fusion of adolescent idiopathic scoliosis. *Spine* 2004; 29(18):2040–2048.
37. Klemme WR, Burkhalter W, Polly DW Jr, Dahl LF, Davis DA. Reversible ischemic myelopathy during scoliosis surgery: a possible role for intravenous lidocaine. *J Pediatr Orthop* 1999; 19(6):763–765.
38. Kostuik JP, Israel J, Hall JE. Scoliosis surgery in adults. *Clin Orthop Relat Res* 1973; 93:225–234.
39. Kostuik JP, Maurais GR, Richardson WJ, Okajima Y. Combined single stage anterior and posterior osteotomy for correction of iatrogenic lumbar kyphosis. *Spine* 1988; 13(3): 257–266.
40. Kuklo TR, Bridwell KH, Lewis SJ, Baldus C, et al. Minimum 2-year analysis of sacropelvic fixation and L5–S1 fusion using S1 and iliac screws. *Spine* 2001; 26(18):1976–1983.
41. Kuklo TR, Lenke LG, Won DS, Graham EJ, et al. Spontaneous proximal thoracic curve correction after isolated fusion of the main thoracic curve in adolescent idiopathic scoliosis. *Spine* 2001; 26(18): 1966–1975.
42. Kuklo TR, Lenke LG, Graham EJ, et al. Correlation of radiographic, clinical and patient assessment of shoulder balance following fusion versus non-fusion of the proximal thoracic curve in adolescent idiopathic scoliosis. *Spine SRS Issue* 2002; 27(18):2013–2020.

43. LaChapelle E. Osteotomy of the lumbar spine for correction of kyphosis in a case of ankylosing spondylarthritis. *J Bone Joint Surg Am* 1946; 28:851–858.

44. Lee CS, Lee CK, Kim YT, et al. Dynamic sagittal imbalance of the spine in degenerative flat back: significance of pelvic tilt in surgical treatment. *Spine* 2001; 26:2029–2035.

45. Lee CK, Denis F, Winter RB, Lonstein JE. Analysis of the upper thoracic curve in surgically treated idiopathic scoliosis: a new concept of the double thoracic curve pattern. *Spine* 1993; 18(12):1599–1608.

46. Lenke LG, Betz RR, Harms J, Bridwell KH, et al. Adolescent idiopathic scoliosis: a new classification to determine extent of spinal arthrodesis. *J Bone Joint Surg Am* 2001; 83A(8): 1169–1181.

47. Levi L, Wolf A, Belzberg H. Hemodynamic parameters in patients with acute cervical cord trauma: description, intervention, and prediction of outcome. *Neurosurgery* 1993; 33(6):1007–1017.

48. Liljenqvist U, Lepsien U, Hackenberg L, Niemeyer T, Halm H. Comparative analysis of pedicle screw and hook instrumentation in posterior correction and fusion of idiopathic thoracic scoliosis. *Eur Spine J* 2002; 11(4):336–343.

49. Lovallo JL, Banta JV, Renshaw TS. Adolescent idiopathic scoliosis treated by Harrington-rod distraction and fusion. *J Bone Joint Surg Am* 1986; 68(9):1326–1330.

50. Lu J, Aswell K, Waite P. Advances in secondary spinal cord injury: role of apoptosis. *Spine* 2000; 25(14):1859–1866.

51. Lynn G, Mukherjee DP, Kruse RN, et al. Mechanical stability of thoracolumbar pedicle screw fixation: the effect of crosslinks. *Spine* 1997; 22(14):1568–1572.

52. McMaster MJ. Luque rod instrumentation in the treatment of adolescent idiopathic scoliosis: a comparative study with Harrington instrumentation. *J Bone Joint Surg Br* 1991; 73(6):982–989.

53. O'Brien MF, Kuklo TR, Blanke KM, Lenke LG. *Spinal Deformity Radiographic Measurement Manual*, 2004.

54. Papadopoulos SM, Selden NR, Quint DJ, Patel N, et al. Immediate spinal cord decompression for cervical spinal cord injury: feasibility and outcome. *Journal of Trauma-Injury Infection and Critical Care* 2002; 52(2):323–332.

55. Polly DW Jr, Klemme WR, Cunningham BW, Burnette JB, et al. The biomechanical significance of anterior column support in a simulated single-level spinal fusion. *J Spinal Disord* 2002; 13(1):58–62.

56. Potter BK, Lenke LG, Kuklo TR. Prevention and management of iatrogenic flatback deformity. *J Bone Joint Surg Am* 2004; 86A(8): 1793–1808.

57. Potter BK, Rosner MK, Lehman RA Jr, Polly DW Jr, et al. Reliability of end, neutral, and stable vertebrae identification in adolescent idiopathic scoliosis. *Spine* 2005; 30(14):1658–1663.

58. Schwab F, El-Fegoun AB, Gamez L, Goodman H, Farcy JP. A lumbar classification of scoliosis in the adult patient: preliminary approach. *Spine* 2005; 30(14):1670–1673.

59. Schwab FJ, Smith VA, Biserni M, Gamez L, et al. Adult scoliosis: a quantitative radiographic and clinical analysis. *Spine* 2002; 27(4):387–392.

60. Smith-Petersen MN, Larson CB, Aufranc OE. Osteotomy of the spine for correction of flexion deformity in rheumatoid arthritis. *J Bone Joint Surg Am* 1945; 27:1–11.

61. Suk SI, Lee CK, Kim WJ, Chung YJ, Park YB. Segmental pedicle screw fixation in the treatment of thoracic idiopathic scoliosis. *Spine* 1995; 20(12):1399–1405.

62. Swank S, Lonstein JE, Moe JH, et al. Surgical treatment of adult scoliosis: a review of two hundred and twenty-two cases. *J Bone Joint Surg Am* 1981; 63(2):268–287.

63. Toyone T, Tanaka T, Kato D, Kaneyama R, Otsuka M. Anatomic changes in lateral spondylolisthesis associated with adult lumbar scoliosis. *Spine* 2005; 30(22):E671–E675.

64. Tveit P, Daggfeldt K, Hetland S, Thorstensson A. Erector spinae lever arm length variations with changes in spinal curvature. *Spine* 1994; 19(2): 199–204.

65. Urist MR. Bone morphogenetic protein: the molecularization of skeletal system development. *J Bone Miner Res* 1997; 12(3):343–346.

66. Vale FL, Burns J, Jackson AB, Hadley MN. Combined medical and surgical treatment after acute spinal cord injury: results of a prospective pilot study to assess the merits of aggressive medical resuscitation and blood pressure management. *J Neurosurg* 1997; 87(2): 239–246.

67. Vauzelle C, Stagnara P, Jouvinroux P. Functional monitoring of spinal cord activity during spinal surgery. *Clin Orthop Relat Res* 1973; 93: 173–178.

68. White AA III, Panjabi MM. Practical biomechanics of scoliosis and kyphosis. In: *Clinical Biomechanics of the Spine*. 2nd ed. Philadelphia: Lippincott Williams & Wilkins, 1990; 127–168.

69. Wirth CR, Jacobs RL, Rolander SD. Neuropathic spinal arthropathy: a review of the Charcot spine. *Spine* 1980; 5:558–567.

53 The Spondyloarthropathies

Mazen Elyan
Muhammad Asim Khan

The spondyloarthropathies (SpA) form an interrelated cluster of clinically overlapping chronic rheumatologic diseases that show a predilection for involvement of the sacroiliac joints, spine, entheses (bony insertion of ligaments and tendons), and peripheral joints, as well as other extraskeletal structures, especially the eye, skin, and gastrointestinal tract; these diseases also have a strong association with the HLA-B27 allele of the major histocompatibility complex (Figure 53.1) (1, 2, 3).

Ankylosing spondylitis (AS) is the archetype of this group, which also includes reactive arthritis (ReA), arthritis associated with psoriasis (psoriatic arthritis [PsA]), inflammatory bowel disease (enteropathic arthritis in association with Crohn's disease and ulcerative colitis), and juvenile spondyloarthropathy. Lastly, there is an entity called "undifferentiated spondyloarthropathy" (uSpA) that encompasses such clinical entities as isolated enthesitis or dactylitis and rheumatoid factor-negative oligoarthritis or polyarthritis, usually involving the lower extremities, without any psoriasis or inflammatory bowel disease. This chapter will focus on the axial manifestation of SpAs.

EPIDEMIOLOGY

The SpAs as a group are more common than previously thought, with a prevalence of 0.5% to 1%, indicating that they might be as common as rheumatoid arthritis. They are more common in men (especially AS), but epidemiologic studies suggest that male predominance almost disappears among psoriatic and enteropathic arthritis, and among undifferentiated spondyloarthropathies. The onset of disease, especially AS, is usually in the second and third decade (4), whereas psoriatic arthritis usually starts later in the fourth or fifth decade in patients who have had psoriasis for some time, although a minority of patients may develop arthritis before or at the time the skin lesions become observable (1).

ETIOLOGY AND PATHOGENESIS

There is a strong genetic predisposition, highlighted by a strong association between HLA-B27, first reported in 1973 (5, 6), and this association holds true almost worldwide. The strength of association with HLA-B27, however, differs according to ethnicity and the specific form of SpAs (7) (Table 53.1). There is an increased incidence of SpAs in families of affected individuals (8). HLA-B27 seems to contribute up to 40% of the total genetic risk in AS, and additional genes predisposing to the disease include IL23r (18%), Arts1 (11%), and 1L-1 (4%); thus, up to 73% of genetic contribution can be explained (9). The role of immune dysregulation has been supported by the finding of T cell and macrophage activation, which leads to local increase in the concentration of the proinflammatory cytokines especially tumor necrosis factor-alpha (TNF-α), interleukin-1, and interferon-gamma (10). The central rule of TNF-α has been supported by discovering its presence at sites of inflammation (11). This was further sustained by the promising response to TNF-α inhibitors in SpAs. In patients with AS and PsA, tensile tissues are most vulnerable to the distorted cellular interactions (12). The role of infection has been demonstrated in reactive arthritis but not in other forms of SpAs. Reactive arthritis is usually set off by genitourinary infection with *Chlamydia trachomatis* or enteritis with bacteria such as *Shigella, Salmonella, Yersinia,* or *Campylobacter* species. Not infrequently, the triggering infection may not be identifiable. When bacterial cultures are performed on synovial samples from inflamed joints, no evidence of actual joint infection is found (13).

The role of bowel inflammation has been suggested by endoscopic findings of subclinical enteric mucosal inflammation in 26% to 69% of patients with AS and related SpAs. The risk of developing clinical inflammatory bowel disease in such patients approaches 6% when the histology is found to be "acute inflammation" and 15 % to 25 % when histologically it is found to be "chronic inflammation" (14).

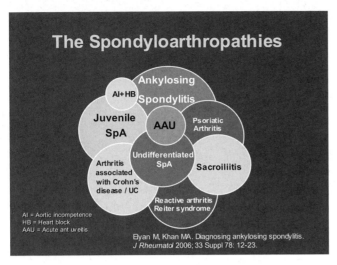

Figure 53.1   An illustration of the overlapping features of SpAs.

Table 53.1   Association of Spondyloarthropathies with HLA-B27 in White Persons*

DISEASE	APPROXIMATE PREVALENCE OF HLA-B27, %
Ankylosing spondylitis	90
Reactive arthritis	40–80
Juvenile spondyloarthropathy	70
Enteropathic spondyloarthritis	35–75
Psoriatic spondyloarthritis	40–50
Undifferentiated spondyloarthropathy	70
Acute anterior uveitis (acute iritis)	50
Aortic incompetence with heart block	80

*Persons of Western European extraction. The prevalence in general healthy populations is approximately 8%.

AS begins with sacroiliitis and later involves the spine in most patients. Inflammation may result in erosions, followed by a healing phase and ossification of the ligaments with resultant bony fusion or ankylosis.

CLINICAL MANIFESTATIONS

The clinical features of the SpAs can be overlapping, especially early on, which sometimes creates some diagnostic confusion. The European Spondyloarthropathy Study Group (ESSG) criteria are the most commonly used classification criteria for SpAs with sensitivity and specificity generally exceeding 85% (15) (Table 53.2).

Ankylosing Spondylitis

Ankylosing spondylitis usually presents with chronic inflammatory low back pain, which is defined by having at least four of the five following characteristics: back pain starting insidiously before the age of 45 years, with duration of at least 3 months,

Table 53.2   The European Spondyloarthropathy Study Group (ESSG) Criteria

CRITERION	DEFINITION
Inflammatory spinal pain with at least four of the following five components: • At least 3 months in duration • Onset before 45 years of age • Insidious (gradual) onset • Improved by exercise • Associated with morning spinal stiffness	History of or current symptoms of spinal pain (low, middle, and upper back, or neck region)
Synovitis	Past or present asymmetric arthritis, or arthritis predominantly in the lower limbs
Spondyloarthropathy	Presence of inflammatory spinal pain OR synovitis AND one or more of the following conditions: • Family history: first-or second-degree relatives with ankylosing spondylitis, psoriasis, acute iritis, reactive arthritis, or inflammatory bowel disease • Past or present psoriasis, diagnosed by a physician • Past or present ulcerative colitis or Crohn's disease, diagnosed by a physician and confirmed by radiography or endoscopy • Past or present alternating buttocks pain • Past or present spontaneous pain or tenderness at examination of the site of the insertion—the Achilles tendon or planter fascia (enthesitis) • Episode of diarrhea occurring within 1 month before onset of arthritis • Nongonococcal urethritis or cervicitis occurring within 1 month before onset of arthritis • Bilateral grade 2–4 sacroiliitis or unilateral grade 3 or 4 sacroiliitis*

*Grades are 0, normal; 1, possible; 2, minimal; 3, moderate; 4, completely fused (ankylosed)

worsening with inactivity and improving with physical exercise, and being associated with back stiffness on waking up in the morning (16). The disease usually involves the axial skeleton including the sacroiliac joints. In very early stages, the patient may complain of alternating buttock pain due to inflammation of the sacroiliac joints. The disease can involve the hip and shoulder joints, and sometimes the more peripheral joints of the limbs can be affected, especially in the presence of associated reactive arthritis, psoriasis, or inflammatory bowel disease.

The back pain results from involvement of the sacroiliac, discovertebral, facet, costovertebral, and costotransverse joints of the spine and the paravertebral ligaments. With disease progression, there is a gradual loss of mobility, flattening of the lumbar spine, and exaggerated thoracic kyphosis. Enthesitis can also result in plantar fasciitis, Achilles tendonitis, or patellar tendonitis (1).

One or more episodes of acute anterior uveitis occurs in 25% to 40% of patients with ankylosing spondylitis (1). Involvement of the gastrointestinal tract, aorta, heart, or lung can also be seen as a part of this disease in some patients (1). Patients with ankylosing spondylitis or related spondyloarthropathies may have an increased risk for coronary artery disease (17).

Physical findings in ankylosing spondylitis include tenderness over the sacroiliac joints and pain with sacroiliac stress tests such as FABERE (hip *f*lexion, *ab*duction, *e*xternal *r*otation, and *e*xtension) (Table 53.3). There might also be tenderness over the spinal processes, heels, iliac crest, anterior chest wall, and other bony prominences due to enthesitis (3). There might be a decrease in chest expansion, which is normally at least 5 cm in healthy young individuals, at the level of the xiphisternum. Measures of spinal mobility such as modified Schober's test and lateral flexion are important in the assessment of the ankylosing spondylitis (3). Occiput-to-wall or tragus-to-wall distances measure forward stooping deformity of cervical spine (3).

Involvement of the cervical spine can gradually result in progressive limitation of the ability to turn or fully extend or laterally bend the neck (Table 53.4).

Psoriatic Arthropathy

Psoriatic arthritis is defined as an inflammatory arthritis associated with psoriasis, which may present in different forms: monoarthritis, asymmetric oligoarthritis (fewer than five joints), polyarthritis, arthritis of distal interphalangeal joints, arthritis mutilans, and spondylitis, although there can be significant overlap among these subtypes (18). The polyarthritis form can clinically resemble rheumatoid arthritis, although psoriatic arthritis patients tend to have less joint pain (19). Arthritis mutilans is a severe destructive arthritis.

Psoriatic arthritis is often associated with tendonitis and/or enthesitis. Axial disease can be similar to ankylosing spondylitis, although it is sometimes asymptomatic with only about one-third of patients developing sacroiliitis. Inflammation of the entire digit involving the joints and the tendon sheaths (dactylitis or "sausage digits") is one of the typical features of psoriatic arthritis.

Inflammatory arthritis occurs in more than 10% of patients with psoriasis (20). It is important to extensively search the whole skin for lesions of psoriasis when evaluating a patient with any form of inflammatory arthritis or spondylitis. This search should include the scalp, ears, umbilicus, pelvic area, perineum, and perianal area. There is no correlation between the severity of skin lesions and the severity of the arthritis (21).

Its onset is usually in the fourth or fifth decade. Patients usually have had psoriasis for some time before the arthritis starts, but some patients may develop arthritis before psoriasis manifests clinically (about 15%) (1). Nail changes of psoriasis such as nail pitting or onycholysis are more common in patients with

---

Table 53.3   Sacroiliac Joint Stress Maneuvers

Maneuver	Description
FABERE* or Patrick's test	• The patient lies supine on the exam table; one hip is flexed, abducted, externally rotated then extended, to form a figure-4 with the ankle on the contralateral knee. • This maneuver stresses the ipsilateral sacroiliac joint. • The test is repeated on the contralateral side. • If this maneuver causes posterior hip pain, mostly overlying the sacroiliac joint, sacroiliitis should be suspected.
Gaenslen's test	• The patient lies supine on the exam table with the side to be tested projecting over the side of the table. • The patient draws his or her knees to the chest. • The physician stabilizes the patient while the side being tested is left to drop off the table, fully extending the hip. • The test can be repeated on the contralateral side. • If this maneuver causes posterior hip pain, sacroiliitis should be suspected.
Lateral pelvic compression test	• The patient lies on his or her side on a firm examining table. • The physician applies pressure on the iliac crest to compress the pelvis down toward the table top. • Pain elicited in the sacroiliac joint area on either or both sides may be indicative of sacroiliitis.
Antero-posterior pelvic compression test	• The patient lies supine on the examining table. • The physician applies pressure on the anterior superior iliac spine bilaterally to compress the pelvis. • Pain elicited in the sacroiliac joint area on either side may be indicative of sacroiliitis.

*FABERE = hip Flexion, Abduction, External Rotation, and Extension.
Source: Elyan M, Khan MA. Diagnosing ankylosing spondylitis. *J Rheumatol Suppl* 2006 Sep; 78:12–23.

Table 53.4   Measures of Spinal Mobility

MEASURE*	DESCRIPTION
Cervical rotation	• Measure the angle of the cervical rotation by using a goniometer. • Another method is to measure with a plastic tape the distance between the tip of the nose and the acromio-clavicular joint at baseline (when the neck is in neutral position) and on maximal ipsilateral rotation. The difference between these two positions measures the rotation and is separately measured for right/left rotations. Smaller difference indicates a more restricted cervical rotation.
Fingertip-to-floor distance	• Distance between tip of right middle finger and the floor following maximal lumbar flexion, while maintaining full extension of the knee. Measured ideally with a rigid tape measure; smaller distances indicate greater movement.
Lumbar lateral flexion	• Distance between tip of ipsilateral middle finger and floor following maximal lumbar lateral flexion, maintaining heel contact with floor and without trunk rotation. Smaller distance indicates greater movement. Measured ideally with a rigid tape measure. • Domjan method: the two marks are placed on the patient's skin in the above two maneuvers and the distance between those two marks reflects lateral flexion.
Modified Schöber's index	• Distance between two marks placed 10 cm apart on the lumbar spine in the midline: the lower mark is at the level of the dimples of Venus or posterior superior iliac spines, with the patient standing upright. The distance between these two marks is measured again while the patient is maximally forward-flexing the spine, with the knees fully extended. There should be an increase of at least 5 cm expansion between the two marks. An expansion of less than 4 cm indicates decreased mobility of the lumbar spine. Measured with a plastic tape measure.
Tragus-to-wall distance	• Horizontal distance between right tragus and wall, when the subject is standing erect with heels and buttocks against the wall (to prevent pivoting), knees fully extended and chin drawn in to keep a horizontal gaze. Larger distance indicates worse spinal/upper cervical posture. Measured with a rigid tape measure.
Occipital-to-wall distance	• Horizontal distance between the posterior convexity of the occiput and the wall, when the subject is standing erect with heels and buttocks against the wall (to prevent pivoting), knees fully extended and chin drawn in to keep a horizontal gaze. Subjects with normal posture show no gap. Larger distance indicates worse spinal/upper cervical posture. Measured with a rigid tape measure.

*All measurements should be recorded after having the patient practice once.
Source: Haywood KL, Garratt AM, Jordan K, Dziedzic K, Dawes PT. Spinal mobility in ankylosing spondylitis: reliability, validity and responsiveness. *Rheumatology (Oxford)* 2004; 43:750–757.

psoriatic arthritis than in psoriasis patients without arthritis (22). There is an association between HIV infection and exacerbation of skin lesions and arthritis; this association is now being noted mostly in sub-Saharan Africa (23).

Reactive Arthritis

Reactive arthritis typically occurs within 1 month from an inciting infection. It usually manifests by acute, asymmetric oligoarthritis and is often associated with conjunctivitis, uveitis, enthesitis, dactylitis, genital psoriasiform lesions (circinate balanitis or circinate vulvitis), urethritis, or cervicitis (18). The term Reiter syndrome has been used to describe the association of reactive arthritis with conjunctivitis and urethritis, although most patients with reactive arthritis do not have the complete triad.

Spondyloarthropathy of Inflammatory Bowel Disease

Inflammatory bowel disease (ulcerative colitis and Crohn's disease) can be associated with a form of inflammatory arthritis called *enteropathic arthritis* or *spondyloarthropathy of inflammatory bowel disease*. Up to 37% of patients with ulcerative colitis or

Crohn's disease may show sacroiliitis, spondylitis, enthesitis, or peripheral arthritis. Definite ankylosing spondylitis is seen in about 10% of these patients (25). Peripheral arthritis is usually self-limited and nondestructive; it, contrary to axial disease, parallels the activity of bowel involvement.

Undifferentiated Spondyloarthropathies

There are undifferentiated forms of spondyloarthropathies, which may include HLA-B27-associated enthesitis, dactylitis, and rheumatoid factor-negative oligoarthritis or polyarthritis. It usually involves the lower extremities, is not preceded by an identifiable infection, and is not associated with psoriasis or inflammatory bowel disease. Some patients may present with episodes of isolated acute anterior uveitis, which may precede the onset of the spondyloarthropathy (1).

IMAGING STUDIES

Radiologic evidence of sacroiliitis on plain pelvis X-rays is the most typical finding for SpAs (Table 53.5) and is required for a definite diagnosis of AS according to the Modified New York criteria (26). If plain pelvis films are not diagnostic and AS is still clinically considered, then an MRI (27) or a CT scan (28) of the

Table 53.5   The New York Criteria for Grading Radiologic Evidence of Sacroiliitis

GRADE	LABEL	DESCRIPTION
0	Normal	Clear margins, uniform width, and no juxta-articular sclerosis
1	Suspicious	Suspicious but not definite abnormality
2	Minimal sacroiliitis	Evidence of some sclerosis and minimal erosions but no marked joint-space narrowing
3	Moderate sacroiliitis	Definite sclerosis on both sides of the joint, erosions and widening of the interosseous space
4	Ankylosis	Complete joint obliteration with or without residual sclerosis

Source: Barozzi L, Olivieri I, De Matteis M, Padula A, Pavlica P. Seronegative spondylarthropathies: imaging of spondylitis, enthesitis and dactylitis. *Eur J Radiol* 1998; 27(suppl 1):S12–S17.

sacroiliac joints can be helpful. MRI is more sensitive than CT and enables assessment of sites of active disease and response to therapy (29). MRI with the Short Tau inversion recovery (STIR) technique, without Gadolinium enhancement, can show evidence of inflammation and bone marrow edema, indicating active inflammation (30, 31).

Conventional X-rays of peripheral joints may reveal soft tissue swelling, erosions, and periostitis in patients with psoriatic arthritis and less often in other spondyloarthropathies. Other typical findings of psoriatic arthritis include pencil-in-cup deformities in the hand and feet joints, and joint ankylosis. There is usually absence of juxta-articular osteopenia in the involved joint.

Osteoporosis is common in AS patients; it can occur relatively early in the disease. Spinal osteoporosis is caused partly by the ankylosis and decreased mobility and is also secondary to the effect of the pro-inflammatory cytokines (32). Measurements of bone density at the spine may be unreliable when there is ligamentous ossification and formation of syndesmophytes. Thus, femoral neck measurements should be relied on for the diagnosis. Sometimes, a peripheral DEXA scan might be needed in patients with bilateral hip arthroplasties.

LABORATORY TESTING

The value of laboratory testing is limited in patients with SpAs. Acute phase reactants such as C-reactive protein (CRP) and erthrocyte sedimentation rate (ESR) may be elevated, especially when there is inflammation of peripheral joints, but they are neither sensitive nor specific in patients with AS (33). The SpAs have been long labeled as seronegative because of lack of association with rheumatoid factor. The synovial fluid analysis is nonspecific, but joints should be aspirated when there is effusion to exclude other possibilities such as septic or crystal-induced arthritis.

HLA-B27 testing is not useful as a routine screening test because SpAs can occur in the absence of HLA-B27, and HLA-B27 can be present in healthy individuals. Nonetheless, HLA-B27 may be helpful in certain clinical situations, especially when the pretest probability of AS approaches 50% (toss-up) with nondiagnostic findings on pelvic films (34).

When there is clinical suspicion of reactive arthritis, bacterial studies such as throat cultures for streptococcal infection and urogenital samples for *Chlamydia* should be obtained. Serologic tests such as for *Salmonella, Yersinia,* and *Campylobacter* may be helpful in the appropriate clinical setting (35). Testing for HIV should be considered in high-risk patients.

DIAGNOSIS

The diagnosis of AS is frequently delayed for years or even missed (36), especially in children, adolescents, women, and HLA-B27-negative patients (37–39). The widely used criteria (modified New York criteria [Table 53.6]) used for diagnosis of AS are classification (not diagnostic) criteria that were designed for research purposes to ensure accuracy of diagnosis in study subjects. The ESSG classification criteria (Table 53.2) are designed to encompass the broad spectrum of SpAs. There are also no diagnostic tests for SpA, and the diagnosis is therefore made based on the interpretation of a combination of clinical, radiological, and laboratory findings.

The diagnosis of AS can be challenging due to the insidious onset with frequently mild and nonspecific symptoms, especially early on. This is further complicated by lack of a specific diagnostic test and the occasional absence of radiological changes in early stages. Decision trees have been proposed for rheumatologists (Figure 53.2A) to aid in diagnosing axial spondyloarthropathies and for primary care physicians to help make referral decisions (Figure 53.2B) to a rheumatologist at early stages (40).

Table 53.6   The Modified New York Classification Criteria for Ankylosing Spondylitis

Clinical criteria
1. Low back pain and stiffness for >3 months that improves with exercise but not with rest
2. Limitation of lumbar spine mobility in both the sagittal and frontal planes
3. Limitation in chest expansion as compared with normal range for age and gender

Radiologic criteria
1. Unilateral sacroiliitis of grade 3–4, OR
2. Bilateral sacroiliitis of grade ≥2

Grading
1. Definite AS if the radiological criterion is associated with at least 1 clinical criterion
2. Probable AS if:
   a. Three clinical criteria are present, OR
   b. The radiological criterion is present without any signs or symptoms satisfying the clinical criteria

AS = ankylosing spondylitis.
Source: van der Linden S, Valkenburg HA, Cats A. Evaluation of diagnostic criteria for ankylosing spondylitis. A proposal for modification of the New York criteria. *Arthritis Rheum.* 1984; 27:361–368.

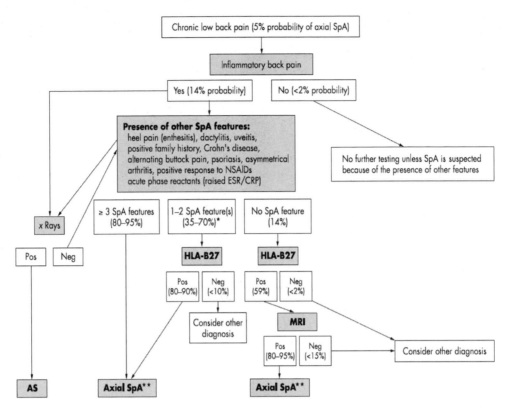

Figure 53.2A Decision tree on diagnosing axial SpA. Starting point is the presence or absence of inflammatory back pain (IBP) in patients presenting with chronic back pain. In general, for making the diagnosis of axial SpA, a disease probability of more than 90% is suggested.
Notes: *Dependent on which features are positive (Table 53.2).
**If the probability of disease exceeds 90%, we consider the diagnosis axial SpA as definite; if the probability is 80%–90%, we consider the diagnosis as probable.
(From Rudwaleit M, van der Heijde D, Khan MA, Braun J, Sieper J. How to diagnose axial spondyloarthritis early. *Ann Rheum Dis* 2004; 63:535–543.)

EVALUATING DISEASE ACTIVITY AND SEVERITY

Distinguishing symptoms that reflect active disease from symptoms of a mechanical or psychological nature impacts specific treatment decisions. Monitoring disease activity by reliable measures enables better assessment of response to treatment. CRP and ESR correlate only moderately with axial disease activity (33). Several instruments have been developed to assess disease activity and severity of AS in a scoring system utilizing symptoms and signs. Examples include the Bath ankylosing spondylitis disease activity index (BASDAI), the Bath ankylosing spondylitis metrology index (BASMI), the Bath ankylosing spondylitis functional index (BASFI), and the health assessment questionnaire (HAQ). The BASDAI is an easy-to-use, reliable, and sensitive-to-change measure that rates the symptoms of fatigue, spinal pain, joint pain and swelling, tenderness, and morning stiffness using a visual analogue scale (41). The BASMI is an easy, reproducible, and sensitive method to assess spinal mobility; it measures cervical extension using tragus-to-wall distance, lumbar flexion using the modified Schöber's test, cervical rotation using a gravity action goniometer, lumbar side flexion using fingertip-to-floor distance in sitting, and intermalleolar distance to measure bilateral hip

abduction (42). The BASFI is an easy, reliable, and sensitive-to-change method to assess degree of disability in patients with ankylosing spondylitis (43). The HAQ has been modified to assess the severity of psoriatic arthritis (44).

TREATMENT

The treatment decisions should be made on an individual basis directed by accepted guidelines and taking into consideration special presentations, disease severity and activity, functional disability, comorbidities, and patients' expectations. The best strategy is implementing a comprehensive plan that includes patient education, exercise, physical therapy, and medications.

Patient Education

Health education for self-management in patients with chronic arthritis produces sustained health benefits and reduces healthcare costs (45). Self-management programs facilitate patients' adherence to drug regimens, decrease their pain, and increase their knowledge about arthritis (46, 47). Patients should be educated about the nature of their illness and their

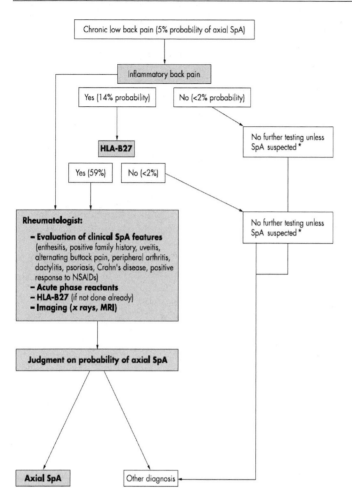

Figure 53.2B Approach to the diagnosis of axial SpA in daily practice for the physician (i.e., GP) less experienced in dealing with patients with rheumatic disease. Percentages in parentheses indicate the probability of axial SpA before (pretest probability) and after a test has been performed (posttest probability). *Suspicions for SpA could be the presence of several other clinical features.
(From Rudwaleit M, van der Heijde D, Khan MA, Braun J, Sieper J. How to diagnose axial spondyloarthritis early. *Ann Rheum Dis* 2004; 63:535–543.)

individual prognosis. The role of pharmacologic and nonpharmacologic therapies should be clearly explained. Smoking cessation should be urged because of the more severe illness, increased incidence of respiratory complications, and numerous other adverse effects of smoking (48). Patients should be always encouraged to assume a central role in managing their illness and should be given information about disease-specific associations in the form of books, pamphlets, videos, or audiotapes. Some useful websites include http://www.arthritis.org, www.spondylitis.org, and http://patients.uptodate.com/. The impact on the family, including familial aggregation, should be discussed with patients and possibly with their family members.

Patients should be advised to sleep on a firm mattress without a pillow, or with a thin or contoured pillow to maintain neck extension and help prevent the development of spinal deformities. They should walk erect, keeping the spine as straight as possible while maintaining normal, reciprocal arm swing and rotational movements of the lower spine and pelvis during walking. Stooped postures such as slouching in chairs or leaning over a desk for prolonged periods should be avoided; adjustable swivel chairs with lumbar support and elevated and inclined writing surfaces may be helpful. Patients should maintain hip extension, for example, by lying prone for a 15-minute period daily (49). Patients should be advised on helpful home and workplace modifications. Fall precaution measures include having nonslippery floors in bathrooms, and having tub or shower grab bars and safety mats. Changing positions frequently and taking breaks for bodily stretching is helpful. Proper head, neck, and back support for driving and installation of wide-angled mirrors improves safety (50).

Exercise and Physical Therapy

Data on the role of exercise and physical therapy are limited, and specific treatment protocols have not been thoroughly studied. Regular exercise and formal sessions of physical therapy are generally underutilized by patients and physicians. Despite the remarkable progress in the pharmacologic therapy of SpAs, these nonpharmacologic modalities remain an essential part of the management plan. Such interventions complement drug therapy to improve function and quality of life and to minimize deformities.

Home-based exercise programs are easily performed and conveniently available to patients at minimal cost. Therefore, physicians should educate patients about the role of exercise and give them instructions about simple exercises in addition to referring them to a physical therapist for specific exercise instructions. Patients who undergo a regular long-term home exercise program supported by educational interventions may improve in exercise self-effectiveness, mobility, and function (51). Patients who undergo supervised comprehensive home physical therapy have shown improvement in spinal mobility and function (52). Improvement can be sustained with maintenance exercises (53). Exercise potentially has other benefits, including less pain and better mood and quality of life (54–56).

Because formal sessions of physical therapy may also have a positive impact on patients, physicians should consider referring patients who may benefit from such intervention. A supervised group physical therapy program combined with home exercises may be better than unsupervised home exercises alone in improving spine mobility, fitness, and overall health (57). A specific protocol of regular strengthening and flexibility exercises supervised by a physical therapist has been shown to improve mobility and function (58), which can be sustained by maintenance exercises (59). Daily passive stretching of the hips may improve and maintain the hip range of motion (60). Supervised physical therapy may have other beneficial effects including improvement in chest expansion and lung vital capacity (61) as well as mood (62).

Hydrotherapy may have a role in the management of AS, and patients should be encouraged to swim and perform water exercises if they can. Such a modality may help improve function (63), spine mobility, pain, and stiffness (64, 65).

Intensive inpatient rehabilitation may be indicated for patients with severe active disease. Such an intervention may provide rapid short-term improvement in pain and stiffness, mobility, function, and quality of life (64, 66–69).

The Cochrane systematic review of physical therapy for AS suggested beneficial effects, in increasing order, of home exercise program, supervised group physical therapy, and combined inpatient spa-exercise therapy followed by supervised outpatient weekly group therapy (70).

Pharmacologic Treatment

Nonsteroidal Anti-inflammatory Drugs (NSAIDs)

NSAIDs are considered the first line of drug therapy for active AS, and they need to be taken on a regular basis in full anti-inflammatory doses to ensure a therapeutic response. Nonselective NSAIDs and cyclo-oxygenase (COX)-2-selective NSAIDs are beneficial for relief of axial and peripheral join pain and for improving function in such patients. Various NSAIDs are of comparable efficacy; however, there are individual variations in response to different NSAIDs (71), in addition to variations in their side effect and drug interaction profiles (72). The risk of gastrointestinal bleeding is dose dependent (73). Selective COX-2 inhibitors carry a lower risk of serious gastrointestinal events than traditional NSAIDs (74). Another way to reduce the risk for gastrointestinal complications is to use a gastrointestinal-protective agent such as misoprostol or a proton pump inhibitor in conjunction with the nonselective NSAID (75).

The cardiovascular toxicity seen with rofecoxib (Vioxx) (76) has also been described in clinical trials of other selective COX-2 inhibitors (77), with some evidence suggesting that it may be an NSAIDs class effect (78). However, a recent meta-analysis did not reveal an increased risk of cardiovascular events with celecoxib (79). Regular therapy with an NSAID may have a mild disease-modifying effect on AS, as shown by retarding the radiographic progression of the disease compared to on demand use (80), although this remains controversial (81).

NSAIDs may also be effective in mild peripheral psoriatic arthritis, when there is no evidence of erosions (82). NSAIDs can also be used in cases of reactive arthritis (83). NSAIDs are relatively contraindicated in patients with inflammatory bowel disease, but selective COX-2 inhibitors may be safer (84).

Tumor Necrosis Factor–Alpha Inhibitors

TNF-α inhibitors have transformed the management of SpAs. Patients who do not respond to conventional therapies can now be offered treatment with these agents. Infliximab (Remicade), etanercept (Enbrel), and adalimumab (Humira) are now approved by the FDA for the treatment of AS and psoriatic arthropathy. TNF-α inhibitors lead to rapid and remarkable improvement in the symptoms and signs of SpAs, including back pain and stiffness, peripheral arthritis, enthesitis, dactylitis, and psoriasis in most patients. Infliximab is FDA approved for treatment of inflammatory bowel disease (ulcerative colitis and Crohn's disease). Adalimumab is FDA-approved for use in patients with Crohn's disease. TNF inhibition may be helpful in refractory cases of reactive arthritis (85).

Infliximab 5 mg/kg at weeks 0, 2, and 6 has shown consistent efficacy in controlling the symptoms and signs of AS (86, 87) as well as in improving productivity and reducing workday loss

(88). Etanercept 50 mg once weekly or 25 mg twice weekly has been shown to be tolerable and efficacious in decreasing signs and symptoms of active AS as well as in improving function, spine mobility, and quality of life (89–91). Adalimumab has been also shown to be safe and efficacious in patients with active AS (92, 93). Treatment with TNF-α inhibitors is associated with decrease in spinal inflammation as detected by MRI (94–96). Treatment with TNF-α inhibitors may slow progression of disease, although this has to be verified in long-term studies (97). A study has shown that treatment with the TNF blocker infliximab increases bone density in patients with AS (98).

For initiation of anti-TNF therapy in AS, patients should fulfill the modified New York Criteria for definitive AS. The disease must be active for at least 1 month, as determined by a BASDAI score of greater than or equal to 4. Initiation of such treatment should be decided by an expert on the subject. The patient must have failed to show satisfactory therapeutic response to at least two different NSAIDs given for at least 3 months at maximal recommended or tolerated anti-inflammatory dose (unless there is intolerance, toxicity, or contraindications to the use of NSAIDs). Those with AS and peripheral arthritis must have failed to respond to adequate therapy with both NSAIDs and sulfasalazine, and those with enthesitis must have failed at least two local steroid injections before anti-TNF therapy is started. The modified United States guidelines do not require therapy with local corticosteroid injections before initiating TNF-α antagonist therapy, compared to the original European guidelines (99) (Table 53.7). When one anti-TNF agent fails or the patient develops side effects that are not related to TNF antagonists as a class, switching to another agent may be an option (100, 101).

Although TNF antagonists are generally well tolerated, they are very expensive and may be associated with potentially serious adverse effects that include allergic and injection-site reactions and increased risk of infections, including reactivation of tuberculosis.

Unfortunately, there are still many patients who meet the criteria for anti-TNF-α treatment according to published guidelines, but who do not receive these agents (102).

Other Therapies

Traditional disease-modifying anti-rheumatic drugs (DMARDs) such as sulfasalazine, methotrexate, and leflunomide have not been proven to be efficacious in the treatment of axial involvement of spondyloarthropathies (103–105). Systemic corticosteroids are not recommended in axial disease because of lack of benefit and significant side effects. Intra-articular or local steroid injection can be used to achieve rapid relief of the active inflammation of the peripheral joints and the enthesitis in the absence of contraindications. Simple analgesics such as acetaminophen, tramadol, and opioids may be used only as an adjunctive short-term treatment until the inflammation is controlled. Caution should be exercised when prescribing narcotics to avoid dependence and abuse. Low-dose tricyclic agents such as amitriptyline may be a helpful adjunctive treatment that helps relieve pain and fatigue, especially in patients with sleep disturbances (106). Adequate calcium and vitamin D intake should be encouraged; the recommended daily intake is 1.0 to 1.5 g of elemental calcium and 400 to 800 IU of vitamin D. Vitamin D deficiency should be

Table 53.7   ASAS Guidelines for the Use of Anti-TNF Therapy in Patients with AS

Diagnosis
- Patients normally fulfilling modified New York criteria for definitive ankylosing spondylitis

Disease Activity
- BASDAI Score ≥4 (scale 0–10 cm)
  and
- Physician Global Assessment by "expert" opinion(yes/no)

Previous Treatment
- All patients should have had adequate therapeutic trials of at least two NSAIDs for at least 3 months at maximum recommended or tolerated anti-inflammatory dose unless contraindicated or treatment was withdrawn because of intolerance, toxicity, or contraindications.
- Patients with pure axial manifestations do not have to take DMARDs before anti-TNF treatment can be started.
- Patients with symptomatic peripheral arthritis should have an insufficient response to at least one local corticosteroid injection if appropriate.
- Patients with persistent peripheral arthritis must have had a therapeutic trial of sulfasalazine.
- Patients with symptomatic enthesitis must have failed appropriate local treatment.

Dosing
- Etanercept 50 mg subcutaneously once a week (or 25 mg twice a week)
- Infliximab 5 mg/kg IV every 6–8 weeks
- Adalimumab 40 mg subcutaneously every other week

Responder Criteria
- 50% improvement of BASDAI or absolute change of 2 on 0–10 cm scale and "expert" opinion

Time of Evaluation
- Between 6 to 12 weeks

TB Precaution
- Use country-specific guidelines

Adapted from Braun J, Davis J, Dougados M, Sieper J, van der Linden S, van der Heijde D; ASAS Working Group. First update of the international ASAS consensus statement for the use of anti-TNF agents in patients with ankylosing spondylitis. Ann Rheum Dis 2006 Mar; 65(3):316–320.

screened for and corrected if present. Prevention and treatment of osteoporosis may help decrease the risk of deformities and fractures and the morbidity and mortality associated with them. Treatment for osteoporosis includes bisphosphonates or sometimes parathyroid hormone. The Assessment in Ankylosing Spondylitis (ASAS) group and the European League against Rheumatism (EULAR) have published recommendations for the management of AS based on available evidence and expert opinion (Table 53.8) (107).

Role of Surgery

Rare surgical emergencies can happen in patients with AS in cases of spinal fractures, cauda equina syndrome, and atlantoaxial subluxation with neurologic compromise. Spinal fractures, instability, and/or psuedoarthrosis should be suspected in AS patients who develop new onset spinal pain even without preceding trauma because of risk that these complications may lead to paraplegia or tetraplegia (108, 109). Cauda equina syndrome, usually manifesting by dull pain in the lower back and upper buttock region; analgesia in the buttocks, genitalia, or thighs (saddle area); and a disturbance of bowel and bladder function are rare neurologic complications of AS, which may result from chronic adhesive arachnoiditis, due to fibrous entrapment and scarring of the sacral and lower lumbar nerve roots (110, 111). Spontaneous atlantoaxial subluxation has been described in patients with AS (112, 113).

Spinal fusion is indicated in cases of atlantoaxial subluxation and to relieve pain and correct deformity resulting from pseudoarthrosis (114). Osteotomy to correct severe kyphosis and uncompensated loss of horizontal vision may provide excellent functional improvement (115).

Total hip replacement is indicated in patients with advanced hip involvement with severe pain or functional disability (116). Similarly, other joint involvement may require joint replacement in advanced cases, especially the knee. General anesthesia can be a challenge due to intubation difficulties resulting from cervical spinal ankylosis and deformity and involvement of the temporomandibular joint. Spinal anesthesia may not be possible due to spinal fusion and ligament ossification. Care should be taken following surgery to avoid pulmonary complications, which may result in decreased vital capacity due to restricted chest wall expansion.

FOLLOW-UP

Patients with SpAs should be followed on a regular basis to monitor disease activity, response to treatment, and medication side effects. Monitoring consists of determining patient symptoms and signs and evaluating laboratory testing and imaging studies. Specific skeletal elements to be monitored include duration of morning stiffness, severity of pain, mobility of the lumbar and cervical spine, chest expansion, enthesopathy, and changes in joint inflammation and range of motion. Measures described

Table 53.8 Experts' Propositions Developed through Three Delphi Rounds—Order According to Topic (General, Non-Pharmacologic, Pharmacologic, Invasive, and Surgical)

NUMBER	PROPOSITION
1	Treatment of AS should be tailored according to: • Current manifestations of the disease (axial, peripheral, entheseal, extra-articular symptoms and signs) • Level of current symptoms, clinical findings, and prognostic indicators —Disease activity/inflammation —Pain —Function, disability, handicap —Structural damage, hip involvement, spinal deformities • General clinical status (age, sex, comorbidity, concomitant drugs) • Wishes and expectations of the patient
2	Disease monitoring of patients with AS should include patient history (for example, questionnaires), clinical parameters, laboratory tests, and imaging, all according to the clinical presentation, as well as the ASAS core set. The frequency of monitoring should be decided on an individual basis depending on symptoms, severity, and drug treatment.
3	Optimal management of AS requires a combination of nonpharmacologic and pharmacologic treatments.
4	Nonpharmacologic treatment of AS should include patient education and regular exercise. Individual and group physical therapy should be considered. Patient associations and self-help groups may be useful.
5	NSAIDs are recommended as first-line drug treatment for patients with AS with pain and stiffness. In those with increased GI risk, nonselective NSAIDs plus a gastroprotective agent, or a selective COX-2 inhibitor could be used.
6	Analgesics, such as paracetamol and opioids, might be considered for pain control in patients in whom NSAIDs are insufficient, contraindicated, and/or poorly tolerated.
7	Corticosteroid injections directed to the local site of musculoskeletal inflammation may be considered. The use of systemic corticosteroids for axial disease is not supported by evidence.
8	There is no evidence for the efficacy of DMARDs, including sulfasalazine and methotrexate, for the treatment of axial disease. Sulfasalazine may be considered in patients with peripheral arthritis.
9	Anti-TNF treatment should be given to patients with persistently high disease activity despite conventional treatments according to the ASAS recommendations. There is no evidence to support the obligatory use of DMARDs before, or concomitant with, anti-TNF treatment in patients with axial disease.
10	Total hip arthroplasty should be considered in patients with refractory pain or disability and radiographic evidence of structural damage, independent of age. Spinal surgery—for example, corrective osteotomy and stabilization procedures, may be of value in selected patients.

AS, ankylosing spondylitis; GI, gastrointestinal; NSAIDs, nonsteroidal anti-inflammatory drugs; DMARDs, disease modifying antirheumatic drugs; TNF, tumor necrosis factor.
Source: Zochling J, van der Heijde D, Burgos-Vargas R, Collantes E, Davis JC Jr, Dijkmans B, Dougados M, Geher P, Inman RD, Khan MA, Kvien TK, Leirisalo-Repo M, Olivieri I, Pavelka K, Sieper J, Stucki G, Sturrock RD, van der Linden S, Wendling D, Bohm H, van Royen BJ, Braun J; "ASsessment in AS" international working group; European League Against Rheumatism ASAS/EULAR recommendations for the management of ankylosing spondylitis. *Ann Rheum Dis* 2006; 65(4):442–452.

above to evaluate disease activity, such as BASDAI, BASMI, BASFI, HAQ, CRP, and ESR, are used in monitoring response to therapy. Radiographic monitoring of axial involvement once every 2 years is usually adequate; radiographs are not sensitive for changes over less than 1 year (117).

References

1. Khan MA. Update on spondyloarthropathies. *Ann Intern Med* 2002; 136(12):896–907.
2. Elyan M, Khan MA. Diagnosing ankylosing spondylitis. *J Rheumatol Suppl* 2006; 78:12–23.
3. Khan MA. *Ankylosing Spondylitis.* New York: Oxford University Press, 2009; 1–147.
4. Akkoc N, Khan MA. Epidemiology of ankylosing spondylitis and related spondyloarthropathies. In: Weisman MH, Reveille JD, van der Heijde D, eds. *Ankylosing Spondylitis and the Spondyloarthropathies: A Companion to Rheumatology.* London: Elsevier, 2006:117–131.
5. Brewerton DA, Hart FD, Nicholls A, Caffrey M, et al. Ankylosing spondylitis and HL-A 27. *Lancet* 1973; 1(7809):904–907.
6. Schlosstein T, Terasaki PI, Bluestone R, Pearson CM. High association of an HL-A antigen, W27, with ankylosing spondylitis. *N Engl J Med* 288:704–706.
7. Khan MA. Prevalence of HLA-B27 in world populations. In: Lopez-Larrea C, ed. *HLA-B27 in the Development of Spondyloarthropathies.* Austin, TX: R.G. Landes Company, 1997:95–112.
8. Said-Nahal R, Miceli-Richard C, Berthelot JM, Duche A, et al. The familial form of spondylarthropathy: a clinical study of 115 multiplex families. Groupe Francais d'Etude Genetique des Spondylarthropathies. *Arthritis Rheum* 2000; 43(6):1356–1365.
9. Wellcome Trust Case Control Consortium, Burton PR, Clayton DG, Cardon LR, et al. Association scan of 14,500 nonsynonymous SNPs in four diseases identifies autoimmunity variants. *Nat Genet* 2007; 39(11):1329–1337.

10. Bollow M, Fischer T, Reisshauer H, Backhaus M, et al. Quantitative analyses of sacroiliac biopsies in spondyloarthropathies: T cells and macrophages predominate in early and active sacroiliitis—cellularity correlates with the degree of enhancement detected by magnetic resonance imaging. *Ann Rheum Dis* 2000; 59:135–140.

11. Braun J, Bollow M, Neure L, Seipelt E, et al. Use of immunohistologic and in situ hybridization techniques in the examination of sacroiliac joint biopsy specimens from patients with ankylosing spondylitis. *Arthritis Rheum* 1995; 38(4):499–505.

12. Benjamin M, Toumi H, Suzuki D, Redman S, et al. Microdamage and altered vascularity at the enthesis–bone interface provides an anatomic explanation for bone involvement in the HLA-B27-associated spondylarthritides and allied disorders. *Arthritis Rheum* 2007; 56(1):224–233.

13. Rahman MU, Schumacher HR, Hudson AP. Recurrent arthritis in Reiter's syndrome: a function of inapparent chlamydial infection of the synovium? *Semin Arthritis Rheum* 1992; 21(4):259–266.

14. Smale S, Natt RS, Orchard TR, Russell AS, Bjarnason I. Inflammatory bowel disease and spondyloarthropathy. *Arthritis Rheum* 2001; 44:2728–2736.

15. Amor B, Dougados M, Listrat V, Menkes CJ, et al. [Evaluation of the Amor criteria for spondylarthropathies and European Spondylarthropathy Study Group (ESSG): a cross-sectional analysis of 2,228 patients.] *Ann Med Interne (Paris)* 1991; 142(2):85–89.

16. Calin A, Porta J, Fries JF, Schurman DJ. Clinical history as a screening test for ankylosing spondylitis. *JAMA* 1977; 237(24):2613–2614.

17. Heeneman S, Daemen MJ. Cardiovascular risks in spondyloarthritides. *Curr Opin Rheumatol* 2007; 19(4):358–362.

18. Moll JM, Wright V. Psoriatic arthritis. *Semin Arthritis Rheum* 1973; 3(1):55–78.

19. Buskila D, Langevitz P, Gladman DD, Urowitz S, Smythe HA. Patients with rheumatoid arthritis are more tender than those with psoriatic arthritis. *J Rheumatol* 1992; 19(7):1115–1119.

20. Gelfand JM, Gladman DD, Mease PJ, Smith N, et al. Epidemiology of psoriatic arthritis in the population of the United States. *J Am Acad Dermatol* 2005; 53(4):573.

21. Cohen MR, Reda DJ, Clegg DO. Baseline relationships between psoriasis and psoriatic arthritis: analysis of 221 patients with active psoriatic arthritis. Department of Veteran Affairs Cooperative Study Group on Seronegative Spondyloarthropathies. *J Rheumatol* 1999; 26:1752–1756.

22. Taylor W, Gladman D, Helliwell P, Marchesoni A, et al. CASPAR Study Group. Classification criteria for psoriatic arthritis: development of new criteria from a large international study. *Arthritis Rheum* 2006; 54(8):2665–2673.

23. Mijiyawa M, Oniankitan O, Khan MA. Spondyloarthropathies in sub-Saharan Africa. *Curr Opin Rheumatol* 2000; 12(4):281–286.

24. Sieper J, Rudwaleit M, Braun J, van der Heijde D. Diagnosing reactive arthritis: role of clinical setting in the value of serologic and microbiologic assays. *Arthritis Rheum* 2002; 46:319 327.

25. de Vlam K, Mielants H, Cuvelier C, De Keyser F, et al. Spondyloarthropathy is underestimated in inflammatory bowel disease: prevalence and HLA association. *J Rheumatol* 2000; 27:2860–2865.

26. van der Linden S, Valkenburg HA, Cats A. Evaluation of diagnostic criteria for ankylosing spondylitis: a proposal for modification of the New York criteria. *Arthritis Rheum* 1984; 27:361–368.

27. Oostveen J, Prevo R, den Boer J, van de Laar M. Early detection of sacroiliitis on magnetic resonance imaging and subsequent development of sacroiliitis on plain radiography: a prospective, longitudinal study. *J Rheumatol* 1999; 26(9):1953–1958.

28. Geijer M, Gothlin GG, Gothlin JH. The clinical utility of computed tomography compared to conventional radiography in diagnosing sacroiliitis: a retrospective study on 910 patients and literature review. *J Rheumatol* 2007; 34(7):1561–1565.

29. Yu W, Feng F, Dion E, Yang H, et al. Comparison of radiography, computed tomography and magnetic resonance imaging in the detection of sacroiliitis accompanying ankylosing spondylitis. *Skeletal Radiol* 1998; 27(6):311–320.

30. Baraliakos X, Hermann KG, Landewe R, Listing J, et al. Assessment of acute spinal inflammation in patients with ankylosing spondylitis by magnetic resonance imaging: a comparison between contrast enhanced T1 and short tau inversion recovery (STIR) sequences. *Ann Rheum Dis* 2005; 64(8):1141–1144.

31. Hermann KG, Landewe RB, Braun J, van der Heijde DM. Magnetic resonance imaging of inflammatory lesions in the spine in ankylosing spondylitis clinical trials: is paramagnetic contrast medium necessary? *J Rheumatol* 2005; 32(10):2056–2060.

32. Gratacós J, Collado A, Pons F, Osaba M, et al. Significant loss of bone mass in patients with early, active ankylosing spondylitis: a followup study. *Arthritis Rheum* 1999; 42(11):2319–2324.

33. Spoorenberg A, van der Heijde D, de Klerk E, Dougados M, et al. Relative value of erythrocyte sedimentation rate and C-reactive protein in assessment of disease activity in ankylosing spondylitis. *J Rheumatol* 1999; 26(4):980–984.

34. Khan MA, Khan MK. Diagnostic value of HLA-B27 testing ankylosing spondylitis and Reiter's syndrome. *Ann Intern Med* 1982; 96:70–76.

35. Sieper J, Rudwaleit M, Braun J, van der Heijde D. Diagnosing reactive arthritis: role of clinical setting in the value of serologic and microbiologic assays. *Arthritis Rheum* 2002; 46:319–327.

36. Kidd BL, Cawley MI. Delay in diagnosis of spondarthritis. *Br J Rheumatol* 1988; 27(3):230–232.

37. Feldtkeller E, Khan MA, van der Heijde D, van der Linden S, Braun J. Age at disease onset and diagnosis delay in HLA-B27 negative vs. positive patients with ankylosing spondylitis. *Rheumatol Int* 2003; 23(2):61–66.

38. Burgos-Vargas R, Pacheco-Tena C, Vazquez-Mellado J. Juvenile-onset spondyloarthropathies. *Rheum Dis Clin North Am* 1997; 23(3):569–98.

39. Ostensen M, Ostensen H. Ankylosing spondylitis: the female aspect. *J Rheumatol* 1998; 25:120–124.

40. Rudwaleit M, van der Heijde D, Khan MA, Braun J, Sieper J. How to diagnose axial spondyloarthritis early. *Ann Rheum Dis* 2004; 63:535–543.

41. Garrett S, Jenkinson T, Kennedy LG, Whitelock H, et al. A new approach to defining disease status in ankylosing spondylitis: the Bath ankylosing spondylitis disease activity index. *J Rheumatol* 1994; 21(12):2286–2291.

42. Jenkinson TR, Mallorie PA, Whitelock HC, Kennedy LG, et al. Defining spinal mobility in ankylosing spondylitis (AS): the Bath AS metrology index. *J Rheumatol* 1994; 21(9):1694–1698.

43. Calin A, Garrett S, Whitelock H, Kennedy LG, et al. A new approach to defining functional ability in ankylosing spondylitis: the development of the Bath ankylosing spondylitis functional index. *J Rheumatol* 1994; 21(12):2281–2285.

44. Husted JA, Gladman DD, Long JA, Farewell VT. A modified version of the health assessment questionnaire (HAQ) in patients with psoriatic arthritis. *Clin Exp Rheumatol* 1995; 13:439–443.

45. Lorig KR, Mazonson PD, Holman HR. Evidence suggesting that health education for self-management in patients with chronic arthritis has sustained health benefits while reducing health care costs. *Arthritis Rheum* 1993; 36(4):439–446.

46. Haywood KL, Garratt AM, Dziedzic K, Dawes PT. Generic measures of health-related quality of life in ankylosing spondylitis: reliability, validity and responsiveness. *Rheumatology (Oxford)* 2002; 41(12):1380–1387.

47. de Klerk E, van der Linden S, van der Heijde D, Urquhart J. Facilitated analysis of data on drug regimen compliance. *Stat Med* 1997; 16(14):1653–1664.

48. Doran MF, Brophy S, MacKay K, Taylor G, Calin A. Predictors of longterm outcome in ankylosing spondylitis. *J Rheumatol* 2003; 30(2):316–320.

49. Helewa A, Stokes B. Spondylarthropathies. In: Robbins L, et al., eds. *Clinical Care in the Rheumatic Diseases.* 2nd ed. Atlanta, GA: Association of Rheumatology Health Professionals, 2001.

50. Eriendsson J. *Car Driving with Ankylosing Spondylitis.* The Ankylosing Spondylitis International Federation and The National Ankylosing Spondylitis Society of Great Britain, 1997.

51. Sweeney S, Taylor G, Calin A. The effect of a home based exercise intervention package on outcome in ankylosing spondylitis: a randomized controlled trial. *J Rheumatol* 2002; 29(4):763–766.

52. Kraag G, Stokes B, Groh J, Helewa A, Goldsmith C. The effects of comprehensive home physiotherapy and supervision on patients with ankylosing spondylitis—a randomized controlled trial. *J Rheumatol* 1990; 17(2):228–233.

53. Kraag G, Stokes B, Groh J, Helewa A, Goldsmith CH. The effects of comprehensive home physiotherapy and supervision on patients with ankylosing spondylitis—an 8-month followup. *J Rheumatol* 1994; 21(2):261–263.

54. Lim HJ, Moon YI, Lee MS. Effects of home-based daily exercise therapy on joint mobility, daily activity, pain, and depression in patients with ankylosing spondylitis. *Rheumatol Int* 2005; 25(3):225–229.

55. Lim HJ, Lee MS, Lim HS. Exercise, pain, perceived family support, and quality of life in Korean patients with ankylosing spondylitis. *Psychol Rep* 2005; 96(1):3–8.

56. Uhrin Z, Kuzis S, Ward MM. Exercise and changes in health status in patients with ankylosing spondylitis. *Arch Intern Med* 2000; 160(19): 2969–2975.

57. Hidding A, van der Linden S, Boers M, Gielen X, et al. Is group physical therapy superior to individualized therapy in ankylosing spondylitis? A randomized controlled trial. *Arthritis Care Res* 1993; 6(3):117–125.

58. Fernandez-de-Las-Penas C, Alonso-Blanco C, Morales-Cabezas M, Miangolarra-Page JC. Two exercise interventions for the management of patients with ankylosing spondylitis: a randomized controlled trial. *Am J Phys Med Rehabil* 2005; 84(6):407–419.

59. Fernandez-de-Las-Penas C, Alonso-Blanco C, Alguacil-Diego IM, Miangolarra Page JC. One-year follow-up of two exercise interventions for the management of patients with ankylosing spondylitis: a randomized controlled trial. *Am J Phys Med Rehabil* 2006; 85(7): 559–567.

60. Bulstrode SJ, Barefoot J, Harrison RA, Clarke AK. The role of passive stretching in the treatment of ankylosing spondylitis. *Br J Rheumatol* 1987; 26(1):40–42.

61. Ince G, Sarpel T, Durgun B, Erdogan S. Effects of a multimodal exercise program for people with ankylosing spondylitis. *Phys Ther* 2006; 86(7):924–935.

62. Analay Y, Ozcan E, Karan A, Diracoglu D, Aydin R. The effectiveness of intensive group exercise on patients with ankylosing spondylitis. *Clin Rehabil* 2003; 17(6):631–636.

63. Van Tubergen A, Boonen A, Landewe R, Rutten-Van Molken M, et al. Cost effectiveness of combined spa-exercise therapy in ankylosing spondylitis: a randomized controlled trial. *Arthritis Rheum* 2002; 47(5):459–467.

64. Helliwell PS, Abbott CA, Chamberlain MA. A randomised trial of three different physiotherapy regimes in ankylosing spondylitis. *Physiotherapy* 1996; 82:85–90.

65. Altan L, Bingol U, Aslan M, Yurtkuran M. The effect of balneotherapy on patients with ankylosing spondylitis. *Scand J Rheumatol* 2006; 35(4):283–289.

66. Band DA, Jones SD, Kennedy LG, Garrett SL, et al. Which patients with ankylosing spondylitis derive most benefit from an inpatient management program? *J Rheumatol* 1997; 24(12):2381–2384.

67. Heikkila S, Viitanen JV, Kautiainen H, Kauppi M. Sensitivity to change of mobility tests: effect of short term intensive physiotherapy and exercise on spinal, hip, and shoulder measurements in spondyloarthropathy. *J Rheumatol* 2000; 27(5):1251–1256.

68. Lubrano E, D'Angelo S, Parsons WJ, Corbi G, et al. Effectiveness of rehabilitation in active ankylosing spondylitis assessed by the ASAS response criteria. *Rheumatology (Oxford)* in press.

69. Lubrano E, D'Angelo S, Parsons WJ, Serino F, et al. Effects of a combination treatment of an intensive rehabilitation program and etanercept in patients with ankylosing spondylitis: a pilot study. *J Rheumatol* 2006; 33(10):2029–2034.

70. Dagfinrud H, Kvien TK, Hagen KB. Physiotherapy interventions for ankylosing spondylitis. *Cochrane Database Syst Rev* 2004; 4:CD002822.

71. Boulos P, Dougados M, Macleod SM, Hunsche E. Pharmacological treatment of ankylosing spondylitis: a systematic review. *Drugs* 2005; 65(15):2111–2127.

72. Garcia Rodriguez LA. Variability in risk of gastrointestinal complications with different nonsteroidal anti-inflammatory drugs. *Am J Med* 1998; 104:30S–34S.

73. Lewis SC, Langman MJ, Laporte JR, Matthews JN, et al. Dose-response relationships between individual nonaspirin nonsteroidal anti-inflammatory drugs (NANSAIDs) and serious upper gastrointestinal bleeding: a meta-analysis based on individual patient data. *Br J Clin Pharmacol* 2002; 54(3):320–326.

74. Deeks JJ, Smith LA, Bradley MD. Efficacy, tolerability, and upper gastrointestinal safety of celecoxib for treatment of osteoarthritis and rheumatoid arthritis: systematic review of randomised controlled trials. *BMJ* 2002; 325(7365):619–623.

75. Hooper L, Brown TJ, Elliott R, Payne K, et al. The effectiveness of five strategies for the prevention of gastrointestinal toxicity induced by non-steroidal anti-inflammatory drugs: systematic review. *BMJ* 2004; 329(7472):948.

76. Juni P, Nartey L, Reichenbach S, Sterchi R, et al. Risk of cardiovascular events and rofecoxib: cumulative meta-analysis. *Lancet* 2004; 364(9450):2021–2029.

77. Solomon SD, McMurray JJ, Pfeffer MA, Wittes J, et al. Adenoma Prevention with Celecoxib (APC) Study Investigators. Cardiovascular risk associated with celecoxib in a clinical trial for colorectal adenoma prevention. *N Engl J Med* 2005; 352(11):1071–1080.

78. Bolten WW. Problem of the atherothrombotic potential of non-steroidal anti-inflammatory drugs. *Ann Rheum Dis* 2006; 65(1):7–13.

79. White WB, West CR, Borer JS, Gorelick PB, et al. Risk of cardiovascular events in patients receiving celecoxib: a meta-analysis of randomized clinical trials. *Am J Cardiol* 2007; 99(1):91–98.

80. Wanders A, Heijde D, Landewé R, Béhier JM, et al. Inhibition of radiographic progression in ankylosing spondylitis (AS) by continuous use of NSAIDs. *Arthritis Rheum* 2005; 52(6):1756–1765.

81. Ward MM. Prospects for disease modification in ankylosing spondylitis: do nonsteroidal antiinflammatory drugs do more than treat symptoms? *Arthritis Rheum* 2005; 52:1634–1636.

82. Sarzi-Puttini P, Santandrea S, Boccassini L, Panni B, Caruso I. The role of NSAIDs in psoriatic arthritis: evidence from a controlled study with nimesulide. *Clin Exp Rheumatol* 2001; 19(1 Suppl 22):S17–S20.

83. Palazzi C, Olivieri I, D'Amico E, Pennese E, Petricca A. Management of reactive arthritis. *Expert Opin Pharmacother* 2004; 5(1):61–70.

84. Mahadevan U, Loftus EV Jr, Tremaine WJ, Sandborn WJ. Safety of selective cyclooxygenase-2 inhibitors in inflammatory bowel disease. *Am J Gastroenterol* 2002; 97(4):910–914.

85. Meador R, Hsia E, Kitumnuaypong T, Schumacher HR. TNF involvement and anti-TNF therapy of reactive and unclassified arthritis. *Clin Exp Rheumatol* 2002; 20(6 Suppl 28):S130–S134.

86. van der Heijde D, Dijkmans B, Geusens P, Sieper J, et al. Ankylosing Spondylitis Study for the Evaluation of Recombinant Infliximab Therapy Study Group. Efficacy and safety of infliximab in patients with ankylosing spondylitis: results of a randomized, placebo-controlled trial (ASSERT). *Arthritis Rheum* 2005; 52(2):582–591.

87. Braun J, Baraliakos X, Brandt J, Listing J, et al. Persistent clinical response to the anti-TNF-alpha antibody infliximab in patients with ankylosing spondylitis over 3 years. *Rheumatology (Oxford)* 2005; 44(5):670–676.

88. van der Heijde D, Han C, DeVlam K, Burmester G, et al. Infliximab improves productivity and reduces workday loss in patients with ankylosing spondylitis: results from a randomized, placebo-controlled trial. *Arthritis Rheum* 2006; 55(4):569–574.

89. Davis JC Jr, Van Der Heijde D, Braun J, Dougados M, et al. Enbrel Ankylosing Spondylitis Study Group. Recombinant human tumor necrosis factor receptor (etanercept) for treating ankylosing spondylitis: a randomized, controlled trial. *Arthritis Rheum* 2003; 48(11): 3230–3236.

90. Braun J, McHugh N, Singh A, Wajdula JS, Sato R. Improvement in patient-reported outcomes for patients with ankylosing spondylitis treated with etanercept 50 mg once-weekly and 25 mg twice-weekly. *Rheumatology (Oxford)* 2007; 46(6):999–1004.

91. Davis JC, van der Heijde DM, Braun J, Dougados M, et al. Sustained durability and tolerability of etanercept in ankylosing spondylitis for 96 weeks. *Ann Rheum Dis* 2005; 64(11):1557–1562.

92. van der Heijde D, Kivitz A, Schiff MH, Sieper J, et al. ATLAS Study Group. Efficacy and safety of adalimumab in patients with ankylosing spondylitis: results of a multicenter, randomized, double-blind, placebo-controlled trial. *Arthritis Rheum* 2006; 54(7):2136–2146.

93. Davis JC Jr, Revicki D, van der Heijde DM, Rentz AM, et al. Health-related quality of life outcomes in patients with active ankylosing spondylitis treated with adalimumab: results from a randomized controlled study. *Arthritis Rheum* 2007; 57(6):1050–1057.

94. Braun J, Landewe R, Hermann KG, Han J, et al. ASSERT Study Group. Major reduction in spinal inflammation in patients with ankylosing spondylitis after treatment with infliximab: results of a multicenter, randomized, double-blind, placebo-controlled magnetic resonance imaging study. *Arthritis Rheum* 2006; 54(5):1646–1652.

95. Baraliakos X, Davis J, Tsuji W, Braun J. Magnetic resonance imaging examinations of the spine in patients with ankylosing spondylitis before and after therapy with the tumor necrosis factor alpha receptor fusion protein etanercept. *Arthritis Rheum* 2005; 52(4):1216–1223.

96. Haibel H, Rudwaleit M, Brandt HC, Grozdanovic Z, et al. Adalimumab reduces spinal symptoms in active ankylosing spondylitis: clinical and magnetic resonance imaging results of a fifty-two-week open-label trial. *Arthritis Rheum* 2006; 54(2):678–681.

97. Baraliakos X, Listing J, Brandt J, Haibel H, et al. Radiographic progression in patients with ankylosing spondylitis after 4 yrs of treatment with the anti-TNF-{alpha} antibody infliximab. *Rheumatology (Oxford)* 2007; 46(9):1450–1453.

98. Demis E, Roux C, Breban M, Dougados M. Infliximab in spondylarthropathy—influence on bone density. *Clin Exp Rheumatol* 2002; 20:S185–S186.

99. Braun J, Davis J, Dougados M, Sieper J, et al. First update of the international ASAS consensus statement for the use of anti-TNF agents in patients with ankylosing spondylitis. *Ann Rheum Dis* 2006; 65(3):316–320.

100. Conti F, Ceccarelli F, Marocchi E, Magrini L, et al. Switching TNF (alpha} antagonists in patients with ankylosing spondylitis and psoriatic arthritis: an observational study over a five-year period. *Ann Rheum Dis* in press.

101. Gomez-Reino JJ, Carmona L. BIOBADASER Group. Switching TNF antagonists in patients with chronic arthritis: an observational study of 488 patients over a four-year period. *Arthritis Res Ther* 2006; 8(1):R29.

102. Barkham N, Kong KO, Tennant A, Fraser A, et al. The unmet need for anti-tumour necrosis factor (anti-TNF) therapy in ankylosing spondylitis. *Rheumatology (Oxford)* 2005; 44(10):1277–1281.

103. Chen J, Liu C. Is sulfasalazine effective in ankylosing spondylitis? A systematic review of randomized controlled trials. *J Rheumatol* 2006; 33(4):722–731.

104. Chen J, Liu C, Lin J. Methotrexate for ankylosing spondylitis. *Cochrane Database Syst Rev* 2006; 4:CD004524.

105. van Denderen JC, van der Paardt M, Nurmohamed MT, de Ryck YM, et al. Double blind, randomised, placebo controlled study of leflunomide in the treatment of active ankylosing spondylitis. *Ann Rheum Dis* 2005; 64(12):1761–1764.

106. Koh WH, Pande I, Samuels A, Jones SD, Calin A. Low dose amitriptyline in ankylosing spondylitis: a short term, double blind, placebo controlled study. *J Rheumatology* 1997; 24:2158–2161.

107. Zochling J, van der Heijde D, Burgos-Vargas R, Collantes E, et al. The Assessment in AS International Working Group and the European League Against Rheumatism. ASAS/EULAR recommendations for the management of ankylosing spondylitis. *Ann Rheum Dis* 2006; 65(4):442–452.

108. Ticó N, Ramon S, Garcia-Ortun F, Ramirez L, et al. Traumatic spinal cord injury complicating ankylosing spondylitis. *Spinal Cord* 1998; 36:349–352.

109. Hitchon PW, From AM, Brenton MD, Glaser JA, Torner JC. Fractures of the thoracolumbar spine complicating ankylosing spondylitis. *J Neurosurg* 2002; 97(2 Suppl):218–222.

110. Bilgen IG, Yunten N, Ustun EE, Oksel F, Gumusdis G. Adhesive arachnoiditis causing cauda equina syndrome in ankylosing spondylitis: CT and MRI demonstration of dural calcification and a dorsal dural diverticulum. *Neuroradiology* 1999; 41:508–511.

111. Ginsburg WW, Cohen MD, Miller GM, Bartleson JD. Posterior vertebral body erosion by arachnoid diverticula in cauda equina syndrome: an unusual manifestation of ankylosing spondylitis. *J Rheumatol* 1997; 24:1417–1420.

112. Shim SC, Yoo DH, Lee JK, Koh HK, et al. Multiple cerebellar infarction due to vertebral artery obstruction and bulbar symptoms associated with vertical subluxation and atlanto-occipital subluxation in ankylosing spondylitis. *J Rheumatol* 1998; 25(12):2464–2468.

113. Thompson GH, Khan MA, Bilenker RM. Spontaneous atlantoaxial subluxation as a presenting manifestation of juvenile ankylosing spondylitis: a case report. *Spine* 1982; 7:78–79.

114. Chen LH, Kao FC, Niu CC, Lai PL, et al. Surgical treatment of spinal pseudoarthrosis in ankylosing spondylitis. *Chang Gung Med J* 2005; 28(9):621–628.

115. van Royen BJ, de Kleuver M, Slot GH. Polysegmental lumbar posterior wedge osteotomies for correction of kyphosis in ankylosing spondylitis. *Eur Spine J* 1998; 7(2):104–110.

116. Sweeney S, Gupta R, Taylor G, Calin A. Total hip arthroplasty in ankylosing spondylitis: outcome in 340 patients. *J Rheumatol* 2001; 28(8):1862–1866.

117. Spoorenberg A, de Vlam K, van der Linden S, Dougados M, et al. Radiological scoring methods in ankylosing spondylitis: reliability and sensitivity to change over one year. *J Rheumatol* 1999; 26:997–1002.

54 Surgical Management of Spondyloarthropathies in the Spinal Cord Injury Patient

Angela E. Downes
Kornelis A. Poelstra

ANKYLOSING SPONDYLITIS

Ankylosing spondylitis (AS), also known as Bekhterev's disease, is the most common spondyloarthropathy and is characterized by ossification of intervertebral disks, joints, and ligaments (1). Greater than 90% of cases are associated with human leukocyte antigen (HLA)-B27 surface antigen in the serum and sacroiliitis. The incidence of AS in the general population is 1 per 1000. The highest prevalence has been reported within Caucasian males in the United States and approaches 1.5%. AS usually starts relatively early in life, between the ages of 10 and 40 years. Juxtaarticular osteitis commonly develops in the sacroiliac (SI) joints at presentation, and the inflammatory [transforming growth factor-β (TGF-β) containing] fibrocartilage subsequently ossifies, leading to bony ankyloses. This process also occurs at the vertebral end plates where syndesmophytes form across the disk space and fuse to create an ankylosed or characteristic "bamboo spine" (Figure 54.1) (1).

Classification

AS is the prototype of the spondyloarthropathies. Other inflammatory conditions in this group are reactive arthritis (Reiter's syndrome), psoriatic arthritis, enteropathic spondyloarthropathy, juvenile-onset spondyloarthropathy, and undifferentiated spondyloarthropathy (2). Of these, AS has the strongest association with the HLA-B27 molecule and there is no generally accepted subclassification within AS.

WORKUP

History

The presenting complaint of AS is often chronic lower back pain. Often symptoms of night pain and morning stiffness that improves with activity are reported. In the other spondyloarthropathies, peripheral joint pain and stiffness usually antedate spinal symptoms. In AS, both SI joints are typically involved, and diffuse pain can then ascend to involve the entire spine (3). Spinal mobility gradually decreases and lumbar lordosis flattens while thoracic kyphosis increases. To compensate for this, the cervical spine must hyperextend to allow the patients to see the horizon. When the neck is unable to compensate for the kyphosis of the thoracic region, the patient loses the ability to look forward at the horizon.

Physical Examination

Decreased mobility of the lumbar spine in spondyloarthropathies can be assessed with the modified Schober's test: The L5 spinous process is marked (the same level as the posterior superior iliac spine on the pelvis), and a mark is made 10 cm superior.

Upon maximal forward bending, the distance between the two sites should increase by 5 cm. An increase less than 2.5 cm is significant.

Spinal Imaging

Anteroposterior (AP) pelvis, modified AP-Ferguson views, and oblique SI joint views may show early involvement of the SI joints when the diagnosis is suspected. Subsequent erosive changes typically begin to appear on the inferior half of the SI joint on the iliac side. Magnetic resonance imaging (MRI) and computed tomography (CT) can be helpful for early recognition, but currently no diagnostic criteria exist for these modalities (1). Erosions at the corners of the vertebral bodies occur early, giving them a squared appearance. Symmetric development of syndesmophytes and continuous paraspinal ligamentous calcification eventually leads to the characteristic "bamboo spine" (Figure 54.1). This should not be confused with diffuse idiopathic skeletal hyperostosis (DISH), which is not an arthropathy but a bone-forming diathesis. However, the classic bamboo spine radiograph actually occurs in only a minority of patients.

Treatment

Because no specific therapy is currently available for the treatment of AS, maintenance of range of motion is of extreme importance. Nonsteroidal antiinflammatory drugs (NSAIDs) and directed

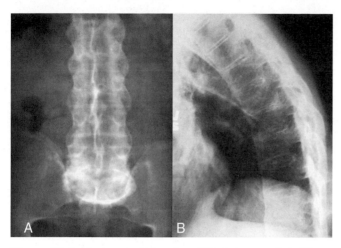

Figure 54.1 Anteroposterior view (**A**) of characteristic "bamboo spine" in AS with fused SI joints. Lateral view (**B**) shows increased kyphosis with bridging bone across the intervertebral disks.

physical activity and stretching are the mainstay of treatment. Sulfasalazine has shown benefit in NSAID nonresponders. Multiple clinical trials, actively supported by patient advocacy groups, are being performed with infliximab, etanercept, thalidomide, and pamidronate. (4–6) Tumor necrosis factor-α (TNF-α) and TGF-β blockade drugs are said to show promising results (5, 6). Surgery is generally considered for patients with severe spinal deformities that result in severe functional consequences. Various spinal osteotomies have been used to treat kyphotic deformities of the AS spine. Radiotherapy has been effective in unresponsive cases of AS, but is linked with increased risk for acute myelogenous leukemia.

Outcome

Patients with AS are prone to spine fractures from even minor trauma. Therefore, the AS patient with pain following trauma should be considered to have a fracture until proven otherwise. With trauma, the spine often fractures through a calcified disk space in between two ankylosed segments, resulting in an unstable injury prone to displacement. Neurologic injury or deterioration is common in AS patients with unstable fractures; therefore, surgical stabilization is generally indicated when an unstable fracture is present (7). Plain films often fail to demonstrate nondisplaced fractures; therefore, computed tomography (CT) or MRI is useful in evaluating the AS patient after trauma (8).

Complications

Vertebroplasty is generally contraindicated in patients with ankylosing disease. The long lever arm mentioned above will cause increased stress over the treated vertebral elements and may prevent healing. Pseudarthrosis develops and spinal instability may result with increased risk for spinal cord or nerve-root compression. Stabilization of unstable fractures with internal fixation of multiple segments is generally successful for allowing fractures to heal, but long constructs may be complicated by subsequent fractures above or below the construct due to the lack of a mobile spinal segment.

DIFFUSE IDIOPATHIC SKELETAL HYPEROSTOSIS

Diffuse idiopathic skeletal hyperostosis (DISH), or Forestier's disease, is a fairly common (up to 28% of elderly patients) degenerative disorder of unknown etiology, affecting mostly older patients (45 to 85 years old), Caucasians, and men (65%) more than women. It was first described in 1950 as a disorder characterized by spinal stiffness, osteophytosis, and "flowing" new bone formation along the margins of the thoracic spine (Figure 54.2A). The anterior longitudinal ligament (ALL) is usually most involved, most commonly in cervical and lower thoracic levels (9).

Although the disease is more prevalent in certain families, no clear genetic association in the human leukocyte antigen (HLA) system has been identified, and no relationships have been found with either rheumatoid arthritis or ankylosing spondylitis, with which it is often confused. DISH can be associated with type II diabetes, obesity, biliary stones, atheromatous vascular disorders, hypertension, and lipid- and purine metabolism disorders.

Classification

DISH is characterized by ossification of the ligamentous insertions (fibro-osteosis) and ossification/calcification of tendons, ligaments, and fascia in both the axial and the appendicular skeleton. This is caused by invasion of blood vessels into cartilage and differentiation of pluripotent cells into osteoblasts. The most common symptoms of DISH are spinal rigidity and decreased joint mobility with occasional dysphagia from esophagus compression (Figure 54.2B). Pain and nerve root irritation due to narrowing of the vertebral foramina rarely occur, but spinal cord compression secondary to ossification of the posterior

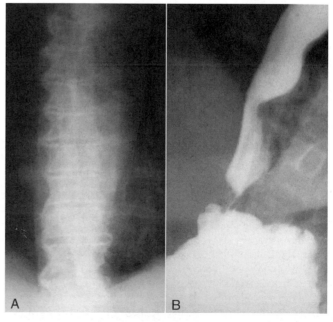

Figure 54.2 (**A**) Characteristic chest X-ray finding of "flowing" bone on right side of the thoracic spinal column. (**B**) Dysphagia due to large DISH-anterior osteophyte compressing the esophagus.

longitudinal ligament can cause myelopathy. The diagnostic criteria for DISH include (1) flowing ossifications along the anterolateral aspect of at least four thoracic vertebrae, and (2) absence of facet-joint ankylosis or sacroiliac sclerosis (these criteria belong to ankylosing spondylitis).(9–12) Interestingly, the right side of the spine is most often affected, most likely due to the aortic pulsation on the left. In addition to the spine, other sites of ossification are involved such as the triceps insertion, Achilles' tendon, plantar aponeurosis, and quadriceps and patellar tendons.

Workup

History

Most patients are asymptomatic, or have short episodes of "periarthritis" due to activation of the enthesopathy process. For the spine, patients usually have a history of stiffness, especially after periods of immobility, but also upon forward bending (9). They also may have mild to moderate pain in the mid to lower back region. Complaints are fairly nonspecific, but radiographic findings may be dramatic. DISH is often discovered incidentally and is predominantly a radiographic diagnosis.

Spinal Imaging

The T7 to T11 levels are most frequently involved and the changes are often visible even on a chest radiograph. Flowing candle wax forms extraarticular ankyloses in DISH as opposed to vertically oriented osteophytes in the "bamboo-spine" in AS that form intra-articular ankyloses (1, 10). Disk space narrowing is minimal and the facet joints are usually preserved. A bone scan generally shows increased uptake and can raise the suspicion of a malignancy. Axial computed tomography (CT) cuts show a thin radiotransparent band between the calcified ALL and the vertebral body wall on the right side of the anterior spine.

Treatment

Because no specific drug therapy has been discovered, simple analgesics or nonsteroidal antiinflammatory drugs (NSAIDs) are usually rendered.

Outcome

Improved flexibility and activities of daily living were successfully maintained for up to two years after the end of an active rehabilitation program (9). Cases associated with symptomatic stenosis may require surgical decompression.

SPINAL TRAUMA IN AS AND DISH

Patients suffering from AS and DISH are at high risk for spine fractures. Delayed diagnosis is frequent because the trauma is often trivial. The AS or DISH patient with pain following trauma should be considered to have a fracture until proven otherwise. Hyperextension injuries occur most frequently through an entire vertebral body, or through a disk space in between the ankylosed segments; the incidence of neurologic compromise is relatively high. The long lever arm that develops as a consequence of the ankylosis of multiple vertebral elements causes fractures to

displace easily. For the same reason, the incidence of three-column injuries is increased in these patients. Involved areas need to be imaged with either CT or magnetic resonance imaging (MRI) to rule out global spinal instability, because this is usually underrepresented on plain radiographs. Neurologic injury or deterioration is common in AS patients with unstable fractures; therefore, surgical stabilization is generally indicated when an unstable fracture is present. Pseudarthrosis develops and spinal instability may result with increased risk for spinal cord or nerve-root compression. Decompression and instrumentation of the involved elements may become complicated by subsequent fractures above or below the construct (stress-riser) due to the lack of mobile motion segments.

In AS, the most affected sites for injury are the lower cervical spine and the thoracolumbar junction. Injuries to the thoracolumbar junction commonly occur as simple compressions, transverse shear fractures, and stress fractures. When evaluating a patient with AS or DISH for spinal fracture, the history should focus on changes in posture, worsening of kyphosis, or alterations in coronal or sagittal alignment. A complete neurologic examination should be performed, as the rate of neurologic injury following spine fracture is up to 50% in these patients. CT should be performed to check for bony alignment and assess for fracture in greater detail. MRI is useful for evaluating ALL and posterior longitudinal ligament (PLL) constitution as well as to determine the presence of a compressive epidural hematoma. An unstable ALL has been found in 87% of cases, and is an important complicating factor.

Radiographic examination and evaluation of AS and DISH patients requires special attention to positioning and the use of backboards or rigid cervical collars. Neutral spine alignment can cause or exacerbate a spinal cord injury. The lateral decubitus position should be used for severe kyphosis. When moving or positioning a patient, particularly during the first 24 hours following an injury, frequent neurological reassessment is necessary to monitor epidural hematoma formation or fracture changes. In patients with nonoperative conditions, immobilization may be achieved with an orthosis, such as a halo vest or custom molded orthoses.

In patients who can medically tolerate surgery for their injuries, early surgical stabilization should be encouraged, especially for unstable three-column fractures, extension type injuries, and shear injuries. Surgery should entail decompression of the cord, stabilization of the spinal column, or both; however, simultaneous deformity correction should not be undertaken. Immediate stabilization and decompression, if neurological deficit is present, are the goals of surgery in the setting of injury.

When preparing for surgery, great care must be taken to ensure proper patient positioning. The lateral decubitus position is recommended in the setting of advanced AS. If posterior cervical stabilization is necessary, a seated position with a halo vest with the posterior half removed may be utilized. Most commonly, anterior-posterior instrumentated fusion with multiple posterior fixation points is necessary in cervical spine injuries in AS and DISH patients. Even if fusion is limited to the anterior column, care must be taken to avoid over-lengthening the spine and causing further injury to the posterior column. Halo vest immobilization is useful in this setting.

In thoracic-level injuries, posterior-only fusions are most commonly performed. However, this poses a risk of over-lengthening the spine, resulting in cord traction and worsening neurologic status. Hook and screw systems are useful for this situation because they balance compression and distraction throughout multiple levels, and they allow instrumentation in the setting of kyphosis. AS and DISH pathology can obscure bony landmarks for screw placement, so intraoperative fluoroscopy is necessary. Fusions from one to four levels above and below the injury have been shown to be successful (8, 9). If the anterior column is injured, such as in a burst fractures, anterior decompression may be required. Cage

devices are contraindicated in the setting of osteoporosis, because implant failure is high in these patients (8, 9). Allograft or iliac crest bone graft should be used instead.

SUMMARY

AS and DISH are distinct pathological processes affecting the spine, but both result in increased susceptibility to fracture, putting the cord at risk with what is even considered to be trivial

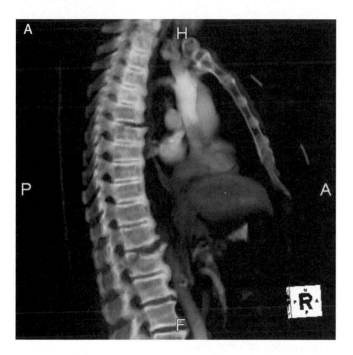

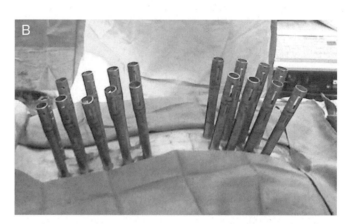

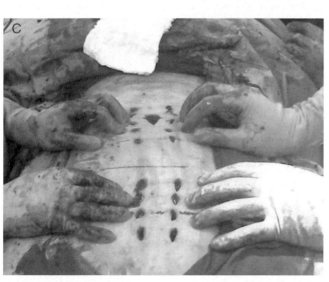

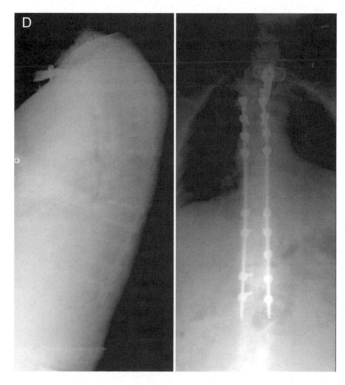

Figure 54.3 (A) CT-scan reconstruction showing T5–T6 and T11–T12 distraction extension injuries with spinal instability in a non-braceable candidate (polytrauma and 320lbs). (B) Intra-operative images showing screw extensions from T4 to L2 on the prone patient for pedicle screw placement at all these levels to address both fractures and bridge the intervening segment to reduce the risk for spinal fracture due to mismatched rigidity of the spine between instrumented and non-instrumented segments. (C) Minimal incisions and minimal blood loss after screw-extension removal and placement of interconnecting rods to stabilize the spine. (D) Four-month post-operative follow-up with AP (left) and lateral (right) radiographs showing excellent alignment and fracture healing without limitations for the patients rehabilitation.

trauma. Patients with these pathologies are difficult to manage because of positioning and surgical cases that demand special care. Whenever there is spine pain associated with even trivial trauma, emergency personnel should have a low threshold to suspected fractures with impending neurologic injury. Neurological checks must be performed after positioning or transporting the patient in the setting of spinal injury, and CT and MRI examinations must be repeated if any neurological change is noted. If neurological deficits are apparent, early surgical intervention with fixation is key to stabilization. Traditional stiff cervical collars and patient positioning are often not appropriate, and forcing the diseased spine into normal alignment can create further issues or worsen the injury. The use of halo vests and placing the patient in lateral decubitus position with surgical beanbags is encouraged in the operating room. The risks of surgery in this patient population are great, and medical management should be attempted if possible, considering the health status of the patient and the experience and skills of the surgeon and operating room team.

Special attention needs to be given to patients that suffer multi-level fractures in an ankylosed spinal column. In case of spinal cord compromise from any of these injury levels (whether tetraplegia or paraplegia is the result), careful attention needs to be focused on the fused spinal segments between the injured vertebral elements. If a patient has compromised mobility, paralysis, or tetraplegia and requires help for transfers, without the ability to use muscles to stabilize the spinal column, the spine is at risk for further fractures. Especially if spinal hardware is used, there is a mismatch in the modulus of elasticity between the rigidly fused spine and the ankylosed segments above and below. If the spine is fractured at two places (floating spine), strong consideration needs to be given to bridging the intermediate segments between the individual fractures. An example of a patient case with DISH is presented in Figure 54.3.

This case represents an example of "Extreme Minimally Invasive Stabilization" or Extreme MIS for patients with SCI and fractures. The patient (320lbs, male) was struck as a pedestrian by a large Sport Utility Vehicle and sustained multiple extremity fractures. Imaging studies also exhibited extension-distraction injuries at T5–T6 and T11–T12 level in the face of ankylosing disease. The spine was reduced and stabilized using only minimally invasive technique across all levels (T4–L2). No formal arthrodesis was performed, because these near "long-bone" fractures typically heal in patients with DISH. They are ideal candidates for treatment with MIS screw fixation only because of their ability to heal these fractures reliably because of the underlying condition.

After 4-month follow-up, there was a solid arthrodesis across both fractures, and patient progressed well with his rehabilitation.

References

1. Bennett DL, Ohashi K, El-Khoury GY. Spondyloarthropathies: ankylosing spondylitis Radiol Clin North Am 2004; 42:121–134.
2. Kataria RK, Brent LH. Spondyloarthropathies. Am Fam Physician 2004; 69:2853–2860.
3. Newman PA, Bruckel JC. Spondylitis association of America: the member-directed, organization addressing the needs of ankylosing spondylitis patients. Rheum Dis 29:561–574.
4. Davis JC Jr, Huang F, Maksymowych W. New therapies for ankylosing spondylitis: etanercept, and pamidronate. Rheum Dis Clin North Am 2003; 29:481–494.
5. Miceli-Richard C, van der Heijde D, Dougados M. Spondyloarthropathy for practicing diagnosis, indication for disease-controlling antirheumatic therapy, and evaluation. Rheum Dis Clin North Am 2003; 29:449–462.
6. Shaikh SA, Clauw DJ. Inflammatory diseases. In: Frymoyer JW, Wiesel SW. *The Adult* 3rd ed., vol 1. Philadelphia: Lippincott Williams & Wilkins, 2004; 141–164.
7. Hitchon PW, From AM, Brenton MD, Glaser JA, Torner JC. Fractures of the thoracolumbar complicating ankylosing spondylitis. J Neurosurg (Spine 2) 2002; 97:218–222.
8. May PJ, Raunest J, Herdmann J, Jonas M. Behandlung der Wirbelsäulenfraktur Spondylitis. Unfallchirurg 2002; 105:165–169.
9. Belanger TA, Rowe DE. Diffuse idiopathic skeletal hyperostosis: musculoskeletal manifestations. J Am Acad Orthop Surg 2001; 9:258–267.
10. Cammisa M, De Serio A, Guglielmi G. Diffuse idiopathic skeletal hyperostosis. Eur J Radiol 1998; 27:S7–S11.
11. Mata S, Hill RO, Joseph L, et al. Chest radiographs as a screening test for diffuse idiopathic skeletal hyperostosis. J Rheumatol 1993; 20:1905–1910.
12. Resnick D, Niwayama G. Diffuse idiopathic skeletal hyperostosis (Dros Inf ServH): ankylosing hyperostosis of Forestier and Rotes-Querol. In: Resnick D, ed. *Diagnosis of Bone and Joint Disorders*, 3rd ed., vol 3. Philadelphia: WB Saunders, 1995; 1436–1495.

VII

REHABILITATION

55 Wheelchairs and Seating for People with Spinal Cord Injuries

Rory A. Cooper
Rosemarie Cooper
Michael L. Boninger
Emily Teodorski
Tricia Thorman
Tamra Pelleschi

Due to the growing populations of people with disabilities and older people, the need for mobility devices is expected to continue to grow (1). Expenditures for mobility devices currently exceed $5 billion annually, with wheelchairs and scooters representing a substantial portion of this market. Wheelchairs allow individuals to complete daily tasks with greater independence and to access school, work, and community environments (2–6). Vital to the individuals who use them, wheelchairs ideally become an extension of self (7). Similar to prosthetic devices, wheelchairs replace the function of a body part, and must be custom fit to the individual. If subsequent changes occur to an individual that alter his or her wheelchair fit, additional adjustments will be required. With the assortment of colors, styles, and features now available, wheelchairs can also serve as a means of self-expression. Depending on their complexity, wheelchairs range in price from about $100 to $35,000 each (8, 9). Wheelchairs have been in use for several hundred years and continue to evolve in their design and use (Figure 55.1). However, much remains to be learned about optimum design and safe use of wheelchairs (10–12).

Models of manual wheelchairs have improved dramatically from a "one size fits all" depot-style design for transport developed during the 1950s (Figure 55.2) (13, 14). Today, custom-fit ultralight manual wheelchairs are available for active wheelchair users (Figure 55.3). Advancements in powered, wheeled mobility continue to enhance functional independence for individuals with more severe disabilities (Figures 55.4 and 55.5).

MANUAL WHEELCHAIRS

Manual wheelchairs have developed rapidly in recent years. A few years ago there was only one style of wheelchair and it came in one color: chrome. Now, there are numerous types of wheelchairs to choose from and they come in a wide range of colors.

Wheelchairs have moved from being chairs with wheels designed to provide some minimal mobility, to advanced orthotics designed to meet the mobility demands of the active user (15). The proper selection and design of a wheelchair depends upon the abilities of the user and on the intended use. Thus, specialized wheelchairs have been, and continue to be developed to yield better performance for the user.

Depot and Attendant-Propelled Wheelchairs

The depot, or institutional wheelchair, is essentially the same wheelchair that was produced in the 1940s. Some depot wheelchairs may be a bit lighter than the 1940s models, but the basic frame design is unchanged. Depot wheelchairs are intended for institutional use, such as in airports, hospitals, and nursing care facilities, where several people may use the same wheelchair. In general, they are inappropriate for active individuals who use wheelchairs for personal mobility. Depot wheelchairs are designed to be inexpensive, to accommodate large variations in body size, to be low maintenance, and to be attendant propelled. Hence, they are generally heavier and their performance is limited.

Many depot wheelchairs are manufactured in developing countries where low labor costs make the manufacture of inexpensive chairs possible (16). The design of a depot wheelchair typically incorporates swing-away footrests, removable armrests, a single cross-brace frame, and solid tires. Swing-away footrests make transferring in to and out of the wheelchair easier; however, they add weight to the wheelchair. Armrests can help to provide some comfort and stability to the depot wheelchair user and they can aid in keeping clothing off of the wheels. Depot chairs typically fold to reduce required storage area and to allow for the chair to fit into an automobile. Solid tires are commonly used to reduce maintenance, but they often dramatically reduce ride

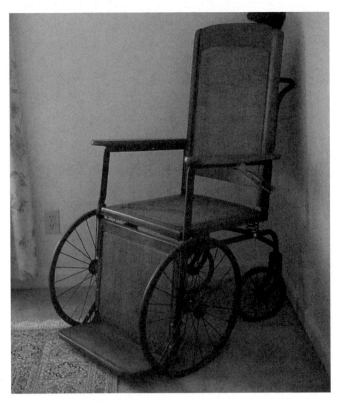

Figure 55.1 Attendant-propelled wheelchair, circa 1920s.

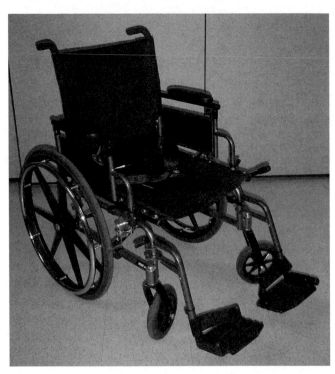

Figure 55.2 Heavy, folding-frame, depot-style wheelchair with no adjustability.

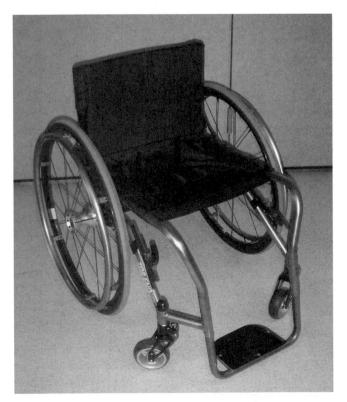

Figure 55.3 Ultralight, adjustable manual wheelchair with rigid frame.

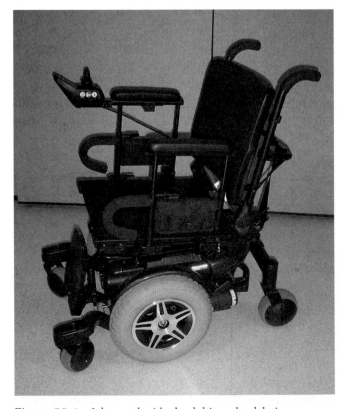

Figure 55.4 Advanced mid-wheel drive wheelchair.

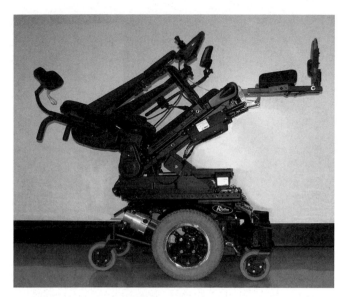

Figure 55.5   Advanced power wheelchair.

comfort and add weight. Therefore, pneumatic tires are recommended when the chair will be used outdoors. Adjustments to the components of a depot chair that help to increase the comfort of the user and to aid in the proper fit are limited. Typically, it is only the length of the legrest that can be adjusted. Depot chairs are available in various seat widths, seat depths, and backrest heights. These dimensions must be specified to the manufacturer or distributor upon order.

Not all wheelchairs are propelled by the person sitting in the wheelchair. In many hospitals and long-term care facilities, wheelchairs are propelled by attendants. The design of these wheelchairs therefore requires special consideration. The primary consideration is that the wheelchair has two users: the rider and the attendant. The rider must be transported safely and comfortably, and the attendant must be able to operate and maneuver the chair safely and easily, with minimum physical strain. The design of the wheelchair must also be such that the attendant can maneuver the chair over obstacles, move in restricted spaces, and be able to assist the rider with transfers. The push handles should be designed in such a way that the attendant experiences no undue stress to the hands, arms, or back. If the wheelchair is to be solely propelled by attendants without any assistance from the rider there may not be a need for large drive wheels. Attendant-propelled chairs are most commonly used by people who are elderly. These types of chairs are sometimes called "Geri" chairs in reference to geriatric users. The chairs are typically designed to minimize the independent mobility of the rider. The rider is seated in a large recliner-type wheelchair with soft padding, reclined position, and small wheels, all of which make it impossible for the rider to move the wheelchair and difficult for most riders to exit the wheelchair. This type of chair helps long-term care facilities to exercise control over their clients. Considerable discussion has occurred regarding the appropriate use of attendant-propelled chairs that significantly impair the rider's independent mobility.

Attendant-propelled wheelchairs may also be designed for use by children. The philosophy behind children's wheelchairs is that the parents of a child can propel the chair until the child is capable of doing so on his/her own or until the child is ready for a powered wheelchair. The design of children's wheelchairs may allow them to be either attendant propelled or rider propelled. For children without severe orthopedic impairments, the chairs are semi-custom fit, and if necessary, specialized seating can be adapted to most children's wheelchairs.

Lightweight and Ultralight Wheelchairs

The rehabilitation wheelchair is designed to be used by an individual as a mobility device. The selection and configuration of a rehabilitation wheelchair involves understanding the needs of the individual intending to use the wheelchair (17, 18, 19). Some rehabilitation wheelchairs can be assigned to a category by their intended use or intended user.

Wheelchair frames built today typically center around tubular construction methods. Manual wheelchairs are generally made out of some lightweight tubing (e.g., aluminum, aircraft steel). The tubing can either be welded together or bolted together using lugs. There are three common frame styles; the box frame, the cantilever frame, and the T or I frame.

These three frame styles stem from slightly different design philosophies. The box frame, named such because the frame tubes that outline the edges form a "box" and its rectangular shape, can be strong, durable, and rigid. The wheels are mounted to a rather rigid frame, and if designed and constructed properly, the frame will deflect minimally during normal loading. Most of the suspension in the box frame design is provided by the seat cushion and the wheels. Many manufacturers who utilize a box frame design do not triangulate (i.e., have tubes crisscrossing) the frame, which allows for some flexibility. A few manufacturers have taken this concept one step further by adding suspension components, such as hinges and elastic elements, to the frame. Hinges are placed at the front of the seat, and elastic elements are placed at the back of the seat. The flexible element for the suspension can be either metal springs or polymer dampeners (elastomers) (20).

The cantilever frame is named so because, when the chair is viewed from the side, the front and rear wheels appear to be connected by only one tube. This is similar to having the front wheels attached to a cantilever beam that is fixed at the rear wheels. Both the box frame and the cantilever frame require cross bracing (i.e., tubes that connect the two halves) to provide adequate strength and stiffness. The design of the cantilever frame is based upon a few basic principles: (1) the frame can act as suspension (i.e., there is some flexibility purposely built into the frame); (2) fewer tubes placed closer to the body of the user may make the chair less conspicuous; and (3) fewer parts and welds makes the frame easier to construct.

The T or I frame is designed to make the frame as light and small as possible and therefore uses a minimal number of tubes. The T-frame uses a single tube called an axle tube to mount the rear wheels. Another tube is welded or mounted to the axle tube, which extends forward to the front caster(s). The frame looks like a T if the wheelchair has only one front caster. The caster of a T-frame is mounted at the end of the tube, which extends forward from the axle tube. The frame appears like an I if another tube is mounted at a right angle to the front of the center tube. The front cross tube holds a caster at either end. In some cases, durability is sacrificed in order to provide a very lightweight and unobtrusive design. The T or I frame is popular among active wheelchair users who enjoy a wheelchair suitable for both daily use and sports. Each of these basic frame types is functional, and each one has its merits.

In addition to frame style, there are two basic frame types: folding and rigid. Three different types of folding mechanisms are frequently used today: cross-brace, parallel brace, and forward folding. Most folding wheelchairs use variations on the cross-brace design; however, each design has its advantages, and selection depends upon the user's preference.

Cross-brace folding wheelchairs are available with either single or double cross-brace mechanisms, which add stiffness to the frame. A cross-brace folding mechanism consists of two frame members connected in the middle and then attached to the bottom of a side frame member on one side of the chair and to the seat upholstery above the top side frame member on the opposite side. The cross members are hinged at the bottom and are pinned together in the middle. When viewed from the back, the cross members form an X. The chair is folded by pulling upward on the seat upholstery. When the seat is lifted, the cross-members move upward, pulling the frame together. The user's weight keeps the frame from folding when the wheelchair frame is extended. Cross member folding mechanisms are simple and easy to use; however, the wheelchair may collapse when tilted sideways. In addition, the frame becomes taller when folded, which may make transporting the chair difficult. Some chairs incorporate over-center locking mechanisms to reduce the problem of frame folding while on a side slope. Folding cross-brace type wheelchairs are available from every major manual wheelchair manufacturer, and there are several variations of this basic design.

The parallel brace folding mechanism allows the frame to fold sideways by having the frame cross member hinge forward. Each cross member is hinged in the center and at each end. When in the extended position, the center hinge is locked. The user releases the lock and pulls forward. The chair folds as the user pulls forward. The cross members can be locked with a pin or a cam mechanism. The advantages of this design are that the frame behaves like a rigid frame in the extended position, and that the chair can fold slightly with the user in it, permitting negotiation of narrow entrances. Parallel brace mechanisms are, however, more difficult to operate and maintain.

Many ultralight wheelchairs incorporate forward-folding backrests, a concept that is extended in the design of a forward-folding wheelchair. The design of a forward-folding wheelchair involves hinging the front end of the wheelchair and the backrest. The backrest can then be folded onto the seat and the front end can be folded under the seat. If the rear wheels are quick release, the unique design of forward-folding wheelchairs allows the chair to become compact, which is a beneficial feature for transporting the chair during travel. One disadvantage of forward-folding wheelchairs is that they require more operations and latches to fold them, which may limit their use by more impaired users.

THE WHEELCHAIR USER INTERFACE

The wheelchair user interface is the least understood but most critical design factor (21–24). As an extension of the user's body, much like an orthotic, the rider and the wheelchair must act as one. Therefore, the chair selected for the user should maximize the user's potential and should not limit them in any way (25, 26, 27). This requires an understanding of the user's ability and the intended use of the wheelchair, as well as careful matching of critical chair dimensions to user's body dimensions (28, 29). Experience has taught that there is a great deal of variability among individual preferences.

Understanding the intentions and abilities of the wheelchair user is an important part of properly recommending a wheelchair (30). Even the best wheelchair will not be successful if it is rejected by the user (31, 32). Therefore, it is imperative that the needs, desires, intended use, and abilities of the user be ascertained and incorporated into the wheelchair selection (33–38). It is no longer acceptable to stock a particular model of wheelchair and to provide it to all new wheelchair users. Manufacturers who fail to determine consumer's intended use of the wheelchair will soon find themselves wanting for business. Additionally, the activities and the environment of the wheelchair and the user must be determined. Obtaining this information will assist with defining the geometry, components, and durability of the wheelchair.

The abilities of the user must be matched with the intended use of the wheelchair. For some users, many of the desired uses can be accomplished simply with the use of existing technology. Others will require custom products, and still others will not be able to achieve their goals with existing designs (39–44). The type of chair and its setup depends upon the interaction between the user and the intended use (person, place, and task) (23, 45–48). The actual abilities of the user as they relate to the intended use must be also be evaluated (49).

Financial and physical resources are required to select and purchase wheelchairs. The limits of the available resources must be weighed against the abilities and desires of the user. Resources are usually limited, and new technology can be costly. The user should be provided the best possible product within the limits of the available resources. Assistive technology is considered to be medical equipment, and thus caution must be taken to insure the safety of all potential users.

Assistive technology clinicians must remain current with respect to new product developments so as not to risk "reinventing the wheel" (50, 51). An existing product can often be adapted to meet the user's needs; however, caution must be observed when making modifications to allow for applications not intended by the manufacturer. Rehabilitation engineers should evaluate possible problems that could result from any modifications. Clinicians should also keep in mind that products from areas outside of traditional sources may prove useful in the selection and development of wheelchairs.

WHEELCHAIR SEATING AND MEASUREMENT

Wheelchair dimensions that closely match the body dimensions of the wheelchair user are a critical component of proper wheelchair seating (13, 49, 50). For many people, the proper dimensions for a wheelchair can be determined by just a few simple measurements. Body measurements are typically made with the consumer in the seated position; however, some therapists prefer to make body measurements on a mat (50). Most therapists prefer to take measurements with the individual in the seated position because it accounts for the effect of gravity on posture. Either method works well, provided the therapist is familiar with the measurements to be made and has adequate experience. Body measurements are best made using a steel or nylon tape measure called an anthropometric tape measure that is designed specifically for making body measurements (52, 53). This type of tape measure incorporates a spring attached to the end that limits the amount of force applied to soft tissue and helps reduce error due to one person applying a small amount of force and causing a small distortion of soft tissue, and another person applying a larger force and causing a larger distortion of soft tissue that results in different measurements for the same consumer. Calipers can also be used to get more accurate breadth and depth measurements. However, calipers are primarily used only by specialized seating clinics and research laboratories. It is also important to determine the individual's range of motion and postural asymmetries.

The individual's height and weight are probably the most obvious body measurements that are necessary when fitting a person for a wheelchair. Weight is a critical measurement for obtaining a wheelchair that is strong enough to accommodate the user's weight. For example, most wheelchairs are tested with 100-kg (220-lb) test dummies (20, 29, 31). The test dummies are made of wood or aluminum and are stiffer than a real person. Nevertheless, the wheelchair needs to be rated for the end user's weight. Many manufacturers claim in their owners and service manuals that their wheelchairs are rated for 250 lb. When selecting a wheelchair for someone who weighs more than 220 lb, it is best to inform the wheelchair manufacturer. The wheelchair provider should also verify that the wheelchair has been tested for a weight greater than the actual weight of the client.

The height of the wheelchair user provides information about the person's size, and can be used to check the final wheelchair measurements. For example, the sum of the sitting height, sitting depth, and lower leg length should be close to the person's supine height. Height and weight also provide information about a person's stature. This is helpful for people building the wheelchair who may never see the end user and for future use by therapists who can use stature as a quick measure of whether the individual's status has changed substantially since the previous wheelchair was selected.

For proper wheelchair seating, the critical body measurements needed are shoulder width, chest width, waist width, and pelvic width. These measurements are essential for determining the seat height, seat angle, seat depth, seat width, backrest height, and backrest angle of the wheelchair. The shoulder width is important when the wheelchair user requires shoulder supports or a shoulder harness. Additional measurements and definitions are used when specialized seating and postural support systems are required.

Backrest height, one of the most critical dimensions of wheelchair seating, is dependent upon the etiology of the user's disability, the intended use, and skills of the user. Comfort, stability, and control of the wheelchair are influenced by backrest height. Backrest heights may vary from 200 to 500 mm. Generally, individuals with lower mobility impairments prefer a lower backrest height. The backrest height is commonly made to be adjustable so that the user can tune it to his or her liking. A lower backrest height permits greater freedom of motion (e.g., leaning, turning) and is less restrictive (i.e., does not interfere with arms when pushing), but provides less support than a high backrest.

The backrest angle is often set so that the backrest is vertical with respect to a level floor. The backrest should be made of a padded, pliable material. If a backrest is made of rigid material it should be padded and it must be mounted in a way that conforms to the user's changing body position. A tapered backrest is sometimes desirable to provide comfortable support for a user with a well-developed upper torso.

The chest width of the individual is important for determining the width of the backrest and backrest supports. The more severely impaired an individual is, the higher the backrest must be to provide adequate sitting balance. A backrest that is too wide can interfere with the individual's ability to propel the wheelchair. If the backrest is too narrow, however, it will cause discomfort. For this reason, the backrest width is more critical for manual wheelchair users than for power wheelchair users. In general, the backrest width should be about 2 cm wider than chest width at the highest point.

The width of the waist of the wheelchair user is important in order to accommodate armrests, side guards, and the wheels on some wheelchairs. Armrests and side guards (i.e., devices used to keep clothing from touching the wheels) are typically at waist width. The distance between the armrests and the waist should be between 5 and 10 cm. This measurement becomes more critical for manual wheelchair users. If the armrests are too far apart, the wheelchair user will have to place the arms in forward flexion to reach the pushrims. This is often described as "chicken winging" because the propulsion stroke resembles a person imitating a chicken.

Seat height, the measurement from the floor to front edge of the seat, will vary depending upon the desired use of the wheelchair for the user and upon the total body length of the user. For optimal mobility, the elbow angle should be between 100 and 120 degrees when the user is sitting upright with their hands resting on the top of the wheels. On average, seat heights vary from about 300 to 600 mm. A user who has long legs will require a higher seat height in order to achieve sufficient ground clearance for the footrests.

Seat angle, a preference of most active users, allows for some flexibility when determining seat height. Seat angle can range from zero to 20 degrees. Tilting the seat towards the backrest allows the user to fit more securely into the chair, and the chair becomes more responsive to the user's movements. Seat angle also gives the user some pelvic tilt, which provides greater trunk stability.

Seat depth, the measurement between the person's backside and the popliteal area behind the knee, is determined from the length of the upper legs. Generally the gap between the front of the seat and the back of the knees of the wheelchair user should be less than 75 mm. This helps to ensure a broad distribution of the trunk weight over the buttocks and upper legs without placing undue pressure behind the knee. Some gap is necessary, however, to allow the user the freedom to adjust position.

Seat width is determined from the person's pelvic width, the intended use, and whether or not the person prefers to use sideguards (pieces of plastic, aluminum, or steel sheet placed between the seat and rear wheels to prevent clothing from rubbing on the rear wheels). Generally, the wheelchair should be as narrow as possible; therefore a chair that is about one inch wider than the user's hips is desirable. This allows the wheelchair user to easily reach the pushrims and places the arm in a position of greater leverage. Active wheelchair users prefer the seat width to be about one centimeter greater than the pelvic width. However, other wheelchair users prefer greater space to accommodate a coat, sweater, or to allow some room to adjust seating position. With manual wheelchairs, a difference between seat width and pelvic width of more than about 3 cm can have a negative impact on stroke biomechanics. Pelvic and seat width measurements for power wheelchair users are also important for maintaining the postural support needed to control the wheelchair. Side guards or armrests can help to keep clothing clean, and allow the user and the chair to mesh better. For adults, seat widths typically range from 250 to 500 mm.

Several important seated measurements are made with respect to the sagittal plane (i.e., side view). When viewing the sagittal plane, the edges from three seat position planes are used as references for defining an individual's wheelchair seating. The back plane is a vertical plane that contacts the posterior-most point of the individual's back. Ideally, the person being measured should be seated as close as possible to vertical torso posture. When the individual being measured can assume an erect sitting posture, the back plane will contact the spine within the thoracic region. The seat plane is a horizontal plane that intersects the back plane and contacts the inferior-most portion of the individuals' seated surface during seated weight bearing. Typically, the point of contact for the seat plane will be the ischial tuberosities. The foot plane is also a horizontal plane that is defined by the point of contact with the base of the feet. It is important to remember that the back plane, seat plane, and foot plane are imaginary planes that are used as references. The actual wheelchair seat may vary substantially from these planes, depending upon the functional anatomy of the individual.

The overall height of the individual in the seated position is the distance between the foot plane and the top of the person's head. This measurement is important when considering a person's interaction with his or her environment. For example, the seated overall height of an individual is going to define whether the roof of a van will need to be elevated, and by how much. The overall height also defines how low a person can sit properly in a wheelchair without having his or her feet contact the ground.

The sitting height is defined as the distance between the seat plane and the top of the head. The sitting height combined with the seat height provides information about how high a person sits. This helps to define the minimum and maximum reach. The sitting depth is the distance between the back plane and the popliteal area behind the knee. The sitting depth is used to determine the depth of the wheelchair seat. The lower leg length is measured from the popliteal fossa to the foot plane. The lower leg length is used to select and adjust the legrest length.

Wheelchair footrests come in various sizes depending upon the size of the individual's foot and the flexibility of the foot and ankle. The foot length is the maximum length of the foot while wearing a shoe. The overall depth for a seated person is defined as the distance between the tips of the toes to the back plane. This distance is important when determining the depth of a table top or desk top required for accommodating a wheelchair user. The overall depth also affects the maneuverability of the wheelchair user. Some people require more support than can be provided by a simple linear seating system.

Headrests are often used to provide support for the head and neck for people with higher levels of impairment. The headrest height is related to the seated height and acromion height. The acromion height is measured from each acromion (lateral tip of the shoulder) to the seat plane. This measurement provides information about postural asymmetry. The distance between the occipital protuberance and the back plane is used to specify the range of the headrest fore and aft adjustment required.

Handling and performance of a wheelchair are affected by wheelbase and width (54, 55). The wheelbase affects caster flutter, rolling resistance, stability, controllability, and obstacle performance. A chair with a longer wheelbase becomes more stable but less controllable. Therefore, a long chair may be less apt to tip over, but the user may not be able to negotiate common terrain. A longer wheelbase makes negotiating obstacles like curbs easier because it reduces the angle of ascent for the center of gravity, which is an important consideration. Active use rehabilitation wheelchairs are typically very controllable and maneuverable, and hence less stable. This is because users prefer control of the chair over stability. A chair with a short wheelbase is more maneuverable and can get the user closer to furnishings. However, a short wheelbase may move more weight over the front wheels, which will increase rolling resistance and reduce the speed at onset of caster flutter. The risk of a forward fall may also be increased with a shorter wheelbase. Obviously, design tradeoffs need to be made in accordance with the skills of the user. The wheelbase of a wheelchair is typically between 250 to 500 mm. The width of the footprint of the wheelchair is also an important design variable, because it helps to determine the stability and maneuverability of the wheelchair.

Camber, the angle that the wheel leans inward toward the seat with respect to vertical, is often variable depending upon the intended use of the wheelchair (56). Some suspension can be gained through the use of wheel camber. By adding camber to the rear wheels, the effective stiffness between the rolling surface and frame is reduced. Camber has several advantages: it widens the footprint of the chair, creating greater side-to-side stability, allows for quicker turns, helps to protect the hands because the bottom of the wheels will scuff the edges of obstacles, which prevents the user's hands from hitting the obstacle, and it positions the pushrims more ergonomically for propulsion (it is more natural to push down and out). Camber angle can either be fixed or adjustable, depending upon the frame design. The width of the chair depends upon the width of the frame and the camber angle. Frame widths for adults range from 300 to 500 mm, and camber angles are usually between 0 and 15 degrees, mostly between 7 and 12 degrees. Thus, total wheelchair widths vary from about 550 to 750 mm. For daily use, the chair should be as narrow as possible without substantially diminishing the handling characteristics. Narrow chairs are easier to maneuver in an environment made for walking. The wheels should be offset enough from the seat to avoid rubbing against the clothing or body.

Ride Comfort and Durability

A wheelchair will typically be used all day, every day for all major life activities (i.e., activities of daily living, work, school, recreation, sports) over a period of three to five years. Ride comfort and durability are both important considerations in wheelchair design (15, 20, 22).

Ride comfort is primarily a function of the stiffness of the frame, wheels, and other components, frame geometry, seat and cushion design, and compliance. Ride comfort is important because people may sit in the chair for 12 to 18 hours per day every day (57, 58). Wheelchairs utilized by active users may be used nearly 10 miles per day over a variety of terrains (e.g., grass, carpet, gravel, concrete, asphalt). The frame design must be durable enough not to break after several thousand miles of road vibration, but should have sufficient flexibility to withstand dropping off of curbs (up to 35 cm high). The frame geometry can be used to reduce the effects of the impulse observed when going off a curb, or to minimize road vibration. Wheelchair suspension, most of which comes from the cushion and the tires, can add to the ride comfort. Typically wheelchairs will use pneumatic tires, and will have foam, gel, or air cushions.

Durability is also an important issue in wheelchair design. Wheelchairs may be used by demanding riders and/or receive little maintenance. Because the same wheelchair is often used for work or school and recreation, the chair must be designed to meet the demands of these activities. The wheelchair must be designed to withstand obstacles (e.g., rocks, curbs, bumps, dips, impacts) encountered during a variety of activities. A frame that is too flexible will absorb the energy of the rider and make the wheelchair inefficient. On the other hand, a frame that is too stiff will reduce ride comfort and may fracture due to shock.

Legrests

Most wheelchair users require support for their feet and lower legs, which is provided by footrests. The footrest must provide sufficient support for the lower legs and feet and must hold the feet in proper position to prevent contractures or other deformities. Footrests may be fixed, folding, or swing-away. The feet must remain on the footrests at all times during propulsion, and therefore some type of cradle is recommended. Some wheelchairs, primarily those with swing-away footrests, use foot stirrups behind the heels of each foot. During active use, a rider's feet may come up over the stirrups, resulting in the feet dragging on the ground or getting caught under the chair, which can be solved by using a continuous strap behind both feet. The feet should not be pinched, trapped, or scratched by the footrests during normal driving activities or when transferring. The frame should be selected and configured so that, with shoes on, the feet sit firmly upon the footrests and do not cause the upper legs to be lifted from the seat cushion. Care must be taken that sufficient ground clearance is maintained. The footrests are commonly placed between 25 and 50 mm from the ground. Footrests are often the first part of the chair to come in contact with an obstacle (i.e., door, wall, another chair). Therefore, they must be durable.

Rigid wheelchairs often use simple tubes across the front of the wheelchair. By using a tubular rigid footrest, the wheelchair becomes stiffer and stronger. Rigid footrests are used during sports activities and work well for people who are very active in their wheelchairs. Forward anti-tip rollers can be mounted to rigid footrests, which are helpful in reducing the risk of some forward-tipping accidents and when playing court sports.

Folding wheelchairs often use footrests that fold up and legrests that swing out of the way to ease transfers. Most people use this type of footrest. Rigid footrests may also be used on folding wheelchairs; however, they will prevent the chair from folding. For individuals who like to use one wheelchair for both daily and recreational use, two sets of legrests (e.g., one rigid and one split) help to allow for multiple uses. Swing-away legrests are not as durable as rigid legrests. In some cases, manufacturers design swing-away legrests so that they will bend upon impact, helping to absorb the energy of the impact and possibly preventing serious injury to the wheelchair user. Elevated legrests can be used for people who cannot maintain a 90-degree knee angle or who need their legs elevated for venous return. Elevating the legrests will make the wheelchair longer, however, which will make the wheelchair less maneuverable by increasing the turning radius.

Armrests

Armrests serve a number of different functions for the wheelchair user. (28) They provide a form of support, are convenient handles when the rider leans to the side, and are helpful when attempting to reach higher places or when nudging items off high shelves. Armrests are commonly used to assist with pressure relief by performing a "push-up." Some wheelchair users are capable of lifting their buttocks from the seat by placing one hand or arm on each armrest and pushing upward. This helps to improve blood flow to the lower extremities and reduces the risk of developing a pressure ulcer.

There are three basic styles of armrest: wrap-around, full-length, and desk-length. A wrap-around armrest gets its name because it mounts on to the frame at the back of the wheelchair below the backrest. The armrest comes up along the back of the backrest canes and wraps around to the front of the wheelchair. Unlike other types of armrests, the major advantage of this design is that it does not increase the width of the wheelchair like other armrest styles. Wrap-around armrests are popular among active wheelchair users. The most significant drawback of this design is that the armrest does not serve as a side guard to keep the rider's clothing away from the wheels.

Full-length and desk-length armrests are similar in design; the main difference being the length of the armrest. Full-length armrests provide support for nearly the entire upper arm. They are popular on electric-powered wheelchairs because they make a convenient and functional location for a joystick or other input device. Full-length armrests provide good support for the arms, but because they can make it difficult to get close to some tables and desks, manufacturers produce desk-length armrests. Both of these types of armrests include clothing guards to protect clothing from the wheels. These types of armrests are mounted to the side of the wheelchair and may add as much as 5 cm (2 inches) to the width of the wheelchair.

Along with different lengths, armrests can also be fixed or adjustable. If they are adjustable, armrests may move up and down to accommodate the length of the rider's trunk and arms. Most armrests can be moved in order to provide clearance for transferring in and out of the wheelchair, and to allow a person to lean over the sides of the wheelchair. To facilitate this movement, armrests are either removed or flipped back. Both styles commonly use a latch that is operated by the user to lock the armrest. Armrests provide a convenient place for people to grasp when attempting to provide assistance, which makes it important to have latches. If designed properly, two people can lift the rider and wheelchair using the armrests. In some cases, armrests are designed to pull-out if any upward force is applied to them, and are therefore not intended to be used for lifting.

Wheel Locks

Wheel locks provide several functions for the wheelchair user, including acting as parking breaks and assisting when transferring to other seats. They help to allow the rider to push things and to be more stable when desired. A variety of wheel locks are used to restrain wheelchairs when the user is transferring or when the chair is parked. High lock brakes, which require the least dexterity to operate, are most common. Extension levers can be added for people with limited reach and/or minimal strength. Some wheel locks are over-center and are either only engaged or disengaged. Other wheel locks allow selection of the braking force. These are sometimes called sweeper brakes because in some positions the wheelchair can still be pushed, allowing the user to push and sweep the floor with a broom. Wheel locks are standard equipment on wheelchairs and are simple to mount if the wheelchair does not come equipped from the manufacturer.

Wheel locks may be push-to-lock or pull-to-lock. In general, wheel locks are more difficult to engage than to disengage. For this reason, push-to-lock wheel locks are preferred by most people because riders often find it easier to push with the palm than pull with the fingers. High wheel locks are often mounted to the upper tube of the wheelchair's side frame. Low wheel locks are usually mounted to the lower tube of the wheelchair's side frame. Low wheel locks require more mobility to operate, but they also alleviate the common problem of hitting the thumb during propulsion that plagues high wheel lock users. High wheel lock users can address this problem by selecting retractable (i.e. scissors or butterfly) wheel locks, which help to prevent jamming the thumbs and can accommodate a wide variety of camber angles. The major drawback of retractable wheel locks is that they are more difficult to use than other types of wheel locks. The wheel lock must be positioned properly with respect to the wheel in order to operate effectively. If the wheels are repositioned then the wheel locks must also be repositioned. Tire pressure will also affect the grip of the wheel locks.

Handrims

Elbow, wrist, and hand pain are common complaints of manual wheelchair users, but little has been done to improve the handrims used on wheelchairs (23, 26, 45). Ergonomic handrims such as the Natural-Fit (Figure 55.6) were designed to directly address the shortcomings of standard handrims (59, 60). These handrims have a wider surface area for the palm of the hand and a contoured trough for the thumb that sits between the rim and wheel. Contact area for gripping the handrim is improved by the combination of these two surfaces. Specially-coated high- and low-friction surfaces to maximize the efficiency of propulsion and braking can also be applied. This design alleviates the need to grip the tire and leaves no place to get fingers caught. Ergonomic handrims such as the Natural-Fit can be easily attached to existing wheels while adding little additional weight and width to the wheelchair. (59) In contrast to standard handrims, the Natural-Fit also includes three other critical features: (1) the addition of a contoured trough between the rim and the

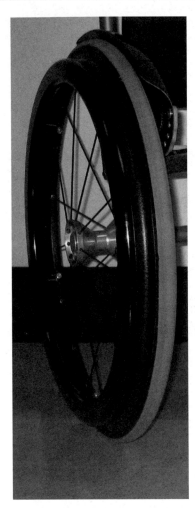

Figure 55.6   Natural-fit handrims.

side of the tire; (2) the laying down of a strip of high-friction vinyl coating on the contoured thumb area; and (3) the addition of a second anodized rim concentrically inside the existing rim.

Individuals with weakness of the upper and lower extremities can gain maximal benefit from wheelchair propulsion by combined use of their arms and legs, or by only using their legs. The design and selection of a foot-drive wheelchair depends greatly upon how the user can take the greatest advantage of their motor abilities. The strength and coordination of the user's legs must be determined to decide whether it is best to pull or to push with the legs, and the design of the chair will be affected by which propulsion method is used. When pushing, the user moves with his/her back to the direction of motion. If this method of foot propulsion is utilized, then a wheelchair with the footrests removed is typically the most effective.

If the person pushes the wheelchair with his or her feet, then modifications to the design of standard wheelchairs are required. When a wheelchair is propelled solely with the feet, the wheels at the front edge of the seat do not swivel. Placing the casters at the back of the seat helps to make the wheelchair easier for the user to control. The casters should lead the rear wheels for the most common direction of travel. This will help to reduce the possibility of the user flipping over if they hit an obstacle and will make the chair more directionally stable. The wheelchair should be set up so that the user/wheelchair center of gravity is well within the footprint of the wheelchair, which will require some consideration when positioning the large wheels.

Seating Bases

The seat base of a wheelchair may be rigid or a cloth sling. In either case, the seat should be stiff and should provide a stable base for the cushion and the user. Rigid seat bases and backrests are advantageous because their properties change little over time. The cushion is, therefore, always properly supported. Rigid seat bases may weigh more than cloth slings; however, as the use of composite materials becomes more widespread, this will cease to be an issue. Currently, aluminum, steel, fiberglass, Kevlar®, carbon fiber, and several types of plastics are used to make seat bases and backrests. As most wheelchairs are available in common sizes, seat bases and backrests only need to be made for those sizes. Rigid and semi-rigid backrests may provide greater lumbar and lateral support over sling seats. Rigid seat bases may be flat or they may incorporate some contouring and hip supports to assist with proper seating and positioning. Rigid seat bases and backrest supports form the foundation for many contoured seating systems, and they are becoming more popular.

Sling seats and backrests are constructed of synthetic materials with high tensile strengths such as nylon, cotton canvas, Kevlar®, or similar materials. In many instances, the structural material may be enclosed in a vinyl, artificial leather, or another water resistant material that forms an exterior shell and acts as the interface to the user. Vinyl and artificial leather, however, deform substantially under load and are not appropriate as structural seating materials. The exterior shell is often vacuum-formed under heat in order to create a bond between the shell material and the structural material.

Seats and backrests may be attached to the wheelchair frame in a variety of ways. One of the more common means is to sew a pocket into each lateral edge of the seat base and backrest upholstery. A metal (steel or aluminum) slat is placed into the upholstery pocket in order to attach the seat base and backrest upholstery to the frame. Screws are then inserted through the slat and into the frame. For backrests, it is not uncommon to insert the backrest canes through the upholstery and to use grommets and oversized contoured washers to secure the backrest upholstery to the canes. A sufficient number of attachment points should be used to prevent an upholstery tear and to prevent the backrest upholstery from sliding down the canes in the event of a screw or grommet failure. Other methods can be used to prevent the backrest upholstery from sliding down the canes in event of component failure. A stiffening material, such as high density foam, can be sewn into the upholstery. The backrest upholstery can also be sewn in a catenary so that equal tension is applied to the canes across the entire surface of the backrest. Seat base and backrest upholstery may also be attached using webbing or lacing.

HYBRID WHEELCHAIRS

A variety of wheelchairs designed to accommodate a wide spectrum of needs are available commercially and represent significant progress in wheelchair design (61, 62, 63). There remains, however, a need for more studies of assistive technology and for improved methods of delivering medical rehabilitation services due to a large and steadily growing number of individuals with a disability and an increasing elderly population (64, 65). Compromises were required with each type of mobility device previously available, and a need arose for a new class of device that was lightweight, maneuverable, and simple to transport. From this need, the pushrim-activated power-assisted wheelchair (PAPAW) was developed (66, 67) (see Figure 55.7).

A PAPAW uses motors and batteries to augment the power applied by the users to one or both pushrims during propulsion or braking (62). Applying a torque to the pushrim activates the motors, which provides additional traveling velocity (68). The PAPAW has been shown to reduce the physiologic demand and biomechanical strain of wheelchair propulsion, which may improve daily driving activities and reduce the strain placed on the upper extremities (69). For these reasons, the PAPAW is a useful mobility tool in the arsenal of rehabilitation professionals working with people with physical impairments. A PAPAW should also be considered when it is necessary to minimize home and vehicle modifications. This is beneficial for most wheelchair users, particularly the aging or those in transitional status between manual and powered chairs. In addition, it eases long-distance propulsion by facilitating less strenuous maintenance of higher speed (63, 66, 69).

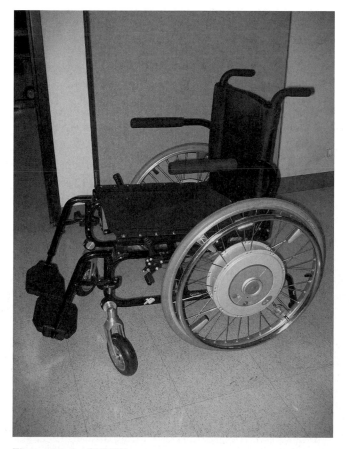

Figure 55.7 PAPAW.

ELECTRIC-POWERED WHEELCHAIRS

People with severe disabilities might need a power wheelchair for mobility purposes (70, 71). Individuals who have a moderate level of trunk control can use a conventional power wheelchair. Conventional power wheelchairs contain a standard seat system. Alternative seating systems have been designed to provide customized seating in the standard power wheelchair seat. Power wheelchairs are distinguishable by their integrated frame and seat. Their appearance is most similar to that of a conventional wheelchair. Power wheelchairs may use a range of drive wheels from 8 inches to 20 inches in diameter. The drive wheels may be driven by either belts or gear boxes. All powered mobility systems are generically lumped under the title "powered wheelchair."

Electric powered wheelchairs were first invented near the turn of the twentieth century, and the first U.S. patent describing an electric powered wheelchair was approved around 1940 (72). Early designs were impractical and did not receive substantial attention. Powered wheelchairs are most beneficial to people with severe disabilities, and because at that time the long-term prognosis of individuals with severe disabilities was poor, there was little demand for powered wheelchairs.

Medical advances occurred and were implemented during World War II enabling more people with severe disabilities to survive (73, 74). The emphasis at this time shifted from acute treatment to long-term rehabilitation. These changes combined to create a demand for better wheelchairs, and more specifically, for powered wheelchairs. The first practical electric powered wheelchairs used starter motors and batteries from automobiles. These early wheelchairs provided limited mobility for some people with upper extremity impairments. Relays were soon used to provide greater control over electric powered wheelchairs. A transistor was added to provide much better control and to allow for the development of specialized control interfaces for the user.

During the 1960s and 1970s, the number of electric powered wheelchairs expanded. However, they remained bulky, inefficient, and unreliable (75, 76, 77). Microprocessors and metal-oxide-semiconductor-field-effect-transistors (MOS-FETs) that helped to improve reliability were introduced during the 1980s. The microprocessor provides improved control and greater ability to match the characteristics of the chair to the abilities of the user. The MOS-FETs help to improve efficiency. Because of their low-cost, extra MOS-FETS have been used to provide some redundancy in the power control circuitry (73).

Considerable changes to the frame design of powered wheelchairs came in the 1990s. Manufacturers began to develop frames designed specifically for electric powered wheelchairs. The most significant change was separating the seat from the frame, which is referred to as a power base design. With the introduction of this concept, other innovations such as rear wheel suspension were developed.

Differentiation of Powered Wheelchairs

Twenty years ago there were few differences between the designs of powered wheelchairs, and most were simply iterations of manual wheelchair design. As the powered wheelchair market grew and products were developed, powered wheelchair designs began to evolve (78, 79). Consumers, clinicians, engineers, and manufacturers eventually began to recognize the need for product differentiation (80, 81, 82, 83). Moreover, as more manufacturers of electric powered wheelchairs emerged to address the specialized needs of the consumer, they began to desire to have their products be distinguishable from those of other manufacturers.

Electric powered wheelchairs are commonly grouped together based upon the functions of the wheelchair and the intended use for the chair. Powered wheelchairs can be grouped into several classes or categories. The intended use of the wheelchair as primarily indoor, both indoor/outdoor, or active indoor/outdoor is a convenient way to group wheelchairs. Indoor wheelchairs have a small footprint (i.e. area connecting the wheels) that allows them to be maneuverable in confined spaces. Consequently, they may not have the stability or power to negotiate obstacles outdoors. Indoor/outdoor powered wheelchairs are used by people who wish to have mobility in the home/school/office and in the community, but who stay on finished surfaces (e.g., sidewalks, driveways, flooring). Wheelchairs that are primarily for indoor use and both for indoor/outdoor use conserve weight by using smaller batteries, which often results in reduced range.

Active indoor/outdoor wheelchairs may be best suited for individuals who want to drive over unstructured environments, travel long distances, and move fast. The active indoor/outdoor use wheelchairs include those with suspension, and manufacturers are increasingly using a power base design. A power base separates the seating system from the main chassis of the wheelchair. The main chassis in a power base consists of the motors, drive wheels, casters, controllers, batteries, and frame. The seating system (i.e., seat, backrest, armrests, legrests, footrests) is a separate, integrated unit, which allows custom systems to be added readily to meet user-specific needs. Seating systems from one manufacturer are often used on a power base from another manufacturer to meet an individual's needs and preferences.

Indoor/outdoor powered wheelchairs can be further divided into categories by the design complexity of the seating system. The simplest form of seating system is a linear seating system. A linear seating system refers to a planar seat and back with fixed angles and orientations. For people who have low sitting tolerance or who need to change posture to perform some activities of daily living, a reclining seating system may be beneficial. A reclining seating system allows the angle of the backrest to be changed (i.e., from upright to reclined). For individuals with a very low sitting tolerance, severe spasticity or hemodynamic problems, a tilt-in-space seating system may be appropriate. Tilt-in-space systems allow the backrest, seat, and legrests to tilt as a unit with respect to the wheelchair's chassis, without changing their orientation with respect to each other. Changing the user's position in space has other advantages: for example, reducing spasticity, improving venous blood flow, and comfort, besides assisting with posture and sitting tolerance.

Stand-up wheelchairs assist users in performing many activities of daily living. They may also have some physiological benefits due to upright posture and have been reported to provide psychological benefits to the user. Individuals may not be able to use a stand-up wheelchair if they do not have good range of motion or if their bones are too fragile. The benefits of a stand-up wheelchair can also be obtained to a certain extent by using a variable seat height wheelchair. The most common function of variable seat height wheelchairs is to provide seat elevation, although some wheelchair models come with seat elevation and seat lowering. Lowering may extend the seat to within a few inches from the floor, and raising the seat can bring it as high as three feet from the floor to the base of the seat.

Power Bases

Power bases are simply powered wheelchairs consisting of the power drive system on a mobile platform. As the conventional powered wheelchair seat system does not fulfill the needs of individuals with minimal trunk control, power bases were developed to allow for a customized seating system to be mounted to the base. Power bases also tend to offer higher performance (i.e., faster, more torque). A significant advantage of some power bases is that the position of the wheels with respect to the seat can be changed. This permits adjustment of the handling of the wheelchair without losing some of the power. The power base includes all wheels, the motors, the batteries, and also often includes the controller. This design allows seating systems to be developed without modifying the power base and provides locations suitable for mounting seating hardware.

In-Wheel Motors

Another means of providing powered mobility to a manual wheelchair is to use in-wheel-motors. In-wheel-motors are wheel hubs made from a motor. The hub is much larger than that of a standard manual wheelchair in order for the motor to be of sufficient size to provide function power. In-wheel-motors use a battery pack that attaches to the frame. The most common means of attaching the battery is to use a small bag slung under the wheelchair. In-wheel-motors are commonly made with quick-release axles in order to simplify transport. Either a joystick or switches can be used to control the motors (i.e., right and left side) to provide electric powered mobility for a manual wheelchair. One must exercise some caution when converting a manual wheelchair to an electric powered wheelchair. Manual wheelchairs are not designed to accommodate the additional weight. This may reduce the stability, durability, and ease of propulsion when in the manual mode. The speeds possible with a powered unit are also likely to be greater than the rider is capable of with a manual chair. Moreover, powered wheelchairs drive much differently than manual wheelchairs. A skilled manual wheelchair rider may pop the casters over small bumps without noticing. However, when the chair is converted to being electrically powered, the caster may be damaged in short order. When used properly with appropriate training and awareness of the trade-offs, power conversion units can provide valuable assistance.

ROBOTIC WHEELED MOBILITY SYSTEMS

Wheeled mobility devices are limited in their functional use (84, 85). Many environments remain inaccessible when using a wheeled mobility device (e.g. stairs, high curbs, steep ramps, high objects, soft surfaces, uneven terrain). The environment of each individual user must be considered and performance trade-offs must be evaluated. The INDEPENDENCE™ 3000™ IBOT Transporter (IBOT), an electronically stabilizing device, provides the opportunity to enhance mobility without some of the traditional performance trade-offs (86, 87).

The IBOT is a result of the recent increase in the use of computer technology in assistive devices. The IBOT is a technologically advanced mobility device designed to overcome many of the limitations of currently available devices. It uses three computers and a number of sensors and actuators to provide a variety of functions. By incorporating state-of-the-art software and hardware, the IBOT responds to changes in terrain. It is controlled by a set of central custom computers that help to maintain stability and provide the user with control. The IBOT incorporates sensors for attitude control, speed control, self-diagnosis, and for changing operational functions. A voting process with the IBOT's redundant computers is used to determine the actions of the device. Software records the operation of the device and maintains a fault log. A pioneering feature of the IBOT is the use of an internal modem that allows the device to communicate with the manufacturer or a service representative at a distance. This provides the potential to download fault logs to determine whether periodic maintenance is necessary and the possibility of uploading software changes.

The IBOT, intended for use as an advanced mobility system, provides the user with five separate functions for operation (88). The functions allow the user the following capabilities:

- Indoor mobility (e.g., driving on finished surfaces: carpet, tile)
- Outdoor mobility (e.g., traversing uneven terrain, steep inclines, grass, sand, gravel, curbs)
- Stair climbing (e.g., independently, assisted)
- Elevated height, with a reduced turning radius (e.g., reaching the top shelf in a cabinet, having an eye-level conversation with someone standing, maneuvering in a confined space)
- Ability to transport the device in some motor vehicles without the use of a motorized lift

The IBOT has four primary drive wheels, each controlled through its own electric motor, and two caster wheels. The two sets of drive wheels on either side of the chair form a cluster. Each cluster may rotate about its central axis, and the wheels may rotate about their hubs. This provides the IBOT with more degrees of freedom than a traditional electric powered wheelchair. The IBOT is operated via a hand-controlled "joystick" and a user panel containing several switches that are attached to an armrest.

The IBOT can be operated in five functions: standard function, four-wheel function, stair function, balance function, and remote function. In standard function the IBOT operates much like an electric powered wheelchair. When driving in "four-wheel function" the clusters are allowed to rotate, providing the freedom to negotiate obstacles or uneven terrain. The IBOT can also be used to negotiate stairs that have at least a single railing. In stair function, the IBOT responds to the reaction forces generated by the user against the stair railing, or an assistant can initiate stair negotiation by using the handles on the back of the device. Cluster rotation is also used to negotiate stairs. The wheels remain fixed at a central axis as the clusters rotate and one wheel from each cluster transitions from one step to the next. During stair climbing there are always two wheels on a step.

The cluster design and the specialized controls incorporated in the IBOT allow the device to be balanced above two wheels. Balance function acts to raise the seat height for reaching high objects or for looking a standing person in the eyes. It also decreases the turning radius for confined spaces. Surface restrictions for balance function include wet floors, ice, and snow. Additionally, driving on areas of soap, oil, or grease spills should be avoided.

ACCESS DEVICES

The primary function of an access device ("interface") is control of the powered mobility system (78, 89). Secondary applications allow for use of environmental control systems and computer access. By using the same control interface for both the powered wheelchair and the secondary systems, the seating position and control selection can be optimized for multiple purposes. A critical consideration when selecting or designing a user interface is that the ability of the user to accurately control the interface is heavily dependent upon their stability within the wheelchair (90). Custom seating and postural support systems are often required for a user interface to be truly effective. The placement of the user interface is also critical to its efficacy as a functional access device.

Joysticks

Joysticks are the most common access device for powered wheelchair systems (91). When a powered wheelchair is ordered and there is no other specification, a joystick is typically supplied by the manufacturer. Joysticks can either be switched or proportional. Switched joysticks respond to discrete positions of the joystick, and usually four switches are implemented. There are eight discrete states with four positions defined by the activation of a single switch and four positions defined by the activation of two switches together. Proportional joysticks get their name because the control output sent to the wheelchair from the joystick is in proportion to how far the joystick is pushed from the center position (92–95).

Another type of joystick called a resistive joystick can also be used. The control output can be one of several electrical signals, and a change in electrical resistance can be used to indicate the position of the joystick (96, 97). As the joystick is moved left, the electrical resistance is increased, and as the joystick is moved to the right, the electrical resistance is decreased. Another independent change in resistance is used to indicate the position of the joystick fore and aft. A change in inductance can also be used to signal the position of the joystick. Two independent inductors (i.e., coils) vary with the position of the joystick in the same manner that the resistance does with resistive type. Digital joysticks based on a new standard called M3S are being introduced, especially in the European market. These joysticks may offer improved immunity to interference from sources such as police radios, cellular phones, ham radios, and even the electric motors of the wheelchair itself.

Sip-&-Puff

Sip-&-Puff access devices consist of a replaceable straw located near the mouth. The wheelchair is controlled by a sequence of pulling and pushing air through the straw with the mouth. These devices are used primarily by people with tetraplegia who do not have functional use of their arms or hands. A variety of configurations can be used to control the wheelchair using a Sip-&-Puff device. Generally, the user will sip a specific number of times to indicate a direction, and puff to confirm the choice and activate the movement of the wheelchair. An auxiliary display providing feedback to the user is commonly used with Sip-&-Puff devices. The display is often a flat panel LCD that is capable of displaying about 20 characters.

Switches

An array of switches can be used for the directional input of a wheelchair (90). The control scheme is similar to that of a switched joystick; however, a combination of switch activations is rarely used for directional input. Switches are indicated for individuals who have good control over an anatomical site that is not usually used to control a wheelchair. An individual with a disability might, for example, have better motor control over their foot rather than their hand. An array of large switches mounted to the footrest could then be used as a direction input.

Switches are also used as a primary means for computer access. Often one switch is used to toggle between the functions of computer access and powered wheelchair control. In computer access mode, the switches are used with any number of coding schemes. International Morse Code, automatic scanning, step scanning, inverse scanning, array scanning, and multi-level scanning are all coding schemes that are used with switches. Morse code has the advantage of only requiring one switch (two switches can be used), but of all of the different types of coding schemes, it generally places the highest cognitive demand on the user. Scanning methods all share a common feature in that the selection choices proceed until the user chooses the correct function or a valid character (13). The act of selection can be through a time delay or the activation of a switch. In automatic scanning, the choices are presented to the user on a computer screen or LCD panel with a preset time delay between each choice. When the desired choice is presented, the user must activate a switch before the next choice is shown. With step scanning the user uses the switch to move from one choice to the next. A delay on any one choice indicates acceptance of that function or character. Inverse scanning is the reverse operation of automatic scanning. The switch is held down until the desired choice is reached and is then released to finalize the selection. All three of the scanning methods can be further modified to allow for the use of more than one method. One such modification would be to use one switch to step through the choices and a second switch to accept the choice.

Array scanning uses four switches to guide a cursor through an x-y grid of choices; a fifth switch with a time delay is used for the selection process. Due to the similarity in the skills necessary to master each task, the switch arrangement in array scanning is highly applicable for both powered wheelchair control and computer access.

Multi-level scanning is similar to the above methods, but after the selection of an option, a new menu is presented. The final function or character is entered from this new menu. The number of levels can also be increased. With all of the possibilities for computer access and the ability to use atypical access sites, switches provide for one of the most versatile powered wheelchair control inputs. As with switched joysticks, however, the disadvantage of a lack of proportional control of the wheelchair speed remains with switched control.

Ultrasonic and Infrared

Many of the input devices described in this section can be used for more than the control of powered wheelchairs. Two common additional uses are environmental control and computer access. In some cases, the computer is mounted to the wheelchair, but often it is at a fixed site. In this case, there must be a method for the linkage of the computer to the control device. Older systems that were used primarily for environmental control used ultrasonic signals to transmit information. Newer designs are based on infrared for both environmental control and computer access.

CUSHIONS

There are two basic types of seating systems used with wheelchairs: linear systems and contoured systems. (98) Linear seating systems are planar in that the seat and back surfaces are flat and only conform to the weight of the user. For many wheelchair users a simple linear seating system or a standard contour is very effective (99, 100). Foam, visco-elastic fluid, dry floatation (air) cushions, and honeycomb are the most common cushion materials (101, 102).

Linear Foam Cushions

Various densities and types (e.g. polyurethane, urethane, T-Foam, Sun-Mate) of foam are commonly used in linear seating systems (Figure 55.8). Foam has been shown to offer the lowest maximum pressure over the seating surface when the appropriate densities and contours are used (103, 104, 105). Foam, over other materials, has the significant advantage of being inexpensive. However, foam has a tendency to deteriorate at an undesirable rate (106, 107, 108). The added cost to make a cushion comes from the sculpting or contouring, which requires clinical skills in order to make foam work most effectively for pressure relief (109).

Standard polyurethane or urethane foams are made from plastic that has been processed to incorporate large numbers of air bubbles. These air bubbles within the foam cause a cross-link type structure. When foam is loaded with small forces and displacement, it behaves like a spring. As greater loads and displacement are applied, the cross-links begin to buckle and the foam begins to behave non-linearly. If further load is applied, the cross-links fully buckle and the foam begins to act like a compressible solid. Little is understood about how these properties are best manipulated to form a pressure relief cushion. For this reason people use foam of various density and stiffness. The cross links of foam changes the force/displacement relationship as force is increased. This nonlinear behavior of foam has not been fully exploited in cushion design.

The density of foam relates to the amount of air trapped within the plastic matrix. Higher density foams contain more plastic and tend to be heavier. As density increases, stiffness also increases; however, stiffness and density are not the same properties. Stiffness refers to the slope of the force-displacement curve during the linear region (i.e. before the cross-links begin to buckle). Foam is also characterized as open cell or closed cell. Closed-cell foam is made such that it is less permeable to fluid.

Foam cushions can be made by contouring a single piece of foam or by combining foams of different stiffness. There are also specialty foams such as T-foam or memory foam. These specialty foams are made to have gel-like properties while maintaining some of the desirable properties of foam. T-foam and memory foam have negligible linear regions; therefore they compress like standard foam, although at a slower rate. These types of foam have memory that retards them from returning to their resting shape. Hence, when a person sits on them, they tend to come in equilibrium with the sitting tissue. The foam then responds slowly to changes in position. T-foam or memory foam can be used to give some additional stability to standard foam cushions. Foam is an excellent material for cushions, but it has low durability and loses its pressure-relieving properties rapidly with use. Most foam cushions will therefore need to be replaced annually.

Air Floatation Cushions

Air floatation cushions provide an excellent example of cushion design based upon the interface pressure theory (Figure 55.9). If one were to simply sit on a balloon full of air, the pressure over

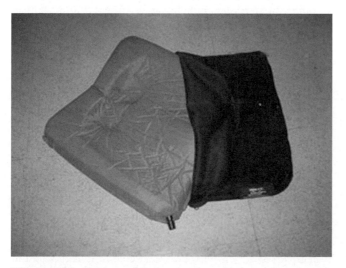

Figure 55.8   Foam cushion.

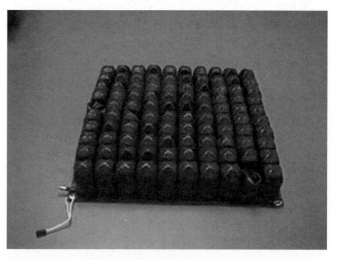

Figure 55.9   Air floatation cushion.

the entire seating surface would be equal. This is because the air in the balloon shifts to conform to the seated surface in order to equalize the internal pressure. A balloon full of air does an excellent job of distributing the pressure over the seating area. However, the pressure would be distributed indiscriminately. In order to better control interface pressure, many air floatation cushions use multiple compartments, contouring, and baffling. Multiple compartments allow interface pressure to be regulated from one compartment to another. The pressure within a particular cell (balloon) will be constant. The pressure at the skin interface may be regulated by shaping the balloon. Balloon shape may lower pressure within the tissue by altering the way in which the body tissue deforms. Some cushions use foam in combination with air bladders to control the pressure within the cushion, and in turn the interface pressure. The combination of foam and air floatation assumes that the compression of the foam within the bladder will regulate pressure to direct it away from low tolerant regions and toward regions of higher pressure tolerance.

A problem with air cushions is that they may lose their air and simultaneously lose their ability to provide pressure relief. This results in some air cushions requiring considerable maintenance. For this reason, it may be recommended that users bring repair kits with them when traveling. Air cushions will also change their properties with changes in altitude. The most common occurrence of this is flying on an airplane when the air pressure within the cushion can change considerably from take-off to cruising altitude.

Visco-Elastic Fluid Cushions

Visco-elastic fluid ("gel") cushions use an electrolyte visco-elastic fluid in a closed plastic or latex pocket. The visco-elastic fluid conforms to the body and provides nearly even pressure distribution (Figure 55.10). Viscosity is used to define a fluid's resistance to flow. Because visco-elastic fluid behaves like a fluid, it will work much like air to equalize pressure over the entire seating surface. This is because the visco-elastic fluid will move to come to a

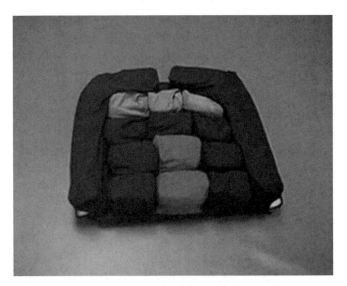

Figure 55.10 Visco-elastic fluid "gel" cushion.

constant pressure within its container. Baffles can be used to control the flow of the visco-elastic fluid just as with air cushions. The pressure distribution can be altered by using a stiff base (e.g., plastic or foam) to provide some contouring. The high viscosity of the visco-elastic fluid prevents it from moving rapidly within its container. This property allows the visco-elastic fluid cushion to provide a more stable seating surface than an air cushion. However, the high viscosity of a visco-elastic fluid cushion also limits its shock-absorbing properties.

The weight of visco-elastic fluid cushions is often a limiting factor for many users. For this reason, some manufacturers have altered the weight of the cushion by developing lightweight visco-elastic fluids. These lightweight fluids may act more like whipped cream and are typically of a lower viscosity, which provides greater shock-absorbing properties. Unlike air floatation cushions, the properties of visco-elastic fluid cushions do not change significantly when there are changes in atmospheric pressure. The properties of the cushion are, however, subject to changes in temperature. If the cushion becomes cold, the user's body may need to exert considerable energy to heat the cushion. Some types of visco-elastic fluids may actually freeze during extremely cold weather. Finally, because visco-elastic fluid cushions may develop leaks with use over time, users should check with manufacturers about possible allergic reactions from contact with the visco-elastic fluid.

Honeycomb

Honeycomb cushion materials have an advantage over foam in that the manufacturer can carefully control the properties of the honeycomb material and resulting cushion. Honeycomb materials are made to exploit the linear properties of some polymers (i.e. types of plastics). When polymers are molded into a honeycomb, they behave like a collection of springs, similar to the linear behavior of foam cushions. Similar to foam cushions, honeycomb cushions can be contoured. Manufacturers will typically contour honeycomb into some standard shapes. Honeycomb cushions, like air and visco-elastic floatation cushions, can be made to simplify cleaning, which makes them more attractive than foam in institutions where multiple people share a single cushion. Honeycomb cushions may have an advantage of increased durability and a larger linear range than foam cushions. However, honeycomb cushions are considerably more expensive and do not come in as many varieties of stiffness as foam.

POSTURAL SUPPORTS

Proper seating can be achieved for many people using standard seating and positioning equipment. The pelvis is often the foundation of the properly aligned seat (110–113). The structure, construction, and dimensions are critical in prescribing or designing a positioning pad or seating cushion (114, 115, 116). Seat cushions may have a squared edge, rolled edge, or beveled edge.

Seat cushions commonly include a cut-out for the ischial tuberosities, an abductor pommel, and hip adductor contours (117–122). For people who require additional positioning or postural support, hip pads and/or hip belts can be used. For people with severe leg abduction or adduction, thin abductor or adductor pads can be attached to the seat pan. A cylinder of low to medium density polyurethane foam on a stainless steel or chrome-plated low-carbon steel pillar will provide adequate support for even the most severe cases. Abductor or adductor pads can be prescribed or designed to be detachable or flip down for easier transfers. Often a single cylinder is adequate; however, some people can benefit from two cylinders that can be independently laterally adjusted. A scissor board (i.e., a wedge of foam adhered to a semi-rigid material) with polyurethane foam can be used to reduce the risk of pressure sores at the knees when a narrow lateral separation is desired.

Custom Contoured Cushions

Contour measurements can be made using vacuum-forming or seating contour measurement systems. Typically such systems are used to create a contour representative of the client's seating profile (117, 123, 124, 125). Vacuum-forming methods are typically based on a flexible bag (e.g. latex, rubber), which is filled with Styrofoam or foam rubber pellets and connected to a vacuum pump. The person to be molded is seated on the bead-bag and positioned in approximately the desired position. Air is drawn from the bag, which becomes ever more rigid. While air is being drawn from the bag the clinician and rehabilitation engineer/technician form the bead bag around the client, pushing and pulling on the bag until the client is in the desired position. Air continues to be withdrawn from the bag until it becomes stiff, at which point the client can be removed from the chair. Vacuum-forming systems are cost effective and relatively simple. Contour measurement systems are more effective when they mimic wheelchair seating (i.e., legrests are attached, armrests are used, backrest is at proper angle and of appropriate height). Once a male mold of the client's contour is completed, it must be transferred from the bead bag to something that can be used to create a cushion. Many commercial contoured cushions are created using computer numerically controlled (CNC) foam milling machines (117, 125). These machines use arrays to represent x, y, and z coordinates of the seating contour. Hence, some companies have developed mechanical or electromechanical panographs to convert the male mold to a graph or directly to a computer file. A panograph may simply consist of a set of bars with rounded tips that glide over the mold surface. The other ends of the shafts are connected to a pen or transducer. The sensors (fingers) of the panograph are indexed over the surface of the mold until a suitable representation has been created.

WHEELCHAIR USAGE

Wheelchairs provide individuals with disabilities access to the community (126, 127, 128). Additionally, it is known that physical activity can positively influence physical and psychological well-being in the unimpaired population. What remains relatively unknown is how this translates to individuals with disabilities.

Using a data-logging device, studies have been conducted to compare wheelchair athletes during participation in events such as the National Veterans Wheelchair Games versus their time at home (85, 129). Unobtrusive devices that measure variables such as distance traveled, hours using the chair, etc. were attached to individuals' wheelchairs for a period of time during their participation at the Games and while they were in their home environment (63). Individuals traveled farther and were more active during their week at the Games than they were at home (85, 129).

THE TEAM APPROACH TO WHEELCHAIR SELECTION

Similar to other areas of rehabilitation, the delivery of assistive technology (AT) services are best provided using a multi-disciplinary team approach. The assessment team will examine the needs of the wheelchair user, the environmental conditions they will encounter, the activities they will perform in the chair, and the amount of training or instruction they might require to use the chair safely and effectively. Ideally, an AT team would include a physician, therapist, AT supplier, and a rehabilitation engineer. Each professional has a unique but complementary role, and in cooperation with the end-user, provides a comprehensive view of the AT needs.

Along with professionals, the individual with SCI and their family members are critical members of the team who determine the goals to be achieved. The decision to accept the chair should ultimately be made by the person spending the most time in it—the wheelchair user. The family and caregiver should also provide input, as they will be the next most affected by the choice of chair.

A physician usually signs the prescription for the wheelchair after determining that an individual is an appropriate candidate. Physiatrists, physicians who complete their residency in Physical Medicine and Rehabilitation, make ideal physicians on AT teams because of their specialized training and knowledge in the ways that AT benefits people with spinal cord injuries. The field of AT has become increasingly more complex and requires specialized knowledge for selection of appropriate AT as well as justification, fitting, tuning, and training.

An occupational and/or physical therapist is also helpful. A rehabilitation engineer or a professional certified in rehabilitation technology by The Rehabilitation Engineering and Assistive Technology Society of North America (RESNA) is crucial to include on the assessment team. Such an individual will have the skills to assess the needs of the user and will take into account the environment the chair will be used in and the activities that will be performed in the wheelchair.

RESNA recognized the need for both consumers and insurers to be able to distinguish individuals with relevant experience and specialized knowledge. Over a period of ten years, RESNA created three credentialing programs that continue to grow throughout the United States each year. These credentialing programs also appear to be slowly becoming a model for several other countries.

The Assistive Technology Supplier (ATS) credential is intended for distributors and representatives of companies that manufacture assistive technology. The ATS is the most important of the credentials offered by RESNA. Prior to the development of the ATS credential, a reliable credential for a supplier or manufacturer representative to demonstrate competency did not exist and consumers were unable to readily identify qualified suppliers, leaving this area of assistive technology largely unregulated.

The Assistive Technology Provider (ATP) credential is geared toward therapists (physical, occupational, speech/language, counselors, and special educators). The ATP provides credentialing for qualified clinicians to be recognized for their specialized knowledge and expertise. For decades, rehabilitation professionals provided clinical services without formal recognition of their expertise, and in many cases their services were not reimbursed by some insurance agencies.

The Rehabilitation Engineering Technology (RET) credential addresses the needs of rehabilitation engineers and provides other professionals and consumers a clear way to recognize clinical rehabilitation engineers. In order to obtain the RET, the engineer must also have obtained the ATP credential. All three of the RESNA credentials require evidence of relevant experience and a passing score on a comprehensive examination. Early indications are that the credentials have improved the quality of services available; however, it is still too soon to tell. Although progress has been made, significant challenges remain. It is often difficult for comprehensive AT clinics to survive solely from reimbursement for their services. Most AT clinics are, therefore, associated with a university, not-for-profit organization (e.g. Easter Seals, United Cerebral Palsy), or a rehabilitation center where other sources can assist in underwriting the costs.

Those involved in the wheelchair selection process should learn about the many wheelchairs available on the market. Magazine articles and commercial database sources such as ABLEDATA are good places to begin research about assistive devices. Wheelchair manufacturers can also be contacted directly or through the Internet for additional information.

The funding agency or third-party payer for the wheelchair should be contacted early to determine the amount and kinds of costs that will be covered. In addition to the purchase price, the chair's long-range maintenance costs should also be considered, as this may be an important factor in making the final decision.

Once the model and pricing options have been investigated, the needs of the individual should be assessed by examining the environment and regular activities of the wheelchair user. Most activities can be placed into one of three categories: daily living, vocational/educational, and leisure. Activities of daily living include those activities done in the home environment, such as transferring in and out of bed, bathing and other toilet activities, and cooking. Access to a range of heights might be important to reach objects in the home and other environments. Other daily living activities include running errands, performing chores, shopping for groceries, and stopping by the post office. Vocational/educational activities can involve maneuvering in an office, outdoor construction site, agricultural setting, or school environment. People's professions are often highly specialized, and specific requirements may exist for mobility within a laboratory, operating room, court room, clean room, or machine shop. Leisure activities, pursued in such places as community centers, restaurants, movie theaters, and recreational environments, often place the most demand on the wheelchair.

The wheelchair model chosen should also be compatible with the public and/or private transportation options available to the wheelchair user, such as a bus, car, or van. If a power wheelchair user plans to travel by air, only modular wheelchairs that operate on sealed gel batteries should be considered, as chairs using other power sources are not permitted on commercial planes. In other countries, access to buses and trains can be an important requirement.

In all environments, the surface conditions will impose the greatest restrictions on the type of wheelchair that is most appropriate. The regularity of the surface and its firmness and stability are important in determining the tire size and wheel diameter. The performance of the wheelchair is often dictated by the need to negotiate grades, as well as height transitions such as thresholds and curbs. The clearance widths in the environment will determine the overall dimensions of the wheelchair. The climate that the chair will be operated in and the need to be able to operate in snow, rain, and changing humidity and temperature levels, among other weather conditions, are important considerations.

A variety of performance characteristics of the wheelchair should be considered with regard to the environment and activities that the individual is trying to perform. The maximum speed of the wheelchair is important when using the wheelchair to travel long distances, such as across campus or across town. The obstacle-climbing ability of the chair will help determine the rider's access to environments that do not meet the Americans with Disabilities Act (ADA) Accessibility Guidelines. Static and dynamic stability characteristics (i.e. the "tippiness" of the chair) will determine how safely the rider will be able to negotiate many of these non-ideal environments.

Additionally, the overall dimensions of the chair will determine how well the wheelchair user can maneuver in tight quarters. The range of the wheelchair will indicate how long and how far the user can go in a given day without having to recharge the batteries. The maximum overall weight of the chair can be an important consideration if the wheelchair user does not have access to mass transit or a van equipped with a lift or ramp. Regardless of functional ability, all users need to develop and tune skills to enable safe operation of a particular wheelchair with its performance characteristics within the restrictions of the environment.

Once an understanding of the individual's need or desire to perform different activities in various environments has been gained, the most important factor in the wheelchair selection process—the user—should be examined. As the kinds of activities that are important to the user have been inventoried, an idea of the individual's level of independence will have been ascertained. An indication of their physical abilities will also have been gained. In order to verify this, some simple tasks can be performed with the person to determine the lateral and frontal stability of their trunk, their hand and arm strength, and the fine motor skills of their fingers (130, 131, 132).

Many powered wheelchair users brace some portion of their hand against the control box and use their hand and arm coordination to operate the joystick. Gross arm function, in many cases, can be used to operate a joystick. If the user does not have the hand function or coordination to operate a joystick input device, other options are available. Other parts of the body, such as the chin or foot, can operate a modified joystick, or a sip-and-puff control can be used.

Be aware, however, that as the physical and functional abilities of the user decrease, the cognitive abilities required to operate an alternative control typically increase, as they are often more advanced and complex. A sense of an individual's cognitive function can be obtained by assessing verbal and visual skills, the rate and accuracy with which they can perform various tasks, their spatial problem-solving abilities, and their understanding of their body's position in space. Visual skills, including sight accuracy and depth perception, are also important for safe operation of a powered wheelchair. In order to encourage safe operation of the chair, programmable controllers allow a lower maximum velocity to be set and acceleration and deceleration rates of the wheelchair to be reduced. To assist persons with more severe cognitive or visual limitations, technologies are being developed that enable the wheelchair to follow walls, navigate through doorways, and stop when other objects are contacted.

Assessment for the presence of spasticity in the user's hands or arms is also important. For persons with spasticity, particularly tremor in the hand, modern controllers have filters that can be adjusted to give smooth wheelchair control. Positioning mechanisms use linkages and adjustable components to enable positioning the joystick in several places to optimize the user's joystick operating function. Finally, once the appropriate choice and technologies in powered mobility have been made, a lot of time will need to be spent optimizing the seating setup to maximize the rider's function.

Before individuals ride away in their new powered mobility, they should go through a wheelchair training program. This is particularly important for younger children. Wheelchair users can first practice basic maneuvers in controlled environments that meet ADA Accessibility Guidelines. They should practice negotiating uneven surfaces, slope transitions (i.e., level to sloped surfaces) in both the uphill and downhill directions, and maneuvering through tight environments. Once these skills are mastered, they should gradually tackle more challenging environments, such as steep grades and transitions that exceed ADA Accessibility Guidelines. The rider should always practice with an appropriate lap belt and chest support in place, as well as with spotters standing by to assist if needed. The wheelchair user should also be given an opportunity to experience the limits of the technology they are using. By setting up and practicing in safe environments, users can experience the limits of the lateral stability, as well as the front and rear stability of their chair so that they have a better understanding of its performance limits.

SUMMARY

Advances in wheelchair technology and options are aimed at improving access to full participation in daily activities, as well as safety during wheelchair use. These advances have provided mobility to individuals who were once unable to independently use mobility devices. The user interface is among the most critical factors determining the function of the user of an electric powered wheelchair. Substantial developments of electric powered wheelchair interfaces have occurred; however, little data or other research on interfaces is available. Accompanying the success of acute medical rehabilitation has been an expectation for greater community integration among people with severe disabilities. Alternative interfaces and complex control algorithms have the potential to fulfill some of the promise for community integration.

The emergence of advanced mobility devices shows promise for the contribution of engineering to the amelioration of mobility impairments for millions of people who have disabilities or who are elderly. The application of advances in power electronics, telecommunications, controls, sensors, and instrumentation has only just scratched the surface. Advancing mobility technology for people with spinal cord injury represents a significant career and business opportunity for professionals who want to serve the public good in a meaningful and tangible way.

Technology plays a critical role in promoting well-being, activity, and participation for individuals with spinal cord injury (SCI). It is one of the few things that can be provided to people with SCI where one can see an immediate and profound benefit. As technology has improved, so has the realm of possibilities open to people with SCI. The range of activities in which people with SCI participate is impressive but still growing. School, work, travel, and leisure activities are all facilitated by technology. Advances in materials have made wheelchairs lighter, and developments in design have made wheelchairs that fit individual needs. Software has made computer interfaces adaptive and in some case intelligent, through learning the user's behavior and optimizing its structure. The trend is certainly taking us in two exciting directions: (1) personalized design where the technology matches and adapts to the user's needs; and (2) aware systems that learn from the user's behavior, the context, and the environment to support the end-user. As participatory action design and aware systems take greater hold, transformational change is likely to take place in the technology available to people with SCI.

References

1. Pearlman, J., Cooper, R.A., Zipfel, E., Cooper, R., McCartney, M. (2006). Towards the development of an effective technology transfer model of wheelchairs to developing countries. *Disability and Rehabilitation: Assistive Technology*, 1(1–2), 103–110.
2. Hubbard, S., Fitzgerald, S.G., Reker, D., Boninger, M.L., Cooper, R.A. (2006). Demographic characteristics of veterans who received wheelchairs and scooters from Veterans Health Administration. *Journal of Rehabilitation Research and Development*, 43(7), 831–844.
3. Chavez, E., Boninger, M.L., Cooper, R., Fitzgerald, S.G., Gray, D., Cooper, R.A. (2004). Application of a participation system to assess the influence of assistive technology on the lives of people with spinal cord injury. *Archives of Physical Medicine and Rehabilitation*, 85(11), 1854–1858.
4. Hunt, P.C., Boninger, M.L., Cooper, R.A., Zafonte, R.D., Fitzgerald, S.G. (2004). Factors associated with wheelchair type and quality among individuals with traumatic spinal cord injury. *Archives of Physical Medicine and Rehabilitation*, 85(11), 1859–1864.
5. Cook, A.M., Hussey, S.M. (1995). *Assistive Technologies: Principles and Practice*. St. Louis, MO: Mosby.
6. Flippo, K.F., Inge, K.J., Barcus, J.M. (1995). *Assistive Technology: A Resource for School, Work and Community*. Baltimore, MD: Paul H. Brookes Publishing.
7. Authier, E.L., Pearlman, J., Allegretti, A., Rice, I., Cooper, R.A. (2007). A sports wheelchair for low income counties. *Disability and Rehabilitation*, 29(11/12), 963–967.
8. Kirby, R.L., Cooper, R.A. (2007). Applicability of the wheelchair skills program to the Indian context. Disability and Rehabilitation, 29(11/12), 969–972.
9. Zipfel, E., Cooper, R.A., Pearlman, J., Cooper, R.M., McCartney, M. (2007). New design and development of a manual wheelchair for India. *Disability and Rehabilitation*, 29(11/12), 949–962.
10. Brubaker, C.E. (1986). Wheelchair prescription: an analysis of factors that affect mobility and performance. *Journal of Rehabilitation Research and Development*, 23(4), 19–26.
11. Cravotta, D. (1991). Mobility for the masses. *Mainstream*, July, 11–17.
12. Department of Veterans Affairs. (1990). Choosing a wheelchair system. *Journal of Rehabilitation Research and Development*, Clinical Supplement No. 2, March.
13. Cooper, R.A. (1995). Rehabilitation engineering applied to mobility and manipulation, Bristol, England: Institute of Physics.
14. Cooper, R.A. (1991). High tech wheelchairs gain the competitive edge. *IEEE Engineering in Medicine and Biology Magazine*, 10(4), 49–55.
15. DiGiovine, M.M., Cooper, R.A., Boninger, M.L., Lawrence, B.L., VanSickle, D.P., Rentschler, A.J. (2000) User assessment of manual wheelchair ride comfort and ergonomics. *Archives of Physical Medicine and Rehabilitation*, 81(4), 490–494.

16. Fitzgerald, S.G., Cooper, R.A., Boninger, M.L., Rentschler, A.J. (2001). Comparison of fatigue life for three types of manual wheelchairs. *Archives of Physical Medicine and Rehabilitation*, 82(10), 1484–1488.

17. Boninger, M.L., Baldwin, M., Cooper, R.A., Koontz, A.M., Chan, L. (2000). Manual wheelchair pushrim biomechanics and axle position. *Archives of Physical Medicine and Rehabilitation*, 81(5), 608–613.

18. Boninger, M.L., Souza, A.L., Cooper, R.A., Fitzgerald, S.G., Koontz, A.M., Fay, B.T. (2002). Propulsion patterns and pushrim biomechanics in manual wheelchair propulsion. *Archives of Physical Medicine and Rehabilitation*, 83(5), 718–723.

19. Boninger, M.L., Cooper, R.A., Fitzgerald, S.G., Lin, J., Cooper, R., Dicianno, B., Liu, B. (2003). Investigating neck pain in wheelchair users. *American Journal of Physical Medicine and Rehabilitation*, 82(3), 197–202.

20. Kwarciak, A.M., Cooper, R.A., Ammer, W.A., Fitzgerald, S.G., Boninger, M.L., Cooper, R. (2005). Fatigue testing of selected suspension manual wheelchairs using ANSI/RESNA standards. *Archives of Physical Medicine and Rehabilitation*, 86(1), 123–129.

21. VanSickle, D.P., Cooper, R.A., Boninger, M.L. (2000). Road loads acting on manual wheelchairs. *IEEE Transactions on Rehabilitation Engineering*, 8(3), 385–393.

22. VanSickle, D.P., Cooper, R.A., Boninger, M.L., DiGiovine, C.P. (2001). Analysis of vibrations induced during wheelchair propulsion. *Journal of Rehabilitation Research and Development*, 38(4), 409–422.

23. Boninger, M.L., Towers, J.D., Cooper, R.A., Dicianno, B.E., Munin, M.C. (2001). Shoulder imaging abnormalities in individuals with paraplegia. *Journal of Rehabilitation Research and Development*, 38(4), 401–408.

24. Cooper, R.A., Wolf, E., Fitzgerald, S.G., Boninger, M.L., Ulerich, R., Ammer, W.A. (2003). Seat and footrest accelerations in manual wheelchairs with and without suspension. *Archives of Physical Medicine and Rehabilitation*, 84(1), 96–102.

25. Fay, B.T., Boninger, M.L., Fitzgerald, S.G., Souza, A.L., Cooper, R.A., Koontz, A.M. (2004). Manual wheelchair pushrim dynamics in persons with multiple sclerosis. *Archives of Physical Medicine and Rehabilitation*, 85(6), 935–942.

26. Boninger, M.L., Impink, B., Cooper, R.A., Koontz, A.M. (2004). Relationship between median and ulnar nerve function and wrist kinematics during wheelchair propulsion. *Archives of Physical Medicine and Rehabilitation*, 85(7), 1141–1145.

27. Souza, A.L., Boninger, M.L., Fitzgerald, S.G., Shimada, S.D., Cooper, R.A. (2005). Upper limb strength in wheelchair users with paraplegia. *Journal of Spinal Cord Medicine*, 28(1), 26–32.

28. Cooper, R.A., Rentschler, A.J., O'Connor, T.J., Ster, J.F. (2000). Technical note: wheelchair armrest strength testing. *Assistive Technology*, 12(2), 106–115.

29. Cooper, R.A., Boninger, M.L., Spaeth, D.M., Ding, D., Guo, S.F., Koontz, A.M., Fitzgerald, S.G., Cooper, R., Kelleher. A., Collins, D.M. (2006). Engineering better wheelchairs to enhance community participation, *IEEE Transactions on Neural Systems and Rehabilitation Engineering*, 14(4), 438–455.

30. Koontz, A.M., Cooper, R.A., Boninger, M.L., Yang, YS, Impink, B., van der Woude, L. (2005). A biomechanical analysis of manual wheelchair propulsion on selected indoor and outdoor surfaces. *Journal of Rehabilitation Research and Development*, 42(4), 447–458.

31. Fitzgerald, S.G., Collins, D.M., Cooper, R.A., Tolerico, M., Kelleher, A.R., Hunt, P.C., Martin, S.G., Impink, B.G., Cooper, R. (2005). Issues in the maintenance and repairs of wheelchairs: a pilot study. *Journal of Rehabilitation Research and Development*, 42(6), 853–862.

32. Galvin, J.C., Scherer, M.J. (1996). *Evaluating, selecting, and using appropriate assistive technology*. Gaitherburg, MD: Aspen Publishers Inc.

33. Ambrosio, F., Boninger, M.L., Souza, A.L., Fitzgerald, S.G., Koontz, A.M., Cooper, R.A. (2005). Biomechanics and strength of manual wheelchair users. *Journal of Spinal Cord Medicine*, 28(5), 407–414.

34. Mercer, J.L., Boninger, M.L., Koontz, A.M., Ren, D., Dyson-Hudson, T., Cooper, R.A. (2006). Shoulder joint kinetics and pathology in manual wheelchair users. *Clinical Biomechanics*, 21(8), 781–789.

35. Collins, T.J., Kauzlarich, J.J. (1988) Directional instability of rear caster wheelchairs. *Journal of Rehabilitation Research and Development*, 25(3), 1–18.

36. Gordon, J., Kauzlarich, J.J., Thacker, J.G. (1989). Tests of two new polyurethane foam wheelchair tires. *Journal of Rehabilitation Research and Development*, 26(1), 33–46.

37. Kauzlarich, J.J., Thacker, J.G. (1987). A theory of wheelchair wheelie performance. *Journal of Rehabilitation Research and Development*, 24(2), 67–80.

38. Kauzlarich, J.J., Bruning, T., Thacker, J.G. (1984). Wheelchair caster shimmy and turning resistance. *Journal of Rehabilitation Research and Development*, 20(2), 15–29.

39. O'Connor, TJ, Cooper, R.A., Boninger, M.L., Glass, L. (2000). Evaluation of a prototype geared pushrim design: comparison with standard manual pushrim and analysis of wheelchair user's physiological data. *Saudi Journal of Disability and Rehabilitation*, 6(2), 114–120.

40. Cooper, R.A., Nakahara, A., Ster, J., Cooper, R. (2002). Design of an internal three speed hub for a manual wheelchair. *Saudi Journal of Disability and Rehabilitation*, 8(3), 143–147.

41. Denison, I., Shaw, J., Zuyderhoff, R. (1994). *Wheelchair selection manual: the effect of components on manual wheelchair performance*. Vancouver, BC: British Columbia Rehabilitation Society.

42. McLaurin, C.A., Brubaker, C.E. (1985). A lever drive system for wheelchairs. *Proceedings RESNA 8th Annual Conference*, Memphis, TN, 48–50.

43. Nashihara, H., Shizukuishi, K., (1992). Development of indoor wheelchair mainly made of wood. *Proceedings RESNA International*, Toronto, Canada, 533–535.

44. Szeto, A.Y.J., White, R.N. (1983). Evaluation of a curb-climbing aid for manual wheelchairs: considerations of stability, effort, and safety. *Journal of Rehabilitation Research and Development*, 20(1), 45–56.

45. Koontz, A.M., Boninger, M.L., Cooper, R.A., Souza, A.S., Fay, B.T. (2002). Shoulder kinematics and kinetics during two speeds of wheelchair propulsion. *Journal of Rehabilitation Research and Development*, 39(6), 635–650.

46. Cooper, R.A., DiGiovine, C.P., Boninger, M.L., Shimada, S.D., Koontz, A.M., Baldwin, M.A. (2002). Filter frequency selection for manual wheelchair biomechanics. *Journal of Rehabilitation Research and Development*, 39(3), 323–336.

47. Boninger, M.L., Dicianno, B.E., Cooper, R.A., Towers, J.D., Koontz, A.M., Souza, A.L. (2003). Shoulder magnetic resonance imaging abnormalities, wheelchair propulsion, and gender. *Archives of Physical Medicine and Rehabilitation*, 84(11), 1615–1620.

48. Lemaire, E.D., Lamontagne, M., Barclay, H., John, T., Martel, G. (1991). A technique for the determination of center of gravity and rolling resistance for tilt-seat wheelchairs. *Journal of Rehabilitation Research and Development*, 28(3), 51–58.

49. Masse, L.C., Lamontagne, M., O'Riain, M.D. (1992). Biomechanical analysis of wheelchair propulsion for various seating positions. *Journal of Rehabilitation Research and Development*, 29(3), 12–28.

50. Trefler, E., Hobson, D.A., Taylor, S.J., Monohan, L.C., Shaw C.G. (1993). *Seating and mobility for persons with disabilities*, Tucson, AZ: Therapy Skill Builders.

51. Wilson, A.B. Jr. (1992). *Wheelchairs: a prescription guide* (2nd Ed.). New York: Demos.

52. Axelson, P., Minkel, J., Chesney, D. (1994). *A guide to wheelchair selection: how to use the ANSI/RESNA wheelchair standards to buy a wheelchair*. Washington, DC: Paralyzed Veterans of America.

53. Jacobs, K., Bettencourt, C.M. (1995). *Ergonomics for therapists*. Boston, MA: Butterworth-Heinemann.

54. Davies, T.D., Beasley K.A. (1988). *Design for hospitality: planning for accessible hotels and motels*. New York: Nichols Publishing.

55. Davies T.D., Beasley, K.A. (1992). *Fair housing design guide for accessibility*. Washington, D.C.: Paralyzed Veterans of America.

56. Veeger, D., Van der Woude, L.H.V., Rozendal R.H. (1989). The effect of rear wheel camber in manual wheelchair propulsion. *Journal of Rehabilitation Research and Development*, 26(2), 37–46.

57. Crane, B.A., Holm, M.B., Hobson, D.A., Cooper, R.A., Reed, M.P., Stadelmeir, S. (2005). Test-retest reliability, internal item consistency, and concurrent validity of the wheelchair seating discomfort assessment tool. *Assistive Technology*, 17(2), 98–107.

58. Crane, B.A., Holm, M.B., Hobson, D., Cooper, R.A., Reed, M.P., Stadelmeier, S. (2004). Consumer involvement in the development of a wheelchair seating discomfort assessment tool (WcS-DAT). *International Journal of Rehabilitation Research*, 27(1).

59. Koontz, A.M., Yang, Y, Boninger, D.S., Kanaly, J., Cooper, R.A., Boninger, M.L., Dieruf, K., Ewer, L. (2006). Investigation of the performance of an ergonomic handrim as a pain-relieving intervention for manual wheelchair users. *Assistive Technology*, 18(2), 123–145.

60. Gaines, R.F., La, W.H.T. (1986). Users' responses to contoured wheelchair handrims. *Journal of Rehabilitation Research and Development*, 23(3), 57–62.

61. Cooper, R.A., Cooper, R., Tolerico, M., Guo, S.F., Ding, D., Pearlman, J. (2006). advances in electric powered wheelchairs. *Topics in Spinal Cord Injury Rehabilitation*, 11(4), 15–29.

62. Algood, S.D., Cooper, R.A., Boninger, M.L., Fitzgerald, S.G., Cooper, R. (2004). Impact of a pushrim activated power assist wheelchair on the metabolic demands, stroke frequency, and range of motion among individuals with tetraplegia. *Archives of Physical Medicine and Rehabilitation*, 85(11), 1865–1871.

63. Fitzgerald, S.G., Arva, J., Cooper, R.A., Spaeth, D.M. (2003). A pilot study on community usage of a pushrim activated power assisted wheelchair. *Assistive Technology*, 15(2), 113–119.

64. Pickles, B., Topping, A. (1994). Community care for Canadian seniors: an exercise in educational planning. *Disability and Rehabilitation*, 16(3), 181–189.

65. Sonn, U., Grimby, G. (1994). Assistive devices in an elderly population studied at 70–76 years of age. *Disability and Rehabilitation*, 16(2), 85–93.

66. Algood, S.D., Cooper, R.A., Fitzgerald, S.G., Cooper, R., Boninger, M.L. (2005). Effect of a pushrim activated power assist wheelchair on the functional capabilities of individuals with tetraplegia. *Archives of Physical Medicine and Rehabilitation*, 86(3), 380–386.

67. Corfman, T.A., Cooper, R.A., Boninger, M.L., Koontz, A.M., Fitzgerald, S.G. (2003). Range of motion and stroke frequency differences between manual wheelchair propulsion and pushrim activated power assisted wheelchair propulsion. *Journal of Spinal Cord Medicine*, 26(2), 135–140.

68. Cooper, R.A., Corfman, T.A., Fitzgerald, S.G., Boninger, M.L., Spaeth, D.M., Ammer, W., Arva, J. (2002). Performance assessment of a pushrim activated power assisted wheelchair. *IEEE Transactions of Control Systems Technology*, 10(1), 121–126.

69. Arva, J., Fitzgerald, S.G., Cooper, R.A., Boninger, M.L., Spaeth, D.M., Corfman, T.J. (2001). Mechanical efficiency and user power reduction with the JWII pushrim activate power assisted wheelchair. *Medical Engineering and Physics*, 23(12), 699–705.

70. Dan, D., Cooper, R.A. (2005). Review of control technology and algorithms for electric powered wheelchairs. *IEEE Controls Systems Magazine*, 25(2), 22–34.

71. Chase, J., Chase, D.M., Bailey, D.M. (1990). Evaluating potential for powered mobility. *American Journal of Occupational Therapy*, 44(12), 1125–1129.

72. Kamenetz, H. (1969). *The wheelchair book: mobility for the disabled*. Springfield, IL: C.C. Thomas.

73. Lipskin, R. (1970). An evaluation program for powered wheelchair control systems. *Bulletin of Prosthetics Research*, 121–129.

74. Scott, C.M., Prior, R.E. (1978). Mobility engineering for the severely handicapped. *Bulletin of Prosthetics Research*, 10(30), 248–255.

75. Shung, J.B., Tomizuka, M., Auslander, D.M., Stout, G. (1983). Feedback control and simulation of a wheelchair. *ASME Journal of Dynamics Systems, Measurement and Control*, 105, 96–100.

76. Shung, J.B., Stout, G., Tomizuka, M., Auslander, D.M. (1983). Dynamic modeling of a wheelchair on a slope. *ASME Journal of Dynamics Systems, Measurement and Control*, 105, 101–106.

77. Stout, G. (1979). Some aspects of high performance indoor/outdoor wheelchairs. *Bulletin of Prosthetics Research*, 10(32), 330–332.

78. Ding, D., Cooper, R.A., Kaminski, B.A., Kanaly, J.R., Allegretti, A., Chaves, E., Hubbard, S. (2003). Integrated control of assistive technology. *Assistive Technology*, 15(2), 89–96.

79. Cooper, R.A., Boninger, M.L., Brienza, D.M., van Roosmalen, L., Koontz, A.M., LoPresti, E., Spaeth, D.M., Bertocci, G.E., Guo, S.F., Buning, M.E., Schmeler, M., Geyer, M.J., Fitzgerald, S.G., Ding, D. (2003). Pittsburgh wheelchair and seating biomechanics research program. *Journal of the Society of Biomechanisms*, 27(3), 144–157.

80. Pearlman, J.L., Cooper, R.A., Karnawat, J., Cooper, R., Boninger, M.L. (2005). Evaluation of the safety and durability of low-cost electric powered wheelchairs. *Archives of Physical Medicine and Rehabilitation*, 86(12), 2361–2370.

81. Fass, M.V., Cooper, R.A., Fitzgerald, S.G., Schmeler, M., Boninger, M.L., Algood, S.D., Ammer, W.A., Rentschler, A.J., Duncan, J. (2004). Durability, value, and reliability of selected electric powered wheelchairs. *Archives of Physical Medicine and Rehabilitation*, 85(5), 805–814.

82. Rentschler, A.J., Cooper, R.A., Fitzgerald, S.G., Boninger, M.L., Guo, S., Ammer, W.A., Vitek, M., Algood, S.D. (2004). Evaluation of selected electric powered wheelchairs using the ANSI/RESNA standards. *Archives of Physical Medicine and Rehabilitation*, 85(4), 611–619.

83. Guo, S., Cooper, R.A., Corfman, T.A., Ding, D. (2003). Influence of wheelchair front caster wheel on the reverse driving stability. *Assistive Technology*, 15(2), 98–104.

84. Simpson, R., LoPresti, E., Hayashi, S., Guo, S., Ding, D., Cooper, R.A. (2005). Smart power assistance module for manual wheelchairs: preliminary results. *Journal of NeuroEngineering and Rehabilitation*, 2(30), 1–11.

85. Cooper, R.A., Thorman, T., Cooper, R., Dvorznak, M.J., Fitzgerald, S.G., Ammer, W., Guo, S.F., Boninger, M.L. (2002). Driving characteristics of electric powered wheelchair users: how far, fast, and often do people drive? *Archives of Physical Medicine and Rehabilitation*, 83(2), 250–255.

86. Cooper, R.A., Boninger, M.L., Cooper, R., Kelleher, A. (2006). Use of the Independence 3000 IBOT™ Transporter at home and in the community: a case report. *Disability & Rehabilitation: Assistive Technology*, 1(1–2), 111–117.

87. Cooper, R.A., Boninger, M.L., Cooper, R., Fitzgerald, S.G., Dobson, A. (2004). Preliminary assessment of a prototype advanced mobility device in the work environment of veterans of spinal cord injury. *Neurorehabilitation*, 19(2), 161–170.

88. Cooper, R.A., Boninger, M.L., Cooper, R., Dobson, A.R., Schmeler, M., Kessler, J., Fitzgerald, S.G. (2003). Technical perspectives: use of the Independence 3000 IBOT Transporter at home and in the community. *Journal of Spinal Cord Medicine*, 26(1), 79–85.

89. Riley, P.O., Rosen, M.J. (1987). Evaluating manual control devices for those with tremor disability. *Journal of Rehabilitation Research and Development*, 24(2), 99–110.

90. Bailey, D.M., DeFelice, T. (1991). Evaluating movement for switch use in an adult with severe physical and cognitive impairments. *American Journal of Occupational Therapy*, 45(1), 76–79.

91. Guo, S.F., Cooper, R.A., Grindle, G. (2003). Development of a compact chin-operated force sensing joystick. *Saudi Journal of Disability and Rehabilitation*, 9(4), 212–218.

92. Dicianno, B.E., Spaeth, D.M., Cooper, R.A., Fitzgerald, S.G., Boninger, M.L., Brown, K.W. (2007). Force control strategies while driving electric powered wheelchairs with isometric and movement-sensing joysticks. *IEEE Transactions on Neural Systems and Rehabilitation Engineering*, 15(1), 144–150.

93. Cooper, R.A., Jones, D.K., Spaeth, D.M., Boninger, M.L., Fitzgerald, S.G., Guo, S.F. (2002). Comparison of virtual and real electric powered wheelchair driving using a position sensing and an isometric joystick. *Medical Engineering and Physics*, 24, 703–708.

94. Cooper, R.A., Jones, D.K., Boninger, M.L., Fitzgerald, S., Albright, S.J. (2000). Analysis of position and isometric joysticks for powered wheelchair driving. *IEEE Transactions on Biomedical Engineering*, 47(7), 902–910.

95. Cooper, R.A., Widman, L.M., Jones, D.K., Robertson, R.N. (2000). Force sensing control for electric powered wheelchairs. *IEEE Transactions on Control Systems Technology*, 8(1), 112–117.

96. Dicianno, B.E., Spaeth, D.M., Cooper, R.A., Fitzgerald, S.G., Boninger, M.L. (2006). Advancements in power wheelchair joystick technology: effects of isometric joysticks and signal conditioning on driving performance. *American Journal of Physical Medicine and Rehabilitation*, 85(8), 631–639.

97. Dicianno, B.E., Spaeth, D.M., Cooper, R.A., Fitzgerald, S.G., Boninger, M.L., Brown, K.W. (2007). Force control strategies while driving electric powered wheelchairs with isometric and movement-sensing joysticks, *IEEE Transactions on Neural Systems and Rehabilitation Engineering*, 15(1), 144–150.

98. Gilsdorf, P., Patterson, R., Fisher, S. (1991). Thirty-minute continuous sitting force measurements with different support surfaces in the spinal cord injured and able-bodied. *Journal of Rehabilitation Research and Development*, 28(4), 33–38.

99. Axelson P. (1993). Wheelchair comparison. *Sports 'N Spokes*, 18(6), 34–40.

100. Gilsdorf, P., Patterson, R., Fisher, S., Appel, N. (1990). Sitting forces and wheelchair mechanics. *Journal of Rehabilitation Research and Development*, 27(3), 239–246.

101. Ferguson-Pell, M., Cochran G. van B., Palmieri, V.R., Brunski, J.B. (1986). Development of a modular wheelchair cushion for spinal cord

injured persons. *Journal of Rehabilitation Research and Development*, 23(3), 63–76.

102. Garber, S., Krouskop, T., Carter, R. (1978). System for clinically evaluating wheelchair pressure-relief cushions. *American Journal of Occupational Therapy*, 32, 565–570.

103. Ferguson-Pell, M.W. (1980). Design criteria for the measurement of pressure at body/support interfaces. *Engineering in Medicine*, 9, 209–214.

104. Garber, S., Krouskop, T. (1982). Body build and its relationship to pressure distribution in the seated wheelchair patient. *Archives of Physical Medicine and Rehabilitation*, 63, 17–20.

105. Goosen, R.H.M., Snijders, C.J. Design criteria for the reduction of shear forces in beds and seats. *Journal of Biomechanics*, 28(2), 225–230.

106. Lim, R., Sirett, R., Conine, T.A. Daechsel, D. (1986). Clinical trial of foam cushions in the prevention of decubitis ulcers in elderly patients. *Journal of Rehabilitation Research and Development*, 25(2), 19–26.

107. Mooney, V., Einbund, M., Rogers, R., Stauffer, E. (1971). Comparison of pressure distribution qualities in seat cushions. *Bulletin of Prosthetics Research*, 129–143.

108. Noble, P.C., Goode, B., Krouskop, T.A., Crisp, B. (1984). The influence of environmental aging upon the loadbearing properties of polyurethane foams. *Journal of Rehabilitation Research and Development*, 21(2), 31–38.

109. Reddy, N.P., Palmieri, V., Cochran, G.V.B. (1981). Subcutaneous interstitial fluid pressure during external loading. *American Physiological Society*, R327–329.

110. Andersson, G.B.J., Oertengren, R. (1974). Lumbar disc pressure and myolectric back muscle activity during sitting. III. Studies on a wheelchair. *Scandinavian Journal of Rehabilitation Medicine*, 3, 122–127.

111. Andersson, G.B.J., Murphy, R.W., Oertengren, R., Nachemson, A.L. (1979). The influence of backrest inclination and lumbar support on the lumbar lordosis in sitting. *Spine*, 4, 52–58.

112. Grieco, A. (1986). Sitting posture: an old problem and a new one. *Ergonomics*, 29, 345–362.

113. Shields, R.K., Cook, T.M. (1988). Effect of seat angle and lumbar support on seated buttock pressure. *Journal of the American Physical Therapy Association*, 68, 1682–1686.

114. Babbs, C.F., Bourland, J.D., Graber, G.P., Jones, J.T., Schoenlein, W.E. (1990). A pressure sensitive mat for measuring contact pressure distributions for patients lying on hospital beds. *Biomedical Instrumentation Technology*, 24, 363–370.

115. Bennet, L., Kavner, D., Lee, B.K., Trainor, F.A. (1979). Shear versus pressure as causative factors in skin blood flow occlusion. *Archives of Physical Medicine and Rehabilitation*, 60, 309–314.

116. Chow, W.W., Odell, E.I. (1978). Deformations and stresses in soft body tissues of a sitting person. *Journal of Biomechanical Engineering*, 100, 79–87.

117. Brienza, D.M., Chung, K.-C., Brubaker, C.E., Kwiatkowski, R.J. (1993). Design of a computer-controlled seating surface for research applications. *IEEE Transactions on Rehabilitation Engineering*, 1(1), 63–66.

118. Bush, C.A. (1969). Study of pressures on skin under ischial tuberosities and thighs during sitting. *Archives of Physical Medicine*, 50, 207.

119. Dinsdale, S. (1974). Decubitis ulcers in swine: role of pressure and friction in causation. *Archives of Physical Medicine and Rehabilitation*, 55, 147–152.

120. Ferguson-Pell, M.W., Cardi, M.D. (1993). Prototype development and comparative evaluation of wheelchair pressure mapping system. *Journal of Assistive Technology*, 5(2), 78–91.

121. Le, K.M., Masden, B.L., Barth, P.W., Ksander, G.A., Angell, J.B., Vistnes, L.M. (1984). An in-depth look at pressure sores using monolithic silicon pressure sensors. *Plastic and Reconstructive Surgery*, 754–756.

122. Levine, S.P., Kett, R.L., Ferguson-Pell, M. (1990). Tissue shape and deformation versus pressure as a characterization of the seating interface. *Assistive Technology*, 2, 93–99.

123. Kadaba, M., Ferguson-Pell, M., Palmieri, B.S., Cochran, G.V.B. (1984). Ultrasound mapping of the buttock-cushion interface contour. *Archives of Physical Medicine and Rehabilitation*, 65, 467–469.

124. Sprigle, S., Schuch, J.Z. (1993). Using seat contour measurements during seating evaluations of individuals with SCI. *Journal of Assistive Technology*, 5(1), 24–35.

125. St-Geoges, M., Valiquette, C., Drouin, G. (1989). Computer-aided design in wheelchair seating. *Journal of Rehabilitation Research and Development*, 26(4), 23–30.

126. Pate, R.R., Pratt, M., Blair, S.N., Haskell, W.L., Macera, C.A., Bouchard, C., et al. (1995). Physical activity and public health: a recommendation from the Centers for Disease Control and Prevention and the American College of Sports Medicine. *Journal of the American Medical Association*, 273(5), 402–407.

127. US Department of Health and Human Services. (1996). *Physical activity and health: a report of the Surgeon General*. Atlanta, GA, US Department of Health and Human Services, Centers for Disease Control and Prevention, National Center for Chronic Disease Prevention and Health Promotion.

128. US Department of Health and Human Services. (2000). *Healthy people 2010: understanding and improving health* (2nd ed.). Washington, DC: US Government Printing Office.

129. Tolerico, M.L. (2005). Investigation of the mobility characteristics and activity levels of manual wheelchair users in two real world environments. Master's Thesis. University of Pittsburgh, Pittsburgh, PA.

130. Chaves, E.S., Cooper, R.A., Collins, D.M., Karmarkar, A., Cooper, R.M. (2007). Review of use of restraints and lap belts with wheelchair users. *Assistive Technology*, 19(2), 94–107.

131. Katz, R.T., Rymer W.Z. (1989). Spastic hypertonia: mechanisms and measurement. *Archives of Physical Medicine and Rehabilitation*, 70(2), 144–155.

132. Keegan, J.J. (1953). Alterations of the lumbar spine related to posture and seating. *Journal of Bone and Joint Surgery*, 35-A, 589.

56 Spinal Orthoses

Edmond Ayyappa
Omid Yousefian

The use of spinal orthotics has been recorded in antiquity through hieroglyphics of the fifth Egyptian dynasty (approximately 2700 BCE) in which are specifically described the application of cervical orthoses (1). Galen, who was a highly celebrated Roman physician to the gladiators, described the use of spinal orthotics in 200 BCE. A spinal orthosis made from tree bark was known to have been used by pre-Columbian cliff dwellers in North America and ascribed to the period of 900 CE. During the nineteenth century, European craftsman migrating to the United States introduced spinal bracing designs, mostly made of leather and steel. Since the 1960s, the utilization of thermoplastics in spinal bracing has evolved and become common practice. Increasingly in the last decade, prefabricated designs have emerged as the more common approach, due to cost considerations. The last decade has seen an increase in the use of computer-aided design and manufacturing (CAD-CAM) for spinal orthotics, and this is a dynamic emerging technology.

EMERGENCY SPINAL TRAUMA

Patients who experience spinal cord injury (SCI) are typically treated in a frontline emergency setting by paramedics, emergency medical technicians, or emergency room staff. Such treatment often utilizes the Sternal Occipital Mandibular Immobilizer (SOMI), rigid collar orthoses, or other prefabricated off-the-shelf bracing (described later). These devices, along with supplemental stabilization through the use of sandbags and backboard taping, provide the kind of temporary immobilization required to carry the patient through the emergency evaluation. Following the initial assessment and any subsequent emergency surgical stabilization and traction that might be indicated, a spinal orthosis will often help to realign the spine, reduce pain and swelling, and provide added stability while fractures and soft tissue injuries heal. When the fracture is stable and soft tissue injuries are minor, the patient may be weaned away from the orthosis when he can tolerate the attendant discomfort without the brace. Depending on the level and severity of injury, a

wide variety of orthoses may be utilized to reduce motion and promote healing.

INDICATORS FOR MECHANISMS OF ACTION

With a few exceptions, spinal orthoses are utilized in two broad areas: cervical and thoracolumbar. The main function of a cervical orthosis is to control motion. Although such motion control is a desirable function in all orthoses, thoracolumbar bracing is as likely to be employed in pain management. In addition, fracture management, muscle weakness, joint displacement, and ligamentous tears are all occasionally addressed with various spinal orthoses. Treatment of patients with SCI may be complicated by such conditions.

The basic principles of motion control in spinal orthotics are the simultaneous application of multiple three-point pressure systems working in concert with circumferential containment, which increases intra-cavitary pressure. In a three-point force system the orthosis provides a force in one direction that is opposed but in equilibrium with two forces in the opposite direction at either end of the spinal segment, thus achieving or sustaining a reduction in movement of the involved segment. Because of a generalized containment of the vertebral bodies, increased intra-abdominal hydraulic forces may ease pressure between nerve and bone. Increased intra-cavitary pressure transfers load from the vertebral disks to the surrounding soft tissue, thus reducing the load borne on the involved spinal segment.

Some spinal orthoses serve as kinesthetic reminders to limit motion or to avoid undesirable posture. The orthoses provides sensory feedback that continuously, or in some cases subconsciously, causes the patient to adapt postural substitutions that relieve adverse pressure. In the orthotic treatment of SCI, including fracture management with attendant loss of sensation, the importance of generous padding and great attention to trim lines to avoid chafing and ulcers cannot be overemphasized. In addition, the treatment team should consider that prolonged use of spinal orthotics can lead to disuse atrophy of the spinal muscle and thus to prolonged impairment. Treatment timed appropriately to the changing conditions of the patient will yield optimal success.

TERMINOLOGY

Orthoses are described primarily in terms of the anatomic regions and joints that are crossed (i.e., CO = cervical orthoses, CTO = cervical thoracic orthoses, LSO = lumbar sacral orthoses). This is a universal system of terminology adhered to by the Medicare coding system and professional organizations such as the American Academy of Orthotists and Prosthetists, American Academy of Physical Medicine and Rehabilitation, and the American Academy of Orthopedic Surgeons (2). Thus, a theoretic orthosis that extended through the full length of the spine would be referred to as a CTLSO. Following such basic terminology a more specific descriptor is often added. For example a CTLSO (Milwaukee) is a historic approach to scoliotic treatment and a CTLSO (body jacket) is commonly used for postsurgical stabilization. In 1983, Medicare and the American Orthotic and Prosthetic Association jointly developed a common procedural coding system, commonly referred to as the "L-code system" that is now universally used by all government agencies, including Veterans Affairs, insurance companies, and other third-party payers to describe specific orthotic treatment. The orthoses outlined in the following pages have thus been identified using this universal technology.

CO SOFT COLLAR

Although the soft collar does not appreciably control motion of the cervical spine, it does provide a kinesthetic reminder to limit motion (Figure 56.1). The increased area of contact may remind

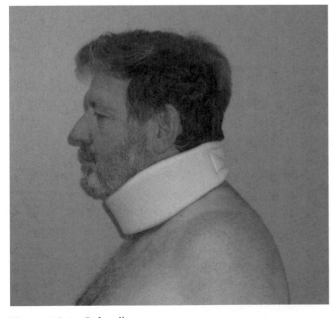

Figure 56.1   Soft collar.

the patient to self-restrict motion, and a soft collar is generally considered the most comfortable of all cervical devices. The soft collar allows up to 75% to 80% of normal cervical motion (3). Therefore, the soft collar is contraindicated for any injury that involves significant damage to the ligamentous or bony structures of the cervical spine during the initial treatment phase. Its use in hyperextension injuries or muscular or ligamentous strain injuries to the cervical spine is controversial at best (4). As a therapy, it may warm the cervical region, which may induce muscle relaxation and contribute to a greater level of comfort. The device is typically used for soft tissue injuries such as muscle strain, and is constructed of prefabricated polyurethane foam, typically covered with cotton stockinet. The soft collar is tolerated well by most patients and is not uncommonly used to transition patients from other more rigid devices to no orthosis, as it provides a sense of security.

CO PLASTIC OR UNIVERSAL COLLAR

The plastic or universal collar is made from less flexible polyethylene and provides some motion control of flexion in the mid-cervical spine. It is not thought to be effective in providing control of extension, lateral flexion, or rotation (5, 6). A similar device is the Pneu-trac®, a plastic collar with an inflatable air compartment that may increase circumferential containment.

CTO PHILADELPHIA COLLAR

The Cervical Thoracic Orthosis (CTO) Philadelphia collar extends more distally and more proximally than the plastic collar. Its soft material is reinforced with more rigid material and, for maximum effectiveness, should encapsulate the mandible and occiput, extending anteriorly well below the sternal notch and posteriorly to approximately the level of T3. With these longer lever arms, the orthosis becomes more effective in controlling cervical motion than the previous designs discussed. The conventional Philadelphia collar allows 30% to 44% of normal flexion and extension, approximately 44% of normal rotation, and up to 66% of lateral flexion (3). The Philadelphia is the low-end version of this basic design, and more effective versions of this design, which provide increased stabilization, include the Marlin Aspen® (formerly the Newport®), Malibu®, and Miami® collars (7), discussed later in this chapter.

OTHER CERVICAL ORTHOSES

With a molded chin and occipital support, these devices are designed to provide more rigid stabilization of the cervical spine than the orthoses previously discussed. All are prefabricated and available off the shelf with limited modifications, but require some custom fitting. A review of research on orthotic control of cervical motion in the sagittal plane compares the control potential of common cervical orthosis with that of no orthosis (Figures 56.2 and 56.3). The severity of physical insult will, at minimum, influence and often dictate the orthotic treatment option (Figure 56.4).

A popular variant of the basic cervical orthotic design is the Johnson's orthosis, also made of thermoplastics with a replaceable liner, and giving perhaps slightly increased comfort

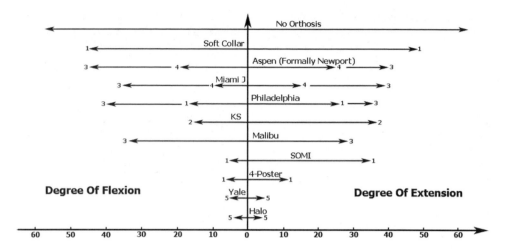

Figure 56.2   Orthotic control of cervical motion in the sagittal plane.

levels. The Philadelphia collar and its variants provide an excellent kinesthetic reminder to limit motion, provide good circumferential adjustability, and in its various versions, nearly all provide tracheotomy access. These devices are generally indicated for stable mid-cervical injuries, strain, sprain, and stable bony and ligamentous insults. The device is also used when weaning a patient off a halo orthosis or other CTLSO following weeks or months of immobilization. These collars are an excellent choice when the pressures exerted by "poster type" orthoses are not well tolerated by the patient.

The Johnson Malibu (Figure 56.5), Miami J. (Figure 56.6), KS, and Aspen Orthoses (formerly called the Newport) are all made of padded thermoplastic, and provide increased cervical control over the soft collar and Philadelphia devices. They are easier to don than the poster orthosis and SOMI, are relatively rigid,

yet flexible at the margins for patient comfort. Pads and shells are removable and washable. All are CTOs in that they do not extend to the thoracic region.

CERVICAL THORACIC ORTHOSIS

Cervical thoracic orthoses include the Yale, SOMI, two-poster, four-poster, and Halo orthosis. The Yale orthosis is largely thermoplastic and extends inferiorly to 2 cm proximal to the xyphoid process, and is very effective in controlling both flexion and extension. The two-poster and four-poster (Figure 56.7) cervical orthoses are generally made of aluminum and thermoplastics. Such poster designs have a sternal plate rigidly connected to a mandibular support. The use of the poster-type orthoses has been largely eclipsed over the last two decades by the rigid

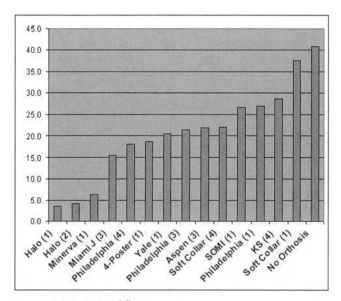

Figure 56.3   Lateral flexion.

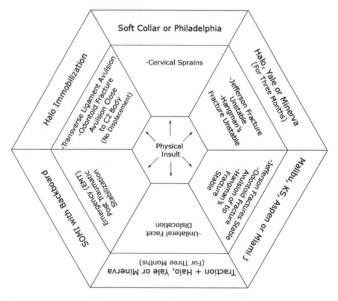

Figure 56.4   Treatment modalities of cervical trauma.

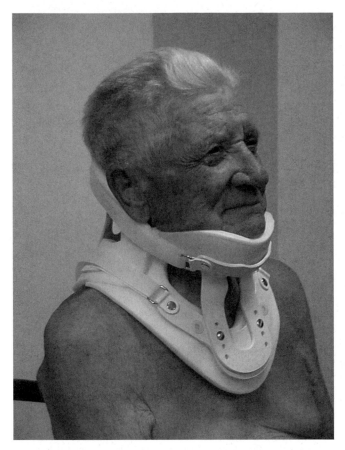

Figure 56.5 The Johnson Malibu cervical orthosis.

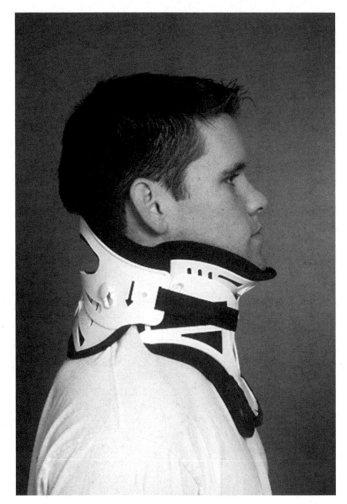

Figure 56.6 Miami J. cervical orthosis.

collars described earlier. A significant amount of orthotic skill and consistent follow-up is paramount to the successful application of the poster designs. The SOMI brace (Figure 56.8) is a highly effective off-the-shelf cervical-thoracic orthosis that can be applied with minimal disturbance while the patient is lying supine. It has a removable mandibular cup and stabilizing headband to allow temporary access for eating, shaving, and personal hygiene. The SOMI may be indicated when significant yet noninvasive cervical, thoracic, and lumbar control is required. The SOMI controls flexion quite well but is less effective in controlling extension and lateral flexion (3).

Custom Molded Minerva

The custom molded Minerva is clinically seen to provide excellent control for thoracic and cervical regions without the need for invasive skull pins. The thermoplastic Minerva made by a skilled orthotist has been shown to be more effective than a Halo in controlling cervical flexion and extension at all levels. However, it is not as effective in controlling lateral flexion (8) (Figure 56.9). The heavier plaster version, reminiscent of old-time orthopedics, cannot be removed, but a lightweight thermoplastic version allows for greater function with increased potential for hygiene and self-care as the patient stabilizes. An off-the-shelf version of the custom Minerva is also available.

Halo

The Halo (Figure 56.10) is generally thought to provide maximum cervical control compared to all other cervical orthoses. The Halo eliminates 90% of normal cervical motion (3). With the conventional Halo, four pins are screwed into the skull and tightened to a recommended torque. The Halo is best applied with both a skilled orthotist and physician in attendance. The orthotist selects a halo-ring size with ½- to ¾-inch of clearance around the total circumference of the head. This allows fingers to palpate and access pin sites for hygienic purposes. The patient is placed in the supine position with the head supported 8 to 10 inches beyond the bed or gurney's edge. Attention must be given to proper placement of the Halo on the head, which should be located ¼-inch above the ears and ⅛-inch above the lateral third of the eyebrows. This is to avoid injuring cranial nerves, damaging the frontal sinus cavity, or penetrating thin cranial bones in the temporal area. Established correctly, the front positioning plate should line up over the bridge of the nose. The patient's eyes should be closed during insertion and tightening of the pins to allow room for the ocular muscles to close when the patient sleeps. After pre-positioning the Halo, a local anesthetic is

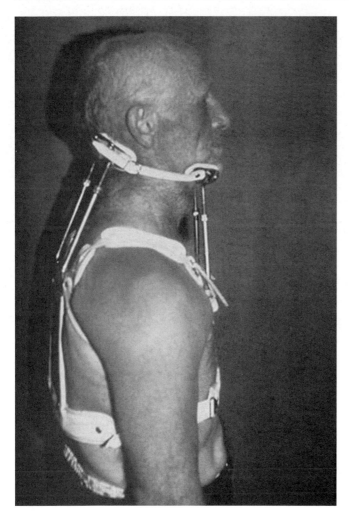

Figure 56.7   Four-poster cervical orthosis.

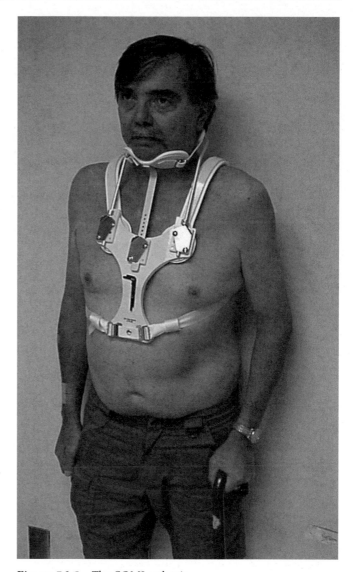

Figure 56.8   The SOMI orthosis.

administered at the pin sites. Then one anterior skull pin and its diagonally opposite posterior counter-pin are selected and simultaneously hand tightened. This should position the pins at a 90-degree angle to the skull. The process is repeated with the other two pins. A sterile lubricant reduces skin friction. Two torque screwdrivers are then used in the same fashion to set the pins directly into the skull. The suggested torque settings are 2 to 4 in/lb for infants, 6 to 8 in/lb for normal adults, and 4 to 6 in/lb for geriatrics (9). Because of competing forces produced by the four anchors, the screws will need to be re-torqued after 10 to 15 minutes. Motion and cellular necrosis may result in loosening and degeneration of the periosteum around the screws, which will need to be inspected after 24 hours and weekly thereafter. After the positioning plates have been removed from the Halo, a circumference measurement of the chest will determine the appropriate vest size. The body jacket may be applied under traction or while the attending physician secures the cervical spine by hand. An effective method for applying a body jacket in cases where patients are experiencing extreme pain or requiring substantial stabilization is to use the Risser Rotating Frame® (Figure 56.11).

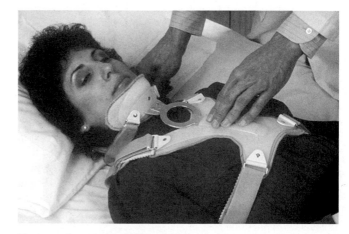

Figure 56.9   A Minerva orthosis.

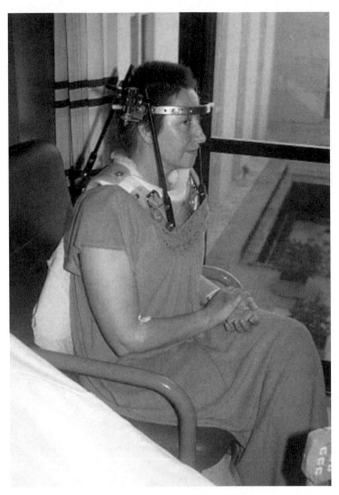

Figure 56.10   The Halo.

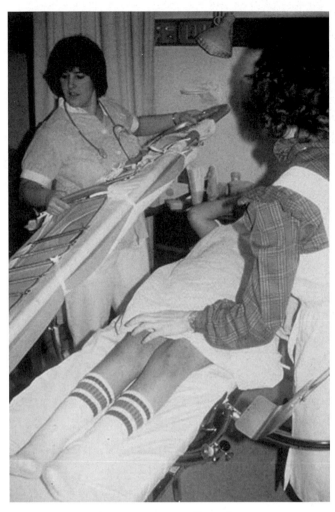

Figure 56.11   The Risser Rotating Frame®.

To provide cardiac access, the adjustment wrench of a Halo should always be taped to the chest plate. The Halo is indicated for severe cervical spine fractures and severe physical spinal instability. The Halo may be contraindicated when the severity of instability does not justify use of the pins, and the noninvasive Halo device is preferable. The noninvasive version of the Halo is considered slightly less effective, whereas the aesthetic advantages are obvious. Although the Halo provides maximum control to the cervical spine to allow for vertebral healing and stabilization to occur, obvious disadvantages are the pins embedded into the skull, which must often be tolerated for long periods and long-term wear, which sometimes results in increased pain at the pin sites. Personal hygiene becomes problematic, and for bedridden patients, ulcers can be a vexing challenge. Generally the Halo has the lowest acceptance rate of any spinal orthosis (10). It has also been associated with a high rate of complications. In a review of 179 Halo patients, Garfin found that pin loosening occurred in 36%: infection in 20%; skin problems in 11%; and urgent complications such as dysphasia, nerve injury, and dural penetration in 1% to 2% of patients reviewed (11). In light of such complications, the treatment team must consider if the implied immobilization potential of the invasive Halo justifies the risk of such complications.

The noninvasive Halo can be used for similar unstable conditions and is especially desirable for patients with high-level spinal fractures needing immediate stabilization for MRI or other imaging studies without use of Halo pins. The Halo has been used to stabilize the head and decrease spinal deformities of ALS patients. The noninvasive version may be applied easily either in or out of surgery and is MRI safe. Medical-grade silicone pads in chin and forehead straps reduce peak pressure areas. Although an excellent alternative, the noninvasive version may not provide an equal degree of stabilization. Objective studies comparing the two variations have not been performed.

THORACOLUMABAR IMMOBILIZATION

Thoracic fractures from T2 to T9 have the advantage of internal immobilization from the rib cage, and in the absence of rib and sternal fractures, fractures of the thoracic spine in this region are inherently stable (10). Fractures from T10 to L2 require either internal surgical stabilization through plates, wires, or cables or external orthotic immobilization to prevent collapse, deformity, and possible neurologic damage (10).

The potential of a lumbar orthosis to limit motion is probably more influenced by the activity of the individual than with a cervical orthosis. Trunk extension is more effectively controlled with a TLSO than is trunk flexion.

TLSO (hyperextension) orthotic stabilization of the low thoracic and lumbar region is addressed by the Jewett (Figure 56.12) and CASH orthoses, the most well-known examples of hyperextension TLSOs. They are lightweight, prefabricated orthoses that limit anterior flexion. When limiting lateral flexion is desirable, the Jewett is the brace of choice, because the CASH (Cruciform Anterior Spinal Hyperextension) orthosis performs poorly at lateral flexion control. The Jewett may require increased hand strength and dexterity to don, compared to its CASH counterpart. The Jewett is most effective in preventing flexion and extension between T6 and L1. The CASH, clinically viewed as slightly less effective than the Jewett, is commonly used for low back pain as well and is tolerated better by most patients compared to the Jewett.

The Taylor TLSO purports to provide anterior flexion control of the thoracic and lumbar region without the weight, bulk, and donning challenges of the TLSO body jacket. However, its effectiveness at motion control compared to the Jewett or TLSO body jacket is controversial at best. The TLSO Milwaukee, used historically for scoliosis, can in theory be an effective means of thoracic immobilization, but patient acceptance is so dismal that it is not a viable option.

The TLSO body jacket (Figure 56.13) is a custom-molded orthosis for maximum balance of comfort and efficiency in motion control of the thoracic region. Of the noninvasive approaches to controlling thoracic motion, it may well be the most effective. The treatment team should keep in mind that limiting thoracic motion may increase lumbar motion. Indications for the custom-molded TLSO body jacket include post-surgical thoracic protection and chronic instability, for which it is an excellent treatment choice. However, it is difficult to don and doff, and because it may migrate on the body, requires frequent positional adjustment. Attention to the trim lines is critical and requires an experienced orthotist. Generally the TLSO body jacket is considered somewhat awkward and bulky. It will migrate proximally as the bed-bound patient raises and lowers the head of the bed. This may diminish comfort levels and increase the risk of orthotic-related ulcers. When it is ordered, the nursing staff should be instructed by the orthotist in the donning and

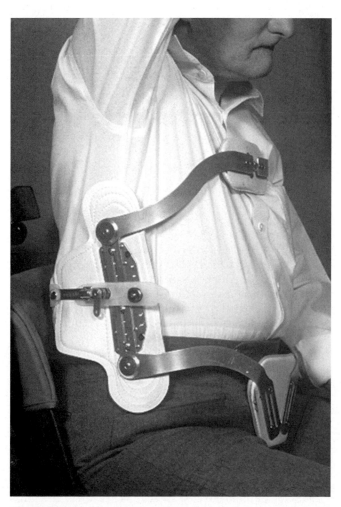

Figure 56.12 The Jewett orthosis.

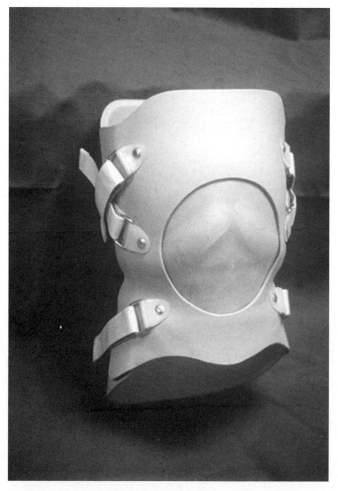

Figure 56.13 The TLSO body jacket.

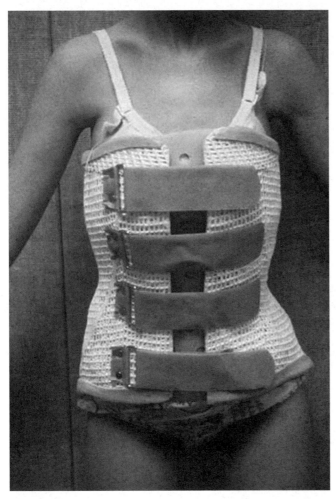

Figure 56.14 The TLSO body jacket is available in temporary and off-the-shelf versions.

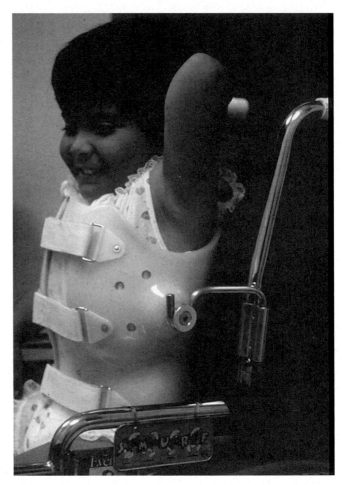

Figure 56.15 Wheelchair suspension is an effective means of un-weighting the seat.

doffing procedure, and the placement should be checked by the nursing staff every 4 hours to ensure that migration has not occurred.

The TLSO body jacket is available in temporary and off-the-shelf versions as well (Figure 56.14). Although the off-the-shelf versions can be fit quickly and at a reduced cost, the attendant complications from poor fit are increased compared to the custom molded versions. In cases of body asymmetries, off-the-shelf body jackets are an inappropriate choice and do not accommodate to all body shapes. The two basic designs are the bivalve and the one piece with chest plate. An advantage of the bivalve is that it can be applied while the patient is reclined in bed. Typically, the patient rolls over to one side and the posterior section of the TLSO is positioned. Then the patient is rolled over to the prone position. At this point the anterior section is keyed to the posterior section. Velcro straps secure the orthosis firmly in place. Donning the one-piece TLSO body jacket is slightly more awkward and may generate some pain in many patients. The bivalve design is easier to don and may provide increased control. The one-piece TLSO with posterior opening might compromise control in the spinal region. Likewise, if the opening is anterior, some efficiency of abdominal containment may be affected and circumferential compression may be less effective.

The TLSO (wheelchair suspension) is a unique concept developed at Newington Children's Hospital, Newington, Connecticut (Figure 56.15). The device partially suspends the patient, and used intermittently in a wheelchair-bound patient, may be helpful in the treatment of sacral ulcers or as a temporary means of partially unweighting the lumbar spine. It is most effective on smaller, lighter adults and children, and when applied as a temporary method of treatment.

Elements of an effective orthotic fit using an LSO or TLSO include obtaining a secure pelvic purchase, application of palpable three-point forces, reduction in lumbar lordosis, comfort in sitting, and postural compensation with improved standing balance.

LUMBAR ORTHOSES

Norton assessed lumbar motion of patients in orthoses using Kirshner wire projections off the spine (12). His team found that locking the thoracic region creates increased lumbar motion. As a result, clinicians treating patients for conditions localized at the lumbar region are advised to address such problems with an LSO rather than a TLSO in any form. Norton also found that whereas some persons achieve forward flexion at the hip, others draw more from the lumbar spine. Forward-flex ROM generally reaches a maximum of 30 degrees. The research also found that maximum lumbar flexion in an LSO occurs between L4–L5 in slouched sitting (12). Patients with problems in the lumbar spine should be counseled in proper sitting posture. Lateral flexion in an LSO is best controlled by high lateral trimlines, which may limit comfort but tend to decrease range of motion. For example, the DeRoyal Ultralign off-the-shelf fabric support LSO is more effective than the DeRoyal Proalign off-the-shelf elastic support with rigid inserts. The trimlines for the Ultralign extend proximal to costal margins, which explains its effectiveness in limiting lateral flexion (13). Tuong et al showed that angular motion is typically decreased by lumbar bracing, but that on occasion lateral translation can increase, specifically at L5, S1 (14).

LSO (Corset)

The LSO (corset) is the most broadly applied orthosis for soft-tissue lumbar problems and low back pain. Compared to other lumbosacral orthoses, the corset has excellent patient acceptance while providing the least effective biomechanics in control of motion. Dorsky et al. has shown that an elastic corset allowed a total mean lumbar sagittal motion of 31% of normal range, and the lace-up corset allowed a total mean sagittal range of 53% of normal. By contrast, a molded TLSO allowed a mean sagittal range of 69% of normal. The lack of effectiveness of a TLSO Body Jacket is attributed to containment of the thoracic region. (15) A simple Velcro® closure abdominal binder, available in common sizes and highly adjustable, is even more convenient and is a popular alternative to the lumbosacral corset. Both are relatively easy to don and doff.

LSO (Body Jacket)

Superior migration is common in LSO bracing. Although perineal straps prevent superior migration, they are almost never tolerated. Circumferential compression unloads vertebral bodies and reduces pain in most cases. The device reminds the patient to limit motion. It is available in both custom-molded and off-the-shelf versions. The custom-molded LSO body jacket or the LSO chairback brace are generally considered to provide a higher level of motion control and comfort than the off-the-shelf versions. However, the LSO off-the-shelf body jacket has a higher degree of acceptance by both patient and orthotist than the TLSO, in part because the rib cage need not be accommodated. There is some evidence that walking and other ADLs performed in an LSO can actually increase motion at the L5–S1 level (12). For maximum effectiveness, a hip spica extension attached to an LSO limits motion in ambulatory patients.

CONCLUSION

Prescription criteria in spinal orthotics based primarily on specific biomechanical control needs. Orthotic designs vary widely in their control capabilities. The prescribing physician and treatment team must often balance a need for biomechanical control with known undesirable side effects and the ever-present potential for patient noncompliance, as well as comfort and aesthetic considerations. Migration of spinal orthoses is common, particularly when the patient is confined to a bed, which can result in ulceration and complications. An informed patient care treatment team is essential for clinical success, primarily among them, a skilled certified orthotist.

References

1. Smith GE. The most ancient splints. *Brit Med J* 1908; 1:732–734.
2. Redford JB. Orthotics and orthotic devices: general principles. *Phys Med Rehabil State of the Art Rev* 2000; 14(3):381–394.
3. Johnson, et al. Cervical orthoses: A study comparing their effectiveness in restricting cervical motion in normal subjects. *Bone Joint Surg* 1977; 59-A.3:332–339.
4. Herkowitz HN, Kurz LT, Samberg LC. Management of cervical spine injuries. *Spine State Art Rev* 1989; 3:231–241.
5. Fischer SV, Bowar JF, Essam AA, Gullikson G. Cervical orthosis effect on cervical spine motion, roentgenographic and geniometric method of study. *Arch Phys Med Rehabil* 1977; 58:109–115.
6. Hartman JT, Palumbo F, Hill BJ. Cineradiography of the braced normal cervical spine. *Clin Orthop Relat Res* 1975; 109:97–102.
7. Lunsford T, The effectiveness of four contemporary cervical orthoses in restricting cervical motion. *Prosthetics Orthotics* 1994; 93–99.
8. Maiman D, et al. The effect of a thermoplastic Minerva body jacket on cervical spine motion. *Neurosurgery* 1985; 25(3):363–368.
9. Lavernia C, Botte M, Garfin SR. Cervical orthoses. *Spinal Orthoses for Traumatic and Degenerative Disease,* Chapter 30. Philadelphia: WB Saunders, 1998; 1197–1223.
10. Brown C, Chow G. Orthoses for spinal trauma and postoperative care. *Atlas of Orthoses and Assistive Devices, American Academy of Orthopedic Surgeons* 3rd ed. St. Louis: Mosby, 1997; 251–258.
11. Garfin SR. Complications in the use of the Halo fixation device. *J Bone Joint Surg* 1986; 68:320–325.
12. Norton PL, Brown T. The immobilizing efficiency of back braces the effect on the posture and motion of the lumbosacral spine. *Bone Joint Surg* 1957; 39-A.1:111–139.
13. Zhang, S, et al. Efficacy of lumbar and lumbosacral orthoses in restricting spinal ROMs. *J Back Musculoskelet Rehabil* 2006; 19:49–56.
14. Tuong, NH, et al. Three-dimensional evaluation of lumbar orthosis effects on spinal behavior. *Rehabil Res Development* 1998; 35:34–42.
15. Dorsky, S, et al. A Three-Dimensional Analysis of Lumbar Brace Immobilization Utilizing a Noninvasive Technique. *33rd Annual Meeting, Orthopaedic Research Society* 1987; 364.

57 Upper Limb Orthoses

Michal S. Atkins
Darrell Clark
Robert L. Waters

People with spinal cord injuries benefit from the use of an appropriately prescribed upper limb orthoses. This chapter describes the common uses of these orthoses primarily in people with tetraplegia. First, the rationale, history, and current trends in the use of splints and orthoses are explored. Next, the orthotic selection as it relates to different levels of injuries is examined. Finally, a comprehensive orthotic program is described and key points in ensuring the successful use of the devices are highlighted.

Upper limb orthoses—devices used to protect, support, and improve the function of the arm and hand—play an important part in the effort to maximize the use of the upper limbs of the person with tetraplegia (1).

Individuals with spinal cord injury, primarily with tetraplegia, are issued upper limb orthoses for the following reasons:

1. To prevent overstretching of muscles, such as the finger flexors (2–4).
2. To correct deformity, such as the claw hand (2, 5).
3. To prevent joint contractures, such as an elbow flexion contracture (3, 6–8).
4. To support the wrist and hand in a more functional, most often tenodesis position (4, 9).
5. To support a flail wrist and/or hand (2, 10).
6. To strengthen weak muscles (9, 10).
7. To facilitate function (3, 4, 9, 11).
8. To relieve pain associated with the injury, muscle weakness, and/or with overuse. (12, 13)

Often several of these goals can be achieved with a single orthosis.

Upper limb orthoses can be prefabricated and commercially available off-the-shelf or custom made. Orthoses that are fabricated by an occupational therapist are mostly made of low-temperature, thermoplastic materials that are relatively easy to mold to the shape of the arm and are most commonly called splints. Orthoses provided by an orthotist are fabricated with more durable materials and are designed for longer-term use. In this chapter, both less expensive, prefabricated options and more permanent and costly orthoses are described. Because orthotists who specialize in upper limb orthotics and institutions that support them are few, occupational therapists find ways to accomplish similar goals with less durable materials. These orthoses are also briefly described.

Orthoses for individuals with spinal cord injury (SCI) can be divided into two broad categories: static orthoses for position, and dynamic orthoses for function. Static hand and wrist-hand orthoses are used to help prevent deformity and are designed to maintain thumb opposition, thumb web space, and palmar arch, as well as proper angulation between the hand and forearm. This is especially important in the first months following injury, when the potential for muscle return is greatest and flexion contractures can develop in the absence of extensor muscle recovery. Although some clients continue to wear static orthoses when no further return is expected, there is no research evidence to support the belief that orthoses can prevent the flattening of hand structures (2, 14). Dynamic orthoses, such as the wrist-driven, wrist-hand orthosis (WDWHO) (also known as the wrist-driven, flexor-hinge splint or tenodesis splint) (Figure 57.1A and B) and the ratchet wrist-hand orthosis (Figure 57.2A and B) provide prehension to increase independence in activities of daily living (ADLs).

HISTORIC BACKGROUND

The designs for upper limb orthoses were often originally developed for persons with conditions other than SCI. One of the earliest of these was the flexor-hinge hand splint. Originally designed for individuals with polio, this orthosis transmitted the force generated by active wrist extension via a mechanical linkage to paralyzed index and long fingers, enabling finger closure against the thumb (15). The design of this orthosis evolved into what today is known as the wrist-driven, wrist-hand orthosis—formerly called flexor-hinge splint or tenodesis splint. This orthosis offered prehension capability that had obvious application for the person with SCI. Individuals with C6 lesions and with strong wrist extensors and paralyzed finger flexors could utilize the

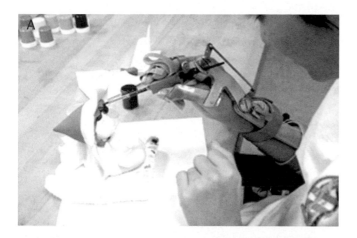

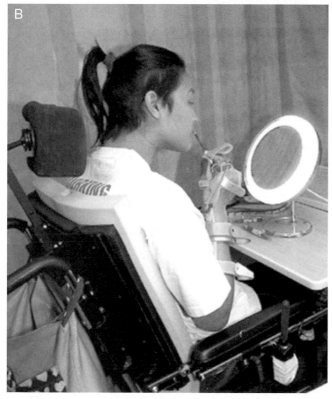

Figure 57.1 (A) Person with C6 tetraplegia using wrist-driven WHO to paint; (B) person with C6 tetraplegia using wrist-driven WHO to apply makeup.

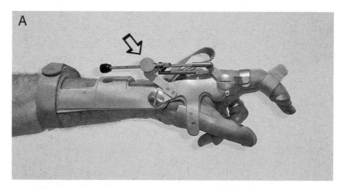

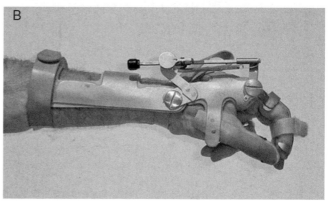

Figure 57.2 Ratchet WHO: (A) opening is achieved by activating a button; (B) grasping an object is achieved by pushing the fingers onto the object with the opposite hand.

WDWHO to improve function. The orthosis harnesses the individual's active wrist extensor power and utilizes the power of wrist extension to flex the fingers at the metacarpophalangeal joints against a stable thumb.

Some patients lack sufficient wrist extensor strength to utilize the WDWHO. The development of external powered designs led to a system that utilized a CO_2-powered "artificial muscle" to provide proportionally controlled prehension. This system was designed in 1957 at Rancho Los Amigos Hospital in collaboration with Dr. Joseph McKibben, a physicist whose daughter contracted polio. Dubbed the "McKibben muscle," it featured a rubber bladder, which was covered with a woven fabric. This unit was attached to the side of the WHO. When

pressurized with CO_2, the bladder would expand against the woven fabric and shorten in length. This in turn operated a linkage bar, which propelled the fingers into flexion against the stable thumb. A two-way valve, operated by shoulder shrugging, released the pressure to allow finger extension (16).

By the mid-1960s, smaller, more powerful electric motors brought a shift away from CO_2 as a source of external power for upper limb orthoses. Electrical external power was coupled to the WDWHO through the use of cables and battery-powered motors. Again, there were obvious potential benefits to the patient with partial upper limb paralysis.

Encouraged by results of the work with the WDWHO, orthotists and biomedical engineers at Rancho Los Amigos Hospital undertook a much more ambitious project—a battery-powered, multidimensional upper extremity orthosis that would attempt to duplicate all major motions of the arm and hand. Designed using anthropometric measurements, this tongue-switch controlled device offered the opportunity for individuals with high-level tetraplegia to achieve greater independence in ADLs.

In practice, however, externally powered systems typically proved difficult to maintain. Without ready access to technical support personnel who could repair delicate electronic parts, the orthoses fell into disrepair and were discarded. Patient training was crucial to the successful use of the orthoses. The complexity of orthotic design required a well-organized training program by occupational therapists. The absence of either of these two factors often proved a deterrent to continued use by all but the most committed patients.

In recent decades, in part propelled by managed care and efforts to control cost, designs have tended to revert to more simple mechanical components, which are less expensive to fabricate and easier to operate and maintain. One design adapted prosthetic harnessing systems to the WDWHO. Upper limb prostheses have long been powered by the use of strapping systems that utilize contralateral shoulder protraction to operate a cable that opens the hand. This principle was applied to the WDWHO with limited success.

Current designs continue to utilize simple mechanical components, which are more easily maintained.

CURRENT TRENDS, PHILOSOPHY, AND PRINCIPLES

Overall, there has been a significant decrease in the use of upper limb orthoses in individuals with SCI since the 1970s (17). This is because of a variety of factors, two of which have combined for greatest impact: general cost-cutting measures resulting in decreased inpatient length of stay (LOS) (18), and evidence of lack of long-term orthotic use in a large percentage of individuals with SCI (19).

Data on long-term use of upper limb orthoses (19) has contributed to the decreased number of prescriptions for these items. An additional factor is simply the philosophy of providing patients with the smallest amount of equipment possible. With emphasis on patient-centered care, consumer feedback has become central in shaping trends. Consumers with SCI have often reported that equipment and orthoses make them look more disabled and often make their life more cumbersome.

The efficacy of static splints in tetraplegia has long been questioned. Because of the obvious difficulty in conducting a scientific study comparing the incidence and severity of joint and muscle contractures in large groups of patients treated with and without splinting, statistically significant evidence to support their use is scarce, yet most authors (3, 14, 19) agree that "there is clinical and intuitive support for the use of splinting for the prevention of joint problems and promotion of function of the tetraplegic hand." (3, pg. 5–0).

Additionally, cost-containment efforts in the United States have resulted in not only decreased LOS, but also a reduction in the numbers and types of equipment that patients receive. Selection criteria have become more restrictive. Some institutions provide equipment only on an outpatient basis. Others utilize patient "contracts," in which patients commit to using equipment for specified time periods or for specific tasks (17). Other cost-cutting measures include the use of prefabricated orthoses on a clinical trial basis. These orthoses cost much less and allow a patient to demonstrate the potential for the long-term usage of a more definitive orthosis.

There is also an ongoing search for new materials and designs that can reduce weight or result in orthoses that are more aesthetically pleasing; that is, less stigmatizing in appearance. This may be accomplished through surface coating of metals, such as aluminum anodizing, or the use of alternative materials, such as plastic or carbon fiber. Designers must always remain aware of the need to maintain an optimum balance between material strength and weight. All of this must be accomplished in a cost-effective way.

The increased use of robotics in industry to perform complex tasks suggests potential applications for the disabled population. Experimental work has been done on robotic arms that can manipulate items such as a computer or feeding utensils. Hillman et al. (20) designed a workstation using a commercially available robot manipulator controlled by a microcomputer. The arm chosen was relatively low in cost and offered a wide range of motion, plus an open/close gripper.

Upper extremity neuroprostheses are orthotic devices with either implanted or external functional electrical stimulation systems mostly used to power hand grasp and pinch. Examples of these systems are the NeuroControl Freehand System, and the NESS 200 (AKA the Handmaster) (21).

The bionic glove, another example of an upper extremity neuroprosthesis, (22) developed at the University of Alberta, utilizes neuromuscular electric stimulation (NMES) to stimulate finger flexors, extensors, and thumb flexors to produce functional prehension through tenodesis action at the wrist. Electrodes are imbedded in a glove worn by the patient. Three channels of electrical stimulation are used to stimulate the thumb and fingers. Control is provided through a wrist position transducer inside the garment. Wrist motion produces prehension through tenodesis action. (See Chapter 63, Functional Electric Stimulation.)

Lastly, orthotics are used to overcome pain and musculoskeletal changes brought about by the aging process. Recent studies on the long-term effects of aging with SCI have demonstrated the adverse effects on the shoulders, wrists, and hands caused by prolonged pushing of a wheelchair, transferring, and reaching overhead (13). Prolonged weight-bearing activities on the hands, wrists, and arms have been shown to cause increased pain, functional loss, and occupational loss. In 2005 the Paralyzed Veterans of America's Consortium for Spinal Cord Medicine published a clinical practice guideline (available on the Internet for a free download) called *Preservation of Upper Limb Function Following Spinal Cord Injury* (12). The manual lists scientific literature about the cumulative negative effects to the wrist, elbow, and shoulder of people with SCI. Along with an extensive recommendation list, the authors recommend the use of resting splints at night for people with carpal tunnel syndrome and for general hand pain relief due to overuse (12). Another example of pain reduction with the use of orthoses is seen with the reduction in neck and shoulder pain achieved by harnessing the upper limbs in mobile arm supports, thus reducing the weight of the arms with people with C4 and C5 weak muscles.

EVALUATION AND TREATMENT PLANNING

To determine which orthoses would best work for an individual, all data gathered by the rehabilitation team must be taken into consideration. Along with physical aspects such as the neurologic level of the injury, ambulatory status, and the presence of pain, psychosocial issues are of great importance. Questions relating to the discharge destination, the presence of significant others, and occupational goals play an important role in choosing the appropriate orthosis for the individual.

In orthosis evaluation and treatment planning, the occupational therapist must consider the following key points:

- Along with objective physical evaluations, the therapist must observe the function of the hand. How does the person pick up objects and manipulate them? Is the tenodesis action functional? Can tenodesis action be enhanced through splinting? Answers to questions like these help the therapist and the patient choose the optimal orthosis for the ultimate goal of enhancing function.

- Some hand tests may prove useful in assessing the efficacy of an orthosis (10). The person with C6 tetraplegia, for example, performs a hand test with and without the WDWHO to determine if the orthosis provides an advantage over using no orthosis for picking up and manipulating objects. Examples of hand tests are the Jebson Hand Test (23), the Sullerman Hand Function Test (24), and the Tetraplegia Hand Activity Questionnaire (THAQ)(25). Other hand tests that might be useful were developed for assessing the outcomes of hand surgeries (see Chapter 48, Functional Restoration of the Upper Extremity in Tetraplegia). When finger and thumb muscles are present, pinch and grip strength are also measured. It is the authors' observation that a simple quick activity-based hand/arm test is needed, a test that would capture current daily activities such as swiping a credit card and using cell phones.
- Along with routine ASIA (26) sensory tests of pain and light touch, proprioception is also checked. In testing sensory dermatomes of the hand (C6–C8), if sensation is present, it is valuable to also check object identification and/or two-point discrimination. These tests allow the therapist to predict the need for visual compensation in manipulating objects. If the patient has a deficit in hand tactile sensory input, a small, less-bulky orthosis may be chosen over a bigger orthosis to allow the patient to have an unobstructed view of the hand and object.
- Choosing orthoses for both upper limbs is common with static, positioning splints. Mobile arm supports are prescribed both unilaterally or bilaterally according to the pattern of upper limb weakness. However, there is a great advantage in fitting both arms with mobile arm supports to allow for upper body symmetry in the wheelchair. With a functional orthosis such as the WDWHO, it may be tempting to fit some patients with bilateral orthoses. However, it is uncommon for patients to achieve a higher level of function with two orthoses. Typically, the patient achieves optimal function using one orthosis and using the other hand as an assist. If sensation in the radial fingers or thumb is impaired or absent, as in the person with C5 tetraplegia, the patient must compensate visually, and this makes bilateral use of the orthoses less effective.
- Patients act as partners in selecting the appropriate orthosis by designating which goals and activities are meaningful to them. The Canadian Occupational Therapy Measure (COPM)(27, 28) is an excellent tool in determining these goals (27–29). The choice of a more permanent orthosis is often made after various orthoses are tried and as a continuing dialog between the team and the patient about fit and functionality takes place.
- To help determine initial orthotic selection, two questions must be answered:
  - What orthoses are needed to prevent further deformity and complications?
  - What orthoses would optimize arm function for achieving the person's functional and occupational goals?
- Mounting data on the pattern and timeline of recovery of people with complete and incomplete tetraplegia helps guide the therapist in choosing the appropriate orthosis before full motor recovery is achieved. A patient with complete (ASIA A) tetraplegia who tests with 1/5 radial wrist extensors 1 month post injury, for example, has a 22% chance of having a 3/5 strength after 1 year (30). This statistical prediction makes it reasonable for the therapist to concentrate on tenodesis training geared toward ordering the WDWHO. At first the orthosis may have an extension assist component. However, as the wrist strengthens over time and endurance improves, the person will be able to use the orthosis effectively without an extension assist component.

ORTHOTIC DESIGN PRINCIPLES BY FUNCTIONAL LEVEL

This section reviews the most common orthoses given to patients by level of injury. It is important to note the small but important difference between the ASIA neurologic level and the functional level.

Functional level, a term often used by occupational and physical therapists, is defined as the lowest segment at which the strength of key muscles is 3+/5 or above and sensation is intact. Key muscles are those that significantly change functional outcomes (31). The distinction between the ASIA neurologic level (26) and functional level is important. Typically, persons with a certain functional level may be stronger than those with the same ASIA neurologic level, because key muscles must have 3+/5 for the functional level vs. 3/5 for the ASIA neurologic level.

The difference between the two scales reflects the difference in their purpose at inception. The ASIA neurologic level was created to assure high interrater reliability. The purpose of determining the functional level, as the name suggests, is to establish an accurate way to predict functional recovery. Functional level depends on more than one key muscle. For example: for an ASIA neurologic level 5, the biceps, the key muscle, must have a grade of 3/5. Functionally, in addition to the biceps, a person must also have some deltoid function in order to bring the hand to the mouth and face. Therefore, both the biceps and deltoids are key muscles at the C5 functional level. Both of these muscles must have a strength of 3+/5 or above. For the purpose of this chapter, the levels described below refer to the functional level of injury.

High Cervical Injuries (C1–C4)

Orthotic management for persons with high tetraplegia focuses on preventing complications in the event of possible motor return, as well as ensuring the patient's comfort and preserving the aesthetic appearance of the arm and hand. It also serves to prevent hygiene problems and skin breakdown.

The person is fitted with a prefabricated, soft, resting hand splint (Figure 57.3A) or with a wrist support splint (Figure 57.3B). The soft, resting hand splint helps maintain the functional position of the hand and wrist, thereby reducing the risk of contracture and deformity. This is accomplished by supporting the wrist in approximately 20 to 30 degrees of extension and holding the thumb in a position of abduction. In the past a metal hand orthosis, the static wrist-hand orthosis (WHO) (Figure 57.3C), was used to maintain the functional position of the hand (9), but

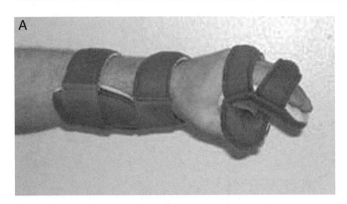

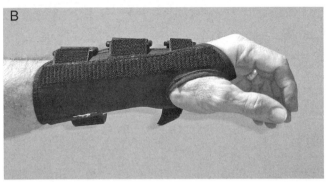

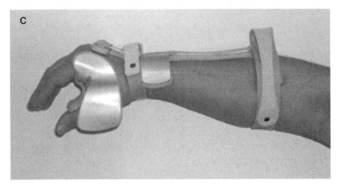

Figure 57.3   **(A)** Soft resting hand splint; **(B)** pre-fab wrist support; **(C)** static wrist-hand orthosis (WHO).

currently this practice is less common because of reasons previously mentioned.

Mouthsticks

Although not an upper limb orthosis, the mouthstick is described here because it is the only simple, low-tech device that is widely available and allows the person with a high cervical injury a way to perform activities.

A mouthstick is a rod that an individual holds in the mouth. Depending on the design, the working end is utilized for various tasks. Mouthsticks may be passive in nature, with a simple rubber tip for pushing or a clamp to hold a utensil; or dynamic, allowing the individual to pick up and move small objects (Figure 57.4). Mouthsticks are typically made from either a wooden or metal rod with attachments designed to accomplish specific functions, such as page turning, typing, or writing. Typical dynamic designs provide a tongue-operated plunger that

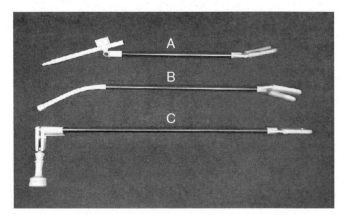

Figure 57.4   Mouthsticks: **(A)** implement holder (pencil, paintbrush, marker, etc.); **(B)** pointer (keyboard operations, page turner); **(C)** pincer (for picking up small, light objects).

allows opening and closing of a pincer mechanism on the distal end. Pushing on the plunger with the tongue opens the pincer. Closure is accomplished with a rubber band or spring, which closes the mechanism when the tongue is relaxed.

Individuals with Functional C4 and Some C5 Return

Persons with this level of injury have minimal arm movement. Biceps and deltoids are present but too weak to support the weight of the arm (in the >2/5 to 3/5 range). Great effort is made to enhance their minimal strength to facilitate upper limb function. A mobile arm support mounted on the wheelchair may provide sufficient antigravity support for a patient with grade >2/5 or 3/5 muscles to attain some functional upper extremity use (9, 32).

To prevent hand deformity, the patient is encouraged to wear a static orthosis at night. This splint may be either a commercially available, prefabricated model or a custom-made resting hand splint or long opponens splint (10, 33). Both the resting hand splint and the long opponens splint support the wrist and allow the fingers and thumb to rest in a functional position (Figure 57.3A). A more durable, permanent orthosis that serves the same purpose is the WHO mentioned previously.

To prevent elbow range-of-motion limitations, an elbow extension orthosis may be worn at night. This orthosis keeps the elbow extended against an unopposed biceps. This commercially available orthosis comes in many styles and materials. A more rigid orthosis is selected for patients with biceps spasticity.

To achieve function, the inexpensive, lightweight universal cuff (Figure 57.5) provides a pouch for inserting utensils such as a fork or toothbrush. Some of the static orthoses also incorporate a similar pouch or another means of attaching tools to allow for increased function. The clinician must be cognizant of the weight of the orthosis, because excessive weight may decrease function.

Mobile Arm Supports (MAS)

The mobile arm support (MAS) is also known as the balanced forearm feeder or ball bearing feeder. It attaches to the patient's

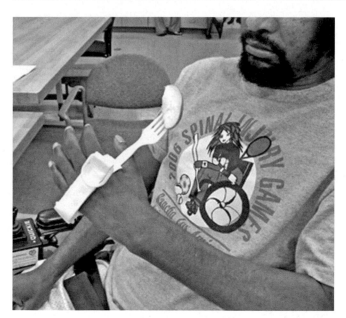

Figure 57.5 Person with no prehension may benefit from a universal cuff.

wheelchair to support the arm and allows horizontal motion at the shoulder and elbow. It thereby allows the hand to be positioned for performing activities (Figure 57.6). The MAS consists of a mounting bracket, proximal arm, distal arm, and forearm support trough. Simple pivot joints are analogous to the shoulder, elbow, and wrist. The component parts are individually fitted and adjusted to assist the patient in gaining maximal functional and therapeutic benefits from the support. For patients with C4 tetraplegia and minimal (in the 2/5 muscle strength range) return of deltoid and biceps, the MAS often allows individuals with otherwise nonfunctional upper limbs to engage in tabletop, hand-to-face activities and to drive a hand-controlled power wheelchair (34). Because this device may provide the only means by which a person can move the upper limbs, it is not surprising that Garber and Gregorio (19) found that, following discharge from rehabilitation, the MAS was retained in use and satisfaction with the use of the device was high.

With deltoids of grade 2/5 or better, the patient may benefit by having an elevating proximal arm added to the mobile arm

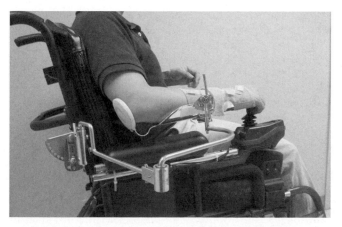

Figure 57.6 Mobile arm support (MAS): JAECO 1950s MAS.

support. This component replaces the standard proximal arm and allows vertical motion of the arm through a rubber band–assisted mechanism. This enables the patient to bring the hand to the face or top of the head to allow for feeding, hygiene, and grooming. It may also help to strengthen the deltoids.

Muscles of the shoulder, elbow, and/or trunk are used to operate the MAS. Varying combinations of muscle strength and coordination will permit the successful manipulation of the device. Patients must have adequate passive range of motion at the shoulder, elbow, and forearm to effectively use the mobile arm support. The ability to contract and relax muscles smoothly is important in obtaining full benefit from the support. Excessive spasticity will interfere with function (9, 34).

As mentioned before, the MAS may provide minimal, yet critical, functional gains to patients who are very weak (combinations of less than 2/5 muscle strength). The MAS may provide the patient with the ability to drive a wheelchair with hand controls versus head-operated controls (34). However, the therapist must make certain that the patient is able to use the MAS on uneven and inclined surfaces, because the MAS is dependent on gravity to keep it stable.

Although the MAS may be adjusted for use in a semireclined wheelchair back position, an upright position is preferable for functional activities. Wheelchair trunk supports are needed to obtain adequate upright position and stability.

A newer commercially available MAS called the JAECO/Rancho Multilink Mobile Arm Support provides for a relatively easy wheelchair setup and solutions to some problems that were encountered with the old 1950s JAECO system. The design is narrower, allowing for an easier clearance through doorways. It allows for mounting to a variety of wheelchairs, has a more pleasing appearance, and is easier to adjust (Figure 57.7) (32). A new arm-height adjustor allows a weak patient to work in multiple vertical planes, reaching the mouth and a table top by a therapist/caregiver pressing a button (Figure 57.7).

Two other newly developed, more expensive MAS systems, not originally designed for people with tetraplegia, may have functional potential for people with tetraplegia; the Wilmington Robotic Exoskeleton (WREX) (35) and a MAS created in the Netherlands (36).

Individuals with C5 Tetraplegia

To maximize the potential for future function as muscle recovery progresses, the wrist is positioned in a static orthosis to help protect against excessive stretch of the weak or absent wrist extensors. In addition, a position of natural finger flexion facilitates the development of flexor tendon tightness, on which tenodesis function relies. Tenodesis is the passive closing of the fingers when the wrist is extended, and the opening of the hand when the wrist is flexed.

If patients have some wrist extension strength—between 2/5 and 3/5—they may benefit from a period of therapeutic strengthening of the wrist extensors, while still maintaining proper wrist-hand position. A wrist-action, wrist-hand orthosis (WAWHO) (Figure 57.8), may be used as a transitional orthosis (9) in the months following the injury. The orthosis allows free-wrist motion and has adjustable stops that limit motion to a prescribed range. The stops may be adjusted to accommodate existing and changing strength in wrist extensors. If extensors are absent, the

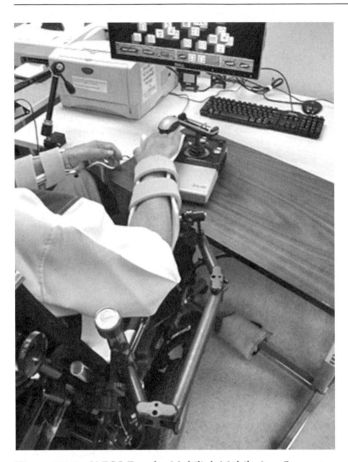

Figure 57.7   JAECO/Rancho Multilink Mobile Arm Support.

stops may be adjusted to eliminate motion and provide static support in the desired position. As strength increases, increased range of motion may be allowed. An extension assist rod with elastic bands may assist in extending the weak wrist (wrist muscle strength range of less than 2/5 to 3/5).

As in individuals with C4 and limited C5 return, the elbow must be maintained in extension to prevent flexion contractures. To achieve this goal, the patient wears an elbow orthosis at night.

There is no optimal functional orthosis for the person with C5 tetraplegia. To stabilize the wrist, a wrist support splint (Figure 57.3B) is worn. The universal cuff, mentioned previously, is often used for feeding and hygiene. However, its uses are limited. The person must use other adaptive equipment for other activities such as

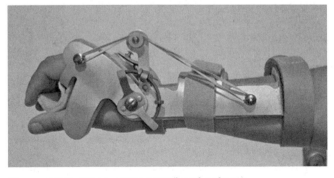

Figure 57.8   Wrist-action wrist-hand orthosis.

writing, grooming, and cooking (see Chapter 59, Activities of Daily Living). The universal cuff is often combined with an orthosis that supports the wrist in a functional position.

Another more expensive custom-made orthosis is the ratchet wrist-hand orthosis (Figures 57.2A and B). Now rarely used, the ratchet WHO is a metal orthosis that is controlled externally by the opposite arm. The ratchet WHO holds the wrist joint in a static position. A thumb post holds the thumb abducted and aligned in opposition to the index and middle fingers to allow prehension. Finger pieces hold the index and middle fingers in enough flexion to allow pad-to-pad contact with the thumb. A "ratchet" bar connects the finger pieces to the main body of the orthosis. Closing is accomplished by motion of the contralateral hand against the ratchet mechanism to flex the fingers against the thumb. Release is accomplished through a return spring, which is activated by pressing a release button. Individual muscle strength and experimentation will determine the easiest way for the patient to manage the operation of the orthosis. This orthosis was more in favor in the past when rehabilitation length of stay was longer, allowing for sufficient time for orthoses evaluation, exploration, and training. Individuals become proficient in a variety of functional activities using the ratchet WHO, including independent feeding, hygiene, writing, and grooming, as well as certain tabletop activities (9).

In select cases, some individuals with C4 tetraplegia and C5 return may use the ratchet WHO in combination with the MAS (37). It must be stressed, however, that when the person requires the use of mobile arm supports with a ratchet WHO, functional capabilities are more limited. The person requires assistance donning and doffing the orthosis, and the work area must be set up carefully. Once the optimal setup is achieved, however, the individual is able to perform a variety of tabletop activities.

In general, it has been the authors' experience that therapists and patients prefer the use of orthoses and adaptive equipment other than the ratchet. This is partially because of its cumbersome operation, appearance, and excessive weight.

In contrast to the limited functional options of the person with C5 tetraplegia, individuals with C6–C7 injuries have significant muscle return, which allows for a more favorable orthosis—the wrist-driven, wrist-hand orthosis (Figures 57.1A and B) described below.

Individuals with C6–C7 Functional Level

The orthotic management of the upper limbs of persons with C6 and C7 lesions is similar, and is therefore jointly discussed. At the C6 level the person will have intact radial wrist extensors, along with some strength in the serratus anterior and clavicular pectoral muscles. Pectoral strength provides the ability to bring the arm across the chest to midline, thereby allowing activities requiring bilateral arm use. Intact wrist extensors allow the individual to harness the tenodesis action at the wrist to accomplish dynamic prehension for feeding, hygiene, and similar activities.

In addition to C6 muscle return, the person with functional C7 has return of the triceps and latissimus dorsi, and some return of the extrinsic finger muscles, most often return of the extensor group.

The focus in managing the hand of persons with C6 or C7 functional level is optimizing the biomechanic dynamics of the wrist and hand to promote effective tenodesis grip and pinch

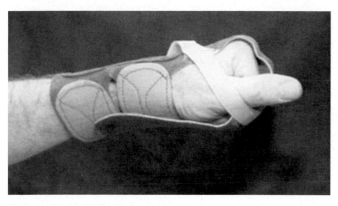

Figure 57.9 Moberg glove.

(2, 4, 11, 14, 38, 39). Because "the effectiveness of the tenodesis grip is determined by the passive properties of the hand" (38, p. 239), great efforts are placed on preserving and encouraging this mechanism, as it is key to optimal function (4). Various static and dynamic orthoses are prescribed by different SCI centers for the purpose of encouraging adaptive shortening of the flexor digitorum profundus, superficialis, flexor pollicis longus, and protecting the web space (38). Such orthoses wrap the fingers as in a boxing glove, and position the thumb in lateral pinch against the index finger. An example of this is the Moberg glove (Figure 57.9), which brings full closure of the fingers. To encourage the dynamic nature of tenodesis, a simple splint like the dynamic tenodesis strap (Figure 57.10) is used (10, 11). Some of

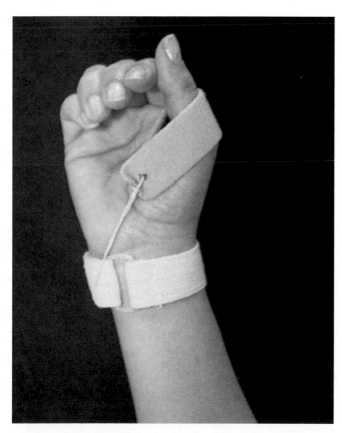

Figure 57.10 Dynamic tenodesis strap.

these splints are worn in combination with others. The person with functional C6 tetraplegia may still need to wear an elbow extension splint at night to preserve full extension of this joint. Such orthoses become unnecessary for the person with C7 tetraplegia. The importance of preventing elbow flexion contractures cannot be overemphasized. C6 and C7 patients who have weak triceps strength may not have sufficient extensor strength to stabilize the elbow and perform independent transfers in the presence of elbow flexion contractures.

A functional dynamic orthosis, such as the wrist-driven wrist-hand orthosis, may substitute for lost pinch and grasp.

Wrist-Driven, Wrist-Hand Orthosis

The wrist-driven, wrist-hand orthosis (WDWHO) (Figures 57.1A and B) is a dynamic orthosis that provides a transfer of power from the wrist extensors to the fingers for the purpose of prehension (9). It requires an experienced orthotist to design and fabricate the orthosis, and a knowledgeable therapist to train the patient in proper use. In the absence of this expertise, and with shortened length-of-stay, patients in many rehabilitation settings do not receive this orthosis. The WDWHO provides for a strong pinch in activities such as self-catheterization or attaching urinal leg-bag tubing. Although some patients use the WDWHO for writing, it is not optimal because it tends to block the patient's view of the paper. Other lightweight and smaller devices are available for writing (see Chapter 59, Activities of Daily Living).

Prehension with the WDWHO is produced by active wrist extension, which operates a mechanical linkage, transferring power from the wrist extensors to flex the index and middle fingers against the thumb. Gravity-assisted wrist flexion creates hand opening. An adjustable actuating lever at the wrist joint allows varying degrees of hand opening and closing. When the actuating lever is in the lowest setting, the hand opening is smaller and firm prehension is accomplished with the wrist slightly flexed. This position is useful for fine activities such as picking up finger foods. With the lever in the highest setting, the hand opening is wider and firm prehension is accomplished with the wrist in extension. This position is useful for grasping large objects such as a cup. Experimentation and practice is required to determine the optimal settings for specific tasks. Wrist extension can be assisted with elastic bands across the wrist joint. This assist may later be discontinued if there is sufficient return in muscle strength (9).

A modified version of the basic design, which utilizes a plastic hand cuff, was developed by Thorkild Engen, C.O. in the 1960s. In recent years, this design has been offered commercially by Dynamic Orthotic Systems in Houston, Texas (www.dynamicorthoticsystems.com).

Another recent iteration of the design, also utilizing plastic cuffs, is an adjustable orthosis that can serve as an evaluation and training device. The orthosis, the Talon, offers adjustability in the tenodesis bar, the wrist-to-metacarpalphalageal axis, and the finger pieces and thumb post (www.beckerorthopedic.com).

Unlike other orthoses, the WDWHO has been investigated by various authors (40–44). In one of the more recent outcome studies (40), Clarke found that of the 30 subjects interviewed, 80% were either using the orthosis at present, used the orthoses for a period following their discharge from acute rehabilitation, or were planning to use the orthosis in the future. Of the functional levels studied (C5 with C6 return, C6 and C7), individuals with C6 tetraplegia used this orthosis most consistently.

According to this study, factors that influence the prolonged use of the WDWHO are the patient having specific functional goals, using the orthosis on a dominant hand, and independently donning and doffing the orthosis (40).

Individuals with C8 Functional Level

The person with C8 functional level has intact finger extrinsic muscles, but has weak or absent intrinsic muscles. The activity of the long flexors, with absent lumbricals, creates a "claw hand." Prehension without initial metacarpalphalangeal flexion is therefore less effective. A static hand orthosis with a metacarpalphalangeal extension stop (lumbrical bar) helps substitute for the intrinsic-minus hand in preventing the clawing of the hand and improving hand opening. Additionally, a thumb post maintains the web space and the thumb in opposition. It is the authors' experience, however, that most individuals with C8 tetraplegia opt to do without orthoses soon after their injury.

The Ambulatory Person with Tetraplegia

The problem of maximizing upper extremity use when equipment cannot be strapped to the wheelchair is a great challenge as more and more individuals with SCI have incomplete injuries and are able to ambulate (37). According to the National Spinal Cord Injury Statistical Center collecting data on approximately 13% of all new SCIs in the United States, as many as 34.1% of all spinal cord injuries had incomplete tetraplegia since the year 2000 (45). These patients with incomplete injuries pose a special challenge, because the proximal muscles of the upper limbs may often be weak. The person may be able to reach a cup or a toothbrush, but may be unable to deliver it to the mouth because shoulder and elbow flexion muscles (C5–C6) are weak. In a sitting position, the arm can be supported with a table or chair-mounted mobile arm support. However, this is not so when the person is standing or walking. Although waist-mounted mobile arm supports are sometimes used, they are heavy and cumbersome. The WREX (previously mentioned) has a mobile unit that attaches to a custom-made back brace for the ambulatory patient, allowing the person to reach their face. This unit has been tried with children with arthrogryposis, and is available through JAECO Orthopedic (Hot Spring, Arkansas) (35). This unit may hold some potential for people with incomplete tetraplegia.

Simpler solutions have been documented, such as the dynamic triceps-driven orthosis (DTDO) (46) invented at the Mayo Clinic. This orthosis assists a person in reaching the mouth and face by extending the contralateral arm. Through the use of a simple dynamic orthosis, a person can accomplish elbow flexion and reach the face. It is important to note, however, that unlike upper limb support systems mounted to a wheelchair, no optimal solutions exist yet for the ambulating patient with weak upper limbs.

ORTHOTIC FITTING

Along with good orthotic design, proper fit is essential. Upon delivery, the orthosis must be carefully evaluated to ensure proper fit and function. A fit that is less than optimal will compromise function. Close communication between the therapist, orthotist, and patient is essential. Other team members are encouraged to provide feedback for best fit and use. The nurse, for example, must learn to assist the patient in putting on a night static orthosis and monitor it for proper fit during the evening and night shifts. The patient must be encouraged to effectively direct care by communicating clearly with staff and significant others about the orthosis.

Initially, the orthosis is placed on the hand for 30 minutes, after which it is removed and any red areas are noted and evaluated again 1 hour later. If the redness has not disappeared, adjustments may be necessary. The patient must be instructed in the importance of skin inspection to prevent excessive pressure and skin breakdown. Wearing tolerance is gradually increased until optimal tolerance is achieved.

PATIENT EDUCATION AND TRAINING

Key to the success of any orthotic management is the patient's participation and understanding of the program. The orthosis must complement the goals and life context of the individual (9, 40).

A systematic approach to orthosis training aids in the successful use of the device. The patient must demonstrate a knowledge of the overall purpose of the orthosis, whether it is positional or functional. This understanding is important in obtaining cooperation and a willingness to use the orthosis consistently. This is especially true of the positional orthosis because functional gains are not always obvious to the patient. It is important that the patient be knowledgeable about wearing tolerance and schedule.

Whereas most static orthoses require less training than dynamic/functional ones, such education should not be overlooked. Family members and caregivers must learn to apply the orthosis correctly and demonstrate the ability to adequately care for the orthosis prior to taking it home.

Functional orthoses, most typically the ratchet and WDWHO, require more lengthy and complex training. The patient may be introduced to the orthosis by watching a video or observing another patient using the device successfully. After demonstrating basic understanding of the operation of the orthosis, training with activities begins.

With both the ratchet WHO and the WDWHO, the patient may begin by practicing opening and closing of the fingers. The person becomes familiar with the components of the orthosis, particularly the actuating lever at the wrist with the WDWHO and the bar of the ratchet WHO. Both the bar and the actuating lever control the size of the opening and the resultant prehension. Experiential learning is by far the best in teaching the patient to handle different size objects and shapes. The fine-tuning of different settings is accomplished through further experimentation.

With the presence of any hand sensory impairment, patients must learn to compensate for sensory impairment with the aid of greater visual attentiveness. Additionally, they must learn the importance of skin inspection in avoiding excessive pressure from either the orthosis itself or from the forceful prehension achieved.

The individual practices grasping, placing, and releasing objects. It is best to start with soft, medium-sized objects. Training involves activities at various heights that require pronation and supination. Board games such as Connect Four are excellent for practicing grasp and release. Patients are given choices that are meaningful and relevant to them.

Once basic manipulation is mastered, functional training may follow. Patients will often have specific tasks they wish to accomplish. For example, patients are typically interested in relearning self-care activities, such as feeding and brushing their teeth. The person can be expected to become independent in these tasks using the wrist-driven, wrist-hand orthosis. The patient using the ratchet WHO may continue to need assistance in setting up for the activity.

Typical activities that training with the WDWHO include are feeding, hygiene and grooming, parts of dressing, self-catheterization, home and community skills such as computer and desktop-related activities, cooking, managing money, and manipulating knobs, switches, and keys.

The opportunity for new patients to interact with experienced and successful users of similar devices is helpful, and this may occur even before patients receive their own orthoses. Group activities such as games with patients using similar orthoses are great opportunities for humorous social interactions, and at the same time for engagement in repetitive use of the functional orthosis.

To achieve optimal independence the person must be able to don and doff the orthosis without assistance. Removal is easier than application, and it is often helpful to start training in this task first. Loops may be added to the ends of the retaining straps to allow the individual to use the thumb of the other hand to unfasten the straps. Then the patient simply pushes or shakes the orthosis off. Success in applying the orthosis influences ultimate acceptance and use of the device (40).

Prior to the patient's discharge, the patient and caregivers are instructed in solving simple problems. With the mobile arm support, for example, the patient will receive a set of Allen wrenches for tightening loose MAS joints. The patient and caregivers must also have easy access to professional help when greater problems arise. Additionally, appointments are arranged for follow-up outpatient visits. Often, the training program must continue following discharge because short inpatient stays do not permit a full and complete orthosis training program.

Periodic follow-up visits are important for the maintenance of the orthoses and for reevaluation of the patient's goals and need for orthoses. With time and practice, individuals often improve in functional strength, and either no longer require the orthoses or may benefit from an upgrade (19, 40).

CONCLUSION

The management of the upper limb in tetraplegia requires the use of orthoses. The purpose of these orthoses is to prevent deformity, maintain proper position, help strengthen weak muscles, and most important, enhance function. The functional level of the patient determines the types of orthoses that are required. Other vital considerations are the person's goals, motivation, support systems, and resources. To ensure the proper use of an orthosis, education of the treatment team, the patient, and significant others is a key concern. Follow-up evaluation and the continued modification of orthoses as the patient's needs and abilities evolve are also key factors in ensuring success with orthoses.

Lastly, studies (2, 8, 10) and textbooks (11) support a regimen of splinting the upper limb of the person with tetraplegia in the acute phase and beyond. However, as some authors point out (2, 19) orthotic management guidelines are based on general knowledge and trends, and largely lack evidence to support the use of one orthosis over another. This is especially true in the area of positioning for preventing deformity. An Australian research group led by Lisa Harvey has published various studies on stretching and properties of the hand in tetraplegia. They state: "We argue that therapists should continue administering stretch for the treatment and prevention of contracture until the results of further studies emerge." (8, p. 1) To support and improve the care of individuals with SCI, more studies are needed, particularly those that demonstrate the outcomes of the use of various splints and orthoses.

GLOSSARY

Long opponens splint (also called wrist-hand orthosis, WHO): A static positioning orthosis that supports the wrist and allows the fingers and thumb to rest in a functional position.

Mobile arm support: A metal device attached to the patient's wheelchair that supports the arm and allows horizontal and vertical arm motion.

Mouthstick: A rod, held in the person's mouth, allowing such tasks as page turning and manipulation of small objects on a tabletop.

Ratchet wrist-hand orthosis: A variation of the wrist-driven wrist-hand orthosis design that allows the individual with C5 tetraplegia some prehension function.

Resting wrist-hand splint: A static positioning splint that keeps the wrist and hand in a functional position. The wrist is at approximately 20–30° of extension, the fingers are in slight flexion, and the thumb is in abduction.

Universal cuff: A simply designed cuff that fastens to the individual's hand. A pocket in the cuff allows attachment of various implements to accomplish feeding, hygiene, etc.

Wrist-driven, wrist-hand orthosis, also called Flexor-hinge hand splint, also called tenodesis splint: A dynamic orthosis that provides a transfer of power from the wrist extensors to the fingers for the purpose of prehension.

References

1. American Board for Certification in Orthotics-Prosthetics. Orthotics-Prosthetics, *Scope of Practice Report*, 1996.
2. Krajnik, S, Bridle, MJ. Handsplinting in quadriplegia: current practice. *American Journal of Occupational Therapy* 1992; 46:149–156.
3. Connolly, S, Aubut, J, Teasell, R, Jarus, T. Upper limb rehabilitation following spinal cord injury. In: Eng, JJ, ed. *Spinal Cord Injury Rehabilitation Evidence*. (Version 2.0) Vancouver, 2006; 5.1–5.58. www.icord.org/scire/pdf/scire _ch5.pdf.
4. Johanson, M, Murray, W. The unoperated hand: The role of passive forces in hand function after tetraplegia. *Hand Clinics.* 2002; 391–398.
5. Moberg, E. *The Upper Limb in Tetraplegia: A New Approach to Surgical Rehabilitation.* Stuttgart, Germany: Thieme, 1978.
6. Hill, J, Presperin, J. Deformity control. In: Hill, J, ed. *Spinal Cord Injury: A Guide to Functional Outcomes in Occupational Therapy.* Rockville, MD: Aspen, 1986; 48–81.
7. Itzkovich, M, Catz, A, Ona, I. A new double-purpose device for elbow extension in tetraplegia with paralysis below C5. *Paraplegia*, 1993; 31:116–118.
8. Harvey, L, Herbert, R. Muscle stretching for treatment and prevention of contracture in people with spinal cord injury. *Spinal Cord* 2002; 40:(1)1–9.

9. Baumgarten, J. Upper extremity adaptations for the person with quadriplegia. In; Adkins, ed., *Spinal Cord Injury Clinics in Physical Therapy.* New York: Churchill Livingston, 1985; 6:219–241.

10. Curtin, M. Development of a tetraplegic hand assessment and splinting protocol. *Paraplegia* 1994; 32:159–169.

11. Hill, J., ed. *Spinal Cord Injury: A Guide To Functional Outcomes in Occupational Therapy.* Rockville, MD: Aspen, 1986.

12. Consortium for Spinal Cord Medicine. *Preservation of Upper Limb Function Following Spinal Cord Injury: Clinical Practice Guidelines for Healthcare Professionals.* Washington, DC: Paralyzed Veterans of America, 2005.

13. Kemp, B, Adkins, R, Thompson, L. Aging with spinal cord injury: what recent research show. *Topics in Spinal Cord Injury Rehabilitation.* 2004; 175–197.

14. DiPasquale-Lehnerz, P. Orthotic intervention for development of hand function with C6 quadriplegia. *American Journal of Occupational Therapy* 1994; 48:138–144.

15. Garrett, A, Perry, J, Nickel, V. Traumatic quadriplegia. *Journal of the American Medical Association* 1964; 187:7–11.

16. Barber, L, Nickel, V. Carbon dioxide-powered arm and hand devices. *American Journal of Occupational Therapy* 1969; 23:215–225.

17. Occupational Therapy Department. *Survey on Upper Limb Orthotic Prescriptions for Persons with Tetraplegia.* Rancho Los Amigos National Rehabilitation Center, Downey, CA: Unpublished, 1999.

18. Ottenbacher, K, Smith, P, Illig, S, Linn, R, Ostir, G, Granger, C. Trends in length of stay, living setting, functional outcome, and mortality following medical rehabilitation. *Journal of the American Medical Association* 2004; 292:1687–1695.

19. Garber, S, Gregorio, T. Upper extremity assistive devices: assessment of use by spinal cord injured patients with Tetraplegia. *American Journal of Occupational Therapy* 1990; 44:126–131.

20. Hillman, M, Jepson, J. Development of a robot arm and workstation for the disabled. *Journal of Biomedical Engineering* 1999; 12:199–204.

21. Knutson, J, Audu, M, Triolo, R. Interventions for mobility and manipulation after spinal cord injury: A review of orthotic and neuroprosthetic options. *Topics in Spinal Cord Injury Rehabilitation.* 2006; 61–81.

22. Popvic, D, Stojanovic, A, Pjanovic, A, Radosavljevic, S, Popvic, M, Jovic, S, Vulovic, D. Clinical evaluation of the bionic glove. *Archives of Physical Medicine and Rehabilitation* 1999; 50:311–319.

23. Jebson, R, Taylor, N, Trieschmann, R, Trotter, M, Howard, L. An objective and standardized test of hand function. *Archives of Physical Medicine and Rehabilitation* 1969; 50:311–319.

24. Sullerman, C, Ejeskar, A. Sullerman hand function test. *Scandinavian Journal of Plastic Reconstructive Hand Surgery* 1995; 29:167–176.

25. Land, J, Odding, E, Duivenvoorden, H, Begen, M, Stam, H. Tetraplegia Hand Activity Questionnaire (THAQ): the development, assessment of arm-hand function-related activities in tetraplegic patients with a spinal cord injury. *Spinal Cord* 2004; 294–301.

26. American Spinal Injury Association/International Medical Society of Paraplegia. *International Standards for Neurological Classification of Spinal Cord Injury,* revised 2000.

27. Law, L, Baptiste, S, Carswell, A, McColl, M, Poplatajko, H, Pollock, N. *Canadian Occupational Performance Measure* (2nd ed.) Ottawa, Ontario: Canadian Assoc. Of Occupational Therapy, 1994.

28. Whalley Hammell, K. *Spinal Cord Rehabilitation: Therapy in Practice.* London, UK: Chapman & Hall, 1995.

29. Donnelly, C, Eng, J, Hall, J, Alford, L, Giachino, R, Norton, K, Kerr, D. Client-centered assessment and the identification of meaningful treatment goals for individuals with spinal cord injury. *Spinal Cord* 2004; 302–307.

30. Waters, R, Adkins, R, Yakura, J, Ien, S. *Recovery Following Spinal Cord Injury: A Clinician's Handbook.* Downey, CA: Los Amigos Research and Education Institute, 1995.

31. Occupational Therapy Department: Functional goals for patients with quadriplegia. (a form) Rancho Los Amigos National Rehabilitation Center, Downey, CA: 1991.

32. Landsberger, S, Leung, P, Vargas, V, Shaperman, J, Baumgarten, J, Yasuda, YL, Sumi, E, McNeal, D, Waters, R. Mobile arm supports: history, application, and work in progress. *Topics in Spinal Cord Injury Rehabilitation* 2005; 74–94.

33. Consortium for Spinal Cord Medicine. *Outcomes following traumatic spinal cord injury: Clinical practice guidelines for healthcare professionals.* Washington, DC: Paralyzed Veterans of America, 1999.

34. Atkins, M, Baumgarten, J, Yasuda, YL, Adkins, R, Waters, R Leung, P, Requejo, P. Mobile arm supports (MAS): evidence-based benefits and criteria for use. The *Journal of Spinal Cord Medicine.* 2008; 31:388–393

35. Rahman, T, Sample, W, Jayakumar, S, King, M, Yong Wee, Seliktar, R, Alexander, M, Scavina, M, Clark, A. Passive exoskeletons for assisting limb movement. *Journal of Rehabilitation Research and Development* 2006; 43(5):583–590.

36. Herder, J, Vrijlandt, N, Antonides, T, Cloosterman, M, Masternbroek, P. Principle and design of a mobile are support for people with muscular weakness. *Journal of Rehabilitation Research and Development* 2006; 43(5):591–604.

37. Ziglar, J, Atkins, M, Resnik, C. Rehabilitation. In: Levine F, Garfin S, Zigler J, eds. *Spine Trauma.* Philadelphia, PA: Saunders 1998; 567–607.

38. Harvey, L. Principles of conservative management for a non-orthotic tenodesis grip in tetraplegics. *J Hand Ther* 1996; 238–242.

39. Curtin, M. An analysis of tetraplegia hand grips. *Brit Journal of Occupational Therapy* 1999; 62:444–450.

40. Carraro-Clarke, D. Wrist-Driven, Wrist-Hand Orthosis use post-discharge by individuals with tetraplegia. Masters Thesis presented to the Department of Occupational Therapy: San Jose State University, California, 1997.

41. Shepherd, C., Ruzika, S. Tenodesis brace use by persons with spinal cord injuries. *American Journal of Occupational Therapy* 1991; 45:82–83.

42. Engel, W, Kmiotek, M, Hohf, J, French, J, Barnerias, M, Siebens, A. A functional splint for grasp driven by wrist extension. *Archives of Physical Medicine and Rehabilitation* 1967; 48:43–52.

43. Knox, C, Engel, W, Siebens, A. Results of a survey on the use of a wrist-driven splint for prehension. *American Journal of Occupational Therapy* 1971; 15(2):109–111.

44. Wise, M, Wharton, G, Robinson, T. Long term use of functional hand orthoses by quadriplegics. *Proceedings of the Twelfth Annual Meeting of the American Spinal Injury Association.* San Francisco, CA: 1986; 111–113.

45. National Spinal Cord Injury Statistical Center. Spinal Cord Injury Facts and Figures at a Glance. University of Alabama. Birmingham, Alabama: June, 2006 (www.uab.edu/show.asp?durki=21446).

46. Lawlor, B, Stolp-Smith, K. A new dynamic triceps-driven orthosis (DTDO): Achieving elbow flexion in patients with C5 deficits. *Archives of Physical Medicine and Rehabilitation* 1998; 79:1309–1311.

58 Lower Limb Orthoses and Rehabilitation

Ann Yamane

Orthoses assist in furnishing a safe and efficient mode of ambulation. The type of orthoses used will vary depending on the biomechanical needs and functional goals of each individual. The orthotic treatment plan used in the management of individuals with a spinal cord injury (SCI) is most effective and beneficial when the functional goals are determined with the entire rehabilitation team. The importance of developing and understanding both short- and long-term goals cannot be over emphasized, as orthoses furnished during an inpatient stay must have the ability to follow the biomechanical changes of the individual over time. This requires the team members to anticipate the level of recovery of function the individual may expect to obtain.

The overall goal of an orthotic treatment plan is to design an orthosis that addresses the biomechanical needs of the client by providing support and substitution for lost muscle function, or providing control of excessive spasticity. One of the orthotist's objectives is to utilize the least amount of control necessary by limiting motion at any joint only if it will assist in providing improved joint stability and creating a stable base of support. A second objective, frequently overlooked, is to provide a stable skeletal alignment to impact the long-term effects of skeletal malalignment leading to the acquisition of pathomechanical deformities (1). For example, a patient may be fitted with an ankle-foot orthosis (AFO) to obtain clearance of the foot during swing phase, but the orthosis may not provide adequate support of the subtalar joint during stance phase. This alignment leads to long-term problems, with a foot and ankle positioned in excessive subtalar eversion, midtarsal pronation, and forefoot abduction during stance phase of gait. In a patient population in which muscle loss and imbalance are common, skeletal alignment as well as stability during ambulation is an important consideration for improved long-term outcomes.

PATIENT EVALUATION

An important aspect in determining an orthotic treatment plan recommendation for a patient with an SCI includes an understanding of the functional goals of the patient. Will the orthosis be used for independent community ambulation, household ambulation, exercise, or only for a specific setting or task? These factors impact the decision-making process and the complexity of the orthotic intervention.

Another significant piece is the information gained from the physical examination consisting of an assessment of range of motion (ROM), manual muscle testing (MMT), sensory testing, postural static and dynamic alignment, and evaluation of gait.

Range of Motion

If ROM limitations are prevented, potential alignment problems can be prevented. For example, in order for an individual with a plantarflexion contracture to have their foot flat on the ground, the subtalar and midtarsal joints distal to the talocrural joint will substitute the necessary range of motion. This long-term malalignment and instability at the subtalar and midtarsal joints can be avoided if addressed early in the treatment process (2). Muscle length evaluation of the gastrocnemius, soleus, hamstrings, rectus femoris, hip flexors, and iliotibial band are routinely included in the patient assessment.

Manual Muscle Testing

Manual muscle testing (MMT) and the evaluation of spasticity and motor control aid in the understanding of the biomechanical controls potentially necessary in an orthosis to produce a stable mode of ambulation. An understanding of the person's muscle weakness or control issues allows the opportunity to surmise the possible compensations the individual will use in developing a pathologic gait pattern. In addressing orthotic intervention we must understand the interaction between the ankle, knee, hip, pelvis, and trunk during both stance and swing phase. For example, an AFO with a plantarflexion stop positioned in dorsiflexion is designed to substitute for inadequate dorsiflexion strength of the tibialis anterior and toe extensors by controlling plantarflexion range of motion during swing phase.

Table 58.1   Manual Muscle Testing (5)

Qualitative Grade	Numerical Grade	Muscle-Testing Criteria
Normal	5	Completes full ROM against gravity, maximum resistance
Good	4	Completes full ROM against gravity, strong resistance
Fair plus	3+	Completes full ROM against gravity, mild resistance
Fair	3	Completes full ROM against gravity
Poor	2	Completes full ROM, gravity minimized
Poor minus	2–	Completes partial ROM, gravity minimized
Trace	1	Contraction palpated/Detect visually
Zero	0	No muscle contraction palpated

ROM = range of motion.

Consideration must be given to the impact this control will have at loading response. Placing the ankle in dorsiflexion within an AFO eliminates controlled plantarflexion and creates a knee flexion moment during loading response (3). In order to determine if the individual will be able to stabilize the knee, we must evaluate the person's muscle strength and control at the knee and hip. Good (4/5) quadriceps strength (Table 58.1) is adequate to control a knee flexion moment (4).

When assessing a person with an incomplete SCI, the MMT evaluation is especially important in determining joint instability in the sagittal and coronal planes, and in predicting any potential pathomechanical deformities. Our MMT examination evaluates the strength at each joint and assesses the agonist and antagonist strength for symmetry. For instance, in a case where the tibialis anterior strength is good (4/5) and the peroneals are not innervated (0/5), the subtalar joint will be maintained in inversion. In addition, if the strength of the gastrocnemius and soleus is poor (2/5), the foot and ankle will be positioned in dorsiflexion and inversion. Although the individual has adequate clearance of the foot during swing phase, the unopposed dorsiflexion and inversion must be addressed or a pathomechanical deformity will develop.

Sensory Testing

Joint proprioception of the ankle and knee is essential for the successful control of the knee. If an individual does not have position sense awareness to place the knee in relationship to the ankle, hip, and trunk, they will have difficulty finding stability in a well-aligned position. As a compensation to gain knee stability during stance phase, an individual may use uncontrolled

knee extension to their end range of motion to prevent knee flexion.

Sensory testing for light touch and pain will assist in determining the type of orthosis design considerations appropriate in distributing the desired forces. It will also furnish us with information regarding the type of patient education necessary to prevent skin breakdown. A person without protective sensation will require education on observing the skin for redness caused by excessive pressure over any bony prominence.

Static Postural Alignment Evaluation

A static postural alignment evaluation without an orthosis offers information with respect to the natural skeletal alignment of the individual. This knowledge assists in developing a hypothesis regarding the impact of muscle weakness or spasticity on joint range of motion, alignment, and ambulation. For example, in observing the static alignment of an individual with a plantarflexion contracture caused by spasticity of the gastrocnemius and soleus, we may see a number of

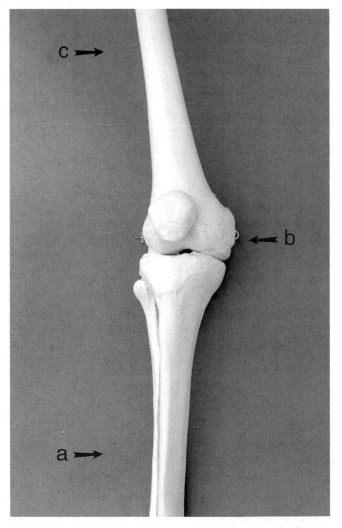

Figure 58.1 Three-point force system for control of genu valgum: (**b**) corrective force; (**a**, **c**) counteractive forces.

compensations distally, including subtalar eversion, midtarsal pronation, and forefoot abduction. Proximally, we may observe knee hyperextension, internal rotation of the tibia and femur, retraction of the pelvis, and an anterior tilt of the pelvis.

Gait Evaluation

If possible, a gait evaluation without use of an orthosis is helpful in assessing the person's dynamic alignment and pathologic gait pattern. If the client does not have the necessary stability to ambulate safely, MMT and ROM results are correlated with the static alignment evaluation to develop an orthotic recommendation. Temporary evaluative orthoses are another available assessment option.

All phases of gait are interwoven, and although one orthosis design may be beneficial during one phase of gait, it may prove to be inadequate or even detrimental during a subsequent phase of gait. The task is to determine the biomechanical needs during both swing and stance phases of gait and develop an orthosis design that addresses the most critical issues without creating any additional problems.

BIOMECHANICAL CONTROLS FOR AFOS

Three-Point Force Systems

The controls incorporated in orthotic systems are based on three-point force systems that affect alignment by controlling two adjacent skeletal segments (Figure 58.1). The corrective force is located on the convex side of the curve at the joint addressed (Figure 58.1B). Two counteractive forces are positioned on the opposite side above (Figure 58.1C) and below (Figure 58.1A) the corrective force. Increasing the distance of the counteractive forces from the corrective force increases the lever arms and therefore the effectiveness. Based on the principle Pressure = Total force/Area of force application, the objective is to distribute the forces over a larger area to decrease the resultant pressures (5). A well-fitting total contact orthosis that avoids bony prominences and utilizes appropriate and effective three-point force systems will assist in achieving this objective.

To provide mediolateral stability at the subtalar joint and control excessive subtalar eversion, the three-point force system

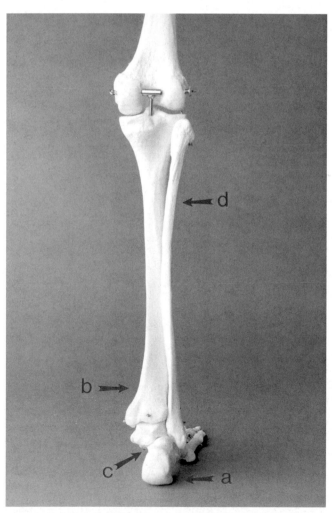

Figure 58.2 Three-point force system for correction of subtalar eversion. Corrective forces: (**b**) proximal medial malleolus, (**c**) sustentaculum tali. Counteractive forces: (**a**) distal lateral calcaneus, (**d**) proximal lateral calf.

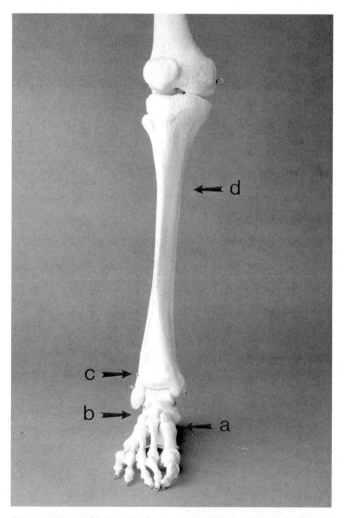

Figure 58.3 Three-point force system for correction of subtalar inversion. Corrective forces: (**c**) proximal lateral malleolus, (**b**) cuboid. Counteractive forces: (**a**) distal medial calcaneus, (**d**) medial tibial flare.

(Figure 58.2) cannot apply pressure directly to the bony medial malleolus, therefore the corrective force must be applied over two adjacent areas: proximal to the medial malleolus (Figure 58.2b) and at the sustentaculum tali (Figure 58.2c). The sustentaculum tali (ST) is located on the calcaneus, and if stabilized correctly by an ST modification or pad, provides a horizontal ledge to support the talus (6). The two counteractive forces at the distal lateral calcaneus (Figure 58.2a) and proximal lateral calf (Figure 58.2d) are above and below the joint and as far away from the joint as possible to produce longer lever arms.

Subtalar inversion motion (Figure 58.3) resulting from the unopposed tibialis anterior is controlled by the corrective force placed proximal to the lateral malleolus (Figure 58.3c) and over the cuboid (Figure 58.3b) if possible. The two counteractive forces are located at the distal medial calcaneus (Figure 58.4a) and the medial proximal tibial flare (Figure 58.3d).

Plantarflexion Stop

The most common use for an AFO is the control of the ankle joint in the sagittal plane. The AFO with a plantarflexion stop

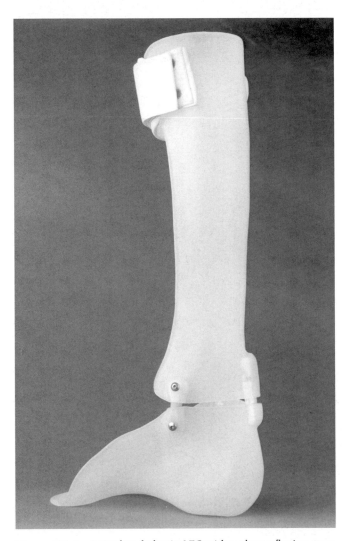

Figure 58.4 Articulated plastic AFO with a plantarflexion stop.

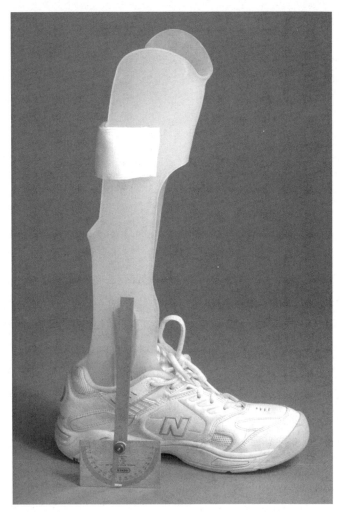

Figure 58.5 The tibial angle to the floor is determined by bisecting the distal one-third of the tibia in relationship to the floor while wearing a shoe.

(Figure 58.4) is designed to provide clearance of the foot during swing phase if there is inadequate strength of the ankle dorsiflexors: the tibialis anterior and extensor digitorum longus. This stop is effective by limiting the plantarflexion ROM of the talocrural joint. An important concept when evaluating the ankle position is the tibial angle to the floor (Figure 58.5). The tibial angle to the floor is determined by bisecting the distal one-third of the tibia in the sagittal plane and measuring this angle in relationship to the floor with the shoe on to establish stability and function during ambulation. For example, a tibia placed in relative dorsiflexion to the floor while wearing a shoe produces a knee flexion moment at loading response and can decrease a mild to moderate knee hyperextension moment during stance phase (Figure 58.6).

Dorsiflexion Stop

A dorsiflexion stop in an AFO (Figure 58.7) is used to limit ankle dorsiflexion and substitutes for weak ankle plantarflexors: the gastrocnemius and soleus. The stop provides stability in the

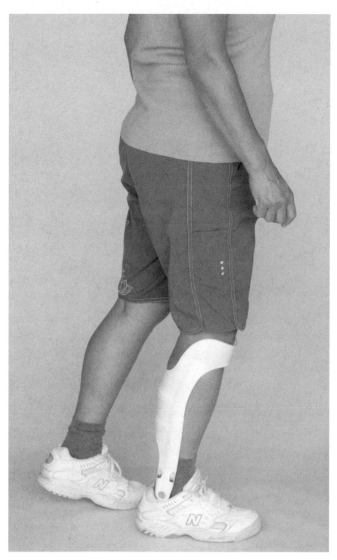

FIGURE 58.6 Tibial angle to floor in relative dorsiflexion causing a knee flexion moment.

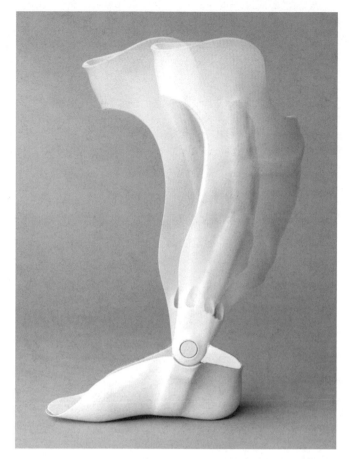

Figure 58.7 Laminated Oregon Orthotic System AFO with double adjustable ankle joints and dorsiflexion stop.

sagittal plane by limiting the dorsiflexion ROM of the talocrural joint. The limitation of dorsiflexion to neutral, or in slight plantarflexion, influences the extension stability of the knee and is of assistance when the quadriceps strength is grade fair minus (3−/5). With restraint of the tibia, the body's center of mass moves anterior to the knee joint axis, and because of the resultant ground reaction force vector, a knee extension moment is created (7).

Dorsiflexion Assist

A dorsiflexion assist joint can be composed of a spring arrangement (Figure 58.8) or a polyurethane flexure joint (Figure 58.9). The joint functions to bring the talocrural joint through dorsiflexion ROM, providing clearance of the foot during swing phase and allowing plantarflexion ROM at loading response, therefore decreasing the knee flexion moment, that may destabilize the knee (8).

With the spring arrangement, the amount of dorsiflexion assist force depends on the length, size, and durometer of the spring. The assist force of the flexure joint is similar to the traditional springs with a maximum of 60 in.-lb (9). Consideration must be given to the size and weight of the individual, as well as the foot and shoe when selecting components for the orthosis.

AFO DESIGNS

Conventional AFO Designs

A conventional design AFO (Figure 58.10) is composed of a shoe, stirrup, ankle joint, sidebar/upright, calfband, and calf closure. The control of the subtalar joint and foot is dependent on the stability and integrity of the shoe; once the shoe is worn, the effectiveness of the AFO decreases. A soleplate or a stirrup must be extended to the metatarsal heads to produce an effective lever arm. Because of the lack of total contact, the conventional AFO is not an effective design for controlling coronal or transverse plane motion.

The "weakest link" in the dorsiflexion assist ankle joint (Figure 58.8) is the durability of the spring; consequently it needs replacement at regular intervals to maintain its effectiveness.

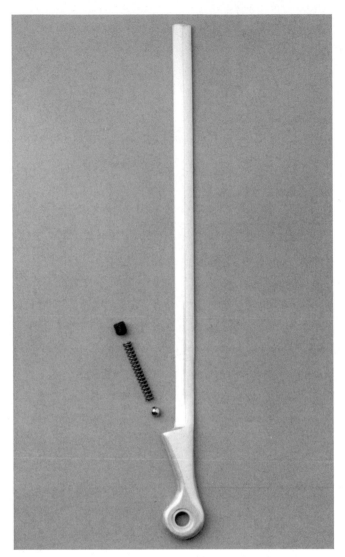

Figure 58.8   Dorsiflexion assist ankle joint.

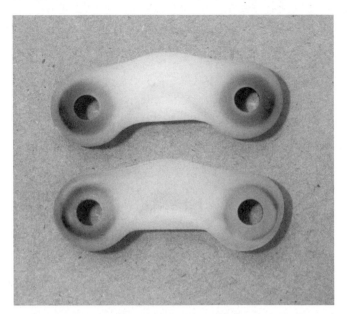

Figure 58.9   Dorsiflexion assist Tamarack flexure joints™ used with thermoplastic AFO designs.

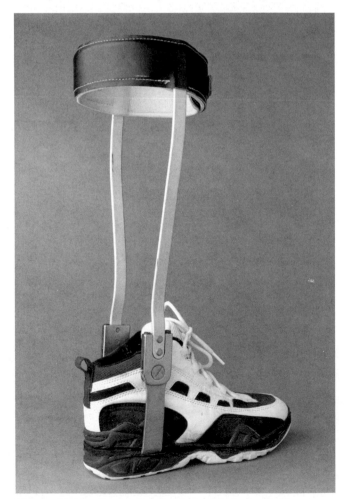

Figure 58.10   Conventional metal ankle-foot orthosis.

A double adjustable ankle joint (Figure 58.11) allows a greater degree of adjustability. The dual-channel system enables the practitioner to utilize the following sagittal plane controls at the ankle: (a) fixed position of the ankle; (b) limited range of motion; and (c) controlled plantarflexion at loading response due to a spring in the posterior channel and a dorsiflexion stop via a pin in the anterior channel.

Thermoplastic AFO Designs

The biomechanical functions of thermoplastic AFOs are described by their trimlines and reflect the motion allowed at the talocrural joint. A solid ankle design (Figure 58.12) with a trimline at the ankle region anterior to the malleoli is used with combined dorsiflexion and plantarflexion muscle loss and positions the ankle in a fixed position. Multiple three-point force systems place the joints in a fixed position, providing maximal

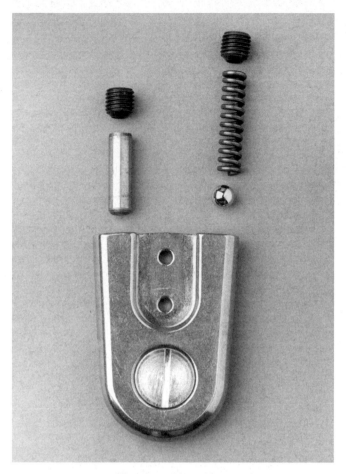

Figure 58.11   Double adjustable ankle joint.

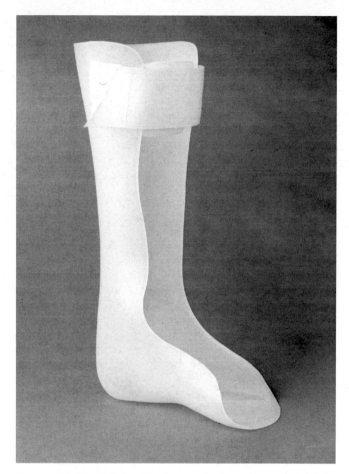

Figure 58.12   Solid ankle thermoplastic ankle-foot orthosis. (AFO).

stability in the sagittal, coronal, and transverse planes at the talocrural, subtalar, and midtarsal joints. To control the knee with this AFO, the individual will need grade fair (3/5) strength of the quadriceps and a tibial angle to the floor of 0 to 5 degrees of relative dorsiflexion.

A posterior leaf spring AFO (Figure 58.13) is trimmed posterior to the malleoli with the flexibility allowing controlled plantarflexion at loading response and dorsiflexion ROM during late midstance and terminal stance. The main function of this AFO design is to limit plantarflexion ROM during swing phase if an individual has weakness of the ankle dorsiflexors. Unfortunately, the inherent flexibility of this design will not control excessive subtalar eversion, midtarsal pronation, and forefoot abduction. The placement of the mechanical axis of the AFO posterior to the anatomic axis leads to migration of the orthosis during plantarflexion and dorsiflexion range of motion, and has the potential for causing skin irritation.

The ground reaction AFO (Figure 58.14) has been used historically to describe the thermoplastic AFO composed of a solid ankle design and a pretibial shell. Ground reaction force vectors induce a knee extension moment from midstance through terminal stance by a dorsiflexion stop that limits dorsiflexion range of motion. When the center of mass of

the individual is moving forward and tibial advancement or dorsiflexion is limited by the AFO, a knee extension moment is created. The knee extension moment is augmented with a tibial angle to the floor of 90 degrees to a slight tilt posteriorly, and a footplate extended distal to the metatarsal heads. The ground reaction AFO design is indicated with quadriceps strength of fair minus (3–/5) (10), and gait training will be necessary to address the knee flexion moment created at loading response.

Articulated thermoplastic AFO designs (Figure 58.4) are widely used because they easily provide a system with a sagittal plane plantarflexion stop and a total contact design offering control in the coronal and transverse planes. Clinically, we observe that the incorporation of an ankle joint decreases the amount of transverse and coronal plane control, with flexibility added to the system by the joint and the interruption in total contact. Common ankle joints include the Tamarack flexure joint™ (Figure 58.15a), Gaffney joint (Figure 58.15b), and the Oklahoma joint (Figure 58.15c). These are articulations only and must be used in conjunction with a plantarflexion stop; the designs do not provide a dorsiflexion stop. Other designs, such as the Camber axis joint® (Figure 58.16a) and the Select joint (Figure 58.16b), provide both plantarflexion and dorsiflexion stops. The disadvantage of these two joints lies in their lack of

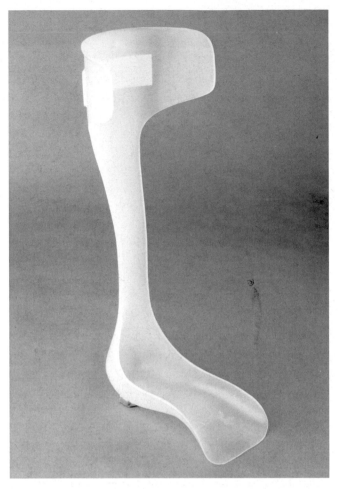

Figure 58.13 Prefabricated posterior leaf spring ankle-foot orthosis.

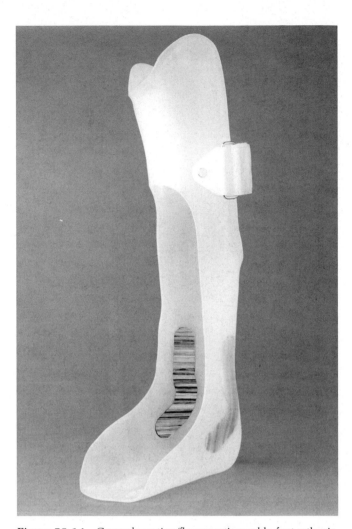

Figure 58.14 Ground reaction/floor reaction ankle-foot orthosis.

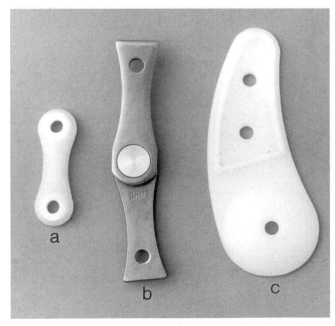

Figure 58.15 Articulated plastic AFO joints: (**a**) Tamarack flexure joint™, (**b**) Gaffney, (**c**) Oklahoma.

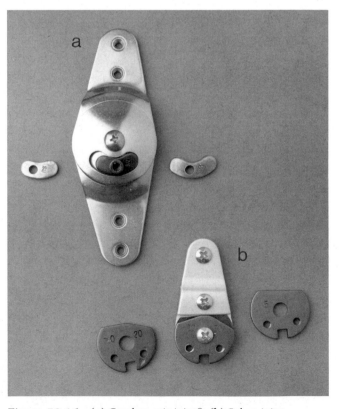

Figure 58.16 (**a**) Camber axis joint®, (**b**) Select joint.

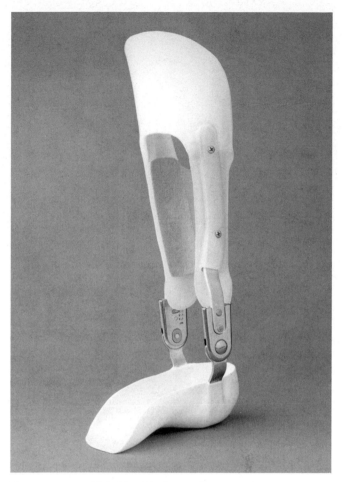

Figure 58.17 Hybrid ankle-foot orthosis.

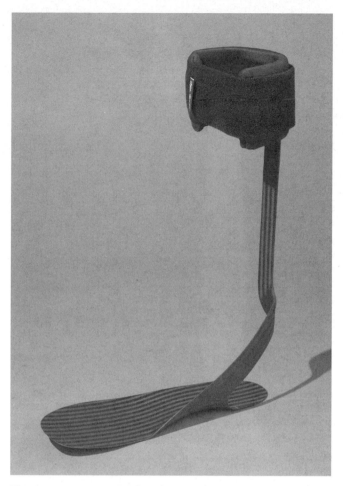

Figure 58.18 Otto Bock carbon composite Walk On® AFO.

durability and control of torsion with the forces exerted on the dorsiflexion stop with larger clients.

Hybrid AFO Designs

A hybrid orthosis is identified by the combined use of a footplate with a metal stirrup, metal ankle joints, sidebars, and a thermoplastic calf section (Figure 58.17). This design enables the patient to use a variety of shoes, and the ankle joints allow biomechanical options for adjustability at the ankle. The incorporation of the metal stirrup and adjustable ankle joints provide an effective dorsiflexion stop that cannot be achieved with the previously mentioned plastic AFO ankle joints. The use of a plastic calf section and a well-designed footplate improves the effectiveness of the three-point force systems used in the orthosis.

Carbon Composite AFO Designs

Prefabricated carbon composite AFO designs (Figures 58.18 and 58.19) are used primarily when there is a lack of adequate dorsiflexion strength and minimal coronal and transverse plane instability. A foot insert can be used in conjunction for increased control of the subtalar joint. Clinical decision-making skills are used to determine the optimal design for each person based on the type of control and motion indicated. An AFO with a thin posterior strut will allow increased dorsiflexion ROM, but a lateral strut may limit dorsiflexion ROM but allow greater flexibility at the metatarsal head region during terminal stance.

GOALS FOR KAFO INTERVENTION

The determining factor for the use of an AFO versus a knee-ankle-foot orthosis (KAFO) lies in the muscle strength of the quadriceps and the presence of any skeletal deformities. KAFOs are indicated when there is (a) grade 2/5 or less quadriceps strength; (b) genu recurvatum; and (c) mediolateral instability of the knee, as in the case of genu valgum or varum.

Conventional KAFOs

Conventional KAFO components include a stirrup, ankle joints, knee joints and sidebars, calf and thigh bands, and infrapatellar and suprapatellar straps (Figure 58.20). The conventional ankle

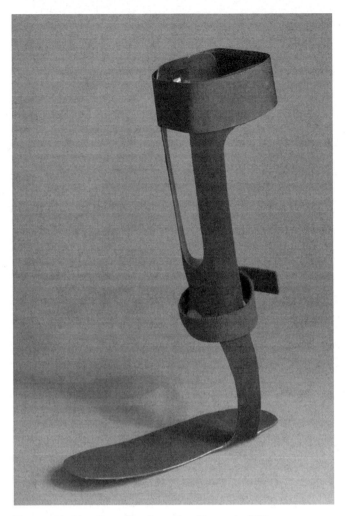

Figure 58.19 Ossur® carbon fiber Dynamic AFO.

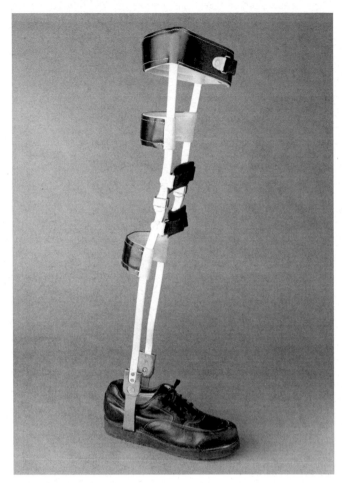

Figure 58.20   Conventional knee-ankle-foot orthosis.

joints provide maximum adjustability at the ankle in respect to dorsiflexion and plantarflexion. A slight change in angulation affects the center of mass in relationship to the lower extremity and base of support. The thigh and calf bands assist in sagittal plane control but do not contribute to coronal or transverse plane control.

Thermoplastic KAFOs

Thermoplastic KAFOs utilize the same types of knee joints used in the conventional designs. The plastic thigh and AFO sections provide improved control over the conventional designs in both the sagittal and coronal planes at the knee, ankle, and foot by allowing increased pressure distribution. The disadvantages of the thermoplastic design with a solid ankle AFO section include the inability to change the ankle controls as the patient's biomechanical needs change, and the inability to alter the plastic shells if there are changes in volume.

Hybrid KAFOs

Hybrid KAFOs (Figure 58.21) are composed of either a plastic or laminated thigh and calf section. The incorporation of a

conventional stirrup and ankle joint system allows maximum sagittal plane adjustment of the ankle position. As in the thermoplastic KAFO designs, the total-contact qualities of the design provide an equivalent degree of control in the sagittal and coronal planes. The laminated systems have improved transverse plane control because of their increased rigidity but require increased fabrication time and expertise.

BIOMECHANICAL CONTROLS FOR KAFOS

Previously the selection in knee joints used in the orthotic treatment plan for individuals with an SCI was divided into offset free motion knee joints and joints with locking mechanisms. Advances in technology have stimulated the development of knee joints termed stance control orthoses. The name describes those knee joints with the ability to allow free knee ROM during swing phase and provide a locked knee during stance phase of the gait cycle. This new technology is indicated for individuals who have sustained an SCI with a unilateral instability. Hussey and Stauffer found individuals with pelvic control, at least fair strength of the hip flexors, and fair or better quadriceps strength of one extremity had a greater opportunity of achieving community ambulation (11).

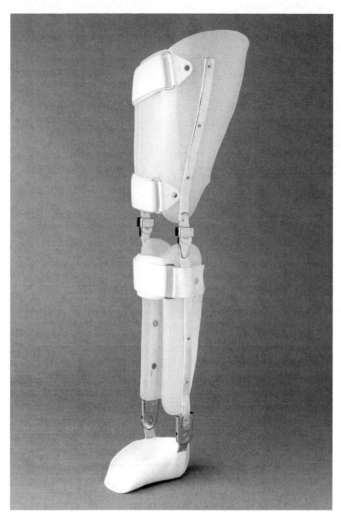

Figure 58.21 Hybrid design knee-ankle-foot orthosis (KAFO).

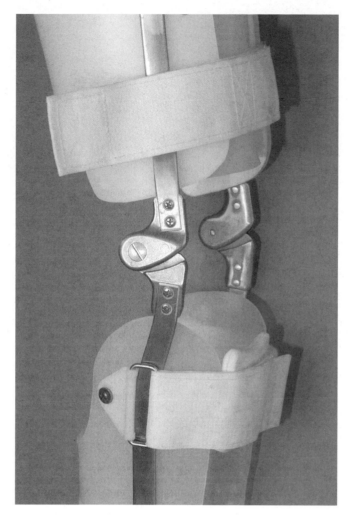

Figure 58.22 Offset free knee joint.

Offset Knee Joint

The offset free knee joint (Figure 58.22) is used if an individual has a unilateral weakness at the knee and at least poor (2/5) hip extensor strength, or the ability to attain passive hip extension range. The knee joint provides increased knee stability by moving the mechanical knee axis posterior to the anatomical knee joint, thus enabling the individual to position their center of mass or weight line anterior to the knee joint axis. The offset free knee joint is used in conjunction with a double adjustable ankle joint with a dorsiflexion stop and a spring in the posterior channel allowing approximately 10 degrees of plantarflexion range of motion at loading response. The advantages for using this type of joint include decreased energy consumption, ease in moving from sitting to standing, and an improved gait appearance. Disadvantages include instability when going down an incline or negotiating uneven terrain. To stabilize the hip, the individual must place their center of mass posterior to the anatomic hip joint axis, and in order to stabilize the knee, maintain their weight line anterior to the knee joint axis (12). This requires joint proprioception, or the ability to maintain a sense of body position and awareness while ambulating, in order to maintain the knee in extension.

Locked Knee Joints

Locked joints such as the Bail lock, drop lock, and lever release maintain the knee in a locked position throughout the gait cycle, creating compensation strategies to clear the floor by circumduction, hip hiking, lateral trunk lean to the contralateral side, and vaulting (13). The bail lock (Figure 58.23) is easy to unlock when moving from standing to sitting. It is useful when an individual is using bilateral KAFOs or has decreased hand function. One disadvantage is the posterior protrusion necessary for clearance during knee flexion. The drop lock (Figure 58.24) is a second method for maintaining the knee locked in extension. It has positive cosmetic qualities, but requires good hand function to operate. A lever release system (Figure 58.25) connecting the medial and lateral locking system unlocks both sides simultaneously with a lever positioned at the proximal lateral trimline.

Stance Control Orthoses

Most of the designs require similar patient criteria for optimal use as that described for an offset free knee joint: (a) full knee extension ROM with a vertical alignment of the trunk, hip,

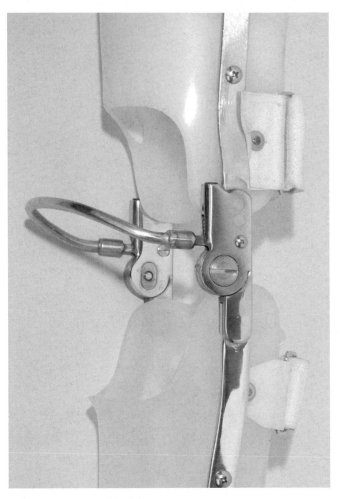

Figure 58.23   Bail lock knee joint.

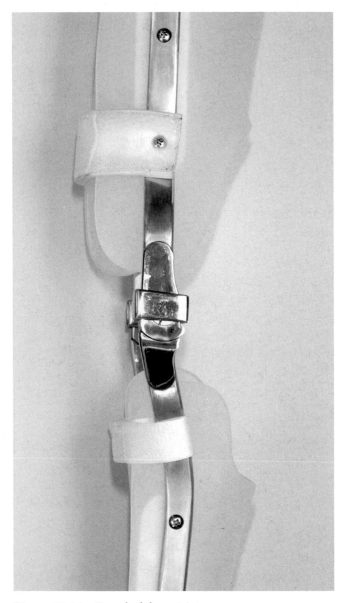

Figure 58.24   Drop lock knee joint.

knee, and ankle; and (b) hip extension strength at least grade 3/5. The advantage of having joint proprioception has been suggested (14).

Less encompassing of the lower extremity and utilizing internal cables connecting the knee and the ankle are the UTX® and the Freewalk™ KAFOs (Figure 58.26). They both require full ROM at the knee to 180 degrees to enable the locking mechanism to engage. Dorsiflexion ROM of 5–10 degrees coupled with a knee extension moment is required at terminal stance to initiate knee flexion of the mechanical knee joint. Fair strength (3/5) of the hip flexors and extensors is recommended for optimal use. These designs are ideal for individuals with a normal alignment of the leg of no greater than 10 degrees of genu valgum or varum.

The Stance Control Orthotic Knee Joint (SCOKJ®) (Figure 58.27) incorporates a cam lock that prevents the knee from flexing during stance phase but does not limit extension. The lock is released mechanically by a linkage controlled most commonly by ankle movement. Three control mode options are available: automatic, used for ambulation when walking with knee flexion during swing phase; unlocked, with unrestricted knee motion; and locked, in full extension (15).

The Stance Phase Lock (SPL) has an internal pendulum mechanism that locks the knee prior to heel strike and unlocks the knee at heel off. It has three modes of control: automatic, unlocked, and locked. This is the only joint that can be used without a footplate, as it is activated by the position of the knee joint in the sagittal plane.

The two additional systems currently available that lock in any degree of flexion are the Electronic-Knee™ (E-Knee™) and the SafetyStride™. The E-Knee™ has a foot-activated sensor and provides positive locking in increments of 8 degrees of flexion when a stumble occurs. There are no ROM or muscle strength requirements for this system. The SafetyStride™ system has no hip strength requirement and needs 3–5 degrees of ankle motion to activate the system.

Bilateral KAFOs

Positioning the individual with bilateral KAFOs in fixed dorsiflexion at the ankle places their center of mass anterior to

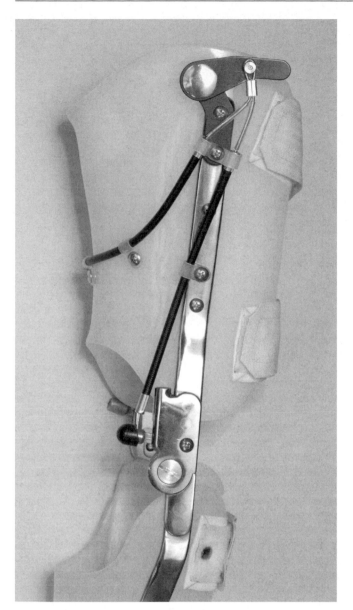

Figure 58.25 Lever release system.

the knee and ankle joints. The individual gains stability at the hip joints by compensating with lumbar lordosis, which positions the weight line posterior to the hip joint and within their base of support.

RECIPROCATING GAIT ORTHOSES

There are several types of reciprocating gait orthoses (RGOs) available to provide stability at the hip, knee, and ankle for individuals with bilateral lower extremity weakness. The orthoses enable the individual to ambulate with a reciprocal gait pattern and initiate hip flexion with either active hip flexion or weight shifting coupled with trunk extension to the contralateral side. The dynamic connection between the two hip joints provides simultaneous mechanical hip flexion and contralateral hip extension stability and control at the hip, enabling the individual to stand with greater ease than with a bilateral KAFO system. The

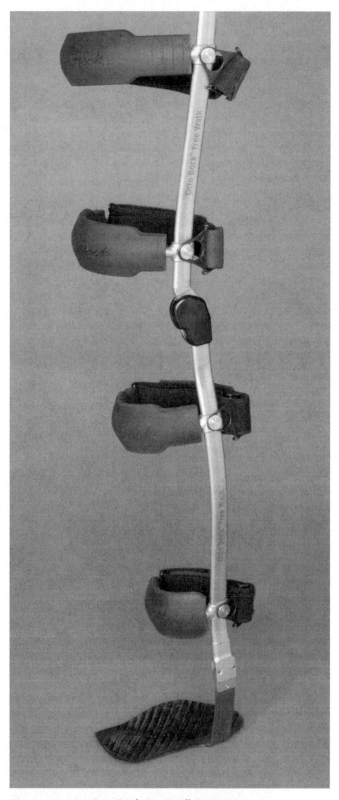

Figure 58.26 Otto Bock FreeWalk™ KAFO.

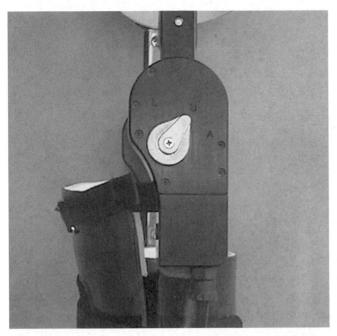

Figure 58.27 Horton Stance Control Orthosis Knee Joint (SCOKJ®).

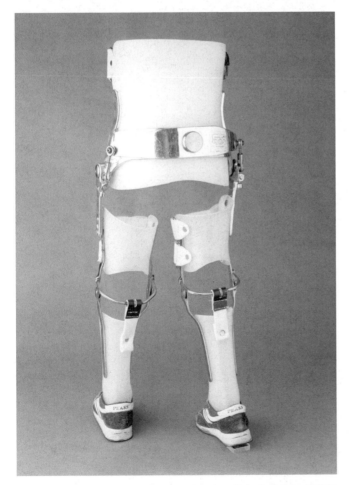

Figure 58.28 Isocentric® Reciprocating Gait Orthosis (RGO) with bilateral thermoplastic KAFOs.

hip joints on an RGO can also be disengaged to allow a traditional swing-through gait pattern. The RGO requires good upper extremity strength for the use of assistive devices.

The Isocentric® RGO (Figure 58.28) is commonly prescribed because of its low-profile design, ease of fabrication, and durability. Alternative Isocentric® RGO designs include a standard AFO with a knee-locking mechanism and no thigh cuff for ease in donning for individuals without knee alignment problems. A second alternative design is an external AFO that allows the person to easily don and doff the system over their regular shoes. This system may be indicated for an individual who plans to use the orthosis to obtain standing balance for only specific activities, and therefore ease of donning is of importance.

CLINICAL SITUATIONS

Dorsiflexion Weakness

The clinical observation of dorsiflexion weakness reveals inadequate clearance of the foot during the swing phase of gait. Compensations observed during swing-phase gait evaluation include increased hip and knee flexion. With the strength of the ankle dorsiflexors less than grade fair (3/5), a heel strike will most likely be absent. Grade fair (3/5) muscle strength of the ankle dorsiflexors may provide adequate clearance of the foot, but a foot slap will be observed at loading response. The lack of adequate inversion strength will decrease coronal plane subtalar joint stability. Our goals for orthotic intervention include (a) adequate clearance of the foot during swing phase; (b) controlled knee flexion during loading response; and (c) balanced alignment with respect to inversion/eversion of the calcaneus or subtalar joint at loading response (10).

Orthotic design options to address dorsiflexion weakness include (a) a dorsiflexion assist AFO (Figure 58.29), or (b) a posterior leaf spring AFO (Figure 58.13). These designs control plantarflexion ROM during swing phase and allow controlled plantarflexion ROM at loading response and dorsiflexion ROM during midstance. Another option is an articulated plastic AFO with a plantarflexion stop (Figure 58.4) that maintains positioning of the dorsiflexion angle and provides clearance during swing phase, allows dorsiflexion ROM during midstance, but does not allow controlled plantarflexion ROM at loading response.

Plantarflexion Weakness

The clinical signs of plantarflexion weakness observed during terminal stance include (a) excessive knee flexion; (b) late heel rise; and (c) short step length on the contralateral side. Orthotic intervention provides a simulated push-off that is accomplished by utilizing a dorsiflexion or anterior stop to limit the amount of dorsiflexion during midstance to terminal stance, thus creating the forefoot rocker described by Perry (16) (Figure 58.30).

Clinical Example

A 33-year-old female involved in an MVA sustained an L3 burst fracture and an L4 SCI. Bilaterally she presents with hip flexors and knee extensors grade 5/5. The following muscles have 4/5 strength: hip extensors and abductors; knee flexors; ankle dorsiflexors and invertors. Toe extensors are 2/5; ankle plantarflexors and evertors are grade 0/5. This profile suggests the person will

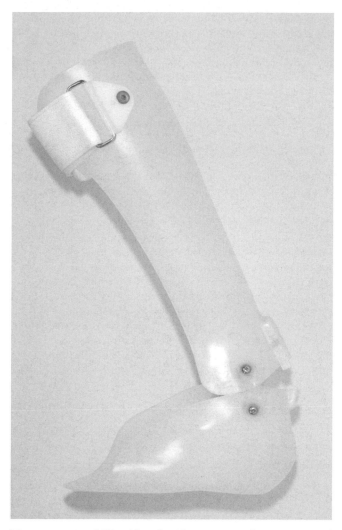

Figure 58.29 AFO with a dorsiflexion assist flexure joint and an adjustable plantarflexion stop.

have a foot ankle positioned in dorsiflexion and inversion, and can be controlled using an AFO. A floor reaction AFO with a dorsiflexion stop meets the biomechanical needs of the person, and the pretibial shell will provide proprioceptive feedback and assist in maintaining control and positioning at the hip.

Plantarflexor Spasticity

Spasticity of the plantarflexors creates an equinovarus positioning. This alignment situation requires the use of a solid ankle design AFO with total contact and effective three-point force systems for sagittal, coronal, and transverse plane stabilization. The solid-ankle AFO is a combination of a plantarflexion stop to prevent plantarflexion range of motion and a dorsiflexion stop to limit dorsiflexion range and decrease the stimulation of a deep tendon reflex.

Quadriceps Weakness

A common compensation observed for quadriceps weakness is a trunk leaning forward to place the weight line anterior to the

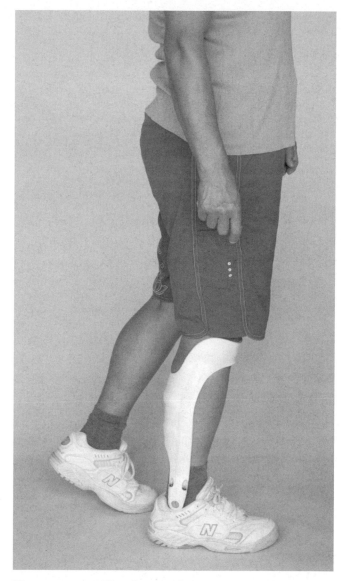

Figure 58.30 AFO with a dorsiflexion stop preventing the tibia from moving into dorsiflexion.

knee joint axis. A second compensation is hyperextension or recurvatum of the knee. For mild to moderate weakness of the quadriceps, compensation may be achieved with the eliminating of knee flexion and maintaining the knee in extension at initial contact (17).

Quadriceps weakness may either be addressed with an AFO with a dorsiflexion stop, or a KAFO with the following options: an offset free knee, a locked knee, or a stance control knee. An AFO designed to control knee flexion instability allows plantarflexion range of motion to position the foot flat on the ground and reduce the knee flexion moment that is produced at loading response (18). The AFO also incorporates a dorsiflexion stop to prevent the tibia from moving into dorsiflexion (Figure 58.30) and thus addresses the quadriceps weakness and potentially substitutes for weakened plantarflexors. The center of mass continues to move forward, although the tibia is restricted and the ground reaction force vector line is positioned anterior to the knee joint axis, thus providing knee extension. This orthotic intervention simulates the body's normal compensation of recruitment of the plantarflexors and/or hip extensors to substitute for the lack of knee control caused by quadriceps weakness.

A KAFO with an offset free knee joint (Figure 58.22) would utilize the same principles as the AFO previously described but the addition of the offset knee joint facilitates knee extension stability by placing the mechanical knee joint axis posterior to the anatomical knee joint axis. A stance control knee orthosis will provide the individual with normal knee flexion during swing phase and greater stability during stance phase of gait.

Combined Quadriceps and Hamstring Weakness

An individual with hamstring weakness using their center of mass to prevent the knee joint from flexing will find that their knee will have a tendency to move into excessive hyperextension during stance phase. An AFO with a plantarflexion stop positioned in dorsiflexion and limiting the amount of posterior tibial angle in relationship to the floor will control minimal to moderate hyperextension problems, but will also create a knee flexion moment at loading response. If moderate or greater hyperextension control is needed, either a KAFO with an offset knee joint or a stance control knee is indicated.

Bilateral Lower Extremity Weakness

For an individual with a complete SCI, ambulation with bilateral lower extremity weakness is dependent on the person's functional level and goals. In the case of a person classified with an L5 ASIA A injury, the individual has functional strength of the hip musculature, knee flexors and extensors, ankle dorsiflexors, and toe extensors. Factors that may influence successful ambulation include normal range of motion of knee extension and ankle dorsiflexion, minimal spasticity, and decreased weight. With this clinical picture, we would expect independent ambulation with bilateral AFOs and forearm crutches or canes using a four-point or two-point gait pattern on level surfaces and elevations (19).

At the ASIA T12–L2 levels, our goal is independent ambulation on level surfaces with bilateral KAFOs using forearm crutches with the option of a swing-to, swing-through, or four-point gait pattern. Good upper extremity and trunk strength is necessary for this pattern of ambulation. Key muscles to check for adequate muscle length are the hip flexors, hamstrings, and ankle plantarflexors. Other limiting factors include increased spasticity and decreased coordination. An RGO is a consideration if reciprocal gait pattern and increased hip stability are desired for individuals with bilateral weakness of the hip and knee extensors.

Goals for the ASIA T9–T11 levels may include independent ambulation on level surfaces with bilateral KAFOs using a walker or forearm crutches with a swing-to or swing-through gait pattern. The individual must have adequate strength of the upper extremity, trunk, and quadratus lumborum. The individual must have adequate range of motion of hip extension, knee extension, and ankle dorsiflexion. Spasticity and coordination are again important considerations. Another alternative for ambulation would include the use of an RGO.

Individuals with ASIA T6–T8 levels may utilize ambulation with bilateral KAFOs and a walker for short distances, or a swing-to gait pattern in the parallel bars. Considerations include upper extremity strength, trunk control, adequate hip extension, knee extension, and ankle dorsiflexion range of motion. A second option is again an RGO. The RGO would include a higher thoracic section to provide increased trunk control to capture trunk motion for initiation of movement.

CONCLUSION

The use of orthotic intervention in an individual with an SCI depends on many factors, including functional level and goals. The most successful outcomes are achieved with an orthotic recommendation based on input from a rehabilitation team that includes the patient, physician, physical and occupational therapists, and the orthotist. A thorough evaluation is crucial to the success and acceptance of the orthoses, along with an accurate understanding of the biomechanical needs in relationship to the functional goals of the individual. In the short- and long-term goals of orthotic intervention, patient education is an important factor in preventing pathomechanical deformities caused by an inadequate or inappropriate orthotic treatment plan.

Through optimal skeletal alignment of the person, along with appropriate biomechanical controls in our orthosis design, we hope to create a stable base of support to allow safe and efficient ambulation and prevent the development of pathomechanical deformities.

*R*eferences

1. Fish DJ, Nielsen JP. Clinical assessment of human gait. *JPO* 1993; 5(2):27–36.
2. Perry J. *Gait Analysis: Normal and pathological function,* 1st ed. Thorofare, NJ: SLACK Inc., 1992; 192–195.
3. Perry J. *Gait Analysis: Normal and pathological function,* 1st ed. Thorofare, NJ: SLACK Inc., 1992; 196–201.
4. Perry J. *Gait Analysis: Normal and pathological function,* 1st ed. Thorofare, NJ: SLACK Inc., 1992; 228–231.
5. Fess EE, Philips CA. *Hand Splinting: Principles and methods,* 2nd ed. St. Louis: C.V. Mosby, 1987; 126.
6. Carlsen MJ, Berglund G. An effective orthotic design for controlling the unstable subtalar joint. *Orthotics and Prosthetics* 1979; 33(1):31–41.
7. Perry J. *Gait Analysis: Normal and pathological function,* 1st ed. Thorofare, NJ: SLACK Inc., 1992; 224, 225.
8. Perry J. *Gait Analysis: Normal and pathological function,* 1st ed. Thorofare, NJ: SLACK Inc., 1992; 60–63.
9. www.oandp.com/products/tamarck/flexurejoint.htm.
10. Yang GW, Chu DS. Floor reaction orthosis: clinical experience. *Orthotics and Prosthetics* 1986; 40(1):33–37.
11. Hussey RW, Stauffer ES. Spinal cord injury: requirements for ambulation. *Arch Phys Med Rehabil,* 1973; 54:544–547.
12. Perry J, Hislop HJ, ed. *Principles of lower-extremity bracing,* New York: APTA, 1967; 36–47.
13. Perry J. *Gait Analysis: Normal and pathological function,* 1st ed. Thorofare, NJ: SLACK Inc., 1992; 224–226.
14. Perry J. *Gait Analysis: Normal and pathological function,* 1st ed. Thorofare, NJ: SLACK Inc., 1992; 175, 176.
15. McMillan G, Kendrick KK, Michael JW, Aronson J, Horton GW. Preliminary evidence for effectiveness of a stance control orthosis. *J Prosthetics Orthotics* 2004; 6(1):6–13.
16. Perry J. *Gait Analysis: Normal and pathological function,* 1st ed. Thorofare, NJ: SLACK Inc., 1992; 30–36.
17. Perry J. *Gait Analysis: Normal and pathological function,* 1st ed. Thorofare, NJ: SLACK Inc., 1992; 272–275.
18. Lehmann JF, deLateur BJ, Price R. Ankle-foot orthoses for paresis and paralysis. *Phys Med and Rehab Clin NA* 1992; 3(1):139–159.
19. Nixon V. *Spinal Cord Injury: A guide to functional outcomes in physical management,* 1st ed., Rockville, MD: Aspen Publishers, 1985.

59 Activities of Daily Living

Andrew L. Sherman
Maria E. Gomez
Diana D. Cardenas

Activities of daily living (ADLs) are a defined set of activities necessary for normal self-care: the activities of personal hygiene, dressing, eating, transfers/bed mobility, functional mobility, and bowel and bladder control (1). The treatment of ADL function specifically as it relates to the rehabilitation service has historically been performed by occupational therapists. However, the modern rehabilitation approaches stress that all members of the rehabilitation team promote a "functional approach" to treatment and share in the ADL treatment responsibility.

The immediate goal of rehabilitation in spinal cord injury (SCI), just as with any other injury, focuses on improving all areas of patient function. The ultimate goal of rehabilitation is to gain independence in each area, regardless of the level of injury. Historically, most if not all of these goals were attained in an inpatient multidisciplinary rehabilitation hospital. However, due to many factors, the inpatient rehabilitation length of stay has had to decrease. Therefore, in many cases of SCI, independence may not be attained in all areas of ADL function during the inpatient stay. The rehabilitation goals must then be expanded to the post acute rehabilitation state, as ADL goals can still be achieved during the outpatient rehabilitation period and beyond.

In order to understand how independence in function is achieved, first we must define the terms that describe the reduction of such independence. The terms most often used to describe a loss of independence are impairment, disability, and handicap. Often used interchangeably, these terms provide sharply different meanings in the world of rehabilitation medicine. Impairment describes the actual injury; the damage or weakening of physiological, psychological, and anatomical function or structure. An example is the spinal cord damage itself. Disability describes the direct basic functional loss, the specific ADL activity that cannot be performed due to the impairment. An example is the inability to walk. Finally, impairment illustrates the (societal) impact of the injury. For example, if the patient is a radio announcer there may be no significant work handicap. However, if the patient is a construction worker, then a work handicap will exist that will need to be overcome—either through job modification or vocational rehabilitation, if the patient can work again.

Providing the means for patients with SCI to achieve their maximum level of function, or maximum ADL status, is important for many reasons. Lund et al. found that the level of life satisfaction in SCI respondents that perceived no severe problems with participation (in life activities) was similar to those of a normal population (2). However, despite aggressive rehabilitation to maximize function, barriers will remain. Whiteneck et al (3) found that barriers placed upon SCI persons by their natural environment, transportation, need for help in the home, availability of health care, and governmental policies negatively impacted their quality of life (3). Thus, the rehabilitation program must be focused on not only the individual but the environment to which they are returning (4).

ADLs can be considered "basic" or "advanced." The basic ADLs make up the basic components of self-care, such as personal hygiene and dressing. Another group of self-care activities exist that can be termed "instrumental (IADL)" (5), "higher-level" ADL (1), "expanded," or "advanced" ADL (6). The activities that make up this group include but are not limited to domestic activities such as shopping, cooking, and cleaning; interpersonal activities (such as regaining a role within the family, community, work force, etc); leisure activities; and learning to access assistive technologies. By seeking improvement in all of these areas, the injured person with SCI will maximize functional independence, often beyond physical limitations. Basic ADLs and IADLs together exist as components of total self-care.

Instruments for quantifying ADL status instruments have been created for a number of reasons. First, rehabilitation physicians were looking for a way to better quantify not only baseline capabilities but improvement in function in order to be able to see how their rehabilitation techniques were working. Additionally, ADL instruments allow the treatment team to set goals for rehabilitation in the language of those instruments (5). Then, clinicians can see quantitatively if the rehabilitation goals were ultimately met. Finally, the rehabilitation third party payers such as insurance companies needed a way to quantify if patients were improving and predict how long it may take for the goals to be achieved. The two most used instruments to measure baseline ADL function are the Functional independence Measure (FIM) and the Katz ADL scale (7–10).

ADL EVALUATION

The first step in the process of any medical treatment begins with proper evaluation. The entire rehabilitation treatment team must assess any new patient for their current baseline and then future potential function that can be achieved with treatment. The components that are essential to be assessed in the comprehensive patient evaluation include physical impairments, ADL function, IADL function, social awareness, and psychological function. These components can then be put together to create a comprehensive treatment plan that the entire inpatient rehabilitation team can focus on.

Currently the most widely used validated ADL evaluation scale is the functional Independence Measure (FIM) (11). The FIM instrument evaluates nine areas of self-care and can be applied multiple times throughout the course of treatment not only to provide a baseline of function but also to chart improvement in these key areas. The areas that the FIM reports on are self-feeding, grooming, bathing, dressing upper and lower body, toileting, and transfer to the toilet, tub, or shower. The FIM has demonstrated a high degree of inter-relater reliability (12). After the SCI patient leaves the hospital, the FIM can be continued in a self-reporting form (FIM-SR). Masedo et al, found that the FIM-SR motor scales and total FIM-SR score are reliable and valid measures of perceived functional independence in individuals with SCI (13). Although some rehabilitation professionals discuss the Katz ADL index as an alternative measure, this index has not been validated as reliable in spinal cord injury patients in long-term care settings.

Despite the advantages that using a validated comprehensive ADL measure creates, there are significant limitations. First, the FIM is not specific to one type of diagnosis. For example, there is no measurement of mastery of assistive devices, such as seen with high-level tetraplegia (C1–C4) when a patient masters an environmental control unit. Specifically, Watson et al reported that despite subjective reports of improved function in a group of patients with high-level tetraplegia, a group of occupational therapists were not able to detect these changes in the FIM (14). Finally, the FIM does not report respiratory function or chart improvement in this area of function.

One alternative in use has been the Minimum Data Set (MDS). This measure has been criticized for its long length, making use on a weekly basis in rehabilitation hospitals to chart progress largely impractical. Therefore, the MDS is more likely to be useful in the nursing home setting (15).

Another alternative measure is the Quadriplegic Index of Function (QIF). This measure is also longer and more time consuming to employ than the FIM. The prohibitive length makes it largely impractical to chart weekly or even monthly progress in acute rehabilitation units. Additionally, some items in the QIF were found to be redundant and the measure not useful in those patients with paraplegia or cauda equina syndrome (16). Marino and Goin then proposed a shorter form QIF (16).

Therefore, the Spinal Cord Independence Measure (SCIM III, revised three times) created a new, more comprehensive measure

applicable to persons with paraplegia and tetraplegia, both complete and incomplete (17, 18). The measure is now under study to see if it is more sensitive or specific for SCI-injured persons than other measures. The SCIM probes three domains: self-care (feeding, bathing, dressing, grooming), respiration and sphincter management, and mobility (mobility in bed and preventing pressure ulcers, and bed-wheelchair and wheelchair-toilet-tub transfers) (18, 19). Itzkovich et al. found total agreement between raters was above 80% in most SCIM III tasks (17). They also found the SCIM III was more responsive to changes than the FIM in the subscales of respiration and sphincter management, and mobility indoors and outdoors.

NEUROMUSCULAR FUNCTIONAL EVALUATION

Upper Extremity Evaluation

The evaluation of the neuromuscular status of a patient with SCI depends directly on the level and severity of injury. For example, Flanders et al found that the imaging characteristics of cervical SCI (hemorrhage and edema) are related to levels of physical recovery as determined by the FIM scale (20). The level of injury, severity of injury, and neuromuscular status have also been found to predict functional outcome given the physical impairment. Imaging factors that correlate with poor functional recovery are hemorrhage, long segments of edema, and high cervical locations (21).

Spinal cord-injured patients can have, in general terms, their potential for independent function predicted in a number of areas based upon their level of injury (see Tables 59.1–59.7). For example, patients with complete high cervical SCI (C1–C4) will have no motor function in their hands and wrists to assist with functional activities, and those with paraplegia will have full use of their upper extremities. Patients with mid-cervical (C5–C6) SCI have limited elbow and wrist function, and the ability to perform functional activities such as manual transfers and wheelchair mobility will be impaired. Those with lower cervical SCI (C7–C8) will retain antigravity elbow extension and more wrist and hand movement that will improve the ability to perform ADLs and IADLs (6). Therefore, expertly assessing the level and severity of injury allows the team to predict ADL outcome and set goals for rehabilitation.

Even within these SCI injury groups, and within patients who have the same level of injury, the impairments of upper limb function may be heterogeneous. For some, shoulder strength will be preserved at a normal level, but for others, the strength may only partially return. Even if strength in muscle groups is identical, functional potential is dependent on other factors such as the range of motion, potential skeletal deformities, respiratory capacity, skin integrity, and psychological motivation and/or pain levels. For example, one person with a C5 injury can potentially control a power wheelchair with shoulder motion and a "U type" joystick, whereas another patient with the same injury but with shoulder pain and lack of motion cannot control the same chair.

The first component of upper limb function a clinician must evaluate is range of motion (ROM). Adequate ROM is important to be able to move the upper limb to perform the activities that are required. For example, a person with SCI may have level 4/5 grip strength, but if they also have a "frozen shoulder" (adhesive capsulitis), they may be unable to bring their hand up to their mouth to eat. The affected patient also might not be able to dress

Table 59.1   Expected Functional Outcomes for Levels C1–C3

	EXPECTED FUNCTIONAL OUTCOME	EQUIPMENT
Respiratory	Ventilator dependent Inability to clear secretions	2 ventilators (bedside, portable) Suction equipment Generator/battery backup
Bowel	Total assist	Padded reclining shower/commode chair
Bladder	Total assist	
Bed mobility	Total assist	Full electric hospital bed with Trendelenburg feature and side rails
Bed/wheelchair transfers	Total assist	Transfer board Power or mechanical lift with sling
Pressure relief/positioning	Total assist; may be independent with equipment	Power recline and/or tilt wheelchair Wheelchair pressure-relief cushion Postural support and head control devices as indicated Hand splints if indicated Specialty bed or pressure-relief mattress if indicated
Eating	Total assist	
Dressing	Total assist	
Grooming	Total assist	
Bathing	Total assist	Handheld shower Shower tray Padded reclining shower/commode chair (if roll-in shower available)
Wheelchair propulsion	Manual: total assist Power: independent with equipment	Power recline and/or tilt wheelchair with head, chin, or breath control and manual recliner Vent tray
Standing/ambulating	Standing: total assist Ambulation: not indicated	
Communication	Total assist to independent, depending on workstation setup and equipment	Mouthstick, high-tech computer access, environmental control unit Adaptive devices everywhere as indicated
Transportation	Total assist	Attendant-operated van or accessible public transportation
Homemaking Assist required	Total assist 24-hour attendant care Able to instruct in all aspects of care	

From: Cardenas DD, Hoffman JM, Stockman PL. Spinal cord injury. In: Robinson LR, ed. *Trauma Rehabilitation*. Philadelphia: Lippincott Williams & Wilkins, 2006; 115–142.

correctly or reach above their shoulder for items. A simple injection followed by aggressive stretching could restore motion in the shoulder and open up a new level of independent function and exercise tasks.

The next component of upper limb function evaluated is gross motor strength. For example, a person with C5 tetraplegia may have adequate deltoid strength but will often have no strength in the hand, elbow extensors, or wrist flexors. A person with C7 tetraplegia usually will have adequate arm, elbow, and wrist strength, but will lack sufficient hand strength to perform many fine motor tasks such as upper extremity dressing with buttons, catheter manipulation, or shoelace tying. A person with C8 tetraplegia may only lack hand intrinsic strength but the functional outcome may be significant. For a lawyer who dictates all letters, the C8 weakness may not result in a work disability, but for a surgeon, musician, or typist, the hand weakness would likely cause obvious work-related disabilities, even though they could otherwise work from a wheelchair.

Finally, sensation is evaluated. Even if strength eventually returns in the limbs of some persons with SCI, any residual lack

Table 59.2   Expected Functional Outcomes for Level C4

	EXPECTED FUNCTIONAL OUTCOME	EQUIPMENT
Respiratory	May be able to breathe without a ventilator	If not ventilator free, see Table 59.1
Bowel	Total assist	Padded reclining shower/commode chair
Bladder	Total assist	
Bed mobility	Total assist	Full electric hospital bed with Trendelenburg feature and side rails
Bed/wheelchair transfers	Total assist	Transfer board Power or mechanical lift with sling
Pressure relief/positioning	Total assist; may be independent with equipment	Power recline and/or tilt wheelchair Wheelchair pressure-relief cushion Postural support and head control devices as indicated Hand splints if indicated Specialty head or pressure-relief mattress if indicated
Eating	Total assist	
Dressing	Total assist	
Grooming	Total assist	
Bathing	Total assist	Handheld shower Shampoo tray Padded reclining shower/commode chair (if roll-in shower available)
Wheelchair propulsion	Manual: total assist Power: independent	Power recline and/or tilt wheelchair with head, chin, or breath control and manual recliner Vent tray
Standing/ambulating	Standing: total assist Ambulation: not indicated	Tilt table Hydraulic standing table
Communication	Total assist to independent depending on work station setup and equipment	Mouthstick, high-tech computer access, environmental control omit
Transportation	Total assist	Attendant-operated van or accessible public transportation
Homemaking	Total assist	
Assist required	24-hour attendant care to include homemaking Able to instruct in all aspects of care	

From: Cardenas DD, Hoffman JM, Stockman PL. Spinal cord injury. In: Robinson LR, ed. *Trauma Rehabilitation*. Philadelphia: Lippincott Williams & Wilkins, 2006; 115–142.

of sensation will still carry functional consequences. For example, humans use sensory feedback in the hands to perform fine motor tasks, among other necessary functions. Without such sensory feedback, the hands and upper limbs may become "clumsy" and lack dexterity (22).

Trunk and Balance Assessment

The trunk in all SCI-injured persons must be evaluated carefully. Adequate trunk strength allows for proper seating mechanics, wheelchair propulsion force and balance, and respiratory

sufficiency. Just as with the upper and lower extremity, an adequate assessment of trunk ability includes a measurement of trunk ROM, strength, and sensation (23).

It is often difficult for non-rehabilitation specialists or the lay public to understand that there is a difference between people with high paraplegia versus low paraplegia. For example, many athletic competitions such as wheelchair tennis place all persons with paraplegia in the same group. However, those with paraplegia above T6 and especially as high as T2, will lack many abilities of a person with paraplegia below T6, despite having full upper extremity strength. Respiratory capacity, transfer strength,

Table 59.3 Expected Functional Outcomes for Level C5

	EXPECTED FUNCTIONAL OUTCOME	EQUIPMENT
Respiratory	Low endurance and vital capacity secondary to paralysis of intercostals; may require assist to clear secretions	
Bowel	Total assist	Padded shower/commode chair or padded transfer tub bench with commode cutout
Bladder	Total assist	Adaptive devices may be indicated (electric leg bag emptier)
Bed mobility	Some assist	Full electric hospital bed with Trendelenburg feature with patient's control and side rails
Bed/wheelchair transfers	Total assist	Transfer board Power or mechanical lift with sling
Pressure relief/positioning	Independent with equipment	Power recline anchor tilt wheelchair Wheelchair pressure-relief cushion Hand splints Specialty bed or pressure-relief mattress if indicated Postural support devices
Eating	Total assist for setup, then independent eating with equipment	Long opponens splint Adaptive devices as indicated
Dressing	Lower extremity: total assist Upper extremity: some assist	Long opponens splint Adaptive devices as indicated
Grooming	Some to total assist	Long opponens splint Adaptive devices as indicated
Bathing	Total assist	Handheld shower Padded tub transfer bench or shower/commode chair
Wheelchair propulsion	Manual: independent to some assist indoors on non-carpeted surface, level surface; some to total assist outdoors Power: independent	Power: power recline and/or tilt with arm drive control Manual: lightweight rigid or folding frame with hand rim modifications
Standing/ambulating	Standing: total assist Ambulation: not indicated	Hydraulic standing frame
Communication	Independent to some assist after setup with equipment	Long opponens splint Adaptive devices as indicated
Transportation	Independent with highly specialized equipment; sonic assist with accessible public transportation; total assist for attendant-operated vehicle	Highly specialized modified van with lift
Homemaking	Total assist	
Assist required	Personal care: 6 h/d Home care: 4 h/d	Able to instruct in all aspects of care

From: Cardenas DD, Hoffman JM, Stockman PL. Spinal cord injury. In: Robinson LR, ed. *Trauma Rehabilitation*. Philadelphia: Lippincott Williams & Wilkins, 2006; 115–142.

Table 59.4   Expected Functional Outcomes for Level C6

	EXPECTED FUNCTIONAL OUTCOME	EQUIPMENT
Respiratory	Low endurance and vital capacity secondary to paralysis of intercostals; may require assist to clear secretions	
Bowel	Some to total assist with commode cutout	Padded shower'/commode chair or padded transfer tub bench
Bladder	Some to total assist with equipment; may be independent with leg bag emptying	Adaptive devices if indicated
Bed mobility	Some assist	Full electric hospital bed w/side rails Full to king standard bed may be indicated
Bed/wheelchair transfers	Level: some assist to independent Uneven: some to total assist	Transfer board Mechanical lift
Pressure relief/ positioning	Independent with equipment and/or adapted techniques	Power recline wheelchair Wheelchair pressure-relief cushion Pressure-relief mattress or overlay if indicated Postural support devices
Eating	Independent with or without equipment, except cutting, which is total assist	Adaptive devices as indicated (e.g., U-cuff, tendinosis splint, adapted utensils, plate guard)
Dressing	Lower extremity: some to total assist Upper extremity: independent	Adaptive devices as indicated (e.g., button, hook, loops on zippers, pants; socks, self-fasteners on shoes)
Grooming	Some assist to independent with equipment	Adaptive devices as indicated (e.g., U-cuff, adapted handles)
Bathing	Upper body: independent Lower body: some to total assist	Handheld shower Padded tub transfer bench or shower/commode chair
Wheelchair propulsion	Manual: independent indoors, some to total assist outdoors Power: independent with standard arm drive on all surfaces	Power: may require power recline or standard upright power wheelchair Manual: lightweight rigid or folding frame with modified rims
Standing/ambulating	Standing: total assist Ambulation: not indicated	Hydraulic standing frame
Communication	Independent with or without equipment	Adaptive devices as indicated (e.g., tendinosis splint; writing splint for keyboard use, button pushing, page turning, object manipulation)
Transportation	Independent driving from Wheelchair Tie-downs	Modified van with lift Sensitized hand controls
Homemaking	Some assist with light meal preparation; total assist for all other homemaking	Adaptive devices as indicated
Assist required	Personal care: 6 h/d Home care: 4 h/d	

From: Cardenas DD, Hoffman JM, Stockman PL. Spinal cord injury. In: Robinson LR, ed. *Trauma Rehabilitation*. Philadelphia: Lippincott Williams & Wilkins, 2006; 115–142.

Table 59.5   Expected Functional Outcomes for Levels C7 through C8

	EXPECTED FUNCTIONAL OUTCOME	EQUIPMENT
Respiratory	Low endurance and vital capacity secondary to paralysis of intercostals; may require assist to clear secretions	
Bowel	Some to total assist	Padded shower/commode chair or padded transfer tub bench with commode cutout
Bladder	Independent to some assist	Adaptive devices if indicated
Bed mobility	Independent to some assist	Full electric hospital bed or full to king standard bed
Bed/wheelchair transfers	Level: independent Uneven: independent to some assist	With or without transfer board
Pressure relief/positioning	Independent Pressure-relief mattress or overlay if indicated Postural support devices	Wheelchair pressure-relief cushion
Eating	Independent	Adaptive devices as indicated
Dressing	Lower extremity: independent to some assist Upper extremity: independent	Adaptive devices as indicated
Grooming	Independent	Adaptive devices as indicated
Bathing	Upper body: independent Lower body: independent to some assist	Handheld shower Padded tub transfer bench or shower/commode chair
Wheelchair propulsion	Manual: independent on all indoors surfaces and level outdoor terrain, some assist with uneven terrain	Manual: lightweight rigid or folding frame with modified rims
Standing/ambulating	Standing: independent to some assist Ambulation: not indicated	Hydraulic or standard standing frame
Communication	Independent	Adaptive devices as indicated
Transportation	Independent car if independent with transfer and wheelchair loading/unloading; independent driving modified van from captain's seat	Modified vehicle Transfer board
Homemaking	Independent with light meal preparation and homemaking; some to total assist for complex meal prep and heavy housecleaning	Adaptive devices as indicated
Assist required	Personal care: 6 h/d Home care: 2 h/d	

From: Cardenas DD, Hoffman JM, Stockman PL. Spinal cord injury. In: Robinson LR, ed. *Trauma Rehabilitation*. Philadelphia: Lippincott Williams & Wilkins, 2006; 115–142.

and balance are all diminished in high-level paraplegia. Additionally, those with injuries above T6 may suffer from repeated bouts of autonomic dysreflexia resulting in diminished function.

Lower Limb Assessment

Even if there is no voluntary movement, the lower limbs play a role in the potential ability to perform many ADLs. Adequate body positioning of the lower limbs is essential to sitting properly in the wheelchair, allowing the injured person to transfer properly, and position the body for IADLs. Persons with incomplete

SCI clearly utilize their lower limbs differently, as they may be full or partial ambulators. The strength of the lower limbs must be properly assessed to not only apply proper rehabilitation techniques and goals but also to order proper braces (24, 25).

Assessment of the lower limbs must begin with motor strength. Lower limbs with no motor function typically cannot assist with gait or transfers. However, they certainly can hinder transfers if there are deformities, contractures, or increased muscle tone (spasticity). Therefore, the next part of the lower limbs assessment must include joint and muscle ROM and tone. Occasionally, persons with complete SCI but a high level of

Table 59.6   Expected Functional Outcomes for Levels T1 through T9

	EXPECTED FUNCTIONAL OUTCOME	EQUIPMENT
Respiratory	Compromised vital capacity and endurance	
Bowel	Independent	Elevated padded toilet seat or padded tub bench with commode cutout
Bladder	Independent	
Bed mobility	Independent	Full to king standard bed
Bed/wheelchair transfers	Independent	May or may not require transfer board
Pressure relief/positioning	Independent	Wheelchair pressure-relief cushion Pressure-relief mattress or overlay if indicated Postural support devices
Eating	Independent	
Dressing	Independent	
Grooming	Independent	
Bathing	Independent	Handheld shower Padded tub transfer bench or shower/commode chair
Wheelchair propulsion	Independent	Manual: lightweight rigid or folding flame
Standing/ambulating	Standing: independent Ambulation: typically not functional	Standing frame
Communication	Independent	
Transportation	Independent in car with transfer and wheelchair loading/unloading	Hand controls
Homemaking	Independent with complex meal preparation and light housekeeping; some to total assist for heavy housecleaning	
Assist required	Home care: 3 h/d	

From: Cardenas DD, Hoffman JM, Stockman PL. Spinal cord injury. In: Robinson LR, ed. *Trauma Rehabilitation*. Philadelphia: Lippincott Williams & Wilkins, 2006; 115–142.

muscle tone can actually use this tone to assist with stand-pivot transfers or other mobility (26). However, other persons with SCI and increased tone will have difficulties with lower limb positioning, dressing, toileting, and hygiene. Therefore, individual impairments present in the person with SCI must be assessed in the context of function, not just the impairment.

Neurological Level and Outcome

In summary, people with SCI are not created equally. Not only do they differ by whether the injury is complete or incomplete, or whether they have a tetraplegia or paraplegia, but they differ even within these groups. For example, two patients with C7 complete injuries can have significantly different functional outcomes and potential based on the "strength" of the C7 recovery, whether there are zones of partial preservation, additional injuries, and body habitus. Still, some attempts have been made to predict functional outcome or expectations based on the neurologic level of injury (Tables 59.1–59.7). Therefore, persons with

SCI will require different levels of resources depending on their goals and potential for improvement given the current status of medical treatment.

ENVIRONMENTAL EVALUATION AND MODIFICATION

As a part of most inpatient rehabilitation treatment programs, the "Home Evaluation" and the "Home Visit" is highly anticipated. The feeling that the home visit must mean the end of the inpatient portion of rehabilitation is near excites and further motivates the SCI patient to reach his or her goals and participate fully. However, evaluating the home environment as early as possible in the rehabilitation process is also important so that appropriate goals can be set, and needed modifications can begin earlier (27).

The environmental evaluation begins with a family history (who is in the home), vocational history, and leisure history. These are the components of the patient's lifestyle that allow the

Table 59.7   Expected Functional Outcomes for Levels T10 through S5

	Expected Functional Outcome	Equipment
Respiratory	Intact respiratory function	
Bowel	Independent	Padded standard or raised toilet seat
Bladder	Independent	
Bed mobility	Independent	Full to king standard bed
Bed/wheelchair transfers	Independent	May or may not require transfer board
Pressure relief/positioning	Independent	Wheelchair pressure-relief cushion
		Pressure-relief mattress or overlay if indicated
		Postural support devices
Eating	Independent	
Dressing	Independent	
Grooming	Independent	
Bathing	Independent	Handheld shower
		Padded tub transfer bench
Wheelchair propulsion	Independent	Manual: lightweight rigid or folding frame
Standing/ambulating	Standing: independent	Standing frame
	Ambulation: functional, some assist to independent	Forearm crutches or walker
		Knee-ankle-foot orthosis (KAFO)
Communication	Independent	
Transportation	Independent in car with transfer and wheelchair loading/unloading	Hand Controls
Homemaking	Independent with complex meal preparation and light housekeeping; sonic assist for heavy housecleaning	
Assist required	Home care: 0-2 h/d	

From: Cardenas DD, Hoffman JM, Stockman PL. Spinal cord injury. In: Robinson LR, ed. *Trauma Rehabilitation*. Philadelphia: Lippincott Williams & Wilkins, 2006; 115–142.

therapist to create a roadmap of where the injured patient was and where they need to get back to, and even beyond, to maximize function. In certain cases the therapist may find that the SCI patient was not functioning at optimal levels even before the injury due to psychiatric illness or other disorders.

The second component of the evaluation concerns the home structure itself. The therapist must create a picture of the home and environment that will allow for an understanding of what impediments might exist that will pose a barrier to maximizing function. By knowing the limitations, the therapist can set therapy goals that may also involve making modifications to the home and environment to maximize function (28).

The home evaluation begins at the front door, known by realtors as the "frontage." This area includes the front walkway, porch, and front door. The therapist must evaluate how accessible these areas are for wheelchair use. Areas that inhibit access are "barriers," and the therapist must work with the patient to create modifications to overcome these barriers. For example, to overcome the barrier of front steps, a ramp must be built to allow access. Ramp grade should be eight degrees or less. The ramp should include a platform for rest and not be longer than 30 feet in length for each segment (1). Curb cuts must be created on the street and sidewalks.

Once inside the home, the evaluation continues as a patient who uses a wheelchair needs to maneuver through the internal environment. Initial areas that must be evaluated include the lobby and hallway dimensions, the interior door width, and the floor type. For example, removal of screen doors and reversing the hinges (swinging door) is often necessary to allow the person with SCI to enter the home independently. Additionally, wider hallway (36 in. minimum) and door widths (32 in. minimum) must be created to accommodate the turning radius of the wheelchair (1). The minimum space required for a standard adult wheelchair is 60 inches (29). Finally, wheelchair propulsion ability will usually be better on a hard or wood floor than on a shaggy rough carpet.

Further in the interior, the therapist must evaluate the kitchen and then recommend modifications. Most conventional kitchens are built so that sinks and countertops are too high for the typical wheelchair. Therefore, counters, tables, and other areas must be lowered to the proper height of around 32 inches (1). Additionally, space must be created so the wheelchair user can place the wheelchair under the counter or sink to perform the cooking, cleaning, etc. Utensil and other storage areas for commonly used items should be moved to the lower levels. Usually, it is helpful if the freezer on the refrigerator is on the bottom. For some items above head, adaptive equipment can assist retrieval of those items. Newer models of "standing wheelchairs" can also allow SCI persons to access conventional kitchen dimensions, although these chairs are not available to most persons with SCI due to the high cost (30).

Bathroom configuration is next to be evaluated and modified. Sink counters must be lowered to around 32 inches (1, 28). Room must be created under the sink for the person with SCI to be able to access the sink, and the pipes must be insulated to prevent leg burns. Tub/shower areas should be modified to allow for roll-in access if possible. A hand-held shower head allows for more complete cleaning. Bars may need to be installed for balance for those with more incomplete injuries. Additionally, a "no slip floor" should be installed for this population because they are more likely to have balance problems. For persons with high-level tetraplegia, a ceiling lift or other transfer unit can improve function and reduce the difficulty of moving into proper cleaning position.

Finally, the bedroom evaluation must take into account not only the comfort needs of the patient, but also any medical needs and monitoring that may need to take place. For example, the person with high-level tetraplegia may need pulmonary monitoring and emergency alert capabilities. A lift device can be installed to assist with transfers. An environmental access device can allow for increased independence within the room and rest of the home.

The therapist involved with the home modification must then evaluate and modify all other areas of the home, including work areas, office areas, and leisure areas with similar thoughts as listed above. Telephones, alarms, and entertainment control units must be moved where they are accessible (31). Outside areas such as the backyard and side areas must also undergo evaluation and modification to improve the ability of the SCI person to function and move independently in these areas. Lastly, the garage area must experience the evaluation and modification process to allow for entry and exit into the vehicle that is being utilized by the SCI-injured person (29, 32).

TREATMENT APPROACHES FOR FUNCTIONAL TRAINING

Functional independence occurs when the patient can perform ADLs without help. Most persons with SCI enter the rehabilitation unit rendered dependent or nearly dependent in most ADLs. Although the entire rehabilitation team takes on the mission to restore functional independence, the occupational therapist (OT) most often takes the lead in providing most of the direct treatment (1). A specialized OT (in SCI) applies proven techniques to the SCI patient to help them improve their functional abilities in the rehabilitation hospital and beyond.

As discussed above, the functional treatment program begins with a comprehensive assessment of the medical impairments, functional deficits, and environmental set up. Then based on the findings, the multi-disciplinary treatment team sets appropriate goals before actual treatment can be initiated. The goals then drive the treatment approach that best allows the injured patient to reach those set short-term and long-term goals. Persons with complete SCI share the common situation that in most cases their impairment remains static or permanent.

Therapists may choose from a number of treatment approaches to achieve the goal of functional independence or achieving maximum function. More than one different type of approach may also be used if felt appropriate by the therapist. Additionally, the occupational therapist may utilize expertise from other specialists on the team, including the physical therapist, speech pathologist, recreational therapist, rehabilitation nurse, and vocational therapist to maximize functional restoration and treatment. Within that framework, treatment can be either restorative or compensatory. The goal of restorative treatment is simply to reverse the disability, even if the

impairment cannot be reversed (33, 34). The individual is encouraged to perform the ADL task the same way as before the injury. Compensatory treatment aims to reverse the disability and even the handicap by finding other means of traversing the divide created by the impairment without directly restoring the function. Either way, the functional task gets done independently or with the least dependence possible.

The choice of which method to use depends on the underlying condition of the patient. Most persons with complete SCI may gain one or two levels of neurological function but are unlikely to gain any more neurological return in their immediate future. Therefore, therapists most often utilize compensatory strategies to create independent function. However, persons with incomplete SCI may see tremendous neurological recovery over time (35, 36). Therefore, therapists must carefully observe their patient and try to project the amount and speed of the recovery. If recovery occurs quickly, restorative treatment strategies; i.e. standing balance strategies at the kitchen when the patient cannot yet ambulate, are more likely to work.

Three recognized "frames of reference" exist when considering restorative ADL therapy treatments (1). The developmental approach assumes recovery occurs in a hierarchical, sequential, predictable manner (37, 38). Therapists then assist this process by sequentially ordering therapy into simple, then more complex tasks. The next approach, biomechanical, assumes that each task is a sum of more basic parts. Each of these "parts" then must undergo repetitive therapy or "remediation" so that they achieve the end result of improved function (1). An example would be strengthening the biceps repetitively in order to help a patient self-feed. The final approach, psychosocial (1), is used along with the other two approaches and recognizes the complex nature of recovery and motivation; the "mind-body" connection. Many therapists will even utilize a psychologist during their physical or ADL recovery treatments to maximize the potential recovery. Emotional well being is essential to motivate the SCI-injured person to not only participate fully on the rehabilitation program but to continue to care for themselves properly after rehabilitation is over.

When considering compensatory rehabilitation strategies, a few common themes can be found in treatments. Therapists may utilize methods that seek to change the way a task is completed that takes into account the permanent impairment. For example, hand tenodesis techniques are taught for self-feeding, dressing, or hygiene. Tenodesis allows a hand to passively form a closed fist (by extending the wrist) even if the forearm has weakened flexor muscles (39). This is possible because wrist extension is controlled by muscles innervated by C6, and the wrist and finger flexor muscles are controlled by C7. Tendon transfer surgery can often create function when distal weakness persists.

Another method of therapy utilized for compensation strategies includes that use of adaptive equipment. "Reachers," modified utensils, and functional splints can all provide improvements in functional independence (40). Adaptive equipment also allows patients to dress more independently, bathe more safely and independently, and walk more safely.

Functional electrical stimulation (FES) had been used to augment therapies and training. FES can be applied to the lower extremities and the upper extremities. Studies are ongoing to investigate how to best apply this modality to conventional therapies to generate the best outcomes in patients with SCI.

Implantable FES systems, the Freehand System to improve hand function hand, and the Vocare system to improve bowel and bladder function showed promise to improve function in these areas, but these systems no longer are available because the company producing them could not sustain itself economically (41).

The last compensation strategy, one already discussed earlier, is to apply home and environmental modifications that can create functional independence when the neurology will not allow motor restoration. For example, although a spinal cord-injured person may be discharged unable to stand, they may have full independence in a modified kitchen when the counters are lowered—or in a less accessible kitchen but with a "standing" wheelchair.

Within this broader scope of treatment strategies, certain treatment techniques have been found to be helpful for certain ADL treatments. These will be discussed below.

VI. ADL TREATMENTS

Self-Feeding

Eating and drinking make up the most basic daily living activity. The ability to self-feed is a skill that must be recreated multiple times per day for the rest of one's life. For persons with paraplegia, the basic activity is not a severe challenge other than possibly accessing the food or accessing the cooking or storage areas. For those with tetraplegia, however, depending on the level of injury, self-feeding can become an onerous activity to master. If needed upper limb strength and dexterity does not return to normal, then the patient can expect that compensatory techniques will need to be taught in rehabilitation.

Basic self-feeding ability begins with the ability to eat, chew, and swallow. All patients must be assessed for dysphagia or aspiration. If no such limitation exists, then treatment can focus on developing the skills necessary for independent self-feeding. This may encompass any of the elements of basic feeding skills, such as upper limb strengthening, dexterity training, and adaptive equipment training. Some of the adaptive equipment commonly seen in persons with spinal cord injury specifically includes plate guards, weighted utensils and cups, rocker knife, utensil cuffs, mobile arm supports and suspension slings, or special non-spill cups (Figures 59.1 and 59.2) (6).

Self-Dressing

SCI persons with injuries at levels up to C7 (weak) or C6 (strong) can gain functional independence in self-dressing with rehabilitation. Predictably, dressing the lower extremities poses the bulk of the challenge faced by injured SCI persons (42). However, persons with tetraplegia and hand weakness will face the challenge of learning to manage buttons, zippers, and other fasteners. Training combines both restorative and compensatory techniques. Psychological intervention may be helpful because learning to dress independently takes time and persistence, and may cause frustration initially.

Restorative techniques rely on eventual neurological improvement that comes from repetitive practice. One technique is to simply persist and encourage the patient to dress themselves regardless of the time it takes. The cooperation of the nursing team is essential because the therapist cannot dress every patient in the

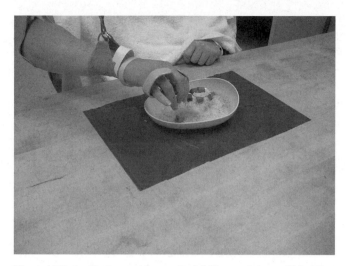

Figure 59.1   Patient with cervical SCI practicing self-feeding techniques with an adaptive hand splint with utensil and mobile arm support.

morning on a particular unit, and the rehabilitation nurse needs to help the SCI patient practice despite the extra time it takes.

Additionally, the therapist can break down self-dressing into component parts and exercise each of these parts to create a whole. For example, if the most difficult part of the dressing program is to slip the left leg into the pants, then this movement needs to be repeated over and over again while possibly assisting the patient with other components until this targeted component is mastered. Additionally, the therapist can recreate the motions necessary in this component with weights, or focus on increasing range of motion in the shoulder or elbow to complete the movement.

The other therapy-driven technique of training that works well utilizes compensatory techniques and assistive devices. For example, a person with complete SCI may find it more practical to dress their lower limbs in bed then in the wheelchair, and thus lower limb dressing would be trained in that manner. Button aids consisting of a wire loop that hooks around the button and pulls

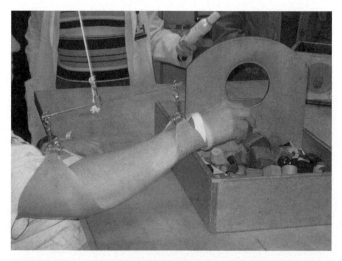

Figure 59.2   Patient with tetraplegia practicing fine hand coordination techniques with mobile arm sling for support.

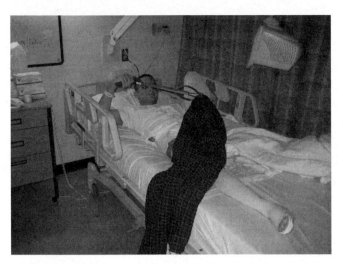

Figure 59.3 Patient with tetraplegia practicing lower body dressing techniques with adaptive device for assistance.

it through, zipper pull aides, and elastic shoelaces are some assistive devices that can facilitate functional independence (1). Other aids include sock reachers and aides, and certain pant dressing sticks that assist with pulling up pants around the legs (Figures 59.3 and 59.4). Therapists must take the time to train the SCI patient in the use of these aids to make them practical for use (43).

Bathing and Grooming

Grooming oneself is extremely important to allow the injured SCI patient to reintegrate into society and participate in vocational and social activities. This area is often the first one a patient will neglect when the psychological impact of the SCI injury results in depression or a lack of motivation. Because this area is personal and intimate, it is often the most important area, along with toileting, where achieving independence becomes essential to restoring the injured patient's self-worth and well being (44).

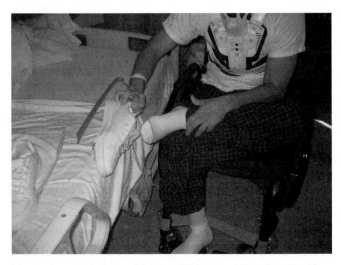

Figure 59.4 Patient with tetraplegia practicing donning shoe with assistive device.

A person with SCI begins each day like any other able-bodied person in that a person typically gets out of bed, goes to the bathroom to brush their teeth, shave, wash at the sink, and then shower. Toileting may or may not occur at this time, or soon thereafter. The key to having a more independent experience in this setting is to have an accessible bathroom facility. The ability to roll up to the sink frontally allows the person with SCI to do many of these ADLs independently. In cases of complete SCI, sinks need to be lowered for access. In cases of incomplete SCI, sinks may need to be raised instead of lowered to support the upright position (1). A shower that allows "roll in" results in possible independent bathing ability. An accessible toilet allows for the possibility of independent toileting. If the accessibility issue is conquered, then rehabilitation training can focus on relearning the techniques essential to independent function (45).

Compensatory tools used for bathing include grab bars, shower chairs, non-slip mats, soap on a rope, and handheld shower heads. Tools for grooming include electric toothbrushes for those who don't have adequate grip strength, and flossing holders. Typically, shaving is accomplished with an electric razor for high-level tetraplegia (6). For those individuals with better hand function, shaving with adapted razors with built-up handles and altered shaving cream dispensers can prove a successful technique. For female patients, shaving armpits or legs proves a much greater challenge, and rehabilitation training must include this training as treatment of the whole patient.

Bowel and Bladder Management

The occupational therapist often combines forces with the rehabilitation nursing team to ensure successful retraining of toileting function. Due to the personal and intimate nature of this ADL, a patient will enjoy both physical and psychological benefits if they can achieve independence in this area (44). Restorative therapies for bladder management focus on improving hand dexterity and function. This allows the patient to manipulate catheter devices, drainage bags, and other bladder function devices.

Restorative therapies for bowel management also include hand dexterity training. The patient must be adept in some cases at rectal digital stimulation, placement of suppositories, or use of a mini enema. Adequate range of motion of the shoulder and scapula may need to be addressed in order for the patient to be able to clean oneself after toileting. Finally, transfer skills on and off a toilet or bedside commode are necessary to ensure a certain level of physical and emotional independence with toileting activities.

Compensatory training makes up the rest of the bowel and bladder rehabilitation efforts (46). Assistive devices can mean the difference between needing help of another person and performing toileting without such help. For example, in some cases, compensatory devices that allow for a weak hand to grab, hold, and insert the catheter safely must augment the bladder catheter insertion process (47). Condom catheter placement may also require compensatory devices to achieve independence. Lower body clothing may need to be altered to allow for easier access during the day. Practical independence in bladder management requires that emptying occurs not only independently, but in a short enough time. Other compensatory devices include adapted suppository inserters, dynamic splints, long-handed

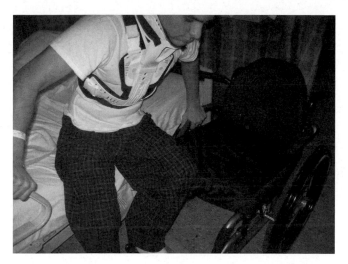

Figure 59.5 Patient with tetraplegia positioning himself for a lateral transfer without a sliding board.

mirror for inspection and hygiene, raised toilet seats, and commode chairs (1).

Functional Mobility

"Functional mobility" is a process that is like a story with a beginning and an end. The process typically must go along "in order" and not skip any stages. The story begins with relearning simple bed mobility. Bed mobility starts with simple shifting, then rolling, then sitting up. From sitting up, the patient can then work on weight shifting and trunk stability and balance. Once trunk stability is achieved, the patient can learn transfers from the bed to the wheelchair. The "hierarchical" process of transfer training usually begins with a "quad" pivot or a sliding board-assisted transfer, then progressing to free transfers if possible (Figures 59.5 and 59.6). From the wheelchair, the patient can then work on transfers to the bathtub, shower chair, car, and even floor to chair. The last stage of mobility to be achieved is then standing, and in appropriate cases, walking.

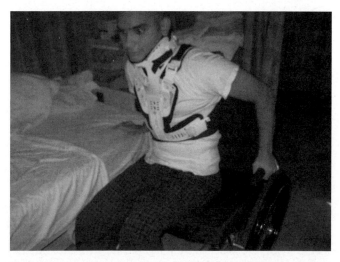

Figure 59.6 Patient with tetraplegia completing a bed-to-wheelchair lateral transfer without a sliding board.

The first stage in achieving functional mobility process is to develop independence in bed mobility (48). Moving around in bed prevents decubitus ulcers and promotes improved respiratory function. The process of training includes restorative rehabilitation with repetitive movements, use of momentum, and repetition of components of movements essential to achieving independence in bed mobility. Compensatory training includes utilizing special mattresses and adaptive equipment. Such equipment may include overhead bars or loops attached to the ends or sides of the bed. Due to the comprehensive nature of learning bed mobility, the training is best accomplished when the physical and occupational therapists team up to provide both restorative and compensatory training at the same time.

Developing independence in transfers is the second stage to achieving independent functional mobility (48). Basic transfer training usually happens with the physical therapy team. However, when all of the therapists from all disciplines work together, much more can be accomplished. For example, "functional transfer training" i.e. bed to toilet, often provided by the occupational therapist, and practiced with the help of the rehabilitation nursing staff, can create more independence than bed to chair transfer training alone.

Independence in transfers combines a three-step training approach. In the first step in transfer training, the SCI patient must build up enough upper trunk and extremity strength to account for the transfer stress. In the second step, the SCI patient develops the balance needed for transfer stability. The final involves creating enough endurance and vasomotor stability to sit long enough in order that the SCI patient may then start to transfer and participate in gym activities.

The type of transfer training depends to a large degree on the level of injury, particularly in patients with complete lesions (49). Those with C1–C5 levels of injury typically require total assistance with transfers using either a sliding board or a mechanical lift. A sliding board is usually required for transferring those patients with lower levels of tetraplegia (C6–C8), although some persons with C6 levels may also require a mechanical lift and total assistance depending on their conduction. Sliding boards exist in multiple shapes and sizes. The board secures across the area to transfer, and the patient slides across. Many patients with paraplegia achieve independent transfers without the use of a sliding board.

Ambulation can be considered in certain cases of incomplete paraplegia and lower-level paraplegia. Many types of ambulation programs have been developed. Often initial training requires first learning how to go from the sit to stand position. Adequate joint range of motion and muscle tone is needed. This is one area that spasticity may actually be helpful! Spasticity can provide the tone necessary to stand. Use of parallel bars can get a new ambulator started. Walking aids such as walkers, platform walkers with elevated handrests, crutches, and canes are provided to assist with relearning ambulation. Functional electrical stimulation is under investigation as a method to augment the ambulation training, and has shown conflicting but promising results (50).

ASSISTIVE DEVICES

The comprehensive rehabilitation program provides both restorative and compensatory training options for SCI patients. A large portion of the compensatory training includes assessment for and provision of assistive devices. These devices provide assistance in all aspects of self-care, including self-feeding, bathing, grooming, hygiene, transfers, ambulation, and more. The key to providing spinal cord-injured persons with the correct devices remains in having the rehabilitation team accurately assess each patient's needs and capabilities (6, 51, 52). The device must accomplish two important criteria:

1. The device is capable of being utilized.
2. The device will increase function significantly enough to justify the cost.

With all devices there are two costs involved. The first cost is the actual dollar cost. Often insurance companies are involved so the justification process is essential to obtaining reimbursement. The second cost is more indirect but still substantial; the cost of training and rehabilitation with the device. Many devices require substantial amounts of repetitive training for the patient to master and benefit from its use (53).

There are many ways to list or classify devices. We will use a functional approach (Listings below modified from Lane AE [1]).

Self-feeding (54–56):
a. Weighted utensils: The extra weight is useful for persons who have tremors. The excess weight increases the stability of eating.
b. Rocker knife: The rocker motion is essential for those who use only one hand.
c. Shallow spoons. Angled spoon or fork.
d. Built-up or custom-handled utensils.
e. Splints with slots for utensils.
f. Tenodesis splint devices.
g. Self-feeding spoon support: A self-feeding device for automatically lifting food off of an eating surface of a plate to an eating position located above the device. May also include a plate with a plate support.
h. Freehand implanted device.
i. Multiple robotic high-tech solutions in development.

Dressing devices (54–58):
a. Button aids: A wire loop that hooks around a button and then pulls the button through the hole.
b. Zipper puller: Typically a loop tied through the zipper puller with or without extensions as needed.
c. Velcro or elastic shoelaces on a Velcro strip.
d. Long shoehorn with handle.
e. Reachers: Reachers can retrieve any item of clothing. A grasper is needed to open and close the end of the reachers, and this may also need to be adapted to if the hand is weaker.
f. Dressing stick.
g. Sock aids: Can assist in putting socks on and off.
h. Balanced forearm orthoses.

Bowel/bladder assistive devices (57–59):
a. Assistive device for hand dexterity such as the "Handhold".
b. Surgical reconstruction of hand.
c. Catheter holder.
d. Electric leg bag opener.
e. Suppository inserter.
f. Rectal sphincter stimulation device.

Home ADL devices (60–63):
a. Reachers.
b. Button pushers.
c. Door knob gripper.
d. Wall switch extension handle.
e. Under counter and other types of jar openers.
f. Big digit timers.
g. Cutting board with corner guard.
h. Key holders.
i. ECUS.
j. Over stove mirrors.

Bathroom/shower/bath (64):
a. Toothpaste squeezer.
b. Grab bars.
c. Shower chair.
d. Commode.
e. Tub rail.
f. Safety (floor) treads.
g. Razor adaptor.
h. Catheter inserters.
i. Suppository inserters.
j. Long-handed mirror.
k. Waterproof timers (with large numbers).

Bed mobility/transfer aids (62–64)
a. Trapeze for bed.
b. Overhead loops for legs.
c. Sliding board for transfers.
d. Ceiling lifts.

Gait aides (65, 66):
a. Walker.
b. Rolling walker.
c. Platform walker.
d. Crutches.
e. Loftstrand crutches (with ergonomic handles).
f. Cane.

INSTRUMENTAL ADLS

Instrumental ADLs include those activities that allow the SCI-injured patient to maintain their living environment (1, 6). This broad definition allows the clinician to include any of those activities that would lead to increasing quality of life beyond just being able to perform the basics of life existence. Some of these indoor activities include expanded cooking, housecleaning, laundry, and computer skills (Figure 59.7). Some outdoor activities would include shopping, outdoor housecleaning or gardening, and leisure activities. Because the major thrust of inpatient rehabilitation in modern times is to return the patient to the home environment as quickly as feasible, these "advanced" ADLs may not be adequately treated or even ignored to some degree in the initial hospital stay. However, the benefits of treating instrumental ADL deficits early in the rehabilitation process cannot be overstated (67–69). Many units have "home simulation" rooms to ease the transition to the home environment, but these have become less utilized in the inpatient setting with the decreased length of stay and other hospital cost-cutting measures.

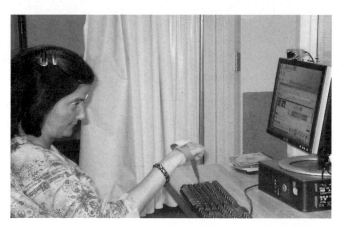

Figure 59.7 Patient with tetraplegia practicing computer skills with adaptive device.

One main household instrumental ADL of great importance is kitchen management. Once the patient accomplishes relearning the ability to feed themselves and move around the kitchen, they still need to prepare food and clean after themselves. The ability to survive in the kitchen independently involves the interplay between the SCI-injured person's physical capabilities and the adapted home environment (28, 29). For example, a person with paraplegia may have the cognitive and motor skills to cook a meal. However, they also need the stove to be accessible for them to operate it, the ingredients to cook the meal within reach, and the utensils needed within reach. A person with tetraplegia may also need adapted handles on the oven or adapted utensils to create their food.

Other challenges met by SCI-injured person include manipulating large pots and mixing bowls, and cleaning up after they are finished. The entire preparation area needs to be accessible for the SCI-injured person. Stabilizers may be necessary for mixing bowls. Finally, sinks and dishwashers need to be accessible, and knobs adapted as needed. People with SCI will need to be able to sit with their legs under the sink if they are going to be able to clean effectively and not spill water on themselves.

After the meal is completed, the last challenge is transporting the meal to the eating area. The meal may be hot, and transporting it on one's lap may be dangerous. So a mechanism should be created to accomplish this delivery safely and without spilling.

Outside the kitchen, many tasks require intensive work. General housecleaning includes vacuuming, mopping, sweeping, window cleaning, furniture dusting, and other activities. Some SCI-injured patients may qualify for assistance in these areas either by paid housecleaner or by a home aide. However, the SCI-injured person may feel psychological satisfaction by regaining the ability to perform these tasks. Restorative therapies would focus on upper limb dexterity, trunk stability, and upper limb strength. Compensatory needs would focus on creating enough accessibility in the home to accomplish these activities.

Another task valued by independent persons, and thus part of ADL rehabilitation in persons with SCI, is the ability to perform their own laundry. A consideration is to have the laundry area on the same floor of the living area and bedroom. Stairs would likely prohibit independence with laundry (6, 28). If there

was a basement or garage laundry, the therapist or family could construct a chute where clothes can be freely sent to the washer area without having to shuttle them constantly. At the laundry itself, front-loading washer and dryer eases placement of clothes for the wheelchair-bound individual. Even when the injured person could reach up to put clothes in, they cannot retrieve items at the bottom of the machine. Top-loading machines are reasonable for those with incomplete injuries who can stand.

Outdoor ADLs are important for many reasons. Many studies show a link between social participation and life satisfaction in SCI-injured persons (70–72). Performing tasks independently that drive a person to go outdoors restores a connection with the outside world that can be lost if the person stays home and has others do these tasks for them. For example, food shopping requires the potential for social interaction, but also ensures that the injured person's personal tastes and needs are met.

To accomplish independence in the community, the injured SCI person must be able to access the community. Transportation must be arranged to the desired locations. Higher functioning persons with paraplegia can usually achieve independence in driving their own car or van and placing a folding wheelchair into the car on their own. Those with tetraplegia often require assistance either in the form of a van retrofitted with lifts and other mechanisms, or with an assistant who helps with the transportation. Even when transportation assistance is required, the payoff of interacting in a community setting is essential to restoring normal function and maximizing quality of life.

Once out in the community, however, however, the SCI-injured person faces new sets of challenges. Despite attempts from agencies and government to improve wheelchair accessibility in many states and cities, there are still many areas where barriers exist for wheelchair users. At the grocery store for example, most of the items at the store are not within their reach. Reachers can reduce some of this impediment, but ultimately the shopper using a wheelchair may be forced to learn to ask for assistance to retrieve desired items. Pushing a standard shopping cart also may not be possible. A power chair may be able to carry items, but usually not a large enough amount to be practical.

Another area where SCI-injured persons will access the community is in their physician and therapy visits. One study revealed that many of these healthcare delivery areas were not accessible or did not meet the SCI-injured person's needs despite the feeling by the healthcare clinicians that the area was accessible (73). Much is written about preserving the dignity of the patient. Often this dignity becomes compromised if the wheelchair-bound person is not able to be cared for like their able-bodied counterparts.

LEISURE AND RECREATION

Achieving functional independence means restoring the whole person. Rehabilitation aims to restore not only a person's ability to perform basic living and instrumental ADL skills but also the ability to perform their entire life activities. Prior to their injury, most SCI-injured persons can relate to a lifestyle that included work or school, homemaking activities, leisure activities outside the home, sports participation, dating or marriage, sexual activity, and family obligations. All of these areas must be addressed and treated to achieve successful rehabilitation and restoration of the person who has been injured (67, 74–76).

Unfortunately, many activities that the patient participated in cannot be restored to the exact nature that was performed prior to the injury. However, compensatory techniques often exist that will allow for partial restoration of independence with most leisure activities.

Most often, the expert on the rehabilitation service in restoring a person's ability to interact with the community in a leisure setting is the recreational therapist (RT). Working in conjunction with all of the other therapists in the rehabilitation team, the RT will often set up internal game nights or movie nights or external trips to local city events such as plays or professional athletic contests. Persons with SCI will be exposed to difficulties common when accessing areas that might not be totally wheelchair accessible. The RT may even choose to access public transportation as part of an excursion for higher-functioning persons.

Another area where persons with SCI can regain a great deal of self-pride and motivation to regain physical strength is in athletics, competitive or leisure (77, 78). At the highest level, SCI-injured persons can participate in Paralympics every four years. At the basic level, SCI patients can participate in a variety of leisure athletics. The sports that can be accessed from a wheelchair include tennis, racing, rugby, basketball, track and field exercises, water sports including sailing, and even skiing. Team sports especially can serve as a peer group outlet for participants.

Art is an area that can be explored even by those with the most severe injuries. For example, many persons with tetraplegia have become quite accomplished independent artists using a mouth-brush to paint. Rehabilitation units can provide many initial opportunities and resources to learn how to perform artistry and some crafts.

Many persons with SCI will desire to return to work. In-depth issues of returning to work will be presented in a separate chapter. Vocational retraining takes a number of forms. Training may include reacquiring the physical skills necessary to return to a previous job or vocation. Alternatively, training may take the form of additional schooling or training to acquire new job skills that are more consistent with one's neurological and functional level (79–83).

One last area of function that is often difficult for many clinicians to discuss with their patients is the area of interpersonal relationships, dating, and sexual activities. Much has been written, including in video format, to educate SCI-injured persons on how to restore their ability to both participate in and enjoy sex. The ability to engage in sexual activity is important not only for the injured person, but for the injured person's spouse or partner as a way of regaining intimacy necessary for a healthy relationship. More in-depth information will be presented in a separate chapter.

CONCLUSION

In summary, the rehabilitation approach to treating spinal cord injury remains a functionally based one. Although research that focuses on improving neurological outcomes for SCI is important, the key to improving functional outcomes is research on how to achieve a higher quality of life after injury. Technological advances in mobility aides and assistive devices have made it possible for persons with SCI to enjoy an increased level of independence regardless of their injury. The trend toward ever decreasing lengths of stay in the acute inpatient rehabilitation hospital has resulted in increased amounts of training that must occur in the outpatient setting. Therefore, the rehabilitation team must begin the process of functional assessment as early as possible in the rehabilitation, and then plan for how training will continue to occur along a "rehabilitation continuum." Ultimately, rehabilitation should encompass all areas of an SCI-injured person's ability to function and encourage the patient to engage the world internally and externally around them with the maximum quality of life and life satisfaction.

ACKNOWLEDGMENTS

The authors wish to acknowledge the tremendous contributions of Catherine LeViseur, O.T.R., and Sherry Sonka-Maarek, M.D., to the first-edition version of this chapter.

References

1. Lane AE. Achieving Functional Independence. In: Braddom RL. *Physical Medicine & Rehabilitation*. Philadelphia: Saunders Elsevier 2007; 581–596.
2. Lund ML, Nordlund A, Bernspång B, et al. Perceived participation and problems in participation are determinants of life satisfaction in people with spinal cord injury. Disabil Rehabil 2007; 29(18):1417–1422.
3. Whiteneck G, Meade MA, Dijkers M, et al. Environmental factors and their role in participation and life satisfaction after spinal cord injury. Arch Phys Med Rehabil 2004; 85(11):1793–803.
4. Richards JS, Bombardier CH, Tate D, et al. Access to the environment and life satisfaction after spinal cord injury. Arch Phys Med Rehabil 1999; 80(11):1501–1506.
5. Andresen EM, Fouts BS, Romeis JC, Brownson CA. Performance of health-related quality-of-life instruments in a spinal cord injured population. Arch Phys Med Rehabil. 1999; 80(8):877–884.
6. LeViseur C, Sonka-Maarek. Activities of daily living. In: Lin VW. *Spinal Cord Medicine Principles and Practice*. New York: Demos, 2003; 693–705.
7. Stineman MG, Shea JA, Jette A, et al. The Functional Independence Measure: tests of scaling assumptions, structure, and reliability across 20 diverse impairment categories. Arch Phys Med Rehabil 1996; 77(11):1101–1108.
8. Stineman MG, Goin JE, Tassoni CJ, et al. Classifying rehabilitation inpatients by expected functional gain. Med Care 1997; 35(9):963–973.
9. Stineman MG, Marino RJ, Deutsch A, et al. A functional strategy for classifying patients after traumatic spinal cord injury. Spinal Cord. 1999; 37(10):717–25.
10. Stineman MG, Maislin G, Williams SV. Applying quantitative methods to the prediction of full functional recovery in adult rehabilitation patients. Arch Phys Med Rehabil 1993 Aug; 74(8):787–795.
11. McKinley W, Santos K, Meade M, Brooke K. Incidence and outcomes of spinal cord injury clinical syndromes. J Spinal Cord Med 2007; 30(3):215–224.
12. Ottenbacher KJ, Hsu Y, Granger CV, Fiedler RC. The reliability of the functional independence measure: a quantitative review. Arch Phys Med Rehabil 1996; 77(12):1226–1232.
13. Masedo AI, Hanley M, Jensen MP, et al. Reliability and validity of a self-report FIM (FIM-SR) in persons with amputation or spinal cord injury and chronic pain. Am J Phys Med Rehabil 2005; 84(3):167–176.
14. Watson AH, Kanny EM, White DM, Anson DK. Use of standardized activities of daily living rating scales in spinal cord injury and disease services. Am J Occup Ther 1995; 49(3):229–234.
15. Doran DM, Harrison MB, Laschinger HS, et al. Nursing-sensitive outcomes data collection in acute care and long-term-care settings. Nurs Res 2006; 55(2 Suppl):S75–S81.
16. Marino RJ, Goin JE. Development of a short-form Quadriplegia Index of Function scale. Spinal Cord 1999; 37(4):289–296.
17. Itzkovich M, Gelernter I, Biering-Sorensen F, et al. The Spinal Cord Independence Measure (SCIM) version III: Reliability and validity in a multi-center international study. Disabil Rehabil 2007; 29(24): 1926–1933.

18. Catz A, Itzkovich M. Spinal Cord Independence Measure: comprehensive ability rating scale for the spinal cord lesion patient. J Rehabil Res Dev 2007; 44(1):65–68.

19. Catz A, Greenberg E, Itzkovich M, et al. A new instrument for outcome assessment in rehabilitation medicine: Spinal cord injury ability realization measurement index. Arch Phys Med Rehabil 2004; 85(3):399–404.

20. Flanders AE, Spettell CM, Friedman DP, et al. The relationship between the functional abilities of patients with cervical spinal cord injury and the severity of damage revealed by MR imaging. AJNR Am J Neuroradiol 1999; 20(5):926–934.

21. Boldin C, Raith J, Fankhauser F, et al. Predicting neurologic recovery in cervical spinal cord injury with postoperative MR imaging. Spine 2006 Mar 1; 31(5):554–559.

22. Iyer MB, Pedretti L. Evaluation of sensation and treatment of sensory dysfunction. In: Pedretti L, Early M, eds. *Occupational Therapy: Practice Skills for Physical Dysfunction*, 10th ed. St Louis: Mosby, 2001; 422–443.

23. Nawoczenski DA, Rinehart ME, Duncanson P, et al. Physical management. In: Buchanan LE, Nawoczenski DA, eds. *Spinal Cord Injury: Concepts and Management Approaches*. Baltimore: Williams & Wilkins, 1987; 123–184.

24. Atrice MB, Morrison SA, McDowell SL, et al. Traumatic spinal cord injury. In: Umphred DA ed. Neurological Rehabilitation. 5th edition. St Louis: Mosby, 2005; 605–657.

25. Fulk G, Schmitz TJ, Behrman AL. In O'Sullivan SB, Schmitz TJ, eds. *Physical Rehabilitation—Assessment and Treatment*. Philadelphia: F.A. Davis Company, 2007; 937–998.

26. Ladouceur M, Pépin A, Norman KE, Barbeau H. Recovery of walking after spinal cord injury. Adv Neurol 1997; 72:249–255.

27. Beck LA, Scroggins LM. Optimizing health of individuals with tetraplegia. SCI Nurs 2001; 18(4):181–186.

28. Culler KH. Home management. In: Crepeau EB, Cohn ES, Schell BAB, eds. *Willard and Spackman's Occupational Therapy*. Philadelphia: Lippincott Williams & Wilkins, 2003; 534–541.

29. Cooper BA, Cohen U, Hasselkus BR. Barrier free design: A review and critique of the occupational therapy perspective. Am J Occupational Ther 1991; 45(4):344–50.

30. Edlich RF, Nelson KP, Foley ML, et al. Technological advances in powered wheelchairs. J Long Term Eff Med Implants. 2004; 14(2):107–130.

31. Holme SA, Kanny EM, Guthrie MR, Johnson K. The use of environmental control units by occupational therapists in spinal cord injury and disease services. Am J Occupational Ther 1997; 51(1):42–48.

32. Story MF. Maximizing usability: The principles of universal design. Assistive Tech 1998; 10:4–12.

33. Pierce S. Restoring competence in mobility. In: Trombly C, Radomski M, eds. *Occupational Therapy for Physical Dysfunction*. 5th ed. Philadelphia: Lippincott Williams & Wilkins, 2002; 665–693.

34. Pedretti L. Muscle strength. In: Pedretti L, Early M, eds. *Occupational Therapy: Practice Skills for Physical Dysfunction*. 10th ed. St Louis: Mosby, 2001; 316–359.

35. Edgerton VR, Tillakaratne NJ, Bigbee AJ, et al. Plasticity of the spinal neural circuitry after injury. Annu Rev Neurosci 2004; 27:145–167.

36. Edgerton VR, Roy RR, Hodgson JA, et al. A physiological basis for the development of rehabilitative strategies for spinally injured patients. J Am Paraplegia Soc 1991; 14(4):150–157.

37. Foster M. Life skills. In: Turner A, Foster M, Johnson SE, eds. *Occupational Therapy and Physical Dysfunction*. Edinburgh: Churchill Livingstone, 2002; 275–314.

38. Behrman AL, Harkema SJ. Physical rehabilitation as an agent for recovery after spinal cord injury. Phys Med Rehabil Clin N Am 2007; 18(2):183–202.

39. Shepherd CC, Ruzicka SH. Tenodesis brace use by persons with spinal cord injuries. Am J Occup Ther 1991; 45(1):81–83.

40. Chen LK, Mann WC, Tomita MR, Burford TE. An evaluation of reachers for use by older persons with disabilities. Assist Technol 1998; 10(2):113–125.

41. Kirshblum S. New rehabilitation interventions in spinal cord injury. J Spinal Cord Med 2004; 27(4):342–350.

42. Runge M. Self-dressing techniques for patients with spinal cord injury. Am J Occup Ther 1967; 21(6):367–375.

43. Mingaila S, Krisciūnas A. Occupational therapy for patients with spinal cord injury in early rehabilitation. Medicina (Kaunas) 2005; 41(10): 852–856.

44. Boss BJ, Pecanty L, McFarland SM, Sasser L. Self-care competence among persons with spinal cord injury. SCI Nurs 1995; 12(2):48–53.

45. Sargant C, Braun MA. Occupational therapy management of the acute spinal cord-injured patient. Am J Occup Ther 1986; 40(5):333–337.

46. Francis K. Physiology and management of bladder and bowel continence following spinal cord injury. Ostomy Wound Manage 2007; 53(12): 18–27.

47. Snoek GJ, IJzerman MJ, Hermens HJ, et al. Survey of the needs of patients with spinal cord injury: impact and priority for improvement in hand function in tetraplegics. Spinal Cord 2004; 42(9):526–532.

48. Kirshblum SC, Priebe MM, Ho CH, et al. Spinal cord injury medicine. 3. Rehabilitation phase after acute spinal cord injury. Arch Phys Med Rehabil 2007; 88(3 Suppl 1):S62–S70.

49. Cardenas DD, Hoffman JM, Stockman PL. Spinal cord injury. In: Robinson LR, ed. *Trauma Rehabilitation*. Philadelphia: Lippincott Williams & Wilkins, 2006; 115–142.

50. Field-Fote EC, Lindley SD, Sherman AL. Locomotor training approaches for individuals with spinal cord injury: a preliminary report of walking-related outcomes. J Neurol Phys Ther 2005; 29(3):127–137.

51. Garber SL, Gregorio TL. Upper extremity assistive devices: assessment of use by spinal cord-injured patients with quadriplegia. Am J Occup Ther 1990; 44(2):126–131.

52. Bell P, Hinojosa J. Perception of the impact of assistive devices on daily life of three individuals with quadriplegia. Assist Technol 1995; 7(2):87–94.

53. Wuolle KS, Bryden AM, Peckham PH, et al. Satisfaction with upper-extremity surgery in individuals with tetraplegia. Arch Phys Med Rehabil 2003 Aug; 84(8):1145–1149.

54. Wyckoff E, Mitani M. The spoon plate: a self-feeding device. Am J Occup Ther 1982; 36(5):333–335.

55. Curtin M. Development of a tetraplegic hand assessment and splinting protocol. Paraplegia 1994; 32(3):159–169.

56. Krajnik SR, Bridle MJ. Hand splinting in quadriplegia: current practice. Am J Occup Ther 1992; 46(2):149–156.

57. Adler US, Kirshblum SC. A new assistive device for intermittent self-catheterization in men with tetraplegia. J Spinal Cord Med 2003 Summer; 26(2):155–258.

58. Hakenberg OW, Ebermayer J, Manseck A, Wirth MP. Application of the Mitrofanoff principle for intermittent self-catheterization in quadriplegic patients. Urology 2001; 58(1):38–42.

59. Kiyono Y, Hashizume C, Ohtsuka K, Igawa Y. Improvement of urological-management abilities in individuals with tetraplegia by reconstructive hand surgery. Spinal Cord 2000 Sep; 38(9):541–545.

60. Rigby P, Ryan S, Joos S, et al. Impact of electronic aids to daily living on the lives of persons with cervical spinal cord injuries. Assist Technol 2005; 17(2):89–97.

61. McKinley W, Tewksbury MA, Sitter P, et al. Assistive technology and computer adaptations for individuals with spinal cord injury. NeuroRehabilitation 2004; 19(2):141–146.

62. Craig A, Tran Y, McIsaac P, Boord P. The efficacy and benefits of environmental control systems for the severely disabled. Med Sci Monit 2005 Jan; 11(1):RA32–RA39.

63. Platts RG, Fraser MH. Assistive technology in the rehabilitation of patients with high spinal cord lesions. Paraplegia 1993; 31(5): 280–287.

64. Stineman MG, Ross RN, Maislin G, Gray D. Population-based study of home accessibility features and the activities of daily living: clinical and policy implications. Disabil Rehabil 2007; 29(15): 1165–1175.

65. Clark BC, Manini TM, Ordway NR, Ploutz-Snyder LL. Leg muscle activity during walking with assistive devices at varying levels of weight bearing. Arch Phys Med Rehabil 2004; 85(9):1555–1560.

66. Youdas JW, Kotajarvi BJ, Padgett DJ, Kaufman KR. Partial weight-bearing gait using conventional assistive devices. Arch Phys Med Rehabil 2005; 86(3):394–398.

67. Tinsley HE, Teaff JD, Colbs SL, Kaufman N. A system of classifying leisure activities in terms of the psychological benefits of participation reported by older persons. J Gerontol 1985; 40(2):172–178.

68. Schönherr MC, Groothoff JW, Mulder GA, Eisma WH. Participation and satisfaction after spinal cord injury: results of a vocational and leisure outcome study. Spinal Cord 2005; 43(4):241–248.

69. Scelza WM, Kirshblum SC, Wuermser LA, et al. Spinal cord injury medicine. 4. Community reintegration after spinal cord injury. Arch Phys Med Rehabil 2007; 88(3 Suppl 1):S71–S75.

70. Chan SC, Chan AP. User satisfaction, community participation and quality of life among Chinese wheelchair users with spinal cord injury: a preliminary study. Occup Ther Int 2007; 14(3):123–143.

71. Carpenter C, Forwell SJ, Jongbloed LE, Backman CL. Community participation after spinal cord injury. Arch Phys Med Rehabil 2007; 88(4):427–433.

72. Kennedy P, Taylor N, Hindson L. A pilot investigation of a psychosocial activity course for people with spinal cord injuries. Psychol Health Med 2006; 11(1):91–99.

73. Trösken T, Geraedts M. Accessibility of doctors' surgeries in Essen, Germany. Gesundheitswesen 2005; 67(8–9):613–619.

74. Stiens SA, Bergman SB, Formal CS. Spinal cord injury rehabilitation. 4. Individual experience, personal adaptation, and social perspectives. Arch Phys Med Rehabil 1997; 78(3 Suppl):S65–S72.

75. Stiens SA, Kirshblum SC, Groah SL, et al. Spinal cord injury medicine. 4. Optimal participation in life after spinal cord injury: physical, psychosocial, and economic reintegration into the environment. Arch Phys Med Rehabil 2002; 83(3 Suppl 1):S72–S81, S90–S98.

76. Charlifue S, Gerhart K. Community integration in spinal cord injury of long duration. NeuroRehabilitation 2004; 19(2):91–101.

77. Gioia MC, Cerasa A, Di Lucente L, et al. Psychological impact of sports activity in spinal cord injury patients. Scand J Med Sci Sports 2006; 16(6):412–416.

78. Muraki S, Tsunawake N, Hiramatsu S, Yamasaki M. The effect of frequency and mode of sports activity on the psychological status in tetraplegics and paraplegics. Spinal Cord 2000; 38(5):309–314.

79. Schönherr MC, Groothoff JW, Mulder GA, Schoppen T, Eisma WH. Vocational reintegration following spinal cord injury: expectations, participation and interventions. Spinal Cord 2004; 42(3):177–184.

80. Schönherr MC, Groothoff JW, Mulder GA, Eisma WH. Participation and satisfaction after spinal cord injury: results of a vocational and leisure outcome study. Spinal Cord 2005; 43 (4):241–248.

81. Lidal IB, Huynh TK, Biering-Sørensen F. Return to work following spinal cord injury: a review. Disabil Rehabil 2007; 29(17):1341–1375.

82. Tomassen PC, Post MW, van Asbeck FW. Return to work after spinal cord injury. Spinal Cord 2000; 38(1):51–55.

83. Krause JS. Years to employment after spinal cord injury. Arch Phys Med Rehabil 2003; 84(9):1282–1289.

60 Sports and Recreation Opportunities*

Andy Krieger
Frank M. Brasile
B. Cairbre McCann
Rory A. Cooper

By participating in the Hawaii Ironman World Championships, I was accomplishing several things at multiple levels. As an example to all amputees, I was able to highlight the great things that anyone can accomplish through training and dedication to fitness. To my soldiers, I showed that heart and determination can serve you through the toughest challenges, and as an Ironman, I was fit to fight. Most importantly, I was proving to myself that I could achieve more as an amputee than I had ever done in my able-bodied life.

—U.S. Army Major David M. Rozelle, the first war amputee ever to complete the grueling Ironman World Championship triathlon in Hawaii, on the impact of sports and recreation on his rehabilitation. The event, held in October 2007, included 2.4 miles of swimming, 112 miles of biking, and 26.2 miles of running.

INTRODUCTION

In spite of their traumatic injuries, individuals who incur amputations as a result of their military service have access to sports and recreation opportunities that enable them to lead active, healthy, and productive lives. Sports and recreation for Americans with disabilities was introduced in the 1870s, when deaf athletes competed in the sport of baseball at a school for the deaf in Ohio. In the late 1940s, at the close of World War II, famed neurosurgeon Sir Ludwig Guttmann of Stoke Mandeville, England, introduced wheelchair sports as a means to rehabilitate veterans with disabilities, including those with amputations (1). Since then, sports and recreation for the disabled has proved to be a powerful tool in the rehabilitation process, providing a number of significant therapeutic benefits (2).

Wheelchair Sports, USA (WSUSA), originally known as the National Wheelchair Athletic Association, was established in 1956 to accommodate athletes with disabilities who wanted to participate in sports other than basketball. Many of the athletes

who helped create the organization were World War II veterans, as well as individuals with quadriplegia. WSUSA now offers sporting events to youth with disabilities, having hosted its first youth competition in 1984 (3).

The National Veterans Wheelchair Games, with 16 events, is the largest annual wheelchair sporting event in the world. It now includes an amputee clinic, developed with emphasis on amputees competing on prostheses in various track and field events and facilitated by athletes and coaches of the U.S. Paralympic team. The U.S. Paralympics is the highest caliber sporting event for elite athletes with disabilities.

THERAPEUTIC BENEFITS

Guttmann stated, "...the aims of sport embody the same principles for the disabled as they do for the able-bodied; in addition, however, sport is of immense therapeutic value and plays an essential part in the physical, psychological, and social rehabilitation of the disabled" (1 [p. 12]). Coyle, Kinney, Riley, and Shank (4) cite a number of studies documenting the following therapeutic benefits related to sports and recreation for the disabled:

- Improvement in physical health status: participation in various exercise and fitness activities resulted in significant improvements in cardiovascular and respiratory functioning, and increased strength, endurance, and coordination for persons with disabilities including paraplegia, cystic fibrosis, and asthma.
- Reduction in complications related to secondary disability: physical activity has been demonstrated to reduce secondary medical complications arising from spinal cord injury and other physical disabilities.
- Improvement in long-term health status and reduction in health risk factors: lowered cholesterol levels, reduced heart

*Adapted from Krieger A, Brasile F, McCann C, Cooper RA. Sports and recreation opportunities. In: Cooper RA, Pasquina PF, eds. *Care of the Combat Amputee.* In: Lenhart MK, ed. Textbooks of Military Medicine. Washington, DC: Department of the Army, Office of the Surgeon General, Borden Institute. In press.

disease risk, and improved ability to manage chronic pain were reported for persons with physical disabilities.

- Improvement in psychosocial health and well-being: decreased depression, improved body image, and increased acceptance of disability have been reported for physically disabled participants in fitness and athletic activities.
- Reduction in reliance on the healthcare system: participation in exercise and other physical recreation interventions by persons with disabilities resulted in reduced use of asthma medication, and in decreased anxiety and stress of a magnitude equal to or greater than that accomplished through medication. A group of wheelchair athletes demonstrated a rehospitalization rate that was one third that of a matched group of nonathletes.

CLASSIFICATION

Classification for disabled athletes including amputees is a concept that applies to competitive sports and not to the wide range of recreation and sport activities encompassed in therapeutic, recreational, or fitness sport. The element of competition introduces such factors as rules and regulations for the sport, fairness, and equal opportunity for success despite great difference in individual impairments. Examples of this concept in able-bodied sport include grouping of participants by gender or age, and in certain sports such as weight-lifting, by body weight. When this concept is applied to amputee sports, it seems obvious, for example, that the competitor with an above-knee level of limb loss will be disadvantaged in competition with a below-knee amputee in a sport in which lower limb function is a factor.

From the earliest days of amputee sport, the process of determining the individual's degree of limb loss, or conversely the degree of residual limb function, was quite familiar in trauma surgery, so the first step in classification was considered a medical one. The language of amputee classification has not changed, based as it is on the anatomical facts of limb loss or preservation. Anatomical details such as extremity or extremities involved and the level of loss within an extremity represent the basic first step in grouping amputees in fair sport competition. This is sometimes described as "general classification."

Organized amputee competitive sports and classification was created and developed within the International Sports Organization for the Disabled (ISOD), founded in 1964. The ISOD classification system changed over time. Originally, amputee competitors internationally were divided into 27 classes according to their individual physical deficits. However, this approach led to insufficient numbers of competitors in each class and was unworkable. A decision to reduce the number of classes to 12 was made after the Toronto Olympiad in 1976, and in the 1992 Barcelona Paralympics the number was further reduced to nine, as follows (1, 5):

Class A1: double above-knee (A/K)
Class A2: single above-knee (A/K)
Class A3: double below-knee (B/K)
Class A4: single below-knee (B/K)
Class A5: double above-elbow (A/E)
Class A6: single above-elbow (A/E)
Class A7: double below-elbow (B/E)
Class A8: single below-elbow (B/E)
Class A9: combined lower and upper limb amputations

As disability sport has developed, the role of the individual sports federations has become more prominent, and the classification process has become incorporated into the rules of individual sports. In sitting volleyball for lower extremity amputation, for example, the regulations allow all eligible competitors to participate as one class. In wheelchair sports, lower extremity amputees are governed by the rules of the wheelchair sports organization that pertains primarily to spinal paralysis. Winter sports classification is based on the amount of technical device assistance used to allow the amputee to ski, such as the use of one or two adapted ski poles or sitting position for sledge racing. As the rules in specific sports change, classification may become more complex, but the anatomical details of amputation have remained the key determinant in amputee sports classification.

ASSISTIVE TECHNOLOGY

Today, the number of sports and recreation opportunities for veterans with disabilities is extensive, due in large part to advances in assistive technology that compensates for impairments. The Department of Veterans Affairs (VA) Veterans Health Administration is exemplary within the United States in the provision of adaptive recreational and sports equipment. The VA provides a variety of adaptive sports and recreation equipment to facilitate healthy living. Devices include sports wheelchairs, handcycles, skiing equipment, bowling equipment, and adaptations for archery, just to name a few. The Clinical Practice Recommendations for Issuance of Recreational and Sports Equipment, written by an interdisciplinary team with the VA Prosthetics Clinical Management Program and approved by the under secretary for health, outlines the recommended approach for providing adaptive equipment to beneficiaries. Key concepts are summarized below. For the entire document, including comprehensive information about recreation and sports equipment provided by the VA and the process for purchasing equipment, see www.prosthetics.va.gov.

Each veteran is entitled to an individualized assessment for adaptive recreation and sports equipment. The evaluation includes examining the veteran's medical diagnoses, prognosis, functional abilities, and goals. Veterans and active duty service members enrolled for VA care with loss or loss of use of a body part or function for which an adaptive recreation device is appropriate may be prescribed and provided equipment. Adaptive sports or recreation technology may be issued to veterans seeking to enhance or maintain their health and attain a higher rehabilitation goal through sports or recreation, and who meet eligibility criteria. Eligibility criteria include (but are not limited to)

- Medical clearance to perform the activity
- Completed education on appropriate activity and equipment options
- Demonstrated commitment to the activity through regular participation
- Opportunity to participate in the activity consistently (for example, snow must be adequate for cross-country skiing)
- Trial of appropriate equipment options configured for specific needs and abilities

- Sports and recreation goals supported by the device
- Demonstrated ability to use, transport, and store the equipment

The VA defines "recreational leisure equipment" as any specialized equipment intended for recreational activities that does not inherently exhibit an athletic or physical rehabilitative nature. Examples include adaptive devices for hobbies and crafts or adaptive fishing or hunting devices. The VA defines "recreational sports equipment" as any specialized equipment intended to be utilized in a physically active or competitive environment. Examples include sports wheelchairs, handcycles, sit skis, and artificial limbs for recreational or sports applications. Powered devices for sport participation can potentially be provided to individuals whose activities are severely limited without their use when the individual meets general criteria for power mobility. An example of powered sports equipment is an electric powered wheelchair for powered wheelchair soccer. Recreation and sports technologies provided by the VA must be adaptive in nature to specifically compensate for loss of or loss of use of a body part or body function. Standard nonadaptive equipment such as skis, boats, and two-wheeled bicycles are not provided by VA.

Accessories for adaptive equipment can also be provided when justified. For example, a car carrier to transport the device to a safe training area, or indoor rollers for handcycles or racing wheelchairs in areas with inclement weather may be considered. Seating interventions for postural support and skin protection or specific adaptations for limited hand function may also qualify. The VA Prosthetics and Sensory Aids Service covers repairs and service on sports and recreation equipment per standard policy and procedure. A knowledgeable clinical professional (recreation therapist, rehabilitation engineer, kinesitherapist, physical therapist, or occupational therapist) must be involved in the comprehensive physical evaluation, equipment trials, selection and modification of devices, and education and training. The clinician works closely with the athlete, other equipment experts, and coaches to support the long-term goals of sports and recreation participation.

ACTIVITIES

The information provided below is intended to be a general introduction to sports and recreation opportunities available to amputees in the United States (6–8).

Aerobics/Physical Fitness

Aerobics is a system of exercise designed to improve respiratory and circulatory function. Disabled Sports, USA (DSUSA), has developed a series of aerobic and strength training videotapes for amputees, paraplegics, quadriplegics, and those with cerebral palsy. DSUSA also has established fitness clinics in several cities across the United States.

Air Guns/Shooting

Air rifle and pistol shooting came onto the U.S. competitive sports scene when WSUSA created a program in 1982. Competition requires shooting from three positions, using a specially

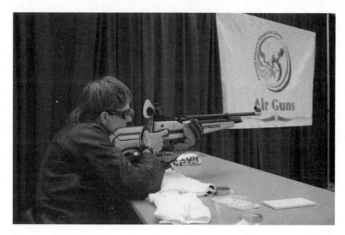

Figure 60.1 Air gun shooting at the National Veterans Wheelchair Games.

designed shooting table or a wheelchair attachment on the athlete's wheelchair. These positions are in accordance with the International Shooting Committee for the Disabled. The sport is organized nationally through the National Wheelchair Shooting Federation/WSUSA. Shooting is a Paralympic sport (Figure 60.1).

Archery

Archery is organized by Disabled Archery USA, in accordance with Fédération Internationale Tir à l'Arc rules. Archers shoot 72 arrows from a distance of 70 m at a target of 122 cm. The National Archery Association has made a commitment to the U.S. Olympic Committee/U.S. Paralympics to act as the national governing body on behalf of archers with disabilities. Archery is a Paralympic sport (Figure 60.2).

Basketball

The National Wheelchair Basketball Association, which organizes the sport nationally, currently consists of 185 teams competing in 21 conferences. Conference play culminates in annual men's,

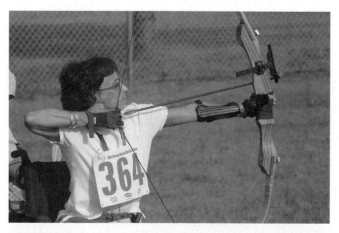

Figure 60.2 Archery at the National Veterans Wheelchair Games.

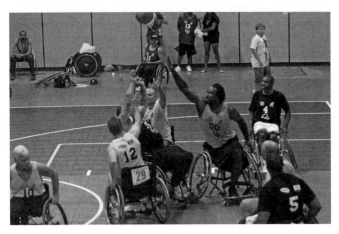

Figure 60.3   Basketball at the National Veterans Wheelchair Games.

women's, youth, and collegiate national tournaments held each spring. Wheelchair basketball rules are a slightly modified form of the National Collegiate Athletic Association rules to accommodate the use of a wheelchair. Wheelchair basketball is a Paralympic sport (Figure 60.3).

Bicycling/Handcycling

Handcycling is a form of adaptive cycling that enables athletes of all abilities to ride a "bike" exclusively using the upper body. Bicycle adaptations for hand propulsion include tandem cycles, units that attach to a wheelchair, and some true bicycles. Some models are designed for children. Handcycling follows the rules of the U.S. Handcycling Federation and is governed by WSUSA. Both cycling and handcycling are Paralympic sports; handcycling, which made its first appearance in Athens, Greece, in 2004, is one of the newest competitions at the Paralympic Games (Figure 60.4).

Billiards

Billiards is regulated by the Wheelchair Poolplayers Association. All players must use a wheelchair for pool competition and must remain seated at all times while at the table (Figure 60.5).

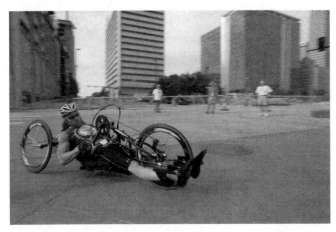

Figure 60.4   Handcycling at the National Veterans Wheelchair Games.

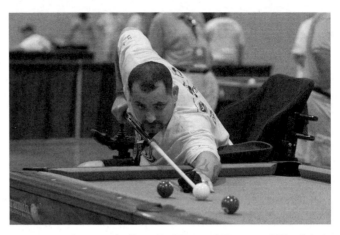

Figure 60.5   Nine ball at the National Veterans Wheelchair Games.

Bowling

Wheelchair bowling is regulated by the American Wheelchair Bowling Association using modified American Bowling Congress rules. The Association hosts an annual national tournament and sanctions numerous other tournaments and local league play (Figure 60.6).

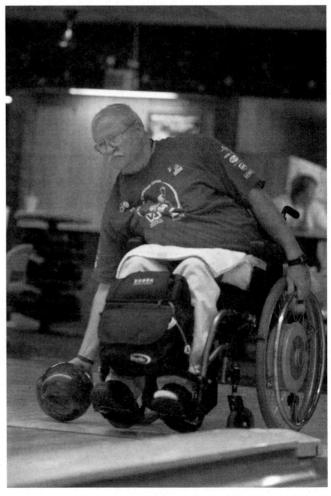

Figure 60.6   Bowling at the National Veterans Wheelchair Games.

Camping

The Office of Special Populations of the National Park Service maintains up-to-date information on accessible parks and offers an individualized search service for a particular geographic area. Many groups organize camping trips into the wilderness for individuals with disabilities.

Canoeing

Canoeing offers freedom to explore areas where a wheelchair will not go. Open canoes offer easy entry and exit, and provide room for friends and gear, including wheelchairs.

Curling

Wheelchair curling is a game of great skill and strategy. The first World Cup in Curling for wheelchair players was held in January 2000 in Crans-Montana, Switzerland. Wheelchair curling had its debut at the Torino 2006 Paralympic Winter Games. The sport is open to male and female athletes with a physical disability in the lower part of the body, including athletes with significant impairments in lower leg/gait function (e.g., spinal injury, cerebral palsy, multiple sclerosis, double leg amputation) who require a wheelchair for daily mobility. Each team must include male and female players. The game is governed by and played according to the rules of the World Curling Federation, with only one modification—no sweeping (Figure 60.7).

Fencing

Through the sport of wheelchair fencing, athletes practice the centuries-old art of swordsmanship. Wheelchair fencing was developed by Sir Ludwig Guttmann at the Stoke Mandeville Hospital and introduced at the 1960 Paralympic Games in Rome. In 2006, 24 countries practiced wheelchair fencing. Requiring a combination of agility, strength, and concentration, fencers compete on one or more of the three weapons, foil, epee, or saber. Athletes compete in wheelchairs that are fastened to the floor. The official governing body is the International Wheelchair and Amputee Sports Federation. Wheelchair fencing is a Paralympic sport.

Fishing

Fishing is a sport that can be fully enjoyed by people with disabilities; a variety of assistive devices are available to meet their needs. Competitive bass fishing tournaments for anglers with physical disabilities are held throughout the United States, including the Paralyzed Veterans of America (PVA) Bass Tour (Figure 60.8).

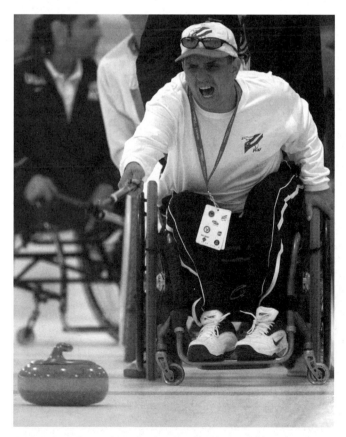

Figure 60.7 Curling at the National Veterans Wheelchair Games.

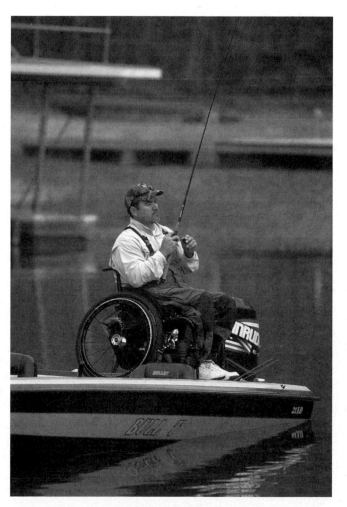

Figure 60.8 Bass fishing at the PVA Bass Tour.

Flying

Hand-controlled flying has grown in popularity since the Federal Aviation Administration approved the use of portable hand controls.

Football

Although it is a fledgling sport in terms of national organization, wheelchair football has been played for many years. Only a few modifications of the National Collegiate Athletic Association rules have been made for the sport. These include a 60-yard surface playing field with 8-yard end zones, 6-person teams, 2-hand touch tackles, down-field throws to simulate kicks, and 15 yards for a first down.

Golf

Golf is easily adapted for people with disabilities through the use of modified golf equipment. Instructional clinics are popular throughout the United States.

Hockey

Sled hockey is played at the regional, sectional, national, international, and Paralympic levels. Ice sled (sledge) hockey was invented at a Stockholm, Sweden, rehabilitation center in the early 1960s by a group of Swedish men who, despite their physical impairment, wanted to continue playing hockey. The group modified a metal-frame sled, or sledge, with two regular-sized ice hockey skate blades that allowed the puck to pass underneath. Just as in ice hockey, sled hockey is played with six players (including a goalie) at a time. Players propel themselves on their sledge by using spikes on the ends of two 3-foot-long sticks, which also allow the player to shoot and pass ambidextrously. Rinks and goals are regulation Olympic-size, and games consist of three 15-minute stop-time periods. Sled hockey is a Paralympic sport.

Horseback Riding

Horseback riding for the disabled is a popular therapeutic activity offered at a number of stables throughout the United States. Equestrian is a Paralympic sport.

Hunting

Hunting with either a bow-and-arrow or gun is regulated by state law. Many states and organizations have programs designed specifically for the disabled. For more information, contact individual state wildlife management services.

Kayaking

Opportunities for competitive kayaking—both whitewater and flat water—are expanding. The sport demands primarily upper-body strength, and athletes with lower level disabilities can compete equally with nondisabled competitors. The Disabled Paddlers Committee of the American Canoe Association governs the sport.

National Disabled Veterans Winter Sports Clinic

The National Disabled Veterans Winter Sports Clinic is currently the largest rehabilitative program of its type in the world and includes adaptive physical activities as well as workshops and educational sessions that aid in the rehabilitation of severely disabled veterans. Activities such as Alpine and Nordic skiing, snowmobiling, scuba diving, fly fishing, wheelchair golf, wheelchair self-defense, rock wall climbing, sled hockey, trapshooting, blues harmonica instruction, dog sledding, goal ball for the visually impaired, curling, wheelchair fencing, and amputee volleyball are only a small sampling of adaptive sports and activities that have been offered over the past 20 years. Set in the Rocky Mountains of Colorado, the Winter Sports Clinic targets disabled veterans with spinal cord injuries, amputations, neurological disorders, and visual impairments to improve physical well-being, mental health, and self–esteem. Co-presented by the VA and Disabled American Veterans, the event hosts over 400 disabled veterans each year.

National Veterans Wheelchair Games

Developed by the VA in conjunction with the International Year of Disabled Persons, the National Veterans Wheelchair Games made its debut on the grounds of the McGuire VA Hospital in Richmond, Virginia, in 1981. There, 74 veterans participated in track, field, swimming, table tennis, slalom, bowling, and billiards. With each successive year, the number of competitors has grown, and now more than 500 veterans compete annually. In 1985 PVA became a co-presenter, lending expertise in sports management and fundraising.

The National Veterans Wheelchair Games is now the largest annual wheelchair sporting event in the world, with 16 core events, including archery, basketball, bowling, handcycling, nine ball, quad rugby, softball, swimming, track and field, and weightlifting, conducted in a 4-day meet. Athletes range in experience from novice to master (age 40 and up), and seven physical classification levels ensure equal competition. In 2006 the VA and the U.S. Olympic Committee signed a memorandum of understanding pledging mutual cooperation on training opportunities for veterans to qualify for future Paralympic teams. In 2007 an amputee clinic emphasizing amputees competing on prostheses was held for the first time, with various track and field events conducted and demonstrated by athletes and coaches of the U.S. Paralympic team.

The National Veterans Wheelchair Games is open to all veterans eligible for healthcare through VA who have a physical disability requiring the use of a wheelchair for sports competition. The secretary of Veterans Affairs can and has made exceptions to this requirement to include active duty service members in their initial stages of rehabilitation who may not have been officially discharged from the service. This could include men and women who served in Operation Iraqi Freedom, Operation Enduring Freedom, or other conflicts. Veterans and service members attending the National Veterans Wheelchair Games for the first time receive an opportunity to gain knowledge from other veteran athletes and to acquire sports skills (9).

Paralympic Games

The Paralympic Games is an international competition among each nation's elite athletes with physical disabilities, including amputees, and is second in size only to the Olympic Games. The Paralympic Games and the Paralympic Winter Games follow the Olympic Games and Olympic Winter Games at the same venues and facilities. The Paralympic Games have been played since 1960 and now feature competition in 19 sports. The Paralympic Winter Games, which showcase four sports, were first held in 1976. The following Paralympic sports include competition for amputees: archery, basketball, curling, cycling, equestrian, fencing, power-lifting, rowing, rugby, sailing, shooting, skiing (Alpine and Nordic), sled hockey, swimming, table tennis, tennis, track and field, and volleyball.

The Paralympic Games has three guiding principles: quality, quantity, and universality. The principle of quality is associated with the Games' grade of excellence, accomplishment, and attainment, achieved by the exciting and inspirational showcasing of elite athletes. Quantity is ensuring that athletes have the support and tools necessary for success, and universality is establishing conditions that reflect the diverse nature of the athletes, including gender and disability types (10, 11).

Power Soccer

With the growth of wheelchair sports, power chair users now have a competitive sport of their own. Power soccer is played with four players on a team trying to push an 18-inch physio-ball over the end line of a regulation basketball court for a score. Thick plexiglas guards protect the players' feet and wheelchairs and allow the player to control the ball (Figure 60.9).

Quad Rugby

Quad rugby is a unique, competitive sport for quadriplegics. The game is played on a basketball court by four-member teams using a volleyball. The objective is to carry the ball across the opponent's goal line. WSUSA is the national governing body for this sport. Quad Rugby is governed by

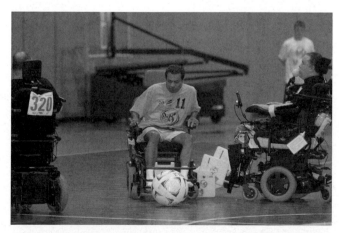

Figure 60.9 Power soccer at the National Veterans Wheelchair Games.

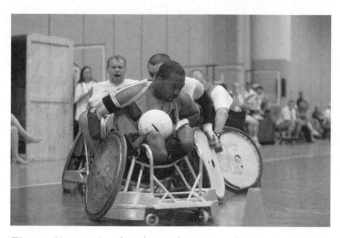

Figure 60.10 Quad rugby at the National Veterans Wheelchair Games.

the U.S. Quad Rugby Association and is a Paralympic sport (Figure 60.10).

Road Racing

Wheelchair road racing is generally run in conjunction with established road races, and wheelchair athletes compete in a separate division against other wheelchair athletes.

Sailing

New designs in sailboats and adaptive equipment allow sailors with disabilities to get on and off and maneuver around sailboats with no or minimal assistance, enabling them to handle a boat much as a nondisabled person would. Sailing is a Paralympic sport.

Scuba Diving

Scuba diving has become readily available to people with disabilities as instructors become more aware of these divers' capabilities.

Skiing

Both competitive and recreation skiing is available for people with disabilities. Athletes can compete in downhill racing, slalom, and giant slalom. Amputees compete standing up in either three- or four-track (i.e., with outriggers skis) competition or use a sit-ski or mono-ski, depending on their disability. Nordic and Alpine skiing are governed by DSUSA and are Paralympic sports.

Slalom

Slalom is a unique wheelchair sport that does not parallel an established able-bodied sport. It is a timed test of speed, dexterity, and maneuverability in which competitors follow an obstacle course clearly marked by arrows, flags, and gates. Slalom competition is governed by Wheelchair Athletics of the USA and WSUSA (Figure 60.11).

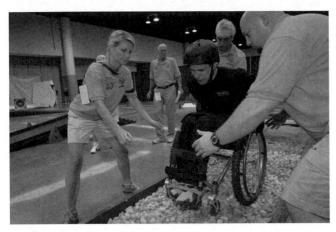

Figure 60.11   Slalom at the National Veterans Wheelchair Games.

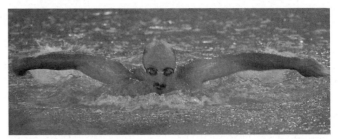

Figure 60.13   Swimming at the National Veterans Wheelchair Games.

Softball

Competitive wheelchair softball is played under the official rules of 16-inch slow-pitch softball as approved by the Amateur Softball Association (Figure 60.12).

Swimming

Competitive and recreational swimming can be enjoyed by those with disabilities. Swimmers compete in a variety of distances in the standard strokes of freestyle, backstroke, butterfly, and breaststroke. Swimming is governed by USA Swimming and is a Paralympic sport (Figure 60.13).

Table Tennis

Singles and doubles competition for men and women is played regionally, nationally, and internationally, in accordance with U.S. Table Tennis Association rules. Quadriplegics and others with impaired hand function play table tennis by strapping or taping the paddle to their hand. Table tennis is governed by the American

Wheelchair Table Tennis Association and is a Paralympic sport (Figure 60.14).

Tennis

Wheelchair tennis can be enjoyed with nondisabled family and friends. The sport follows the rules of the US Tennis Association with one exception: the wheelchair tennis player is allowed two bounces instead of one. Athletes are classified according to their performance in competition. Introductory lessons are often available at community tennis programs. Wheelchair tennis is a Paralympic sport.

Track and Field

Track events are run on a hard surface, 400-m oval tack, ranging from 100 m to 10,000 m. Field events include the javelin, shot put, and discus. Track and field is governed by Wheelchair Track & Field, USA, and is a Paralympic sport (Figures 60.15 and 60.16).

Trap and Skeet Shooting

Trap and skeet shooting are two sports that allow wheelchair users to compete alongside nondisabled shooters under the same rules. Tournaments are held throughout the United States, including the PVA National Trapshoot Circuit (Figure 60.17).

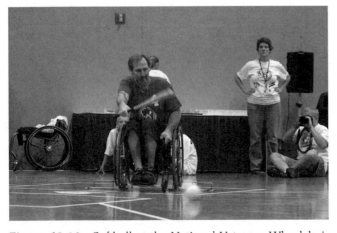

Figure 60.12   Softball at the National Veterans Wheelchair Games.

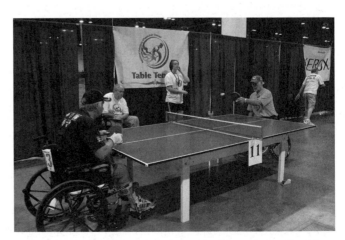

Figure 60.14   Table tennis at the National Veterans Wheelchair Games.

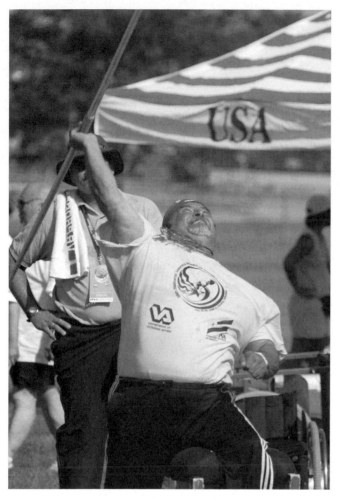

Figure 60.15 Javelin at the National Veterans Wheelchair Games.

Waterskiing

People with disabilities who have the desire to learn to water ski can do so using a modified ski or technique.

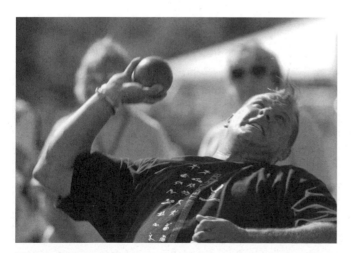

Figure 60.16 Shot put at the National Veterans Wheelchair Games.

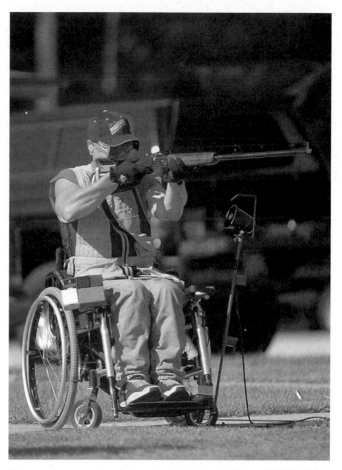

Figure 60.17 Trapshooting at the PVA National Trapshoot circuit.

Weightlifting

Athletes competing in the conventional bench press are placed in divisions based on body weight. Weightlifting is governed by U.S. Wheelchair Weightlifting Association, and powerlifting is a Paralympic sport (Figure 60.18).

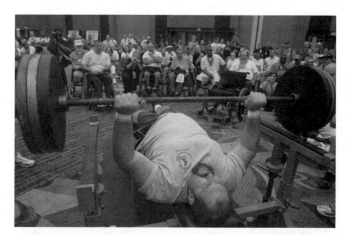

Figure 60.18 Weightlifting at the National Veterans Wheelchair Games.

SUMMARY

Originating in the wheelchair games developed by World War II veterans, a wide variety of sports and recreational opportunities are available today to veterans and others with disabilities. Both recreational and competitive activities have documented therapeutic benefits for participants. Athletes participate in competitive sports according to classification systems based on the extent of their disabilities. Ongoing development of assistive technology increases the capabilities of amputees to engage in recreational as well as practical activities. An extensive list of organizations dedicated to promoting access to these activities for all Americans follows in the attachment to this chapter

R*eferences*

1. Guttmann L. *Textbook of Sport for the Disabled*. Aylesburg, England: HM&M Publishers; 1976.

2. Winnick JP, ed. *Adapted Physical Education and Sport*. 4th ed. Champaign, IL: Human Kinetics Publishers; 2005.

3. About Wheelchair Sports, USA. Wheelchair Sports, USA Web site. http://www.wsusa.org/. Accessed January 4, 2008.

4. Coyle CP, Kinney WB, Riley B, Shank JW, eds. *Benefits of Therapeutic Recreation: A Consensus View*. Philadelphia, Pa: Temple University; 1991.

5. Scruton J. *Stoke Mandeville: Road to the Paralympics*. Aylesbury, England: Peterhouse Press; 1998.

6. Paralyzed Veterans of America. *A Guide to Wheelchair Sports and Recreation*. Waldorf, MD: PVA Distribution Center; 1997.

7. Sports associations. *Sports 'N Spokes*. 2007; 33(1):40.

8. Sports & recreation programs. *Active Living*.2007; 15(1): 87–88

9. National Veterans Wheelchair Games face sheet. National Veterans Wheelchair Games Web site. http://www1.va.gov/vetevent/nvwg/2008/default.cfm. Accessed January 6, 2008.

10. Paralympic Games principles. Paralympic Games Web site. http://www.paralympic.org/release/Main_Sections_Menu/Paralympic_Games/Games_Principles/. Accessed January 4, 2008.

11. Steadward R, Peterson C. *Paralympics: Where Heroes Come*. Edmonton, Alberta, Canada: One Shot Holdings; 1997.

61 Vocational Rehabilitation and Spinal Cord Injury

Kurt L. Johnson

Spinal cord injury (SCI) presents significant barriers to employment. In this chapter, these barriers will be reviewed, along with the strategies and systems available to promote vocational rehabilitation. Although some of the barriers confronted by people living with SCI are related to the associated functional limitations, many are related to economic disincentives due to lack of universal health care, lack of appreciation of vocational potential by individuals with SCI, their families, employers, and others, and inaccessible environments.

Based on their analysis of the 2000 U.S. Census data, approximately 55% of people of working age with disabilities are employed (1). This is in marked contrast to unemployment rates in general which, are around 5% (2). Not surprisingly, disability status puts people at high risk for poverty (3). In repeated surveys, most people with disabilities report that they would prefer to work (4), and with appropriate intervention and support, most can successfully maintain employment.

For people living with SCI, the picture is no different. At the time of their injury, about 58% of 3,756 people with SCI enrolled in the Model Spinal Cord Injury Systems nationally were employed, but at follow-up 1–25 years later, fewer than 27% are employed (5). In their 25-year longitudinal study, Krause and Broderick found that over time, employment rates increased somewhat as did satisfaction with employment and life in general (6). People with SCI who are employed report higher levels of psychologic adjustment, satisfaction with life, independence, and general health than those who are unemployed (7).

The employment picture is complicated by the fact that over half of all traumatic SCI occurs in young, predominantly male adults between the ages of 15 and 25 (8). In addition to the functional limitations secondary to their SCI, these young adults often lack a history of sustained employment, have not completed high school, begun or completed post-secondary education, or embarked on a path of career development. In their follow-up study, Krause et al. (5) found that for people with SCI who had completed less that 12 years of education, the employment rate was 5%, as compared to over 60% for people who had completed

at least 16 years of education. This is further complicated by the co-occurrence of traumatic brain injury for some people with traumatic SCI (9). For these young adults, vocational rehabilitation requires multiple and sustained services. As Roessler (10) has observed, not only is it critical to assist in the initial efforts to obtain employment, but also on an ongoing basis. Periodic interventions may be required to address additional impairment and aging, functional changes, career development issues, technology, and changes in the labor market.

KEY LEGISLATION

In response to the desire of people with SCI and other disabilities to work, and the clear economic, health, psychologic, and social benefits associated with participation in employment, significant federal legislation has been enacted to support employment for people with disabilities. Beginning with the civil rights movement of the 1960s, advocates attempted unsuccessfully to include people with disabilities as a protected class in the key civil rights legislation. In the 1974 amendments to the Rehabilitation Act of 1973, civil rights for people with disabilities were protected in employment and education when the entity (e.g., employer, school) received federal dollars (11, 12, 13).

Americans with Disabilities Act

In 1990, the Americans with Disabilities Act (ADA) was passed, providing true civil rights protection under most circumstances. The ADA prohibits discrimination in employment against qualified individuals with disabilities who are able to perform the essential functions of the job with or without accommodation (14). It also prohibits discrimination against individuals with disabilities in the areas of transportation, public accommodations, state and local governments, and telecommunications. Title I of the ADA which took effect on July 26, 1992 prohibits private employers, state and local governments, employment agencies and labor unions from discriminating against qualified individuals with disabilities in job application procedures, hiring, firing, advancement, compensation, job training, and other terms, conditions, and privileges of employment. Because of a series of U. S. Supreme Court decisions limiting the scope of the ADA, Congress passed the ADA Amendments Act, also known as the ADA Restoration Act, in 2008 to ensure that coverage of the ADA is broadly construed.

ADA does not extend protection to every individual with a disability. Protection is limited to those individuals with disabilities that limit major life activities. Under ADA, a qualifying disability is defined as

- A physical or mental impairment that substantially limits one or more of the major life activities of such an individual;
- A record of such an impairment;
- Being regarded as having such an impairment.

Reasonable accommodation may include but is not limited to

- Making existing facilities used by employees readily accessible to and usable by persons with disabilities;
- Job restructuring, modifying work schedules, reassignment to a vacant position;
- Acquiring or modifying equipment or devices, adjusting or modifying examinations, training materials, or policies, and providing qualified readers or sign language interpreters.

An employer must make an accommodation to the known disability of a qualified applicant or employee if it would not impose an undue hardship on the business. Undue hardship is defined as significant difficulty or expense in light of factors such as the employer's size, financial resources, and the nature and structure of its operation. Employers are not required to lower quality or production standards to make an accommodation, or to provide personal use items such as glasses or hearing aids.

Employers may not ask job applicants about the existence, nature, or severity of a disability but may ask about the applicant's ability to perform specific job functions. A job offer may be contingent on the results of a medical examination only if the examination is required for all entering employees in similar jobs. Medical examinations of employees must be job-related and consistent with the employer's business needs.

The U.S. Equal Employment Opportunity Commission (EEOC) has issued regulations to enforce the provisions of Title I of the ADA for employers with more than 15 employees. Many states have laws that complement or exceed ADA requirements. Complaints of discrimination may be made to the EEOC (see Resource Note #6).

Individuals with Disabilities Education Act

Another key piece of federal legislation is the Individuals with Disabilities Education Act (IDEA), which mandates that children with disabilities must be provided Free and Appropriate Public Education (FAPE) in the least restrictive environment (15). Section 504 of the Rehabilitation Act guarantees students with disabilities in K-12 schools equal access to education and prohibits discrimination, and IDEA covers students with disabilities who require modifications of the curriculum such as additional remedial or educational services or specialized related services such as physical or occupational therapy in order to achieve FAPE. When a student is covered under IDEA, an Individualized Education Plan (IEP) is developed that stipulates the outcomes to be achieved, the services to be provided, and who will provide those services. Goals can be both academic and practical. For example, it would be quite appropriate to include on an IEP for a 17-year-old student with newly acquired C5 tetraplegia a goal to increase competence with respect to specific independent living and work-related skills. By law, students may continue in the K–12 system until the year in which they turn 22, if that is necessary for them to achieve their IEP goals. Because educational activities can include training in independent living, vocational skills, and community mobility skills in addition to literacy and other academic subjects, it may be in the best interests of some young adults to continue in the K–12 system beyond the time when they would ordinarily graduate based on completion of academic credits.

IDEA requires that Individualized Transition Plans be developed for each student on an IEP by the time that student reaches 16 years of age. The Transition Plan identifies transition goals, the services necessary to achieve those goals, and who will provide those services. As part of a transition plan, a student might participate in various kinds of career exploration, work tryouts, or perhaps vocational training. Transition goals might include post-secondary education (e.g., community or technical college, university), employment, or community living. It is the intent of IDEA that the transition process includes a collaboration between schools and other key agencies, including state Departments of Vocational Rehabilitation.

Physiatrists can play a key role as advocates in the transition process by ensuring that the functional limitations of their patients with SCI are addressed, but perhaps more importantly, that their functional strengths are addressed. Physiatrists will have important information about the impact of new assistive technology to enhance performance, seating, and positioning modifications for employment, management of bowel and bladder issues, etc. Transition is a difficult time as students anticipate moving into the world of work, employment, higher education, and community with far fewer supports in place and a fragmented service delivery system. For those students who have concurrent brain injuries or other cognitive or emotional issues, transition can be even more difficult. Families who do not feel they have received appropriate services and have not found the school district to be responsive may file complaints through the U.S. Department of Education Office of Civil Rights, which has offices in each state.

THE PROFESSION OF REHABILITATION COUNSELING

Rehabilitation Counselors provide vocational rehabilitation and other counseling services to people with disabilities, and provide consultation to families, employers, and health care providers (16). Professional Rehabilitation Counselors have master's degrees in rehabilitation counseling from graduate programs in rehabilitation counseling accredited by the Council on Rehabilitation Education, or closely related degrees. They have training in applied psychology; individual, group, and family counseling; medical, psychosocial, and vocational issues in disability; individual and career assessment; career development; labor market and employment issues; job placement; case management; and service delivery systems. They complete internships and acquire the Certified Rehabilitation Counselor credential (17). In many states, they will sit for state exams to become Licensed Professional Counselors.

THE VOCATIONAL REHABILITATION PROCESS

Many people with SCI have a history of employment and may even have a job to which they may return. As noted earlier, others will have had a marginal history of employment, have worked in physical labor jobs and have few transferable skills, or have no employment history at all. In either case the process of vocational rehabilitation begins on the first day of admission to the inpatient rehabilitation setting when the expectation is set that with appropriate intervention, many people with SCI can work at meaningful jobs with acceptable pay, and that the skills the newly injured person acquires in the early stages of rehabilitation are the building blocks for employment and independence later on. At the University of Washington Medical Center and Harborview Medical Center, a staff of professional rehabilitation counselors provides vocational rehabilitation and other counseling services to inpatients and outpatients. Newly injured SCI patients are seen on admission and throughout their inpatient stay. As a member of the interdisciplinary team, the rehabilitation counselor assists in the identification of educational and career interests, assessment of academic and vocational potential, review of existing skills, and counseling around issues related to adjustment, perceived competence, etc. On discharge, the counselor continues following the patient, often in collaboration with a state or community agency to support efforts to enter and maintain employment.

Whenever the process begins, it includes the following steps:

Referral

The physiatrist is often in an ideal position to identify a person with SCI who can profit from vocational rehabilitation services. Not only should individuals who are not working be considered for referral, but so should individuals who are working if there is an indication that they are dissatisfied with their employment or are at risk for losing their job. The vocational rehabilitation process should be driven by the person with SCI and supported by the rehabilitation counselor and others.

Assessment

The assessment begins with a review of records and an interview with the client, significant others, family members, and other key informants. The assessment process includes a review of functional limitations and strengths and an investigation of current and potential barriers to employment. A careful review of educational, vocational, and avocational history will yield a list of transferable skills as well as an employment history (e.g.,

a resume). An appraisal of the career interests may be useful either through the counseling process or with career assessment instruments such as the Strong Interest Inventory® (see reference note #7). Generally, people are more satisfied in employment that is consistent with their career interests, including, for example, preferences for working with data versus people, or in activities requiring creative problem solving versus routine activities. Similarly, it may be useful to understand an individual's temperament or personality style. This can be evaluated by a review of history, interview with the client and other key informants, observation, and/or psychologic assessment such as the Jackson Personality Inventory—Revised® (see Resource 8 at end of chapter).

If potential rehabilitation goals include return to school or pursuit of occupations that require certain levels of educational attainment, then it is necessary to evaluate achievement by a review of educational records, interview, and perhaps through achievement testing using instruments such as the Wide Range Achievement Test 4® (see Resource 9 at end of chapter). When inadequate evidence is available to predict the client's potential to benefit from education or to acquire or perform certain kinds of occupational skills, assessment of aptitude may be appropriate. Generalized aptitude for higher education (e.g., community college) may be estimated from standard intelligence tests, or many community college systems offer an assessment.

When possible, the best assessment involves review of actual performance, interview, and real-world tryouts. The validity of paper and pencil tests is limited. For example, only 9% of the variance in freshman college grades can be accounted for by students' scores on the Scholastic Aptitude Test ® (18). Nevertheless, paper and pencil assessment instruments may be useful as part of the career exploration process.

Another approach to vocational evaluation involves the use of work samples (19). Work samples are either organized along various tasks common to many jobs or tasks thought to represent a specific job. For example, one might have activities that sample the individual's ability to manipulate small objects or demonstrate eye-hand coordination as in the Valpar® system (see Resource 10 at end of chapter). Commercially available vocational evaluation systems using work samples often include norms that purport to allow the evaluator to compare the performance of the person being evaluated with a standard necessary for successful occupational performance. These predictions do not hold up well, however, the vocational evaluation systems may provide a useful way for people with disabilities to try out a variety of occupational activities and for the evaluator to collect observational data about the way the client engages in the task.

Situational Assessment

Situational assessment is the generic term for using real-life situations to assess performance. In vocational rehabilitation, job stations or paid employment may serve this purpose. Job stations may be created by collaborating with employers to have the client try out elements of a job for a period of time. For example, a 25-year-old with paraplegia had worked as a welder prior to injury and was interested in returning to that line of work. The rehabilitation counselor set up a job station in the hospital metal shop where the client worked three hours a day, five days a week, for three weeks at metal fabrication and welding. The shop supervisor worked with the client and the rehabilitation counselor to evaluate the client's ability to perform various tasks, and to develop potential accommodations that would allow the client to work more independently. At the conclusion of the job station, the client had increased his endurance for work, his confidence, and had an employment reference from the shop supervisor as he began his search for paid employment. Federal law allows up to 160 hours of unpaid employment as part of the vocational assessment process. Some clients, particularly those who have had concurrent brain injuries, will require on-site supervision and training from a job coach during their job station. Under these circumstances, the job coach can collect data about rate of acquisition of skill, responsiveness to supervisory feedback, and other variables.

Labor Market Analysis

As part of the assessment process, the outlook for employment in various occupations is evaluated. The U.S. Department of Labor and state Departments of Employment Security maintain statistics on trends in occupations including the number of people currently employed part time and full time in each occupational group, and the percent growth or decline predicted during the next five years. Clients can identify the number of jobs currently available in an occupational group within their immediate geographical area. They can also find out the wages, tasks, educational preparation, and other characteristics of occupations. This information is readily available on the U.S. Department of Labor and other governmental websites.

Counseling

Many clients with SCI will find counseling useful to help them reevaluate their expectations, enhance their personal adjustment, and understand and react to the perceptions and biases of others around them, including family members, potential employers, and coworkers. As part of the counseling process the clients may take stock of the resources they bring to bear on the issues, the barriers they confront, and compensatory strategies to which they have access or can learn.

Selecting a Goal

Through the counseling process, the client evaluates the assessment data and develops a terminal goal and intermediate steps. For example, a 19-year-old with tetraplegia might choose working as an attorney as her long-term goal. To achieve this goal, she might develop intermediate steps that include (1) increasing sitting tolerance; (2) applying for readmission to an undergraduate program; (3) finding accessible housing; (4) finding and training a personal care attendant; (5) identifying transportation options; (6) obtaining and learning to use adaptive equipment, including voice recognition software; (7) beginning classes; (8) choosing a college major; (9) reappraising her long-term goal—interviewing lawyers, law school faculty, conducting research on work in the legal profession; (10) taking the Law School Admissions Test; (11) researching various law schools; (12) applying to law schools; (13) applying for scholarship and financial aid; (14) accepting admission; and (15) finishing law school, finding employment, etc. Having tetraplegia has reduced this student's flexibility in planning. She must complete the same steps she would have prior to her injury, but will require additional planning to achieve success.

Educational or Vocational Reentry

Once the goal setting and planning is completed, the next step in the vocational rehabilitation process is educational reentry as in the example above, or vocational reentry. In vocational reentry, the client may be able to secure a job independently, but often may require assistance in job development and placement from the rehabilitation counselor. Although discrimination against qualified individuals with disabilities is illegal, discrimination at the point of hiring is difficult to prove and may not be intentional on the part of the employer. Employers may not have experience interacting with people with significant disabilities and may not be able to imagine them working productively. Advocacy and assistance in obtaining employment is often an appropriate role for the rehabilitation counselor.

Take for example a 34-year-old man with C5 tetraplegia. After discharge from inpatient treatment and six months of outpatient rehabilitation, he began college taking only one course the first quarter, and in six years graduated with a BA in business with a specialization in accounting. One year after graduation, he passed his Certified Public Accountant exam. Over the next three years, he applied for nearly 700 jobs, had numerous interviews, and worked in volunteer positions, with no offers of employment. His faculty advisor at the college reported that he was an excellent student and when prospective employers were contacted they reported that he had interviewed competently, impressed them as bright and capable, but that they were unable to imagine how he could accomplish the essential functions of the job they had open because of his limited dexterity and inability to manipulate print materials. With the intervention of a rehabilitation counselor and an assistive technology specialist, he was able to secure employment and has been working successfully since then.

Supported Employment

Some people with SCI will require ongoing support in the workplace in order to sustain employment. For some, such as persons with high-level tetraplegia, that support may involve assistance in positioning in relation to a task, manipulating materials, etc. They may also require personal care assistance in the workplace. Others, particularly those who have significant concurrent brain injuries, may require ongoing support in the form of job coaching. This support may be provided either by a coworker or by a professional job coach.

Job Placement

When the rehabilitation counselor is assisting with the job placement process, he or she begins by searching for jobs that will meet elements of the client's goal. When potential jobs are identified, the rehabilitation counselor conducts a job analysis to determine the actual kinds of work done in that particular job, the cognitive, social, and physical demands of the job, and potential accommodations. Then in collaboration with the client and the employer, the fit of the job with the client is evaluated.

- Is this job a good match for what the client was seeking in terms of interest, skills, distance from home, social environment, pay, and benefits?
- Can the client do the essential functions of the job with or without accommodation?
- Given the size of the employer and the employer's resources, are the accommodations reasonable?
- If the client cannot perform the essential functions of the job, is the employer willing to modify the job or create a job the client could do by merging components of other jobs?
- Could the client do the job with additional accommodations not paid for by the employer, such as the support of a job coach?

Job Accommodation

Dowler et al. reviewed the requests for information on accommodation made by 1,000 people with SCI who called the national Job Accommodation Network (20). They reported that callers with tetraplegia most frequently reported difficulties with gross and fine motor skills such as keyboarding, manipulating small parts, holding pens, and sorting. Those with paraplegia reported difficulty with driving, heavy lifting, carrying objects, reaching work areas, etc. As noted earlier, job accommodations can include modification in work schedules, modification of tasks, and modification of the environment to make it more accessible (e.g., installing electric door openers, or a ramp). Some accommodations are as simple as removing a desk drawer or raising the height of a desk with four wood blocks to permit wheelchair access. Other accommodations are high tech and involve designing computer interface software and hardware, or writing scripts to allow a user to control multiple applications using voice recognition. Still other accommodations are practical, such as providing a private changing area and storage for a change of clothing for a male employee with tetraplegia who uses a condom catheter in case of bladder accidents when the condom becomes disconnected during transfers. In many cases, the need for additional accommodations will become apparent as the employee begins settling into the job.

Although accommodations for people with SCI may often seem self-evident, this is not the case for individuals with concurrent brain injuries. For these individuals, special attention must be paid to designing accommodations that serve as compensatory tools for lost cognitive function. These may include prosthetic memory devices but also may include changes in supervision to include explicit and concrete instruction to the employee, using both verbal and written instructions, and so forth.

Long-Term Employment Issues

Employment rates for individuals with disabilities in general and individuals with SCI in particular decline with age more rapidly than for people without disabilities (21). This represents the accelerated morbidity associated with aging with SCI. It is critical that vocational rehabilitation not be considered to be complete once a job has been obtained (10). Proactive, strategic planning with periodic intervention will reduce the occurrence of additional disability and employment problems in the future.

VOCATIONAL REHABILITATION SYSTEMS

In the past, rehabilitation counseling services at some inpatient and outpatient rehabilitation programs were provided as part of the program fee. Increasingly, hospital-based rehabilitation counselors and those in the private sector provide fee-for-service rehabilitation counseling. Some services can be paid for by health insurance policies and others are paid directly by the recipient. It is not unusual for personal injury policies and long-term disability policies to provide for vocational rehabilitation benefits. For people with SCI who are employed, the employer may pay for some services to meet their obligation to provide reasonable accommodations. Finally, many legal settlements rising from traumatic SCI include funding for vocational rehabilitation. In addition to these individual options, there are several major social service systems that provide vocational rehabilitation.

Federal/State Vocational Rehabilitation Programs

The Rehabilitation Act of 1973 funds a vocational rehabilitation program in each state with four federal dollars for each dollar appropriated by the state. Some Native American groups have also established federally funded vocational rehabilitation programs. State vocational rehabilitation programs are designed to help people with disabilities prepare for, obtain, and retain employment. The goal is not to simply obtain employment, but to assist the person with a disability to maximize his or her employment potential. The state vocational rehabilitation agencies work in collaboration with program participants, employers, and the community. To be eligible for services, applicants must have a significant disability that limits their ability to work. Services include

- *Medical Evaluation*: determination of a person' strengths and vocational limitations through expert medical, psychiatric, social, and psychologic evaluation.
- *Vocational Assessment*: identification of a person's interests, readiness for employment, work skills, and job opportunities in the community.
- *Counseling and Guidance*: rehabilitation counselor and participant establish an ongoing relationship in which they explore evaluation results and labor market opportunities and develop a realistic plan for employment.
- *Restoration*: increase work potential and ability to retain a job through use of medical and assistive technologies.
- *Job Preparation*: build work skills through services such as volunteer experience, on-the-job training, vocational and technical education, and higher education.
- *Support Services*: support the participant through services such as transportation assistance; the purchase of tools, equipment, books, or work clothing; job coaching; and independent living support.
- *Job Placement*: develop work opportunities and obtain and maintain a job suited to the participant's interests and capabilities.
- *Follow-up*: follow the progress of the participant for at least 90 days to ensure that employment is satisfactory.
- *Post-employment*: provide short-term services from time to time necessary to help a participant sustain employment.

State Worker's Compensation Programs

Each state has a worker's compensation program for workers who sustain work-related injuries. In many states, the program is regulated by a state agency but implemented by commercial insurance carriers that cover the employer. Larger employers may often be self-insured. In some states, all phases of the process are conducted by the state agency or its contractors. Worker's compensation programs in most states include a vocational rehabilitation component. In worker's compensation rehabilitation, the goal is to return the injured worker to his or her previous job, or a similar job. If neither of these is possible, then depending on the state, the goal may be to return the injured worker to any suitable employment. Covered services are similar to those described for the federal–state system, but usually services are only provided with respect to the work-related injury. Worker's compensation vocational rehabilitation programs typically have two phases. The first is characterized by the continuing recovery and rehabilitation of the injured worker. The second phase begins when the injured worker reaches "maximum medical improvement." Wage replacement is typically paid during both phases. When the injured worker cannot return to previous employment or a similar job, and does not have the transferable skills necessary to perform other suitable work, retraining can be authorized. If a worker is determined to not have the potential to resume employment, he or she is typically awarded a settlement or pension.

Veteran's Administration

Individuals with SCI who are eligible for services through the Veteran's Administration (VA) have access to vocational rehabilitation services at many comprehensive VA system rehabilitation centers and through other community access points. VA services are similar to those provided through the federal/state system.

Other Vocational Rehabilitation Systems

A variety of other systems with similar features exist for workers who sustain disabling work related injuries in federal government, off-shore, maritime, and railroad settings.

KEY DISABILITY BENEFIT SYSTEMS

For some people with SCI, an extended period of education, retraining, and/or rehabilitation will be necessary prior to return to work, and they will be considered totally disabled for at least a year or two. Other people with SCI will not ever return to work. These include people who cannot resolve health insurance issues, or who live in rural areas without access to transportation or employment, or older workers who had relied on their ability to perform physical labor and who do not have sufficient transferable skills to work in another field. Under these circumstances, it is the responsibility of the rehabilitation counselor, the physiatrist, and other rehabilitation professionals to advocate for disability benefits and assist in the application process. Some individuals will have long-term disability insurance policies where the premiums have been deducted from their pay, but most will not and will rely on various state and federal programs.

Social Security Administration

The Social Security Administration (SSA) pays disability benefits under two programs: Social Security Disability Insurance (SSDI) and Supplementary Security Income (SSI). The medical requirements for disability payments are the same under both programs, and a person's disability is determined by the same process. However, eligibility for SSDI benefits is based on history of employment covered by SSA, and eligibility for SSI disability payments is determined by financial need. SSDI is a federal long-term disability insurance program funded by payroll taxes, but SSI is a federal welfare program for, among others, people with disabilities who are unable to work and are poor.

The SSA considers a person disabled if he or she is unable to perform any kind of work at a level of "substantial and gainful" activity, and the disability is expected to last at least a year or to result in death. Applicants should contact a Social Security office as soon as they become disabled because there is a waiting period before some types of disability benefits begin. This waiting period starts with the first full month after the onset of the disability as determined by SSA. Filing for disability benefits can be done by phone, by mail, or in person at any office. Spouses and children who are financially dependent on the disabled worker may also qualify for disability benefits under certain conditions.

Newly injured individuals with SCI should consider applying for SSA benefits immediately if it seems likely that they will not return to work for at least a year. Once eligibility is established, depending on the program, recipients are immediately eligible for state Medicaid benefits, or after a waiting period, federal Medicare benefits. Under the Ticket to Work legislation of 2000, many recipients of SSA benefits will be able to continue their Medicare coverage after they return to work. SSA also has several work incentive programs where a person with a disability who must purchase services or goods in order to work can deduct those expenses from his or her income. If as a result his or her income after deductions is below the threshold, he or she can continue to receive SSA benefits including Medicare. This can be a powerful tool for someone with a high-level SCI who has a strong desire to work but requires personal care assistance on the job, must make lease payments on a van, and needs other services in order to work.

CONCLUSION

Many people with SCI would like to work and can work with appropriate vocational rehabilitation services, but they face numerous barriers to achieving that goal. They achieve many benefits from employment, including economic self-sufficiency, health care benefits, and improved quality of life. People with disabilities feel that access to employment is a basic civil right, and federal laws have been enacted to support that belief. Physiatrists and other rehabilitation professionals can play a key role in advocating for full participation in employment for their patients by understanding the benefits of employment and the potential for their patients to participate in employment, and by taking concrete steps to document both functional limitations and strengths, identify compensatory strategies including assistive technology and accommodations, and by making appropriate referrals to vocational rehabilitation professionals.

References

1. Office of Disability Employment Policy, U. S. Department of Labor (2008). (http://www.dol.gov/odep/pubs/fact/stats.htm)
2. Bureau of Labor Statistics, U. S. Department of Labor (2008). (http://www.bls.gov/)
3. She, P., & Livermore, G. (2006). Long-term poverty and disability among working-age adults (Research Brief). Ithaca, NY: Rehabilitation Research and Training Center on Employment Policy for Persons with Disabilities, Cornell University. (http://digitalcommons.ilr.cornell.edu/edicollect/1226)
4. National Council on Disability (2000). *Achieving independence. The challenge of the 21st century*. Washington, DC: Author.
5. Krause JS, Kewman D, DeVivo M, Maynard F, Coker J, Roach J, et al. Employment after spinal cord injury: An analysis of cases from the Model Spinal Cord Injury Systems. *Arch Phys Med Rehabil* 1999; 80: 1492–1500.
6. Krause J, Broderick L. A 25 year longitudinal study of the natural course of aging after spinal cord injury. *Spinal Cord* 2005; 43: 349–356.
7. Hess D.W, Meade M.A, Forchheimer M, Tate, D. G. Psychological well-being and intensity of employment in individuals with spinal cord injury. *Top Spinal Cord Inj Rehabil*, 2004; 9: 1–10.
8. Britell K, Hammond M. Spinal cord injury. In: R. Hays, G. Kraft, & Stolov, W., Eds. *Chronic disease and disability*. New York: Demos, 1994; 142–160.
9. Strubreither W, Hackbusch B, Hermann-Gruber M, Stahr G, Jonas H. Neuropsychological aspects of the rehabilitation of patients with paralysis from a spinal injury who also have a brain injury. *Spinal Cord* 1997; 35:487–492.
10. Roessler R. Job retention services for employees with spinal cord injuries: A critical need in vocational rehabilitation. *J Applied Rehabil Couns* 2001; 32(1):3–9.
11. Rehabilitation Act of 1973, 87 Stat.355, 29 U.S.C. § 701 *et seq.*
12. Rehabilitation Act Amendments of 1974, 89 Stat.2.
13. Pennell F, Johnson J. Legal and civil right aspects of vocational rehabilitation. In: Johnson K, Haselkorn J, eds. *Vocational Rehabilitation: Physical Medicine and Rehabilitation Clinics of North America*. Philadelphia: Richard Saunders, 1997; 245–266.
14. Americans with Disabilities Act of 1990, 42 U.S.C. § 12101 *et seq.*
15. Individuals with Disabilities Education Act of 1990, 20 U.S.C. § 1400 *et seq.*
16. National Council on Rehabilitation Education (2008). (http://www.rehabeducators.org/)
17. Commission on Rehabilitation Counselor Certification (2008). (http://www.crccertification.com/)
18. Anastasi A, Urbina S. *Psychological assessment*. 7th ed. Upper Saddle River, NJ: Prentice Hall; 1997.
19. Brown C, McDaniel KR, Couch R. *Vocational evaluation systems and software*. Menomonie, WI: Stout Vocational Rehabilitation Institute, University of Wisconsin–Stout; 1994.
20. Dowler lD, Batiste L, Whidden E. Accommodating workers with spinal cord injury. *J Voc Rehabil* 1998; 10:115–122.
21. Mitchell JM, Adkins RH, Kemp BJ. The effects of aging on employment of people with and without disabilities. *Rehabil Counsel Bull* 2006; 49: 157–165.

Bibliography

Johnson, K. L., & Haselkorn, J., eds. (1997). *Vocational Rehabilitation: Physical Medicine and Rehabilitation Clinics of North America*. Philadelphia: Saunders.

Chan, F., Berven, N., & Thomas, K. (2007). *Counseling Theories and Techniques for Rehabilitation Professionals*. New York: Springer Publishing.

Resources

1. Disability and Business Technical Assistance Centers, 1–800–949–4232, www.adata.org.
2. Job Accommodation Network, 1–800–526–7234, www.janwebicdi.wvu.edu
3. Department of Justice, 1–800–514–0301, www.usdoj.gov/crt/ada/adahom1.htm.
4. President's Committee on Employment of People with Disabilities, 1–202–376–6200, www.pcepd.gov.
5. America's Career Infonet, http://www.acinet.org/acinet/
6. U.S. Equal Employment Opportunity Commission (EEOC). For the nearest field office, call 800–669–4000 (voice), 800–669–6820 (TTY). http://www.eeoc.gov/.
7. Strong Interest Inventory is published by Consulting Psychologists Press, Palo Alto, CA. http://www.cpp.com/products/strong/index.asp,
8. Jackson Personality Inventory—Revised is published by Sigma Assessment Systems, Port Huron, MI. http://www.sigmaassessmentsystems.com/assessments/jpir.asp,
9. Wide Range Achievement Test 3 can be purchased from Psychological Assessment Resources, Lutz, FL. http://www3.parinc.com/products/product.aspx?Productid=WRAT3,
10. Valpar is published by Valpar International, Tucson, AZ. http://www.valparint.com/,

62 Driving with a Spinal Cord Disorder

Greg Paquin
Norman F. Simoes
Laurie B. Lindblom

Although driving may not be the primary concern of the rehabilitation staff during the initial rehabilitation process of a patient with a spinal cord disorder, it often becomes of vital importance to the patient shortly after discharge (1). As soon as the person with a spinal cord injury (SCI) becomes engaged in shopping, school, vocational pursuits, and medical appointments, independent transportation becomes very important. In most areas of our society, driving is the ultimate form of independent transportation and is needed to carry out the functions of our lives. The knowledge, for physicians and other rehabilitation staff, of some aspects of driving for people with SCI can make a significant difference in the success these individuals achieve in their pursuit of driving and in the cost of the equipment needed.

This chapter discusses the criteria for determining who can drive, what kind of equipment and training such people may need to drive independently, how such equipment and training needs are determined, and what physicians and other rehabilitation staff can do to improve patients' potential for driving. The scope of alternatives available to drivers with SCI should make physicians and consumers more aware of the importance of driving evaluators.

PHYSICAL REQUIREMENTS

For equivalent levels of spinal cord function, the driving needs of most people with spinal cord disorders are similar, whether the disorder resulted from spinal cord trauma or from other causes, such as tumors or cardiovascular disorders. A person with a spinal cord disorder resulting in intact shoulder girdle innervation (both motor and sensory), and no other complicating factors, has a fair chance to drive. Intact biceps and forearm innervation greatly increase a person's potential for driving.

One must consider the functional abilities presented by the individual and not solely the level of injury when evaluating a person's driving potential. Factors such as nerve root return, variations in the types of injury to the cord itself (central cord syndrome, Brown-Séquard syndrome, etc.), the type and extent of

rehabilitation and personal motivation all play important roles in determining the ability to drive. Some people with C5–6 complete SCI are able to transfer into a car, load their wheelchairs manually, and drive using standard hand controls. Others with the same level of SCI need very sophisticated driving modifications and can operate the controls only after extensive therapy using a specially constructed exercise device. In this chapter, the term *driving* is used to describe the ability to drive safely in all conditions expected to be encountered in normal urban and rural driving; driving is not just the ability to operate the controls of a vehicle in order to move from one location to another at low speed in little or no traffic.

ADAPTIVE EQUIPMENT

The equipment needed may range from $1,200 for a basic hand control in a car for a consumer with paraplegia to $110,000 for a joystick-type control system in a van for a consumer with high-level tetraplegia. The cost difference lies in the type and amount of equipment needed to substitute for the loss of function.

More complex driving systems are normally needed by people with less function, but can be driven by people with more function. Even the most sophisticated driving systems can be driven by able-bodied individuals, as long as they receive training in their use. Less complex systems are often installed in parallel to Original Equipment Manufacturer (OEM) systems, and a driver can use either. More advanced systems replace the OEM systems; some utilize a switch to change from one system to another, and others require that the able-bodied driver use the adaptive system. Adaptive equipment should be matched with the level of individual function to provide sufficient assistance for safe control of the vehicle while reducing cost and the potential for inadvertent overcontrol. There is more than a semantic difference between the equipment people need and the equipment people use. Whereas underequipped consumers are likely to be unsafe drivers, overequipped consumers may also be unsafe drivers, and will have paid far too much for their modifications. Four basic categories of modifications enable people with spinal injuries (or other disabilities) to drive: modifications to provide access to the vehicle and the driving station, modifications to control the speed and direction of the vehicle, modifications to stabilize the driver and protect him or her in the event of an accident, and modifications to control everything else, including shifting, horn, and lights (often called secondary controls).

Vehicle Access

Persons with paraplegia are typically able to transfer into a car independently and to load their wheelchairs into the car (2, 3). Folding wheelchairs can be put into the foot space between the back and front seats. Rigid wheelchairs, after removal of the wheels, can be loaded into the back seat or the passenger seat. Some persons with paraplegia transfer in on the passenger side, slide over to the driver's side, and pull the wheelchair into the passenger seat. The increased use of consoles between front seats has made this option less feasible. A wheelchair stored on the passenger seat should be secured to keep it from falling onto the driver during rapid vehicle maneuvers. Some persons with tetraplegia are able to transfer into a car, but are not able to load the wheelchair. If they have a folding wheelchair, they can use a car top loader (3). After transferring into the vehicle, the consumer attaches a device to the wheelchair that lifts and folds the wheelchair and stows it in a box atop the car. Devices are also available to load scooters into the trunks of cars. If the individual cannot transfer into a car or has a wheelchair (such as a powered wheelchair) that cannot be accommodated in the above manner, a van is usually required.

Consumers who cannot use a car generally choose between minivans and full-sized vans. Minivans are smaller and more economical to operate and fit into home garages. Ground clearance can be a problem, because van floors are typically lowered 10 inches to accommodate a driver in a wheelchair. There is less room to adjust hand controls to take advantage of leverage. Full-sized vans have more room for the storage of vocational or personal items, are based on a truck chassis for durability, and support a greater variety of modifications.

Minivans typically require a combination of a lowered floor and a rear suspension that lowers the vehicle for loading and raises it for driving, thus allowing a wheelchair user to enter and exit the vehicle using a ramp. The ramp either folds out from inside the vehicle or slides from under the floor. Persons with tetraplegia using manual wheelchairs may have difficulty negotiating a ramp. Minivan access modifications typically cost between $15,000 and $18,000.

Full-sized vans require a wheelchair lift to raise the consumer and wheelchair from ground level to van floor level. If only additional headroom is needed, the roof and doorway can be raised. If improved visibility out of the windows or additional headroom is needed, the floor is lowered. Whereas most minivans modified for wheelchair users have side entry (especially for wheelchair drivers), full-sized vans may have the entry on the side or rear. Side entry allows more functional passenger seating, especially in the rear of the vehicle. Rear entry typically allows greater freedom in parking lots, because the wheelchair driver need not rely on neighboring cars' leaving enough room for reentry into the van. Most vans with side lifts (and minivans with ramps) require almost 8 feet next to the van for the consumer to enter or exit. Both minivans and full-sized vans typically use powered doors for independent access for consumers in wheelchairs. Although most consumers depend on interior and exterior switches for the doors and lifting device, consumers who cannot operate the switches can purchase wireless controls. Access modifications to full-sized vans vary considerably, because there are many types available. Costs range from $9,000 to $22,000.

Great care must be exercised by the consumer in the selection of the vehicle, not just for function but for availability of modifications (4). Only certain minivans are modified by large companies, called *second stage manufacturers*. Consumers must always check on the feasibility of the installation of the modifications needed before purchasing a vehicle. Many consumers have been very frustrated upon finding that they purchased a vehicle that could not be modified to meet their needs.

Once inside the van, the consumer may transfer out of the wheelchair into the driver's seat using a device called a *transfer seat*. A wheelchair seat is normally about 6 inches higher than a typical van seat. The transfer seat uses a van seat mounted on a special seat base that moves back several inches, raises about 6 inches and, if necessary, swivels to facilitate the transfer (2). Many consumers who cannot transfer into a car with a standard seat can use a transfer seat in a van, because it reduces the horizontal and vertical distance required during the transfer.

If the consumer cannot use a transfer seat, he or she must drive from the wheelchair. There are wheelchair securement devices designed (and crash-tested) specifically to hold a particular wheelchair in the driver's position (5). An individual who drives from a wheelchair and wants to purchase a new wheelchair will need to determine whether a securement device is available for that chair model. The selection of an appropriate wheelchair is one area in which physicians and other rehabilitation staff can make significant contributions to the success of the consumer in the vehicle purchase (3, 4). Because the wheelchair sits higher than a van seat, the vehicle floor will usually need to be lowered to allow proper visibility out of the windshield and better access to the driving controls. A lower wheelchair seat height may lead to fewer structural modifications in a full-size van but may leave a shorter consumer sitting too low in a minivan. Floor lowering gives rise to many technical issues, such as positioning of the fuel tank and structural integrity of the vehicle (6).

In general, exiting the vehicle is the reverse of entering, with one significant exception. Regardless of how the vehicle is entered, consumers should never exit vehicles by backing onto the lift or the ramp. They should always face out from the vehicle. Consumers have been injured, even killed, because they backed out over the edge of the van doorway and fell after the lift had been lowered to the ground. Newly established Federal Motor Vehicle Safety Standards address this issue with the manufacture and installation of wheelchair lifts.

Speed and Direction Control

If leg function is sufficiently affected by the SCI to prevent safe operation of the gas and brake pedals, the consumer normally uses some type of hand control. A hand control is simply a device that allows the operation of the gas and brake pedals with the hands. Some of the first hand controls were made for the Model A Fords (2, 7). In 1967, 35–40% of the approximately 6,000 members of the Paralyzed Veterans of America were tetraplegic.

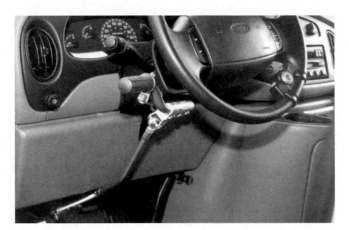

Figure 62.1 Push-right angle-pull hand control.

Of these, about 20 members had "devised means of independent highway travel" (8). This was about the time hand controls and wheelchair lifts became commercially available.

The most common hand control is called the *push-right angle-pull hand control*, seen in Figure 62.1. With this control, which is mounted under the steering column, the consumer pushes forward on a handle to operate the brakes. For gas, the handle is pulled down toward the leg (at a right angle to the direction of the application of the brake). Other varieties of the standard hand control include a twist grip (as on a motorcycle) for the accelerator or push-pull (push forward to brake, pull back to accelerate). Floor-mounted push-pull controls are available and can provide improved leverage. These types of hand control sell for $1,200–$2,000 installed. There are several varieties of hand controls designed to suit special purposes (9).

Many people with tetraplegia find it difficult to push down on or twist a handle for the accelerator. A push-pull hand control can have a *terminal device* (a term used in the industry to refer to the part used by the consumer to interface with the control system) to accommodate the person's limited grip strength, mounted on a rod attached to the hand control. The consumer pushes forward to brake and pulls back to accelerate. The forces are in the 5- to 12-pound range, but the motions are in a direction more favorable to the functional abilities of a person with tetraplegia. These controls often use a device called a *tri-pin* for the terminal device. The tri-pin has three vertical posts. The rear two posts fit on either side of the wrist (in the neutral position), and the forward post goes across the palm of the hand and into the thumb web space. Tri-pins are frequently used for drivers without a functional grip.

If the forces needed to operate a mechanical hand control exceed a consumer's functional abilities, the consumer may use a powered hand control. Figure 62.2 shows a powered control (with the terminal device left off to provide a better view of the control). Powered hand controls use power from the vehicle (vacuum, hydraulic, electric, etc.) to translate the driver's input to the terminal device into forces from an actuator that then pushes on the gas and brake pedals as appropriate. The forces needed to operate this control are measured in ounces (usually under 1 pound), with a total travel length from full gas to full brake of approximately 4 inches. A powered hand control costs between $6,000 and $20,000, depending on brand and features.

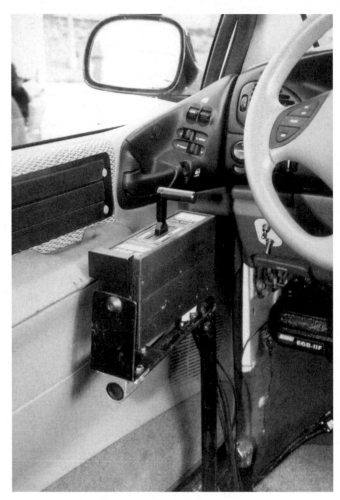

Figure 62.2 Powered hand control.

Most drivers control the direction of the vehicle using the OEM steering wheel. Because most spinal-injured consumers use hand controls, which occupy one hand, only one hand remains for steering. Most hand control users need a terminal device attached to the steering wheel, such as a knob, a cuff, or a tri-pin, which can spin freely while maintaining constant contact with the wheel during rapid movements, such as a swerve in an evasive maneuver. Some consumers prefer to "palm" the wheel, but this can result in a loss of control when it is most needed. If the consumer has difficulty turning the steering wheel, the OEM power steering system can be modified for low-effort steering (reducing the force by half) or zero-effort steering (reducing the force to only about a tenth of that originally needed). Minivans are about 50% harder to steer than full-sized vans, and the effort needed to steer them cannot be reduced as much as on a full-sized van. Reducing the effort costs $1,500–$2,500, with an additional $2,000–$3,000 for a backup system designed to take over in the event of certain types of power steering failures.

If contractures or kyphosis position the driver's sternum within 10 inches from the steering wheel, the air bag should be turned off. However, the vehicle must be equipped with a switch to turn the air bag back on, making it available for able-bodied drivers. The consumer may need a letter from a physician documenting this physical functional limitation in order to have an air bag switch installed. The steering column can also be extended to accommodate wheelchair size and configuration. Steering wheel diameter is a factor if the consumer has elbow flexion contractures. Although reduced-diameter steering wheels are available, they do not have air bags. The consumer is no longer required to obtain permission from the National Highway Traffic Safety Administration (6) for removal of the air bag, but may need a letter from a physician documenting this physical functional limitation in order to drive without an air bag. Smaller steering wheels and steering column extensions generally cost under $500.

If the use of the OEM steering wheel is not functionally feasible, remote steering systems can be used. Figure 62.3 shows a remote steering control system with a knob-type terminal device. The driver turns a small steering wheel, attached to a small box, which uses computer technology to operate the steering system. The OEM steering wheel is often left in place for the air bag and for able-bodied drivers. The box can be placed in any location in the vehicle and at any orientation necessary for safe operation by the consumer. Remote steering systems cost $10,000–$22,000.

Some consumers lack the strength in one arm to operate either the gas/brake system or the steering system. They need a complete system that can be operated with only one hand (2). One-handed control systems generally require less force to operate than other systems and allow the driver to lay the hand not used for steering on an armrest, greatly increasing stability and control. There are two systems currently available: tri-pin or joystick-controlled. Figure 62.4 shows a one-handed steering system with a tri-pin terminal device: the driver pushes to accelerate, pulls back to brake, and rotates the forearm to turn. Diminished range of motion anywhere in the elbow or wrist can affect a consumer's ability to operate the system. This system has been successful with relatively high-level tetraplegics and has been commercially available since 1974 (10).

The other one-handed operation system uses a joystick-type control not unlike those used on electric wheelchairs. This type of joystick control does not provide feedback to the driver about the rate of turn of the vehicle. Whereas this system has been used with great success for consumers with weak shoulders and elbows but good hands (e.g., from muscular dystrophy, from multiple sclerosis, post polio, etc.) who are able to make rapid, small, precise inputs to the control lever, consumers with higher-level tetraplegia who have little muscular strength or proprioception

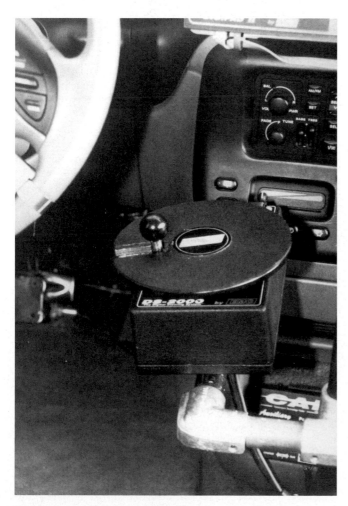

Figure 62.3 Remote steering control.

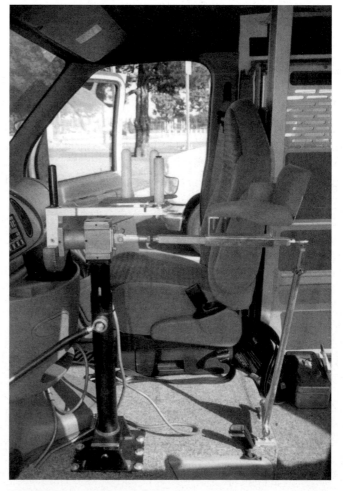

Figure 62.4 One-handed driving system.

below the shoulder and upper arm find it more difficult to control. Both of these one-handed control systems cost $40,000–$70,000.

Driver Stability

Individuals with diminished upper extremity function as a result of an SCI usually also lack trunk stability. They do not have the musculature to maintain their body upright (5) or the sensation (except through the inner ear) to know that they are beginning to fall. Consumers with low thoracic paraplegia have trunk control and strong shoulders and hands to assist in balance. Those with tetraplegia must depend on the wheelchair for stability while driving. Having one hand on a steering wheel with very low forces needed to move the wheel and a powered hand control with very low forces needed to accelerate and brake leaves the driver with tetraplegia "floating" in his or her wheelchair. It also leaves this driver entirely dependent on a chest harness for trunk stability—and, therefore, vehicle control. If the chest harness is not attached to a stable wheelchair back, the person's trunk stability may be inadequate for safe driving. Sometimes, the addition of shoulder pads provides stability during turns.

The driver must also use safety belts. Although the OEM shoulder/lap belt combinations work for able-bodied drivers, disabled drivers may not be able to use such safety belts. Common practice in the industry has been to use a shoulder belt under which the consumer can drive in the wheelchair, as well as a lap belt attached to the wheelchair. Although this method has proved effective, the means of attaching the belt ends to the vehicle and wheelchair have not been standardized at this time. The vehicle modification industry, SAE (11), and NHTSA (12) are working on the problem of standards in this area.

Secondary Controls

Once it has been determined how the consumer with a SCI will access the driver's station and accelerate, brake, and steer, all other controls must be considered. Although the alternatives are numerous, some items should be highlighted. Specific knobs and levers can be modified for the consumer's use simply by extending them or putting wire loops on them (13). Powered shifters and powered parking brakes allow these manual functions to be controlled by push buttons. The consumer must be able to reach some controls while driving (horn, signals, etc.). Others can be operated when the vehicle is stopped (doors, windows, etc.) (14). If only a few controls must be moved, it is sometimes possible to add an additional switch. Newer vehicles may require specially manufactured control panels, each of which costs $2,000–$10,000.

DRIVING PROGRAMS

The scope of the alternatives should suggest the complexity of selecting modifications for a driver with a SCI. Because of this, the profession of *driving evaluator* has been recognized as an essential component to providing proper equipment for the consumer with a SCI. There have been driving evaluators since the mid-1970s; however, the criteria required for this role have only been agreed on in the last 10–15 years and are still being revised (4). The leading organization for driving evaluators in the nation is the Association of Driver Educators for the Disabled (ADED) (15), which certifies driving rehabilitation specialists. Despite the availability of a certification system, there is still little information in the literature about the current assessment techniques used in these evaluation programs (16). In the ADED model, the driving evaluator is normally an occupational therapist. Many occupational therapists have also become driving instructors and can fulfill both roles. Driving instructors are usually unable to perform the functional assessment portion of the evaluation unless they are registered therapists of some type.

Many driver rehabilitation programs operate with a team, which may include an occupational therapist as a driving evaluator, a rehabilitation engineer, and a driving instructor. The physician is the primary referral source and must write a prescription requesting the evaluation.

A proper driving evaluation (4) has three main components: pre-driving evaluation, vehicle selection and evaluation, and behind-the-wheel training. The pre-driving evaluation is usually performed by an occupational therapist or driving evaluator and consists of a review of the candidate's medical and driving history and a clinical assessment. The clinical assessment determines the functional capabilities of the person and obtains information in a number of areas. The visual portion assesses acuity, depth perception, field of vision, and other parameters important for driving. Cognitive functions, such as judgment, problem solving, memory, attention, and the recognition of signs and symbols, are screened. Range of motion, hand function, mobility skills, strength, balance, muscle tone, and other physical examination features are evaluated. A driving simulator may be used to assess coordination, brake reaction time, and potential equipment needs. Simulators are no longer used for all portions of the evaluation, because the effects of the dynamic aspects of driving (acceleration, deceleration, and lateral acceleration when cornering) on the driver and wheelchair are extremely difficult and expensive to simulate. The existence of higher technologies in driving has made an on-the-road portion of the evaluation increasingly important (17).

The vehicle selection process involves team members' forming recommendations about the type of vehicle needed. An equipment evaluation is performed, and a prescription (a specific report of equipment and training needed) is formulated. A vehicle modifier company must be selected, keeping in mind that the modifiers have vast variations in experience, especially with high-technology modifications. Often this decision is made by the third-party payer (18). After the vehicle is modified, the driving instructor ensures that the driver can use the controls as installed and assesses the fit of the equipment. A final mechanical inspection should be based on local (19) or national standards (11, 12).

The final component is the behind-the-wheel training by a driving instructor. The driver needs a valid license or learner's permit to undergo this training. The evaluations for higher-level consumers with tetraplegia are made longer not only because the equipment is more complex, but because that complexity requires more training to enable instructors to subject the consumer to conditions (freeways, construction zones, evasive maneuvers, etc.) that cannot be tested immediately. Consumers must learn to drive the system well enough to cope with situations in which balance and dynamic forces will affect driving (4). To send a consumer on the road with a modern sophisticated driving system and only the experience of driving in a parking lot is not sufficient to determine whether he or she has the strength required to move the controls through all possible necessary motions; to do so can lead to disastrous results. Another consideration is the new driver. The evaluator's observations of perceptual and cognitive limitations may be tainted by the driver's lack of experience behind the wheel. In these situations, training can be conducted as part of the evaluation to remove that possibility from the conjecture.

Some people do not feel that a complete evaluation is necessary for lower-level SCI and instead are of the opinion that if a consumer with paraplegia has no other disabilities, a vehicle modifier can simply install a hand control. Most vehicle modifiers, however, will not install any driving modifications without an evaluation, owing to liability considerations. Most people in the industry agree that training is needed after the purchase of almost all vehicle modifications. A consumer with a SCI learning to use a hand control may confuse the accelerator and the brake. Despite significant progress in learning new skills, a person subjected to an emergency situation will often revert to long-established habits and patterns. The simplest of control modifications, a left-foot gas pedal, is the device that carries with it the highest liability, for drivers often think they need no training to operate it.

ADED (15) has a website (www.driver-ed.org), and the American Automobile Association (AAA) keeps a file, listing driving evaluation programs and instructors. Many state departments of vocational rehabilitation have active programs for funding modifications to allow consumers to return to work and can be resources for finding local driving evaluation programs and instructors. The National Mobility Equipment Dealers Association (NMEDA) (12) can provide information about local vehicle modifiers. Many auto manufacturers (e.g., Ford, General Motors, Toyota, Chrysler) have mobility programs to provide drivers who have disabilities information about their products and about sources of driving evaluations and vehicle modifications.

PREPARATION FOR DRIVING

The physician and other members of the rehabilitation team can prepare a patient who has SCI to drive. Preparations include physical rehabilitation and training, recommendation and prescription of durable medical equipment, and the furnishing of the patient's history. It is important that the rehabilitation team become familiar with local driving programs, equipment suppliers, and other resources for potential drivers.

The secondary effects of a spinal cord disorder, such as decubiti and contractures, weigh heavily on driving equipment needs or even the ability to drive. Other aspects of normal rehabilitation training take on special significance if the patient with an SCI becomes a driver. Awareness of the lack of thermal sensation in the hands can help prevent injury from a metal or plastic part of a driving control system that has been sitting in the sun for hours. The consumer's specific awareness of pressure relief during long drives or potential scrapes while transferring may keep him out of the hospital. Learning safe car transfer techniques under a knowledgeable therapist's supervision can prevent injuries. Because driving allows consumers to be independent, they may be alone when they encounter problems. They need to be aware of the effects of heat when first entering a closed vehicle on a hot day. They should be aware of the potential for autonomic dysreflexia, and of what interventions should be followed. Some consumers with tetraplegia carry a note from their physician or a wallet card describing the most appropriate treatment for their autonomic dysreflexia as information for emergency care professionals who are not familiar with the condition. Most phone services have special rates for cell phones for consumers with disabilities.

Patients whose SCI resulted from trauma should have a careful neurologic check for head trauma. Many consumers with SCI receive a blow to the head either as a cause of or secondary to their SCI, and perceptual problems severe enough to affect or even prevent driving can result from such head trauma (20). Consumers with spina bifida are also known to have a high incidence of perceptual problems that can affect the processing of visual information and even the awareness of which side of the road they are on. A major concern with respect to consumers with perceptual problems is that they are usually not aware of the existence of such problems. Even when written and on-the-road tests indicate such a problem, they may exhibit strong denial, because they cannot sense the problem. Early diagnosis and counseling about such problems may reduce the number of consumers who attempt to drive yet should not be driving. With the proper equipment and training, however, drivers with SCI who do not have perceptual problems can be safe drivers (21).

As regards driving, important actions the physician can take including informing the patient about the existence of driving evaluation programs and referring the consumer to such programs when appropriate. The physician should also inform patients of the need for professional driver training before use of any adaptive equipment. Many accidents have occurred when appropriate equipment has been installed that has then been used by a consumer who has not been trained to use the modifications.

Most driving evaluation programs (especially hospital-based programs) need a physician's referral for a driving evaluation. Although a note on a prescription pad stating "Evaluate for driving" has been the basis for many evaluations, much more information is needed. An accurate diagnosis is a vital starting point, including whether the injury is complete or incomplete. Any secondary conditions, such as contractures, spasticity, or perceptual difficulties, should be described. Medical stability, the effects of medications, and any planned surgeries, such as tendon transfers, are important factors to communicate as well.

WHEELCHAIR SELECTION

The wheelchair is the basic support platform for any consumer with spinal cord tetraplegia who wishes to drive (22). The more stable the platform, the greater the likelihood of success. A reclining wheelchair may seem necessary while the consumer is an inpatient and has not yet learned other means of pressure relief. The motion allowed by the multiple joints of the recliner mechanism may, however, prevent a consumer from being a driver. The physician and rehabilitation staff must weigh the immediate alternatives of preventing pressure ulcers in that manner against the later need to be a safe driver. Wheelchair back height is also a frequent cause of driving problems. The driver with tetraplegia is dependent on a belt-type chest harness that attaches to his or her wheelchair and passes just under the axilla and across the sternum, for maximum support (5). The physician must assess the consumer's request for a lower wheelchair back for cosmetic appearance. They must consider access to back packs or the patient's ability to hook her elbow on the back upright for trunk support against the actual need for trunk support in driving. It should be noted that lateral trunk supports attached to wheelchairs are often not effective in driving. They tend not to be high enough, or to interfere with the arm movements needed for driving. Proper wheelchair back support is also important in the prevention of scoliosis, which can cause problems in reaching controls and steering. It can also affect the fitting of a chest harness, needed to provide trunk stability for cornering.

Physicians should evaluate and describe the patient's spasticity. Spasticity in the upper extremities can be a difficult obstacle to overcome. The consumer's ability to handle the driving controls (normally, in a driving evaluation) is the final determinant of the effect on driving. Drivers may be able to cope with mild spasticity, but severe spasticity can prevent them from driving safely. There is also a difference in the effects of increased tone caused by spasticity (which can affect both reaction time and the force that is applied to the controls) and actual spasms (which can cause inadvertent control inputs or prevent intended inputs). Unfortunately, many of the drugs prescribed to reduce the effects of spasticity in daily activities adversely affect the alertness of the driver.

The driver's destinations are a factor when considering the choice of a wheelchair. If the consumer is only marginally able to use a manual wheelchair but prefers the manual wheelchair for exercise, her ability to be truly independent in the community (including by using ramps, etc.) becomes more critical when driving to unknown destinations. There may be indications (23) that these individuals are putting excessive stress on their shoulders and should thus consider a powered wheelchair. Driving from the wheelchair is often indicated for marginal manual wheelchair users to avoid the extra transfers, but the extra weight of the wheelchair securement device, added to the manual wheelchair, can cause additional problems. Manual wheelchairs having extreme camber in the rear wheels may be too wide to fit on lifts and into lowered floor areas for wheelchair driving.

CONCLUSION

Many people with spinal cord disorders at the C4–5 level can drive, as can most people with spinal cord disorders at the C5–6 level. Whereas lack of the funds required to purchase the high-level technology needed for safe driving is probably the most frequent reason that those with higher levels of SCI do not drive, secondary disabilities such as perceptual problems, contractures, pressure ulcers, and other injuries can also diminish driving potential. For all these consumers, a driving evaluation by a professional evaluator is needed; for the higher-level injuries, it is no less than essential. The primary role of the physician and rehabilitation staff, with respect to the driving consumer, is to maximize the patient's rehabilitation progress, prevent complications from the spinal cord disorder, and identify and treat secondary disabilities. It is also important to ensure that the consumer leaves the hospital with a wheelchair that is appropriate for driving, as well as suitable to the needs of daily life. Informing patients about evaluation programs and referring them to such programs can save patients money by helping them avoid inappropriate modifications.

References

1. Dip R. COT. An investigation into the employment and occupation of patients with a spinal cord injury. *Paraplegia* 1994; 32:182–187.
2. Koppa R. State of the art in automotive adaptive equipment. *Human Factors* 1990; 32(4):439–455.
3. Pierce S. Driver's needs. *Team Rehab Report* 1992; Jan/Feb:20–22, 38.
4. Pierce S. A roadmap for driver rehabilitation. *OT Practice* 1996; Oct:31–38.
5. Babirad Juergen MSA. Considerations in seating and positioning severely disabled drivers. *Assist Tech* 1989; 1:31–37.
6. National Highway Traffic Safety Administration. Exemption from the make inoperative prohibition; final rule (2001). Federal Motor Vehicle Safety Standards, 49 CFR, part 595. Washington D.C.
7. Murphy, Eugene (Ph.D.). Reflections on automotive adaptive equipment. *Bull Prosth Res* Fall 1979; 10–32:191–207.
8. Bray P, Cunningham DM. Vehicles for the severely disabled. *Rehabilitation Literature* 1967; Apr:28(4):98–109.
9. Reichenberger A. Licensed motor vehicles for handicapped drivers; report of a workshop. *National Academy of Sciences* 1975; 69–75.
10. Gacioch M. Vans, vans and more vans. *Mainstream* 1989; Dec:7–17.
11. Society of Automotive Engineers. *SAE Handbook*. Warrendale PA.
12. National Mobility Equipment Dealers Association Guidelines. Tampa: National Mobility Equipment Dealers Association, 1999.
13. Sklar J. An introduction to van modifications for the disabled. *J Traf Safe Edu* 1981; July:11–12, 27.
14. Roush L, Koppa R. A Survey of activation importance of individual secondary controls in modified vehicles. *Assist Technol* 1992; 4:66–99.
15. Association of Driver Rehabilitation Specialists (ADED), P.O. Box 49, Edgerton, WI 53534.
16. French D, Hanson C. Survey of driver rehabilitation programs. *Am J Occup Ther* 1999; 53(4):394–397.
17. Britell C. Van modifications for wheelchair accommodation, transportation I. *A State of the Art Conference on Personal Transportation for Persons with Disabilities.* NIDRR and University of Virginia, 1991; 1–3.
18. Rogers J. Adaptive devices for automobiles. *J Traf Safe Edu* 1975; 9–11.
19. State of California, Department of Rehabilitation requirements for adaptive driving equipment, 1998 (part of Master Agreement with vehicle modifiers).
20. Sivak M, Olson PL, Kewman DG, Hosik W, Henson DL. Driving and perceptual/cognitive skills: behavioral consequences of brain damage. *Arch Phys Med Rehabil* 1981; 62:476–483.
21. Katz RT, Golden RS, Tepper D, Rothke S, Holmes J, Sahgal V. Driving safety after brain damage: follow-up of twenty-two patients with matched controls. *Arch Phys Med Rehabil* 1990; 71:133–137.
22. Simoes NF. Van modifications for wheelchair accommodation, Transportation I. *A State of the Art Conference on Personal Transportation for Persons with Disabilities.* NIDRR and University of Virginia, 1991; 12–14.
23. Smith I. Aging with spinal cord injury. *Rehab Management* 1989; June/July:28–35.

63 Functional Electrical Stimulation

Peter H. Gorman
Chester H. Ho

Functional electrical stimulation (FES) is the technique of applying safe levels of electric current to activate the damaged or disabled nervous system. FES is sometimes referred to as *functional neuromuscular stimulation* (FNS) or *neuromuscular electrical stimulation* (NMES). In practice and in the literature, the terms FES, FNS, and NMES are often used interchangeably. The term *neuroprosthesis* refers to a device that uses electrical stimulation to activate the nervous system.

Therapeutic electrical stimulation is used often in practice by physical therapists. Their goals when using this modality include muscle strengthening, improving range of motion, facilitation and reeducation of voluntary motor function, and temporary inhibition of spasticity. True FES—that is, the use of electricity to restore functional movement that has been lost due to neurologic impairment—is a less common application and has only recently become clinically relevant. This chapter examines both the therapeutic and functional aspects of the application of electricity as applied to individuals with spinal cord injury (SCI) and disease.

Although modern FES is a relatively recent technology, the use of electricity for medicinal purposes dates back to the beginning of the Common Era. The electrical discharges of the torpedo fish were used for treatment of headache and gout in 46 AD. With the advent of electrical generators and storage devices (i.e., capacitors) in the eighteenth century, practitioners (including Benjamin Franklin) reported on the involuntary contraction of muscle, and some touted the use of electrical charges to cure paralytic disease (1). However, until recently, the applicability to persons with disability had not been demonstrated. In more modern times, Liberson et. al. proposed the first FES aid for ambulation in the form of a foot-drop peroneal stimulator in 1961 (2). Later in the same decade, Wilemon first used implanted electrodes and the technique of radio frequency coupling for stimulation across the skin (3). Further escalation of biomedical engineering research during the 1970s and 1980s led to prototypes of clinical FES systems for restoring function in various paralytic conditions. This work then led to multicenter clinical trials in the 1990s that have culminated in regulatory approval of several commercial devices. Clearly, with the advent of both advanced microelectronics and the explosion of knowledge in both basic and clinical neuroscience, rehabilitation medicine has now been provided with the technology and the scientific basis to achieve clinically relevant applications for modern FES (4).

MECHANISM OF FES ACTIVATION

Both nerve and muscle cells have excitable membranes with internal negative resting potentials. When an external electric field is applied to a nerve via two electrodes (there must always be at least two electrodes to complete an electrical circuit), depolarization of the axon below the cathode, or negative electrode, occurs. As the potential decreases under the cathode, the membrane becomes more permeable to sodium (Na^+) ions, which in turn causes further depolarization of the nerve as Na^+ moves into the cell. If this depolarization occurs with sufficient intensity and at a rapid enough rate, the membrane reaches its threshold and an action potential occurs. Thus, the *voltage gated Na^+ channel* is responsible for the generation of the all-or-none action potential. A separate *voltage gated potassium (K^+) channel* is in turn responsible for subsequent repolarization of the nerve. Further description of this topic can be found in standard neurophysiology textbooks such as that by Kandel, Schwartz, and Jessell (5).

Motor units, which consist of axons and the nerve fibers that they innervate, are activated electrically by depolarization of the motor axons or the terminal nerve branches at the neuromuscular junction. Electrical current can directly depolarize muscle fibers, but the amount of current necessary for this to occur is considerably greater than that required for depolarization of nerve axons (6). Therefore, for practical purposes, FES systems stimulate nerves, not muscles. Some literature exists on the electrical stimulation of denervated muscle, but the clinical effect of this remains controversial (7). One concern is that direct muscle stimulation, although it retards muscle atrophy, may (at least theoretically and in some animal models) prevent reinnervation through the inhibition of terminal sprouting and the reformation of neuromuscular junctions (8).

Current density, or the amount of current injected per unit area, is the ultimate determinant of whether a given stimulation will generate action potentials and therefore recruit motor units. Electrode size helps determine the current density, because the smaller electrodes have the greatest current densities under or around them. For surface electrodes, the electrode–skin interface is also quite important, because changes in impedance of this interface can considerably alter the current density under the electrode.

Several important parameters can be adjusted during the application of FES. These include *pulse amplitude* and *duration, frequency, waveform,* and *duty cycle* (9). Pulse amplitude (in milliamps) and duration (in microseconds) are parameters that determine the size of individual pulses provided by a stimulator through a set of electrodes. As either is increased above threshold, spatial recruitment of additional motor units occurs, thereby increasing the number of nerve axons activated and, subsequently, the muscle force output. The product of the amplitude and duration, or the area under the square wave pulse (if that is the type of pulse being used) represents the net charge injected into the tissue. A direct linear relationship does not usually exist between the amount of charge injected and the force output of the muscle being stimulated. Rather, there is often an S-shaped curve describing this strength–duration relationship. Within this recruitment curve exists a section in which there is a very high gain—that is, for very small changes in pulse width or amplitude, large changes in force output occur. This relationship is important when attempting gradual proportional recruitment of motor strength.

Pulse frequency determines the rate at which the nerve fires. Increasing pulse frequency provides for temporal summation of force output. For most applications, it is desirable to have a fused or tetanic contraction of muscle. This occurs at 20–30 Hertz (Hz, cycles per second) physiologically, although some fusion of contraction can be obtained at externally applied frequencies as low as 12 Hz. For FES, the tradeoff as stimulating frequency is increased (thereby obtaining a smoother contraction) is more rapid muscle fatigue.

Waveforms available for use in FES applications include monophasic, asymmetric biphasic, and symmetric biphasic. *Monophasic stimulation,* wherein ion flow is unidirectional, is generally not appropriate for long-term FES use, because it can cause electrode and tissue breakdown (10). A balanced pulse, wherein ion flow occurs in both directions sequentially, avoids these problems and allows for stimulation at both electrodes. Commonly, square waves are used for the first of the two pulses, and then a capacitively coupled discharge is employed as the balancing second pulse.

The *duty cycle* is the percentage of time that the stimulator is on, and is sometimes expressed as a ratio of "on" time to "off" time. The greater the duty cycle, the more profound the problem with muscle fatigue, because the time of rest is reduced. Duty cycles play a role in devices such as the bladder neuroprosthesis, in which intermittent stimulation is desirable to achieve the desired result (see subsequent further discussion of this topic).

Just like muscles undergoing voluntary exercise, FES-stimulated muscles change morphologically and physiologically. Type II ("fast twitch," fatigable) glycolytic fibers convert to Type I ("slow twitch," fatigue-resistant) oxidative fibers over weeks to months, depending on the intensity and frequency of stimulation.

This phenomenon, which is associated with changes in vascular supply, increases the fatigue resistance of the muscle (10). One question that remains only incompletely answered is how much FES exercise is adequate to achieve the fiber changes and therefore allow for fatigue resistant functional use. This is important clinically as one sets up conditioning protocols for patients using FES devices.

COMPONENTS OF FES SYSTEMS

FES systems typically consist of multiple components, including an electronic stimulator, a control mechanism, cabling, and electrodes.

The electronic stimulator is usually battery-powered, although it can be powered from electrically or optically isolated power sources (the isolation being necessary for safety reasons). Stimulators range in sophistication and in number of channels; such devices are as complex as the movement they are designed to produce. Most portable FES neuroprostheses are built around a microprocessor-controlled set of stimulators. The microprocessor may be preprogrammed or may allow software modification of the stimulator output. The number of stimulator channels varies with application from one to twenty-four or more. Various channels are activated sequentially or in unison to allow microprocessor orchestration of complex movements.

Control systems for therapist-operated FES systems consist of dials and switches to control stimulus parameters. For subject-controlled FES systems (i.e., neuroprostheses), control can come in the form of switches, buttons, joysticks, joint position sensors, EMG electrodes, voice-activated controls, sip-and-puff devices, heel switches, and the like.

Electrodes provide the interface between the electrical stimulator and the nervous system. Different types of electrodes that have been used include surface, percutaneous intramuscular, implantable intramuscular, epimysial, and nerve cuff electrodes. In routine physical therapy practice, *surface electrodes* are exclusively used. Options are available with regard to material, size, and means of application. The key criteria are that the electrode–skin interface be of low impedance, that the electrode be flexible enough to accommodate contours, and that the electrode be easy to put on and take off. *Percutaneous intramuscular electrodes* travel across the skin to insert into muscle. They are usually inserted through the use of a hypodermic needle and have a barbed end to ensure stability inside the muscle. Percutaneous electrodes have been used, primarily in developmental research protocols or where temporary application of FES is anticipated. Their long-term survival has not been as great as that for implanted electrodes (11). *Implantable intramuscular electrodes* are more robust than the percutaneous versions, mainly because of their thicker lead wires. *Epimysial electrodes* are surgically sewn onto the epimysial surface of a muscle. They typically have a conductive core or disc (made from metal alloys such as platinum-iridium) and a surrounding silicone elastomer skirt that allows for surgical stabilization. *Nerve cuff electrodes*, as their name implies, directly stimulate nerves by surrounding them circumferentially. Implanted intramuscular, epimysial, and nerve cuff electrodes require surgical placement. Implanted cables (or leads) link the stimulator and the stimulating electrode and are complex in design to withstand bending stresses and to remain insulated in the body's saline environment.

Subject control of an FES system can be either *open loop* or *closed loop*. These terms are borrowed from the engineering literature and describe the mechanism of feedback that is provided. In open-loop control, the electrical output of the FES system is dependent not on the muscular force or joint movement produced by the stimulation, but rather on the stimulator itself. In closed-loop control, real-time information on muscle force and/or joint position or movement is fed back into the FES system and allows for the modification of its electrical output. This allows for a more responsive result that can accommodate for external variables such as irregularities in the environment or muscle fatigue. Practical problems are associated with closed-loop FES, however, that relate to the need for sensors to measure force and joint position or angular velocity in a physiologically reproducible and cosmetically acceptable way (12).

GENERAL SELECTION CRITERIA FOR FES SYSTEMS IN SCI

SCI damages both the long tracts and the spinal-level neurons—or, in terms of the motor system, both upper and lower motor neurons. When anterior horn cells or motor nerve roots are injured, corresponding muscular denervation inevitably follows. If this denervation involves a significant quantity of musculature, then FES will no longer be effective. This is principally because of the profound increase in charge density (by a factor of approximately thirty) required to directly depolarize muscle versus nerve, as previously mentioned. For specific applications, the "significant quantity" of denervated musculature required to render FES ineffective varies. For phrenic nerve pacing, nerve conduction studies (looking at response latencies) or fluoroscopy of the diaphragm during supramaximal tetanic stimulation can be used to screen candidates for diaphragmatic denervation (13). In the case of upper extremity devices, the possibility exists for the associated use of tendon transfer surgery (for implanted devices) to replace one or two crucial denervated muscles with paralyzed but innervated muscles to provide specific aspects of motor movement. For the lower extremity and in bladder neuroprostheses, denervation is less frequently a problem, because the anterior horn cells often lie below the level of the SCI, and therefore are physiologically intact. Individuals with conus medullaris or cauda equina injuries, however, are not good FES candidates, because of the considerable extent of denervation associated with those injury levels.

Contractures can often develop in the hands or the legs of individuals post-SCI. If they are severe enough, these contractures can be a severe impediment to implementation of a neural prosthesis. The prevention of these contractures and tendon shortenings early in the rehabilitation process is crucial to maintaining later candidacy for neuroprostheses.

The time post-injury is not as crucial a criterion for candidacy as once thought. It has been standard practice in upper extremity reconstructive surgery for tetraplegia to wait at least 1 year post-injury before performing any surgical procedures in order to allow time for natural recovery. Recently, this philosophy has been challenged, and individuals have had implant procedures as early as 6 months post-injury. On the other side of the spectrum, there is no outer limit as to the time post-injury for neuroprosthetic consideration. Often, however, individuals who are many years post-SCI have become accustomed to their way of performing tasks, and therefore are less receptive to a neuroprosthetic approach, especially if it requires an invasive procedure.

CONTRAINDICATIONS

Although no absolute contraindications exist for the use of externally applied FES, a patient with a cardiac demand pacemaker or an automatic implanted defibrillator should be approached with extreme caution. There have been some reports that electrical stimulation applied anywhere on the body has the potential to interfere with the sensing portion of the demand pacemaker, thereby suppressing activation of the device (14). Some of the relative contraindications for FES include patients with cardiac arrhythmias, congestive heart failure, pregnancy, electrode sensitivity, and patients with healing wound(s) that could be stressed during stimulation (i.e., muscle stimulation would adversely move healing tissues).

For implanted FES systems, the presence of an implanted cardiac pacemaker, active or recurrent sepsis, or uncontrolled spasticity are absolute contraindications to the surgery. As with any implant in the body, individuals with implanted FES systems need to obtain antibiotic prophylaxis when undergoing invasive procedures such as oral surgery (15). Some FES implants (e.g., the Freehand® hand grasp and the Vocare® bladder systems described in later sections) have been shown to be compatible with magnetic resonance imaging, and the FDA-approved label has been changed to reflect this. This was previously a concern in the SCI population, in light of the relatively frequent use of MRI for evaluation in those patients suspected of having a syringomyelia.

The Medtronic Corporation issued a safety alert regarding the use of short wave diathermy, microwave diathermy, and therapeutic ultrasound diathermy for patients implanted with any of its neurostimulation systems (16). The concern raised was that the use of diathermy could cause heating at the electrode–tissue interface that could produce tissue or nerve damage. Neuro-Control Corporation, the company previously responsible for the Freehand® and the Vocare® system, had also indicated that these modalities should not be performed over the area of their implanted stimulators or electrodes lest doing so damage the components (17). In general, therefore, it is prudent to avoid these modalities in patients with implanted electrical stimulators.

FES APPLICATIONS IN SPINAL CORD DYSFUNCTION

Therapeutic FES can be used for muscle strengthening and cardiac conditioning. Other potential benefits of this type of electrical exercise are improvement in venous return from the legs, reduction of osteoporosis, improvement in bowel function, and psychologic benefits (18).

Functional uses for FES after SCI include applications in standing; walking; hand grasp (and release); bladder, bowel, and sexual function; respiratory assist; electroejaculation for fertility; pressure sore treatment; and swallowing therapy. Each of these technologies has been developed and implemented to various degrees over the course of the past few decades, and many continue to be refined further (19, 20). These applications will be discussed separately. Table 63.1 lists the commercial devices that have been developed for each of these applications and indicates for each the current stage of regulatory approval and availability. The devices listed are not used exclusively for people with spinal cord injury, as there is some overlap with the use of these technologies in patients with hemiparetic stroke, among other

Table 63.1   Commercial FES Systems for Use in Spinal Cord Injury

INDICATION	DEVICE NAME	MANUFACTURER	REGULATORY APPROVAL OR STATUS	AVAILABILITY BY PRESCRIPTION
Cardiovascular and Muscle Exercise	REGYS	Therapeutic Alliances, Inc., Fairborn, OH	FDA	No
	ERGYS 2	Therapeutic Alliances, Inc., Fairborn, OH	FDA (1996)	Yes (primarily in rehab centers)
	SpetraSTIM 4 channel surface stimulator	Therapeutic Alliances, Inc, Fairborn, OH	FDA	Yes, for use by physical therapist
	RT300	Restorative Therapies, Inc., Baltimore, MD	FDA (2005) CE (2006) Canada (2006)	Yes
Breathing Assist	Avery Breathing Pacemaker System (formerly Mark IV)	Avery Biomedical Devices, Commack, NY	FDA (1986) CE (1995)	Yes
	Atrostim Phrenic Nerve Stimulator v2	Atrotech Ltd., Tampere, Finland	IDE (USA) CE approved (Europe)	No
	NeuRx RA/4 Respiratory System	Synapse Biomedical, Inc., Oberlin, OH	IDE research device (US)	No
Hand Grasp and Movement	Freehand	Neurocontrol Corp. (no longer in business)	FDA (1997)	No
	H200™ (formerly Handmaster)	Bioness, Inc., Valencia, CA	FDA (2001)	Yes
	Bionic Glove	Neuromotion (no longer in business)	FDA	No
	STIMuGrip	FineTech Medical, Ltd., Herts, UK	Unknown	No, will be primarily for stroke
	NeuroMove NM900 Biofeedback device	Zynex Medical, Littleton, CO	FDA (2001)	Yes, through physical therapy clinics
Standing and Walking	Parastep I®	Sigmedics, Inc., Fairborn, OH	FDA (1994) CMS coverage (2003)	Yes
	Implantable FES devices	CWRU/ VA research laboratory	IDE research device (US)	No
	WalkAide®	Hanger Orthopedics, Inc., Bethesda, MD	FDA (2006) CE (2006)	Yes
	NESS L300™	Bioness, Inc., Valencia, CA	FDA	Yes
	ActiGait®	Otto Bock®, Dunderstadt, Germany	CE (2006)	In Europe
	Odstock Dropped Foot Stimulator	Odstock Medical Ltd., Salisbury, UK	FDA (2005) CE	Yes, primarily in the UK
	STIMuSTEP	Finetech Medical Ltd., Herts, UK	CE	In Europe; primarily for stroke
Standing and Walking	NeuroStep	Victhom Human Bionics, Quebec, Canada	Clinical trials	No, will be primarily for stroke
Bladder/Bowel	FineTech Brindley (formerly Vocare)	FineTech Medical, Inc., Herts, UK	CE (Europe), FDA (1998)	Yes in Europe; pending in US
	Minnova Pelvic Floor Stimulation Device (noninvasive)	Empi, St. Paul, MN	FDA	Yes, for incontinence from various causes

continued on next page

Table 63.1   *(Continued)*

Indication	Device Name	Manufacturer	Regulatory Approval or Status	Availability by Prescription
	NeoControl Pelvic Floor Therapy Stimulation System (noninvasive)	Neotonus, Marietta, GA	FDA (1998)	Yes, for incontinence
	InterStim III	Medtronic, Minneapolis, MN	FDA (1997)	Yes, Primarily for urge incontinence
	NeuroBionix Urinary Implant	Victhom Human Bionics, Quebec, Canada	Pre-clinical trials	No
	Conti4000 (noninvasive)	Zynex Medical, Littleton, CO	Yes	Yes
Electroejaculation	Seager Model 14 Electro Power Unit	Dalzell USA Medical Systems	FDA	Yes (for fertility clinic use only)
Tissue Health and Skin Care	Percutaneous FES devices	CWRU/VA research laboratory	IDE research device (US)	No
Acute Spinal Cord Injury Treatment	Andara Oscillating Field Stimulator Therapy	Andara Life Science, Indianapolis, IN Cyberkinetics, Foxborough, MA	Humanitarian Use Device for acute SCI (US)	Clinical trial only at Purdue–Indianapolis
Other Devices of Interest	BIONs (miniature injectable electrical stimulation devices)	Alfred Mann Institute, USC, Los Angeles, CA	IDE research device (US, Canada, Italy)	Clinical trials only at USC–LA and Alberta, Canada
	Wearable Therapy	Bioflex Electromedicine, Columbus OH	FDA	Yes
	VitalStim	Chattanooga Group, Hixson, TN	FDA (2002)	Yes, for swallowing disorders

Device manufacture, extent of regulatory approval, and clinical availability are indicated. Not all devices are discussed in the text. Some devices listed may be used primarily for subjects with other diagnoses, but can also be used in spinal cord injury if desired. Updates can be found at http://www.neurotechnetwork.org/educate_neuro_technology.htm. FDA= Food and Drug Administration, CE= European Conformity, IDE= Investigational Device Exemption

diagnoses. Because of space limitations, not all devices presented in the table are discussed in this chapter. Additional updated information on commercial products can be found at www.neurotechnetwork.org/educate_neuro_technology.htm, a site maintained by a nonprofit organization called the Neurotech Network, whose mission is to help the disabled consumer access these sorts of technologies.

Therapeutic Exercise

Persons who have SCI are generally forced to become more sedentary. Paralysis is compounded by impaired autonomic nervous system function, which limits the cardiovascular response to exercise, especially in individuals with lesions above T5. Muscle bulk, strength, and endurance all decrease after SCI, and muscle fibers have been shown to convert primarily to anaerobic metabolism after injury. Paralysis of intercostal musculature reduces vital capacity. In addition, there is reduced peripheral circulation, lean body mass, and bone mineral density, as well as an altered endocrine response.

One way to combat these secondary consequences of paralysis is the use of FES as an exercise modality. The most common type of system for lower extremity FES exercise is the bicycle

ergometer. Several common commercially available ergometers are in use. One is the ERGYS2 Clinical Rehabilitation System® made by Therapeutic Technologies, Inc. This computer-controlled FES exercise ergometer uses six channels and surface electrodes to sequentially stimulate quadriceps, hamstrings, and glutei bilaterally. Another more recently introduced device is the RT300, made by Restorative Therapies, Inc. This device allows a person to perform FES exercise while sitting in his or her own wheelchair. It can also offer variable passive motion that can be set to decrease as patient effort and capability increases. The Restorative Therapies device is available in an adult and a pediatric size. It is also available with an arm crank attachment, although for this device the arm crank and leg FES system cannot work concurrently. There are other systems prototyped, however, that can allow paraplegic individuals to participate in hybrid exercise (i.e., concurrent voluntary arm and electrically stimulated leg activity). One such device is a commercial rowing machine that has been modified to allow for FES exercise of the legs while allowing the participant to voluntarily row with the arms (21).

Cardiac capacity and muscle oxidative capacity have both been shown to improve with FES ergometry. Some subjects can train with FES ergometry up to a similar aerobic metabolic rate (measured by VO_2max, or maximum oxygen consumption during peak exercise) as that achieved in the able-bodied population (22). Electrical exercise also increases peripheral venous return and fibrinolysis. Indeed, one study has indicated that FES in conjunction with heparin therapy is more effective in preventing deep venous thrombosis than heparin therapy alone (23). There are limits to the cardiovascular benefits of FES ergometry, however, especially in those with lesions above T5. In those patients, there is loss of supraspinal sympathetic control, which in turn limits the body's ability to increase heart rate, stroke volume, and cardiac output (24). Evidence is mixed regarding whether FES ergometry can retard or reverse the osteoporosis and bone demineralization seen in patients with SCI. In one study of ten spinal cord injured individuals who underwent 12 months of FES cycling 30 minutes per day, 3 days per week, bone mineral density of the proximal tibia increased 10%. Unfortunately, after a further 6 months of exercise, but at a frequency of only one session per week, the bone mineral density reverted to pretraining levels (25). It is also unclear whether FES ergometry can improve carbohydrate metabolism and insulin sensitivity in the same way that voluntary exercise does in the able-bodied. It has been reported that the majority of SCI individuals involved in a FES ergometry program had an improved self-image after participation. FES ergometry has also been associated with increased plasma endorphins, normalization of the cortisol level, and improved depression scores (24). One must keep in mind the availability and cost of these ergometry devices before prescribing FES exercise either in a hospital/clinic setting or at home. Consistent use must be demonstrated, and a plan for ongoing regular exercise is required for the maintenance of therapeutic effects.

Breathing Assistance in High Tetraplegia

Phrenic nerve pacing was developed in the early 1960s by Glenn and colleagues (26). This technique has been used successfully in over 1,000 individuals with respiratory failure (27). In appropriate candidates, phrenic nerve pacing has the potential to improve mobility, speech, and overall health, as well as to reduce anxiety and the volume of respiratory secretions, to improve the level of comfort, and to reduce required nursing care in ventilator-dependent tetraplegic individuals (28). Unfortunately, many individuals who have high tetraplegia caused by traumatic injury have injury to the anterior horn cells, located at the C3–C5 spinal levels, that innervate the diaphragm. Bilateral phrenic nerve conduction studies are necessary before considering phrenic nerve stimulation and diaphragmatic pacing. In these studies, the conduction velocity is actually a more reliable indicator of phrenic nerve function than is the response amplitude (29). Verification of phrenic nerve function can also be done by observing diaphragm movement under fluoroscopy.

The implanted components of neuroprosthetic systems for phrenic nerve pacing consist of nerve electrodes placed around or adjacent to the phrenic nerves, radio-frequency receivers, and wiring connecting the two. The external components are the radio frequency transmitter and the antenna. The two companies that currently manufacture these devices are Avery and Atrotech; both devices are available in the United States. The Avery device has received premarket approval by the FDA as well as approval from the Center for Medicare & Medicaid Services for Medicare reimbursement, and is the one most widely used. The Atrotech system, manufactured in Finland, is available under an FDA

Investigational Device Exemption. The Atrotech has a more sophisticated four-pole electrode system that is thought to reduce the chance for fatigue. All these systems allow for changes in stimulus frequency, amplitude, and train rate. Surgically, the electrodes are placed on or around the phrenic nerve in the neck or thorax. The cervical approach is much less complicated and risky, but the thoracic approach has advantages with regard to relative lack of electrode movement once implanted and the ability to stimulate the more distal contributions to the nerve. The receiver is placed in a subcutaneous pocket on the anterior chest wall, and the leads are tunneled through the third or fourth intercostal space.

Stimulation is initiated approximately two weeks postoperatively, to allow inflammation and edema of the perineurium to subside. Reconditioning is then required to improve the fatigue resistance of the diaphragm, which is usually atrophied in the ventilator-dependent tetraplegic individual. Low-frequency stimulation (7–12 Hz) is required to help convert the diaphragm to primarily oxidative, slow-twitch type I fibers (30). The respiratory rate usually lies within 8–14 breaths/minute during initiation of therapy, and later is reduced somewhat to 6–12 breaths/minute.

The potential advantages of phrenic nerve pacing over ventilator support include an improved ability to speak and the use of less bulky and less cosmetically obvious equipment. The possible complications of phrenic nerve pacing include infection, mechanical injury to the phrenic nerve, upper airway obstruction, reduction in ventilation caused by altered respiratory system mechanics, and technical malfunctions leading to failure (31). Most patients using electrophrenic respiration maintain their tracheostomy stoma to be used at night and for suctioning, although many of them can plug the sites during the day.

The traditional method of phrenic nerve implantation does involve bilateral thoracotomy. It is more invasive and is associated with a higher surgical risk. Furthermore, direct stimulation of the phrenic nerve has the potential to cause nerve damage. Onders et. al. (32) are currently developing a new approach to diaphragmatic pacing that requires only laparoscopy and percutaneous implantation of the stimulators into the diaphragm itself. The electrodes would stimulate the diaphragm directly, without direct contact with the phrenic nerve. The advantages are that the procedure would be minimally invasive and the risk of damaging the phrenic nerve would be lower. This diaphragmatic intramuscular pacing system, commercially called the NeuRx RA/4 Respiratory System, is available under an FDA Investigational Device Exemption (www.synapsebiomedical.com).

FES for Standing and Walking in Paraplegia

Over twenty-four centers worldwide have participated over the years in investigation of the use of FES for lower extremity standing and walking in paraplegia, and at least twenty-one centers have clinically implemented walking systems (33). Standing alone is a goal of some systems. The potential physiologic benefits of standing include a beneficial effect on digestion, bowel, and bladder function. The functional goals of standing to reach for high objects and face-to-face interaction with other people are also important. The muscles usually stimulated to provide standing function are the quadriceps, which provide for knee locking in a biomechanical way similar to that of knee–ankle–foot orthoses. The majority of effort in lower extremity FES development has focused, however, on functional ambulation.

Several different approaches have been used in helping paraplegics walk. Orthotic approaches without the use of FES have historically included the use of long leg braces and the Vannini–Rizoli boot (34). The latter is a thigh-high leather boot that stabilizes the ankle and places the foot in a 15-degree posterior to anterior slope. For those with good trunk stability and upper extremity strength, this has been shown to be a functional orthosis, but widespread acceptance has not been achieved. Hybrid approaches, such as the reciprocating gait orthosis (RGO), originally developed at Louisiana State University, and modified at Wright State University, use both mechanical bracing and surface FES. Specifically, FES hip extension on one side provides contralateral leg swing through the RGO mechanism. As mentioned above, quadriceps stimulation then provides knee lock (35).

SCI patients who are potential candidates for FES standing or walking systems vary greatly with regard to their injury level. In general, patients with injuries between T4 and T12, with upper body strength and stability as well as intact lower motor neurons in the lumbar and upper sacral myotomes, are appropriate for consideration, although some patients with injuries above T4 have been involved in some protocols. Individuals with significant joint contractures, dysesthetic pain syndromes, uncontrollable spasticity, osteopenia, lack of cardiopulmonary reserve, and lack of motivation may be excluded from participation.

At this writing, one FDA-approved surface FES walking system is available for use in the United States. Sigmetics, Inc., makes the Parastep System®, at an approximate cost (including training provided by a physical therapist) of $11,000. The Parastep System® is a four- or six-channel surface stimulation device for ambulation with the aid of a walker. Patients considered eligible for use of this device have upper motor neuron injuries at the C5–C8 (incomplete) or T1–T12 (complete or incomplete) levels. It is required that the users have adequate trunk control for stability. The Parastep System® uses the triple flexion response elicited by peroneal nerve stimulation as well as knee and hip extensor surface stimulation to construct the gait cycle. The patient controls the gait with switches integrated into a rolling walker (which is also needed for stability and safety). The electronic controller is housed in a cassette-sized box mounted on the patient's belt. The Parastep System® and other similar systems have been used by paraplegics not only for functional standing and walking but also for aerobic exercise (36).

Implantable lower extremity FES has also been developed. The rationale for use of implanted electrodes is the difficulty in activating deep musculature from the surface, as well as problems with reproducibility of surface electrode placement. Both percutaneous electrodes and implantable stimulator–receivers with epimysial or intramuscular electrodes have been tested, although neither is currently available commercially. The most advanced implanted system is the one undergoing ongoing testing at the Cleveland Veterans Affairs Medical Center and Case Western Reserve University. The system was originally used in individuals with complete SCI for standing and transfer. To date, seventeen subjects have received this system. Apart from the clinical utility, the safety profile and user satisfaction have been favorable. Users have reported other additional benefits with the use of this system, including a decrease in the rates of muscle spasticity, urinary tract infections, and pressure ulcers (37).

The Cleveland implantable system is also currently being investigated for the use in individuals with motor incomplete SCI

for ambulation. An initial case report demonstrated that community ambulation was possible for a previously nonambulatory subject with a motor incomplete SCI. In addition, there were benefits with cardiovascular health and energy cost (38).

The following general statements can be made concerning lower extremity FES systems and their potential for clinical use in the near future. First, all of the pure FES systems require the use of a walker for stability and safety. (The hybrid systems achieve proximal leg stability through bracing.) Second, the energy expenditure required for continuous FES walking is at least twice (if not more) that for normal upright ambulation. The speed of ambulation achievable—although it is improving—is not that of normal ambulation. Third, liability issues limit production and raise costs. However, it has been demonstrated that there are many beneficial effects of FES standing and walking systems, as well as the obvious clinical utility of the use of the FES system for standing, transfer, and ambulation. Further exploration of these additional benefits is anticipated.

FES for Hand Grasp and Release

In the past, the main methods employed to address the problem of motor paralysis in the upper extremities of tetraplegic SCI individuals have been the use of adaptive equipment and assistive devices. Surgical interventions, such as tendon transfers, have also been used (39, 40). Technology for the restoration of hand function in tetraplegic individuals has been under development in the United States, Europe, and Japan for over three decades (41). A variety of neuroprosthetic devices for hand function have entered the clinical environment (4, 42). The objective of the use of FES in the hands of tetraplegic individuals is to restore grasp, hold, and release, thereby increasing independence in the performance of functional tasks and minimizing the use of other adapted equipment.

Patient Evaluation and Selection

Physiologically, patients to be considered for hand grasp systems must have adequate motor innervation of forearm and hand muscles to allow for FES grasp synthesis. The electrical activation of muscle must provide sufficient strength and fatigue resistance to allow for use in functional movement. If one or two muscles are not electrically available, surgical adjuncts can be employed to overcome this problem (in the case of the implanted system). For instance, if the extensor digiti communus (EDC) is denervated, the extensor carpi ulnaris can be transferred to the EDC and powered by a FES electrode. Upper extremity passive range of motion must be adequate to allow for functional movements such as bringing the hand up to the mouth. Spasticity must be adequately controlled. Individuals must be in generally good health, have adequate trunk support, and have intact vision to ensure feedback on what the partially or completely insensate hand is doing. Best results occur with motivated people who have good social support systems.

Tetraplegic hand grasp systems have focused on the C5- and C6-level complete SCI patient populations. These individuals have adequate voluntary strength in the proximal muscles of the arm (i.e., deltoid, rotator cuff, biceps) to move their hand in a functional space and therefore benefit from the provision of hand grasp and release. Those with C4-level injury (and therefore no deltoid or biceps strength) have also participated in limited laboratory-based investigations of FES systems (43, 44), but the results of these studies have been limited. Patients injured at the C7 and lower levels have multiple voluntarily active forearm muscles (e.g., brachioradialis, extensor carpi radialis longus and brevis, pronator teres). These muscles can be used to motor new functions without sacrificing current function by means of tendon transfer surgery (45).

Upper Extremity Systems

Three upper extremity neuroprostheses have received FDA regulatory approval and have been used clinically. Two of these systems utilize surface electrodes, and the third utilizes implanted electrodes. Each of these devices will be discussed separately.

FREEHAND SYSTEM.   The Freehand System® has been developed, researched, functionally evaluated, and clinically implemented more extensively than any other upper extremity neuroprosthesis (46–55). In addition, more scientific literature has been published on this device than on either of the other systems. There are approximately 200 spinal cord injured individuals who have the implanted Freehand System.

The Implantable Functional Neuromuscular Stimulator, or Freehand System®, was initially developed at Case Western Reserve University and the Cleveland VA Medical Center, and was commercialized by NeuroControl Corporation. It consists of (1) an external joint position transducer/controller, (2) a rechargeable programmable external control unit (ECU), and (3) an implantable eight-channel stimulator/receiver attached via flexible wires to epimysial disc electrodes (Figure 63.1). The user controls the system through small movements of either the

shoulder or wrist. The joint position transducer, which operates somewhat like a computer joystick, is typically mounted on the skin from sternum to contralateral shoulder or across the ipsilateral wrist and senses these movements. The ECU uses this signal to power proportional control of hand grasp and release. Communication between the ECU and the implantable stimulator, which is located in a surgical pocket created in the upper chest, is through an inductive link. The system can be programmed through a personal computer interface by a trained therapist to individualize the grasps as well as the shoulder control for each patient (46).

Individuals can choose to use either palmar or lateral prehension grasp patterns at any given time with the Freehand System® (Figure 63.2). This is helpful in handling either large objects (e.g., books, telephone receivers) or small objects (e.g., pens, forks), respectively. The original system provided unilateral hand grasp only. An evaluation of the system in a multicenter clinical trial was completed, and in 1997, the FDA approved this

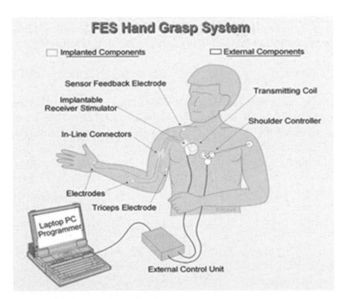

Figure 63.1 Components of an implantable neuroprosthesis. On the left are the implanted components, which include the implant stimulator, electrode leads, epimysial electrodes, and, in some cases, a sensory electrode to provide a form of sensory feedback. Not shown are implantable intramuscular electrodes that are an option available to the surgeon. On the right are the external components of the neuroprosthesis, which include a shoulder position controller incorporating the device's on/off switch, an external control unit, and a transmitting coil. The system is programmable via a PC interface, also shown. (Diagram courtesy of Ronald Hart, Cleveland FES Center.)

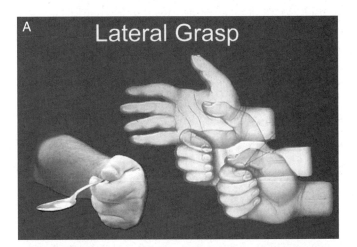

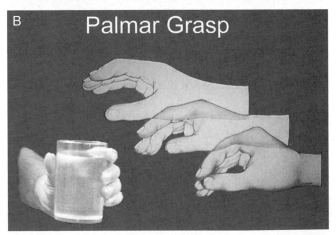

Figure 63.2 Grasp configurations for the Freehand® neuroprosthesis. The user can choose to use either a lateral grasp pattern (left), also known as key grip, or a palmar grasp (right). The lateral grasp is more effective for handling smaller objects such as a spoon or a pen, whereas the palmar grasp is more helpful for handling larger objects, such as a glass or an electric razor. The user chooses between the two grasps by using the switch incorporated into the shoulder position controller. (Figures courtesy Ronald Hart, Cleveland FES Center.)

device for clinical use. Results from the multicenter trial are presented here (51, 56).

A total of sixty-one patients were enrolled in the study. Of the original sixty-one, 69% of patients had C5-level injuries and 25% had C6-level injuries. All of the patients had had one or more surgical procedures to augment hand function. These procedures included tendon transfers (e.g., posterior deltoid-to-triceps, brachioradialis-to-wrist extensors) and joint fusions (e.g., thumb–interphalangeal fusion). A total of 128 cumulative implant years were evaluated during the study. The following adverse events requiring surgical management and the percent of patients involved in each type of event were reported: repositioning or replacement required by receiver (5%), skin openings requiring repair (7%), electrode breakage (5%), infection requiring electrode removal (5%), infection requiring system explant (2%), and tendon adhesion (2%). The major nonsurgical adverse events included swelling or discomfort over the implantable components (21%), skin irritation from external products (23%), irritation from incisions or sutures (16%), and skin irritation from splints or casts (10%). In a follow-up study of these electrodes implanted for a minimum of three years (maximum 16 years), the overall failure rate for any cause was less than 2% (57).

In the evaluation of any assistive technology, two key questions need to be asked: (1) What *can* users do with the device? and (2) What *do* users do with the device? To answer these questions as they apply to the Freehand System®, three tests were devised. The first two, pinch force measurement and the grasp release test (GRT), were aimed at answering the first question. The third set of evaluative tools, namely the activities of daily living (ADL) abilities, assessment, and follow-up tests, were aimed at answering the second question. Finally, a user satisfaction survey was also performed at the time of 6-month or later follow-up.

Summary pinch force measurements with and without the neuroprosthesis are shown in Figure 63.3. Clearly, pinch force in both lateral and palmar prehension improved with the neuroprosthesis. The small improvement seen postoperatively with the neuroprosthesis turned off can be attributed to tendon synchronization performed as an adjunct during the implant procedure. It should also be noted that all patients realized some improvement in pinch force measurement in at least one grasp pattern with the neuroprosthesis.

The GRT was a timed test that evaluated each subject's ability to grasp, move, and release six standardized objects. Three objects (peg, fork, and paperweight) were used with lateral prehension, and three objects (block, can, and videotape) were used with palmar prehension. The number of completed moves achieved by subjects in 30 seconds increased significantly for the heavier objects (paperweight, fork, can, and videotape) with the neuroprosthesis. No improvement was seen in manipulation of the lightest objects, namely the peg and the blocks, except in the weakest users.

The ADL abilities test evaluated whether the neuroprosthesis decreased the amount of assistance required to perform various ADLs (e.g., eating with utensils, brushing teeth, shaving, loading a floppy disk in a computer). Furthermore, subjects were asked whether they preferred to perform the task with or without the neuroprosthesis. All patients (49/49) tested showed improvement in independence in at least one task, and 80% (39/49) showed improvement in at least three tasks. Ninety-eight percent (48/49) of the patients reported that they preferred to use the neuroprosthesis to perform three or more activities. The user satisfaction survey consisted of thirty-eight questions regarding satisfaction, impact on ADLs, occupation, and need for external assistance. Patients reported overall satisfaction with the performance of the system, indicated that the system had a positive impact on their lives, and said that the system provided them with less dependence on other adaptive equipment (58).

Unfortunately the Freehand system is no longer commercially available, as NeuroControl Corporation is no longer in business. The financial failure of this company was likely a direct consequence of the difficulty in providing a very sophisticated and surgically implanted device to a relatively small clinical market (see subsequent further discussion of this topic).

H200.   Another device available for the restoration of hand function in individuals with C5 tetraplegia is marketed by Bioness. Formerly termed the Handmaster®, it is now called the H200™ (59) (Figure 63.4). The device is composed of a hinged shell with a spiral splint that stabilizes the wrist. Surface electrodes

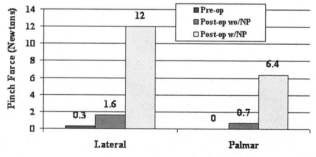

Figure 63.3   Pinch force for lateral and palmar prehension with and without the Freehand® neuroprosthesis (NP). The histogram family on the left represents lateral grasp; palmar grasp is on the right. Force is represented in newtons. There is some increase in force produced postoperatively, even with the neuroprosthesis turned off. This is probably related to the increase in tone produced by surgical tightening of the flexor tendons.

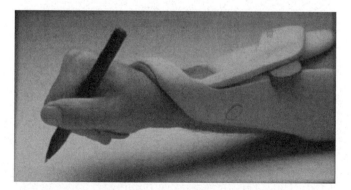

Figure 63.4   The H200™ external orthosis, formerly termed the Handmaster®, manufactured by Bioness, Inc. The device incorporates three surface stimulation electrodes into the molded orthosis to provide pinch grip. Not shown is the controller box, which contains a trigger button to start stimulation and a mode button to choose between preprogrammed patterns of muscle activation. (Photograph courtesy of Bioness, Inc.)

built into the shell stimulate the finger flexors and extensors and the thenar musculature. A trigger button mounted on a separate control unit allows the user to start the stimulation sequence. A separate mode button allows the user to choose different preprogrammed patterns of muscle activation. The device is designed to be used by C5 and C6 tetraplegic individuals as well as by individuals who have hemiplegia from cerebral injury. The Bioness device has been studied clinically in pilot investigations in Israel (60) and in the United States (61, 62). Two of these studies involved individuals with cerebral damage from stroke or traumatic brain injury. In the latter study, twenty subjects with hemiplegia and no functional use of the hemiparetic hand underwent an accelerated outpatient stimulation program that ultimately led to an average daily device use time of 3.4 hours over an average of 13.1 weeks. Significant improvements in passive wrist extension, active elbow flexion, wrist flexion and extension, degree of spasticity, and ability to hold a 1-kg weight were noted after the treatment regimen. With the exception of the lifting of the weight, these measurements were made after treatment without the Handmaster®/H200™ in place, so the impact of the device in the hemiplegic setting was more in the role of a therapeutic electrical stimulation device than of a functional neuroprosthesis or orthoses. A pilot clinical trial of the use of the Handmaster®/H200™ in the SCI population has also been performed (62). Using grip strength, active finger motion, Fugl–Meyer scores, and a survey with regard to ADL performance as outcome measures, investigators showed that hand function significantly improved using the NESS device in subjects with C5 level SCI. Overall, the advantages of the Handmaster®/H200™ are its noninvasiveness, cost, and relative ease of application. Disadvantages include cosmesis because external splinting is required, and the fact that the device is less customizable than the Freehand System®. The H200 remains commercially available for clinical use.

BIONIC GLOVE. The Bionic Glove®, developed at the University of Alberta, uses three channels of surface stimulation to activate finger flexors and extensors and thumb flexors (63). A wrist-position transducer mounted in the fabric of the customized garment provides control. Although the device is described as being usable for C5–C7-level injuries, candidates must have some voluntary wrist extension to activate it. The glove is designed to be put on and taken off by tetraplegic subjects unaided. Control of the hand grasp and release does not employ a proportional paradigm such as that used in the Freehand System®; rather, a mechanism known as trigger hysteresis is used to produce all-or-none hand opening or closing. As the subject flexes his wrist past approximately 20 degrees, the finger and thumb extensors are activated to their full extent. They are kept active until the subject brings his wrist back to only 10 degrees of flexion. At that point, the extensor muscle stimulation will shut off. Similarly, when the wrist is extended to 20 degrees, the finger and thumb flexors will be activated fully. This stimulation will be turned off only when the wrist comes back to 10 degrees of flexion. The hysteresis built into this design allows the user to better control the grasp functionally.

An initial trial of eight men with C6–C7 spinal cord injury, employing the Bionic Glove® prototype, showed that an initial grasp force of 11.3 newtons, on average, could be generated. The force fatigued rapidly, however, and after 5 seconds, the force being generated averaged 8.6 newtons. When subjects repeated their grasps five consecutive times, the initial grasp force decreased to 9.3 newtons and then fatigued to 6.8 newtons after 5 seconds. These forces, although only a fraction of that seen in able-bodied grasp, can be considered adequate for most ADLs. A clinical trial involving twelve people with C5–C7 tetraplegia who used the device for over 6 months has been reported (64). The investigators showed an increase in the power of grasp and range of motion with daily use. Manual tasks completion, as measured by the FIM and the Quadriplegia Index of Function, significantly improved by 24% and 49%, respectively, especially with larger objects. Activity logs indicated that after 6 months, the number of hours per week that the device was used increased to up to 14 hours from an initial level of 4–6 hours/week. Of the original twelve subjects, only six chose to use the device after completion of the 6-month study. The investigators concluded that the device was most beneficial as a therapeutic aide, although for some it is also useful as an assistive device. As of this writing, the device is no longer commercially available.

Future Directions for Hand-Grasp Neuroprostheses

Future developments and improvements in tetraplegic hand grasp systems will include implantable controllers involving both joint angle and myoelectric signal transducers (65, 66), closed-loop feedback with improved sensor technology, proximal muscle control (i.e., shoulder musculature [67] and triceps [68] control of the pronation/supination axis), addition of finger intrinsics to improve finger extension (69), and bilateral implementation of grasp in C6-level individuals. In addition, systems that provide whole arm function for individuals with C4- and higher-level injuries will be developed (70). Ultimately, technologies such as the development of injectable electrodes (for example the BION technology—see subsequent discussion) and cortical control of movement (such as that used with the Braingate system; see www.cyberkinetics.com) may also work with neuroprosthetic hand grasp devices.

Control of Micturition with FES

Electrical stimulation to control bladder function after suprasacral SCI has also been under investigation for several decades. Stimulation at various levels of the neurourologic axis has been attempted, including the lumbar spinal cord, the anterior sacral nerve roots, the pudendal nerve, and the bladder/detrusor itself.

In the United Kingdom, Brindley et al. (71) have had the most experience and success with S2–S4 anterior sacral nerve root stimulation in combination with posterior rhizotomy. This system is surgically implanted through lumbar laminectomy and employs either epidural or intradural electrodes. These electrodes are connected via cable to an implanted radio receiver, which couples to an external stimulator/transmitter. Pulsed stimulation is used to take advantage of the differences between activation of the slow-response smooth musculature of the detrusor (bladder) and activation of the fast-twitch striated sphincter musculature (Figure 63.5). Bladder pressure gradually increases

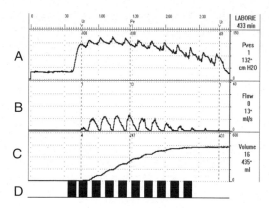

Figure 63.5 Physiology of micturition produced by the Vocare® sacral nerve stimulator, as identified by cystometrogram recording. The x-axis represents time in minutes and seconds, with the total tracing lasting approximately 3 minutes. (**A**) Intravesicular pressure in cm water from 0 to 150. (**B**) Urine flow rate in ml/seconds with the scale from 0 to 40 ml/sec. (**C**) Cumulated volume of urine voided in ml with the scale from 0 to 600 ml. (**D**) Approximate timing of the sacral nerve stimulation used to produce this intermittent voiding pattern.

in a tetanic fashion, while sphincter pressure rapidly falls after the end of each stimulation pulse. This produces short spurts of urination, but can result in nearly complete bladder emptying.

Over 1,500 sacral anterior root stimulators have been implanted throughout the world. Of those, approximately 90% are in regular use four to six times per day. In the United States, the clinical trials of this device in humans started in 1992. As of December 1997, twenty-six extradural sacral root stimulators had been implanted in a United States multicenter trial. In the United States, an extradural surgical technique has been used. The FDA approved the implantation of the device for clinical use in 1998 under the trade name Vocare®, also marketed by the NeuroControl Corporation. Unfortunately, at this writing, the device is not currently available commercially in the United States. It is available in Europe under the name FineTech Brindley Bladder Control System.

To provide continence of urine with this electrical stimulation device, one has to consider ways by which to abolish the reflex incontinence caused by the activation of the sensory reflex pathway. This has been done in most cases by performance of a posterior rhizotomy at the sacral levels. This procedure, done concurrently with the sacral stimulator implant, abolishes uninhibited reflex bladder contractions and restores bladder compliance. Detrusor–sphincter dyssynergia is also reduced, thereby avoiding the chance of autonomic dysreflexia as well. The downside of this procedure, however, is loss of perineal sensation in sensory incomplete individuals, and loss of reflex erection and ejaculation if present.

Patient Evaluation and Selection

Potential candidates for the Vocare® implant must have intact parasympathetic efferent neurons to the detrusor musculature. This can be ascertained by cystometrogrametric recording of bladder pressure, which should be 35 cm water in women and 50 cm water in men. Individuals will likely have other sacral

reflexes intact, such as the bulbocavernosus and anal wink along with ankle tendon stretch reflexes. Patients should be neurologically stable and be motivated to use this device. Concurrent sepsis or pressure sores should be treated prior to implant (72).

Results of Bladder Stimulator Implant

There has been considerable documentation of success in terms of residual volumes after micturition using this implanted device. In a study of twenty patients, post-void residual volumes were reduced on average from 212 cc ± 106 to 22 cc ± 14 (73). A significant reduction in the number of symptomatic urinary tract infections has also been seen. Continence has been achieved in more than 85% of implant recipients, probably because of the concurrent posterior rhizotomy (74, 75). Improved health of the upper urinary tracts, as demonstrated by a decreased incidence of bladder trabeculation, hydronephrosis, and the like, has been seen in patients post implantation.

Interestingly, the sacral anterior root stimulators have also been shown to improve bowel care (i.e., increased defecation, reduced constipation). About half of implant recipients can use the stimulator to defecate. Even in those patients who cannot use the electrical stimulation to defecate, the amount of time spent in bowel evacuation has been shown to be considerably less (76). A slower stimulation time sequence is used for defecation than for micturition. Approximately 60% of men can also produce penile erection using the device (75).

Long-term follow-up from Europe has documented the safety of this implant device and procedure. Like the upper extremity neuroprosthetic system, there is no implanted power source in the sacral nerve root stimulator. Therefore, there is no need to replace the internal componentry. Electronic failure rates have been extremely low. Economic analysis of the long-term cost savings of this device, due to the decreased use of catheters, antibiotics, medical resources, and the like, indicates that the implant pays for itself within 5 to 7 years (77, 78).

Electroejaculation

Originally developed within veterinary medicine, electroejaculation now provides a mechanism by which spinal cord injured men can father children. Electrically stimulated rectal probes are used to produce seminal emission. After serial electroejaculation procedures, the quality of the semen produced (as measured by sperm count, motility, and morphology) generally improves to the point where artificial insemination or in vitro fertilization is possible. Because of the great deal of coordination required to achieve successful pregnancies with this technique, multidisciplinary expertise is required for the establishment of a fertility center for couples with spinal cord injured men (79). It should be noted that electroejaculation is one of several techniques now available to harvest viable sperm for the purposes of artificial insemination or in vitro fertilization.

NMES and Tissue Health/Pressure Ulcer Prevention

Regular use of NMES for functional applications can produce changes in regularly stimulated muscles that may increase the health of the muscle and surrounding soft tissues. The Skin

Care Research Team (SCRT) at the Cleveland VAMC is investigating the unique ability of NMES to affect intrinsic factors that can prevent pressure ulcer development for people with SCI. Surface electrical stimulation has limited efficacy in this application, both clinically and practically. Implanted NMES systems for long-term therapeutic use reduce the charge required to elicit a contractile response and ensure that the response is repeatable and predictable. Utilization of a semi-implanted gluteal stimulation system (Figure 63.6) specifically to improve tissue health has been shown to have a positive impact on multiple indirect indicators of tissue health. Over the long term, increased muscle thickness and blood flow, together with reduced regional interface pressures, have been observed (80–84). In addition, alternating gluteal NMES dynamically alters conditions at the seating support interface owing to periodic changes in interface pressure facilitated by stimulated muscular contractions. This dynamic effect increases over time as the paralyzed muscles become stronger with regular use of gluteal NMES. Daily use of NMES is indicated in order to maintain hypertrophy of paralyzed muscles. This feasibility study implies that therapeutic NMES provides a unique intrinsic approach to reducing the risk of pressure ulcer development for people with compromised tissue health and decreased independent mobility.

Acute Spinal Cord Injury Treatment

There is a considerable body of evidence that the growth of neurites in both amphibian and mammalian models can be influenced by an applied electrical field (85). In a rat model, a direct current field was found to improve recovery after moderately severe experimental SCI (86). Because of these types of finding, an investigation has been initiated to see if oscillating electrical field stimulation applied to the area of the acutely damaged spinal cord could improve sensorimotor outcome in patients with nontransected, ASIA A spinal cord injury. The oscillating field stimulator developed for this purpose is 11 cm long and 1 cm in diameter, and was surgically implanted in the paraspinous musculature at the level of the injury. The initial phase I trial report which involved implantation of ten patients within the first 18 days after traumatic SCI, indicated that the technique was safe, reliable, and possibly efficacious in improving ASIA score outcomes (87). Further work is planned on ten additional subjects.

Other FES Applications

Additional approaches to FES are under ongoing development. One of the most innovative is the manufacture of BION®s (short for BIOnic Neurons), which are hypodermically implantable microstimulators that can be electronically addressable and externally powered by an external device through radio frequency coupling. The devices are currently undergoing clinical trials for treatment of foot drop (88) and may in future be useful for a myriad of possible FES applications in spinal cord injury.

A company called Bioflex Electromedicine has developed a line of garments within which surface electrodes are embedded. These garments can then be hooked into various electrical stimulation devices for the purposes of exercise, functional activity, or pain management. The benefit claimed for the wearable system is that placement of the electrodes is faster, simpler, and more reproducible. Clinical studies have not been published specifically using these devices, although the garments are approved by the FDA for clinical use.

Surface FES has been used recently in people with dysphagia, including those with concurrent SCI and brainstem involvement. A device called Vital Stim has been developed for this application. Several clinical trails have been performed, although the jury is still out on the optimal techniques implemented and the efficacy of the program.

ECONOMIC AND AVAILABILITY ISSUES FOR FES DEVICES

Costs associated with the implementation of FES systems for people with spinal cord injury are quite high. This is due to a combination of factors, including the sizeable costs associated with research, development, and regulatory approval. Furthermore, each type of device can only be applied to a relatively small number of patients, so the ability to distribute R&D costs across subjects is rather limited. For instance, in the case of implantable FES for hand grasp in tetraplegic individuals, it has been estimated that only approximately 12,000 people in the United States would be eligible for this type of technology (89). The consequence of this disparity between cost of development and market size has been that neuroprostheses such as the Freehand® system have not been economically viable for the companies that manufactured them. Indeed NeuroControl Corporation, the former maker of both Freehand and the Vocare® system, is now

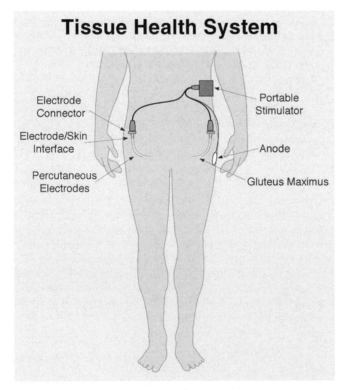

Tissue Health System

Electrode Connector

Electrode/Skin Interface

Percutaneous Electrodes

Portable Stimulator

Anode

Gluteus Maximus

Figure 63.6 Percutaneous gluteal stimulation system (previously published in *Archives of Physical Medicine & Rehabilitation*, and reprinted with permission).

out of business. The picture is not completely bleak, however. In an economic analysis of the comparative costs of bowel and bladder management with and without a bladder neuroprosthesis, Creasey and Dahlberg (77) determined that after five years of use, the bladder neuroprosthesis would actually pay for itself and then subsequently cost less for ongoing care than the use of traditional methods of management with catheters. Using a life care plan analysis, it has also been determined that if a hand grasp system could reduce the need for attendant care two hours per day, then the up-front costs of the system would be paid for over the lifetime of the tetraplegic individual (78). This type of information provides third-party payers with a greater incentive to consider supporting the use of these devices, even when they might be considered "orphan products" given the size of the patient population. The problem is that even if reimbursement is available, the long-term viability of companies producing relatively small numbers of neuroprosthetic devices remains uncertain. Ultimately, society will have to determine whether the costs associated with FES devices are worth it given the benefits received by the individuals living with the consequences of spinal cord injury.

CONCLUSION

This chapter has provided an overview of the current field of FES and its use in individuals who have SCI. Clearly, the field has come a long way from the early use of electricity in medicine. The intense scientific research and developmental work that has occurred over the last half-century has finally borne clinical fruit. During this last two decades, several neuroprosthetic devices have gone through regulatory review and have finally become available for use with patients. This has been a remarkable achievement, but it is somewhat tainted by the marketplace realities associated with some of these products. Further development and refinement of this technology will likely enhance the lives of a greater number of patients with disability caused by spinal cord dysfunction, as well as those of other individuals with neurologic impairment. Although obstacles such as cost, liability, and regulatory burden will have to be addressed as these devices become more commonplace, the future remains promising for their use with spinal cord injury.

Acknowledgements: The authors would like to acknowledge the contributions made by the following people to this chapter: Kath Bogie, Mary Jo Elmo, Jennifer French, Kevin Kilgore, Raymond Onders, and Ronald Triolo.

*R*eferences

1. Franklin B. On the effects of electricity in paralytic cases. *Phil Trans* 1757; 50:481–483.
2. Liberson WT, et al. Functional electrotherapy stimulation of the peroneal nerve synchronized with the swing phase of the gait of hemiplegic patients. *Arch Phys Med Rehabil* 1961; 42:101.
3. McNeal DR. 2000 years of electrical stimulation. In: Reswick JB HF, ed. *Functional Electrical Stimulation*. New York: Dekker; 1977.
4. Grill WM, Kirsch RF. Neuroprosthetic applications of electrical stimulation. *Assist Technol* 2000; 12(1):6–20.
5. Kandel E, Schwartz J, Jessel T. *Principles of Neural Science*, 4th ed. New York: McGraw-Hill; 2000.
6. Crago PE, Peckham PH, Mortimer JT, Van der Meulen JP. The choice of pulse duration for chronic electrical stimulation via surface, nerve, and intramuscular electrodes. *Ann Biomed Eng* 1974; 2(3):252–264.
7. Eichhorn KF, Schubert W, David E. Maintenance, training and functional use of denervated muscles. *J Biomed Eng* 1984; 6(3):205–211.
8. Lomo T, Slater CR. Control of acetylcholine sensitivity and synapse formation by muscle activity. *J Physiol* 1978; 275:391–402.
9. Mortimer J. Motor Prostheses. In: Brooks VB, ed. *Handbook of Physiology: The Nervous System II, Motor Control*. Bethesda, MD: Amer Physiol Soc. 1981:158–187.
10. Munsat TL, McNeal D, Waters R. Effects of nerve stimulation on human muscle. *Arch Neurol* 1976; 33(9):608–617.
11. Memberg WD, Peckham PH, Thrope GB, Keith MW, Kicher TP. An analysis of the reliability of percutaneous intramuscular electrodes in upper extremity FNS applications. *IEEE Trans Rehab Eng* 1993; 1(2):126–132.
12. Crago PE, Nakai RJ, Chizeck HJ. Feedback regulation of hand grasp opening and contact force during stimulation of paralyzed muscle. *IEEE Trans Biomed Eng* 1991; 38(1):17–28.
13. Glenn WW, Phelps ML. Diaphragm pacing by electrical stimulation of the phrenic nerve. *Neurosurgery* 1985; 17(6):974–984.
14. Chen D, Philip M, Philip PA, Monga TN. Cardiac pacemaker inhibition by transcutaneous electrical nerve stimulation. *Arch Phys Med Rehabil* 1990; 71(1):27–30.
15. Segreti J. Is antibiotic prophylaxis necessary for preventing prosthetic device infection? *Infect Dis Clin North Am* 1999; 13(4):871–877, vii.
16. http://medtronic.com/neuro/diathermy_alert/alert_physicians.html (accessed February 12, 2008).
17. NeuroControl Corporation. *VOCARE Bladder System Clinician Manual* Document ID 300–1003-E; 2000.
18. Baker LL, McNeal DR, Benton LA, et al. *Neuromuscular Electrical Stimulation: A Practical Guide*, 3rd ed. Downey, CA: Rancho Los Amigos Medical Center; 1993.
19. Yarkony GM, Roth EJ, Cybulski G, Jaeger RJ. Neuromuscular stimulation in spinal cord injury. I. Restoration of functional movement of the extremities. *Arch Phys Med Rehabil* 1992; 73(1):78–86.
20. Peckham PH, Creasey GH. Neural prostheses: clinical applications of functional electrical stimulation in spinal cord injury. *Paraplegia* 1992; 30(2):96–101.
21. Davoodi R, Andrews BJ, Wheeler GD, Lederer R. Development of an indoor rowing machine with manual FES controller for total body exercise in paraplegia. *IEEE Trans Neural Syst Rehabil Eng* 2002; 10(3):197–203.
22. Glaser RM. Physiology of functional electrical stimulation-induced exercise: basic science perspective. *J Neuro Rehab* 1991; 5(1–2):49–61.
23. Merli GJ, Herbison GJ, Ditunno JF. Deep vein thrombosis: prophylaxis in acute spinal cord injured patients. *Arch Phys Med Rehabil* 1988; 69:661–664.
24. Ragnarsson KT, Pollack SF, Twist D. Lower limb endurance exercise after spinal cord injury: implications for health and functional ambulation. *J Neuro Rehab* 1991; 5(1–2):37–48.
25. Mohr T, Podenphant J, Biering-Sorensen F, Galbo H, Thamsborg G, Kjaer M. Increased bone mineral density after prolonged electrically induced cycle training of paralyzed limbs in spinal cord injured man. *Calcif Tissue Int* 1997; 61(1):22–25.
26. Glenn WW, Hageman JH, Mauro A, Eisenberg L, Flanigan S, Harvard M. Electrical stimulation of excitable tissue by radio-frequency transmission. *Ann Surg* 1964; 160:338–350.
27. Glenn WW, Hogan JF, Phelps ML. Ventilatory support of the quadriplegic patient with respiratory paralysis by diaphragm pacing. *Surg Clin North Am* 1980; 60(5):1055–1078.
28. DiMarco AF. Neural prostheses in the respiratory system. *J Rehabil Res Dev* 2001; 38(6):601–607.
29. MacLean IC, Mattioni TA. Phrenic nerve conduction studies: a new technique and its application in quadriplegic patients. *Arch Phys Med Rehabil* 1981; 62(2):70–73.
30. Oda T, Glenn WW, Fukuda Y, Hogan JF, Gorfien J. Evaluation of electrical parameters for diaphragm pacing: an experimental study. *J Surg Res* 1981; 30(2):142–153.
31. DiMarco AF. Diaphragm pacing in patients with spinal cord injury. *Top Spinal Cord Inj Rehabil* 1999; 5(1):6–20.
32. Onders RP, DiMarco AF, Ignagni AR, Aiyar H, Mortimer JT. Mapping the phrenic nerve motor point: the key to a successful laparoscopic diaphragm pacing system in the first human series. *Surgery* 2004; 136(4):819–826.
33. Kantor C, Andrews BJ, Marsolais EB, Solomonow M, Lew RD, Ragnarsson KT. Report on a conference on motor prostheses for

workplace mobility of paraplegic patients in North America. *Paraplegia* 1993; 31(7):439–456.

34. Kent HO. Vannini-Rizzoli stabilizing orthosis (boot): preliminary report on a new ambulatory aid for spinal cord injury. *Arch Phys Med Rehabil* 1992; 73(3):302–307.

35. Solomonow M. Biomechanics and physiology of a practical functional neuromuscular stimulation powered walking orthosis for paraplegics. In: Stein RB PP, Popovic DB, eds. *Neural Prostheses: Replacing Motor Function after Disease or Disability.* New York: Oxford University Press; 1992:202–232.

36. Groupe D, Kohn KH. *Functional Electrical Stimulation for Ambulation by Paraplegics: Twelve Years of Clinical Observations and System Studies.* Malabar, FL: Kreiger; 1994.

37. Mushahwar VK, Jacobs PL, Normann RA, Triolo RJ, Kleitman N. New functional electrical stimulation approaches to standing and walking. *J Neural Eng* 2007; 4(3):S181–S197.

38. Hardin E, Kobetic R, Murray L, et al. Ambulation after incomplete spinal cord injury with an implanted FES system: a case report. *Journal of Rehabilitation Research and Development* 2007; 44(3):333–346.

39. Keith MW, Kilgore KL, Peckham PH, Wuolle KS, Creasey G, Lemay M. Tendon transfers and functional electrical stimulation for restoration of hand function in spinal cord injury. *J Hand Surg* [Am] 1996; 21(1):89–99.

40. Hentz VR, Ladd AL. Functional restoration of the upper extremity in tetraplegia. In: Young RR, Woolsey RM, eds. *Diagnosis and Management of Disorders of the Spinal Cord.* Philadelphia: WB Saunders Co.; 1995.

41. Gorman PH, Peckham PH. Upper extremity functional neuromuscular stimulation. *J Neuro Rehab* 1991; 5:3–11.

42. Peckham PH, Keith MW, Kilgore KL. Restoration of upper extremity function in tetraplegia. *Topics in Spinal Cord Injury Rehabilitation* 1999; 5:133–143.

43. Nathan RH, Ohry A. Upper limb functions regained in quadriplegia: a hybrid computerized neuromuscular stimulation system. *Arch Phys Med Rehabil* 1990; 71(6):415–421.

44. Yu DT, Kirsch RF, Bryden AM, Memberg WD, Acosta AM. A neuroprosthesis for high tetraplegia. *J Spinal Cord Med* 2001; 24(2):109–113.

45. Keith MW, Lacey SH. Surgical rehabilitation of the tetraplegic upper extremity. *J Neuro Rehab* 1991; 5(1–2):75–87.

46. Kilgore KL, Peckham PH, Keith MW, et al. An implanted upper-extremity neuroprosthesis: follow-up of five patients. *J Bone Joint Surg Am* 1997; 79(4):533–541.

47. Davis SE, Mulcahey MJ, Smith BT, Betz RR. Outcome of functional electrical stimulation in the rehabilitation of a child with C-5 tetraplegia. *J Spinal Cord Med* 1999; 22(2):107–113.

48. Carroll S, Cooper C, Brown D, Sormann G, Flood S, Denison M. Australian experience with the Freehand system for restoring grasp in quadriplegia. *Aust N Z J Surg* 2000; 70:563–568.

49. Biering-Sorensen F, Gregersen H, Hagen E, et al. Improved function of the hand in persons with tetraplegia using electric stimulation via implanted electrodes. *Ugeskr Laeger* 2000; 162:2195–2198.

50. Fromm B, Rupp R, Gerner HJ. The Freehand system: an implantable neuroprosthesis for functional electrical stimulation of the upper extremity. *Handchir Mikrochir Plast Chir* 2001; 33:149–152.

51. Peckham PH, Keith MW, Kilgore KL, et al. Efficacy of an implanted neuroprosthesis for restoring hand grasp in tetraplegia: a multicenter study. *Arch Phys Med Rehabil* 2001; 82(10):1380–1388.

52. Taylor P, Esnouf J, Hobby J. The functional impact of the Freehand System on tetraplegic hand function: clinical results. *Spinal Cord* 2002; 40(11):560–566.

53. Degnan GG, Wind TC, Jones EV, Edlich RF. Functional electrical stimulation in tetraplegic patients to restore hand function. *J Long Term Eff Med Implants* 2002; 12(3):175–188.

54. Cornwall R, Hausman MR. Implanted neuroprostheses for restoration of hand function in tetraplegic patients. *J Am Acad Orthop Surg* 2004; 12(2):72–79.

55. Rupp R, Gerner HJ. Neuroprosthetics of the upper extremity—clinical application in spinal cord injury and future perspectives. *Biomed Tech* [Berl] 2004; 49(4):93–98.

56. NeuroControl Corporation. Summary of the safety and effectiveness (SS&S), PMA Application to the FDA; September 26, 1997.

57. Kilgore KL, Peckham PH, Keith MW, et al. Durability of implanted electrodes and leads in an upper-limb neuroprosthesis. *J Rehabil Res Dev* 2003; 40(6):457–468.

58. Wuolle KS, Bryden AM, Peckham PH, Murray PK, Keith M. Satisfaction with upper-extremity surgery in individuals with tetraplegia. *Arch Phys Med Rehabil* 2003; 84(8):1145–1149.

59. Ijzerman MJ, Stoffers TS, Groen I, et al. The NESS Handmaster orthosis: restoration of hand function in C5 and stroke patients by means of electrical stimulation. *J Rehab Sciences* 1996; 9:86–89.

60. Weingarden HP, Zeilig G, Heruti R, et al. Hybrid functional electrical stimulation orthosis system for the upper limb: effects on spasticity in chronic stable hemiplegia. *Am J Phys Med Rehabil* 1998; 77:276–281.

61. Alon G, Dar A, Katz–Behiri D, Weingarden H, Nathan R. Efficacy of a hybrid upper limb neuromuscular electrical stimulation system in lessening selected impairments and dysfunctions consequent to cerebral damage. *J Neuro Rehab* 1998; 12:73–79.

62. Alon G, McBride K. Persons with C5 or C6 tetraplegia achieve selected functional gains using a neuroprosthesis. *Arch Phys Med Rehabil* 2003; 84(1):119–124.

63. Prochazka A, Gauthier M, Wieler M, Kenwell Z. The bionic glove: an electrical stimulator garment that provides controlled grasp and hand opening in quadriplegia. *Arch Phys Med Rehabil* 1997; 78(6):608–614.

64. Popovic D, Stojanovic A, Pjanovic A, et al. Clinical evaluation of the bionic glove. *Arch Phys Med Rehabil* 1999; 80(3):299–304.

65. Johnson MW, Peckham PH, Bhadra N, et al. An implantable transducer for two-degree-of freedom joint angle sensing. *IEEE Trans Rehab Engin* 1999; 7:349–359.

66. Peckham PH, Kilgore KL, Keith MW, Bryden AM, Bhadra N, Montague FW. An advanced neuroprosthesis for restoration of hand and upper arm control using an implantable controller. *J Hand Surg* [Am] 2002; 27(2):265–276.

67. Kameyama J, Handa Y, Hoshimiya N, Sakurai M. Restoration of shoulder movement in quadriplegic and hemiplegic patients by functional electrical stimulation using percutaneous multiple electrodes. *Tohoku J Exp Med* 1999; 187(4):329–337.

68. Crago PE, Memberg DW, Usey MK, et al. An elbow extension neuroprosthesis for individuals with tetraplegia. *IEEE Trans Rehab Engin* 1998; 6:1–6.

69. Lauer RT, Kilgore KL, Peckham PH, Bhadra N, Keith MW. The function of the finger intrinsic muscles in response to electrical stimulation. *IEEE Trans Rehab Engin* 1999; 7:19–26.

70. Bryden AM, Kilgore KL, Kirsch RF, Memberg WD, Peckham PH, Keith MW. An implanted neuroprosthesis for high tetraplegia. *Top Spinal Cord Inj Rehabil* 2005; 10(3):38–52.

71. Brindley GS, Rushton DN. Long-term follow-up of patients with sacral anterior root stimulator implants. *Paraplegia* 1990; 28(8):469–475.

72. Creasey G. Restoration of bladder, bowel, and sexual function. *Top Spinal Cord Inj Rehabil* 1999; 5(1):21–32.

73. Kerrebroeck PV, Koldewijn E, Debruyne F. Worldwide experience with the Finetech-Brindley sacral anterior root stimulator. *Neurourol Urodyn* 1993; 12:497–503.

74. Koldewijn EL, Van Kerrebroeck PE, Rosier PF, Wijkstra H, Debruyne FM. Bladder compliance after posterior sacral root rhizotomies and anterior sacral root stimulation. *J Urol* 1994; 151(4):955–960.

75. Brindley G. The first 500 patients with sacral anterior root stimulator implants: general description. *Paraplegia* 1994; 32:795–805.

76. MacDonagh RP, Sun WM, Smallwood R, Forster D, Read NW. Control of defecation in patients with spinal injuries by stimulation of sacral anterior nerve roots. *British Med J* 1990; 300(6738):1494–1497.

77. Creasey GH, Dahlberg JE. Economic consequences of an implanted neuroprosthesis for bladder and bowel management. *Arch Phys Med Rehabil* 2001; 82(11):1520–1525.

78. Creasey GH, Kilgore KL, Brown-Triolo DL, Dahlberg JE, Peckham PH, Keith MW. Reduction of costs of disability using neuroprostheses. *Assist Technol* 2000; 12(1):67–75.

79. Ohl D. Electroejaculation. *Urologic Clinics of North America* 1993; 20(1):181–188.

80. Triolo R, Bogie K. Lower extremity applications of functional neuromuscular stimulation after spinal cord injury. *Topics in SCI Rehab* 1999; 5(1):44–65.

81. Bogie K, Reger S, Levine S. Therapeutic applications of electrical stimulation: wound healing and pressure sore prevention. *Assistive Technology* 2000; 12(1):50–66.

82. Bogie KM, Triolo RJ. Effects of regular use of neuromuscular electrical stimulation on tissue health. *J Rehabil Res Dev* 2003; 40(6):469–475.

83. Bogie K, Ho C, Chae J, Triolo R. Dynamic therapeutic neuromuscular electrical stimulation for pressure relief. *Am J Phys Med Rehabil* 2004; 83(3):240.

84. Bogie KM, Wang X, Triolo RJ. Long-term prevention of pressure ulcers in high-risk patients: a single case study of the use of gluteal neuromuscular electric stimulation. *Arch Phys Med Rehabil* 2006; 87(4):585–591.

85. McCaig CD. Dynamic aspects of amphibian neurite growth and the effects of an applied electric field. *J Physiol* 1986; 375:55–69.

86. Fehlings MG, Tator CH, Linden RD. The effect of direct-current field on recovery from experimental spinal cord injury. *J Neurosurg* 1988; 68(5):781–792.

87. Shapiro S, Borgens R, Pascuzzi R, et al. Oscillating field stimulation for complete spinal cord injury in humans: a phase 1 trial. *J Neurosurg Spine* 2005; 2(1):3–10.

88. Weber DJ, Stein RB, Chan KM, et al. Functional electrical stimulation using microstimulators to correct foot drop: a case study. *Can J Physiol Pharmacol* 2004; 82(8–9):784–792.

89. Gorman PH, Wuolle KS, Peckham PH, Heydrick D. Patient selection for an upper extremity neuroprosthesis in tetraplegic individuals. *Spinal Cord* 1997; 35(9):569–573.

64 Cardiovascular Fitness and Exercise Prescription after Spinal Cord Injury

Mark S. Nash

Clinical reports and research studies published over the past several decades have strongly encouraged persons who have SCI to adopt habitual exercise as part of a healthy lifestyle (1–5). This need has been underscored by many investigations that have documented an association between fitness and all-cause cardiovascular diseases (CVD) in persons without disability (6, 7). Public and private policies have now been influenced to the point that routine physical activity is considered both an indispensable lifestyle choice and an effective countermeasure for functional decline and CVD progression (8).

The aging of persons who have SCI underscores the need for global lifestyle intervention and adoption of healthy living standards. Of some 179,000 SCI survivors in the United States, 40% are now forty-five years or older, and one in four has lived twenty or more years with disability (9). Although SCI was once viewed as a "static medical condition" unaffected by time, it is now seen as a dynamic circumstance with continuously changing needs, abilities, and limitations (10). Such needs are hastened or intensified by cumulative stresses imposed by performance of daily activities needed to maintain an independent, healthy lifestyle (11). As fatigue, pain, weakness, skeletal decline, and even incipient neurological deficits appear (12), the performance of these essential daily activities, first mastered after injury, may again become challenging. These challenges, and the secondary disabilities they may impose, ultimately test the undertaking of active, satisfying, productive, and rewarding pursuits. Many believe that prudent exercise programs instituted soon after SCI represent one important way in which fated decline associated with longstanding paralysis might be prevented, or at least slowed.

CARDIOVASCULAR DECONDITIONING AFTER SCI

A sedentary lifestyle either imposed upon or adopted by persons who have SCI almost certainly explains both their poor levels of physical fitness and heightened risk of early CVD morbidity and mortality (13, 14). Reports first appearing in the mid-1980s placed persons living with SCI near the lowest end of the human fitness continuum (15), with more recent evidence suggesting that their sedentary profiles have remained unchanged. As evidence, nearly one of four healthy young persons with paraplegia fails to achieve levels of peak fitness on an arm exercise test sufficient to perform many essential activities of daily living. (16). While those with paraplegia have far greater capacities for activity and more extensive choices for exercise conditioning, they are barely more fit than their SCI counterparts with tetraplegia (15, 17). No evidence suggests that levels of fitness for those who have SCI will improve without a committed effort to increase daily physical activity.

Accelerated CVD (18), dyslipidemia (19), diabetes (20, 21), insulin resistance (21, 22), metabolic syndrome (20, 22, 23), exaggerated post-prandial lipemia (24), elevated inflammatory mediators (22), musculoskeletal decline (9), and either truncal obesity or morbidly elevated body mass indices (25–27) are all widely reported secondary complications in persons who have SCI, although their onset occurs earlier in life than observed in those without disability. These barriers to optimal health and function lend themselves to successful treatment through improved fitness. However, the undertaking of exercise conditioning after SCI is often more complicated, and the conditioning benefits potentially counterbalanced by irreversible consequences of imprudent exercise. It is thus important to identify effective and available exercise activities that reduce the risks of physical dysfunction and CVD sustained by persons who have SCI while not incurring multisystem injury or hastening musculoskeletal decline. This chapter will address exercise conditioning options for individuals who have SCI and the common risks of their exercise participation.

ALTERED CIRCULATORY FUNCTIONS AFTER SCI

Heart Structure and Function

Individuals with chronic SCI experience various types of circulatory dysregulation depending on the level of their lesion (28). This dysregulation influences the dynamics of blood flow at rest and during exercise, as well as the risk for CVD. When injury occurs above the level of spinal sympathetic outflow at the T1 spinal level, resting hypotension and mean arterial pressures of 70 mmHg are common (29). In addition to challenging effective orthostatic pressure regulation, severely low pressures also alter heart structure and function after SCI. As size and architecture of the human heart are profoundly influenced by peripheral circulatory volume and systemic pressures (30, 31), withdrawal from normal activity levels and altered circulatory dynamics transform the structure of the heart and alter its pumping efficiency (32). For those with tetraplegia, a chronic reduction of cardiac preload and myocardial volume, coupled with pressure underloading, causes the left ventricle to atrophy (33, 34). By contrast, those with paraplegia are normotensive and have normal left ventricular mass and resting cardiac output, but shift the elements of their cardiac output to a higher heart rate (HR) and smaller resting stroke volume (SV) (33, 35). This lowered SV is explained by a diminished venous return from the immobile lower extremities or frank venous insufficiency of the paralyzed limbs (35, 36).

Peripheral Vascular Structure and Function

The volume and velocity of lower extremity arterial circulation is significantly diminished after SCI within 6 weeks of SCI (37, 38), with volume flow of about half to two-thirds that reported in matched subjects without paralysis (39, 40). This "circulatory hypokinesis" results from impaired redistribution of blood after SCI and suboptimal ventricular filling pressures caused by pooling of venous blood, inactivity of the skeletal muscle pump in the legs, lack of sympathetic vasoconstriction below the lesion, and diminished regulation of local blood flow by vascular endothelium (39). The lowering of volume and velocity contribute to heightened thrombosis susceptibility commonly reported in those with acute and subacute SCI (31, 41). Contributing factors to thrombosis disposition include a markedly hypofibrinolytic response to venous occlusion of the paralyzed lower extremities (42, 43), low blood flow in the paralyzed lower extremities (39, 44–47), and from interruption of adrenergic pathways that typically regulate fibrinolysis in the presence of intact neuraxis (48). Reduced arterial circulation is also an established cause for skin breakdown in persons who have SCI (47).

EXERCISE PRESCRIPTION AFTER SCI

While the design of exercise training programs varies from individual to individual, a well-considered plan of conditioning-related activities plays an important role in achieving specific fitness and health goals, as well as reversing circulatory dysregulation occurring after SCI. The exercise prescriptions encompass an exercise mode, intensity, duration, and frequency whose interplay and varying degrees of complexity have been critically addressed by various authors (1, 14, 49, 50). While societal pressures often dictate that fitness is achieved through arduous programs of intense, prolonged work, the undertaking of any activity at all is the simplest of plans and is preferable to a sedentary lifestyle. In reality, most persons improve their protection against heart and vascular disease by attaining low and moderate levels of fitness, while high fitness levels typically afford little additional health benefit and impose risks of overuse and

injury that may require interruption or termination of activity. Moreover, persons who have lived a sedentary lifestyle generally become fit quite easily, which suggests that *any* physical activity performed above levels needed for daily activities would be beneficial.

Exercise Mode

Accessible and engaging exercise is the cornerstone of a well-designed exercise program, as other facets of exercise programming become trivial without a compliant conditioning effort. Selection should thus be based upon an ability to undertake uninterrupted activity for at least a few minutes' duration, which for persons who have SCI sometimes excludes ambulation, treadmills, or other exercise modes that require the bearing of weight. Unloading of the lower extremities during ambulation remains an option for those with incomplete injuries but requires specialized equipment to carry out. This leaves modes that are dominated by upper extremity exercise, such as arm ergometry, swimming, wheelchair locomotion, or resistance activities, as more widely accessible and practical exercise options. Availability of resources, costs, and pleasure derived from an activity all determine whether persons who have SCI will be compliant with long-term exercise.

Exercise Frequency and Duration

The elements of exercise frequency and duration are generally considered together, as they are inversely related. Authorities such as the American College of Sports Medicine recommend that persons perform 30–60 minutes of physical activity on most days of the week, although these guidelines are typically developed for persons without disability and fail to consider risks and consequences of upper extremity injury (51). Although exercise conditioning guidelines often warn of generic training risks including muscle strain and injury, they seldom caution that overuse or injury might profoundly diminish personal independence. Thus, restricting exercise frequency to two to three times weekly for 30 minutes is a prudent decision, especially early in training, when performance skills are still being acquired. More frequent exercise and longer periods of activity may be needed to attain high levels of fitness, although once these are attained, the incorporation of shorter, less frequent conditioning sessions into the lifestyle will be required to maintain it. Those exercising for competition will probably need more frequent and longer exercise sessions, although the risk of overuse or injury increases with prolonged exercise activity. Preservation of upper extremity function should be considered within the exercise plan so that chronic fatigue and injury do not interrupt the consistency of daily activities and independent lifestyle.

Exercise Intensity

Exercise intensities between 50–80% of peak capacity are usually sufficient to significantly improve fitness and to reduce CVD risks. Lower intensities may assist the most deconditioned of individuals in starting a program and ingraining an exercise habit, allowing progression to intensities above 50% of peak levels when tolerance is established. Under laboratory conditions, exercise intensity can be measured by the oxygen uptake derived from an exercise test using metabolic analysis. Concurrent measurement of oxygen uptake and HR allows the determination of HR targets that correspond to selected exercise intensities. However, upper limb activities generally elicit higher HR responses than lower extremity work, and the linear intensity-HR relationships are sometimes compromised in persons who have SCI (52). Further, individuals with injuries above the level of sympathetic outflow at T1 may experience incompetent rise of HR during exercise, which imposes peak HR at levels similar to those invoked by pharmacological adrenergic blockade. Therefore, HR might not be an accurate index of exercise intensity for all individuals who have SCI, and the use of simple "age-adjusted" (e.g., 220 − Age) methods commonly adopted for field-based assessment of exercise intensity in persons without disability may overestimate true work intensity in those who have SCI.

An alternative to the use of HR as a surrogate for work intensity is Borg's Rating of Perceived Exertion (RPE) scale (53), which is based upon somatic ratings of effort. The Borg range model postulates a relationship between somatic sensations and HR response but assumes a body habitus uncompromised by loss of sensation and cardiovascular dysregulation. Limited evidence suggests that it is valid and reliable for use by persons who have SCI, and a recent study has challenged its use as an index of work intensity in persons with both paraplegia and tetraplegia (54).

An underused yet simple method of intensity determination is the "talk test" (55), which is grounded in the observation that "a person who is active at a *light* intensity level should be able to sing while doing the activity. One who is active at a *moderate* intensity level should be able to carry on a conversation comfortably while engaging in the activity. If a person becomes winded or too out of breath to carry on a conversation, the activity can be considered *vigorous*." Other methods of intensity determination include use of the Karvonen equation, which bases exercise intensity on a percentage of the HR reserve (HRR = [HR max − HR rest] + HR rest), rather than estimation of an age-adjusted maximal HR. Unless a metabolic analyzer is used to establish the individual-specific intensity–HR relationship, use of the Karvonen is probably the simplest and best method for ensuring that training is performed within the appropriate intensity range, which is generally set in the 50–85% range of HRR (51).

EXERCISE MODES AND CONDITIONING BENEFITS

Electrically Stimulated Exercise

Various forms of electrically stimulated exercise are available for use by persons who have SCI. These include site-specific stimulation of the lower extremities (56–58) and upper extremities (59–62), leg cycling (63–65), leg cycling with upper extremity assist (66–68), lower body rowing (69), electrically assisted arm ergometry (70), electrically stimulated standing (71, 72), and electrically stimulated bipedal ambulation, either with an orthosis (73, 74) or without (75). Some of these applications can be used to strengthen muscles whose motor function is partially spared by SCI (76), whereas others use electrical current as a neuroprosthesis for the lower extremities (75) and upper extremities (59, 77–79). While electrical stimulation of local muscle sites stimulates hypertrophy and increases fiber endurance (58, 80), these muscle contractions promote adaptation of the heart in only the most deconditioned of subjects. Notwithstanding, they have been successfully used in

subjects with acute SCI to improve the pressor response to orthostatic repositioning (81) and promote a transitory fibrinolysis (82). Electrically stimulated contractions also increase resting and peak blood flow (39, 44–46), a response recently shown to be mediated by Endothelin(ET)-1 and its ET(A) receptors (83).

Most electrical stimulation devices currently approved for use by the U.S. Food and Drug Administration (FDA) employ surface electrical stimulation. The most common uses of surface electrical stimulation for system exercise in those who have SCI include electrically stimulated cycling, either with or without upper extremity assistive propulsion, and electrically stimulated ambulation. Qualifications necessary to safely participate in exercise programs have been described (63, 84).

Cycling Exercise

Electrically stimulated cycling uses electrically activated contractions of the bilateral quadriceps, hamstrings, and gluteus muscles under computer microprocessor command (85). Control of pedal rate and muscle stimulation intensity is exerted by feedback provided from position sensors placed in the pedal gear (86).

Enhanced levels of fitness (65, 67, 87), improved gas exchange kinetics (88), and increased muscle mass (89) have been reported after training using electrically stimulated cycling. For those with neurologically incomplete injuries, gains in lower extremity mass, isometric strength, and muscle endurance have been reported (89). Reversal of the adaptive left ventricular atrophy reported in persons with tetraplegia has also been observed, with near normalization of pretraining cardiac mass (90). This change may be associated with significantly improved lower extremity circulation following training, which is also accompanied by a more robust hyperemic response to experimental occlusion ischemia (39). Attenuation of paralytic osteopenia has been observed by some investigators (91, 92), and an increased rate of bone turnover by another researcher (93), although the sites benefiting from training are the lumbar spine and proximal tibia, not the proximal femur (92). Not all studies have found a posttraining increase in mineral density for bones located below the level of the lesion (94), although those that fail to do so have usually studied subjects with longstanding paralysis, in whom reversal of osteopenia has seen more limited success. Notwithstanding, a study examining the appearance of lower extremity joints and joint surfaces using magnetic resonance imaging reported no degenerative changes induced by cycling, and less joint surface necrosis than previously reported in sedentary persons who have SCI (95). Improved body composition favoring increased lean mass and decreased fat mass (96), and an enhancement of whole-body insulin uptake, insulin-stimulated 3–0-methyl glucose transport, and increased expression of GLUT4 transport protein in the quadriceps muscle have been observed (97). In a recent report, this training has resulted in improved profiles of insulin resistance. All of these benefits are important in treating the clustering of medical complications that are co-morbid with CVD.

Bipedal Ambulation Using Electrical Stimulation

Complex electrical stimulation to achieve bipedal ambulation has been used as a neuroprosthesis for those with motor-complete injuries (75, 98) and as an assistive neuroprosthesis accompanying body weight support for those who have incomplete injuries and lack the strength required to support independent ambulation (99–101). Surface and implantable neuroprostheses for those without spared motor function have received several decades of research attention (102), although the sole method currently approved by the FDA (Parastep-1) uses surface electrical stimulation of the quadriceps, hamstring, and gluteus muscles (98). Muscle activation is sequenced by a microprocessor worn on the belt, with step activation initiated by a control switch located on a rolling walker used by ambulating subjects. When pressed, the electrical stimulator sends current to the stance limb, initiating contraction of the quadriceps and gluteus muscles (75). Contralateral hip flexion is then achieved by exploiting an ipsilateral flexor withdrawal reflex obtained by introducing a nociceptive electrical stimulus over the common peroneal nerve at the head of the fibula. This allows the hip, knee, and ankle to move into flexion, followed by extension of the knee joint by electrical stimulation to the quadriceps. As muscle fatigue occurs, increasing levels of stimulation can be provided by a switch mounted on the handle of the rolling walker.

Rates of ambulation are relatively slow, and distances of ambulation relatively limited when using the system (98, 103) (Figure 64.1). Despite the limitations of ambulation velocity and distance, ambulation distances of up to 1 mile have been reported after training in some subjects (75, 104) and upper extremity fitness is enhanced after ambulation training (75, 104). Other adaptations to training include significantly increased lower extremity muscle mass, (105) improved resting blood flow (44), and an augmented hyperemic response to an experimental ischemic stimulus (44).

Arm Endurance Training

Persons who have SCI who adopt arm crank exercise, reciprocating arm exercise, wheelchair ergometry, and swimming for exercise conditioning significantly improve their levels of fitness (4, 8, 49, 106–113), with the magnitude of improvement inversely proportional to the level of spinal lesion. Endurance exercise has also been incorporated into virtual "gameplay" environments that serve as a countermeasure to boredom, which is often experienced during prolonged arm exercise (Figure 64.2).

While it is possible for persons with tetraplegia to train on an arm ergometer, special measures must be taken to affix the hands with special handles or gloves, and in these cases a reciprocal motion may be favored over a circular one (Figure 64.3). Clinically meaningful gains in peak oxygen uptake can still be achieved, although not as great as those of their spinal cord injured counterparts with paraplegia (114, 115). These gains in fitness are shown in Table 64.1. Level of SCI is generally the key determinant in predicting fitness enhancement after arm endurance training (116, 117).

Benefits of arm training are widely reported for persons with paraplegia, although their peak performance is limited by circulatory dysregulation accompanying thoracic SCI (118–120). As noted, individuals with injuries below the level of sympathetic outflow at T6 have significantly lower resting SV and higher resting HR than persons without paraplegia (119–121). The exaggerated HR response during exercise is thought to compensate for a lower cardiac SV imposed by pooling of blood in the

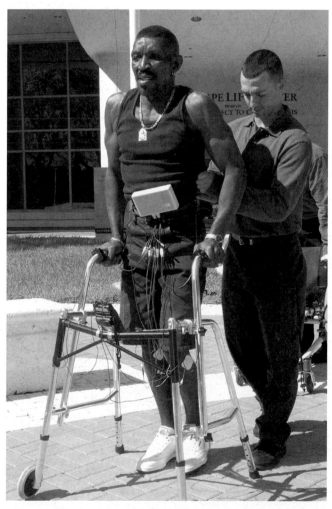

Figure 64.1 Parastep® electrically stimulated ambulation performed by an individual with paraplegia.

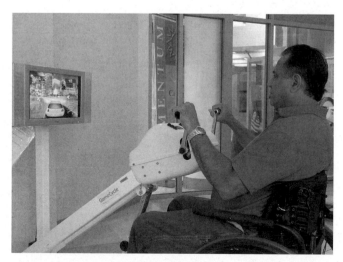

Figure 64.2 An individual with paraplegia experiencing "gameplay" exercise on a GameCycle®. The arm ergometer is a controller for speed and direction of a race car displayed by a Nintendo® GameCube®.

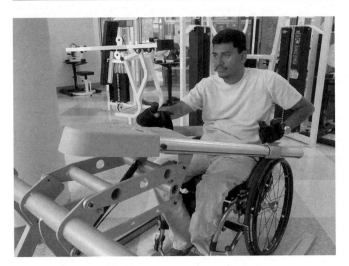

Figure 64.3 Arm exercise on a VitaGlide® reciprocating ergometer performed by an individual with C5–C6 tetraplegia using gloves to improve grasp.

lower extremity venous circuits, diminished venous return and cardiac end-diastolic volumes, or frank circulatory insufficiency (122, 123). Adjustments to the adrenergic systems after SCI may also regulate the excessive chronotropic response to work, as higher resting catecholamine levels and exaggerated catecholamine responses to physical work have been reported in paraplegics with middle thoracic (T5) cord injuries (124). These

exceed resting and exercise levels of both high level paraplegics and healthy persons without SCI (124, 125). Hypersensitivity of the supralesional spinal cord is believed to regulate this unusual adrenergic state, which contrasts the downregulation of adrenergic functions observed in persons with high thoracic and cervical cord lesions (93).

An exaggerated HR response is experienced during physical activity by persons with paraplegia (126). This finding is consistent with reports in which subjects with paraplegia require higher levels of oxygen consumption to perform the same work intensity as subjects without SCI (118, 120, 127, 128), and may represent a limiting factor in the performance of activities of daily living (120, 129, 130). As the sympathetic nervous system regulates hemodynamic and metabolic changes accompanying exercise (131), the elevated oxygen consumption and HR response to work in paraplegics with injuries below T5 may be due to adrenergic overactivity accompanying their paraplegia (124, 125).

Despite these hemodynamic and metabolic limitations, significant improvements in blood lipid profiles and CVD risks accompany their exercise training. In a cross-sectional study of persons with paraplegia, a significant inverse relationship was reported between VO_2 peak and the total cholesterol (TC) to high-density lipoprotein cholesterol (HDL-C) ratio, serum triglycerides, and the low-density lipoprotein cholesterol (LDL-C) to HDL-C ratio, as well as significant direct association between VO_2 peak and the HDL-C to Apoprotein A-1 ratio (17). These findings suggest a direct association between CVD risk indices and fitness similar to that observed for persons without SCI. In prospective analysis, persons who have SCI who

Table 64.1 Typical Improvements in Fitness and Power Output Accompanying Resistance and Endurance Exercise Conditioning

Participants/Activity	Program Duration	Exercise Duration	Frequency	Intensity	Fitness Gains
Para/ACE	12–32 weeks	30–40 min	3–5/wk	50%–70% VO_2 peak; 80% HR peak	7%–16% VO_2 peak; 16%–36% PO peak
Para/WCE	4–6 weeks	30–40 min	3/wk	50%–80% PO peak; 80% HR peak	14%–16% VO_2 peak; 20%–22% PO peak
Para/CRT	12–16 weeks	40 min	3/wk	50%–60% 1-RM plus unloaded, intermittent ACE	10–30% VO_2 peak; 13–59% 1-RM
Tetra/ACE	8–10 weeks	15–30 min	3/wk	HR = 96; 50%–60% HRR; 60% PO peak	8% VO_2 peak; 14%–24% PO peak
Tetra/WCE	8 weeks	20 min	7/wk	75%–85% HR peak	9% VO_2 peak

Abbreviations: ACE = armcrank ergometry; WCE = wheelchair ergometry; CRT = circuit resistance training; HR = heart rate; PO = power output; HRR = heart rate reserve.

underwent wheelchair ergometry training at 70–80% but not 50–60% of the HRR reserve improved their fasting HDL-C and decreased TG, LDL-C, and TC-to-HDL-C ratio (132). Thus, higher intensities, durations, and frequencies of exercise training may be required to invoke significant exercise-related lipid/lipoprotein changes, as is the case for persons without paraplegia, who often fail to alter their lipid profiles after low-intensity exercise training, but do so at higher intensities (133).

Arm Resistance Exercise

Increasing attention is being paid to the use of resistance activities as an endurance training tool and a countermeasure to CVD risk (51). These studies are especially important for persons who have SCI, as their susceptibility to upper limb decline has been widely reported, (134–141) and insufficient shoulder strength, range, and muscle endurance commonly cited as potential causes (139–143).

Studies examining effects of resistance exercise on the cardiovascular system and on strengthening of the upper extremities have received less attention for persons with paraplegia than their non-disabled counterparts. Nonetheless, studies have reported successful strengthening, enhanced function, reduced pain, and an improvement in CVD risks. Resistance training for triceps strengthening needed for elbow extension during crutch walking was successful in persons who have SCI (144), as was strengthening of the shoulder joint extensors and elbow flexors by high intensity (70% VO_2 peak) arm ergometry (145). These results, however, suggest that arm crank exercise is less effective as a training mode for upper extremity strengthening, because it fails to target the muscles most involved in performance of ADLs.

Targeted resistance training in persons who have SCI has been undertaken by several investigators. Conditioning of the chest and upper back were targeted in subjects with paraplegia and tetraplegia undergoing nine weeks of thrice-weekly resistance on a hydraulic fitness machine (146). Significant increases in average fitness and power output were observed after training, although testing was dedicated to general fitness, not measurement of strength gain. Another study focused training on concentric strengthening of the scapular retractor muscles (147), resulting in higher levels of retractor activation during backward wheelchair propulsion.

Despite gains in strength and power output using targeted resistance exercise, more global conditioning benefits and reduction of CVD risks have been achieved through use of circuit resistance training (CRT), which targets a wider range or resistance activities but requires that the exercises be rapidly sequenced without rest. Examples of these activities are shown in Figure 64.4. In the first of these studies, young, healthy persons with paraplegia improved muscle strength and cardiopulmonary endurance to a greater degree than was achieved by either strengthening or endurance conditioning programs (148). A similar protocol performed by "middle-aged" individuals who began training with shoulder pain resulted in similar gains in strength and endurance and enhanced anaerobic power, which were accompanied by reduced shoulder pain (149). These training-targeted benefits were reproduced in a similar exercise protocol using elastic bands (150), which would allow home-based implementation of a CRT program without need for resistance equipment. Benefits of training reported in these studies were replicated in a twice-weekly training program in which significant

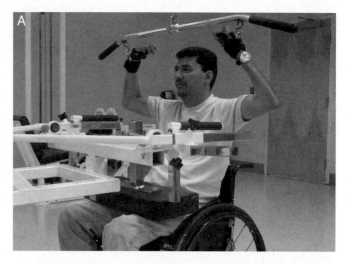

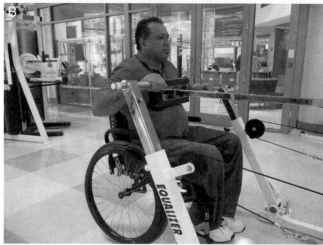

Figure 64.4 Resistance exercises performed by persons with tetraplegia (**A**) and paraplegia (**B**). Wrist wraps with "D" rings can function as handholds where grasp cannot provide safety and control.

improvements in subpeak power and upper body strength were accompanied by reduction of pain, stress, and depression, as well as by improved indices of satisfaction with physical function, perceived health, and overall life quality (151). Benefits documented in this study were reversed if participants failed to maintain long-term compliance with the conditioning regimen (152).

UNIQUE EXERCISE COMPLICATIONS AND CAVEATS

Special attention to avoiding exercise hazards and injuries is required when designing exercise programs for persons who have SCI. Many of their potential exercise risks will mirror those experienced by persons without paralysis, although complications such as general overuse may have more exaggerated outcomes in those who have SCI. Their occurrence will also complicate performance of daily activities to a far greater extent than similar injuries arising in persons without SCI.

Special medical complications may be experienced by individuals exercising under the control of electrical current. The foremost of these complications involves episodes of autonomic hyperreflexia, which can occur in individuals having injuries at and above the T6 spinal cord level (28, 153). Recognition of these episodes, withdrawal of the offending stimulus, and the possible administration of a fast-acting peripheral vasodilator may be critical in preventing serious medical complications. Prophylaxis with a slow calcium channel blocker or an α_1-selective adrenergic antagonist may be needed before exercise if electrical current consistently evokes symptoms of adrenergic hyperstimulation (37, 154). It is widely known that wheelchair racers have intentionally induced this response as an ergogenic aid by restricting urine outflow through an indwelling catheter (155), a practice widely viewed as dangerous, and one that should be discouraged.

Fracture and joint dislocation have been noted as a consequence of electrically stimulated exercise and may be caused by asynergistic movement of limbs against the force imposed by either electrical stimulation or the device used for exercise (156). This explains why these activities are contraindicated for individuals with severe spasticity, or spastic response to the introduction of electrical current (63). Small risks of post-exercise hypotension (29) are associated with lost vasomotor responses to orthostatic repositioning (81), although these episodes can abate after upper limb training.

Special precautions must be taken by those participating in upper extremity exercise to prevent overuse injuries of the arms and shoulders (148, 157, 158). These include adoption of conservative exercise intensities at the start of training. If a wheelchair is used for exercise training, it should be designed to provide efficiency and safety at higher repetition rates, and to provide greater exercise stability. Because the shoulder joints are ill designed to perform locomotor activities, but must do so nonetheless in individuals unable to walk, injuries may compromise essential activities of wheelchair propulsion (159), weight relief (160), and depression transfers (161) and may profoundly influence essential daily activities for persons who have SCI.

Individuals who have SCI often lack sudomotor responses below their level of injury and are thus challenged to maintain thermal stability (38, 162, 163). Mean body temperature and body heat content increase more in persons who have SCI than in those who do not (164, 165). These effects are less pronounced as the level of SCI descends (166), and when exercising in an environment controlled for temperature and humidity (2, 167, 168). Thus, attention should be paid to pre-exercise hydration and, if possible, to limiting the duration and intensity of activities performed in intemperate environments.

CONCLUSIONS

Persons who have spinal cord injuries often lead sedentary lifestyles. Sedentary behaviors can be imposed by choice, limited sparing of muscle, or restricted exercise options. Irrespective of cause, these lifestyles compromise health and function as persons age with their disability. Although exercise injuries need to be anticipated, and special caveats observed, many exercise options are available for persons who have SCI that reverse effects of immobilization deconditioning and sedentary living. Beneficial multisystem adaptations accompany these exercise programs, including reduction of CVD risks and attenuation of conditions considered to be co-morbid with all-cause CVD progression.

Improved cardiovascular fitness enhances the ability of persons who have SCI to lead healthy, active, satisfying, and productive lives. Greater emphasis on the effects of conditioning exercise across the spectrum of injuries after complete and incomplete spinal cord paralysis is needed to better examine functional and health changes resulting from increased physical activity and exercise pursuits as persons age with SCI.

References

1. Nash MS. Exercise as a health-promoting activity following spinal cord injury. *J Neurol Phys Ther* 2005; 29:87–103, 106.
2. Myers J, Lee M, Kiratli J. Cardiovascular disease in spinal cord injury: an overview of prevalence, risk, evaluation, and management. *Am J Phys Med Rehabil* 2007; 86:142–152.
3. Glaser RM. Exercise and locomotion for the spinal cord injured. *Exerc Sport Sci Rev* 1985; 13:263–303.
4. Valent L, Dallmeijer A, Houdijk H, Talsma E, van der Woude L. The effects of upper body exercise on the physical capacity of people with a spinal cord injury: a systematic review. *Clin Rehabil* 2007; 21:315–330.
5. Phillips WT, Kiratli BJ, Sarkarati M, et al. Effect of spinal cord injury on the heart and cardiovascular fitness. *Curr Probl Cardiol* 1998; 23:641–716.
6. Adult participation in recommended levels of physical activity—United States, 2001 and 2003. *MMWR Morb Mortal Wkly Rep* 2005; 54:1208–1212.
7. Proceedings of the 5th International Conference on Nutrition and Fitness, Athens, Greece, June 9–12, 2004. Part 1. *World Rev Nutr Diet* 2005; 94:XIV-XLVI, 1–188.
8. Marcus BH, Williams DM, Dubbert PM, et al. Physical activity intervention studies: what we know and what we need to know: a scientific statement from the American Heart Association Council on Nutrition, Physical Activity, and Metabolism (Subcommittee on Physical Activity); Council on Cardiovascular Disease in the Young; and the Interdisciplinary Working Group on Quality of Care and Outcomes Research. *Circulation* 2006; 114:2739–2752.
9. Gerhart KA, Bergstrom E, Charlifue SW, Menter RR, Whiteneck GG. Long-term spinal cord injury: functional changes over time. *Arch Phys Med Rehabil* 1993; 74:1030–1034.
10. Menter RR. Spinal cord injury and aging: exploring the unknown. 1993 Heiner Sell Lecture of the American Spinal Injury Association. *J Am Paraplegia Soc* 1993; 16:179–189.
11. Ohry A, Shemesh Y, Rozin R. Are chronic spinal cord injured patients (SCIP) prone to premature aging? *Med Hypotheses* 1983; 11:467–469.
12. Waters RL, Sie IH, Adkins RH. The musculoskeletal system. In: Whiteneck GG, Charlifue SW, Gerhart KA (eds.), *Aging with Spinal Cord Injury.* New York: Demos Medical Publishers 1993:53–72.
13. Washburn RA, Figoni SF. Physical activity and chronic cardiovascular disease prevention in spinal cord injury: a comprehensive literature review. *Top Spinal Cord Injury Rehabil* 1998; 3:16–32.
14. Nash MS. Exercise reconditioning of the heart and peripheral circulation after spinal cord injury. *Top Spinal Cord Inj Rehabil* 1997; 3:1–15.
15. Dearwater SR, LaPorte RE, Robertson RJ, Brenes G, Adams LL, Becker D. Activity in the spinal cord-injured patient: an epidemiologic analysis of metabolic parameters. *Med Sci Sports Exerc* 1986; 18:541–544.
16. Noreau L, Shephard RJ, Simard C, Pare G, Pomerleau P. Relationship of impairment and functional ability to habitual activity and fitness following spinal cord injury. *Int J Rehabil Res* 1993; 16:265–275.
17. Bostom AG, Toner MM, McArdle WD, Montelione T, Brown CD, Stein RA. Lipid and lipoprotein profiles relate to peak aerobic power in spinal cord injured men. *Med Sci Sports Exerc* 1991; 23:409–414.
18. Bauman WA, Spungen AM, Raza M, et al. Coronary artery disease: metabolic risk factors and latent disease in individuals with paraplegia. *Mt Sinai J Med* 1992; 59:163–168.
19. Bauman WA, Spungen AM. Disorders of carbohydrate and lipid metabolism in veterans with paraplegia or quadriplegia: a model of premature aging. *Metabolism* 1994; 43:749–756.
20. Bauman WA, Spungen AM. Metabolic changes in persons after spinal cord injury. *Phys Med Rehabil Clin N Am* 2000; 11:109–140.
21. Duckworth WC, Solomon SS, Jallepalli P, Heckemeyer C, Finnern J, Powers A. Glucose intolerance due to insulin resistance in patients with spinal cord injuries. *Diabetes* 1980; 29:906–910.

22. Lee MY, Myers J, Hayes A, et al. C-reactive protein, metabolic syndrome, and insulin resistance in individuals with spinal cord injury. *J Spinal Cord Med* 2005; 28:20–25.

23. Nash MS, Mendez AJ. A guideline-driven assessment of need for cardiovascular disease risk intervention in persons with chronic paraplegia. *Arch Phys Med Rehabil* 2007; 88:751–757.

24. Nash MS, DeGroot J, Martinez-Arizala A, Mendez AJ. Evidence for an exaggerated postprandial lipemia in chronic paraplegia. *J Spinal Cord Med* 2005; 28:320–325.

25. Zlotolow SP, Levy E, Bauman WA. The serum lipoprotein profile in veterans with paraplegia: the relationship to nutritional factors and body mass index. *J Am Paraplegia Soc* 1992; 15:158–162.

26. Spungen AM, Adkins RH, Stewart CA, et al. Factors influencing body composition in persons with spinal cord injury: a cross-sectional study. *J Appl Physiol* 2003; 95:2398–2407.

27. Haisma JA, van der Woude LH, Stam HJ, et al. Complications following spinal cord injury: occurrence and risk factors in a longitudinal study during and after inpatient rehabilitation. *J Rehabil Med* 2007; 39:393–398.

28. McKinley WO, Jackson AB, Cardenas DD, DeVivo MJ. Long-term medical complications after traumatic spinal cord injury: a regional model systems analysis. *Arch Phys Med Rehabil* 1999; 80:1402–1410.

29. King ML, Lichtman SW, Pellicone JT, Close RJ, Lisanti P. Exertional hypotension in spinal cord injury. *Chest* 1994; 106:1166–1171.

30. Grossman W, Jones D, McLaurin LP. Wall stress and patterns of hypertrophy in the human left ventricle. *J Clin Invest* 1975; 56:56–64.

31. Grossman W, Braunwald E, Mann T, McLaurin LP, Green LH. Contractile state of the left ventricle in man as evaluated from end-systolic pressure-volume relations. *Circulation* 1977; 56:845–852.

32. Cooper G IV, Tomanek RJ. Load regulation of the structure, composition, and function of mammalian myocardium. *Circ Res* 1982; 50:788–798.

33. Kessler KM, Pina I, Green B, et al. Cardiovascular findings in quadriplegic and paraplegic patients and in normal subjects. *Am J Cardiol* 1986; 58:525–530.

34. Nash MS. Exercise and immunology. *Med Sci Sports Exerc* 1994; 26:125–127.

35. Hopman MT. Circulatory responses during arm exercise in individuals with paraplegia. *Int J Sports Med* 1994; 15:126–131.

36. Hopman MT, van Asten WN, Oeseburg B. Changes in blood flow in the common femoral artery related to inactivity and muscle atrophy in individuals with long-standing paraplegia. *Adv Exp Med Biol* 1996; 388:379–383.

37. de Groot PC, Bleeker MW, Hopman MT. Magnitude and time course of arterial vascular adaptations to inactivity in humans. *Exerc Sport Sci Rev* 2006; 34:65–71.

38. de Groot PC, Bleeker MW, van Kuppevelt DH, van der Woude LH, Hopman MT. Rapid and extensive arterial adaptations after spinal cord injury. *Arch Phys Med Rehabil* 2006; 87:688–696.

39. Nash MS, Montalvo BM, Applegate B. Lower extremity blood flow and responses to occlusion ischemia differ in exercise-trained and sedentary tetraplegic persons. *Arch Phys Med Rehabil* 1996; 77:1260–1265.

40. Taylor PN, Ewins DJ, Fox B, Grundy D, Swain ID. Limb blood flow, cardiac output and quadriceps muscle bulk following spinal cord injury and the effect of training for the Odstock functional electrical stimulation standing system. *Paraplegia* 1993; 31:303–310.

41. Fitzgerald RH Jr. Post-discharge prevention of deep vein thrombosis following total joint replacement. *Orthopedics* 1996; 19 Suppl:15–18.

42. Winther K, Gleerup G, Snorrason K, Biering-Sorensen F. Platelet function and fibrinolytic activity in cervical spinal cord injured patients. *Thromb Res* 1992; 65:469–474.

43. Boudaoud L, Roussi J, Lortat-Jacob S, Bussel B, Dizien O, Drouet L. Endothelial fibrinolytic reactivity and the risk of deep venous thrombosis after spinal cord injury. *Spinal Cord* 1997; 35:151–157.

44. Nash MS, Jacobs PL, Montalvo BM, Klose KJ, Guest RS, Needham-Shropshire BM. Evaluation of a training program for persons with SCI paraplegia using the Parastep 1 ambulation system. Part 5. Lower extremity blood flow and hyperemic responses to occlusion are augmented by ambulation training. *Arch Phys Med Rehabil* 1997; 78:808–814.

45. Thijssen DH, Ellenkamp R, Smits P, Hopman MT. Rapid vascular adaptations to training and detraining in persons with spinal cord injury. *Arch Phys Med Rehabil* 2006; 87:474–481.

46. Thijssen DH, Heesterbeek P, van Kuppevelt DJ, Duysens J, Hopman MT. Local vascular adaptations after hybrid training in spinal cord-injured subjects. *Med Sci Sports Exerc* 2005; 37:1112–1118.

47. Deitrick G, Charalel J, Bauman W, Tuckman J. Reduced arterial circulation to the legs in spinal cord injury as a cause of skin breakdown lesions. *Angiology* 2007; 58:175–184.

48. el-Sayed MS. Extrinsic plasminogen activator response to exercise after a single dose of propranolol. *Med Sci Sports Exerc* 1992; 24:327–332.

49. Hoffman MD. Cardiorespiratory fitness and training in quadriplegics and paraplegics. *Sports Med* 1986; 3:312–330.

50. Jacobs PL, Nash MS. Exercise recommendations for individuals with spinal cord injury. *Sports Med* 2004; 34:727–751.

51. Haskell WL, Lee IM, Pate RR, et al. Physical activity and public health: Updated recommendation for adults from the American College of Sports Medicine and the American Heart Association. *Med Sci Sports Exerc* 2007; 39:1423–1434.

52. Valent LJ, Dallmeijer AJ, Houdijk H, et al. The individual relationship between heart rate and oxygen uptake in people with a tetraplegia during exercise. *Spinal Cord* 2007; 45:104–111.

53. Borg G. Perceived exertion as an indicator of somatic stress. *Scand J Rehabil Med* 1970; 2:92–98.

54. Lewis JE, Nash MS, Hamm LF, Martins SC, Groah SL. The relationship between perceived exertion and physiologic indicators of stress during graded arm exercise in persons with spinal cord injuries. *Arch Phys Med Rehabil* 2007; 88:1205–1211.

55. Persinger R, Foster C, Gibson M, Fater DC, Porcari JP. Consistency of the talk test for exercise prescription. *Med Sci Sports Exerc* 2004; 36:1632–1636.

56. Figoni SF, Glaser RM, Rodgers MM, et al. Acute hemodynamic responses of spinal cord injured individuals to functional neuromuscular stimulation-induced knee extension exercise. *J Rehabil Res Dev* 1991; 28:9–18.

57. Rodgers MM, Glaser RM, Figoni SF, et al. Musculoskeletal responses of spinal cord injured individuals to functional neuromuscular stimulation-induced knee extension exercise training. *J Rehabil Res Dev* 1991; 28:19–26.

58. Greve JM, Muszkat R, Schmidt B, Chiovatto J, Barros Filho TE, Batisttella LR. Functional electrical stimulation (FES): muscle histochemical analysis. *Paraplegia* 1993; 31:764–770.

59. Scott TR, Peckham PH, Keith MW. Upper extremity neuroprostheses using functional electrical stimulation. *Baillieres Clin Neurol* 1995; 4:57–75.

60. Mulcahey MJ, Betz RR, Smith BT, Weiss AA, Davis SE. Implanted functional electrical stimulation hand system in adolescents with spinal injuries: an evaluation. *Arch Phys Med Rehabil* 1997; 78:597–607.

61. Billian C, Gorman PH. Upper extremity applications of functional neuromuscular stimulation. *Assist Technol* 1992; 4:31–39.

62. Bryden AM, Memberg WD, Crago PE. Electrically stimulated elbow extension in persons with C5/C6 tetraplegia: a functional and physiological evaluation. *Arch Phys Med Rehabil* 2000; 81:80–88.

63. Ragnarsson KT, Pollack S, O'Daniel W Jr, Edgar R, Petrofsky J, Nash MS. Clinical evaluation of computerized functional electrical stimulation after spinal cord injury: a multicenter pilot study. *Arch Phys Med Rehabil* 1988; 69:672–677.

64. Nash MS, Bilsker MS, Kearney HM, Ramirez JN, Applegate B, Green BA. Effects of electrically-stimulated exercise and passive motion on echocardiographically-derived wall motion and cardiodynamic function in tetraplegic persons. *Paraplegia* 1995; 33:80–89.

65. Hooker SP, Figoni SF, Rodgers MM, et al. Physiologic effects of electrical stimulation leg cycle exercise training in spinal cord injured persons. *Arch Phys Med Rehabil* 1992; 73:470–476.

66. Raymond J, Davis GM, Climstein M, Sutton JR. Cardiorespiratory responses to arm cranking and electrical stimulation leg cycling in people with paraplegia. *Med Sci Sports Exerc* 1999; 31:822–828.

67. Mutton DL, Scremin AM, Barstow TJ, Scott MD, Kunkel CF, Cagle TG. Physiologic responses during functional electrical stimulation leg cycling and hybrid exercise in spinal cord injured subjects. *Arch Phys Med Rehabil* 1997; 78:712–718.

68. Krauss JC, Robergs RA, Depaepe JL, et al. Effects of electrical stimulation and upper body training after spinal cord injury. *Med Sci Sports Exerc* 1993; 25:1054–1061.

69. Laskin JJ, Ashley EA, Olenik LM, et al. Electrical stimulation-assisted rowing exercise in spinal cord injured people: a pilot study. *Paraplegia* 1993; 31:534–541.

70. Cameron T, Broton JG, Needham-Shropshire B, Klose KJ. An upper body exercise system incorporating resistive exercise and neuromuscular electrical stimulation (NMS). *J Spinal Cord Med* 1998; 21:1–6.

71. Davis R, Houdayer T, Andrews B, Emmons S, Patrick J. Paraplegia: prolonged closed-loop standing with implanted nucleus FES-22 stimulator and Andrews' foot-ankle orthosis. *Stereotact Funct Neurosurg* 1997; 69:281–287.

72. Triolo RJ, Bieri C, Uhlir J, Kobetic R, Scheiner A, Marsolais EB. Implanted Functional Neuromuscular Stimulation systems for individuals with cervical spinal cord injuries: clinical case reports. *Arch Phys Med Rehabil* 1996; 77:1119–1128.

73. Ferguson KA, Polando G, Kobetic R, Triolo RJ, Marsolais EB. Walking with a hybrid orthosis system. *Spinal Cord* 1999; 37:800–804.

74. Phillips CA, Gallimore JJ, Hendershot DM. Walking when utilizing a sensory feedback system and an electrical muscle stimulation gait orthosis. *Med Eng Phys* 1995; 17:507–513.

75. Graupe D, Kohn KH. Functional neuromuscular stimulator for short-distance ambulation by certain thoracic-level spinal-cord-injured paraplegics. *Surg Neurol* 1998; 50:202–207.

76. Carroll SG, Bird SF, Brown DJ. Electrical stimulation of the lumbrical muscles in an incomplete quadriplegic patient: case report. *Paraplegia* 1992; 30:223–226.

77. Dimitrijevic MM. Mesh-glove. 1. A method for whole-hand electrical stimulation in upper motor neuron dysfunction. *Scand J Rehabil Med* 1994; 26:183–186.

78. Kameyama J, Handa Y, Hoshimiya N, Sakurai M. Restoration of shoulder movement in quadriplegic and hemiplegic patients by functional electrical stimulation using percutaneous multiple electrodes. *Tohoku J Exp Med* 1999; 187:329–337.

79. Mulcahey MJ, Smith BT, Betz RR. Evaluation of the lower motor neuron integrity of upper extremity muscles in high level spinal cord injury. *Spinal Cord* 1999; 37:585–591.

80. Dudley GA, Castro MJ, Rogers S, Apple DF Jr. A simple means of increasing muscle size after spinal cord injury: a pilot study. *Eur J Appl Physiol Occup Physiol* 1999; 80:394–396.

81. Lopes P, Figoni SF, Perkash I. Upper limb exercise effect on tilt tolerance during orthostatic training of patients with spinal cord injury. *Arch Phys Med Rehabil* 1984; 65:251–253.

82. Katz RT, Green D, Sullivan T, Yarkony G. Functional electric stimulation to enhance systemic fibrinolytic activity in spinal cord injury patients. *Arch Phys Med Rehabil* 1987; 68:423–426.

83. Thijssen DH, Ellenkamp R, Kooijman M, et al. A causal role for endothelin-1 in the vascular adaptation to skeletal muscle deconditioning in spinal cord injury. *Arterioscler Thromb Vasc Biol* 2007; 27:325–331.

84. Phillips CA. Medical criteria for active physical therapy. Physician guidelines for patient participation in a program of functional electrical rehabilitation. *Am J Phys Med* 1987; 66:269–286.

85. Glaser RM. Functional neuromuscular stimulation. Exercise conditioning of spinal cord injured patients. *Int J Sports Med* 1994; 15:142–148.

86. Petrofsky JS, Phillips CA. The use of functional electrical stimulation for rehabilitation of spinal cord injured patients. *Cent Nerv Syst Trauma* 1984; 1:57–74.

87. Hooker SP, Scremin AM, Mutton DL, Kunkel CF, Cagle G. Peak and submaximal physiologic responses following electrical stimulation leg cycle ergometer training. *J Rehabil Res Dev* 1995; 32:361–366.

88. Barstow TJ, Scremin AM, Mutton DL, Kunkel CF, Cagle TG, Whipp BJ. Changes in gas exchange kinetics with training in patients with spinal cord injury. *Med Sci Sports Exerc* 1996; 28:1221–1228.

89. Scremin AM, Kurta L, Gentili A, et al. Increasing muscle mass in spinal cord injured persons with a functional electrical stimulation exercise program. *Arch Phys Med Rehabil* 1999; 80:1531–1536.

90. Nash MS, Bilsker S, Marcillo AE, et al. Reversal of adaptive left ventricular atrophy following electrically-stimulated exercise training in human tetraplegics. *Paraplegia* 1991; 29:590–599.

91. BeDell KK, Scremin AME, Perell KL, Kunkel CF. Effects of functional electrical stimulation-induced lower extremity cycling on bone density of spinal cord-injured patients. *Am J Phys Med Rehabil* 1996; 75:29–34.

92. Mohr T, Podenphant J, Biering-Sorensen F, Galbo H, Thamsborg G, Kjaer M. Increased bone mineral density after prolonged electrically induced cycle training of paralyzed limbs in spinal cord injured man. *Calcif Tissue Int* 1997; 61:22–25.

93. Bloomfield SA, Jackson RD, Mysiw WJ. Catecholamine response to exercise and training in individuals with spinal cord injury. *Med Sci Sports Exerc* 1994; 26:1213–1219.

94. Leeds EM, Klose KJ, Ganz W, Serafini A, Green BA. Bone mineral density after bicycle ergometry training. *Arch Phys Med Rehabil* 1990; 71:207–209.

95. Nash MS, Tehranzadeh J, Green BA, Rountree MT, Shea JD. Magnetic resonance imaging of osteonecrosis and osteoarthrosis in exercising quadriplegics and paraplegics. *Am J Phys Med* 1994; 73:184–192.

96. Hjeltnes N, Aksnes AK, Birkeland KI, Johansen J, Lannem A, Wallberg-Henriksson H. Improved body composition after 8 wk of electrically stimulated leg cycling in tetraplegic patients. *Am J Physiol* 1997; 273:R1072–R1079.

97. Hjeltnes N, Galuska D, Bjornholm M, et al. Exercise-induced overexpression of key regulatory proteins involved in glucose uptake and metabolism in tetraplegic persons: molecular mechanism for improved glucose homeostasis. *FASEB J* 1998; 12:1701–1712.

98. Klose KJ, Jacobs PL, Broton JG, et al. Evaluation of a training program for persons with SCI paraplegia using the Parastep 1 ambulation system. Part 1. Ambulation performance and anthropometric measures. *Arch Phys Med Rehabil* 1997; 78:789–793.

99. Remy-Neris O, Barbeau H, Daniel O, Boiteau F, Bussel B. Effects of intrathecal clonidine injection on spinal reflexes and human locomotion in incomplete paraplegic subjects. *Exp Brain Res* 1999; 129:433–440.

100. Stein RB, Belanger M, Wheeler G, et al. Electrical systems for improving locomotion after incomplete spinal cord injury: an assessment. *Arch Phys Med Rehabil* 1993; 74:954–959.

101. Norman KE, Pepin A, Barbeau H. Effects of drugs on walking after spinal cord injury. *Spinal Cord* 1998; 36:699–715.

102. Graupe D, Salahi J, Kohn KH. Multifunctional prosthesis and orthosis control via microcomputer identification of temporal pattern differences in single-site myoelectric signals. *J Biomed Eng* 1982; 4:17–22.

103. Gallien P, Brissot R, Eyssette M, et al. Restoration of gait by functional electrical stimulation for spinal cord injured patients. *Paraplegia* 1995; 33:660–664.

104. Jacobs PL, Nash MS, Klose KJ, Guest RS, Needham-Shropshire BM, Green BA. Evaluation of a training program for persons with SCI paraplegia using the Parastep 1 ambulation system. Part 2. Effects on physiological responses to peak arm ergometry. *Arch Phys Med Rehabil* 1997; 78:794–798.

105. Jaeger RJ. Lower extremity applications of functional neuromuscular stimulation. *Assist Technol* 1992; 4:19–30.

106. Cowell LL, Squires WG, Raven PB. Benefits of aerobic exercise for the paraplegic: a brief review. *Med Sci Sports Exerc* 1986; 18:501–508.

107. Davis GM, Shephard RJ, Leenen FH. Cardiac effects of short term arm crank training in paraplegics: echocardiographic evidence. *Eur J Appl Physiol* 1987; 56:90–96.

108. Franklin BA. Aerobic exercise training programs for the upper body. *Med Sci Sports Exerc* 1989; 21:S141–S148.

109. Miles DS, Sawka MN, Wilde SW, Durbin RJ, Gotshall RW, Glaser RM. Pulmonary function changes in wheelchair athletes subsequent to exercise training. *Ergonomics* 1982; 25:239–246.

110. Pollock ML, Miller HS, Linnerud AC, Laughridge E, Coleman E, Alexander E. Arm pedaling as an endurance training regimen for the disabled. *Arch Phys Med Rehabil* 1974; 55:418–424.

111. Sedlock DA, Knowlton RG, Fitzgerald PI. The effects of arm crank training on the physiological responses to submaximal wheelchair ergometry. *Eur J Appl Physiol* 1988; 57:55–59.

112. Taylor AW, McDonell E, Brassard L. The effects of an arm ergometer training programme on wheelchair subjects. *Paraplegia* 1986; 24:105–114.

113. Yim SY, Cho KJ, Park CI, et al. Effect of wheelchair ergometer training on spinal cord-injured paraplegics. *Yonsei Med J* 1993; 34:278–286.

114. DiCarlo SE. Effect of arm ergometry training on wheelchair propulsion endurance of individuals with quadriplegia. *Phys Ther* 1988; 68:40–44.

115. DiCarlo SE, Supp MD, Taylor HC. Effect of arm ergometry training on physical work capacity of individuals with spinal cord injuries. *Phys Ther* 1983; 63:1104–1107.

116. Drory Y, Ohry A, Brooks ME, Dolphin D, Kellermann JJ. Arm crank ergometry in chronic spinal cord injured patients. *Arch Phys Med Rehabil* 1990; 71:389–392.

117. Hjeltnes N. Cardiorespiratory capacity in tetra- and paraplegia shortly after injury. *Scand J Rehabil Med* 1986; 18:65–70.

118. Hooker SP, Greenwood JD, Hatae DT, Husson RP, Matthiesen TL, Waters AR. Oxygen uptake and heart rate relationship in persons with spinal cord injury. *Med Sci Sports Exerc* 1993; 25:1115–1119.

119. Hopman MT, Pistorius M, Kamerbeek IC, Binkhorst RA. Cardiac output in paraplegic subjects at high exercise intensities. *Eur J Appl Physiol* 1993; 66:531–535.

120. Van Loan MD, McCluer S, Loftin JM, Boileau RA. Comparison of physiological responses to maximal arm exercise among able-bodied, paraplegics and quadriplegics. *Paraplegia* 1987; 25:397–405.

121. DeBruin MIBRA. Cardiac output of paraplegics during exercise. *Int J Sports Med* 1984; 5:175–176.

122. Hopman MT, Kamerbeek IC, Pistorius M, Binkhorst RA. The effect of an anti-G suit on the maximal performance of individuals with paraplegia. *Int J Sports Med* 1993; 14:357–361.

123. Hopman MT, Oeseburg B, Binkhorst RA. Cardiovascular responses in paraplegic subjects during arm exercise. *Eur J Appl Physiol* 1992; 65:73–78.

124. Schmid A, Huonker M, Barturen JM, et al. Catecholamines, heart rate, and oxygen uptake during exercise in persons with spinal cord injury. *J Appl Physiol* 1998; 85:635–641.

125. Schmid A, Huonker M, Stahl F, et al. Free plasma catecholamines in spinal cord injured persons with different injury levels at rest and during exercise. *J Auton Nerv Syst* 1998; 68:96–100.

126. Hjeltnes N. Oxygen uptake and cardiac output in graded arm exercise in paraplegics with low level spinal lesions. *Scand J Rehabil Med* 1977; 9:107–113.

127. Knutsson E, Lewenhaupt-Olsson E, Thorsen M. Physical work capacity and physical conditioning in paraplegic patients. *Paraplegia* 1973; 11:205–216.

128. Davis GM, Shephard RJ. Cardiorespiratory fitness in highly active versus inactive paraplegics. *Med Sci Sports Exerc* 1988; 20:463–468.

129. Janssen TW, van Oers CA, van der Woude LH, Hollander AP. Physical strain in daily life of wheelchair users with spinal cord injuries. *Med Sci Sports Exerc* 1994; 26:661–670.

130. Janssen TW, van Oers CA, Veeger HE, Hollander AP, van der Woude LH, Rozendal RH. Relationship between physical strain during standardised ADL tasks and physical capacity in men with spinal cord injuries. *Paraplegia* 1994; 32:844–859.

131. Ehsani AA, Heath GW, Martin WH 3d, Hagberg JM, Holloszy JO. Effects of intense exercise training on plasma catecholamines in coronary patients. *J Appl Physiol* 1984; 57:155–159.

132. Hooker SP, Wells CL. Effects of low- and moderate-intensity training in spinal cord-injured persons. *Med Sci Sports Exerc* 1989; 21:18–22.

133. Blair SN, Kohl HW III, Paffenbarger RS Jr, Clark DG, Cooper KH, Gibbons LW. Physical fitness and all-cause mortality. A prospective study of healthy men and women. *JAMA* 1989; 262:2395–2401.

134. Gellman H, Sie I, Waters RL. Late complications of the weight-bearing upper extremity in the paraplegic patient. *Clin Orthop* 1988; 132–135.

135. Sie IH, Waters RL, Adkins RH, Gellman H. Upper extremity pain in the postrehabilitation spinal cord injured patient. *Arch Phys Med Rehabil* 1992; 73:44–48.

136. Escobedo EM, Hunter JC, Hollister MC, Patten RM, Goldstein B. MR imaging of rotator cuff tears in individuals with paraplegia. *AJR Am J Roentgenol* 1997; 168:919–923.

137. Goldstein B, Young J, Escobedo EM. Rotator cuff repairs in individuals with paraplegia. *Am J Phys Med Rehabil* 1997; 76:316–322.

138. Nichols PJ, Norman PA, Ennis JR. Wheelchair user's shoulder? Shoulder pain in patients with spinal cord lesions. *Scand J Rehabil Med* 1979; 11:29–32.

139. Pentland WE, Twomey LT. The weight-bearing upper extremity in women with long term paraplegia. *Paraplegia* 1991; 29:521–530.

140. Pentland WE, Twomey LT. Upper limb function in persons with long term paraplegia and implications for independence. Part I. *Paraplegia* 1994; 32:211–218.

141. Burnham RS, May L, Nelson E, Steadward R, Reid DC. Shoulder pain in wheelchair athletes: the role of muscle imbalance. *Am J Sports Med* 1993; 21:238–242.

142. Curtis KA, Roach KE, Applegate EB, et al. Reliability and validity of the Wheelchair User's Shoulder Pain Index (WUSPI). *Paraplegia* 1995; 33:595–601.

143. Curtis KA, Tyner TM, Zachary L, et al. Effect of a standard exercise protocol on shoulder pain in long-term wheelchair users. *Spinal Cord* 1999; 37:421–429.

144. Nilsson S, Staff PH, Pruett ED. Physical work capacity and the effect of training on subjects with long-standing paraplegia. *Scand J Rehabil Med* 1975; 7:51–56.

145. Davis GM, Shephard RJ. Strength training for wheelchair users. *Br J Sports Med* 1990; 24:25–30.

146. Cooney MM, Walker JB. Hydraulic resistance exercise benefits cardiovascular fitness of spinal cord injured. *Med Sci Sports Exerc* 1986; 18:522–525.

147. Olenik LM, Laskin JJ, Burnham R, Wheeler GD, Steadward RD. Efficacy of rowing, backward wheeling and isolated scapular retractor exercise as remedial strength activities for wheelchair users: application of electromyography. *Paraplegia* 1995; 33:148–152.

148. Jacobs PL, Nash MS, Rusinowski JW. Circuit training provides cardiorespiratory and strength benefits in persons with paraplegia. *Med Sci Sports Exerc* 2001; 33:711–717.

149. Nash MS, van de Ven I, van Elk N, Johnson BM. Effects of circuit resistance training on fitness attributes and upper-extremity pain in middle-aged men with paraplegia. *Arch Phys Med Rehabil* 2007; 88:70–75.

150. Nash MS, Jacobs PL, Woods JM, Clark JE, Pray TA, Pumarejo AE. A comparison of 2 circuit exercise training techniques for eliciting matched metabolic responses in persons with paraplegia. *Arch Phys Med Rehabil* 2002; 83:201–209.

151. Hicks AL, Martin KA, Ditor DS, et al. Long-term exercise training in persons with spinal cord injury: effects on strength, arm ergometry performance and psychological well-being. *Spinal Cord* 2003; 41:34–43.

152. Ditor DS, Latimer AE, Ginis KA, Arbour KP, McCartney N, Hicks AL. Maintenance of exercise participation in individuals with spinal cord injury: effects on quality of life, stress and pain. *Spinal Cord* 2003; 41:446–450.

153. Bergman SB, Yarkony GM, Stiens SA. Spinal cord injury rehabilitation. 2. Medical complications. *Arch Phys Med Rehabil* 1997; 78:S53–S58.

154. Sadowsky CL. Electrical stimulation in spinal cord injury. *NeuroRehabilitation* 2001; 16:165–169.

155. Sairyo K, Katoh S, Sakai T, Mishiro T, Ikata T. Characteristics of velocity-controlled knee movement in patients with cervical compression myelopathy: what is the optimal rehabilitation exercise for spastic gait? *Spine* 2001; 26:E535–E538.

156. Field-Fote EC. Combined use of body weight support, functional electric stimulation, and treadmill training to improve walking ability in individuals with chronic incomplete spinal cord injury. *Arch Phys Med Rehabil* 2001; 82:818–824.

157. Donaldson N, Perkins TA, Fitzwater R, Wood DE, Middleton F. FES cycling may promote recovery of leg function after incomplete spinal cord injury. *Spinal Cord* 2000; 38:680–682.

158. Nyland J, Quigley P, Huang C, Lloyd J, Harrow J, Nelson A. Preserving transfer independence among individuals with spinal cord injury. *Spinal Cord* 2000; 38:649–657.

159. Mulroy SJ, Gronley JK, Newsam CJ, Perry J. Electromyographic activity of shoulder muscles during wheelchair propulsion by paraplegic persons. *Arch Phys Med Rehabil* 1996; 77:187–193.

160. Reyes ML, Gronley JK, Newsam CJ, Mulroy SJ, Perry J. Electromyographic analysis of shoulder muscles of men with low-level paraplegia during a weight relief raise. *Arch Phys Med Rehabil* 1995; 76:433–439.

161. Perry J, Gronley JK, Newsam CJ, Reyes ML, Mulroy SJ. Electromyographic analysis of the shoulder muscles during depression transfers in subjects with low-level paraplegia. *Arch Phys Med Rehabil* 1996; 77:350–355.

162. Sawka MN, Latzka WA, Pandolf KB. Temperature regulation during upper body exercise: able-bodied and spinal cord injured. *Med Sci Sports Exerc* 1989; 21:S132–S140.

163. Muraki S, Yamasaki M, Ishii K, Kikuchi K, Seki K. Relationship between core temperature and skin blood flux in lower limbs during prolonged arm exercise in persons with spinal cord injury. *Eur J Appl Physiol* 1996; 72:330–334.

164. Boot CR, Binkhorst RA, Hopman MT. Body temperature responses in spinal cord injured individuals during exercise in the cold and heat. *Int J Sports Med* 2006; 27:599–604.

165. Gass GC, Camp EM, Nadel ER, Gwinn TH, Engel P. Rectal and rectal vs. esophageal temperatures in paraplegic men during prolonged exercise. *J Appl Physiol* 1988; 64:2265–2271.

166. Muraki S, Yamasaki M, Ishii K, Kikuchi K, Seki K. Effect of arm cranking exercise on skin blood flow of lower limb in people with injuries to the spinal cord. *Eur J Appl Physiol* 1995; 71:28–32.

167. Ishii K, Yamasaki M, Muraki S, et al. Effects of upper limb exercise on thermoregulatory responses in patients with spinal cord injury. *Appl Human Sci* 1995; 14:149–154.

168. Price MJ, Campbell IG. Thermoregulatory responses of spinal cord injured and able-bodied athletes to prolonged upper body exercise and recovery. *Spinal Cord* 1999; 37:772–779.

65 Architectural Considerations for Improving Access

Ian Hsiao
Thomas Hodne

The disabled population in the United States has increased from 36 million in the 1970s (1) to close to 50 million toward the end of twentieth century (2). This number includes 1.5 million who use wheelchairs, 7.4 million who use assistive devices for mobility impairments, 4.6 million who use back braces, 596,000 who use leg braces, and 199,000 who use artificial limbs (2). Including temporary disablement, it is estimated that close to 60% of the U.S. population has experienced mobility problems at some point during life (3). As the aging of baby boomers looms, the elderly population will continue to increase, as will these statistics—both in number and percentage of the overall population. Among all disabled people, persons with spinal cord injury (SCI) (a group estimated to number 230,000 [4]) particularly suffer from mobility impairments. For them, satisfaction with life after SCI (5, 6) has much to do with access to the environment. One study pointed out that access to the environment is positively and linearly associated with satisfaction with life (7). Results from another survey showed that difficulty with access to many facilities was the fifth most common problem out of forty associated with having a disability. Those who responded also rated problems with access as one of the most troublesome results of having a disability (8, 9).

A person's lifestyle can be changed enormously with an occurrence of spinal cord injury. Ability to participate in nearly all activities of daily living is greatly affected by mobility limitations, and quality of life has also been shown to be affected (10). To avoid deterioration of health, a person with SCI should be involved in self-care and health care activities and should maintain appropriate participation in productive activities (11). Participation is defined as the extent of a person's involvement in life situations in relation to impairments, activities, health condition, and contextual factors (12). Studies of patients who have SCI have found that environmental barriers can detrimentally affect social activities and life satisfaction (13, 14). On the other hand, better environmental access increases the likelihood that a person with SCI will engage in a variety of meaningful activities (15). In fact, with moderate modifications, such as the addition of ramps, wider doors, and wheelchair lifts as equipment,

many patients with SCI can enjoy much more accessible homes (16). The physical environment can determine what tasks need to be performed and can affect the individual's ability to live more independently (17, 18).

In contrast to those of just two decades ago, today's regulations and building codes recognize the need for access and include provisions that are intended to allow people with disabilities to be able to approach, enter, exit, and otherwise make use of new buildings and buildings undergoing substantial renovation (19). The underlying goal of barrier-free design is the provision of opportunities for handicapped people equal to those available to everyone else (20). Barrier-free design allows disabled people to perform day-to-day tasks at home and at work. The most appropriate designs to facilitate disabled people are those that are inconspicuous (21). Although these barrier-free design requirements are readily understood by architects and builders who work with them every day, other interested parties, such as doctors, nurses, administrators, therapists, and social workers who deal with people who have spinal cord disorders, may benefit from a further discussion of the subject in layman's terminology. The scope of barrier-free design is broad and lengthy. This chapter concentrates on discussing considerations that are necessary in the design and construction of buildings to improve access for those who must use wheelchairs, especially those with spinal cord injury and disease

BACKGROUND

Historically, architecture has been intended for the able-bodied person. For example, steps are the most obvious and prevalent architectural impediment to access for wheelchair users. Ancient temples, gothic cathedrals, and even fairly recent houses of worship usually have steps as a major design element. Palaces, mansions, courthouses, banks, universities, and other public and private buildings were also intended to be impressive, with grand stairs and entrances in keeping with their importance. On a practical note, the floors of more mundane buildings and residences were set above ground on pilings and foundations for a number of good reasons, such as to raise the living space and entrances above sewage paths, possible floods, and snow blockage, and to keep animals out of the house. Steps were ubiquitous and entirely fitting and appropriate in societies where people with disabilities were virtually non-existent. The result today is an environment that is inaccessible to many (3, 22). For example, one study showed that in some rural areas, at least 40% of churches, local parks and recreation areas, county office buildings, libraries, and post offices were only partially accessible, or not accessible at all (23).

World War II, which ended more than half a century ago and cost many millions of lives, is also recognized as the turning point that has saved and extended the lives of countless numbers of people who have SCI. World War II saw many young men become paraplegic and quadriplegic because of battlefield wounds. The timely medical treatment they received, along with better patient management techniques and the advent of "miracle" drugs to control infections, helped many of these men who otherwise would have died to survive and return to civilian life. With gratitude and recognition for the severity of their disabilities in the service of the country, the 80th Congress passed Public Law 702 on June 19, 1948. This law, known as the Specially Adapted Housing (SAH) Act, established compensation in the form of a grant of assistance from the Veterans Administration (VA) to help severely disabled veterans (when such disability is service-connected) purchase a "wheelchair" home especially adapted for their needs.

Forty-two years later, President George Bush Sr. signed the Americans with Disabilities Act (ADA) into law as Public Law 101–336 on July 26, 1990. The act builds on and expands the rights created by the Rehabilitation Act of 1973, Title V. ADA provides people with disability with an expansion of protections and basic civil rights, defining *disability* as a physical or mental impairment that substantially limits one or more of an individual's major activities of daily living, such as walking, hearing, speaking, learning, or performing manual tasks. The law prohibits discrimination based on physical or mental handicap and requires the removal of barriers for all covered entities so that disabled persons have equal access to the facilities. The prohibition of discrimination includes in employment, in services provided by public agencies, in public accommodations, and in telecommunications. Concerning environmental accessibility, Title III, Section 302{9} of ADA prohibits any owner, lessee, or operator of an establishment offering service to the public from discriminating based on a person's disability in the "full and equal" enjoyment of goods, services, or accommodations offered by the establishment. This prohibition includes all organizations, such as hotels, motels, restaurants, retail stores, theaters, banks, offices of professionals (including physicians and lawyers), parks, zoos, golf courses, and other recreational facilities. Failure to remove architectural barriers is considered discrimination unless removal is "not easily accomplishable and unable to be carried out without much difficulty or expense." Under Section 303, new public facilities or places of employment built 30 months or more after July 1989 must be accessible to disabled people unless accessibility is structurally impractical.

Along with the passage of Public Law 702, the Department of Veterans Affairs, formerly the Veterans Administration, and more commonly known as the VA, helped to further improve the lives of disabled people through the funding of *702 homes*—homes especially built for paralyzed, amputee, or blinded veterans eligible through the Specially Adapted Housing grant. One of the statutory requirements for a 702 home is that "the home must be so adapted as to be suitable to the veteran's needs for dwelling purposes." It is believed that the VA developed the very first set of design criteria anywhere for people with disabilities when, more than 50 years ago, it set forth the list of requirements for specially adapted housing. This list can currently be found in paragraph 3.03, Minimum Property Requirements, of the Department of Veterans Benefits Manual M26–12, Loan Guaranty Operations for Regional Offices—Specially Adapted Housing Grant Processing Procedure, and in VA Pamphlet 26-69-1 "Questions and Answers on Specially Adapted Housing for Veterans." In 1978, based on these design criteria, the VA published VA Pamphlet 26–13 "Handbook For Design: Specially Adapted Design," which contains excellent illustrations for these criteria.

Another early publication dealing with accessible design criteria is ANSI A117.1–1986 (American National Standard for Buildings and Facilities—Providing Accessibility and Usability for Physically Handicapped People), hereinafter simply referred to as ANSI A117.1. ANSI A117.1 is the definitive standard for accessible design and has been referred to in and even adopted by state and local building codes. This national standard resulted from research conducted more than 40 years ago at the University of Illinois under a grant from the Easter Seal Research Foundation, culminating in a set of design criteria for accessibility that was approved and issued as a design standard of the ANSI in 1961. ANSI is a nongovernmental national organization that publishes a wide variety of recommended standards. ANSI's standards for barrier-free design are developed by a committee made up of fifty-two organizations representing associations of handicapped people, rehabilitation professionals, design professionals, builders, and manufacturers. The standard was reaffirmed in 1971, expanded to include residential environments in the 1980 edition, and revised in the 1986 edition. The current edition of this standard is American National Standard CABO/ANSI A117.1–2003 Accessible and Usable Buildings and Facilities. New to the 2003 edition are criteria for elements and fixtures primarily for children's use, enhanced reach range criteria, transportation facilities, additional provisions for assembly areas, and an addition and rearrangement for accessible dwelling and sleeping units. These new criteria are intended to provide a level of coordination between the accessible provisions of this standard and the Fair Housing Accessibility Guidelines and the Americans with Disabilities Act Accessibility Guidelines (ADAAG). It is highly recommended that the reader obtain a copy for an in-depth reference source dealing with access for people who have disabilities.

Further development came from ADAAG and the Uniform Federal Accessibility Standards (UFAS). ADAAG contains scoping and technical requirements for accessibility to buildings and facilities by individuals with disabilities under the ADA of 1990. These requirements are to be applied during the design, construction, and alteration of buildings and facilities covered by titles II and III of ADA to the extent required under ADA by regulations issued by federal agencies, including the Department of Justice and the Department of Transportation. ADAAG outlines the building requirements for all areas of newly designed or newly constructed buildings and altered portions of existing buildings and for facilities in general. This includes restaurants, cafeterias, medical care facilities, businesses, libraries, and transportation facilities. UFAS was published in the *Federal Register* on August 7, 1984 (49 FR 31528). UFAS presents uniform standards for the design, construction, and alteration of buildings so that physically handicapped persons will have ready access and use of public facilities in accordance with the Architectural Barriers Act, 42 U.S.C. 4151–4157. The UFAS sets the rules for facility accessibility by physically handicapped persons for federal and federally funded facilities. These standards are to be applied during the design, construction, and alteration of buildings and facilities to the extent required by the Architectural Barriers Act of 1968. These standards were jointly developed by the General Services Administration, the Department of Housing and Urban Development, the Department of Defense, and the U.S. Postal Service. These four standard-setting agencies determined that, as much as possible, the uniform standards adopted by them would not only comply with the guidelines adopted by the Architectural and Transportation Barriers Compliance Board, but also be consistent with the standards published by the ANSI for general use. Both the UFAS scope provisions, which establish the minimum number of elements and spaces required to comply with standards, and the UFAS technical requirements, meet or exceed the comparable provisions of the ANSI Guidelines.

The above publications have withstood the test of time, but whereas the VA criteria have remained essentially unchanged, ANSI A117.1 and UFAS have been revised, expanded, and greatly improved over the years to influence and reflect changes to building codes that improve access for people with disabilities. The VA criteria are very general, whereas the ANSI A117.1 and UFAS materials are very detailed, and although they differ slightly in some aspects, they complement each other well in addressing architectural considerations for people with spinal cord disorder. The remainder of this chapter discusses the operating environment for mobility aids, especially wheelchairs; accessibility in an indoor environment; and how architectural design standards enable persons with SCI to approach, enter, exit, and otherwise use buildings. All the illustrative figures in the following sections are in compliance with the standards in ANSI A117.1.

OPERATING ENVIRONMENT FOR MOBILITY AIDS

To discuss accessibility in the built environment for people with SCI, one must first look at how mobility aids limit access. People who experience SCI undergo tremendous life-changing experiences. Activities as simple as walking, climbing stairs, carrying grocery bags, and operating doors become daunting—if not insurmountable—tasks that are no longer to be taken for granted. The majority of people with SCI depend on mobility aids such as wheelchairs and, to a lesser extent, crutches, braces, and walkers, all of which affect where they can go and what they can do. Wheelchairs have contributed significantly to improved environmental accessibility for people with impaired mobility. In recent years, powered wheelchairs have become increasingly popular, and although they provide great mobility for many

severely disabled persons, their size, weight, and maneuvering characteristics can have a limiting effect on accessibility. Unquestionably, modern wheelchairs are better than ever, but they still have the same dynamic limitations they have always had in that they can only go where wheeled conveyances can go. Basically, a person using a wheelchair, being not as tall as a standing adult person, does not require any special vertical height considerations for mobility but does require a horizontal space wide enough for passage and a surface pathway that is free of changes in level, steps, bumpy surfaces, potholes, and other obstructions. If we look down from above, an average-sized standing person measures about 1 foot or so, front to back, and about 2 feet or so from side to side. Conversely, a wheelchair with occupant is at least 2 feet wide and about 4 feet from front to back. The wheelchair user occupies roughly three to four times the floor area taken up by an average-sized person; weighs more (the wheelchair plus his own weight); is restricted to flat, stable, relatively level paths of travel; and has to use comparatively smaller arm and shoulder muscles to do the work intended for the much larger leg muscles.

Although certain wheelchair dimensions have gained widespread acceptance as standard measurements (24), as illustrated in Figure 65.1, one must also bear in mind that people come in all different shapes and sizes, and wheelchairs are custom-fitted according to the person's physical dimensions. Wider people and taller people have wheelchairs that are proportionately larger in those dimensions, and may not necessarily be able to negotiate accessible routes meeting the minimum criteria. Other people

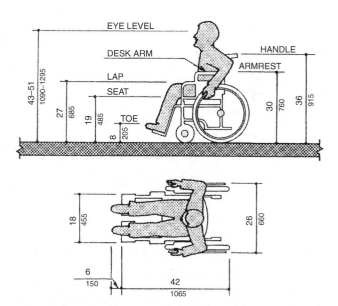

Note: Footrests may extend further for very large people.

Figure 65.1 Dimensions of adult-sized wheelchairs. The height of the handle is 36 inches. The armrest is 30 inches high. Eye level is between 43 and 51 inches. The lap is at 27 inches. The seat is at 19 inches. The toe is at 8 inches. The width of a wheelchair measured from the outer edges of the back wheels is 26 inches, and its length is 42 inches measured from the outer edges of the footrests.

have attachments, such as ventilators for breathing, or wheelchair and environmental controls on their wheelchairs that project to the side, front, and back, and require larger clearances for accessibility. Still others need wheelchairs that recline or leg rests that are extended and raised, which further complicate accessibility. Proper seating cushions in a wheelchair are important because undue elevation of the legrests can cause postural alterations that result in excessive pressure on the sacrum, with the attendant risk of pressure sores (25). The point is that the accessibility standards discussed herein meet the needs of the majority of wheelchair users, but some individuals have size and dynamic considerations that require greater dimensions and clearances for access purposes. (It should be mentioned that, although life in a wheelchair does have its limitations, there are always exceptions to the rules.) Doorways must have a clear opening width of 32 inches (815 mm) minimum. Clear opening width of doorways with swinging doors must be measured between the face of door and stop, with the door open 90 degrees. Openings, doors, and doorways without doors more than 24 inches (610 mm) in depth must provide a clear opening width of 36 inches (915 mm) minimum. Closing speed of doors must be adjusted so that from an open position of 90 degrees, the time required to move the door to an open position of 12 degrees must be 5 seconds minimum.

The ideal floor or ground surface for wheelchairs and other mobility aids is dry, flat, level, firm, stable, and slip-resistant (26). The running slope of walking surfaces cannot be steeper than 1:20. In fact, a surface with these characteristics is the easiest and safest path of travel for anyone, able-bodied or otherwise, to traverse. A wet surface can be slippery and make it difficult for a wheelchair to be propelled in a controllable manner and is extremely hazardous for anyone using crutches or a walker. A person may fall when a crutch tip lands on a wet spot on a highly polished floor of any material. The path of travel for SCI persons must be as level as possible and have maneuvering space for turning, opening doors, and passing other people while using a wheelchair. The basic operating environment for wheelchairs becomes readily understandable when an able-bodied individual has the opportunity to spend some time in a wheelchair and attempts to go about his daily activities. In this manner wheelchair sensitivity and awareness training for able-bodied people gives them an immediate education to the problems faced by wheelchair users and can create instantaneous advocates for people with disabilities in the process.

OUTDOOR ENVIRONMENTS AND ACCESSIBILITY

Accessibility relating to outdoor environments has been described in some publications, and guidelines have been developed (27, 28). If possible, accessible facilities should be located on level sites adjacent to a firm path with a stable surface. A study suggested that cardiopulmonary stresses for wheelchair locomotion are higher than for walking, and that a softer surface, such as a carpet, can pose a greater obstacle to wheelchair locomotion than a hard surface, such as tile (29). An objective method is proposed and tested to assess the accessibility of walking and wheeling surfaces, and thus to improve accessibility for people with mobility limitations (30). By and large, the type of a path's surface determines the accessibility of activities subserved by the access

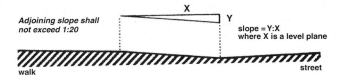

Figure 65.2 Measurement of curb ramp slopes. The ramp slope is a ratio equal to the vertical rise (Y) divided by the horizontal run (X). It is equal to the tangent of the angle that the plane of the ramp surface makes with a horizontal (level) plane. For a curb ramp, the adjoining slope at walk or street must not exceed 1:20.

route. In order of decreasing accessibility, possible choices include concrete, asphalt, wood planking (which tends to be used over wet, fragile, or sandy areas), well-packed fine-grade rock, well-compacted pea-sized gravel, bound wood chips, coarse gravel, rock, unbound wood chips, and sand (31). A curb ramp should be provided wherever an accessible route crosses a curb. The slopes of curb ramps must comply with the requirements of ramps. Ramps allow for easier access for people in wheelchairs, but can cause difficulties for people using walkers or crutches. Any part of an accessible route with a slope greater than 1:20 should be considered a ramp. The least possible slope should be used for any ramp. The slope of a ramp in new construction should be no more than 1:12, whereas the rise for any run should be 30 inches (760 mm) maximum (see Figure 65.2). Disabled people not in wheelchairs sometimes have difficulty with ramps, particularly lengthy ones, and often prefer to use steps. Wherever possible, a ramp should be situated within a reasonable distance of steps to allow for a real choice.

Parking spaces for physically disabled people are to be at least 96 inches (2,440 mm) wide and should have an adjacent access aisle of at least 60 inches (1,525 mm) minimum width. Parked vehicle overhangs should not reduce the clear width of an accessible route. Two accessible parking spaces may share a common access aisle, but should be part of an accessible route to the building or facility entrance. Parking spaces designated for physically handicapped people and accessible passenger loading zones that serve a particular building are best located on the shortest possible accessible circulation route to an accessible entrance. Parking spaces and access aisles should be level with surface slopes, not exceeding 2.1% (1:48) in all directions per section 502-3 ANSI A117.1-2003. Passenger loading zones must provide a vehicular pull-up space 96 inches (2,440 mm) minimum in width and 20 feet (6,100 mm) minimum in length. Passenger loading zones must provide a vehicular pull-up space 96 inches (2,440 mm) minimum in width and 20 feet (6,100 mm) minimum in length. Passenger loading zones must have an adjacent access aisle. Access aisles serving vehicle pull-up spaces must be 60 inches (1,525 mm) minimum in width. Access aisles must be 20 feet (6,100 mm) minimum in length.

INDOOR ACCESSIBILITY

The indoors, including home environments, pose obstacles for the disabled person, such as passageways, entranceways, and small rooms, and so require their own set of construction standards to comfortably accommodate the disabled. The emphasis of this section is placed on the home environment, because it is the place people spend the most time. Because the VA was in the forefront of accessible design for the home environment to begin with and has more than 50 years of experience in specially adapted housing, the VA criteria are primarily used as the basis for this section in dealing with indoor access. However, the VA criteria and those of ANSI A117.1 are comparable, but not equal, as will be clearly seen in the following paragraphs.

One of the first considerations for any wheelchair user in purchasing a building lot or an existing home is the property itself. If one plans to use it for outdoor relaxation and recreation, the property should be fairly level, and firm enough to allow for comfortable wheelchair handling. At the same time, the ground surface should slope away from the house on all sides so that water doesn't accumulate and penetrate the walls. The general building code requirement for positive surface drainage is that the ground should fall away at least 3 inches within 6 feet of the perimeter of the house (a slope of 4.17%), and can have a gentler slope beyond that distance, with 2% as the absolute minimum. Because the maximum comfortable slope for wheelchair walkways is 5%, it should be easy to accommodate hard surface walkways, patios, and recreational activities and still provide proper site drainage without any special considerations. Building codes also specify that any wood component of the house structure must be no less than 8 inches above the adjoining grade level for protection against water and insects. For a concrete slab home with wood framing, the interior floor should be at least 8 inches above the ground outside, whereas a house with wood floor framing should be another 10 to 12 inches higher, for a total of 18 to 20 inches above grade. Obviously, a concrete floor slab home on a level site would need less ramping for accessibility than a wood floor house on the same site.

Unfortunately, not many people can afford the new, ideal, wheelchair-accessible home described, so they must look at other options for accessible living, such as existing, smaller homes or apartments. When one is looking to make existing homes more accessible, feasibility and cost are two important factors to consider. Can a short ramp provide entrance accessibility, or is a long switchback ramp, or even a vertical wheelchair platform lift, necessary to gain access to the home? Long ramps and wheelchair lifts can add $10,000 or more to the cost of a home—and this only gets the individual to the outside of the front door! Two-story and split-entry, multilevel homes are less expensive than comparably sized ranch homes because they require less property to build on, less foundation, and less roof. Therefore, these homes would be more affordable if access improvements to them could be accomplished in a cost-effective manner. Many of these homes have all the bedrooms on the upper level, which is not good for the typical SCI person, but if a room on the main level can be converted to a bedroom and a bathroom can be made accessible, it may prove worthwhile. Often the best solution is to determine whether the property is large enough to build a bedroom and bathroom addition on the main floor level.

Once these site conditions and cost feasibility issues have been addressed, other considerations must be resolved, such as maneuvering space for wheelchairs both inside the house and leading from parking locations to entry points of the home, and vehicular parking. Wider hallways and doorways are probably the first things people associate with wheelchair accessibility. The VA criteria and ANSI A 117.1 are comparable but differ somewhat

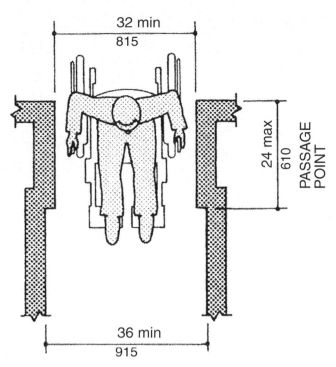

Figure 65.3 Minimum clear width for single wheelchair. The minimum clear passage width for a single wheelchair must be 36 inches minimum along an accessible route but may be reduced to 32 inches minimum at a point for a maximum depth of 24 inches, such as at a doorway.

on this subject. The VA requires that hallways in new construction be 48 inches wide and that doorways be 36 inches wide, whereas existing houses may have hallways 42 inches wide and doorways 32 inches wide. ANSI says that an accessible route (hallway) must have 36 inches clear width and doorways must have 32 inches clear width. However, although 48-inch-wide hallways and 36-inch-wide doors allow for great accessibility in the home, some feel that a 36-inch-wide hallway with appropriate maneuvering spaces at doorways is sufficient and allows the rooms along the hallway to be larger. Either way works for the wheelchair user, but the deciding factor will probably end up being a matter of personal preference and cost-effectiveness.

ANSI A117.1 is more detailed on the subject of passageways, and continues with additional standards. The minimum clear width for single wheelchair passage should be 32 inches (815 mm) at a point for a maximum depth of 24 inches (610 mm) and 36 inches (915 mm) continuously, as shown in Figure 65.3. The minimum width for two wheelchairs to pass is 60 inches (1,525 mm), as illustrated in Figure 65.4. Continuing, to facilitate a turn sharper than 90 degrees around an obstruction, it is necessary to increase the width of the accessible route to allow for the wheelchair's size. An able-bodied person can completely reverse direction in a very small area, whereas a wheelchair user, having a much larger footprint, must take into account the wheelchair's length, width, wheelbase, and tracking characteristics when making turns. ANSI calls for an accessible route between 42 and 48 inches wide when it is necessary to maneuver around an obstruction within a distance of less than 4 feet (Figure 65.5), although it must be noted that, as mentioned earlier, the VA

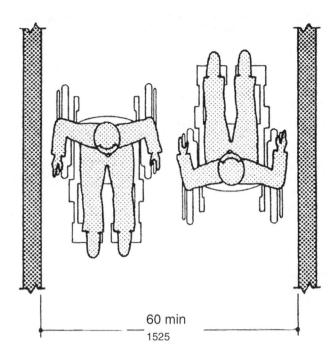

60 min
1525

Figure 65.4   Minimum clear width for two wheelchairs.

always requires a minimum clear width of 42 inches for any walk or ramp.

Door hardware, such as door handles, can also present a problem for some persons with SCI. The VA criteria do not mention door hardware, whereas ANSI states that handles, pulls, latches, locks, and other operating devices on accessible doors should have a shape that is easy to grasp with one hand and that does not require tight grasping, pinching, or twisting of the wrist to operate. Lever-operated mechanisms or push-type mechanisms are acceptable designs. Lever-type door handles really do make a difference in making doors easier to open and close. Persons having quadriplegia and a negligible grip function can usually manage to operate a lever handle on a door, but find it impossible to operate the typical round handle found on most

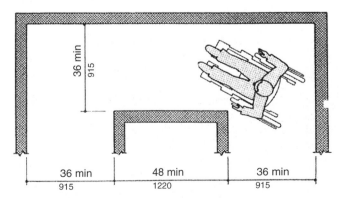

36 min
915

36 min
915

48 min
1220

36 min
915

Figure 65.5   Accessible route for a 90-degree turn. A 90-degree turn can be made from a 36-inch-wide passage into another 36-inch passage if the depth of each leg is a minimum of 48 inches on the inside dimensions of the turn.

doors in this country. Other nations prefer lever handles; however, the United States continues to utilize the rounded doorknob in residential construction.

In addition, the type of floor on which a wheelchair moves is important. Current research indicates that for normal walking, a coefficient of static friction greater than 0.4 produces the safest walking surfaces. It has been reported that, in assessing the biomechanical factors that cause slipping accidents, dynamic friction is more significant than static friction. In switching from tile to carpet locomotion, significant increases in energy expenditure occur for wheelchair users that are not noted in bipedal ambulators. It is hoped that additional studies of energy expenditure during ambulation will be forthcoming in the near future. The tops of the handrails are recommended to be mounted between 34 and 38 inches (864 to 965 mm) above surfaces and to have a clear space away from the adjacent wall of 1.5 inches (38 mm). People who have suffered strokes with hemiparesis, as well as amputees, may have only one arm with the functional capability to use a handrail. Therefore, handrails should be provided on both sides of passageways. The VA also gives regulations for stairways. Each stairway adjacent to an area of rescue assistance should have a minimum clear width of 48 inches between handrails.

On any given flight of stairs, all steps should have uniform riser heights and uniform tread depth. Stair treads should be no less than 11 inches (280 mm) in depth, as measured from consecutive risers. Stairs are designed best with sloping risers angled outward to meet the leading edge of the tread, to minimize the hazard of tripping. The sloping angle of the underside of the nosing is recommended to be within at least 60 degrees of horizontal. The radius of curvature at the leading edge of the tread should be no greater than 0.5 inch (13 mm). Nosings should project no more than 1.5 inches (38 mm). People with lower extremity prostheses, orthoses, or difficulties of coordination often use risers to provide guidance, support, and balance for their limbs or crutches during ascent. For these reasons, open risers are not permitted on accessible stairways. Pictures and other objects on stairway walls are discouraged, because distraction may occur. When carpeting is used on stairways, large patterns which could cause problems of depth perception or confusion are not recommended. Carpeting also reduces the size of steps and may cause heels to catch and soles to slide; thus, it is to be avoided if possible. Lighting sources are best provided at both the top and bottom of stairways, to minimize shadows. It is suggested that gradual changes in levels of lighting be provided between stairways and surrounding areas to allow time for the eyes to accommodate. These safety measures are of heightened importance for people with visual impairments, and for senior citizens.

KITCHENS AND BATHROOMS

Probably the most challenging spaces in any home for accessibility considerations are the kitchen and the bathroom. Again, if a new home is being designed, there is a wealth of information and a growing number of design professionals available to help develop accessible designs for these important functional areas. The accessibility issues arise with existing homes already occupied by wheelchair users. Kitchens generally have wall cabinets that are too high, base cabinets that can be too low, no accessible work counter space, dangerous cooking equipment, and inaccessible sinks; bathrooms have narrow doors (and hallways leading to them), no maneuvering space inside, and inaccessible plumbing fixtures.

For the wheelchair user who only uses the kitchen to eat meals, the problem is sitting at the kitchen table, which may be too low to wheel under. The simple solution is to put blocks under each leg that will raise the table enough to get under, or to cut the skirt out at the wheelchair seating location. Old style refrigerators had freezers at the top that were therefore out of reach, but new models come in many configurations. Side-by-side refrigerator freezers with double doors having ice and cold water dispensers might be the answer to good accessibility to shelves and having cold storage within easy reach. Raising the toe space of base cabinets can increase the maneuvering space to some extent, but one may have to consider removing a base cabinet and lowering the countertop to gain an accessible work counter surface about 30 inches above the floor (standard countertops are 36 inches high). The recommended clear height from the floor to the bottom of the countertop is 29 inches, so the countertop itself would be only 1 inch thick. The width of the seating space below the counter should be 30 inches. The kitchen sink would be more usable if there was no base cabinet below preventing the wheelchair from a head on approach, but the depth of the sink might preclude lowering the countertop. A new sink with the drain offset and to the rear would place the drain away from legs and decrease potential injuries from hot water. A new sink should probably have less depth to gain knee space below. The faucet control should be easy to reach and use; a single lever control works well. Some people have even mounted the sink sideways to place the faucet and control to the side instead of at the rear of the countertop. The stove should have all controls at the front or side so that one does not have to reach over cooking surfaces or hot pots and pans. Stoves, ovens, ranges and microwaves should be at a height that allows access to wheelchair users without bending or stretching and possibly losing balance with harmful consequences. Side-opening doors may be a consideration to allow closer approach to the cooking appliances, but there should always be a heat-resistant surface within easy reach onto which to immediately transfer hot foods. Storage has always been a problem in the kitchen, but some solutions are available. There are motorized wall cabinets that can be lowered within reach and raised when not needed, and there are pullout storage and waste containers for base cabinets that eliminate hard to reach corners, as well as lazy susans and door-mounted shelving to bring items close to hand. If space allows, a floor-mounted pantry can be a very useful and accessible storage space. A standalone pantry consisting of a series of 8- to 10-inch-wide pullout vertical shelving units or a double door cabinet with door-mounted shelves and vertical swingout shelves can be very accessible.

Traditionally, bathrooms have had narrow doors, with 24 inches' width being typical; the door needs to be wider for wheelchair access. While some individuals can pass through a 30-inch door opening with their wheelchair, most require a 32- to 36-inch door for access to any room. Even with a wider door, the space inside the bathroom is typically still limited, and it may be necessary to have the door swing outward instead of into the bathroom to avoid maneuvering problems around the door. Bathrooms are usually around 5 feet by 8 feet and contain a bathtub, a commode, and a sink with a wall-mounted medi-

cine cabinet. If the sink has a cabinet below, the first access improvement would be to replace the vanity with a wall-hung sink or a countertop with a drop-in sink having a 27-inch-high by 30-inch-wide clear space below for the wheelchair. The sink should have an offset rear drain for knee space and the hot water and drain pipes need to be insulated to prevent burns. Removing the base cabinet below the sink will greatly improve access to the sink and increase floor space for maneuvering as well. The faucet must have easy-to-operate controls; single-lever controls seem to work well for most people. Angle the mirror or lower it to place the bottom edge no more than 40 inches above the floor so that it may be useful for a seated person. If the sink is near a corner of the room, consider putting a medicine cabinet on the side wall within wheelchair reach. Some people will use a commode wheelchair, which has a hole in the seat and is made to back up over the commode for toileting, thus allowing the use of a standard commode. If the individual transfers to the toilet, the toilet seat height should be at the same height as the wheelchair seat, around 19–20 inches. Transferring from the side will require about 30 inches of clear floor space alongside the toilet; if the space is not available, a commode chair may be necessary (see Figures 65.6 and 65.8). Standard commodes are about 14 to 15 inches high, so manufacturers now make commodes that have elongated bowls and that are 19 inches high for wheelchair use. A less expensive way to raise the toilet seat height is by means of a filler, which is essentially a very thick (4 to 5 inches) plastic toilet seat. A toilet base filler piece is also available that raises the entire toilet to wheelchair seat height. Grab bars are essential items at the toilet, and shower/bathtub locations and should be mounted 33 to 36 inches above the

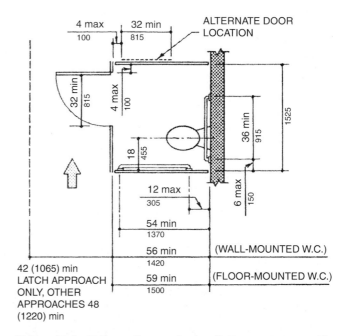

Figure 65.6 Toilet stalls: standard stall. Door swings out. The location of the door is illustrated in front of the clear space (next to the water closet), with a maximum stile width of 4 inches. An alternate door location is illustrated on the side of the toilet stall with a maximum stile width of 4 inches. The minimum width of the standard stall is 60 inches. The centerline of the water closet must be 18 inches from the side wall.

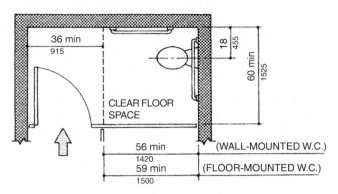

Figure 65.7 Toilet stalls: alternate stalls; door swing in.

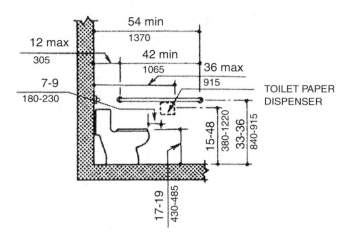

Figure 65.9 Toilet stalls.

floor (see Figures 65.6, 65.7, 65.8, and 65.9). Horizontal grab bars are suitable for those in wheelchairs, whereas vertical grab bars are usually intended for people who have some ability to stand; an L-shaped grab bar can be beneficial to a greater range of people of varying degrees of disability. Grab bars are recommended to be 1.25 to 1.5 inches in diameter and must be securely anchored to wood or metal blocking inside the wall to be effective and safe. Bathing or showering is a personal preference, but a curbless shower can be a very effective means of increasing maneuvering space for wheelchairs in a bathroom. Installing a curbless shower will almost always result in a 5-foot by 5-foot wheelchair maneuvering space in an existing bathroom. Manufacturers have developed shower modules that are designed to replace existing bathtubs and to be wheelchair accessible. Standard bathtubs are 2 feet 6 inches by 5 feet, and prefabricated wheelchair showers are the same size, to fit into the same space. Plumbing codes require showers to have 2-inch-diameter drains, while bathtubs only need 1.5-inch drains, so the existing tub drain has to be replaced with a 2-inch shower drain. Newer models of accessible prefabricated showers do not require structural modifications to lower the floor but may require a larger hole in the floor at the drain location where the plastic is thicker. The shower entrance threshold will be flush

or very minimal depending on the thickness of the existing bathroom flooring material. Keeping the water inside a shower without an entrance step can be addressed by means of a collapsible 1.5-inch-high neoprene threshold. The neoprene threshold is glued to the floor across the shower entrance and prevents the water from running onto the rest of the bathroom floor because of its height. A wheelchair can easily enter the shower because the soft neoprene collapses under the wheel to become almost flat and springs back to its original shape after the wheel passes over. The shower should have grab bars on all three sides if possible, and there should be a handheld shower head mounted on a slide bar that allows the person to easily adjust the showerhead height with a large lever or wing nut. Shower controls must be no higher than 48 inches above floor for a frontal approach, or 54 inches high for a side approach. The shower must have a thermostatic control valve to keep a constant temperature and prevent sudden temperature changes that can cause scalding injuries. If an SCI person prefers a bathtub instead of a shower, grab bars must be provided for safety, and the means of transfer to the tub must be decided upon. A strong individual may transfer directly into the tub water using only grab bars and the wheelchair or tub for support but may benefit from additional grab bars at various heights to get out of the tub after bathing. Some people will transfer from the wheelchair to a bench inside the tub, or to a transfer bench that extends outside the tub, and use a slide mounted hand-held shower for bathing. Ceiling-mounted hoists that can raise a person seated in a sling and carry him into the bathing area to be lowered into a bathtub or shower bench are also readily available. Bathroom floors must be nonslip; matte finish ceramic tile is commonly used. In many cases, existing bathrooms are simply too small for accessibility and must be expanded into adjacent spaces, such as bedrooms. Bedroom closets are prime candidates for bathroom expansion plans, but try to avoid moving walls containing plumbing, if possible, for economic reasons.

ENTRANCES AND GARAGES

The next area of attention is the entranceway. A walkway should always connect the driveway and the front entrance, and

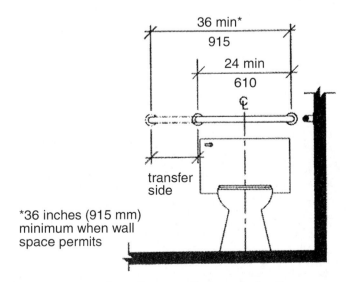

Figure 65.8 Toilet stalls: rear wall of standard wall.

the entrance should be protected from the elements by a roof overhang. For personal safety and security, the outside parking area, path to the entrance, and entrance platform should be well illuminated. Remote controls, motion-sensing lights, and low-voltage pathway lighting are readily available means of providing illumination effectively and efficiently. The walkway must be at least 42 inches wide and have a hard, stable, nonslip surface with a maximum slope of 5% (1:20). Concrete with a broom texture finish is an excellent material for walks. Asphaltic concrete is frequently used, but requires annual maintenance and can stick to shoes and wheelchair tires, leaving black marks inside the house. Concrete pavers come in a variety of patterns and colors and are very popular and attractive, but can prove to be somewhat bumpy to a wheelchair user. Bear in mind that smaller pavers with recessed, chamfered joints are going to be bumpier than large pavers with flush, square butt joints.

While on the subject of entranceways, it should be mentioned that every effort should be made to eliminate, or at least to minimize, thresholds—more commonly known as *sills* or *door saddles*. Thresholds are the raised, shaped wood or marble pieces at the bottom of doorways that separate different floor types and thicknesses; these can be quite troublesome for wheelchairs to negotiate, especially manual wheelchairs with small front wheels. ANSI A117.1 addresses the threshold issue by stating "Changes in level up to $1/4$ inch (6 mm) may be vertical and without edge treatment. Changes in level between $1/4$ inch and $1/2$ inch (6 mm and 13 mm) shall be beveled with a slope no greater than 1:2. Changes in level greater than $1/2$ inch shall be accomplished by means of a ramp."

Continuing with the subject of ramps, the VA criteria call for "[a]t least two ramps suitable for entry and exit, one of which shall be located so as not to expose the veteran to a potential fire hazard, such as placement necessitating passage through a kitchen or garage or utility room containing heating equipment." It must be noted that walkways are perfectly acceptable, although ramps are specifically indicated for entry and exit. If at all possible, always use a walkway instead of a ramp to approach a residential entrance; it's a lot easier to negotiate in all kinds of weather, and your client or spouse will generally appreciate the noninstitutional look of the entry without the railings and balusters a ramp requires.

If the path of travel to the front door does require a ramp instead of a walkway, the VA states that the ramp must be at least 42 inches wide and have a maximum slope of 8%. Because ANSI calls for a minimum width of 36 inches and a maximum slope of 8.33%, the SAH requirements are a little more favorable to wheelchairs, because ramps are wider and have a slightly gentler maximum slope. Without being very specific, the VA criteria state "railings must be provided if the height and length of the ramp indicate any question of a hazard." Perhaps the VA defers to local building codes in this matter. Both the International One and Two Family Dwelling Code and the CABO One and Two Family Dwelling Code state that "handrails shall be provided on at least one side of all ramps exceeding a slope of 1 unit vertical in 12 units horizontal (8.33% slope)."

Technically speaking, because the VA maximum ramp slope is only 8%, an argument could be made that the building code would not even require handrails. Nevertheless, it is always a good idea to provide handrails on both sides of a ramp for utilitarian, if not safety, reasons. Many individuals with SCI will use handrails to pull themselves up the ramp instead of using the wheelchair

handrims, and many simply appreciate the security of having a handrail available just in case they may need it. Bear in mind, however, that since platforms 30 inches or more above adjoining grade require guardrails, the same would apply for ramps that rise more than 30 inches above the adjoining surfaces. "Ramp platforms and entrance platforms must be generous in area to allow for turning the wheelchair." Again, the VA does not specify any minimum size for a platform, but the generally accepted minimum size for wheelchair use is 5 feet by 5 feet. A 5-foot by 5-foot entrance platform should accommodate any wheelchair if the entrance door swings inward, which is almost always the case; and because the standard width for main entrance doors is 36 inches, gaining access to the inside of the house should not be a problem. There could be a problem, however, if the entrance has a storm or screen door that swings outward, over the platform.

Another consideration for the entrance ramp is the materials of which it is comprised. At least one of the ramps must be within the following regulations, to avoid any threat of a fire hazard. The requirements state that ramps must be constructed of fireproof material and be treated to prevent slipping when wet. Although it would seem that only concrete or other masonry products would meet the fireproof specification for ramps, treated fire-retardant lumber is allowable. Concrete ramp surfaces should never be hard-troweled to a smooth finish. The most common treatment for preventing a slippery surface is to draw a stiff-bristled broom across the surface perpendicular to the path of travel soon after the concrete has been poured. This creates a textured surface into which wheels can bite on rainy days. Wood ramps can be treated with textured paint or have special textured strips or matting applied to prevent slipping. In addition to concrete and wood, plastics have become an important construction material in the residential homebuilding industry. New materials and manufacturing processes have created plastic extrusions simulating wood decking, posts, balusters, and railings; these are becoming increasingly popular for decks and ramps. The plastic decking comes with a textured nonslip surface, which should be very useful for safety reasons when utilized for ramps.

The final area of consideration is the problem presented by vehicular parking for the disabled. Many SCI wheelchair users will have an automobile, van, or minivan for personal transportation, usually depending on the type of wheelchair they use. People with paraplegia and highly functional quadriplegia who use manual wheelchairs can make use of any of these vehicles, because their wheelchairs can be folded and stored behind the seat or in the trunk. High-level injury people with quadriplegia tend to use powered wheelchairs and so will generally require a full-size van or minivan to accommodate the greater bulk of the wheelchair. Vans and minivans can be modified with ramps or battery-powered lifts for access, and the driver's seat may be removed for the wheelchair user to drive using hand controls.

Garages with enough interior space to allow wheelchairs direct entry to the house are most desirable, because they afford protection from the elements and from extremes of hot or cold. Some local building codes require a 4-inch minimum step up from the garage to the living space. If such is the case, providing a ramp at least 3 feet, 6 inches wide with a level landing at least 5 feet by 5 feet is necessary for maneuvering space at the door. At least 5 feet must be provided between the side of the vehicle used by the SCI patient and the garage wall or another car to allow for wheelchair maneuvering and opening of the car doors.

SCI individuals who use powered wheelchairs and vans equipped with wheelchair lifts need even larger side wall clearances, up to 8 feet, to deploy a van's wheelchair lift and to maneuver the powered wheelchair. Note that wheelchair-adapted vans may have a raised roof, requiring a garage door higher than the 7-foot standard height. The SCI patient should also consider allowing a 4-foot-wide passage at the front and rear of the vehicle for maximum utilization of the garage. A garage suitable for wheelchair use approaches the size of a two-car garage, especially if the vehicle it will house is a lift-equipped van.

CONCLUSION

Many persons who have SCI prefer to return to their homes after initial injury, but many homes are inaccessible (8). This is especially true in rural areas. The consequences are that the quality of life is lowered and the healthcare costs are higher. A study to determine the frequency with which the need to find accessible housing delays discharge from a rehabilitation unit found that the lack of accessible housing resulted in delay of discharge in 10% of patients in a rehabilitation hospital (32). These patients stayed in the hospital beyond the planned date of discharge while accessible housing was found for them. The delays ranged from 6 to 210 days, with an average delay of 60 days and an average cost of $29,280. The average savings, had the patient been transferred to a transitional living unit when ready for hospital discharge, would have been $27,660. Nevertheless, there has been steady progress in the construction of barrier-free environments since ADA was signed more than a decade ago. Along with the advancements of technology, the facilitation of community reintegration for disabled persons has been demonstrated successfully in a few studies. For example, one report stated that environmental barriers do not prohibit a return to school for young people aged 18 years or younger who sustained SCI, even though such returns are problematic (33). It is the purpose of this chapter to reinforce social perception and promote general understanding of the needs of the disabled persons. Ensuring the greater participation of all facets of our society in this field will require the combined efforts of medical professionals in rehabilitation centers and disabled members of the community, as well as other interested parties.

References

1. Stephens S. Hidden barriers. *Progressive Architecture* 1978; 59:94–95.
2. National Health Interview Survey on Disability (NHIS–D). Center for Disease Control and Prevention, 1998.
3. Jones M, Catlin JH. Design for access. *Progressive Architecture* 1978; 59(4):65–71.
4. Go BK, DeVivo Ml, Richards S. The epidemiology of spinal cord injury. In: Stover SL, DeLisa JA, Whiteneck GG (eds.), *Spinal Cord Injury: Clinical Outcomes from the Model Systems.* Gaithersburg, MD: Aspen Publishers, 1995.
5. Post MW, Van Dijk AJ, Van Asbeck FW, Schrijvers AJ. Life satisfaction of persons with spinal cord injury compared to a population group. *Scand J Rehabil Med* 1998; 30(1):23–30.
6. McColl MA, Stirling P, Walker J, Corey P, Wilkins R. Expectations of independence and life satisfaction among aging spinal cord injured adults. *Disabil Rehabil* 1999; 21(5–6):231–240.
7. Richards JS, Bombardier CH, Tate D, Dijkers M, Gordon W, Shewchuk R, DeVivo MJ. Access to the environment and life satisfaction after spinal cord injury. *Arch Phys Med Rehabil* 1999; 80(11):1501–1506.

8. Hagglund KJ, Clay DL, Acuff M. Community reintegration for persons with spinal cord injury living in rural America. *Topics in Spinal Cord Injury* 1998; 4(2):28–49.
9. Seekins T, Clay J, Ravesloot C. A descriptive study of secondary conditions reported by a population of adults with physical disabilities served by three independent living centers in a rural state. *J Rehabil* 1994; 60:47–51.
10. Putzke JD, Richards JS, Hicken BL, DeVivo MJ. Predictors of life satisfaction: a spinal cord injury cohort study. Arch Phys Med Rehabil 2002;83:555–561.
11. Treischmann RB. Spinal cord injuries: psychological, social and vocational rehabilitation, 2nd ed. New York: Demos; 1988.
12. Chaves ES, Boninger ML, Cooper R, Fitzgerald SG, Gray DB, Cooper RA. Assessing the influence of wheelchair technology on perception of participation in spinal cord injury. *Arch Phys Med Rehabil* 2004; 85(11):1854–1858.
13. Keysor JJ, Jette AM, Coster W, Bettger JP, Haley SM. Association of environmental factors with levels of home and community participation in an adult rehabilitation cohort. *Arch Phys Med Rehabil* 2006; 87(12):1566–1575.
14. Whiteneck G, Meade MA, Dijkers M, Tate DG, Bushnik T, Forchheimer MB. Environmental factors and their role in participation and life satisfaction after spinal cord injury. *Arch Phys Med Rehabil* 2004; 85(11):1793–1803.
15. Richards JS, Bombardier CH, Tate D, et al. Access to the environment and life satisfaction after spinal cord injury. *Arch Phys Med Rehabil* 1999; 80:1501–1506.
16. Harrison C, Kuric J. Community reintegration of SCI persons: problems and perceptions. *SCI Nurs* 1989; 6(3):44–47.
17. Gray D, Gould M, Bickenbach JE. Environmental barriers and disability. *J Architectural Plann Res* 2003; 20:29–37.
18. Rogers J, Holm M. Task performance of older adults and low assistive technology devices. *Int J Technol Aging* 1991; 4:93–106.
19. Green NR. The state of the art of design for accessibility. *Am Inst Arch J* 1987; 76:58–61.
20. Steinfeld E. Barrier-free design begins to react to legislation, research. *Architectural Record* 1979; 69–71.
21. Jordan JJ. Recognizing and designing for the special needs of the elderly. *Am Inst Arch J* 1977; 66:50–55.
22. Stephens, S.: Hidden barriers. *Progressive Architecture* 1978; 59:94–95.
23. Breaking New Ground Resource Center. *Assistive Technology Needs Assessment of Farmers and Ranchers with Spinal Cord Injury: Final Report.* West Lafayette, IN: Breaking New Ground Resource Center, 1992.
24. *General Services Administration, Department of Defense, Department of Housing and Urban Development, U.S. Postal Service, Secretariat, Uniform Federal Accessibility Standards*, published originally in the Federal Register, August 7, 1984; available from the U.S. Architectural and Transportation Barriers Compliance Board, Suite 501, 1111 18th St., NW, Washington, D.C., 20036–3894.
25. Nelham RL. Principles and practice in the manufacture of seating for the handicapped. *Physiotherapy* 1984; 70:54–58.
26. Nesmith L. Designing for special populations. *Am Inst Arch J* 1987; 76:62–64.
27. Bunin NM, Jasperse D, Cooper S. *A Guide to Designing Accessible Outdoor Recreation Facilities*, a publication of the Heritage Conservation and Recreation Service, U.S. Department of the Interior, Lake Central Regional Office, Ann Arbor, MI, Jan. 1980.
28. Plourde RM. *Recreation.* Access Information Bulletin, November 1980; available from Paralyzed Veterans of America, 801 18th St., NW, Washington, D.C., 20006.
29. Glaser RM, Sawka MN, Wilde SW, Woodrow BK, Suryaprasad AG. Energy cost and cardiopulmonary responses for wheelchair locomotion and walking on tile and on carpet. *Paraplegia* 1981; 19(4):220–226.
30. Chesney DA, Axelson PW. Preliminary test method for the determination of surface firmness. *IEEE Trans Rehabil Eng* 1996; 4(3):182–187.
31. Welner AH. Environmental accessibility for physically disabled people. *Krusen's Handbook of Physical Medicine and Rehabilitation*, 4th ed. 1992; 1273–1290.
32. Sandford PR, Falk-Palec DJ, Spears K. Return to school after spinal cord injury. *Arch Phys Med Rehabil* 1999; 80(8):885–888.
33. Forrest G, Gombas G. Wheelchair accessible housing: its role in cost containment in spinal cord injury. *Arch Phys Med Rehabil* 1995; 76:450–452.

VIII

RECENT ADVANCES IN
SPINAL CORD RESEARCH

66 Mechanisms and Natural History of Spinal Cord Injury: Morphological, Cellular, and Molecular Features

Sandra K. Kostyk
Philip G. Popovich

Our understanding of the mechanisms that underlie the acute and chronic responses to spinal cord injury (SCI) and the implications that these processes have for long-term neurologic function continues to evolve. As we develop greater understanding of these processes, we are identifying more avenues and time points where interventions to improve recovery may be possible. Over the years, it has become increasingly clear that the solution to the problem of residual deficits after SCI will not involve a single treatment for all, but rather is likely to involve individualized approaches, and often a "cocktail approach" with different classes of interventions over time. It is the goal of current research efforts to identify these opportunities for intervention.

The current state of knowledge in the field is primarily the result of what we have learned from postmortem studies in humans, more recently from MRI studies, and the inferences we have made from studies in rodents and other mammals. Human autopsy studies are subject to marked variation in injury type and interval from injury to death, as well as variability in the quality of tissue fixation. Conventional techniques used to prepare human tissues for histology are often incompatible with the procedures that are required to perform detailed immunohistochemical studies of the molecular and cellular responses to injury. Consequently, anatomic analyses of injured human tissues are limited in their scope. Animal studies allow us to more accurately control the type of injury and the duration of the postinjury interval. However, variations between species and strains suggest that extrapolation to the human situation must be undertaken with caution. Nonetheless, there are numerous parallels between experimental and human SCI that validate our efforts to pursue controlled animal models to study the injury and regenerative response of the spinal cord. We focus here on various aspects of traumatic mammalian SCI—both on the secondary pathologic mechanisms that contribute to delayed neuronal and glial cell loss and on the intrinsic mechanisms of repair.

THE MECHANISM OF INJURY: MECHANICS AND ANATOMIC RELATIONSHIPS IN SCI

Traumatic SCI generally results from flexion, extension, rotation, compression, traction, or compound injuries to the vertebral column that result in varying degrees of compression of the spinal cord. Less commonly, penetrating injuries result in laceration of the spinal cord. Spinal cord impingement by bone fragments; subdural, extradural, or subarachnoid hemorrhage; and disc fragments contribute to the etiology of the injury. The peculiarities of spinal cord anatomy play a role in the nature of the injury response. The elongated slender spinal cord is enclosed within a relatively tight and confining bony structure and is surrounded by adherent meningeal and dural sheaths. The size of the spinal canal and the subarachnoid space and components of the spinal cord vary greatly across its length. The number of ascending and descending axons within the cord is greatest at the cervical level, where the "free" space around the spinal cord is minimal. At C5, the most frequent location of cervical SCI, the difference between the diameter of the spinal cord and the bony canal is approximately 0.65 cm (1). Thus, there is little room for extraneous material such as blood or bone fragments, and little room to accommodate swelling. A key determinant of the degree of injury is the energy transfer through this heterogeneous tissue and fluid system. The energy transferred during injury has been equated to a pressure pulse or strain gradient that travels along the spinal compartments, its speed and properties modified by the tissue components and physical properties specific to each location (2, 3). Biological composition and susceptibility to strain and force favors early gray matter destruction, with relative sparing of white-matter tracts (4).

The resulting SCI clinical syndromes are also influenced by the peculiarities of the mechanics and anatomy of the spinal column. Hyperflexion injuries result in compression of the posterior aspect of the vertebral body on the anterior aspect of the spinal cord. Hyperextension injuries predominantly cause a central cord syndrome. Ischemic cord syndromes depend on the specific vascular territory involved. Most injuries result from rapid contusion or compression, leaving a bridge of tissue connecting the proximal and distal parts of the spinal cord (5, 6, 7, 8). Crush or hyperflexion injuries more commonly result in clinically complete SCI, whereas hyperextension and contusion/compression injuries are more commonly associated with clinically incomplete injuries (9). A small percentage of individuals surviving traumatic injuries sustain complete transections of the spinal cord (10). The percentage of complete transections may be higher among those dead at the scene of injury, but they are less commonly accessible in spinal cord pathology tissue banks.

The velocity and force of the injury are also important. Sudden compressive injury is believed to result in more significant injury with hemorrhage, swelling, and greater secondary damage and scarring. This hypothesis is supported by the observations of Hayes and Kakulas (9), who completed comparative pathologic studies of sports-related injuries and high-velocity injuries caused by motor vehicle accidents. Similarly, in rodent models of SCI, the rate and magnitude of tissue displacement at the time of injury correlates with degree of tissue damage and functional outcome (2, 11–14). Slowly growing tumors (e.g., ependymomas) and slowly induced compressive injuries, such as those caused by the bony encroachment of cervical spondylosis or from progressive ossification of the posterior longitudinal ligament, result in less scarring and respond better to decompression surgery.

NEUROPATHOLOGY OF HUMAN SPINAL CORD INJURIES

How the spinal cord is injured determines the nature of the neuropathologic response. In general, neuropathologists have classified subacute and chronic histopathology into four or five broad categories (Table 66.1), identified by Bunge et al. (6):

1. Contusion/cyst injuries. Cords with central cysts or cavitations with varying amounts of spared white matter rim tissue. There is no disruption of the dura, and the surface anatomy is intact.
2. Massive compression injuries. Cords with severe compression injuries with disruption of the pial surface and a predominantly collagenous scar with or without some preserved axonal tracts.

3. Laceration injuries. Cords with partial lacerations, such as injuries caused by knife or gunshot wounds. The surface pia and dura are disrupted, and the lesions have variable amounts of collagenous connective tissue.
4. Complete transection. These lesions involve complete severing of the meninges and cord parenchyma with infiltration of fibrous scar tissue.
5. Solid cord injury. The spinal cord retains its surface continuity with less apparent central cord gray matter necrosis, with no cyst formation, and with preservation of most central gray matter structure. These lesions may be more commonly found in cords from individuals with shorter survival times after injury (i.e., before the onset of progressive secondary tissue degeneration seen in more chronic injuries). The main clinical defect in this category is believed to be caused by demyelination and disruption of axons in lateral white-matter tracts.

It is difficult to accurately determine the frequency of occurrence of the various categories of injuries and the various pathologic responses. The data in Table 66.1 are frequency estimates summarized from data obtained from literature describing pathological tissue samples from the Miami Project to Cure Paralysis (Florida), the Royal Perth Hospital (Perth, Australia), and the London Health Science Center (London, England) (6–10, 15–17). However, many social and environmental factors affect the etiology and the frequency of injury type, including locality (e.g., urban, suburban, rural), cultural customs, frequency and type of behaviors with increased risk (e.g., skiing, diving), and peace versus wartime exposure. The estimates listed in Table 66.1 are provided to help emphasize the variety of lesion pathology that can be seen. Not all therapeutic options and advances are likely to help individuals with each type of injury. To effectively manage each form of injury, clinical and research interventions must address the predominant mechanisms that underlie the unique pathologic presentation in each case.

The primary cause and mechanics of injury determine the immediate pathology observed within minutes to hours after an SCI. In the absence of penetrating or severe tissue disruption, microscopic analysis of cross sections of spinal cord early after injury, from victims "dead on arrival," may reveal little obvious damage or only scattered petechial hemorrhages (7, 8, 18). This finding emphasizes the role that secondary pathological mechanisms play in the determination of lesion extent. This early period is considered a "window of opportunity" for clinical intervention.

Table 66.1   General Patterns of Neuropathology Following SCI

CLASSIFICATION OF CHRONIC PATHOLOGY	CLINICAL FUNCTION	ESTIMATED FREQUENCY
Contusion/cyst	Complete or incomplete	~45–65%
Massive compression	Usually complete	~20–25%
Laceration	Usually incomplete	~14–21%
Complete transection	Complete	<5–10%
Solid cord/lateral colum injury	Usually incomplete	~10%

These rough estimates of the frequency of the general classes of injury were derived primarily from summaries of the pathologic findings from the databases of the Royal Perth Hospital at the University of Western Australia, the Miami Project to Cure Paralysis in Florida, and the hospitals of the London Health Science Center (6–10, 15–17). Frequency of type of injury is likely to vary between various locales: urban, suburban, rural, and so forth.

Within hours of injury there is evidence of an increasingly recognizable injury zone, with the area of necrosis increasing from days to months after the injury (7). Examination of postmortem tissue often reveals central hemorrhagic necrosis and edema several segments rostral and caudal to the injury site (7, 8, 18). The area of necrosis is usually localized to the gray matter. Within 3 to 4 hours of injury, polymorphonuclear leukocytes (i.e., neutrophils) appear in and around the injury zone (7). By 1 to 3 days after injury, evidence of early activation of resident microglia has been observed in postmortem specimens (7). Four to 10 days after injury, numerous macrophages and other inflammatory cells have invaded the region (5–8). Evidence of phagocytic "foamy macrophages" can still be observed weeks to months after the SCI (7). In contrast to infiltration by cells of myeloid lineage, lymphocytic invasion of extravascular tissue in human injuries is modest (7, 19).

Astrocytes, a predominant glial subtype, play a significant role in the human injury response. Within days, and peaking by 2 to 3 weeks, astrocytes hypertrophy and send out long processes forming part of the "glial scar" that surrounds injured tissue (8). In injuries that involve a break in the glial limitans (e.g., lacerations and complete transections) there is an invasion of mesenchymal cells leading to dense fibrous collagenous scar tissue. In the case of complete transections, the severed ends of the spinal cord retract and are then encapsulated by a dense glial scar that is further encased by a dense cap of fibrous tissue (17). The subarachnoid space surrounding the cord at the level of the lesion may be infiltrated by fibrous tissue. Collagenous and fibrous tissue may also comprise a part of the residual connecting bridge of spinal tissue, most commonly in lacerations and massive compression injuries (6, 8, 10).

Eventually, blood and necrotic tissue are cleared, frequently leaving a residual fluid-filled cavity. Cavities, or posttraumatic cysts, may extend several segments rostral and caudal to the site of impact and are often multiloculated. The cavities are surrounded by thin gliotic walls and by varying amounts of potentially dysfunctional yet anatomically preserved residual ascending and descending fibers. Although a cystic lesion may develop as a subacute consequence of SCI over weeks or months, some patients may develop new cysts or expand former cysts years after their initial injury. This may occur subsequent to an additional, but more subtle injury. For example, slow progressive neurologic deterioration in previously stable SCI patients may occur after a fall or minor car accident or because of vertebral instability or spinal stenosis secondary to osteophytic overgrowth at the injury zone. These cysts often can be visualized on magnetic resonance imaging (MRI) and can sometimes be followed as they expand in diameter or in rostral–caudal extent. There have been attempts to use fetal tissue transplants to arrest expanding cyst formation in chronically injured SCI patients (20–22). However, it is not clear if this approach yields significant long-term benefits.

In many lesions there is a spared rim of connecting white matter. The percentage of these axons that remain functional probably varies. Oligodendrocytes at the site and border of lesions are susceptible to injury, leading to demeylination. Although there is abundant evidence of segmental demyelination and remyelination in experimental models of SCI, the degree to which this occurs subsequent to human SCI has been harder to quantitate from human postmortem tissue. Signs of demyelination have been reported in some pathological studies (6, 10) but in others have not been observed (7). However, convincing evidence of demyelination and remyelination in chronic human tissue has been demonstrated recently using immunohistologic techniques and confocal imaging (23). Numerous Schwann cells and peripheral nerve axons are found in chronic lesions in a process referred to as Schwannosis (24). This is essentially a neuroma formation within the cord. There is no evidence to suggest that these peripheral axons contribute to recovery; rather, it appears that they are more likely to exacerbate pathological responses (25).

Attempts have been made to correlate functional outcome in humans with the amount of white matter in the residual rim of spared tissue. In one study of eleven clinically complete patients, eight showed no residual white matter at all (15). The majority of the residual tissue consisted of connective tissue (13.3% to 100%), hypertrophied glia (56% to 94.2%), and regenerating dorsal nerve roots (5.8% to 44%) (15). No axons of central origin were clearly identified in these cases. Of the ten clinically incomplete cases studied, seven had cavities, and most had significant gliosis. White-matter tracts accounted for 2.1% to 40.4% of the residual tissue in the injury zone (15). In the remaining three cases, residual white matter tracts were apparent but were without corresponding clinical functional correlates. This category of anatomically incomplete but clinically complete individuals has been termed by some as "discomplete" (26). The amount of white matter sparing in ten clinically incomplete patients in the same study was not necessarily more than in the "discomplete" group, nor did the amount of spared tissue correlate with the amount of preservation of clinical function. Clearly, the location and functional nature of preserved axons, and perhaps the integrity of their myelin sheaths, hold more clinical relevance than the total amount of white matter spared. In fact, using high-resolution MRI images, Metz et al. (27) found that the best functional outcome was associated with the preservation of the ventral white matter tracts. Aside from the laterally located corticospinal and rubrospinal tracts, the bulk of descending spinal pathways is located in the ventral funiculi (including tectospinal, anterior corticospinal, vestibulospinal, and medial reticulospinal tracts).

MECHANISMS OF TISSUE REPAIR IN THE INJURED SPINAL CORD

Through safety education and the implementation of protective devices such as air bags and seat belts, we have made progress in reducing the frequency and severity of SCI. Based on preclinical experimentation in animal models, acute clinical interventions (i.e., methylprednisolone) have been studied in the hope of minimizing the final extent of injury (28–30). The efficacy, benefits and risks of these clinical interventions are debatable. In human necropsy specimens obtained within 3 months of injury, there is still significant swelling, petechial hemorrhage, and ongoing liquefaction of tissue with evidence of active macrophage phagocytosis (9, 10). The potential for intervention immediately after and during the first few months post-SCI appears great. A more complete understanding of the evolving interplay between cells, soluble molecules, and extracellular matrices is needed to develop better clinical interventions to decrease secondary injury and promote the wound healing process.

Table 66.2   Features of the Wound Healing: Response in the Spinal Cord

WOUND INJURY RESPONSES	WOUND REPAIR PROCESSES
Hemorrhage/ edema	Angiogenesis
Inflammation/bystander damage	Inflammation/remove debris
Macrophage (pro-inflammatory cytokines)	Macrophages (growth factors/oncomodulin/cytokines)
Cytokines/chemokines	Cytokines/chemokines
Glial cell proliferation/scarring	Glial cell/stem cell proliferation/re-population/tissue integrity
Oxygen radicals/ Lipid breakdown	Growth factors
Extracellular matrix deposition/barriers	Extracellular matrix modification/scaffolding (MMPs)
Apoptosis/excitotoxicity/Ca$^+$ influx	Synaptogenesis/plasticity
Demyelination	Remyelination
Syrinx	Axon regeneration/functional recovery

Source: Adapted from McTigue et al., 2000 (31).

A key emerging concept is that the very processes that are essential for repairing injured spinal cord may also contribute to secondary injury and create a hostile environment for functional recovery (31). For example, inflammatory cells and mediators (e.g., cytokines, chemokines) are critical for the removal of debris and in triggering the early phases of tissue repair and preserving structural integrity of the cord (32). However, these same cells and mediators can adversely affect the survival of neurons and glia, thereby leading to increased secondary injury and scar formation (33, 34). Table 66.2 outlines a few of these processes, emphasizing the simultaneous dynamic between the "good" versus the "bad" aspects of the injury response. Advances in understanding the acute dynamics of the pathologic changes that occur immediately following injury have been made primarily through careful studies of animal models of SCI. These studies have formed the basis of the theory that there is often residual tissue that is not directly injured during the initial insult but that becomes anatomically or physiologically compromised as a result of swelling, excitotoxicity, and perhaps acute inflammation (35–37). The area of compromised tissue expands, circumferentially as a function of time after injury, but also rostral and caudal to the initial injury zone (Figure 66.1). Thus, acute inter-

ventions that minimize tissue injury over time may have significant implications for prospective recovery of function given that there is evidence that considerable functional recovery can be achieved if even only 10% of spinal axons survive the injury (38).

Animal Models of SCI

As discussed, various factors are important in determining the final extent of injury in humans, including velocity, peak force, and tissue displacement. Several animal models of SCI have been developed that allow for controlled and reproducible injuries that correlate well with human injuries. In most animal models of contusion injury, a thoracic laminectomy is performed and a force transiently impacted on the exposed spinal cord. In weight drop models, which have been used extensively in cats and rats, a small weight is dropped from a predetermined height onto the exposed spinal cord (11, 17, 38). A contusion device that includes a small impounder controlled by an electromagnet computer interface has also been developed that produces graded injuries in both rats and mice and shows excellent correlation between histologic and behavioral outcomes (14, 39). The use of models such as these has begun to allow us to tease apart the cellular and molecular response to SCI (40). With the advent of transgenic mice and controlled SCI models, more rapid elucidation of the molecular events that influence mechanisms of secondary injury and repair will be forthcoming (34, 41). Figure 66.1 represents a schematic of the injury zone and regions of secondary damage.

The Inflammatory Response

The role that cells and mediators of the immune system play in central nervous system (CNS) injury is fascinatingly complex. Neuroinflammation likely contributes to tissue repair, but paradoxically can exacerbate the secondary injury response. The latter might contribute to the failure of complete functional recovery. The earliest response of the immune system involves the coordination of communication between phagocytic cells (neutrophils, macrophages, microglia); lymphocytes, soluble molecular mediators (complement, cytokines, chemokines, matrix metalloproteinases); and extracellular matrix molecules. Some of the byproducts of the exuberance of the inflammatory response, for example oxygen free radicals, proteolytic enzymes,

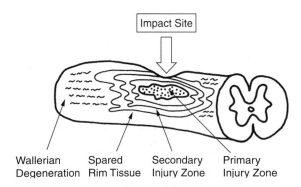

Impact Site

Wallerian Degeneration   Spared Rim Tissue   Secondary Injury Zone   Primary Injury Zone

Figure 66.1 Schematic representation of a contusion injury to spinal cord. The primary injury zone, at the site of impact, is surrounded by "at-risk" tissue, the secondary injury zone. Depending on interventions and the exuberance of the injury response, the extent of this secondary zone may vary. Spared tissue, although not necessarily functional tissue, may partially or completely surround the injury zone. Wallerian degeneration occurs both above and below the impact site.

lipid peroxidation, and excitotoxins, can damage neurons and glial cells. Unfortunately, the result of the response to injury in the spinal cord is the extension of the injury zone and the production of a scar that patches the injury site rather than stimulating epimorphic regeneration of the original tissue structure.

The Sequential Involvement of Inflammatory Cells

The intricate synchronization of the various inflammatory cells in the injury response after SCI has been a focus of intense study in the rodent (42–47). Figure 66.2 provides an overview schematic overview of the time course of some of the inflammatory responses observed in the rodent. Microglia (resident CNS macrophages) surrounding the injury zone are activated almost immediately, with peak morphologic activation of the cells near the epicenter occurring within hours to days after injury. As the injury zone expands over time, microglia express new molecules on their cell surface along axonal tracts rostral and caudal to the injury zone. Thus, peak activation of microglial cell surface markers is a protracted process occurring over several days, weeks, and perhaps months or years following injury. It is believed that the acute activation of microglia and subsequent microglial–astroglial signaling cascades establish a chemotactic gradient for calling peripheral blood leukocytes into the injured spinal cord.

In all species studied, within hours of the initial insult, neutrophils invade the injury zone and then, just as quickly, within the first day or two, die or are removed by the next wave of inflammatory cells. Circulating monocytes do not infiltrate the primary injury zone in significant numbers until after 2 to 3 days postinjury (48). T-cells can be identified in the injury zone by 3 days and peak in number by 1 week. A more robust and protracted lymphocytic response maybe associated with fibrotic lesions such as those seen in mouse SCI models (45). Figure 66.2 summarizes the temporal appearance of inflammatory cells in a

rodent model of SCI. The figure is meant to emphasize the variable range of expression and time course between strains and species. The extent to which these cellular responses generalize to other species or to human SCI remains to be seen. Because the pathology associated with SCI in different species is distinct (43, 45, 49), unique inflammatory cascades could play a role in differentially influencing mechanisms of secondary injury or repair. Studies comparing different strains of mice with varying degrees of inflammatory responses have shown inconsistent correlations between the inflammatory response, axonal plasticity, lesion pathology, and functional recovery (45, 47).

Cytokines and Chemokines

Cytokines are a family of regulatory proteins that help orchestrate the immune response. They can be generated by immune cells themselves and also by other cell types, including astrocytes, microglia, and injured endothelia (50). They are generally divided into two classes: proinflammatory cytokines (including TNF-α, IL-1, and IL-6) that initiate and perpetuate immune activation; and anti-inflammatory cytokines (including IL-4, IL-10, and IL13) that are essential for dampening the immune response. The cellular responses described above correspond closely with the time course of expression of a variety of chemokines and cytokines in the same injury model (31, 51–55).

TNF-α (a proinflammatory cytokine) enhances the permeability of endothelial cells and promotes the binding of leukocytes to the endothelial cell surface, thus facilitating infiltration of the spinal cord by circulating cells. Some evidence exists that TNF-α may be neuroprotective *in vitro*; however, there is also confounding evidence that suggests that when macrophages or microglial are simultaneously present *in vitro* or *in vivo*, TNF-α promotes neurotoxicity (56–58). Elevated levels of TNF-α protein and mRNA have been detected as early as 1 hour after SCI, with persisting elevations for at least 7 days after injury (53, 59). Attenuation of TNF-α is associated with improved SCI outcome (59, 60).

IL-10 is a potent anti-inflammatory cytokine that blocks or decreases the production of various cytokines and chemokines and suppresses monocyte function. An injection of IL-10 shortly after an SCI contusion injury decreases the induction of TNF-α in the spinal cord and improves functional recovery (59). However, it appears that whereas early suppression of inflammation may be beneficial, further alteration of the endogenous response with a second dose of IL-10 at 3 days after injury leads to no effect on tissue sparing or recovery (59). Findings of this sort emphasize the complicated and multifaceted role of the immune system in the response to injury in the CNS. It has been suggested that the timing of the delivery of this cytokine is critical and that reduction of the early inflammatory response is neuroprotective, whereas prolonged or delayed suppression may antagonize intrinsic repair processes in which the immune system plays a pivotal role (61). The importance of the timing of a cytokine-regulated inflammatory response was similarly noted when comparing the effects of the injection of a cocktail of proinflammatory cytokines at 1 day or 4 days subsequent to experimental SCI. In this paradigm, delayed injections resulted in improved tissue preservation, although acute administration of these cytokines resulted in greater tissue loss (62). The production of cytokines at one time point after injury may be

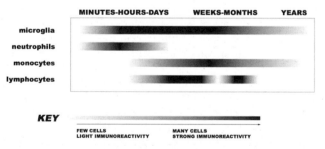

KEY

FEW CELLS LIGHT IMMUNOREACTIVITY   MANY CELLS STRONG IMMUNOREACTIVITY

Figure 66.2 Overview of the inflammatory reaction subsequent to experimental spinal cord injury. Although the inflammatory reaction is more complex than depicted in this figure, the primary cellular components of the reaction are illustrated. Cellular reactions are graded on a continuum from reactions that occur immediately to those observed for months or even years after injury. The intensity of shading (from weakest to darkest) corresponds with documented changes in the magnitude of the cellular reaction. Note the acute involvement of microglia and neutrophils followed by monocytes and lymphocytes, as well as the biphasic response of lymphocyte infiltration as observed in rat. Similar studies have not been completed for other species or humans after spinal cord injury.

neuroprotective and promote tissue repair, whereas the effect of the same cytokines at other time points in the sequence of the injury response may be destructive. Understanding when components of the immune response are beneficial versus when they are detrimental should ultimately facilitate manipulation of the injury response in the clinical setting.

Macrophages: Divergent Roles in Inflammation and Repair

The importance of timing and specificity is also critical to the positive or negative effects of the macrophage response in SCI. Microglia are the resident macrophages of the CNS and are among the first cells to respond to spinal cord trauma. There appears to be significant phenotypic heterogeneity, as determined by cell surface markers, among spinal cord microglia (43, 63). As these surface markers may play a role in intracellular signaling, phenotypic heterogeneity may imply functional heterogeneity (64). This, in itself, may contribute to some of the differences seen in the injury responses in white matter (delayed demyelination) versus gray matter (acute necrotization) (33). The heterogeneity of the macrophage response to SCI is further complicated by the fact that resident microglial reactions are bolstered by blood monocytes that are recruited to the site of injury during the first few days postinjury. Although there is likely considerable overlap in the functional potential of hematogenous macrophages and resident CNS microglia, there is sufficient evidence to support a divergent role for these macrophage subsets in the injured spinal cord. In an effort to tease apart the roles of endogenous macrophages (microglia) that are activated almost immediately after injury and the hematogenous derived macrophages (monocytes) that arrive after several days, anatomic and neurologic outcome has been evaluated in a rat model of spinal contusion injury after selective depletion of peripheral monocytes (65). In the absence of monocyte-derived macrophages, reduced necrosis and cavitation occur at the lesion epicenter concomitant with increased axon sprouting. This suggests that acute monocyte infiltration of the injury site contributes to secondary neuronal and glial injury. Similarly, the inhibition of the infiltration of leukocytes into the injury using and anti-integrin treatment limits secondary damage and improves outcome (66). The reduction of consequences of the inflammatory infiltrate also resulted in improvement in a guinea pig model of SCI (67).

However, other studies suggest that, under the appropriate conditions, activated macrophages may promote CNS repair. Oncomodulin, a protein released by activated macrophages has been shown to promote regeneration of CNS axons (68). Macrophages activated with specific proteins and then transplanted into the rodent spinal cord have been shown to promote axonal regeneration and improve functional recovery (69, 70). In animal studies, macrophages that were activated by exposure to peripheral but not optic nerve supported axonal regeneration (69, 71). The key to the success of this paradigm appears to be the specific molecule that has activated the macrophage. However, given the mixed neuropromoting and neurotoxic potential of macrophages, attempts at modulation or transplantation in human studies must be approached with caution. A phase I clinical trial using autologous activated

macrophages in humans with spinal cord injury has been completed, and further treatments and studies are under consideration (72, 73).

T-Cells and Autoimmunity

In addition to discriminating between "self" and "nonself" molecules, activated T-cells have many physiologic tasks, including modulating macrophage function, maintaining microvascular endothelial integrity, and stimulating antibody-producing B-cells. The full extent of the role that these cells play in the evolution of tissue injury or repair after SCI is not yet clear, but the sequential appearance of activated T-cells in the injured spinal cord suggests that they have a defined role in the orchestration of the normal wound response. The activation and response of these cells very much depends on local cytokine and glucocorticoid levels. Glucocorticoid levels are modified by SCI (74, 75) and clearly are affected by the exogenous administration of methylprednisolone in the clinical situation. It has been postulated that T-cells become sensitized to peptides of CNS origin after injury and that an autoimmune response to these self-peptides (e.g., fragments of myelin basic protein [MBP], or proteolipid protein) may amplify or dampen the injury response (76).

MBP-reactive T-cells can be isolated from peripheral lymph nodes 7 days after SCI in the rat. When these cells are injected into intact animals, the animals develop a paralytic disorder similar to the acute neuroinflammatory disorder experimental allergic encephalomyelitis (EAE) (77). Interestingly, T-cells isolated at later time points after SCI (i.e., after more than 7 days) do not induce a similar deficit, suggesting that endogenous regulatory mechanisms suppress this potentially injurious autoimmune reaction. The absence of a sustained autoimmune response after traumatic SCI in humans suggests that if a similar phenomenon of T-cell activation against self-antigens occurs, it is suppressed, perhaps by other T-cells that are not CNS-reactive (43, 78, 79). Still, it is possible that, during the transient phase of T-cell activation, autoreactive T-cells could contribute to neurodestruction or demyelination.

Just as controversy surrounds the primary function of macrophages in the injured spinal cord, autoreactive T-cells are garnering similar attention. For example, recent evidence suggests that the exogenous administration of MBP-reactive T-cells may lead to increased neural protection and behavioral improvement (80, 81). Because all individuals normally possess a low frequency of myelin-reactive T-cells, manipulation of these cells in human SCI may be of therapeutic benefit (76). However, as is the case with variously activated macrophages discussed above, we still do not have sufficient understanding of the multiple functions and potential of T-cells in the human setting. Indeed, the development of therapeutic vaccines to treat human Alzheimer's disease relies on select activation of CNS-reactive lymphocytes. A similar therapy may be a candidate for treating human SCI (82, 83).

Apoptosis, Demyelination, and Remyelination

Immediately after SCI, necrotic cell death occurs within the primary injury zone. In addition, apoptotic cell death occurs acutely within the lesion epicenter and also extends rostral and caudal from the impact zone over time (84–87). This extension of the postinjury cell death process lasts for more than 6 weeks, and likely for much longer. It involves primarily oligodendrocytes and microglia along the axonal pathways undergoing progressive Wallerian degeneration (88, 89). This process presumably contributes to delayed post-SCI demyelination.

In animal models, many demyelinated axons become remyelinated. It appears that expanding populations of oligodendrocyte progenitor cells, and possibly infiltrating Schwann cells, participate in this process (90–93). Observers have identified axons in the injured cord, both in human postmortem tissue and in animal models, that stain for both central and peripheral myelin, suggesting that Schwann cells infiltrate the cord and promote remyelination of demyelinated axons (23, 95–97). Schwann cells form a basement membrane that can be stained even in poorly fixed tissue, whereas oligodendrocytes do not, thus facilitating their distinction. In a study from the Royal Perth Hospital in Australia, out of twenty-seven cases studied at least 6 months postinjury, sixteen showed remyelination of central axons by Schwann cells (15). Axons were found coated with Schwann cells near the lesion site and, in continuity with oligodendrocyte myelin, further from the lesion site. Recovery of function has been demonstrated in animal models when demyelinated axons have been remyelinated by Schwann cells, and these axons conduct impulses similar to normal CNS axons (98, 99).

Whereas Schwann cell remyelination of denuded axons occurs via invasion of the injured spinal cord by peripheral Schwann cells, oligodendrocyte remyelination is likely the result of proliferation and differentiation of progenitor cells found throughout the spinal cord, which are stimulated to multiply by factors produced after SCI (90, 100, 101). However, the combined efforts of the Schwann cells and oligodendrocytes are in general not sufficient to support clinically significant functional recovery. Studies have demonstrated that the internodes in remyelinated sections are not as thick or as long as they are in normal tissue (102, 103). Studies have begun to explore interventions, such as the provision of growth factors such as the neurotrophins to amplify proliferation of oligodendrocyte precursors cells in SCI models to improve myelination (90).

Extracellular Matrix Molecules: Facilitation and Inhibition

Understanding the participation of the deposition of extracellular matrix molecules in the SCI wound healing process is as problematic as the participation of the other processes described earlier. On the one hand, the formation of a glial scar and deposition of these molecules is part of the wound healing process that is essential for responding to the destruction imposed by the injury. On the other hand, the exuberance of the response and the types of matrices laid down may, in the long term, inhibit the regenerative efforts of injured axons (104–106). The type of scar tissue found at the injury zone depends in part on the mechanism of spinal tissue destruction and, in the case of animal models, on the species under study. As described earlier, penetrating injuries that disrupt the dural–meningeal interface tend to result in greater fibrous scarring with significant

collagen deposition (5, 107, 108). Nonpenetrating injuries tend to result in greater cavitation, with increased deposition of glial and macrophage-derived extracellular matrix molecules (109, 110). Interestingly, the rat SCI contusion injury models result in wounds with marked cavitation, whereas the mouse models have wounds filled with solid scar tissue (2, 14, 111). The differences between the SCI wound healing responses in each species provide different advantages for further exploration of the responses found in different types of human wounds (2).

Evidence suggests that extracellular matrix molecules in the injury zone, even in the absence of a significant physical scar, may halt the growing tips of regenerating axons (106, 112, 113). Molecules, particularly those up-regulated by activated astrocytes (including tenascin-C and several forms of chondroitin sulfate proteoglycan), associate with laminins to form a new matrix in the injury zone (114, 115). Although the laminins are generally considered supportive of axon growth, proteoglycans are more commonly considered to be inhibitory (116, 117). However, the situation is actually significantly more complicated. Extracellular matrix molecules are complex multidomain structures. Subregions or domains of the molecules may be growth inhibitory, whereas other regions on the same molecule are stimulatory. For example, laminins are composed of three chains, but tenascin-C is composed of six arms with multiple epidermal growth factor (EGF) and fibronectin domains (118). It has been hypothesized that fragments of these molecules may assume new conformations in the setting of CNS injury, and that these may have unique effects on neurons (118–120). Several interventions to alter the composition of the ECM or adhesion molecules following SCI are currently being explored (121–127). Chondroitinase ABC removes chondroitin sulphate proteoglycan glycosaminoglycan side chains and decreases chondroitin sulphate proteoglycan inhibitory activity on axon growth and, when injected into the injured spinal cord, promotes sprouting and functional recovery (126–129). Altering the inhibitory nature of the extracellular matrix in combination with other interventions to promote regeneration is one of the more promising approaches for therapeutic intervention (129–130). A variety of molecules expressed on the surface of mature CNS cells, particularly on mature oligodendrocytes (including myelin-associated glycoproteins, Nogo-A, and ephrin-B3) are intrinsically inhibitory to axon regeneration and, along with some of the extracellular matrix molecules, decrease the injured tissue's ability to support axon regeneration. Simultaneous therapeutic manipulation of the multiple inhibitors of axon growth may be needed to achieve functional recovery (131).

A recent approach directed at altering the extracellular matrix has been to investigate the role of the matrix metalloproteinases (MMPs) in SCI (132). MMP-2 and MMP-9 are two of the proteolytic enzymes that are produced by inflammatory cells and are involved in modifying the extracellular matrix in injury and repair mechanisms in the CNS. Blockade of MMPs in the first 1 to 3 days after SCI improves recovery, but if the blockade is maintained for longer than a few days, the beneficial response is obviated. MMP-2 appears to promote wound healing in the spinal cord (132). Discovering how to balance the expression and timing of these different enzymes may facilitate functional recovery.

Stem Cells and Progenitor Cells

In amphibian models of successful spinal cord regeneration, a critical source for cells in the reparative and regenerative process appears to be a robust proliferative response from the ependymal cells that line the central spinal canal (133–135). In mammalian injuries, a proliferative response also occurs near the central canal that contributes to the formation of tissue bridges that fill the injury zone (136–138). However, this proliferative response does not result in epimorphic regeneration of the mammalian cord. Although there is a recovery of gross structural connectivity, the substructure and cellular organization does not reform the typical adult pattern of neuronal, glial, and cellular layers and organization. Nevertheless, there may be potential for a more successful regenerative response than have been suspected in the past. Recent studies in mammals have demonstrated that multipotent progenitor cells exist throughout the adult CNS, including the spinal cord, suggesting prospects for further enhancement of the recovery response (139–140). Harvested adult rat spinal cord progenitor cells can be induced to proliferate *in vitro* in the presence of fibroblast growth factor-2 into cells expressing differentiation markers of astrocytes, oligodendrocytes, and occasionally neurons (141). A recent study has demonstrated ongoing cell proliferation in the intact adult rodent spinal cord, with the majority of proliferating cells maturing into astrocytes and oligodendrocytes (140). In the uninjured cord, division of these cells appears to occur throughout the cord rather than as a result of migration from progenitors in the ependymal zone (140). In the rodent spinal cord, proliferation and migration and differentiation of ependymal progenitor cells has been observed after minor trauma (142). It is not yet clear how or whether progenitor cells contribute to the repair process or whether they can be manipulated in vivo to participate in a more functionally successful repair of the injury zone. The demonstration of multipotent stem cells with proliferative potential throughout the nervous system suggests promise for further experimental interventions to augment the endogenous repair process in SCI.

CHRONIC SCI

Late Pathologic Complications of SCI

It is not uncommon to find slow progressive neurologic deterioration years after an injury (143). Long-term spinal cord injured individuals may begin complaining of fatigue, new weakness, sensory disturbances, and functional loss. Common causes include the late development of syringomyelia, perhaps caused by tethering of the cord by fibrous scarring and arachnoidal pathology. A recent study of spinal thecal sac constriction in rodents supports the theory that induced constrictive pressure gradients contribute to cyst formation (144). Hypertrophy of injured bony tissues (spondylosis) at the old injury site can lead to spinal stenosis and cord flattening, thus leading to further neurologic deterioration over time. A study of seventy-five SCI patients in France demonstrated a significant correlation of the occurrence of syrinx with spinal canal stenosis and argues for early surgical intervention and spinal realignment (145). It has been suggested that some of the deficit resulting from the compression of cervical spondylosis may involve demyelination of the pathways in the spinal cord (6). A similar phenomenon has been described in animal models, with additional demonstration of

remyelination after decompression (146). Occasionally, one can find a patient who does not show significant recovery immediately subsequent to decompression but who regains some sensory or motor function many months after decompression. One can postulate that this late recovery might be caused by the subsequent remyelination of intact axons.

Synaptic Plasticity

The loss of projections to distal targets following SCI affords the adjacent circuitry and terminals the opportunity to sprout and form new synapses and alter synaptic strength at other sites (143). Several studies have demonstrated reorganization within the brain after SCI (147–151). Central changes in cortical circuitry may be particularly important in orchestrating recovery after incomplete injuries. Marked changes in cortical activity levels have been noted bilaterally early after a unilateral cord injury, with increasing contralateral activity over the next few months as functional motor recovery improves, in the macaque (152). Recent studies suggest that reorganization of cortical and subcortical circuitry may be responsible for the phenomena of phantom sensations frequently observed after SCI (153–155). Acute and chronic changes can also be demonstrated in dorsal horn primary afferents and descending spinal pathways after SCI and may also be involved in the development of chronic pain syndromes in SCI (156–158). Sprouting of motor axons terminals directly at muscle synapses following SCI can also lead to altered functional plasticity (159). The demonstration of reorganization of supraspinal and intraspinal circuitry after SCI suggests potential avenues for further enhancing synaptic modifications subsequent to behavioral interventions to improve outcomes (160–166). Some of these changes mentioned above presumably occur shortly after injury, others over months. Additional synaptic changes may occur over the course of years as the nervous system adapts to continuously varying challenges. While much attention is focused on stimulating axon regeneration across the lesion site, it has become increasingly clear that there are multiple sites along the neuraxis where potential interventions may be targeted to attempt to enhance the inherent plasticity of the nervous system and improve functional outcome. Figure 66.3 provides a schematic representation of potential sites for focused interventions to affect neuronal plasticity.

CONCLUSION

It has become increasingly clear that the natural evolution of each spinal cord injury depends on multiple factors. Numerous simultaneous and synchronous processes orchestrate the wound healing response, some beneficial and some, perhaps, harmful in their exuberance. To effect more successful functional recovery, it will be necessary to anticipate the type of ongoing injury response and consider the appropriate timing of the targeted intervention. As more information has accumulated about both the acute and the prolonged and ongoing molecular and cellular changes and adaptations that occur subsequent to spinal cord injury, increasing efforts are being considered to combine multiple interventions simultaneously and sequentially over extended periods of time. Facilitating the safe translation of treatments to human spinal cord injury will be the next step to improving outcome (166).

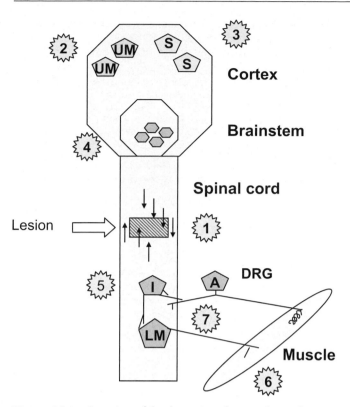

Figure 66.3 Overview of the dynamics of neuroplastic changes and potential points for intervention after spinal cord injury. The majority of SCI lesions are incomplete (1). A portion of axons may survive the initial injury, and a portion of axons may have the potential to grow around or possibly through the scar at the injury site (indicated by ascending and descending arrows). Sprouting, plasticity, and possibly alterations in neurotransmitters occur at other sites along the neuraxis and may affect outcome. Supraspinal changes in connectivity in upper motor neurons in motor cortex (2), in somatosensory cortex (3), and also within the thalamus and other parts of the brainstem (4) occur following SCI. Some of these changes may play a role in phantom sensations and pain following SCI, and some may participate in the recovery process that occurs in the months and years after SCI. Altered connectivity and sprouting below the level of the injury may affect interneurons and lower motorneurons affecting motor function and spasticity (5). Changes in synaptic contacts and spouting, especially when lower motor neurons are directly injured, may also occur at neuromuscular junctions (6) and in sensory afferents (7). (Abbreviations: UM = Upper motor neuron; S = Sensory cortex neurons; I = Spinal interneuron; LM = Lower motor neuron; A = Afferent neuron.) (Adapted from Little and Stiens, 1994 [ref. 159].)

ACKNOWLEDGMENTS

This work was supported in part by funds supplied by the National Institutes of Health, NS37846 and NS047175.

References

1. Meyer PR, Cybulski GR, Rusin JJ, Haak MH. Spinal cord injury. In: Young RR, Woolseyed RM (eds.), *Diagnosis and Management of Disorder of the Spinal Cord*. Philadelphia; W.B. Saunders, 1995; 103–134.
2. Stokes BT, Jakeman LB. Experimental modeling of human spinal cord injury: a model that crosses the species barrier and mimics the spectrum of human cytopathology. *Spinal Cord* 2002; 40(3):101–109.
3. Greaves CY, Gadala MS, Oxland TR. A three-dimensional finite element model of the cervical spinal with spinal cord: an investigation of three injury mechanisms. *Annals of Biomedical Engineering* 2008; 36(3): 396–405.
4. Blight AR. Mechanical factors in experimental spinal cord injury. *J Am Paraplegia Soc* 1988; 11:26–34.
5. Kakulas BA. Pathology of spinal injuries. *Central Nervous System Trauma* 1984; 1:117–129.
6. Bunge RP, Puckett WR, Becerra JL, Marcillo A, Quencher RM. Observations of the pathology of human spinal cord injury: a review and classification of 22 new cases with details from a case of chronic cord compression with extensive focal demyelination. In: Seil FJ (ed.), *Neural Injury and Regeneration*. New York: Raven Press, 1993; 59:75–89.
7. Fleming JC, Norenberg MD, Ramsay DA, Dekaban GA, Marcillo AE, Saenz AD, Pasquale-Styles M, Dietrich WD, Weaver LC. The cellular inflammatory response in human spinal cords after injury. *Brain* 2006; 129:3249–3269.
8. Norenberg MD, Smith J, Marcillo A. The pathology of human spinal cord injury: defining the problems. *J Neurotrauma* 2004; 21(4):429–440.
9. Hayes KC, Kakulas BA. Neuropathology of human spinal cord injury sustained in sport-related activities. *J Neurotrauma* 1997; 14:235–248.
10. Kakulas BA. A review of the neuropathology of human spinal cord injury with emphasis on special features. *J Spinal Cord Med* 1999; 22:119–124.
11. Nobel L, Wrathall J. Spinal cord contusion in the rat: morphometric analyses of alteration in the spinal cord. *Exp Neurol* 1985; 88:135–149.
12. Behrmann DL, Bresnahan JC, Beattie MS, Shah BR. Spinal cord injury produced by consistent mechanical displacement of the cord in rats: behavioral and histologic analysis. *J Neurotrauma* 1992; 9:197–217.
13. Basso DM, Beattie MS, Bresnahan JC. Graded histological and locomotor outcomes after spinal cord contusion using the NYU weight-drop device versus transection. *Exp Neurol* 1996; 139:244–256.
14. Ma M, Basso DM, Walters P, Stokes BT, Jakeman LB. Behavioral and histological outcome following graded contusion injury in C57Bl/6 mice. *Exp Neurol* 2001; 169:239–254.
15. Kakulas BA. A quantitative study of tissue elements in human spinal cord injuries. *Ann Rev International Spinal Research Trust* 1996; 28:329–339.
16. Bunge RP. Clinical implications of recent advances in neurotrauma research. In: Salzman SK, Faden AI (eds.), *The Neurobiology of Central Nervous System Trauma*. New York: Oxford University Press, 1994; 329–339.
17. Bunge RP, Pucket WR, Hiester ED. Observations of the pathology of several types of human spinal cord injury, with emphasis on the astrocyte response to penetrating injuries. In: Seil FJ (ed.), *Neuronal Regeneration, Reorganization and Repair*. Philadelphia: Lippincott-Raven Publishers, 1997; 305–315.
18. Kakulas BA. The clinical neuropathology of spinal cord injury: a guide to the future. *Paraplegia* 1987; 25:212–216.
19. Chang HT. Subacute human spinal cord contusion: few lymphocytes and many macrophages. *Spinal Cord* 2007; 45(2):174–182.
20. Falci S, Holtz A, Akesson E, Azizi M, Ertzagaard P, Hultling C, Kjaeldgaard A, Levi R, Ringden O, Westgren M, Lammertse D, Seiger A. Obliteration of a posttraumatic spinal cord cyst with solid human embryonic spinal cord grafts: first clinical attempt. *J Neurotrauma* 1997; 14:875–884.
21. Thompson FJ, Reier PJ, Uthman B, Mott S, Fessler RG, Behrman A, Trimble M, Anderson DK, Wirth ED. Neurophysiological assessment of the feasibility and safety of neural tissue transplantation in patients with syringomyelia. *J Neurotrauma* 2001; 18:931–945.
22. Wirth ED, Reier PJ, Fessler RG, Thompson FJ, Uthman B, Behrman A, Beard J, Vierck CJ, Anderson DK. Feasibility and safety of neural tissue transplantation in patients with syringomyelia. *J Neurotrauma* 2001; 18:911–929.
23. Guest JD, Hiester ED, Bunge RP. Demyelination and Schwann cell responses adjacent to injury epicenter cavities following chronic human spinal cord injury. *Experimental Neurology* 2005; 192:384–393.
24. Bruce JH, Norenberg MD, Kraydieh, Puckett W, Marcillo A, Deitrich D. Schwannosis: role of gliosis and proteoglycan in human spinal cord injury. *J Neurotrauma* 2000; 17:781–788.
25. Ackery AD, Norenberg MD, Krassioukov A. Calcitonin gene-related peptide immunoreactivity in chronic human spinal cord injury. *Spinal Cord* 2007; 45:678–686.
26. Dimitrijevic MR. Residual motor functions in spinal cord injury. *Adv Neurol* 1988; 47:138–155.

27. Metz GAS, Durt A, Van De Meent H, Klusman I, Schwab ME, Dietz V. Validation of the weight-drop contusion model in rats: a comparative study of human spinal cord injury. *J Neurotrauma* 2000; 17:1–17.

28. Bracken MB, Shepard MJ, Collins WF, et al. A randomized controlled trial of methylprednisolone or naloxone in the treatment of acute spinal-cord injury: results of the second National Acute Spinal Cord Injury Study. *N Engl J Med* 1990; 322:1405–1411.

29. Geisler FH, Dorsey FC, Coleman WP. Recovery of motor function after spinal cord injury: a randomized, placebo-controlled trial with GM-1 ganglioside. *N Engl J Med* 1991; 324:1829–1838.

30. Braken MB, Shepard MJ, Holford TR, et al. Administration of methylprednisolone for 24 or 48 hours or tirilazad mesylate for 48 hours in the treatment of acute spinal cord injury: results of the third national acute spinal cord injury randomized controlled trial. *JAMA* 1997; 277:1597–1604.

31. McTigue DM, Popovich PG, Jakeman LB, Stokes BT. Strategies for spinal cord repair. In: Seil FJ (ed.), *Progress in Brain Research*. New York: Elsevier, 2000; 128:3–8.

32. Popovich PG. Inflammation and repair of the injured spinal cord: lessons from peripheral wound healing and evolution. In: Bondy SC, Campbell A (eds.), *Inflammatory Events in Neurodegeneration*. New York, Prominent Press, 2001; 276–290.

33. Popovich PG. Immunological regulation of neuronal degeneration and regeneration in the injured spinal cord. In: Seil FJ (ed.), *Progress in Brain Research*. New York: Elsevier, 2000; 128:43–58.

34. Jakeman LB, Stokes BT. Considering the use of transgenic mice in spinal cord injury research. In: Marwah J, Dixo E, Banik N (eds.), *Traumatic CNS Injury*. Scottsdale: Prominent Press, 2001; 180–202.

35. Young W. Secondary injury mechanisms in acute spinal cord injury. *J Emerg Med* 1993; 11(S1):13–22.

36. Blight AR. An overview of spinal cord injury models. In: Narayan RK, Wilberger JE, Povlishock JT (eds.), *Neurotrauma*. New York: McGraw-Hill, 1996; 1367–1379.

37. Schwab ME, Barholdi D. Degeneration and regeneration of axons in the lesioned spinal cord. *Physiol Rev* 1996; 76:319–370.

38. Blight AR, DeCrescito V. Morphometric analysis of experimental spinal cord injury in the cat: The relation of injury intensity to survival of myelinated axons. *Neuroscience* 1986; 19:321–341.

39. Jakeman LB, Guan Z, Wei P, Ponnappan R, Dzwonczyk R, Popovich PG, Stokes BT. Traumatic spinal cord injury produced by controlled contusion in mouse. *J Neurotrauma* 2000; 17:299–319.

40. Scheff, SW, Rabchevsky AG, Fugaccia I, Main JA, Lumpp JE Jr. Experimental modeling of spinal cord injury: characterization of a force-defined injury device. *J Neurotrauma* 2003; 20:179–193.

41. Kuhn Pl, Wrathall JR. A mouse model of graded contusive spinal cord injury. *J Neurotrauma* 1998; 15(2):125–140.

42. Dusart I, Schwab ME. Secondary cell death and the inflammatory reaction after dorsal hemisection of the rat spinal cord. *Eur J Neurosci* 1994; 6:712–724.

43. Popovich PG, Wei P, Stokes BT. The cellular inflammatory response after spinal cord injury in Sprague–Dawley and Lewis rats. *J Comp Neurol* 1997; 377:443–464.

44. Carlson SL, Parrish ME, Springer JE, Doty K, Dossett L. Acute inflammatory response in spinal cord following impact injury. *Exp Neurology* 1998; 151:77–88.

45. Kigerl KA, McGaughy VM, Popovich PG. Comparative analysis of lesion development and intraspinal inflammation in four strains of mice following spinal cord injury. *J Comp Neurol* 2006; 494:578–594.

46. Donnelly DJ, Popovich PG. Inflammation and its role in neuroprotection, axonal regeneration and functional recovery after spinal cord injury. *Exp Neurol* 2008; 378–388.

47. Ma M, Wei P, Ransohoff RM, Jakeman LB. Enhanced axonal growth into a spinal cord contusion injury site in a strain of mouse (129Xl/SvJ) with a diminished inflammatory response. *J Comp Neurol* 2004; 469–486.

48. Popovich PG, Hickey WF. Bone marrow chimeric rats reveal the unique distribution of resident and recruited macrophages in the contused rat spinal cord. *J Neuropath Exp Neurol* 2001; 60:676–685.

49. Guth L, Zhang Z, Steward O. The unique histopathological responses of the injured spinal cord: implications for neuroprotective therapy. *Ann N Y Acad Sci* 1999; 890:366–384.

50. Benveniste EN. Inflammatory cytokines within the central nervous system: sources, function and mechanism of action. *Am J Physiol* 1992; 263:C1–C16.

51. Semple-Rowland SL, Mahatme A, Popovich PG, Green DA, Hassler G, Stokes BT, Streit WJ. Analysis of TGF-b1 gene expression in contused rat spinal cord using quantitative RT-PCR. *J Neurotrauma* 1995; 12:1003–1014.

52. McTigue DM, Tani M, Kricac K, Chernosky A, Kelner GS, Maciejewski D, Maki R, Ransohoff RM, Stokes BT. Selective chemokine mRNA accumulation in the rat spinal cord after contusion injury. *J Neurosci Res* 1998; 53:368–376.

53. Streit WJ, Semple-Rowland SL, Hurley SD, Miller RC, Popovich PG, Stokes BT. Cytokine mRNA profiles in contused spinal cord and axotomized facial nucleus suggest a beneficial role for inflammation and gliosis. *Exp Neurol* 1998; 152:74–87.

54. Pineau I, Lacroix S. Proinflammatory cytokine synthesis in the injured mouse spinal cord: multiphasic expression pattern and identification of the cell types involved. *J Comp Neurol* 2007; 500:267–285.

55. Rice T, Larsen J, Rivest S, Yong VW. Characterization of the early neuroinflammation after spinal cord injury in mice. *J Neuropath Exp Neurol* 2007; 66:184–195.

56. Cheng B, Christakos S, Mattson MP. Tumor necrosis factor protects against metabolic–excitotoxic insults and promote maintenance of calcium homeostasis. *Neuron* 1994; 12:139–152.

57. Barger SW, Horster D, Furukawa K, Goodman Y, Kreiglstein J, Mattson MP. Tumor necrosis factor a and b protect neurons against amyloid-b peptide toxicity: evidence for involvement of a MB-binding factor and attenuation of peroxide and Ca2+ accumulation. *Proc Natl Acad Sci USA* 1995; 92:9328–9332.

58. Toulamond S, Parnet P, Linthorst ACE. When cytokines get on your nerves: cytokine networks and CNS pathologies. *Trends Neurosci* 1996; 19:409–410.

59. Bethea JR, Nagashima H, Acosta MC, Briceno C, Gomez F, Marcillo AE, Loor K, Green J, Dietrich WD. Systemically administered interleukin-10 reduces tumor necrosis factor-alpha production and significantly improves functional recovery following traumatic spinal cord injury in rats. *J Neurotrauma* 1999; 16:851–863.

60. Taoka Y, Okajima K, Uchiba M, Harada N, Johno M, Naruuo M. Activated Protein C reduces the severity of compression injury in rats by inhibiting activation of leukocytes. *J Neurosci* 1998; 18:1393–1398.

61. Bethea JR. Spinal cord injury–induced inflammation: a dual-edged sword. In: Seil FJ (ed.), *Progress in Brain Research*. New York: Elsevier, 2000; 128:33–42.

62. Klusman I, Schwab ME. Effects of pro-inflammatory cytokines in experimental spinal cord injury. *Brain Res* 1997; 762:173–184.

63. Perry VH, Anderson PB, Gordon S. Macrophages and inflammation in the central nervous system. *Trends Neurosci* 1993; 16:268–273.

64. Streit WJ, Graeber MB, Kreutzberg GW. Functional plasticity of microglia: a review. *Glia* 1988; 5:501–507.

65. Popovich PG, Guan Z, Wei P, Huitinga I, van Rooijen N, Stokes BT. Depletion of hematogenous macrophages promotes partial hindlimb recovery and neuroanatomical repair after experimental spinal cord injury. *Exp Neurol* 1999; 158:351–365.

66. Weaver LC, Gris D, Saville LR, Oatway MA, Chen Y, Marsh DR, Hamilton EF, Dekaban GA. Methylprednisolone causes minimal improvement after spinal cord injury in rate, contrasting with benefits of anti-integrin treatment. *J Neurotrauma* 2005; 22:1375–1387.

67. Yates JR, Heyes MP, Blight AR. 4-cholor-3hydroxyanthranilate reduces local quinolinic acid synthesis, improves functional recovery and preserves white matter after spinal cord injury. *J Neurotrauma* 2006; 23:866–881.

68. Yin Y, Henzel MT, Lorber B, Nakazawa T, Thomas TT, Jiang F, Langer R, Benowitz LI. Oncomoduline is a macrophage-derived signal for axon regeneration in retinal ganglion cells. *Nat Neurosci* 2006; 9(6):843–852.

69. Rapalino O, Lazarov-Spiegler O, Agranov E, Velan GJ, Yoles E, Fraidakis M, Solomon A, Gepstein R, Katz A, Belkin A, Hadani M, Schwartz M. Implantation of stimulated homologous macrophages results in partial recovery of paraplegic rats. *Nat Med* 1998; 4:814–821.

70. Rabchevsky AG, Streit WJ. Grafting of cultured microglial cells into the lesioned spinal cord of adult rats enhances neurite outgrowth. *J Neurosci Res* 1997; 47:34–48.

71. Zeev-Brann AB, Lazarov-Spiegler O, Brenner T, Schwartz M. Differential effects of central and peripheral nerves on macrophages and microglial. *Glia* 1998; 23:181–190.

72. Knoller, N Auerbach G, Fulga V, Zelig G, Attias J, Bakimer R, Marder JB, Yoles E, Belkin M, Schwartz; Hadani M. *J Neurosurg Spine* 2005; 3:173–181.

73. Kigeri K, Popovich P. Drug Evaluation: ProCord—a potential cell-based therapy for spinal cord injury. *IDrugs* 2006; 9:354–360.

74. Cruse JM, Keith JC, Bryant ML Jr, Lewis RE Jr. Immune system-neuroendocrine dysregulation in spinal cord injury. *Immunol Res* 1996; 15:306–314.

75. Popovich PG, Stuckman S, Gienapp IE, Whitacre CC. Alterations in immune cell phenotype and function after experimental spinal cord injury. *J Neurotrauma* 2001; 18:957–966.

76. Schwartz M, Kipnis J. Protective autoimmunity: regulation and prospects for vaccination after brain and spinal cord injuries. *Trends Mol Med* 2001; 7:252–258.

77. Popovich PG, Stokes BT, Whitacre CC. Concept of autoimmunity following spinal cord injury: possible roles for T lymphocytes in the traumatized central nervous system. *J Neurosci Res* 1996; 45:349–363.

78. Popovich PG, Whitacre CC, Stokes BT. Is spinal cord injury an autoimmune disorder? *Neuroscientist* 1998; 4:71–76.

79. Jones TB, Hart RP, Popovich PG. Molecular control of physiological and pathological T-cell recruitment after mouse spinal cord injury. *J Neurosci* 2005; 25:6576–6583.

80. Moalem G, Leibowitz-Amit R, Yoles E, Mor F, Cohen IR, Schwartz M. Autoimmune T-cells protect neurons from secondary degeneration after central nervous system axotomy. *Nat Med* 1999; 5:49–55.

81. Hauben E, Yoles E, Nevo U, Moalem G, Agranov G, Neeman M, Axelrod S, Mor F, Cohen I, Schwartz M. Autoimmune T-cells are neuroprotective in spinal cord injury. *J Neurotrauma* 1999; 16:980.

82. Hauben E, Schwartz M. Therapeutic vaccination for spinal cord injury: helping the body to cure itself. *Trends Pharmacol Sci* 2003; 24:7–12.

83. Schwartz M, Yoles E. Immune-based therapy for spinal cord repair: autologous macrophages and beyond. *J Neurotrauma* 2006; 23:360–370.

84. Beattie MS, Shuman SL, Bresnahan JC. Apoptosis and spinal cord injury. *Neuroscientist* 1998; 4:163–171.

85. Springer JE, Azbill RD, Knapp PE. Activation of the capsase-3 apoptotic cascade in traumatic spinal cord injury in rats. *Nat Med* 1999; 5:943–946.

86. Beattie MS, Farooqui AA, Bresnahan JC. Review of current evidence for apoptosis after spinal cord injury. *J Neurotrauma* 2000; 17:915–925.

87. Kim GM, Xu J, Xu J, Song SK, Yan P, Xu XM, Hsu CY. Tumor necrosis factor receptor deletion reduces nuclear factor-kappaB activation, cellular inhibitor of apoptosis protein 2 expression, and functional recovery after traumatic spinal cord injury. *J Neurosci* 2001; 21:6617–6625.

88. Crowe MJ, Bresnahan JC, Shuman SL, Masters JN, Beattie MS. Apoptosis and delayed degeneration after spinal cord injury in rats and monkeys. *Nat Med* 1997; 3:73–76.

89. Shuman SL, Bresnahan JC, Beattie MS. Apoptosis of microglia and oligodendrocytes after spinal cord contusion in rats. *J Neurosci Res* 1997; 50:798–808.

90. McTigue DM, Horner PJ, Stokes BT, Gage FH. Neurotrophin-3 and brain-derived neurotrophic factor induce oligodendrocyte proliferation and myelination of regenerating axon in the contused adult rat spinal cord. *J Neurosci* 1998; 18:5354–5365.

91. McTigue DM, Wei P, Stokes BT. Proliferation of NG2-positive cells and altered oligodendrocyte numbers in the contused rat spinal cord. *J Neurosci* 2001; 21:3392–3400.

92. Tripahi R, McTigue DM. Prominent oligodendrocyte genesis along the border of spinal contusion lesions. *Glia* 2007; 55:698–711.

93. Lytle JM, Vicini S, Wrathall JR. Phenotypic changes in NG2+ cells after spinal cord injury. *J Neurotrauma* 2006; 1726–1738.

94. Gledhill RF, Harrison BM, McDonald WI. Demyelination and remyelination after acute spinal cord compression. *Exp Neurol* 1973; 38:472–487.

95. Smith PM, Jeffery ND. Histological and ultrastructural analysis of white matter damage after naturally-occurring spinal cord injury. *Brain Pathol* 2006; 16:99–109.

96. Hagg T, Oudega M. Degenerative and spontaneous regenerative processes after spinal cord injury. *J Neurotrauma* 2006; 23:264–280.

97. Ludwin SK. Remyelination in the central nervous system and the peripheral nervous system. In: Waxman SG (ed.), *Advances in Neurology*, Vol. 47: *Functional Recovery in Neurological Disease*. New York: Raven Press, 1988; 251–254.

98. Blight AR, Young W. Central axons in injured cat spinal cord recover electrophysiological function following remyelination by Schwann cells. *J Neurol Sci* 1989; 91:15–34.

99. Honmou O, Felts PA, Waxman SG, Kocsis JD. Restoration of normal conduction properties in demyelinated spinal cord axons in the adult rat by transplantation of exogenous Schwann Cells. *J Neurosci* 1996; 16:3199–3208.

100. Keirstead HS, Levine JM, Blakemore WF. Response of the oligodendrocyte progenitor cell population (defined by NG2 labeling) to demyelination of the adult spinal cord. *Glia* 1998; 22:161–170.

101. Schonberg Dl, Popovich PG, McTigue DM. Oligodendrocyte generation is differentially influenced by Toll-like receptor (TLR)2 and TLR4-mediated intraspinal macrophage activation. *J Neuropathol Exp Neurol* 2007; 66:1124.

102. Gledhill RF, McDonald WI. Morphological characteristics of central demyelination and remyelination: a single fiber study. *Ann Neurol* 1977; 1:552–560.

103. Harrison BM, McDonald WI. Remyelination after transient experimental compression of the spinal cord. *Ann Neurol* 1977; 1:542–551.

104. Fitch MT, Silver J. Activated macrophages and the blood–brain barrier: inflammation after CNS injury leads to increases in putative inhibitory molecules. *Exp Neurol* 1997; 148:587–603.

105. Fitch MT, Silver J. CNS injury, glial scars and inflammation: inhibitory extracellular matrices and regenerative failure. *Exp Neurol* 2008; 209:294–301.

106. Pizzi MA, Crowe MJ. Matrix metalloproteinases and proteoglycans in axonal regeneration. *Exp Neurol* 2007; 204:496–511.

107. Spilker MH, Yannas IV, Kostyk SK, Norregaard TV, Hsu H-P, Spector M. The effects of tubulation on healing and scar formation after transection of the adult rat spinal cord. *Restorative Neurology Neurosci* 2001; 18:23–38.

108. Iannotti C, Zhang YP, Shields LB, Han Y, Burke DA, Xu XM, Shields CB. Dural repair reduces connective tissue scar invasion and cystic cavity formation after acute spinal cord laceration injury in adult rats. *J Neurotrauma* 2006; 23:853–865.

109. Nobel LJ, Wrathall JR. Spinal cord contusion in the rat: morphometric analyses of alterations in the spinal cord. *Exp Neurol* 1985; 88:135–149.

110. Bresnahan JC, Beattie MS, Stokes BT, Conway KM. Three dimensional computer analysis studies of graded contusion lesions in spinal cord or the rat. *J Neurotrauma* 1991; 8:91–101.

111. Jakeman LB, Guan Z, Wei P, Ponnappan R, Dzwonczyk R, Popovich PG, Stokes BT. Traumatic spinal cord injury produced by controlled contusion in mouse. *J Neurotrauma* 2000; 17:303–323.

112. Davies SJ, Field PM, Raisman G. Regeneration of cut adult axons fails even in the presence of continuous aligned glial pathways. *Exp Neurol* 1996; 142:203–216.

113. Bush SA, Silver J. The role of the extracellular matrix in CNS regeneration. *Curr Opin Neurobiol* 2007; 17:120–127.

114. Brodkey JA, Laywell ED, O'Brien TF, Faissner A, Stefansson K, Dorries HU, Schachner M, Steindler DA. Focal brain injury and up-regulation of a developmentally regulated extracellular matrix protein. *J Neurosurg* 1995; 82:106–112.

115. McKeon RJ, Höke A, Silver J. Injury induced proteoglycans inhibit the potential for laminin-mediated axon growth on astrocytic scars. *Exp Neurol* 1995; 136:32–43.

116. Lein PJ, Banker GA, Higgins D. Laminin selectively enhances axonal growth and accelerates the development of polarity by hippocampal neurons in culture. *Dev Brain Res* 1992; 69:191–197.

117. Zuo J, Neubauer D, Dyess K, Ferguson TA, Muir D. Degradation of chondroitin sulfate proteoglycan enhances the neurite-promoting potential of spinal cord tissue. *Exp Neurol* 1998; 154:654–662.

118. Meiners S, Mercado ML, Geller HM. The multi-domain structure of extracellular matrix molecules: implications for nervous system regeneration. In: Seil FJ (ed.), *Progress in Brain Research*. New York: Elsevier, 2000; 128:23–31.

119. Meiners S, Mercado ML, Kamal MS, Geller HM. Tenacin-C contains domains that independently regulate neurite outgrowth and neurite guidance. *J Neurosci* 1999; 19:8443–8453.

120. Chen ZL, Strickland S. Neuronal death in the hippocampus is promoted by plasmin-catalyzed degradation of laminin. *Cell* 1997; 91:917–925.

121. Lemons ML, Howland DR, Anderson DK. Chondroitin sulfate proteoglycan immunoreactivity increases following spinal cord injury and transplantation. *Exp Neurol* 1999; 160:51–65.

122. Yick LW, Wu W, So KF, Yip HK, Shum DK. Chondroitinase ABC promotes axonal regeneration of Clarke's neurons after spinal cord injury. *Neuroreport* 2000; 11:1063–1067.

123. Plant GW, Bates ML, Bunge MB. Inhibitory proteoglycan immunore-activity is higher at the caudal than the rostral Schwann cell graft-transected spinal cord interface. *Mole Cell Neurosci* 2001; 17:471–487.

124. Jakeman LB, Chen Y, Lucin KN, McTigue DM. Mice lacking L1 cell adhesion molecule have deficits in locomotion and exhibit enhanced corticospinal tract sprouting following mild contusion injury to the spinal cord. *Eur J Neurosci* 2006; 23: 1997–2011.

125. Klapka N, Hermanns S, Straten G, Masanneck C, Duis S, Hamers FP, Muller D, Zuschratter W, Muller HW. Suppression of fibrous scarring in spinal cord injury of rat promotes long-distance regeneration of cor-ticospinal tract axons, rescue of primary motor neurons in somatosen-sory cortex and significant functional recovery. *Eur J Neurosci* 2005; 22:3047–3058.

126. Bradbury EJ, Moon LD, Popat RJ, King VR, Bennet GS. Patel PN, Fawcett JW, McMahon SB. Chondroitinase ABC promotes functional recovery after spinal cord injury. *Nature* 2002; 416(6881): 636–640.

127. Cafferty WB, Yang SH, Duffy PJ, Li S, Strittmatter SM. Functional axonal regeneration through astrocytic scar genetically modified to digest chondroitin sulfate proteoglycans. *J Neurosci* 2007; 27:2176–2185.

128. Barritt AW, Davies M, Marchand F, Hartley R, Grist J, Yip P, McMahon SB, Bradbury EJ. Chondroitinase ABC promotes sprouting of intact and injured spinal systems after spinal cord injury. *J Neurosci* 2006 26:10856–10867.

129. Massey JM, Amps J, Viapiano MS, Mathews RT, Wagoner MR, Whitaker CM, Alilain W, Yonkof AL, Khalyfa A, Cooper NG, Silver J, Onifer SM. Increased chondroitin sulfate proteoglycan expression in denervated brainstem targets following spinal cord injury creates a barrier to axonal regeneration overcome by chondroitinase ABC and neurotrophin-3. *Exp Neurol* 2008; 209:426–445.

130. Houle JD, Tom VJ, Mayes D, Wagoner G, Phillips N, Silver J. Combin-ing an autologous peripheral nervous system "bridge" and matrix mod-ification by chondroitinase allows robust, functional regeneration beyond a hemisection lesion of the adult rat spinal cord. *J Neurosci* 2006; 26: 7405–7415.

131. Liu BP, Cafferty WBJ, Budel SO, Strittmatter SM. Extracellular regula-tors of axonal growth in the adult central nervous system. *Phil Trans R Soc B* 2006; 361:1593–1610.

132. Hsu J-Y C, McKeon R, Goussev S, Werb Z, Lee J-U, Trivedi A, Nobel-Haeusslein LJ. Matrix Metalloproteinase-2 facilitates wound healing events that promote functional recovery after spinal cord injury. *J Neurosci* 2006; 39:9841–9850.

133. Michel ME, Reier PJ. Axonal-ependymal associations during early regeneration of the transected spinal cord in Xenopus Laevis tadpoles. *J Neurocytol* 1979; 8:529–548.

134. Beattie MS, Lopate G, Bresnahan JC. Metamorphosis alters the response to spinal cord transection in Xenopus Laevis frogs. *J Neurobiol* 1990; 21:1108–1122.

135. Chernoff EA, Stocum DL, Nye HL, Cameron JA. Urodele spinal cord regeneration and related processes. *Devel Dynam* 2003; 226: 295–307.

136. Matthews MA, St Onge MF, Faciane CL. An electron microscopic analy-sis of abnormal ependymal cell proliferation and envelopment of sprouting axons following spinal cord transection in the rat. *Acta Neuropathol* 1979; 45:27–37.

137. Vaquero J, Ramiro M, Oya S, Cavezudo JM. Ependymal reaction after experimental spinal cord injury. *Acta Neurochir* 1981; 55:295–302.

138. Beattie, MS, Bresnahan JC, Koman J, Tovar CA, Van Meter M, Anderson DK, Faden AI, Hsu CY, Noble LJ, Salzman S, Young W. Endogenous repair after spinal cord contusion injuries in the rat. *Exp Neurol* 1997; 148:453–463.

138. Shihabuddin LS, Palmer TD, Gage FH. The search for neural progeni-tor cells: prospects for the therapy of neurodegenerative disease. *Mol Med Today* 1999; 5:474–480.

140. Horner PJ, Power AE, Kempermann G, Kuhn HG, Palmer TD, Winkler J, Thal LJ, Gage FH. Proliferation and differentiation of progenitor cells throughout the intact adult rat spinal cord. *J Neurosci* 2000; 20: 2218–2228.

141. Shihabuddin LS, Ray J, Gage FH. FGF-2 is sufficient to isolate progen-itors found in the adult mammalian spinal cord. *Exp Neurol* 1997; 148: 577–586.

142. Mothe AJ, Tator CH. Proliferation, migration, and differentiation of endogenous ependymal region stem/progenitor cells following

minimal spinal cord injury in the adult rat. *Neuroscience* 2005; 131: 177–187.

143. Little JW, Burns SP, James J, Steins. Neurological recovery and neuro-logical decline after spinal cord injury. *Phys Med Rehabil Clin N Am* 2000; 11:73–89.

144. Josephson A, Greitz D, Klason T, Olson L, Spenger C. A spinal thecal sac constriction model supports the theory that induced pressure gradients in the cord cause edema and cyst formation. *Neurosurgery* 2001; 48:636–645.

145. Perrouin-Verbe B, Lenne-Aurie K, Robert R, Auffray-Calvier E, Richard I, Mauduyt del la Greve I, Mathe JF. Post-traumatic syringomyelia and post-traumatic spinal canal stenosis: A direct relationship: review of 75 patients with a spinal cord injury. *Spinal Cord* 1998; 36:137–143.

146. Waxman SG, Demyelination in spinal cord injury. *J Neurol Sci* 1989; 91:1–14.

147. Jain N, Catania KC, Kass JH. Deactivation and reactivation of somatosensory cortex after dorsal spinal cord injury. *Nature* 1997; 386:495–498.

148. Kass JH. The reorganization of somatosensory and motor cortex after peripheral nerve or spinal cord injury in primates. In: Seil FJ (ed.), *Progress in Brain Research.* New York: Elsevier, 2000; 128:173–182.

149. Hubscher CH, Johnson RD. Chronic spinal cord injury induced changes in the response of thalamic neurons. *Exp Neurol* 2006; 197:177–188.

150. Lotze M, Laubis-Herrmann U, Topka H. Combination of TMS and fMRI reveals a specific pattern of reorganization in M1 in patients after complete spinal cord injury. *Restor Neurol Neurosci* 2006; 24:97–107.

151. Nishimura Y, Onoe H, Morichika Y, Perfiliev S, Tsukada H, Isa T. Time-dependent central compensatory mechanisms of finger dexterity after spinal cord injury. *Science* 2007; 16:1150–1157.

152. Cohen L, Topaka H, Cole R, Hallet M. Paresthesias induced by mag-netic brain stimulation in patients with thoracic spinal cord injury. *Neurology* 1991; 41:1283–1288.

153. Bruehlmeier M, Dietz V, Leenders K. How does the human brain deal with a spinal cord injury? *Eur J Neurosci* 1998; 10:3918–3922.

154. Moore CI, Stern CE, Dunbar C, Kostyk SK, Gehi A, Rosen BR, Corkin S. Referred phantom sensations and cortical reorganization after spinal cord injury in humans. *PNAS* 2000; 97(20):14703–14708.

155. Kalous A, Osborne PB, Keast JR. Acute and chronic changes in dorsal horn innervation by primary afferents and descending supraspinal pathways after spinal cord injury. *J Comp Neurol* 2007; 504:238–253.

156. Golderger ME, Murray M, Tessler A. Sprouting and regeneration in the spinal cord: their roles in recovery of function after spinal injury. In: Gorio A (ed.), *Neuroregeneration.* New York: Raven Press, 241–264.

157. Tai Q, Goshgarian HG. Ultrastructural quantitative analysis of gluta-matergic and GABAeregic synaptic terminals in the phrenic nucleus after spinal cord injury. *J Comp Neurol* 1996; 372:343–355.

158. Little JW, Stiens SA. Electrodiagnosis in spinal cord injury. *Phys Med Rehabil Clin North Am* 1994; 5:571–593.

159. Holmes GM, Rogers RC, Bresnahan JC, Beattie MS. External anal sphincter hyper-reflexia following spinal transection in the rat. *J Neu-rotrauma* 1998; 15:451–457.

160. Chen XY, Wolpaw JR, Jakeman LB, Stokes BT. Operant conditioning of H-reflex increase in spinal cord-injured rats. *J Neurotrauma* 1999; 16:175–186.

161. Dobkin BH. Spinal and supraspinal plasticity after incomplete spinal cord injury: correlations between functional magnetic resonance imaging and engaged locomotor networks. *Prog Brain Res* 2000; 128: 99–111.

162. Little JW, Harris RM, Lerner S. Immobilization impairs recovery after spinal cord injury. *Arch Phys Med Rehabil* 1991; 72: 408–412.

163. Raineteau O, Schwab ME. Plasticity of motor systems after incomplete spinal cord injury. *Nat Rev Neurosci* 2001; 2(4):263–273.

164. Wolpaw JR, Tennissen AM. Activity-dependent spinal cord plasticity in health and disease. *Ann Rev Neurosci* 2001; 24:807–843.

165. Endo T, Spenger C, Westman E, Tominaga T, Olson L. Reorganization of sensory processing below the level of spinal cord injury as revealed by fMRI. *Exp Neurol* 2008; 209:155–160.

166. Courtine Greoire, Bunge MB, Fawcett JW, Grossman RG, Kaas JH, Lemon R, Maier I, Martin J, Nudo RJ, Ramon-Cueto A, Rouiller EM, Schnell L, Wannier T, Schwab ME, Edgerton VR. Can experiments in non-human primates expedite the translation of treatment for spinal cord injury in humans? *Nature Med* 2007; 13:561–566.

67 Acute Treatment Strategies for Spinal Cord Injury: Pharmacologic Interventions, Hypothermia, and Surgical Decompression

Edward D. Hall

Although spinal cord injury (SCI) can victimize active individuals at any age, most cases of SCI occur in young adults in the second and third decades of life. Those who survive their initial injuries can now expect to live long lives because of improvements in medical and surgical care, although intensive rehabilitation and prolonged disability exacts a significant toll on the individual, the individual's family, and society. Effective ways of maintaining or recovering function could markedly improve the outlook for those with traumatic SCI by enabling higher levels of independence and productivity.

The potential for pharmacological intervention to either preserve or recover neurological function after SCI exists because most traumatic injuries do not involve actual physical transection of the cord, but rather the spinal cord is damaged as a result of a contusive, compressive, or stretch injury. Typically, residual white matter containing portions of the ascending sensory and descending motor tracts remains intact, allowing for the possibility for functional recovery. However, during the first minutes and hours after injury, a secondary degenerative process is initiated by the primary mechanical injury that is proportional to the magnitude of the initial insult. Nevertheless, the initial anatomical continuity of the injured spinal cord in the majority of cases, together with our present knowledge of many of the factors involved in the secondary injury process, has led to the notion that pharmacological treatments that interrupt the secondary cascade, if applied early, could improve spinal cord tissue survival, thus preserving the anatomic substrates necessary for functional recovery to take place.

POSTTRAUMATIC SECONDARY SPINAL CORD INJURY: MECHANISMS OF CONTINUED TISSUE DAMAGE

Several reviews of post-SCI secondary injury have been published to which the reader is referred (1–6). Figure 67.1 displays some of the key players and the complex interrelationships involved in the secondary cascade of events occurring during the first minutes, hours, and days after traumatic SCI. The most immediate event is mechanically-induced depolarization and the consequent opening of voltage dependent ion channels (i.e., Na^+, K^+, Ca^{++}). The depolarization leads to massive release of a variety of neurotransmitters, including glutamate, which can cause the opening of glutamate receptor-operated ion channels (e.g., NMDA, AMPA). The most important consequence of these rapidly evolving ionic disturbances is the accumulation of intracellular Ca^{++} (i.e., Ca^{++} overload), which initiates several damaging effects. The first of these is mitochondrial dysfunction which leads to a failure of aerobic energy metabolism, shift to glycolytic (i.e., anaerobic) metabolism and the accumulation of lactate. The second is activation of mitochondrial and cytoplasmic nitric oxide synthase (NOS) and nitric oxide production. The third is activation of phospholipase A_2, which liberates arachidonic acid (AA) that is then converted by cyclooxygenases (COX 1, 2) to a number of deleterious prostanoids. These include the potent vasoconstrictor prostaglandin $F_{2\alpha}$ ($PGF_{2\alpha}$) and the vasoconstrictor/platelet aggregation promoter thromboxane A_2 (TXA_2). In addition, activated lipoxygenases lead to an increase in tissue leukotrienes (LTs), some of which are chemoattractants for inflammatory polymorphonuclear leukocyte and macrophage influx, which can invade the injured or ischemic tissue and amplify the secondary injury process. The fourth consequence of intracellular Ca^{++} overload is the activation of the calcium-activated protease calpain, which degrades a variety of cellular substrates including cytoskeletal proteins.

One of the byproducts of mitochondrial dysfunction, COX and lipoxygenase activity, and NOS activation is the formation of reactive oxygen species (ROS), including peroxynitrite (PON; ONOO−). Peroxynitrite is a product of the reaction of superoxide radical with nitric oxide. Although PON can trigger cellular damage by a variety of mechanisms (Figure 67.2), cell membrane (plasma and organellar) lipid peroxidation (LP) has been conclusively demonstrated to be a key mechanism (3, 7, 8).

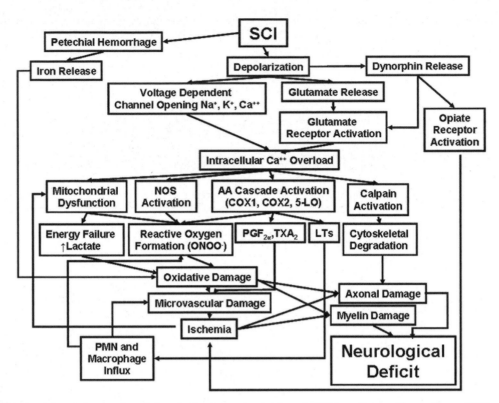

Figure 67.1 Pathophysiology of secondary injury in the injured spinal cord. NOS = nitric oxide synthase; COX = cyclooxygenase; 5-LO = 5-lipoxygenase; ONOO$^-$ = peroxynitrite anion; PGF$_{2\alpha}$ = prostaglandin F$_{2\alpha}$; TXA$_2$ = thromboxane A$_2$; LTs = leukotrienes; PMN = polymorphonuclear leukocyte. Modified with permission from Ref. 31.

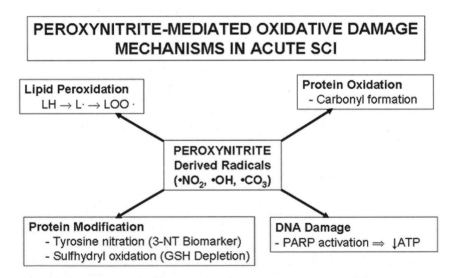

Figure 67.2 Mechanisms of peroxynitrite (PN)-mediated oxidative damage in acute SCI. The PN-derived radicals, including nitrogen dioxide radical (•NO$_2$), hydroxyl radical (•OH) and carbonate radical (•CO$_3$), can, first of all, initiate lipid peroxidation by removal of an electron from an polyunsaturated fatty acid (LH) in the phospholipid bilayer of neuronal and other cellular membranes, leading to the production of an lipid alkyl radical (L•), which can convert to a lipid peroxyl radical (LOO•) that then reacts with neighboring polyunsaturated fatty acids in a chain reaction. Ultimately, the peroxidized lipids undergo breakdown to form aldehydic products such as malondialdehyde (MDA) and 4-hydroxynonenal (4-HNE), each of which can bind to proteins and be measured by immunoblotting or immunohistochemistry. Second, the radicals can induce protein carbonylation by reaction with highly susceptible amino acids such as lysine and histidine. These can also be measured by immunoblotting/immunohistochemistry. Third, •NO$_2$ can react with the 3 position of tyrosine residues, forming 3-nitrotyrosine (3-NT), which is a fairly selective biomarker for PN-mediated oxidative damage, or it can cause oxidation of protein sulfhydryl groups (e.g., cysteine residues), an example of which is glutathione oxidation (2GSH → 2 GS• → GSSG). Fourth, PN can cause DNA oxidative damage that then leads to overactivation of a DNA repair enzyme poly-ADP ribose polymerase (PARP), which depletes ATP levels and cellular metabolic failure.

However, iron is a powerful catalyst that accelerates the propagation of LP reactions. "Initiation" of LP occurs when a radical species attacks and removes an allylic hydrogen from a polyunsaturated fatty acid (LH), resulting in a radical chain reaction (LH + R• → L• + RH). In the case of PON, the LP-initiating radicals formed include nitrogen dioxide ($\cdot NO_2$), hydroxyl radical ($\cdot OH$), and carbonate radical ($\cdot CO_3$). Upon initiation, the initiating radical is quenched by receipt of an electron (hydrogen) from the polyunsaturated fatty acid. This, however, converts the latter into a lipid or alkyl radical. This sets the stage for a series of "propagation" reactions that begin when the alkyl radical takes on a mole of oxygen creating a lipid peroxyl radical (LOO•): (L• + O_2 → LOO•). The peroxyl radical then reacts with a neighboring LH within the membrane and steals its electron, forming a lipid hydroperoxide (LOOH) and a second alkyl radical (LOO• + LH → LOOH + L•). Peroxyl radicals are normally quenched by tissue vitamin E (LOO• + Vitamin E → LOOH + Vitamin E•). However, when the rate of LP becomes too great, as has been shown to occur in the acutely injured spinal cord, the levels of the active antioxidant form of vitamin E become rapidly depleted (9). Once lipid peroxidation begins, iron may participate in driving the process as lipid hydroperoxides (LOOH) formed through initiation are decomposed by reactions with either ferrous iron (Fe^{++}) or ferric iron (Fe^{+++}). In the case of Fe^{++}, the reaction results in the formation of a lipid alkoxyl radical (LO•) (LOOH + Fe^{++} → LO• + OH^- + Fe^{+++}). If, however, the reaction involves Fe^{+++}, the lipid hydroperoxide is converted back into a lipid peroxyl radical (LOO•) (LOOH + Fe^{+++} → LOO• + Fe^{++}). Both reactions of LOOH with iron have acidic pH optima, and thus posttraumatic LP is facilitated when the pH of the injured tissue becomes acidic, as it does in the injured spinal cord due to increased glycolytically generated lactate formation (10, 11). Either alkoxyl (LO) or peroxyl (LOO) radicals arising from LOOH decomposition by iron can initiate so-called lipid hydroperoxide–dependent lipid peroxidation, resulting in "chain branching" reactions (LOO• + LH → LOOH + L• or LO• + LH → LOH + L•). Lactate accumulation also promotes LP by stimulating the release of iron from storage sites (e.g., ferritin). In addition, primary and secondary petechial hemorrhages supply hemoglobin-bound iron. Lipid peroxidation occurs in all spinal cord cell types, including neurons, oligodendroglia, astroglia, and blood vessels. The latter causes microvascular damage, microthrombosis, vasoconstriction, and secondary ischemia that indirectly contributes to the secondary neural injury (12).

In the case of SCI, the secondary events occur initially in the central gray matter and then spread to the surrounding white matter. As implied above, the key issue in predicting recovery of function is the degree of preservation of the ascending and descending white-matter tracts. Many of the axons that do survive, however, do not conduct impulses due to posttraumatic demyelination. Therefore, the goal of neuroprotective pharmacotherapy in the context of SCI is to preserve as many of the white-matter axons and as much of their investing myelin as possible. However, it should be realized that a significant factor in influencing the extent of neural injury after SCI is a decrease in spinal cord microvascular perfusion (i.e., secondary ischemia). When this occurs, the result is an exacerbation of the injury process due to superimposed tissue ischemic hypoxia. Moreover, deficiencies in CNS hypoperfusion can be aggravated by systemic hypotension or hypoxia. Thus, it is important to note that secondary injury involves both neuronal and microvascular events.

GLUCOCORTICOID STEROIDS: EMPIRICAL USE IN NEUROSURGERY AND INITIAL EVALUATION OF METHYLPREDNISOLONE THERAPY FOR SCI

The glucocorticoid steroids, mainly dexamethasone and methylprednisolone (MP), were extensively employed in the clinical treatment of spinal cord trauma beginning in the mid-1960s and continuing throughout the 1970s. The mechanistic rationale for their use initially centered on the expectation that they would reduce posttraumatic spinal cord edema. This notion was based upon the rather remarkable reduction of peritumoral brain edema that glucocorticoids can induce in brain tumor patients (13). Furthermore, steroid pretreatment became a standard of care prior to neurosurgical procedures to prevent intra- and postoperative brain swelling. A limited amount of experimental evidence supported the possibility that glucocorticoid dosing in animal SCI models might be neuroprotective (13).

In the mid-1970s, a randomized, multicenter clinical trial was organized to determine whether steroid dosing was beneficial in improving neurological recovery in humans after SCI. This trial was named the National Acute Spinal Cord Injury Study (NASCIS I). It compared the efficacy of "low-dose" MP (100 mg intravenous bolus/day for 10 days) and "high-dose" MP (1,000 mg intravenous bolus/day for 10 days) in affecting outcome after spinal cord injury (14, 15). The trial, which began in 1979, did not involve a placebo group due to the prevailing belief that glucocorticoid dosing probably was beneficial and could not ethically be withheld. However, the results failed to show any difference between the low- and high-dose groups at either 6 months (14) or 1 year (15), suggesting to the investigators that steroid dosing was of little benefit. Additionally, there was a suggestion that the 10-day high-dose regimen increased the risk of infections, a predictable side effect of sustained glucocorticoid dosing. Based upon the negative results of NASCIS I, as well as waning neurosurgical enthusiasm for steroid treatment of CNS injury in general, the majority of neurosurgeons concluded after NASCIS that the conventional use of steroids in the acute management of spinal trauma was not beneficial, and indeed was fraught with the potential for serious side effects.

HIGH DOSE METHYLPREDNISOLONE THERAPY: FOCUS ON INHIBITION OF POSTTRAUMATIC LIPID PEROXIDATION

Increasing knowledge of the posttraumatic LP mechanism in the 1970s and early 1980s prompted the search for a neuroprotective pharmacologic strategy aimed at antagonizing oxygen radical-induced LP in a safe and effective manner. Attention was focused on the hypothetical possibility that glucocorticoid steroids might be effective inhibitors of posttraumatic LP, a supposition based upon their high lipid solubility and their known ability to intercalate into artificial membranes between the hydrophobic polyunsaturated fatty acids of the membrane phospholipids, and thereby to limit the propagation of LP chain reactions throughout the phospholipid bilayer (16–19).

The author's laboratory became interested in the LP hypothesis of secondary SCI during parallel investigations of the effects of high-dose MP (15–90 mg/kg i.v.) on spinal cord electrophysiology (as those might serve to improve impulse conduction and recovery of function in the injured spinal cord) (20). Consequently, it was decided to test the possibility that a similar high dose of MP, which enhanced spinal neuronal excitability and impulse transmission, might also be required to inhibit posttraumatic spinal cord LP. In an initial set of experiments in cats, it was observed that the administration of an IV bolus of MP could indeed inhibit posttraumatic LP in spinal cord tissue (18), but that the doses required for this effect were much higher (30 mg/kg) than previously hypothesized, than empirically employed in the clinical treatment of acute CNS injury, and than tested in the NASCIS trial. Further experimental studies, also conducted in cat SCI models, showed that the 30 mg/kg dose of MP not only prevented LP, but in parallel inhibited posttraumatic spinal cord ischemia (21, 22), supported aerobic energy metabolism (i.e., reduced lactate and improved ATP and energy charge) (11, 23, 24), improved recovery of extracellular calcium (i.e., reduced intracellular overload) (22), and attenuated calpain-mediated neurofilament loss (24). However, the central effect in this protective scenario is the inhibition of posttraumatic LP. With many of these therapeutic parameters (LP, secondary ischemia, aerobic energy metabolism), the dose–response for MP follows a sharp U-shaped pattern. The neuro- and vasoprotective effect is partial with a dose of 15 mg/kg, is optimal at 30 mg/kg, and diminishes at higher doses (60 mg/kg) (17). In vitro studies using neuronal membranes have shown MP to be more effective than DEX for inhibiting in neuronal membranes (25).

The antioxidant neuroprotective action of MP is closely linked to the drug's tissue pharmacokinetics (11, 17, 26, 27). For instance, when MP tissue levels are at their peak subsequent to administration of a 30 mg/kg IV dose, lactate levels in the injured cord are suppressed. When tissue MP levels decline, spinal tissue lactate rises. However, the administration of a second dose (15 mg/kg IV) at the point at which the levels after the first dose have declined by 50% acts to maintain the suppression of lactate seen at the peak of the first dose, and to more effectively maintain ATP generation and energy charge and protect spinal cord neurofilaments from degradation (11, 24). This prompted the hypothesis that prolonged MP therapy might better suppress the secondary injury process and lead to better outcomes than a single large IV dose. Indeed, subsequent experiments in a cat spinal injury model demonstrated that animals treated with MP using a 48-hour antioxidant dosing regimen had improved recovery of motor function over a 4-week period (28, 29). Table 67.1 summarizes the neuroprotective pharmacology of high doses MP derived from acute SCI models.

Although it is believed that much of the vaso- and neuroprotective effect of MP is indeed due to inhibition of LP, this glucocorticoid has recently been shown to decrease oligodendroglial apoptosis in the injured rat spinal cord via a mechanism related to glucocorticoid receptor activation since a glucocorticoid receptor antagonist blocks the oligodendroglial protection (30). It has also been proposed that some of MP's protective effects may be due to its well-known anti-inflammatory effects, although these are believed to be less important since those actions are seen at much lower doses than those required to protect the injured spinal cord via LP inhibitory effects (31).

Table 67.1 Pharmacologic Characteristics of High-Dose Methylprednisolone (MP) Therapy for Acute SCI (Reproduced with permission from Ref. 31)

- Inhibition of posttraumatic lipid peroxidation appears to be the principal neuroprotective mechanism, and this is unrelated to glucocorticoid receptor-mediated actions.
- Microvascular and neuroprotective effects are both involved.
- Large intravenous doses are required (30 mg/kg).
- Antioxidant protective effects of MP follow a biphasic (U-shaped) dose-response curve: doubling the dose from 30 to 60 mg/kg results in a loss of the protective efficacy.
- Early treatment is required because lipid peroxidation develops rapidly and is irreversible.
- Time course of antioxidant protection parallels the spinal cord tissue pharmacokinetics: there is consequently a need for constant i.v. infusion to maintain effective tissue concentrations.
- Optimal treatment duration is uncertain, but must continue as long as conditions within the injured spinal cord favor lipid peroxidative reactions (i.e., at least 24–48 hr).
- Glucocorticoid receptor-mediated anti-inflammatory effects play only a minor role in comparison to lipid antioxidant effects.

NASCIS II CLINICAL TRIAL OF HIGH-DOSE METHYLPREDNISOLONE: IMPROVED FUNCTION IF STARTED BEFORE 8 HOURS POST-INJURY

The above-reviewed experimental studies with high-dose MP inspired the second National Acute Spinal Cord Injury Study (NASCIS II) (32), even though the earlier NASCIS trial, which came to be known as NASCIS I, had failed to show any efficacy of lower MP doses even when administered over a 10-day period (14, 15). The NASCIS II trial compared 24 hours of dosing with MP versus placebo for the treatment of acute SCI. A priori trial hypotheses included the prediction that SCI patients treated within the first 8 post-injury hours would respond better to pharmacotherapy than patients treated after 8 hours. Indeed, the results demonstrated the effectiveness of 24 hours of intensive MP dosing (30 mg/kg IV bolus plus a 23-hour infusion at 5.4 mg/kg per hour) when treatment was initiated within 8 hours. Significant benefit was observed in individuals with both neurologically complete (i.e., "plegic") and incomplete (i.e., "paretic") injuries. Moreover, the functional benefits were sustained at 6-week, 6-month, and 1-year follow-up (32–35). The high dose regimen actually improved function below the level of the injury and lowered the level of the functional injury (34). Subsequent to NASCIS II, two other groups of investigators in Japan (36) and France (37) reported successful replications of the therapeutic efficacy of the NASCIS II MP protocol in SCI patients.

Although predictable side effects of steroid therapy were noted in NASCIS II, including GI bleeding, wound infections, and delayed healing, these were not significantly more frequent than those recorded in placebo-treated patients (32). Another finding was the fact that delay in the initiation of MP treatment until after 8 hours had elapsed was actually associated with decreased neurological recovery (34). Thus, treatment within the 8-hour window is beneficial, whereas dosing after 8 hours have elapsed can be detrimental. Possible explanations for this effect are discussed below.

TIRILAZAD: A 21-AMINOSTEROID WITHOUT GLUCOCORTICOID EFFECTS

Methylprednisolone is a potent glucocorticoid that possesses a number of glucocorticoid receptor-mediated anti-inflammatory and cytoprotective actions. Despite the above-mentioned possible role of these effects of MP in the injured spinal cord, the principal neuroprotective mechanism appears to be the inhibition of posttraumatic LP that is not mediated via glucocorticoid receptor-mediated activity (38–40). This knowledge prompted speculation that modifying the steroid molecule to enhance the anti-LP effect while eliminating the steroid's glucocorticoid effects would result in more targeted antioxidant therapy devoid of the typical side effects of steroid therapy. This rationale led to the discovery and development of more potent steroidal LP inhibitors, the 21-aminosteroids or "lazaroids," which lack the glucocorticoid receptor-mediated side effects that limit the clinical utility of high-dose MP. One of these, tirilazad, was selected for development based upon its beneficial effects in animal SCI models (41–43). Figure 67.3 compares the structures of the glucocorticoid MP and the non-glucocorticoid 21-aminosteroid tirilazad.

NASCIS III.   The demonstrated efficacy of a 24-hour dosing regimen of MP in human SCI in NASCIS II (32), as well as the discovery of tirilazad (38–40), led to NASCIS III (44, 45). In the NASCIS III trial, three groups of patients were evaluated. The first (active control) group was treated with the 24-hour MP dosing regimen that had previously been shown to be effective in NASCIS II. The second group was also treated with MP, but the duration of MP infusion was prolonged to 48 hours. The purpose was to determine whether extension of the MP infusion from 24 to 48 hours resulted in greater improvement in neurological recovery in acute SCI patients. The third group of patients was treated with a single 30 mg/kg IV bolus of MP followed by the 48-hour administration of tirilazad. No placebo group was included, because it was deemed ethically inappropriate to withhold at least the initial large bolus of MP. Another objective of the study was to ascertain whether treatment initiation within 3 hours of injury was more effective than therapy that was delayed until 3 to 8 hours after SCI.

Upon completion of the NASCIS III trial, it was found that all three treatment arms produced comparable degrees of recovery when treatment was begun within the shorter 3-hour window. When the 24-hour dosing of MP was begun more than 3 hours after SCI, recovery was poorer than in the cohort treated within 3 hours of SCI. However, in the 3- to 8-hour post-SCI cohort, when MP dosing was extended to 48 hours, significantly better recovery was observed than with the 24-hour dosing. In the comparable tirilazad cohort (3 to 8 hours after SCI), recovery was slightly, but not significantly better than in the 24-hour MP group, and poorer than in the 48-hour MP group. These results showed that (1) initiation of high dose MP treatment within the first 3 hours is optimal, (2) the non-glucocorticoid tirilazad is as effective as 24-hour MP therapy, and (3) if treatment is initiated more than 3 hours post-SCI, extension of the MP dosing regimen is indicated, from 24 hours to 48 hours. However, in comparison with the 24-hour dosing regimen, significantly more glucocorticoid-related immunosuppression-based side effects were seen with more prolonged dosing (i.e., the incidence of severe sepsis and pneumonia significantly increased). In contrast, tirilazad showed no evidence of steroid-related side effects, suggesting that this non-glucocorticoid 21-aminosteroid would be safer for extension of dosing beyond the 48-hour limit used in NASCIS III (44, 45).

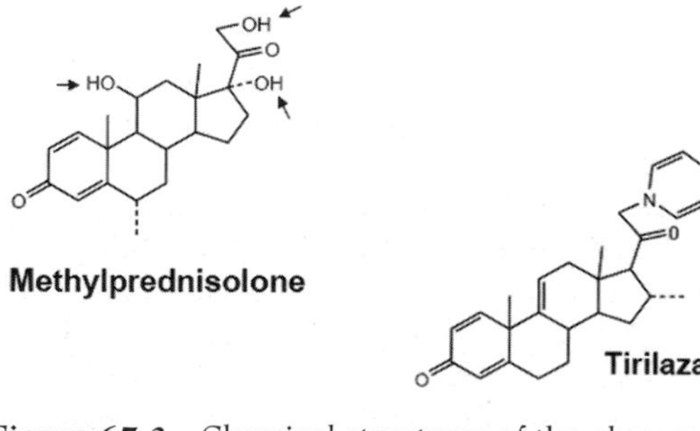

POTENTIAL ADVERSE REACTIONS AND OTHER LIMITATIONS TO THE USE OF HIGH DOSE METHYLPREDNISOLONE IN ACUTE SCI

The use of large doses of glucocorticoid steroids in SCI patients has appropriately been referred to as a "two-edged sword" (46). This is derived from the fact that the neuroprotective properties of MP can be offset by the potential of the necessary high doses of MP to elicit glucocorticoid receptor-mediated side effects that could compromise the neurological outcome and even the survival of acute SCI patients (Table 67.2). This is most apparent when treatment is extended beyond the apparently safe limit of 24 hours demonstrated in NASCIS II to 48 hours, as examined in NASCIS III—for example, in the increased risk of pneumo-

Figure 67.3 Chemical structures of the glucocorticoid steroid methylprednisolone and the non-glucocorticoid 21-aminosteroid tirilazad. Tirilazad does not have glucocorticoid activity due to the lack of the three hydroxyl moieties (arrows) in methylprednisolone and other glucocorticoid steroids that are essential for producing glucocorticoid receptor-mediated effects (e.g., immunosuppression, gluconeogenesis).

Table 67.2 Limitations and Difficulties Associated with High-Dose MP Therapy of Acute SCI (Reproduced with permission from Ref. 31)

- Risk of glucocorticoid steroid receptor–mediated side effect
  - Infection—pneumonia and septic shock
  - Diabetic complications
  - Delayed wound healing
- Sharp biphasic dose-response curve requires care in dose calculation and administration (i.e., little room for error).
- Needed duration of dosing (24 vs. 48 hours) dependent upon time to initiation of treatment.
- Initiation of treatment beyond the 8-hour window can exacerbate damage—inhibition of membrane phospholipase A_2 can impede clean-up of peroxidized lipids and perhaps aggravate peroxidative damage.
- Glucocorticoid dosing can inhibit axonal sprouting and synaptogenesis: attenuation of regenerative responses.

nia (2.6% of patients treated with the 24-hour NASCIS II protocol vs. 5.8% of patients treated with the 48-hour NASCIS III protocol, $p < 0.02$) (44). Predictable complications of high-dose MP, including increased incidence of pneumonias, pressure sores, GI bleeding, and deep vein thrombosis, have also been documented when the 24-hour NASCIS II dosing protocol is used as a prophylactic neuroprotectant for spinal surgery (47). However, there are other glucocorticoid-related actions that are not necessarily life-threatening but that could potentially complicate the steroid's proper usage in SCI patients or counteract its neuroprotective actions: (1) a sharp biphasic dose–response relationship that creates the potential for miscalculations as regards the precise dosing protocol needed for individual patients, (2) the need to administer the steroid within the first 8 hours (preferably, the first 3 hours) after injury, and definitely not after 8 hours, which can worsen secondary damage, and (3) possible negative effects of MP on axonal sprouting and synaptic plasticity, which glucocorticoids have been shown in experimental studies to be capable of producing.

Biphasic (U-Shaped) Neuroprotective Dose Response.

The sharp U-shaped dose–response curve for the neuroprotective properties of MP and the need for repeated dosing (i.e., continuous infusion) in order to maintain these effects (17) make the administration of MP in SCI patients difficult, even tricky. For instance, although optimal doses of MP can lessen posttraumatic anaerobic metabolism in the injured spinal cord and lessen lactate accumulation (11, 24, 27), inadequate or excessive MP dosing has been shown to aggravate posttraumatic lactate accumulation (11, 24, 27). This is a consequence of glucocorticoid receptor-mediated gluconeogenesis stimulatory actions of MP and similar steroids. As a result, there is an opposition between the beneficial effects of optimal MP doses to support aerobic metabolism and those given to lessen lactate accumulation, while nonoptimal doses can enhance lactate production via an increase in blood glucose levels. These can potentially drive up anaerobic glycolysis in the injured cord, thus aggravating, rather than inhibiting, LP reactions. Because of this, considerable care is required, including an actual measurement (or fairly accurate estimate) of the patient's body weight to enable accurate calculation of the optimal 30 mg/kg i.v. bolus followed by the 5.4 mg/kg/hr i.v. infusion. If the mg/kg i.v. bolus is too low or the 24- or 48-hour infusion rate is too slow, the needed levels of MP may not be achieved. On the other hand, if the bolus is too high or the infusion too fast, the levels may overshoot the optimal neuroprotective concentration and result in a loss of the antioxidant neuroprotection.

During the last 18 post-NASCIS II years of widespread use of high-dose MP (NASCIS II 24-hour or NASCIS III 48-hour protocols), there have undoubtedly been many dose miscalculations that have resulted in less than or more than optimal MP dosing in many SCI patients. As Bracken (48) notes, there are only ad hoc reports of compliance with the 24-hour NASCIS II MP dosing protocol in routine practice. However, these include reports of therapy commencing later than the recommended 8-hour cutoff, discontinuation of therapy before 24 hours have elapsed, accidental administration of the full 24-hour dose within the first hour, maintenance infusion at rates faster or slower than the recommended 5.4 mg/kg/hr, and inaccurate estimates of patient body weight. The rather narrow U-shaped dose–response curve mandates that great care be taken in calculating and administering the NASCIS II or III MP protocols. Based upon the experimentally determined U-shaped dose–response curve, the need for initiation of treatment as soon as possible, and the requirement for maintenance dosing to maintain the neuroprotective effects during the first 24–48 hours, it is likely that MP will have no benefit if the protocol is erroneously calculated for a particular patient.

Duration of Treatment Dependent on Treatment Initiation Time.

The results of the NASCIS III study show that if treatment cannot be initiated until after the first 3 posttraumatic hours, it would be better to extend the infusion phase of the treatment from 24 hours to 48 hours. On the other hand, if treatment is begun within the first 3 hours, the 24-hour NASCIS II protocol is sufficient (44, 45). Thus, attention to injury time versus treatment initiation time is an important consideration that adds a small but significant complication to the therapy.

Late Treatment Initiation May Exacerbate Damage.

Initiation of MP therapy beyond the 8-hour therapeutic window determined in NASCIS II may actually exacerbate the posttraumatic secondary injury and lessen the expected neurological outcome when compared with no therapy all (34). Therefore, the need to take into account the exact time of injury in making the decision to treat or not treat the SCI patient using high-dose MP is yet another complicating factor. Treatment later than 8 hours after injury should absolutely be avoided. The most likely reason for this is that late treatment after significant LP has already occurred may be due to glucocorticoid receptor-mediated inhibition of membrane phospholipase A_2. This enzyme serves an antioxidant function by removing peroxidized lipids from the oxidatively damaged membranes. If this is not able to take place, the oxidative damage process may be extended, worsening secondary SCI.

Possible Negative Effects on Neuronal Survival and Plasticity.

Glucocorticoids have been repeatedly shown to inhibit axonal sprouting and synaptogenesis in various CNS areas (49–52). Although it is not known whether these actions will occur concomitantly with the acute antioxidant neuroprotective effects, the potential of the steroid to attenuate posttraumatic plasticity mechanisms is perhaps the most serious concern about the administration of high doses of MP for any longer than necessary. Although the beneficial neurological effects of 24, and even 48, hours of dosing seen in NASCIS II and III, respectively, might suggest that the antiplasticity effects are not a problem with short-term high-dose MP therapy, this has not been thoroughly investigated. However, it is encouraging as regards the safety and neuroprotective value of the ongoing clinical use of high doses of MP in SCI therapy that high doses of MP have actually been reported as lessening axonal dieback of vestibulospinal fibers and promoting their terminal sprouting in transected rat spinal cords (53). The same group has shown that identical high doses of MP can improve axonal regeneration into Schwann cell grafts (54) and lessen caspase 3 activation (55) in transected rat spinal cords. In regards to the latter anti-apoptotic action, other labs have also shown that 30 mg/kg i.v. dose MP therapy can lessen apoptotic neurodegeneration after traumatic (56) or ischemic (57) SCI in rats. As noted above, the 30 mg/kg i.v. dose of MP has been shown to protect oligodendroglia via a glucocorticoid receptor-mediated action (30). These effects were achieved with acute MP administration within the first 4 hours after injury.

In any event, the potential for steroid side effects, inhibition of plasticity mechanisms, and even neurotoxic actions underscores the fact that glucocorticoids such as MP are far from an ideal approach to dealing with the posttraumatic oxidative stress and LP-related damage and the consequent need for antioxidant dosing that continues beyond the first 24 to 48 hours. The realization of these limitations was the impetus for the discovery of the non-glucocorticoid steroid tirilazad (38, 39), which aimed to provide a LP-inhibiting steroid that would be easier to use and that would be devoid of the detrimental CNS and non-CNS aspects of glucocorticoid steroids. Tirilazad's ability to improve neurological recovery in NASCIS III at least as well as MP (i.e., treatment within 3 hours of injury) while producing fewer side effects (44, 45) strongly suggests that it is worthy of additional trials in acute SCI that could ultimately show greater efficacy and safety in comparison to high-dose MP.

THE METHYLPREDNISOLONE CONTROVERSY: CRITICAL APPRAISALS OF A CLINICALLY AND FUNCTIONALLY EFFECTIVE TREATMENT

Prior to the completion of NASCIS II, there was no treatment for acute SCI that had ever been demonstrated in a placebo-controlled clinical trial to have a beneficial effect on neurological outcome. In the wake of the publication of NASCIS II (32–34, 58), high-dose MP became the standard of treatment for acute SCI and was officially registered for that indication in many countries. In the United States, because the FDA requires two randomized trials that show similar results, the SCI indication for MP was never officially sought by the drug's sponsor, and thus its widespread use in the United States for SCI is technically "off label." In 2000, three separate reviews appeared in the literature criticizing the NASCIS trials and the resulting view that high-dose MP therapy should be considered the standard of care for acute SCI (59–61). The first critical review (59) was written by a single author who was a member of the "American Association of Neurological Surgeons/Congress of Neurological Surgeons Practice Guidelines Subcommittee for the Pharmacological Treatment of SCI." However, he was the sole author, and a Disclosure was included at the end of the paper: "The views expressed in this paper do not represent the final consensus of the committee." It could be perceived that the other AANS/CNS committee members did not agree with the negative assessment of high-dose MP therapy for SCI patients.

The first criticism was that the overall analysis of the effects of either MP versus placebo was negative when all patients were included in the analysis (i.e., no split of patients treated within 8 hours vs. after 8 hours). The further claim was made that the stratified analysis on the basis of time to treatment was a post hoc decision rather than an a priori analysis plan. However, this was not the case in the design of NASCIS II. The rule for subgroup analysis is that if the subgroup is prespecified in the study protocol then that becomes the primary endpoint. Indeed, the NINDS proposal that funded NASCIS II specified that two dichotomies would be studied. The first was that the effects of early versus late treatment with MP or naloxone would be analyzed by splitting the patient population, which was randomized (treatment initiation) to one of the three treatment arms within 14 hours after SCI, at the median randomization time deter-

mined at the end of the trial (48). The precise time of the data cut was not prespecified, because going into the trial, there was no way to know what the median treatment initiation time would be. After the final patient was enrolled, it turned out that the 8 hours was the nearest whole number to the median treatment initiation time (8.5 hours), and thus 8 hours was selected for the data split (48). This approach has similarly been used and widely accepted in establishing the 3-hour cutoff for the safe and effective use of tissue plasminogen activator in acute stroke therapy (62, 63). Thus the frequently repeated claim that the NASCIS II trial did not reach its primary endpoint in regards to the efficacy of MP is not consistent with the documented trial design in which the intention to look at early versus late treatment was pre-specified. Second, it was prespecified in the design of NASCIS II that the investigators would also examine the influence of injury severity on the efficacy of MP or naloxone by comparing the neurological outcomes in sensor-motor incomplete and complete SCI patients (48).

Additional criticisms of NASCIS II put forth by Hurlbert (59) were that the MP effect sizes were small, that their functional importance was uncertain because of the reliance on neurological sensory and motor assessments rather than functional improvement scales, and that effects on long tract function were not established. Each of these has been addressed by additional analyses of the NASCIS II data set carried out by Bracken and colleagues. Concerning the size of the effect, it has indeed been acknowledged that the benefits of MP in the context of NASCIS II were "modest, but (MP) does appear to have the potential to result in important clinical recovery in some patients," and that "[e]ven small changes in motor recovery, typically assessed in the MPSS trials on one side of the body, have the potential to be amplified into meaningful improvements in the quality of life" (48). Regarding the issue of long tract versus segmental recovery effects, further analysis of the NASCIS II data revealed that the greatest degree of motor function recovery within patients receiving MP within the 8-hour window occurred in long spinal tracts as recorded below the level of the injury, although significant segmental recovery was also found at the level of the lesion (34, 48). The criticism that the clinical significance of the functional improvement was not assessed by inclusion of functional or quality of life measures such as the Functional Independence Measure (FIM) in NASCIS II is valid. However, the NASCIS II principal investigator has published an estimate of functional recovery in NASCIS II from results modeled in the NASCIS III study, which did include FIM assessments (64). In that report, it is claimed that "[t]he extent of MP therapy-related motor function recovery observed in NASCIS II predicted clinically important recovery in the FIM."

The final NASCIS II critique by Hurlbert (59) concerning the questionable safety of high dose MP therapy in SCI patients is difficult to reconcile with the NASCIS II data set, which found no significant differences in adverse reactions between placebo- and MP-treated patients (32, 33). Because NASCIS II represents the only placebo-controlled trial of a 24-hour high-dose regimen in SCI patients, it is difficult to understand the claim that this particular regimen is unsafe. In contrast, the NASCIS III trial did show that extension of the duration of dosing from 24 hours to 48 hours did result in an increased incidence of pneumonias and a nearly significant ($p < 0.07$) increase in the occurrence of severe sepsis, undoubtedly manifestations of the immunosuppressive properties of intensive glucocorticoid dosing (44). Therefore, the available data that directly addresses the safety of high-dose MP in SCI patients in a controlled context shows that the 24-hour regimen is not associated with an increase in adverse reactions, whereas the 48-hour regimen does carry some risk of serious glucocorticoid-related problems. However, this has to be balanced against the results of NASCIS III, showing that in patients not treated until after the first 3 post-SCI hours, the extension of dosing to 48 hours produces a significantly better neurological outcome than the 24-hour regimen. Considering the devastating nature of most SCIs, it seems that the risk of MP treatment would be outweighed by the potential benefits to the patient's neurological recovery, especially since no other acute pharmacological treatments are presently available.

Hurlbert (59) also criticized the NASCIS III trial on five counts, including the lack of a placebo group and the claims that the overall analysis was negative, that the stratification of patients treated within 3 hours versus between 3 and 8 hours was a post hoc analysis, that the improvement in the FIM score in 48-hour MP treated patients compared to the 24-hour MP cohort was modest, and that MP treatment is unsafe based upon the increased incidence of sepsis and pneumonias. The first of these criticisms (the lack of a placebo group) has already been addressed. The next two (regarding the statistical analysis) are identical to those leveled against NASCIS II. Here again, the NASCIS III investigators have gone on record as stating that the dichotomized analysis of the NASCIS III data on the basis of time to treatment (early versus late) was a preplanned, not a post hoc, analysis; these therefore qualify as primary endpoints (44, 48). The issue of the significance of the FIM score improvement shown in 48-hour MP patients in NASCIS III requires a careful viewing of the data. Hurlbert (59) focuses on the fact that in the intent to treat analysis, the improvement in the Total FIM score only reached a level of $p < 0.08$ (44). However, a look at the subscores reveals a significantly better self-care score in the 48-hour treated patients ($p < 0.03$) and a better sphincter control score ($p < 0.01$). If, however, the analysis is redone including only those patients in which the dosing protocols were completely followed, even the Total FIM score in the 48-hour treated patients reaches the 0.05 level, unlike the 24-hour MP cohort. As regards the safety criticism, the 48-hour MP group displayed a significant increase in pneumonias and a nearly significant increase in severe sepsis in comparison to the 24 hour group. As noted above, these are predictable risks of high-dose glucocorticoid therapy in critically ill patients. The risk–benefit ratio is a matter of personal opinion.

The other two critiques (60, 61) have multiple authors and, similar to Hurlbert (59), criticize more than only the NASCIS trial design, analysis, and reporting. As already discussed above, the PI of the NASCIS trials has addressed the various criticisms and misunderstandings put forth in these in the form of a recent meta-analysis of the NASCIS and non-NASCIS trials of MP in acute SCI, and their overall statistically significant support of the efficacy and safety of high-dose MP therapy for acute SCI (48). He concludes from the meta-analysis that "high dose MP given within 8 hours of acute spinal cord injury is a safe and modestly effective therapy that may result in important clinical recovery for some patients. Further trials are needed to identify superior pharmacological therapies and to test drugs that may sequentially influence the postinjury cascade."

This view is generally endorsed in a summary statement in the journal *Spine* given by the Spine Focus Panel (65), in which it was stated by Dr. Michael Fehlings (Toronto, Ontario) that "[m]embers of the Spine Focus Panel extensively discussed the role of methylprednisolone in acute spinal cord injury but could not reach agreement on key points. While it was acknowledged that the NASCIS trials represent landmark clinical studies, no clear consensus could be reached on the appropriate use of steroids in acute spinal cord injury. Many members of the Spine Focus Panel acknowledged that although methylprednisolone is only modestly neuroprotective, this drug is clearly indicated in acute spinal cord injury because of its favorable risk/benefit profile and the lack of alternative therapies. However, a significant minority was of the opinion that the evidence supporting the use of steroids in spinal cord injury was weak and did not justify the use of this medication. The Spine Focus Panel did agree that given the devastating impact of spinal cord injury and the modest efficacy of methylprednisolone, clinical trials of other therapeutic interventions are urgently needed." After the summary statement, Dr. Fehlings presented an *Editorial: Recommendations Regarding the Use of Methylprednisolone in Acute Spinal Cord Injury; Making Sense Out of the Controversy* (66), in which he first summarizes the criticisms of NASCIS II and III, followed by a presentation of the "Suggested Indications for the Use of Methylprednisolone in Acute SCI." These are reproduced in Table 67.3. He closes the editorial by stating, "Given the devastating impact of SCI and the evidence of a modest, beneficial effect of MP, clinicians should consciously consider using this drug despite the well-founded criticisms that have been directed against the NASCIS II and III trials. With great understanding of the biomolecular events contributing to the pathogenesis of SCI, it is hoped that other neuroprotective agents will enter into clinical practice in the next 5–10 years."

However, the recently published guidelines for *Early Acute Management in Adults with Spinal Cord Injury: A Clinical Practice Guideline for Health Care Professionals*, put out by the Consortium for Spinal Cord Medicine Clinical Practice Guidelines (67), simply indicates that "[n]o Clinical evidence exists to definitively recommend the use of any neuroprotective pharmacological agent, including steroids, in the treatment of acute spinal cord injury to improve functional recovery." Unfortunately, in the relatively brief section of the guidelines dealing specifically with MP, the guideline authors present an oversimplified assessment of the NASCIS II and III findings that simply repeats the incorrect

---

Table 67.3   Suggested Indications for the Use of Methylprednisolone in Acute SCI

1. For acute nonpenetrating SCI (<3 hours after injury), MP should be given as per NASCIS II protocol (i.e., 24 hours of treatment).
2. For acute nonpenetrating SCI (>8 hours after injury), MP should not be used.
3. For acute nonpenetrating SCI (after 3 hours, within 8 hours), MP should be given as per NASCIS III protocol (i.e., 48 hours of treatment).
4. For acute penetrating SCI, MP is not recommended.

Source: Fehlings 2001 (ref. 65).

assertions put forth in the critiques discussed above (59–61). These views unfairly discount the fact that the conclusions that high-dose MP is able to significantly improve neurological recovery when initiated within 8 hours postinjury were based upon a prospective study design, in the case of the NASCIS II trial (32, 33), and not a post hoc analysis, as claimed in the critical reviews. Moreover, the statement in the guidelines that "[b]oth the NASCIS II and III studies documented serious complications such as higher infection and sepsis rates, respiratory complications and gastrointestinal hemorrhage," is incorrect. To the contrary, NASCIS II involving 24 hours of treatment with MP did not show any significant increase in these particular side effects (33). Even with 48 hours of MP treatment studied in NASCIS III, a statistically significant ($p < 0.05$ vs. 24-hour MP) increase was only seen in the incidence of "severe pneumonias" (5.6% in the 48-hour MP cohort, compared to 2.6% in the 24-hour MP group) (44). The only other side effect parameter that trended close to significance was the incidence of "severe sepsis," which increased from 0.6% to 2.6% ($p < 0.07$). None of the other "documented serious complications associated with MP administration" claimed in the guidelines to be increased came anywhere close to statistical significance. Thus, the recently published guidelines, similar to the previously published NASCIS critiques (59, 61, 68), exaggerate the dangers of high-dose MP treatment while inaccurately downplaying the evidence of a significant neurological recovery benefit when applied with the first 8 hours after SCI. Considering the typically devastating nature of acute SCI to the patient and the patient's family, and the fact that no other neuroprotective approach is currently available, the misleading assessments of high-dose MP treatment are likely a disservice to SCI patients. However, the guidelines do correctly state that "MP therapy should not be initiated more that 8 hrs after the SCI." Early treatment within 8 hours appears to have benefit, whereas treatment after that time window has elapsed may be detrimental, as also discussed earlier in this chapter.

CURRENT AND FUTURE SPINAL CORD INJURY DRUG DEVELOPMENT: FOCUS ON VARIED THERAPEUTIC MECHANISMS AND CONSIDERATION OF COMBINATION THERAPIES

At present, high-dose MP therapy, although not officially approved in the United States for acute SCI treatment, continues to be the unofficial U.S. standard of care, as it is in most countries where MP is marketed. This appears to be the case even though some clinicians believe that the NASCIS II and III trials are unconvincing, and that the risks high-dose MP therapy outweighs the modest neurological benefits (59, 61, 69). In any event, it is likely that future trials of new drug treatments may have to be evaluated on top of high-dose MP since the majority of clinicians who treat acute SCI patients are not prepared to withhold MP from their patients. The only situation in which this may be avoidable will be one in which preclinical studies show that the neuroprotective effects of MP or a second drug are offset when the two are used simultaneously, or one in which there is a documented dangerous interaction of the two drugs. For instance, it has been reported that the coincident use of MP and the GM1 ganglioside in a preclinical SCI model resulted in an attenuation of MP's neuroprotective efficacy and an increase in post-SCI

mortality (70). This future development scenario wherein a second neuroprotective or neurorestorative drug is administered at the same time as or in series with high-dose MP, obviously raises a significant challenge as regards preclinical evaluation of the combination in order to demonstrate at least additive, if not supra-additive, benefit and safety (71).

NEUROPROTECTIVE STRATEGIES UNDER INVESTIGATION: EFFORTS TO DEVELOP CLINICALLY SIGNIFICANT TREATMENTS TO COMPLEMENT CURRENT CARE STANDARDS

NEWER ANTIOXIDANT STRATEGIES. In view of the clear role of reactive oxygen or oxygen radical–induced LP in the pathophysiology of posttraumatic spinal cord degeneration, and the demonstrated benefits of antioxidant compounds with neuroprotective activity such as MP and tirilazad, it is logical to pursue the development of improved antioxidant compounds that could more safely and effectively inhibit posttraumatic LP when compared with high-dose MP. Recent work suggests that the most critical reactive oxygen species in acute SCI may be peroxynitrite (72–74), which is formed from the combination of superoxide and nitric oxide radicals (75, 76). Peroxynitrite is capable of causing widespread damage to lipids, proteins, and nucleic acids (Figure 67.2). Figure 67.4 provides immunohistochemical evidence of intense peroxynitrite-mediated oxidative damage in the contused rat spinal cord during the first 6 postinjury hours. Prototypical scavengers of peroxynitrite, such as penicillamine or its derived oxygen radicals (such as tempol), are neuroprotective in in vivo models of acute brain injury (77–79) and SCI (80). In addition, the peroxynitrite decomposition catalyst FeTSPP has been recently reported to be neuroprotective in a mouse SCI model (81). Still another promising antioxidant-based approach concerns the design of dual inhibitors of LP and neuronal nitric oxide synthase (an enzyme that contributes to the production of peroxynitrite). Such a dual inhibitor compound, BN-80933, has been reported to attenuate posttraumatic and post-ischemic degeneration in in vivo models (82). Importantly, in comparison with a neuronal nitric oxide synthase inhibitor

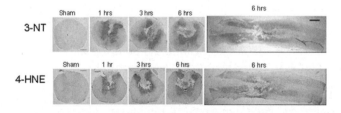

Figure 67.4 Immunohistochemistry of oxidative damage in the injured rat thoracic spinal cord following moderately severe contusion injury. Top row: transverse and sagittal sections showing intense staining for the PN biomarker 3-nitrotyrosine (3-NT). Bottom row: staining for the lipid peroxidation marker 4-hydroxynonenal (4-HNE). Very little immunostaining was seen in noninjured (Sham) animals, in contrast to the intense staining for 3-NT and 4-HNE in the gray matter and immediately surrounding white matter. The longitudinal sections show that the oxidative damage staining extends for some distance away from the injury epicenter. Scale bars = 1 mm. Photomicrographs are taken from Xiong et al., 2007 (74), with permission.

alone, BN-80933 has been shown to have superior neuroprotective efficacy.

ANTI-INFLAMMATORY STRATEGIES.   As discussed above in the context of the discussion of the possible anti-inflammatory mechanisms of action of MP, inflammatory processes play an important, although incompletely understood, role in the pathophysiology of acute SCI. Understanding this role is complicated by the observations that while some aspects of posttraumatic inflammation in the spinal cord are clearly detrimental, other delayed inflammatory aspects may facilitate repair mechanisms (83). As regards the negative aspects of inflammation in the injured cord, the best developed therapeutic approach has been aimed at the observations that COX2 activation is involved in the secondary injury process (Figure 67.1) and that inhibitors of COX2 are neuroprotective and enhance neurological recovery in animal models of SCI (84–88). Considering that multiple COX2 inhibitors (rofecoxib, celecoxib) have been approved for certain rheumatic inflammatory conditions in the United States and most countries, the potential application of one of these to acute SCI therapy should probably be pursued. However, at present parenteral formulations for IV use have not been marketed.

Another promising agent that has been shown to be neuroprotective in rodent SCI models is semisynthetic tetracycline antibiotic minocycline. It has been reported by multiple laboratories as reducing oligodendroglial cell death, astrogliosis, and microgliosis and producing an improvement in neurological recovery (89–95). It also acts to inhibit mitochondrial cytochrome C release, indicative of a mitochondrial-protective action. The precise neuroprotective mechanism has not been clearly defined. However, it appears to inhibit the release of inflammatory cytokines and free radicals and to inhibit matrix metalloproteinases (94). Furthermore, one report has indicated that it may be superior to MP in its neuroprotective activity. More study is needed to fully define the optimum dosing and therapeutic time window for this compound in SCI models, even though it shows considerable promise.

A recent experimental study has also demonstrated that the administration of the immunomodulator interferon-β immediately after contusion SCI in rats can improve neurological recovery and spinal cord tissue preservation. This effect is associated with a reduction in posttraumatic neutrophil infiltration, as measured by myeloperoxidase levels, along with a decrease in LP in the injured spinal tissue (96). If replicated and shown to have a clinically practical therapeutic window, this could be another anti-inflammatory neuroprotective approach for acute SCI.

CALPAIN INHIBITORS.   Another very strong candidate mechanism for neuroprotective intervention is the calcium-activated enzyme calpain (97, 98). Multiple laboratories and studies have demonstrated an important role of calpain activation in mediating posttraumatic axonal damage in acute SCI models (74, 99–106). Several of these studies have reported neuroprotective efficacy of prototype calpain inhibitors. However, the translation of calpain inhibition into SCI neuroprotective clinical trials has been precluded by the lack of small-molecule inhibitors with sufficient CNS penetration and appropriate pharmaceutical and pharmacokinetic properties. Hopefully, these limitations will be overcome with future inhibitors in view of the clear role of calpain in SCI pathophysiology. One of the relatively newer calpain inhibitors MDL28170 has been recently reported to modestly improve the neurological recovery of rats after contusion SCI (107).

PRESERVATION OF MITOCHONDRIAL FUNCTION.   Very recent work has demonstrated the time course of mitochondrial dysfunction in the contused rat spinal cord to be a critically important neuroprotective target (108). The peak of the mitochondrial failure was shown to be delayed until 24 hours postinjury, suggesting a possibly extended therapeutic window for approaches that might inhibit mitochondrial failure. The mitochondrial pathophysiology is accompanied by an increase in mitochondrial oxidative damage markers, suggesting that antioxidants may serve to protect mitochondria after injury. Another approach that has been shown to protect mitochondria in TBI models is the immunosuppressive drug cyclosporine A (CsA) (109, 110). This effect is the result of an inhibition of the mitochondrial permeability transition phenomenon that heralds the collapse of mitochondrial respiratory function. Specifically, CsA acts by binding to the cyclophilin D protein, which is a component of the mitochondrial permeability transition pore. However, only one study has examined CsA in a rat contusion SCI model, and it has found that a dose level that protects mitochondrial function in mouse and rat TBI models (109, 110) is not effective in achieving neuroprotective effects in a rat SCI model (111). However, a broader dose–response curve needs to be studied in the SCI model to accurately assess whether the compound will be potentially useful in SCI. In any event, the preservation of spinal cord mitochondrial function is essential to cell survival. High- dose MP therapy has been shown to improve spinal cord energy metabolism, presumably by acting to protect mitochondria (11, 23, 24). Another approach under investigation that may show promise for achieving mitochondrial protection involves the use of "mild uncoupling agents" to enhance the resistance of mitochondrial-to-posttraumatic damage (112).

OPIATE RECEPTOR ANTAGONISM AND THYROTROPIN RELEASING HORMONE (TRH) AND TRH ANALOGS.   The opiate receptor antagonist naloxone was shown many years ago to be neuroprotective in models of acute SCI (113, 114) and showed evidence of some efficacy in the NASCIS II trial (34). This has been interpreted as an indication that opiate receptor mechanisms are involved in the acute pathophysiology of SCI, although these are rather poorly understood. Another indirect opiate receptor antagonist approach that has been intensively explored by Faden and colleagues concerns the use of TRH, which can act as a physiological antagonist of opiate receptor activation by injury-induced endorphin release (115). TRH administration has been shown to improve neurological recovery in cats (116) and rats (117) and has been preliminarily tested in a phase II safety trial in a small number of SCI patients (118). Based on the knowledge that TRH may possess multiple neuroprotective actions, TRH analogs with improved pharmaceutical and brain penetration properties have been discovered and are actively being evaluated for possible entry into future SCI trials (117, 119, 120).

ANTI-APOPTOTIC THERAPEUTIC STRATEGIES—PREVENTING DELAYED CELL DEATH.   A potentially promising area of neuroprotective drug discovery for treating acute SCI is the development of agents targeting apoptotic (aka "programmed") cell death mechanisms. A number of studies have documented that apoptosis contributes to both acute and delayed cell loss subsequent to traumatic SCI. Apoptotic cell death can be detected hours to several weeks after SCI and occurs in numerous cell types, including neurons, oligodendroglia, and inflammatory cells such as neutrophils, microglia, and macrophages (121–128). Oligodendroglial apoptosis has been proposed to be the key contributor to axonal demyelination and dysfunction in areas distant from the injury epicenter. This, of course, would exacerbate long-term post-SCI neurological deficits. In spite of these observations, the role of apoptosis as a contributing factor in limiting functional recovery compared to "necrotic" cell death mechanisms has not been well established. This is largely because (1) the apoptotic cascade is extremely complex, with many potential drug targets to explore, (2) it is increasingly realized that necrosis and apoptosis are not totally distinct processes, but, rather, the two ends of a continuum, and (3) it is now recognized that similar cellular signals such as glutamate excitotoxicity, intracellular calcium overload, reactive oxygen species formation, mitochondrial dysfunction, and inflammatory mediators can elicit both types of cell death. This issue can only be addressed by elucidating the extracellular and intracellular signaling events regulating this cell death process. Therefore, the application of some of the previously discussed acute treatment strategies, including antioxidants, anti-inflammatory compounds, and mitochondrial protective agents, may attenuate apoptotic as well as necrotic cell death mechanisms in the injured spinal cord. For a more detailed discussion of the apoptotic cascade and potential treatment strategies, the reader is referred to the recent review by Hall and Springer (31).

Hypothermia—Whole-Body and Localized Spinal Cord Cooling.

One of the oldest experimental approaches aimed at achieving neuroprotection and improved neurological recovery after acute SCI involves the induction of spinal cord hypothermia in order to reduce the intensity of the secondary injury mechanisms (129). This has been attempted in various studies by either local cooling of the injured spinal cord involving superfusion of the exposed spinal cord with cold saline or artificial cerebrospinal fluid or by total-body hypothermia achieved by external cooling or intravenous infusion of cold physiological solutions. In a recent review by Inamasu et al. (130) on the topic of hypothermic treatment for acute SCI, the authors tentatively concluded that this approach may be useful for mild to moderate SCI, but will likely not be useful in the context of severe injuries unless it is combined with pharmacological neuroprotection. Nevertheless, one of the attractions to hypothermia as a neuroprotective strategy is that it has been shown to attenuate several aspects of the secondary injury cascade simultaneously. Consistent with that idea, contemporary reports have demonstrated that moderate hypothermia (e.g., 32–33°C) induced at 30 min. postinjury and maintained for 4 hours can reduce inflammatory mediators (131), decrease apoptotic cell death (132), and improve neurological recovery (133). On the other hand, localized cooling of the injured spinal cord down to as low as 24°C by perfusion of cold saline into the epidural space beginning at 30 min. postinjury and then continued for 3 hours did not improve tissue sparing or neurological recovery (134). It is clear that much more work is needed to define the best cooling approach for acute SCI as regards the optimal degree of cooling, the therapeutic window for its application, the duration for which it is maintained, and whether or not its use is additive or synergistic with pharmacological neuroprotection.

IMPORTANCE OF EARLY SPINAL CORD DECOMPRESSION AND STABILIZATION SURGERY

It should be noted that the full potential of neuroprotective therapies, whether pharmacological or the use of hypothermia, would be logically enhanced by early spinal cord decompression and stabilization surgery to lessen the primary physical damage to spinal cord, improve spinal cord blood flow at the injury site, and decrease the risk of further damage caused by an unstable spinal column. The removal of bony fragments that are often compressing the spinal cord would serve to lessen ischemic damage and would also improve the systemic delivery of systemically administered neuroprotective agent(s) to the injury site. Despite the logic of early surgery, it is probably rarely done in the first few post-SCI hours. This is troubling in view of a recent study showing that decompression of the compression-injured rat spinal cord needs to take place within the first 6–12 hours, and preferably in the first 2 hours (135). A clinical trial called Surgical Treatment of Acute Spinal Cord Injury Study (STASCIS) is currently being conducted to examine the relative benefits of early (<24 hours post-injury) versus late (>24 hours) surgical decompression in spinal cord injured patients (136).

SUMMARY

The pathophysiology of acute spinal cord injury involves a complex cascade of secondary neurodegenerative events that are set in motion by the primary injury. This cascade includes molecular events that are often referred to as necrotic and apoptotic. The increasingly successful definition of the SCI secondary injury process has led to the pursuit of a number of pharmacological neuroprotective strategies that have been shown to interrupt the secondary injury process at selected points and to improve neurological recovery in acute SCI animal models. The glucocorticoid steroid MP and the non-glucocorticoid 21-aminosteroid tirilazad have been examined in phase III clinical trials in SCI patients and show some evidence of benefit, although the effects appear, on average, to be modest. Although the use of MP and the NASCIS trial design and statistical analysis has sparked intense criticism and debate, the majority of clinicians who treat SCI believe that MP has value, and that it should be employed. In the opinion of the author, the magnitude of MP's neuroprotective effects is at least sufficient to validate the concept of acute pharmacotherapy for SCI and to inspire continued efforts to discover and develop improved therapies. The primary neuroprotective mechanism of MP, and more so tirilazad, is believed to be inhibition of posttraumatic free radical–induced lipid peroxidation. Thus, the continued search for safer and more effective antioxidant agents seems warranted. One such mechanistic approach would be to scavenge peroxynitrite, which may be the preeminent reactive oxygen species involved in secondary injury in the injured spinal cord. However, several other promising approaches could either replace or be built upon high-dose MP therapy. Leading candidates include COX 2 inhibitors, minocycline, interferon-β, calpain inhibitors, mitochondrial protectants, inhibitors of the apoptotic cascade, and multi-mechanistic TRH analogs. These could possibly be used in combination with either local or systemic hypothermia to achieve an even greater effect. However, it seems likely that the full expression of the neuroprotective potential of these approaches will be enhanced by early spinal cord decompression surgery when appropriate. Although the design of future clinical trials that look at multiple therapies will be complex, the devastating consequences of SCI to the patient, the patient's family, and society strongly support our continued efforts to develop safe and effective neuroprotective therapies that will lessen secondary injury and result in clinical significant neurological recovery.

References

1. Anderson DK, Hall ED. Pathophysiology of spinal cord trauma. *Ann Emerg Med* 1993; 22(6):987–992.
2. Hall E. Mechanisms of secondary CNS injury. In: Palmer J, ed. *Neurosurgery 96: Manual of Neurosurgery*. New York: Churchill-Livingstone; 1995:505–510.
3. Hall ED, Braughler JM. Central nervous system trauma and stroke. II. Physiological and pharmacological evidence for involvement of oxygen radicals and lipid peroxidation. *Free Radic Biol Med* 1989; 6(3):303–313.
4. Tator CH, Fehlings MG. Review of the secondary injury theory of acute spinal cord trauma with emphasis on vascular mechanisms. *J Neurosurg* 1991; 75(1):15–26.
5. Faden AI. Therapeutic approaches to spinal cord injury. *Adv Neurol* 1997; 72:377–386.
6. Faden AI, Salzman S. Pharmacological strategies in CNS trauma. *Trends Pharmacol Sci* 1992; 13(1):29–35.
7. Braughler JM, Hall ED. Central nervous system trauma and stroke. I. Biochemical considerations for oxygen radical formation and lipid peroxidation. *Free Radic Biol Med* 1989; 6(3):289–301.
8. Hall ED, Braughler JM. Free radicals in CNS injury. *Res Publ Assoc Res Nerv Ment Dis* 1993; 71:81–105.
9. Hall ED, Yonkers PA, Andrus PK, Cox JW, Anderson DK. Biochemistry and pharmacology of lipid antioxidants in acute brain and spinal cord injury. *J Neurotrauma* 1992; May (9 Suppl 2):S425–S442.
10. Anderson DK, Means ED, Waters TR, Spears CJ. Spinal cord energy metabolism following compression trauma to the feline spinal cord. *J Neurosurg* 1980; 53(3):375–380.
11. Braughler JM, Hall ED. Lactate and pyruvate metabolism in injured cat spinal cord before and after a single large intravenous dose of methylprednisolone. *J Neurosurg* 1983; 59(2):256–261.
12. Hall ED, Wolf DL. A pharmacological analysis of the pathophysiological mechanisms of posttraumatic spinal cord ischemia. *J Neurosurg* 1986; 64(6):951–961.
13. Reulen HJ, Schurmann K. *Steroids and Brain Edema*. Berlin: Springer-Verlag; 1972.
14. Bracken MB, Collins WF, Freeman DF, et al. Efficacy of methylprednisolone in acute spinal cord injury. *JAMA* 1984; 251(1):45–52.
15. Bracken MB, Shepard MJ, Hellenbrand KG, et al. Methylprednisolone and neurological function 1 year after spinal cord injury: results of the National Acute Spinal Cord Injury Study. *J Neurosurg* 1985; 63(5):704–713.
16. Demopoulos HB, Flamm ES, Pietronigro DD, Seligman ML. The free radical pathology and the microcirculation in the major central nervous system disorders. *Acta Physiol Scand Suppl* 1980; 492:91–119.
17. Hall ED. The neuroprotective pharmacology of methylprednisolone. *J Neurosurg* 1992; 76(1):13–22.
18. Hall ED, Braughler JM. Acute effects of intravenous glucocorticoid pretreatment on the in vitro peroxidation of cat spinal cord tissue. *Exp Neurol* 1981; 73(1):321–324.
19. Hall ED, Braughler JM. Glucocorticoid mechanisms in acute spinal cord injury: a review and therapeutic rationale. *Surg Neurol* 1982; 18(5):320–327.
20. Hall ED. Glucocorticoid effects on central nervous excitability and synaptic transmission. *Int Rev Neurobiol* 1982; 23:165–195.
21. Hall ED, Wolf DL, Braughler JM. Effects of a single large dose of methylprednisolone sodium succinate on experimental posttraumatic spinal cord ischemia: dose-response and time-action analysis. *J Neurosurg* 1984; 61(1):124–130.
22. Young W, Flamm ES. Effect of high-dose corticosteroid therapy on blood flow, evoked potentials, and extracellular calcium in experimental spinal injury. *J Neurosurg* 1982; 57(5):667–673.
23. Anderson DK, Means ED, Waters TR, Green ES. Microvascular perfusion and metabolism in injured spinal cord after methylprednisolone treatment. *J Neurosurg* 1982; 56(1):106–113.
24. Braughler JM, Hall ED. Effects of multi-dose methylprednisolone sodium succinate administration on injured cat spinal cord neurofilament degradation and energy metabolism. *J Neurosurg* 1984; 61(2):290–295.
25. Braughler JM. Lipid peroxidation-induced inhibition of gamma-aminobutyric acid uptake in rat brain synaptosomes: protection by glucocorticoids. *J Neurochem* 1985; 44(4):1282–1288.
26. Braughler JM, Hall ED. Correlation of methylprednisolone levels in cat spinal cord with its effects on $(Na^{+}K^{+})$-ATPase, lipid peroxidation, and alpha motor neuron function. *J Neurosurg* 1982; 56(6):838–844.
27. Braughler JM, Hall ED. Uptake and elimination of methylprednisolone from contused cat spinal cord following intravenous injection of the sodium succinate ester. *J Neurosurg* 1983; 58(4):538–542.
28. Anderson DK, Saunders RD, Demediuk P, et al. Lipid hydrolysis and peroxidation in injured spinal cord: partial protection with methylprednisolone or vitamin E and selenium. *Cent Nerv Syst Trauma* 1985; 2(4):257–267.
29. Braughler JM, Hall ED, Means ED, Waters TR, Anderson DK. Evaluation of an intensive methylprednisolone sodium succinate dosing regimen in experimental spinal cord injury. *J Neurosurg* 1987; 67(1):102–105.
30. Lee J-M, Yang P, Xiao Q, Chen S, Lee K-Y, Hsu CY, Xu J. Methylprednisolone protects oligodendrocytes but not neurons after spinal cord injury. *J Neurosci* 2008; 28(12):3141–3149.
31. Hall D, Springer JE. Neuroprotection and acute spinal cord injury: a reappraisal. *NeuroR$_x$: The Journal of the American Society for Experimental NeuroTherapeutics* 2004; 1(1):80–100.
32. Bracken MB, Shepard MJ, Collins WF, et al. A randomized, controlled trial of methylprednisolone or naloxone in the treatment of acute spinal-cord injury: results of the second National Acute Spinal Cord Injury Study. *N Engl J Med* 1990; 322(20):1405–1411.
33. Bracken MB, Shepard MJ, Collins WF Jr., et al. Methylprednisolone or naloxone treatment after acute spinal cord injury: 1-year follow-up data. Results of the second National Acute Spinal Cord Injury Study. *J Neurosurg* 1992; 76(1):23–31.
34. Bracken MB, Holford TR. Effects of timing of methylprednisolone or naloxone administration on recovery of segmental and long-tract neurological function in NASCIS 2. *J Neurosurg* 1993; 79(4):500–507.
35. Bracken MB. Pharmacological treatment of acute spinal cord injury: current status and future projects. *J Emerg Med* 1993; 11 (Suppl 1):43–48.
36. Otani K AH, Kadoya S. Beneficial effect of methylprednisolone sodium succinate in the treatment of acute spinal cord injury. *Sekitsui Sekizui* [in Japanese] 1994; 7:633–647.
37. Petitjean ME, Pointillart, V, Dixmerias F. Medical treatment of spinal cord injury in the acute stage. *Ann Fr Anesth Reanim* [in French] 1998; 17:114–122.
38. Hall ED. Lazaroid: mechanisms of action and implications for disorders of the CNS. *The Neuroscientist* 1997; 3:42–51.
39. Hall ED, McCall JM, Means ED. Therapeutic potential of the lazaroids (21-aminosteroids) in acute central nervous system trauma, ischemia and subarachnoid hemorrhage. *Adv Pharmacol* 1994; 28:221–268.
40. Braughler JM, Chase RL, Neff GL, et al. A new 21-aminosteroid antioxidant lacking glucocorticoid activity stimulates adrenocorticotropin secretion and blocks arachidonic acid release from mouse pituitary tumor (AtT-20) cells. *J Pharmacol Exp Ther* 1988; 244(2):423–427.
41. Anderson DK, Braughler JM, Hall ED, Waters TR, McCall JM, Means ED. Effects of treatment with U-74006F on neurological outcome following experimental spinal cord injury. *J Neurosurg* 1988; 69(4):562–567.
42. Anderson DK, Hall ED, Braughler JM, McCall JM, Means ED. Effect of delayed administration of U74006F (tirilazad mesylate) on recovery of locomotor function after experimental spinal cord injury. *J Neurotrauma* 1991; 8(3):187–192.

43. Hall ED. Effects of the 21-aminosteroid U74006F on posttraumatic spinal cord ischemia in cats. *J Neurosurg* 1988; 68(3):462–465.

44. Bracken MB, Shepard MJ, Holford TR, et al. Administration of methylprednisolone for 24 or 48 hours or tirilazad mesylate for 48 hours in the treatment of acute spinal cord injury: results of the third National Acute Spinal Cord Injury randomized controlled trial, National Acute Spinal Cord Injury Study. *JAMA* 1997; 277(20):1597–1604.

45. Bracken MB, Shepard MJ, Holford TR, et al. Methylprednisolone or tirilazad mesylate administration after acute spinal cord injury: 1-year follow up: results of the third National Acute Spinal Cord Injury randomized controlled trial. *J Neurosurg* 1998; 89(5):699–706.

46. Galandiuk S, Raque G, Appel S, Polk HC Jr. The two-edged sword of large-dose steroids for spinal cord trauma. *Ann Surg* 1993; 218(4):419–425, discussion 425–417.

47. Molano Mdel R, Broton JG, Bean JA, Calancie B. Complications associated with the prophylactic use of methylprednisolone during surgical stabilization after spinal cord injury. *J Neurosurg* 2002; 96(3 Suppl):267–272.

48. Bracken MB. Methylprednisolone and acute spinal cord injury: an update of the randomized evidence. *Spine* 2001; 26(24 Suppl):S47–S54.

49. Scheff SW, Benardo LS, Cotman CW. Hydrocortisone administration retards axon sprouting in the rat dentate gyrus. *Exp Neurol* 1980; 68(1):195–201.

50. Scheff SW, Cotman CW. Chronic glucocorticoid therapy alters axon sprouting in the hippocampal dentate gyrus. *Exp Neurol* 1982; 76(3):644–654.

51. Scheff SW, DeKosky ST. Steroid suppression of axon sprouting in the hippocampal dentate gyrus of the adult rat: dose-response relationship. *Exp Neurol* 1983; 82(1):183–191.

52. Scheff SW, DeKosky ST. Glucocorticoid suppression of lesion-induced synaptogenesis: effect of temporal manipulation of steroid treatment. *Exp Neurol* 1989; 105(3):260–264.

53. Oudega M, Vargas CG, Weber AB, Kleitman N, Bunge MB. Long-term effects of methylprednisolone following transection of adult rat spinal cord. *Eur J Neurosci* 1999; 11(7):2453–2464.

54. Chen A, Xu XM, Kleitman N, Bunge MB. Methylprednisolone administration improves axonal regeneration into Schwann cell grafts in transected adult rat thoracic spinal cord. *Exp Neurol* 1996; 138(2):261–276.

55. Li X, Oudega M, Dancausse HA, Levi AD. The effect of methylprednisolone on caspase-3 activation after rat spinal cord transection. *Restor Neurol Neurosci* 2000; 17(4):203–209.

56. Ray SK, Wilford GG, Matzelle DC, Hogan EL, Banik NL. Calpeptin and methylprednisolone inhibit apoptosis in rat spinal cord injury. *Ann N Y Acad Sci* 1999; 890:261–269.

57. Kanellopoulos GK, Kato H, Wu Y, et al. Neuronal cell death in the ischemic spinal cord: the effect of methylprednisolone. *Ann Thorac Surg* 1997; 64(5):1279–1285, discussion 1286.

58. Bracken MB. Treatment of acute spinal cord injury with methylprednisolone: results of a multicenter, randomized clinical trial. *J Neurotrauma* 1991; 8 Suppl 1:S47–S50, discussion S51–S42.

59. Hurlbert RJ. Methylprednisolone for acute spinal cord injury: an inappropriate standard of care. *J Neurosurg* 2000; 93(1 Suppl):1–7.

60. Short DJ, El Masry WS, Jones PW. High dose methylprednisolone in the management of acute spinal cord injury—a systematic review from a clinical perspective. *Spinal Cord* 2000; 38(5):273–286.

61. Coleman WP, Benzel D, Cahill DW, et al. A critical appraisal of the reporting of the National Acute Spinal Cord Injury Studies (II and III) of methylprednisolone in acute spinal cord injury. *J Spinal Disord* 2000; 13(3):185–199.

62. Marler JR, Tilley BC, Lu M, et al. Early stroke treatment associated with better outcome: the NINDS rt-PA stroke study. *Neurology* 2000; 55(11):1649–1655.

63. Kwiatkowski TG, Libman RB, Frankel M, et al. Effects of tissue plasminogen activator for acute ischemic stroke at one year: National Institute of Neurological Disorders and Stroke Recombinant Tissue Plasminogen Activator Stroke Study Group. *N Engl J Med* 1999; 340(23):1781–1787.

64. Bracken MB, Holford TR. Neurological and functional status 1 year after acute spinal cord injury: estimates of functional recovery in National Acute Spinal Cord Injury Study II from results modeled in National Acute Spinal Cord Injury Study III. *J Neurosurg* 2002; 96(3 Suppl): 259–266.

65. Fehlings MG. Summary statement: the use of methylprednisolone in acute spinal cord injury. *Spine* 2001; 26(24 Suppl):S55.

66. Fehlings MG. Editorial: recommendations regarding the use of methylprednisolone in acute spinal cord injury: making sense out of the controversy. *Spine* 2001; 26(24 Suppl):S56–S57.

67. Wing P, Consortium for spinal Cord Medicine. *Early Acute Management in Adults with Spinal Cord Injury: A Clinical Practice Guideline for Health Care Providers.* Washington, D.C.: Paralyzed Veterans of America; 2008.

68. Short D. Use of steroids for acute spinal cord injury must be reassessed. *BMJ* 2000; 321(7270):1224.

69. Hurlbert RJ. Methylprednisolone for acute spinal cord injury: reevaluating the NASCIS trials. *The Journal of Spinal Cord Medicine* 2002; 25(3):206.

70. Constantini S, Young W. The effects of methylprednisolone and the ganglioside GM1 on acute spinal cord injury in rats. *J Neurosurg* 1994; 80(1):97–111.

71. Hall ED. Drug development in spinal cord injury: what is the FDA looking for? *J Rehabil Res Dev* 2003; 40(4 Suppl 1):81–91.

72. Bao F, Liu D. Peroxynitrite generated in the rat spinal cord induces apoptotic cell death and activates caspase-3. *Neuroscience* 2003; 116(1):59–70.

73. Xu J, Gyeong-Moon K, Chen S, et al. iNOS and nitrotyrosine expression after spinal cord injury. *J Neurotrauma* 2001; 18(5):523–532.

74. Xiong Y, Rabchevsky AG, Hall ED. Role of peroxynitrite in secondary oxidative damage after spinal cord injury. *J Neurochem* 2007; 100(3):639–649.

75. Beckman JS. The double-edged role of nitric oxide in brain function and superoxide-mediated injury. *J Dev Physiol* 1991; 15(1):53–59.

76. Radi R, Beckman JS, Bush KM, Freeman BA. Peroxynitrite-induced membrane lipid peroxidation: the cytotoxic potential of superoxide and nitric oxide. *Arch Biochem Biophys* 1991; 288(2):481–487.

77. Carroll RT, Galatsis P, Borosky S, et al. 4-Hydroxy-2,2,6,6-tetramethylpiperidine-1-oxyl (Tempol) inhibits peroxynitrite-mediated phenol nitration. *Chem Res Toxicol* 2000; 13(4):294–300.

78. Hall ED, Kupina NC, Althaus JS. Peroxynitrite scavengers for the acute treatment of traumatic brain injury. *Ann N Y Acad Sci* 1999; 890:462–468.

79. Beit-Yannai E, Zhang R, Trembovler V, Samuni A, Shohami E. Cerebroprotective effect of stable nitroxide radicals in closed head injury in the rat. *Brain Res* 1996; 717(1–2):22–28.

80. Hillard VH, Peng H, Zhang Y, et al. Tempol, a nitroxide antioxidant, improves locomotor and histological outcomes after spinal cord contusion in rats. *J Neurotrauma* 2004; 21(10):1405–1414.

81. Genovese T, Mazzon E, Esposito E, et al. Beneficial effects of FeTSPP, a peroxynitrite decomposition catalyst, in a mouse model of spinal cord injury. *Free Radic Biol Med* 2007; 43(5):763–780.

82. Chabrier PE, Auguet M, Spinnewyn B, et al. BN 80933, a dual inhibitor of neuronal nitric oxide synthase and lipid peroxidation: a promising neuroprotective strategy. *Proc Natl Acad Sci USA* 1999; 96(19):10824–10829.

83. Popovich PG, Jones TB. Manipulating neuroinflammatory reactions in the injured spinal cord: back to basics. *Trends Pharmacol Sci* 2003; 24(1):13–17.

84. Tonai T, Taketani Y, Ohmoto Y, Ueda N, Nishisho T, Yamamoto S. Cyclooxygenase-2 induction in rat spinal cord injury mediated by proinflammatory tumor necrosis factor-alpha and interleukin-1. *Adv Exp Med Biol* 2002; 507:397–401.

85. Schwab JM, Brechtel K, Nguyen TD, Schluesener HJ. Persistent accumulation of cyclooxygenase-1 (COX-1) expressing microglia/macrophages and upregulation by endothelium following spinal cord injury. *J Neuroimmunol* 2000; 111(1–2):122–130.

86. Resnick DK, Graham SH, Dixon CE, Marion DW. Role of cyclooxygenase 2 in acute spinal cord injury. *J Neurotrauma* 1998; 15(12):1005–1013.

87. Hoffmann C. COX-2 in brain and spinal cord implications for therapeutic use. *Curr Med Chem* 2000; 7(11):1113–1120.

88. Hains BC, Yucra JA, Hulsebosch CE. Reduction of pathological and behavioral deficits following spinal cord contusion injury with the selective cyclooxygenase-2 inhibitor NS-398. *J Neurotrauma* 2001; 18(4):409–423.

89. Festoff BW, Ameenuddin S, Arnold PM, Wong A, Santacruz KS, Citron BA. Minocycline neuroprotects, reduces microgliosis, and inhibits caspase protease expression early after spinal cord injury. *J Neurochem* 2006; 97(5):1314–1326.

90. Hains BC, Waxman SG. Activated microglia contribute to the maintenance of chronic pain after spinal cord injury. *J Neurosci* 2006; 26(16): 4308–4317.

91. Lee SM, Yune TY, Kim SJ, et al. Minocycline reduces cell death and improves functional recovery after traumatic spinal cord injury in the rat. *J Neurotrauma* 2003; 20(10):1017–1027.

92. Stirling DP, Khodarahmi K, Liu J, et al. Minocycline treatment reduces delayed oligodendrocyte death, attenuates axonal dieback, and improves functional outcome after spinal cord injury. *J Neurosci* 2004; 24(9): 2182–2190.

93. Teng YD, Choi H, Onario RC, et al. Minocycline inhibits contusion-triggered mitochondrial cytochrome c release and mitigates functional deficits after spinal cord injury. *Proc Natl Acad Sci USA* 2004; 101(9): 3071–3076.

94. Wells JE, Hurlbert RJ, Fehlings MG, Yong VW. Neuroprotection by minocycline facilitates significant recovery from spinal cord injury in mice. *Brain* 2003; 126(Pt 7):1628–1637.

95. Yune TY, Lee JY, Jung GY, et al. Minocycline alleviates death of oligodendrocytes by inhibiting pro-nerve growth factor production in microglia after spinal cord injury. *J Neurosci* 2007; 27(29):7751–7761.

96. Gok B, Okutan O, Beskonakli E, Palaoglu S, Erdamar H, Sargon MF. Effect of immunomodulation with human interferon-beta on early functional recovery from experimental spinal cord injury. *Spine* 2007; 32(8): 873–880.

97. Yuen P, Wang KW. Therapeutic potential of calpain inhibitors in neurodegenerative disorder. *Exp Opin Invet Drugs* 1996; 5:1291–1304.

98. Yuen P, Wang KW. Calpain inhibitors: novel neuroprotectants and potential anticataract agents. *Drugs of the Future* 1998; 23:741–749.

99. Wingrave JM, Schaecher KE, Sribnick EA, et al. Early induction of secondary injury factors causing activation of calpain and mitochondria-mediated neuronal apoptosis following spinal cord injury in rats. *J Neurosci Res* 2003; 73(1):95–104.

100. Ray SK, Hogan EL, Banik NL. Calpain in the pathophysiology of spinal cord injury: neuroprotection with calpain inhibitors. *Brain Res Brain Res Rev* 2003; 42(2):169–185.

101. Ray SK, Matzelle DD, Wilford GG, Hogan EL, Banik NL. Inhibition of calpain-mediated apoptosis by E-64 d-reduced immediate early gene (IEG) expression and reactive astrogliosis in the lesion and penumbra following spinal cord injury in rats. *Brain Res* 2001; 916(1–2):115–126.

102. Ray SK, Matzelle DD, Wilford GG, Hogan EL, Banik NL. Cell death in spinal cord injury (SCI) requires de novo protein synthesis. Calpain inhibitor E-64-d provides neuroprotection in SCI lesion and penumbra. *Ann NY Acad Sci* 2001; 939:436–449.

103. Ray SK, Matzelle DD, Wilford GG, Hogan EL, Banik NL. Increased calpain expression is associated with apoptosis in rat spinal cord injury: calpain inhibitor provides neuroprotection. *Neurochem Res* 2000; 25(9–10):1191–1198.

104. Shields DC, Schaecher KE, Hogan EL, Banik NL. Calpain activity and expression increased in activated glial and inflammatory cells in penumbra of spinal cord injury lesion. *J Neurosci Res* 2000; 61(2):146–150.

105. Banik NL, Shields DC. The role of calpain in neurofilament protein degradation associated with spinal cord injury. *Methods Mol Biol* 2000; 144:195–201.

106. Zhang SX, Bondada V, Geddes JW. Evaluation of conditions for calpain inhibition in the rat spinal cord: effective postinjury inhibition with intraspinal MDL28170 microinjection. *J Neurotrauma* 2003; 20(1): 59–67.

107. Yu CG, Geddes JW. Sustained calpain inhibition improves locomotor function and tissue sparing following contusive spinal cord injury. *Neurochem Res* 2007; 32:2046–2053.

108. Sullivan PG, Krishnamurthy S, Patel SP, Pandya JD, Rabchevsky AG. Temporal characterization of mitochondrial bioenergetics after spinal cord injury. *J Neurotrauma* 2007; 24(6):991–999.

109. Sullivan PG, Thompson MB, Scheff SW. Cyclosporin A attenuates acute mitochondrial dysfunction following traumatic brain injury. *Exp Neurol* 1999; 160(1):226–234.

110. Sullivan PG, Rabchevsky AG, Hicks RR, Gibson TR, Fletcher-Turner A, Scheff SW. Dose-response curve and optimal dosing regimen of cyclosporin A after traumatic brain injury in rats. *Neuroscience* 2000; 101(2):289–295.

111. Rabchevsky AG, Fugaccia I, Sullivan PG, Scheff SW. Cyclosporin A treatment following spinal cord injury to the rat: behavioral effects and stereological assessment of tissue sparing. *J Neurotrauma* 2001; 18(5): 513–522.

112. Sullivan PG, Springer JE, Hall ED, Scheff SW. Mitochondrial uncoupling as a therapeutic target following neuronal injury. *J Bioenerg Biomembr* 2004; 36(4):353–356.

113. Faden AI, Jacobs TP, Holaday JW. Opiate antagonist improves neurologic recovery after spinal injury. *Science* 1981; 211(4481):493–494.

114. Flamm ES, Young W, Demopoulos HB, DeCrescito V, Tomasula JJ. Experimental spinal cord injury: treatment with naloxone. *Neurosurgery* 1982; 10(2):227–231.

115. Faden AI, Holaday JW. A role for endorphins in the pathophysiology of spinal cord injury. *Adv Biochem Psychopharmacol* 1981; 28:435–446.

116. Faden AI, Jacobs TP, Holaday JW. Thyrotropin-releasing hormone improves neurologic recovery after spinal trauma in cats. *N Engl J Med* 1981; 305(18):1063–1067.

117. Faden AI, Sacksen I, Noble LJ. Structure-activity relationships of TRH analogs in rat spinal cord injury. *Brain Res* 1988; 448(2):287–293.

118. Pitts LH, Ross A, Chase GA, Faden AI. Treatment with thyrotropin-releasing hormone (TRH) in patients with traumatic spinal cord injuries. *J Neurotrauma* 1995; 12(3):235–243.

119. Faden AI. TRH analog YM-14673 improves outcome following traumatic brain and spinal cord injury in rats: dose-response studies. *Brain Res* 1989; 486(2):228–235.

120. Faden AI, Fox G, Fan L, Knoblach S, Araldi GL, Kozikowski AP. Neuroprotective and cognitive enhancing effects of novel small peptides. *Ann NY Acad Sci* 1999; 890:120.

121. Beattie MS, Farooqui AA, Bresnahan JC. Review of current evidence for apoptosis after spinal cord injury. *J Neurotrauma* 2000; 17(10): 915–925.

122. Crowe MJ, Bresnahan JC, Shuman SL, Masters JN, Beattie MS. Apoptosis and delayed degeneration after spinal cord injury in rats and monkeys. *Nat Med* 1997; 3(1):73–76.

123. Emery E, Aldana P, Bunge MB, et al. Apoptosis after traumatic human spinal cord injury. *J Neurosurg* 1998; 89(6):911–920.

124. Liu XZ, Xu XM, Hu R, et al. Neuronal and glial apoptosis after traumatic spinal cord injury. *J Neurosci* 1997; 17(14):5395–5406.

125. Lou J, Lenke LG, Ludwig FJ, O'Brien MF. Apoptosis as a mechanism of neuronal cell death following acute experimental spinal cord injury. *Spinal Cord* 1998; 36(10):683–690.

126. Shuman SL, Bresnahan JC, Beattie MS. Apoptosis of microglia and oligodendrocytes after spinal cord contusion in rats. *J Neurosci Res* 1997; 50(5):798–808.

127. Takagi T, Takayasu M, Mizuno M, Yoshimoto M, Yoshida J. Caspase activation in neuronal and glial apoptosis following spinal cord injury in mice. *Neurol Med Chir* [Tokyo] 2003; 43(1):20–29, discussion 29–30.

128. Yong C, Arnold PM, Zoubine MN, et al. Apoptosis in cellular compartments of rat spinal cord after severe contusion injury. *J Neurotrauma* 1998; 15(7):459–472.

129. Martinez-Arizala A, Green BA. Hypothermia in spinal cord injury. *J Neurotrauma* 1992; 9 Suppl 2:S497–S505.

130. Inamasu J, Nakamura Y, Ichikizaki K. Induced hypothermia in experimental traumatic spinal cord injury: an update. *J Neurol Sci* 2003; 209(1–2):55–60.

131. Dietrich WD, Chatzipanteli K, Vitarbo E, Wada K, Kinoshita K. The role of inflammatory processes in the pathophysiology and treatment of brain and spinal cord trauma. *Acta Neurochir Suppl* 2004; 89:69–74.

132. Shibuya S, Miyamoto O, Janjua NA, Itano T, Mori S, Norimatsu H. Post-traumatic moderate systemic hypothermia reduces TUNEL positive cells following spinal cord injury in rat. *Spinal Cord* 2004; 42(1):29–34.

133. Yu CG, Jimenez O, Marcillo AE, et al. Beneficial effects of modest systemic hypothermia on locomotor function and histopathological damage following contusion-induced spinal cord injury in rats. *J Neurosurg* 2000; 93(1 Suppl):85–93.

134. Casas CE, Herrera LP, Prusmack C, Ruenes G, Marcillo A, Guest JD. Effects of epidural hypothermic saline infusion on locomotor outcome and tissue preservation after moderate thoracic spinal cord contusion in rats. *J Neurosurg Spine* 2005; 2(3):308–318.

135. Shields CB, Zhang YP, Shields LB, Han Y, Burke DA, Mayer NW. The therapeutic window for spinal cord decompression in a rat spinal cord injury model. *J Neurosurg Spine* 2005; 3(4):302–307.

136. Baptiste DC, Fehlings MG. Update on the treatment of spinal cord injury. *Prog Brain Res* 2007; 161:217–233.

68

Traversing Barriers in the Spinal Cord Microenvironment that Prevent Functional Recovery: Interventions to Prevent Cell Death and Promote Neuroplasticity and Regeneration

Yu-Shang Lee
Ching-Yi Lin
Henrich Cheng

RECENT EXPERIMENTAL FINDINGS AND REGENERATIVE MEDICINE: POTENTIAL THERAPEUTIC OPTIONS

Functional recovery of the injured spinal cord represents one of the most formidable challenges in regenerative medicine. Regenerative medicine is a new, multidisciplinary field that employs combinatorial approaches of cell replacement, trophic support, protection from oxidative stress, and neutralization of the growth-inhibitory components to replace or rescue injured tissues (1, 2). The National Spinal Cord Injury Statistical Center in Birmingham, Alabama, reported the annual incidence of traumatic spinal cord injury (SCI), not including those who die in the accident, as being approximately forty cases per million people in the United States, producing approximately 12,000 new cases each year, with a prevalence of approximately 255,700 persons in 2007. The surviving patients living with spinal cord dysfunction are challenged and live with severe activity limitations that threaten to compromise their fullest personal potential. These continued functional deficits, healthcare needs, and costs, as well as caregiver burden and stress, often remain tremendous. It is clear that the injury physically and psychologically affects not only the patient, but also the family and society (http://www.spinalcord.uab.edu/).

The attainment of an optimal intervention for SCI is hindered by the complexity of the SCI pathophysiologic conditions and the unpredictability of the patient's prognosis. Over the last two decades, numerous advances have been made in the basic science of axon regeneration, leading to a greater collective understanding of the cellular and molecular biology of acute and chronic spinal cord trauma (3, 4). In addition, spinal lesion models have become more sophisticated and reproducible, and behavioral analysis qualifies a greater spectrum of the structural and functional consequences of various motor, sensory, and autonomic systems after SCI (5, 6). Particularly notable has been the development of reproducible spinal cord contusion injuries (7), which provide an experimental approach that better approximates human traumatic SCI (8, 9). Eventually, it would be ideal to develop adjunct neurophysiologic, pharmacologic, imaging, transplant, and exercise protocols to define the most rational therapeutic approach required on a patient-by-patient basis. This might enhance recovery and cure of each individual with SCI (10). This chapter reviews aspects of the microenvironment that impede and intrinsic changes that promote neural plasticity and regeneration. Neural plasticity is the ability of the nervous tissue to reorganize itself, by forming new neural connections or activities in response to injury, disease, exercise, or experience. Regeneration is the process of neuron substitute and/or neurite grown from the rest of the remaining neurons to replace damaged, interrupted, or lost neural circuits. This chapter reviews current neural plasticity and reparative strategies that are being explored and their potential clinical applications to prevention and cure of the devastating effects of SCI (Figure 68.1).

TISSUE RESPONSES AND NEURAL PLASTICITY AFTER SCI: ATTEMPTS TO RESTORE FUNCTION FOR BETTER OR WORSE

A traditional concept of neuroscience has been that the mature central nervous system (CNS) has relatively little ability to adaptively respond to injury. Surprisingly, however, recent data have

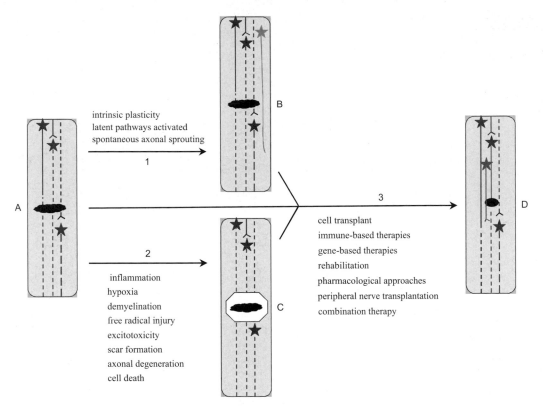

Figure 68.1 A sequential diagram illustrates neural interactions, cellular responses, and therapeutic approaches to acute spinal cord injury. Acute spinal cord injury (**A**), caused by traumatic or nontraumatic damage; responses to compensate for lost tissue (**B**) by intrinsic plasticity (**1**) or experiences negative responses (**2**) that lead to secondary injury (**C**). Several therapeutic approaches (**3**) have been shown to benefit the neural regeneration and recovery (**D**) following injury.

uncovered a significant amount of structural plasticity and intrinsic regeneration capability in mature neurons in the adult CNS when they are exposed to a facilitative environment (11). Additionally, it must be emphasized that injury itself may represent a powerful external stimulus, which simultaneously modifies the microenvironment of the nervous tissue as well as the functional interaction between neural circuits and the surrounding milieu (12). For example, traumatic or vascular brain injuries induce complex changes in the expression of intrinsic neuronal growth molecules and extrinsic growth-regulatory cues (13, 14), as well as producing peculiar patterns of electrical activity (15, 16). These responses are primarily aimed to restore homeostatic conditions (17, 18) but also have a compensatory character to stimulate growth processes that serve to encourage repair (19). Furthermore, neural plasticity that includes the reorganization of the supraspinal level and increases nerve sprouting plays an important role to facilitate a certain degree of recovery (Figure 68.2) (20, 21). However, both in vitro (22) and in vivo (23) experimental studies suggest that postinjury sprouting may not always be functionally appropriate. Aberrant axonal connectivity can possibly be maladaptive and can contribute to the development of epilepsy following SCI (24, 25). Therefore, an understanding of the stereotypical reaction to injury of different CNS neurons, and how to overcome inhibitory mechanisms that block regeneration and promote mechanisms that enhance neuronal plasticity (26), may open new doors of hope for therapeutic interventions for a range of

neurodegenerative diseases and CNS injuries, especially spinal cord injury (27).

The Negative Environment Following SCI: Inhibitory Mechanisms to Prevent Reconnection at the Injured Site

A traumatic spinal cord injury is produced by a primary mechanical disruption to spinal cord tissues from direct impact and shock waves (28, 29). Immediately, there is a prolonged period of secondary cellular and biochemical pathophysiologic alterations, including hemorrhage, edema, inflammation, disturbances in ionic homeostasis, oxidative damage, glutamate excitotoxicity, ischemia-reperfusion, metabolic perturbation, axonal and neuronal necrosis, and apoptosis and demyelination followed by cyst formation and infarction (30, 31). The progression of these secondary injury processes contributes to the gradual expansion of the initial lesion, both radically and longitudinally, from the epicenter of the initial impact (32). Although the spinal cord is rarely completely transected from the initial impact (33), secondary processes can expand damage to produce a clinical syndrome indistinguishable from complete transection (34, 35). Thus, acute traumatic SCI results in a devastating and irreversible loss of neurologic function below the level of injury and adversely damages multiple tissues within the body. Recovery of function is dependent on the degree of tissue loss and the preservation and/or engagement of neuronal networks

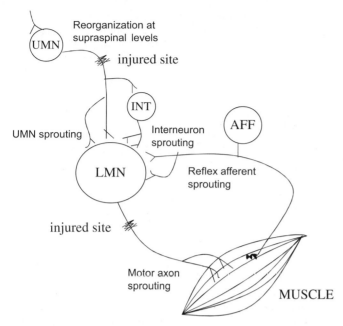

Figure 68.2 Neural plasticity may contribute to functional recovery after spinal cord injury (SCI). Two major events may occur in neural plasticity including reorganization at supraspinal levels and increasing the nerve sprouting from upper motoneurons (UMN) or lower motoneurons (LMN) or interneurons. The reorganization of the brain involves the topography of the affected neural populations by SCI being replaced or compensated for by the adjacent neurons to maintain certain functions. Nerve sprouting is the response of nerve fibers to reestablish the appropriate connection or to compensate for other nerve functions after SCI. INT = interneurons; AFF = afferent neurons.

that serve as substrates for the restoration of lost spinal cord functions (36).

The inflammatory response is a complex process starting immediately after SCI, which involves vascular changes, cellular responses, and chemical reactions. Neutrophils invade the spinal parenchyma from the circulatory system within 24 hours; they are followed by lymphocytes that invade and reach peak numbers within 48 hours. The invading inflammatory cells increase the local concentrations of cytokines and chemokines. Hemorrhage continues, with localized edema, loss of microcirculation by thrombosis, vasospasm and mechanical damage, and loss of vasculature autoregulation. All of these further exacerbate the spinal cord injury (3). Several weeks after injury to the spinal cord, macrophages have cleared the tissue debris at the lesion site, resulting in a posttraumatic cyst surrounded by scar tissue (35). However, the complex interplay between inflammatory cells and astrocytes as well as the glial cells is still poorly understood. Excitotoxicity starts after the initial insult; the injured neurons respond with an injury-induced barrage of action potentials attributed to local ionic disturbances, such as increased intracellular sodium, extracellular potassium, and intracellular calcium concentrations (37). The ensuing depolarization stimulates calcium entry at the somatic level and glutamate release at spared synapses (38), which appears to trigger regen-

eration but also to cause excitotoxicity (39), leading to spinal shock, neuronal death, and even functional deficits.

Demyelination occurs soon after SCI. All fast-conducting nerve fibers in the CNS are surrounded by myelin, a sheath produced by oligodendrocytes. Myelin damage occurs early following SCI and may result from delayed apoptotic death of oligodendrocytes (40). Demyelination always contributes to the functional deficit following SCI, because it causes the disruption of electrical impulse conductivity, leading to axons that remain anatomically intact and physiologically nonfunctional, and which fail to conduct action potentials due to an imbalanced distribution of sodium and potassium channels (35). The demyelinated axons are partly responsible for the delayed sensory-motor dysfunction. Although the literature suggests that, in experimental animals, primary demyelination may be an important factor in SCI (41), this does not seem to be the case in humans. Extensive areas of primary demyelination have never been seen except in trauma associated with chronic spinal cord compression (42).

Fortunately, there appear to be several interesting ways in which this inhibition might be overcome (such as using the monoclonal antibody IN-1) (43, 44). Other alternatives to avoid this nonpermissive microenvironment of CNS white matter also are worth exploring. One possibility is to reroute pathways from nonpermissive white to permissive gray matter (45). In the gray matter of the spinal cord, which contains nerve cell bodies and many nonmyelinated fibers, less Nogo activity occurs. Long-distance 5-HT regeneration in the spinal cord has been demonstrated to occur to over 95% in gray matter after either chemical (46) or surgical lesioning (47). Moreover, in using in vitro explant coculture of postnatal sensorimotor cortex and spinal cord, the corticospinal fibers are noted to arborize within the gray matter of spinal cord explants (48). Reimplantation of the severed dorsal roots in the adult rat spinal cord has revealed axonal regeneration and terminal arborization when the roots are reinserted into the gray matter, whereas regeneration is limited when insertion is into the white matter (49).

Therefore, a full understanding of the roles of subpopulations of neuronal and nonneuronal cells in the SCI, as well as mechanisms that overcome inhibitory environments and enhance neuronal plasticity, will provide important new avenues that will inhibit aberrance and promote adaptive and regenerative neuronal alterations (50).

The role of oligodendrocytes in blocking regeneration has been well established in recent years. It is likely that these inhibitory influences restrict axonal growth both at the lesion site and within the host nervous system distal to the lesion. This inhibitory mechanism is crucial for the stabilization of axon sprouting (i.e., for prevention of subsequent dysfunctional collateral branching) after functional axonal connections in CNS myelination during development. This is suggested by the temporal correlation between the developmental onset of myelination and the completion of primary axonal growth (51, 52). Axonal sprouting within the adult CNS has been reported to occur more readily in lightly myelinated regions such as the substantia gelatinosa of the spinal cord (53), the olfactory system (54), the hippocampus (55), the septum (56), and the cerebellum. This indicates that neuronal plasticity involving axonal sprouting is inversely related to the extent of CNS myelination. Consequently, the corticospinal tract of the spinal cord becomes severely restricted in its ability to sprout after myelination. The inhibitory nature of myelin toward axonal regeneration in the CNS has been further explored by studies of inhibitory molecules. Myelin-associated glycoprotein (MAG) is a potent inhibitor of axonal regeneration (57, 58). Soluble MAG is released from myelin and potently inhibits axonal regeneration. A comparison of neurite growth in contact with CNS or peripheral nervous system (PNS) constituents has revealed that PNS myelin is a positive substrate for neurite growth, whereas CNS myelin has strong inhibitory properties (59–61). In Aguayo's bridging studies, regenerating fibers could elongate throughout the whole distance of a PNS graft. However, the fibers usually fail to enter the spinal cord for any significant distance beyond the distal nerve–cord interface (62). Pioneering work by Schwab and associates has demonstrated that oligodendroglial cells produce proteins, such as neurite growth inhibitors NI-35 and NI-250, components of central myelin, which inhibit axon regeneration (63, 64). The neurite growth inhibitors were isolated and characterized as Nogo proteins and were subgrouped into A, B, and C. A single Nogo gene has been elucidated after differential splicing and gives rise to these three different proteins.

As damage to the CNS continues, glial proliferation produces a dense scar (65), stimulated by the increased expression of glial fibrillary acidic protein (GFAP), which is found for some distance surrounding the injury site. Two other intermediate filaments, vimentin and nestin, are found exclusively within and immediately surrounding the lesion site with connexion-43. The subsequent proliferation and hypertrophy of astrocytes around the injury site is denoted by increased immunoreactivity to GFAP (66–69). This increased number of astrocytes may result from cell migration and/or division (70). Increased expression of GFAP has been attributed to neuron-glia interactions, and in particular, to a response to microglia (71–73). After damage, many of the astrocytes proliferate throughout the scar and bind together with tight junctions, which makes it difficult for axons and migrating cells to traverse the scar. This physical barrier assembled as a glial scar is accompanied by a significant biochemical barrier, which forms through the production of inhibitory molecules such as Nogo-A, MAG, oligodendrocyte-myelin glycoprotein (Omgp), tenascin-R, NG2, chondroitin sulfate proteoglycans (CSPGs), free radicals, nitric oxide, and arachidonic acid (69,74). Clearly, this dense glial scar, along with all the associated inhibitory molecules, stands as a formidable impediment to neural repair (75).

The pathobiology of SCI produces axonal degeneration and cell death initially with mechanical insults (compression, contusion, lacerations, shear, etc.) to the spinal cord and secondarily with activation of a delayed secondary cascade of events (edema, ischemia, inflammation, excitotoxicity, demyelination, scar formation, axonal degeneration, apoptosis, necrosis, etc.), which ultimately causes progressive degeneration of the spinal cord (76). Unfortunately, the most reactive neural cell populations are more likely to die if regeneration fails (77), as a result of devastating secondary damages. However, this continuously occurring and irreversible cell death offers an opportunity for therapeutic intervention to rescue those neurons that are at risk of dying during the first few hours after injury.

Both intrinsic neuronal and extrinsic environmental factors can impede regeneration after trauma in the mammalian CNS.

In comparison, an axotomy in the PNS triggers an up-regulation of specific cellular and molecular programs that lead to regeneration. However, similar cellular programs are either not up-regulated, or are up-regulated only transiently, after axotomy of CNS neurons. Wallerian degeneration and retrograde cell death occur in these neurons after axotomy.

Regeneration of damaged axons within the CNS has often been suggested to be inhibited by reactive astrocytes, which activate a physiologic "stop pathway" that is built into the axon and normally operates when axons from stable connections interact with target cells (78–84). Astrocytes not only present a physical barrier to growth, but also a chemical barrier; after injury, they also express a boundary molecule that is able to restrict axonal growth (80, 83–86). Through their production of proteoglycans within the extracellular matrix, astrocytes are directly associated with failure of axon regrowth (80). Certain serum factors and/or inflammatory cytokines may play a role in the molecular cascade that produces the extracellular matrix. The breakdown of the blood–brain barrier and the infiltration of macrophages at the lesion site are associated with the deposition of chondroitin sulfate proteoglycans close to the so-called glial scar (86).

Regardless of whether astrocytes play a complete inhibitory role or a partially supportive role, their use for regeneration is still controversial. Some evidence suggests that embryonic astrocytes can act as conductive substrates for growing axons, whereas adult astrocytes or reactive astrocytes are inhibitory to axonal growth (71, 82, 87, 88). Astrocytes can potentially express molecules that are both growth permissive and growth inhibitory. Some molecules can be growth permissive at one time but growth inhibitory at another time. Throughout development, astrocyte-related molecules are present. They include tenascin, phosphacan, heparin sulfate proteoglycan (HSPG), CSPG, and dermatan/keratan sulfate proteoglycan (KSPG) (67, 68, 82, 85). These molecules have different expression patterns at various stages. Recent findings suggest that in the adult CNS, tenascin, CSPG, and HSPG may be inhibitory, whereas KSPG is a supportive substrate for neuronal differentiation (68, 80, 83, 85). Although tenascin is a permissive molecule for axonal outgrowth during the early stages of development, it may have a nonpermissive or repulsive role later (89). A high ratio of HSPG to CSPG expression appears during the early stage of spinal cord development, which is more permissive for axonal growth; however, this is reversed during later stages of development (68). Many aspects relating to the expression of cell adhesion molecules at different developmental stages remain to be clarified. For example, the role of families of glial receptors for axon adhesion and the actual glial cell adhesion systems that function in the spinal cord are still unknown. Although it is known that astrocytes can synthesize several growth factors in vitro and/or express mRNA in vivo (90–92), it is still unknown whether or not they secrete neurotrophic factors in vivo to facilitate regeneration or act as mediators of neurotrophic factor transport.

Spontaneous Plasticity Following SCI: Enhancement Mechanisms

Lesioned nerve fibers in the CNS of the adult are often characterized by a spontaneous, but short-lived and ultimately abortive, attempt at repair, called regenerative sprouting (93). However, a more complete understanding of developmental neurobiology has provided many insights into possible ways in which neuronal regeneration in the CNS may be encouraged (35). Current efforts are aimed at blocking growth-inhibitory molecules by the in vivo application of antibodies against these molecules or the receptors to which they bind, or rather by pharmacologically manipulating the downstream signaling pathways induced by these inhibitory molecules in neurites following SCI (94, 95).

Spontaneous axonal sprouting and regeneration often occur following SCI, although these sprouts usually do not lead to functional connection. Additionally, enhanced axonal growth in the vicinity of the lesion is correlated with functional recovery following SCI (26, 96, 97). Such recovery may depend on synaptic plasticity within spinal circuitries below the hemisection injury as well (16). In fact, after spinal cord sections of animals and humans, significant function can be achieved with the sparing of only about 10%–15% of the white matter (98). This suggests that only a small degree of regeneration may be required to restore meaningful function. Notably, it is difficult to determine whether sprouting axons in vivo are derived from undamaged or damaged neurites.

Remyelination can occur spontaneously after CNS injury and plays a role in recovery of function. However, this spontaneous remyelination is inconsistent or malfunctional, and in many cases, it fails to occur because the adult spinal cord seems unable to efficiently replace either lost myelin or lost oligodendrocytes (93). Therefore, optimizing remyelination through transplantation of myelin-producing cells offers a more pragmatic approach to the restoration of meaningful neurologic function (35).

Although spontaneous regeneration of injured nerve fibers is limited in the mature CNS, many people who suffer incomplete SCI show clear functional recovery. This recovery process can continue for many years after the injury and probably depends on the reorganization of damaged circuits and the formation of new circuits through collateral sprouting of both lesioned and unlesioned fibers (35). The new synapse growth with the appropriated connection to the target neurons or the increases of the synapse formation between nerve fibers and muscles can lead to maximization of functional recovery (Figure 68.3) (99). However, the "Kennard principle" (or "early lesion effect") points out that the ability of one group of nerve fibers to take over the role of another injured group is much less prominent in the adult CNS (98) than just after birth. One mechanism for this phenomenon is the activation and strengthening of previously silent synapses by feedback inhibition and feed-forward sprouting. For example, when axons are severed, the remaining intact nerve fibers react to the imbalance of the neural circuitry by sprouting compensatory fibers (93), and the destroyed, vacated synaptic sites are reoccupied by compensatory growth of spared, intact nerve fibers above and below the lesion. This way, the spinal motor pools receive some input from the brain, and trace movements can occur (100). Several interventions (neurotrophic factors, antibodies, etc.) that promote regeneration of damaged nerve fibers will almost certainly also enhance compensatory growth of nonlesioned nerve fibers in the partially lesioned brain stem and spinal cord of the adult rat (101). Functional and anatomical evidence indicates that spontaneous plasticity can be potentiated by activity and by specific experimental

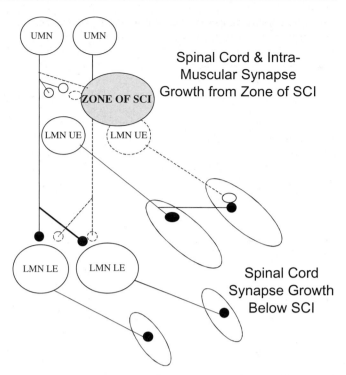

Spinal Cord & Intra-Muscular Synapse Growth from Zone of SCI

Spinal Cord Synapse Growth Below SCI

Figure 68.3 Appropriated connections of nerve fibers and target neurons after SCI. In addition to the initiation of nerve sprouting after the injury, neural plasticity also involves synapse growth to achieve functional recovery. As in the incomplete cervical spinal cord injury shown here, the spared motoneuron units may have synapse growth or provide the input to compensate for the function of the injured site. (UMN = upper motoneurons; LMN = lower motoneurons; UE = upper extremities; LE = lower extremities.)

manipulations. Nevertheless, the bulk of the compensatory processes may actually end in aberrant circuit reorganization and maladaptive functional outcomes (12). Together, these observations indicate that, although axon regeneration or reorganization may produce aberrant connections and functional abnormalities, the degree of anatomical reconstruction and the ensuing recovery of adaptive function can be significantly improved by specific experience or training paradigms.

Intrinsic Control of Neuronal Regeneration: Mechanisms to Be Understood

Classically, CNS neurons were thought to be incapable of regeneration. However, in the chronic phase of SCI, primarily unmyelinated cut and nearby uncut axons have been found to exhibit regenerative and sprouting responses. Studies indicate that central neurons have an intrinsic capacity for regenerative sprouting in the spinal cord if exposed to a facilitative environment. This intrinsic ability of CNS neurons for axonal regeneration is enhanced by the presence of growth factors and regeneration-related proteins/molecules, such as growth-associated protein (GAP)–43 and cyclic AMP (cAMP), among others (102). Growth factor production is triggered by environmental changes, which initiate signaling cascades to sustain the growth of neurites. The developmental time course of the decrease in endogenous cAMP temporally coincides with the lack of regeneration in lesioned branches in older neurons (103). The differences in the growth capacities of embryonic and adult neurons could be attributable to changes in the internal machinery for axon growth or simply to changes in responsiveness to the inhibitory molecules induced by injury and disease (35). Such an inhibitory adult CNS milieu and the maladaptive responses cause limited spontaneous regeneration with development (62, 104). Different types of axons vary greatly in their ability to regenerate. In the adult CNS, substantial regeneration occurs only in restricted regions, and the phenomenon of growth is actually sustained by the structural plasticity of neurites, and most notably axons (12). For example, the axons of the Purkinje cells in the cerebellum appear to have no regenerative response to axotomy. However, the spinal motor neurons probably have the best chance for regenerating in the CNS, especially when cut close to the cell body (35). Such variability suggests that distinct neuron populations are subjected to differential regulation by combining type-specific intrinsic features with different extrinsic signaling molecules. In contrast to axons of the PNS, the distance of the injury from the cell body influences the regenerative potential of CNS axons. Unfortunately, many of the critical axonal tracts that need to be repaired after SCI are long. Thus, it is critical to identify the mechanisms behind this phenomenon and to find methods that induce long-tract regeneration in axons severed far from the cell body (35).

Spontaneous Regrowth of Descending Fibers after SCI: The Challenge of Connecting to Targets

Several major descending axon tracts including the corticospinal, rubrospinal, coerulospinal, vestibulospinal, reticulospinal, and raphespinal tracts have been studied on the basis of their contribution to motor function. For example, the corticospinal tract axons have been demonstrated to sprout and regrow as early as 2 weeks after SCI and to persist largely until at least 13 weeks after injury (105, 106). Consequently, the corticospinal axon terminals remain rostral to the lesion area. Although all of these descending fibers make initial attempts to regrow after injury, the severed axons are unsuccessful in regrowing into and across the lesion site because of the inhibitory environment in the injured site (107).

STRATEGIES TO RESCUE NEURONS: PREPARATIONS FOR NEUROPLASTICITY

The major goal of neuroprotective therapy is to prevent secondary cell death from occurring within hours, days, or even weeks following injury. Cell death after SCI is caused by a variety of mechanisms. These include the following:

- *Excitotoxicity*—overprotection of and stimulation by normal physiologic neurochemicals, such as glutamate
- *Cell destruction*—caused by release of high levels of free radicals
- *Inflammation*—intervention by the immune system
- *Swelling*—mass effect caused by cytotoxic and vasogenic edema (108)

Neuroprotective effects can be provided in several ways. For example, the application of corticosteroids, antioxidative agents, intracellular signaling manipulators, and trophic factors is beneficial.

Corticosteroids: Anti-inflammation, Free Radical Scavengers

In general, neuroprotection research has progressed much further than research focusing on transplantation. However, despite all the research being conducted, the only real advance that has been made is the North American Spinal Cord Injury Study (NASCI) on glucocorticosteroids. Over ten clinical trials on neuroprotective agents, not including the NASCI study, failed in last decade. In 1979, Dr. Wise Young discovered, in a cat model, that methylprednisolone in high doses resulted in neurophysiologic recovery. This discovery has led to more than 10 years of research and the mobilization of the drug from the laboratory to clinical application. Currently, high doses of methylprednisolone have become standard neuroprotective therapy for SCI. Methylprednisolone probably acts as a free radical scavenger as well as an anti-inflammatory agent. Provided that the patient is available within 24 hours after injury, it is given in an initial IV bolus dose, followed by infusion over 24 to 48 hours. During the 1990s, researchers conducted considerable experiments to find a drug that was superior to methylprednisolone. Many drugs have been tested, but none has so far proven superior to methylprednisolone. Examples include GM 1 ganglioside (Syngen®) and 21 aminosterois from J7J (Triclozad®), both of which were found to be less efficacious than glucocorticoids.

Antioxidants: Reducing Oxidative Stress on Cells

Oxidative stress plays a key role both in primary damage following acute traumatic SCI and in secondary deleterious processes associated with inflammatory mediators and neutrophil-mediated inflammation (109, 110). Reactive oxygen species (ROS) and reactive nitrogen species (RNS) are postulated to contribute to CNS injury through oxidative damage to membrane lipids, proteins, and DNA. ROS include superoxide anions, hydrogen peroxide, and hydroxyl radicals, whereas RNS include nitric oxide and peroxinitrite, potent derivatives of nitric oxide (NO) and superoxide.

Nitric oxide (NO), a radical synthesized from L-arginine by NO synthase (NOS), can be protective or destructive depending on its redox state and cellular source (111–113). Studies suggest that the activities of both neuronal NOS (nNOS) and inducible NOS (iNOS) are detrimental to the ischemic brain or spinal cord and that endothelial NOS (eNOS) activity may be protective (112, 114, 115). Furthermore, intraspinal injection of L-NAME induced a dose-dependent loss of neurons in the spinal cord, further supporting the protective effect of constitutive NO (116).

Superoxide is produced under physiologic conditions as a byproduct of mitochondrial respiration. Other such byproducts are xanthine oxidase, NADPH-oxidase, and cyclooxygenase (COX) (117, 118). Inhibition of COX-2 and iNOS has been reported to exert neuroprotective effects (119). Superoxide dismutase (SOD) converts superoxide into H_2O_2; H_2O_2 is reduced to H_2O by catalase and selenium-dependent glutathione peroxidase. A disruption of the balance between oxidative damage and antioxidant defense can produce excess superoxide and H_2O_2, thereby producing OH. In cases of familial amyotrophic lateral sclerosis (ALS), a dysfunction of copper/zinc SOD (Cu/Zn-SOD) is thought to be a causative agent for death of motoneurons (120, 121). It was demonstrated that superoxide, hydroxyl, and peroxinitrite radicals increase in the CNS following traumatic brain injury and SCI (122–124). Apoptosis in rat motor neurons, induced by the withdrawal of a trophic factor, also involves the combined effects of NO and superoxide (125). An increased level of nitrotyrosine, a product of peroxinitrite, was recently found present in sections of injured spinal cord and ischemic brain (124). Induction of magnesium-containing SOD has been reported for a variety of oxidative stress conditions. Increased expression of Mn-SOD could limit the formation of peroxinitrite (126). SOD prevents the secondary injury of SCI and improves neurologic recovery and infarction in rabbits following ischemia and reperfusion injury (127). Two synthetic SOD/catalase mimetics, EUK-8 and EUK-134, have been shown to reduce oxidative stress and prolong survival in an ALS mouse model (128). Mn-SOD has been shown to be a major protective factor in NO-mediated neurotoxicity (92). On the other hand, several reports have shown that constitutive overexpression of Cu/Zn SOD or Mn-SOD in cells and animals causes oxidative damage (129–131). When activity of Cu/Zn SOD increases and accumulates, its reaction with transition metals (Fenton's reaction) is facilitated. This may occur when H_2O_2 comes into contact with the reduced form of copper (Cu^+).

Although various experimental treatments have been tried, the only clinically proven treatment now available for spinal cord trauma is the administration of methylprednisolone (MP). MP sodium succinate (MPSS), a water-soluble derivative of MP, is usually used in animal experiments and in humans. MPSS may improve neurologic outcome through its anti-inflammatory effect while activating glucocorticoid receptors (132). The application of MPSS reduces lipid hydrolysis and peroxidation in response to experimental SCI (124, 133, 134); it was further revealed that MPSS blocked the pathways for producing toxic prostaglandin $F_{2\alpha}$ ($PGF_{2\alpha}$) and $PGF_{2\alpha}$-induced hydroxyl radical formation during spinal cord impact.

In previous studies, other antioxidants showed a modest effect. Vitamin E delayed onset, but did not extend survival, in ALS mouse models (135). Recent studies with vitamin E indicate that high doses can slow the progression of Alzheimer's disease (136). The brain possesses a very effective system of vitamin E recycling through ascorbate- and ascorbate/GSH-dependent pathways (137). Dehydroascorbate, the oxidized form of vitamin C, increases glutathione levels through stimulation of the pentose phosphate pathway (138). A carboxyfullerent having antioxidant properties, continuously infused, prolonged the survival of mice having a high-expressing strain of ALS by around 8 days, and no effects on tissue oxidative stress were demonstrated (139). Stobadine is an effective scavenger of hydroxyl, peroxyl, and alkoxyl radicals and an effective quencher of a singlet of oxygen. The antioxidant effect of stobadine has been demonstrated in spinal cord homogenates (140). The nitrone-based antioxidant phenyl-N-tert-butylnitrone (PBN) has been found to be efficacious in preventing ischemia and reperfusion injury, septic shock, and other trauma.

The tripeptide glutathione (GSH) is known to scavenge both inorganic and organic peroxides. In addition, it regenerates vitamin E from the vitamin E radical (141, 142). Astrocytic GSH peroxidase activity is 3.5-fold higher than its neuronal counterpart (143). It suggests that the cytoplasm of astrocytes is better able than neurons to metabolize hydrogen peroxide at the expense of GSH. In normal cells, the availability of cysteine is a limiting factor in GSH production. By providing this amino acid, N-acetylcysteine (NAC) clinicians can substantially increase intracellular GSH levels (144). The promotion of de novo GSH synthesis is critical, because the glutathione (GSSG) that is oxidized after SCI forms glutathiyl-protein adducts, which are no longer available to be reduced back to GSH. Evidence supporting this is reported by Kamencic et al. (145), who state that promoting GSH synthesis after SCI decreases secondary damage. In the case of SCI, spinal cord neurons can be exposed to high concentrations of arachidonic acid (AA) because of the release of a free fatty acid, 4-hydroxynonenal (HNE). HNE is one of the major biologically active products of AA peroxidation (146). Malecki reported that pretreating spinal cord neurons with NAC or ebselen, a molecule with GSH peroxidase–like activity, reduced the cytotoxic effect of HNE. Ebselen shows protection in clinical stroke and subarachnoid hemorrhage. It can consume hydrogen peroxide and is regenerated by GSH. GSH peroxidase, thioredoxin reductase, and selenoprotein P have been shown to play a potential role in protection against peroxynitrite (147). Overexpression of GSH peroxidase has been shown to increase the resistance of cortical neurons to amyloid beta-peptide-mediated neurotoxicity (148).

Previous studies indicate that impaired mitochondrial function, ROS, and lipid peroxidation occur soon after SCI, whereas the compensatory activation of catalase and GSH levels occurs at later times (149). Therefore, therapeutic strategies aimed at facilitating the actions of antioxidant enzymes or inhibiting ROS formation and lipid peroxidation in the CNS may prove beneficial in treating SCI.

Intracellular Signaling Manipulators: Preventing Injury and Promoting Growth

Not until the last decade have we learned how intracellular mediators work in response to the many diffusible and substrate-bound factors vital to cell survival and axonal growth. By altering the intracellular signals that a cell uses to transduce responses to injury-causing or growth-inhibiting substrates, cell death after SCI might be prevented. After SCI, necrosis occurs during the acute phase and is followed by apoptosis in the latent injured spinal cord. Hence, developing apoptosis-preventing strategies should be worthwhile. Several transcription factors such as fas, p53, c-Jun, bax, and bcl-2 are involved in apoptotic pathways (150). By blocking the ionic changes that occur near the cell, apoptotic cell death can be inhibited through an increase in protease inhibitors that block the downstream effectors of cell death signals (151) or up-regulation of antiapoptotic genes (152). Additionally, manipulation of growth-related intracellular factors such as growth-associated proteins, Ca^{2+} concentrations, transcription factors, and second messengers such as the cyclic nucleotides and inositol triphosphate also appears to have some beneficial effects (153–157). One hypothesis to identify the mechanism of either growth promotion or inhibition via various ligand receptor systems is suggested by the studies on intracellular concentrations of cAMP and cyclic GMP (cGMP) (158, 159). It appears that raising intracellular cyclic nucleotide concentrations is sufficient to convert an inhibitory response to a promotional one (160). The modification of intracellular responses has the benefit of generating a broad and generalized response from the cell. However, this application should be modified with specified measures in accordance with tissue and time, to prevent adverse systemic side effects such as a release of Ca^{2+} channel blockers and cyclic nucleotide analog, which can be lethal when systemically applied (160).

Trophic Factors: Supporting Axonal Growth

The limited regrowth of injured nerve fibers in the mammalian CNS has been known since the turn of the century. This regenerative failure is thought to be caused by lack of trophic substances and lack of permissiveness in the immediate microenvironment supporting axonal regrowth (161). Despite extensive animal experimentation in various SCI models and the grafting of various cell and tissue types, significant functional recovery in adult animals after complete transection has not been achieved (162). Recently, however, the astounding developments in molecular biology, particularly the expanding knowledge regarding growth factors and neurotrophic factors and their receptors in the CNS, allow us to develop a slightly more positive view regarding the possibilities of reaching the ultimate goal of repairing the damaged spinal cord.

The role of neurotrophic factors during neuronal development is well known. In SCI, regeneration can only occur if the involved neurons survive after axotomy. Recent studies indicate that neurotrophic factors also play a significant role in the development of the adult nervous system and help to increase the chance of survival after axotomy (163). Researchers have thus investigated opportunities to use neurotrophic growth factors to enhance cell survival. At the Miami Project to Cure Paralysis (164), tissue cultures with basic fibroblast growth factor (bFGF) have been shown to protect against damage from both glutamate and free radicals. In animal studies, bFGF decreases the size of injuries caused by trauma or loss of blood flow (165) and improves locomotor function via axonal regeneration in the transected rat spinal cord (166). Acidic fibroblast growth factor (aFGF) is a normal constituent of the spinal cord, expressed in motor neurons and primary sensory neurons (167, 168). Because aFGF lacks a signal sequence, it is thought to be sequestered within synthesizing cells, perhaps reaching the extracellular milieu only after damage to the cell membrane. Consequently, aFGF may be involved in repair after tissue damage (169, 170). It has been shown that aFGF prevents a die-back phenomenon of the corticospinal tract and promotes its sprouting and regeneration across the injured site after complete thoracic cord transection in adult rats, using Schwann cell guidance channels or peripheral nerve grafts (44).

Trophic factors from the NGF family, such as neurotrophins, rescue immature and mature axotomized CNS neurons from retrograde cell death (44). Several studies suggest that neurotrophins may have influences on both the survival and gene expression of the axotomized neurons and thus shift intracellu-

lar balance from growth restriction toward regeneration (44). The application of neurotrophins alone, or together with nerve grafts, increases the expression of regeneration-associated genes such as c-Jun, GAP-43, and Ta1-tubulin (171–173). In terms of axonal regeneration across complete transection of the spinal cord, no evidence for long-tract regeneration in adults has yet been demonstrated using neurotrophins (174–176). Studies in hemisected spinal cords have shown that increases in neurotrophin levels within tissue using neurotrophic factors (44) or factor-producing fibroblasts (177, 178) may facilitate the regeneration of descending tracts. In these studies, tract tracing has shown axons that regenerated around the lesion site and several millimeters into the target region, with a correlated improvement in behavior. However, when hemisection is conducted, other possible mechanisms beyond authentic regeneration from the injured tracts, such as axonal sprouting of noninjured axons, activation of redundant pathways, and alterations in the receptor number or phenotype and excitability of surviving neurons or glia, cannot be excluded. In addition to FGFs and neurotrophins, other trophic factors may also be important for the survival and regeneration of an injured spinal cord (179, 180). They include ciliary neurotrophic factor (CNTF), epidermal growth factor (EGF), glial-derived neurotrophic factor (GDNF), platelet-derived growth factor (PDGF), insulin-like growth factor (IGF), and vascular endothelial growth factor (VEGF).

RECONNECTIONS WITHIN THE INJURED SITE: NEURAL REGENERATION ENHANCEMENT STRATEGIES

Although at present the complete repair of the SCI remains a distant prospect, a number of experimental treatments have demonstrated partial return of function from spinal cord levels immediately below the injury (Table 68.1). Full recovery in the damaged spinal cord is hindered by the limited ability of the CNS to replace lost cells, repair damaged myelin, regenerate long-tract axons, and reestablish functional neural connections (35). However, improved functional recovery can be obtained by forced use or specific training (181), which increases the regenerative capabilities of injured axons and promotes plastic reorganization of the cortical circuits involved in the control of the disrupted behavior (182). Repair processes in the injured nervous system are aimed at rewiring or replacing the interrupted connections through boosting intrinsic/extrinsic neuronal regeneration of severed axons or structural reorganization of spared neurites. These strategies rely on the main methodological approaches described below, including reducing the inhibitory environment; promoting CNS regeneration by peripheral axotomy; treating demyelination; and offering immune-based therapies, gene-based therapies, and nerve graft therapies. Neurotrophic factors and pharmacologic approaches may be pursued as well.

Overcoming Environmental Barriers: Traversing Scar Tissue with Neural Bridges

Scar formation is a natural reaction of the lesioned CNS tissue and one of the major impediments to neural repair (75). Attempts to prevent it have not been successful, although previous data have shown that a reduction in scar formation is accompanied by the regeneration of numerous corticospinal axons and notable functional motor recovery (183, 184). Scar formation is

Table 68.1   Function Recoveries through Neuroregenerative Strategies in SCI Rodent Models

A variety of approaches, such as reduction of inhibitory factors and combination therapies, have been investigated in different SCI rodent models including contusion, T-shape lesion, complete transection, and hemisection. Differential benefits of functional outcome, such as partial recovery of motor, bladder, and sensory function, have been demonstrated after application of different treatments.

RECOVERY STRATEGIES	SCI MODEL	FUNCTIONAL OUTCOME
Reduction of inhibitory factors		
Delayed Nogo receptor therapy	Contusion	Motor
Nogo A antibody	T-shape lesion	Motor
Chondroitinase ABC	Contusion	Motor/bladder
EGFR inhibitor	Contusion	Motor/sensory/bladder
Semaphorin3A inhibitor	Complete transection	Motor
RGMa	Hemisection	Motor
Combination therapies		
OEC with FK506	Complete transection	Motor
OEC/SC/Chondroitinase ABC	Complete transection	Motor
HUCBC/ BDNF	Contusion	Motor
Embryonic spinal tissue/rolipram	Hemisection	Motor
SC/rolipram	Contusion	Motor
MP/Nogo-66 receptor	Hemisection	Motor
BDNF/NT-3	Contusion	Motor/bladder

EGFR = epidermal growth factor receptor; RGMa = repulsive guidance molecule; HUCBC = human umbilical cord blood stem cell; NGRP = neuronal and glial restricted precursors; HESC-DOPC = human embryonic stem cell–derived oligodendrocyte progenitor cell; SC = Schwann cell; OEC = olfactory ensheathing cell; BDNF = brain-derived neutrophic factor; MP = methylprednisolone; NT-3 = neurotrophin-3.

associated with the creation of a nonpermissive biochemical environment containing specific inhibitory molecules, many of which are up-regulated following injury that can block neurite outgrowth (35). There have been many attempts to overcome these inhibitions by antibodies directed toward the Nogo protein (185), by using peptides that block the Nogo receptor or by genetically depleting the Nogo or Nogo66 receptor (186) in order to promote regenerative sprouting of the lesioned spinal cord (97, 187). Bridges that form a growth-permissive scaffold within the lesion site should greatly facilitate regenerative axon growth (93). Many types of cells, tissues, and artificial materials have been implanted as bridges into the injured spinal cord (188). The success of these experiments is limited, often because proliferating astrocytes form the barrier to restrict access of regenerating fibers to the implants. Fibrin or hydrogels loaded with growth factors that attract regenerating neurites and keep scar formation under control show promise in the repair of spinal cord tissues (189–191). The principal obstacle to be overcome with all of these material bridges is how to integrate them into the spinal cord tissue without inducing scar formation. This can be achieved by noninvasive low-dose X-ray irradiation (192), by injection of ethidium bromide into the lesion area to remove all proliferating cells generated in response to the CNS injury, or by injection of specific antibodies (193) or interleukin-10 (IL-10) (194) to remove those cytokines that promote scar formation. Bacterial chondroitinase ABC, applied at the site of injury, digests the glycosaminoglycan side chains of the CSPGs, up-regulated in glial scar tissue and inhibitory to axon growth, which promotes both axon regeneration and functional recovery in rats with partial

spinal transection (195, 196) and promotes both axon regeneration and plasticity in crush injury models (197). Attempts to limit the formation of the astrocytic scars with 7b-hydroxycholesterol-oleate, a cholesterol derivative (198), have proven successful not only in reducing astrocyte levels, but also in enhancing local sprouting in serotonergic axons below the lesion. Bridges that form a growth-permissive scaffold within the lesioned spinal cord should greatly facilitate regenerative axon growth across the injured area, leading to the growth of regenerative axons into the remaining intact parenchyma and to the return of substantial neurologic function.

Promoting CNS Regeneration: Peripheral Axotomy and Activating Growth Factors

Conditioning lesions have been primarily applied to boost regeneration of the central neurite of dorsal root ganglia neurons (12). Observations confirm that a lesion of the peripheral axon induces a strong regenerative response; paradoxically, transection of central axons does not (199). Some have suggested that the CNS cell body responses, triggered by a peripheral axotomy, could enhance the intrinsic growth capacity and sustain the regeneration of the central neurite (12). The growth-promoting action of peripheral axotomy is associated with recruitment of macrophages in dorsal root ganglia (200) as well as trophic factors released by PNS tissue. The outcome of this priming lesion can be efficiently mimicked by injection of inflammogens or macrophages in the intact ganglia (201). Direct application of cAMP (202) or IL-6 (203) to the ganglia mimics the conditioning lesions by activating growth factor expression and enhancing regeneration of the central neurite (204). However, the timing of the priming lesion is critical, as the effective regeneration is induced only by priming lesions made before SCI, which definitely has no clinical utility, and a priming lesion made after SCI generally results in an abortive regenerative response (205, 206).

Restoring Conduction along Demyelinated Axons: Remyelination and Restoration of Action Potential/Conduction

Many CNS nerve fibers are insulated by a myelin sheath. Local demyelination often occurs in surviving bundles of nerve fibers at the spinal cord lesion (207, 208), leading to disruption of electrical impulse conductivity due to the malfunctions of sodium and potassium channels and the inhibitory influences of Nogo-A, MAG, and Omgp (35). The adult spinal cord seems unable to efficiently replace either lost myelin or lost oligodendrocytes (93). However, the presence of conduction deficits in myelinated fibers raises the possibility that chronic SCI might be treated by improving the function of surviving nerve fibers, even in the absence of regeneration (209). Neural stem cells primed with a growth factor cocktail to become oligodendrocytes have thus been implanted into injured spinal cords in order to promote remyelination in adult rats (210–212). Current efforts continue to focus on blocking Nogo-A and other growth-inhibitory molecules by applying antibodies against these molecules, by blocking the receptors to which they bind, or by pharmacologically manipulating the downstream signaling pathways induced by these inhibitory molecules in growing neurites (213, 214). Two approaches are in clinical development. The first is pharmacologic treatment with 4-aminopyridine, or fampridine, a potassium channel blocker that can restore action potential conduction in demyelinated, or partially myelinated, axons in the injured spinal cord (215). This can lead to a modest improvement of motor and sensory function. Large-scale human trials of the drug have already begun. The extent of benefit provided to an individual will be expected to rely on the particular surviving pathways within the spinal cord and the states of myelination. A more challenging, though possibly permanent, method of treating demyelination may be through the cellular transplantation of oligodendrocytes, Schwann cells, or neural stem cells, which could be primed to become oligodendrocytes or Schwann cells (211, 212). Repair of the demyelination and restoration of electrical conductivity in nerve fibers would enable patients to make much better use of their surviving nerve tracts (93).

Immune-based Therapies: Modulating the Inflammatory Response and Supporting Injured Neurons

The immune system plays important roles in neural cell repair, removal of cellular debris, and tissue healing after acute spinal cord SCI. The early inflammatory response starts with invasion of neutrophils, which can be unfavorable for injured nerve cell survival. This is followed by a response of the resident innate immune cells (microglia), but these cannot supply all the needs of the damaged tissue. Moreover, once evoked, and for as long as the damage persists, the microglial response remains beyond

the capacity of the CNS to tolerate it (216). One study has shown that poor macrophage response can cause regeneration in the spinal cord (217). Augmenting the endogenous inflammatory response with grafts of activated macrophages that had been preincubated in the presence of peripheral nervous (PN) tissue (218, 219) elicited regeneration in an optic nerve injury model. Other studies also have shown that activated macrophages may be capable of enhancing regeneration in the CNS (83). The details of how the continued regenerative response is sustained have not been explained. However, the lengthy processes of cell purification and expansion of autologous cells limits the cell transplant techniques that can be used in acute injuries unless cell lines or cells from donors are used (35). Therefore, there is an interest in designing cell-free grafts of biocompatible bridging materials that can be positioned within the injury site to control inflammatory and glial reactions and promote axonal regeneration (220). The substrate required will ideally be easily manipulated, exhibit immuno-tolerance, possess a porous scaffold to enable nerve regeneration and cell repopulation, and be easily integrated into the CNS (35). Fibrin, or freeze-dried alginate, gels loaded with growth factors that attract regenerating neurites and keep scar formation under control, show much promise in this respect and are attractive options because of their reabsorbable properties (221). In addition, rapidly absorbable substrates such as poly-a-hydroxyacids, vinyl chloride, and acrylonitrile porous tubes are currently being tested in the transected spinal cord (222) with some success, although there are some concerns over mechanical hindrance.

Therapies and Neurotrophic Factors: Promoting Neuroprotection and Neuroregeneration

The neurotrophic factors contribute to recovery of function by producing increased trophic activity after acute SCI. These neurotrophic factors promote axonal growth and prevent cellular death (223). One class of neurotrophic factors is the neurotrophin family. Several neurotrophins, including nerve growth factor (NGF), BDNF, and neurotrophin 3 (NT-3), show their capacity for supporting the survival of neurons after SCI both in vitro and in vivo. Moreover, they facilitate and guide neurite outgrowth and reestablish the network of the injured CNS. The mechanisms of the neurotrophins' effects are through specific high-affinity Trk receptors (Trk A, B, C) and through a common low-affinity receptor designated p75NGFR. The other class of neurotrophic factors also includes recovery-promoting polypeptides, such as the heparin-binding growth factors aFGF and bFGF. Normally, aFGF is produced in the spinal cord by motor neurons and primary sensory neurons (224). In studies using a rat model, aFGF was demonstrated to promote axonal regeneration and reduce death of neurons after spinal cord injury (45, 225). Within the injured neocortex, aFGF has been shown to induce NGF production, and NGF has been shown to promote the growth of adult axons across reactive scar tissue in the brain and spinal cord (226). Also, aFGF may down-regulate the expression of, or allow axons to overcome, the known inhibitors of axon regeneration such as proteoglycan (227) or tenascins (65). In addition to the regeneration effects of neurotrophic factors mentioned above, other molecules have been shown to boost intrinsic neuronal growth potentialities when applied systemically or locally to the injured nerve cells (12).

A number of promising pharmacologic therapies are currently under investigation for neuroprotective abilities in animal models of SCI (228). These include methylprednisolone, 21-aminosteroids, gangliosides (GM-1), the sodium channel blocker riluzole, the calcium channel blocker Nimodipine, calpain antagonists CEP-4143, the tetracycline derivative minocycline, the fusogen copolymer polyethylene glycol (PEG), and the tissue-protective hormone erythropoietin (EPO). Moreover, clinical trials investigate the putative neuroprotective and neuroregenerative properties for the Rho pathway antagonist Cethrin® (BioAxone Therapeutic, Inc.) and for implantation of activated autologous macrophages (ProCord®, Proneuron Biotechnologies) in patients with cervical and thoracic SCI. These studies will lead to a new era in translational clinical trials to repair SCI (12, 229). Therefore, improving drug treatment strategies aimed at attenuating early trauma-induced pathophysiology will be of great clinical value for the victims of SCI, especially in acute cases (35).

Gene-based Therapies: Transplants that Promote Increased Neurotrophin Synthesis at Lesion Sites

Growth-associated genes have been stably overexpressed in neurons with a variety of different techniques. For example, methods such as generation of transgenic animals and virus-mediated gene transfer (230) can locally produce growth factors where they are needed. Implanting cells engineered to secrete these factors directly into the lesion site (93) in order to repair an injured spinal cord (12) is effective as well. Spontaneous sprouting, but not regeneration (231), has been obtained in vitro by inducing expression of different integrins (232) or SPRR1A (233) and in vivo by overexpressing either GAP-43 or CAP-23 (234) in transgenic mice. These results indicate that up-regulation of individual genes may enhance axon plasticity but may not be sufficient to induce a full switch to the axon elongating mode.

CONCLUSIONS

Exciting advances are occurring in the field of neural regeneration for the treatment of the injured CNS. An increased understanding of CNS development, the nature of neuronal injury, the mechanisms that cause neuronal death and malfunctions, and the factors that direct or facilitate neuronal/axonal regeneration demonstrates that neuronal injury can be treated more effectively clinically. However, as reports of functional regeneration become more numerous, it is important to critically evaluate the mechanisms of the observed functional changes and to clinically challenge the interpretation of in vivo regeneration in animal models as well as to carefully pattern the clinical trials. For example, one difficult challenge is to successfully translate the same techniques used in animal models to human patients. The current concerns center around ensuring reproducibility for animal experiments designed to promote regeneration following SCI and determining whether rodent animal models are sufficient or whether alternative large-animal models, such as dogs, cats, and even primates, are needed for evaluating treatments prior to applying them to humans. Also under discussion is the timeframe (acute or chronic) during which patients should be treated with specific interventions. Future technological advances will allow us to address many unanswered questions and identify the most promising therapeutic interventions for SCI patients. These endeavors and advances will make functional repair for SCI patients soon become attainable in clinical therapeutics.

References

1. Polak JM, Mantalaris S. Stem cells bioprocessing: an important mile stone to move regenerative medicine research into the clinical arena. *Pediatr Res* 2008; 63:461–466.
2. Chang YC, Shyu WC, Lin SZ, Li H. Regenerative therapy for stroke. *Cell Transplant* 2007; 16:171–181.
3. Hulsebosch CE. Recent advances in pathophysiology and treatment of spinal cord injury. *Adv Physiol Educ* 2002; 26:238–255.
4. Bareyre FM, Schwab ME. Inflammation, degeneration and regeneration in the injured spinal cord: insights from DNA microarrays. *Trends Neurosci* 2003; 26:555–563.
5. Kesslak JP, Keirstead HS. Assessment of behavior in animal models of spinal cord injury. *J Spinal Cord Med* 2003; 26:323–328.
6. Schallert T, Fleming SM, Leasure JL, Tillerson JL, Bland ST. CNS plasticity and assessment of forelimb sensorimotor outcome in unilateral rat models of stroke, cortical ablation, parkinsonism and spinal cord injury. *Neuropharmacology* 2000; 39:777–787.
7. Scheff SW, Rabchevsky AG, Fugaccia I, Main JA, Lumpp JE Jr. Experimental modeling of spinal cord injury: characterization of a force-defined injury device. *J Neurotrauma* 2003; 20:179–193.
8. Stokes BT, Jakeman LB. Experimental modelling of human spinal cord injury: a model that crosses the species barrier and mimics the spectrum of human cytopathology. *Spinal Cord* 2002; 40:101–109.
9. Young W. Spinal cord contusion models. *Prog Brain Res* 2002; 137:231–255.
10. Lim PA, Tow AM. Recovery and regeneration after spinal cord injury: a review and summary of recent literature. *Ann Acad Med Singapore* 2007; 36:49–57.
11. Chuckowree JA, Dickson TC, Vickers JC. Intrinsic regenerative ability of mature CNS neurons. *Neuroscientist* 2004; 10:280–285.
12. Rossi F, Gianola S, Corvetti L. Regulation of intrinsic neuronal properties for axon growth and regeneration. *Prog Neurobiol* 2007; 81:1–28.
13. Carmichael ST, Archibeque I, Luke L, Nolan T, et al. Growth-associated gene expression after stroke: evidence for a growth-promoting region in peri-infarct cortex. *Exp Neurol* 2005; 193:291–311.
14. Marklund N, Fulp CT, Shimizu S, Puri R, et al. Selective temporal and regional alterations of Nogo-A and small proline-rich repeat protein 1A (SPRR1A) but not Nogo-66 receptor (NgR) occur following traumatic brain injury in the rat. *Exp Neurol* 2006; 197:70–83.
15. Carmichael ST, Chesselet MF. Synchronous neuronal activity is a signal for axonal sprouting after cortical lesions in the adult. *J Neurosci* 2002; 22:6062–6070.
16. Gulino R, Dimartino M, Casabona A, Lombardo SA, Perciavalle V. Synaptic plasticity modulates the spontaneous recovery of locomotion after spinal cord hemisection. *Neurosci Res* 2007; 57:148–156.
17. Silver J, Miller JH. Regeneration beyond the glial scar. *Nat Rev Neurosci* 2004; 5:146–156.
18. Rhodes KE, Fawcett JW. Chondroitin sulphate proteoglycans: preventing plasticity or protecting the CNS? *J Anat* 2004; 204:33–48.
19. Calabrese EJ. Enhancing and regulating neurite outgrowth. *Crit Rev Toxicol* 2008; 38:391–418.
20. Little JW, Stiens SA. Electrodiagnosis in spinal cord injury. *New Developments in Electrodiagnostic Medicine* 1994; 5:571–593.
21. Nishimura Y, Onoe H, Morichika Y, Perfiliev S, et al. Time-dependent central compensatory mechanisms of finger dexterity after spinal cord injury. *Science* 2007; 318:1150–1155.
22. McKinney RA, Debanne D, Gahwiler BH, Thompson SM. Lesion-induced axonal sprouting and hyperexcitability in the hippocampus in vitro: implications for the genesis of posttraumatic epilepsy. *Nat Med* 1997; 3:990–996.
23. Salin P, Tseng GF, Hoffman S, Parada I, Prince DA. Axonal sprouting in layer V pyramidal neurons of chronically injured cerebral cortex. *J Neurosci* 1995; 15:8234–8245.
24. Kruitbosch JM, Schouten EJ, Tan IY, Veendrick-Meekes MJ, de Vocht JW. Cervical spinal cord injuries in patients with refractory epilepsy. *Seizure* 2006; 15:633–636.

25. Kalous A, Osborne PB, Keast JR. Acute and chronic changes in dorsal horn innervation by primary afferents and descending supraspinal pathways after spinal cord injury. *J Comp Neurol* 2007; 504:238–253.

26. Cafferty WB, McGee AW, Strittmatter SM. Axonal growth therapeutics: regeneration or sprouting or plasticity? *Trends Neurosci* 2008; 31: 215–220.

27. Beck H, Yaari Y. Plasticity of intrinsic neuronal properties in CNS disorders. *Nat Rev Neurosci* 2008; 9:357–369.

28. Tator CH, Fehlings MG. Review of the secondary injury theory of acute spinal cord trauma with emphasis on vascular mechanisms. *J Neurosurg* 1991; 75:15–26.

29. Behrmann DL, Bresnahan JC, Beattie MS, Shah BR. Spinal cord injury produced by consistent mechanical displacement of the cord in rats: behavioral and histologic analysis. *J Neurotrauma* 1992; 9:197–217.

30. Banik NL, Hogan EL, Hsu CY. The multimolecular cascade of spinal cord injury: studies on prostanoids, calcium, and proteinases. *Neurochem Pathol* 1987; 7:57–77.

31. Wallace MC, Tator CH, Lewis AJ. Chronic regenerative changes in the spinal cord after cord compression injury in rats. *Surg Neurol* 1987; 27:209–219.

32. Guizar-Sahagun G, Grijalva I, Madrazo I, Franco-Bourland R, Salgado H, Ibarra A, Oliva E, Zepeda A. Development of post-traumatic cysts in the spinal cord of rats-subjected to severe spinal cord contusion. *Surg Neurol* 1994; 41:241–249.

33. Bunge RP, Puckett WR, Becerra JL, Marcillo A, Quencer RM. Observations on the pathology of human spinal cord injury. A review and classification of 22 new cases with details from a case of chronic cord compression with extensive focal demyelination. *Adv Neurol* 1993; 59:75–89.

34. Tator CH, Rowed DW. Current concepts in the immediate management of acute spinal cord injuries. *Can Med Assoc J* 1979; 121:1453–1464.

35. Verma P, Fawcett J. Spinal cord regeneration. *Adv Biochem Eng Biotechnol* 2005; 94:43–66.

36. Tian DS, Xie MJ, Yu ZY, Zhang Q, et al. Cell cycle inhibition attenuates microglia induced inflammatory response and alleviates neuronal cell death after spinal cord injury in rats. *Brain Res* 2007; 1135:177–185.

37. Berdan RC, Easaw JC, Wang R. Alterations in membrane potential after axotomy at different distances from the soma of an identified neuron and the effect of depolarization on neurite outgrowth and calcium channel expression. *J Neurophysiol* 1993; 69:151–164.

38. Sattler R, Tymianski M, Feyaz I, Hafner M, Tator CH. Voltage-sensitive calcium channels mediate calcium entry into cultured mammalian sympathetic neurons following neurite transection. *Brain Res* 1996; 719:239–246.

39. Chu GK, Tator CH. Calcium influx is necessary for optimal regrowth of transected neurites of rat sympathetic ganglion neurons in vitro. *Neuroscience* 2001; 102:945–957.

40. Crowe MJ, Bresnahan JC, Shuman SL, Masters JN, Beattie MS. Apoptosis and delayed degeneration after spinal cord injury in rats and monkeys. *Nat Med* 1997; 3:73–76.

41. Salgado-Ceballos H, Guizar-Sahagun G, Feria-Velasco A, Grijalva I, et al. Spontaneous long-term remyelination after traumatic spinal cord injury in rats. *Brain Res* 1998; 782:126–135.

42. Norenberg MD, Smith J, Marcillo A. The pathology of human spinal cord injury: defining the problems. *J Neurotrauma* 2004; 21:429–440.

43. Schnell L, Schneider R, Kolbeck R, Barde YA, Schwab ME. Neurotrophin-3 enhances sprouting of corticospinal tract during development and after adult spinal cord lesion. *Nature* 1994; 367:170–173.

44. Bregman BS, Kunkel-Bagden E, Schnell L, Dai HN, et al. Recovery from spinal cord injury mediated by antibodies to neurite growth inhibitors. *Nature* 1995; 378:498–501.

45. Cheng H, Cao Y, Olson L. Spinal cord repair in adult paraplegic rats: partial restoration of hind limb function. *Science* 1996; 273:510–513.

46. Nygren LG, Fuxe K, Jonsson G, Olson L. Functional regeneration of 5-hydroxytryptamine nerve terminals in the rat spinal cord following 5,6-dihydroxytryptamine induced degeneration. *Brain Res* 1974; 78: 377–394.

47. Cheng H, Olson L. A new surgical technique that allows proximodistal regeneration of 5-HT fibers after complete transection of the rat spinal cord. *Exp Neurol* 1995; 136:149–161.

48. Kuang RZ, Merline M, Kalil K. Topographic specificity of corticospinal connections formed in explant coculture. *Development* 1994; 120: 1937–1947.

49. Siegal JD, Kliot M, Smith GM, Silver J. A comparison of the regeneration potential of dorsal root fibers into gray or white matter of the adult rat spinal cord. *Exp Neurol* 1990; 109:90–97.

50. Cullheim S, Thams S. The microglial networks of the brain and their role in neuronal network plasticity after lesion. *Brain Res Rev* 2007; 55:89–96.

51. Okado N, Oppenheim RW. The onset and development of descending pathways to the spinal cord in the chick embryo. *J Comp Neurol* 1985; 232:143–161.

52. Jhaveri S, Erzurumlu RS, Friedman B, Schneider GE. Oligodendrocytes and myelin formation along the optic tract of the developing hamster: an immunohistochemical study using the Rip antibody. *Glia* 1992; 6:138–148.

53. McMahon SB, Kett-White R. Sprouting of peripherally regenerating primary sensory neurones in the adult central nervous system. *J Comp Neurol* 1991; 304:307–315.

54. Devor M. Neuroplasticity in the rearrangement of olfactory tract fibers after neonatal transection in hamsters. *J Comp Neurol* 1976; 166:49–72.

55. Cotman CW, Nieto-Sampedro M, Harris EW. Synapse replacement in the nervous system of adult vertebrates. *Physiol Rev* 1981; 61:684–784.

56. Raisman G, Field PM. A quantitative investigation of the development of collateral reinnervation after partial deafferentation of the septal nuclei. *Brain Res* 1973; 50:241–264.

57. McKerracher L, David S, Jackson DL. Identification of myelin associated glycoprotein as a major myelin derived inhibitor of neurite growth. *Neuron* 1994; 13:805–811.

58. Tang S, Woodhall RW, Shen YJ, deBellard ME, et al. Soluble myelin-associated glycoprotein (MAG) found in vivo inhibits axonal regeneration. *Mol Cell Neurosci* 1997; 9:333–346.

59. Paino CL, Bunge MB. Induction of axon growth into Schwann cell implants grafted into lesioned adult rat spinal cord. *Exp Neurol* 1991; 114:254–257.

60. Bunge MB, Pearse DD. Transplantation strategies to promote repair of the injured spinal cord. *J Rehabil Res Dev* 2003; 40:55–62.

61. Schwab ME, Kapfhammer JP, Bandtlow CE. Inhibitors of neurite growth. *Annu Rev Neurosci* 1993; 16:565–595.

62. Aguayo A, David S, Bary G. Influence of the glial environment on the elongation of axons after injury: transplantation studies in adult rodents. *J Exp Biol* 1981; 95:231–240.

63. Savio T, Schwab ME. Lesioned corticospinal tract axons regenerate in myelin-free rat spinal cord. *Proc Natl Acad Sci U S A* 1990; 87: 4130–4133.

64. Schwab ME. Myelin associated inhibitors of neurite growth and regeneration in the CNS. *Trends Neurosci* 1990; 13:452–456.

65. Fawcett JW, Asher RA. The glial scar and central nervous system repair. *Brain Res Bull* 1999; 49:377–391.

66. Logan A, Berry M, Gonzalez AM, Frautschy SA, et al. Effects of transforming growth factor beta 1 on scar production in the injured central nervous system of the rat. *Eur J Neurosci* 1994; 6:355–363.

67. Snow DM, Lemmon V, Carrino DA, Caplan AI, Silver J. Sulfated proteoglycans in astroglial barriers inhibit neurite outgrowth in vitro. *Exp Neurol* 1990; 109:111–130.

68. Dow KE, Ethell DW, Steeves JD, Riopelle RJ. Molecular correlates of spinal cord repair in the embryonic chick: heparin sulfate and chondroitin sulfate proteoglycans. *Exp Neurol* 1994; 128:233–238.

69. Ridet JL, Malhotra SK, Privat A, Gage FH. Reactive astrocytes: cellular and molecular cues to biological function. *Trends Neurosci* 1997; 20: 570–577.

70. Snow DM, Letourneau PC. Neurite outgrowth on a step gradient of chondroitin sulfate proteoglycan (CS-PG). *J Neurobiol* 1992; 23: 322–336.

71. Hatten ME, Liem RK, Shelanski ML, Mason CA. Astroglia in CNS injury. *Glia* 1991; 4:233–243.

72. Svensson M, Eriksson P, Persson JK, Molander C, et al. The response of central glia to peripheral nerve injury. *Brain Res Bull* 1993; 30: 499–506.

73. Svensson M, Mattsson P, Aldskogius H. A bromodeoxyuridine labelling study of proliferating cells in the brainstem following hypoglossal nerve transection. *J Anat* 1994; 185(Pt 3):537–542.

74. Fitch MT, Doller C, Combs CK, Landreth GE, Silver J. Cellular and molecular mechanisms of glial scarring and progressive cavitation: in vivo and in vitro analysis of inflammation-induced secondary injury after CNS trauma. *J Neurosci* 1999; 19:8182–8198.

75. Caroni P, Schwab ME. Antibody against myelin-associated inhibitor of neurite growth neutralizes nonpermissive substrate properties of CNS white matter. *Neuron* 1988; 1:85–96.

76. Hagg T, Oudega M. Degenerative and spontaneous regenerative processes after spinal cord injury. *J Neurotrauma* 2006; 23:264–280.

77. Dusart I, Ghoumari A, Wehrle R, Morel MP, et al. Cell death and axon regeneration of Purkinje cells after axotomy: challenges of classical hypotheses of axon regeneration. *Brain Res Rev* 2005; 49: 300–316.

78. Liuzzi FJ, Lasek RJ. Astrocytes block axonal regeneration in mammals by activating the physiological stop pathway. *Science* 1987; 237: 642–645.

79. Tessier-Lavigne M. Eph receptor tyrosine kinases, axon repulsion, and the development of topographic maps. *Cell* 1995; 82:345–348.

80. Davies SJ, Fitch MT, Memberg SP, Hall AK, et al. Regeneration of adult axons in white matter tracts of the central nervous system. *Nature* 1997; 390:680–683.

81. McKeon RJ, Schreiber RC, Rudge JS, Silver J. Reduction of neurite outgrowth in a model of glial scarring following CNS injury is correlated with the expression of inhibitory molecules on reactive astrocytes. *J Neurosci* 1991; 11:3398–3411.

82. Fawcett J. Astrocytes and axon regeneration in the central nervous system. *J Neurol* 1994; 242:S25–S28.

83. Rapalino O, Lazarov-Spiegler O, Agranoc E. Implantation of stimulated homologous macrophages results in partial recovery of paraplegic rats. *Nat Med* 1998; 4:814–821.

84. Fitch MT, Silver J. Glial cell extracellular matrix: boundaries for axon growth in development and regeneration. *Cell Tissue Res* 1997; 290: 379–384.

85. Norenberg MD. Astrocyte responses to CNS injury. *J Neuropathol Exp Neurol* 1994; 53:213–220.

86. Fitch MT, Silver J. Activated macrophages and the blood brain barrier: inflammation after CNS injury leads to increase in putative inhibitory molecules. *Exp Neurol* 1997; 148:587–603.

87. Kawaja MD, Gage FH. Reactive astrocytes are substrates for the growth of adult CNS axons in the presence of elevated levels of nerve growth factor. *Neuron* 1991; 7:1019–1030.

88. Kliot M, Smith GM, Siegal JD, Silver J. Astrocyte-polymer implants promote regeneration of dorsal root fibers into the adult mammalian spinal cord. *Exp Neurol* 1990; 109:57–69.

89. Bartsch S, Husmann K, Schachner M, Bartsch U. The extracellular matrix molecule tenascin: expression in the developing chick retinotectal system and substrate properties for retinal ganglion cell neurites in vitro. *Eur J Neurosci* 1995; 7:907–916.

90. Nishi R. Neurotrophic factors: two are better than one. *Science* 1994; 265:1052–1053.

91. Schaar DG, Sieber BA, Dreyfus CF, Black IB. Regional and cell-specific expression of GDNF in rat brain. *Exp Neurol* 1993; 124:368–371.

92. Schmidt-Kastner R, Tomac A, Hoffer B, Bektesh S, et al. Glial cell–line derived neurotrophic factor (GDNF) mRNA upregulation in striatum and cortical areas after pilocarpine-induced status epilepticus in rats. *Brain Res Mol Brain Res* 1994; 26:325–330.

93. Schwab ME. Repairing the injured spinal cord. *Science* 2002; 295: 1029–1031.

94. Brosamle C, Huber A, Fiedler M, Skerra A, Schwab ME. Regeneration of lesioned corticospinal tract fibers in the adult rat induced by a recombinant, humanized IN-1 antibody fragment. *J Neurosci* 2000; 20: 8061–8068.

95. Brittis PA, Flanagan JG. Nogo domains and a Nogo receptor: implications for axon regeneration. *Neuron* 2001; 30:11–14.

96. Metz GA, Antonow-Schlorke I, Witte OW. Motor improvements after focal cortical ischemia in adult rats are mediated by compensatory mechanisms. *Behav Brain Res* 2005; 162:71–82.

97. Wieloch T, Nikolich K. Mechanisms of neural plasticity following brain injury. *Curr Opin Neurobiol* 2006; 16:258–264.

98. Raineteau O, Schwab ME. Plasticity of motor systems after incomplete spinal cord injury. *Nat Rev Neurosci* 2001; 2:263–273.

99. Little JW, Burns SP, James JJ, Stiens SA. Neurologic recovery and neurologic decline after spinal cord injury. *Topics in Spinal Cord Injury Medicine* 2000; 11:73–89.

100. Fouad K, Pedersen V, Schwab ME, Brosamle C. Cervical sprouting of corticospinal fibers after thoracic spinal cord injury accompanies shifts in evoked motor responses. *Curr Biol* 2001; 11:1766–1770.

101. Raineteau O, Fouad K, Noth P, Thallmair M, Schwab ME. Functional switch between motor tracts in the presence of the mAb IN-1 in the adult rat. *Proc Natl Acad Sci U S A* 2001; 98:6929–6934.

102. Johansson BB. Regeneration and plasticity in the brain and spinal cord. *J Cereb Blood Flow Metab* 2007; 27:1417–1430.

103. Spencer T, Filbin MT. A role for cAMP in regeneration of the adult mammalian CNS. *J Anat* 2004; 204:49–55.

104. David S, Aguayo AJ. Axonal elongation into peripheral nervous system "bridges" after central nervous system injury in adult rats. *Science* 1981; 214:931–933.

105. Hill CE, Beattie MS, Bresnahan JC. Degeneration and sprouting of identified descending supraspinal axons after contusive spinal cord injury in the rat. *Exp Neurol* 2001; 171:153–169.

106. Li Y, Raisman G. Sprouts from cut corticospinal axons persist in the presence of astrocytic scarring in long-term lesions of the adult rat spinal cord. *Exp Neurol* 1995; 134:102–111.

107. Ramon-Cueto A, Cordero MI, Santos-Benito FF, Avila J. Functional recovery of paraplegic rats and motor axon regeneration in their spinal cords by olfactory ensheathing glia. *Neuron* 2000; 25:425–435.

108. Zhang ZG, Zhang L, Jiang Q, Zhang R, et al. VEGF enhances angiogenesis and promotes blood-brain barrier leakage in the ischemic brain. *J Clin Invest* 2000; 106:829–838.

109. Anderson DK, Hall ED. Pathophysiology of spinal cord trauma. *Ann Emerg Med* 1993; 22:987–992.

110. Juurlink BH, Paterson PG. Review of oxidative stress in brain and spinal cord injury: suggestion for pharmacological and nutritional management strategies. *J Spinal Cord Med* 1998; 21:309–334.

111. Lipton SA, Choi YB, Pan ZH, Lei SZ, et al. A redox-based mechanism for the neuroprotective and neurodestructive effects of nitric oxide and related nitroso-compounds. *Nature* 1993; 364:626–632.

112. Iadecola C. Bright and dark sides of nitric oxide in ischemic brain injury. *Trends Neurosci* 1997; 20:132–139.

113. Feil R, Kleppisch T. NO/cGMP-dependent modulation of synaptic transmission. *Handb Exp Pharmacol* 2008; 529–560.

114. Huang Z, Huang PL, Panahian N, Dalkara T, et al. Effects of cerebral ischemia in mice deficient in neuronal nitric oxide synthase. *Science* 1994; 265:1883–1885.

115. Wu W, Li L. Inhibition of nitric oxide synthase reduces motoneuron death due to spinal root avulsion. *Neurosci Lett* 1993; 153:121–124.

116. Dora CD, Koch S, Sanchez A, Ruenes G, et al. Intraspinal injection of adenosine agonists protect against L-NAME induced neuronal loss in the rat. *J Neurotrauma* 1998; 15:473–483.

117. Freeman BA, Crapo JD. Biology of disease: free radicals and tissue injury. *Lab Invest* 1982; 47:412–426.

118. Halliwell B. Free radicals, antioxidants, and human disease: curiosity, cause, or consequence? *Lancet* 1994; 344:721–724.

119. Lopez-Vales R, Garcia-Alias G, Guzman-Lenis MS, Fores J, et al. Effects of COX-2 and iNOS inhibitors alone or in combination with olfactory ensheathing cell grafts after spinal cord injury. *Spine* 2006; 31: 1100–1106.

120. Deng HX, Hentati A, Tainer JA, Iqbal Z, et al. Amyotrophic lateral sclerosis and structural defects in Cu,Zn superoxide dismutase. *Science* 1993; 261:1047–1051.

121. Rowland LP. Amyotrophic lateral sclerosis: human challenge for neuroscience. *Proc Natl Acad Sci U S A* 1995; 92:1251–1253.

122. Mesenge C, Charriaut-Marlangue C, Verrecchia C, Allix M, et al. Reduction of tyrosine nitration after N(omega)-nitro-L-arginine-methylester treatment of mice with traumatic brain injury. *Eur J Pharmacol* 1998; 353:53–57.

123. Scott GS, Jakeman LB, Stokes BT, Szabo C. Peroxynitrite production and activation of poly (adenosine diphosphate-ribose) synthetase in spinal cord injury. *Ann Neurol* 1999; 45:120–124.

124. Liu D, Li L, Augustus L. Prostaglandin release by spinal cord injury mediates production of hydroxyl radical, malondialdehyde and cell death: a site of the neuroprotective action of methylprednisolone. *J Neurochem* 2001; 77:1036–1047.

125. Estevez AG, Spear N, Manuel SM, Radi R, et al. Nitric oxide and superoxide contribute to motor neuron apoptosis induced by trophic factor deprivation. *J Neurosci* 1998; 18:923–931.

126. Beckman JS, Koppenol WH. Nitric oxide, superoxide, and peroxynitrite: the good, the bad, and ugly. *Am J Physiol* 1996; 271:C1424–C1437.

127. Cuevas P, Carceller-Benito F, Reimers D. Administration of bovine superoxide dismutase prevents sequelae of spinal cord ischemia in the rabbit. *Anat Embryol (Berl)* 1989; 179:251–255.

128. Jung C, Rong Y, Doctrow S, Baudry M, Malfroy B, Xu Z. Synthetic superoxide dismutase/catalase mimetics reduce oxidative stress and prolong survival in a mouse amyotrophic lateral sclerosis model. *Neurosci Lett* 2001; 304:157–160.

129. Peled-Kamar M, Lotem J, Okon E, Sachs L, Groner Y. Thymic abnormalities and enhanced apoptosis of thymocytes and bone marrow cells in transgenic mice overexpressing Cu/Zn-superoxide dismutase: implications for Down syndrome. *EMBO J* 1995; 14:4985–4993.

130. Bar-Peled O, Korkotian E, Segal M, Groner Y. Constitutive overexpression of Cu/Zn superoxide dismutase exacerbates kainic acid-induced apoptosis of transgenic-Cu/Zn superoxide dismutase neurons. *Proc Natl Acad Sci U S A* 1996; 93:8530–8535.

131. Kamsler A, Segal M. Control of neuronal plasticity by reactive oxygen species. *Antioxid Redox Signal* 2007; 9:165–167.

132. Xu J, Fan G, Chen S, Wu Y, et al. Methylprednisolone inhibition of TNF-alpha expression and NF-kB activation after spinal cord injury in rats. *Brain Res Mol Brain Res* 1998; 59:135–142.

133. Saunders RD, Dugan LL, Demediuk P, Means ED, et al. Effects of methylprednisolone and the combination of alpha-tocopherol and selenium on arachidonic acid metabolism and lipid peroxidation in traumatized spinal cord tissue. *J Neurochem* 1987; 49:24–31.

134. Koc RK, Kurtsoy A, Pasaoglu H, Karakucuk EI, et al. Lipid peroxidation and oedema in experimental brain injury: comparison of treatment with methylprednisolone, tirilazad mesylate and vitamin E. *Res Exp Med (Berl)* 1999; 199:21–28.

135. Gurney ME, Cutting FB, Zhai P, Doble A, et al. Benefit of vitamin E, riluzole, and gabapentin in a transgenic model of familial amyotrophic lateral sclerosis. *Ann Neurol* 1996; 39:147–157.

136. Sano M, Ernesto C, Thomas RG, Klauber MR, et al. A controlled trial of selegiline, alpha-tocopherol, or both as treatment for Alzheimer's disease: the Alzheimer's Disease Cooperative Study. *N Engl J Med* 1997; 336:1216–1222.

137. Packer JE, Slater TF, Willson RL. Direct observation of a free radical interaction between vitamin E and vitamin C. *Nature* 1979; 278:737–738.

138. Puskas F, Gergely P Jr., Banki K, Perl A. Stimulation of the pentose phosphate pathway and glutathione levels by dehydroascorbate, the oxidized form of vitamin C. *FASEB J* 2000; 14:1352–1361.

139. Dugan LL, Turetsky DM, Du C, Lobner D, et al. Carboxyfullerenes as neuroprotective agents. *Proc Natl Acad Sci U S A* 1997; 94:9434–9439.

140. Lukacova N, Chavko M, Halat G. Effect of stobadine on lipid peroxidation and phospholipids in rabbit spinal cord after ischaemia. *Neuropharmacology* 1993; 32:235–241.

141. Christman JW, Blackwell TS, Juurlink BH. Redox regulation of nuclear factor kappa B: therapeutic potential for attenuating inflammatory responses. *Brain Pathol* 2000; 10:153–162.

142. Juurlink BH. Management of oxidative stress in the CNS: the many roles of glutathione. *Neurotox Res* 1999; 1:119–140.

143. Huang J, Philbert MA. Distribution of glutathione and glutathione-related enzyme systems in mitochondria and cytosol of cultured cerebellar astrocytes and granule cells. *Brain Res* 1995; 680:16–22.

144. Toborek M, Malecki A, Garrido R, Mattson MP, et al. Arachidonic acid-induced oxidative injury to cultured spinal cord neurons. *J Neurochem* 1999; 73:684–692.

145. Kamencic H, Griebel RW, Lyon AW, Paterson PG, Juurlink BH. Promoting glutathione synthesis after spinal cord trauma decreases secondary damage and promotes retention of function. *FASEB J* 2001; 15:243–250.

146. Malecki A, Garrido R, Mattson MP, Hennig B, Toborek M. 4-Hydroxynonenal induces oxidative stress and death of cultured spinal cord neurons. *J Neurochem* 2000; 74:2278–2287.

147. Sies H, Arteel GE. Interaction of peroxynitrite with selenoproteins and glutathione peroxidase mimics. *Free Radic Biol Med* 2000; 28:1451–1455.

148. Barkats M, Millecamps S, Abrioux P, Geoffroy MC, Mallet J. Overexpression of glutathione peroxidase increases the resistance of neuronal cells to Abeta-mediated neurotoxicity. *J Neurochem* 2000; 75:1438–1446.

149. Azbill RD, Mu X, Bruce-Keller AJ, Mattson MP, Springer JE. Impaired mitochondrial function, oxidative stress and altered antioxidant enzyme activities following traumatic spinal cord injury. *Brain Res* 1997; 765:283–290.

150. Bredesen DE. Neural apoptosis. *Ann Neurol* 1995; 38:839–851.

151. Harvey NL, Kumar S. The role of caspases in apoptosis. *Adv Biochem Eng Biotechnol* 1998; 62:107–128.

152. Blomer U, Kafri T, Randolph-Moore L, Verma IM, Gage FH. Bcl-xL protects adult septal cholinergic neurons from axotomized cell death. *Proc Natl Acad Sci U S A* 1998; 95:2603–2608.

153. Bisby MA, Tetzlaff W. Changes in cytoskeletal protein synthesis following axon injury and during axon regeneration. *Mol Neurobiol* 1992; 6:107–123.

154. Skene JH. Axonal growth-associated proteins. *Annu Rev Neurosci* 1989; 12:127–156.

155. Benowitz LI, Routtenberg A. GAP-43: an intrinsic determinant of neuronal development and plasticity. *Trends Neurosci* 1997; 20:84–91.

156. Hopker VH, Shewan D, Tessier-Lavigne M, Poo M, Holt C. Growth-cone attraction to netrin-1 is converted to repulsion by laminin-1. *Nature* 1999; 401:69–73.

157. Zheng JQ, Poo MM. Calcium signaling in neuronal motility. *Annu Rev Cell Dev Biol* 2007; 23:375–404.

158. Qiu J, Cai D, Filbin MT. Glial inhibition of nerve regeneration in the mature mammalian CNS. *Glia* 2000; 29:166–174.

159. Song HJ, Ming GL, Poo MM. cAMP-induced switching in turning direction of nerve growth cones. *Nature* 1997; 388:275–279.

160. Hannila SS, Filbin MT. The role of cyclic AMP signaling in promoting axonal regeneration after spinal cord injury. *Exp Neurol* 2008; 209:321–332.

161. Hou ST, Jiang SX, Smith RA. Permissive and repulsive cues and signalling pathways of axonal outgrowth and regeneration. *Int Rev Cell Mol Biol* 2008; 267:125–181.

162. Olson L, Bjorklund H, Hoffer BJ, Palmer MR, Seiger A. Spinal cord grafts: an intraocular approach to enigmas of nerve growth regulation. *Brain Res Bull* 1982; 9:519–537.

163. Lykissas MG, Batistatou AK, Charalabopoulos KA, Beris AE. The role of neurotrophins in axonal growth, guidance, and regeneration. *Curr Neurovasc Res* 2007; 4:143–151.

164. Eriksson PS, Perfilieva E, Bjork-Eriksson T, Alborn AM, et al. Neurogenesis in the adult human hippocampus. *Nat Med* 1998; 4:1313–1317.

165. Horner PJ, Power AE, Kempermann G, Kuhn HG, et al. Proliferation and differentiation of progenitor cells throughout the intact adult rat spinal cord. *J Neurosci* 2000; 20:2218–2228.

166. Furukawa S, Furukawa Y. [FGF-2-treatment improves locomotor function via axonal regeneration in the transected rat spinal cord.] *Brain Nerve* 2007; 59:1333–1339.

167. Elde R, Cao Y, Cintra A. prominent expression of acidic fibroblast growth factor in motor and sensory neurons. *Neuron* 1991; 7:349–364.

168. Koshinaga M, Sanon HR, Whittemore SR. Altered acidic and basic fibroblast growth factor expression following spinal cord injury. *Exp Neurol* 1993; 120:32–48.

169. Mcneil PL, Muthukrishnan L, Warder E. Growth factors are released by mechanically wounded endothelial cells. *J Cell Biol* 1989; 109:811–822.

170. Klagsbrun M. The fibroblast growth factor family: structural and biological properties. *Prog Growth Factor Res* 1989; 1:207–235.

171. Kobayashi NR, Fan DP, Giehl KM, Bedard AM, et al. BDNF and NT-4/5 prevent atrophy of rat rubrospinal neurons after cervical axotomy, stimulate GAP-43 and Talpha1-tubulin mRNA expression, and promote axonal regeneration. *J Neurosci* 1997; 17:9583–9595.

172. Bregman BS, Broude E, McAtee M. Transplants and neurotrophic factors prevent atrophy of mature CNS neurons after spinal cord injury. *Exp Neurol* 1998; 149:13–27.

173. Broude E, McAtee M, Kelley MS, Bregman BS. c-Jun expression in adult rat dorsal root ganglion neurons: differential response after central or peripheral axotomy. *Exp Neurol* 1997; 148:367–377.

174. Jakeman LB, Wei P, Guan Z, Stokes BT. Brain-derived neurotrophic factor stimulates hindlimb stepping and sprouting of cholinergic fibers after spinal cord injury. *Exp Neurol* 1998; 154:170–184.

175. Houweling DA, Lankhorst AJ, Gispen WH, Bar PR, Joosten EA. Collagen containing neurotrophin-3 (NT-3) attracts regrowing injured corticospinal axons in the adult rat spinal cord and promotes partial functional recovery. *Exp Neurol* 1998; 153:49–59.

176. Ribotta MG, Provencher J, Feraboli-Lohnherr D, Rossignol S, et al. Activation of locomotion in adult chronic spinal rats is achieved by transplantation of embryonic raphe cells reinnervating a precise lumbar level. *J Neurosci* 2000; 20:5144–5152.

177. Grill R, Murai K, Blesch A, Gage FH, Tuszynski MH. Cellular delivery of neurotrophin-3 promotes corticospinal axonal growth and partial functional recovery after spinal cord injury. *J Neurosci* 1997; 17:5560–5572.

178. Liu Y, Kim D, Himes BT, Chow SY, et al. Transplants of fibroblasts genetically modified to express BDNF promote regeneration of adult rat rubrospinal axons and recovery of forelimb function. *J Neurosci* 1999; 19:4370–4387.

179. Sharma HS. A select combination of neurotrophins enhances neuroprotection and functional recovery following spinal cord injury. *Ann N Y Acad Sci* 2007; 1122:95–111.

180. Blesch A, Tuszynski MH. Transient growth factor delivery sustains regenerated axons after spinal cord injury. *J Neurosci* 2007; 27:10535–10545.

181. Tomov TL, Guntinas-Lichius O, Grosheva M, Streppel M, et al. An example of neural plasticity evoked by putative behavioral demand and early use of vibrissal hairs after facial nerve transection. *Exp Neurol* 2002; 178:207–218.

182. Peeva GP, Angelova SK, Guntinas-Lichius O, Streppel M, et al. Improved outcome of facial nerve repair in rats is associated with enhanced regenerative response of motoneurons and augmented neocortical plasticity. *Eur J Neurosci* 2006; 24:2152–2162.

183. Kalderon N, Fiuks Z. Structural recovery in lesioned adult mammalian spinal cord by x-irradiation of the lesion site. *Proc Natl Acad Sci U S A* 1996; 93:11179–11184.

184. Ridet JL, Pencalet P, Belcram M, Giraudeau B, et al. Effects of spinal cord X-irradiation on the recovery of paraplegic rats. *Exp Neurol* 2000; 161:1–14.

185. Seymour AB, Andrews EM, Tsai SY, Markus TM, et al. Delayed treatment with monoclonal antibody IN-1 1 week after stroke results in recovery of function and corticorubral plasticity in adult rats. *J Cereb Blood Flow Metab* 2005; 25:1366–1375.

186. Lee JK, Kim JE, Sivula M, Strittmatter SM. Nogo receptor antagonism promotes stroke recovery by enhancing axonal plasticity. *J Neurosci* 2004; 24:6209–6217.

187. Walmsley AR, Mir AK. Targeting the Nogo-A signalling pathway to promote recovery following acute CNS injury. *Curr Pharm Des* 2007; 13:2470–2484.

188. Verhoeven K, Villanova M, Rossi A, Malandrini A, et al. Localization of the gene for the intermediate form of Charcot-Marie-Tooth to chromosome 10q24.1-q25.1. *Am J Hum Genet* 2001; 69:889–894.

189. Lee YS, Hsiao I, Lin V. Peripheral nerve graft and aFGF restore partial hindlimb function in adult paraplegic rats. *J Neurotrauma* 2002; 19:1203–1216.

190. Lee YS, Lin CY, Robertson RT, Hsiao I, Lin VW. Motor recovery and anatomical evidence of axonal regrowth in spinal cord-repaired adult rats. *J Neuropathol Exp Neurol* 2004; 63:233–245.

191. Lee YS, Lin CY, Robertson RT, Yu J, et al. Re-growth of catecholaminergic fibers and protection of cholinergic spinal cord neurons in spinal repaired rats. *Eur J Neurosci* 2006; 23:693–702.

192. Kalderon N, Fuks Z. Severed corticospinal axons recover electrophysiologic control of muscle activity after X-ray therapy in lesioned adult spinal cord. *Proc Natl Acad Sci U S A* 1996; 93:11185–11190.

193. Ridet I, Privat A. Volume transmission. *Trends Neurosci* 2000; 23:58–59.

194. Balasingam V, Yong VW. Attenuation of astroglial reactivity by interleukin-10. *J Neurosci* 1996; 16:2945–2955.

195. Bradbury EJ, Moon LD, Popat RJ, et al. Chondroitinase ABC promotes functional recovery after spinal cord injury. *Nature* 2002; 416:636–640.

196. Moon LD, Asher RA, Rhodes KE, Fawcett JW. Regeneration of CNS axons back to their target following treatment of adult rat brain with chondroitinase ABC. *Nat Neurosci* 2001; 4:465–466.

197. Pizzorusso T, Medini P, Berardi N, Chierzi S, et al. Reactivation of ocular dominance plasticity in the adult visual cortex. *Science* 2002; 298:1248–1251.

198. Privat A, Pencalet P, Gimenez-Ribotta M, Mersel M, Rajaofetra NU. [Spinal cord injuries: comments on preventive and curative strategy.] *Agressologie* 1993; 34(Spec No 2):64.

199. Schreyer DJ, Skene JH. Injury-associated induction of GAP-43 expression displays axon branch specificity in rat dorsal root ganglion neurons. *J Neurobiol* 1993; 24:959–970.

200. Lu X, Richardson PM. Responses of macrophages in rat dorsal root ganglia following peripheral nerve injury. *J Neurocytol* 1993; 22:334–341.

201. Lu X, Richardson PM. Inflammation near the nerve cell body enhances axonal regeneration. *J Neurosci* 1991; 11:972–978.

202. Neumann S, Bradke F, Tessier-Lavigne M, Basbaum AI. Regeneration of sensory axons within the injured spinal cord induced by intraganglionic cAMP elevation. *Neuron* 2002; 34:885–893.

203. Cao Z, Gao Y, Bryson JB, Hou J, et al. The cytokine interleukin-6 is sufficient but not necessary to mimic the peripheral conditioning lesion effect on axonal growth. *J Neurosci* 2006; 26:5565–5573.

204. Qiu J, Cai D, Dai H, McAtee M, et al. Spinal axon regeneration induced by elevation of cyclic AMP. *Neuron* 2002; 34:895–903.

205. Neumann S, Woolf CJ. Regeneration of dorsal column fibers into and beyond the lesion site following adult spinal cord injury. *Neuron* 1999; 23:83–91.

206. Neumann S, Skinner K, Basbaum AI. Sustaining intrinsic growth capacity of adult neurons promotes spinal cord regeneration. *Proc Natl Acad Sci U S A* 2005; 102:16848–16852.

207. Schwab ME, Bartholdi D. Degeneration and regeneration of axons in the lesioned spinal cord. *Physiol Rev* 1996; 76:319–370.

208. Kakulas BA. A review of the neuropathology of human spinal cord injury with emphasis on special features. *J Spinal Cord Med* 1999; 22:119–124.

209. Blight AR. Miracles and molecules—progress in spinal cord repair. *Nat Neurosci* 2002; 5(Suppl):1051–1054.

210. Uchida N, Buck DW, He D, Reitsma MJ, et al. Direct isolation of human central nervous system stem cells. *Proc Natl Acad Sci U S A* 2000; 97:14720–14725.

211. Liu S, Qu Y, Stewart TJ, Howard MJ, et al. Embryonic stem cells differentiate into oligodendrocytes and myelinate in culture and after spinal cord transplantation. *Proc Natl Acad Sci U S A* 2000; 97:6126–6131.

212. Sasaki M, Honmou O, Akiyama Y, Uede T, et al. Transplantation of an acutely isolated bone marrow fraction repairs demyelinated adult rat spinal cord axons. *Glia* 2001; 35:26–34.

213. Simonen M, Pedersen V, Weinmann O, et al. Systemic deletion of the myelin-associated outgrowth inhibitor Nogo-A improves regenerative and plastic responses after spinal cord injury. *Neuron* 2003; 38:201–211.

214. GrandPre T, Li S, Strittmatter SM. Nogo-66 receptor antagonist peptide promotes axonal regeneration. *Nature* 2002; 417:547–551.

215. Shi R, Blight AR. Differential effects of low and high concentrations of 4-aminopyridine on axonal conduction in normal and injured spinal cord. *Neuroscience* 1997; 77:553–562.

216. Popovich PG, Longbrake EE. Can the immune system be harnessed to repair the CNS? *Nat Rev Neurosci* 2008; 9:481–493.

217. Hirschberg DL, Schwartz M. Macrophage recruitment to acutely injured central nervous system is inhibited by a resident factor: a basis for an immune-brain barrier. *J Neuroimmunol* 1995; 61:89–96.

218. Lazarov-Spiegler O, Solomon AS, Zeev-Brann AB, Hirschberg DL, et al. Transplantation of activated macrophages overcomes central nervous system regrowth failure. *FASEB J* 1996; 10:1296–1302.

219. Lazarov-Spiegler O, Solomon AS, Schwartz M. Peripheral nerve-stimulated macrophages simulate a peripheral nerve-like regenerative response in rat transected optic nerve. *Glia* 1998; 24:329–337.

220. Geller HM, Fawcett JW. Building a bridge: engineering spinal cord repair. *Exp Neurol* 2002; 174:125–136.

221. Tobias CA, Dhoot NO, Wheatley MA, Tessler A, et al. Grafting of encapsulated BDNF-producing fibroblasts into the injured spinal cord without immune suppression in adult rats. *J Neurotrauma* 2001; 18:287–301.

222. Gautier SE, Oudega M, Fragoso M, Chapon P, et al. Poly(alpha-hydroxyacids) for application in the spinal cord: resorbability and biocompatibility with adult rat Schwann cells and spinal cord. *J Biomed Mater Res* 1998; 42:642–654.

223. Mocchetti I, Wrathall J. Neurotrophic factors in central nervous system trauma. *J Neurotrauma* 1995; 12:853–870.

224. Koshinaga M, Sanon HR, Whittemore SR. Altered acidic and basic fibroblast growth expression following spinal cord injury. *Exp Neurol* 1993; 120:32–48.

225. Guest JD, Hesse D, Schnell L. Influence of IN-1antibody and acidic FGF-fibrin glue on the response of injured corticospinal tract axons to human Schwann cell grafts. *J Neurosci Res* 1997; 50:888–905.

226. Oudega M, Hagg T. Nerve growth factor promotes regeneration of sensory axons into adult rat spinal cord. *Exp Neurol* 1996; 140:218–229.

227. Hoke A, Silver J. Proteoglycans and other repulsive molecules in glial boundaries during development and regeneration of the nervous system. *Prog Brain Res* 1996; 108:149–163.

228. Baptiste DC, Fehlings MG. Update on the treatment of spinal cord injury. *Prog Brain Res* 2007; 161:217–233.

229. Baptiste DC, Fehlings MG. Pharmacological approaches to repair the injured spinal cord. *J Neurotrauma* 2006; 23:318–334.

230. Koda M, Hashimoto M, Murakami M, Yoshinaga K, et al. Adenovirus vector-mediated in vivo gene transfer of brain-derived neurotrophic factor (BDNF) promotes rubrospinal axonal regeneration and functional recovery after complete transection of the adult rat spinal cord. *J Neurotrauma* 2004; 21:329–337.

231. Mason MR, Campbell G, Caroni P, Anderson PN, Lieberman AR. Over-expression of GAP-43 in thalamic projection neurons of transgenic mice does not enable them to regenerate axons through peripheral nerve grafts. *Exp Neurol* 2000; 165:143–152.

232. Condic ML. Adult neuronal regeneration induced by transgenic integrin expression. *J Neurosci* 2001; 21:4782–4788.

233. Bonilla IE, Tanabe K, Strittmatter SM. Small proline-rich repeat protein 1A is expressed by axotomized neurons and promotes axonal outgrowth. *J Neurosci* 2002; 22:1303–1315.

234. Caroni P, Aigner L, Schneider C. Intrinsic neuronal determinants locally regulate extrasynaptic and synaptic growth at the adult neuromuscular junction. *J Cell Biol* 1997; 136:679–692.

69 Reconstructing the Microenvironment of the Injured Spinal Cord: Cell Transplantation and Bridge Building to Enhance Functional Recovery

Henrich Cheng
Yu-Shang Lee
Ching-Yi Lin

THE INJURED SPINAL CORD: CHALLENGES FOR REPAIR AND FUNCTIONAL RECOVERY

The fully functional recovery of the traumatic central nerve system (CNS) is a great clinical challenge, especially for a patient with spinal cord injury (SCI). Some CNS-injured patients may show significant functional recovery without intervention, depending on the severity of the injury. Recovery has been observed in SCI patients with severe motor or sensory deficits within several days to weeks after injury. These successes may be due to a reduction of edema, or to improvement of blood flow and metabolism at the injured site to allow the return of spinal cord–related functions. However, most SCI patients still suffer from irreversible functional deficits because of different pathophysiologic changes leading to an environment that will not permit axonal regeneration following injury (1). Reconnection of neural activity between brain and peripheral organs is one of the keys to restoring function. Many strategies have been developed to target these pathophysiologic factors to further enhance axonal regeneration or reorganization of spinal cord circuit to achieve maximal recovery. For example, recent progress in cell-based therapies has demonstrated the replacement of lost neurons or oligodendrocytes and the establishment of an environment conducive to axonal regeneration, with functional recovery in animal models of SCI (2, 3). In addition, strategies to remove glia scarring and inhibitory molecules also have shown the ability to enhance axonal regeneration beyond the damage site (4, 5). In this chapter, we focus on two strategies: (i) replacement of nerve cells after neuronal death/axonal regeneration, and (ii) reconnection and promotion of recovery of normal function in the neural pathways.

ENHANCING FUNCTIONAL RECOVERY OF PATIENTS AFTER SCI: COMBINING PHARMACOLOGIC, TRANSPLANT, AND EXERCISE THERAPIES

Clinical treatment for a CNS lesion has been based on the principle of decompression and bone stabilization. For the damaged CNS per se, no definite mode of therapy exists, except general supportive methods. For example, treatment that promotes functional regeneration across a complete spinal cord transection in man does not exist. Complete transection of the adult mammalian spinal cord leads to irreparable, permanent loss of connectivity. The execution of coordinated movements depends on control exerted by higher centers in the brain. After a transection in the spinal cord, the networks responsible for the generation of locomotion, which are located in the cervical and lumbar enlargements of the cord, are left intact but cannot be used because of lack of connections with the supraspinal control pathways.

However, by applying the knowledge of neural regeneration that has developed quickly in the last decade, we are now standing on a new platform looking toward an era of novel CNS repair and functional recovery. As a result, the major goals of spinal cord regeneration research are to find ways to stimulate axonal regrowth, to reestablish functional supraspinal descending connections with the isolated spinal cord segment, and, concurrently, to reestablish sensory input from the isolated spinal cord to the brain (6). The challenges include learning the mechanisms for SCI and repair, developing a therapy in this sensitive and multifaceted environment, and clinically documenting it. Most of spinal cord research today is performed on lower animals;

researchers must first take the leap to higher animals, and then to humans, facing substantially increased complexity along the way.

Most researchers agree it is unlikely that any single therapeutic intervention will facilitate complete functional repair, whether it promotes neuron survival, stimulates axonal outgrowth, or transiently blocks inhibitory signals. In this case the best potential strategy to encourage axonal regeneration, to achieve functional recovery, to attenuate the glial scar formation, to provide an appropriate environment that is "permissive" for regeneration and preventing neuronal/glial death is a combination of treatments. An example is to transplant cells that are permissive for growth, and to elevate cAMP and neurotrophins at the lesion site (7–9). With the use of this concept, inactivation of Rho and EGFR and digestion of CSPGs with chondroitinase should lead to many more axons growing long distances (10). Such a strategy is supported by the ensuring optimal neuroprotection following SCI. This is likely to be achieved by a combination of pharmacologic compounds directed to different pathophysiologic targets: free radical scavengers (11), AMPA kainite antagonist and inhibitors or activators of cytokines (12, 13), and NMDA antagonists (14). Additionally, tissue protectors IL-10, together with Schwann cells or OECs, significantly improved motor performance in a contused spinal cord rat model (15). It is obvious that this must be a combinatorial approach.

Furthermore, delicately adjusting the balance between those factors that promote regeneration with those endogenous mechanisms inhibiting adult CNS repair may be sufficient to drive recovery in a functionally positive direction. Finally, determining the spatial and temporal organization of experimental therapies is critical to designing an integrated approach to neurotrauma recovery. The rapidly expanding body of information regarding CNS development will continue to provide valuable data for creating the necessary conditions within the injured adult CNS that are more conducive to functional repair, perhaps in part by approximating the favorable growth state of initial development. Minimizing death of the injured neuron from retrograde degeneration will be helpful in function recovery. The cell body in the cerebral cortex (as in the descending corticospinal tract); in the brainstem (as in the descending rubrospinal tract); or in the lower spinal cord level (as in the ascending dorsal column) should be prevented from dying back. The damaged axon must then extend its disrupted processes to its proper neuronal targets for functional recovery. After synaptic contact is made, remyelination of the pathway and plasticity change in accordance with the functional connection will follow.

According to the above scenario, functional recovery for a patient with SCI can be classified into two strategies. Strategy A focuses on the replacement of cells after neuronal death. Strategy B strives to reconnect and recover normal function in the neural pathway, and involves reactivation of dysfunctional pathways, reestablishment of normal connections, and regrowth of pathways with surviving upper and lower neurons.

In the strategy to replace cells after neuronal death, cellular transplantation is necessary to restore neural networks and/or chemical function. Sources for cellular replacement may be from embryonic tissues, adult neural progenitor cells, adult cells transformed by certain factors, adult ensheathing cells, and transgenic cells with specific functions. In an effort to reconnect and recover normal function in the neural pathway, a repair strategy using neural grafts together with trophic factors has been shown to result in meaningful functional recovery in rodent spinal cord transection models (16). Functional reactivation of the dysfunctional pathways in the spinal cord was noted after the application of trophic factors. Studies in this strategy cover neurotrophic factor delivery, axon guidance, removal of growth inhibition, bridging and artificial substrates, and modulation of the immune response. Results from these studies indicate that functional recovery can be attained to some extent in the discontinuous CNS by either increasing the permissive cues or decreasing the non-permissive cues of the existing environment around the sprouting nerves. However, many mechanisms that do not include regeneration may account for observed functional recovery. Functional recovery may be attained from reactivation of the dysfunctional pathways, increased sprouting or synaptogenesis of the remaining survival pathways, or regeneration and correct path finding from the disrupted pathways (Figure 69.1). For better functional recovery, all these mechanisms are important, although some are not authentic regenerative mechanisms.

STRATEGY TO REPLACE NERVE CELLS AFTER NEURONAL DEATH/AXONAL REGENERATION (CELL-BASED THERAPIES)

Neuronal death occurs to various extents after SCI, with or without neuroprotection. Nerve cell replacement is very critical in certain SCI lesions, especially when the spared systems cannot take over the function of lost cells. For example, the motor neuron pools in the cervical or lumbar enlargement are degraded to such a degree that they are inadequate to support essential lower motor neuronal functions. No matter how well the lesion is bridged or reinnervated, the target motor neurons that project to the muscles are irrevocably lost. As mature neurons can barely divide to heal the injured site, a strategy of cell replacement may be required with the hope that the grafted neurons will mature and integrate into the host nervous system. One benefit of cellular transplantation is the possibility of neutralizing the neurochemical factors present in the injured tissue that inhibit regeneration. The regenerated nerve fibers may migrate across the injured area and grow into the spinal cord distal to the injury after the inhibitory environment has been neutralized. The other benefit of cellular transplantation is to remyelinate the axons that have lost their myelin sheaths, and consequently have worsened or lost signal transmission. In transplantation, the ideal cellular candidate for a cell-based repair strategy should be able to (a) support axonal regeneration in adult CNS, (b) restore myelin in demyelinated spared axons, (c) freely migrate and integrate into the injured CNS parenchyma, and (d) coexist with astrocytes (17). For experimental and ultimately clinical purposes of SCI repair, methods have been developed and many sources of transplantable cells have been used and are continuing to be refined to obtain purified and well-characterized populations of these cells, which can be prepared for autologous transplantation (17, 18). Currently, the most promising research directions in cell-based therapies for SCI include fetal cells, stem cells, Schwann cells, olfactory ensheathing glia (OEG), and activated macrophages

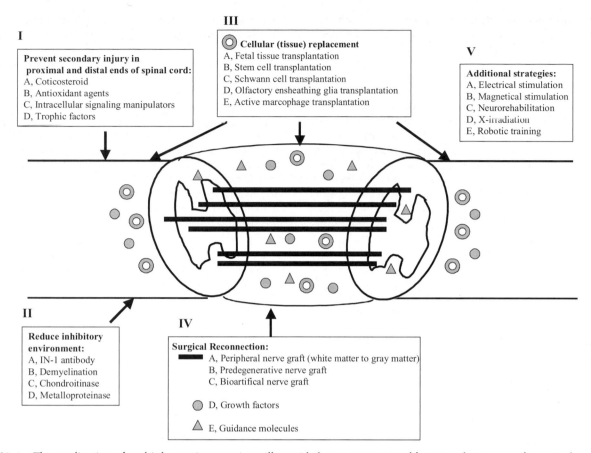

Figure 69.1   The application of multiple repair strategies will provide better outcomes of functional recovery after spinal cord injury. (**I**) Reducing the secondary injury can make more nerve cells survive. (**II**) Removing the inhibitory environment (e.g., myelin, scar tissue) after injury can promote more axonal regrowth. (**III**) Nerve cells or tissue transplantation can make up for the loss of nerve cell after spinal cord injury. (**IV**) Peripheral nerve grafts, the application of guidance molecules, and growth factors can reconnect the neural pathway. (**V**) In addition to the intraspinal cord repair strategies, rehabilitation approaches can physically help to attain better functional improvement.

that can provide different benefits for the enhancement of functional recovery.

Fetal Cell Transplantation

Recognizing the need for cell replacement, several laboratories have taken advantage of fetal tissue grafts to replace cells in the CNS after a variety of insults (19). This is perhaps the only transplantation technique that has already been tested on humans with CNS disorders, as well as patients with Parkinson's disease and syringomyelia. Ideally, a cell replacement source should be homogeneous, readily obtainable, and synergetic. However, fetal tissue grafting usually requires multiple donor sources in a very short period of time for collection. Hence, the mechanical, physical, and ethical hurdles of using this therapy limit its large-scale use. Nevertheless, knowledge from the studies on fetal cell transplantation provides valuable insight on neural regeneration.

The capacity of axonal regrowth across spinal cord transections exists during a small time window early in development, which occurs during the time of initial axonal elongation and before the build-up of inhibitory mechanisms in the spinal cord (20–23). After complete transection in the newborn rat or kitten spinal cord, supraspinal projections to the spinal cord caudal to

the lesion are abolished. Transplantation of fetal spinal cord tissue into the lesion can restore some supraspinal projections and result in improved locomotor function (24, 25). Fetal spinal cord tissue transplantation in the lesioned neonatal spinal cord has been shown to increase axonal growth and improve both skilled forelimb reaching and posture, as well as locomotor function (25–27). In the adult spinal cord, changes in the regenerative potential of the neurons and the cellular and molecular environments limit the capacity of the mature cord to regrow after injury. Mature CNS cells are post-mitotic and do not divide in culture, making it difficult to replicate and replace the lost/injured cells (28). The amount of axonal growth and the extent of recovery of function decrease drastically in adult animals after fetal cell transplantation. After SCI, the descending axons from the adult's supraspinal centers project into a fetal spinal cord tissue transplant, but terminate near the host/transplant border, despite the fetal cord environment within the transplant (29, 30). Very little evidence has shown that nerve fibers emit from the transplant to the host tissue. Application of an exogenous trophic factor may increase the regrowth of nerve fibers in the fetal tissue transplant. Administration of neurotrophins (BDNF, neurotrophin-3 [NT-3], and neurotrophin 4/5 [NT-4/5]) increases the amount of supraspinal axonal growth into the transplant and the extent of branching within the transplant after spinal cord hemisection and fetal spinal cord transplantation (30).

Stem Cell Technology

Stem cells, obtained by expanding a small biopsy of brain or bone marrow tissue in culture, are undifferentiated cells that have the capability to divide and differentiate into many other types of cells induced by the priming of optimal growth factors. Several unique features of embryonic stem cells make them excellent candidates for transplantation (28). These features include their pluripotentiality and relative lack of immune reaction. Because of their stem cell–like attributes and pluripotency (31), bone marrow cells have become a very interesting subject in recent years (32) for repairing SCI. These attributes, however, have not been corroborated (33), and they are even subject to challenges based on issues pertaining to cell fusion and transdifferentiation (34, 35), as well as the absence of distinct neuronal morphological features, despite their expression of some neuronal markers (36, 37). The transplantation of bone marrow cells and stem cells remains appealing for autologous transplantation and spinal cord repair because they can be very easily procured, expanded in culture, and delivered via intramedullary or intravenous routes, among other reasons (38, 39).

Stem cells hold great promise as a source for introducing new neurons or glial cells to the damaged spinal cord. Stem cell transplantation involves three stages. First, the stem cells are purified. Next, they are grown in cell cultures. Then they are transplanted back into the spinal cord. Stem cells are genetically unmodified cells with a multipotent character that adapts itself to its environment. Thus, after transplantation, the graft hopefully "takes" and the cells subsequently differentiate into the appropriate neuronal and glial subpopulations (40–43). Previous studies utilized stem cells that had been isolated and cultured from diverse regions of the developing and adult rodent brain as well as other tissues. Neural cells for replacement may transdifferentiate from adult non-neuronal tissue, such as bone marrow stromal cells, using an appropriate growth factor (44). Stem cells can be propagated and genetically tagged with markers or therapeutic genes in vitro before grafting in vivo (45–47). Several studies have reported that stem-cell grafts can lead to neurogenesis in animal models of neural degeneration (48). Despite these encouraging data, however, the functional implication for this approach is still dim. A recent report by McDonald et al. has shown transplantation with embryonic stem (ES) cells into the contused spinal cord of a rat (49) to improve locomotion ability. Whether the improvement was derived from the surviving ES cells that contributed to the reestablishment of the neural network, or only from their chemical effects, is uncertain. Furthermore, embryonic stem cells exhibit certain degrees of genetically manipulability (50). Not only are the cells remarkably plastic—adult stem cells in the hippocampus, olfactory bulb, cerebellum, and retina can give rise to regionally specific cell types—they can also migrate considerable distances (28). Endogenous neural progenitor cells are susceptible to many of the same injury processes as mature cells, and their response to nervous system injury is inadequate in replacing lost tissue.

The existence of neural stem cells has recently been shown in nonhuman primates and humans (51, 52). The adult brain (44) and spinal cord (53) have been shown to contain stem cells that continuously divide throughout adult life. Neural progenitor cells proliferate and migrate in the spinal cord after trauma or other stress (54–56). In an acute demyelination model, progenitor cells are able to proliferate and become oligodendrocytes, thus remyelinating the lesioned area (57–59). In another model of pyramidal cell apoptosis of brain, the progenitor cells are capable of replacing the dead cortical neurons and extending their axons through the intact CNS (60). These findings suggest that an endogenous self-repair potential, albeit trivial, exists in the adult spinal cord. However, it is clear that endogenous stem cells do not produce complete recovery in cases of severe trauma. To determine whether a strategy that uses endogenous or exogenous stem cell replacement can be successfully applied to repair the injured spinal cord, further studies must be conducted, to clarify the molecules and genes that govern cell proliferation, migration, and differentiation; the methods of increasing the survival of proliferated stem cells in the lesioned area; and how these cells can be functionally integrated into the remaining circuitry.

Schwann Cell, Olfactory Ensheathing Glia, and Activated Macrophages Transplantation

Much work has been done with Schwann cells, another type of neural support cell. For instance, researchers at the Miami Project have developed methods to cultivate human Schwann cells and to produce millions of cells for transplantation from biopsies of peripheral nerves in adults. Schwann cells have neurotrophin, extracellular matrix (ECM), and cell adhesion properties that are favorable to axonal regeneration in the peripheral nervous system (61, 62). Additionally, Schwann cells are good for genetic manipulation and are thus useful cellular vehicles for *ex vivo* gene delivery and other combination therapies (63–65). However, Schwann cells often fail to become completely integrated into the CNS (66), because they interact unfavorably with CNS elements (67, 68). There is experimental (69) and human clinical (70) evidence suggesting that Schwann cells may even promote gliosis and the deposition of non-permissive ECM molecules, such as chondroitin sulfate proteoglycans (71, 72). To circumvent this inhibitory milieu, brain-derived neurotrophic factors (BDNF)-expressing Schwann cells were seeded 5 mm below the site of complete spinal cord transection (73) and shown to facilitate axon elongation to more caudal regions. Even under these conditions, the distance traveled by axons exiting the Schwann cell environment is very limited (74).

Besides transplants using Schwann cells as the supporting cells, olfactory ensheathing glia (OEG) has been tested in injury sites to observe regeneration in CNS. OEGs are neurosensory cells of the olfactory epithelium that are continuously replaced in the adult; their newly formed axons grow into the olfactory bulb. OEG have many growth-promoting properties for neurons and are able to migrate extensively within the CNS. OEGs could promote long-distance axonal regeneration after transplantation to partial or complete spinal cord lesions (75–78). OEG-induced axonal regrowth led to the recovery of forepaw reaching in rats after partial spinal cord lesions at the cervical level (79). In adult rats, OEG transplants successfully led to functional and structural recovery after complete spinal cord transection at T8 (76). These recoveries may demonstrate that OEGs produce a variety of growth-permissive ECM molecules and growth factors, intimately interact with host astrocytes (80, 81), align themselves with the lesion site, migrate long distances into the anterior and posterior spinal cord stumps, and guide regenerating axons through the lesion (82, 83). As with other cell types used to modify the environment at the injury site, it is critical to identify the molecular characteristics of the changes after OEG transplantation that lead to increases in axonal growth. In future clinical applications, it is also important to make sure that the human OEG has properties similar to rodent OEG.

The limitation of immune responsiveness in the mammalian CNS may be due to the intricate nature of neuronal networks, which appear to be more susceptible than other tissues to the threat of permanent disorganization during massive inflammation. For example, macrophages promote wound healing in most body tissues, but are normally unable to enter the spinal cord in large numbers. It has been demonstrated that the innate immune system, represented by activated macrophages, can facilitate the processes of regeneration in the severed spinal cord (84). From a clinical perspective, activated macrophages for immunomodulation constitute an approach that consists of taking white blood cells (known as macrophages) from the injured patient's own blood and activating them in a laboratory for a short period. The therapy must be started within a few days of the injury and cannot be applied to chronically paralyzed SCI patients. Additional areas having the potential of supporting transplantation therapy include the use of gene therapy to stimulate neurons; work is also ongoing to develop synthetic guidance tubes that could replace peripheral nerve grafts as conduits for axonal regeneration.

STRATEGY TO RECONNECT AND RECOVER NORMAL FUNCTION IN NEURAL PATHWAYS

Reestablishing neural function after SCI requires transplantation techniques to set up a cellular bridge at the point of injury, thus allowing damaged axons to regenerate over the gap created by the injury and reestablish connection of the appropriate nerve circuits. It is clear that an inhibitory environment in the spinal cord must be overcome in some way. Ways now exist to identify those inhibitors and the methods by which they can be blocked (56). The main problem is for the regenerated nerve fibers to migrate across the point where they must grow into the spinal cord distal to the injury.

Studies of developing chick embryos have indicated that their regenerating ability after SCI disappears later in the developmental period. Thoracic cord transection, prior to E13, results in relatively complete neuroanatomic axonal regeneration and functional recovery (85–87). On the other hand, transection after E13 results in sparse axonal regrowth and little or no functional recovery (85–88). Thus, the transition from a permissive to a restrictive period for CNS repair correlates with the developmental onset of myelination in the embryonic chick spinal cord (89). Similar findings were observed in mammals. Recovery after complete lesions has been shown in neonates before myelination (90).

Researchers have used many different animal models of SCI. Spinal cords are typically not transected: they are bruised or crushed. Whereas incomplete spinal cord lesions have generated valuable information about reactive and compensatory changes, lesions such as hemisections, weight-dropping contusion models, compressions, and different chemical or mechanical partial lesions are less suitable for the studies of functional recovery through regeneration of cut axons (91–94). Many examples in previous studies show recovery data that have been difficult to interpret because the exact degree of axonal injury cannot be determined. To avoid all ambiguities of interpretation and to model the worst possible clinical scenario, one with complete discontinuity in the lesion area, some researchers have chosen to study only animals in which a complete surgical transection of the spinal cord has been carried out (16, 76). The thoracic cord between T8 and T9 has been frequently chosen as the major transection site in these studies because (a) the descending pathways to the hindlimbs are definitely interrupted, (b) the innervation to the forelimbs is not disturbed, (c) the rib cage can assist the stability of the spinal column in this condition, and (d) the distance to the lumbar enlargement is long enough to allow retrograde tracing studies. Although animal studies aim at regeneration and functional recovery under the condition of complete pathway interruption, most SCI patients have incomplete anatomic interruption. To pursue a comprehensive functional recovery for an SCI patient, all mechanisms involved in the functional improvement are important, even if some are not authentic regenerative processes. In terms of functional recovery in patients with incomplete pathway interruption SCI, neuroprotective measures and the reactivation of the dysfunctional spinal cord may be more important than regeneration of the interrupted nerve fibers.

In the 1980s Aguayo and colleagues showed that axotomized spinal cord neurons, brain-stem neurons, and retinal ganglion cells of adult rats were capable of growing axons into the regions of the regenerating axon and its microenvironment (95–98). In the peripheral nervous system (PNS), Schwann cells are the critical elements that provide several factors beneficial to regeneration (99, 100). Schwann cells undergo a series of changes in response to axotomy, which include not only the initiation of myelin breakdown, but also a massive upregulation of the synthesis of NGF, BDNF, CNTF, and several presumptive growth-promoting components (N-CAM, tenascin, L1, etc.) (101). Comparing neurite growth in contact with CNS or PNS constituents has revealed that PNS myelin is an acceptable substrate for neurite growth, whereas CNS myelin has strong inhibitory properties (102). In Aguayo's bridging studies, regenerating fibers could elongate throughout the whole distance of a PNS graft. However, the fibers usually failed to enter the spinal cord for any significant distance beyond the distal nerve–cord interface (95). Pioneering work by Schwab and associates has demonstrated that oligodendroglial cells produce proteins, such as Nogo gene–related proteins NI-35 and NI-250, that can inhibit axon regeneration (103–105). Although there appear to be several interesting ways in which this inhibition might be overcome, such as the use of monoclonal antibody IN-1 (91, 92), other alternatives to avoid the non-permissive microenviroment of CNS white matter should also be explored.

White Matter to Gray Matter Rerouting in Peripheral Nerve Bridges

In the gray matter of the spinal cord, which contains nerve cell bodies and many nonmyelinated fibers, less NI activity occurs to allow more permissive environment for axonal regeneration. For example, long-distance regeneration of 5-HT fibers (neuronal cell bodies originating from raphe magnus, obscurus, and pallidus) in the spinal cord has been demonstrated to occur in over 95 percent of gray matter after either chemical (94) or surgical lesioning (106). Moreover, using in vitro explant coculture of postnatal sensorimotor cortex and spinal cord, the corticospinal fibers were noted to arborize within the gray matter of spinal cord explants (107). Reimplantation of the severed dorsal roots in the adult rat spinal cord revealed axonal regeneration and terminal arborization when the roots were reinserted into the gray matter, whereas regeneration was limited when insertion was into the white matter (108). Based on these findings, rerouting pathways from nonpermissive white to permissive gray matter was chosen as a major strategy in Cheng's repair strategy to evade those oligodendroglial proteins that inhibit axon regeneration (16). The peripheral nerve bridges thus redirected descending motor pathways from proximal white to distal gray matter, and ascending pathways from distal white to proximal gray matter, taking into account the specific anatomy of rat descending and ascending pathways (109). Grafting intercostal nerve segments to the rat spinal cord was carried out after removal of 5 mm of the cord at T8. Paraplegic rats that were subjected to the full repair strategy (18 white-to-gray bridges, fibrin glue with aFGF, compressive wiring) demonstrated a return of hindlimb positioning, followed by return of hindlimb movements and partial weight bearing. None of these changes was noted in any of several different types of paraplegic control animals. Structural analysis using anterograde and retrograde wheat-germ agglutinin horseradish peroxiclase (WGA-HRP) axonal tracing revealed many regenerated descending fiber tracts, including the corticospinal tract. Detailed analysis of gait demonstrated that the repaired animals were able to use their forelimbs in controlled order and patterns similar to those found in normal rats. Although the repaired animals remain functionally inferior to normal animals, the data demonstrate that it is possible to regain some hindlimb function after complete SCI (16, 77). The above research demonstrated for the first time that this grafting strategy could result in limited but definitive functional improvement in locomotor activity on rats with transected spinal cords.

Predegenerative Nerve Graft

The difficulty of regeneration within the CNS can be caused by a lack of growth-promoting substances. The activities of these substances decrease in the mature CNS. However, it is necessary to have these substances for regeneration; they act as natural neurite growth stimulators. In addition to growth-promoting substances, it is necessary to have a sufficient level of trophic factors and an extracellular matrix, such as laminine and collagen, to support axonal regeneration. For example, predegenerated peripheral nerve segments, which are collected from a transected sciatic nerve before the application, are one of the platforms to stimulate neuritis outgrowth. In the predegenerative nerve, there are no neuronal elements or myelin. Also, a larger number of Schwann cells are present, when compared to the fresh nerve. Schwann cells are active and able to produce a range of known growth factors, such as NGF, BDNF, and CNTF, as well as unknown growth factors (110–112). Several studies have shown

that predegenerated peripheral nerve grafts facilitate neurite outgrowth from the injured hippocampus in a more effective way than freshly taken grafts. This effect was particularly distinct when grafts that were predegenerated for 7 days and 35 days were used (78, 113). The role of predegenerative nerve grafts is not restricted to the previously mentioned uses. The predegenerative nerve may have valuable substances that have not yet been identified. These substances also secrete numerous extracellular matrix components that can build pathways for regenerating axons and are able to bind adhesive molecules in the basement membrane and on the surface of the Schwann cells (114, 115).

Previous studies indicate that nerve grafts that have been destroyed by freeze-thaw treatments contain Schwann cell basal lamina tubes, which are similar to Schwann cells and are apparently favorable scaffolds (116). The empty basal lamina tubes are in the shape of a tunnel. These tunnels can be favorable for axonal growth. The inner surfaces of these tunnels contain adhesion molecules on which the axons can securely adhere. Also, acellularbasal lamina allografts are immunologically advantageous (117). The infiltration of macrophages after nerve injury, and subsequently in vitro, as seen in the predegenerated cultures, seems to be a further promoter of Schwann cell proliferation, because macrophages participate in the production of mitogenic factors for Schwann cells (118) and induce NGF expression through interleukin-1 stimulation (119).

Biomaterial Conduit and Axonal Regeneration

To accomplish regrowth and reconnection of damaged axons is the major goal of research in spinal cord repair. Currently, bioengineering strategies for the repair of the peripheral nervous system are focused on alternatives to the nerve graft, whereas investigations for spinal cord injury are focused on producing a permissive environment for regeneration. The technologies of tissue engineering (120) provide an opportunity to repair spinal cord injury through promoting axonal growth and functional recovery. Development of tissue-engineering strategies to facilitate nerve growth through an injured spinal cord use a scaffold of either cellular or cell-free bridges or a combination of both. Such a scaffold can be of a synthetic or biological nature and can be resorbable or non-resorbable. The potential cellular transplantation and peripheral nerve graft can provide a favorable environment, as mentioned previously. Moreover, combined strategies of implants of cells either attached to the outside (121) or contained within formed tubes (122) have also been demonstrated with some degree of success.

Several investigations have focused on using (i) cell-free bridges made of biocompatible materials (e.g., for neural reconstruction applications, the material possesses favorable mechanical property and degradation characteristics) (123, 124), and (ii) synthetic polymers such as hydrogels based on crosslinked poly hydroxyethyl-methacrylate (pHEMA) and poly N-(2-hydroxypropyl)-methacrylamide (pHPMA) (125, 126) have also been studied for their ability to serve as scaffolds for spinal nerve regeneration. Furthermore, a poly N-(2-hydroxypropyl)-methacrylamide (pHPMA) hydrogel containing the cell-adhesive region of fibronectin Arg-Gly-Asp (RGD) has also been demonstrated to have the capability to provide angiogenesis, axonal growth, and tissue-reducing necrosis in SCI rats (127). Other synthetic materials that have been investigated in the CNS include poly (lactic acid) or poly (D, L-lactide) (128); poly (2-hydroxyethyl methacrylate), or pHEMA (124); poly (lactic-co-glycolic acid) (PLGA) and block copolymer of poly (lactic-co-glycolic acid)-poly(lysine) (129); and poly (ethylene glycol) "glue" (130). Most of the results from these various investigations provide the alternative permissive substrate to facilitate axonal regrowth. In order to overcome the inhibitory environment and have proper synaptic connection at the distal end of the spinal cord, the combination of tissue-engineering technologies with other advanced biomolecular therapies such as neurotrophic factors is necessary to develop better functional outcomes.

CONCLUSION

Complete loss of function occurs in an area distal to a complete SCI. It has been a dogma in the field of spinal cord medicine that such a lesion will not heal and cannot be repaired in an adult mammal. Despite this negative outlook, previous studies have shown that further studies focusing on spinal cord repair might nevertheless be worthwhile. For example, long-distance regeneration of certain descending tracts (NA and 5-HT) does indeed occur after chemical lesion, and appear to take place in gray matter. Also, many types of CNS neurons can be stimulated to extend processes through a free graft of peripheral nerve. In addition, growth and trophic factors have potent stimulatory effects. Finally, refined surgical protocols could be implemented, using fibrin glue as a stabilization component. Furthermore, it is important to study whether the repair strategy can be applied to animals with chronic SCI. Special additional measures might be necessary to achieve functional effects in a chronic paraplegia situation. The final goal is obviously to develop a method worthy of clinical trials.

References

1. Neumann S, Skinner K, Basbaum AI. Sustaining intrinsic growth capacity of adult neurons promotes spinal cord regeneration. *Proc Natl Acad Sci USA* 2005; 102:16848–16852.
2. Kim BG, Hwang DH, Lee SI, Kim EJ, Kim SU: Stem cell-based cell therapy for spinal cord injury. *Cell Transplant* 2007; 16:355–364.
3. Tang BL, Low CB: Genetic manipulation of neural stem cells for transplantation into the injured spinal cord. *Cell Mol Neurobiol* 2007; 27:75–85.
4. Galtrey CM, Fawcett JW. The role of chondroitin sulfate proteoglycans in regeneration and plasticity in the central nervous system. *Brain Res Rev* 2007; 54:1–18.
5. Walmsley AR, Mir AK. Targeting the Nogo-A signalling pathway to promote recovery following acute CNS injury. *Curr Pharm Des* 2007; 13:2470–2484.
6. Bareyre FM, Schwab ME. Inflammation, degeneration and regeneration in the injured spinal cord: insights from DNA microarrays. *Trends Neurosci* 2003; 26:555–563.
7. Lu P, Yang H, Jones LL, Filbin MT, Tuszynski MH. Combinatorial therapy with neurotrophins and cAMP promotes axonal regeneration beyond sites of spinal cord injury. *J Neurosci* 2004; 24:6402–6409.
8. Nikulina E, Tidwell JL, Dai HN, Bregman BS, Filbin MT. The phosphodiesterase inhibitor rolipram delivered after a spinal cord lesion promotes axonal regeneration and functional recovery. *Proc Natl Acad Sci USA* 2004; 101:8786–8790.
9. Pearse DD, Pereira FC, Marcillo AE, Bates ML, Berrocal YA, Filbin MT, Bunge MB. cAMP and Schwann cells promote axonal growth and functional recovery after spinal cord injury. *Nat Med* 2004; 10:610–616.
10. Filbin MT. Recapitulate development to promote axonal regeneration: good or bad approach? *Philos Trans R Soc Lond B Biol Sci* 2006; 361:1565–1574.
11. Pencalet P, Ohanna F, Poulat P, Kamenka JM, Privat A. Thienylphencyclidine protection for the spinal cord of adult rats against extension of lesions secondary to a photochemical injury. *J Neurosurg* 1993; 78:603–609.
12. Rosenberg LJ, Teng YD, Wrathall JR. 2,3-Dihydroxy-6-nitro-7-sulfamoylbenzo(f)quinoxaline reduces glial loss and acute white matter pathology after experimental spinal cord contusion. *J Neurosci* 1999; 19:464–475.
13. Bethea JR, Nagashima H, Acosta MC, Briceno C, Gomez F, Marcillo AE, Loor K, Green J, Dietrich WD. Systemically administered interleukin-10 reduces tumor necrosis factor-alpha production and significantly improves functional recovery following traumatic spinal cord injury in rats. *J Neurotrauma* 1999; 16:851–863.
14. Gaviria M, Privat A, d'Arbigny P, Kamenka J, Haton H, Ohanna F. Neuroprotective effects of a novel NMDA antagonist, Gacyclidine, after experimental contusive spinal cord injury in adult rats. *Brain Res* 2000; 874:200–209.
15. Lim PA, Tow AM. Recovery and regeneration after spinal cord injury: a review and summary of recent literature. *Ann Acad Med Singapore* 2007; 36:49–57.
16. Cheng H, Cao Y, Olson L. Spinal cord repair in adult paraplegic rats: partial restoration of hindlimb function. *Science* 1996; 273:510–513.
17. Barnett SC. Olfactory ensheathing cells: unique glial cell types? *J Neurotrauma* 2004; 21:375–382.
18. Franklin RJ. Obtaining olfactory ensheathing cells from extra-cranial sources a step closer to clinical transplant-mediated repair of the CNS? *Brain* 2002; 125:2–3.
19. Kordower JH, Tuszynski MH. CNS regeneration: In: Kordower JH, Tuszynski MH (eds.), *Basic Science and Clinical Advances*. San Diego: Academic, 1999; 159–182.
20. Keirstead HS, Dyer JK, Sholomenko GN, McGraw J, Delaney KR, Steeves JD. Axonal regeneration and physiological activity following transection and immunological disruption of myelin within the hatching chick spinal cord. *J Neurosci* 1995; 15(10):6963–6974.
21. Keirstead HS, Pataky DM, McGraw J, Steeves JD. In vivo immunological suppression of spinal cord myelin development. *Brain Res Bull* 1997; 44:727–734.
22. Nicholis JG, Saunders NR. Regeneration of immature mammalian spinal cord after injury. *Trends Neurosci* 1996; 19:229–234.
23. Hasan SJ, Keirstead HS, Muir GD, Steeves JD. Axonal regeneration contributes to repair of injured brainstem-spinal neurons in embryonic chick. *J Neurosci* 1993; 13:492–507.
24. Bregman BS. Spinal cord transplants permit the growth of serotonergic axons across the site of neonatal spinal cord transection. *Dev Brain Res* 1987; 34:265–279.
25. Miya D, Giszter S, Mori F, Adipudi V, Tessler A, Murray M. Fetal transplants alter the development of function after spinal cord transection in newborn rats. *J Neurosci* 1997; 17:4856–4872.
26. Diener PS, Bregman BS. Fetal spinal cord transplants support growth of supraspinal and segmental projection after cervical spinal cord hemisection in the neonatal rat. *J Neurosci* 1998; 18:779–793.
27. Diener PS, Bregman BS. Fetal spinal cord transplants support the development of target reaching and coordinated postural adjustments after neonatal cervical spinal cord injury. *J Neurosci* 1998; 18:763–778.
28. Verma P, Fawcett J. Spinal cord regeneration. *Adv Biochem Eng Biotechnol* 2005; 94:43–66.
29. Bregman BS, Diener PS, McAtee M, Dai HN, James CV. Intervention strategies to enhance anatomical plasticity and recovery of function after spinal cord injury. *Adv Neurol* 1997; 72:257–275.
30. Bregman BS, Diener PS, McAtee M, Dai HN, Kuhn PL. Neurotrophic factors increase axonal growth after spinal cord injury and transplantation in adult rat. *Exp Neurol* 1997; 148:475–494.
31. Pittenger MF, Mackay AM, Beck SC, Jaiswal RK, Douglas R, Mosca JD, Moorman MA, Simonetti DW, Craig S, Marshak DR. Multilineage potential of adult human mesenchymal stem cells. *Science* 1999; 284:143–147.
32. Reier PJ. Cellular transplantation strategies for spinal cord injury and translational neurobiology. *NeuroRx* 2004; 1:424–451.
33. Castro RF, Jackson KA, Goodell MA, Robertson CS, Liu H, Shine HD. Failure of bone marrow cells to transdifferentiate into neural cells in vivo. *Science* 2002; 297:1299.
34. Terada N, Hamazaki T, Oka M, Hoki M, Mastalerz DM, Nakano Y, Meyer EM, Morel L, Petersen BE, Scott EW. Bone marrow cells adopt the phenotype of other cells by spontaneous cell fusion. *Nature* 2002; 416:542–545.

35. Camargo FD, Chambers SM, Goodell MA. Stem cell plasticity: from transdifferentiation to macrophage fusion. *Cell Prolif* 2004; 37:55–65.

36. Hofstetter CP, Schwarz EJ, Hess D, Widenfalk J, El Manira A, Prockop DJ, Olson L. Marrow stromal cells form guiding strands in the injured spinal cord and promote recovery. *Proc Natl Acad Sci USA* 2002; 99:2199–2204.

37. Svendsen CN, Bhattacharyya A, Tai YT. Neurons from stem cells: preventing an identity crisis. *Nat Rev Neurosci* 2001; 2:831–834.

38. Jendelova P, Herynek V, Urdzikova L, Glogarova K, Kroupova J, Andersson B, Bryja V, Burian M, Hajek M, Sykova E. Magnetic resonance tracking of transplanted bone marrow and embryonic stem cells labeled by iron oxide nanoparticles in rat brain and spinal cord. *J Neurosci Res* 2004; 76:232–243.

39. Azizi SA, Stokes D, Augelli BJ, DiGirolamo C, Prockop DJ. Engraftment and migration of human bone marrow stromal cells implanted in the brains of albino rats—similarities to astrocyte grafts. *Proc Natl Acad Sci USA* 1998; 95:3908–3913.

40. Gaiano N, Fishell G. Transplantation as a tool to study progenitors within the vertebrate nervous system. *J Neurobiol* 1998; 36:152–161.

41. Brustle O, Jones KN, Learish RD, Karram K, Choudhary K, Wiestler OD, Duncan ID, McKay RD. Embryonic stem cell-derived glial precursors: A source of myelinating transplants. *Science* 1999; 285:754–756.

42. Ono K, Takii T, Onozaki K, Ikawa M, Okabe M, Sawada M. Migration of exogenous immature hematopoietic cells into adult mouse brain parenchyma under GFP-expressing bone marrow chimera. *Biochem Biophys Res Comm* 1999; 262:610–614.

43. Bartlett PF. Pluripotential hemopoietic stem cells in adult mouse brain. *Proc Natl Acad Sci USA* 1999; 79:2722–2725.

44. Gage FH. Mammalian neural stem cells. *Science* 2000; 287:1433–1438.

45. Flax JD, Aurora S, Yang C, Simonin C, Wills AM, Billinghurst LL, Jendoubi M, Sidman RL, Wolfe JH, Kim SU, Snyder EY. Engraftable human neural stem cells respond to developmental cues, replace neurons, and express foreign genes. *Nature Biotechnol* 1998; 16:1033–1438.

46. Gage FH, Coates PW, Palmer TD, Kuhn HG, Fisher LJ, Suhonen JO, Peterson DA, Suhr ST, Ray J. Survival and differentiation of adult neuronal progenitor cells transplanted to the adult brain. *Proc Natl Acad Sci USA* 1995; 92:11879–11883.

47. Liu Y, Himes BT, Solowska J, Moul J, Chow SY, Park KI, Tessler A, Murray M, Snyder EY, Fischer I. Intraspinal delivery of neurotrophin-3 using neural stem cells genetically modified by recombinant retrovirus. *Exp Neurol* 1999; 158:9–26.

48. Snyder EY, Yoon C, Flax JD, Macklis JD. Multipotent neural precursors can differentiate toward replacement of neurons undergoing targeted apoptotic degeneration in adult mouse neocortex. *Proc Natl Acad Sci USA* 1997; 94:11663–11668.

49. McDonald JW, Liu XZ, Qu Y, Liu S, Mickey SK, Turetsky D, Gottlieb DI, Choi DW. Transplanted embryonic stem cells survive, differentiate and promote recovery in injured rat spinal cord. *Nature Med* 1999; 5:1410–1412.

50. McDonald JW, Sadowsky C. Spinal-cord injury. *Lancet* 2002; 359:417–425.

51. Kornack DR, Rakic P. Continuation of neurogenesis in the hippocampus of the adult macaque monkey. *Proc Natl Acad Sci USA* 1999; 96:5768–5773.

52. Eriksson PS, Perfilieva E, Björk-Eriksson T, Alborn AM, Nordborg C, Peterson DA, Gage FH. Neurogenesis in the adult human hippocampus. *Nature Med* 1998; 4:1313–1317.

53. Horner PJ, Power AE, Kempermann G, Kuhn HG, Palmer TD, Winkler J, Thal LJ, Gage FH. Proliferation and differentiation of progenitor cells throughout the intact adult rat spinal cord. *J Neurosci* 2000; 20:2218–2228.

54. Gould E, Tanapat P. Stress and hippocampal neurogenesis. *Biol Psychiatry* 1999; 46:1472–1479.

55. Kempermann G, Kuhn HG, Gage FH. More hippocampal neurons in adult mice living in an enriched environment. *Nature* 1997; 386:493–495.

56. van Praag H, Kempermann G, Gage FH. Running increases cell proliferation and neurogenesis in the adult mouse dentate gyrus. *Nature Neurosci* 1999; 2:266–270.

57. McTigue DM, Horner PJ, Strokes BT, Gage FH. Neurotrophin-3 and brain-derived neurotrophic factor induce oligodendrocyte proliferation and myelination of regenerating axons in the contused spinal cord. *J Neurosci* 1998; 18:5354–5365.

58. Franklin RJ, Gilson JM, Blakemore WF. Local recruitment of remyelinating cells in the repair of demyelination in the central nervous system. *J Neurosci Res* 1997; 50:337–344.

59. Gensert JM, Goldman JE. Endogenous progenitors remyelinate demyelinated cells in the repair of demyelinated axons in adult CNS. *Neuron* 1997; 19:197–203.

60. Magavi SS, Leavitt BR, Mackliss JD. Induction of neurogenesis in the neocortex of adult mice. *Nature* 2000; 405:951–955.

61. Scott GS, Jakeman LB, Stokes BT, Szabo C. Peroxinitrite production and activation of poly (adenosine phosphate-ribose) synthase in spinal cord injury. *Ann Neural* 1999; 45:120–124.

62. Liu D, Li Liping, Augustus L. Prostaglandin release by spinal cord injury mediates production of hydroxyl radical, malongialdehyde and cell death: a site of the neuroprotective action of methylprednisolone. *J Neurochem* 2001; 77:1036–1047.

63. Estevez AG, Spear N, Manuel SM, Radi R, Henderson CE, Barbieto L, Beckman JS. Nitric oxide and superoxide contribute to motor neuron apoptosis induced by trophic factor deprivation. *J Neurosci* 1998; 18:923–931.

64. Beckman JS, Koppenol WH. Nitric oxide, superoxide and peroxynitrite: the good, the bad, and ugly. *Am J Physiol* 1996; 271:C1424–C1437.

65. Cuevas P, Reimers D, Carceller F, Jimenez A. Ischemic reperfusion injury in rabbit spinal cord: protective effect of superoxide dismutase on neurological recovery and spinal infarction. *Acta Anat* 1990; 137:303–310.

66. Cuevas P, Carceller-Benito F, Reimers D. Administration of bovine supcroxide dismutase prevents sequelae of spinal cord ischemia in the rabbit. *Anat Embryol* 1989; 179:251–255.

67. Jung C, Rong Y, Doctrow S, Baudry M, Malfroy B, Xu Z. Synthetic superoxide dismutase/catalase mimetecs reduce oxidative stress and prolong survival in a mouse amyotrophic lateral sclerosis model. *Neurosci Letter* 2001; 304:157–160.

68. Zulueta MG, Ensz LM, Mukhina M, Lebovitz RM, Zwacka RM, Engelhardt JF, Oberley LW, Dawson VL, Dawson TM. Manganese superoxide dismutase protects nNOS neuron from NMDA and nitric oxide–mediated neurotoxicity. *J Neurosci* 1998; 18:2040–2055.

69. Rowland LP. Amyotrophic lateral sclerosis: human challenge for neuroscience. *Proc Natl Acad Sci USA* 1995; 92:1251–1253.

70. Peled-Kamar M, Lotem J, Okon E, Sachs L, Groner Y. Thymic abnormalities and enhanced apoptosis of thymocytes and bone marrow cells in transgenic mice overexposing Cu/Zn-superoxide dismutase: implications for Downs syndrome. *EMBO J* 1995; 14:4985–4993.

71. Norenberg MD. Astrocyte responses to CNS injury. *J Neuropathol Exp Neurol* 1994; 53:213–220.

72. Steg G, Johnels B. Physiological mechanisms and assessment of motor disorders in Parkinson's disease. *Adv Neurol* 1993; 60:358–364.

73. Kelner MJ, Bagnell R, Montoya M, Estes L, Uglick SF, Cerutti P. Transfection with human copper-zinc superoxide dismutase induces bi-directional alterations in other antioxidant enzymes, proteins, growth factor response, and paraquat resistance. *Free Rad Biol Med* 1995; 18:497–506.

74. Bar-Peled O, Korkotian E, Segal M, Groner Y. Constitutive overexpression of Cu/Zn superoxide dismutase exacerbate kainic acid-inuded apoptosis of transgenic Cu/Zn superoxide dismutase neurons. *Proc Natl Acad Sci USA* 1996; 93:8530–8535.

75. Bregman BS, Boude E, McAtee M, Kelley MS. Transplants and neurotrophic factors prevent atrophy of mature CNS neurons after spinal cord injury. *Exp Neurol* 1998; 149:13–27.

76. Ramon-Cueto A, Cordero M, Santos-Benito F, Avila J. Functional recovery of paraplegic rats and motor axon regeneration in their spinal cords by olfactory ensheathing glia. *Neuron* 2000; 25:425–435.

77. Cheng H, Almstrom S, Gimenez-Lort L, Cheng R, Orgren S, Hoffer B, Olson L. Gait analysis of adult paraplegic rats after spinal cord repair. *Exp Neurol* 1997; 148:544–557.

78. Lewin-Kowalik J, Sieron AL, Krause M, Kwiek S. Predegenerated peripheral nerve grafts facilitate neurite outgrowth from the hippocampus. *Brain Res Bull* 1990; 25:669–673.

79. Li Y, Field PM, Raisman G. Repair of adult rat corticospinal tract by transplants of olfactory ensheathing cells. *Science* 1997; 277:2000–2002.

80. Ditelberg JS, Sheldon RA, Epstein CJ, Ferriero DM. Brain injury after perinatal hypoxia-ischemia is exacerbated in copper/zinc superoxide dismutase transgenic mice. *Neurology* 1995; 45(4):A391.

81. Xu J, Fan G, Chen S, Wu Y, Xu XM, Hsu CY. Methylprednisolone inhibition of TNF-alpha expression and NF-kB activation after spinal cord injury in rats. *Mol Brain Res* 1998; 59(2):135–142.

82. Logan A, Berry M, Gonzalez AM, Frautschy SA, Sporn MB, Baird A. Effects of transforming growth factor beta 1 on scar production in the injured central nervous system of the rat. *Eur J Neurosci* 1994; 6:355–363.

83. Saunders RD, Dugan LL, Demediuk P, Means ED, Horrocks LA, Anderson DK. Effects of methylprednisolone and the combination of alpha-tocopherol and selenium on arachidonic acid metabolism and lipid peroxidation in traumatized spinal cord tissue. *J Neurochem* 1987; 49(1):24–31.

84. Rapalino O, Lazarov-Spiegler O, Agranov E, Velan GJ, Yoles E, Fraidakis M, Solomon A, Gepstein R, Katz A, Belkin M, Hadani M, Schwartz M. 1998. Implantation of stimulated homologous macrophages results in partial recovery of paraplegic rats. *Nat Med* 1998; 4(7):814–821.

85. Hasan SJ, Keirstead HS, Muir GD, Steeves JD. Axonal regeneration contributes to repair of injured brainstem-spinal neurons in embryonic chick. *J Neurosci* 1993; 13:492–507.

86. Keirstead HS, Dyer JK, Sholomenko GN, McGraw J, Delaney KR, Steeves JD. Axonal .regeneration and physiological activity following transection and immunological disruption of myelin within the hatchling chick spinal cord. *J Neurosci* 1995; 15:6963–6974.

87. Shimizu I, Oppenheim RW, O'Brian M, Schneiderman A. Anatomical and functional recovery following spinal cord transaction in the chick embryo. *J Neurobiol* 1990; 21:918–937.

88. Steeves JD, Keirstead HS, Ethell DW, Hasan SJ, Muir GD, Pataky DM, McBride CB, Petrausch B, Zwimpfer TJ. Permissive and restrictive periods for brainstem-spinal regeneration in the chick. *Prog Brain Res* 1994; 103:243–262.

89. Keirstead HS, Hasan SJ, Muir GD, Steeves JD. Suppression of the onset of myelination extends the permissive period for the functional repair of embryonic spinal cord. *Proc Natl Acad Sci USA* 1992; 89:11664–11668.

90. Iwashita Y, Kawaguchi S, Murata M. Restoration of function by replacement of spinal cord segments in the rate. *Nature* 1994; 367:167–170.

91. Schnell L, Schnelder R, Kolbeck R, Barde Y, Schwab M. Neurotrophin-3 enhances sprouting of corticospinal tract during development and after adult spinal cord lesion. *Nature* 1994; 367:170–173.

92. Bregman B, Kunkel-Bagden E, Schnell L, Dai H, Gao D, Schwab M. Recovery from spinal cord injury mediated by antibodies to neurite growth inhibitors. *Nature* 1995; 378:498–501.

93. Nygren L, Fuxe K, Jonsson G, Olson L. Functional regeneration of 5-hydroxytryptamine nerve terminals in the rat spinal cord following 5,6–dihydroxytryptamine induced degeneration. *Brain Res* 1974; 78:377–394.

94. Young W, Flamm E. Effect of high-dose corticosteroid therapy on blood flow, evoked potentials, and extracellular calcium in experimental spinal injury. *J Neurosurg* 1982; 57:667–673.

95. Aguayo A, David S, Bary G. Influence of the glial environment on the elongation of axons after injury: transplantation studies in adult rodents. *J Exp Biol* 1981; 95:231–240.

96. David S, Aguayo A. Axonal elongation into peripheral nerve system "bridges" after central nervous system injury in adult rats. *Science* 1981; 214:931–933.

97. Benfey AM, Aguayo A. Extensive elongation of axons from rat brains into peripheral nerve grafts. *Nature* 1982; 296:150–152.

98. Richardson P, McGuinness U, Aguayo A. Peripheral nerve autografts to the rat spinal cord: studies with axonal tracing methods. *Brain Res* 1982; 237:147–162.

99. Paino C, Bunge M. Induction of axon growth into Schwann cell implants grafted into lesioned adult rat spinal cord. *Exp Neurol* 1991; 114:254–257.

100. Bunge R. Expanding roles for the Schwann cell: ensheathment, myelination, trophism and regeneration. *Curr Opin Neurobiol* 1993; 3:805–809.

101. Schachner M. Neural recognition molecules in disease and regeneration. *Curr Opin Neurobiol* 1994; 4:726–734.

102. Schwab M, Kapfhammer J, Bandtlow C. Inhibitors of neurite growth. *Ann Rev Neurosci* 1993; 16:565–595.

103. Savio T, Schwab M. Lesioned corticospinal tract axons regenerate in myelin-free rat spinal cord. *J Neurosurg* 1967; 5:638–646.

104. Schwab M. Myelin-associated inhibitors of neurite growth and regeneration in the CNS. *Trends Neurosci* 1990; 13:452–456.

105. Broesamle C, Schwab M. Axonal regeneration in the mammalian CNS. *Sem Neurosci* 1996; 8:107–113.

106. Cheng H, Olson L. A new surgical technique that allows proximodistal regeneration of 5-HT fibers after complete transection of the rat spinal cord. *Exp Neurol* 1995; 136:149–161.

107. Kuang R, Merline M, Kalil K. Topographic specificity of cortospinal connections formed in explant coculture. *Development* 1994; 120: 1937–1947.

108. Siegal J, Kliot M, Smith G, Silver J. A comparison of the regeneration potential of dorsal root fibers into grey or white matter of the adult rat spinal cord. *Exp Neurol* 1990; 109:90–97.

109. Brown L. Projections and termination of the corticospinal tract in rodents. *Exp Brain Res* 1971; 13:432–450.

110. Blexrud MD, Lee DA, Windebank AJ, Brunden KR. Kinetics of production of a novel growth factor after peripheral nerve injury. *J Neurol Sci* 1990; 98:287–299.

111. Brummendorf T, Rathjen FG. Structure/function relationships of axon-associated adhesion receptors of the immunoglobulin superfamily. *Curr Opin Neurobiol* 1996; 6:584–593.

112. Windebank A J, Poduslo JF. Neuronal growth factors produced by adult peripheral nerve after injury. *Brain Res* 1986; 385:197–200.

113. Lewin-Kowalik J, Sieron AL, Krause M, Barski JJ, Grka D. The influence of peripheral nerve graft's predegeneration stage on the regrowth of hippocampal injured neuritis and concomitant changes in grafts submicrosomal fraction proteins. *Acta Physiol Hung* 1992; 79:219–231.

114. Brummendorf T, Rathjen FG. Structure/function relationships of axon-associated adhesion receptors of the immunoglobulin superfamily. *Curr Opin Neurobiol* 1996; 6:584–593.

115. Cadelli D, Schwab ME. Regeneration of lesioned septohippocampal acetylcholinesterase–positive axons is improved by antibodies against the myelin–associated neurite growth inhibitors NI-35/250. *Eur J Neurosci* 1991; 3:825–832.

116. Ide C, Osawa T, Tohyama K. Nerve regeneration through allogenic nerve grafts, with special reference to the role of the Schwann cell basal lamina. *Prog Neurobiol* 1990; 34:1–38.

117. Gulati AK. Immunological fate of Schwann cell–populated acellular basal lamina nerve allografts. *Transplantation* 1995; 59:1618–1622.

118. La Fleur M, Underwod JL, Rappolee DA, Werb Z. Basement membrane and repair of injury to peripheral nerve: defining a potential role for macrophages, matrix metalloproteinases, and tissue inhibitor of metalloproteinases-1. *J Exp Med* 1996; 184:2311–2326.

119. Brown MC, Perry VH, Lunn ER, Gordon S, Heumann R. Macrophages dependence of peripheral sensory nerve regeneration: possible involvement of nerve growth factor. *Neuron* 1991; 6:554–557.

120. Tresco PA. Tissue engineering strategies for nervous system repair. *Prog Brain Res* 2000; 128:349–363.

121. Steuer H, Fadale R, Müller E, Müller HW, Planck H, Schlosshauer B. Biohybride nerve guide for regeneration: degradable polylactide fibers coated with rat Schwann cells. *Neurosci Lett* 1999; 277:165–168.

122. Pinzon A, Calancie B, Oudega M, Noga BR. Conduction of impulses by axons regenerated in a Schwann cell graft in the transected adult rat thoracic spinal cord. *J Neurosci Res* 2001; 64: 533–541.

123. Plant GW, Woerly S, Harvey AR. Hydrogels containing peptide or aminosugar sequences implanted into the rat brain: influence on cellular migration and axonal growth. *Exp Neurol* 1997; 143:287–299.

124. Giannetti S, Lauretti L, Fernandez E, Salvinelli F, Tamburrini G, et al. Acrylic hydrogel implants after spinal cord lesion in the adult rat. *Neurol Res* 2001; 23:405–409.

125. Lesny P, De Croos J, Pradny M, Vacik J, Michalek J, et al. Polymer hydrogels usable for nervous tissue repair. *J Chem Neuroanat* 2002; 23:243–247.

126. Friedman JA, Windebank AJ, Moore MJ, Spinner RJ, Currier BL, et al. Biodegradable polymer grafts for surgical repair of the injured spinal cord. *Neurosurgery* 2002; 51:742–751.

127. Woerly S, Pinet E, de Robertis L, Van Diep D, Bousmina M. Spinal cord repair with PHPMA hydrogel containing RGD peptides (NeuroGel). *Biomaterials* 2001; 22:1095–111.

128. Maquet V, Martin D, Scholtes F, Franzen R, Schoenen J, et al. Poly(D, Lactide) foams modified by poly(ethylene oxide)-block-poly(D,L-lactide) copolymers and a-FGF: in vitro and in vivo evaluation for spinal cord regeneration. *Biomaterials* 2001; 22:1137–1146.

129. Teng YD, Lavik EB, Qu X, Park KI, Ourednik J, et al. Functional recovery following traumatic spinal cord injury mediated by a unique polymer scaffold seeded with neural stem cells. *Proc. Natl. Acad. Sci. USA* 2002; 99:3024–3029.

130. Borgens RB, Shi R. Immediate recovery from spinal cord injury through molecular repair of nerve membranes with polyethylene glycol. *FASEB J* 2000; 14:27–35.

70

A Review of Clinical Trials and Future Directions for Clinical Studies in Acute Spinal Cord Injury

Alexandre Rasouli
Daniel P. Lammertse
Michael Y. Wang

B ecause of the devastating social, economic, and medical consequences of traumatic spinal cord injury (SCI) there has been great enthusiasm and resources directed toward identifying potential treatments for SCI. Over the past three decades, an unprecedented number of well-designed clinical trials have been conducted to assess treatments intended to improve the neurologic outcome from both acute and chronic SCI.

Although many of these trials have been the subject of controversy, the knowledge gleaned from them in terms of the epidemiology, natural history, and unique medical consequences of SCI have been vital. In addition, valuable experience has been gained in the arenas of logistics of conducting clinical trials in this population, costs associated with these efforts, and optimal scientific methodologies for trial design.

In the acute setting, SCI clinical trials can be subdivided into interventions for pharmacologic neuroprotection, surgical treatment, neural regeneration, and rehabilitative technologies (1). This chapter reviews the history of clinical trials for acute SCI, outlines some of the lessons learned from this experience, and discusses studies that are ongoing or soon to begin.

NEUROPROTECTIVE STRATEGIES

Although physical trauma to the spinal cord undoubtedly causes direct physical injury to the neural tissues, it has become clear that a cascade of events follows the inciting episode that can both inhibit recovery and cause additional neural damage. This concept of secondary injury has been validated in both animal and clinical studies, and secondary injuries have been the target of the bulk of pharmacologic interventions to date (2). These processes begin immediately following the injury and continue for weeks. The exacerbating factors include astroglial scarring, posttraumatic cavitation, deprivation of trophic support, lack of permissive cues at axonal growth cones, progressive demyelination, decreased cyclic adenosine monophosphate (cAMP) levels, and a strong inhibitory environment established by extracellular matrix molecules (keratan sulfate proteoglycans and

chondroitin sulfate proteoglycans NG2, neurocan, brevican, versican, phosphocan) and by glial and myelin components (myelin-associated glycoprotein, α-myelin, Nogo, semaphorins) (3–12). Depending on the specific biochemical target of the therapy, these interventions need to be initiated within a certain time window following injury.

Methylprednisolone

During the 1970s there was an intense enthusiasm for steroid therapies in the fields of neuroscience and neurologic surgery. This led to a number of trials to assess the effects of steroids on a variety of central nervous system disorders. At the time, the general sentiment of the medical community was that corticosteroids would be beneficial for SCI, and treatment, either with dexamethasone or methylprednisolone, had become commonplace by the early 1980s. It was in this environment that pharmacologic trials for SCI began.

The first randomized, controlled, multicenter trial of a neuroprotective agent was the National Acute Spinal Cord Injury (NASCIS) I Study, which attempted to assess the clinical efficacy and optimal dosing for Methylprednisolone sodium succinate (MPSS) (13, 14). Although its precise mechanism of action is still unclear, MPSS was thought to exert either a cell-stabilizing effect via the glucocorticoid receptor or a stabilizing effect via free radical inhibition (15–17). The trial was predicated on several animal studies, which suggested improved neurologic recovery when the corticosteroid was administered promptly after experimental injury (18). Published in 1984, the NASCIS I study included 330 patients with acute SCI (defined as any loss of sensation or motor function below the level of injury), who were randomized to two groups at nine centers within 48 hours of injury: a "low-dose group," receiving a 100-mg IV of methylprednisolone bolus and then 25 mg every 6 hours for 10 days, and a "high-dose" group, receiving bolus and maintenance doses ten times those of the low-dose group every 6 hours for 10 days. Outcome measures consisted of motor and sensory indices of fourteen muscle groups and twenty-nine dermatomes. The follow-up periods were 6 weeks and 6 months. Although there was no difference in between the two groups in terms of neurologic outcome, there was an increased incidence of wound infection and even fatality in the higher-dose group, with the former achieving statistical significance. Of note, the trial did not include a placebo or control arm.

One year later, NASCIS II was launched as the first randomized, prospective, placebo-controlled trial of a candidate therapy for SCI (19, 20). The study was designed to address the lack of a placebo control in NASCIS I and to incorporate new basic-science findings regarding effective methylprednisolone dosing and mechanisms of action (17). The study involved 487 patients who were randomized into three groups at ten centers within 12 hours of sustaining either complete or incomplete SCI: (1) a methylprednisolone group receiving an unprecedented 30-mg/kg IV bolus, followed by a maintenance infusion of 5.4 mg/kg/hour over 23 hours; (2) a placebo group; and (3) a group receiving a 5.4-mg/kg bolus and a 4.0-mg/kg/hour maintenance infusion of the opioid antagonist naloxone, the neuroprotective effects of which had been suggested by animal studies (21). The outcome measurement methodology was similar to that in NASCIS I, utilizing novel motor-sensory composite index scores (summed for only one side of the body) and subclassification of SCI severity as "plegic" (complete) and "paretic" (motor incomplete). It should be noted that these outcome measurement parameters were developed specifically for the NASCIS trials and did not conform to the now widely adopted ASIA international standards.

When all members of the methylprednisolone group in NASCIS II were compared to placebo, there were no statistically significant improvements in sensory or motor function at 6 weeks. However, when the steroid group was stratified according to timing of administration, patients receiving treatment within 8 hours of injury did show significant improvement in sensory and motor function by 6 weeks versus placebo. The relative improvement was sustained through the 6-month follow-up point. Within the steroid group treated within 8 hours, further subgroup analysis with respect to injury severity revealed that "plegic" SCI patients had the greatest statistically significant improvement in motor and sensory measures versus placebo. Patients with "paresis" had only motor improvement, and "plegic" patients with partial sensory loss had neither sensory nor motor improvement that reached statistical significance (19, 20, 22). The complication of wound infection was more frequent but statistically insignificant in the steroid group despite the high dosing. There were no differences in motor or sensory outcomes between the naloxone and placebo groups at either of the follow-up points. The release of the NASCIS II study outcomes established the now widely applied "steroid protocol."

The results of NASCIS II were corroborated several years later in a Japanese multicenter trial, in which 177 patients were prospectively randomized to receive either the NASCIS II steroid protocol (a 30-mg/kg methylprednisolone bolus followed by a 5.4-mg/kg/hour infusion for 24 hours) or placebo (23). Follow-up points at 1.5 and 6 months both showed patients exhibiting enhanced functional recovery (measured in terms of NASCIS motor and sensory scores, as well as in bowel/bladder function) in the steroid group.

Although NASCIS II was a landmark trial, several factors made the trial controversial (1, 17). Much of the controversy surrounded the public release of the study conclusions in an NIH bulletin before the data could be objectively reviewed by the clinical and scientific communities at large. This created a premature de facto standard of care for acute SCI. The original study data has also never been made available to the scientific community, and there have been allegations of possible nontransparency and data misinterpretation. In addition, the acceptance by the medical treatment community of the NASCIS protocol as a "standard of care" for SCI created an environment in which subsequent clinical trials following in its wake were obligated to have an MPSS treatment arm.

The objective of the third and final NASCIS was to investigate the interplay between timing of steroid administration and duration of therapy, and to evaluate the efficacy of a Lazaroid, 21-aminosteroid tirilazad mesylate (Tirilazad), which purportedly had a better safety profile than methylprednisolone. These Lazaroid compounds were experimentally demonstrated to have many of the neuroprotective effects of MPSS without some of the glucocorticoid effects that were responsible for the adverse side effects from high-dose MPSS treatment. In NASCIS III 499 patients at sixteen centers were randomized into three treatment groups within 6 hours of injury: the first group received methylprednisolone according to the NASCIS II dosing for 24 hours, the second group received this dosing for 48 hours, and the third group received an MPSS bolus of 5.4 mg/kg/hour followed by a maintenance infusion of tirilazad at 2.5 mg/kg IV every 6 hours for 48 hours (24). With outcome measures including motor function, sensory function, and functional independence, the NASCIS III trial revealed that increased duration of steroid administration (48 hours) resulted in a statistically significant clinical benefit only if treatment was initiated between 3 and 8 hours of injury. Infectious complications were more common in the 48-hour corticosteroid group but approached or met criteria for statistical significance only for severe sepsis and severe pneumonia. Because there was no significant difference in mortality between treatment groups, the investigators opined that the added risk of infection-related morbidity was acceptable in light of the improved neurologic outcomes. This led to the conclusion that patients who received MPSS within 3 hours of injury should receive 24 hours of MPSS dosing, whereas those treated at 3 to 5 hours following injury should receive a full 48 hours of MPSS. There were no differences between the Tirilazad group and the 24-hour methylprednisolone group (25).

Since the publication of these steroid trials, the general application of high-dose MPSS treatment has been called into question. Due largely to the higher complication rates associated with this intervention, along with questions about the validity and applicability of the NASCIS II and III studies, a number of academic centers have ceased using the "steroid protocol." The controversy over the use of high-dose steroid therapy has mounted in the years since publication of NASCIS II, culminating in the publication of a clinical practice guideline by the American Association of Neurological Surgeons and the Congress of Neurological Surgeons in 2002 on pharmacologic therapy after acute cervical spinal cord injury. This guideline specifically states that evidence for the use of methylprednisolone fell short of that required to establish a standard of care, classifying the use of methylprednisolone as a clinical option "that should be undertaken only with the knowledge that evidence suggesting harmful side effects is more consistent than any suggestion of clinical benefit (26–30)."

GM-1 Ganglioside

Trials of the glycosphingolipid ganglioside GM-1 followed closely on the heels of the methylprednisolone studies. Gangliosides are mammalian neuronal cell membrane constituents that play a substantial role in neuronal plasticity, axonal recovery after experimental SCI, and cell preservation after ischemia (31–35). The Maryland GM-1 ganglioside trial was a prospective, randomized, placebo-controlled pilot study of thirty-seven patients with SCI who were assigned to one of two groups: GM-1 100-mg IV per day for 30 days, and placebo (36). The Frankel scale served as a major outcome measure, and the follow-up point was at 6 months. Overall, the patients treated with GM-1 had more improvement, as assessed by Frankel grade, than their placebo-treated counterparts. In those patients whose injury was severe enough to make a 2 grade Frankel scale improvement possible, 50% of the GM-1 treated patients achieved this degree of change compared to only 7% of those receiving placebo. Despite the small sample size, this difference was statistically significant. The pilot study was then expanded into the largest clinical trial of SCI therapy to date, known as the Sygen Multicenter Acute Spinal Cord Injury Study (SMASCIS) (37). The study randomized 797 patients with SCI into three groups, two treatment groups receiving GM-1 (300-mg IV bolus + 100-mg IV daily for 56 days versus 600-mg IV bolus + 200-mg IV daily for 56 days) and one placebo group. The treatment was initiated within 72 hours of injury, and all groups received NASCIS II protocol methylprednisolone prior to initiation of the study drug. Outcome measures included ASIA sensory and motor scores, ASIA impairment scale rating, and Benzel scale rating. At 8 weeks, patients exhibited dose-related, statistically significant improvements in impairment scale ratings relative to placebo, but by the 6-month endpoint, these differences (defined as at least a 2-grade improvement in the impairment index) became insignificant. SMASCIS had revealed that GM-1 ganglioside was ultimately no better than placebo in improving long-term outcomes in SCI.

Nonetheless, the multicenter Sygen trial remains the largest well-documented cohort of prospectively enrolled, rigorously examined SCI patients available for analysis. This database thus serves as a valuable source of information on the natural history of neurologic recovery following these injuries and may be useful in the design and interpretation of future clinical trials.

Thyrotropin-Releasing Hormone

Thyrotropin-releasing hormone (TRH) and its analogs have been shown in multiple animal models of acute SCI to improve functional recovery by acting as neuroprotective partial opioid antagonists (38–43). The prospective trial evaluating its efficacy in human subjects involved twenty patients at two hospitals at the University of California San Francisco with acute SCI, who were randomly assigned within 12 hours of injury into one of two groups: a TRH group receiving a 0.2-mg/kg bolus IV dose followed by a 0.2-mg/kg/hour infusion for 6 hours, and a placebo group (44). NASCIS motor and sensory indices and the Sunnybrook system were used as outcome measures. Follow-up time points were at 24 hours, 72 hours, 7 days, 1 month, 4 months, and 1 year after injury. Patients with complete injuries did not demonstrate a benefit from TRH administration relative to placebo group patients; however, patients with incomplete injuries did show statistically significant improvement in outcome measures after TRH treatment versus placebo despite the small sample size. Although the results were encouraging, the authors were cautious with their conclusions. It remains unclear as to why a larger clinical trial of TRH for SCI was never performed.

Nimodipine and Gacyclidine

In a number of animal models of SCI, the calcium channel blocker nimodipine effected improved neurological recovery by increasing spinal cord blood flow and limiting vasospasm, ischemia, and secondary infarction (45–47). A prospective clinical trial of the antihypertensive in France involved 106 patients with complete or incomplete SCI who were randomized to one of four groups: a nimodipine 0.015-mg/kg/hour IV loading dose for 2 hours plus a 0.03-mg/kg/hour infusion for 7 days, methylprednisolone according to NASCIS II protocol, both agents, and placebo (48). Outcomes were measured with ASIA grade and ASIA motor and sensory scores. At 1-year follow-up, none of the treatment groups demonstrated efficacy over placebo, but increased rates of medical complications were associated with MPSS administration. Interestingly, a large number (80 of the 106 patients) of enrollees were surgically treated early (within 24 hours of injury), and a subgroup analysis revealed that surgery within 8 hours of injury and between 8 to 24 hours of injury yielded identical outcomes.

Posttraumatic glutamate toxicity is the target of the novel N-methyl-D-aspartate antagonist (NMDA) receptor antagonist gacyclidine, which in rat models has been shown to enhance recovery after contusion SCI (49, 50). In a prospective, controlled clinical trial 272 patients were randomized to one of four groups within 2 hours of SCI: gacyclidine at 0.005 mg/kg IV within two hours of trauma and once again at 6 hours after trauma, two doses of gacyclidine at 0.001 mg/kg IV, two doses of gacyclidine at 0.02 mg/kg, and placebo. Outcome measures were the ASIA motor and sensory scores. At 1-year follow-up, there were no statistical differences in outcomes between any of the groups (51).

Ongoing Trials

The synthetic antimicrobial analog minocycline is postulated to counteract many of the principal cytotoxic responses after cord injury that culminate in neuronal death, including the release of various cytokines, free radicals, and matrix metalloproteinases. Studies in murine contusion models showed superior locomotor recovery relative to methylprednisolone and placebo groups (52). The current prospective, double-blinded human trial is in progress at the University of Calgary; patients are randomly assigned to receive a minocycline 200-mg IV twice daily for 1 week or a placebo injection. A subset of the patients will also be randomized to assess the efficacy and safety of blood pressure management to optimize spinal cord perfusion pressure. Outcome measures will include ASIA motor and sensory index scores, ASIA impairment scale scores, and radiographic assessments; the endpoint will be at 1 year postinjury (53).

Early intravascular hypothermia trials are being initiated at the University of Miami and the Miami Project to Cure Paralysis to assess the effects of moderate hypothermia to reduce the effects of secondary injury. The single-center pilot study involves placement of an intravascular cooling catheter within 8 hours of injury and cooling to 33°C for 48 hours, followed by a rewarming period.

SURGICAL INTERVENTION

Most surgeons agree that patients with mechanical compression of the neural elements who are either incomplete or deteriorating neurologically require surgical intervention for decompression and stabilization. However, there is little consensus or scientific evidence on the urgency of surgery.

The first prospective, randomized clinical trial addressing the utility and timing of decompressive spinal surgery after SCI was undertaken at the Rothman Institute in Philadelphia (54). Sixty-two patients with complete or incomplete cervical SCI were randomized into one of two groups: decompression within 72 hours of injury (early group) and decompression after at least 5 days (late group). Outcomes, which were measured in terms ASIA grade and motor score, were no better in the early group after 1 year, nor were there differences between length of stay in the intensive care or acute rehabilitation units between the two groups. The major criticism of this study was that the average time to surgery in the acute group was 1.82 days (compared to 16.75 days in the late group), a period of time that in the modern era would not be considered to be early enough to result in a high likelihood of neurologic improvement.

A larger prospective, but nonrandomized, trial in Canada involved 208 patients with SCI who were treated with either decompression and fusion or nonoperative management. The operative group featured lower mortality rates but higher thromboembolic complications versus the control group; there were no differences between the groups in terms of hospital length of stay or neurologic recovery (55).

The Surgical Trial in Acute Spinal Cord Injury Study (STASCIS) is the largest clinical trial effort to date to assess neurologic recovery as a function of surgical decompression, and specifically, of the timing of decompression. In addition to an exhaustive retrospective review of nearly 1,000 surgical cases to assess study feasibility, STASCIS included three phases. STASCIS 1 was a multicenter, retrospective review of surgical timing trends in North American centers and involved approximately 600 patients (56). The results revealed that the most common intervention period was after 5 days of injury; the second most common trend was to intervene within 24 hours. STASCIS 2 established the safety of early decompression (within 12 hours), in which half of the patients underwent early decompression and had no increase in complications relative to the case-matched controls (1). STASCIS 3 is the current and most important component of the trial series: a nonrandomized, prospective, multicenter cohort study that will evaluate the association of neurologic outcomes with the efficacy and timing of decompressive surgery. It will only involve cervical SCI resulting in paresis or plegia and will be one of the first to include correlative assessment of MRI and computed tomographic studies (57).

REGENERATION STRATEGIES

Whereas neuroprotective strategies are directed primarily at limiting secondary neural injury, regeneration strategies involve repair of the damaged tissues. This, of course, is more theoretically appealing due to the potential for greater degrees of neurologic improvement. However, any such therapeutic strategy must also somehow modify the nonideal local milieu of the injured cord (58–60), as biochemical, cellular, and extracellular matrix perturbations may limit the potential for axonal repair. Although a number of laboratory investigations have reported remarkable success utilizing such strategies, translation to the clinical setting has been difficult, and clinical trials of regenerative strategies are just beginning.

Immune-Mediated Neural Repair and Autologous Macrophage Transplantation

A controlled inflammatory response is essential to proper tissue repair in any part of the body, including the CNS. The brain and spinal cord are naturally sequestered from the inflammatory cells of systemic circulation by highly selective basement membranes (the blood–brain barrier). Therefore, the injured CNS often will not elicit a bona fide immune response, and its innate healing capacity will thus be stultified (61). The concept of immune-mediated neural repair is based on several laboratory studies that demonstrated protective autoimmunity with macrophages: animals with transection SCI treated with autologous macrophages at the lesion site had enhanced functional and histologic recovery (62, 63).

This strategy was translated to the clinical setting in an Israeli pilot trial utilizing autologous activated macrophages, which were injected into the lesion sites of SCI. The macrophages were activated in vitro with autologous dermis. The results from the pilot trial demonstrated that three of eight ASIA A patients converted to ASIA C at one year of follow-up (64, 65). Based on these encouraging results, a Phase II randomized, controlled clinical trial of autologous incubated macrophage treatment of SCI patients with complete injuries was initiated in 2003 at six SCI treatment centers in Israel and North America (sponsored by ProNeuron Biotechnologies, Ness Ziona, Israel). The trial had enrolled fifty patients by the spring of 2006 but was stopped for financial reasons. This trial was remarkable for a number of reasons. The enrollment window of 14 days allowed patients who had been stabilized and received acute treatment at a referring trauma center to be transported to one of the study sites. At these facilities the patients were then consented, assessed, and randomized. They then underwent blood and skin harvest for cell processing, followed by surgical implantation of the incubated autologous macrophages into the caudal boundary of the spinal cord contusion. In addition, the patient selection process included radiographic criteria: those with intramedullary lesions larger than 3 cm on MRI were excluded. This strategy of excluding patients with severe radiographic spinal cord abnormalities may be helpful for determining the efficacy of an intervention with smaller numbers of patients.

Rho Antagonist

Several inhibitors of nerve regeneration have been identified, including Nogo, myelin-associated glycoprotein (MAG), and myelin-oligodendrocyte glycoprotein (OMgp). These factors act commonly through the GTPase Rho, an enzyme that orchestrates a potent inhibitory cascade after injury that culminates in growth cone disintegration, neurite sprouting inhibition, and neuronal and glial cell apoptosis (66, 67). The naturally occurring inhibitor of the Rho enzyme, C3 transferase from *C. botuliinum,* has been shown to effect remarkably rapid functional recovery in hemisection SCI rats (68). Histologic analysis of C3-treated rats treated within 24 hours of injury showed increased neuronal sprouting, and functional analysis revealed enhanced locomotor recovery and limb coordination (68–71).

A recombinant pharmaceutical version of C3 transferase known as Cethrin (Alseres Pharmaceuticals, Hopkinton, Massachusetts), in which the enzyme is linked to a protein that facilitates blood–brain barrier penetration, has undergone phase I/IIa trials at nine North American centers to establish safety and efficacy. Preliminary results of this trial have been discussed at scientific meetings and published in abstract form (71). The study included thirty-seven patients with complete (ASIA A) SCI at either the cervical or thoracic level who were given increasing doses of extradurally applied Cethrin (0.3, 1.0, 3.0, and 6.0 mg). Outcome measures (ASIA international standards) were collected at 1.5, 3, 6, and 12 months. The investigators documented no adverse effects of the treatment, and by the 1.5-month follow-up period, they observed improvement of at least one ASIA impairment scale grade in 30% of patients. Initial data from the 6-month follow-up period suggest similar rates of recovery.

A phase II/III multicenter clinical trial of the drug Cethrin was due to begin in 2008. The study is anticipating enrollment of complete SCI (ASIA A) patients to undergo surgery for epidural application of the soluble enzyme antagonist at the time of early surgical decompression (17). Study enrollment will incorporate a Bayesian trial design in an effort to determine optimal dosing while keeping sample numbers to a minimum.

Anti-Nogo Antibody

Nogo is an oligodendrocyte-expressed soluble factor that is potent in its ability to thwart axonal regeneration (72). Investigators have been able to restore corticospinal axonal regeneration and locomotion in rat and primate SCI models in which Nogo was neutralized with the monoclonal antibody IN-1 (73–76). A phase I clinical trial of intrathecally administered Nogo-A antibody (Novartis International AG, Basel, Switzerland) in acute, complete (ASIA A) SCI is currently under way in European SCI centers with expansion of the trial to Canadian centers anticipated in 2008. Results of the phase I trial have yet to be published (53).

Oscillating Field Stimulation

The embryonic neural tube develops its cranial and caudal orientation due in part to axonal migration toward the cathode of an electrical field. This concept was investigated in the experimental setting by Borgens at Purdue University, who demonstrated not only that axonal regrowth following injury could be spatially oriented by an electrical field, but also that the speed and extent of axonal regrowth could be enhanced with the optimal electrical field of 500–600 mV/mm (77). Axonal tropism to electrical fields is the principle behind oscillating field stimulation, in which the polarity of an implanted electrical field generator is periodically alternated to attract outgrowth of both descending (motor) and ascending (sensory) axons at the lesion site of SCI. The efficacy of this technique has been shown in canine and rodent models (77, 78). An open-label phase I pilot clinical trial of ten human subjects with complete SCI at cervical or thoracic levels was recently completed at the University of Indiana, in which oscillating field stimulators were implanted within 18 days and removed at 4 months. No control subjects were included in this trial. Six electrodes were implanted. At 1 year, all subjects showed some improvement in motor and sensory ASIA index scores (78).

Peripheral Nerve and Schwann Cell Transplantation

Inducing the CNS to mimic the natural regenerative ability of the peripheral nervous system (PNS) is a pillar of current SCI research. The injured peripheral nerve expresses a permissive environment for axonal regrowth, which is engendered primarily by its myelin-forming cell, the Schwann cell, and its basal lamina. Schwann cells secrete trophic factors, express cell adhesion molecules, and produce extracellular matrix molecules that are requisite for axonal growth and regeneration (79–81). The permissive features of Schwann cells may prove valuable in the treatment of spinal cord injury. Several groups have demonstrated improved axonal regeneration and functional recovery after Schwann cell transplantation to the site of spinal cord injury (SCI) in rats (79, 81–85). Furthermore, the grafting of peripheral nerves with varying combinations of growth factors in SCI rats has resulted in significant axonal and functional recovery (60, 86–93). Most of the ongoing clinical studies involving peripheral nerve grafts that are used to bridge lesional sites in the spinal cord are phase 1 trials and currently involve very few patients. Some have shown neurologic improvement, whereas others have not; none of these yet are prospective, randomized trials (94, 95). Other studies have involved the injection of Schwann cells to the area of cord lesion. A recent review of current clinical trials documents a Chinese clinical trial utilizing a Schwann cell delivery strategy to treat forty-seven patients with SCI and reports improvement in ASIA motor and sensory scores (1).

Olfactory Ensheathing Glial Cell Transplantation

The olfactory ensheathing glial (OEG) cell spans both the PNS and CNS and thus has a unique role in regenerative SCI therapy; several preclinical studies have shown the OEG to have permissive capabilities similar to that of the Schwann cell (96). A nonrandomized, noncontrolled clinical trial of OEG transplantation in 171 patients with SCI showed patients having modest improvement in ASIA motor and sensory scores after 8 weeks (97). The study was criticized for its short duration, potential for bias, and lack of control. Neurologic outcomes in the first seven chronic (>6 months postinjury) SCI patients treated with surgical implant of olfactory mucosal autograft in an ongoing surgical case series in Lisbon, Portugal, were recently published (98). The investigators claimed to show a modest improvement in ASIA motor and sensory scores in the treated patients. Preliminary safety results of a small Australian controlled clinical trial of surgical implantation of cultured autologous olfactory cells in patients with chronic SCI have recently been published (98). The investigators reported no significant safety concerns at 1 year after implant and plan to report efficacy outcomes after 3 years of follow-up.

Bone Marrow Transplantation

The pluripotency of bone marrow stem cells make them attractive options for neural regeneration after injury. Rat models of SCI have evinced autologous stromal bone marrow cells as having the capacity to differentiate into glial cells and to enhance functional recovery after transplantation (99). A pilot clinical trial of bone marrow transplantation with granulocyte-macrophage colony-stimulating factor (GM-CSF) in six patients with SCI was recently completed; it revealed the safety of the technique and resulted in improvement of two ASIA scale grades in four of the patients by 18 months. A larger randomized, controlled study is in the planning stage (100).

CHALLENGES FOR TRIALS IN ACUTE SPINAL CORD INJURY

Despite the tremendous enthusiasm and financial support for trials in acute SCI, numerous logistical barriers exist. In addition to the challenges associated with determining which interventions are most likely to effect an improved outcome, clinical researchers must overcome problems with regard to trial design, multicenter collaboration, patient enrollment, adequate sample size, regulatory compliance, and financial considerations. Awareness of these challenges led to an international effort to establish guidelines for the conduct of clinical trials in SCI, sponsored by the International Campaign for Cures for Spinal Cord Injury Paralysis (ICCP) (101–104).

Proper trial design is critical to the success of any randomized, prospective, controlled trial (RPCT). Legitimate disagreements between investigators over the necessary sample size, number of participating centers, randomization scheme, control group, outcome measures, and timing of intervention are often difficult to resolve and can affect the outcome of the trial. The aforementioned RPCTs performed over the past three decades have provided invaluable experience into the potential pitfalls associated with studies of adequate magnitude.

In order to ensure an adequate sample size and to control for institutional bias, trials on acute SCI beyond the pilot phase are necessarily multi-institutional. This presents obvious barriers and requires significant commitment to collaboration between centers. Fortunately, coordination between recognized acute care hospitals and rehabilitation centers has been developing due to prior interactions on RPCTs and also through emerging trial networks (1).

Patient enrollment and treatment within a critical "Golden window" of intervention to reduce secondary injury presents unique challenges. Because SCIs occur at any hour of the day or night, evaluation requires an on-call team to perform a precise neurologic examination and then properly determine if inclusionary and exclusionary conditions are met. Furthermore, proper consent must be obtained from the patient or a surrogate, which can be complicated by intracranial trauma, distracting injuries, sedative medications, and the availability of family members (105).

The recruitment of an adequate number of patients to definitively demonstrate a treatment effect has been one of the largest barriers to clinical trials for acute SCI. A wealth of experience on the sample numbers needed for both incomplete and complete patients was obtained from the GM-1 ganglioside trial, which enrolled 760 patients. This database was used by the ICCP SCI Clinical Trials Workgroup to derive estimates of the number of enrolled subjects required to show statistically significant improvement of a treatment with various trial conditions, including enrollment timing postinjury, estimated magnitude of treatment effect, and severity of injury (101). Depending on the trial design and these key patient variables, the number of enrolled patients required to achieve statistical significance can range from less than 100 to over 1,000, with earlier interventions, enrollment of less severe (incomplete) injuries, and lower magnitude of treatment effect necessitating larger numbers of enrolled subjects. These large sample numbers multiply the costs associated with properly conducting such studies.

Adding to these difficulties has been the substantially greater degree of governmental and institutional regulation associated with conducting a large multicenter trial. Although these regulatory processes have been appropriately instituted to enhance patient safety and confidentiality, there is no question that they result in added expenditures for clinical trials (106).

Finally, the costs associated with conducting clinical trials for acute SCI have been a significant barrier to studies designed to gather class I data in First World countries. Over the last 15 years, the National Institutes of Health (NIH) have not funded a RPCT for acute SCI, and trials have either been limited in enrollment or funded through nongovernmental organizations, such as the pharmaceutical industry.

FUTURE DIRECTIONS

SCI remains a challenging clinical problem, and to date no definitive evidence exists for an acute intervention that will enhance neurologic outcomes. Ultimately, the plethora of promising interventions being studied in the laboratory will have to be validated in the clinical setting, and thus the creation of a streamlined and financially feasible mechanism for clinical trials will be necessary. There exists great enthusiasm for this in the SCI community, composed of SCI patients and their advocates, basic science researchers, and clinicians from a variety of disciplines; this support will hopefully push this process forward. Ultimately, combination therapies incorporating interventions to limit secondary injury, along with surgical treatment, regenerative therapies, and rehabilitation, will likely be necessary to impact the outcomes of this devastating disease.

References

1. Tator CH. Review of treatment trials in human spinal cord injury: issues, difficulties, and recommendations. *Neurosurgery* 2006; 59(5):957–987.
2. Ramon-y-Cajal S. *Degeneration and Regeneration of the Nervous System.* May RM, translator. New York: Oxford University Press, 1928.
3. De Winter F, Oudega M, Lankhorst AJ, et al. Injury-induced class 3 semaphorin expression in the rat spinal cord. *Exp Neurol* 2002; 175(1):61–75.
4. Fitch MT, Silver J. Activated macrophages and the blood–brain barrier: inflammation after CNS injury leads to increases in putative inhibitory molecules. *Exp Neurol* 1997; 148(2):587–603.
5. Jones LL, Tuszynski MH. Spinal cord injury elicits expression of keratan sulfate proteoglycans by macrophages, reactive microglia, and oligodendrocyte progenitors. *J Neurosci* 2002; 22(11):4611–4624.
6. Lemons ML, Howland DR, Anderson DK. Chondroitin sulfate proteoglycan immunoreactivity increases following spinal cord injury and transplantation. *Exp Neurol* 1999; 160(1):51–65.

7. McKerracher L, David S, Jackson DL, et al. Identification of myelin-associated glycoprotein as a major myelin-derived inhibitor of neurite growth. *Neuron* 1994; 13(4):805–811.

8. Moon LD, Asher RA, Rhodes KE, et al. Relationship between sprouting axons, proteoglycans and glial cells following unilateral nigrostriatal axotomy in the adult rat. *Neuroscience* 2002; 109(1):101–117.

9. Pasterkamp RJ, Anderson PN, Verhaagen J. Peripheral nerve injury fails to induce growth of lesioned ascending dorsal column axons into spinal cord scar tissue expressing the axon repellent Semaphorin3A. *Eur J Neurosci* 2001; 13(3):457–471.

10. Pearse DD, Pereira FC, Marcillo AE, et al. cAMP and Schwann cells promote axonal growth and functional recovery after spinal cord injury. *Nat Med* 2004; 10(6):610–616.

11. Woolf CJ. No Nogo: now where to go? *Neuron* 2003; 38(2):153–156.

12. Zheng B, Ho C, Li S, et al. Lack of enhanced spinal regeneration in Nogo-deficient mice. *Neuron* 2003; 38(2):213–224.

13. Bracken MB, Collins WF, Freeman DF, et al. Efficacy of methylprednisolone in acute spinal cord injury. *JAMA* 1984; 251(1):45–52.

14. Bracken MB, Shepard MJ, Hellenbrand KG, et al. Methylprednisolone and neurological function 1 year after spinal cord injury. Results of the National Acute Spinal Cord Injury Study. *J Neurosurg* 1985; 63(5):704–713.

15. Ducker TB, Hamit HF: Experimental treatments of acute spinal cord injury. *J Neurosurg* 1969; 30(6):693–697.

16. Hall ED, Braughler JM. Glucocorticoid mechanisms in acute spinal cord injury: a review and therapeutic rationale. *Surg Neurol* 1982; 18(5): 320–327.

17. Lammertse DP. Update on pharmaceutical trials in acute spinal cord injury. *J Spinal Cord Med* 2004; 27(4):319–325.

18. Campbell JB, DeCrescito V, Tomasula JJ, et al. Experimental treatment of spinal cord contusion in the cat. *Surg Neurol* 1973; 1(2):102–106.

19. Bracken MB. Treatment of acute spinal cord injury with methylprednisolone: results of a multicenter, randomized clinical trial. *J Neurotrauma* 1991; 8(Suppl 1):S47–S52.

20. Bracken MB, Shepard MJ, Collins WF, et al. A randomized, controlled trial of methylprednisolone or naloxone in the treatment of acute spinal-cord injury. Results of the Second National Acute Spinal Cord Injury Study. *N Engl J Med* 1990; 322(20):1405–1411.

21. Faden AI, Jacobs TP, Holaday JW. Opiate antagonist improves neurologic recovery after spinal injury. *Science* 1981; 211(4481):493–494.

22. Bracken MB, Shepard MJ, Collins WF Jr., et al. Methylprednisolone or naloxone treatment after acute spinal cord injury: 1-year follow-up data. Results of the second National Acute Spinal Cord Injury Study. *J Neurosurg* 1992; 76(1):23–31.

23. Otani K, Abe H, Kadoya S, et al. Beneficial effect of methylprednisolone sodium succinate in the treatment of acute spinal cord injury. *Sekitsui Sekizui J* 1994; 7633–7647.

24. Bracken MB, Shepard MJ, Holford TR, et al. Administration of methylprednisolone for 24 or 48 hours or tirilazad mesylate for 48 hours in the treatment of acute spinal cord injury. Results of the Third National Acute Spinal Cord Injury Randomized Controlled Trial. National Acute Spinal Cord Injury Study. *JAMA* 1997; 277(20):1597–1604.

25. Bracken MB. High dose methylprednisolone must be given for 24 or 48 hours after acute spinal cord injury. *BMJ* 2001; 322(7290):862–863.

26. Hurlbert RJ. Methylprednisolone for acute spinal cord injury: an inappropriate standard of care. *J Neurosurg* 2000; 93(1 Suppl):1–7.

27. Hurlbert RJ: The role of steroids in acute spinal cord injury: an evidence-based analysis. *Spine* 2001; 26(24 Suppl):S39–S46.

28. Hurlbert RJ. Strategies of medical intervention in the management of acute spinal cord injury. *Spine* 2006; 31(11 Suppl):S16–S21; discussion S36.

29. Hurlbert RJ, Moulton R. Why do you prescribe methylprednisolone for acute spinal cord injury? A Canadian perspective and a position statement. *Can J Neurol Sci* 2002; 29(3):236–239.

30. Hadley MN, Walters BC, Grabb PA, et al. Guidelines for the management of acute cervical spine and spinal cord injuries. *Clin Neurosurg* 2002; 49:407–498.

31. Agnati LF, Fuxe K, Calza L, et al. Further studies on the effects of the GM1 ganglioside on the degenerative and regenerative features of mesostriatal dopamine neurons. *Acta Physiol Scand Suppl* 1984; 53:237–244.

32. Bose B, Osterholm JL, Kalia M. Ganglioside-induced regeneration and reestablishment of axonal continuity in spinal cord–transected rats. *Neurosci Lett* 1986; 63(2):165–169.

33. Toffano G, Agnati LF, Fuxe KG. The effect of the ganglioside GM1 on neuronal plasticity. *Int J Dev Neurosci* 1986; 4(2):97–100.

34. Toffano G, Savoini G, Moroni F, et al. GM1 ganglioside stimulates the regeneration of dopaminergic neurons in the central nervous system. *Brain Res* 1983; 261(1):163–166.

35. von Euler G, Fuxe K, Agnati LF, et al. Ganglioside GM1 treatment prevents the effects of subacute exposure to toluene on N-[3H]propylnorapomorphine binding characteristics in rat striatal membranes. *Neurosci Lett* 1987; 82(2):181–184.

36. Geisler FH, Dorsey FC, Coleman WP. Recovery of motor function after spinal-cord injury—a randomized, placebo-controlled trial with GM-1 ganglioside. *N Engl J Med* 1991; 324(26):1829–1838.

37. Geisler FH, Coleman WP, Grieco G, et al. The Sygen multicenter acute spinal cord injury study. *Spine* 2001; 26(24 Suppl):S87–S98.

38. Faden AI. New pharmacologic approaches to spinal cord injury: opiate antagonists and thyrotropin-releasing hormone. *Cent Nerv Syst Trauma* 1985; 2(1):5–8.

39. Faden AI. Opiate antagonists and thyrotropin-releasing hormone. II. Potential role in the treatment of central nervous system injury. *JAMA* 1984; 252(11):1452–1454.

40. Faden AI, Hallenbeck JM, Brown CQ. Treatment of experimental stroke: comparison of naloxone and thyrotropin releasing hormone. *Neurology* 1982; 32(10):1083–1087.

41. Faden AI, Jacobs TP, Holaday JW. Thyrotropin-releasing hormone improves neurologic recovery after spinal trauma in cats. *N Engl J Med* 1981; 305(18):1063–1067.

42. Faden AI, Jacobs TP, Smith MT. Thyrotropin-releasing hormone in experimental spinal injury: dose response and late treatment. *Neurology* 1984; 34(10):1280–1284.

43. Vink R, McIntosh TK, Faden AI. Treatment with the thyrotropin-releasing hormone analog CG3703 restores magnesium homeostasis following traumatic brain injury in rats. *Brain Res* 1988; 460(1): 184–188.

44. Pitts LH, Ross A, Chase GA, et al. Treatment with thyrotropin-releasing hormone (TRH) in patients with traumatic spinal cord injuries. *J Neurotrauma* 1995; 12(3):235–243.

45. Gambardella G, Collufio D, Caruso GN, et al. Experimental incomplete spinal cord injury: treatment with a combination of nimodipine and adrenaline. *J Neurosurg Sci* 1995; 39(1):67–74.

46. Guha A, Tator CH, Piper I. Effect of a calcium channel blocker on posttraumatic spinal cord blood flow. *J Neurosurg* 1987; 66(3):423–430.

47. Pointillart V, Gense D, Gross C, et al. Effects of nimodipine on posttraumatic spinal cord ischemia in baboons. *J Neurotrauma* 1993; 10(2):201–213.

48. Pointillart V, Petitjean ME, Wiart L, et al. Pharmacological therapy of spinal cord injury during the acute phase. *Spinal Cord* 2000; 38(2):71–76.

49. Feldblum S, Arnaud S, Simon M, et al. Efficacy of a new neuroprotective agent, gacyclidine, in a model of rat spinal cord injury. *J Neurotrauma* 2000; 17(11):1079–1093.

50. Gaviria M, Privat A, d'Arbigny P, et al. Neuroprotective effects of a novel NMDA antagonist, Gacyclidine, after experimental contusive spinal cord injury in adult rats. *Brain Res* 2000; 874(2):200–209.

51. Lepeintre JF, D'Arbigny P, Mathe JF, et al. Neuroprotective effect of gacyclidine: a multicenter double-blind pilot trial in patients with acute traumatic brain injury. *Neurochirurgie* 2004; 50(2–3 Pt 1):83–95.

52. Wells CE, Spillane JD, Bligh AS. The cervical spinal canal in syringomyelia. *Brain* 1959; 82(1):23–40.

53. Jha A, Lammertse DP, Charlifue SW, et al. Topics in spinal cord injury rehabilitation. *Top Spinal Cord Inj Rehabil* 2006; 11(3):86–100.

54. Vaccaro AR, Daugherty RJ, Sheehan TP, et al. Neurologic outcome of early versus late surgery for cervical spinal cord injury. *Spine* 1997; 22(22):2609–2613.

55. Tator CH, Duncan EG, Edmonds VE, et al. Comparison of surgical and conservative management in 208 patients with acute spinal cord injury. *Can J Neurol Sci* 1987; 14(1):60–69.

56. Tator CH, Fehlings MG, Thorpe K, et al. Current use and timing of spinal surgery for management of acute spinal surgery for management of acute spinal cord injury in North America: results of a retrospective multicenter study. *J Neurosurg* 1999; 91(1 Suppl):12–18.

57. Dvorak MF, Fisher CG, Fehlings MG, et al. The surgical approach to subaxial cervical spine injuries: an evidence-based algorithm based on the SLIC classification system. *Spine* 2007; 32(23):2620–2629.

58. Fawcett JW. Overcoming inhibition in the damaged spinal cord. *J Neurotrauma* 2006; 23(3–4):371–383.

59. Dinh P, Bhatia N, Rasouli A, et al. Transplantation of preconditioned Schwann cells following hemisection spinal cord injury. *Spine* 2007; 32(9):943–949.

60. Rasouli A, Bhatia N, Suryadevara S, et al. Transplantation of preconditioned Schwann cells in peripheral nerve grafts after contusion in the adult spinal cord: improvement of recovery in a rat model. *J Bone Joint Surg Am* 2006; 88(11):2400–2410.

61. Perry VH, Brown MC, Gordon S. The macrophage response to central and peripheral nerve injury: a possible role for macrophages in regeneration. *J Exp Med* 1987; 165(4):1218–1223.

62. Rapalino O, Lazarov-Spiegler O, Agranov E, et al. Implantation of stimulated homologous macrophages results in partial recovery of paraplegic rats. *Nat Med* 1998; 4(7):814–821.

63. Schwartz M, Lazarov-Spiegler O, Rapalino O, et al. Potential repair of rat spinal cord injuries using stimulated homologous macrophages. *Neurosurgery* 1999; 44(5):1041–1046.

64. Lazarov-Spiegler O, Solomon AS, Schwartz M. Peripheral nerve-stimulated macrophages simulate a peripheral nerve–like regenerative response in rat transected optic nerve. *Glia* 1998; 24(3):329–337.

65. Lazarov-Spiegler O, Solomon AS, Zeev-Brann AB, et al. Transplantation of activated macrophages overcomes central nervous system regrowth failure. *FASEB J* 1996; 10(11):1296–1302.

66. Dubreuil CI, Winton MJ, McKerracher L. Rho activation patterns after spinal cord injury and the role of activated Rho in apoptosis in the central nervous system. *J Cell Biol* 2003; 162(2):233–243.

67. Sung JK, Miao L, Calvert JW, et al. A possible role of RhoA/Rho-kinase in experimental spinal cord injury in rat. *Brain Res* 2003; 959(1):29–38.

68. Dergham P, Ellezam B, Essagian C, et al. Rho signaling pathway targeted to promote spinal cord repair. *J Neurosci* 2002; 22(15):6570–6577.

69. Baptiste DC, Fehlings MG. Update on the treatment of spinal cord injury. *Prog Brain Res* 2007; 16:1217–1233.

70. Fehlings MG, Baptiste DC. Current status of clinical trials for acute spinal cord injury. *Injury* 2005; 36(Suppl 2):B113–B122.

71. Lehmann M, Fournier A, Selles-Navarro I, et al. Inactivation of Rho signaling pathway promotes CNS axon regeneration. *J Neurosci* 1999; 19(17):7537–7547.

72. Schwab ME, Caroni P. Oligodendrocytes and CNS myelin are nonpermissive substrates for neurite growth and fibroblast spreading in vitro. *J Neurosci* 1988; 8(7):2381–2393.

73. Atalay B, Bavbek M, Cekinmez M, et al. Antibodies neutralizing Nogo-A increase pan-cadherin expression and motor recovery following spinal cord injury in rats. *Spinal Cord* 2007; 12:780–786.

74. Bregman BS, Kunkel-Bagden E, Schnell L, et al. Recovery from spinal cord injury mediated by antibodies to neurite growth inhibitors. *Nature* 1995; 378(6556):498–501.

75. Chen MS, Huber AB, van der Haar ME, et al. Nogo-A is a myelin-associated neurite outgrowth inhibitor and an antigen for monoclonal antibody IN-1. *Nature* 2000; 403(6768):434–439.

76. Weinmann O, Schnell L, Ghosh A, et al. Intrathecally infused antibodies against Nogo-A penetrate the CNS and downregulate the endogenous neurite growth inhibitor Nogo-A. *Mol Cell Neurosci* 2006; 32(1–2): 161–173.

77. Borgens RB, Toombs JP, Breur G, et al. An imposed oscillating electrical field improves the recovery of function in neurologically complete paraplegic dogs. *J Neurotrauma* 1999; 16(7):639–657.

78. Shapiro S, Borgens R, Pascuzzi R, et al. Oscillating field stimulation for complete spinal cord injury in humans: a phase 1 trial. *J Neurosurg Spine* 2005; 2(1):3–10.

79. Bixby JL, Lilien J, Reichardt LF: Identification of the major proteins that promote neuronal process outgrowth on Schwann cells in vitro. *J Cell Biol* 1988; 107(1):353–361.

80. Bryan DJ, Wang KK, Chakalis-Haley DP: Effect of Schwann cells in the enhancement of peripheral-nerve regeneration. *J Reconstr Microsurg* 1996; 12(7):439–446.

81. Fawcett JW, Keynes RJ. Peripheral nerve regeneration. *Annu Rev Neurosci* 1990; 13:43–60.

82. Blakemore WF, Crang AJ. The relationship between type-1 astrocytes, Schwann cells and oligodendrocytes following transplantation of glial cell cultures into demyelinating lesions in the adult rat spinal cord. *J Neurocytol* 1989; 18(4):519–528.

83. Gilmore SA, Sims TJ. Patterns of Schwann cell myelination of axons within the spinal cord. *J Chem Neuroanat* 1993; 6(4):191–199.

84. Martin D, Robe P, Franzen R, et al. Effects of Schwann cell transplantation in a contusion model of rat spinal cord injury. *J Neurosci Res* 1996; 45(5):588–597.

85. Xu XM, Chen A, Guenard V, et al. Bridging Schwann cell transplants promote axonal regeneration from both the rostral and caudal stumps of transected adult rat spinal cord. *J Neurocytol* 1997; 26(1):1–16.

86. Aguayo AJ, David S, Bray GM. Influences of the glial environment on the elongation of axons after injury: transplantation studies in adult rodents. *J Exp Biol* 1981; 95:231–240.

87. Bunge MB. Bridging the transected or contused adult rat spinal cord with Schwann cell and olfactory ensheathing glia transplants. *Prog Brain Res* 2002; 137:275–282.

88. Cheng H, Cao Y, Olson L. Spinal cord repair in adult paraplegic rats: partial restoration of hind limb function. *Science* 1996; 273(5274): 510–513.

89. David S, Aguayo AJ. Axonal elongation into peripheral nervous system "bridges" after central nervous system injury in adult rats. *Science* 1981; 214(4523):931–933.

90. Hagg T. Collateral sprouting as a target for improved function after spinal cord injury. *J Neurotrauma* 2006; 23(3–4):281–294.

91. Keirstead HS, Morgan SV, Wilby MJ, et al. Enhanced axonal regeneration following combined demyelination plus Schwann cell transplantation therapy in the injured adult spinal cord. *Exp Neurol* 1999; 159(1): 225–236.

92. Takami T, Oudega M, Bates ML, et al. Schwann cell but not olfactory ensheathing glia transplants improve hindlimb locomotor performance in the moderately contused adult rat thoracic spinal cord. *J Neurosci* 2002; 22(15):6670–6681.

93. Zingale A. An experimental model to study axonal regeneration of the rat spinal cord. *J Neurosurg Sci* 1989; 33(4):329–331.

94. Cheng H, Liao KK, Liao SF, et al. Spinal cord repair with acidic fibroblast growth factor as a treatment for a patient with chronic paraplegia. *Spine* 2004; 29(14):E284–E288.

95. Tadie M, Liu S, Robert R, et al. Partial return of motor function in paralyzed legs after surgical bypass of the lesion site by nerve autografts three years after spinal cord injury. *J Neurotrauma* 2002; 19(8):909–916.

96. Pearse DD, Sanchez AR, Pereira FC, et al. Transplantation of Schwann cells and/or olfactory ensheathing glia into the contused spinal cord: survival, migration, axon association, and functional recovery. *Glia* 2007; 55(9):976–1000.

97. Huang H, Chen L, Wang H, et al. Influence of patients' age on functional recovery after transplantation of olfactory ensheathing cells into injured spinal cord injury. *Chin Med J (Engl)* 2003; 116(10):1488–1491.

98. Lima C, Pratas-Vital J, Escada P, et al. Olfactory mucosa autografts in human spinal cord injury: a pilot clinical study. *J Spinal Cord Med* 2006; 29(3):191–206.

99. Akiyama Y, Radtke C, Kocsis JD. Remyelination of the rat spinal cord by transplantation of identified bone marrow stromal cells. *J Neurosci* 2002; 22(15):6623–6630.

100. Park HC, Shim YS, Ha Y, et al. Treatment of complete spinal cord injury patients by autologous bone marrow cell transplantation and administration of granulocyte-macrophage colony stimulating factor. *Tissue Eng* 2005; 11(5–6):913–922.

101. Fawcett JW, Curt A, Steeves JD, et al. Guidelines for the conduct of clinical trials for spinal cord injury as developed by the ICCP panel: spontaneous recovery after spinal cord injury and statistical power needed for therapeutic clinical trials. *Spinal Cord* 2007; 45(3):190–205.

102. Steeves JD, Lammertse D, Curt A, et al. Guidelines for the conduct of clinical trials for spinal cord injury (SCI) as developed by the ICCP panel: clinical trial outcome measures. *Spinal Cord* 2007; 45(3):206–221.

103. Tuszynski MH, Steeves JD, Fawcett JW, et al. Guidelines for the conduct of clinical trials for spinal cord injury as developed by the ICCP Panel: clinical trial inclusion/exclusion criteria and ethics. *Spinal Cord* 2007; 45(3):222–231.

104. Lammertse D, Tuszynski MH, Steeves JD, et al. Guidelines for the conduct of clinical trials for spinal cord injury as developed by the ICCP panel: clinical trial design. *Spinal Cord* 2007; 45(3):232–242.

105. Robertson C, McCullough L, Brody B. Finding family for prospective consent in emergency research. *Clin Trials* 2007; 4:631–637.

106. Kaiser J. Privacy policies take a toll on research. *Science* 2007; 318:1049.

71 Considerations for the Translation of Preclinical Discoveries and Valid Spinal Cord Injury Clinical Trials

John D. Steeves

Never before have there been so many scientific discoveries describing an approach to improve outcomes after a spinal cord injury (SCI). Likewise, there has never been such avid reporting by the popular press of these initial discoveries, with the attendant premature pressure that the intervention may have imminent benefit for humans. The translation process from discovery to human application can be arduous, tedious, and mysterious, but it is nevertheless necessary (1–5).

The overall goals for treatment of SCI might be summarized as a series of temporally overlapping targets (Table 71.1). The timelines for effective treatment are necessarily vague, as there is limited human efficacy data. However, it is not the intent of this chapter to describe the details of the underlying mechanisms or experimental treatment strategies. Instead, the focus is on the principled pathway for translation and the factors that may confound the accurate interpretation of trial results.

Protection strategies are directed against the mechanical, pathologic, and inflammatory effects on spinal cord tissues immediately following the primary injury and throughout the first few weeks, when secondary cell death processes are most active. Surgical decompression of the cord and mechanical stabilization of the spine is standard acute care so that the spinal column does not impinge on the cord and cause further damage. Other acute goals are maintenance of adequate vascular perfusion of the spinal cord, reduction of spinal edema, and minimization of secondary cell death (e.g., apoptosis).

Repair includes endogenous cellular and tissue responses that are spontaneously activated after injury or need appropriate stimulation to provide a benefit. For example, stimulation of appropriate angiogenesis or decreasing widespread demyelination is likely to be beneficial. Current thinking suggests that astrogliosis after SCI is maladaptive to functional recovery and that limiting such responses by astrocytes may be a worthy therapeutic target. Interventions that enhance the expression of required growth factors, stimulate the proliferation and differentiation of resident neural progenitors, or activate endogenous "developmental programs" to facilitate intrinsic neuronal outgrowth are also areas of active preclinical investigation.

Regeneration is often used as a synonym for repair, but here the emphasis is on interventions that specifically stimulate or facilitate outgrowth from severed axons, as well as strategies, such as cell and biocompatible material transplants that replace lost tissue and/or provide scaffolds for neural growth. Obvious approaches include transplantation of autologous or allografted neural stem cells or neural progenitors. Although cell transplantation is a most promising therapeutic intervention, there is still little scientific consensus as to what are the most appropriate cellular candidates for transplantation after SCI. Further studies are essential before this approach will have meaningful application.

Recovery of a clinically meaningful functional capacity is the overall goal and may necessarily involve all the above approaches, but activity-dependent training alone can provide benefit. The underlying mechanisms are often collectively referred to as neuroplasticity, which includes a variety of mechanisms, such as formation of novel synaptic connections by axonal sprouts from existing (i.e., preserved) fibers, alterations in synaptic strength, or rewiring of functional circuits within intact (uninjured) spinal and brain regions. Treatments, such as weight-supported walking, robot-assisted training, and functional electric stimulation capitalize on and facilitate plasticity. Activity-dependent efforts are also important to consolidate any anatomical repair induced by any intervention that protects, repairs, or regenerates the injured cord.

Many of the preclinical neural repair findings examine the combined or sequential manipulations of promoters, inhibitors, and intracellular modulators of axonal growth, cell transplants, and/or activity-dependent training (6, 7).

Research laboratories often use in vitro cell cultures to initially examine responses to molecules and then use in vivo rodent models of traumatic SCI to identify and study mechanisms of injury and repair. These tightly controlled experiments will not necessarily provide a direct transition to clinical studies. Finding the most appropriate trail to translate a finding from cellular discovery to community-level adoption (i.e., from bench to bed or backyard) is not a well-traveled path for SCI. There are

Table 71.1 Overall Goals for Improving Functional Capacity after SCI

THERAPEUTIC TARGETS OR CLINICAL GOALS	TIMELINE FOR HUMAN APPLICATION	SELECTED UNDERLYING BIOLOGICAL MECHANISMS
Protection	First few weeks	Edema Secondary cell death Inflammation Immune system responses
Repair/ Regeneration	Weeks to months	Angiogenesis Myelination Astrocyte reactions
	Weeks to years	Cell transplants Biocompatible substrates Axonal outgrowth
Recovery	Weeks to years	Axonal sprouting Synaptic plasticity Neuronal circuit rewiring

a multitude of challenges that must be addressed, confounding factors to be controlled, and choices to be made before a therapeutic intervention can move confidently forward for introduction in a human study. For many scientists and clinical investigators, the translation process is a puzzling path. This review will attempt to identify some of the translational elements, as well as some of the confounding factors, that can alter the accurate interpretation of clinical trial outcomes.

REPLICATION AND VALIDATION OF PRECLINICAL SCIENTIFIC DISCOVERIES

Most everyone would agree that the translation of a scientific discovery through the appropriate clinical trial programs to approval as a treatment can be a very expensive process, sometimes amounting to more than half a billion dollars before regulatory approval is ever granted. Thus, at the preclinical stage, it is important to develop a high degree of confidence that an experimental therapeutic is likely to have clinically meaningful benefit for humans. There is no regulatory body that can (or wishes to) comprehensively oversee the conduct of scientists or validate a preclinical discovery. Nevertheless, as outlined below, there are principles that have been suggested in previous reviews (cf., 5, 8, 9) as processes for objectively validating any preclinical scientific discovery; these are summarized as follows:

1. Independent replication (validation) of preclinical finding
   a. Using different types of SCI or variations of treatment (to demonstrate the *robustness* of the initial finding)
   b. Using different species (to demonstrate the *fundamental nature* of the therapeutic target and/or intervention)
   c. Using a clinically appropriate type of SCI injury to mimic the human condition (to demonstrate *relevance*)
2. Adoption of high-quality preclinical protocols, similar to human studies, which include blinded assessments, power analysis, and a preclinical "functional" outcome measure similar to one that could be used in a human clinical trial

Of all the above points, independent replication (i.e., validation) of a discovery is a universal desire of the scientific community. Initially, independent verification of the initial findings, using the same experimental protocol, is the one accomplishment that inspires the greatest confidence among the scientific community. Thus, it is important that all aspects of the scientific protocol be provided to the group undertaking the replication study. Due to space considerations by journals, it is often difficult to publish detailed methodologies, but these should be retained and made available upon request.

Validation through exact replication of the initial experiments is further augmented by additional evidence for the "robustness" of the therapy, where variations in the formulation of the therapy and/or the type of experimental SCI investigated still provide a similar benefit to the initial discovery. Obtaining similar results from different animal species provides evidence for the fundamental (e.g., universal) nature of the therapeutic intervention and increases confidence that human application will also achieve beneficial outcomes. Most initial discoveries are made in rodent models (rat or mouse), which are usually inbred research species; thus, similar findings using an outbred species, such as cat, dog, pig, or monkey, provide further assurance to the community of the potential human safety and benefit of the treatment. Last but not least, any evidence that can be gathered from an animal model that closely mimics the human disorder and pathology (i.e., the clinical target for the therapy) is of high value.

Initial discoveries in SCI research often utilize homogeneous incomplete spinal injuries, including partial laceration (e.g., hemisection) or mild-to-moderate forms of contusive injury, whereas the human condition is more heterogeneous, often severe, and involves complex forms of mechanical trauma that include simultaneous three-dimensional mechanical forces causing contusion, dislocation, and distraction of the spinal cord.

A continuing evolution in the objective quality of preclinical experimental protocols is under way. Similarly, researchers in other neuroscience disciplines, such as stroke, have found it helpful to develop guidelines for good laboratory practices, or

GLP (10–13). Over the past decade or so, there have been a number of failed stroke clinical trials, which have undermined the confidence of the pharmaceutical industry to undertake clinical development. These failures stimulated stroke investigators to reexamine the preclinical animal models and the quality of experimental studies used to model human stroke. Unintended experimental bias and the lack of sustained quality in the preclinical translation process have been identified as the most likely contributors to stroke trial failures (10–13).

The inclusion of control animals, within any experimental protocol, has long been an established practice of preclinical researchers. Less common, but growing in practice, is the use of trained, "naive" evaluators to record the anatomical or behavioral outcomes (i.e., blinded assessments). Likewise, an understanding of the potential magnitude of the experimental effect, along with the use of statistical power analysis, can help determine the appropriate number of animals for each study arm in an experiment (as opposed to completing an underpowered experiment). In short, wherever possible, scientists should consider satisfying the rigorous standards of human study protocols when designing their preclinical experiments.

A disconnect between preclinical and clinical results is something no one wishes to see, especially after there has been an extensive investment of time and money in a translation process. One problem identified from past studies was the use of different outcome measurements in preclinical versus clinical studies (e.g., an anatomical outcome at the preclinical level versus a functional human outcome, such as an activity of daily living). Thus, if the human study does not find the same benefit as noted in the preclinical experiments, is this a true result or is it because one of the preclinical or clinical outcome tools is inaccurate or insensitive?

The quality of the outcome tool and the rigor of the outcome assessment can alter results. As an example, many scientists quickly adopted the BBB scale for preclinical (functional) behavioral assessments of rats (14), in part because it requires minimal equipment and appears to be easy to undertake. The BBB scale involves the observation of open-field ambulatory movements by a rat that is rated against criteria and scored on a 21-point scale for stance, intralimb joint movement, and interlimb coordination (gait). It is a nonlinear scale that requires reliance on subjective interpretation, and without proper training, the reliability of reported BBB scores is suspect. The closest human approximation to the BBB is the second version of the Walking Index for Spinal Cord Injury (WISCI II, 15). Once again, the quality of WISCI assessment training is critical for accurate data, but this is sometimes underemphasized.

More demanding quantitative outcome measures that involve kinematic and/or electrophysiological analysis can be completed in a similar manner for both animals and humans. However, these outcome tools are often expensive, and accurate utilization requires in-depth training with sophisticated equipment. Furthermore, such assessment tools are not routinely available in most clinical centers. This may not be a problem for early phase clinical trials (e.g., phase II), where the number of subjects is small and the trials are likely confined to well-equipped clinical research centers. However, by the pivotal phase III trial, the larger number of required subjects will require more participating centers, which are likely to have limited infrastructure and a limited number of highly trained investigators. At this point, a "simpler" functional outcome measure is likely to be the only way

forward, with the hope that it is no less accurate or less sensitive to detecting a clinically meaningful change.

CHARACTERISTICS OF HUMAN SCI AND CONFOUNDING FACTORS INFLUENCING CLINICAL TRIALS

It is also not the intent of this chapter to review specific SCI clinical trials; please see other review articles (16–19). Recently, a multinational panel published guidelines for the conduct of clinical trials for SCI, which detailed the degree of spontaneous recovery after SCI (20), outlined approaches for trial outcome measures (21), discussed inclusion/exclusion criteria and ethics (6), as well as outlined various trial designs and protocols (22). Other articles have also provided outlines of some of the issues associated with SCI clinical trials (1, 4). These articles provide a basis for a more informed assessment of trial results.

In the transition from preclinical animal experiments to human studies, there are a number of new considerations to contemplate. As mentioned above, human SCI is not the relatively homogenous situation created in an experimental setting. Although the design of special impact devices has allowed scientists to create animal spinal injuries within the same relative timeframe of most human spinal injuries (<10 ms), human SCI often involves mechanical damage that simultaneously compresses, dislocates, and distracts the spinal cord (i.e., disruption is created along three different axes). Human SCI can also be acquired from a variety of nontraumatic incidents, including infection, vertebral stenosis, or spinal tumors. SCI is heterogeneous in terms of the following:

- Spinal levels of injury (from ventilator-dependent, high cervical SCI to ambulatory, cauda equina injury)
- Severity of injury (from incomplete spinal damage to complete sensory and motor loss below the level of injury)
- Temporal circumstance (from the acute stage, through subacute, to more chronic time points after SCI)

From a clinical study perspective, it is usually wise to minimize the variability between study subjects. In other words, one should enroll a homogeneous population of subjects should one want to more clearly document a therapeutic action. If the enrolled subjects range from incomplete to sensorimotor complete, then the potentially different outcomes may offset or cancel each other in the statistical analysis, leading an investigator to erroneously conclude that there is no treatment effect. Likewise, if subjects can achieve significant spontaneous recovery after SCI, it might obscure any beneficial action of the therapy being examined. Finally, the greater the variability of SCI allowed within a study, the more stratification that is likely to be required, and thus, the lower the statistical power (significance) of any analyses. The only way to overcome subject heterogeneity in a study is to increase the number of enrolled participants or to start again; either way, it will mean more time and money. In every possible respect, the (placebo) control group should be matched to the composition of the experimental study group.

Other confounding factors that could jeopardize the accurate interpretation of outcomes in a clinical trial include the following:

1. Prior emergency or primary care, intensive care treatment and management, surgical decompression, and spine stabilization

2. Medical complications and/or damage to other organs (infection; respiratory, cardiovascular, autonomic, or bladder/bowel problems; pressure sores; neuropathic pain)
3. Onset, type, and extent of rehabilitation activity
4. Unsuitable protocol design or statistical analysis
5. Investigator and/or subject expectations and bias, because they know the type of treatment that has been provided
6. Lack of randomization of subjects and/or treatment allocation sequence
7. Inappropriate inclusion/exclusion criteria for subject participation
8. Lack of appropriate control subjects (matching criteria of experimental treatment group)
9. Inappropriate, insensitive, or unreliable clinical outcome tool and/or primary outcome (clinical endpoint)
10. Lack of independent, blind assessments of outcomes
11. Poor intra- or interrater reliability of outcome assessments
12. Lack of sufficient long-term assessment (at least 6–12 months after treatment)

More detailed discussions of SCI subject inclusion/exclusion criteria and ethics (6) or SCI clinical trial design (22) have been published.

SPONTANEOUS RECOVERY AFTER HUMAN SCI

The magnitude of spontaneous functional recovery after SCI, without any experimental intervention (e.g., a placebo control), can influence both the selection of an outcome measure and the threshold for determining a clinically significant benefit in an experimentally treated group. For any trial, there is always a desire to have a simple, easily measured primary outcome (e.g., length of survival), or at least an endpoint that is routinely used by clinicians, as long as the outcome is accurate, sensitive, reliable, and not subject to a large amount of spontaneous change. When it comes to SCI, this is easier said than done.

The International Standards for Neurological Classification of SCI (ISNCSCI), including the ASIA impairment scale (AIS), has become a standardized diagnostic and is a routinely applied neurologic assessment and classification scale for patients suspected of suffering a spinal injury (23,24). The major classifications of SCI range over five grades:

A *Complete sensory and motor loss,* below spinal cord injury level
B *Complete motor loss, sensory incomplete,* with S4–S5 sacral sensation being spared
C *Sensory and motor incomplete,* but half the key muscles below injury have *less than functional* muscle strength (i.e., muscle grade < 3/5)
D *Sensory and motor incomplete,* but more than half the key muscles below injury have *functional* muscle strength (i.e., muscle grade ≥ 3/5)
E *Normal sensory and motor function*

Using three different datasets, the following spontaneous changes in ASIA grades were reported over the first year after SCI

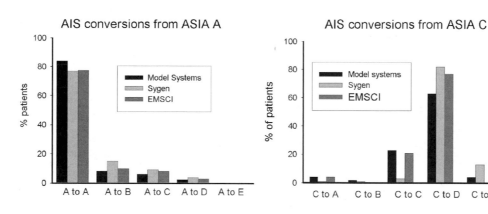

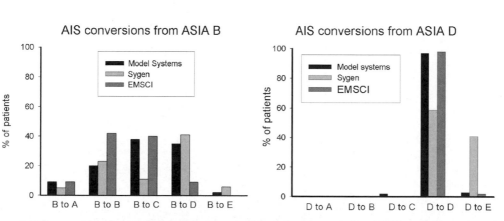

Figure 71.1 Percent AIS conversion from initial examination (within 3 days to 4 weeks of SCI) to the 1-year anniversary date after SCI. Data are from the U.S. Model Systems, Sygen, and European Multicentre Spinal Cord Injury (EMSCI) databases (20).

(Figure 71.1, (20)). Sensorimotor complete (AIS A) subjects show little spontaneous improvement over the first year after SCI, with about 75% of the subjects remaining as AIS A. Conversely, in two of the three datasets, about 80% of AIS B or AIS C patients naturally improve by one or two grades (without any treatment). Finally, most AIS D patients remain as AIS D, which is likely a "ceiling effect" of the classification system.

Several studies have also noted that most of these "natural history" changes in AIS scores occur within the first 3 months after SCI, but may take as long as 12–18 months to stabilize (Figure 71.2). From a study design point of view, the highest probability for readily detecting a clinical benefit due to a therapeutic intervention is during the "chronic" stage of SCI (>12 months), when spinal function has stabilized and spontaneous improvement is diminished. However, this is potentially the most difficult time point for a therapy to biologically influence the injured spinal cord in a beneficial manner.

Conversely, in (early) acute trials, subjects may have to be enrolled (within hours of injury) before an accurate assessment and classification of SCI can be completed. This can make interpretation of results difficult (or impossible), as the possibility of a type 1 error increases (i.e., a false positive result, due to error in classification of a subject as AIS A when he or she was actually an AIS B or AIS C subject). Thus, the investigator could conclude there was a clinically meaningful benefit from a therapeutic intervention when actually it was more likely a mistake in initial classification. Likewise, the influence of "spinal shock" on the AIS classification cannot be easily ignored when very early AIS assessments are required. Once again, the transient neurologic sensorimotor hypoactivity, associated with spinal shock, could lead the investigator to conclude that a subject is AIS A when he or she is actually an AIS B or AIS C subject.

Thus, an accurate assessment, using the international standards (ISNCSCI), is of great importance, not only to the accurate classification of SCI, but also to the correct enrollment of subjects who satisfy the specific inclusion criteria of the study. When there are multiple study sites, the demands for standardized training increase, as does the need for ongoing verification that the assessors continue to undertake their examinations in the same consistent manner throughout the trial, with adequate intra- and interrater reliability being maintained.

CLINICAL ENDPOINTS (OUTCOME MEASURES)

It is easy to state that any outcome tool (i.e., evaluation) used in a trial be appropriate to the clinical target for that therapy, as well as have the sensitivity and reliability to detect a significant difference from appropriate (placebo) control subjects. It is a much greater challenge to precisely define and validate what that tool should be for each and every SCI clinical trial (21, 26, 27). If the clinical target of the therapy is an improvement in bladder function, then the primary outcome tool and clinical endpoint will naturally be different from that used to determine a change in motor function.

The primary endpoint for different phases of a clinical study may also differ. Demonstration of safety is the primary goal of a phase I trial, whereas demonstration of an enhanced functional capacity or clinically meaningful improvement, due to the intervention being examined, is the usual endpoint of a pivotal phase III trial. Phase II trials may focus on the intermediate demonstration that the therapy has triggered an appropriate biologic or neurologic activity and may use a surrogate marker, such as a well-defined biochemical assay or neurologic measure. Thus, a single outcome measurement tool may not answer the varying demands and goals of each trial phase.

For pivotal phase clinical trials, the primary clinical outcome should provide the most clinically relevant and convincing evidence directly related to the primary objective of

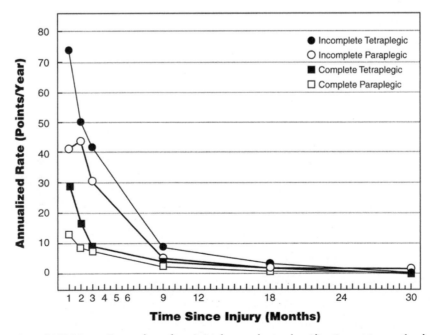

Figure 71.2   Recovery rates of AIS Motor Scores based on initial neurologic classification at 1 month after SCI (25).

the trial, usually a functional efficacy measure with distinct thresholds. A primary outcome measure should have "face validity" (i.e., there should be general agreement among knowledgeable experts that the variable or construct is appropriate and adequate to measure the intended outcome and that it measures a magnitude of change that would be expected to have a meaningful impact on the subject's level of functional capacity). For every pivotal SCI study, the primary endpoint needs to be justified, as does the reason for its selection and the statistical threshold that will be used to demonstrate a significant difference from the control situation. Once the primary outcome for a pivotal clinical trial has been selected and approved by the regulatory agency, the success or failure of that trial will rely solely on the experimental therapeutic intervention providing the stated endpoint; in other words, choose wisely! Finally, the primary outcome measure can also be used to estimate sample size in power analysis.

Secondary outcome measures include supportive or ancillary measures. Secondary outcome measures in early phase trials could be very useful in defining a valid primary outcome and clinically meaningful endpoint for the pivotal phase III study.

STANDARD NEUROLOGIC CLASSIFICATION OF SCI (AIS) AS AN OUTCOME TOOL

Outcome measurement tools that require sophisticated equipment and/or expertise can be pragmatically difficult to adopt and accurately utilize across multiple study sites. This is probably why aspects of the AIS diagnostic exam have been used and will continue to be used in SCI trials. Many clinical investigators are familiar and comfortable with this assessment tool. A change in AIS grade has been used as a clinical endpoint in past trials (NASCIS and GM1 trials), but to date, no therapeutic intervention has been validated using AIS grades as a clinical tool. Unless the treatment effect is large, AIS grades are unlikely to have the sensitivity to differentiate a clinically meaningful difference from control subjects (20, 21). The sensory or motor subscores of the AIS may have greater sensitivity or discriminative powers and might be used in early phase clinical trials (i.e., phase II).

The standard AIS neurologic examination does not assess C1–C4, T2–L1, or S2–S4/5 motor function, nor does it evaluate autonomic nervous system activity. It has been argued that the testing of light touch and pinprick sensations has a limited scoring range, that it can be time consuming when all dermatomes are assessed, and that there can be a high degree of variability in the patient's report from one test to the next. Nevertheless, preservation of sensory perception below the level of SCI, as well as S4–S5 sensation, correlates with a better prognosis for some motor recovery after SCI (23, 28).

The AIS motor score is based on manual muscle testing (Table 71.2), using a grading of muscle strength from 0 to 5 (see below) of ten key muscle actions on each side of the body, representing motor function for that spinal segment (score of 50 for the upper limbs and 50 for the lower limbs). The muscle grading scores for upper limb and lower limb should be tabulated separately, as upper extremity motor score (UEMS) or lower extremity motor score (LEMS). The key muscle actions and muscle grading criteria are as shown in Table 71.2.

From the "raw" muscle and sensory grading scores, an investigator can calculate the neurologic level (lowest spinal segment where muscle and sensory function is normal on both sides), motor level, sensory level, and zone of partial preservation (ZPP, only calculated for AIS A patients). A consistent and statistically significant improvement in the AIS motor score is more likely to be viewed as functionally significant and clinically meaningful, as it will often correlate with improved activities of daily living and a reduced burden of care. However, this will not always be the case. A consistent 5–10 point improvement in the AIS motor score for an experimental group may provide a statistically significant difference from the control group, but there may not be a clinically meaningful benefit if the motor improvement is a small, nonfunctional increase in muscle grade (e.g., from grade 1 to grade 2) across a widely distributed number of spinal segments (21). Careful forethought on all possible outcomes for a clinical endpoint is important. To illustrate possible (albeit extreme) limitations for different aspects of the AIS, consider the following two hypothetical scenarios:

Table 71.2   Key Representative Muscles for Individual Spinal Segments of AIS

PRINCIPAL SPINAL SEGMENT	KEY MUSCLE ACTION	SPINAL SEGMENT	KEY MUSCLE ACTION
C5	Elbow flexion	L2	Hip flexion
C6	Wrist extension	L3	Knee extension
C7	Elbow extension	L4	Ankle dorsiflexion
C8	Finger flexion (distal phalanx of middle finger)	L5	Toe extension
T1	Finger abduction (little finger)	S1	Ankle plantar flexion

Grading Strength of Muscle Action: 0 = total paralysis; 1 = palpable or visible contraction (nonfunctional); 2 = active movement, full range of motion, gravity eliminated (nonfunctional); 3 = active movement, full range of motion, against gravity (first potentially functional grade); 4 = active movement, full range of motion, against some resistance (functional); 5 = active movement, full range of motion, against normal resistance.

Example 1

Trial Primary Endpoint—Two-grade change in AIS (e.g., A to C) is the primary endpoint to demonstrate a clinical benefit of the therapy (e.g., as previously used in Sygen trial)

Baseline Assessment—Subject is a C5 AIS A tetraplegic who only has *functional* bilateral contraction of elbow flexors (C5 representative muscle). Initial examination yields UEMS = 15/50; LEMS = 0/50.

End of Study Assessment—With experimental treatment *X*, subject acquires functional voluntary movement of wrist extensors, elbow extensors, and finger flexors (C6, C7, and C8) on both sides (UEMS = 42/50), but has no muscle contraction or sensation below T1 (LEMS = 0/50). Subject is now a functional paraplegic and capable of many independent activities of daily living.

Trial Outcome—Failure. Even though subject showed a 27-point improvement in UEMS and regained significant independence, the subject would still be classified as AIS A. Thus, according to the declared primary endpoint (two-grade change in AIS), the subject would be deemed a treatment failure.

Example 2

Trial Primary Endpoint—10-point improvement in AIS motor point score is the threshold for achieving the primary endpoint.

Baseline Assessment—C4 AIS A tetraplegic subject only has *nonfunctional* (muscle score <3) bilateral contraction of elbow flexors (UEMS = 4, LEMS = 0).

End of Study Assessment—With experimental treatment *Y*, subject acquires sensation at S4–S5 level and contraction of anal sphincter, and several representative muscle groups achieve nonfunctional muscle contraction scores of 1–2 (UEMS = 14, LEMS = 10). Subject is still a functional tetraplegic and incapable of most independent activities of daily living.

Trial Outcome—Success. The subject is still a functional tetraplegic but has attained a 20-point improvement in motor point score and is now classified AIS C. According to the primary endpoint for this hypothetical trial, the subject would be deemed a treatment success.

Discussion of Scenarios

If the above outcomes are consistent across a sufficient sample size (and statistically different from placebo control outcomes), then which therapeutic intervention is most likely to provide the greatest clinically meaningful difference (i.e., improvement in functional outcome)? In summary, caution should be used when choosing clinical endpoints for trials. A change in AIS motor points is a possible primary outcome measure for early phase SCI trials, but the motor point change should correlate with a functional improvement in relevant activities of daily living.

FUNCTIONAL OUTCOME MEASURES

Due to the large degree of spontaneous and/or variable neurologic improvement for AIS C and AIS D subjects (Figure 71.1), it would be challenging to use a neurologic measure, such as the AIS, for these incomplete SCI subjects. Studies involving subjects with preserved sensory and motor function (AIS C and AIS D) would likely use a functional outcome tool, such as the spinal cord independence measure (SCIM, 29–31), as a measure of therapeutic efficacy. The latest version of SCIM (SCIM III, 31) is recommended, and in an evidence-based review, it was preferred over the functional independence measure (FIM) for assessing global disability after SCI (cf., 27). SCIM was found to be more sensitive to change than FIM and had strong correlations with AIS scores and rehabilitation outcomes.

There are also a number of more specific functional outcome measures directed to assessing either upper limb or lower limb function. The Action Research Arm Test (ARAT) has been used for several decades in the study of stroke (32, 33), but it has been introduced for the study of arm and hand function after cervical SCI. The Quadriplegia Index of Function (QIF) was also developed in the 1980s (34), and a short form version is available (35) as a scale for evaluating upper limb function in ten areas of self-care and mobility for people living with tetraplegia. It does not test any lower limb functions. It has strong correlations with SCIM, UEMS, and ASIA motor scores (27). A new upper limb outcome tool (Graded Refined Assessment of Strength, Sensibility and Prehension [GRASSP]) is currently being evaluated and validated for its clinical use in a multinational study.

Several tests of ambulatory performance have been developed and validated and have undergone evidence-based review (36, 37). They include the most recent version of the Walking Index for Spinal Cord Injury (WISCI II, 15, 38, 39) and a number of timed walking tests (cf., 40). WISCI is a 21-level hierarchical scale of walking, based on physical assistance and need of braces and devices, with an ordinal range from 0 (unable to walk) to 20 (walking without assistance for at least 10 minutes). It is an example of a more sensitive and precise scale for rating a specific functional activity in people with incomplete SCI. WISCI is currently a valid outcome measure for strategies directed to improving ambulation in subjects with incomplete SCI. Although the WISCI has been validated as a qualitative outcome measure for the assessment of standing and walking after incomplete SCI, a more detailed assessment may be provided by a combination of WISCI and some of the other quantitative timed walking tests. Such ambulatory tests include the timed up and go (TUG), the time taken for a 10-m walk test (10MWT), and the distance traversed during a 6-minute walk test (6mWT).

TRIALS WITH CERVICAL SENSORIMOTOR COMPLETE (AIS A) SUBJECTS

For obvious reasons of safety and not wanting to cause any harm, it is unlikely that any investigator would want to begin a new clinical trial program (phase I) for an experimental drug or cell transplant using subjects with spared sensory or motor function below the level of SCI. Thus, AIS A (sensorimotor complete) subjects remain an important and valuable clinical trial population.

From many perspectives, improving the functional outcome for cervical injured AIS A patients is also a high priority. Therefore, understanding the natural history of neurologic and functional changes after cervical AIS A is fundamental to SCI trial programs (20). In addition, many pharmacologic and cell-based therapeutics are likely to be infused or applied near the SCI site. Thus, in early phase studies, it would be useful to be able to track

Table 71.3 Differences in Activities between AIS Motor Level of C4 and C6

C4 INDEPENDENT ACTIVITY	C4 ASSISTED ACTIVITY	C4 DEPENDENT ACTIVITY
Talking	Coughing	Feeding
Swallowing	Telephone (*with adaptation*)	Turning
Breathing	Drinking (*with assistance*)	Transfers
		Washing
		Dressing
		Bowels
		Urination
		Car

C6 INDEPENDENT ACTIVITY	C6 ASSISTED ACTIVITY	C6 DEPENDENT ACTIVITY
Feeding	Coughing	Bowels—some
Teeth cleaning	Turning	Urination—some
Bathing and hair washing		
Dressing—some	Dressing—some	
Some cooking and kitchen work		
Writing—some with minimal aids		
Transfers—some, *sliding board*	Transfers—some, *hoist*	
Push *wheelchair* up incline (5%)	Standing—in *frame*	
Car—some using hand controls		Car—some

both safety and efficacy (i.e., to track changes in neurologic function or local effects) within spinal segments adjacent to the level of SCI (24; Steeves et al., in preparation).

One parameter, often noted, is a spontaneous improvement (recovery) of one motor level (i.e., one spinal segment) below the initial motor level (41). This can spontaneously occur in more than 40% of cervical AIS A subjects; fortunately, a spontaneous degradation of one neurologic level is observed in less than 15% of patients (Steeves et al., in preparation). Perhaps of greater functional significance, a spontaneous two–spinal segment improvement in motor function or neurologic level is also less common (5%–20%) after an AIS A cervical SCI. However, a two–spinal segment improvement in motor function can be accompanied by a significant change in activities of daily living (ADL), which could be argued as having clinically meaningful benefit (e.g., improving from an AIS motor level of C4 to C6; see Table 71.3). Thus, in comparison to placebo control subjects, any therapeutic intervention that could consistently stimulate a two–spinal level improvement in more than 20% of cervical AIS A subjects might be clinically meaningful.

SUMMARY OF CONSIDERATIONS FOR SCI CLINICAL TRIALS

There are many confounding factors that can influence the conduct of a trial program and any data collected. Many of these factors can be controlled or eliminated with careful prospective trial design and precise study protocols. However, human SCI studies are often forced to compromise between what is ideal and what can practically be achieved. Unless the therapeutic treatment effect is large, which is not usually the case, a change in AIS grade alone will not reliably identify those subjects receiving a clinically meaningful benefit. Likewise, in comparison to appropriate controls, a significant difference in AIS motor points alone may not reliably identify a therapeutic benefit. Tracking and com-

paring local spinal segmental changes in the AIS neurologic or motor level may identify important effects (either deleterious or beneficial). Nevertheless, a functional outcome tool will likely be more valuable to demonstrate face validity in a pivotal (phase III) trial.

An important and incompletely answered question is what should be the minimally acceptable clinical endpoint in a pivotal SCI clinical trial examining a therapy (drug, cell transplant, or rehabilitation training)? The word *performance* is often used interchangeably with the words *capability* or *capacity*, but they involve different elements when referring to human function. Performance of an ADL, successful community integration, or improved quality of life is subject to the influence of a variety of factors (e.g., motivation) that are independent and beyond the influence of most SCI experimental treatments. By the end of a phase III trial, an intervention should provide improved functional capacity in a relevant activity (i.e., it should provide a meaningful, clinically important difference, regardless of whether it is sensorimotor, autonomic, or relating to another function). However, whether the person makes use of any improved capacity by also improving his/her performance is up to the individual and beyond the control of a clinical study.

ACKNOWLEDGMENT

The input and constructive comments of Dr. Steven Stiens are appreciated.

*R*eferences

1. Steeves J, Fawcett J, Tuszynski M. Report of international clinical trials workshop on spinal cord injury February 20–21, 2004, Vancouver, Canada. *Spinal Cord* 2004; 42:591–597.

2. Kleitman N. Keeping promises: translating basic research into new spinal cord injury therapies. *J Spinal Cord Med* 2004; 27:311–318.

3. Ramer LM, Ramer MS, Steeves JD. Setting the stage for functional repair of spinal cord injuries: a cast of thousands. *Spinal Cord* 2005; 43:134–161.

4. Blight A, Tuszynski M. Clinical trials in spinal cord injury. *J Neurotrauma* 2006; 23:586–593.

5. Blesch A, Tuszynski M. Spinal Cord injury: plasticity, regeneration and the challenge of translational drug development. *Trends Neurosci* 2008; 32:41–47.

6. Tuszynski MH, Steeves JD, Fawcett JW, Lammertse D, et al. Guidelines for the conduct of clinical trials for spinal cord injury as developed by the ICCP panel: clinical trial inclusion/exclusion criteria and ethics. *Spinal Cord* 2007; 45:222–231.

7. Benowitz LI, Yin Y. Combinatorial treatments for promoting axon regeneration in the CNS: strategies for overcoming inhibitory signals and activating neurons' intrinsic growth state. *Dev Neurobiol* 2007; 67: 1148–1165.

8. Reier PJ. Cellular transplantation strategies for spinal cord injury and translational neurobiology. *NeuroRx* 2004; 1:424–451.

9. Dobkin BH. Curiosity and cure: translational research strategies for neural repair-mediated rehabilitation. *Dev Neurobiol* 2007; 67:1133–1147.

10. Dirnagl U. Bench to bedside: the quest for quality in experimental stroke research. *J Cereb Blood Flow Metab* 2006; 26:1465–1478.

11. Sena E, van der Worp HB, Howells D, Macleod M. How can we improve the pre-clinical development of drugs for stroke? *Trends Neurosci* 2007; 30:433–439.

12. Crossley NA, Sena E, Goehler J, Horn J, et al. Empirical evidence of bias in the design of experimental stroke studies: a metaepidemiologic approach. *Stroke* 2008; 39:929–934.

13. Macleod MM, Fisher M, O'Collins V, Sena ES, et al. Good laboratory practice: preventing introduction of bias at the bench. *Stroke* 2009; 40:e50–e52.

14. Basso DM, Beattie MS, Bresnahan JC. A sensitive and reliable locomotor rating scale for open field testing in rats. *J Neurotrauma* 1995; 12:1–21.

15. Ditunno PL, Ditunno JF Jr. Walking index for spinal cord injury (WISCI II): scale revision. *Spinal Cord* 2001; 39(12):654–656.

16. Amador MJ, Guest JD. An appraisal of ongoing experimental procedures in human spinal cord injury. *J Neurol Phys Ther* 2005; 29:70–86.

17. Baptiste DC, Fehlings MG. Update on the treatment of spinal cord injury. *Prog Brain Res* 2007; 161:217–233.

18. Knafo S, Choi D. Clinical studies in spinal cord injury: moving towards successful trials. *Br J Neurosurg* 2008; 22:3–12.

19. Hawryluk GW, Rowland J, Kwon BK, Fehlings MG. Protection and repair of the injured spinal cord: a review of completed, ongoing, and planned clinical trials for acute spinal cord injury. *Neurosurg Focus* 2008; 25:E14.

20. Fawcett JW, Curt A, Steeves JD, Coleman WP, et al. Guidelines for the conduct of clinical trials for spinal cord injury as developed by the ICCP panel: spontaneous recovery after spinal cord injury and statistical power needed for therapeutic clinical trials. *Spinal Cord* 2007; 45:190–205.

21. Steeves JD, Lammertse D, Curt A, Fawcett JW et al. Guidelines for the conduct of clinical trials for spinal cord injury (SCI) as developed by the ICCP panel: clinical trial outcome measures. *Spinal Cord* 2007; 45:206–221.

22. Lammertse D, Tuszynski MH, Steeves JD, Curt A, et al. Guidelines for the conduct of clinical trials for spinal cord injury as developed by the ICCP panel: clinical trial design. *Spinal Cord* 2007; 45:232–242.

23. Marino RJ, Barros T, Biering-Sorensen F, et al. International standards for neurological classification of spinal cord injury. *J Spinal Cord Med* 2003; 26:S50–S56.

24. Furlan JC, Fehlings MG, Tator CH, Davis AM. Motor and sensory assessment of patients in clinical trials for pharmacological therapy of acute spinal cord injury: psychometric properties of the ASIA Standards. *J Neurotrauma* 2008; 25:1273–1301.

25. Burns AS, Ditunno JF. Establishing prognosis and maximizing functional outcomes after spinal cord injury: a review of current and future directions in rehabilitation management. *Spine* 2001; 26(24 Suppl):S137–S145.

26. Johnston MV, Graves DE. Towards guidelines for evaluation of measures: an introduction with application to spinal cord injury. *J Spinal Cord Med* 2008; 31:13–26.

27. Alexander MS, Anderson K, Biering-Sorensen F, Blight AR, et al. Outcome measures in spinal cord injury: recent assessments and recommendations for future directions. *Spinal Cord* 2009; 47:582–591.

28. Marino RJ, Ditunno JF, Donovan WH, Maynard F. Neurologic recovery after traumatic spinal cord injury: data from the Model Spinal Cord Injury Systems. *Arch Phys Med Rehabil* 1999; 80:1391–1396.

29. Catz A, Itzkovich M, Agranov E, Ring H, Tamir A. SCIM—spinal cord independence measure: a new disability scale for patients with spinal cord lesions. *Spinal Cord* 1997; 35:850–856.

30. Catz A, Itzkovich M, Agranov E, Ring H, Tamir A. The spinal cord independence measure (SCIM): sensitivity to functional changes in subgroups of spinal cord lesion patients. *Spinal Cord* 2001; 39:97–100.

31. Itzkovich M, Gelernter I, Biering-Sorensen F, et al. The Spinal Cord Independence Measure (SCIM) version III: reliability and validity in a multicenter international study. *Disabil Rehabil* 2007; 29:1926–1933.

32. Lyle, RC. A performance test for assessment of upper limb function in physical rehabilitation treatment and research. *Int J Rehabil Res* 1981; 4:483–492.

33. Yozbatiran N, Der-Yeghiaian L, Cramer SC. A standardized approach to performing the action research arm test. *Neurorehabil Neural Repair* 2008; 22:78–90.

34. Gresham GE, Labi ML, Dittmar SS, Hicks JT, et al. The Quadriplegia Index of Function (QIF): sensitivity and reliability demonstrated in a study of thirty quadriplegic patients. *Paraplegia* 1986; 24:38–44.

35. Marino RJ, Goin JE. Development of a short-form Quadriplegia Index of Function scale. *Spinal Cord* 1999; 37:289–296.

36. Lam T, Noonan VK, Eng JJ, SCIRE Research Team. A systematic review of functional ambulation outcome measures in spinal cord injury. *Spinal Cord* 2008; 46:246–254.

37. Jackson AB, Carnel CT, Ditunno JF, Read MS, et al. Outcome measures for gait and ambulation in the spinal cord injury population. *J Spinal Cord Med* 2008; 31:487–499.

38. Morganti B, Scivoletto G, Ditunno P, Ditunno JF, Molinari M. Walking index for spinal cord injury (WISCI): criterion validation. *Spinal Cord* 2005; 43:43–71.

39. Ditunno JF, Scivoletto G, Patrick M, Biering-Sorensen F, et al. Validation of the Walking Index for Spinal Cord Injury in a US and European clinical population. *Spinal Cord* 2008; 46:181–188.

40. van Hedel HJ, Wirz M, Dietz V. Assessing walking ability in subjects with spinal cord injury: validity and reliability of 3 walking tests. *Arch Phys Med Rehabil* 2005; 86:190–196.

41. Fisher CG, Noonan VK, Smith DE, Wing PC, et al. Motor recovery, functional status, and health-related quality of life in patients with complete spinal cord injuries. *Spine* 2005; 30:2200–2207.

72

Retraining the Human Spinal Cord: Exercise Interventions to Enhance Recovery after a Spinal Cord Injury

V. Reggie Edgerton
Susan J. Harkema
Roland R. Roy

GENERAL CONCEPTS: CONTROL OF STANDING AND STEPPING

Investigators and clinicians have been continually inspired to pursue methods that achieve recovery of gait in humans after a spinal cord injury (SCI). Repeated demonstrations of spinal stepping on the treadmill by the hindlimbs of cats after a complete SCI suggest such latent neural circuitry in humans could coordinate recovery of function. It is well documented that the details of the neural control of stepping and standing can be generated by neural pathways within the lumbosacral spinal cord in quadrupeds (1–3). Qualitatively, the potential for the same type of detailed control is present in the human lumbosacral spinal cord, although the level of complete independence from supraspinal control is not as clear as has been observed in some quadrupedal animals (4, 5).

It appears that the detailed coordination of all the muscles of the lower limbs needed to execute effective stepping is present in the human lumbosacral spinal cord, but unlike the recovery of full weight-bearing stepping in the cat with the appropriate step training therapy, humans with a clinically complete SCI at the thoracic level can perform only partially weight-bearing steps (4, 5). The importance of this concept is that the brain generates the commands to step or stand and, in the process of generating these commands, continues to update itself as to how these motor tasks are being performed under any given environmental condition. Once the decision is made and as long as this decision persists, most of the detailed modulation of the activation patterns of the musculature of the lower limbs to step or stand is controlled largely automatically by spinal networks and the ongoing peripheral input (2). It remains unclear just how automatically the human spinal cord can perform this function without some assistance from supraspinal centers. Rehabilitative strategies in the past have largely overlooked the significant level of fine motor control that can be achieved at the spinal level in rats, cats, and humans after an SCI. This chapter focuses on this perspective and on some of the underlying concepts. Two of these concepts are that the spinal cord is an important

information processing and decision-making center and that its information processing ability is experience dependent (i.e., the properties and potential of the spinal networks are shaped by the motor tasks that are practiced).

Let us compare the theoretical models of the neural control of stepping in uninjured (control) subjects and in individuals with an incomplete or a complete SCI (Figure 72.1A). After an incomplete injury at the thoracic level, there is a significant loss of synapses, particularly from descending axons that have been interrupted and that normally project to spinal interneurons and motor pools (6). This loss of synapses results in a significant change in the functional properties of the remaining neurons and their synapses. Although multiple factors contribute to this change, the adaptations and the relative importance of the remaining functional synapses alone must result in a novel sharing of the excitable neuronal membrane surfaces. In addition, the remaining synapses are modified in number, size, and synaptic surface relative to their original and even novel neuronal targets (6–8).

Changes in the spinal pathways after an SCI seem to occur also because of the newly imposed patterns or levels of activity, even without any anatomical reorganization. These activity-related changes seem to be learned (i.e., the functionality of the pathways either can be reinforced or depressed depending on the pattern of activity that predominates). After a severe SCI, there is little or no voluntary control of the stepping patterns, but the remaining spinal networks can generate effective stepping patterns. These networks seem to acquire the ability to function more independently of supraspinal control than normally occurs, particularly when a motor task is practiced (Figure 72.1B). For example, individuals with an incomplete SCI were able to improve their stepping ability by step training without having any improvement in their voluntary control of leg movement (9, 10). Supraspinal changes also occur in individuals with an incomplete SCI (11). It appears that a relatively small amount of remaining descending functional input distal to a lesion can become highly effective, probably as a result of concomitant adaptations at the

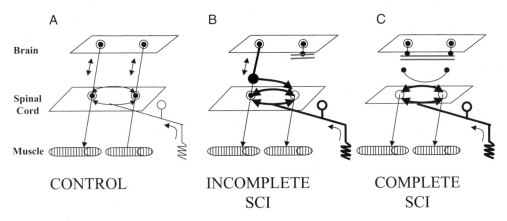

Figure 72.1 A general conceptual model of the control of locomotion and the adaptive events that may occur in the spinal cord after an incomplete (**B**) or a complete (**C**) disruption of ascending and descending signals to and from the brain compared to the uninjured (control) state (**A**). The bolder lines imply pathways that are probably at least functionally adapted after an SCI. In the incomplete model (**B**), both supraspinal and spinal components most likely adapt in ways that can improve function. Significant adaptations, however, also occur in the spinal cord without any input to the spinal cord from the brain (**C**).

spinal and supraspinal levels. Similar changes seem to occur in the spinal cord below the lesion after a complete SCI (Figure 72.1C).

There is more than a loss of neural function after an SCI. Muscle atrophy results in a concomitant reduction in force-generating potential (12). Interestingly, the amount of atrophy that occurs differs substantially among individuals after an SCI, with no obvious explanation existing for this variability. Some of this variability may be the result of differing degrees of spasticity or medication usage, but this has not been studied carefully. Changes in the potential of muscles to generate forces also define the ability to control movements. For any level of neural function remaining, the larger the muscle fibers (or motor units) that can be recruited, the more force that can be generated (13).

SENSORY INFORMATION: MONITORED AND PROCESSED BY THE SPINAL CORD

All modes of sensory input, such as from muscle spindles, Golgi tendon organs, free nerve ending in muscles, joint receptors, and skin receptors, probably provide information that can be used to recognize the specific temporal events associated with a step cycle or a given standing posture. This sensory information seems to be sufficient for the spinal cord to "anticipate" what should happen next, based on the excitatory and inhibitory events that have occurred immediately preceding a given time point. It seems reasonable to assume that the spinal cord has evolved so that its neural pathways can readily recognize appropriate patterns of sensory cues (e.g., when one leg is beginning the swing phase and the other is in the early stance phase during a step cycle). We propose that the spinal cord interprets a complete or "gestalt" pattern of afferent input from all peripheral sensors in a dynamically appropriate pattern. In essence, this enables the spinal cord to make context-dependent decisions.

In effect, the ensemble pattern of sensory information projected to the spinal cord at any given instant during a step provides precise information as to the kinematics and kinetics events of the lower limbs. In turn, the spinal circuitry recognizes this pattern and responds by generating the appropriate motor signals sufficient for initiating and sustaining the next phase of

the step cycle. When considering the millions of years of evolution of the locomotor systems in a 1G environment, one can more easily understand how the spinal circuitry has been designed to routinely address and utilize the highly predictable patterns of sensory input associated with locomotion. Implied within this concept is the likelihood that the spinal circuitry can not only correct movements in response to sensory information, but also anticipate what the correct patterns should be. In other words, from an engineering perspective the spinal circuitry responds with the characteristics of a feed-forward control system.

The meaningful components of the sensory information relayed through the spinal cord during stepping or standing can be compared conceptually to the alphabet, words, phrases, and sentences. For example, activation of different combinations of individual sensory receptors in a muscle might represent a "word," and information inclusive of the actions of synergists and antagonists might provide a "phrase" among joint segments. Finally, this sensory ensemble among muscles controlling all joints of both legs might send a complex pattern of information in the form of a "sentence" to the spinal cord. Thus, different combinations of sources and modes of receptor information formulate meaningful words, phrases, and sentences for the spinal cord to interpret. In response, the sequence of motor activation patterns can be generated in part by anticipating and recognizing the "words," "phrases," and "sentences" of proprioception. The spinal cord may recognize not only the presence or absence of sensory input, but also the dynamics of multiple combinations of inputs. The spinal networks seem to recognize and anticipate temporal patterns and detect and correct patterns of movement and mechanical events that are inconsistent with effective stepping or "ineffective" sensory patterns.

As helpful as sensory information can be in providing a source of "control" for the spinal cord, it also can have highly undesirable consequences that must be managed. After an SCI, a common feature is the emergence of aberrant connections throughout the sensorimotor circuitry, whereby a given source of sensory input can reflexively generate uncoordinated contractions among multiple muscles, a phenomenon which falls into the category of spasticity. The initial and consistent response of the clinician is to prescribe antispastic medication. This is a crucial decision that is likely to have long-term consequences on the eventual level of functional recovery of the patient. For example, while reducing spasticity, the administration of baclofen also will reduce the amount of sensory information available to the spinal circuitry that generally controls posture and locomotion. Given the absence or near absence of supraspinal control in SCI subjects, the control that can be derived from the sensory system becomes very crucial. Therefore minimizing this input has severe consequences (i.e., the level of performance of postural and locomotor activities will be compromised further). Furthermore, the spinal circuitry will adapt to a more nonfunctional state when it is deprived of sensory input, most likely resulting in the formation of more extensive aberrant connections. A decision that must be made, therefore, is whether or not to use an interventional strategy to attempt to normalize the sensory input to the spinal cord by providing intermittent load-bearing exercise in the form of standing and/or stepping. The choice becomes one of tolerating disruptive and spontaneous contractions while trying to maximize the functional potential of the spinal circuitry versus the convenience of suppressing these spontaneous contractions. The strategy chosen should be based on a discussion of all of the pros and cons between the patient and the physician, with both being fully aware of the long-term consequences.

What is effective stepping? The uninjured individual has numerous ways to step successfully (i.e., to progress over some distance without falling and to traverse diverse terrains). Although one need not assume that all afferent input associated with stepping will be precise at every instant, the more closely the pattern of input approximates normal stepping, the more likely the stepping patterns will be executed effectively and successfully. In more severely injured individuals, there are fewer neural control options available for stepping, making it more critical for

the remaining sources of sensory information to function effectively in guiding a motor response (i.e., to match the input normally associated with load-bearing stepping). As noted earlier the afferent input to the spinal cord (and to the brain, if the injury is incomplete) after an SCI generates a new, or at least a modified, "experience." The newly acquired properties of the spinal cord will reflect the sensory experience during and after the period of spontaneous anatomical and functional reorganization that occurs after an SCI.

CENTRAL PATTERN GENERATION: SPINAL CORD CONTROL OF LOCOMOTION

Up to this point, we have emphasized the importance of sensory information processing to generate stepping. The same neurons that perform the central processing of sensory information as discussed above, however, generate the coordination of alternating flexion and extension movements in SCI subjects by activating the appropriate muscle nerves of the lower limbs bilaterally, as occurs during locomotion in uninjured subjects. By definition, central pattern generation is the generation of these alternating patterns of movement without any sensory input or supraspinal input, as would occur during locomotion in uninjured subjects (14). One can surgically isolate the lumbosacral spinal cord of a mouse, rat, or cat and induce repetitive step-like patterns by administering one or more of a number of pharmacologic agents (serotonergic, noradrenergic, and dopaminergic agonists and glycinergic and GABAergic antagonists) associated with neurotransmitters involved in the motor output of these spinal segments (1, 15–17) (Figure 72.2). In this experimental preparation, repetitive step-like cycles can be generated for hours by groups of neurons without any phasic descending or afferent input. This cyclic generation of a step-like pattern is called *fictive*

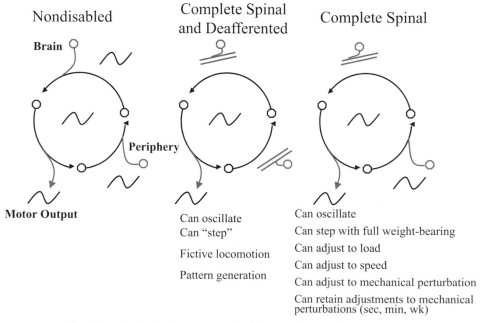

Figure 72.2 Conceptual models of the spinal circuitry in a nondisabled, a spinal isolated (no supraspinal or peripheral afferent input to the spinal cord), and a complete spinal (elimination of supraspinal connections only) animal are shown. Some of the functional capabilities of the two injury models are listed below, indicating the much greater functional capacity when the afferents are intact.

locomotion (Figure 72.2). Although the level of activation of a motor pool can vary from cycle to cycle, the motor output cannot be matched to the external environment or any kinematics or kinetics events of the limbs because there is no afferent feedback from the periphery. To generate successful load-bearing stepping and standing, afferent information must be available to the spinal cord. Thus, an important functional property of some of the same spinal pathways that generate fictive locomotion is the ability to effectively process the sensory information associated with the continuously changing phases of the step cycle.

HOW SMART IS THE SPINAL CORD?: EVIDENCE FOR COMPLEX SENSORY AND MOTOR PROCESSING

What do we mean when we say the spinal cord is *smart*? We use the term here to emphasize that the spinal cord can process sensory information in the context of the combination of events occurring at any given time. We often refer to this as *state-dependent processing*, reflecting the ability of the spinal cord to "decide" how to respond to a given sensory input. For example, a given pattern of sensory input can be processed (interpreted) such that ipsilateral flexion and contralateral extension can be generated in the hindlimbs when the dorsal surface of the foot is mechanically perturbed during the swing phase of a step. If the same stimulation is applied during the stance phase of that same limb, however, then an ipsilateral extension and contralateral flexion response will be induced (1, 18). Thus, the spinal cord interprets the stimulus differently, depending on the phase of the step cycle. These are examples of useful "decision-making" abilities of the spinal cord because both of these responses are positive adaptive events to assure that stepping continues with minimal disruption.

A number of other examples exist in animals and in humans that illustrate that the spinal cord responds to proprioceptive input in a "state-dependent" manner. One of the most functional illustrations of this phenomenon is when the level of loading on the limbs during stepping is altered. For example, in individuals with a complete SCI, the level of activation of extensor muscles increases as the level of load-bearing increases (19). A similar response to loading also has been observed in nondisabled and incomplete SCI subjects (Figure 72.3). In most cases, these responses to loading intuitively appear "teleologically correct," in the sense that it would seem to be an advantage for the response to loading to be automatic or programmed in the lower (spinal cord) control circuits.

CAN THE SPINAL CORD LEARN A MOTOR TASK?: REPETITIVE PRACTICE IMPROVES GAIT

In adult cats whose spinal cords were surgically transected at a mid- or low-thoracic level, the ability to step or stand is a function of whether these motor tasks are practiced (2, 20–23). If adult spinal cats are trained daily to step with full load-bearing on a treadmill over a period of 3 to 12 weeks, then their stepping ability improves. If they are trained daily to stand, then their standing ability is improved. The specificity of this training or experience is illustrated by the fact that the animals trained to stand will learn to stand, but their stepping ability remains poor or even worsens. It is not known, however, whether a complete spinal animal can

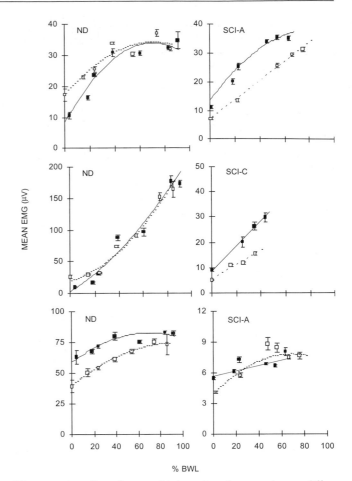

Figure 72.3 Data from multiple series of steps taken at different levels of loading, as regulated by a body weight support system, are shown. Exemplary data from a nondisabled (ND) subject and from SCI subjects are shown. In general, extensor and flexor EMG activity increased with higher peak limb loading conditions independent of the level of available supraspinal input. Averaged soleus (**top**), medial gastrocnemius (**middle**), and tibialis anterior (**bottom**) surface EMG mean amplitude per burst (μV; rectified, high pass filtered at 32 Hz) versus limb peak load (percent of body weight load, % BWL) from ND, clinically incomplete (SCI-C) and clinically complete (SCI-A) subjects. Each point represents the average of EMG mean amplitudes (±SEM) within a 10% interval of the BWL range (0%–10%, 10%–20%, etc.). Data from the right limb (**open symbols**) and left limb (**closed symbols**) of each subject are shown separately. (From ref. 19.)

be trained simultaneously to step and stand during the same training period. Two other features of learning are present in these trained spinal animals. If step training is stopped, their ability to step declines, as if they "forget" how to perform the motor task. If these same spinal animals then are retrained to step after they have "forgotten," they learn to step much more quickly than when trained the first time after the SCI. This response is another learning-related phenomenon (i.e., relearning a motor task occurs faster than during initial training) (for review, see 22, 24). Similar studies have been and are still being performed in humans with an SCI (4, 5, 9, 10, 25). It appears that the essential learning features described above for laboratory animals also apply to humans.

Greater gains in performing a specific motor task after an SCI occur when that motor task is practiced compared to no or limited practice. Thus, it seems that motor training should be used in concert with interventions designed to repair or regenerate tissue via growth factor modulation, cell implants, and so forth (26, 27). If the spinal cord pathways have not learned to step, then new axonal growth or the incorporation of new or modified cells may not become functional if the spinal pathways can no longer recognize the postural and locomotor cues to generate the motor patterns that correspond to a given set of sensory inputs. In general, it seems likely that greater recovery in motor function after an SCI will occur by combining the interactive or complementary effects of multiple interventions. At the same time, it is possible for the activity-dependent changes from one intervention to interfere with the individual effect. For example, it has been reported that initiation of an activity-dependent rehabilitative strategy immediately after a brain injury can result in less recovery than will occur without any such treatment (28). In general, activity-dependent interventions potentially can induce cellular and systemic modulation in either a negative or a positive direction, as can any specific pharmacologic intervention. Thus, more is not always better. It seems likely that one could easily impose too many stressors for any physiological system to adapt to simultaneously, particularly after a severe SCI.

NEUROPLASTICITY: SPINAL AND SUPRASPINAL CONTROL SYSTEMS

Remarkable levels of recovery have been reported in some individuals who have some residual descending input after an SCI (9, 10). In a clinical trial involving 146 subjects 8 weeks post-SCI who were considered clinically incomplete (ASIA B, C, or D) and had a locomotor score (FIM-L) of less than 4, near normal walking speed overground was attained after 3 months of weight-bearing step training (29). A four-and-a-half-year-old child who was nonambulatory and wheelchair dependent received locomotor training for seventy-six sessions, beginning 16 months after a C5 SCI that left only a small amount of preserved cord tissue dorsally and ventrally (30). After 1 month of locomotor training, the child was able to use his legs for community ambulation using a roller walker. By the end of the training period, an average of 2,488 community-based steps per day and a maximum speed of 0.48 meters/second were obtained. In a 1-month follow-up after the completion of seventy-six sessions, the level of performance was sustained, and the preferred walking speed had increased significantly beyond that recorded at the end of training. These changes occurred in spite of no change in the clinical lower motor scores, reflecting no change in the level of voluntary control. The child now attends kindergarten full time using a walker. Although this is a case study, it points out several important issues. First, the level of reorganization that can occur both supraspinally and spinally within the sensorimotor system is far greater than usually assumed. Second, the number of therapy sessions needed to initiate and continue to improve motor function is significantly more than is generally allowed for a given patient. These observations point out the importance of knowing which individuals with a given kind and severity of SCI can be expected to improve and to what level they will improve as a result of a given amount of locomotor training. Based on postmortem analysis of the spinal cord of individuals with long-term SCI, it was

concluded that a high level of motor control seems possible with relatively few descending axons extending below the level of the lesion (31). Rhesus monkeys have been shown to regain very effective bilateral locomotor function within 3 months after a unilateral thoracic corticospinal tract lesion (32). As suggested earlier, all of these observations probably reflect a synergistic effect of adaptive responses in the spinal cord and supraspinal motor control centers. The ability of motor control centers in the brain to adapt after an SCI is dramatic. It appears that the brain has the ability to reorganize itself so that novel pathways can control movement as a result of the combined and concomitant adjustments occurring at the supraspinal and spinal levels (33, 34).

PHARMACOLOGIC INTERVENTIONS: ENHANCEMENT OF FUNCTIONAL PERFORMANCE

Reducing Motor Output: Diminishing Spasticity

Pharmacologic interventions are frequently used to reduce muscle spasms in SCI subjects. For example, baclofen, a gamma aminobutyric acid (GABA) B receptor blocker, and clonidine and tizanidine, α-2 adrenergic receptor agonists, can reduce the incidence and magnitude of these involuntary contractions. One possible negative effect when using these pharmacologic interventions, however, is a reduction in the sensory information that can be processed by the spinal cord to control posture and locomotion. The tradeoffs in maintaining more motor control versus less frequent and severe spontaneous contractions, which can be disruptive, should be considered in the pharmacologic management of spasticity as discussed previously (see the section on Sensory Information Monitored and Processed by the Spinal Cord).

Little progress has been made in developing a solution to the dichotomy of spasticity suppression vs. preservation of neuromotor control, largely because the etiology of spasticity is so poorly understood. A working hypothesis is that spontaneous, uncoordinated contractions after an SCI are manifestations of a learned chronic dysfunction of the sensorimotor pathways of the spinal cord (35). Inappropriate activation patterns might be expected if the SCI subject does not step or stand. On the other hand, if locomotor-like activation patterns are induced by locomotor training using manual assistance and body weight support on a treadmill (BWST), then perhaps more appropriate activation patterns can be "learned" (2, 22). In conjunction with this concept, fewer pharmacologic interventions may be needed to minimize spasticity if appropriate sensorimotor patterns are learned. No carefully documented quantitative data, however, have been obtained to date to stringently address these possibilities. A recent randomized clinical trial, however, reported significant recovery of walking in individuals with an acute incomplete SCI who received intense repetitive practice of weight-bearing in the absence of antispasticity medication (36). The role of antispasticity medication in the rehabilitation of standing and walking after an SCI warrants further investigation.

Enhancing Information Processing within the Spinal Cord: Improved Motor Output

Another approach on the horizon is the administration of adrenergic and serotonergic agonists intrathecally to the lumbosacral spinal cord segments to facilitate locomotion. Activation of either the adrenergic or serotonergic neurotransmitter system can generate fictive locomotion in cats and rats (37, 38). In the lumbosacral spinal cord of uninjured individuals the only effective source of these transmitters is from the synapses of axons descending from supraspinal neurons. After a complete SCI, little or no norepinephrine (NE) or 5-hydroxytryptamine (5-HT) persists in the spinal cord. When chronic spinal animals are given an agonist of these neurotransmitters, however, locomotion is improved in some animals, but depressed in others (1). Although the explanation for this variability is not fully understood, it probably reflects the highly dynamic feature of the responsiveness of the spinal cord, often referred to as the "pharmacologic state," which can change over time.

From a clinical viewpoint, there are some practical challenges to pharmacologically facilitating stepping (39). We have little understanding of how NE or 5-HT modulates sensory processing within the spinal cord. If the effectiveness of sensory processing to generate patterns of effective motor output could be enhanced, then pharmacologic interventions might be helpful. This appears to be the case at least when the level of inhibition is limited by blocking glycine receptors with strychnine (i.e., disinhibiting, and thus facilitating) (40, 41). If the drug itself must induce the rhythmic pattern, however, then a pharmacologic approach has less promise. This pharmacologic "enabling," rather than "inducing," effect has the potential advantage of letting the individual decide exactly when he/she would like to step or stand by manipulating the proprioceptive information from the lower limbs, as opposed to a drug inducing a step-like motion with the subject having no control as to when to start or to stop.

Although improvements in locomotion have been achieved using pharmacologic interventions in laboratory animals, in virtually all cases, there also is evidence of dysfunction. This variation in response may reflect different pharmacologic sites in the spinal cord as well as the criticality of the dosage administered. In all cases, the side effects of drugs that manipulate these neurotransmitter systems can make their use clinically prohibitive. This might be expected for 5-HT and NE, unless the dosages can be very low and localized, given the ubiquitous nature of their distribution throughout the nervous system.

As noted previously, another potential pharmacologic strategy for improving motor function is to manage the excitability of the spinal pathways so that afferent input associated with stepping and standing can excite the appropriate motor pathways. One such drug that seems to facilitate sensory processing is strychnine, a specific blocker of glycine receptors. Glycine is a major inhibitory neurotransmitter in the spinal cord, playing a role in the reciprocal inhibition of antagonistic motor pools via interneurons. Experiments in spinal cats suggest that modulation of inhibitory pathways can be used to improve locomotion. In spinal cats that were trained to stand and could not step, strychnine facilitated stepping when the animal was placed on a treadmill (40). Strychnine seemed to facilitate information processing rather than directly inducing step-like oscillations. Perhaps analogous drugs can be developed so that this approach can be used in humans.

REHABILITATION GOALS IN TREATING SKELETAL MUSCLES: METHODS TO PREVENT AND REVERSE ATROPHY

The motor output of any given muscle at any given time is largely a function of how many motor units within a motor pool are activated and of the total cross-sectional area of all of the muscle

fibers of those units. Within a few weeks after an SCI, muscles are likely to have atrophied (12, 42). Interestingly, however, the severity of the atrophy varies among subjects and among muscles within a subject (12, 43–46). The reasons for this varied response are poorly understood.

Muscle atrophy can be a limiting factor in regaining mobility simply because the reduction in force output is at least proportional to the loss in muscle mass, and it is usually much greater. For example, if there is a 50% loss in muscle mass and muscle fiber cross-sectional area, and assuming no other changes, then there will be at least a 50% loss in the force that can be generated. Although only a small proportion of a muscle's force potential is needed when walking, severe muscle atrophy can preclude effective mobility. Indeed, one normally only activates a small proportion of the motor units within a given motor pool to walk at a comfortable speed, but if there is a 50% atrophy of all fibers in a muscle, then those motor units that are recruited will generate half the normal force that would have been generated without atrophy. This effect alone may be sufficient to prevent a subject with an SCI from executing a motor task, such as stepping or standing.

To walk "normally" after 50% muscle atrophy, more motor units will have to be recruited to generate the same kinematics and kinetics of a given movement. For example, a subject with 50% muscle atrophy might have to recruit 40%, as opposed to the normal 20%, of his motor units to generate the force needed to step (Figure 72.4A). The recruitment of additional motor units in each of the contributing motor pools has consequences with respect to the onset of fatigue, because the higher threshold units are more fatigable (Figure 72.4B). The larger motor units with higher thresholds for excitation have lower levels of metabolic support via oxidative phosphorylation and have a lower potential to sustain metabolic homeostasis than do the smaller, lower-threshold units. Thus, in a rehabilitative strategy to maximize motor performance involving muscles controlled by neurons

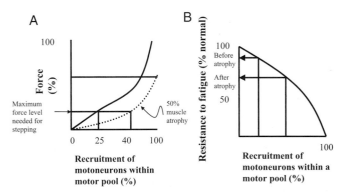

Figure 72.4 The theoretical relationship between the percentage of motoneurons recruited within a given motor pool and the net force that can be generated by those motoneurons recruited (**A**). Note the nonlinear increase in force with recruitment because, in general, the smaller motor units are recruited before the larger motor units. When the muscle atrophies, the same percent recruitment generates less force. Thus, to accomplish a given task, more units must be recruited in the atrophied muscle. The larger motoneurons recruited the latest (having a higher threshold level) also are the most fatigable. Therefore, when more motor units are required to perform a task, the population as a whole will be more susceptible to fatigue (**B**).

distal to the spinal lesion, it will be an advantage to minimize muscle atrophy.

How can we prevent or minimize muscle atrophy? Some combination of electrical stimulation, treadmill training, diet, and use of anabolic growth factors could contribute to the preservation of muscle mass after an SCI (47, 48). Only modest, and in some cases no, gains in muscle mass have been observed with electrical stimulation of a muscle. This may be related to the fact that, in most cases, the muscles are being activated under minimal or no load conditions (42). If the muscles in spinal patients are loaded when stimulated, then some muscle mass is preserved (46, 49). Subjects trained on a treadmill using BWST show an increase in muscle mass as indicated by magnetic resonance imaging (MRI)–derived muscle volume measurements after step training (50, 51). The development of an effective way to avoid or to minimize muscle atrophy after an SCI could have a very significant effect on the motor tasks that can be performed.

It is also clear that muscle phenotypes change after an SCI, with an increase in the percentage of muscle fibers expressing fast myosin phenotypes in both laboratory animals and human subjects (see 12 for review). The functional consequences of this are not clear, but theoretically this could make the muscles more fatigable and less efficient in generating force per unit of ATP. Locomotor training and muscle stimulation also can reduce the magnitude of the transition of expressing more fast myosin isoforms and less slow myosin after an SCI (52–55).

REHABILITATIVE STRATEGIES FOR AMBULATION: LOCOMOTOR TRAINING

Procedures typically used in conventional therapy after an SCI vary depending on the severity and level of the injury. In general, ASIA A and B subjects have not been provided with any form of step training after their injury. Traditionally the most functionally important skills needed to compensate for the loss of mobility using the unaffected muscle groups take precedence in therapy. For example, inpatient and outpatient therapies for paraplegics may include work on trunk support, upper extremity strengthening, transfers, and wheelchair mobility. For many ASIA C and D subjects, those skills also may be important. Rehabilitation strategies focused on facilitating recovery below the level of injury more recently have received much more consideration. These strategies have been defined and implemented as activity-based therapy that involves activation of the neuromuscular system below the level of lesion with task-specific retraining (10, 56, 57).

A general principle to follow is that the injured neuromotor system can regain considerable skill with practice. In essence, the neuromotor system has to relearn how to execute a motor task because, after an injury, new neural strategies must be allowed and should be facilitated to reemerge with the new spinal cord. Apparatuses that enable one to relieve the level of weight bearing and facilitate kinematically more correct reciprocal stepping should be employed in a systematic and progressive manner after an injury.

The use of motor scores to plan a rehabilitation strategy, as is routinely done clinically, is useful only as a blunt indicator of one's motor capacity. It is important to note that one cannot tell in either spinal animals or humans with an SCI the degree to which the activation of different muscles can be attributed to voluntary versus involuntary control (Figure 72.5). For example, the level of excitation of lower limb muscles in

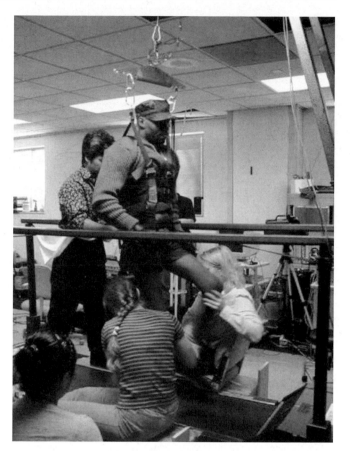

Figure 72.5 An individual with an SCI suspended in a harness by a body weight support system over a treadmill (BWST) is illustrated. Physical therapists assist each limb when necessary to facilitate the normal kinematics of stepping. Other therapists may be needed to assist at the hips to facilitate balance and trunk control in patients with more severe injuries.

individuals with an SCI during stepping using BWST substantially exceeds that when they voluntarily attempt to activate the same muscles (33). Furthermore, ambulatory ability often improves after step training without any change in the lower extremity motor score (9).

The most prominent and well-developed activity-based therapy to date is "locomotor training" (56). A series of guiding principles for training has emerged in the translation of findings from basic science to the human condition that focuses on optimizing normative stepping parameters, including the speed of stepping and the appropriate kinematics and kinetics (57, 58). Locomotor training using manual assistance and BWST has a number of advantages over more conventional approaches for the recovery of walking after an SCI. For example, the use of orthotics can be avoided. The BWST system allows step training to proceed without any dependence on upper extremity loading on parallel bars or other assistive devices (Figure 72.5). The harness assists in maintaining an upright trunk and, in the early practice of standing and stepping, in activating the trunk musculature. This intervention can rapidly enable independence in holding an upright posture. Repetitive activation of the segmental sensorimotor pathways used during the normal gait cycle appears to improve the probability of generating more effective stepping over a period of weeks (Figure 72.6). Based on

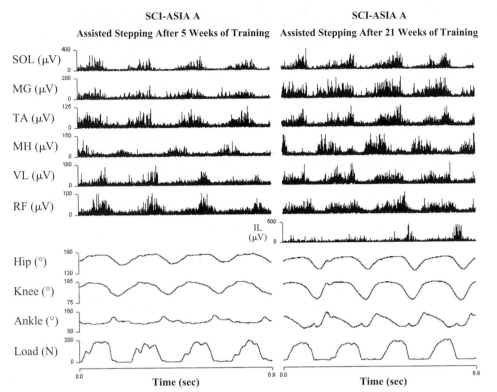

SCI-ASIA A

Assisted Stepping After 5 Weeks of Training   **Assisted Stepping After 21 Weeks of Training**

SCI-ASIA A

Figure 72.6   EMG activity (rectified, high-pass filtered at 32 Hz) from the soleus (SOL), medial gastrocnemius (MG), tibialis anterior (TA), MH (medial hamstrings), vastus lateralis (VL), rectus femoris (RF), and iliopsoas (IL); hip, knee, and ankle angles; and limb load from the left limb during stepping at 0.54 meters/second with BWST after 5 weeks and after 21 weeks of training from an individual with a clinically complete SCI (ASIA A). This subject generated EMG bursts in the lower limbs synchronized with the kinematics of stepping. Within several weeks of step training, joint excursions and EMG burst amplitudes increased. These changes were muscle specific and remained linked to the kinematics and kinetics of the step cycle. These data were collected in collaboration with Anton Wernig, MD (Department of Physiology, University of Bonn) and Sabina Müeller, PT (Rehabilitation Clinics, Langensteinbach, Karlsbad, Germany).

numerous EMG recordings as shown in Figure 72.6, it appears that the spinal cord can learn to activate a greater percentage of motor units and/or activate them at a higher frequency as a result of step training.

Early clinical evidence indicating that locomotor training can improve the potential for ambulation is based on the studies of acute and chronic, clinically incomplete SCI subjects (9, 10). Subjects have undergone locomotor training using BWST and manual assistance, and their functional outcomes have been compared to a matched group of subjects selected from historical records who had been treated with conventional therapies in the same clinic (Figure 72.7). A greater number of individuals achieved higher levels of ambulation in both the acute and chronic SCI groups using BWST than in the conventional groups. After training on a treadmill, ten of thirteen chronic subjects who were wheelchair dependent regained locomotor function by at least one level on a motor score ranging from 0 to 4. Some actually regained independent walking ability. There was no difference, however, in the recovery of voluntary muscle activity determined by manual muscle testing between the BWST and conventional groups. This suggests that the ability to ambulate in the locomotor training group was not attributable to an improved ability to generate voluntary force in a given muscle group, as is tested routinely to obtain "motor scores," but to the force that occurs as a result of neurally modulating "automatic" pathways that

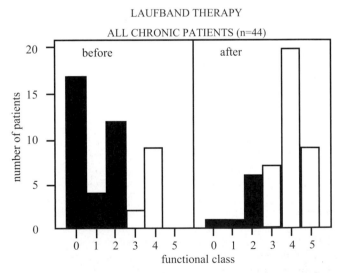

Figure 72.7   The locomotor capabilities of chronic incomplete SCI subjects (*n* = 44) before and after Laufband therapy (training locomotion on a treadmill) are shown. Six functional groups (0–5 [see ref. 9 for definitions]) contain wheelchair-bound (classes 0–2; black columns) and non-wheelchair-bound (classes 3–5; white columns) subjects. Note the significant shift in the distribution toward greater mobility observed after 12 weeks of training.

normally execute postural and locomotor movements. A large percentage of individuals who undergo appropriate locomotor training will improve their ability to walk overground.

Wernig has emphasized the importance of adhering to his "rules of locomotion" in efforts to regain locomotor function after an SCI (9). Although these "rules" have general applicability to rehabilitative approaches for a variety of neuromuscular disorders, therapists need to acquire not only considerable skill in the general methods of progressively enhancing locomotor function, but also in seemingly minor details that can make significant differences in succeeding in improving locomotor function. Thus, in many cases, the skill and experience of the therapists will determine the level of success of the rehabilitation. Variability in this level of expertise may explain the differences in the success of improvement in locomotor function at different rehabilitation centers (59, 60). In a 0.5- to 6.5-year follow-up of the subjects tested originally by Wernig (10), all subjects had at least maintained the same level of function, and some continued to improve, after completion of the step-training program. This encouraging result probably reflects the fact that when a rehabilitating subject reaches a critical functional level of motor control that is useful to daily life, the individual will be essentially practicing this locomotor function on a daily basis while performing routine daily activities.

Recently, a single-blinded, parallel-group, multicenter randomized clinical trial compared two interventions for walking that utilized key principles of locomotor training in incomplete (ASIA B, C, or D) acute SCI individuals (36). The BWST group received step and stand training with BWST and manual assistance, had overground practice for at least 1 hour for five sessions per week for a total of sixty sessions, and avoided antispasticity medication. The control group received the same intensity of treatment and avoided antispasticity medication, but all stand and step practice occurred overground. The individuals in both groups achieved walking abilities beyond that expected and reported in the literature when tested at 6 months after entering into the trial and 3 months after the interventions were initiated. Approximately 90% of these individuals recovered the ability to walk in the home and community (median speed of 1.1 meters/second) regardless of whether they trained overground or on the treadmill.

There are many factors that should be considered in the interpretation of these results. First, the inclusion and exclusion criteria eliminated over 1,330 individuals and may have preselected those individuals who had a higher probability of recovery because of age, overall health, and lower incidence of comorbidities. The two treatment groups received a much higher intensity of weight-bearing standing and stepping than is usual in acute rehabilitation centers, and they avoided antispasticity medication. It is possible that, by allowing the spinal circuitry to remain active and by introducing intense weight-bearing, the potential for function reorganization of the spinal cord after the SCI was optimized. We cannot distinguish among these possibilities from the current data, and future studies are needed to better understand the potential recovery after an SCI with task-specific retraining of the nervous system below the level of injury. These results, however, clearly show that early, intense repetitive task-specific practice with weight-bearing can result in significant recovery in motor incomplete SCI individuals beyond that realized using conventional therapies.

One advantage of using BWST for locomotor training is that it allows step training to begin safely as soon as a patient is medically stable. This may be important because muscle atrophy occurs very rapidly, particularly within the initial 2 months after an SCI. There also are losses of neural function when motor function is minimized. The BWST system allows the therapist to approximate the kinematics and temporal parameters of stepping more easily and accurately than when the injured individual uses parallel bars or steps overground with assistive devices. Locomotor training permits repetitive task-oriented practice over a range of normal walking speeds, and the practice parameters can be varied to optimize motor learning (e.g., by selecting the most effective level of weight bearing and speed at any given training state). This facilitates the sensorimotor processing associated with weight-bearing stepping, whereas conventional gait training may impose repetitive practice of inefficient and less-effective stepping.

Other potential general health benefits that theoretically could be associated with locomotor training using BWST include reducing the risk or severity of osteoporosis, metabolic diseases, heart disease, and skin lesions. For example, improved glucose tolerance has been reported in complete SCI subjects after stimulation of the quadriceps muscles for two sessions per week over a period of 12 weeks when there is high resistance to movement (49). Some efforts are being made to determine what benefit individuals with an SCI can gain from activity-dependent therapies in some of the secondary deficiencies associated with the absence of normal weight-bearing activity (61–65). Significant progress in obtaining robust sets of clinical data related to some of these issues is beginning to emerge, particularly through the Neural Recovery Network, as described below. At the present time, it is very obvious that some individuals with a severe SCI, even years after the injury, can regain significant postural and locomotor function with the appropriate therapy. The key questions are which individuals are likely to gain from such therapy, how much gain can be predicted with a given amount of therapy, and what will be the input-output ratio in terms of human and economic costs? Only after generating these types of data can an individual patient make a well-informed decision about his or her rehabilitative strategy. Similarly, the same data should be considered by those institutions that define the level of access that a patient will have to such therapy.

The degree to which activity-dependent interventions, in addition to weight-bearing locomotor training, can be used to improve ambulatory function in SCI subjects is beginning to be considered. For example, efforts are continuing in attempting to use high-resistance training (66) or muscle stimulation (67) combined with locomotor training to facilitate locomotion as well as to prevent muscle atrophy. The approaches used to gain some locomotor function have been highly varied, and the success of these interventions differs depending on the level of locomotor dysfunction in the individual. A thorough review of these combinatorial approaches is beyond the scope of the present chapter. It seems almost inevitable, however, that the most successful rehabilitative strategies will consist of a combination of interventions.

Locomotor training as a rehabilitative strategy has been successful for many people with acute and chronic incomplete SCI, with varied results. This may be due to differences among therapists in their relative level of knowledge of the principles underlying retraining of the nervous system and in their skill in applying these principles, as well as in the intensity and duration of the intervention. Therapists who are aware of the potential of the spinal networks and sensory signals to modulate muscle activation patterns will have the best chance of optimizing locomotor training for their patients. Implementing locomotor training in the clinic is in the relatively early stages of development, and future efforts should focus on education, training, and establishing of standards. Accessibility to effective locomotor training remains limited in the United States. Recently, the Neural Recovery Network, composed of rehabilitation centers across the United States, has begun to provide consistent activity-based therapy, including locomotor training, and training of therapists in surrounding regions.

CONCLUSIONS

This chapter summarizes the evolution of a new generation of clinical concepts applicable to rehabilitative strategies to improve ambulation after an SCI. These concepts are based on data derived from extensive animal experimentation, mostly over the last 35 years. One concept is that a high level of processing of complex proprioceptive input occurs in the spinal cord, including in humans. The spinal cord is not a simple relay station for transmitting information to and from supraspinal centers. It is an integrated component of networks of neurons continually and steadily making "online" decisions with great detail.

A second concept of fundamental importance is that, although many elements of fine motor control can be derived from the brain, we now know that most of the details associated with the neural control of standing and stepping can be processed within the spinal circuitry.

A third concept is that the level of motor function that emerges after an SCI is defined in large part by use-dependent mechanisms. Although some functional and anatomical reorganization will occur spontaneously, the efficacy of the neural pathways that generate locomotion are use dependent. Through these use-dependent mechanisms, there may be an unrecognized capacity within the spinal cord to functionally "rewire" itself (i.e., the spinal cord is highly plastic).

Fourth, it is feasible to modulate the "physiologic state" of the spinal cord via training, epidural stimulation, and pharmacologic agents to "enable," as opposed to directly impose, the spinal cord to execute weight-bearing stepping.

Finally, the spinal cord is smart. Our understanding of the concepts of spinal "smartness," however, remains rudimentary. We are only beginning to formulate the best strategies to utilize motor training paradigms (i.e., how much time per day to train, how often to train, how specific the training tasks should be, and so forth). We also must learn to individualize the strategies and learn how to change them with and according to the changes that occur in the individual. The resolution of some of these seemingly minor details can have a significant impact on the success of a program for rehabilitating walking after an SCI.

ACKNOWLEDGMENTS

We are grateful for the support of the National Institute of Neurological Disorders and Stroke (NINDS), the National Institute of Child Health and Development (NICHD), the National Aeronautics and Space Administration (NASA), the Kent Waldrep National Paralysis Foundation, the Craig Neilsen Foundation, and the Christopher and Dana Reeve Paralysis Foundation.

References

1. Rossignol S. Neural control of stereotypic limb movements. In: Rowell LB, Shepherd JT, eds. *Handbook of Physiology Section 12. Exercise: Regulation and Integration of Multiple Systems.* New York: American Physiological Society, 1996.
2. Edgerton VR, Roy RR, de Leon RD. Neural Darwinism in the mammalian spinal cord. In: Grau J, Patterson M, eds. *Spinal Cord Plasticity: Alterations in Reflex Function.* Kluwer Academic Publishers, 2001: 185–206.
3. Edgerton VR, et al. Retraining the injured spinal cord. *J Physiol (Lond)* 2001; 533:15–22.
4. Harkema SJ. Neural plasticity after human spinal cord injury: application of locomotor training to the rehabilitation of walking. *Neuroscientist* 2001; 7:455–468.
5. Dietz V, Curt A, Colombo G. Locomotor pattern in paraplegic patients: training effects and recovery of spinal cord function. *Spinal Cord* 1998; 36:380–390.
6. Nacimiento W, Sappok T, Brook GA, Toth L, et al. Structural changes of caudal to a low thoracic spinal cord hemisection in the adult rat: a light and electron microscopic study. *Acta Neuropathol* 1995; 90:552–564.
7. Ichiyama RM, Broman J, Edgerton VR, Havton LA. Ultrastructural synaptic features differ between alpha- and gamma-motoneurons innervating the tibialis anterior muscle in the rat. *J Comp Neurol* 2006; 499:306–315.
8. Ichiyama RM, Broman J, Roy RR, Zhong H, et al. Synaptic plasticity of alpha and gamma motoneurons after spinal cord injury and locomotor training. *Abstr Soc Neurosci* 2006; Program No. 646.4.
9. Wernig A, Muller S, Nanassy A, Cagol E. Laufband therapy based on 'rules of spinal locomotion' is effective in spinal cord injured persons. *Eur J Neurosci* 1995; 7:823–829.
10. Wernig A, Nanassy A, Muller S. Laufband (treadmill) therapy in incomplete paraplegia and tetraplegia. *J Neurotrama* 1999; 16:719–726.
11. Thomas SL, Gorassini MA. Increases in corticospinal tract function by treadmill training after incomplete spinal cord injury. *J Neurophysiol* 2005; 94:2844–2855.
12. Roy RR, Baldwin KM, Edgerton VR. The plasticity of skeletal muscle: effects of neuromuscular activity. In: Holloszy J, ed. *Exercise and Sports Sciences Reviews*, Volume 19. Baltimore, MD: Williams and Wilkins, 1991:269–312.
13. Bodine SC, Roy RR, Eldred E, Edgerton VR. Maximal force as a function of anatomical features of motor units in the cat tibialis anterior. *J Neurophysiol* 1987; 57:1730–1745.
14. Grillner S. Control of Locomotion in bipeds, tetrapods, and fish. In: Brooks VB, ed. *Handbook of Physiology, The Nervous System, Motor Control.* Bethesda, MD: American Physiological Society, 1981:1179–1236.
15. Edgerton VR, Tillakaratne NJ, Bigbee AJ, de Leon RD, Roy RR. Plasticity of the spinal neural circuitry after injury. *Annu Rev Neurosci* 2004; 27:145–167.
16. Edgerton VR, Courtine G, Gerasimenko YP, Lavrov I, et al. Training locomotor networks. *Brain Res Rev* 2008; 57:241–254.
17. Rossignol S, Barbeau H. Pharmacology of locomotion: an account of studies in spinal cats and spinal cord injured subjects. *J Am Paraplegia Soc* 1993; 16:190–196.
18. Forssberg H, Grillner S, Rossignol S. Phasic gain control of reflexes from the dorsum of the paw during spinal locomotion. *Brain Res* 1977; 132:121–129.
19. Harkema SJ, Hurley SL, Patel UK, Requejo PS, et al. Human lumbosacral spinal cord interprets loading during stepping. *J Neurophysiol* 1997; 77:797–811.
20. de Leon RD, Hodgson JA, Roy RR, Edgerton VR. Locomotor capacity attributable to step training versus spontaneous recovery following spinalization in adult cats. *J Neurophysiol* 1998; 79:1329–1340.
21. de Leon RD, Hodgson JA, Roy RR, Edgerton VR. Full weight-bearing hindlimb standing following stand training in the adult spinal cat. *J Neurophysiol* 1998; 80:83–91.
22. Edgerton VR, Roy RR, de Leon R, Tillakaratne N, Hodgson JA. Does motor learning occur in the spinal cord? *Neuroscientist* 1997; 3:287–294.

23. Lovely RG, Gregor RJ, Roy RR, Edgerton VR. Effects of training on the recovery of full weight bearing stepping in the adult spinal cat. *Exp Neurol* 1986; 92:421–435.

24. de Leon RD, Hodgson JA, Roy RR, Edgerton VR. Retention of hindlimb stepping ability in adult spinal cats after the cessation of step training. *J Neurophysiol* 1999; 81:85–94.

25. Barbeau H, McCrea DA, O'Donovan MJ, Rossignol S, et al. Tapping into spinal circuits to restore motor function. *Brain Res* 1999; 30:27–51.

26. Thuret S, Moon LD, Gage FH. Therapeutic interventions after spinal cord injury. *Nat Rev Neurosci* 2006; 7:628–643.

27. Buchli AD, Rouiller E, Mueller R, Dietz V, Schwab ME. Repair of the injured spinal cord: a joint approach of basic and clinical research. *Neurodegener Dis* 2007; 4:51–56.

28. Griesbach GS, Hovda DA, Molteni R, Wu A, Gomez-Pinilla F. Voluntary exercise following traumatic brain injury: brain-derived neurotrophic factor upregulation and recovery of function. *Neuroscience* 2004; 125:129–139.

29. Dobkin B, Apple D, Barbeau H, Basso M, et al. Spinal Cord Injury Locomotor Trial Group. Weight-supported treadmill vs over-ground training for walking after acute incomplete SCI. *Neurology* 2006 66:484–493.

30. Behrman AL, Nair P, Bowden M, Dauser RC, et al. Locomotor training restores walking in a nonambulatory child with severe, chronic, cervical incomplete spinal cord injury. *Phys Ther* in press.

31. Kakulas BA. A review of the neuropathology of human spinal cord injury with emphasis on special features. *J Spinal Cord Med* 1999; 22:119–124.

32. Courtine G, Roy RR, Raven J, Hodgson J, et al. Performance of locomotion and foot grasping following a unilateral thoracic corticospinal tract lesion in monkeys (Macaca mulatta). *Brain* 2005; 128:2338–2358.

33. Maegele M, Muller S, Wernig A, Edgerton VR, Harkema SJ. Recruitment of spinal motor pools during voluntary movements versus stepping after human spinal cord injury. *J Neurotrama* 2002; 19:1217–1229.

34. Humphrey DR, Mao H, Griffith RW. Brain reorganization continues for 25 years after spinal injury: changing patterns of activation in human cerebral cortex during attempts to move. *Abstr Soc Neurosci* 2006; Program No. 88.9.

35. Beres-Jones JA, Johnson TD, Harkema SJ. Clonus after human spinal cord injury cannot be attributed solely to recurrent muscle-tendon stretch. *Exp Brain Res* 2003; 149:222–236.

36. Dobkin B, et al. Weight-supported treadmill vs over-ground training for walking after acute incomplete spinal cord injury. *Neurology* 2006; 66:484–493.

37. Kiehn O. Locomotor circuits in the mammalian spinal cord. *Annu Rev Neurosci* 2006; 29:279–306.

38. Rossignol S, Dubuc R, Gossard JP. Dynamic sensorimotor interactions in locomotion. *Physiol Rev* 2006 86:89–154.

39. Barbeau H, Norman KE. The effect of noradrenergic drugs on the recovery of walking after spinal cord injury. *Spinal Cord* 2003; 41:137–143.

40. de Leon RD, Tamaki H, Hodgson JA, Roy RR, Edgerton VR. Hindlimb locomotor and postural training modulates glycinergic inhibition in the spinal cord of the adult spinal cat. *J Neurophysiol* 1999; 82:359–369.

41. Talmadge RJ, Roy RR, Edgerton VR. Alterations in the glycinergic neurotransmitter system are associated with stepping behavior in neonatal spinal cord transected rats. *Abstr Soc Neurosci* 1996; 22:1397.

42. Edgerton VR, Bodine-Fowler S, Roy RR, Ishihara A, Hodgson JA. Neuromuscular adaptation. In: Rowell LB, Shepherd JT, eds. *Handbook of Physiology. Section 12. Exercise: Regulation and Integration of Multiple Systems*, New York: Oxford University Press, 1996:54–88.

43. Castro MJ, Apple DF Jr, Rogers S, Dudley GA. Influence of complete spinal cord injury on skeletal muscle mechanics within the first 6 months of injury. *Eur J Appl Physiol* 2000; 81:128–131.

44. Castro MJ, Apple DF Jr, Staron RS, Campos GE, Dudley GA. Influence of complete spinal cord injury on skeletal muscle within 6 mo of injury. *J Appl Physiol* 1999; 86:350–358.

45. Castro MJ, Apple DF Jr, Hillegass EA, Dudley GA. Influence of complete spinal cord injury on skeletal muscle cross-sectional area within the first 6 months of injury. *Eur J Appl Physiol Occup Physiol* 1999; 80:373–378.

46. Shields RK, Dudley-Javoroski S. Musculoskeletal adaptations in chronic spinal cord injury: effects of long-term soleus electrical stimulation training. *Neurorehabil Neural Repair* 2007; 21:169–179.

47. Edgerton VR, Kim SJ, Ichiyama RM, Gerasimenko YP, Roy RR. Rehabilitative therapies after spinal cord injury. *J Neurotrauma* 2006; 23:560–570.

48. Edgerton VR, Roy RR, Allen DL, Monti RJ. Adaptations in skeletal muscle disuse or decreased-use atrophy. *Am J Phys Med Rehabil* 2002; 81(Suppl 11):S127–S147.

49. Mahoney ET, Bickel CS, Elder C, Black C, et al. Changes in skeletal muscle size and glucose tolerance with electrically stimulated resistance training in subjects with chronic spinal cord injury. *Arch Phys Med Rehabil* 2005; 86:1502–1504.

50. Giangregorio LM, et al. Body weight supported treadmill training in acute spinal cord injury: impact on muscle and bone. *Spinal Cord* 2005; 43:649–657.

51. Giangregorio LM, et al. Can body weight supported treadmill training increase bone mass and reverse muscle atrophy in individuals with chronic incomplete spinal cord injury? *Appl Physiol Nutr Metab* 2006; 31:283–291.

52. Kim SJ, et al. Electromechanical stimulation ameliorates inactivity-induced adaptations in the medial gastrocnemius of adult rats. *J Appl Physiol* 2007; 103:195–205.

53. Roy RR, Talmadge RJ, Hodgson JA, Oishi Y, et al. Differential response of fast hindlimb extensor and flexor muscles to exercise in adult spinalized cats. *Muscle Nerve* 1999; 22:230–241.

54. Roy RR, et al. Influences of electromechanical events in defining skeletal muscle properties. *Muscle Nerve* 2002; 26:238–251.

55. Talmadge RJ, Garcia ND, Roy RR, Edgerton VR. Myosin heavy chain isoform mRNA and protein levels after long-term paralysis. *Biochem Biophys Res Commun* 2004; 325:296–301.

56. Behrman AL, Harkema SJ. Physical rehabilitation as an agent for recovery after spinal cord injury. *Phys Med Rehabil Clin N Am* 2007; 18:183–202.

57. Dietz V, Harkema SJ. Locomotor activity in spinal cord–injured persons. *J Appl Physiol* 2004; 96:1954–1960.

58. Harkema SJ. Neural plasticity after human spinal cord injury: application of locomotor training to the rehabilitation of walking. *Neuroscientist* 2001; 7:455–468.

59. Wernig A. Long-term body-weight supported treadmill training and subsequent follow-up in persons with chronic SCI: effects on functional walking ability and measures of subjective well-being. *Spinal Cord* 2006; 44:265–266.

60. Hicks AL, Adams MM, Martin Ginis K, Giangregorio L, et al. Long-term body-weight-supported treadmill training and subsequent follow-up in persons with chronic SCI: effects on functional walking ability and measures of subjective well-being. *Spinal Cord* 2005; 43:291–298.

61. Mahoney ET, Bickel CS, Elder C, Black C, et al. Changes in skeletal muscle size and glucose tolerance with electrically stimulated resistance training in subjects with chronic spinal cord injury. *Arch Phys Med Rehabil* 2005; 86:1502–1504.

62. Effing TW, van Meeteren NL, van Asbeck FW, Prevo AJ. Body weight–supported treadmill training in chronic incomplete spinal cord injury: a pilot study evaluating functional health status and quality of life. *Spinal Cord* 2006; 44:287–296.

63. Latimer AE, Ginis KA, Hicks AL, McCartney N. An examination of the mechanisms of exercise-induced change in psychological well-being among people with spinal cord injury. *J Rehabil Res Dev* 2004; 41:643–652.

64. Kerstin W, Gabriele B, Richard L. What promotes physical activity after spinal cord injury? An interview study from a patient perspective. *Disabil Rehabil* 2006; 28:481–488.

65. Myslinski MJ. Evidence-based exercise prescription for individuals with spinal cord injury. *J Neurol Phys Ther* 2005; 29:104–106.

66. Edwards LC, Layne CS. Effect of dynamic weight bearing on neuromuscular activation after spinal cord injury. *Am J Phys Med Rehabil* 2007; 86:499–506.

67. Gregory CM, Bowden MG, Jayaraman A, Shah P, et al. Resistance training and locomotor recovery after incomplete spinal cord injury: a case series. *Spinal Cord* 2007; 45:522–530.

68. Thrasher TA, Flett HM, Popovic MR. Gait training regimen for incomplete spinal cord injury using functional electrical stimulation. *Spinal Cord* 2006; 44:357–361.

73 Epidural Spinal Cord Stimulation to Facilitate Functional Recovery after Spinal Cord Injury: Combinations of Therapies for Synergistic Outcomes

Jiping He
Richard Herman

MOTOR INCOMPLETE SCI AND OPTIONS FOR LOCOMOTOR AMBULATION: CONTEMPORARY TREATMENT AND NEXT STEP OPTIONS

Natural History of Spinal Cord Injury: Enhancement with Neural Rehabilitation

Clinical observations indicate that during the first year following incomplete spinal cord injury (ISCI), substantial improvements in motor function may occur, but patterns of recovery and the sequence of motor function differ within a population. Functional recovery after ISCI depends on several factors: the nature and extent of the injury, intrinsic changes in spinal chemistry and applied pharmacologic treatment, and rehabilitative interventions completed. Adaptive neural responses occur at multiple sites (1, 2) and involve variable and complex processes. Multiple interventional strategies can be used to accelerate these various processes and enhance functional recovery. They include traditional physical therapy, pharmacologic interventions, genetic therapy, and other treatments either individually or in combination. These approaches should be designed to enhance adaptive responses and plasticity of the spinal and supraspinal nervous system.

The foundation of any neurorehabilitation therapy is a working understanding of the underlying mechanisms that neural structures use to recover. As discussed below, research on animals has demonstrated that the spinal cord possesses the ability to generate locomotion without supraspinal input and has the ability to adapt or "learn" when exposed to appropriate afferent input produced by sensorimotor training. These findings provide the basis for the application of locomotor treadmill training following ISCI, a therapy that appears to be augmented with the addition of peripheral electrical stimulation as well as stimulation of the spinal cord.

Spinal Locomotion: Recovery with Enhanced Activation of Central Pattern Generators

Numerous studies have demonstrated that the neuronal circuitry of the spinal cord is capable of generating rhythmic, locomotor output in the absence of supraspinal input. Such "spinal locomotion" is perhaps most convincingly demonstrated by the recovery of coordinated and alternating patterns of muscle activity and limb movements in chronic low spinal cats undergoing training on a moving treadmill (3, 4). This pattern of recovery is also described in vertebrates such as the lamprey, neonatal and other animal models, and in vitro preparations (5–10). The locomotion expressed in these animal models can be characterized as innate, spinal cord–mediated, initiated and modulated by monoaminergic (e.g., noradrenergic) substances, plastic, and adaptable. This adaptability is particularly important, suggesting that the pattern can be modified by treadmill speed, tonic afferent inputs (limb position, visceral stimulation), or phasic afferent inputs (perturbation of position) (6, 11).

Grillner et al. (9) postulate that such generation of locomotion implies that a spinal neural network is recruited as a component of most goal-directed patterns of vertebrate behavior. They suggest that, in all classes of vertebrates, the overall locomotor control system is designed in a similar way. Activation of lower brainstem reticulospinal neurons by higher centers (e.g., basal ganglia) activates spinal networks of nerve cells, which generate the motor pattern. Sensory feedback acting on the spinal locomotion circuits is an integral part of the control system and helps adapt the motor pattern to environmental demands.

Locomotor recovery following chronic spinal cord injury can be ascribed to enhanced activation of locomotion rhythm, generating circuits in the spinal cord. Spinal locomotor generation can occur in spinal cats when sensory feedback is abolished ("fictive locomotion"), particularly when locomotion is initiated and/or sustained by pharmacotherapy (12) and/or functional electrical stimulation of muscles, sensory nerves, or spinal cord (13, 14). Fictive locomotion is a phenomenon observed under special experimental preparations—rhythmic flexor and extensor muscle activities and alternating leg movement similar to locomotion patterns, either recording electroneurograms (ENG) directly from the exposed spinal cord outputs or electromyograms (EMG) from major muscles—but under both conditions, the sensory feedback pathways are blocked or severed, so no sensory modulation of the rhythmic pattern is elicited (13). Because this phenomenon can also be observed in decerebrate preparations from lampreys to cats, it demonstrates the existence of a rhythmic pattern generator in the spinal cord of these animal preparations.

There is evidence to support the existence of locomotor rhythm-generating circuitry in the human spinal cord as well. Coordinated leg movements and EMG activity have been observed in patients with clinically complete (not necessarily anatomically complete) spinal lesions. Such movements have been expressed spontaneously (15), have been induced by electrical stimulation (15–21), or have occurred with treadmill training with partial body weight support (22–29). This would suggest that spinal circuitry for the generation of locomotor output exists within the human spinal cord and can be modulated in a manner similar to the chronic spinal animal following interactive treadmill training (3, 4). Whether all these features of the locomotor patterns discovered in spinal cats can be elicited from spinal humans has yet to be determined, but most certainly have been identified (19, 20, 25, 30–34).

Spinal Learning: Can Repetitive Stimulation Change Spinal Circuitry and Response?

Following ISCI, repetitive sensorimotor stimuli can induce changes in spinal circuitry by altering supraspinal and spinal plasticity. These types of changes have been observed in humans with complete and with incomplete lesions in studies that have utilized a locomotor training paradigm (14, 22–25, 27, 35–40), as well as in animals models (3, 4, 6, 38, 41–43). Unfortunately, even the most innovative techniques have not to date resulted in recovery of voluntary motor control in persons with *complete* spinal cord injury (24).

Spinal reflex gains may be modulated by inputs from spinal circuits as well as supraspinal centers. This concept of "sensorimotor gain control" (44) appears to be widely used in the nervous system for a variety of movements, and it has been widely observed during locomotion as well as other cyclic activities in humans and in several animal models (33, 45–55). This modulation has been observed in reflex gains from muscle afferents (56), cutaneous afferents (57, 58), and proprioceptors (59). Reconfiguration of reflex pathways can occur (e.g., group Ib reflex pathways for extensors from inhibitory to excitatory) (60). It is further noted that spinal reflexes can be conditioned even after spinalization (61, 62).

Spinal cord reorganization or "spinal learning" can occur with sensorimotor training and depends strongly upon the patterns of neural signals that are presented to the residual circuits. With "appropriate" phasic excitation of afferents (24, 25, 36, 39, 63) via sensorimotor stimuli producing locomotor-like limb

motion and loading (64), long-term plastic changes can be induced in spite of limited or no supraspinal input (3, 4, 24, 39, 56, 65, 66). Such spinal learning appears to be quite task specific and depends upon repetitive activation of the appropriate pathways through persistent training, as demonstrated by the animal studies of De Leon et al. (36, 39).

Partial Weight Bearing Therapy (PWBT)

As described in more detail in the chapter by Edgerton in this section of the textbook, the developmental evidence and recent experimental reports on spinal locomotion and spinal learning provide the rationale for the application of locomotion training programs in humans with incomplete spinal cord injury. Specifically, the reintroduction of locomotion-related afferent activity facilitates favorable plastic changes in the spinal cord circuitry and induces locomotion rhythm generation. As an extension of their previous work in spinalized cats, Barbeau and colleagues were the first to develop and utilize this method in human subjects (67, 68). In the decade and a half since, treadmill training with partial body weight support has emerged as a promising technique for improving locomotor function in individuals with incomplete spinal cord injury (ISCI) (11, 23–27, 37, 68–71). Termed partial weight bearing therapy (PWBT) for the purpose of discussion, this technique has been applied in individuals with acute and chronic ISCI, with mixed results.

To date, the successful application of PWBT *alone* for recovery of functional overground walking in humans has been best demonstrated in individuals with ISCI designated as ASIA D. PWBT has been applied with some limited success in individuals with higher or bilaterally asymmetric motor scores within the ASIA C category. Improvements in locomotion in individuals with motor complete injuries, however, have been limited to the expression of rhythmic EMG activity when the limbs were driven through a pattern of joint angles consistent with locomotion and rhythmic loading of the feet (22, 25). This has been observed with manual assistance by therapists, as well as with driven motions applied using robotic training devices (71).

PWBT, applied in combination with functional electrical stimulation (6, 40, 72) and pharmacologic agents (73), has been shown to facilitate locomotor function in individuals with ISCI, improving coordination, speed, and endurance, and reducing reliance on assistive devices. More importantly, these benefits have not been limited to treadmill ambulation, but have been shown to be transferable to overground walking and to continue beyond the period of treadmill training (70).

One technique that has been used to enhance PWBT involves the application of functional electrical stimulation (FES) of skin/nerves of the distal lower limb to induce a flexion-withdrawal response (6, 38, 40, 67, 72, 74–76). This response can generally be obtained via electrical stimulation of the peroneal nerve in individuals with upper motoneuronal spinal cord injury (13). Appropriate stimulus training induces strong activation of the ipsilateral limb flexors and can be manipulated to generate a functional swing motion of the limb. Although this type of reflex-FES has been applied for decades in an effort to overcome locomotor deficits in subjects with upper motoneuronal lesions (13, 77, 78), it has only recently been combined with treadmill gait training (40, 79).

Peripheral Nerve Electrical Stimulation for Ambulation: Current Results and Outcome Limits

Electrical stimulation has been used to activate paralyzed muscles for a variety of applications, primarily as a tool for long-term use in rehabilitation of persons with neurologic disorders such as spinal cord injury, head injury, stroke, and so forth (80–83). Computer-controlled sequences of electrical pulses are delivered to selected muscles via either implanted or surface electrodes. Implanted electrical stimulation devices for restoration of hand grasp in tetraplegia were reported with certain success (84). Stimulation devices that utilize percutaneous electrodes (thin wires that cross the skin) have also been developed for restoration of standing and stepping function in thoracic-level spinal cord–injured patients (82, 85, 86) and stroke patients (87). Other devices that utilize electrodes that are implanted on the surface of the skin have also been used for restoration of standing and locomotor function in spinal cord–injured and other patients (88–90). These research programs have clearly demonstrated that neuromuscular stimulation can be effectively used to activate paralyzed muscles for performing motor activities of daily living. Much of the current research is focused on making these systems practical for everyday use at home and in the workplace by making them easier to use, more reliable, and more functional.

The major challenges facing FNS for restoration of ambulation include the effect of muscle fatigue from stimulation parameters and the need to maintain proper gait patterns over functional ambulation ranges in different community settings. When stimulating a nerve bundle (which is the usual mechanism involved in stimulating muscles), the number of fibers recruited by a given pulse can be varied by modifying stimulus pulse amplitude or pulse width. The firing frequency of fibers is determined by stimulus pulse period. Recent research has shown that these parameters can be adjusted adaptively according to the task at hand and muscle status (91) and in studies on human subjects (92–96).

Spinal Cord Electrical Stimulation for Functional Ambulation Recovery: Theory and Methods

An additional approach that has been receiving increasing attention and has shown promise for facilitating functional locomotor recovery is that offered by epidural spinal cord stimulation (ESCS). ESCS has been used in clinical application for chronic pain therapy since the 1960s. The technique is to place electrodes along the dorsal side of dural space at the spinal level corresponding to the dermatome mapping (97). This dermatome mapping defines the relative relation of the spinal cord level where the electrical stimulation is applied and the skin area where the effect of the stimulation is normally felt. The stimulation intensity is normally above the sensory threshold, with frequency of electrical pulses generating a pleasant tingling sensation. In 1973, Cook and Weinstein first introduced the technique of ESCS for motor disorder therapy associated with gait disturbance among multiple sclerosis (MS) subjects and for treatment of spasticity (98, 99).

The use of ESCS for augmenting motor function has intensified over time. The pioneering work of Garcia-Rill and his colleagues demonstrated the application of ESCS for possible locomotion recovery. Iwahara et al. (16, 17) demonstrated that active and fictive hindlimb locomotion could be induced in decerebrate cats, using nonpatterned surface stimulation of the dorsal lumbar spinal cord. Although not weight bearing, the resulting locomotor patterns were well organized and expressed in the absence of afferent input. In this experiment, a continuous electrical stimulation training was delivered to the lumbar enlargement section of cat spinal cord through the electrodes placed on the dorsal dura surface of the cord. A key finding from this study is that the stimulation parameters were different from those used for chronic pain therapy. The stimulation intensity was much higher (near or at motor threshold instead of just above sensory threshold), and the required pulse width (or pulse duration) was also much larger, 1 ms or more, instead of a maximum of 420 us used for pain treatment.

Promising results have also been reported in human studies by Dimitrijevic et al. (19, 20). These investigators have shown that tonic, nonpatterned stimulation of the posterior lumbar spinal cord can induce "locomotor-like" muscle activity and rhythmic limb movement in supine individuals with chronic complete spinal cord injury. Finally, ESCS has shown potential for improving locomotion among ASIA D ISCI patients (100) and in patients with MS (98, 100–102). Collectively, these results suggest that impaired descending control of rhythmic locomotion circuits from higher CNS centers (e.g., arising due to ISCI) can be modified by ESCS. Furthermore, there are some indications that motor learning may proceed with amplified descending control when conducted in conjunction with electrical stimulation of the spinal cord (6, 99, 103–104).

Assembling these concepts, Herman and He initiated an FDA-monitored protocol to evaluate the use of ESCS for facilitating locomotor recovery in ISCI subjects who required wheelchairs for ambulation. The protocol required proper subject screening to maximize the impact of treatment, selection of a stimulation system to provide the range of required stimulation parameters, a surgical procedure to implant the device, and a training regimen to activate the system for the therapeutic purpose of functional ambulation recovery.

This locomotor stimulation system is derived from existing technology used to electrically stimulate the spinal cord for the pain relief. For more than three decades, spinal stimulation has been an effective treatment for chronic intractable pain from various causes. For illustration purposes, a Medtronic system (X-TREL™) was used here (http://www.neuromodulation.com/), but there are several other epidural spinal cord stimulation systems with similar functionalities. They are available from major medical device companies such as Advanced Neuromodulation Systems, Boston Scientific, and Medtronic.

The technique involves surgically implanting a receiver (X-TREL™), under local anesthesia, subcutaneously in the flank/waist area of the subject. The receiver has an antenna that accepts radio frequency signals from an external transmitter. This transmitter has a nominal voltage of up to 14 V and a pulse width of up to 1000 μsec. These signals then program the spinal cord stimulator to produce electrical pulses that travel along a wire to a set of electrodes.

During surgical implantation, a pair of quadrapolar electrodes are threaded into the dorsal epidural space and grossly positioned via fluoroscopy. Figure 73.1 shows the position of electrodes and stimulator/receiver.

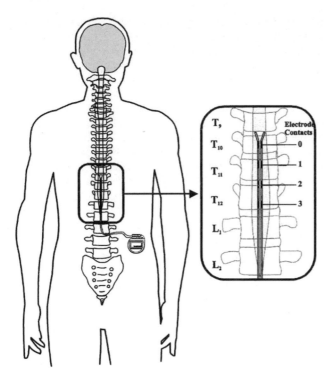

Figure 73.1 The stimulating electrodes are placed at T10–T12 along the midline of the dorsal spinal cord in the epidural space. The four pairs of electrodes are numbered 0 to 3, and each can be set as anode (+) or cathode (−). The receiver/stimulator is placed in the abdominal area under soft tissue for comfort.

In the study, the bifurcated electrode assembly was positioned on both sides of the midline of the dorsal spinal cord in a rostrocaudal orientation (the #0 electrode pair superiorly and the #3 pair inferiorly). To identify corresponding ipsilateral segmental innervations of muscle, bipolar (cathode/anode) arrangement of electrodes over each posterior spinal cord structure was ascertained. It was anticipated that cathodal current at the L2 segment, 3–4 mm from midline, coupled with the anode at the #3 or #1 contact, would provide the best opportunity for stimulating L2-innervated muscles (105–107). Stimulation of the dorsal roots produced phasic muscle twitches. It was contemplated that, at a lower voltage (and perhaps increased frequency), stimulation of the dorsal root might excite the locomotor pattern generator in the premotor area of the ventral spinal cord (16, 19, 103).

The results from the study demonstrated that ESCS facilitated the recovery of functional ambulation, improving coordination, speed, endurance, sense of effort, and energy cost and fuel selection during overground walking (108, 112). Importantly, these investigators demonstrated that the application of ESCS during PWBT permitted training intensity (e.g., treadmill speed, body support, and duration) to be increased, and greatly facilitated the transfer of spinal locomotion learned during PWBT to functional overground ambulation. Furthermore, the application of ESCS during ambulation produced immediate performance enhancements even after extensive exposure to PWBT and ESCS. Recently, some research results have been reported in rat models for SCI on possible neural mechanisms responsible for the ESCS-induced positive results of ambulation recovery (113–114).

Whole Body Metabolic Response to Locomotion Training: A Novel Observation

In a small-scale study of human subjects with ISCI using ESCS to facilitate recovery of functional walking, a remarkable reduction in sense of effort associated with a twofold increase in preferred walking speed was noted (110–111). With the assistance of Professor Wayne Willis (Department of Kinesiology, ASU), such modifications in gait behavior with ESCS led to the assessment of whole body metabolic activity. These studies demonstrated that ESCS reduced the O_2 (or energy) cost of transport (cost to transport a unit mass a unit distance) by only about 25% when subjects walked at preferred rates. In fact, ESCS reduced CO_2 production by a much greater relative extent. If one assumes normal whole-body acid–base balance, then the gas exchange data indicated that ESCS increased the exercise-induced fat oxidation rate by two- to eightfold, to walk the same distance. Concomitantly, carbohydrate (CHO) oxidation was decreased by over 50%. An alternative interpretation of the gas exchange data is that the lower CO_2 production during ESCS-assisted walking could have reflected less accumulation of blood lactate and associated bicarbonate titration. Both interpretations imply that ESCS somehow reduced the dependence of the exercising muscle on glycolysis, an interpretation that is entirely consistent with the marked improvement in muscle endurance observed in the ESCS condition. The subject's "sensation of lightness" associated with a sensation of "a low sense of effort" was certainly a feature in the difference between the stimulation and nonstimulation conditions. These behaviors were also noted by Cook and Weinstein (98), who used ESCS to facilitate locomotion in MS patients.

Herman et al. (110) concluded that ESCS elicits a greater activation of an oxidative motor unit pool, thereby reducing the subject's sense of effort and energy cost of walking and increasing preferred walking speeds.

These observations led to the temptation to challenge the time-honored concept that preferred rates of walking were intimately related to least energy expenditure and, by implication, a low sense of effort. It has been long believed that a fundamental feature of human motor behavior is as follows: "In freely chosen rate of activity, a rate is chosen that represents minimal energy expenditure per unit task" (115). Discussing only locomotion, Alexander (116) states that vertebrate animals adjust their patterns of locomotion so as to minimize power requirements at their chosen speeds. He also comments that horses and humans each choose the gait that requires the least oxygen consumption for their current speed. However, this time-honored concept regarding minimization of energy cost is not generalizable to all forms of locomotion, or indeed to all cycling activities (for example, bicycling and arm crank ergometry (117). In fact, Ganley et al. (118) and Herman et al. (110) reported that the principles of least energy expenditure, as outlined by Ralston and Alexander, are not confirmed by normal and ISCI subjects during treadmill and overground walking. Rather, these investigators reported that preferred rates of walking were dependent on minimizing carbohydrate metabolism and that increasing sense of effort at increasing gait velocities was directly associated with progressively enhanced carbohydrate metabolism. It has also been demonstrated that the increasing sense of effort at speeds above the preferred walking rate was robustly related to carbohydrate oxidation with a small relationship to the speed of walking.

Epidural Electrical Stimulation of the Spinal Cord: Rationale for Use

ISCI cases account for approximately 50% of all SCI cases. The ambulation ability of patients with ISCI is often permanently impaired. Therapeutic rehabilitation modalities that can enable the recovery of functional ambulation are urgently needed to offer these people greater independence and a higher quality of life. Recent research results in animals and human subjects suggest that the best therapeutic approach should make maximum use of the neural control system that remains functional. Furthermore, in order for the rehabilitation outcome to be truly "functional" in a quality-of-life sense, the therapeutic intervention should minimize the perception of effort and actual metabolic cost associated with the trained ambulation.

A review of the literature documents that the mammalian spinal cord can generate ambulation even when isolated from supraspinal structures. In addition, the spinal cord of animals and humans can adapt or learn in a manner that improves locomotor function when appropriate sensorimotor training paradigms are applied. When these strategies are augmented with electrical stimulation of peripheral nerves and/or the dorsal spinal cord, the benefits of treadmill training can be extended, enabling individuals with more profound motor deficits to achieve more benefits from treadmill training. Collectively, these research findings provide the basis for the application of a combined program of PWBT (augmented by peripheral FES as a rehabilitation adjunct, if needed) and ESCS to facilitate the recovery of *functional* ambulation in individuals with ISCI (110, 111). Although invasive, the use of ESCS is a practice that has been widely adopted for the treatment of chronic pain since it was first reported by Shealy et al. over 30 years ago (119). Epidural stimulation systems have evolved substantially in the past two decades, with current systems featuring multiple electrodes having multiple contacts (120). Such electrode configurations were developed in an effort to improve stimulus recruitment of dorsal columns in pain control applications (120) and have been demonstrated to improve long-term device reliability (121), reduce the need for surgical repositioning (120), and improve stimulation "coverage" when applied for chronic pain applications (122). Moreover, these multicontact, multichannel systems are appropriate for locomotion applications, where the programmable delivery of focused stimulation to an extended region of the posterior lumbar cord is desirable. Neuromodulation system implantation requires only minor surgery, and the risks associated with chronic implantation of current generation devices are minimal.

Subject Selection and Preparation for Trials: Potential for Recovery and Capacity for Compliance

The combination therapy of ESCS and PWBT as an approved protocol by the U.S. FDA provides a promising rehabilitation approach to promote functional ambulation in the ISCI patient, even in the presence of depressed lower extremity motor scores. When implementing this therapy, there are several issues important to its success. First is the prognosis of the patient population in which this therapy may be effective (i.e., selection of subjects to receive the therapy, using criteria including wheelchair dependence and/or impaired endurance that restricts

at-home and community ambulation). Second, attention needs to be paid to preparation of the subjects to acclimate them to the demanding physical activity during the therapy. Third, it is critical to determine the set of proper parameters for stimulation. Finally, an objective evaluation of the outcome and an adjustment of therapy strategy need to be performed.

In general, a candidate subject to receive coordinated ESCS+PWBT should meet the following criteria: he or she should be emotionally stable and compliant with doctor's instruction, have an injury level above T8 vertebra, have sufficient upper body strength to hold a walker for balance and body weight support during gait training, have a suitable range of motion and signs of voluntary muscle contraction, and be without medical issues specifically regarding pulmonary and cardiovascular dysfunction. Prior to locomotion training, each subject needs to go through tilt table–standing training to ensure that the cardiopulmonary system can tolerate the sustained standing posture required for PWBT. During this training, blood pressure, pulse, and respiration rates are monitored as the subject is tilted upright at 15-degree increments until vertical. Tilt table training is continued until the subject is able to maintain an upright position for 30 minutes without abnormal variations in cardiorespiratory measures.

Starting Gait Training with Coordinated Epidural Spinal Cord Stimulation

After demonstration of the ability to undergo a partial weight bearing training (PWBT) program, as outlined in the chapter by Edgerton in this section, ESCS electrodes are surgically implanted. Subjects are monitored postoperatively for at least 3 days as inpatients to optimize wound healing and return the patients to presurgery independence. Wound healing should be routinely monitored over an additional 2–3 weeks to ensure the stabilization of electrodes. Complete wound healing is required before subjects can resume PWBT. The subjects restart PWBT without stimulation until presurgical performance has been reached. At this stage, the subject will undergo PWBT, while the strength of stimulation, determined by measuring sensory and motor thresholds, is incrementally adjusted, with the frequency and pulse duration maintained at a constant level. When the quality of walking is deemed optimal, these parameters of stimulation will be continued in conjunction with treadmill training with and without weight support for a period of time until the subject attempts independent walking. If the amplitude of the current is insufficient, there will be a systematic assessment of the effects of frequency and pulse duration.

Enhancing PWBT with ESCS by Functional Electrical Stimulation

The gait training under the PWBT program is the same as described in the chapter by Edgerton. The therapist will use standard physical therapy techniques as needed to assist subjects in obtaining the best gait possible. This may include interventions using commonly employed techniques for enhancing the subject's walking ability with PWBT and/or with overground walking. One potential technique is called functional electrical stimulation (FES). FES devices provide transcutaneous stimulation of peripheral nerves (e.g., tibial and popliteal nerves) to promote a withdrawal reflex during the swing phase of the subject's walking cycle.

PWBT training continues at 5 days per week for 1–2 hours daily depending on the subject's physical condition, including endurance. The first adjustment of stimulation parameters for ESCS is to identify both the sensory and motor thresholds. The sensory threshold is the stimulation intensity at which stimulation-induced sensation is felt at the appropriate dermatome area. The motor threshold is the stimulation intensity at which muscles at the proper spinal segmental level are recruited by the stimulation. The stimulation intensity is the function of three parameters modulating the electrical pulse trains: amplitude (voltage), pulse width (duration), and number of pulses per second (frequency or rate). Among the three parameters, the frequency is best to be synchronized with the nerve firing rates in the spinal cord, and the most effective range is between 40 and 60 Hz; the pulse width is most effective at 1 ms; and the voltage is the final parameter adjustable to achieve the desired intensity. Notice that the pulse width is much higher than that used for chronic pain therapy and that the frequency is lower.

Chronologic Subject Evaluation: Neurophysiologic, Metabolic, Strength, Effort, and Gait Performance Measures

A battery of measurement and tests can be performed regularly to monitor physical and physiologic conditions and functional gait improvement. The evaluation can be either on a treadmill or of overground walking and can be performed at least once a month. All or selected subsets of the tests listed below can be adopted for objective evaluation, depending on the availability of the system and expected outcome of the rehabilitation.

1. Electrophysiology (EP)
   A. The Hoffman (H-reflex test): The tibial nerve in the popliteal fossa is stimulated once every 5 seconds by a current consisting of a pulse width of 0.1–0.2 ms and an intensity sufficient to induce a peak long-latency EMG response (H-reflex) in the gastrocnemius (medial) muscle as well as a short latency (direct) motor (M) response. Peak H reflex activity represents excitability of the motoneuron pool and can be quantified by its amplitude, relationship with M response, and period of inhibition by stimuli 1–5 seconds apart. These tests can be conducted with/without ESCS to examine the effect of ESCS on reflex pathways.
   B. Somatosensory evoked potentials (SEP): This consists of stimulation of the common peroneal nerve of each of the lower limbs and recording averaged EEG activity via scalp electrodes placed according to the international 10/20 EEG system, covering the left and right hemispheres. The stimuli are of short duration (e.g., 0.1–0.2 ms) and low frequency (e.g., 4–6 Hz). Current intensity is set to induce a minimal motor contraction. Averaged EEG responses, "N" and "P" for negative and positive, should yield short- and middle-latency (recording window of 300 ms) reactions, suggesting intact pathways to the somatosensory cortex. Moreover, we posit that EEG responses recorded during swing or stance phases of the walking cycle will reveal somatosensory responses only to the stance phase, implying gating of afferent pathways during the swing phase.

2. Whole body energetics and metabolism (fuel consumption): This is measured by a conventional technique of indirect calorimetry. Expired air is collected in meteorologic balloons for a timed period, analyzed for O_2 and CO_2 concentrations with gas analyzers (Parvo, Salt Lake City, Utah), and measured for volume with a gas meter. Alternatively, gas analysis may be carried out using a portable calorimeter (Cosmed System, see below). Expired air is continuously obtained after 2 minutes of walking (treadmill or overground) for fixed durations or until fatigue. The research staff will not allow the subject to go above his/her age-adjusted peak pulse rate. If the subject's pulse rate goes above the peak pulse rate, then he/she will rest until the baseline pulse rates are obtained. During the walk, the subject's "sense of effort" is determined using the "modified" Borg scale. The results indicate how effectively electrical stimulation reduces energy requirements, sense of effort, and fuel oxidation of skeletal muscle. Fingertip blood samples are also collected prior to, during, and after walking for the analysis of blood glucose and lactate concentrations. These blood samples are taken a maximum of four times each day for at least 2 days per month. These tests could be performed one to four times for this stage.

3. Sense of effort: Walking episodes can be related to the subject's perception of effort (work) according to the validated scale (Borg) of 1–10. Pulse rates can be correlated with perceptual values. This parameter is most useful when applied daily during overground evaluation. Pulse rates are obtained before, during, and after treadmill walking. Blood pressure and respiratory rates are obtained before and after walking on the treadmill.

4. Tests of maximum voluntary contraction (MVC): This procedure involves the measurement of muscle forces when a subject is voluntarily contracting one or more muscle groups with maximum effort while the limb is held in a constant position. The subject can be in either a sitting or supine position. The subject is instructed to extend or flex the knee with maximal force for 10 seconds while electromyographic signals (EMG) are recorded. The objective of this measurement is to quantify maximal isometric force at midrange of motion as an impairment measure.

5. Digital video recordings: These provide gross assessment for the research staff but are insufficient to obtain accurate spatiotemporal data at baseline and transition points of weight support and treadmill rates. For overground analysis, the Gaitmat™ system can be utilized to provide this data. This linear walkway provides a sensitive assessment of ambulation rate, double support time, foot alignment at ground contact, and relative weight distribution. The data reflect bilateral swing time, stance time, and stride time. These quantitative data can be used in part to specify intra- and interlimb coordination.

6. Gait performance assessment: A more comprehensive assessment of functional performance and physical improvement can be regularly performed at a well-equipped gait lab. This evaluation should be performed at the onset of PWBT training and at regular time intervals to provide a quantitative analysis of gait performance for improvement. Metabolism and sense of effort will be measured, in addition to the following:
   A. Bilateral surface EMG activity of the *vastus medialis, rectus femoris, biceps femoris long head, biceps femoris short head, gastrocnemius and soleus*, and *tibialis anterior*.
   B. Gait kinematics (a minimum of two markers per rigid body segment to quantify the motion of the feet, shanks, thighs, pelvis, and torso bilaterally).
   C. Ground reaction force/plantar pressure.
   D. Vertical support force provided by the LiteGait apparatus (treadmill) or exerted on an instrumented walker (overground).

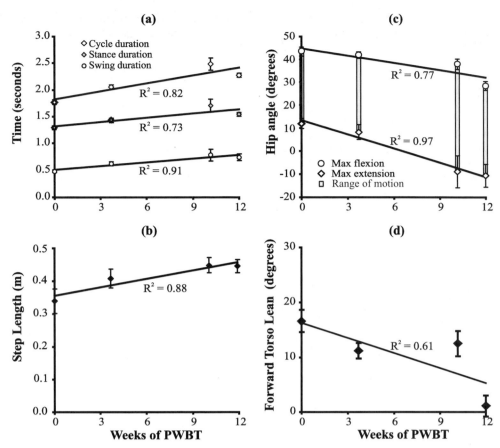

Figure 73.2   Progressive improvement in gait measures following 3 months of PWBT: (**a**) step cycle duration, (**b**) step length, (**c**) range of motion for the hip joint, and (**d**) torso upwardness (reduced forward leaning). The horizontal axis is weeks.

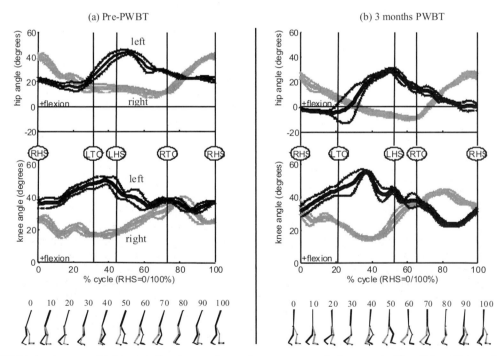

Figure 73.3   PWBT also improved joint coordination and stepping symmetry during treadmill walking. Comparing the joint angles shown on the left (before training) to those shown on the right (after 3 months of training), the range of motion for both hip and knee improved and became much more symmetrical. As the stepping became more symmetrical and step length increased, the patient could follow the speed of the treadmill, and this led to regular patterns of joint motion, most notably in the posture during treadmill stepping and joint coordination.

E. H-reflex.

7. Maximum distance a subject can walk with the assistance of a walker: Overground walking assessments can be performed in subjects who are able to ambulate over a minimum of 15 meters with a sense of effort below 7 (no ESCS) on the modified Borg scale. The use of a walker is to provide balance support and alleviate the concern of falling. The ultimate objective of locomotion rehabilitation is for persons with ISCI to recover functional ambulation over ground. This assessment is to examine the extent of recovery of this ability. The subject will be instructed to walk, with the assistance of a walker for balance support and prevention of falling, as long and as far as he/she can tolerate the activity. The force inserted on the walker by the subject during overground walking can be recorded by embedded load cells, if available.

RESULTS OF POSITIVE IMPACT OF ESCS ON RECOVERY OF FUNCTIONAL WALKING

A summary of reported results is given below to illustrate the impact of coordinated therapy of ESCS and PWBT for synergistic improvement of functional ambulation in people with ISCI. These results are obtained from two men in their mid forties with chronic incomplete spinal cord injury who use wheelchairs for community transport. One patient had a low-level ASIA C lesion at C5–C6 with lower extremity motor scores (LEMS) of 15/50

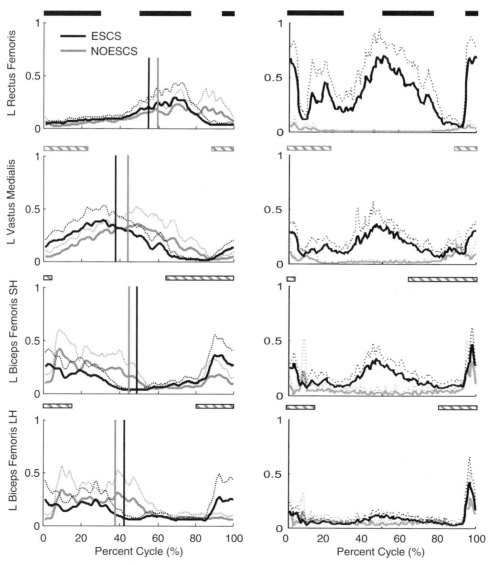

Figure 73.4 Alterations in EMG activity with application of ESCS in S1 (**left panel**) and S2 (**right panel**). Comparisons of amplitude and time-normalized data are derived from same-day treadmill walking with ESCS (**black traces**) and without (**gray**). Dark solid lines denote the average, and dotted lines indicate the standard deviation. ESCS produced statistically significant changes in EMG timing in S1 (black and gray vertical lines denote the mean centroid time for each condition), and robust alterations in EMG timing and amplitude in S2. Overbars denote periods of typical activity in able-bodied individuals.

(subject one, S1), and the other patient was more pronounced in his LEMS of 10/50 caused by injury at T8 (subject two, S2).

The protocol called for (1) PWBT applied alone (S1) or with the assistance of reflex FES (S2) until the participant reached a plateau in treadmill walking performance, followed by (2) surgical implantation of an epidural spinal cord stimulation system, (3) PWBT retraining to presurgical performance levels (with FES in S2), (4) coordinated training with PWBT and ESCS (and FES in S2), and (5) overground training with ESCS (and FES in S2).

A short communication describing results from S1 was reported by Herman et al. (110). The main findings from this report are (1) that PWBT improved physical strength and condition; (2) that PWBT improved walking kinematics on a treadmill but not overground; (3) that ESCS induced additional improvement in gait kinematics beyond PWBT; and (4) that ESCS improved endurance significantly during overground ambulation. Additional details regarding acute and chronic changes in kinematics, muscle activity, speed, and endurance are described in Carhart et al. (111). Furthermore, results of indirect calorimetry are emphasized in Herman et al. (110) and Carhart et al. (123). Some important findings are highlighted above and below.

PWBT Improves Locomotion in Low-Level Asia C Participants, but Utility of the Trained Gait is Limited

As reported by other investigations involving PWBT (23, 25, 27, 69, 124), both patients enjoyed significant improvement in their ability to generate coordinated stepping movements with tread-mill training alone (Figures 73.2 and 73.3). However, following several months (4 months in S1, 3.5 months in S2) of PWBT, the subjects still required extensive body weight support. In addition, neither participant was able to perform independent treadmill walking with body weight support at speeds greater than 0.68 m/s. Finally, overground ambulation in these "low-level" ASIA C subjects was still hampered by slow speeds, near maximal effort, and rapid exhaustion while traversing short distances. Thus, the appearance of a coordinated, rhythmic gait pattern induced by PWBT remained nonfunctional as the attempt to transfer the learned movements to efficient and functional overground walking failed.

ESCS Facilitates PWBT

Evaluation of muscle activity during treadmill walking revealed that ESCS increased muscle recruitment and improved the synergy behavior of muscles during walking. This was manifested as statistically significant shifts in EMG timing in S1, and a change in pattern and increase in the amplitude of EMG activity in S2 (Figure 73.4). Accompanying changes in joint kinematics were subtle in S1, but more pronounced in S2 (Figure 73.5). Both participants enjoyed significant improvements in step execution.

When ESCS was applied in conjunction with PWBT, the electrical current appeared to provide the modulation/amplification of the neural circuits responsible for locomotion rhythm generation. More importantly, the addition of ESCS permitted treadmill training intensities to be increased. In both participants, this

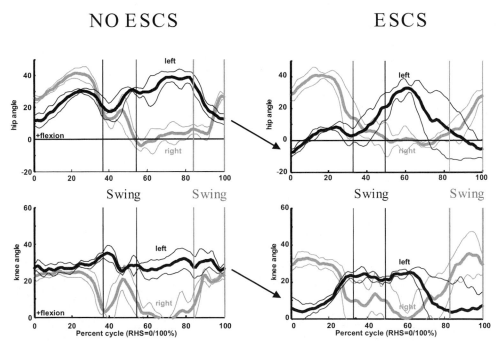

Figure 73.5   Comparison of kinematics during walking over ground with and without ESCS in S2. Gray curves denote joint angles on the right side, whereas black curves denote those of the left. Solid lines show the mean and dotted lines for the standard deviation. With ESCS on, kinematics was substantially improved in S2, and he was able to generate knee extension bilaterally. This was ascribed to enhanced extensor activity in the more paretic left limb during stance phase. Hip motion was also improved, and both limbs exhibited an alternating pattern of flexion and extension more prominently.

(a)

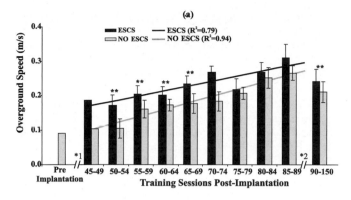

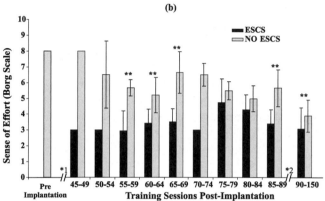

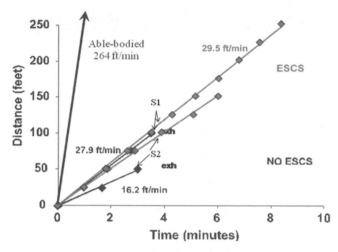

Figure 73.7 After 4 months of ESCS-assisted walking training, both subjects demonstrated significant improvement in walking ability, but it is the effect of ESCS on endurance and speed that propelled the eventual functional walking overground.

Figure 73.6 Chronological performance measures for overground walking in an ISCI person during coordinated PWBT and ESCS therapy. There is the immediate effect of turning on ESCS to improve endurance, speed, and sense of effort on a daily basis, as seen by the big difference between black (ESCS) and gray bars on individual testing days. There is also significant improvement chronologically on performance. Please note that the test is on different training sessions (one session a day) to remove the fatigue effect.

was manifested as an ability to train on the treadmill at greater intensities (e.g., at 0.9 m/s versus 0.65 m/s with PWBT alone in S1), with a lower level of perceived exertion, and for longer durations. In this sense, it appears that ESCS facilitated PWBT and enhanced the training effects provided by sensorimotor therapy.

ESCS Enhances the Effects of PWBT and Provides Acute Improvements in Ambulation

With continued PWBT and ESCS, both participants were able to transfer the learned coordinated movements into functional overground ambulation. The application of ESCS significantly improved speed, reduced sense of effort, and enhanced endurance during overground walking, as demonstrated by longitudinal tracking of these performance measures of S1 (Figure 73.6).

As shown, ESCS produced the greatest changes in speed and sense effort early in the overground training process, yet produced the greatest enhancement in endurance after extensive treadmill and overground training. A similar effect is observed for S2; Figure 73.6 summarizes the chronic and instant effect of ESCS on endurance and speed over the period of therapy.

Although S2 obtained modest maximum speeds and endurance with ESCS, his increase in performance with ESCS were much more dramatic. That is, ESCS produced a doubling of maximum overground walking speed and a fivefold increase in maximum endurance (Figure 73.7). This was accompanied by a significant reduction in the patient's reliance on an instrumented walker for vertical support.

ESCS Alters the Metabolic Response and Substrate Oxidation

Among the most intriguing findings in our previous work are the apparent alterations in metabolic fuel consumption produced by the acute application of ESCS. Following the transition to overground walking, we evaluated the metabolic responses of both participants while walking overground using a front-wheeled walker. Results for S1 are shown in Figure 73.8 and demonstrate that ESCS reduced the energy cost of walking in this subject by roughly 20% to 30%. Moreover, analysis of CO_2 production implied (1) a large increase in fat oxidation with ESCS, and/or (2) less accumulation of blood lactate. Both findings imply that ESCS reduced dependence of the exercising muscle on glycolysis, and hence accounted for the marked improvement in muscle endurance observed in the ESCS condition. Similar, yet more profound, differences in oxygen cost of transport and metabolic fuel consumption were exhibited by S2. For example, experiments comparing overground walking performance between the ESCS and NOESCS conditions showed that the activation of the epidural implant reduced the oxygen cost of walking in S2 by a remarkable 57%. This was accompanied by a fivefold increase in maximal walking distance, a doubling of average walking speed, and a statistically significant reduction in reliance on a wheeled walker for body weight support (as shown in Figure 73.9). Furthermore, ESCS reduced respiratory exchange ratio to a value reflecting a reliance on fat oxidation roughly similar to that of able-bodied subjects walking at preferred speed.

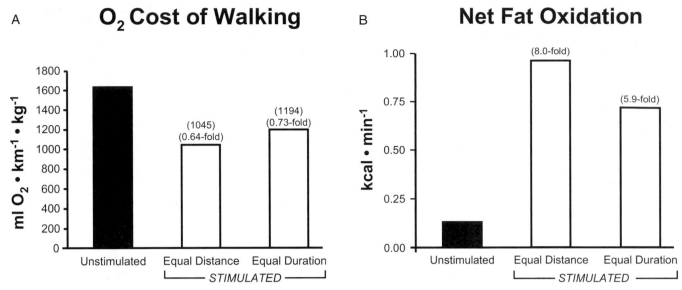

A **O₂ Cost of Walking**

B **Net Fat Oxidation**

Figure 73.8   Changes in the oxygen cost of walking (**A**) and metabolic fuel consumption (**B**) indicate that ESCS induces improvement in overground walking by improving walking energy efficiency and stimulating more usage of fat, rather than carbohydrates, as the source of fuel. The fat oxidation process will not be perceived and does not contribute to the sense of effort.

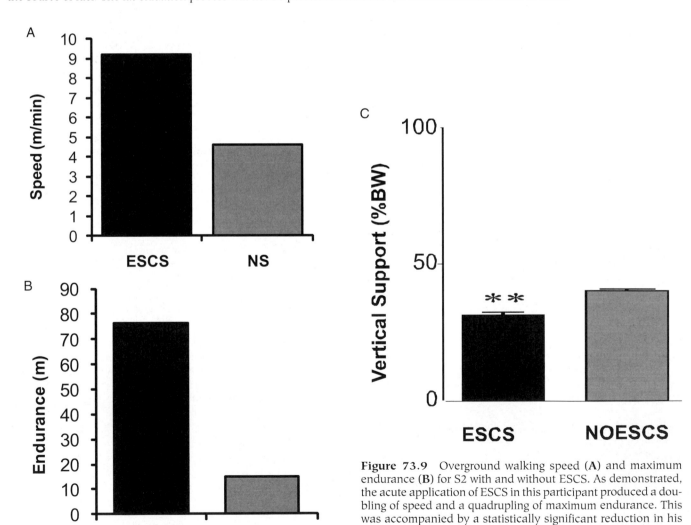

Figure 73.9   Overground walking speed (**A**) and maximum endurance (**B**) for S2 with and without ESCS. As demonstrated, the acute application of ESCS in this participant produced a doubling of speed and a quadrupling of maximum endurance. This was accompanied by a statistically significant reduction in his reliance on an instrumented walker for vertical body weight support, reflected by the gait cycle average vertical support force (**C**).

Table 73.1 Endurance,[a] O₂ Cost of Transport,[b] and the Respiratory Exchange Ratio (RER)[c] during Overground Walking in S2 with Different Approaches

CONDITION	ENDURANCE (m)	O₂ COST (ml/kg/km)	RER (VCO₂/VO₂)
NS	15.2	3276	0.902
FES	60.9	1814	0.871
ESCS	76.2	1400	0.783
FES + ESCS	68.6	1299	0.836

[a]Distance to volitional exhaustion.
[b]Mass specific O_2 consumption rate divided by average speed.
[c]An RER of 0.70 suggests complete reliance on fat as the oxidative fuel, and an RER of 1.00 suggests that carbohydrate is the exclusive fuel.

The relative performance enhancements offered by FES, ESCS, and a combination of these approaches in S2 were also evaluated. Some results of this work are summarized in Table 73.1, which demonstrates that stimulation greatly improved endurance and oxygen cost of walking in this participant. Interestingly, ESCS yielded a lower O_2 cost of walking than FES and was associated with a much greater reliance on fat oxidation. Superimposing FES and ESCS yielded the greatest improvement in walking speed, the lowest O_2 cost of transport, and the lowest reliance on the walker for support, but apparently at the expense of greater carbohydrate dependence and a slight decrease in endurance.

SUMMARY

As described in this chapter, epidural spinal cord stimulation can be an effective therapy to improve functional walking in the incomplete spinal cord–injured population when used properly with PWBT. The stimulating electrodes should deliver the current to cover the cord segments between lower thoracic and upper lumbar regions. The most effective stimulation parameters are long pulse duration (above 0.5 ms), low to mid-range frequency (20–60 pulses per second), and intensity level between sensory and motor thresholds. We posited that a number of mechanisms may be contemplated to explain our results. These include (1) that ESCS facilitates locomotion recovery by augmenting use-dependent plasticity created by PWBT, and (2) that ESCS elicits a greater activation of an oxidative motor unit pool, thereby reducing the subject's sense of effort, energy cost of walking, and dependence on carbohydrate oxidation of skeletal muscle.

References

1. Raineteau O, Schwab ME. Plasticity of motor systems after incomplete spinal cord injury. *Nat Rev Neurosci* 2001; 2(4):263–273.
2. Wolpaw JR, Tennissen AM. Activity-dependent spinal cord plasticity in health and disease. *Annu Rev Neurosci* 2001; 24:807–843.
3. Barbeau H, Rossignol S. Recovery of locomotion after chronic spinalization in the adult cat. *Brain Res* 1987; 412(1):84–95.
4. Lovely RG, Gregor RJ, et al. Weight-bearing hindlimb stepping in treadmill-exercised adult spinal cats. *Brain Res* 1990; 514:206–218.
5. Grillner S, Wallén P. Central pattern generators for locomotion, with special reference to vertebrates. *Annu Rev Neurosci* 1985; 8:233–261.
6. Barbeau H, Rossignol S. Enhancement of locomotor recovery following spinal cord injury. *Curr Opin Neurol* 1994; 7(6):517–524.
7. Cazalets JR, Borde M, et al. Localization and organization of the central pattern generator for hindlimb locomotion in the newborn rat. *J Neurosci* 1995; 15:4943–4951.
8. Kjaerulff O, Kiehn O. Distribution of networks generating and coordinating locomotor activity in the neonatal rat spinal cord in vitro: a lesion study. *J Neurosci* 1996; 16:5777–5794.
9. Grillner S, Parker D, et al. Vertebrate locomotion: a lamprey perspective. *Ann N Y Acad Sci* 1998; 860:1–18.
10. Wang H, Jung R. Variability analyses suggest that supraspino-spinal interactions provide dynamic stability in motor control. *Brain Res* 2002; 930(1–2):83–100.
11. Rossignol S. Locomotion and its recovery after spinal injury. *Curr Opin Neurobiol* 2000; 10(6):708–716.
12. Rossignol S, Barbeau H. Pharmacology of locomotion: an account of studies in spinal cats and spinal cord injured subjects. *J Am Paraplegia Soc* 1993; 16(4):190–196.
13. Kralj A, Bajd T. *Functional Electrical Stimulation: Standing and Walking after Spinal Cord Injury.* Boca Raton, FL: CRC Press, 1989.
14. Bajd T, Kralj A, et al. Use of functional electrical stimulation in the lower extremities of incomplete spinal cord injured patients. *Artif Organs* 1999; 23(5):403–409.
15. Calancie B, Needham-Shropshire B, et al. Involuntary stepping after chronic spinal cord injury: evidence for a central rhythm generator for locomotion in man. *Brain* 1994; 117(5):1143–1159.
16. Iwahara T, Atsuta Y, et al. Locomotion induced by spinal cord stimulation in the neonate rat in vitro. *Somatosens Mot Res* 1991; 8(3):281–287.
17. Iwahara T, Atsuta Y, et al. Spinal cord stimulation-induced locomotion in the adult cat. *Brain Res Bull* 1992; 28(1):99–105.
18. Bussel B, Roby-Brami A, et al. Evidence for a spinal stepping generator in man: electrophysiological study. *Acta Neurobiol Exp (Warsz)* 1996; 56(1):465–468.
19. Dimitrijevic MR, Gerasimenko Y, et al. Evidence for a spinal central pattern generator in humans. *Ann N Y Acad Sci* 1998; 860:360–376.
20. Pinter MM, Dimitrijevic MR. Gait after spinal cord injury and the central pattern generator for locomotion. *Spinal Cord* 1999; 37(8):531–537.
21. Pinter MM, Gerstenbrand F, et al. Epidural electrical stimulation of posterior structures of the human lumbosacral cord: 3. Control of spasticity. *Spinal Cord* 2000; 38(9):524–531.
22. Dobkin B, Edgerton V, et al. Training induces rhythmic locomotor EMG patterns in subjects with complete SCI. *Neurology* 1992; 42(Suppl 3): 207–208.
23. Wernig A, Muller S. Laufband locomotion with body weight support improved walking in persons with severe spinal cord injuries. *Paraplegia* 1992; 30(4):229–238.
24. Hodgson JA, Roy RR, et al. Can the mammalian lumbar spinal cord learn a motor task? *Med Sci Sports Exerc* 1994; 26(12):1491–1497.
25. Dietz V, Colombo G, et al. Locomotor capacity of spinal cord in paraplegic patients. *Ann Neurol* 1995; 37:574–582.
26. Dobkin BH, Harkema S, et al. Modulation of locomotor-like EMG activity in subjects with complete and incomplete spinal cord injury. *J Neurol Rehabil* 1995; 9(4):183–190.
27. Wernig A, Muller S, et al. Laufband therapy based on "rules of spinal locomotion" is effective in spinal cord injured persons. *Eur J Neurosci* 1995; 7(4):823–829.
28. Tuszynski M, Edgerton V, et al. Recovery of locomotion after experimental spinal cord injury: axonal regeneration or modulation of intrinsic spinal cord walking circuitry? *J Spinal Cord Med* 1999; 22(2):143.
29. Dobkin BH. Spinal and supraspinal plasticity after incomplete spinal cord injury: correlation magnetic resonance imaging and engaged locomotor networks. *Prog Brain Res* 2000; 128:99–111.
30. Illis LS. Is there a central pattern generator in man? *Paraplegia* 1995; 33(5):239–240.
31. Rosenfeld JE, Halter JA, Dimitrijevic MR. Evidence of a pattern generator in paralyzed subjects with spinal cord injury during spinal cord stimulation. *Abstr Soc Neurosci* 1995; 21:688.
32. Duysens J, Van de Crommert HW. Neural control of locomotion: the central pattern generator from cats to humans. *Gait Posture* 1998; 7(2):131–141.
33. Van de Crommert HW, Mulder T, et al. Neural control of locomotion: sensory control of the central pattern generator and its relation to treadmill training. *Gait Posture* 1998; 7(3):251–263.
34. Dietz V, Nakazawa K, et al. Level of spinal cord lesion determines locomotor activity in spinal man. *Exp Brain Res* 1999; 128(3):405–409.

35. Dietz V, Colombo G, et al. Locomotor activity in spinal man. *Lancet* 1994; 344:1260–1263.

36. de Leon RD, Hodgson JA, et al. Locomotor capacity attributable to step training versus spontaneous recovery after spinalization in adult cats. *J Neurophysiol* 1998; 79:1329–1340.

37. Barbeau H, Ladouceur, et al. Walking after spinal cord injury: evaluation, treatment, and functional recovery. *Arch Phys Med Rehabil* 1999; 80(2):225–235.

38. Barbeau H, McCrea DA, et al. Tapping into spinal circuits to restore motor function. *Brain Res Brain Res Rev* 1999; 30(1):27–51.

39. de Leon RD, Hodgson JA, et al. Retention of hindlimb stepping ability in adult spinal cats after the cessation of step training. *J Neurophysiol* 1999; 81(1):85–94.

40. Field-Fote EC. Combined use of body weight support, functional electric stimulation, and treadmill training to improve walking ability in individuals with chronic incomplete spinal cord injury. *Arch Phys Med Rehabil* 2001; 82(6):818–824.

41. Basso DM, Beattie MS, et al. A sensitive and reliable locomotor rating scale for open field testing in rats. *J Neurotrauma* 1995; 12:1–21.

42. Feraboli-Lohnherr D, Orsal D, et al. Recovery of locomotor activity in the adult chronic spinal rat after sublesional transplantation of embryonic nervous cells: specific role of serotonergic neurons. *Exp Brain Res* 1997; 113:443–454.

43. Bernstein DS, Jung R. Perturbation analysis of a model of brain and central pattern generator in the lamprey. Proceedings of the 17th Southern Biomed. Eng. Conference, San Antonio, Texas, 1998.

44. Prochazka A. Sensorimotor gain control: a basic strategy of motor systems? *Prog Neurobiol* 1989; 33:287–307.

45. Capaday C, Stein RB. Amplitude modulation of the soleus H-reflex in the human during walking and standing. *J Neurosci* 1986; 6(5): 1308–1313.

46. Capaday C, Stein RB. Difference in the amplitude of the human soleus H-reflex during walking and running. *J. Physiol* 1987; 392:513–522.

47. Sillar KT, Roberts A. A neuronal mechanism for sensory gating during locomotion in a vertebrate. *Nature* 1988; 331:262–265.

48. Stein RB, Capaday C. The modulation of human reflexes during functional motor tasks. *Trends Neurosci* 1988; 11:328–332.

49. Duenas SH, Loeb GE, et al. Monosynaptic and dorsal root reflexes during locomotion in normal and thalamic cats. *J Neurophysiol* 1990; 63(6):1467–1476.

50. Edamura M, Yang JF, et al. Factors that determine the magnitude and time course of human H-reflexes in locomotion. *J Neurosci* 1991; 11(2):420–427.

51. Koerber JR, Mendell LM. Modulation of synaptic transmission as Ia-afferent connections on motorneurons during high-frequency afferent stimulation: dependence on motor task. *J Neurophysiol* 1991; 65(6):1313–1320.

52. Murphy PR, Martin HA. Fusimotor discharge patterns during rhythmic movements. *Trends Neurosci* 1993; 16(7):273–278.

53. Pearson KG, Collins DF. Reversal of the influence of group 1b afferents from plantaris on activity in medial gastrocnemius muscle during locomotor activity. *J Neurophysiol* 1993; 70:1009–1017.

54. Hiebert GW, Whelan PG, et al. Contribution of hind limb flexor muscle afferents to the timing of phase transitions in the cat step cycle. *J Neurophysiol* 1996; 75(3):1126–1137.

55. McCrea DA. Neuronal basis of afferent-evoked enhancement of locomotor activity. *Ann N Y Acad Sci* 1998; 860:216–225.

56. Dietz B, Quintern J, et al. Afferent control of human stance and gait: evidence for blocking of group I afferents during gait. *Exp Brain Res* 1985; 61:153–163.

57. Forssberg H, Grillner S, et al. Phase dependent reflex reversal during walking in chronic spinal cats. *Brain Res* 1975; 85:103–107.

58. Yang JF, Stein R. Phase-dependent reflex reversal in human leg muscles during walking. *J of Neurophysiol* 1990; 63(5):1109–1117.

59. Hasan Z, Stuart DG. Animal solutions to problems of movement control: the role of proprioceptors. *Annu Rev Neurosci* 1988; 11:199–223.

60. McCrea DA, Shefchyk SJ, et al. Disynaptic group1 excitation of synergist ankle extensor motorneurons during fictive locomotion. *J Physiol* 1995; 487:527–539.

61. Shurrager PS, Culler E. Conditioning in the spinal dog. *J Exp Psychol* 1940; 26:133–149.

62. Durkovic R. The spinal cord: a simplified system for the study of neural mechanisms of mammalian learning and memory. In: Goldberger ME, Gorio A, Murray M, eds. *Development and Plasticity of the Mammalian Spinal Cord.* New York: Springer-Verlag, 1986:183–192.

63. Wolpaw JR, Tennissen AM. Activity-dependent spinal cord plasticity in health and disease. *Annu Rev Neurosci* 2001; 24:807–843.

64. Dietz V, Muller R, et al. Locomotor activity in spinal man: significance of afferent input from joint and load receptors. *Brain* 2002; 125(Pt 12):2626–2634.

65. Edgerton V, Roy RR, et al. Potential of adult mammalian lumbrosacral spinal cord to execute and acquire improved locomotion in the absence of supraspinal input. *J Neurotrama* 1992; 9:S119–S128.

66. Rossignol S, Chau C, et al. Locomotor capacities after complete and partial lesions of the spinal cord. *Acta Neurobiol Exp (Warsz)* 1996; 56(1):449–463.

67. Barbeau H, Wainberg M, et al. Description and application of a system for locomotor rehabilitation. *Med Biol Eng Comput* 1987; 25(3):341–344.

68. Visintin M, Barbeau H. The effects of body weight support on the locomotor pattern of spastic paretic patients. *Can J Neurol Sci* 1989; 16(3):315–325.

69. Dietz V, Wirz M, et al. Locomotion in patients with spinal cord injuries. *Phys Ther* 1997; 77(5):508–516.

70. Wernig A, Nanassy A, et al. Maintenance of locomotor abilities following Laufband (treadmill) therapy in para- and tetraplegic persons: follow-up studies. *Spinal Cord* 1998; 36(11):744–749.

71. Colombo G, Wirz M, et al. Driven gait orthosis for improvement of locomotor training in paraplegic patients. *Spinal Cord* 2001; 39(5):252–255.

72. Barbeau H, Norman K, et al. Does neurorehabilitation play a role in the recovery of walking in neurological populations? *Ann N Y Acad Sci* 1998; 860:377–392.

73. Fung J, Barbeau H. Effects of conditioning cutaneomuscular stimulation on the soleus H-reflex in normal and spastic paretic subjects during walking and standing. *J Neurophysiol* 1994; 72(5):2090–2104.

74. Wieler M, Stein RB, et al. Multicenter evaluation of electrical stimulation systems for walking. *Arch Phys Med Rehabil* 1999; 80(5):495–500.

75. Ladouceur M, Barbeau H. Functional electrical stimulation-assisted walking for persons with incomplete spinal injuries: longitudinal changes in maximal overground walking speed. *Scand J Rehabil Med* 2000; 32(1):28–36.

76. Mirbagheri MM, Ladouceur M, et al. The effects of long-term FES-assisted walking on intrinsic and reflex dynamic stiffness in spastic spinal-cord-injured subjects. *IEEE Trans Neural Syst Rehabil Eng* 2002; 10(4):280–289.

77. Liberson WT, Holmquest HJ, et al. Functional electrotherapy: stimulation of peroneal nerve synchronized with the swing phase of the gait of hemiplegic patients. *Arch Phys Med Rehabil* 1961; 42:101–105.

78. Bajd T, Kralj A, et al. The use of a four-channel electrical stimulator as an ambulatory aid for paraplegic patients. *Phys Ther* 1983; 63(7):1116–1120.

79. Barbeau H, Ladouceur M, et al. The effect of locomotor training combined with functional electrical stimulation in chronic spinal cord injured subjects: walking and reflex studies. *Brain Res Brain Res Rev* 2002; 40(1–3):274–291.

80. Bajd T, Andrews BJ, et al. Restoration of walking in patients with incomplete spinal cord injuries by use of surface electrical stimulation: preliminary results. *Prosthet Orthot Int* (1985). 9:109–111.

81. Stein RB, Gordon T, et al. Optimal stimulation of paralyzed muscle after human spinal cord injury. *J Appl Physiol* 1992; 72(4):1393–1400.

82. Chizeck HJ, Kobetic, et al. Control of functional neuromuscular stimulation systems for standing and locomotion in paraplegics. *Proc IEEE* 1988; 76(9):1155–1165.

83. Yarkony GM, Roth EJ, et al. Neuromuscular stimulation in spinal cord injury: I: restoration of motor functional movements of the extremities. *Arch Phys Med Rehabil* 1992; 73:78–86.

84. Peckham PH, Keith MW. Motor prostheses for restoration of upper extremity function. In: Stein RB, Peckham PH, Popovic DB, eds. *Neural Prostheses: Replacing Motor Function after Disease or Disability.* New York: Oxford University Press, 1992:162–190.

85. Abbas JJ, Chizeck HJ. A neural network controller for functional neuromuscular stimulation systems. Proceedings of the 13th IEEE/EMBS Conference, Orlando, Florida, 1991.

86. Marsolais EB, Kobetic R. Development of a practical electrical stimulation system for restoring gait in the paralyzed patient. *Clin Orthop Rel Res* 1988; 233:64–74.

87. Jacobs M-CL, Jacques WM, Kapma JA, et al. Effect of chronic smoking on endothelium-dependent vascular relaxation in humans. *Clin Sci* 1993; 85:51–55.

88. Graupe D, Kohn KH. *Functional Electrical Stimulation for Ambulation by Paraplegics*. Melbourne, FL: Krieger Publishing Co., 1994.

89. Solomonow M. Biomechanics and physiology of a practical functional neuromuscular stimulation walking orthosis for paraplegics. In: Stein RB, Popovic DP, eds. *Neural Prostheses: Replacing Motor Function after Disease or Disability*. New York: Oxford University Press, 1992:202–232.

90. Stein RB, Belanger M, et al. Electrical systems for improving locomotion after incomplete spinal cord injury: an assessment. *Arch Phys Med Rehabil* 1993; 74:954–959.

91. Abbas J, Chizeck HJ. Neural network control of functional neuromuscular stimulation systems: computer simulation studies. *IEEE Trans Biomed Eng* 1995; 42(11):1117–1127.

92. Abbas J, Triolo RJ. Experimental evaluation of an adaptive feedforward controller for use in functional neuromuscular stimulation systems. IEEE/EMBS Conference Proceedings 1993; 15:1326–1327.

93. Abbas J, Triolo RJ. Experimental evaluation of an adaptive feedforward controller for use in functional neuromuscular stimulation systems. *IEEE Trans Rehab Eng* 1997; 5(1):12–22.

94. Riess JA, Abbas JJ. Evaluation of adaptive neural network controller in cyclic movement using functional neuromuscular stimulation. Proceedings of RESNA, Minneapolis, Minnesota, 1998.

95. Ou J, Riess JA, et al. Adaptive control of cyclic movements in a multisegment system. IFESS, Cleveland, Ohio, 2001.

96. Dutta A, Kobetic R, et al. Ambulation after incomplete spinal cord injury with emg-triggered functional electrical stimulation. *IEEE T Biomed Eng* 2008; 55(2):791–794.

97. Borg G, Hassmen P, et al. Perceived exertion related to heart rate and blood lactate during arm and leg exercise. *Eur J Appl Physiol Occup Physiol* 1987; 56(6):679–685.

98. Cook AW, Weinstein SP. Chronic dorsal column stimulation in multiple sclerosis: preliminary report. *N Y State J Med* 1973; 73(24):2868–2872.

99. Mushahwar V, Horch K. Muscle recruitment through electrical stimulation of the lumbo-sacral spinal cord. *IEEE Trans Rehabil Eng* 2000; 8(1):22–29.

100. Davis R, Gray E, et al. Beneficial augmentation following dorsal column stimulation in some neurological diseases. *Appl Neurophysiol* 1981; 44(2):37–49.

101. Tallis RC, Illis LS, et al. The quantitative assessment of the influence of spinal cord stimulation on motor function in patients with multiple sclerosis. *Int Rehabil Med* 1983; 5(1):10–16.

102. Davis R, Emmonds SE. Spinal cord stimulation for multiple sclerosis: quantifiable benefits. *Stereotact Funct Neurosurg* 1992; 58(1–4):52–58.

103. Mushahwar V, Collins D, et al. Spinal cord microstimulation generates functional limb movements in chronically implanted cats. *Exp Neurol* 2000; 163(2):422–429.

104. Mushahwar V, Gillard DN, et al. Spinal cord microstimulation generates locomotor and target directed movements. *Abstr Soc Neurosci* 2000; 26(260.9):696.

105. Holsheimer J, Struijk JJ, et al. Contact combinations in epidural spinal cord stimulation: a comparison by computer modeling. *Stereotact Funct Neurosurg* 1991; 56(4):220–233.

106. Barolat G, Massaro F, et al. Mapping of sensory responses to epidural stimulation of the intraspinal neural structures in man. *J Neurosurg* 1993; 78(2):233–239.

107. He J, Barolat G, et al. Perception threshold and electrode position for spinal cord stimulation. *Pain* 1994; 59(1):55–63.

108. Willis W, He J, et al. Epidural spinal cord stimulation (ESCS) improves physical work capacity and reduces CO_2 production in chronic spinal cord injured during walking. *Abstr Soc Neurosci* 2001; 8:935.

109. Carhart MR, He J, et al. Epidural spinal cord stimulation and partial weightbearing therapy for the restoration of locomotion. Proceedings of the 2nd Joint Conference of the IEEE Engineering in Medicine and Biology Society and the Biomedical Engineering Society, Houston, Texas, 2002.

110. Herman R, He J, et al. Spinal cord stimulation facilitates functional walking in a chronic, incomplete spinal cord injured. *Spinal Cord* 2002; 40(2):65–68.

111. Carhart M, He J, et al. Epidural spinal cord stimulation and partial weight bearing therapy: a novel approach to rehabilitation of spinal cord injured. *IEEE Transaction on Neural Systems and Rehabilitation Engineering* 2004; 12(1):32–42.

112. Willis W, Carhart M, et al. Influence of two electrical stimulation modes on walking performance in a spinal cord injured individual. Annual Meeting of Experimental Biology, San Diego, California, 2003.

113. Edgerton VR, Courtine G, et al. Training locomotor networks. *Brain Res Rev* 2008; 57(1):241–254.

114. Gerasimenko Y, Roy RR, et al. Epidural stimulation: comparison of the spinal circuits that generate and control locomotion in rats, cats and humans. *Exp Neurol* 2008; 209(2):417–425.

115. Ralston HJ. Energetics of human walking. In: Herman R, Grillner S, Stein PSG, Stuart D, eds. Neural Control of Locomotion. New York: Plenum Press, 1976:77–98.

116. Alexander RM. Optimization and gaits in the locomotion of vertebrates. *Physiol Rev* 1989; 69(4):1199–1227.

117. Martin PE, Sanderson DJ, et al. Factors affecting preferred rates of movement in cyclic activities. In Zatsiorsky VM, ed. *Biomechanics in Sport: Performance Enhancement and Injury Prevention*. Oxford: Blackwell Science Ltd., 2000:147–160.

118. Ganley K, Willis W, et al. Epidural spinal cord stimulation improves locomotor performance in low ASIA C wheelchair-dependent, spinal cord–injured individuals: insights from metabolic response. *Top Spinal Cord Inj Rehabil* 2005; 11(2):50–63.

119. Shealy C, Mortimer J, et al. Electrical inhibition of pain by stimulation of the dorsal columns: preliminary clinical report. *Anesth Analg* 1967; 46:489–491.

120. Alo KM, Holsheimer J. New trends in neuromodulation for the management of neuropathic pain. *Neurosurgery* 2002; 50(4):690–704.

121. Kumar K, Toth C, et al. Epidural spinal cord stimulation for treatment of chronic pain—some predictors of success: a 15-year experience. *Surg Neurol* 1998; 50(2):110–121.

122. Law J. Targeting a spinal stimulator to treat the "failed back surgery syndrome." *Appl Neurophysiol* 1987; 50:437–438.

123. Carhart MR, Willis W, et al. Mechanical and metabolic changes in gait performance with spinal cord stimulation and reflex-FES. Submission, 25th Annual International Conference of the IEEE-EMBS, Cancun, Mexico, 2003.

124. Protas EJ, Holmes SA, et al. Supported treadmill ambulation training after spinal cord injury: a pilot study. *Arch Phys Med Rehabil* 2001; 82(6):825–831.

74 Functional Magnetic Stimulation

Vernon W. Lin
Ian Hsiao

Functional magnetic stimulation (FMS) can be defined as a technique that uses magnetic stimulation to produce useful bodily function (1). Although magnetic stimulation of the human body has been tried for over a century, most advances in FMS, especially on the application of using FMS for improving bodily function in patients with spinal cord injury (SCI), has been made within the last 20 years. Magnetic stimulation is a technique that can activate nerves or muscles from a distance. Unlike electric stimulation, magnetic stimulation does not rely on the passage of electric current through the tissue. The basic difference between electric and magnetic stimulation is that the former injects current into the body via electrodes. In the case of magnetic stimulation, the magnetic field generated from the magnetic coil (MC) is able to pass through high-resistance structures such as skin, fat, or bone to stimulate underlying nerves, including brain tissues. This magnetic field, if with time-varying and sufficient amplitude, induces an electrical field, which in turn causes ions to flow and results in depolarization of the nerve. The mechanism of stimulation at the neuronal level is thought to be the same for both magnetic and electric stimulation; that is, current passes across a nerve membrane and into the axon, resulting in depolarization and the initiation of an action potential that propagates by the normal mechanism of nerve conduction. The considerable advantage of magnetic stimulation is the remarkable absence of painful sensations when compared to stimulation with skin-surface electrodes. With such electrodes, a high current density develops under the electrode, thereby favoring stimulation of skin receptors. With magnetic stimulation, there is no localized high-current density at the skin surface under the MC.

The scientific principle governing magnetic stimulation was discovered by Michael Faraday in 1831. He observed that a changing magnetic field induced a current in a conductor lying in the field. Just a few years before the end of nineteenth century, Arsenne d'Arsonval first demonstrated that a changing magnetic field could stimulate excitable tissue. In 1965 Bickford and Fremming (2) demonstrated that human peripheral nerves could be excited by a magnetic coil. In 1982 Polson et al. (3) produced a magnetic stimulator capable of peripheral stimulation and recorded the first muscle-evoked potential. Subsequent improvements in the magnetic stimulator design by Barker et al. (4) gave way to numerous possibilities for clinical neurophysiologic investigation (5). Motor cortical stimulation using MC was first performed by Barker et al. (4). At that time, compound muscle-action potentials were recorded from the abductor digiti minimi from magnetic stimulus applied to the opposite motor cortex. Since then, there have been a number of reports comparing cortical stimulation by MC versus electric stimulation (6). There have also been reports demonstrating the utility and safety of cortical magnetic stimulation in conditions such as SCI (7), multiple sclerosis, and amyotrophic lateral sclerosis (8). Transcranial magnetic stimulation is beyond the scope of this chapter, and can be found in Chapter 7 of this text.

Since early 1990s, FMS of the spinal nerves has been applied to patients with SCI as a therapeutic tool. FMS of the cervical and upper thoracic nerves was demonstrated to produce significant inspired volume and pressure (9, 10), and was thought to be useful in high cervical tetraplegics for enhancing inspiratory function and muscle conditioning. Similarly, FMS of the lower thoracic nerves in both able-bodied subjects and patients with SCI was demonstrated to produce significant expired volume, pressure, and flow that would simulate an effective cough, also called functional magnetic cough (FMC) (11–13). FMS of the sacral nerves were also shown to raise bladder and colonic pressures, and induced micturition (functional magnetic micturition or FMM) and defecation (functional magnetic defecation or FMD) in selected SCI subjects with neurogenic bladder and bowel (14–16).

Nerve Activation by Magnetic Stimulation

Cell membrane maintains a potential difference between intra- and extracellular space. In static cells the trans-membrane potential ranges from -40 to -90 mV. An externally applied electric field (such as the one induced through magnetic stimulation) may alter the cell's cross membrane potential, that is, depolarize the membrane and activate excitable tissue. The time-varying magnetic field generated by current flowing through the wire loops of a circular magnetic coil is in the shape of a torus in which the coil is contained, and the torus is elongated perpendicularly to the plane of the coil. When a volume conductor is intersected by this magnetic field a current flow is generated. If the coil is held parallel to the surface of a volume conductor, current will flow in the conductor in a circular path parallel to the coil, but in the opposite direction. When the coil is held at right angles to the surface of the volume conductor, current will flow in a circular path in the same plane as the coil and in the same circular direction. The induced currents and their paths in the body will also depend on any inhomogeneity in conductivity due to different anatomical structures and their electric anisotropy. The presence of these structures will cause a buildup of charges at conductivity variant boundaries, and the electric fields associated with these charges will combine with that produced by the time-varying magnetic field, thus distorting the concentric-induced current loops that would occur in an infinite homogeneous medium. Hence, the precise distribution of currents in the body is complex and can only be accurately predicted by extensive modeling and detailed knowledge of the electrical properties of the tissue in the vicinity of the coil (17).

Magnetic Stimulator

Magnetic stimulators for nerve activation typically consist of two components: a high-current pulse generator producing discharge currents of 5,000 amps or more, and a stimulating coil producing magnetic pulses with field strengths of 2 Tesla or more with a pulse duration around 250 μs. The magnetic field strengths of up to several Tesla required in magnetic stimulation are achieved by driving the stimulating coil with brief current pulses of several kiloamperes. The first commercial magnetic stimulators were produced in Sheffield, UK, in 1985. The magnetic stimulator consists of a capacitor charge/discharge system together with the associated control and safety electronics. Using the charging circuitry, the energy storage capacitor is charged to a set level up to several thousand volts determined by front panel controls. When the magnetic stimulator receives a trigger input signal, the energy stored in the capacitor is discharged into the stimulating coil. The stored energy, apart from that lost in the wiring and capacitor, is transferred to the coil and then returned to the instrument to reduce coil heating. The discharge switch consists of an electronic device, called a thyristor, which is capable of switching large currents in a few microseconds.

Magnetic Coil

The stimulating coil, normally housed in molded plastic covers, consists of one or more tightly wound and well-insulated copper coils together with other electronic circuitry such as temperature sensors and safety switches. A circular 90-mm-mean-diameter coil is the most common design. This is very effective in the stimulation of the human motor cortex controlling the upper limbs with a large cortical representation, and also in the stimulation of spinal nerve roots. To date, circular coils with a mean diameter of 90–120 mm are still widely used in magnetic stimulation. Although the circular coils are very useful for general purposes, the site of stimulation is not well defined. To improve focal stimulation, magnetic coil design becomes one of the most important aspects of the FMS technique when a coil is needed to stimulate a small area of tissue for local stimulation. The planar "butterfly" coil was the first major improvement over the conventional planar

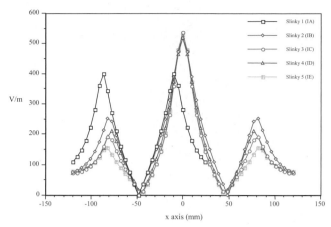

Figure 74.1 Electric field strength distribution of slinky-1 though slinky-5 coils from computer modeling results. Slinky-1 had two peaks of the same magnitude at the windings of the coil, and slinky-2 to slinky-5 had primary peaks at the center of the coil and two secondary peaks at the coil windings. All of the primary peaks for these four coils demonstrated similar magnitudes, and their secondary peaks decreased as slinky number increased. The ratios between the primary and secondary peaks from slinky-2 to slinky-5 were 2.0, 2.8, 2.5, and 3.4, respectively.

circular coil, followed more recently by the planar "four-leaf" coil (18). Lately, the three-dimensional (3-D) MC design has shown even greater promise. Early work on the 3-D "slinky" MC design using computer simulations has demonstrated improved focality for the field distributions (19, 20) as demonstrated in Figure 74.1. On the other hand, there are also many other applications when simultaneous stimulation and even stimulation of multiple nerves in a broad area is desired (e.g., stimulating expiratory muscles to mimic a cough in patients with SCI). In these cases, as demonstrated in Figure 74.1, the size and shape of coils are important factors in determining the range of stimulation; larger coils can certainly cover a larger area of stimulation.

CLINICAL APPLICATIONS IN PATIENTS WITH SPINAL CORD INJURY

The majority of the FMS applications in individuals with SCI have adopted the technique for noninvasive stimulation of the spinal and other peripheral nerves. FMS is used for diagnosis, conditioning of the muscles, and monitoring recovery over time. For example, the stimulation of the spinal nerves would result in the activation of the phrenic nerves, if the MC is placed near C3 to C5. Similarly, upper extremities will be stimulated if the MC is located at the lower cervical region. Upper intercostal nerves are activated if the MC is placed at the upper thoracic region, and lower intercostal nerves will be activated if MC is placed at lower thoracic region (Figure 74.2).

In terms of spinal nerve activation, the point of activation of the spinal nerve when magnetic stimulation was applied had been a controversial issue for some time. Using a cadaver thoracic spine model (17), Maccabee et al. measured the voltages across the neural foramen during magnetic stimulation and determined that the highest voltages were measured within the foramen, suggesting that the most probable site of nerve activation was at the intervertebral foramen.

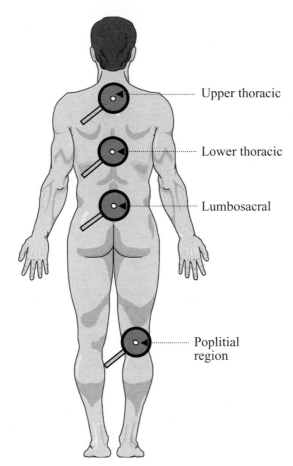

Upper thoracic

Lower thoracic

Lumbosacral

Poplitial region

Figure 74.2   Location of magnetic coils on human body for various clinical applications: upper thoracic for inspiration (augmentation)/ventilation (10,58,59,73); lower thoracic for cough/gastric emptying/GI transit (11,12,13,40,60,61,99); lumbosacral for micturition/defecation/colonic transit (14,15,16,97,98); lower limb for fibrinolysis (113).

FMS of the Respiratory Muscles

Respiratory Muscle Dysfunction in Patients with SCI and Current Management

Major muscles of inspiration include the diaphragm (C3–C5), parasternal, and external intercostal muscles (T1–T6). Able-bodied subjects are usually capable of generating approximately 100 cmH_2O of inspired pressure during a maximal effort, to which the diaphragm contributes 55–60%, and intercostal muscles contribute 20–25%. Major muscles of expiration include the abdominal muscles (T7–L1) and the internal intercostal muscles. Able-bodied subjects generate approximately 150 cmH_2O of maximal expiratory pressure. Respiratory dysfunction is a major cause of mortality and morbidity in subjects with SCI (21–23). Respiratory dysfunction arises partly from paralysis of the expiratory muscles, which leads to difficulties in clearing airway secretions effectively. High cervical SCI may result in loss of supraspinal control over the diaphragm and inspiratory muscles as well, resulting in ventilatory failure. Respiratory dysfunction measured by pulmonary function tests (PFT) in SCI patients is characteristic of restrictive lung disease, defined as a breathing disorder resulting from impairment of the elastic properties of the lung and chest wall, and marked by static or reduced lung volumes and capacities (23, 24). Patients with cervical cord injury have paralysis of both inspiratory and expiratory muscles, and therefore have marked reduction of vital capacity (VC), little or no expiratory reserve volume (ERV), and an inspiratory capacity equivalent to VC (25–27). The reduction of VC is most severe in tetraplegic patients. Vital capacities in individuals with acute cervical lesions range from 24–31% of predicted VC (27, 28). The total lung capacity (TLC) is reduced, and the ratio between residual volume and total lung capacity (RV/TLC) is increased in subjects at all injury levels. The lung function of patients tested more than 12 months after injury is not significantly different from the function in those tested 6–12 months after injury (29). Decreases of both static-inspired and expired breathing pressure measured at the mouth indicate the impairment of respiratory muscle functions.

Improvement of early surgical spine stabilization, pharmacological treatment, and chest physical therapy has improved survival of SCI patients (30, 31). Adequate alveolar ventilation can be maintained in most SCI patients until the recruitment of respiratory muscles, which occurs during the acute rehabilitation period of SCI. Chest physical therapy techniques include bronchial hygiene, postural draining, chest percussion, quad cough, and high frequency chest wall oscillation (32–34). Application of some of these techniques in a timely manner has decreased mortality in SCI. In addition to chest physical therapy, functional exercise of respiratory and accessory muscles has been used effectively in the treatment of many SCI patients. Functional exercise includes the use of glossopharyngeal breathing and breathing against resistance (35, 36).

Historically, functional electric stimulation (FES) of the respiratory muscles has been an active area of research in the last several decades. Please refer Chapter 63 in this book for an in-depth description of the state-of–the-art development of FES of the respiratory muscles. Various types of electrical implants have been employed to generate inspired and expired pressures. These include electrodes on the phrenic nerve, ventral roots, intercostal nerves, diaphragm, and abdominal muscles (37–42). Electrical phrenic nerve pacing is a technique used to assist mechanical ventilation in subjects with bilateral diaphragm paralysis, such as in cervical SCI above C6 (39, 42, 43). The criteria for electrical phrenic nerve stimulation include chronic ventilatory insufficiency secondary to paralysis that has been stable for at least one month, viable phrenic nerves, and a diaphragm that responds well to a diaphragmatic pacemaker (44). Upper intercostal muscles (T1–T6) were demonstrated to act as inspiratory agonists by lifting and expanding the rib cage (45, 46). Intercostal muscle pacing was achieved in human subjects via ventral root stimulation, and inspired volumes between 600–900 ml were generated (47). FES of the abdominal muscles also generated significant expiratory pressures. By placing percutaneous electrodes on the abdominal wall motor points, significant expiratory flow and pressure were measured in patients with SCI (41, 42, 48). DiMarco et al. (49) demonstrated significant expiratory pressure when stimulating ventral roots at the T9–T10 level in canines in 1995. A quadripolar-stimulating electrode was inserted epidurally and on the ventral surface of the lower thoracic spinal cord. At functional residual capacity (FRC), significant positive airway pressures were generated. These results showed that a major portion of the expiratory muscles can be activated reproducibly and in concert using electrical stimulation, and the resulting pressure can be comparable to that of a manually assisted cough (49, 50).

FMS of the Expiratory Muscles and Functional Magnetic Cough (FMC)

FMS of the respiratory muscles is effective and has many advantages when compared with the existing FES technology. FMS is easier to use, and does not require surgery or electrode implants, thus preventing complications such as infection, bleeding, wire breakage, implant failures, etc. FMS is not as painful as FES, and is well tolerated by conscious individuals. FMS can be applied over clothing, because it does not require skin contact or the use of electrode gel. There are also disadvantages of the FMS technology when compared with FES. One disadvantage is the bulky size of the stimulator. There are still significant technical challenges before FMS units can be modified into portable and affordable devices.

Magnetic stimulation has been applied to stimulate the cerebral cortex to evaluate the nerve conduction velocity for the respiratory system. Using transcranial brain stimulation, diaphragm compound muscle action potential (CMAP) had a latency of 16.21 ± 0.33 ms, an amplitude of 3.52 ± 2.40 mV, and a central motor conduction time of 8.39 ± 0.41 ms (51). Similarly, nerve conduction studies of the thoracic nerves using magnetic stimulation (52) and transcranial stimulation for determining the central conduction time for upper intercostal muscles were reported by Lissens et al. (53). Magnetic stimulation of the phrenic nerve was first reported by Similowski et al. (54). The MC was positioned above the spinous process of the seventh cervical vertebra (C7) to stimulate both phrenic nerves with a single stimulus. They were able to obtain reproducible supramaximal CMAP in five of six subjects. Wragg et al. (55) compared magnetic stimulation of the phrenic nerve with electric stimulation, and showed that mean twitch transdiaphragmatic pressure (Pdi) obtained by magnetic stimulation was significantly higher than electrical twitch Pdi. The researchers speculated that magnetic stimulation might have resulted in stimulation of extradiaphragmatic musculature. Mills et al. (56) also showed that cervical magnetic stimulation in patients with known diaphragmatic paralysis could not generate transdiaphragmatic pressure. The stimulation of the extradiaphragmatic musculature most likely played a role in stiffening the upper thoracic cage to allow the diaphragm to act efficiently. Additionally, Laghi et al. (57) also reached the same conclusion that cervical magnetic stimulation recruited both extradiaphragmatic and diaphragmatic muscles, whereas electric stimulation had a more selective action on the diaphragm. They further concluded that magnetic stimulation could be an equally effective method for detecting diaphragmatic fatigue.

FMS of the respiratory muscles was first demonstrated in animals (40, 58, 59). FMS of the phrenic nerves, upper intercostal nerves, and lower intercostal nerves was first demonstrated in a canine study (40); the resultant inspired/expired pressures were -20 ± 1.99 cmH$_2$O, -10 ± 1.03 cmH$_2$O, and 11 ± 2.25 cmH$_2$O, respectively. The inspired/expired volumes were 373 ± 20.5 ml, 219 ± 12.2 ml, and -119 ± 22.5 ml, respectively. The graphical results are displayed in Figure 74.3. The stimulation profile was 30 Hz frequency, 1-second burst length, and 70% intensity. These animal studies demonstrated the efficacy for FMS to generate significant inspired or expired volumes and pressures, and also established the foundation for FMS as a potential technology for

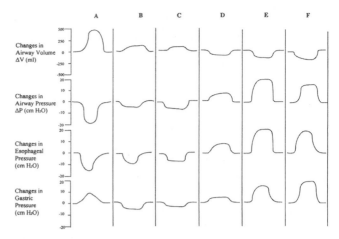

Figure 74.3 A representative tracing of a recording showing changes in volume, airway, esophageal, and gastric pressures by placing the magnetic coil at the carotid region before phrenectomies (**A**), and at the C6–C7 (**B**), T2–T3 (**C**), T6–T7 (**D**), T9–T10 (**E**), and L2–L3 (**F**) spinous processes after phrenectomies were performed (40).

inspiratory/expiratory muscle training, ventilatory assistance, and cough production.

Expiratory functions produced in humans by FMS were first demonstrated by stimulating the lower thoracic spinal nerve roots (60). A 12.5-cm round MC was placed in the lower thoracic region for stimulating the lower intercostal muscles and the abdominal muscles as shown in Figure 74.2. Maximal expired pressure, volume, and flow rate generated by FMS were 83.6 ± 16.39 cmH$_2$O, 1.54 ± 0.18 L, and 4.75 ± 0.35 L/s, respectively. These values corresponded to 73.2%, 100%, and 90% of the maximal voluntary expired pressure, volume, and flow, respectively. The optimal coil placement observed was at T7, and the optimal stimulation parameters were with a frequency of 25 Hz and an intensity of 70–80%. When similar stimulation protocol was applied to patients with SCI, FMS of the expiratory muscles also produced a substantial maximal expired pressure (68.2 ± 24.1 cmH$_2$O), volume (0.77 ± 0.48 L), and flow rate (5.27 ± 1.49 L/s) (12). These values corresponded to 121%, 167%, and 110% of their voluntary maximum, respectively. Like other respiratory muscle exercise trainings such as diaphragmatic breathing, lateral costal breathing, and inspiratory resistive breathing, FMS can be used as a device for conditioning of the intercostal, diaphragm, and the abdominal muscles. In a study involving patients with SCI (61), a 4-week FMS of expiratory muscle training showed significant improvement in voluntary maximal expired pressure (116%), volume (173%), and flow rate (123%) when compared with their baseline data. The improved expiratory function was maintained for at least another two weeks after the termination of the FMS conditioning period.

Functional Magnetic Stimulation of the Inspiratory Muscles

Phrenic pacers have been used for patients with high cervical SCIs for maintaining ventilatory support. Although the application of mechanical ventilation has reduced death rates of patients in the intensive care units, mechanical ventilation accelerates disuse of respiratory muscles, and therefore leads to difficulty in weaning from mechanical ventilation. FES of the phrenic nerves involves placement of electrodes directly on the phrenic nerves in the neck or thorax (62–64) or placement of intramuscular electrodes in the diaphragm (65–68) using a laparoscopic procedure. In addition, upper intercostal muscle pacing by electric ventral root stimulation facilitates inspiratory function in subjects with partial phrenic function (69–70). More recently, FES was also applied to abdominal muscles as a method of enhancing ventilation in human subjects with SCI (71). The above FES methods are invasive, require surgery for electrode implants, and expose patients to the risks associated with chronic implants, such as infection and hemorrhage (72). Functional magnetic ventilation (FMV) is a newly developed mode of noninvasive negative pressure ventilation that employs a magnetic stimulator. This mode of ventilation has similarities to electrophrenic pacing because the phrenic nerves are electrically stimulated, yet without surgical interventions.

Magnetic stimulation for ventilation (FMV) was successfully demonstrated in a canine study for duration of two hours after a complete C2 spinal cord transection. The averaged tidal volume (V_T) produced during FMV was 0.35 ± 0.05 L with a maximum of 0.8 L and a minimum of 0.2 L. The V_T and tracheal pressure (P_{tr}) over time during FMV are shown in Figure 74.4, the mean V_T increased from 0.31 L to 0.49 L at 15 minutes, and fluctuated between 0.49 L to 0.43 L until the termination of FMV. At the end of FMV, the mean V_T (0.42 L) produced by magnetic stimulation was higher than the mean spontaneous V_T of 0.31 L. The average P_{tr} was −6.3 ± 1.51 cmH$_2$O after 15 minutes of FMV, which is more negative than the spontaneous P_{tr} of −2.0 ± 0.23 cmH$_2$O. After the first 15 minutes, the P_{tr} ranged from 3.95 to 4.78 cmH$_2$O for the remaining two hours of FMV. The baseline mean arterial blood PCO$_2$ of the dogs was 33.2 ± 0.71 mmHg. At 15 minutes of FMV, mean PCO$_2$ increased to 66.0 ± 2.9 mmHg. For the rest of the 2-hour period of FMV, the mean PCO$_2$ fluctuated from a low of 59.1 ± 2.8 mmHg at 30 minutes to a high of 80.9 ± 8.1 mmHg at 90 minutes and decreased to 74.5 ± 6.2 mmHg at the end of FMV. The changes in mean pH reflected the corresponding increases and decreases in arterial PCO$_2$. The mean pH changed from a baseline level of 7.33 ± 0.01 to 6.99 ± 0.03 during 2 hours of FMV. The corresponding rise in K$^+$ most likely occurred due to an extracellular shift of K$^+$ as the pH decreased. The modified tension-time index dropped from 0.17 to 0.14 ± 0.05 during the same period, suggesting that FMV did not induce inspiratory muscle fatigue. The only chemistry values that demonstrated significant changes over the 2-hour-long period were CK and K$^+$.

This study demonstrated a new mode of noninvasive negative pressure ventilation using magnetic stimulation. FMV was achieved for two hours in dogs with C2 spinal cord transection. Sufficient tidal volumes with elevated PCO$_2$ were produced during FMV. Though FMV is only in its infancy, with further technical improvements, this novel application may prove to be a practical clinical tool for patients needing ventilatory support. Other than ventilatory support, FMS can also be used for inspiratory muscle conditioning for patients with SCI. Clinical trials applying FMS for conditioning the inspiratory muscles in patients with SCI are currently underway at our institution.

FMS of the Gastrointestinal Tract

Neurogenic Bowel and Current Management

Deficits in gastrointestinal (GI) transit are prevalent in many patient populations, particularly patients who have undergone surgical procedures or who have neurological disorders. In

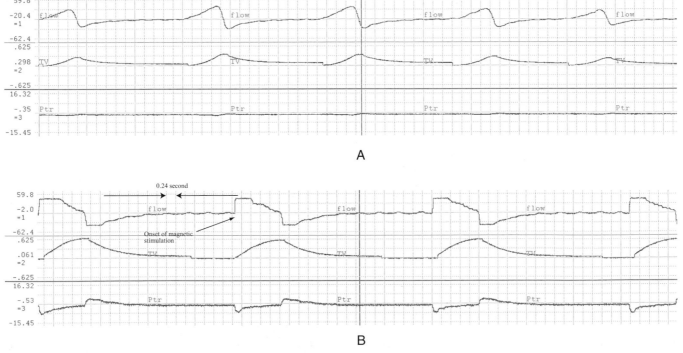

Figure 74.4 VT and Ptr during spontaneous breathing of a dog and the pattern during FMV. Data acquisition samples of flow (L/min), VT (L), and Ptr (cmH$_2$O) for (**A**) spontaneous breathing and (**B**) FMV.

postoperative patients, decreases in gastric motility can hinder the absorption of nutrients and oral medications, resulting in a delay in recovery (73) and increased morbidity (74). Neurological disorders affecting the gastrointestinal tract result primarily in abnormalities in motor function (75). Neurogenic bowel is also a common source of morbidity and mortality among patients with acute and chronic SCI (76). Signs and symptoms include fecal impaction, (77) constipation, abdominal distention (78, 79), prolonged bowel care, (78, 80) and delayed colonic transit (81–85). The prevalence of chronic gastrointestinal symptoms also appears to increase with time after SCI (79). Bowel management for patients with SCI includes a balanced diet, judicial use of oral and rectal medications, and digital stimulation (86). Some SCI patients with long transit times find bowel care to be complicated, laborious, and difficult to adhere to. These patients often spend several hours a day emptying their colons, contributing to a decreased quality of life and independence. In addition, for patients with very difficult bowel evacuation and/or severe GI dysfunctions, colostomies have been a necessary procedure to simplify their care (79, 87).

Electrical stimulation of visceral organs is not a new concept. Hymes et al. (88) used surface electrical stimulation of the abdomen, and noted a striking decrease in postoperative ileus in a prospective, randomized study of 213 patients. Richardson and Cerullo (89) followed this with a study of 21 patients with neurogenic bowel disease from a variety of etiologies and found a marked reduction in the incidence of ileus among those patients treated with abdominal neurostimulation. In addition, Richardson et al. (90) used transabdominal neurostimulation on 44 acute SCI patients. None of the patients developed paralytic ileus, whereas 15% of 43 control subjects with similar injuries did. Frost et al. (91) used electrical stimulation of the sacral dermatomes in SCI patients, and concluded that electrical stimulation of the S2 dermatome caused a significant rise in the number of rectal pressure spikes, but no significant change in the time required for patients to initiate bowel movement.

Advances in ventral sacral root stimulation demonstrated increased colorectal contractions in patients with SCI (92–96). Sacral anterior root stimulation brought significant progress for both electromicturition and electrodefecation. Varma et al. (92) used Brindley stimulators with sequential electrical stimulation of the anterior sacral roots (S2, S3, S4) on five SCI patients. Reproducible results were obtained: S2 stimulation provoked isolated low-pressure colorectal contractions, S3 stimulation initiated high-pressure colorectal motor activity, which appeared peristaltic and was enhanced with repetitive stimuli, and S4 stimulation increased colonic and rectal tone. MacDonagh et al. (93) used Brindley-Finetech stimulators on 12 SCI patients, and demonstrated contractions of both rectosigmoid and the anal sphincter at the beginning of the stimulation. This was followed by a period where the anal sphincter relaxed while the rectum was still contracting; which resulted in defecation. Of the 12 patients tested, six achieved complete evacuation of feces using the stimulator alone, and the remaining had to perform manual evacuation. In 1991 Binnie et al. (94) used the same Brindley S2–S4 anterior sacral nerve root stimulator on 10 SCI patients, and demonstrated a significant increase in frequency of defecation as compared to 10 SCI controls without the stimulators.

FMS of the GI tract

In two recent animal investigations (97, 98), by applying a smaller figure-8 coil near the thoracolumbar region, FMS produced significant improvement in gastric emptying at one hour post orogastric gavage (90.4% in the experimental group vs. 69.6% in the control group). The effect of FMS on gastrointestinal transit time showed a similar pattern. A significant decrease on gastrointestinal transit time was observed between groups ($p < 0.05$). Post-hoc t-tests showed a significantly increased geometric center in the group that received stimulation of both anterior cervical and thoracolumbar regions (7.8 ± 0.3), and the group that received anterior cervical stimulation alone (7.3 ± 0.3), when compared with the control group (6.1 ± 0.4; $p < 0.005$). This information and the absence of gastric myoelectrical activity in chronic SCI led to the postulation that the weakness of the abdominal musculature might be an important factor associated with delayed gastric emptying in patients with chronic SCI. The induction of abdominal muscle contractions may bring about improved gastric emptying and gastrointestinal transits, in a manner similar to other physical examples of external compressions that produce compressions of the internal organs, such as the compression of the heart due to chest compressions during cardiac pulmonary resuscitation and the compressions of the bladder from abdominal compressions to produce more effective bladder emptying.

FMS of the Colon and Functional Magnetic Defecation (FMD)

Placing MC at the lumbosacral region (Figure 74.2), FMS was shown to activate the colon and improved colonic transit and gastric emptying in human studies. In a clinical trial in patients with SCI (16), significant changes in rectal pressure and colonic transit time due to FMS were observed. Rectal pressures increased from 26.7 ± 7.44 to 48.0 ± 9.91 cmH$_2$O with lumbosacral stimulation, and from 30.0 ± 6.35 to 42.7 ± 7.95 cm H$_2$O with transabdominal stimulation. Using FMS, the mean colonic transit time decreased from 105.2 hours to 89.4 hours. The rectosigmoid transit times decreased from 50.4 ± 9.79 to 34.8 ± 9.39 hours. This study demonstrated that FMS could activate the colon and resulted in improvement in colonic transit. FMS of the colon can be performed either by placing the MC at the lower abdomen for transabdominal stimulation, or by placing the MC at the lumbosacral region for sacral nerve stimulation. With transabdominal stimulation, tensing of the abdominal musculature was observed along with an increase in rectal pressure. With lumbosacral stimulation (Figure 74.2), a significant elevation of rectal pressure was observed, and frequently we observed defecation in response to magnetic stimulation, known as functional magnetic defecation (FMD).

FMS Facilitating Gastric Emptying

Furthermore, when placing the MC at T9 (Figure 74.2), gastric emptying was enhanced by FMS in both able-bodied subjects and SCI patients (99). The gastric emptying half-time (GE$_{t1/2}$) shortened more than 8% for able-bodied subjects, and shortened 33% for SCI subjects, respectively. Figure 74.5 shows an example of gastric emptying curves of a SCI subject at baseline and with

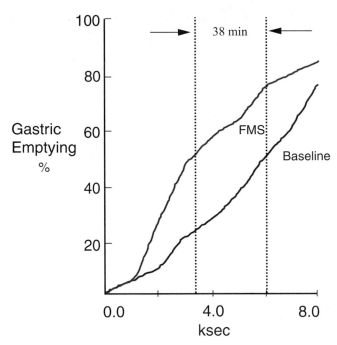

Figure 74.5 An example of the gastric emptying curves versus time with and without FMS in one SCI subject.

FMS. The $GE_{t1/2}$ of gastric emptying with FMS was accelerated by approximately 38 minutes when compared with the baseline values. One possible mechanism is that FMS functions similarly to electrical stimulation to accelerate gastric emptying through direct activation of the underlying gastric neuromuscular apparatus. Instead of stimulating at the stomach level, the thoracic spinal nerves are activated as they exit the neuroforamen (17). FMS may be acting in a similar manner as gastric pacing, which uses electrodes implanted on the surface of the stomach muscle to cause rhythmic gastric contractions. Another postulation is related to the fact that rhythmic abdominal muscle contractions may bring about improvement in gastric emptying. This is because the abdominal muscles (major expiratory agonists) are innervated by the lower thoracic spinal nerves.

FMS of the Bladder

Neurogenic Bladder and FES of the Bladder

Neurogenic bladder is considered one of the most common sources of morbidity and mortality in patients with SCI. FES of the bladder has been examined by many investigators. Various types of electrical implants have been tried for emptying the bladder. These have employed electrodes on the bladder wall (100–103), on the sacral nerves (104), on the conus medullaris (105, 106), or on the pudendal nerve (107). Direct bladder stimulation requires strong current pulses, which may cause a lower extremity flexion reflex and may be painful if the spinal lesion is incomplete. Electrode breakage is common because of the considerable movement that accompanies bladder contraction.

Sacral nerve root stimulation has offered the greatest success in producing voiding without prohibitive side effects. Brindley et al. (108) used sacral anterior stimulator implants (the FineTech

Brindley Bladder Control System, Finetech Medical Ltd., UK) in producing micturition, reducing residual urine, and vesicourethral reflux. These implants are placed around the anterior roots of S2, S3, and S4 spinal nerves and are capable of generating bursts of stimulation. During the gap between each successive burst of impulses, the sphincter and pelvic floor rapidly relax while the detrusor is still contracting. Thus, voiding occurs in spurts after each burst of stimulation. Out of 50 implanted patients, Brindley et al. demonstrated that 40 had a significant decrease in residual urine volumes to less than 60 ml, with a strong subjective approval rating in 40 of the 50 patients. The 5–11-year follow-up of this group indicated that of the 48 surviving individuals, 41 were using the implant for micturition and 37 were generally continent. One of the disadvantages of the technique of sacral nerve root stimulation for voiding was the disruption of the dura to place the electrodes. Cerebrospinal fluid leakage at the point where the electrode cables exited the dura was a significant risk. The FineTech Brindley Bladder Control System, or VOCARE bladder control system in United States, has been implanted in more than 2,500 patients worldwide (109).

In patients with SCI, the normal coordination of bladder contraction and sphincter relaxation is lost. The FES of the sacral nerve does not reproduce the normal coordination of detrusor and sphincter; the bladder response produced has to work against varying degrees of outlet resistance. The sphincteric resistance could be reduced through direct surgical sphincter resection or through pudendal neurectomy. Pudendal neurectomy is a drastic way to diminish urethral resistance, because rhizotomy and/or neurectomy are usually associated with an interference with the competence of the urinary or anal sphincter as well as sexual function.

Functional Magnetic Micturition (FMM)

The first clinical study investigating the efficacy of FMS of the bladder in SCI individuals was reported in 1994 (14). In that study, micturition by FMS was observed in 17 out of 22 subjects. All subjects, except the one with lower motor neuron lesion and areflexic bladder, responded well to FMS of the bladder. The mean changes in bladder pressure (Pves) by sacral stimulation (Figure 74.2) were 24.4 ± 4.88 cmH$_2$O. The sacral FMS produced a greater increase in Pves than did suprapubic stimulation ($p < 0.05$). Higher intensities and frequencies of sacral stimulation are associated with greater changes in Pves. Micturition by FMS was observed in 17 subjects. Micturition observed was reproducible, either via suprapubic or sacral FMS (Figure 74.2). Complete bladder emptying was observed in one subject using a water-cooled coil applied suprapubically. With 100 ml of water in the bladder, and a sequence of intermittent stimulation that lasted 4.5 minutes, complete bladder emptying occurred. Bladder emptying was also observed when using a 12-cm MC by sacral stimulation. Figure 74.6 demonstrates that the bladder of one subject was emptied with three brief magnetic stimulation bursts after the bladder was filled with 232 ml of water. Other important findings included detrusor modulation by sacral FMS, external urethral sphincter muscle fatigue by suprapubic FMS, and the usefulness of an intermittent sacral FMS sequence to facilitate micturition. In addition, it was found that patients with reflex bladders were ideal candidates for FMS of the bladder, and patients with lower motor neuron lesions, or flaccid bladders, were not good candidates.

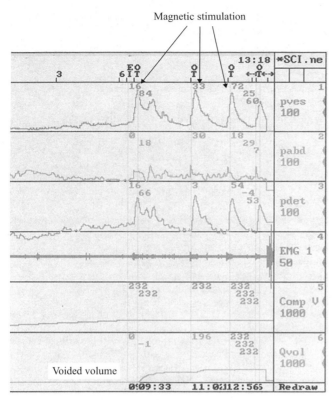

Magnetic stimulation

Figure 74.6 FMS of the sacral nerve was performed with one subject lying in a supine position, and the magnetic coil placed at the L2–L4 region. Magnetic stimulation parameters were set at 70% of maximal intensity, 20 Hz frequency, and 2-second burst length. The changes in Pves and voided volume in response to FMS was demonstrated. After three stimulations, the bladder was emptied.

FMS and FES of the Sacral Nerves/ Roots in Animals

In a separate canine study, micturition by FMS was observed in 10 animals (15). The stimulation parameters were 30 Hz, 70% of maximal intensity, and 2-second burst length. The mean increase in ΔPves (change in bladder pressure) by suprapubic magnetic stimulation, 40.7 ± 8.08 cmH$_2$O, was significantly lower when compared with lumbosacral stimulation, 68.0 ± 12.96 cmH2O ($p < 0.05$). Voiding was achieved in an additional three animals in one protocol using the water-cooled coil. With the intermittent stimulation sequence applied to the lumbosacral spine, significant micturition can be observed repeatedly and reliably. This animal study demonstrated the effectiveness of FMS on micturition. Another study comparing sacral root FMS and FES was performed. Electric stimulation was achieved at the following three locations along the sacral nerves/roots: (1) proximal ventral sacral root using the Cortac platinum contact electrode near the L4 vertebrae; (2) distal right S2 root (intraforaminal) by using a bipolar hook electrode placed around the right S3 root at L6 vertebrae, 2 cm proximal to the foramen; and (3) right S2 sacral nerve (extraforaminal) at 2 cm distal to the neuroforamen. The magnetic stimulation was applied by placing the 9-cm MC at L3 to L5. The results showed that the

latency for FMS when placing the MC between L3 and L5 was 1.8 ± 0.06 ms, which was exactly between the latencies obtained for extra- and intra-foramina stimulation (1.7 ± 0.03 ms and 1.9 ± 0.23 ms) using hook electrodes placed along the right S2 sacral root/nerve. This corresponds with earlier studies that predicted the foci of stimulation would be located at the foramen (17). Moreover, the average amplitude obtained by FMS (1.4 ± 0.26 mV) was similar to that obtained from the contact electrode (1.5 ± 0.43 mV). These amplitudes are more than double those obtained by unilateral S2 stimulation. This illustrates that FMS could stimulate multiple sacral nerves simultaneously, producing similar CMAP as ventral sacral root stimulation. Similar levels of ΔPves and ΔPur (change in urethral pressure) produced by FMS and FES in this study confirmed this result.

FMS of the Lower Limb for Enhancing Fibrinolysis

Thromboembolism is one of the most common complications in acute SCI and postoperative patients. Complications of deep venous thrombosis (DVT) that lead to significant morbidity include post-thrombotic syndrome, prolonged edema, and pressure ulcers, and may be a source of spasticity or autonomic dysreflexia. The importance of prophylaxis with these patients cannot be underestimated. The widely used prophylactic modalities for DVT include medications, external pneumatic compression, intermittent pneumatic compression, gradient elastic stocking (110), and FES (111). Application of FES to the tibialis anterior and gastrocnemius soleus muscle group has been proposed as a means of preventing DVT in patients with acute SCI. FES was shown to increase plasma fibrinolytic activity as well as venous blood flow (111). When FES was combined with low-dose heparin in one clinical trial, there was a substantial decrease in the incidence of DVT when compared with placebo or low-dose heparin alone (112). FES has not gained popularity as a prophylactic modality, partly because it is cumbersome, requires direct contact with the skin, and is painful in patients with good sensation.

FMS as a noninvasive and potentially more effective method of stimulating endogenous fibrinolysis was performed in 20 normal subjects (113). This FMS study was designed to test changes in fibrinolysis in blood samples of patients taken before, 15 minutes after, and one hour after FMS. The test for fibrinolysis was a modified dilute whole-blood clot lysis method, and was performed on site. The subject was placed in the prone position, with the MC placed on the popliteal region (Figure 74.2), alternating from side to side every 30 seconds. The frequency of stimulation, burst length, and burst interval were 30 Hz, 4 seconds, and 26 seconds, respectively. Fibrinolysis was tested by the dilute whole blood clot lysis time (WBCLT) in the tube by the method of Sirridge, and a modified semi-automated method by using a Sonoclot Coagulation Analyzer.

The effect of the FMS protocol on fibrinolytic response for individual subjects was that the mean WBCLT values decreased from 17 ± 1.3 hours at baseline to 12 ± 1.0 hours and 11 ± 0.8 hours at 10 minutes and 60 minutes post-FMS, respectively. The post-FMS values, 10 minutes and 60 minutes, were significantly different, p = 0.0001 and p < 0.0001, respectively, from the pre-FMS lysis time measurement. The degree of fibrinolytic enhancement at 10 and 60 minutes post-FMS was not uniform in all individuals. This study demonstrated that FMS of the leg muscles could produce an enhancement of systemic fibrinolysis that exceeded the increase in fibrinolytic activity accounted for by changes in posture and the influence of the circadian rhythm. This enhancement was apparently sustained for at least 60 minutes after cessation of the stimulation protocol. Using similar protocol on 22 patients with SCI, preliminary results showed that the WBCLT values at 10 minutes post-FMS (15 ± 1.6 hr) and 60 minutes post-FMS (16 ± 1.5 hr) were significantly decreased from pre-FMS (19 ± 1.2hr; $p < 0.001$). The values of WBCLT at 10 minutes and 60 minutes post-FMS did not change significantly ($P < 0.45$). These results showed that FMS provided a more rapid enhancement of systemic fibrinolysis than modalities such as FES and a more sustained enhancement than voluntary exercise. It can be an excellent tool for use in situations where voluntary exercise cannot be performed, such as in patients who have SCI, multiple sclerosis, stroke, central nervous system tumors, or in spinal dysraphias.

FMS-Induced Analgesia

Analgesic medications can provide transient pain relief, but the chronic use of both opioid and non-opioid analgesics is associated with a plethora of limiting side-effects. Increasingly, patients are turning to "alternative" pain treatments, including nonpharmacologic analgesic modalities such as electrical stimulation. Electric stimulation-induced analgesia has been widely used in the management of chronic pain for over 30 years. Transcutaneous electrical nerve stimulation (TENS), percutaneous electrical nerve stimulation (PENS), and electroacupuncture (EA) have been used for the treatment of chronic musculoskeletal and neuropathic pain. Spinal column stimulation (SCS), a more invasive procedure requiring the permanent implantation of an epidural electrical stimulator, has been widely used for the treatment of patients with severe and intractable chronic pain. Clinical data suggest that TENS is the least effective form of electrical stimulation analgesia (114–116), PENS is more effective (117–118), and SCS is most effective (119–120). The invasive electrical stimulation techniques such as PENS, EA, and SCS can stimulate deeper nerves or spinal cord neurons, but require needle electrodes to overcome skin impedance or surgical implantation of stimulation systems, which are prone to breakdown.

An earlier animal study investigated the antinociceptive effect of FMS when applied over the lumbosacral spine of rats (121). The effects of FMS on acute mechanical and thermal hindpaw withdrawal thresholds were determined, and neuroablative and pharmacologic manipulations were utilized to further characterize the mechanism and anatomic site of FMS antinociceptive action. Immediately after 5 minutes of FMS, the mechanical withdrawal threshold increased from 66 ± 3 g to 160 ± 9.8 g and the heat withdrawal threshold increased from $50.1 \pm 0.1°C$ to $51.7 \pm 0.2°C$. The frequency of stimulation, burst length, and burst interval were 20 Hz, 5 s, and 15 s respectively. The FMS effect gradually diminished, lasting 30 minutes for mechanical antinociception and 40 minutes for heat antinociception as shown in Figure 74.7. Sham-treated rats had no significant changes over time for mechanical or heat withdrawal thresholds. When the nociceptive thresholds of the FMS-treated rats were compared to the sham-treated rats, there was a significant difference between groups over time ($p < .01$, for both mechanical and heat, two-way repeated measures ANOVA), which persisted 30 minutes after FMS for both mechanical and heat antinociceptive effects.

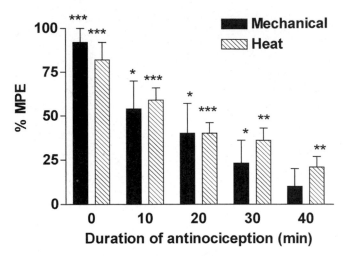

Figure 74.7   All antinociceptive effects on the rat hindpaws are presented as the percentage of the maximum possible effect (%MPE). % MPE = ([post-treatment threshold—pre-treatment threshold]/[cutoff threshold—pre-treatment threshold] × 100). The cutoff thresholds were 52°C for heat nociception and 170 g of force for mechanical nociception. Immediately after 5 minutes of lumbosacral magnetic stimulation, there was a robust antinociceptive effect for mechanical ($92 \pm 8\%$ MPE) and heat ($82 \pm 10\%$ MPE) stimuli applied to the hindpaw (N = 10). This effect gradually diminished, persisting for 30 minutes for mechanical antinociception and 40 minutes for heat antinociception. (*$p < .05$, **$p < .01$, ***$p < .001$ vs. baseline thresholds.)

In order to determine the possible role of endogenous neurotransmitters in mediating FMS antinociceptive effects, attempts to block FMS antinociception were made by using the opiate receptor antagonist naloxone (5 mg/kg) and the α_2 adrenoceptor antagonist atipamezole (5 mg/kg). The drugs were administered by the intraperitoneal route (volume of 1 mL/kg). Systemic naloxone completely blocked FMS-evoked antinociceptive effects, indicating that FMS activates an endogenous opioidergic analgesic mechanism to induce antinociception. When naloxone (5 mg/kg, i.p.) was injected 25 minutes before FMS, the FMS

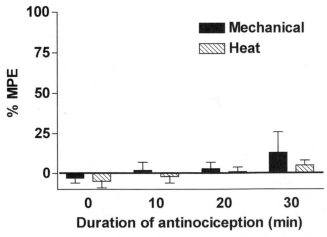

Figure 74.8   The opiate receptor antagonist naloxone (5 mg/kg, i.p.) completely blocked the antinociceptive effect of FMS (N = 9).

treatment had no effect on mechanical and heat thresholds as shown in Figure 74.8. Saline-injected rats had FMS antinociceptive responses similar to naïve animals, with elevated withdrawal thresholds persisting for 30 minutes post-stimulation. Control rats injected with naloxone (5 mg/kg, i.p.) and not treated with FMS had stable pre- and post-injection withdrawal thresholds over a 60 minutes period, indicating that this dose of naloxone did not affect nociceptive thresholds. Naloxone completely antagonized FMS antinociception, indicating that an endogenous opiate mechanism mediated this effect.

Systemic atipamezole did not block the antinociceptive effect of FMS, suggesting that endogenous adrenergic analgesic mechanisms did not play a major role in FMS antinociception. When atipamezole (5 mg/kg, i.p.) was injected 25 minutes before FMS, the FMS treatment still evoked long-lasting mechanical (10 minutes) and heat (30 minutes) antinociception. There was no significant difference in the mechanical nociceptive thresholds between the atipamezole and saline treatment groups over time, but there was a significant difference between these treatment groups for heat stimuli (p < .05). The saline-treated rats had a greater FMS-evoked heat antinociceptive effect than the atipamezole-treated rats, and this difference persisted for 20 minutes after FMS. These data suggested that the FMS heat antinociceptive effect might be partially mediated by activation of the α_2 adrenoceptor. Control rats injected with atipamezole (5 mg/kg, i.p.) and not treated with FMS had stable pre- and post-injection withdrawal thresholds over a 60-minute period, indicating that this dose of atipamezole did not affect nociceptive thresholds. The attempt to reverse FMS-evoked antinociception with the α_2 adrenoceptor antagonist atipamezole only resulted in a partial reversal of FMS antinociception for heat stimuli, and had no effect on FMS antinociception for mechanical stimuli. These results suggested that endogenous noradrenergic mechanisms did not play major roles in FMS antinociception, and that FMS utilized different analgesic mechanisms than that mediating stress analgesia.

This study demonstrated that 5 minutes of FMS over the lumbosacral spine at an intensity high enough to evoke a slight motor response in the tail could induce a long-lasting, robust antinociceptive effect that resembled the antinociception produced by EA, requiring endogenous opioidergic mediation. These results indicate that FMS can provide a transcutaneous method of evoking action potentials in the deeper nerves or spinal cord neurons, resulting in analgesia. The magnitude and duration of this analgesic effect is comparable to that reported in other studies measuring electroanalgesia to acute nociceptive stimuli in animals and humans (122–127). Further animal and clinical investigations are required to determine the optimal treatment parameters for FMS-evoked analgesia, and to determine whether FMS is more effective than transcutaneous, percutaneous, or spinal electrical stimulation in analgesia trials.

FMS vs. Electrical Acupuncture on the Cardiovascular Reflex Responses

Cardiovascular disease is a leading cause of morbidity and mortality in middle-aged and older-age individuals in both Western and Eastern societies, and is the leading cause of death in patients with SCI in the United States (128). In particular, hypertension resulting in substantial morbidity and mortality is an independent risk factor for ischemic cardiovascular diseases.

Treatments for cardiovascular disorders include risk factor reduction, pharmacologic therapy, invasive and interventional therapies, and electrical acupuncture (EA). Clinical and experimental studies suggest that acupuncture may be beneficial in severe cardiovascular disease manifestation, including hypertension, arrhythmias, and angina pectoris (129–131). Each of these conditions can be exacerbated by cardiovascular reflexes that lead to changes in heart rate, blood pressure, myocardial contractility, and/or myocardial oxygen demand during stress. As an alternative to EA, magnetic stimulation potentially can offer a noninvasive method of stimulating somatic nerves to achieve the same beneficial effects as EA (130) and with the unique benefit of not using the acupuncture needle. For example, magnetic stimulation-evoked antinociceptive effects through the opioid system (129, 131); and the underlying mechanism was demonstrated to be similar to EA (131).

The magnetic stimulator with a butterfly-shaped coil was driven by a stimulator through an isolation unit at a frequency of 2 Hz. The stimulation intensity was fixed at 30% of the maximal intensity for all experiments. Stimulation durations were three sets of eight minutes, interrupted by two five-minute rest periods without stimulation; the total duration of stimulation was 24 minutes for all experiments. In eight rats, after recording two reproducible control responses to gastric distension, magnetic stimulation (2 Hz, 30% of maximal intensity) was applied unilaterally at the Jianshi-Neiguan (P5–P6) acupoints for 24 minutes. In six control rats, after recording two reproducible control responses to gastric distension, the median nerve was transected and magnetic stimulation was applied (2 Hz, 30% intensity) unilaterally at P5–P6 for 24 minutes, to determine if the median nerve served as the afferent pathway for the magnetic stimulation response. To evaluate the role of the endogenous opioid system in the inhibitory effects of magnetic stimulation, we intravenously administrated the nonspecific opioid receptor antagonist naloxone. Gastric distension was repeated at 10 minutes intervals over 90 minutes.

After 24 minutes of magnetic stimulation at P5–P6, the pressor reflex during distension of the stomach was reduced from 23 ± 5 to 16 ± 4 mmHg, a response that persisted for 10 minutes after termination of the procedure. The extent of inhibitory effects during magnetic stimulation and EA was similar (32% vs. 35%, respectively). In another group of six animals in which magnetic stimulation at P5–P6 inhibited the reflex response to gastric distension (22 ± 4 to 13 ± 3 mmHg), it was found that intravenous naloxone partially restored the pressor response to 18 ± 4 mmHg, a value not significantly different from the pre-magnetic stimulation control period, and one which was significantly higher than the response to magnetic stimulation at P6 without naloxone. Intrathecal injection of δ and K-opioid receptor antagonists, ICI 174,864 and nor-BNI, immediately after termination of magnetic stimulation largely reversed its inhibition of the cardiovascular reflex. In contrast, the μ-opioid antagonist CTOP failed to alter the cardiovascular reflex.

FMS over the P5–P6 acupoint modulated the cardiovascular excitatory response induced by gastric distension in rats (132). The influence of EA at P5–P6 acupoints lasted longer than magnetic stimulation, suggesting differences in somatic input to the central nervous system. The inhibitory effects of magnetic stimulation were abolished by median nerve transection, indicating that this nerve served as the somatic afferent pathway in this response. The inhibitory effect of magnetic stimulation was reversed by intravenous naloxone as well as by δ and K but not by μ opioid receptor blockade at T4–T5 in the spinal cord, suggesting that opioids, especially enkephalins and dynorphin, contributed to the magnetic stimulation-mediated modulation of cardiovascular reflex responses.

SAFETY CONSIDERATIONS

The issue of safety of magnetic stimulation of the human nervous system has received significant attention, due to its clinical applications. Thus, many of the safety issues discussed here have been derived from studies using the skull and brain as a model. Consideration of the safety of magnetic stimulation can be divided into the following five main areas: magnetic effects, electrical effects, power dissipation, clinical side effects, and cardiac effects.

Magnetic Effects

The peak fields 5 cm below a 9-cm mean diameter coil, which is the common size for spinal nerve stimulation, are 1.4 T under the winding and 1.1 T on the axis of the coil. Current U.S. guidelines for whole body exposure to static magnetic fields during MRI imaging are 2 T. In 1987, a task group commissioned by the World Health Organization reported that there was no evidence of any adverse effects on human health due to short-term exposure to static fields of up to 2 T (133). The output from a magnetic stimulator is a brief pulse of magnetic field rather than a static field. Safety study and guidelines of exposure to pulsed magnetic fields have been studied in two recent reports (134, 135). However, there are no known reasons why purely magnetic effects should be greater in a pulsed field than a static one; hence, it could be argued that any clinically harmful properties of magnetic stimulation will be linked to the induced electric fields. Metal implants will have mechanical forces exerted on them due to induced currents. Patients with metal implants in the abdomen or the spine are not suitable for magnetic stimulation.

Electric Effects

A safety study that used a human brain as its model was conducted; calculations were based on a mean stimulating coil diameter of 9 cm, a stimulator figure of merit of $F = 19 \, J(1/2)$, and a pulse rise time of 140 ms. The maximum induced electric field was 260 V/m, with a maximum induced current density of 9.1 mA/cm^2. The induced electric fields were comparable with those used for peripheral stimulation. The maximum induced charge density per phase was 0.8 mC/cm^2. Agnew and McCreery (136) found no evidence of neural damage when stimulating at 50 Hz with a charge density of less than 10 mC/cm^2. Magnetic stimulation of the spinal nerves is similar to the stimulation of peripheral nerves in extremities, except when the neural foraminae are involved. Wherever foraminae exist, there is an opportunity to channel the current flow creating more focal stimulation. Current focusing makes stimulation of spinal nerves more precise and effective.

Power Dissipation

To raise the temperature of 1 cm^3 of water by 1°C, 4.2 J of energy is required. Assuming a similar specific heat capacity of water

for tissue and no thermal losses, the maximum temperature rise anywhere in the human tissue per stimulus will be less than 2×10^{-6}°C, which is two times lower than the value established by international standards for safety (137). Cumulative effects are also small. There is an enormous inherent amount of energy/heat (250 Joules/pulse) generated by the magnetic coil, however, that needs to be dissipated effectively for prolonged stimulation. The best solution to this concern is to use a water-cooled magnetic coil. It is able not only to carry away the heat generated by the coil, but it is also able to dissipate the heat generated by the human tissue.

Clinical Side Effects

Due to the absence of contact with the stimulated structure, magnetic stimulation is free of any traumatic risk, unlike needle electrode stimulation. At present, no side effects of magnetic stimulation have been reported; however, the technique does remain under some scrutiny when used for brain stimulation. It should be noted that the maximal charge induced by magnetic stimulation is 50 μC/pulse (corresponding to 0.05–0.0005% of the charges used in electro-convulsive therapy), and that the peak magnetic field is similar to the static fields used in some magnetic resonance imaging scanners. No hazard due to these fields has yet been reported despite many minutes of continuous exposure (133, 136) and weeks of transcranial magnetic stimulation (137). A few reports have shown that repetitive transcranial magnetic stimulation may result in increased seizure activities (138–140). Personal experience with long-term FMS of the respiratory muscles, bladder, or bowel did not yield significant adverse side effects (3, 141).

Cardiac Effects

Ventricular fibrillation did not occur in rats (3) when a coil was placed over the heart using a clinical stimulator, nor in experiments with anaesthetized dogs (142–144) using a clinical stimulator. Ventricular ectopic beats were produced in dogs using a purpose-designed stimulator with approximately 10 kJ of stored energy, a figure some 20 times greater than the capacity from clinical machines. It is possible that a magnetic stimulator could induce sufficient current and voltage in a cardiac pacemaker to damage its internal electronics if the stimulating coil was placed close to the implant. Thus, we would regard the presence of a pacemaker as a possible contra-indication and would never place a coil over such a device or directly over the heart.

SUMMARY

FMS is clearly an emerging technology with many potential clinical applications. This chapter has reviewed the basic principles of magnetic stimulation and clinical applications for patients with SCI. This chapter has also reviewed relevant clinical applications that FMS may be applied in patients with SCI or spinal cord disorders. FMS of the lower spinal nerves can produce substantial expiratory function that would mimic cough, or result in functional magnetic cough (FMC). FMS of the upper throracic nerves and/or the phrenic nerves can produce substantial inspiratory function; functional magnetic ventilation (FMV) has also been demonstrated to maintain ventilation for hours in canines.

FMS of the lower thoracic spinal nerves and/or lumbosacral nerves also demonstrated efficacy in improving bladder emptying, gastric emptying, gastrointestinal motility, and clonic transit in SCI; and successful functional magnetic micturition (FMM) and functional magnetic defecation (FMD) were also demonstrated in our subjects. Furthermore, our clinical studies also showed that using FMS, significant fibrinolytic activities were observed in normal and SCI; and FMS of the lower limb may eventually be proven to be an effective clinical alternative to current thromboembolism preventive measures.

In our recent animal investigations, FMS showed significant analgesic effects for pain relief. When applied to acupoints, FMS produced beneficial effects as EA. FMS has distinctive advantages when compared with the existing FES technology. FMS is able to stimulate multiple spinal nerves simultaneously for useful physiological functions. FMS is easy to use and does not require surgery or electrode implants, thus preventing complications such as infection, bleeding, wire breakage, implant failures, etc. FMS is not as painful as FES and is well tolerated by conscious individuals. FMS can be applied over clothing because it does not require skin contact or the use of electrode gel. FMS can be used as a tool for muscle conditioning. The applications of FMS in patients with SCI and other neurologically impaired individuals are expected to grow significantly in the future. The main limitations of the FMS technology are the size of the magnetic stimulator, the high power demand, and the stimulator's cost. We envision that home or portable FMS units will be available in the near future. We also expect that many patients and family members will find this technology and its many clinical applications can improve their function and quality of life.

References

1. Lin VWH, Hsiao I. *Functional magnetic stimulation. In: Lin V, ed. Spinal Cord Medicine: Principles and Practice.* New York: Demos Medical Publishing 749–764, 2003.
2. Bickford RG, Fremming BD. Neuronal stimulation by pulsed magnetic fields in animals and man. Digest of the 6th International Conference on Medical Electronics and Biological Engineering 1965; 112:6–7.
3. Polson MJR, Barker At, Gardiner S. The effect of rapid rise-time magnetic fields on the ECG of the rat. Clin Phys Physiol Meas 3:231–234, 1982.
4. Barker AT, Jalinous R, Freeston IL. Non-invasive magnetic stimulation of human motor cortex. Lancet 1:1106–1107, 1985.
5. Hess CW, Murray NM, Mills KR, Schriefer TN. Motor Evoked Potentials During Slow Wave Sleep and REM sleep. In: Non Invasive Stimulation of Brain and Spinal Cord: Fundamentals and Clinical Applications. Alan R. Liss, Inc. 1988; 85–92.
6. Amassian VE, Cracco RQ, Maccabee PJ. Focal stimulation of human cerebral cortex with the magnetic coil: A comparison with electrical stimulation. Electroenceph Clin Neurophysiol 74:401–416, 1989.
7. Katz B. Electric Excitation of Nerve. London: Oxford University Press. 1939.
8. Barker AT, Jalinous R, Freeston IL, Jaratt JA. Clinical evaluation of conduction time measurements in central motor pathways using magnetic stimulation of human brain. Lancet 1:1324–1326, 1986.
9. DiMarco AF, Kovvuri S, Pedtro J, Romaniuk JR, Supinski GS. Intercostal muscle pacing in quadriplegic patients. Am Rev Resp Dis 143:A473, 1991.
10. Lin VWH, Romaniuk JR, Supinski GS, DiMarco AF. Inspired volume production via direct intercostal muscle stimulation, Muscle & Nerve, 1992.
11. Lin VWH, Hsieh C, Hsiao IN, Canfield J. Functional magnetic stimulation of the expiratory muscles- A non-invasive and new method for restoring cough. J Appl Physiol 84:1144–1150, 1998.
12. Lin, VWH. Singh, R, Chitkara, I, Perkash. Functional magnetic stimulation for restoring cough in patients with tetraplegia. Arch Phys Med Rehabil 79:517–522, 1998.
13. Singh H, Magruder M, Bushnik T, Lin VWH. Expiratory muscle activation by functional magnetic stimulation of thoracic and lumbar spinal nerves. Crit Care Med 27(10):2201–05, 1999.
14. Lin VWH, Wolfe V, Perkash I. Micturition by functional magnetic stimulation. J Spinal Cord Med 20:218–226, 1997.
15. Lin VWH, Hsiao I, Perkash I. Micturition by functional magnetic stimulation in dogs—a preliminary report. J Neurourology Urodynamics 16(4):305–313, 1997.
16. Lin VWH, Nino-Murcia M, Frost F, Wolfe V, Hsiao I, Perkash I. Functional magnetic stimulation of the colon in patients with spinal cord injuries. Arch PM&R 82:167–173, 2001.
17. Maccabee PJ, Amassian VE, Eberle L, Rudell A, Cracco RQ, Lai KS. Measurement of the electric field induced into inhomogeneous volume conductors by magnetic coil: Applications to human spinal geometry. Electroenceph Clin Neurophysiol 81:224–237, 1991.
18. Roth BJ, Maccabee PJ, Eberle LP, Amassian VE, Hallett M, Cadwell J, Anselmi GD, Tatarian GT. In vitro evaluation of a 4-leaf coil design for magnetic stimulation of peripheral nerve. Encephalography Clin Neurophysiol 93:68–74, 1994.
19. Hsiao IN, Lin VWH. Improved coil design for functional magnetic stimulation of expiratory muscles. IEEE Trans Biomed Engineer, 48(6):684–94, 2001.
20. Lemons VR, Wagner FC Jr. Respiratory complications after cervical spinal cord injury. Spine 19(20):2315–20, 1994.
21. Fishburn MJ, Marino RJ, Ditunno JF. Atelectasis and pneumonia in acute spinal cord injury. Arch Phys Med Rehabil 1:197–200, 1990.
22. McMichan JC, Michel L, Westbrook PR. Pulmonary dysfunction following traumatic quadriplegia. JAMA 243: 528–531, 1980.
23. Roth EJ, Nussbaum SB, Berkowitz M, Primack S, Oken J, Powley S, Lu A. Pulmonary function testing in spinal cord injury: correlation with vital capacity. Paraplegia 33(8):454–457, 1995.
24. Hemingway A, Bors E, Hobby RP. An investigation of the pulmonary function in paraplegics. J Clin Invest 37:773–782, 1985.
25. James WS, Minh V, Minteer A, Moser KM. Cervical accessory respiratory muscles: function in a patient with a high cervical cord lesion. Chest 71:59–64, 1977.
26. Gausch PA, Linder SH, Williams T, Ryan S. A functional classification of respiratory compromise in spinal cord injury. Sci Nursing 8(1): 4–10, 1991.
27. Ledsome JR, Sharp JM. Pulmonary function in acute cervical cord injury. Am Rev Resp Dis 124:41–44, 1981.
28. Anke A, Aksnes AK, Stanghelle JK, Hjeltnes N. Lung volumes in tetraplegic patients according to cervical spinal cord injury level. Scan J of Rehab Med 25(2):73–77, 1993.
29. Hachen HJ. Idealized care of the acutely injured spinal cord in Switzerland. J Trauma 17:931–936, 1977.
30. O'Donohue WJ Jr, Baker JP, Bell GM, Muren O, Parker CL, Patterson JL Jr. Respiratory failure in neuromuscular disease. Management in a respiratory intensive care unit. JAMA 235(7):733–735, 1976.
31. Connors GL, Hilling L. Prevention, not just treatment. (Review) Respir Care Clin of North Am 4(1):1–12, 1998.
32. Braun SR, Giovannoni R O'Connor M. Improving the cough in patients with spinal cord injury. Am J Physical Med 63(1):1–10, 1984.
33. Chiappetta A, Bakerman R. High-frequency chest-wall oscillation in spinal muscular atrophy. J Respir Care Prac 8(4):112–114, 1995.
34. Dail CAW, Afield JE, Collier CR. Clinical aspects of glossopharyngeal breathing. JAMA 158: 445–469, 1955.
35. Gross D, Ladd HW, Riley EJ, Macklem PT, Grassino A. The effect of training on strength and endurance of the diaphragm in quadriplegia. Am J Med 68(1):27–35, 1980.
36. DiMarco AF, Altose MD, Cropp A. Activation of the inspiratory intercostal muscles by electrical stimulation of the spinal cord. Am Rev Respir Dis 136:1385–1390, 1987.
37. DiMarco AF, Budzinska K, Supinski G. Artificial ventilation by means of electrical activation of the intercostal/accessory muscles alone. Am Rev Respir Dis 139:961–967, 1989.
38. DiMarco AF, Onders RP, Ignagni A, Kowalski KE, Stefan SL, Mortimer JT. Phrenic nerve pacing via intramuscular diaphragm electrodes in tetraplegic subjects, Chest 127:671–678, 2005.
39. Lin VWH, JR Romaniuk, A DiMarco. Functional magnetic stimulation of the respiratory muscles in dogs. Muscle Nerve 21:1048–1057, 1998.

40. Linder SH. Functional electrical stimulation to enhance cough in quadriplegia. Chest 103:166–169, 1993.
41. Jaeger RJ, Langbein EW, Kralj AR. Augmenting cough by FES in tetraplegia: a comparison of results at three clinical centers. Basic & Applied Myology 4(2):195–200, 1994.
42. Glenn WW, Holcomb WG, Hogan J, Matano I, Gee JB, Motoyama EK, et al. Diaphragm pacing by radiofrequency transmission in the treatment of chronic ventilatory insufficiency. Present status. J Thorac Cardiovasc Surg 66(4):505–520, 1973.
43. Glenn WWL. The treatment of respiratory paralysis by diaphragm pacing. Ann Thorac Surg 30:106–109, 1980.
44. Campbell EMJ. The role of scalene and sternomastoid muscles in breathing in normal subjects: An electromyographic study. J Anat 89:378–386, 1955.
45. Taylor A. The contribution of the intercostal muscles to the effect of respiration in man. J Physiol 151:390–402, 1960.
46. DiMarco AF, Supinski GS, Petro JA, Takaoka Y. Evaluation of intercostal pacing to provide artificial ventilation in quadriplegics. Am J Respir Crit Care Med 150(4):934–940, 1994.
47. Stani U, Kandare F, Jaeger R, Sorli, J. Functional electrical stimulation of abdominal muscles to augment tidal volume in spinal cord injury. IEEE Trans Rehab Eng 8:30–34, 2000.
48. DiMarco AF, Romaniuk JR, Supinski GS. Electrical activation of the expiratory muscles to restore cough. Am J Respir Crit Care Med 151(5):1466–1471, 1995.
49. DiMarco AF, Kowalski KE, Geertman RT, Hromyak DR. Spinal cord stimulation: a new method to produce an effective cough in patients with spinal cord injury. Am J Respir Crit Care Med. 173(12):1386–1389, 2006.
50. Lissens MA. Motor evoked potentials of the human diaphragm elicited through magnetic transcranial brain stimulation. J Neurolog Sci 124:204–207, 1994.
51. Chokroverty S, Deutsch A, Guha C, Gonzalez A, Kwan P, Burger R, Goldberg J. Thoracic spinal nerve and root conduction: a magnetic stimulation study. Muscle Nerve 18(9):987–991, 1995.
52. Lissens MA, Vanderstraeten GG. Motor evoked potentials of the human respiratory muscles. Muscle Nerve 19:1204–1205, 1996.
53. Similowski T, Fleury B, Launois S, Cathala HP, Bouche P, Derenne JP. Cervical magnetic stimulation: a new painless method for bilateral phrenic nerve stimulation in conscious humans. J Appl Physiol. 67:1311–1318, 1989.
54. Wragg S, Aquiline R, Moran J, M. Ridding M, et al. Comparison of cervical magnetic stimulation and bilateral percutaneous electrical stimulation of the phrenic nerves in normal subjects. Eur Respir 7:1778–1792, 1994.
55. Mills GH, Kyroussis D, Hamnegard CH, Polkey MI, Green M, Moxman J. Bilateral magnetic stimulation of the phrenic nerves from an anterolateral approach. Am J Respir Crit Care Med 154:1099–1105, 1996.
56. Laghi F, Harrison MJ, Tobin MJ. Comparison of magnetic and electrical phrenic nerve stimulation in assessment of diaphragmatic contractility. J Appl Physiol 80:1731–42, 1996.
57. Lin VWH, Romaniuk JR, Supinski GS, DiMarco AF. Inspiratory volume production via direct intercostal muscle stimulation. Muscle Nerve 15:1088, 1992.
58. Lin VWH, Romaniuk JR, Allen C, Cadwell J, DiMarco AF. High frequency magnetic stimulation of the inspiratory muscles. Muscle Nerve 16:1088, 1992.
59. Lin VWH, Hsieh C, Hsiao IN, Canfield J. Functional magnetic stimulation for cough. Am J Respir Crit Care Med 155:A917, 1997.
60. Lin VWH, Hsiao I, Zhu E. Functional magnetic stimulation for conditioning respiratory muscles. Arch PM&R, 82:162–6, 2001.
61. Glenn WW, Hogan JF, Phelps ML. Ventilatory support of the quadriplegic patient with respiratory paralysis by diaphragm pacing. Surgical Clinics of North America 60:1055–1078, 1980.
62. Garrido-Garcia H, Martin-Escribano P, Palomera-Frade J, Arroyo O, Alonso-Calderon JL, Mazaira-Alvarez J. Transdiaphragmatic pressure in quadriplegic individuals ventilated by diaphragmatic pacemaker. Thorax 51:420–423, 1996.
63. Glenn WWL, Phelps ML, Elefteriades JA, Dentz B, Hogan JF. Twenty years of experience in phrenic nerve stimulation to pace the diaphragm. PACE 9:780–783, 1986.
64. Peterson DK, Nochomovitz M, DiMarco AF, Mortimer JT. Intramuscular electrical activation of the phrenic nerve. IEEE Trans Biomed Eng. BME 33:342–351, 1986.
65. Nochomovitz ML, DiMarco AF, Mortimer JT, Chemiack NS. Diaphragm activation with intramuscular stimulation in dogs. Am. Rev. Resp. Dis 127:325–329, 1983.
66. Peterson DK, Nochomovitz ML, Stellato TA, Mortimer JT. Long-term intramuscular electrical activation of the phrenic nerve: efficacy as a ventilatory prosthesis. IEEE Trans. Biomed. Eng 41:1127–1135, 1994.
67. DiMarco AF, Onders RP, Kowalski KE, Miller ME, Ferek S, Mortimer JT. Phrenic nerve pacing in a tetraplegic patient via intramuscular diaphragm electrodes. Am J Respir Crit Care Med 166:1604–1606, 2002.
68. DiMarco AF, Budzinska K, Supinski GS. Artificial ventilation by means of electrical activation of the intercostal/accessory muscles alone in anesthetized dogs. Am Rev Resp Dis 139:961–967, 1989.
69. DiMarco AF, Kovvuri S, Pedtro J, Romaniuk JR, Supinski GS. Intercostal muscle pacing in quadriplegic patients. Am Rev Resp Dis 143:A473, 1991.
70. Stanic U, Kandare F, Jaeger R, Sorli J. Functional electrical stimulation of abdominal muscles to augment tidal volume in spinal cord injury. IEEE Trans Rehab Eng 8:30–34, 2000.
71. Glenn WW. Diaphragm pacing: present status. Pacing Clin Electrophysiol 1:357–370, 1978.
72. Goldhill DR, Whelpton R, Winyard JA, Wilkinson KA. Gastric emptying in patients the day after cardiac surgery. Anaesthesia 50: 122–125, 1995.
73. Condon RE, Cowles VE, Schulte WJ, Frantzides CT, Mahoney JL, Sarna SK. Resolution of postoperative ileus in humans. Ann Surg 203: 574–581, 1986.
74. Camilleri M, Bharucha AE. Gastrointestinal dysfunction in neurological disease. Sem Neurol 16: 203–216, 1996.
75. Apple DF. A chronicle of progress. Paraplegia 28:535–536, 1990.
76. Gore RM, Mintzer RA, Calenoff L. Gastrointestinal complications of spinal cord injury. Spine 6:538–544, 1981.
77. Harari D, Sarkarati M, Gurwitz JH, McGlinchey-Berroth G, Minaker KL. Constipation-related symptoms and bowel program concerning individuals with spinal cord injury. Spinal Cord 35:394–401, 1997.
78. Stone JM, Nino-Murcia M, Wolfe VA, Perkash I. Chronic gastrointestinal problems in spinal cord injury patients: a prospective analysis. Am J Gastroenterol Sep 85(9):114–119, 1990.
79. Glickman S, Kamm MA. Bowel dysfunction in spinal cord injury patients. Lancet 347:1651–1653, 1996.
80. Menardo G, Bausano G, Corazziari E, Fazio A, Marangi A, Genta V, et al. Large-bowel transit in patients with paraplegia. Gut 25:1314, 1984.
81. Nino-Murcia M, Stone JM, Chang PJ, Perkash I. Colonic transit in spinal cord-injured patients. investigative radiology 25(2):109–112, 1990.
82. Keshavarzian A, Barnes WE, Bruninga K, Nemchausky B, Mermall H, Bushnell D. Delayed colonic transit in spinal cord-injured patients measured by indium-111 amberlite scintigraphy. Am J Gastroenterol 90 (8):1295–1300, 1995.
83. Beuret-Blanquart F, Weber J, Gouverneur JP, Demangeon S, Denis P. Colonic transit time and anorectal manometric anomalies in 19 patients with complete transection of the spinal cord. J Auton Nerv Syst 30:199–207, 1990.
84. Menardo G, Bausano G, Corazziari E, Fazio A, Marangi A, Genta V, et al. Large-bowel transit in paraplegic patients. Dis Colon Rectum 30(12):924–928, 1987.
85. Stein RB, Gordon T, Jefferson J, Sharfenberger A, Yang JF, Totosy de Zepetnek J, Belanger M. Optimal stimulation of paralyzed muscle after human spinal cord injury. Amer Physiol Soc 72(4):1393–1400, 1992.
86. Kelly SR, Shashidharan M, Borwell B, Tromans AM, Finnis D, Grundy DJ. The role of intestinal stoma in patients with spinal cord injury. Spinal Cord 37(3):211–214, 1999.
87. Hymes AC. Electrical surface stimulation for treatment and prevention of ileus and atelectasis. Surg Forum 25:222–224, 1974.
88. Richardson RR, Cerullo LJ. Transabdominal neurostimulation in treatment of neurogenic ileus. Appl Neurophysiol 42:375–382, 1979.
89. Richardson RR, Meyer RR, Raimondi AJ. Transabdominal neurostimulation in acute spinal cord injuries. Spine 4(1):47–51, 1979.
90. Frost F, Hartwig D, Jaeger R, Leffler E, Wu Y. Electrical stimulation of the sacral dermatomes in spinal cord injury: effect on rectal manometry and bowel emptying. Arch Phys Med Rehabil 74:696–701, 1993.
91. Varma JS, Binnie N, Smith AN, Creasey GH, Edmond P. Differential effects of sacral anterior root stimulation on anal sphincter and colorectal motility in spinally injured man. Brit J Surg 73:478–482, 1986.

92. MacDonagh RP, Sun WM, Smallwood R, Forster DMC, Read NW. Control of defecation in patients with spinal injuries by stimulation of sacral anterior nerve roots. Brit Med J 300:1494–1497, 1990.

93. Binnie, NR, Smith AN, Creasey GH, Edmond P. Constipation associated with chronic spinal cord injury: the effect of pelvic parasympathetic stimulation by the Brindley stimulator. Paraplegia 29:463–469, 1991.

94. Van der Sijp JRM, Kamm MA, Nightingale JMD, Britton KE, Mather SJ, Morris GP, Kermans LMA, Lennard-Jones JE. Radioisotope determination of regional colonic Transit in severe constipation: comparison with radiopaque markers. Gut 34:402–408, 1993.

95. Varma JS. Autonomic influences on colorectal motility and pelvic surgery. World J Surg 16(5):811–9, 1992.

96. Lin VWH, Hsiao I, Xu, H, Bushnik T, Perkash I. Functional magnetic stimulation facilitates gastrointestinal transit in rats. Muscles Nerve, 23:919–924, 2000.

97. Lin VWH, Hsiao, I, Perkash I, Goodwin D. Functional magnetic stimulation facilitates colonic transit in rats. Arch Phys Med Rehabil 82(7):969–72, 2001.

98. Lin VWH, Kim K, Hsiao I, Brown W. Functional magnetic stimulation facilitates gastric emptying. Arch Phys Med Rehabil;83(6):806–810, 2002.

99. Bradley WE, et al. Use of a radio transmitter receiver unit for the treatment of neurogenic bladder. a preliminary report. J Neurosurgery 19:782–786, 1962.

100. Hald T, et. al., Clinical experience with a radio-linked bladder stimulator. J Urol 39:73–83, 1967.

101. Stenberg CC, Burnette HW, Bunts RC. Electrical stimulation of human neurogenic bladder: experience with four patients. J Urol 140(12):1331–1339, 1988.

102. Halverstadt DB, Parry WL. Electronic stimulation of the human bladder: nine years later. J Urol 13:341–344, 1975.

103. Habib HN. Experience and recent contributions in sacral nerve stimulation for voiding in both human and animal. Brit J Urol 39:73–83, 1967.

104. Nashold BS, et al. Electromicturition in paraplegia. Arch Surg 104:195–202, 1972.

105. Sarramon JP, et al. Neurostimulation medullaire dans les vessies neurogenes centrales. Acta Urol Belg 47:129–138, 1979.

106. Li US, et al. Role of electric stimulation in bladder evacuation following spinal cord trauma. J Urol 147:1429–1434, 1992.

107. Brindley GS, et al., Sacral anterior root stimulators for bladder control in paraplegia: the first 50 cases. J Neurol Neurosurg Psychiatry 49:1104–1114, 1986.

108. Rijkhoff NJ. Neuroprostheses to treat neurogenic bladder dysfunction: current status and future perspectives. Childs Nerv Syst 20:75–86, 2004.

109. Agu O, Hamilton G, Baker D. Graduated compression stockings in the prevention of venous thromboembolism. Br J Surg 86(8), 992–1004, 1999.

110. Katz RT, Green D, Sullivan T, Yarkony G. Functional electric stimulation to enhance systemic fibrinolytic activity in spinal cord injury patients. Arch Phys Med Rehabil 68, 423–426, 1987.

111. Merli GJ, Herbison GJ, Ditunno JF, Weitz HH, Henzes JH, Park CH, Jaweed MM. Deep vein thrombosis: prophylaxis in acute spinal cord injured patients. Arch Phys Med Rehabil 69(9):661–664, 1988.

112. Lin VWH, Perkash A, Liu H, Todd D, Hsiao I, Perkash I. Functional magnetic stimulation—A new modality for enhancing systemic fibrinolysis. Arch Phys Med Rehab 80:545–550, 1999.

113. Carroll, C, Tramer, M, McQuay, H, Nye, B, Moore, A. Transcutaneous electrical nerve stimulation in labour pain: a systematic review. Br J Obstet Gynaecol 104:169–175, 1997.

114. Carroll, D, Tramer, M, McQuay, H, Nye, B, Moore, A. Randomization is important in studies with pain outcomes: systematic review of transcutaneous electrical nerve stimulation in acute postoperative pain. Br J Anaesth 77: 798–803, 1996.

115. Gadsby JG, Flowerdew, MW. Transcutaneous electrical nerve stimulation and acupuncture-like transcutaneous electrical nerve stimulation for chronic low back pain. Cochrane Database Syst Rev CD000210, 2000.

116. Ghoname, EA, Craig, WF, White, PF, Ahmed, HE, et al. Percutaneous electrical nerve stimulation for low back pain; a randomized crossover study. JAMA 281:818–823, 1999.

117. Ghoname EA, White PF, Ahmed HE, Hamza MA, Craig WF Noe CE. Percutaneous electrical nerve stimulation: an alternative to TENS in the management of sciatica. Pain 83:193–199, 1999.

118. Long DM. The current status of electrical stimulation of the nervous system for the relief of chronic pain. Surg Neurol 49:142–144, 1998.

119. Simpson, BA. Spinal cord stimulation. Br J Neurosurg 11:5–11, 1997.

120. Lin VWH, Kingery WS, Hsiao IN. Functional magnetic stimulation over the lumbosacral spine evokes a prolonged analgesic response in rats. Clin Neurophysiol. 113(7):1006–1012, 2002.

121. Danziger N, Rozenberg S, Bourgeois P, Charpentier G, Willer JC. Depressive effects of segmental and heterotopic application of transcutaneous electrical nerve stimulation and piezo-electric current on lower limb nociceptive flexion reflex in human subjects. Arch Phys Med Rehabil 79:191–200, 1998.

122. Garrison DW, Foreman RD. Effects of transcutaneous electrical nerve stimulation (TENS) on spontaneous and noxiously evoked dorsal horn cell activity in cats with transected spinal cords. Neurosci Lett 216(2):125–128, 1996.

123. McDowell BC, McCormack K, Walsh DM, Baxter DG, Allen JM. Comparative analgesic effects of H-wave therapy and transcutaneous electrical nerve stimulation on pain threshold in humans. Arch Phys Med Rehabil 80(9):1001–1004, 1999.

124. Romita VV, Henry JL. Intense peripheral electrical stimulation differentially inhibits tail vs. limb withdrawal reflexes in the rat. Brain Res 720:45–53, 1996.

125. Woolf CJ, Mitchell D, Barrett GD. Antinociceptive effect of peripheral segmental electrical stimulation in the rat. Pain 8: 237–252, 1980;.

126. Ellis WV. Pain control using high-intensity pulsed magnetic stimulation. Bioelectromagnetics 14:553–556, 1993.

127. Myers J, Lee M, Kiratli J. Cardiovascular disease in spinal cord injury: an overview of prevalence, risk, evaluation, and management. Am J Phys Med Rehabil. 86(2):142–152, 2007.

128. Cheung LL, Li P, Wong C. The Mechanism of Acupuncture Therapy and Clinical Case Studies. New York: Taylor and Francis, 2001.

129. Li P, Rowshan K, Crisostomo M, Tjen-A-Looi SC, Longhurst JC. Effect of electroacupuncture on pressor reflex during gastric distension. Am J Physiol Regul Integr Comp Physiol 283:R1335-R1345, 2002.

130. Zhou W, Fu LW, Tjen-A-Looi SC, Li P, Longhurst JC. Afferent mechanisms underlying stimulation modality-related modulation of acupuncture-related cardiovascular responses. J Appl Physiol 98:872–880, 2005.

131. Zhou W, Hsiao I, Lin V, Longhurst J. Modulation of cardiovascular excitatory responses in rats by magnetic stimulation: role of the spinal cord. J Appl Physiol 100:926–932, 2006.

132. Saunders RD. Task group on static and slowly varying magnetic fields (up to 300 Hz). Radio Protect Bull 78:11–14, 1987.

133. Schaefer DJ, Bourland JD, Nyenhuis JA. Review of patient safety in time-varying gradient fields. J Magn Reson Imaging 12(1):20–29, 2000.

134. Schulze-Bonhage A, Scheufler K, Zentner J, Elger CE. Safety of single and repetitive focal transcranial magnetic stimuli as assessed by intracranial EEG recordings in patients with partial epilepsy. J Neurol 246(10):914–919, 1999.

135. Agnew WF, McCreery. Considerations for safety in the use of extracranial stimulation for motor evoked potential. Neurosurgery 20:143–147, 1987.

136. Loo C, Sachdev P, Elsayed H, McDarmont B, Mitchell P, Wilkinson M, Parker G, Gandevia S. Effects of a 2- to 4-week course of repetitive transcranial magnetic stimulation (rTMS) on neuropsychologic functioning, electroencephalogram, and auditory threshold in depressed patients. Biol Psychiatry 49(7):615–623, 2001.

137. Barker AT, Freeston IL, Jalinous R, Jaratt JA. Magnetic stimulation of the human brain and peripheral nervous system: an introduction and the results of an initial clinical evaluation. Neurosurgery 20:100–109, 1987.

138. Classen J, Witte OW. Epileptic seizures triggered directly by focal transcranial magnetic stimulation. Electroencephalogr Clin Neurophysiol 94:19–25, 1995.

139. Wassermann EM, Cohen LG, Flitman SS, Chen R, Hallett M. Seizures in healthy people with repeated "safe" trains of transcranial magnetic stimuli. Lancet 347:825–826, 1996.

140. Pascual-Leonè A, Vals-Sole J, Brasil-Neto JP, Cohen LG, Hallett M. Seizure induction and transcranial magnetic stimulation. Lancet 339:997, 1992.

141. McRobbie DM, Foster MA. Cardiac responses to pulsed magnetic fields with regard to safety in NMR imaging. Phys Med Biol 30:695–702, 1985.

142. Bourland JD, Nyenhuis JA, Schaefer DJ. Physiologic effects of intense MR imaging gradient fields. Neuroimaging Clin N Am 9(2):363–77, 1999.

143. Yamaguchi M, Andoh T, Goto T, Hosono A, Kawakami T, Okumura F, Takenaka T, Yamamoto I. Effects of strong pulsed magnetic fields on the cardiac activity of an open chest dog. IEEE Trans Biomed Eng 41(12):1188–1191, 1994.

75 Restoration of Ventilation and Cough with Functional Electrical Stimulation: Patient Evaluation and Comparison of Currently Available Systems

Anthony F. DiMarco

Individuals with spinal cord injury (SCI) often suffer from respiratory muscle paralysis resulting in severe compromise of their pulmonary function. The significance of this loss in motor function is reflected in the fact that a substantial portion of the morbidity and mortality in the SCI population occurs secondary to pulmonary complications (12, 13, 23, 96, 116, 128, 131). Moreover, loss of respiratory muscle function results in significant discomfort, inconvenience, and much greater health care costs (55, 71, 79, 84, 96, 119). Patients with high cervical SCI are often dependent upon mechanical ventilatory support, as interruption of the descending bulbospinal respiratory tracts to the inspiratory motoneurons in the spinal cord results in paralysis of the diaphragm and inspiratory intercostal muscles. Although effective in maintaining life support, mechanical ventilation is associated with significant complications, including pneumonia, atelectasis, barotrauma, and higher rate of hospitalization (19, 55, 58, 110). Respiratory failure secondary to SCI is also associated with a significantly higher mortality (23, 116). Individuals with paralysis of the major expiratory muscles lack an effective cough mechanism, reducing their ability to clear airway secretions (22, 55, 83). Consequently, these patients are at a significantly higher risk of developing respiratory tract infections, including bronchitis and pneumonia (14, 79, 96), a leading cause of death in patients with SCI (24, 25, 58, 71, 84, 118, 119). These disadvantages have led clinicians to seek alternative methods of ventilatory support (4–7) and airway clearance (34–36, 80, 81, 86, 90, 91).

The degree of respiratory muscle impairment resulting from SCI can be predicted by the level of injury and knowledge of the innervations of the major respiratory muscles. Each hemidiaphragm is innervated by a single phrenic nerve, which is formed by the cervical rootlets from the C3–C5 spinal cord segments. The inspiratory intercostal muscles, innervated primarily by the upper thoracic intercostal nerves (T1–T6), are also an important muscle group, contributing 35–40% of the inspiratory capacity. As the diaphragm is the major inspiratory muscle, ventilation can be maintained easily by contraction of this muscle alone. Therefore, patients with spinal cord lesions below C5 can generally breathe spontaneously without ventilatory assistance. The expiratory intercostal and abdominal muscles are the major expiratory muscles and are innervated primarily by the thoracic roots (T6–T12). Therefore, patients with mid-thoracic spinal cord injuries and higher have significant expiratory muscle paralysis impairing their ability to generate an effective cough.

Fortunately, except for the interruption of nervous input from the respiratory centers in the medulla, the somatic neuromuscular and mechanical functions of the respiratory apparatus including the lungs, respiratory muscles, and their respective nervous innervations below the level of spinal cord injury remain intact in most patients with SCI. For this reason, these motor axons and their respective muscle targets are amenable to stimulation techniques to restore function.

Although there has been significant progress in the restoration of both inspiratory and expiratory muscle function, the greatest emphasis and clinical success has been on restoration of ventilation via electrical activation of the diaphragm (26, 28, 30, 63, 64, 66). In fact, bilateral phrenic nerve stimulation to activate the diaphragm, a form of functional electrical stimulation (70), has been a clinically accepted modality in the management of patients with ventilator-dependent tetraplegia for several decades (67, 68). The major portion of this chapter is therefore devoted to this subject. Methods to activate the inspiratory intercostal muscles to restore breathing and expiratory muscles to restore cough are still under development and are also reviewed.

DIAPHRAGMATIC PACING (DP): RHYTHMIC PHRENIC NERVE STIMULATION TO MAINTAIN VENTILATORY SUPPORT

Respiratory failure requiring some form of artificial ventilatory support is common in patients with cervical spinal cord injury. In fact, in the acute phase of injury, 15–20% of patients develop respiratory insufficiency (119). Fortunately, neurologic function improves in most patients such that long-term ventilatory

978

support is not required. Nonetheless, ~5% require life-long ventilatory assistance (15) and are subject to the associated restrictions in lifestyle, physical discomfort, higher medical costs, and significantly higher morbidity and mortality (25, 58, 71, 116, 119, 129). It is also important to recognize that the average age at the time of injury is in the fourth decade and many patients can be expected to live 20 years or longer with this impairment, assuming they survive the first year (119). As a form of artificial ventilatory support, diaphragmatic pacing (DP) mimics natural physiology more closely and alleviates many of the disadvantages of mechanical ventilation.

Electrical activation of the phrenic nerves to restore breathing is not a new concept. In fact, over two centuries ago, Caldani demonstrated that diaphragm contraction could be achieved by the application of electrical stimulation to the phrenic nerve (11). In the early nineteenth century, Ure applied electrical stimulation on a condemned criminal shortly after his execution (123). Small incisions were made in the neck and beneath the fifth costal cartilage thru which wires of a voltaic battery were applied. The diaphragm was noted to contract and ventilation restored. In the latter half of the nineteenth century, Duchenne proclaimed that phrenic nerve stimulation was the best method of restoring natural ventilation (49). Electrical stimulation applied over the posterior borders of the sternocleidomastoid muscles via moistened sponges resulted in activation of the diaphragm and was deemed an effective method of artificial ventilation. In the 1940s, Sarnoff demonstrated that percutaneous stimulation of the phrenic nerves could maintain adequate levels of ventilation even in patients with respiratory failure secondary to poliomyelitis (112, 130). These primitive techniques, however, were not reliable for long-term use, limiting their broad application.

Glenn and co-investigators in the 1960s and 1970s at Yale University performed the necessary basic science and clinical studies that allowed DP to become a clinical reality (60, 61, 63–65). It was this work that first demonstrated that artificial ventilatory support could be provided safely and effectively to support ventilation for people with spinal cord injury. They developed a fully implantable receiver that could be activated via radiofrequency waves transmitted through the chest wall. By this method, the receiver detects the radiofrequency signal and triggers electrical impulses that stimulate the phrenic nerves and activate the diaphragm. These investigators also developed preoperative assessment methods, surgical techniques for electrode placement, and appropriate stimulation parameters necessary to maintain complete ventilatory support.

Subsequent studies have been performed refining the concept with improved electrode design (59, 63, 64, 66-68, 102, 120, 121) and less invasive methods of electrode placement (38, 39, 104, 115). In fact, recent studies indicate that the phrenic nerve branches can be activated with electrodes positioned in the diaphragm near the motor points by laparoscopic surgery, obviating the need for more invasive surgery (1, 37, 115).

DIAPHRAGMATIC PACING COMPARED WITH MECHANICAL VENTILATION: BENEFITS, PROBLEMS, AND POTENTIAL INNOVATIONS

Mechanical ventilation has been and remains a life-saving modality for patients with acute and chronic respiratory failure, including those with cervical spinal cord injury. Although cumbersome,

mechanical ventilators easily provide sufficient inspired volumes to maintain blood gas homeostasis. In fact, many patients find comfort in the high degree of reliability these time-tested machines provide. Built-in alarm systems provide an additional safety measure by alerting health care providers of respiratory system abnormalities (92). The specificity of alarms also assist health care personnel in pinpointing problems, which can then be readily addressed (92). Unfortunately, the rapid rise and fall of tracheal pressure during mechanical ventilation via a tracheostomy limits the spontaneity and capacity for sustained speech (10). With utilization of positive end-expiratory pressure (PEEP) and prolonged inspiratory time, however, swings in tracheal pressure can be reduced to improve speech quality (73, 75). Alternatively, speech can be improved by placing a one-way speaking valve fitted to the tracheostomy. With this modality, the cuff must be maintained in a deflated state to allow exhaled air to pass across the vocal cords. Although most patients with ventilator-dependent tetraplegia are ventilated via tracheostomy, Bach and colleagues (4, 5) have shown that many of these patients can be decannulated and treated with noninvasive mechanical ventilation. Patients use their epiglottises and vocal cords to modulate inspired volume and expectorate secretions. This method results in an overall reduction in secretions, fewer hospitalizations, and reductions in health care costs. Possibly secondary to concerns of safety and reliability, however, most individuals with ventilator-dependent tetraplegia are still managed with a tracheostomy.

Although extremely reliable, mechanical ventilation is associated with significant morbidity, mortality, and inconvenience (19, 55, 58, 110). Some of the disadvantages associated with mechanical ventilation include physical discomfort, fear of disconnection, and difficulty with speech (10, 26). Mobility is of particular concern. The requirement for connection to a large mechanical box with attached tubing is cumbersome, precarious, and extremely restrictive. Other important issues stem from patient and caregiver anxiety and embarrassment associated with the ventilator and attached tubing. Although DP has not been shown to reduce long-term morbidity or mortality, this modality provides significant and distinct advantages compared to mechanical ventilation (Table 75.1).

Most patients that use DP realize an improved sense of well being and overall health (10, 20, 26, 27, 51, 68, 78, 99). It is not surprising that they describe feeling "more normal" since the noise of the ventilator and attached tubing are eliminated. Although of little concern in the home setting, elimination of ventilator noise is important while in public, particularly at social events. Because ventilator tubing is unnecessary, tension on the tracheostomy tube and fear of ventilator disconnection are eliminated. Moreover, the fact that an individual is maintained on artificial ventilatory support is not detectable to the casual observer. In a recent prospective study over a 20-year period (72), the incidence of respiratory tract infections was found to be significantly lower in patients treated with DP compared to those treated with mechanical ventilation. Although not statistically significant, there was also a tendency for improved survival in the DP group (72).

DP results in more physiologic negative pressure breathing. Negative pressure ventilation may reduce the incidence of barotrauma and may also have beneficial cardiovascular effects (52, 87, 125). Because the size of the breath is smaller and speech can only take place during expiration with DP compared to

Table 75.1   Potential Benefits of Diaphragmatic Pacing

A. Improved Quality of Life
  1. Subjective sense of more normal breathing
     a. Utilization of breathing muscles
     b. Negative pressure respiratory support
  2. Reduced anxiety and embarrassment
     a. Elimination of ventilator noise
     b. Elimination of fear of ventilator disconnection
     c. Elimination of ventilator tubing
     d. Daytime closure of tracheostomy
  3. Improved comfort level
     a. Elimination of pull of ventilator tubing
     b. Negative pressure breathing
  4. Improved speech
  5. Restoration of olfactory sensation
  6. Increased mobility
     a. Easier transport outside the home
     b. Easier transfer to and from bed
B. Reduced Overall Costs
  1. Reduction or elimination of ventilator supplies
  2. Reduced level of nursing and respiratory therapy
     services

Reproduced with permission of Thomas Land Publishers, Inc. from DiMarco AF. Diaphragm pacing in patients with spinal cord injury. Top Spinal Cord Inj Rehabil 1999; 5:6–20. www.thomasland.com.

mechanical ventilation, speech is usually characterized by low volume, short phrases, and long inspiratory pauses (10). The quality of speech, however, is often improved because ventilator noise is eliminated. In the upright postures, speech can be improved with use of an abdominal binder (74), which elastically compresses the abdominal contents, thereby lengthening the diaphragm and increasing its contractile force, resulting in an increase in tidal volume. As a result of the increase in tidal volume, voice amplitude and quality improve. The quality of olfaction is also poor with mechanical ventilation. With DP and the redirection of airflow around the nasal mucus membranes, the sense of smell is restored. Moreover, improved olfaction contributes to improved life quality measures (2).

Perhaps one of the most important benefits of DP compared to mechanical ventilation, however, is a marked improvement in patient mobility (30, 48, 52, 53, 122). Patient travel outside the home is much easier, allowing greater participation in social events, rehabilitation programs, and in some cases has facilitated achievement of gainful employment (28, 37, 38). Even activity at home, such as transfers from bed to chair, is much less difficult and cumbersome. It should be noted, however, that the benefits of DP may vary considerably between individuals. Careful screening must be performed, therefore, before undertaking DP.

Initiation of DP is very expensive. With earlier devices requiring a thoracotomy and implantation of electrodes on the phrenic nerves, cost exceeded $100,000 US. With the institution of intramuscular DP, which can be performed as an out-patient (37, 38), however, the costs are significantly lower. Even with the higher figure associated with conventional DP, however, cost comparisons with mechanical ventilation are quite favorable, as patients can be transferred to less intensive and therefore less expensive care settings (26, 29, 57, 72). Moreover, most patients

undergoing DP can be expected to live many years on ventilatory support (119). Long-term, therefore, the high initial costs of DP are more than offset by the savings associated with the maintenance supplies required for mechanical ventilation.

PATIENT REQUIREMENTS FOR DIAPHRAGMATIC PACING: VENTILATOR-DEPENDENT WITH INTACT PHRENIC NERVE FUNCTION

Individuals with ventilator-dependent tetraplegia and intact phrenic nerve and diaphragm function are candidates for DP. Unfortunately, many patients with cervical spinal cord injury have also sustained injury to the phrenic motoneuron pools and/or the phrenic nerves directly and therefore are not candidates for pacing (26, 45). It is imperative, therefore, that the integrity of phrenic nerve function be established. The presence of significant lung, chest wall, or primary muscle diseases may also prevent successful pacing (63, 66–68, 103).

As mentioned previously, many patients with cervical spinal cord injury and respiratory failure can eventually be weaned from mechanical ventilation (15). Although the time course of recovery of respiratory function varies among patients, the degree of impairment is most likely permanent at one year post-injury (105). Given the high cost and invasive nature of conventional DP, this procedure is not generally performed prior to this time.

In all patients, attempts should be made to wean ventilator-dependent patients off mechanical support. Weaning parameters, including vital capacity and maximum inspiratory pressure (MIP) generation, should be assessed. Vital capacity values of <10 ml/kg and MIP measurements of <20 cmH$_2$O suggest inadequate inspiratory muscle function to support spontaneous breathing (105). In some patients with sufficient inspiratory muscle function, it is possible that noninvasive ventilation may be a suitable alternative to DP (6, 7).

Psychosocial factors should also be considered in the evaluation of the patients being considered for DP (26, 38, 52). Goal-oriented individuals with the desire to improve mobility and function more independently are optimal candidates for this modality. Depending upon individual circumstances, the level of motivation and cooperation of family members may also be important. DP is most likely to be successful in situations in which the patient and family seek to improve the overall health, social interaction, and occupational potential of the spinal cord-injured individual. Prior to a formal technical evaluation, therefore, psychosocial assessments should be performed. The evaluation process for DP is shown in Figure 75.1.

DIAPHRAGMATIC PACING: EVALUATION OF PHRENIC NERVE FUNCTION

The technical success of DP is highly dependent upon adequate phrenic nerve function. Consequently, phrenic nerve function must be assessed in all prospective patients (37, 59, 66). This assessment should include measurements of phrenic nerve conduction times (68, 93, 95). This method entails electrical stimulation of the phrenic nerves in the cervical region with surface electrodes or monopolar needle electrodes positioned near the posterior border of the sternocleidomastoid muscle at the level of the cricoid cartilage. During stimulation, diaphragm action

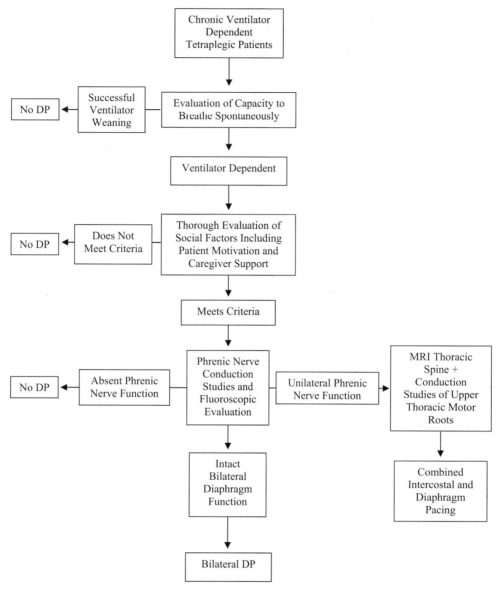

Figure 75.1 Schema for evaluation of potential candidates with cervical spinal cord injury for diaphragmatic pacing. (Reproduced with permission of The McGraw-Hill Companies from DiMarco AF. Diaphragmatic Pacing. In: Tobin MJ, ed. Principles and Practices of Mechanical Ventilation, 2nd Edition. New York: McGraw Hill, 2006; 1263–1275.)

potentials are monitored with surface electrodes placed between the seventh and ninth intercostal spaces in the anterior axillary line. Single pulses of gradually increasing intensity are applied until a supramaximal M-wave is generated. Phrenic nerve conduction time can be calculated as the time interval between the applied stimulus and the first appearance of the compound motor action potential (CAP). Cervical magnetic stimulation of the phrenic nerve can also be used to assess phrenic nerve function (117). Normal conduction times in adults range between 7 and 9 ms (68, 93, 95). Mild prolongation up to 14 ms is acceptable, however, and does not preclude successful DP (68). In children, mean latencies are shorter at 2.2 ms at 6 months of age and increase to 4.2 ms between 5 and 11 years of age (9, 98). The magnitude of the CAP is a reflection of the number of stimulated diaphragm motor units in the vicinity of the

recording electrode. Although low amplitude may reflect a low number of functional phrenic nerve fibers, the magnitude of the CAP may also be reduced secondary to technical factors or reversible atrophy. Compared to conduction times, therefore, this measurement is a much less reliable indicator of phrenic nerve function (29, 93).

Although generally considered the gold standard in the assessment of phrenic nerve function, the measurement procedure for phrenic nerve conduction times is fraught with both false positives and false negatives. This test therefore should be performed by a physician experienced in electrodiagnosis, and more specifically in the assessment of phrenic nerve function. In addition, the visual estimate of diaphragm descent of at least 3–4 cm under fluoroscopic guidance during phrenic nerve stimulation is a useful confirmatory test (26, 66).

An additional but more cumbersome test to evaluate phrenic nerve function is the assessment of diaphragm force development during phrenic nerve stimulation. This test requires the placement of small balloon-tipped catheters in the stomach and esophagus to measure the pressure difference across the diaphragm (trans-diaphragmatic pressure, Pdi). Unilateral single-shock stimulation results in Pdi values of ~10 cmH_2O in normal subjects (97). Due to the development of diaphragm atrophy, however, this value may be lower in ventilator-dependent individuals.

DIAPHRAGMATIC PACING SYSTEMS: OPTIMAL DESIGN, BASIC CONFIGURATION, AND POTENTIAL VARIATIONS

Optimal design of an inspiratory muscle stimulation system would consist of a closed-loop system employing command signals from the central nervous system to activate the inspiratory muscles. Currently available stimulation systems and those under development, however, involve open-loop systems. Inspired volumes and respiratory rates are fixed at predetermined levels. The pattern of ventilation achieved during stimulation, therefore, is not amenable to changes in metabolic needs or other adjustments that are normally made during speech and swallowing. This is not a major limitation, however, because the metabolic requirements

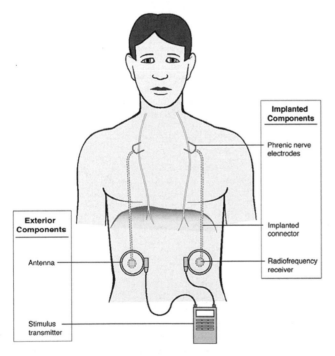

Figure 75.2 Basic design of commercially available diaphragmatic pacing systems utilizing radio-frequency transmission. The internal components consist of a single electrode implanted on each phrenic nerve in the thorax; each electrode is connected by wires to subcutaneously implanted radio-frequency receivers. The external components consist of a stimulus transmitter and attached rubberized antennas. For proper transmission, the antennas must be positioned over the radio-frequency receivers. The receiver converts radio-frequency signals from the transmitter to electrical signals, which stimulate the phrenic nerves to activate the diaphragm.

are relatively constant in tetraplegia due to muscle paralysis, and patients learn to adapt their speech and swallowing within the constraints of the fixed ventilatory pattern.

The basic configuration of all DP pacing systems is similar, being comprised of both implanted materials and external components (Figure 75.2) (37). With the exception of intramuscular diaphragm stimulation in which electrode wires exit the skin (37–39), each system employs radiofrequency transmission. The electrodes, radio-frequency receivers and connecting wires comprise the surgically implanted components. The power supply, radio-frequency transmitter, and antenna wires comprise the external components outside the body. The following is a brief review of inspiratory muscle pacing systems, including those that involve placement of electrodes directly on the phrenic nerves (conventional diaphragmatic pacing systems), newer devices that involve placement of electrodes directly into the diaphragm, and combined intercostal and diaphragm stimulation (which can be applied in patients with only unilateral diaphragm function). The technical features of each commercially available system are provided in Table 75.2.

DIAPHRAGMATIC PACING SYSTEMS IN USE: AVAILABLE CONTEMPORARY PRODUCTS

With each of these systems, a thoracotomy is performed to place a single electrode on each phrenic nerve. Unipolar systems require subcutaneous implantation of an indifferent electrode as well (66). An alternative site of electrode placement is in the cervical region (48). Although less invasive surgically, placement in this location is generally discouraged for the following reasons (29, 121, 123). First, cervical phrenic nerve stimulation may result in incomplete diaphragm activation because an accessory branch from a lower segment of the cervical spinal cord may join the main trunk of the phrenic nerve in the lower neck or within the thorax (51, 64). Second, neck movement may place significant mechanical stress on the phrenic nerve and electrode, resulting in nerve injury or poor electrode contact. Finally, other nerves in the cervical region in close vicinity to the phrenic nerve may also be stimulated, resulting in undesirable movement and/or discomfort (57).

The most commonly used surgical approach for thoracic placement is the second intercostal space (62, 65, 66). Although some centers prefer to place the electrodes in two separate procedures, they are generally placed in one operation (65). It is critically important that the phrenic nerves are carefully manipulated during surgery (64, 66, 67). Excessive stretching may compromise the network of blood vessels within the perineurium, resulting in ischemic injury. The wires are tunneled subcutaneously to connect each electrode to a separate radio-frequency receiver positioned over the anterior portion of the chest wall. The site of receiver placement should be selected in advance, following consultation with the patient and caregivers, to ensure easy accessibility. The lower anterior rib cage, just above the costal margin in the mid-clavicular line, provides a firm surface over which the receivers can be palpated and external antennas secured (45, 46, 64, 66, 67). Some patients, however, may prefer placement over the anterior abdominal wall. Although pressure injury may be less common, receiver location may be more difficult, particularly with weight gain. In some instances, tattoos may be useful for easier identification of receiver location. Details of the surgical procedure can be found in previous reviews (62, 65, 66).

Table 75.2   Technical Features of Diaphragmatic Nerve Pacing Systems

	CONVENTIONAL			INTRAMUSCULAR
	MANUFACTURER			
IMPLANTED COMPONENTS	AVERY BIOMEDICAL DEVICES*	ATROTECH OY	MEDIMPLANT	SYNAPSE BIOMEDICAL
Receiver	Model I-110A (Monopolar) Model I-110 (Bipolar)	RX44-27-2		
Specifications				
Size (mm)	30 (diam) × 8	44 (diam) × 6	56 × 53 × 14	
Number needed to provide bilateral stimulation	2	2	1	
Electrodes	E-377-05 (Monopolar)	TF 4-40		Peterson Electrode
Specifications	E-325 (Bipolar)	(Quadripolar)	(Quadripolar)	(Monopolar)
Number needed to provide bilateral stimulation	2	2	8	2–4
External Components				
Transmitter (stimulus generator)	Mark IV**	PX 244 V2.1	Medimplant 8-channel stimulator	NeuRx RA/4
Specifications				
Size (mm)	146 × 140 × 25	185 × 88 × 28	170 × 130 × 51	150 × 80 × 40
Transmitter/battery weight (kg)	0.54	0.45 + 0.6 (12V) 0.45 + 0.045 (9V)	1.42	0.26
Battery life (hr)	400	160–320 (12V) 8 (9V)	24	500
Parameters				
Rate (breaths/min)	6–28	8–35	5–60	8–18
Inspiratory Period (s)	1.0–2.8	0.5–4	0–4	0.8–1.5
Amplitude (mA)	0–10	0–6		5–25
Pulse width (µs)	160–1000	200	100–1200	20–200 Yes
Pulse interval (ms)	25–130	10–100		
Sigh possible	Yes	Yes	Yes	Yes
Ramp	Amplitude	Amplitude and Frequency	Amplitude	Pulse Width
Antenna	902A	TC 27-250/80	RF transmission coil	

*Formerly known as Avery Laboratories, Inc.

**The Mark IV supersedes all earlier versions manufactured by Avery Laboratories. Most patients implanted with earlier models have been upgraded to the Mark IV.

Reproduced with permission of American Paraplegia Society from DiMarco AF, Onders RP, Ignagni A, Kowalski KE. Inspiratory muscle pacing in spinal cord injury: case report and clinical commentary. J Spinal Cord Med 2006;29:95–108.

Prior to closure of the surgical incisions, threshold current values of each electrode should be evaluated. This is performed by gradually increasing stimulus amplitude until a diaphragm twitch is observed or palpated. With conventional systems, high threshold values (>1 mA) may indicate poor electrode contact with the nerve and require electrode repositioning. The application of suprathreshold current should result in forceful diaphragm contraction and the generation of large inspired volumes.

The external, battery-powered transmitter generates radio-frequency signals, which are inductively coupled to the receivers via circular rubberized antennas. Each antenna should be posi-tioned over each receiver and secured in place to allow proper transmission of the signal. The transmitter signal is demodulated by the receiver, converting the radio-frequency signal to an electrical one, which is transmitted to the electrode to stimulate the phrenic nerve and activate the diaphragm.

Phrenic nerve stimulation causes descent of the diaphragm and a fall in intra-thoracic pressure resulting in inspiratory air-flow. With cessation of stimulation, the diaphragm relaxes, result-ing in passive exhalation. Adequate levels of ventilation are provided by cyclic phrenic nerve stimulation, 8–14 times/minute. Each breath is generated by delivery of a train of electrical pulses at a specified amplitude. The number of pulses/sec within each train is referred to as the stimulus frequency (typically 20 Hz or less). The size of inspired volumes can be adjusted by changes in stimulus amplitude and frequency, and breathing frequency can be adjusted by the rate of train delivery. Inspiratory time and inspiratory flow rate can be adjusted, in tandem, by changes in stimulation on-time. Because normal inspiration usually proceeds with a gradual increase in inspired volume, most stimulation systems employ a ramp delivery system with gradual increases in stimulus amplitude or frequency. Sigh breaths can also be provided by increases in stimulus frequency. An example of the changes in intra-thoracic (esophageal), intra-abdominal (gastric), and airway pressures during DP are shown in Figure 75.3.

There are three commercially available conventional DP systems. These include the Avery, Atrotech, and Medimplant systems. Only the Avery system is available in the United States and worldwide. The Medimplant system is available only in Europe. The intramuscular diaphragm stimulation system manufactured by Synapse Biomedical was recently approved by the FDA and is also commercially available. The specific features of each system are briefly reviewed; the technical characteristics of each are provided in Table 75.2.

Avery Laboratories Mark IV: Worldwide Availability and Optional Biofeedback Control

The basic science and clinical studies performed by Glenn et al (61, 63, 64, 66-68, 82) led to the development of the first available phrenic nerve pacing systems by Avery Laboratories in the 1960s. The Avery system has been the most widely employed device and is commercially available worldwide. The Avery electrode consists of a semicircular platinum-iridium ribbon embedded in molded silicone rubber. The nerve is placed in a shallow trough in the electrode, which must be fixed to surrounding tissues with sutures. Monopolar and bipolar electrodes are available; bipolar electrodes are recommended for patients with cardiac pacemakers (48, 66). The most recently developed Mark IV transmitter (Commack, NY) provides a wide range of stimulus amplitudes (48). The transmitter is portable with flexibility in terms of control of respiratory rate, inspiratory time, stimulus amplitude, and pulse interval. An optional interface allows biofeedback control from pulse oximetry and CO_2 monitoring (48). Electronic output and neurophysiologic response of the pacing system can be monitored via telephone (3).

Atrotech OY: Unique Four-Pole Electrode System

A major difference between the Atrotech (Tampere, Finland) and Avery devices relates to developments in electrode technology (8, 120). The Atrotech electrode consists of two identical strips of Teflon fabric with two platinum buttons mounted onto each strip (Figure 75.4). One strip is placed above and the other behind the nerve. The buttons are positioned symmetrically around the nerve along its long axis. This four-pole electrode system divides the phrenic nerve equally into four stimulation compartments.

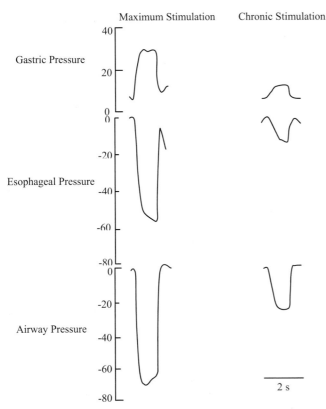

Figure 75.3 Representative gastric, esophageal, and airway pressures during maximum (24 mA, 50 Hz) and chronic (24 mA, 11 Hz) bilateral phrenic nerve stimulation. Pressure measurements are represented in cmH_2O. Data were collected following a reconditioning period, ~10 weeks after electrode implantation. (Reproduced with permission of Elsevier Limited from DiMarco AF. Restoration of respiratory muscle function following spinal cord injury: review of electrical and magnetic stimulation techniques. Respir Physiol Neurobiol 2005; 147:273–287.)

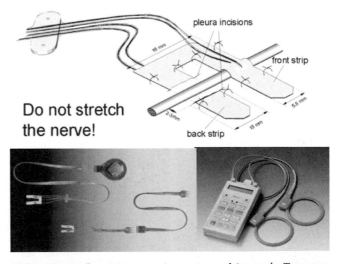

Figure 75.4 Respiratory pacing system of Atrotech, Tampere, Finland, consisting of two electrode arrays and one implantable stimulator (left) and external controller with two antenna coils (right). (Reproduced with permission of Pasi Talonen on behalf of Atrotech Oy from Creasey G, Elefteriades J, DiMarco A, Talonen P, Bijak M, Girsch W, Kantor C. Electrical stimulation to restore respiration. J Rehabil Res Dev 1996; 33:123–132.)

In theory, each quadrant of the phrenic nerve, which supplies a specific set of diaphragm motor units, is stimulated sequentially during the inspiratory phase at a stimulus frequency of 5–6 Hz. During one stimulus sequence, which consists of four current combinations, one pole acts as a cathode and one pole on the opposite side as an anode. Combined stimulation of all quadrants of the nerve, each at 5–6 Hz, results in activation of the diaphragm at a frequency of 20–25 Hz (8, 120).

With this method, the stimulation frequency of individual phrenic nerve axons is thought to be less than with monopolar stimulation. The reduced stimulus frequency should provide more time for recovery, lessen the risk of diaphragm fatigue, and shorten the conditioning process. Compared with unipolar stimulation, the slower frequency of the four-pole sequential stimulation system should enhance the transformation of muscle fibers into slow-twitch, fatigue-resistant fibers and shorten the conditioning process (8, 120, 127).

The transmitter is powered by two types of batteries: a 12 V, which is the main power source, and a back-up 9 V NiCd, which are rechargeable. The transmitter is also relatively small and quite flexible. Pulse width is fixed at 0.2 ms. Attachment of the external programming unit allows for parameter adjustments.

The Atrotech OY system had been approved by the FDA through an investigational device exemption (IDE). As of October 2005, however, the IDE has been terminated. This device therefore is no longer available in the United States.

Medimplant Biotechnisches Labor: Unique Four-Electrode Lead System Allowing 16 Electrode Combinations

This system (Vienna, Austria) also utilizes a unique electrode design (Figure 75.5) (121). Four electrode leads are positioned around each phrenic nerve, requiring a complex microsurgical technique. The electrodes are sutured to the epineurum of the phrenic nerve and the nerve tissue between each electrode lead comprises different stimulating compartments, only one of which is stimulated during any single inspiratory phase, functioning similarly to the bipolar Avery electrode. The various compartments are stimulated in sequence during subsequent inspirations. The control unit generates the stimulating sequence for both phrenic nerves. As many as sixteen different electrode combinations can be adjusted individually for each nerve. Similar to the Atrotech device, only a portion of the nerve is stimulated at any given time. This form of sequential stimulation, also referred to as carousel stimulation, is also thought to allow more recovery time and therefore less chance for fatigue compared to monopolar stimulation (94). As with the other devices, stimulus amplitude, stimulus frequency, train rate, and inspiratory time can be independently adjusted.

This system has limited availability, predominantly in Austria and Germany, and is not available in the United States.

Intramuscular Phrenic Nerve Stimulation System (Synapse Biomedical, Oberlin, Ohio): Motor Point Electrodes Placed via Abdominal Laparoscopic Approach

Phrenic nerve stimulation can also be accomplished by electrodes positioned within the diaphragm (38, 39, 100, 107). This technique has several important advantages compared to

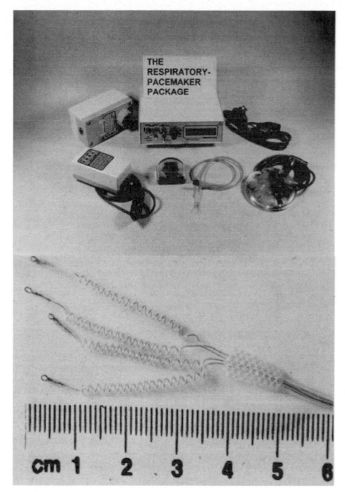

Figure 75.5 Top: Medimplant Respiratory Pacemaker System (Vienna, Austria). Bottom: Complete four prongs of electrode for placement against one phrenic nerve. (Reproduced with permission of Manfred Bijak on behalf of Medimplant from Creasey G, Elefteriades J, DiMarco A, Talonen P, Bijak M, Girsch W, Kantor C. Electrical stimulation to restore respiration. J Rehabil Res Dev 1996; 33:123–132.)

conventional phrenic nerve pacing. Importantly, the electrodes can be placed less invasively and with less overall risk by laparoscopic surgery rather than thoracotomy (106). Consequently, this procedure can be performed on an outpatient basis, resulting in a significant reduction in cost (38). Moreover, the potential of phrenic nerve injury is virtually eliminated because this procedure does not involve manipulation of the nerve. A common misperception is that this technique functions via direct diaphragm muscle stimulation. However, this method stimulates phrenic nerve branches in the muscle at motor points. Therefore, as with conventional phrenic nerve stimulation, bilateral intact phrenic nerve function is required for successful application.

By this technique, four laparoscopic ports are made through the abdominal wall to provide access to the abdominal cavity. These ports are utilized for visualization, insufflation of the abdominal cavity, diaphragm mapping, and insertion of the implant tool (Figure 75.6). With use of specially designed surgical

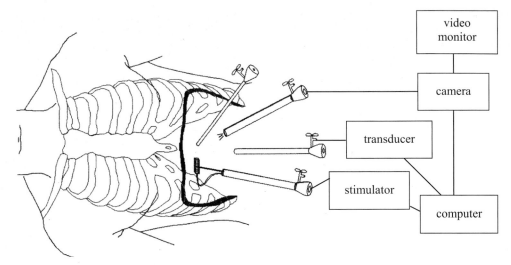

Figure 75.6 Schematic illustration of laparoscopic implant materials required for implantation of intramuscular diaphragm electrodes. Four laparoscopic ports are necessary to provide access to the abdominal cavity. Ports are necessary for visualization, insufflation of the abdominal cavity, diaphragm mapping, and insertion of the electrode implant tool. (Reproduced with permission of the American Thoracic Society from DiMarco AF, Onders RP, Kowalski KE, Miller ME, Ferek S, Mortimer JT. Phrenic nerve pacing in a tetraplegic patient via intramuscular diaphragm electrodes. Am J Respir Crit Care Med 2002; 166:1604–1606.)

tools (1, 38, 39, 104, 108, 109), two intramuscular electrodes are implanted into each hemi-diaphragm near the phrenic nerve motor points (Figure 75.7) (113, 114). A mapping procedure is necessary to achieve appropriate electrode placement (38, 39, 104). If the electrode is not positioned in the immediate vicinity of the nerve, a very limited portion of the phrenic nerve branches will be activated resulting in only small inspired volume generation. In most instances, stimulation of both electrodes in each hemi-diaphragm is necessary to achieve adequate inspired volumes to support ventilation. Because the phrenic nerve is activated through current spread through the diaphragm, high stimulus currents in the range of 24–25 mA are necessary to achieve adequate phrenic nerve stimulation. In contrast, only 1–2 mA is required with direct phrenic nerve stimulation. Importantly, success rates, in terms of maintaining ventilator support, appear similar to those achieved with conventional DP systems (38, 39, 52, 112).

Because this system is relatively new, there is much less clinical experience with this method compared to conventional diaphragmatic pacing systems. In addition, this system entails electrode wires exiting the skin, and therefore carries some risk of infection and potential for the stimulating wires to be damaged. This system has recently been approved by the FDA (2008).

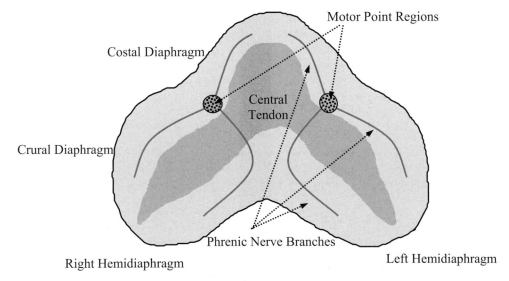

Figure 75.7 Schematic representation of entrance points of each phrenic nerve into each hemidiaphragm (phrenic nerve motor points). (Reproduced with permission of the College of Chest Physicians from DiMarco AF, Onders RP, Ignagni A, Kowalski KE, Mortimer JT. Phrenic nerve pacing via intramuscular diaphragm electrodes in tetraplegic subjects. Chest 2005; 127:671–678.)

DIAPHRAGMATIC PACING WITH COMBINED THERAPIES: INTERCOSTAL AND DIAPHRAGMATIC PACING

Unfortunately, many ventilator-dependent patients with cervical spinal cord injury have damage to the phrenic motoneurons and/or the phrenic nerves, and therefore are not candidates for DP (26, 45, 46, 105). The upper thoracic nerves, which innervate the inspiratory intercostal muscles, however, usually remain intact. The intercostal muscles, which contribute ~35% of the inspiratory capacity, therefore are also amenable to electrical stimulation. In fact, previous studies have demonstrated that electrical stimulation applied to the upper thoracic ventral roots results in activation of this muscle group and the generation of large inspired volumes (27, 31, 32, 45, 46). To stimulate the ventral roots, a hemi-laminectomy incision is necessary to place 4-mm disc electrodes on the ventral surface of the upper thoracic spinal cord. Gas exchange during intercostal muscle breathing alone by this method is comparable to that achieved with phrenic nerve stimulation (33).

In patients with ventilator-dependent tetraplegia and absent phrenic nerve function, activation of the intercostal muscles by this technique results in the generation of inspired volumes of similar magnitude to those resulting from unilateral diaphragmatic stimulation (45). Inspired volumes achieved by this technique, however, are not sufficient to maintain ventilation for more than a few hours. However, in patients with only unilateral diaphragm function, and therefore not candidates for DP, combined intercostal muscle and unilateral diaphragm activation is successful in providing ventilatory support (46). As with DP, these individuals could be comfortably maintained off mechanical ventilatory support from 16 to 24 hours/day. Importantly, these patients achieve similar benefits as those with DP, including improvements in mobility, sense of smell, speech quality, and overall sense of well being. Side effects of intercostal muscle stimulation include mild flexion of the hands and contraction of the muscles of the upper torso, which are generally well tolerated (45, 46). This method may also prove to be a useful adjunct to enhance inspired volume in cases in which phrenic nerve pacing alone is suboptimal.

This technique has received approval by the FDA through an IDE but is not commercially available.

DIAPHRAGMATIC PACING WITH INITIATION OF THERAPY: STIMULUS THRESHOLD DETERMINATION, DIAPHRAGM STRENGTH ASSESSMENT, AND THE CONDITIONING PROCESS

Phrenic nerve pacing is a life support system and should be instituted with careful supervision. DP is usually started about 2 weeks after surgical implantation to provide sufficient time for resolution of inflammation and edema at the electrode/nerve interface and initial healing of surgical wounds (66). To assess the integrity of the pacing system, several parameters should be assessed initially and monitored on a regular basis. These include the minimum stimulus amplitude that results in visible or palpable diaphragm contraction (stimulus threshold) and lowest stimulus parameters that result in maximum inspired volume generation (supramaximal amplitudes and frequencies). The

magnitude of diaphragm force generation can also be assessed by measuring the changes in airway pressure during tracheal occlusion. This latter parameter is useful in instances in which there are significant airway secretions or atelectasis, which are likely to reduce inspired volume.

Prior to initiation of DP, arterial blood gasses should be measured. Many patients are maintained in a hyperventilated state with relatively large tidal volumes while on mechanical ventilation (27, 44, 45). Chronic hyperventilation results in a reduction in bicarbonate stores. Therefore, with initiation of pacing, which is designed to maintain eucapnea, an acidosis may develop secondary to the rise in PCO_2 values into the normal range. Patients may experience dyspnea secondary to this acidosis despite inspired volume generation sufficient to maintain eucapnea. To prevent this development, ventilator settings should be gradually adjusted to restore eucapnea prior to initiation of pacing. To provide a smooth transition to pacing, the ventilator should also be adjusted to provide the approximate respiratory rates and inspired volumes expected during pacing.

With each DP system, threshold and supramaximal amplitudes should be determined for each lead or lead combination. Inspired volume generation is initially adjusted by changing stimulus frequency at supramaximal stimulus amplitudes. At respiratory rates between 8 and 14 breaths/minute, stimulus frequency should be set to achieve inspired volumes sufficient to maintain PCO_2 values in the low normal range (~35 mmHg). To minimize the potential of muscle injury, stimulus frequency should be maintained at the lowest possible level and not exceed 20 Hz. Previous studies have shown that chronic diaphragmatic stimulation at high frequencies is associated with myopathic changes in the diaphragm resulting in reductions in force generation (18, 52, 53). Fine tuning of specific respiratory rates and inspired volumes should then be individualized for patient comfort.

Because the diaphragm has likely undergone significant atrophic changes, full-time ventilatory support cannot be achieved immediately with the pacing system (38, 39, 59, 67, 101). Initially, pacing is likely to be associated with the development of diaphragm fatigue. Therefore, the diaphragm must be reconditioned with gradually increasing amounts of stimulation to improve strength and endurance (101). The specific methods of transition from mechanical ventilation to DP are arbitrary. The primary goal is to achieve full-time pacing as soon as possible without the development of significant diaphragm fatigue. One approach is to determine the initial time to onset of fatigue. DP is initiated with the above-mentioned stimulus parameters until either reductions in inspired volume (monitored every 5–10 min) or oxygen saturation (monitored continuously by pulse oximetry) are observed, or the patient experiences dyspnea. Increasing accessory muscle use is also a useful physical finding indicating diaphragm fatigue. Pacing is then applied for a somewhat shorter time period (~5 min) every hour during the day, for the first week. The time to onset of fatigue is then reevaluated weekly and a new pacing schedule determined accordingly. After full-time pacing has been comfortably achieved during the day, pacing is provided during sleeping hours. The tracheostomy should remain patent during sleep to prevent the development of upper airway obstruction. This may occur secondary to the lack of activation of the upper airway muscles in synchrony with the diaphragm, which is common during sleep (59, 76). In some patients, initial inspired volumes may be inadequate to comfortably maintain adequate ventilation for even short periods. In these instances, the initial conditioning phase can be performed in conjunction with mechanical ventilation (45). By setting the ventilator in the assist mode, the negative inspiratory pressure generated at the tracheal opening by pacing can be used to trigger the ventilator.

During the course of the conditioning phase, stimulus frequencies and respiratory rates should be reduced to the lowest values necessary to maintain adequate ventilation and patient comfort. With the Avery system, stimulation frequency can be reduced to as low as 7–9 Hz with respiratory rates in the 6–12 breaths/minute range (63). With the Synapse system, stimulation is usually initiated with four electrodes at 20 Hz. With conditioning of the diaphragm, stimulation frequency can be reduced to as low as 11 Hz with stimulation of only two electrodes (38). Conditioning time is variable between patients, ranging between 4 weeks and several months. However, most patients achieve significant ventilator-free time within a few weeks. A plateau in inspired volume generation is generally reached within 8–12 weeks, signaling completion of the conditioning process.

The application of low-frequency stimulation during the initial phases of the conditioning process often results in diaphragm vibration, observed as shaking of the anterior abdominal wall. This is due to diaphragm stimulation below its intrinsic fusion frequency (102). However, with continued stimulation during the conditioning process, vibrating contractions are replaced by smooth coordinated contractions, even at very low stimulus frequencies (63, 64). This occurs as a result of the gradual transformation of the diaphragm, which is normally constituted with nearly equal populations of both Type I and Type II fibers, to one consisting of a uniform population of Type I fibers (63, 111). Type I fibers have a lower fusion frequency, are highly oxidative, and are fatigue-resistant (61). High-endurance characteristics are desirable for a muscle expected to contract 8 to 15 times/minute for life. It should be noted, however, that conversion of the diaphragm to a Type I muscle results in reductions in maximum force generating capacity and thereby maximum inspired volume generation. However, this is not a concern in most patients because coincident generalized muscle paralysis restricts the need of spinal cord individuals for higher levels of ventilation.

Higher levels of stimulation may be required in the sitting compared to the supine posture. In the upright posture, the gravitational effects of the abdominal contents on the diaphragm are markedly reduced, resulting in diaphragm shortening. At a shorter length, diaphragm force-generating capacity is less, and therefore inspired volume generation is reduced for a given level of stimulation. The application of a snug-fitting binder, however, reduces postural-related changes in diaphragm length such that changes in stimulus parameters may not be required.

DIAPHRAGMATIC PACING IN CHRONIC USE: LONG-TERM PATIENT OUTCOMES

Inspiratory muscle pacing is clearly an effective method of maintaining artificial ventilatory support in many patients with ventilator-dependent tetraplegia (38, 52, 63, 67). There are numerous reports of successful long-term pacing in individual patients for 10 years or longer (52, 67). The actual success rate is somewhat difficult to determine, however, as most patients have

undergone these techniques at centers where total patient numbers were small (57, 76, 122).

In one of the largest series of patients (reported at a time when diaphragmatic pacing was still in development), DP was considered successful in only ~50% of patients (59). Some of the failures in this report were attributable to the damaging effects of high-frequency stimulation (18, 63). Reduced lung and chest wall compliance was also thought to be a factor leading to reduced success in the elderly (69). It is apparent that many of the patients who were deemed failures were not good candidates for this technique. In one report of 14 tetraplegics in whom only chronic low-frequency stimulation was applied (50), some patients used the device successfully for as long as 15 years, with a mean use of 7.6 years. Importantly, threshold and amplitude of stimulation required for maximum diaphragm excursion and tidal volume were maintained unchanged over the period of follow-up. Pathologic specimens were available in some cases, and there was no evidence of nerve or diaphragm injury. In another investigation (52), the clinical outcome of patients whose phrenic nerves were implanted before 1981 were compared to patients implanted between 1981 and 1987. In the latter group, low-frequency stimulation was universally applied at low respiratory rates, and pacing was successful in each of the 12 patients evaluated. Six patients continued pacing for a mean duration of ~15 years. The remaining patients did not achieve sustained long-term pacing due to lack of adequate financial and social support or medical comorbidities. This analysis serves to emphasize the importance of adhering to strict criteria for patient selection.

Use of the term success with regard to DP is not well defined and open to interpretation. One approach is to define success in the context of each individual patient's goals. For example, some patients may tolerate pacing for only 15–20 minute periods. This small degree of independence from mechanical ventilation, however, may allow much easier bed-to-chair or chair-to-vehicle transfers, possibly increasing mobility. Albeit small, this may be considered successful by some. Most patients, however, will have expectations of more meaningful time off mechanical ventilation. This may be as short as 4–6 hours, but full-time, 24 hours/day, may be anticipated by others. Based upon an analysis of 64 patients with the Atrotech device in whom the average duration of pacing was 2 years (127), about 50% were able to maintain a full-time (24 hours/day) pacing regimen, and ~80% were able to pace throughout the day. Interestingly, with the more recent Synapse Biomedical intramuscular diaphragmatic pacing device, about 50% of patients are also able to maintain full-time pacing. In patients not using the device full-time however, the duration of use may be as short as 4–5 hours (127). The reasons why a substantial percentage of patients do not use the device full-time most likely relate to the lack of long-term maintenance of adequate inspired volumes (38, 46). Other factors may also play a role, however, including greater sense of security with mechanical ventilation, a device that is equipped with more alarm systems. When counseling individuals considering DP as an alternative to mechanical ventilation, therefore, individual patient's goals and expectations should be thoroughly assessed in relation to potential outcomes.

The effects of DP on long-term survival are unknown. Complicating any comparison between patients managed with mechanical ventilation vs. DP is the fact that there are multiple prognostic factors impacting survival, including age, level and completeness of injury and time since injury (116). It is conceivable, however, that mechanical ventilation is associated with a higher incidence of serious complications, including respiratory tract infections, barotrauma, and other mechanical issues related to ventilator use.

CLINICAL MONITORING OF PATIENTS WITH DIAPHRAGMATIC PACING: COMPLICATIONS AND SIDE EFFECTS

Due to technical developments and clinical experience garnered over the past several decades, the incidence of serious complications and side effects with modern day pacing devices is quite low (127). Important factors impacting the incidence of complications include the proper use of stimulus parameters, adequacy of patient monitoring, and appropriate patient selection. Because inspiratory muscle pacing is a life support system, back-up mechanical ventilation or other means of providing ventilatory support, e.g. use of an Ambu bag, should be readily available. A summary of the complications and side effects is presented in Table 75.3.

SURGICAL COMPLICATIONS. At the time of surgery, damage to the phrenic nerve can occur as a result of direct mechanical trauma or compromise of nerve blood supply (59, 67). As the nerve is quite fragile, surgical dissection should be carefully performed by an experienced surgeon. Excessive tension on the nerve and extremes of temperature will result in nerve injury resulting in inadequate inspired volume generation (51). Late injury to the phrenic nerve can also occur due to mechanical injury and/or the development of fibrosis around the nerve (46, 59, 67). Mechanical tension on the nerve is more likely to occur with cervical electrode placement because most patients have motor control of their cervical muscles; extremes of neck motion may result in undue stretching of the nerve/electrode assembly (49, 55). Nerve injury and fibrosis was fairly common with the previous use of bipolar cuff electrodes that encircled the nerve (59, 67, 126). The introduction of the monopolar electrodes by Avery significantly reduced the incidence of this complication (115, 116). The Atrotech and Medimplant electrodes do not encircle the nerve, and the incidence of nerve injury related to the electrode itself is thought to be low (127). Tissue reaction around the electrode may result in a gradual reduction in inspired volume production, and in some instances, vibration during diaphragm stimulation (59, 67). Fibrosis at the electrode site may also result in changes in stimulus threshold values. With use of the intramuscular electrode system of Synapse Biomedical in which the electrodes are not in direct contact with the nerve, these risks are virtually eliminated.

There are infection risks with any surgical procedure, particularly those involving implantation of a foreign body. Since the institution of this technique in the 1970s, reported infection rates have been relatively constant in the range of ~3–5% (59, 126, 127). However, with modern surgical techniques and use of preoperative antibiotics, this rate may be significantly lower (51). Infection involving any of the implanted materials generally requires their removal. Placement of intramuscular diaphragm electrodes carries a small risk of pneumothorax and infection at the exit site of the electrode wires.

TECHNICAL MALFUNCTION. The most common cause of mechanical failure of the pacing device is loss of battery power. This problem is completely avoidable, however, by adherence to battery changes at regular intervals and recharging schedules. Low battery alarms are also present on most systems. The external antenna wires are also subject to breakage at stress points, either near the connection to the transmitter or near their attachment to the chest wall. With careful application and avoidance of excessive torque at stress points, antenna wires may have a useful life of several years before their replacement becomes necessary. With the percutaneous Synapse system, there is also a risk of wire breakage at the exit site, which can result in pacer failure.

With regard to the implanted components, the radiofrequency receiver may fail. This was a fairly common problem with older systems due to leakage of body fluids through the epoxy encapsulation (59, 65, 67, 78). With these systems, receiver failure often occurred within 5 years. With improvement in housing materials, receiver life has been extended to at least 10 years. Although uncommon, electrode breakage or malfunction can also occur and result in failure of the pacing system. In a recent analysis of the quadripolar Atrotech system in patients who had undergone pacing for about 2 years, electrode failure rate was ~3% (115). Failure of one or more of the four electrode combinations, although fairly common, usually did not interfere with successful pacing (115).

UPPER AIRWAY OBSTRUCTION. Diaphragm contraction without coincident upper airway muscle contraction results in collapse of the upper airway and the development of apnea. Because the state of wakefulness results in synchronous activation of the upper airway muscles during DP, this is not a concern while

---

Table 75.3 Complications and Side-Effects of Diaphragmatic Pacing

A. Mechanical Injury to the Phrenic Nerve
1. Iatrogenic injury at the time of surgery
2. Late injury due to scar formation and/or tension on the nerve
B. Infection
1. Receiver site
2. Electrode site
C. Technical Malfunction
1. External components
a. Battery failure
b. Breakage of antenna wires
2. Implanted components
a. Receiver failure
b. Electrode malfunction
c. Breakage of implanted connecting wires
D. Upper Airway Obstruction after Tracheostomy Closure
E. Paradoxical Movement of the Upper Rib Cage, particularly in children

Reproduced with permission of The McGraw-Hill Companies from DiMarco AF. Diaphragmatic Pacing. In: Tobin MJ, ed. Principles and Practices of Mechanical Ventilation, 2nd Edition. New York: McGraw-Hill, 2006:1263–1275.

awake. During sleep, however, activation of the upper airway dilator muscles is reduced, resulting in a much greater tendency for asynchronous upper airway and chest wall muscle contraction (60, 76). To prevent the development of obstructive apneas, therefore, most patients maintain a patent tracheostomy stoma during sleep. The maintenance of a tracheostomy is also useful for the easy application of ventilatory support in the event of pacemaker failure or instances of severe respiratory tract infection during which the pacing system is not capable of meeting metabolic demands.

In some cases, patients utilizing the Medimplant pacing system were able to close their tracheostomies (94). Patients first underwent a training program to ensure that spontaneous breathing could be tolerated for at least 20 minutes. Potential benefits of tracheostomy closure include reductions in the incidence of respiratory tract infections and decreases in the volume of respiratory secretions. The potential for tracheostomy closure in most patients undergoing full-time DP, however, has not been systematically evaluated.

EXPOSURE TO MAGNETIC AND RADIOFREQUENCY FIELDS. According to the Patient Manual for the Atrostim Jukka (Atrotech, Tampere, Finland), the electronic circuitry of pacing systems can be damaged by exposure to strong magnetic fields, which occurs with magnetic resonance imaging. Moreover, the phrenic nerve could be damaged by potentially high levels of energy transmission to the electrode. Electrotherapeutic devices that generate strong radio-frequency fields may also interfere with the pacing system.

PARADOXICAL RIB CAGE MOVEMENT. Young children have a very high chest wall compliance, resulting in marked inward movement of the rib cage consequent to the negative intrathoracic pressure generated by diaphragm contraction. This paradoxical rib cage movement significantly reduces inspired volume generation (59, 125). Consequently, these patients are often unable to maintain full-time ventilatory support. Because rib cage compliance gradually decreases between 10 and 15 years of age, the performance of the pacing system gradually improves and pacing can be maintained for longer periods.

ROUTINE ASSESSMENT OF DIAPHRAGMATIC PACING: CLINICAL EVALUATION DURING FUNCTIONAL USE

Physicians and caregivers should evaluate pacemaker function on a routine basis and also in situations in which patients are experiencing dyspnea. It should be noted that most patients, despite their spinal cord injury, are readily able to detect small changes in inspired volume (47). Increase in accessory muscle contraction, when present, is a useful physical finding suggesting inadequate inspired volume generation by the pacing system. Diaphragm contraction can also be assessed by palpation of the chest wall. Inspiration is associated with lateral expansion of the lower rib cage and outward movement of the anterior abdominal wall. Reductions in the degree of chest wall movement indicate reductions in inspired volume. Finally, use of a spirometer attached to the tracheostomy tube can provide a direct measurement of inspired volume generation. Adjustments of the transmitter allow separate stimulation of each hemidiaphragm such that the function of each hemidiaphragm can be evaluated

separately. Adequacy of ventilation can be assessed with pulse oximetry and end-tidal CO_2 measurements.

If inspired volume is found to be inadequate and the patient is experiencing any respiratory distress, mechanical ventilation should be instituted promptly until the problem is corrected. The batteries should be replaced initially, as this is the most common cause of pacemaker malfunction. If function is not restored, the antenna should be replaced and the back-up transmitter employed, in sequence.

Increases in airway resistance or reductions in respiratory system compliance can also result in reductions in inspired volume generation. Most patients have an ineffective cough mechanism due to expiratory muscle paralysis and therefore require suctioning or some alternative method of secretion removal. Retained secretions may increase airway resistance and cause atelectasis, resulting in reductions in lung compliance. Evacuation of secretions generally results in prompt reversal of these mechanical derangements and improvement in symptoms. Respiratory tract infections such as bronchitis and pneumonia may also result in abnormal lung mechanics and cause reductions in inspired volume. If reductions in inspired volume persist, therefore, chest radiography should be performed.

If inspired volumes remain low despite functional external components, the internal components should be assessed. This evaluation should be performed at medical centers with the proper equipment, expertise, and familiarity with pacing systems. Briefly, this assessment can be performed by placing surface electrodes at the costal margin to record the pacemaker stimulus pulse and diaphragmatic action potential (126). These signals should be amplified and recorded on an oscilloscope. If the pacing system is functioning properly, the radio-frequency signal from the transmitting antenna, stimulus pulse from the phrenic nerve electrode, and diaphragmatic action potential are seen on the oscilloscope. If only the radio-frequency signal and stimulus pulse are seen but not the action potential, this suggests that the wire insulation is not intact, the phrenic nerve is not in contact with the electrode, or the phrenic nerve is damaged. If the stimulus pulse and action potential are both not seen, this suggests receiver malfunction.

EXPIRATORY MUSCLE STIMULATION: FUNCTIONAL ELECTRICAL STIMULATION TO RESTORE COUGH

Patients with upper thoracic and cervical spinal cord injury suffer from paralysis of a major portion of their expiratory muscles, and therefore cannot generate an effective cough mechanism (22, 54, 83). As a result, most of these patients are not able to adequately clear airway secretions and are dependent upon caregiver support for secretion management. Lack of an effective cough is also a contributing factor to the high incidence of atelectasis and recurrent respiratory tract infections in this patient population (14, 79, 96). Current airway management techniques include mechanical suctioning, manually assisted coughing, use of the mechanical insufflation/exsufflation device and other methods. Many patients find these techniques uncomfortable, cumbersome, embarrassing, and of limited effectiveness. Importantly, respiratory complications remain a major cause of morbidity and mortality in spinal cord-injured patients despite their use (24, 58, 71, 84).

Restoration of expiratory muscle function and the generation of an effective cough have several important potential

Table 75.4 Potential Benefits of Expiratory Muscle Stimulation to Restore Cough

A. Reduced level of required nursing care

B. Improved sense of well-being and overall health
   1. Reduction in incidence of respiratory tract infections

C. Reduced anxiety and embarrassment
   1. Elimination of need for suctioning
   2. Possible closure of tracheostomy

D. Improved comfort level
   1. More natural means of secretion removal

E. Reduced overall costs
   1. Reduction and/or elimination of suction supplies

benefits (Table 75.4). These include a reduced level of nursing care. If patients could trigger an effective cough and evacuate secretions on demand, the need for caregiver support would be reduced or possibly eliminated. Perhaps the most important potential benefit, however, is the reduction in the incidence of respiratory complications including pneumonia, bronchitis, and atelectasis. Theoretically, engagement of the expiratory muscles to produce a cough would provide a more natural and effective means of secretion removal. Most mechanical methods to remove secretions result in the evacuation of secretions in the upper airway, whereas a normal cough may result in clearance of more distal airways. Because this method is a more natural method of secretion removal, it should be more comfortable and reduce or eliminate the anxiety and embarrassment associated with current methods. Finally, the reduction in caregiver requirements and suction supplies should result in an overall reduction in cost.

There are several potential methods by which the expiratory muscles can be stimulated. These include high-frequency magnetic stimulation, surface abdominal muscle stimulation, and electrical stimulation applied in the region of the lower thoracic spinal cord. It should be remembered, however, that cough is a complex reflex with several components, including an initial inspiration and subsequent glottic closure followed by expiratory muscle contraction. Fortunately, many patients with spinal cord injury are able to control their upper airway and inspiratory muscles, and lack only control of expiratory muscle function. These patients, therefore, can be trained to activate their expiratory muscles in phase with the other components of the cough response. In the case of patients on mechanical ventilation, the ventilator can be used to provide the inspiratory component of the cough reflex.

Magnetic stimulation of the expiratory muscles is achieved by placement of a stimulation coil over the lower back to activate the neural pathways innervating the expiratory muscles (86, 90). Several recent studies have demonstrated that this method results in the generation of large positive airway pressures and expiratory flow rates when applied in normal subjects (86, 90). When applied in tetraplegic individuals, however, airway pressures and flow rates were not significantly different than those that could be generated during spontaneous efforts (90). It is likely that muscle atrophy contributed, at least in part, to these low values and would improve with reconditioning. One

significant advantage of this technique, however, is that activation of the expiratory muscles can be achieved by noninvasive means.

Magnetic stimulation also has several disadvantages limiting its practical application. First, the device is large, requires an external power source, and is not easily portable, restricting its application in mobile patients. Second, the device generates considerable heat at the stimulating coil and therefore carries some risk of thermal injury. Third, the presence of large amounts of adipose tissue may interfere with successful stimulation due to the greater distance between the stimulating coil and motor roots. Finally, because the point of stimulation is not precise, there may be difficulty obtaining reproducible activation of the expiratory muscles. Nonetheless, with further study this device may be useful in selected patients.

The abdominal muscles can also be activated by electrodes placed directly over the surface of the abdominal wall (80, 81, 91). In previous studies in tetraplegic patients, maximum expiratory pressure could be increased by only ~30 cmH$_2$O during assisted cough to 55–60 cmH$_2$O (81). Peak flow rates with surface stimulation are also not significantly different than volitional cough. In addition, no significant abdominal muscle contraction could be elicited in over 20% of patients (81). In a more recent study in normal subjects employing surface electrodes with much larger surface areas, however, pressure generation was quite substantial in the range of that generated with magnetic stimulation (88). Although this method also has the advantage of being noninvasive, the repeated application of electrodes over the skin may lead to irritation and breakdown. Also, significant adipose tissue may interfere with its successful application in obese patients due to the high electrical resistance of fatty tissue. Repeated application of electrodes to the skin surface may also prove to be quite tedious and cumbersome.

Spinal cord stimulation involves the placement of electrodes on the dorsal surface of the lower thoracic spinal cord via laminotomy incisions at the T9, T11, and L1 spinal cord levels (34–36, 41–43). Electrode wires are connected to a radio-frequency receiver placed over the anterior chest wall. Similar to the conventional inspiratory muscle pacing systems, stimulation is applied by activating a small portable external control box (9.5 × 6 × 2.5 cm) connected to a rubberized transmitter, which is secured to the skin with tape over the implanted receiver (34, 35). This method results in marked activation of the abdominal and internal intercostal muscles, resulting in positive airway pressures similar to those achieved by normal subjects during a maximal cough effort (34, 35). The effects of stimulation at the T9 and L1 levels each alone and combined at both spinal cord levels is shown for one subject in Figure 75.8. Large airway pressures and peak expiratory flow rates in the range of 70–80 cmH$_2$O and 5–6 L/s, respectively could be achieved during stimulation at either the T9 or L1 levels. With combined stimulation at both sites, airway pressure and flow rates increased to 140 cmH$_2$O and 8 L/s, respectively.

Major advantages of this method are that the device is portable and allows the patient to generate a cough on demand without caregiver assistance. Recent studies also indicate that the effects of stimulation are highly reproducible and that fatigue does not occur despite repeated stimulation (34). Some patients have now used this device successfully for more than 3 years. Importantly, this technique has provided significant short-term benefits in terms of airway management, reductions in need for

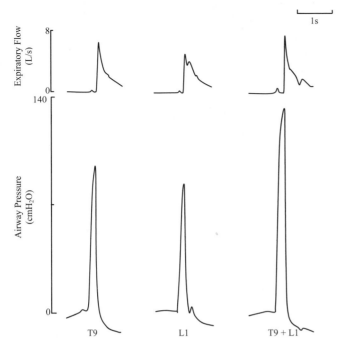

Figure 75.8 Representative tracings of expiratory flow and airway pressure generation during stimulation at the T9 (40 V, 53 Hz, 150 μs), L1 (40 V, 53 Hz, 200 μs) and combined T9 + L1 spinal cord levels, at TLC. (Reproduced with permission of the American Thoracic Society from DiMarco AF, Kowalski KE, Geertman RT, Hromyak DR. Spinal cord stimulation: a new technique to produce an effective cough in patients with spinal cord injury. Am J Respir Crit Care Med 2006; 173:1386–1389.)

caregiver assistance, and improvement in overall quality of life (36). The need for caregiver assistance while traveling with family or for recreational activities may be eliminated (36).

Because this technique results in generalized stimulation of the lower thoracic and upper lumbar motor roots, there is coincident activation of the paraspinal muscles and secondary trunk motion. Although patients are generally aware of lower body movement during stimulation, the brief period of stimulation (0.4–0.6 ms) is well-tolerated without pain or discomfort. In some instances, lower limb movement is observed, but this is easily controlled by reducing stimulus parameters. In some patients, signs of autonomic dysfunction, including increases in blood pressure and reductions in pulse rate can occur. However, following a period of acclimatization to electrical stimulation, this response resolves completely such that the frequent application of stimulation elicits no hemodynamic responses. Importantly, bowel leakage does not occur during stimulation.

FUTURE DIRECTIONS: IMPROVED VOLUNTARY CONTROL, NEW TECHNIQUES, AND FULLY IMPLANTABLE SYSTEMS

As mentioned, current inspiratory muscle pacing systems are open-loop in design, i.e. the diaphragm is activated independent of the spontaneous generation of electrical signals in the brainstem. Consequently, the upper airway muscles may not be activated in synchrony with the diaphragm, resulting in upper airway

obstruction during sleep. It is conceivable that diaphragm activation could be triggered by a signal from an upper airway muscle (61). This type of closed-loop system would eliminate the need for a tracheostomy and allow for ventilatory adjustments to speech and changes in metabolic demand. An alternative approach to the issue of upper airway obstruction and need for a tracheostomy is the use of continuous positive airway pressure (CPAP) delivered through a nasal or full face mask as is currently used to manage obstructive sleep apnea.

DP is generally reserved for patients with chronic tetraplegia (i.e., 12 months following injury). This delay occurs for several reasons, including the fact that the phrenic nerve may recover over this time period. Moreover, the procedure is expensive and the placement of electrodes on the phrenic nerve carries the risk of injury. Implantation of intramuscular diaphragm electrodes, however, which is less expensive and requires a less invasive procedure with little to no risk of nerve injury, may be an attractive alternative to mechanical ventilation in the acute phase of spinal cord injury (39). In patients who subsequently develop sufficient recovery of phrenic nerve function to breathe spontaneously, the electrodes can be removed. This approach would significantly reduce the need for diaphragm reconditioning. Prior to implementation, however, this alternative approach should be investigated prospectively in clinical trials, including both risk-benefit and cost-benefit analyses.

Many patients have suffered significant injury to both phrenic nerves and therefore cannot be offered DP. Further development of intercostal nerve to phrenic nerve transfer has the potential to restore phrenic nerve viability and allow these patients the option of diaphragmatic pacing as well (85). Newer techniques to activate the intercostal muscles also have the potential to extend ventilator free time with activation of this muscle group alone (27, 31, 32, 45, 46). Development of a totally implantable system, as with cardiac pacemaker devices, would increase patient convenience and eliminate the need to attach materials to the body surface.

With regard to activation of the expiratory muscles to restore cough, a significant limitation of epidural spinal cord stimulation is that electrode implantation requires an invasive procedure. It is possible, however, that wire electrodes may also be effective in activating the expiratory muscles. Use of a wire electrode, which can be inserted through a needle, would significantly reduce the risks and cost associated with the more invasive laminotomy procedure.

Recent studies in animals (89) also suggest that the expiratory muscles can be activated by electrical stimulation via multiple wireless microstimulators implanted percutaneously near the neuroforamen to activate the spinal nerves. Further investigation will be necessary to determine the efficacy and safety of this technique in humans.

ACKNOWLEDGMENT

The author would like to acknowledge the assistance of Ms. Dana Hromyak, RRT for her invaluable assistance in the preparation of this chapter.

References

1. Aiyar H, Stellato TA, Onders RP, Mortimer JT. Laparoscopic implant instrument for the placement of intramuscular electrodes in the diaphragm. IEEE Trans Rehabil Eng 1999; 7:360–371.

2. Alder D, Gonzalez-Bermejo J, Duguet A, Demoule A, Le Pimpec-Barthes F, Hurbault A, Morelot-Panzini C, Similowski T. Diaphragm pacing restores olfaction in tetraplegia. Eur Respir 2009; 34:365–370.

3. Auerbach AA, Dobelle WH. Transtelephonic monitoring of patients with implanted neurostimulators. Lancet 1987; 1:224–225.

4. Bach JR. Alternative methods of ventilatory support for the patient with ventilatory failure due to spinal cord injury. J Am Paraplegia Soc 1991; 14:158–174.

5. Bach JR. Noninvasive alternatives to tracheostomy for managing respiratory muscle dysfunction in spinal cord injury. Top Spinal Cord Injury Rehabil 1997; 2:49–58.

6. Bach JR, Alba AS. Management of chronic alveolar hypoventilation by nasal ventilation. Chest 1990; 97:52–57.

7. Bach JR, Alba AS. Noninvasive options for ventilatory support of the traumatic high level tetraplegic patient. Chest 1990; 98:613–619.

8. Baer GA, Talonen PP, Shneerson J M, Markkula H, Exner G, Wells FC. Phrenic nerve stimulation for central ventilatory failure with bipolar and four-pole electrode systems. Pacing Clin Eletrophysiol 1990; 19:1061–1072.

9. Brouillette RT, Ilbawi MN, Hunt CE. Phrenic nerve pacing in infants and children: A review of experience and report on the usefulness of phrenic nerve stimulation studies. J Pediatr 1983; 102:32–39.

10. Brown R, DiMarco AF, Hoit JD, Garshick E. Respiratory dysfunction and management in spinal cord injury. Respir Care 2006; 51:853–870.

11. Caldani LMA. Institutiones physiologicae, Venezia, 1786. Cited by Schechter DC: Application of electrotherapy to noncardiac thoracic disorders. Bull NY Acad Med 1970; 46:932–951.

12. Carter RE. Experience with high tetraplegia. Paraplegia 1979; 17:140–146.

13. Carter RE. Experience with ventilator dependent patients. Paraplegia 1993;31:150–153.

14. Carter RE. Respiratory aspects of spinal cord injury management. Paraplegia 1987; 25:262–266.

15. Carter RE, Donovan WH, Halstead L, Wilkerson MA. Comparative study of electrophrenic nerve stimulation and mechanical ventilatory support in traumatic spinal cord injury. Paraplegia 1987; 25:86–91.

16. Chae J, Triolo RJ, Kilgore KL, Creasey GH, DiMarco AF. Neuromuscular electrical stimulation in spinal cord injury. In: Kirshblum S, Campagnolo DI, DeLisa JA, eds. Spinal Cord Medicine. Philadelphia: Lippincott Williams & Wilkins, 2002; 360–388.

17. Chen CF, Lien IN. Spinal cord injuries in Taipei, Taiwan, 1978–1981. Paraplegia 1985; 23:364–370.

18. Ciesielski TE, Fukuda Y, Glenn WW, Gorfien J, Jeffery K, Hogan JF. Response of the diaphragm muscle to electrical stimulation of the phrenic nerve. A histochemical and ultrastructural study. J Neurosurg 1983; 58:92–100.

19. Claxton AR, Wong DT, Chung F, Fehlings MG. Predictors of hospital mortality and mechanical ventilation in patients with cervical spinal cord injury. Can J Anaesth 1998; 45:144–149.

20. Creasey G, Elefteriades J, DiMarco A, et al. Electrical stimulation to restore respiration. J Rehabil Res Dev 1996; 33:123–132.

21. de Haan A, de Jong J, van Doorn JE, Huijing PA, Woittiez RD, Westra HG. Muscle economy of isometric contractions as function of stimulation time and relative muscle length. Pfluegers Arch 1986; 407:445–450.

22. DeTroyer A, Estenne M, Heilporn A. Mechanism of active expiration in tetraplegic subjects. N Engl J Med 1986; 314:740–744.

23. DeVivo MJ, Ivie CS III. Life expectancy of ventilator-dependent persons with spinal cord injuries. Chest 1995; 108:226–232.

24. DeVivo MJ, Krause JS, Lammertse DP. Recent trends in mortality and causes of death among persons with spinal cord injury. Arch Phys Med Rehabil 1999; 80:1411–1419.

25. DeVivo MJ, Stover SL. Long-term survival and causes of death. In: Stover SL, DeLisa JA, Whiteneck GG, eds. Spinal cord injury: clinical outcomes from the model systems. Gaithersburg MD: Aspen Publishers, 1995; 289–316.

26. DiMarco AF. Diaphragm pacing in patients with spinal cord injury. Top Spinal Cord Inj Rehabil 1999; 5:6–20.

27. DiMarco AF. Neural prostheses in the respiratory system. J Rehabil Res Dev 2001; 38:601–607.

28. DiMarco AF. Phrenic nerve stimulation in patients with spinal cord injury. Respir Physiol Neurobiol 2009; 169:200–209.

29. DiMarco AF. Respiratory muscle stimulation in patients with spinal cord injury. In: Horch KW, Dhillon GS, eds. Neuroprosthetics: Theory and Practice. Hackensack, NJ: World Scientific, 2004; 951–978.

30. DiMarco AF. Restoration of respiratory muscle function following spinal cord injury: review of electrical and magnetic stimulation techniques. Respir Physiol Neurobiol 2005; 147:273–287.

31. DiMarco AF, Altose MD, Cropp A, Durand D. Activation of intercostal muscles by electrical stimulation of the spinal cord. Am Rev Respir Dis 1987; 136:1385–1390.

32. DiMarco AF, Budzinska K, Supinski GS. Artificial ventilation by means of electrical activation of intercostal/accessory muscles alone in anesthetized dogs. Am Rev Respir Dis 1989; 139:961–967.

33. DiMarco AF, Connors AF, Kowalski KE. Gas exchange during separate diaphragm and intercostal muscle breathing. J Appl Physiol 2004; 96:2120–2124.

34. DiMarco AF, Kowalski KE, Geertman RT, Hromyak DR. Lower thoracic spinal cord stimulation to restore cough in patients with spinal cord injury: results of a National Institutes of Health-sponsored clinical trial. Part I: methodology and effectiveness of expiratory muscle activation. Arch Phys Med Rehabil 2009; 90:717–725.

35. DiMarco AF, Kowalski KE, Geertman RT, Hromyak DR. Spinal cord stimulation: a new technique to produce an effective cough in patients with spinal cord injury. Am J Respir Crit Care Med 2006; 173: 1386–1389.

36. DiMarco AF, Kowalski KE, Geertman RT, Hromyak DR, Frost FS, Creasey GH, Nemunaitis GA. Lower thoracic spinal cord stimulation to restore cough in patients with spinal cord injury: results of a National Institutes of Health-sponsored clinical trial. Part II: clinical outcomes. Arch Phys Med Rehabil 2009; 90:726–732.

37. DiMarco AF, Onders RP, Ignagni A, Kowalski KE. Inspiratory muscle pacing in spinal cord injury: case report and clinical commentary. J Spinal Cord Med 2006; 29:95–108.

38. DiMarco AF, Onders RP, Ignagni A, Kowalski KE, Stefan SL, Mortimer JT. Phrenic nerve pacing via intramuscular diaphragm electrodes in tetraplegic subjects. Chest 2005; 127:671–678.

39. DiMarco AF, Onders RP, Kowalski KE, Miller ME, Ferek S, Mortimer JT. Phrenic nerve pacing in a tetraplegic patient via intramuscular diaphragm electrodes. Am J Respir Crit Care Med 2002; 166: 1604–1606.

40. DiMarco AF, Romaniuk JR, Kowalski KE, Supinski GS. Efficacy of combined intercostal and expiratory muscle pacing to maintain artificial ventilation. Am J Respir Crit Care 1997; 156:119–126.

41. DiMarco AF, Romaniuk JR, Kowalski KE, Supinski GS. Mechanical contribution of individual expiratory muscles to pressure generation during spinal cord stimulation. J Appl Physiol 1999; 87:1433–1439.

42. DiMarco AF, Romaniuk JR, Kowalski KE, Supinski GS. Pattern of expiratory muscle activation via spinal cord stimulation. J Appl Physiol 1999; 86:1881–1889.

43. DiMarco AF, Romaniuk JR, Supinski GS. Electrical activation of the expiratory muscles to restore cough. Am J Respir Crit Care Med 1995; 151:1466–1471.

44. DiMarco AF, Supinski G, Petro J, Takaoka Y. Artificial respiration via combined intercostal and diaphragm pacing in a quadriplegic patient. Am Rev Respir Dis 1994; 149:A135.

45. DiMarco AF, Supinski GS, Petro J, Takaoka Y. Evaluation of intercostal pacing to provide artificial ventilation in quadriplegics. Am J Respir Crit Care Med 1994; 150:934–940.

46. DiMarco AF, Takaoka Y, Kowalski KE. Evaluation of intercostal and diaphragm pacing to provide artificial ventilation in tetraplegics. Arch Phys Med Rehabil 2005; 86:1200–1207.

47. DiMarco AF, Wolfson DA, Gottfried SB, Altose MD. Sensation of inspired volume in normal subjects and quadriplegic patients. J Appl Physiol 1982; 53:1481–1486.

48. Dobelle WH, D'Angelo MS, Goetz BF, Kiefer DG, Lallier TJ, Lamb JI, Yazwinsky JS. 200 cases with a new breathing pacemaker dispel myths about diaphragm pacing. ASAIO J 1994; 40:M244–M252.

49. Duchenne G. De l'Electrisation localisee et de son application a la pathologie et a le therapeutique, 3d Edition. Paris: J. B. Bailliere, 1872.

50. Elefteriades JA, Hogan JF, Handler A, Loke JS. Long-term follow-up of bilateral pacing of the diaphragm in quadriplegia. N Engl J Med 1992; 326:1433–1434.

51. Elefteriades JA, Quin JA. Diaphragm pacing. Chest Surg Clin N Am 1998; 8:331–357.

52. Elefteriades JA, Quin JA, Hogan JF, Holcomb WG, Letsou GV, Chlosta WF, Glenn WW. Long-term follow-up of pacing of the conditioned diaphragm in quadriplegia. Pacing Clin Electrophysiol 2002; 25:897–906.

53. Esclarin A, Bravo P, Arroyo O, Mazaira J, Garrido H, Alcaraz MA. Tracheostomy ventilation versus diaphragmatic pacemaker ventilation in high spinal cord injury. Paraplegia 1994; 32:687–693.

54. Estenne M, DeTroyer A. Cough in tetraplegic subjects: an active process. Ann Intern Med 1990; 112:22–28.

55. Fishburn MJ, Marino RJ, Ditunno JF Jr. Atelectasis and pneumonia in acute spinal cord injury. Arch Phys Med Rehabil 1990; 71:197–200.

56. Flageole H. Central hypoventilation and diaphragmatic eventration: diagnosis and management. Semin Pediatr Surg 2003; 12:38–45.

57. Fodstad H. The Swedish experience in phrenic nerve stimulation. Pacing Clin Electrophysiol 1987; 10:246–251.

58. Frankel HL, Coll JR, Charlifue SW, Whiteneck GG, Gardner BP, Jamous MA, Krishan KR, Nuseibeh I, Savic G, Sett P. Long-term survival in spinal cord injury: a fifty year investigation. Spinal Cord 1998; 36:266–274.

59. Glenn WW, Brouillette RT, Dentz B, et al. Fundamental considerations in pacing of the diaphragm for chronic ventilatory insufficiency: A multi-center study. Pacing Clin Electrophysiol 1988; 11:2121–2127.

60. Glenn WWL, Gee JB, Cole DR, Farmer WC, Shaw RK, Beckman CB. Combined central alveolar hypoventilation and upper airway obstruction. Treatment by tracheostomy and diaphragm pacing. Am J Med 1978; 64:50–60.

61. Glenn WWL, Hageman JH, Mauro A, Eisenberg L, Flanigan S, Harvard M. Electrical stimulation of excitable tissue by radiofrequency transmission. Ann Surg 1964; 160:338–350.

62. Glenn WWL, Hogan JF. Technique of transthoracic placement of phrenic nerve electrodes for diaphragm pacing. Chicago, Film Library, American College of Surgeons. 1982.

63. Glenn WWL, Hogan JF, Loke JS, Ciesielski TE, Phelps ML, Rowedder R. Ventilatory support by pacing of the conditioned diaphragm in quadriplegia. N Engl J Med 1984; 310:1150–1155.

64. Glenn WW, Hogan JF, Phelps ML. Ventilatory support of the quadriplegic patient with respiratory paralysis by diaphragm pacing. Surg Clin North Am 1980; 60:1055–1078.

65. Glenn WWL, Holcomb WG, Hogan JF, et al. Diaphragm pacing by radiofrequency transmission in the treatment of chronic ventilatory insufficiency: present status. J Thorac Cardiovasc Surg 1973; 66:505–520.

66. Glenn WWL, Phelps ML. Diaphragm pacing by electrical stimulation of the phrenic nerve. Neurosurgery 1985; 17:974–984.

67. Glenn WWL, Phelps ML, Elefteriades JA, Dentz B, Hogan JF. Twenty years experience in phrenic nerve stimulation to pace the diaphragm. Pacing Clin Electrophysiol 1986; 9:780–784.

68. Glenn WW, Sairenji H. Diaphragm pacing in the treatment of chronic ventilatory insufficiency. In: Roussos C, Macklem PT, eds. The thorax: lung biology in health and disease. New York: Marcel Dekker, 1985; 29:1407–1440.

69. Goldenthal S. Bilateral and unilateral activation of the diaphragm in the intact human: External electrical stimulation by capacitive coupling as recorded by cineradiography. Conn Med 1961;25: 236–238.

70. Gorman P, Ho C. Functional electrical stimulation. In: Lin V, ed. Spinal Cord Medicine: Principles and Practice, 2nd Edition, chapter 63.

71. Hartkopp A, Bronnum-Hansen H, Seidenschnur AM, Biering-Sorensen F. Survival and cause of death after traumatic spinal cord injury: a long-term epidemiological survey from Denmark. Spinal Cord 1997; 35:76–85.

72. Hirschfeld S, Exner G, Luukkaala T, Baer GA. Mechanical ventilation or phrenic nerve stimulation for treatment of spinal cord injury-induced respiratory insufficiency. Spinal Cord 2008; 46:738–742.

73. Hoit JD, Banzett RB. Simple adjustments can improve ventilator-supported speech. Am J Speech Lang Pathol 1997; 6:87–96.

74. Hoit JD, Banzett RB, Brown R. Binding the abdomen can improve speech in men with phrenic nerve pacers. Am J Speech Lang Pathol 2002; 11:71–76.

75. Hoit JD, Banzett RB, Lohmeier HL, Hixon TJ, Brown R. Clinical ventilator adjustments that improve speech. Chest 2003; 124:1512–1521.

76. Hunt CE, Brouillette RT, Weese-Mayer DE, Morrow A, Ilbawi MN. Diaphragm pacing in infants and children. Pacing Clin Electrophysiol 1988; 11:2135–2141.

77. Hunt CE, Matalon SV, Thompson TR, et al. Central hypoventilation syndrome:. experience with bilateral phrenic nerve pacing in 3 neonates. Am Rev Respir Dis 1978; 118:23–28.

78. Ilbawi MN, Idriss FS, Hunt CE, Brouillette RT, DeLeon SY. Diaphragmatic pacing in infants: techniques and results. Ann Thorac Surg 1985; 40:323–329.

79. Jackson AB, Groomes TE. Incidence of respiratory complications following spinal cord injury. Arch Phys Med Rehabil 1994; 75:270–275.

80. Jaeger RJ, Langbein EW, Kralj A. Augmenting cough by FES in tetraplegia: a comparison of results at three clinical centers. BAM 1994; 4:195–200.

81. Jaeger RJ, Turba RM, Yarkony GM, Roth EJ. Cough in spinal cord injured patients. A comparison of three methods to produce cough. Arch Phys Med Rehabil 1993; 74:1358–1361.

82. Judson JP, Glenn WWl. Radio-frequency electrophrenic respiration: Long-term application to a patient with primary hypoventilation. JAMA 1968; 203:1033–1037.

83. Kelly BJ. Luce JM. The diagnosis and management of neuromuscular diseases causing respiratory failure. Chest 1991; 99:1485–1494.

84. Kiwerski JE. Factors contributing to the increased threat of life following spinal cord injury. Paraplegia 1993; 31:793–799.

85. Krieger LM, Krieger AJ. The intercostal to phrenic nerve transfer: an effective means of reanimating the diaphragm in patients with high cervical spine injury. Plast Reconstr Surg 2000; 105:1255–1261.

86. Kyroussis D, Polkey MI, Mills GH, Hughes PD, Moxham J, Green M. Simulation of cough in man by magnetic stimulation of the thoracic nerve roots. Am J Respir Crit Care Med 1997; 156,1696–1699.

87. Langou RA, Cohen LS, Sheps D, Wolfson S, Glenn WW. Odine's curse: hemodynamic response to diaphragm pacing (electrophrenic respiration). Am Heart J 1978; 95:295–300.

88. Lim J, Gorman RB, Saboisky JP, Gandevia SC, Butler JE. Optimal electrode placement for noninvasive electrical stimulation of human abdominal muscles. J Appl Physiol 2007; 102:1612–1617.

89. Lin VW, Deng X, Lee YS, Hsiao IN. Stimulation of the expiratory muscles using microstimulators. IEEE Trans Neural Syst Rehabil Eng 2008; 16:416–420.

90. Lin VWH, Hsieh C, Hsiao IN, Canfield J. Functional magnetic stimulation of the expiratory muscles: a noninvasive and new method for restoring cough. J Appl Physiol 1998; 84:1144–1150.

91. Linder SH. Functional electrical stimulation to enhance cough in quadriplegia. Chest 1993; 103:166–169.

92. MacIntyre Nr, Day S. Essentials for ventilator alarm systems. Respir Care 2001; 46:874–896.

93. MacLean IC, Mattioni TA. Phrenic nerve conduction studies: a new technique and its application in quadriplegic patients. Arch Phys Med Rehabil 1981; 62:70–73.

94. Mayr W, Bijak M, Girsch W, et al. Multichannel stimulation of phrenic nerves by epineural electrodes. ASAIO J 1993; 39:M729–M735.

95. McKenzie DK, Gandevia SC. Phrenic nerve conduction times and twitch pressures of the human diaphragm. J Appl Physiol 1985; 58:1496–1504.

96. McMichan JC, Michel L, Westbrook PR. Pulmonary dysfunction following traumatic quadriplegia: recognition, prevention and treatment. JAMA 1980; 243:528–531.

97. Miller JM, Moxham J, Green M. The maximal sniff in the assessment of diaphragm function in man. Clin Sci (London) 1985; 69:91–96.

98. Moosa A. Phrenic nerve conduction in children. Dev Med Child Neurol 1981; 23:434–448.

99. Moxham J, Shneerson JM. Diaphragmatic pacing. Am Rev Respir Dis 1993; 148:533–536.

100. Nochomovitz ML, DiMarco AF, Mortimer JT, Cherniack NS. Diaphragm activation with intramuscular stimulation in dogs. Am Rev Respir Dis 1983; 127:325–329.

101. Nochomovitz ML, Hopkins M, Brodkey J, Montenegro H, Mortimer JT, Cherniack NS. Conditioning of the diaphragm with phrenic nerve stimulation after prolonged disuse. Am Rev Respir Dis 1984; 130:685–688.

102. Oda T, Glenn WWL, Fukuda Y, Hogan JF, Gorfien J. Evaluation of electrical parameters for diaphragm pacing: An experimental study. J Surg Res 1981; 30:142–153.

103. Oliven A. Electrical stimulation of the respiratory muscles. In: Cherniack NS, Altose MD, Homma I, eds. Rehabilitation of the patient with respiratory disease. New York: McGraw-Hill, 1999; 535–542.

104. Onders RP, DiMarco AF, Ignagni AR, Aiyar H, Mortimer JT. Mapping the phrenic nerve motor point: the key to a successful laparoscopic diaphragm pacing system in the first human series. Surgery 2004; 136:819–826.

105. Oo T, Watt JWH, Soni BM, Sett PK. Delayed diaphragm recovery in 12 patients after high cervical spinal cord injury. A retrospective review of the diaphragm status of 107 patients ventilated after acute spinal cord injury. Spinal Cord 1999; 37:117–122.

106. Paw P, Sackier JM. Complications of laparoscopy and thoracoscopy. J Intensive Care Med 1994; 9:290–304.

107. Peterson DK, Nochomovitz ML, DiMarco AF, Mortimer JT. Intramuscular electrical activation of the phrenic nerve. IEEE Trans Biomed Eng 1986; 33:342–352.

108. Peterson DK, Nochomovitz ML, Stellato TA, Mortimer JT. Long-term intramuscular electrical activation of the phrenic nerve: efficacy as a ventilatory prosthesis. IEEE Trans Biomed Eng 1994; 41:1127–1135.

109. Peterson DK, Nochomovitz ML, Stellato TA, Mortimer JT. Long-term intramuscular electrical activation of the phrenic nerve: safety and reliability. IEEE Trans Biomed Eng 1994; 41:1115–1126.

110. Pugin J, Oudin S. Cellular and molecular basis for ventilator-induced lung injury. In: Dreyfuss D, Saumon G, Hubmayr RD, eds. Lung Biology in Health and Disease: Ventilatory-induced Lung Injury. New York: Taylor and Francis Group, 2006; 205–222.

111. Salmons S, Henriksson J. The adaptive response of skeletal muscle to increased use. Muscle Nerve 1981; 4:94–105.

112. Sarnoff SJ, Hardenberg E, Whittenberger JL. Electrophrenic respiration. Am J Physiol 1948; 155:1–9.

113. Schmit BD, Mortimer JT. The effects of epimysial electrode location on phrenic nerve recruitment and the relation between tidal volume and interpulse interval. IEEE Trans Rehabil Eng 1999; 7:150–158.

114. Schmit BD, Stellato TA, Miller ME, Mortimer JM. Laparoscopic placement of electrodes for diaphragm pacing using stimulation to locate the phrenic nerve motor points. IEEE Trans Rehabil Eng 1998; 6:382–390.

115. Shaul DB, Danielson PD, McComb JG, Keens TG. Thoracoscopic placement of phrenic nerve electrodes for diaphragmatic pacing in children. J Pediatr Surg 2002; 37:974–978.

116. Shavelle RM, DeVivo MJ, Strauss DJ, Paculdo DR, Lammertse DP, Day SM. Long-term survival of persons ventilator dependent after spinal cord injury. J Spinal Cord Med 2006; 29:511–519.

117. Similowski T, Fleury B, Launois S, Cathala HP, Bouche P, Derenne JP. Cervical magnetic stimulation: a new painless method for bilateral phrenic nerve stimulation in conscious humans. J Appl Physiol 1989; 67:1311–1318.

118. Soden RJ, Walsh J, Middleton JW, Craven ML, Rutkawki SB, Yeo JD. Causes of death after spinal cord injury. Spinal Cord 2000; 38:604–610.

119. Spinal cord injury: facts and figures at a glance 2008. The National Spinal Cord Injury Statistical Center, University of Alabama, Birmingham, AL. www.spinalcord.uab.edu.

120. Talonen PP, Baer GA, Hakkinen V, Ojala JK. Neurophysiological and technical considerations for the design of an implantable phrenic nerve stimulator. Med Biol Eng Comput 1990; 28:31–37.

121. Thoma H, Gerner H, Holle J, et al. The phrenic pacemaker: substitution of paralyzed functions in tetraplegia. ASAIO Trans 1987; 33: 472–479.

122. Tibballs J. Diaphragmatic pacing: An alternative to long-term mechanical ventilation. Anaesth Intensive Care 1991; 19:597–601.

123. Ure, A: Experiments made on the body of a criminal immediately after execution, with physiological and philosophical observations J. Sciences Arts 12:1, 1818.

124. Vanderlinden RG, Epstein SW, Hyland RH, Smythe HS, Vanderlinden LD. Management of chronic ventilatory insufficiency with electrical diaphragm pacing. Can J Neuro Sci 1988; 15:63–67.

125. Weese-Mayer DE, Hunt CE, Brouillette RT, Silvestri JM. Diaphragm pacing in infants and children. J Pediatr 1992; 120:1–8.

126. Weese-Mayer DE, Morrow AS, Brouillette RT, Ilbawi MN, Hunt CE. Diaphragm pacing in infants and children. A life-table analysis of implanted components. Am Rev Respir Dis 1989; 139:974–979.

127. Weese-Mayer DE, Silvestri JM, Kenny AS, et al. Diaphragm pacing with a quadripolar phrenic nerve electrode: an international study. Pacing Clin Electrophysiol 1996; 19:1311–1319.

128. Whiteneck G. Long-term outlook for persons with high quadriplegia. In: Whiteneck G, Alder C, Carter RE, et al, eds. The Management of High Quadriplegia. New York: Demos Publications, 1989; 353–361.

129. Whiteneck GG, Charlifue SW, Frankel HL, Fraser MH, Gardner BP, Gerhart KA, et al. Mortality, morbidity, and psychosocial outcomes of persons spinal cord injured more than 20 years ago. Paraplegia 1992; 30:617–630.

130. Whittenberger JL, Sarnoff SJ, Hardenberg E. Electrophrenic respiration. II. Its use in man. J Clin Invest 1949; 28:124–128.

131. Wick AB, Menter RR. Long-term outlook in quadriplegic patients with initial ventilator dependency. Chest 1986; 90:406–410.

IX

SPECIAL TOPICS IN SPINAL CORD MEDICINE

76 History of Spinal Cord Medicine

Ibrahim M. Eltorai

The history of spinal cord medicine, like other branches of medicine, entails so many topics: for example, anatomy; physiology; pathophysiology; clinical manifestations; investigative procedures; management; and medical, surgical, and rehabilitative aspects. This text focuses mainly on spinal cord injury (SCI), the history of which will be detailed in this chapter. The history of the diseases of the spinal cord can be consulted in textbooks covering neurology, the history of neurology, and the founders of neurology (1–3).

Although spinal cord injury was documented in history ca. 3000 BCE, it did not receive much attention until the fourth decade of the twentieth century, and from then on, it progressed rapidly and continues to do so. The history of SCI will be subdivided into the following categories:

1. Ancient History
2. The Middle Ages
3. The Renaissance: Early and Late
4. The Dawn of the Scientific Revolution
   a. The eighteenth century
   b. The nineteenth century
   c. The twentieth and twenty-first centuries
      i. Establishment of SCI care and rehabilitation in the United States and overseas
      ii. Medical and surgical management
5. Special Topics in the Care of SCI
   a. Spinal shock
   b. Autonomic dysreflexia
   c. Heterotopic ossification
   d. Urodynamics
   e. SCI urology
   f. Pressure ulcers
6. Spinal Cord Repair and Regeneration

ANCIENT HISTORY OF SCI

Ancient Egypt

The first and most authentic description of cervical vertebral injury resulting in tetraplegia was documented in an Egyptian papyrus, which provided some level of detail. The Edwin Smith surgical papyrus was written between 3000 and 2500 BCE by an Egyptian physician, most probably Imhotep (Figure 76.1), and translated by the famous Egyptologist Dr. James Breasted, of the University of Chicago (4–6). It is the most authentic surgical document in ancient human history. Of the spinal cord injury cases, 29–33 and 48 (Figure 76.2) are the most specific; these cases contain clear descriptions of a complete cervical cord injury. The most typical is case 31, which states

> If thou examinest a man having a dislocation of a vertebra of his neck, shouldst thou find him unconscious of his two arms and his two legs on account of it (and) urine drips from his member without his knowing it, his flesh has received wind, his two eyes are blood shot: it is a dislocation of a vertebra of his neck extending to his backbone, which causes him to be unconscious of his two arms and his two legs. If, however, the middle vertebra of the neck is dislocated, has an emissio seminis which befalls his phallus, thou shouldst say concerning him, "one having dislocation of vertebra of his neck while he is unconscious of his two legs and his two arms and his urine dribbles, 'an ailment not to be treated (cured).'"

Case 33 has almost the same picture. These cases describe the cardinal symptoms of complete cervical cord injury secondary to a dislocation, fracture, or fracture dislocation of cervical spine causing tetraplegia, complete sensory loss, loss of micturition control, priapism, involuntary seminal emission, or conjunctival congestion due to the loss of vasomotor tone. The ancient physician gave no hope of cure in such cases, a pessimistic prognosis that continued throughout thousands of years across the world. In the twenty-first century CE, however, this theory may be changing, at least partially. The ancient physician did, however, realize the necessity of physical rest and support of the injured vertebrae, and that advice has remained unchanged through the ages.

Greece

Spinal history is very sketchy between the Egyptian and Greek periods, and the records are very fragmentary. The religious cult

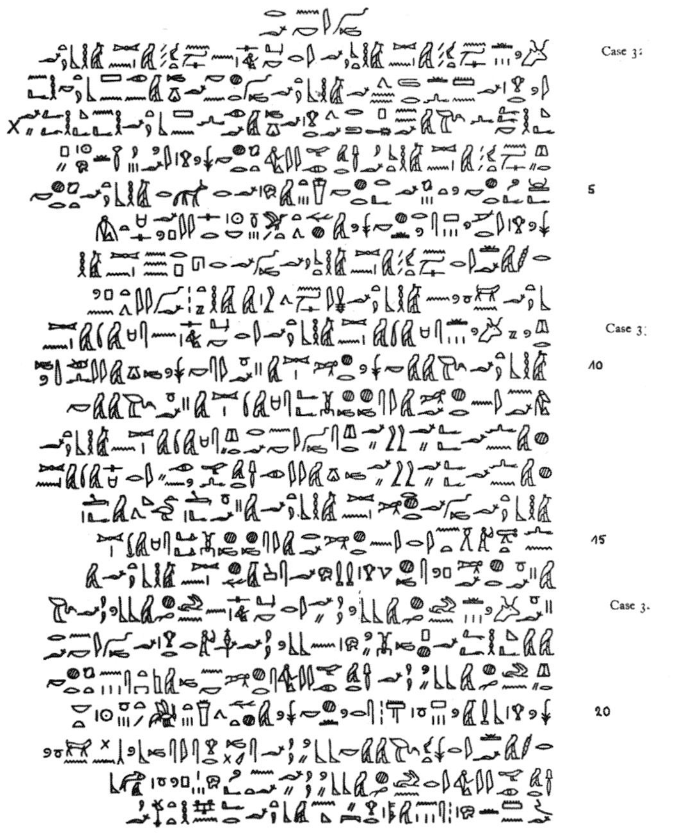

Figure 76.1   Edwin Smith papyrus.

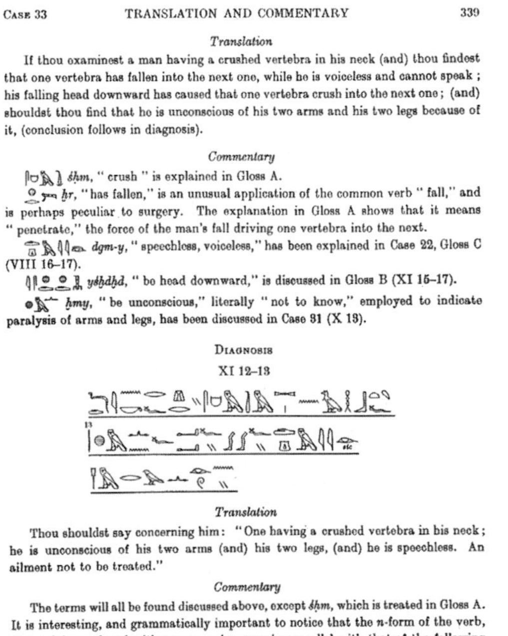

CASE 33   TRANSLATION AND COMMENTARY   339

Translation

If thou examinest a man having a crushed vertebra in his neck (and) thou findest that one vertebra has fallen into the next one, while he is voiceless and cannot speak; his falling head downward has caused that one vertebra crush into the next one; (and) shouldst thou find that he is unconscious of his two arms and his two legs because of it, (conclusion follows in diagnosis).

Commentary

𓉐𓂧𓏏 *shm*, "crush" is explained in Gloss A.

𓂝 𓏤 *hr*, "has fallen," is an unusual application of the common verb "fall," and is perhaps peculiar to surgery. The explanation in Gloss A shows that it means "penetrate," the force of the man's fall driving one vertebra into the next.

𓊪 *dgm-y*, "speechless, voiceless," has been explained in Case 22, Gloss C (VIII 16–17).

𓇋𓏏 *yshdhd*, "be head downward," is discussed in Gloss B (XI 16–17).

𓂝 *hmy*, "be unconscious," literally "not to know," employed to indicate paralysis of arms and legs, has been discussed in Case 31 (X 19).

DIAGNOSIS

XI 12–13

Translation

Thou shouldst say concerning him: "One having a crushed vertebra in his neck; he is unconscious of his two arms (and) his two legs, (and) he is speechless. An ailment not to be treated."

Commentary

The terms will all be found discussed above, except *shm*, which is treated in Gloss A. It is interesting, and grammatically important to notice that the *n*-form of the verb, *hmy-n-f*, is employed with a permansive meaning parallel with that of the following pseudo-participle (*dgm-y*).

Verdict 3 indicates that there is no hope of recovery. See Case 5 (II 15). It is therefore, as usual, followed by no directions for treatment.

z 2

Figure 76.2   Translation of the Edwin Smith papyrus.

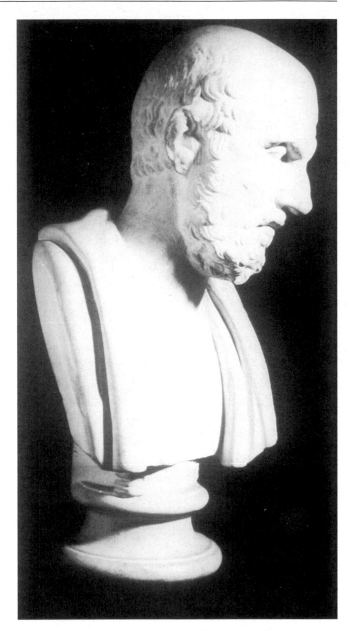

Figure 76.3   Hippocrates.

of Aesculapius took the place of scientific medicine. Aesculapius is believed to be the son of Apollo, god of medicine. The culmination of Greek medicine came between 462 and 429 BCE, due to the writings of Hippocrates (460–370 BCE) (7) (Figure 76.3) He started to disassociate medicine from religion. He traveled extensively in Greece and went to Egypt. For treatment of spinal injuries he used a method he invented called "suspension on a ladder," as well as other methods of traction. He described paraplegia with bowel and bladder dysfunction, as well as pressure ulcers. He did not discriminate between paralysis due to trauma or disease and considered the same treatment to be appropriate for either of them. However, his contribution lived after him through the ages. He elaborated on gibbosity at different levels and mentioned paralysis accompanied by cold abscess due to Pott's disease. For traumatic gibbosity, he indicated that it was uncorrectable, stating that, "wherefore succession on a ladder has never straightened any gibbus, as far as I know, it is principally practiced by those physicians who seek to astonish the mob. . . . But the physicians who follow such practice, as far as I have known them, are all stupid." In *Anatomy of the Spine,* Hippocrates mentioned details of articulations, nerves and vessels, sheaths (meninges) of the spinal marrow (cord), ligaments, and muscles. He was the first to describe the spinal cord as vertebral marrow, "Rückenmark" in German. Regarding spinal injuries, he stated in his book *On the Articulations,* part 46 (page 235):

> In cases of displacement backward along the vertebrae, it does not often happen, in fact, it is very rare, that one or more vertebra are torn from one another and displaced. For such injuries do not readily occur, as a spine could not easily be displaced backward but by a severe injury on the fore part through the belly (which would prove fatal) or if a person falling from height should pitch on the nates, or shoulders (and even in this case would die, but not immediately); and the spinal marrow would suffer, if from the displacement of a vertebra it were to be bent even to a small extent; for the displaced vertebra would compress the spinal marrow, if it did not break it; and if compressed and strangled, it would induce insensibility of many great and important parts, so that the physician need not give himself any concern about rectifying the displacement of the vertebra, accompanied, as it is, by many other ill consequences of a serious nature.

He knew that both anterior and posterior dislocations would damage the spinal marrow (spinal cord). He condemned open reduction of such cases and favored spontaneous callus formation. He mentioned that displacement of vertebrae forward was mostly fatal, or that the patients, if they were to survive, would lose the power of their legs and arms (quadriplegia) and have torpor of the body and retention of urine. He introduced various methods of reduction of deformities, particularly the gibbus, especially by using the extension bench. Greek medicine spread, especially from the school of Alexandria to the Roman Empire, although it was not easily accepted initially.

The Roman Epoch

Aulus Cornelius Celsus (8) lived in the first century of the Common Era. His treatise *De Medicina* had a brief discussion on spinal cord injuries, especially on the fractures of the spinous processes. For dislocations of vertebrae, he recommended Hippocrates' traction method for incomplete lesions. For complete lesions, death usually ensued.

Galen, the Greco-Roman physician (131–201 CE) (8) practicing in Rome in the second century as a physician to Emperor Marcus Aurelius, followed Hippocratic methods and added very little of his own. But Galen, one of the greatest physicians of antiquity, was a founder of experimental physiology. He wrote over 400 separate treatises. Not only did he describe the brain anatomy, but he also discussed the spinal cord and the brachial and lumbosacral plexuses. He anticipated Brown-Séquard's hemisection. He described injuries of the first and second cervical vertebrae, stating that they were fatal and that respiration stops with injuries, especially at the third or fourth

vertebrae. He experimented on animals and did sections of the spinal cord at different levels to see their pathophysiology. He described other lower-level injuries. There was no change in methodology for 200 years after his work.

Oribasius, who lived in the fourth century (324–400 CE), was born Greek and went to Rome at the invitation of the Emperor Julian the Apostate to compile his knowledge of Greek medicine. He modified the Hippocratic table to correct spinal deformity by forceful and brisk procedures (9).

Paul of Aegina (Greco-Roman also) (625–690 CE) (10) compiled several books. *Book VI* describes Hippocrates' technique and adds to it spinal splinting after reduction of dislocations. Paul of Aegina is considered the originator of laminectomy for decompression and removal of the offending bones.

Mesopotamian Medicine

There is no specific record from history references in relation to spinal injuries in Mesopotamia, although the Assyrians had a great civilization and complex theology, as documented in the thousands of tablets found in museums (11a).

Hebraic Medicine

Talmudic medicine notes spinal injuries in men and animals, with resulting paralysis. More scientific practice was conducted by Maimonides in the Middle Ages (see section on the Middle Ages) (11b).

Early Hindu Medicine

The most documented surgical practices were written in the *Sushruta Samhita* (12) in the third or fourth centuries CE. Regarding spinal injuries, the cervical dislocations were manually manipulated and reduced, and then bandages and a splint were applied; bed rest was also prescribed. For lower fractures of the spine, the patient was placed on a board and tied with ropes to five pegs for immobilization. Sushruta believed that spinal fractures were not curable.

Chinese Medicine

Documented history of spinal cord injuries has not been found in the available old texts of Chinese medicine, although Chinese physicians were aware of them. Likely, Chinese medicine, especially acupuncture, was applicable for management of pain, spasticity, bladder issues, and perhaps paralysis. Chinese herbology was practiced for general care and treatment in hospitals, but there is no mention of spinal cord paralysis. Early in the twentieth century, western medicine (English, Russian, and American) penetrated China, and an orthopedic hospital was established in 1913.

THE MIDDLE AGES (700–1400 CE)

With the gradual infiltration of the Roman Empire by barbarian tribes, there was stagnation and decline of science, which was replaced by superstition and intellectual degeneration. Jewish medicine was probably the only medicine in practice (13). In the

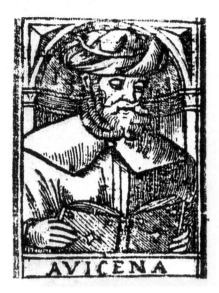

İbni Sıma'ya aid bu resim Avrupa-
da çok taammüm eden resimlerden-
dir. Yalnız eserler bunun menşe'ini
göstermiyorlar. Ufak farklarla bir-
birine benzeyen bu resimlerin sayısı
az değildir. Bu resim La Medicina
de los Arabes, namı altında 9 Mart
1770 de Madridde açılan Tıb aka-
demisinin senei devriyesinde D. A.
Piquer tarafından verilen koferansın,
Madridde 1935 de X uncu beynel-
milel Tıb Tarihi kongresine verilen
tezler meyanında basıldığından ilâve
olunmuştur

Figure 76.4 Avicenna.

seventh century, with the rise of Arab and Islamic civilization, translations from the Greek and Roman and the Persian and Hindu medical sciences flourished, with the work of many eminent physicians to numerous to be cited here. Avicenna (980–1037) (14–15), who was the most eminent, compiled about 100 books. The most comprehensive is his *Cannon in Medicine,* in five volumes, which was translated into Latin and remained the main reference of European schools for about six centuries (Figure 76.4).

In relation to spinal injuries, he followed the method of Paul of Aegina, reducing dislocations of the thoracolumbar spine by putting the patient prone on the floor. The physician stood with his heels on the gibbosity. He also reduced cervical dislocation by extension in the supine position followed by fixation of the neck through splints. Among the Arabists was the Hebrew physician Moses Maimonides (11) (Figure 76.5), whose works were on diet, hygiene, and toxicology. He practiced in Cairo and followed the same system as Avicenna. His book, published in 1199, mentioned paraplegia with some neurologic signs.

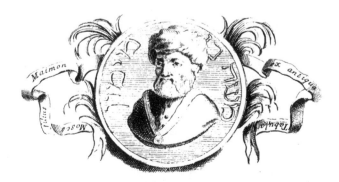

Figure 76.5 Moses Maimonides.

Western medicine was very primitive at this stage and was in the hands of the monks using religious rites, herbs, salves, and brews. Nothing was mentioned about spinal injuries.

THE RENAISSANCE

By the thirteenth century, the school of Salerno pulled European medicine out of the dark ages. Constantinus Africanus (16) learned Arabic and used Greco-Arabic medicine. Roland of Parma, in Salerno, wrote his book *Chirurgia* (17) in 1210. He used different methods for treating spinal injuries, discarding Hippocrates' bench. He performed reduction of cervical injuries with the patient in the sitting position using traction from the hair or a cloth sling under his jaw. In thoracic and lumbar dislocations, the patient was placed supine; the physician exerted traction on the legs, with counter-traction by an assistant on the upper half of the body. Many famous authors in Italy and France wrote about spinal injuries and published several books. This went hand in hand with the gradual transition from the Latin and Greek to French and English and with the development of science, mathematics, and philosophy.

The Fifteenth and Sixteenth Centuries

Paul of Aegina's book, written 1465, was adopted by Serefeddin Sabuncuaglu, a Turk, and was republished by Uenver in 1939 (18). Reduction of a fracture of the spine was done by two assistants pulling the upper and lower extremities and the physician exerting direct pressure at the fracture site.

Ambroise Paré, born in 1510, became a barber-surgeon and joined the army, where he progressed to be the chief surgeon of the army to four successive Kings. This was due to his progressive and courageous techniques and to his books, *Dix Livres de Chirurgie* (*Ten Books of Surgery*), published in 1564 (19). He adopted, but modified, Hippocratic techniques by reducing the fracture in the prone position, but he cautioned against causing more damage by this manipulation. He splinted the spine with lead splints, and then turned the patient on his back, leaving him in bed for a long time. He went back to the work of Paul of Aegina, reviving laminectomy for fractures causing compression of the cord. For fractures of the spinous process, he removed them for pain only. In absence of pain, and when still attached by the periosteum, he set them in position and splinted the back until full healing occurred. For cervical dislocation, he had an attendant press hard on the shoulders while he pulled up the head by two hands close to the ears, and with some turning of the head, the dislocation was reduced. A stabilizing bandage was then applied around the shoulders. France followed Paré's technique for a long time. In the nineteenth century, Jean Francis Calot used the same techniques (20).

THE DAWN OF THE SCIENTIFIC REVOLUTION

The Seventeenth and Eighteenth Centuries

In this period, anatomical dissection was permitted in Europe, but management of spinal injuries was still primitive. Paré's technique was used with some modifications in Germany, Holland, Italy, and England. In 1762 Antrine Louis (21) removed a bullet lodged in the spine. In 1793 J. Soemmering wrote a book about dislocations and fractures of the spine, *Bemerkungen ueber Verrenkung und Bruch des Ruckgraths.* Jean Louis Petit (22), in the second half of the eighteenth century, wrote his treatise, *Les Maladies des Os (Diseases of the Bones)*, and his method was used almost exclusively in that century. He reduced fractures by hyperflexion of the spine, trying to disengage the spinous processes.

In the German school, Lorenz Heister (23) was a leading surgeon, using Petit's method for thoracic and lumbar injuries, but he used the extension for cervical injuries. Petit's technique was avoided by Hunczovsky in Germany by using hyperextension techniques, suspending the patient from the ceiling by the neck (24).

The Nineteenth Century

The history of spinal cord medicine was reviewed by Ohry and Ohry-Kossy (25) in a monograph published as *Paraplegia Supplement.* The review states:

> With the advent of the century the old-fashioned medical practice was slowly changed into scientific medicine. The progress is based on the knowledge of the anatomy and physiology of the spinal cord by pioneers of that century (Garrison's History of Neurology) [1]. Sir Astley Cooper described cauda equina lesions and their management. He described fractures and dislocations of the spine with the resulting paralysis [26]. In 1860 Brown-Séquard described different kinds of spinal paralysis based on vascular changes [27–30]. The injuries were divided into thoracolumbar and cervical paraplegia until 1881, when Sir William Gull coined the term Quadriplegia . . . . The outlook was generally very gloomy, and this was carried into the 20th century through World War I.

Two famous leaders had spinal cord injuries by bullets, and both died: Lord Nelson, who was injured in the Battle of Trafalgar,

died a few hours after the injury in 1805 (31, 32). In 1881, James A. Garfield, the 20th president of the United States, was shot and died in less than 3 months (33, 34).

The 20th Century

With developments in bacteriology, the invention of disinfection by Pasteur and Lister, Roentgen's discovery of X-rays, and the invention of ether anesthesia by William Morton, the outlook on SCI changed to some extent, although the prognosis was still poor.

In the Balkan wars, the mortality rate from SCI was 95%. Harvey Cushing (35) reported that 80% of battlefield casualties with cervical spine injuries died in the first 2 weeks. Those who survived were the ones with incomplete and lower injuries. The British army reported the same results. In the interwar period, the prognosis was still poor. The patients who survived were crippled, miserable, and unwanted, even by their families, who wished for their demise (after D. Munro).

Progress in the Twentieth Century

DEVELOPMENT OF MEDICAL TECHNOLOGY. Numerous advances in orthopedic surgery can be reviewed in the orthopedic and neurosurgical literature (36–38), as well as in chapters in this text. Surgical and orthopedic instrumentation such as rods, fixators, wires, screws, meshes, plates, clamps, hooks, and cements were developed. Different surgical approaches to the spine came into use, including thoracoabdominal, transoral, transthoracic, transabdominal, throascopic, and laparoscopic approaches. Laminotomy, laminoplasty, laminectomy, foraminectomy, arthrodesis, and bone grafting were introduced, to mention just a few. Recent advances in transportation and first aid, management of traumatic shock, antibiotics, and the development of laser beam and microsurgery have contributed to more survival.

In 1929, Alfred Taylor of New York used a traction halter fitted to the occiput and the mandible for cervical spinal injuries. In 1933, William A. Crutchfield devised cranial skeletal traction (39). Other traction devises were made by Barton (1938), Vinke (1948), and Gardner (1970s). In 1959, Perry and Nickel introduced halotraction, which is still in use today. After World War I, the German experiences were recorded by Foerster (40), and the French experiences by Lhermitte and Roussy (41).

ESTABLISHMENT OF SCI CARE CENTERS. In the United States, dramatic changes occurred when Dr. Donald Munro (42–45) (Figure 76.6) developed a great interest in the care of spinal cord injury patients in the early 1930s. As a neurosurgeon with a background in general and urological surgery, he was an ideal leader and a master of all aspects of para- and tetraplegia. He made great efforts toward the rehabilitation of spinal cord injury patients, as well as working to meet their socioeconomic needs. He was the true creator of modern spinal cord injury care and deserves to bear the title of "Father of Paraplegia Care." A large number of neurosurgeons and orthopedic surgeons have significantly contributed to a better outcome in spinal injuries.

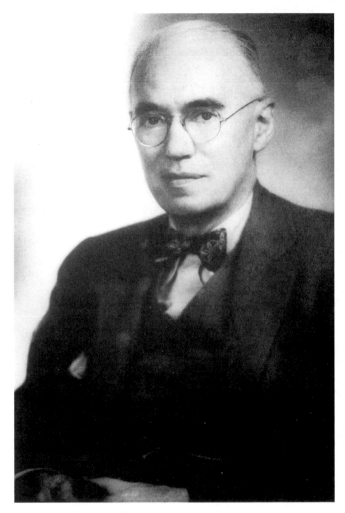

Figure 76.6 Donald Munro, MD.

On the other side of the Atlantic, Sir Ludwig Guttmann (Figure 76.7) established a unit in Stoke Mandeville (46), in Ayelsbury, on February 1, 1944, for comprehensive treatment and rehabilitation with multidisciplinary staffing. Under his leadership, the unit became a world-renowned center for teaching and research as well as care management, not to forget Hans Frankel. Because of the influence of these two units on either side of the Atlantic, many other units were established. Drs. Ernest Bors and A. Estin Comarr in Long Beach, California, pioneered the rehabilitation and urology protocols that were followed in all the centers (Figure 76.8). H. Talbot in Boston, Eric Kreuger in the Bronx, and B. Moeller in Memphis are other notable figures to mention. In the United Kingdom, the following centers are to be mentioned: Lodgemoor in Sheffield; the Robert Jones and Agnes Hunt Orthopedic Hospital at Oswestry, Shropshire; the Pinderfield Hospital, Wakefield, Yorkshire; the Liverpool Spinal Unit at Promenade Hospital; the Edenhall Unit in Musselburgh, Scotland; the Phillipshall Hospital near Glasgow; and the Rookwood Hospital, Cardiff, Wales. Centers in Europe included the following: in Austria, Tobelbad; in France, Fontainebleau (Paris) and Invalides (Paris), Mulhouse; in Belgium, Brugman in Brussels; in Germany, Koblenz, Bochum, Amsburg, Frankfurt, Murnau, Tübingen, Ludwigshafen,

Heidelberg, Cologne, and Berlin; in Holland, Aardenburg, Amsterdam; and in Ireland, Dublin. A list of other centers in Europe, Canada, Australia, the Middle and Far East, and South America can be obtained from The International Spinal Cord Society. In the United States, the Department of Veterans Affairs has twenty-three centers, which are discussed in Chapter 83 of this text. The Department of Health and Human Services has established regional centers in different states. In Canada in 1945, Lyndhurst Lodge was established in Toronto, and the Canadian Paraplegic Association was also founded. The Canadian Veterans Administration established some wards for spinal cord injury care. There are numerous private centers throughout the country.

SCI REHABILITATION MEDICINE. In a three-volume textbook published in 1939, entitled *Principles and Practice of Physical Therapy* (46), spinal cord injury rehabilitation was not covered in the chapter on physical therapy of the nervous diseases, probably due to the high mortality at this time, which was 80%. A detailed history of rehabilitation medicine was written by J. DeLisa (47); other texts include Guttmann (48).

Dr. Donald Munro established a comprehensive SCI rehabilitation center in Boston City Hospital, which was a model

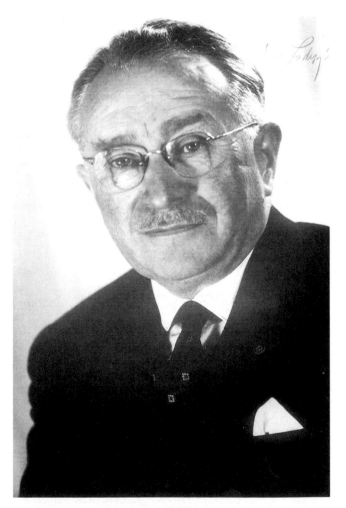

Figure 76.7 Sir Ludwig Guttmann.

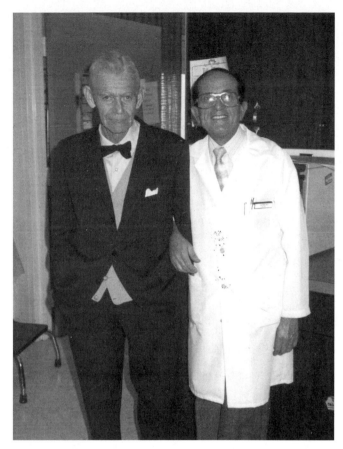

Figure 76.8 Ernest Bors, MD. (**left**), and Ibrahim Eltorai, MD. (**right**).

unit in the United States. Under his care, the SCI patient was treated physically, neurologically, and urologically, as he developed tidal drainage; in addition pychosocial rehabilitation and vocational orientation were included. Among the contributors who established SCI rehabilitation programs were Howard Rusk, Arthur Abramson, and Harry Kessler.

Rehabilitation aspects now include efforts toward physical, psychologic, behavioral, sexual, vocational, and functional independence (49).

SCI EDUCATION. Before Donald Munro, the care of SCI was not taught in medical schools as an independent subject. Teaching began in the VA centers under the leadership of Eric Krueger, who instituted comprehensive programs. His follower Emanuele Manerino initiated the fellowship program, which continues until now; this position was filled by Joseph Binard and is currently held by Margaret Hammond.

The American Paraplegia Society was founded by Comarr (1954) and was later supported greatly by Mr. James J. Peters. Both societies held annual meetings with numerous teaching programs and workshops. In England, Sir Ludwig Guttmann founded the International Society of Paraplegia (now known as the International Spinal Cord Society), which held meetings annually in different countries. There have been combined meetings between the three societies. There are countless others, including the Cervical Spine Research Society based in Illinois

and the Miami Project to Cure Paralysis based in Miami, Florida.

Journals have become the media for spreading knowledge everywhere, especially *Spinal Cord* (formerly called *Paraplegia*), the journal of the International Spinal Cord Society; the *Journal of Spinal Cord Medicine* (previously the *Bulletin of the APS*); and the *Journal of Neurotraumatology,* founded by the International Societies of Neurotraumatology. Great information can also be obtained from the *American Journal of Physical Medicine and Rehabilitation;* journals of the spine, urology, orthopedic surgery, neurosurgery, plastic surgery, and hand surgery; and numerous other journals.

Many books have been printed in English, as well as in many other languages. However, this text is the most eminent.

Medical schools have both undergraduate and postgraduate courses for teaching spinal cord medicine.

RECOGNITION IN THE FIELD. DeLisa was instrumental in approving SCI care as a subspecialty under the Board of Physical Medicine and Rehabilitation, by which SCI care came to stand on equal ground with other subspecialties and to be finally accepted after many years. (See Chapter 86 in this book.)

SPECIAL TOPICS IN THE CARE OF SCI

Spinal Shock

In 1874 Goltz and Freusberg in Strasbourg described spinal shock on the dog in a masterly way (50). Sherrington did his work on spinal shock on the monkey by cervical transection of the cord. He specified it primarily as a neurogenic condition. He referred to the rise of blood pressure after the disappearance of shock by skin stimulation, but he did not describe it as autonomic dysreflexia (51).

Autonomic Dysreflexia

Head and Riddoch first described autonomic dysreflexia in 1917 (52). Its significance and dangers were described by Whitteridge (1946–1947) (53), Guttmann and Whitteridge (1947) (54), Thompson and Whitham (1948) (55), Pollock et al. (1951) (56), Bors and French (1952) (57), Schreibert (1955) (58), and Arieff et al. (1962) (59). Many others followed from Europe, America, and Australia. (See Eltorai [60].)

Heterotopic Ossification

Para-articular osteoarthropathy was first described by Riedel (1883) (61) and Reichert (1845) (62). A detailed description in paraplegics was elaborated by Klumpke-Dejerine and Cellier (1918) (63) and by Dejerine et al. (1919) (64). This was followed by many other writers, among them Soule (1945) (65), Abramson (1948) (66), Abramson and Komberg (1949) (67), Liberson (1953) (68), Damanski (1961) (69), Hardy and Dickson (1963) (70), Paeslack (1965) (71), Freehafer and Yurick (1966) (72), Roussier et al. (1973) (73), and the chapter in this text.

Urodynamics

Galen believed that bladder evacuation was by contraction of the abdominal muscles, and eminent people, such as Vesalius and Albrecht von Haller, stressed this for centuries. The first measurement of intravesical pressure was done by Rudolph

Haidenhain (1837–1897) in Breslau. He and Colberg focused on sphincter tone. De Wittich and Rosenplanter (1867) recorded intravesical pressure. Julius Budge (1811–1888) studied the neurophysiology of the bladder and concluded that the sacral third and fourth anterior roots were the motor nerves of the bladder. Goltz experimentally transected the spinal cord at the thoracolumbar level in dogs and noted reflex bladder evacuation and eviction, which disappeared by ablation of the lower cord.

Human studies were initiated by F. Schatz (1841–1920). Dubois (1848–1918) measured bladder pressure in normal controls and paraplegics and also measured rectal pressure. Other names in this field are Quinke and Adler in Germany, Angelo Mosso and Paul Pellacani in Italy, Fritz Born in Switzerland, and Guyon and Duchastelet in France.

In Germany, Adler studied manometry in the neurogenic bladder and differentiated conal from supraconal lesions. In Vienna, Schwartz studied cystometry in gunshot wounds of the spinal cord. In the United States, Walker, Dalton, Roussy, and Rossi also made advances. In Baltimore, Walker proposed simple devices for cystometry. In St. Louis, Dalton coined the term cystometry and described the different types of neurogenic bladder. Roussy and Rossi studied cystometry in SCI at different levels. In England, Henry Head and George Riddoch studied neurogenic bladders and described automatic micturition as a part of the mass reflex in supraconal lesions. Sir Gordon Holmes studied neurogenic bladders in soldiers in France (1915–1916). In 1933 in London, Denny-Brown and Robertson measured bladder pressure, urethral pressure at the bladder neck, external sphincter pressure, and rectal pressure. In 1935, Kenneth Watkins described reflexic and areflexic bladders in cord injuries. Donald Munro, who in 1947 introduced tidal drainage, described the atonic cord bladder early in injury, the autonomous cord bladder, the hypertonic cord bladder, and the inhibited cord bladder. Many others contributed to the field in the early years, including Nesbit, Lapides, Tang, Ruch, Bors, Comarr, and Bradley. There are also neurourology and urodynamic societies and their publication, the *Journal of Neurourology and Urodynamics*.

History of SCI Urology

1. Earliest description of urinary incontinence due to vertebral injury in Edwin Smith Papyrus, 2500 BC, translated by James Breasted in 1930 (4).
2. Ancient catheters of metal used by the ancient Egyptians and Chinese. They used metal (gold and bronze) or hollow plant stems (clover) (75–77).
3. In 1036, Avicenna created the flexible catheter. For more details in the Renaissance, see Mattehlover and Billet (78).
4. In 1937, Foley introduced his cuffed catheter (79).
5. See below for devices for incontinence; for further details, see Schultheiss et al. (80), Bors and Comarr (81), Lindsmyer (82), and Bodner and Perkash in this text.
6. Intermittent catheterization was originated, in 1898 Wagner and Stolper who used intermittent catheterization for spine and spinal cord injuries (83). In 1944, Sir Ludwig Guttmann used intermittent catheterization for acute SCI (84). In 1951, Pollock et al. published a short report on intermittent catheterization (85). Other reports include Brussatis in 1953 (86); Guttmann 1954, 1955, and 1958; Comarr in 1965 (87); and many others (see Bors and Comarr [81]). Other catheters include those made of red rubber (Lewis, 1945 [88]), polyvinyl (Gibbon, 1958 [89]; Walsh, 1960 [90]), silicone (Sherwood, 1965 [91]), and polyethylene (Gibbon). For condom drainage, see Bors and Comarr, Chapter 7 (81).
7. Tidal drainage was developed by Munro in 1937 (43).
8. Bladder training was developed by Comarr in 1959, using a straight catheter at night and hourly emptying and drinking of fluids during the day (92).

Incontinence Devices

1. Phallic sheath of ancient Egyptians: Bitschai, 1956 (75).
2. Ambroise Paré Urinal (1510–1590) (93).
3. SA Vincent's (1960) perineal cushion to compass the urethra (94).
4. Cunningham's penile clamp (95).
5. Electrical stimulation for neurogenic bladder (presented later).
6. Alloplastic sphincter, originated by Fredric E. B. Foley (1891–1966), published in 1947 (79). There is separation of the corpora cavernosa from the corpus spongiosus; they are isolated by skin sutures until they heal. Then, a pneumatic cuff is put around the corpus spongiosus, already covered by skin. The cuff is inflated and deflated at will.
7. J.R. Berry's (1961) acrylic implant on the bulbar urethra (96).
8. Joseph Kaufman's (1973) silicone gel prosthesis (97).
9. Rosen's (1976) inflatable compression prosthesis (98).
10. Jonas's (1983) clamp, implanted at the penile scrotal angle to be opened by external manipulation (99).
11. Brantley and Scott's (1972) device, called Scott's sphincter (100).
12. Ultzmann (1842–1889) used electrical stimulation in 1890; this was the first use of this therapy (101). In 1898, Frankl-Hochwarth and Zuckerlandl used electrical therapy in neurogenic bladder (102). In 1930, Kowarschik used pelvic floor stimulation, through plug electrodes (103). In 1964, Boyce et al. implanted electrodes on the bladder wall (104). In 1963 Caldwell used a weak sphincter stimulation to fatigue it (105). In 1967 Burghele et al. attached stimulators to the splanchnic nerves (106). In 1967 Habib used a sacral nerve stimulator (107). In 1976 Brindley used spinal anterior root stimulation (108).

Urinary Diversion

Suprapubic cystostomy with or without the tube:

1. With a tube—used before World War II for SCI (Boyd, 1948 [109]; Hertzman, 1963 [110]).
2. Tubeless cystostomy by Blocksom, 1957 (111).
3. Suprapubic vesicostomy by Lapides, 1960 (112): skin and bladder flap.

Supravesical Diversion

1. Ileal conduit: Bricker, 1957 (113).
2. Colonic or cecal conduit: Mogg, 1965 (114a); Cook et al., 1968 (114b).
3. Cutaneous ureterostomy, pyelostomy, nephrostomy: Talbot et al., 1953 (115); Wossnitzer and Lattimer, 1960 (116); Thompson and Ross, 1962 (117).

Surgery for Retention or Narrow Outlet of the Bladder

1. Transurethral resection (TUR) of the vesical neck: Emmett, 1954 (118).
2. External sphincterotomy: Nourse, 1947 (119); Baumrucker, 1948 (120); Dees, 1948 (121).
3. Open procedures at vesicle neck and external sphincter:
a. Y-V plasty of the bladder neck: Young, 1953 (122).
b. Added removal of posterior lip: Jeejeebhoy, 1962 (123).
4. When the retention is due to weak dartus, transplantation of the bilateral rectus muscle flaps to the dartus for the neurotization: Thevenot, 1913 (124):
   a. Use of gracilis muscles: Ingelman-Sundberg, 1957 (125).
   b. Transfer of the latissimus dorsi: Stenzl, 2003 (126).
5. Transurethral sphincterotomy: Perkash, 1978 (127).

Bladder Augmentation

For contracted bladder:

1. Autoaugmentation by bladder myectomy: Stöhrer et al., 1997 (128).
2. Augmentation by bowel loop:
   a. Ileocystoplasty: Hanley, 1956 (129).
   b. Colocystoplasty: Pelot and Vaggtalin, 1961 (130).
   c. Cecocystoplasty (rare): Menville et al., 1958 (131).
   d. Nonintestinal augmentation: Norris et al. (1982), using amniotic membrane (132).

Dialysis

Another milestone in SCI management is dialysis for renal failure. Before 1972, SCI patients with renal failure were left to die peacefully. In 1972, Bors and Comarr opened the first and only SCI dialysis unit in the nation, with the help of fundraising by an SCI dialysis society headed by Bonnie Saxston. The unit worked very actively, and it surely prolonged the span of life of patients in its care. Research was also active and was headed by Dr. N. Vaziri of UCI, whose publications on SCI nephrology are tremendous; they can be accessed by e-mailing ndvaziri@uci.edu.

Neurological Treatment

1. Mucosal anesthesia: Bors et al., 1962 (133).
2. Pudendal nerve block: Bors, Comarr, and Mouton, 1950 (134).
3. Sacral nerve block: Heimburger et al., 1948 (135).
4. Closed irreversible measures:
   a. Subarachnoid alcohol: Dogliotti, 1931 (136).
   b. Phenol block: Kelly et al., 1959 (137).
   c. Electrocoagulation of the conus: Dossman, 1965 (138).
5. Open procedures:
   a. Pudendal neurotomy: Rochet, 1899 (139).
   b. Sacral neurotomy: Moulder and Meirowsky, 1956 (140).
   c. Pelvic neurectomy: Thiermann, 1952 (141).
   d. Presacral hypogastric neurectomy: Learmonth, 1931 (142).
   e. Presacral and pelvic neurectomy: Richer and Ginestie, 1948 (143).
   f. Posterior sacral rhizotomy: Bohm and Franksson, 1965 (144).
6. Spinothalamic tractotomy: Grant and Wood, 1957 (145).

7. Botulinum toxin (BTX) blockages of the external sphincter: Dykstra et al. (146).

These subjects are vast. For further details on the history of urology, please see Murphy's *History of Urology* (147), Schultheiss (80), and Kutzenberger et al. (148).

A remarkable therapeutic modality of urinary calculi is by ESWL, developed by Chaussy et al. in 1980 (149).

Pressure Ulcers

In the Egyptian period, ulcers were described and were treated by a variety of remedies (e.g., honey, molded loaf, raw meat, animal and botanical extracts, and minerals such as copper sulfate, zinc oxide, alum, and many others) (Edwin Smith and Eber's Papyri). Incantations were read before the dressings were applied (150–152).

During the Greek period, Hippocrates recommended keeping ulcers dry, except when wine was applied, and preferred to keep the ulcer exposed to air except when a cataplasm was applied. He used juices, honey, vinegar, oil, lead, alum, lotus, and many other topical applications. He recommended wound irrigation with clean water or boiled river water (153, 154). Celsus advised cleaning with vinegar and suturing small ulcers with women's hair.

Indian medicine (Vaidya, 400 BCE) distinguished different types of ulcers with clinical diagnosis even by auscultation (Majno [155]).

Chinese medicine featured physicians who specialized in treating ulcers. They fortified ulcers with five modalities. They fortified the bones with acid principle, the nerves with stinging principle, the pulse with salty principle, and respiration with bitter principle (Fu et al. [156]).

In the Middle East, Avicenna used a variety of topical applications (157), and Maimonides added nutrition as an aspect of ulcer healing (158).

During the Renaissance, there was no eminent physician until the time of Ambroise Paré, who insisted on gentle handling of wounds, advocated for meticulous cleanliness, and recommended good diet and medicines for healing (159).

In the Industrial Revolution of the nineteenth century, the discovery of bacteria by Pasteur and antisepsis by Lister improved the outlook of wounds in general. Discovery of X-rays by Roentgen helped diagnose bone pathology. In the nineteenth century, Charcot supported the trophic theory of pressure ulcers, which was opposed by Brown-Séquard (Levine [160]).

In the twentieth century, antibacterial chemotherapies appeared, first with sulfonamide (Prontosil) by K. Domag (1935). Penicillin was discovered by Alexander Fleming in 1929, but was clinically applied by Florey and Chain in 1940. Since then, a tremendous number of antibiotics have been developed to help control wound infection. Nutritional elements (i.e., proteins, vitamins, and minerals) and their contribution to wound healing were perfected in the United States. Biomechanics of bedsores received great attention (Kennedi et al. [161]).

Topical Applications

It is impossible to enumerate these. A brief list is presented:

- Antisepsis and antibiotics (162, 163)
- Antibacterials, but not cytotoxins (164,165)

- Debriding agents: enzymes, maggots, synthetic materials (166)
- Healing agents
- Animal products: placenta (167)
- Plant products: aloe vera (168)
- Growth factors (168)

Physical agents:

- Electrostimulation (Wolcott [169])
- Magnetic stimulation (Wood, Cameron, Drzewinska [170–172])
- Low-intensity laser therapy (Ceschino et al. [173])
- Ultraviolet therapy (heliotherapy) (174)
- Topical oxygen therapy (Fischer [175])
- Hyperbaric oxygen therapy (Eltorai [176])
- Ultrasound (Paul et al. [177])
- Ozone (Takahova et al. [178])
- Dry air (Denholm [179])
- CO_2 laser (Stellar [180])
- Occlusive dressing (Ryan [181])

Biological and biochemical agents:

- Xenografts (Grotenderst, Eresk [182, 183])
- Dermografts: still experimental (Phan et al. [184])
- Topical hyperalimentation (Niinikoski et al. [185])
- Surgical repair flaps (186–189)
- Grafts (Thiersh [190])

For further details, see the chapter on pressure ulcers in this textbook.

Regeneration

This field has received tremendous attention from scientists and research workers nationally and internationally. There are uncountable avenues for accomplishing spinal cord repair. Funds seem to be adequate, and enthusiasm is a driving power. The dictum of Imhotep, "an ailment not to be treated (cured)," is now fading, and the future will show the victory of science.

There is an uncountable number of research papers and symposia, which cannot be summarized in this chapter. There is a comprehensive chapter in this text, and there are many review papers. A few of the topics are as follows (also see the chapter in this text regarding regeneration):

Pharmacotherapy in Spinal Cord Regeneration

1. Methylprednisolone, alone or combined with alphatocopherol and selenium (antioxidants): Sanders et al., 1987 (191).
2. Methylprednisolone sodium succinate (Solu-Medrol): Bracken, 1985 (192); Bracken, 1990 (193); De La Torre, 1972 (194).
3. Alphamethyltyrosine: Osterholm et al., 1971 (195).
4. Aspirin, dipyridamol: Fujita et al., 1985 (196).
5. Calcium channel antagonists: Faden et al., 1984 (197)— Nimodipine (L-type calcium channel blocker): Fehlings and Tator, 1995 (198); Petitjean et al., 1998 (199).

6. Dimethylsulfoxide (DMSO): Ruigrak et al., 1981 (200); De La Torre et al., 1972 (201); Kajihara et al., 1973 (202).
7. Enzyme therapy—hyaluridinase, trypsin, and elastase: Matinian and Windle, 1975 (203).
8. Gacyclidine (GK-11) antiglutamatergic agent: Tadi et al., 1999 (204).
9. Gangliosides (GM-1, Sygen): Geisler et al., 1991 (205); Baptiste and Fehlings, 2006 (206).
10. Genetic strategies: Tator, 1996 (207).
11. Immunosuppressive drugs: Faringa et al., 1974 (208).
12. Lidocaine: Siavash et al., 1987 (209).
13. Naloxone: Black et al., 1986 (210).
14. Opioid antagonism: Bracken, 1990 (193).
15. Dynorphin A: Kunihara, 2004 (211).
16. Minocycline: He et al., 2001 (212); Festoff et al., 2006 (213).
17. Nerve growth factor: Scott et al., 1964 (214).
18. Neurotrophic factors: Tator, 1996 (207).
19. Pregnenolone combined with lipopolysaccarides and endothacin: Guth et al., 1994 (215).
20. Nitric oxide inhibitors: Hitchon et al., 1996 (216).
21. Thyrotropin releasing hormone (TRH): Pitts et al., 1995 (217).
22. Tirilazad mesylate: Bracken et al., 1998 (218).
23. Riluzole: Mu, 2000 (219).
24. Melatonin: Fujimoto et al., 2000 (220); Samantaray et al., 2008 (221).
25. Antimyelin inhibitors of regeneration:
    a. NOGO antibody: Freund et al., 2006 (222); Freund et al., 2007.
    b. Cethrin to antagonize the myelin inhibitors and facilitate axonal growth: McKerracher et al., 2006 (224).

Physical Therapy of SCI

1. Cooling (hypothermia): Negrin, 1975 (225); Hansebout, 1984 (226); Kwon, 2008 (227).
2. Oscillating field stimulation: Shapiro et al., 2005 (228).
3. X-rays: Turbes et al., 1960 (229).
4. Electromagnetic stimulation: Young et al., 1984 (230); Wilson and Jagadeesh, 1976 (231); Wilson, 1986 (232).
5. Hyperbaric oxygen therapy: Higgins et al., 1981 (233); Asamoto et al., 2000 (234).
6. Revascularization: Goldsmith and De La Torre, 1991 (235).
7. Acupuncture: Politis and Korchinski, 1990 (236).
8. CSF drainage: Coselli et al., 2002 (237).

Cellular Transplantation

1. Activated autologous macrophages (PROCORD): Rapalino et al., 1998 (238).
2. Schwann cells from autologous source (e.g., sural nerve): Richardson et al., 1980 (239).
3. Olfactory ensheathing cells, which are autologous and can be obtained from aborted fetuses: Ramón-Cueto et al., 2000 (240); Dobkin et al., 2006 (241).
4. Bone marrow stromal cells, autologous, intrathecal, or intravascular: Paul et al., 2009 (242).
5. Human embryonic stem cells: Keirstead et al., 2005 (243); Lebkowski et al., 2001 (244). From human umbilical cord blood: Dasari et al., 2009 (245).

6. Glial scar–associated inhibitors—use of a bacterial enzyme known as ChABC (chondroitinase ABC), which causes degradation of the CSPGs (chondroitin sulfate proteoglycan): Barritt et al., 2006 (246); Garcia-Alias et al., 2007 (247); Bradbury et al., 2002 (248); Caggiano et al., 2005 (249); Yick et al., 2003 (250).

7. Self-renewal of the nervous system through cells in the adult mammalian CNS. These cells can promote repair, are found in the subventricular zone throughout the CNS, and can be isolated surgically: Reynolds and Weiss et al., 1992 (251)

The historical review given offers only a brief overview of the evolution of spinal cord medicine. No single review can be comprehensive due to the multiplicity of fields researching SCI and the rapid progress being made in each of them. Specific references will have to be consulted. For reviews on regeneration, please see Ramer et al., 2005 (252); Hawryluk et al., 2008 (253); Rowland et al., 2008 (254); and the chapter in this text on regeneration.

EPILOGUE

Through advances in all areas of spinal cord medicine, the mortality rate associated with this condition has come down, and survival has risen. This chapter has offered a brief exposé of the history of spinal cord medicine, especially with regard to the injury and to enumerating leaders in this field, who have toiled heavily and who deserve remembrance. Through efforts of the past and present, the picture has changed markedly from pessimism to optimism, and the door of despair is closing while the door of hope is opening. Look to the future, but forget not the past!

References

1. Lawrence C. *Garrison's History of Neurology*. Springfield: Charles C. Thomas Pub. Ltd., 1969.
2. Haymaker W, Schiller F. *Founders of Neurology: One Hundred Forty Six Biographical Sketches by Eighty Nine Authors*. Springfield: Charles C. Thomas Pub. Ltd., 1970.
3. Jacob MD, Stanley W, et al. *History of Neurology: Handbook of Clinical Neurology*. Amsterdam: Elsevier, 2010.
4. Breasted JH. *The Edwin Smith Surgical Papyrus*. Vol. I. Chicago, 1930:316–342, 425–428.
5. Elsberg C. The Edwin Smith Surgical Papyrus: the diagnosis and treatment of injuries to the skull and spine 5000 years ago. *Ann Med Hist* 1931:271–279.
6. Hughes JT. The Edwin Smith Surgical Papyrus: an analysis of the first case reports of spinal cord injuries. *Paraplegia* 1988; 2:71–82.
7. Adams F. *The Genuine Works of Hippocrates* [translated from the Greek]. Baltimore, MD: Williams and Wilkins, 1939:231–242.
8. Galen. *Omnia Opera* [Carolus Kuhn edition]. Leipzig, 1821:170–174, 237–250.
9. Oribasius. *Oeuvres d'Oribase* [Daremberg edition]. Vol IV. Paris, 1862: 242–243, 394–395, 449–451.
10. Adams F. *Paulus Aeginata*. Vol II. London, 1846:455–456, 493–497.
    a. Lyons AS, Petrucelli RJ. *Medicine: An Illustrated History*. New York: Harry N. Abrams, 1997:59.
    b. Rambam (Maimonides). *Medical Aphorisms of Moses*. Hebrew translation by Hameathi RN, 1283; 2nd ed. edited by Bosner F, Muntner S. Jerusalem: Yeshiva University Press, 1982.
11. Kaviraj, KLB. *Sushutra Samhita*. Vol II. Calcutta, 1911; 100:284–285.
12. Ohry A, Ohry-Kossoy K. Spinal cord injuries in the nineteenth century. A monograph published as a supplement to *Paraplegia* 1989:123–124.
13. Avicenna [Abu Ali Al Hussein]. *Avicennae Operum de Rex Medica* [in Arabic]. Vol II, Book IV, Chapters XXI–XXII. Venice, 1564.
14. Avicenna [Ibn Sina]. *Al Quanom FIT Tibb* [in Arabic]. Cairo: Government Press, Boulaque, 1877.
15. Howorth B, Petrie JG, Bennett G. *Injuries of the Spine*. Baltimore, MD: Williams and Wilkins, 1964:1–13.
16. Carbonelli G. *La Chirurgia de M. Rolando da Parma*. Rome, 1927.
17. Uenver AS. Serefeddin Subuncuoglu's *Album des Dessins de Cerrahiyei Ilhaniye*. Istanbul, 1939:38–42, 58, 66.
18. Paré A. *Oeuvres*. Paris, 1598: 528, 554, 559.
19. Guttmann L. *Spinal Cord Injuries: Comprehensive Management and Research*. Oxford: Blackwell Scientific, 1976:1–3.
20. Louis A. *Remarques et Observation sur la Fracture et la. Luxation des Vertebras*. Memoires lu a la séance publique de l'Académie Royale de Chirurgie, le 18 avril 1774. *Arch Gen Med* (2nd series) 1836; 11:397–429.
21. Petit JL. Traité des maladies chirurgicales et des opérations qui leur conviennent, 3 vol. P Fr Didot. In: Greenblatt S, Dagi TF, Epstein M, eds. *A History of Neurosurgery in Its Scientific and Professional Contexts*. Park Ridge, IL: American Association of Neurological Surgeons, 1997:75.
22. Heister L. Chirurgie, 5th ed. Nürnberg: Raspe, 1747.
23. Hunczovsky JH. *Anweisung zu chirurgischen Operationen für seine Vorlesungen bestimmt*. Wien R Graeffer, 1787:249–295, 325–326.
24. Ohry A, Ohry-Kossoy K. Spinal cord injuries in the nineteenth century. A monograph published as a supplement in *Paraplegia* 1989:1–39.
25. Cooper A. Lecture 181 of injuries of the spine. *Lancet* 1823; 1:303–306.
26. Brown–Séquard E. Possibility of repair and of return of function after a partial or a complete division of the spinal cord in man and animals. *Lancet* 1859; 1:96–97.
27. Brown–Séquard CE. Lecture III: diagnosis and treatment of paraplegia due to myelitis, meningitis or a simple congestion. *Lancet* 1860; 2:27–28.
28. Brown–Séquard CE. Lecture III, part II. *Lancet* 1860; 2:77–78.
29. Horsley, V. Chronic spinal meningitis. *Brit Med J* 1909; 1:513.
30. Trunkey D. The admiral's wounds. *Amer Coll Surg Bull* 1994; 79(2):19–27.
31. Beatty W. Nelson's fatal wound. *Lancet* 1906; 6:68.
32. Ridpath JC. *The Life and Work of James A. Garfield, 20th President of the United States*. Cincinnati: James Brothers, 1882.
33. Eltorai IM. Fatal spinal cord injury of the 20th president of the United States: day-by-day review of his clinical course, with comments. *J Spinal Cord Med* 2004; 27(4):330–341.
34. Guttmann L. *Spinal Cord Injuries: Comprehensive Management and Research*. Oxford: Blackwell Scientific, 1976:5.
35. Livshits AV. *Surgery of the Spinal Cord*. [Translated from Russian by Tator-Chenko, VE.] Madison, CT: International Press, Inc., 1991.
36. Chapman MW, Madison M. *Operative Orthopedics*. Vol. 4. Philadelphia: JB Lippincott, 1993.
37. Meyer P Jr. *Surgery of Spinal Trauma*. New York: Churchill Livingston, 1989.
38. Barnett GH, Hardy RW. Gardner tongs and cervical traction. *Med Instrum* 1982; 16:291–292.
39. Foerster O. *Handbuch der Neurologie Ergangungsband*. Berlin: Springer, 1929.
40. Munro D. The rehabilitation of patients totally paralyzed below the waist, with special reference to making them ambulatory and capable of earning their own living. *New Eng J Med* 1954; 233(16):453–461.
41. Munro D. The cord bladder: its definition, treatment, and prognosis, when associated with spinal cord injury. *New Eng J Med* 1936; 215(17):766–777.
42. Munro D. Tidal drainage of the urinary bladder. *New Eng J Med* 1935; 212(6):229–239.
43. Munro D. The treatment of the urinary bladder in cases with injury of the spinal cord. *Am J Surg* 1937; 38(1):120–136.
44. Munro D. *The Treatment of Injuries to the Nervous System*. Philadelphia: W. B. Saunders, 1952.
45. Mock HE, Pemberton R, Coulter JS. *Principles and Practice of Physical Therapy*. Hagerstown, MD: WF Prior, 1939.
46. DeLisa J, ed. *Rehabilitation Medicine*. Philadelphia: JP Lippincott, 1993:3–39.
47. Guttmann L. *Spinal Cord Injuries: Comprehensive Management and Research*. Oxford: Blackwell Scientific, 1976.
48. Krueger EG. Birth of holistic spinal neurotraumatology in America. Donald Munro Memorial Lecture. *J Am Paraplegia Soc* 1984; 7:10–12.
49. Goltz P. Die Funktionen des Lendenmarkes des Hundes. *Arch Ges Physio* 1874; 8:460.

50. Denny-Brown D. *Selected Writings of Sir Charles Sherrington.* London: Hamish Hamilton, 1939:120–154.

51. Guttmann L. *Spinal Cord Injuries: Comprehensive Management and Research.* Oxford: Blackwell Scientific, 1976:354–363.

52. Silver JR. Historical review: the history of Guttmann's and Whitteridge's discovery of autonomic dysreflexia. *Spinal Cord* 2000; 38:581–596.

53. Guttmann L, Whitteridge D. Effects of bladder distention on autonomic mechanism after spnal cord injuries. *Brain* 1947; 70:361–404.

54. Thompson CE, Witham AC. Paroxysmal hypertension in spinal cord injuries. *N Engl J Med* 1948; 239(2):291–294.

55. Pollock LJ. Defects in regulatory mechanism of autonomic function in injuries to the spinal cord. *J Neurophysiol* 1951; 14:85–93.

56. Bors E, French JD. Management of paroxysmal hypertension following injury to cervical and upper thoracic segments of the spinal cord. *Arch Surg* 1952; 64:803–812.

57. Schreibert CD. Studies on the sacral reflex arc in paraplegic surgical therapy of autonomic hyperreflexia in cervical and upper thoracic myelopathy. *J Neurosurg* 1955; 12:468–474.

58. Arieff AJ, Tigay EL, Ryzik SW. Acute hypertension induced by urinary bladder distention, headache and its correlates in quadriplegic patients. *Arch Neurol* 1962; 6:88–96.

59. Eltorai IM. *Autonomic Dysreflexia.* Angiology, 2003 (reprinted by APS).

60. Riedel B. Demonstration eines durch achttägiges Umhergehen total destruirten Kniegelenkes von einem Patienten mit Stichverletzung des Rückens. *Verh Dtsch Ges Chir* 1883; 12:93.

61. Reichert C. Bemerkungen zur vergleichenden Naturforschung im Allgemeinen und vergleichende Beobachtungen bei das Bindegewebe und die verwandten Gebilde. Dorpat: W. Gl ser. Brailsford, JF. *The Radiology of Bones and Joints.* London: J. & A. Churchill Ltd, 1948:591.

62. Klumke-Dejerine C. Arthropathies du genou chez les paraplègiques. *Rev Neurol* 1918; 25:159, 207, 348.

63. Klumke-Dejerine C, Cellier A. Para-osteo-arthropathies de para-plégiques par lésions médullaires. *Am Med* 1919; 34:399.

64. Soule AB. Neurogenic ossifying fibromyopathies. *J Neurosurg* 1945; 2:485.

65. Abramson AS. Bone disturbances in injuries to spinal cord and cauda equina (paraplegia): their prevention by ambulation. *J Bone Joint Surg* 1947; 30:982–991.

66. Abramson A, Kamberg G. Spondylitis, pathological ossification, and calcification associated with spinal-cord injury. *J Bone Joint Surg* 1949; 31A:982.

67. Liberson M. Soft tissue calcifications in cord lesions. *Am Med Ass*1953; 152:1010.

68. Damanski M. Paraheterotopic ossification in paraplegia *J Bone Joint Surg* 1961; 43B:286.

69. Hardy A, Dickson JW. Pathological ossification in traumatic paraplegia. *J Bone Joint Surg* 1963; 4B:76.

70. Paeslack V. Internistische Störungen bein Paraplegiker. Stuttgart: Georg Thieme, 1965.

71. Freehafer A, Yurick R, Mast A. Para-articular ossification in spinal cord injury. *Med Services J Can* 1966; 22:471–477.

72. Rossier AB, et al. Current facts on paraosteoarthropathy (POA). Proceedings of the Annual Meeting of the International Medical Society of Paraplegia, Heidelberg. *Paraplegia* 1973; 2(1):36–78.

73. Anders EK, Bradley WE. History of cystometry. *Urology* 1983; 12(3):335–350.

74. Bitschai B. *History of Urology in Egypt.* Privately printed. Riverside Press, 1956.

75. Herman JR. *Urology: A View through the Retrospectroscope.* Hagerstown, MD: Harper and Row, 1973:3–4.

76. Hanafy M, Saad M, Al-Ghorab M. Ancient Egyptian medicine. *Urology* 1974; 6:114–120.

77. Mattelaer JJ, Billiet I. Catheters and sounds: history of bladder catheter-isation. *Paraplegia* 1995; 33:429–433.

78. Foley FEB. An artificial sphincter: a new device and operation for control of enuresis and urinary incontinence. *J Urol* 1947; 58:250–259.

79. Schultheis D, et al. Historical aspects of the treatment of urinary incontinence. *Eur Urol* 2000; 38:352–362.

80. Bors E, Comarr AE. *Neurological Urology.* Basel: S. Karger, 1971.

81. Lindsenmeyer TA. Neruogenic bladder following spinal cord injury. In: Kirshblum S, Campagnolo DI, DeLisa JA, eds. *Spinal Cord Medicine.* Philadelphia: Lippincott, Williams and Wilkins, 2001.

82. Wagner W, Stolper P. Die Verletzungen der Wirbelsäule und des Rückenmarks. Verlag von Ferdinand Enke: Stuttgart, 1898:111–125.

83. Guttmann L, Frankel H. The value of intermittent catheterization in the early management of traumatic paraplegia and tetraplegia. *Paraplegia* 1966; 4:63–84.

84. Pollock LJ, et al. Management of residuals of injuries to spinal cord and cauda equina. *JAMA* 1951; 46:1551–1552.

85. Brussatis F. Moderne paraplegiker behandlung. *Dtsch Med Wochenschr* 1953; 78:1654–1657, 1705–1707.

86. Comarr AE. Traumatic cord bladder and its managements. *J Int Coll Surg* 1955; 32:38–45.

87. Lewis LG. Treatment of bladder dysfunction after neurologic trauma. *J Urol* 1945; 54:284–295.

88. Gibbon N. A new type of catheter for urethral drainage of the bladder. *Br J Urol* 1958; 30:1–7.

89. Walsh A. Catheter drainage and infection in acute retention of urine. *Lancet* 1960; 1:708.

90. Sherwood NS. Experience with a new silastic catheter. *J Urol* 1965; 93:307–308.

91. Comarr AE. The practical urological management of the patient with spinal cord injury. *BJU* 1959; 31:1–46.

92. Paré A. *Dix livres de la Chirurgie.* Paris: Royer, 1564.First English translation by Johnson T: *The collected works of Ambroise Paré.* London: Cotes and Young, 1634.

93. Vincent SA. Mechanical control of urinary incontinence. *Lancet* 1960; 2:292–294.

94. Cunningham JH. The diagnosis of stricture of the urethra by the Roentgen rays. *Trans Am Assoc Genitourin Surg* 1910; 5:369.

95. Berry JL. A new procedure for correction of urinary incontinence: preliminary report. *J Urol* 1961; 85:771–775.

96. Kaufman JJ. History of surgical correction of male urinary incontinence. *Urol Clin North Am* 1978; 5:265–278.

97. Rosen M. A simple artificial implantable sphincter. *Br J Urol* 1976; 48:675.

98. Jonas U. Operative behandlung der männli-chen sphinkterinsuffizienz: experimente zur entwicklung eines neuartigen alloplastischen sphinkters. *Akt Urol* 1984; 15:280–286.

99. Scott FB, Bradley WE, Timm GW. Treatment of urinary incontinence by implantable prosthetic sphincter. *Urology* 1973; 1:252–259.

100. Ultzmann R. *Die Krankheiten der Harnblase.* Stuttgart: Enke, 1890:343–356.

101. Frankl-Hochwart L, Zuckerkandl O. *Die Nervösen Erkrankungen der Harnblase.* Wien: Hölder, 1898.

102. Kowarschik J. *Die Diathermie.* Berlin: Springer, 1930:168–170.

103. Boyce WH, Lathem JE, Hunt LD. Research related to the development of an artificial electrical stimulator for the paralyzed human bladder: a review. *J Urol* 1964; 91:41–51.

104. Caldwell KPS. The electrical control of sphincter incontinence. *Lancet* 1963; 2:174–175.

105. Burghele T, Ichim V, Demetresco M. Etude expérimentale sur la physiologie de la miction et l'évacuation électrique de la vessie chez les traumatisés médullaires. *Exp Surg* 1967; 1:156.

106. Habib HN. Experience and recent contributions in sacral nerve stimulation for voiding in both human and animal. *Br J Urol* 1967; 39:73.

107. Brindley GS. History of the sacral anterior root stimulator. *Neurourol Urodyn* 1993; 12:481–483.

108. Boyd ML. The advantage of suprapubic drainage over catheter or other methods of urinary drainage in acute bladder paralysis which result from traumatic injuries of the spinal cord. *J Urol* 1948; 60:922–932.

109. Hirtzman C. Présentation d'un système de drainage vésical applicable dans les premier jours de la paraplégie à l'exclusion de tout sondage. *Ann Med Phys* 1963; 6:197–202.

110. Blocksom BH. Bladder pouch for prolonged tubeless cystostomy. *J Urol* 1957; 78:398–401.

111. Lapides J, Ajemian EP, Lichtwardt JR. Cutaneous vesicostomy. *J Urol* 1960; 84:609–614.

112. Bricker EM, Butcher HR, McAfee CA. Reappraisal of ileal segment substitution for the urinary bladder. *Surgery* 1957; 42:581.
   a. Mogg RA. Urinary diversion using the colonic conduit. *Br J Urol* 1967; 39:687–692.
   b. Cook RCM, Lister J, Zachary RB. Operative management of the neurogenic bladder in children: diversion through intestinal conduits. *Surgery* 1967; 63:825–831.

113. Talbot HS, Paull DP, Read GR. Late renal complications of paraplegia. III. Treatment of vesico-uretheral reflux by skin ureterostomy through a pedicle flap. *J Urol* 1953; 70:216–222.

114. Wosnitzer M, Lattimer JK. Comparison of permanent nephrostomy and permanent cutaneous ureterostomy. *J Urol* 1960; 83:553–560.

115. Thompson IM, Ross G. Single stoma skin flap interposition cutaneous ureterostomy. *Surg Gynecol Obstet* 1962; 115:363–368.

116. Emmett JL. Neurogenic vesical dysfunction (cord bladder) and neuromuscular ureteral dysfunction. In: Campbell M, ed. *Urology*. Vol 2, Section XI, Chapter 1. Philadelphia: W.B. Saunders, 1954:1285–1383.

117. Nourse MH, Bumpus HC. Care of paraplegics' urinary tract. *J Urol* 1947; 57:495–497.

118. Baumrucker GO. Management of the paralyzed bladder. *Arch Surg* 1948; 56:484–507.

119. Dees JE. Transurethral resection for neurological bladder. *J Urol* 1948; 60:907–914.

120. Young BW. The retropubic approach to vesical neck obstruction in children. *Surg Gynecol Obstet* 1953; 96:150–154.

121. Jeejeebhoy H. A new approach to the management of the spastic external sphincter. *J Urol* 1962; 88:506–510.

122. Thevenot L. Essais de traitement chirurgical des retentions d'urine sans obstacle méchanique. *Progr Méd* 1913; 41:651–652.

123. Ingelman-Sundbert A. An operation for relief of urinary retention caused by paralysis of the detrusor muscle. *Urol Int* 1957; 4:247–253.

124. Stenzl A. Neue operationmethode bei Blasenlähmung. Zum Urinieren den Latissimus kontrahieren. *MMW Fortschr Med* 2003; 145:12.

125. Perkash I. Detrusor-sphincter dyssynergia and dyssynergia responses: recognition and rational for early modified transurethral sphincterotomy in complete spinal cord injury lesion. *J Urol* 1978; 120:469.

126. Stöhrer M, Kramer G, Goepel M, Löchner-Ernst D, et al. Bladder autoaugmentation in adult patients with neurogenic voiding dysfunction. *Spinal Cord* 1997; 35(7):456–462.

127. Hanley HG. The emptying mechanisms of various ileal loops studied with the X-ray image amplifier. *Br J Urol* 1956; 28:402–405.

128. Pélot G, Voegtlin R. Colocystoplastie chez les traumatizés médullaires. *J Urol Néprhol* 1961; 67:180–188.

129. Menville JG, Nix T, Prat AM. Cecostystoplasty. *J Urol* 1958; 79:819–823.

130. Norris MA, et al. Bladder reconstruction in rabbits with glutaraldehyde-stabilized amniotic membranes. *Urology* 1982; 19:631–633.

131. Bors E, Rossier A, Sullivan FJ. Urological and neurological observations following anesthetic procedures of patients with spinal cord injuries. II. Cystometric and electromyographic effects of topical anesthesias. *Urol Surv* 1962; 12:205–222.

132. Bors E, Comarr AE, Mouton SH. The role of nerve blocks in management of traumatic cord bladders: spinal anesthesia, subarachnoid alcohol injections, pudendal nerve anesthesia and vesical neck anesthesia. *J Urol* 1950; 63:653–666.

133. Heimburger RF, Freeman LW, Wilde NJ. Sacral nerve innervention of the human bladder. *J Neurosurg* 1948; 5:154–164.

134. Dogliotti AM. Anesthesia, narcosis, local, regional, spinal. Chicago: SB Debour, 1939.

135. Kelly RE, Gauther-Smith PC. Intrathecal phenol in the treatment of reflex spasms and spasticity. *Lancet* 1959; 2:1102–1105.

136. Dossman WF. Electrocoagulation of cord and nerve roots in the treatment to spasms of bladder and lower limbs. *J Neurosurg* 1965; 22:352–353.

137. Rochet V. Résection de la branche des nerfs honteaux internes dans certaines affections spasmsodiques de l'urétre et du périnée. *Arch Provincials Cir* 1899; 312–321.

138. Moulder MK, Meirowsky AM. The management of Hunner's ulcer by differential sacral neurotomy: preliminary report. *J Urol* 1956; 75:261–262.

139. Thiermann E. Zur operative behandlung der neurologisch gestörten blase. *Z Urol Sonderhef* 1952:249–255.

140. Learmonth JR. A contribution to the neurophysiology of the urinary bladder. *Brain* 1931; 54:147–176.

141. Richer V, Ginestié J. Chirugie du systéme nerveux vésical. *Presse Méd* 1948; 62:742–743.

142. Bohm E, Franksson C. Interstitial cystitis and sacral rhizotomy. *Acta Chir* Scand 1957; 113:63–67.

143. Grant FC, Wood FA. Experiences with cordotomy. *Clin Neurosurg* 1958; 5:38–65.

144. Dykstra D, Enriquez A, Valley M. Treatment of overactive bladder with botulinum toxin type B: a pilot study. *Int Urogynecol J Pelvic Floor Dysfunct* 2003; 14(6):424–426.

145. Murphy LJT. *The History of Urology*. Springfield: Thomas, 1972.

146. Kutzenberger J, Pannek J, Stöhrer M. Neurourology. current developments and therapeutic strategies [in German]. *Urologe A* 2006; 45(2):158–160, 162–166.

147. Chaussy C, Brendel W, Schmied E. Extracorporeally induced destruction of kidney stones by shock waves. *Lancet* 1980; 2(8207):1265–1268.

148. Constantian MB. *Pressure Ulcers: Principles and Technique Management*. Boston: Little Brown, 1980:4.

149. Ebbell B. *The Papyrus Ebers: The Greatest Egyptian Medical Document*. London: Oxford University Press, 1937.

150. Ebers A, Stern L. *Papyrus Ebers: Das Hermetische Buch über die Arzneimittel der alter Aegypten*. Vol. 1–3. Leipzig: JC Henriches, 1875.

151. Ibid., 325–336.

152. Ibid., 289–306.

153. Majno A. *The Healing Hand: Man and Wound in the Ancient World*. Cambridge, MA: Harvard University Press, 1975.

154. Fu X, Wang Z, Sheng Z. Advances in wound healing research in China: from antiquity to the present. *Wound Repair Regen* 2001; 9(1):2–10.

155. Avicenna [Ibn Sina]. *Al Knun Fi'l Tibb* [in Arabic]. Cairo Government Press, 1877:168–180.

156. Rosner F, Munter S. *The Medical Aphorisms of Moses Maimonides*. Vol. II. New York: Yeshiva University Press, 1971:28.

157. Paré A. The works of Ambrose Paré translated out of Latin and compared with the French by Th. Johnson. London: Th. Coates and R. Young, 1634.

158. Levine JM. Historical perspective: the neurotrophic theory of skin ulceration. *J Am Geriatr Soc* 1991; 40:1281–1283.

159. Kennedi RM, et al. *Bedsore Biomechanics*. Baltimore, MD: University Park Press, 1976.

160. Morgan J. Topical therapy of pressure ulcers. *Surg Gynecol Obstet* 1975; 141:945–947.

161. Michael J. Topical use of PVP (Betadine) preparations in patients with spinal cord injury. *Drugs Exp Clin Res* 1985; 11(2):107–109.

162. Lineaweaver W, et al. Cellular and bacterial toxicities of topical antimicrobials. *Plast Reconstr Surg* 1985; 75(3):394–396.

163. Dakin HD. The antiseptic action of hypochlorites. *BMJ* 1915; 2:809–810.

164. Teich S, et al. Maggot therapy for severe skin infections. *S Med J* 1986; 79(1):153–155.

165. Kumar N. Evaluation of the effect of placental extracts on bedsores. *Indian Med J* 1994; 88(5):145.

166. Wiseman DM, et al. Wound dressing: design and use. In: Cohen IK, Diegelmann RF, Lindblad EJ, eds. *Wound Healing: Biochemical and Clinical Aspects*. Philadelphia: W. B. Saunders, 1992.

167. Wolcott HE, et al. Accelerated healing of skin ulcers by electrotherapy. *South Med J* 1969; 62:795.

168. Wood JM, et al. Multicenter study on the use of pulsed low intensity direct current for healing of Stage II and Stage III decubitus ulcers. *Arch Dermatol* 1993; 129:999–1009.

169. Cameron B. Experimental acceleration of wound healing. *Am J Orthop* 1961; 336–343.

170. Duma-Drzewinska A. Pulsed high frequency currents applied in treatment of bedsores [in Polish, with English translation]. *Pol Tyg Lek* 1978; 33(22):1–2.

171. Ceschino M, et al. Helium neon soft laser in the treatment of decubitus ulcer. *Minerva Clinic* 1988; 43(1–2):49–56.

172. High S, High JP. Treatment of infected wounds using ultraviolet radiation. *J Physio Therap* 1983; 69(10):359–360.

173. Fischer BH. Topical hyperbaric oxygen treatment of pressure sores and skin ulcers. *Lancet* 1969; 2:405–409.

174. Eltorai I. Hyperbaric oxygen in the management of pressure sores in patients with injuries of the spinal cord. *J Dermatol Surg Oncol* 1981; 7(9):737–740.

175. Paul BJ, Lafratte CW, et al. Use of ultrasound in the treatment of pressure sores in patients with spinal cord injury. *Arch Phys Med Rehabil* 1960; 41:438.

176. Tahakova MA. Die ozonatherapie bei obliterierenden arteriellen gefaeserkrankungen und atomische geschwuren. *Med Heute* 1967; 9:272–274.

177. Denholm DH. The hair dryer treatment for decubiti. *Can Nurse* 1974; 10:33.

178. Stellar S, et al. Carbon dioxide laser debridement of decubitus ulcers followed by immediate rotation flap or skin graft closure. *Ann Surg* 1974; 179:230–237.

179. Ryan TJ. Beyond occlusive wound care. Royal Society of Medicine International Congress and Symposium 136. Royal Society of Medical Services, London, New York, 1988.

180. Grotendorst AR. Chemattractants and growth factor. In: Cohen IK, Diegelmann RF, Lindblad EJ, eds. *Wound Healing: Biochemical and Clinical Aspects.* Philadelphia: W. B. Saunders, 1992.

181. Eresk RA, Lario J. The most indolent ulcers of the skin treated with porcine xenografts and silver ion. *Surg Gynecol Obstet* 1984; 158:431–436.

182. Pham H, et al. Evaluation of human skin equivalent for treatment of diabetic foot ulcers in a prospective randomized clinical trial. *Wounds* 1999; 11(4):79–86.

183. Niinikoski J, et al. Local hyperalimentation of experimental granulation tissue. *Curr Surg* 1978; 394–418.

184. Davis JS. The operative treatment of scars following bedsores. *Surg* 1938; 3:1.

185. Conway H, et al. Plastic surgical closure of decubitus ulcers in patients with paraplegia. *Surg Gynecol Obstet* 1947; 85:321.

186. Constantian, MB. *Pressure Ulcers: Principles and Technique of Management.* Boston: Little Brown, 1989:149–246.

187. Mathes SJ, Nahai F. *Clinical Atlas of Muscle and Myocutaneous Flaps.* St Louis: CV Mosby, 1979.

188. Thiersch K. *Orthopedic Operations of General Surgery.* Philadelphia: W. B. Saunders, 1944:55.

189. Sanders RD, Dugan LL, Demedink P, et al. Effect of methylprednisolone and combinations of alpha-tocopherol and selenium on arachidonic acid metabolism and lipid peroxidation in traumatized spinal cord tissue. *J Neurochem* 1987; 49(1):24–31.

190. Bracken MB, Shepard MJ, Hellenbrand KG, Collins WF, et al. Methylprednisolone and neurological function 1 year after spinal cord injury: results of the National Acute Spinal Cord Injury Study. *J Neurosurg* 1985; 63:704–713.

191. Bracken MB, Shepard MJ, Collins WF, Holford TR, et al. A randomized, controlled trial of methylprednisolone or naloxone in the treatment of acute spinalcord injury. Results of the Second National Acute Spinal Cord Injury Study. *N Engl J Med* 1990; 322:1405–1411.

192. de la Torre, et al. Modification of experimental head and spinal cord injury using DMSO. *Trans Am Neurol Assoc* 1972; 97:230–233.

193. Osterholm JL, et al. A review of altered norepinephrine metabolism attending severe spinal injury. Results of alphamethyltyrosine treatment. *Proceedings of the Eighteenth Spinal Cord Injury Conference,* 1971:17–20.

194. Fujita Y, et al. Evaluation of low dose aspirin, dipyridamole and steroid therapeutic effects on motor function. *Paraplegia* 1985; 23:56–57.

195. Faden A, Jacobs TP, Smith MT. Evaluation of calcium channel antagonist nimodepine in experimental spinal cord ischemia. *J Neurol Surg* 1984; 60:796–799.

196. Fehlings MG, Tator CH. The relationships among the severity of spinal cord injury, residual neurological function, axon counts, and counts of retrogradely labeled neurons after experimental spinal cord injury. *Exp Neurol* 1995; 132:220–228.

197. Petitjean ME, Pointillart V, Dixmerias F, Wiart L, et al. Medical treatment of spinal cord injury in the acute stage. *Ann Fr Anesth Reanim* 1998; 17:114–122.

198. Ruigrak TJC, et al. The effect of dimethylsulfoxide on the calcium paradox. *Am J Pathol* 1981; 103:390–403.

199. de la Torre, et al. Modification of experimental head and spinal cord injury using DMSO. *Trans Am Neurol Assoc* 1972; 97:230–233.

200. Kajihara K, et al. Dimethylsulfoxide in the treatment of experimental spinal cord injury. *Surg Neurol* 1973; 1:16–22

201. Matinian LA, Windle WF. Functional structural restitution after transection of the spinal cord. *Ann Res* 1975; 181:423.

202. Tadie M, D'Arbigny P, Mathé J, Loubert G, et al. Acute spinal cord injury: early care and treatment in a multicenter study with gacyclidine. *Soc Neurosci* 25:1090, 1999.

203. Geisler FH, Dorsey FC, Coleman WP. Recovery of motor function after spinal cord injury: a randomized placebo controlled trial with GM-1 ganglioside. *N Eng J Med* 1991; 324:1829–1838.

204. Baptiste DC, Fehlings MG: Pharmacological approaches to repair the injured spinal cord. *J Neurotrauma* 2006; 23:318–334.

205. Tator CH. Experimental and clinical studies of the pathophysiology and management of acute spinal cord injury. *J Spinal Cord Med* 1996; 19(4):206–214.

206. Faringa R, et al. Immunosuppressive treatment to enhance spinal cord regeneration in rats. *Neurology* 1974; 24:287–303.

207. Siavash S, et al. Effect of lidocaine treatment on acute spinal cord injury. *Neurosurgery* 1987; 20(4):536–541.

208. Black P, et al. Naloxone and experimental spinal cord injury. Part I. Neurosurgery 1986; 19(6):905–908.

209. Kunihara T, Matsuzaki K, Shiiya N, Saijo Y, Yasuda K. Naloxone lowers cerebrospinal fluid levels of excitatory amino acids after thoracoabdominal aortic surgery. *J Vasc Surg* 2004; 40:681–690.

210. He Y, Appel S, Le W. Minocycline inhibits microglial activation and protects nigral cells after 6-hydroxydopamine injection into mouse striatum. *Brain Res* 2001; 909:187–193.

211. Festoff BW, Ameenuddin S, Arnold PM, Wong A, et al. Minocycline neuroprotects, reduces microgliosis, and inhibits caspase protease expression early after spinal cord injury. *J Neurochem* 2006; 97:1314–1326.

212. Scott D, Liu CN. Factors promoting regeneration of spinal neurons: positive influence of nerve growth factor. *Prog Brain Res* 1964; 131:127–150.

213. Guth L, et al. Key role for pregnenolone in combination therapy that promotes recovery after spinal cord injury. *Proc Natl Acad Sci USA* 1994; 91:12308–12312.

214. Hitchon PW, et al. Response of spinal cord blood flow to nitric oxide inhibitor. *Neurosurgery* 1996; 39(4):795–803.

215. Pitts LH, Ross A, Faden AP. Treatment with thyrotropin releasing hormone (TRH) in patients with traumatic spinal cord injury. *J Neurotrauma* 1995; 12:235–243.

216. Bracken MB, Shepard MJ, Holford TR, Leo-Summers L, et al. Methylprednisolone or tirilizad mesylate administration after acute spinal cord injury: 1-year follow-up. *J Neurosurg* 1998; 89:699–706.

217. Mu X, Azbill RD, Springer JE. Riluzole and methylprednisolone combined treatment improves functional recovery in traumatic spinal cord injury. *J Neurotrauma* 2000; 17:773–780.

218. Fujimoto T, Nakamura T, Ikeda T, Takagi K. Potent protective effects of melatonin on experimental spinal cord injury. *Spine* 2000; 25:769–775.

219. Samantaray S, et al. Melatonin attenuates calpain upregulation, axonal damage and neuronal death in spinal cord injury in rats. *J Pineal Res* 2008; 44:348–357.

220. Freund P, Schmidlin E, Wannier T, Bloch J, et al. Nogo-A-specific antibody treatment enhances sprouting and functional recovery after cervical lesion in adult primates. *Nat Med* 2006; 12:790–792.

221. Freund P, Wannier T, Schmidlin E, Bloch J, et al. Anti-Nogo-A antibody treatment enhances sprouting of corticospinal axons rostral to a unilateral cervical spinal cord lesion in adult macaque monkey. *J Comp Neurol* 2007; 502:644–659.

222. McKerracher L, Higuchi H. Targeting Rho to stimulate repair after spinal cord injury. *J Neurotrauma* 2006; 23:309–317.

223. Negrin J. Local hypothermia in spinal cord traumatic lesions. Third International Congress of Neurological Surgery, Copenhagen. *Excerpta Med Int Con* 1975; Series 110:377–381.

224. Hansebout RR, Tanner JA, Romero-Sierra C. Current status of spinal cord cooling in the treatment of acute spinal cord injury. *Spine* 1984; 9:508–511.

225. Kwon BK, Mann C, Sohn HM, Hilibrand AS, et al. Hypothermia for spinal cord injury. *Spine J* in press.

226. Shapiro S, Borgens R, Pascuzzi R, Roos K, et al. Oscillating field stimulation for complete spinal cord injury in humans: a phase 1 trial. *J Neurosurg Spine* 2005; 2:3–10.

227. Turbes CC, et al. X-radiation of experimental lesions of the spinal cord. *Neurology* 1960; 10:84–89.

228. Young W, et al. Pulsed electromagnetic field (PEMF) and methylprednisolone (MP) alter calcium and functional recovery in spinal cord injury. Paper 67, presented at Annual Meeting of American Association of Neurological Surgeons, San Francisco, April 8–12, 1984.

229. Wilson DH, Jagadeesh P. Experimental regeneration in peripheral nerves and spinal cord in laboratory animals exposed to a pulsed electromagnetic field. *Paraplegia* 1976; 14:12–20.

230. Wilson DH. The use of peripheral nerve grafts in spinal cord repair: In: Glusta EDN, Frankel HL, eds. *Spinal Cord Medical Engineering.* Springfield, IL: Charles Thomas Publishers, 1986:115–130.

231. Higgins A, et al. Effects of hyperbaric oxygen therapy on long tract neural conduction in the acute phase of spinal cord injury. *J Neurosurg* 1981; 55:501–510.

232. Asamoto S, et al. Hyperbaric oxygen (HBO) therapy for acute traumatic cervical spinal cord injury. *Spinal Cord* 2000; 38:538–540.

233. Goldsmith HS, de la Torre JC. Axonal regeneration after spinal cord injury and reconstruction. *Brain Res* 1991; 589:217–224.
234. Politis MJ, Korchinski MA. Beneficial effects of acupuncture treatment following experimental spinal cord injury: a behavioral morphological and biochemical study. *Acupunct Electrother Res* 1990; 15:37–49.
235. Coselli JS, Lemaire SA, Köksoy C, Schmittling ZC, Curling PE. Cerebrospinal fluid drainage reduces paraplegia after thoracoabdominal aortic aneurysm repair: results of a randomized clinical trial. *J Vasc Surg* 2002; 35:631–639.
236. Rapalino O, Lazarov-Spiegler O, Agranov E, Velan GJ, et al. Implantation of stimulated homologous macrophages results in partial recovery of paraplegic rats. *Nat Med* 1998; 4:814–821.
237. Richardson PM, McGuinness UM, Aguayo AJ. Axons from CNS neurons regenerate into PNS grafts. *Nature* 1980; 284:264–265.
238. Ramón-Cueto A, Cordero MI, Santos-Benito FF, Avila J. Functional recovery of paraplegic rats and motor axon regeneration in their spinal cords by olfactory ensheathing glia. *Neuron* 2000; 25:425–435.
239. Dobkin BH, Curt A, Guest J. Cellular transplants in China: observational study from the largest human experiment in chronic spinal cord injury. *Neurorehabil Neural Repair* 2006; 20:5–13.
240. Paul C, et al. Grafting of human bone marrow stromal cells into spinal cord injury. *Spine* 2009; 34:328–334.
241. Keirstead HS, Nistor G, Bernal G, Totoiu M, et al. Human embryonic stem cell–derived oligodendrocyte progenitor cell transplants remyelinate and restore locomotion after spinal cord injury. *J Neurosci* 2005; 25:4694–4705.
242. Lebkowski JS, Gold J, Xu C, Funk W, et al. Human embryonic stem cells: culture, differentiation, and genetic modification for regenerative medicine applications. *Cancer J* 2001; 7:83–93.
243. Dasari VR, et al. Neuronal apoptosis inhibited by cord blood stem cells after spinal cord injury. *J Neurotrauma* (in press).
244. Barritt AW, Davies M, Marchand F, et al. Chondroitinase ABC promotes sprouting of intact and injured spinal systems after spinal cord injury. *J Neurosci* 2006; 26:10856–10867.
245. Garcia-Alias G, Lin R, Akrimi SF, et al. Therapeutic time window for the application of chondroitinase ABC after spinal cord injury. *Exp Neurol* 2007; 210:331–338.
246. Bradbury EJ, Moon LD, Popat RJ, et al. Chondroitinase ABC promotes functional recovery after spinal cord injury. *Nature* 2002; 416:636–640.
247. Caggiano AO, Zimber MP, Ganguly A, et al. Chondroitinase ABCI improves locomotion and bladder function following contusion injury of the rat spinal cord. *J Neurotrauma* 2005; 22:226–239.
248. Yick LW, Cheung PT, So KF, et al. Axonal regeneration of Clarke's neurons beyond the spinal cord injury scar after treatment with chondroitinase ABC. *Exp Neurol* 2003; 182:160–168.
249. Reynolds BA, Weiss S. Generation of neurons and astrocytes from isolated cells of the adult mammalian central nervous system. *Science* 1992; 255:1707–1710.
250. Ramer LM, Ramer MS, Steeves JD. Setting the stage for functional repair of spinal cord injuries: a cast of thousands. *Spinal Cord* 2005; 43:134–161.
251. Hawryluk GW, Rowland J, Kwon BK, Fehlings MG. Protection and repair of the injured spinal cord: a review of completed, ongoing, and planned clinical trials for acute spinal cord injury. *Neurosurg Focus* 2008; 25(5):E14.
252. Rowland JW, Hawryluk GW, Kwon B, Fehlings MG. Current status of acute spinal cord injury pathophysiology and emerging therapies: promise on the horizon. *Neurosurg Focus* 2008; 25(5):E2.

77 Psychological Factors in Spinal Cord Injury

Robert A. Moverman

In attempting to detail the complex multitude of factors that can be involved in coping with spinal cord injury (SCI), it is perhaps best to first acknowledge that each individual (a) has many issues and reactions that are similar to others with SCI and (b) has unique personal, interpersonal, and cultural factors that contribute to their situation. Both are important considerations for the healthcare professional, but it is (b) that ultimately matters. It is extremely important to treat each patient as an individual so as to best guide them on their journey through rehabilitation and beyond. With this caveat in mind, this chapter will focus on premorbid personality considerations, issues in the rehabilitative setting, post-rehab issues, and psychotherapeutic interventions.

PREMORBID PSYCHOLOGICAL ISSUES

SCI is primarily a condition that occurs in young adults. The majority of cases involve individuals in the 16- to 30-year-old age group, and more than 80% are male (1). The most frequent etiology of injury involves a motor vehicle accident. These young adult males who sustain an SCI are likely to be more impulsive and sensation seeking than the general population. Conflicts with or disregard for authority figures may also be common. Many of these young adult males have a considerable amount of their self-esteem centered on their physical strength and self-reliance. Therefore, dependency on others after an SCI and loss of the usual outlets of self-expression can lay the groundwork for significant emotional and behavioral obstacles.

It is also important to note some of the demographic factors related to violence and SCI. It has been said that gunshot wounds in the United States have reached epidemic proportions (2). To begin, the national figures vary considerably by state. In Louisiana, for instance, gunshot constitutes the primary cause of SCI. Furthermore, the rates vary by ethnicity. Among Hispanics and African Americans, for instance, approximately half of all SCI cases involve gunshot wounds, whereas less than 10% of all Caucasian cases are so caused. The regional, cultural, and environmental influences are thus quite distinct

and warrant careful consideration in any psychosocial intervention (2).

False Patients

In the natural course of assessment and treatment of new patients, one will invariably encounter a particular type of case: an individual with reported loss of function, typically involving one or both of the lower extremities, in the absence of any specific neurological findings. In other words, there is no clear explanation for the presenting problem. Although some may truly have a medical condition that simply defies initial detection, a sizable number of these cases involve nonmedical etiology. The condition may reflect a subconscious psychological conflict (conversion disorder) or a deliberate feigning of symptoms (factitious disorder; malingering). Although psychological treatment may prove helpful for these persons with significant characterological deficits, these "patients" interestingly may respond well to traditional rehabilitation team services (3).

ISSUES IN THE REHAB PHASE

Premorbid Personality Style

A person's psychological and social style of interacting with the world can be a fairly good benchmark indicator of subsequent coping with and adjusting to SCI. Although the psychological impact of disability can radically alter one's perspective on life, most persons with SCI eventually conform to their basic personality styles. However, minor deficits may become more problematic in the rehabilitation process.

Denial is a basic defense mechanism. It is common for a person with a newly diagnosed SCI to maintain unrealistic expectations for a cure, especially when a reliable and accurate prognosis cannot be made early on. Moreover, rehabilitation professionals may contribute to this misperception by shrinking from confronting the patient with bad news about the chances for recovery. This is not necessarily problematic, provided the patient is taking appropriate steps to deal with life after rehabilitation. For example, someone may be allowed to hold onto the hope of walking again if discharge plans include planning for any necessary home modifications, personal care assistants, and so forth. While in the rehabilitation phase of treatment, there may well be an intrinsic value to not being burdened by the potentially stressful concerns of permanent disability.

Projection (blaming staff for one's difficulties or lack of progress); intellectualization (losing oneself in all the latest SCI research); and avoidance (a number of SCI patients do not want to use a mirror to view themselves, for example, in learning to self-catheterize) are other examples of defense mechanisms against psychological distress. Research has particularly shown that individuals with avoidant coping styles including disengagement, withdrawal, etc. tend to cope less well with adversity than do persons with other coping styles. This seems to be true for people in general as well as for those with SCI (4, 5).

One of the most difficult problems with which the rehab team must cope involves the projection of anger onto the staff. This may be at least partially due to the unavailability of customary outlets for affect ventilation. Occasional yelling, blaming, and otherwise directing anger toward the staff is certainly unwelcome but understandable. Taking such attacks as a personal affront, or as an indication of a job poorly done, is unnecessarily sensitive or egocentric. It is therefore helpful for the staff psychologist or social worker to counsel the team on such cases.

Another salient personality dimension involves introversion versus extroversion. Introverts typically do not feel particularly comfortable in a social or group-oriented environment, whereas extroverts are much more outgoing and people-focused. One needs to consider this sensitivity in dealing with SCI, because a rehab setting places many staff, patients, and visitors in rather close proximity. Although some patients may not feel comfortable in this milieu, others may thrive on it:

An SCI unit once had several extraverted young males with spinal cord injury who banded together to engage in a variety of antics throughout the hospital. They called themselves the "quad squad." Although their behavior at times irked some staff and patients, they maintained a tight bond of peer support and participated well in their program.

Locus of control (LC) involves the concept of whether one views oneself as the source of one's own consequences in life. Individuals with an internal LC feel that their own actions determine various outcomes, whereas those with an external LC view themselves more as the recipients of such events. LC has an obvious connection to defense mechanisms and coping styles. Although one may prefer patients to feel empowered and directive of their life (internal LC), an external LC may also have some advantages. For instance, such patients may feel less anxious or tense about future achievements. Nonetheless, as is the case in studies of other populations, individuals with SCI who have an internal LC seem to have more successful psychosocial adaptation than those with an external LC (6).

Self-esteem plays an important role when it comes to adjustment to SCI. The significance of a healthy self-concept is evident in the frequent finding that poor self-esteem leads to a higher incidence of adjustment problems. As noted above, many young adult males with SCI have a common premorbid focus on physical strength and ability as the defining feature of their self-worth. The loss of physical function can thus leave these individuals depleted of their customary means of feeling good about themselves. They may thus be less well equipped to deal with the psychological challenges of SCI.

Although one's level of psychosocial and community support is not a personality style, it is usually a key factor in the adjustment to SCI. A healthy amount of caring, concern, and unconditional positive regard from others can often counteract some of the negative influences on one's ability to cope with SCI. Specifically, a close and supportive family can be instrumental in this regard. Similarly, persons with a strong religious faith or sense of spirituality may find it easier to cope with SCI.

Stages of Adjustment

Some have argued that the adjustment to SCI conforms to the well-known stage theory initially proposed for adjustment to the loss of a loved one. In general, empirical research is not supportive of the stage model of disability adjustment (7) and suggests that every person with SCI goes through his or her own unique adjustment process, which may or may not involve stages. A coping mechanism that is natural for one person may feel foreign to another. Additionally, a number of factors can influence an individual's coping process, such as the frequency and timing of medical complications, rate of recovery (if any), idiosyncratic side effects of medications, and so forth. One's basic temperament may not return until several months post-injury, and the adjustment process may continue for years. Olkin (8) asserts that the concept of "adjustment to disability" is inaccurate, because it implies a response curve that eventually levels off at some mythical stage. She recommends the phrase "response to disability" in recognition of the continuous process of responses through one's lifetime.

Emotional Effects of Physical Issues

Psychological responses to SCI can be quite varied. Many types of emotional reactions have been noted, including depression, anger, anxiety, and indifference. In some cases, no psychological dysfunction is evident at all. Nonetheless, it has been estimated that between 20% and 40% of individuals with SCI have some type of psychological disorder, in comparison to about 5% in the general population (9).

The highest level of distress often takes place 2 to 3 weeks post-injury and may be more a condition of sadness than a clinical syndrome. However, a minority of those with SCI do develop depressive disorders (as many as 25% of males and close to 50% of females) (10). In one study of thirty individuals with SCI, the frequency of depression was higher among those with complete injuries. This may be caused by a higher level of hope among those with incomplete injuries (11). The risk is also correlated with physical factors such as pain, fatigue, and decreased sleep. Furthermore, indications exist that a number of medications or metabolic changes can potentiate depressed mood (12).

Anxiety is another prevalent condition among those in rehab with SCI. Among the situations influencing anxiety are the uncertainty of prognosis, a heightened sense of vulnerability, fear of further injury (either through complications or through physical therapy activities, such as fear of falling), decreased activity, and an increased time to think about oneself.

One interesting study found that the most distressing situation for SCI patients in rehab was not related to personal difficulties, but rather to the perception that the staff expected them to be distressed (13). In terms of social psychology theory, people tend to react in a manner in which they believe others expect them to react. Thus, it is important for staff to be cognizant of any such bias and to strive to avoid it.

A decrease in quality of sleep is one of the most significant factors that can lead to emotional difficulties in rehab. Hospitals can be uncomfortably noisy, and the typical semiprivate room arrangement can be fraught with inconveniences such as nursing checks, medications, and charting of vital signs. In addition to the emotional changes that lack of sleep can bring, other complications could include decreased energy and attention during the daytime therapy regimen. It has also been noted that insomnia, which may be caused by concomitant respiratory difficulties among SCI patients, can lead to a greater utilization of general medical and psychiatric services, decreased pain threshold, increased risk of coronary events, and reduced quality of life (14).

Decreased physical activity may also cause problems. Unlike able-bodied persons whose mobility can allow various ways to "burn off steam," SCI individuals do not have the same degree of this healthy release available to them. The development of alternative stress-relieving approaches, though perhaps elusive at first, can be quite therapeutic.

An increased physical dependence on other individuals can be another major source of emotional distress for many SCI patients. In addition to the general need for assistance in a variety of daily activities, many people with SCI find the need for help with bowel and bladder elimination, along with its concomitant loss of modesty, particularly disturbing. A prolonged stay in a medical facility, as is common with SCI, can produce the added psychological discomfort of being out of one's familiar environment.

Post-traumatic stress disorder (PTSD) has been considered a possible byproduct of SCI. The initial injury, if life-threatening or perceived by the patient as potentially life-threatening, can in some cases lead to typical PTSD symptoms such as easy irritability, startle response, rage, phobias relating to events and objects associated with the accident, and so forth. One study of 126 persons with SCI found that one-third met the diagnostic criteria for PTSD, which is comparable to the figures for persons in other traumatized groups (15). One author has encouraged clinicians to consider PTSD an important diagnostic possibility in working with persons with SCI (16).

Lastly, the issue of neuropsychological impairment among persons with SCI can sometimes be of critical significance. Research has found that traumatic brain injury (TBI), which often includes neurocognitive deficits, can be a frequent concomitant of SCI, remaining undiagnosed throughout the course of rehabilitation (17). Decreased cognitive functioning can in turn lead to increased stress and emotional unrest.

Physical Effects of Emotional Issues

In addition to difficult physical or medical factors that can produce psychological challenges, emotional distress can itself lead to physical or medical problems. For example, depression often involves a loss of energy or concentration skills, which can impede the rehabilitation process. Depression among those with SCI has also been noted to be associated with an increased risk of urinary tract infections, pressure sores, and overall poor health and recovery (18). Essentially, the body functions better when the mind is functioning well.

A number of persons with SCI have persistent problems with pain. Much has been written about the role of psychological factors in the maintenance of chronic pain, so it is no surprise that psychosocial issues (such as depressed mood and a negative psychosocial environment) have been found to be associated with greater pain problems among those with SCI (34, 35). Furthermore, one researcher found that an internal locus of control was associated with decreased pain perceptions, whereas anger was more associated with perceptions of greater pain (35).

It is well known that stress can suppress the body's immune function. Emotional stress can also increase muscular tension, increasing the likelihood of spasm problems. Furthermore, stress levels can occasionally have an impact on excretory function, as evidenced by cases of persons for whom deep relaxation training can help promote a bowel movement.

Perhaps one of the most consequential psychological factors that can affect the health and physical functioning of a person with SCI is the defense mechanism of denial, along with its frequent accompaniment, behavioral noncompliance and self-neglect. Unhealthy behaviors such as smoking, drinking, or poor diet can complicate medical care. For example, cigarette smoking can increase the risk of skin breakdown and interfere with bone healing. Self-neglect as well can have deleterious consequences. The SCI-related conditions of autonomic dysreflexia and skin breakdown are preventable through heightened self-awareness and proper self-care. Self-neglect of this sort can insidiously and seriously erode one's health.

Lastly, there is a potential for "a vicious circle" involving the interaction of emotional and physical problems. For instance, a pattern of chronic sleep impairment or "sleep fragmentation" may result from the ongoing interactions of stress, spasms, fatigue, and nocturnal interruptions for nursing care. This in turn can produce further emotional and/or medical difficulties.

ISSUES IN THE POST-REHAB PHASE

"Fitting In"

Upon leaving the safe and supportive milieu of a rehabilitation facility, a person with SCI enters a new stage of adjustment—dealing with the "real world." It is not uncommon for doctor and patient alike to avoid the question of long-term prognosis, particularly regarding ambulatory function. Although some amount of day trips or home visits may have already occurred as a component of rehab, the day-to-day realities of life after rehab can nonetheless prove quite challenging. Numerous architectural barriers such as narrow aisles in stores, and having to remain seated while everyone else is standing can all make a striking contrast to the rehab setting. Other issues can also come into play. For instance, support and attention from friends and family may diminish. Being subject to the stigma or ignorance of others can occur in the form of staring, shunning, and assumptions of additional (even mental) impairments. Variation in attitude towards people with disability exists among different cultures. In the United States, for instance, a relatively more positive attitude exists in comparison to other countries (19).

Trying to reestablish connections with friends may prove frustrating if there are transportation limitations. Relationships are often altered because of dependency needs and the physical requirements of many social or recreational activities. Fortunately, technological advances in mobility assistance have made it possible for some nonambulating persons to independently navigate uneven terrain, reach high shelves and counters, and even climb stairs (the INDEPENDENCE® iBOT® 4000 Mobility System).[1] The iBOT® Mobility System also allows its users to communicate at eye level with others who are standing, and this is likely to provide considerable psychological benefit.

A major interpersonal theme for someone with SCI involves the area of assertive communication. When one needs to request help, set limits on the behavior of others, or otherwise deal with a sensitive disability-related occurrence (bowel accidents have been reported to be among the most difficult situations to deal with on a social level), doing so can be as difficult as it is important. Developing a comfortable manner of openly addressing one's SCI-related issues when they arise may be a challenge, especially if it is not in keeping with the individual's premorbid interactional style. Even when one deals calmly and directly with his or her concerns, situations such as the following may nonetheless take place:

A patient with paraplegia drove to watch his son play in a Little League game. When he arrived, the designated handicap parking spot behind the backstop was occupied by another vehicle. Sitting inside was an able-bodied woman; her car had no visible handicap plate or placard. The man attempted to get her attention with his horn, but she remained there for the entire game. He thus parked directly behind her and essentially had an obstructed view of the game. When it ended, he remained parked, refusing to let her leave. She got out of her car and approached him. When she asked why he was not backing up to let her out, he replied, "Ma'am, I have a spinal cord injury. I could not enjoy the game because you parked in the only handicap spot, and I want you to know that this was very upsetting to me." The woman replied, "Well, I suggest that you learn to walk!"

Family Challenges

In a marriage or other significant relationship, the redistribution of domestic responsibilities may need to be worked out, and honest communications without unnecessary sensitivity to hurting the other's feelings may require considerable skill. Another home-based issue involves the fact that getting up and out the door each day may no longer be a streamlined operation. Additional time is typically required for not only the person with SCI but also for any designated helpers. Finally, effective parenting may require the development of new skills. For example, someone with an SCI may not be able to use their previous physical methods to manage a child's behavior or provide affection. Better marital adjustment has been found among couples who were married post-injury than pre-injury (20). This might be due to the fact that each partner willingly entered the union aware and

accepting of the reality of the SCI and the impact it might have on their relationship.

Particular note should be given to the concept of caregiver stress. Persons with SCI may require considerable assistance in areas such as bathing, dressing and transportation. It is often the partner or another loved one who provides much of this care, and the possibility of eventual "burnout" exists. Although there is some evidence that spouses of persons with SCI experience stress levels comparable to their injured partners' (21), research on caregiver stress is generally inconclusive. Richards, Shewchuk, and Elliott state, "We need to learn what these individuals face in terms of stress and how best they can benefit from support" (22).

Sexual Challenges

Sexual functioning is among the most significant concerns for many persons with SCI, yet it is addressed in rehab far less than other, less-urgent issues. Discomfort over discussing sexuality is common not only among patients, but among many members of the rehab team as well. Moreover, sexual functioning has been found to be a frequently cited area of dissatisfaction among those with SCI. A change in desire as well as function may occur. Among males, learning how to feel sexual in the absence of traditional "performance measures" of sexual adequacy can be a daunting challenge. New patterns and methods of discovering erotic pleasures require flexibility, patience, self-confidence, and perhaps a more relaxed attitude toward modesty concerns (e.g., discussing the possibility of a bowel or bladder accident in advance may dispel some of the anxiety if one occurs). In addition to the myriad of techniques and devices available to assist with sexual performance (Chapter 32), sexual counseling can also assist couples in gaining a heightened awareness of physical pleasure and sensuality. Finally, questions about fertility may arise concerning the acquisition and preservation of sperm, the likelihood of pregnancy, and the feasibility of performing parenting skills.

Research in this area has revealed encouraging data that might temper some couples' concerns. For instance, one researcher found that partners with pre- and post-injury onset of their relationship had comparable satisfaction with their current sex lives (23). In another study, men with paraplegia and tetraplegia obtained similar results on the scales of a sexual function inventory (24), and obtained scores comparable to those of men in the normative samples in the area of sexual satisfaction.

Work and Leisure Challenges

A number of work- and leisure-related stresses can arise following SCI. The stigma surrounding persons with a disability can increase the stress associated with returning to the working world. Additionally, persons with SCI often need to find a new career (i.e., one with fewer physical demands). Architectural barriers in the workplace may also be a source of difficulties. A more insidious issue involves the vicious circle that can develop during the challenge of finding a new job, in which emotional distress or depression over vocational issues leads to poor self-presentation on job interviews, rejection by potential employers, and further distress.

Research has shown that people need to be able to "play" in order to maintain good mental health. Recreational and leisure

---

[1]®INDEPENDENCE and iBOT are registered trademarks of Independence Technology, LLC.

activities offer time for positive distraction, release of stress, and a general enhancement of quality of life. The inability to return to sport and other recreational pursuits can be quite frustrating to those with SCI. Fortunately, a number of programs have developed over the past 10 years or so that offer viable alternatives to those with SCI (Chapter 60). For instance, organizations exist that offer adaptive devices for skiing, golfing, kayaking and even bungee jumping!

Aging

Because paraplegia involves a proportional increase in upper body use, the risk of that part of the body's wearing out with age is increased. Thus, the more one strives to remain independent, the greater the risk becomes for problems in maintaining that level over the years. Increased difficulty in overcoming the disability may thus arise, requiring new adjustments after years of successful adaptation to SCI. The ability to perform on the job may likewise become more challenging and lead to worry about one's livelihood. Financial stress can also develop over factors such as the need to replace an aging wheelchair. Concerns about an aging or increasingly less able-bodied spouse/caretaker may arise. In short, a number of vulnerabilities can manifest themselves over time.

Recidivism

One of the more relevant issues in the area of long-term adjustment to SCI involves the return of unhealthy or unsafe behaviors, particularly smoking and substance abuse. Although persons with SCI may previously have had a problem with this and then "swore off" alcohol or drugs after their injury, the urge to resume this pattern may return. It has been found that persons with SCI are most susceptible to relapse in the three to six months following discharge from the hospital (25). Additionally, the incidence of substance abuse among the SCI population is higher than that of the general population. This may be due to an effort at self-medicating to deal with emotional struggles, the sensitivity to peer pressure, or a weakening of the resolve to quit in the face of other emotional challenges. Substance use can impair one's cognitive function, which is relevant because persons with SCI must be especially cognizant of bodily needs. The inadequate performance of pressure relief maneuvers because of inattention or impaired judgment could lead to problems with skin integrity. Other results of tobacco or substance use could include greater likelihood of respiratory or balance difficulties, bladder and kidney problems, dysreflexia, skin breakdown, and deleterious interactions with medications (38).

The previously cited likelihood of neuropsychological deficits, such as memory, concentration, or executive function impairment represents another factor that could compromise health and well-being. Whatever the obstacles may be, individuals with SCI need to maintain a high level of insight, judgment, and attention in order to attend properly to the various areas of physical management. Similarly, health and mental health care professionals need to be aware that patients who had given up smoking or substance use after their injury may nonetheless remain "at risk" for some time. Periodic inquiry at follow-up appointments is recommended, and those who continue to abstain may be given positive verbal reinforcement.

Depression and Suicide

Although mental health services are available in the rehab setting, problems involving emotional distress in the months or years after injury may go undetected. It has been estimated that less than 10% of those people in the general population who are clinically depressed actually receive treatment. Many of those who receive treatment (medication and/or psychotherapy) do in fact improve. Those who do not get treatment often show little improvement; untreated depression can cause secondary problems in those with SCI, such as decreased nutrition, concentration, and motivation. In one study, almost half of all persons with traumatic SCI showed symptoms of clinically significant depression at least one year post-injury (26), so clinical attention to this issue is clearly warranted.

Suicide or unplanned self-harm ranks as the primary cause of death in SCI for up to 6 months post-injury (27), and there is a five- to tenfold increased suicide rate for persons with SCI in comparison to non-injured peers (28). The loss of life may be sudden or insidious (e.g., long-term effects of poor nutrition or poor attention to physical functions). Risk factors include age group (under 40, as opposed to teens or forty-plus in the general population), family fragmentation, prior episodes of depression, lack of social support, and a variety of other risk factors also found in the general population (12).

Quality of Life

Perhaps the ultimate issue regarding adjustment to SCI is that of quality of life, or how to enjoy living with a significant disability. Victor Frankl, in his landmark book, *Man's Search for Meaning* (29), wrote: "A man's concern, even his despair, over the worthwhileness of life is an existential distress but by no means a mental disease." And, "Mental health is based on a certain amount of tension between what one is and what one should become." In other words, there is no psychopathology in struggling over the purpose of living, and indeed this struggle reflects a sound mind. For those with SCI to wrestle with quality of life concerns is "normal." The outcome of this struggle, however, is of critical significance. Each person must find a personal path leading to life satisfaction.

It is not uncommon to hear people without SCI make comments such as, "I could never go on living if I were paralyzed." Yet the quality-of-life ratings for SCI and non-SCI individuals are actually comparable, particularly after some time has elapsed since the injury (30). The process of finding quality of life is an adaptive process. Mitigating factors may include severe pain, spasticity, incontinence, and other medical factors (31). A person's medical and psychosocial level of functioning can be far better predictors of quality of life than the mere presence or absence of SCI. Moreover, it is not necessarily the loss of ambulation that causes the most angst among those with SCI. Equally and perhaps more distressing can be other issues such as bowel and bladder problems (32).

Despite all the physical and mental challenges that individuals with SCI face, a number of benefits may also be accrued. Developing a greater sense of patience, flexibility, and appreciation for the love and concern of others might not otherwise take place. Being able to triumph over adversity, to learn alternative or adaptive means of meeting one's goals, and to turn suffering into an achievement can be powerful sequelae of SCI.

One particularly remarkable story comes from a young woman who became paraplegic but went on to become a professional athlete in the field of wheelchair marathons. She found so much inner strength and richness in her new disabled life that she exclaimed to an audience at our hospital, "If I could turn back the clock and make this injury have never happened, I would not do it." Likewise, a man with tetraplegia who found the means to continue reading, writing, and eventually get a college education said, "I broke my neck; it didn't break me!"

PSYCHOTHERAPEUTIC INTERVENTIONS

The Rehab Team

Assisting a patient in the psychological adjustment to SCI involves a team, which by way of its time and interest can convey a therapeutic sense of caring and support. The team members need to be ever-mindful of regular communication not only with the patient, but among themselves as well. Consider the following personal vignette:

I was asked to speak with a patient whose SCI left him with no control of his lower extremities and limited use of his upper extremities. The nursing staff informed me that he was becoming excessively needy and demanding. They noted that his call light never went on when he had visitors in the room, but would frequently be turned on when he was alone in his room. Furthermore, his requests to the nurses that responded to his calls were invariably trivial or inconsequential (requests to fluff his pillow, angle the television better, and so forth). This was "proof" that he was taking advantage of the staff through this dependent behavior. I was asked to help him deal with this issue in our therapy sessions.

I approached the patient about a concern some of the staff had about his use of the call button. His was a disc-shaped device placed by his chest. He had sufficient upper extremity control to tap it with his hand, but a problem with involuntary arm movement resulted in occasional inadvertent hitting of the disc. His guests were aware of this situation and would remove the disc from his reach during their stay. They assumed that any needs for a nurse could be handled by their verbal request. The patient, meanwhile, felt bad for any nurse that took the time to come to his room when the call light mistakenly went on. He did not want their effort to be for naught, so he would "create" a need when they arrived (e.g., to fluff his pillow). This is a rather dramatic example of the problems arising out of inadequate communication—the patient, his visitors, and the nurses all had the opportunity to solve this problem by simply addressing it, but nobody did. Of course, once the reality of the situation was revealed to all, a new call system was arranged and the patient's "reputation" among the nursing staff was restored.

Many facets of life with SCI demand clear communication. A number of false assumptions can occur among patients because they often lack a basic understanding of their condition. For example, they may consider their disability to be progressive, or that their life expectancy must now be much shorter (in fact, it is only slightly less so than the general population). Others have needlessly feared being released from the hospital with nowhere to go. Education and reassurance on such matters is critical in helping individuals adjust to their condition, and can only take place in an environment focused on open sharing of information and concerns.

All staff must be aware of social and professional boundaries when relating to hospitalized patients. When working closely with patients on a daily basis, there is a natural tendency to develop a sense of closeness, to take verbal liberties, or to have fondness develop between patient and staff. Patients may also mistakenly interpret caring, compassion, and physical closeness as a personal attraction. Asking a treating therapist or nurse out for a date, for instance, is not uncommon among patients. Additionally, staff may invite patients to casual functions not meant for staff-patient socializing. A clear set of guidelines is invaluable in maintaining professional conduct and clarity surrounding boundary issues among patients and staff. Ongoing education and discussion among staff is important to ensure that no such complicating violations occur.

Another area of communication that can be as subtle as it is important involves the maintenance of a positive focus. If a treatment team believes that an SCI patient has a productive future as well as general rehab potential, the patient will sense this and may develop an increase in motivation and confidence. If on the other hand a patient senses that the staff has low expectations or assumes the individual is depressed or globally dependent, this message too will be conveyed. It is important to retain hope, optimism, and confidence in the person with SCI so as to model and encourage a favorable reaction to the injury. Arranging for frequent passes into the community helps convey the importance of reconnecting with and facing the outside world.

The Psychotherapist

The role of the mental health professional is pivotal in the overall success of SCI rehab patients. The outcome of rehabilitation can easily be jeopardized by factors such as anxiety, depression, and unstable or unclear family communication and relationships. These factors can impede the patient's overall motivation, progress, and outcome. Other areas that psychotherapy can address include stress and anger management, pain control, insomnia, motivation problems, family, marital, and sexuality issues, tobacco/substance abuse, and conflicts or behavior problems involving the patient and staff. This latter factor may be appropriately managed with "behavior rounds," in which the team, led by the mental health professional, discusses roadblocks to optimal recovery. For instance, when a patient expresses frustration through rude or oppositional behavior toward staff, each of whom may have a different manner of responding, discussing these responses as well as formulating a consistent and assertive approach, can be quite beneficial.

Not all persons are open to the idea of receiving mental health services, and this writer has had many patients on our SCI unit refuse to be evaluated or treated. Although this may be due to an instinctual aversion to the idea of being in therapy, it could also reflect a desire to conserve their energy and effort for the more physical areas of recovery. This is certainly within their rights, and it is often wiser to accede to this wish for the time being and only make another attempt if and when psychological issues are found to be impeding the physical rehabilitation process. It may nonetheless be helpful to "set the stage" by explaining that psychological treatment can include training in many self-help techniques to better manage problems in such areas as pain, insomnia, and effective communication with staff.

Specific Techniques

Psychological Testing

Psychologists are particularly well suited to conduct personality assessments because of their familiarity with psychometric assessment. Tests such as the Minnesota Multiphasic Personality Inventory (MMPI-2), Beck Anxiety and Depression Scales, and other instruments can be useful in clarifying the nature and extent of psychological difficulties. Furthermore, discussion of test results with the client can pave the way for more open discussion of the role and benefits of psychological counseling. One newer instrument, the Millon Behavioral Medicine Diagnostic (MBMD), is used by rehab teams because of its focus not only on psychopathology but on negative health patterns, coping styles, stress moderators, and treatment prognostics (how a person's behavioral and emotional styles may influence interactions with healthcare providers). The MBMD also contains a unique and often-relevant measure: the extent to which spiritual factors may be helpful in the coping process. Cushman & Scherer (37) have provided a thorough review of the many psychological assessment tools available to the medical rehabilitation professional.

The subspecialty field of neuropsychological assessment is also very useful in the SCI setting. Information concerning premorbid and post-injury deficits in memory, attention, and learning ability can help promote optimal rehabilitation efforts.

Supportive Counseling

Any effective psychotherapeutic endeavor requires an open and comfortable rapport. Providing a safe haven—a trusting environment in which to explore problematic issues—can itself be an important contribution to the process. Allowing the patient and family a place to ventilate frustrations, explore conflicting feelings, or take time to process their situation is an important aspect of counseling.

Behavior Therapy

Many effective behavioral interventions are useful in the SCI rehab setting. These include assertion training (clear and effective expression of needs, feelings, or concerns); relaxation training (for insomnia, pain, and muscle tension, fear, or anxiety) and reinforcement strategies (for motivation enhancement). Behavioral interventions are also useful in addressing specific behavioral problems. For example, a patient who is failing to complete his or her morning routine on a satisfactory level may be given a therapeutic pass contingent on improving in this area. A schedule of behavior rounds meetings, led by the staff mental health professional, may be helpful in bringing team members together to formulate a consistent strategy for effectively eliminating counter-therapeutic behaviors.

Cognitive Therapy

Training a person with SCI to realistically appraise situations while minimizing self criticism (negative "self-talk") can be a key component of good coping technique. It is common for a disabled person to subscribe to beliefs such as, "I'm no longer attractive," "I'm not a real man (woman) anymore," "I may as well give up on amounting to anything anymore," and so forth. Cognitive therapy involves evaluating one's thinking in a way that creates logical and affirmative self-statements to replace the emotional and negative ones. For instance, thought stopping is a technique that enables one to "turn off" intrusive fears, worries, or depressing ideation that intrude into consciousness. Cognitive therapy meshes well with the repetitive practice and problem-solving orientation of other therapies. One specific area where cognitive therapy could be useful is among persons with chronic SCI pain, as their pain intensity and pain-related disability seems to be influenced by "catastrophizing," a specific type of negative thinking (36). Another example of cognitive therapy would be the use of a self-report "checklist" to determine why a patient may not be actively participating in his or her therapies or displaying recommended behaviors. Although the patient may be deemed oppositional or passive-aggressive, it is also possible that he or she forgets, does not grasp the rationale for the activity, does not feel it will make a difference, or assumes there is no way to "find the time." Developing a collaborative awareness of the thinking or assumptions underlying the problematic behavior can often lead to insight and behavior change. An example of a form that allows the patient to identify "reasons for not doing self-help assignments" is available in Beck (32, p. 408).

Strategic Interventions

In particularly difficult situations, specific interventions or staff responses may be called for. This is especially likely to be necessary and effective with oppositional or controlling patients. Paradoxical intention is an example of this style of treatment. For instance, a patient who vents his anger at a therapist to the point that very little gets accomplished in the session might be told to begin the session by venting his anger for a full five minutes with the expressed notion of "getting it out of the system." Clearly, these high-risk strategies need to be carefully conceptualized and considered before being implemented. However, in this writer's experience, the payoff in terms of behavior change can be remarkable.

Group/Peer Therapy

One of the most powerful psychotherapeutic agents of change involves the impact of someone with SCI sharing thoughts and feelings with another person with SCI. Whether in the context of formal group therapy or a single peer visitor, patients should be given the opportunity to share time with other persons with a similar history. SCI patients are sometimes reluctant at first to participate in such meetings, but they often acknowledge later that these interactions were helpful. Finally, sessions that involve patient and family, or even multiple families, are a useful format for discussing family conflicts and for sharing feelings. This is particularly relevant during the change of roles and expectations between the SCI person and his or her significant others.

Psychopharmacology

Although not in the realm of psychological treatment, prescription of psychopharmacological agents can be useful in the management of psychiatric symptoms. Antidepressant medication may be particularly helpful in reducing neurovegetative symptoms (e.g., decreased appetite or energy), as well as features of PTSD and some pain conditions. Short-term use of anxiolytic medication may prove useful in the reduction of anxiety symptomatology. Preferably, a rehab team will include a staff or consulting psychiatrist for evaluation and treatment in this domain.

CONCLUSION

In short, each case of SCI is both unique and similar to others. Despite a multitude of potential psychosocial challenges, persons with SCI clearly can enjoy a satisfying and productive life. The challenge of reshaping or redefining one's life goals and identity can be most successfully met with the support of a helpful staff that maintains a realistic and positive perspective. The rehab team's role in open communication with each other, as well as with the patient, can serve as a valuable model for patients, families, and their community.

References

1. National Spinal Cord Injury Statistical Center. Spinal cord injury: Facts and figures at a glance. *J Spinal Cord Med* 2000; 23:153–155.
2. Gittler MS, Thornton LS. Violently acquired spinal cord injury: A horse of a different color. AASCIPSW Conference, Las Vegas, 2000.
3. Moverman RA. Assessment and intervention in cases of "the false patient." *SCI Psychosocial Process* 1997; 10:53–57.
4. Woods TE, Sherman JE, Sperling KB. Coping with spinal cord injury: Different strategies are associated with distress and life satisfaction. AAS-CIPSW Conference, Las Vegas, 2001.
5. Kennedy P, Lowe R, Grey N, Short E. Traumatic spinal cord injury and psychologic impact: A cross sectional analysis of coping strategies. *Br J Clin Psychol* 1995; 34:627–639.
6. Livneh H. Psychosocial adaptation to spinal cord injury: The role of coping strategies. *J Applied Rehabil Counseling* 2000; 31:3–10.
7. Olkin R. *What Psychotherapists Should Know about Disability.* New York: Guilford, 1999.
8. Olkin R. Crips, gimps and epileptics explain it all to you. *Readings* 1993; 8:13–17.
9. Howell T, Fullerton DT, Harvey RF, Klein M. Depression in spinal cord injured patients. *Paraplegia* 1981; 19:284–288.
10. Fuhrer MR, Rintala DH, Hart KA, et al. Depressive symptomatology in persons with spinal cord injury. *Arch Phys Med Rehabil* 1993; 74:255–260.
11. Fullerton DT, Harvey RF, Klein MH, et al. Psychiatric disorders in patients with spinal cord injuries. *Arch Gen Psychiat* 1981; 38:1369–1371.
12. Consortium for Spinal Cord Medicine. *Depression Following Spinal Cord Injury: A Clinical Practice Guideline for Primary Care Physicians.* Washington, DC: Paralyzed Veterans of America, 1998.
13. Tucker SJ. The psychology of spinal cord injury: Patient-staff interaction. *Rehabil Lit* 1980; 41:114–121.
14. Buzan R. Management of Sleep Disorders in SCI: A Psychiatric Perspective. AASCIPSW Conference, Las Vegas, 2000.
15. Radnitz C, et al. The prevalence of posttraumatic stress disorder in veterans with spinal cord injury. *SCI Psychosocial Process* 1995; 8:145–149.
16. Butt L. Post-traumatic stress disorder and spinal cord injury: Part I. *SCI Psychosocial Process* 1998; 11:48–51.
17. Fee F, Fee V. Psychologic consequences of concomitant spinal cord injury and traumatic brain injury. *Psychosocial Process* 1995; 8:106–111.
18. Consortium for Spinal Cord Medicine. Depression: *What You Should Know.* Washington, DC: Paralyzed Veterans of America, 1999.
19. Westbrook MT, Legge V, Pennay M. Attitudes towards disabilities in a multicultural society. *Social Science Medicine* 1993; 36:615–623.
20. Crewe N, Krause J. Marital relationships and spinal cord injury. *Arch Phys Med Rehabil* 1988; 69:435–438.
21. Chan RCK. Stress and coping in spouses of persons with spinal cord injuries. *Clin Rehabil* April 2000; 137–144.
22. Richards JS, Shewchuk RM, Elliott TR. Caregivers of persons with spinal cord injury: The forgotten half? *Top Spinal Cord Inj Rehabil* 2000; 6(Suppl):222–223.
23. Kreuter M, Sullivan M, Siosteen A. Sexual adjustment after spinal cord injury-comparison of partner experiences in pre- and postinjury relationships. *Paraplegia* 1994; 32:759–770.
24. Romeo AJ, Wanlass R, Arenas S. A profile of psychosexual functioning in males following spinal cord injury. *Sexuality and Disability* 1993; 11:269–276.
25. Lebenberg IC. Substance Abuse Prevention after SCI: Essentials for Healthcare Providers. AASCIPSW Conference, Las Vegas, 2000.
26. Krause JS, Kemp B, Coker J. Depression after spinal cord injury: Relation to gender, ethnicity, aging, and socioeconomic status indicators. *Arch Phys Med Rehabil* 2000; 81:1099–1109.
27. DeVivo M, Stover S. Cause of death for patients with spinal cord injury. *Arch Internal Medicine* 1989; 149:1761–1766.
28. Rish et al. SCI: 25–year morbidity and mortality study. *Milit Med* 1997; 162:141–148.
29. Frankl V. *Man's Search for Meaning.* New York: Washington Square Press, 1984.
30. Krause JS. Life satisfaction after spinal cord injury. *Rehabil Psychol* 1992; 37:61–71.
31. Westgren N, Levi R. Quality of life and traumatic spinal cord injury. *Arch Phys Med Rehabil* 1998; 79:1433–1439.
32. Rogers B, Kennedy P. A qualitative analysis of reported coping in a community sample of people with spinal cord injuries: The first year post discharge. *SCI Psychosocial Process* Summer 2000, 41.
33. Beck AT, Rush AJ, et al. *Cognitive Therapy of Depression,* New York: Guilford, 1979.
34. Richards JS, Meredith RL, Nepomuceno C, Fine PR, Bennett G. Psychosocial aspects of chronic pain in spinal cord injury. *Pain.* 1980 Jun; 8(3):355–66.
35. Conant LL. Psychological Variables Associated with Pain Perceptions Among Individuals with Chronic Spinal Cord Injury Pain. *Journal of Clinical Psychology in Medical Settings.* V 5 no. 8 1998, pp. 1068–9583.
36. Turner JA, Jensen MP, Warms CA, Cardenas DD. Catastrophizing is associated with pain intensity, psychological distress, and pain-related disability among individuals with chronic pain after spinal cord injury. *Pain.* 2002 Jul; 98(1–2):127–34.
37. Cushman, LA, Scherer, MJ *Psychological Assessment in Medical Rehabilitation.* Washington, DC: American Psychological Association, 1995.
38. Toronto Rehabilitation Institute, *Healthy Living after Spinal Cord Injury,* Toronto, Ontario: Toronto Rehab, 2003.

78 Social Issues in Spinal Cord Injury

E. Jason Mask
Helen Bosshart

The onset of a spinal cord injury (SCI) creates tremendous changes throughout many aspects of life for individuals and their families. Although rehabilitation programs include psychosocial services to begin to prepare persons with SCI for life after returning home, many of the social and environmental issues are not realized until after discharge from the rehabilitation setting. As lengths of stay have decreased in the last decade, this has become even more of a reality. There is precious little time to learn the basic skills for physical functioning, let alone time for adaptation to the myriad of very real social consequences of SCI. Despite the time constraints, it is imperative that rehabilitation professionals assist the individual and family in exploring resources and alternatives for managing the social impact of SCI.

FAMILY RELATIONSHIPS

SCI creates a devastating impact on the family, as well as for the individual. In addition to the stresses and uncertainties of this life-threatening event for a loved one, the day-to-day responsibilities of caring for a family must also be managed. The disruption of roles, especially during the initial phases post-injury, may create a sense of disequilibrium within the family. When the individual receives rehabilitation services in a distant community as opposed to the home community, the issues are further magnified. How does a spouse continue to work and manage a family, yet be available and supportive? Are children left with other family members or friends for extended periods of time? How do elderly relatives arrange travel and coordination for visits? How is the balance of support for the family and support for the person with SCI achieved? The emotional needs and the toll of SCI for family members must be acknowledged and addressed not only during the initial rehabilitation process, but throughout the continuum of care as follow-up services are provided. Peer support can assist the individual and family in learning new coping strategies from individuals who have experienced similar catastrophic situations (1).

The importance of family relationships and social support as they relate to rehabilitation outcomes must also be considered.

For those individuals who have burned bridges with family members long ago, there may be limited incentive and motivation to get better in rehabilitation. If the only discharge prospect is nursing home placement because of a lack of family support and the physical inability to live independently, one can understand why some of these individuals do not achieve the rehabilitation outcomes anticipated. Conversely, those individuals with good family support are more likely to adapt well to SCI. In a study of thirty-four individuals in SCI rehabilitation in which the family was incorporated in the treatment program, Moore et al. reported better outcomes on six of seven dependent measures when compared to the control group without family involvement (2).

Marriage and Divorce

A marital or couples relationship is subjected to the ultimate test as a result of SCI. Many times, the spouse may be in a dual role of caregiver and partner. This may lead to conflicts and a negative impact on the couple's relationship (3). Spouses who serve as caregivers have reported higher levels of depression, physical stress, emotional stress, fatigue, anger, and resentment than the individual with SCI and other spouses who are not caregivers (4). The importance of respite care and peer support must be acknowledged and appropriately addressed with individuals with SCI and caregivers in an effort to minimize the burden of caregiving. Just as importantly, spouses are in need of ongoing emotional support as a mitigating factor to cope with the stress of dealing with the relationship changes triggered by an SCI (5).

The studies examining the prevalence of divorce are conflicting. El Ghatit and Hanson found a divorce rate of 27% in 333 marriages that were intact at the time of the husband's injury—no different from the divorce rate of the general population (6). DeVivo and Fine (7) found that their sample of 276 persons had more divorces 3 years after injury than would be predicted by population base rates. DeVivo and Richards (8) found that 81% of persons who were married at the time of their injury were still married 5 years later, compared to an expected 89%. In the more recent studies, there does appear to be a slightly higher rate of divorce for persons with SCI than in the general population.

Some studies examining marriages after SCI have found fewer problems and higher levels of marital satisfaction. Crewe et al. (9) found life satisfaction to be higher in post-injury marriages. Crewe and Krause (10) conducted a questionnaire follow-up study of 300 subjects and reported that better adjustment in post-injury marriages persisted over time. Kreuter et al. found no differences in pre-injury and post-injury marriages from the perspective of emotional attachment and satisfaction with the marriage (11). Phelps found that for married or partnered men with SCI, relationship factors including partner satisfaction and relationship quality are significantly related to sexual satisfaction (12).

There is also the question of meeting new people and forming new relationships after SCI. Some people have expressed difficulties in meeting new people and attracting a partner while in a wheelchair. Crewe and Krause (13) found that persons with SCI who get married after their SCI were more active both socially and vocationally while single, when compared to those who remain single. This suggests that those individuals who increase their activity level and do not succumb to social isolation after an SCI increase their chances of finding a partner. The importance of community reintegration during the initial rehab program cannot be emphasized enough to help individuals develop a sense of confidence and appropriate social skills for successful relationships post-injury.

Parenting

Buck and Hohmann (14, 15) found no difference in the emotional stability of children raised by a disabled father when compared with a group raised by a family without a physical disability. There were also no differences in the child's adjustment based on severity of SCI, specifically paraplegia versus quadriplegia. They also found that the children of disabled fathers reported more physical and verbal affection from the father than the children of nondisabled fathers reported. Alexander (16) also found that SCI in mothers does not appear to affect their children adversely in terms of individual adjustment, attitudes toward their parents, self-esteem, gender roles, and family functioning. The onset of SCI often prompts the individual to reexamine values and priorities in life, placing greater emphasis on the importance of a satisfying family life.

FINANCIAL ISSUES

Although Chapter 80 is devoted to the cost of SCI, it is indeed a critical social issue that impacts many aspects of the individual's life post-injury. We would be remiss if the importance of adequate finances to meet basic life needs were not briefly addressed in the context of this chapter. Treischmann reports, "Life with a physical disability imposes a financial penalty on the individual and the family because the cost of adaptive equipment, medical expenses, home modifications, and the purchase of services reduces the discretionary income for vacations, new clothing and furniture, recreational equipment and activities, dining out, and socializing. The standard of living for the entire family is reduced in comparison to a family without a disability with the same income" (1). The financial burden associated with life after SCI

cannot be overemphasized. Brown and Giesy (17) report that financial security is a major factor in marriage and divorce rates. Ernst et al. (18) conducted a survey of 253 long-term survivors of SCI, individuals who were at least 25 years post-injury and a minimum of 45 years of age. Of these individuals, 63% reported inadequate financial resources to meet their needs, 28% reported financial difficulties in obtaining medical equipment, and 19% reported that a lack of finances prevented them from leading more active lives. A definite financial impact exists across the spectrum of social issues for individuals with SCI. Recreation and leisure, housing, medications and medical supplies, personal assistance services, transportation, and quality of life all are negatively affected for individuals with inadequate financial resources.

It is essential that rehabilitation professionals assist the individual and family in exploring all of the resources (state, local, federal) that may be of benefit to them. There may also be alternative support opportunities in local communities, such as churches, veteran service organizations, civic clubs, and other nonprofit organizations. Every effort should be made to assist in decreasing the environmental and financial barriers that compromise quality of life. As health professionals, we should also advocate for health policies that eliminate barriers to equitable access to quality services.

PRODUCTIVITY

Although many rehabilitation programs look at return to school or employment as a measure of successful rehabilitation outcomes, for many individuals financial disincentives may counter a return to gainful employment. For those individuals who are injured after they have already retired from the workforce, certainly returning to work would not be a goal or personal choice. As a result, it may be more appropriate to focus on productivity and meaningful use of time rather than employment as we examine outcomes in this area. Webster's (19) defines productivity as follows: "producing abundantly; fertile; prolific; yielding favorable or useful results; constructive; involved in the creation of goods and services to produce wealth or value." If we look at productivity after SCI, it seems that a key ingredient is that there are some goal-directed activities for which the individual achieves a sense of accomplishment. This may be in many forms, including employment, vocational rehabilitation, and return to school, volunteerism, activities in the home, and recreation and leisure pursuits. Fuhrer et al. (20) found those individuals with less involvement in employment, school, volunteer work, or other self-improvement activities reported higher degrees of depressive symptomatology.

Employment

The National SCI Statistics Center reports that 60.5% of individuals admitted to a Model SCI Care System reported being employed at the time of their injury. Return to work post-injury is higher for individuals with paraplegia as opposed to tetraplegia. By post-injury year 10, 35.3% of individuals with paraplegia are employed, as opposed to 24.3% of individuals with tetraplegia (21). Being at a younger age at time of injury (under age 30) and being able to drive independently were identified as key factors in return to employment, as were being in a higher-scale pre-injury occupation and having a higher level of education (22, 23). The pre-injury physical intensity of the occupation is also predictive of return to employment, with persons having less physically demanding pre-injury occupations more likely to be employed post-injury (24). Lack of transportation and personal assistance needs are variables that limit employment opportunities for some individuals. Financial disincentives are also very real for many individuals, because they may face the reality of receiving less income from gainful employment than their current disability benefits. As a result, in the veteran population, service-connected veterans who are not at risk of losing financial benefits are more likely to work than nonservice connected veterans.

Vocational rehabilitation services often play a vital role in return to the workforce after SCI. Timing in the provision of these services is especially important. McAweeney et al. (25) reported that 64% of their study participants identified a need for a vocational assessment after SCI. How soon should the individual "adapted" to living with SCI be ready to focus energies on return to school or work? Should vocational rehabilitation be an integral component of the initial rehabilitation experience, or is it better to pursue vocational rehabilitation a year or two after onset of SCI? The key to success is the individual's readiness, and it is important for rehabilitation professionals to assist in providing basic education about what services may be available, as well as completing a vocational assessment and assisting with referrals for services. Follow-up assessments of vocational readiness must be incorporated in rehabilitation follow-up visits. In view of the evidence that those with lower levels of pre-injury education and onset above age 30 are least likely to return to work or school after their injury, it would seem especially important for rehab professionals to target interventions in vocational rehabilitation programs to assist these individuals. The importance of long-term support in finding a job, as opposed to the traditional approaches in vocational rehabilitation, must also be addressed.

Recreation and Leisure

Participation in meaningful activities is important to all of us if we are to have any level of life satisfaction. After SCI, the individual may find that there are a number of pre-injury recreation and leisure options that either are no longer available or must be modified as a result of physical limitations. Assisting the individual in exploring leisure options after SCI is an important component of the rehabilitation process. Satisfaction with leisure activities has been positively correlated with successful adjustment for individuals with severe disabilities (10). Elliott and Shewchuk (26) found depressive behavior to be directly associated with less leisure activity. McAweeney et al. (25) reported that 37.1% subjects in a study with 122 participants had unmet needs in the area of peer recreation. Kerstin found that physical activity in people with SCI is important for maintaining physical health and for increasing the possibility of living an independent life (27). The importance of assisting individuals in finding their niche in leisure activities, whether sedentary or physical, cannot be overemphasized. Some individuals elect to become involved in competitive sports; the numbers of participants in the Paralympics and National Wheelchair Games are increasing steadily. The success stories of individuals who participate for the first time and blossom are very common on rehab units, because team activity and competition

enhance self-image and a sense of physical and mental well-being. Giola reported that sports activity is associated with better psychological status in persons with SCI, irrespective of tetraplegia and paraplegia, and that psychological benefits are not emphasized by demographic factors (28).

SOCIOECONOMIC STATUS AND CULTURAL ISSUES

How an individual adapts to SCI is inherently correlated with socioeconomic status and cultural background. Although there is little published in the literature on this topic, there is increasing evidence that race and ethnicity, as well as socioeconomic status, affect social participation (29). Kerr and Thompson (30) reported that those with less education and greater financial hardships had difficulties in adjusting to SCI. Education is a strong predictor of employment for African-Americans (31). Individuals from Latino backgrounds reported higher overall depression scores than African-American or Caucasian participants in a recent study reported by Kemp et al. (32). American Indians reported elevated levels of depression and diminished social well being in five of eight areas when compared with previous studies on other populations (33). Some express concern that the psychometric instruments used in rehabilitation may not be culturally sensitive. This is an issue that researchers must address, because the SCI minority population is expected to grow. It is also especially important for rehab professionals to be sensitive to the cultural differences of patients to ensure that services are designed to address areas where we know individuals from different ethnic backgrounds have increased susceptibility to problems.

PERSONAL ASSISTANCE SERVICES (PAS)

Finding and keeping reliable personal assistance services is consistently listed as one of the most difficult problems for individuals with SCI. Entire textbooks and patient education manuals (34–36) are devoted to this topic, so we will focus briefly on some of the key issues that rehabilitation professionals should be prepared to address during the rehab process. For those individuals who are functionally dependent in some aspects of activities of daily living, it is essential that the rehab program provide training in the management of personal assistance services. Needs can range from personal grooming, toileting, and transfers to grocery shopping, running errands, and housekeeping. Although in some cases the services are provided through home health agencies, with increasing frequency individuals are finding and hiring their own attendants, controlling and directing the services that they need. Frost et al. (37) report that the demand for personal care assistants has made this position the fastest-growing occupation monitored by the government. They also report that the Federal Bureau of Labor Statistics predicts the number of people working in this occupation will increase from 347,000 in 1992 to 827,000 in 2005.

The training programs should at a minimum cover the following topics: defining personal assistance needs; advertising and recruitment of a personal assistant; interviewing skills and strategies; training the personal assistant; managing the employee/employer relationship; and back-up plans. Role play and rehearsals are encouraged to assist in skills development.

Rehabilitation professionals also must assist in exploring funding options, because they vary widely from state to state. There is also the issue of the individual's eligibility for various programs. Exchange of services, such as providing a place to stay in lieu of payment, has proven to be a viable alternative for many.

Access to reliable personal assistance services has been fraught with problems. Services are often severely limited as a result of funding sources. The low wages typically provided for these services are considered precipitating factors in the high turnover rate in agencies, as well as individuals hired directly. There have also been reports of patients being abused or neglected both physically and verbally by the attendant, an especially high-risk concern for individuals who are physically dependent on these individuals and often unable to physically protect themselves. It is important for training programs to strongly address patient rights and the steps to take to deal with potentially abusive situations.

COMMUNITY REINTEGRATION

Marcel Dijkers defined community reintegration as "a term used in human service fields to refer to being part of the mainstream of family and community life, discharging normal roles and responsibilities, and being an active and contributing member of one's social groups and of society as a whole" (38). This definition aptly describes what community reintegration means for individuals following SCI. The term reintegration as opposed to integration is used, because in most cases this is a return to community living after SCI. Resuming old roles or modifying them as needed is a part of the process of adaptation following SCI.

Rehabilitation programs must provide community reentry activities to assist the individual with SCI in testing the community and society and developing the skills needed for success. How to maneuver in a wheelchair, how to open doors, and how to deal with curbs or other architectural barriers are only a few of the essential mobility skills. How to interact with the nondisabled public and put them at ease may require the development of new skills. Dunn (39) identified situations of social discomfort for individuals following SCI and advocated for the provision of social skills training to assist in mastering these situations. Social skills training must be a component of patient and family education programs so that there is opportunity to develop skills for the potentially uncomfortable or embarrassing situations often experienced by individuals after SCI. Anecdotally, former patients tell stories of their recall of how to manage new problematic situations when they occur, as a result of the role plays and behavioral rehearsals during their rehabilitation. Song emphasized the importance of individual coping strategies. He found that the social integration of persons with SCI was influenced most by emotion-focused coping followed by family support, informational support, perceived stress, and dealing with social barriers (40).

Community reentry outings prior to discharge from the rehab setting are requisite. Trips to the mall, the grocery store, the movies, and other recreational or sports activities allow patients opportunities to practice the skills they have developed in rehab. Although the activity planned might not be of particular interest to all participants, the value of the community outing should be emphasized in preparation for resuming roles in the community.

Many real activity participation barriers persist in the environment for individuals with disabilities. Wheelchair-accessible housing is limited, and long waiting lists are common for handicap-accessible apartments through federal or local programs. People who lack the financial resources to modify their homes for wheelchair accessibility may well experience a significant compromise in quality of life as a result of their living conditions and home environment. Lack of accessible, reliable, and affordable transportation severely limits the activity level of many individuals with SCI. This is especially true for those living in rural areas without access to any public transportation. Several studies report that transportation services are an unmet need for individuals with SCI (25, 41, 42). Lack of transportation was reported to prevent seeking medical care (13%); interfere with independence (48%); and prevent socialization (31%) in a long-term care needs survey conducted by the American Association of SCI Psychologists and Social Workers (18).

Patient-education programs also must have a component focusing on community resources and community involvement. It is important for individuals to have a knowledge of available resources, as well as good problem-solving skills to address their unmet needs in the community. Involvement in independent living center activities may afford opportunities for expanding social support networks and developing new skills. Volunteering in the community can provide a sense of satisfaction by giving to others. Participation in peer support groups may help facilitate community reintegration by learning from others who have been there. Gerhart et al. (43) emphasizes the value of independent living services in adaptation to SCI.

QUALITY OF LIFE

In recent years, increased attention has been given to the concept of quality of life as it relates to people with disabilities. A high degree of consensus concurs that quality of life is an important attribute, but defining the concept has not been an easy task. Edlund and Tancredi (44) postulated several different meanings—fulfillment; the ability to lead a "normal life;" and the social usefulness of an individual from a rational objective point of view, or from an individualistic, subjective point of view. Hornquist (45) sees the degree of need satisfaction as the driving principle. Cohen (46) defines quality of life as the capacity of the individual to realize life plans. Campbell (47) states, "quality of life is a vague and ethereal entity, something that many people talk about but which nobody very clearly knows what to do about." Although defining the concept is difficult, determining what contributes to a high level of life satisfaction and quality of life for individuals with SCI has found some interesting results.

Time since injury has been noted to have a positive correlation with life satisfaction in some studies (48, 49), reflecting that quality of life improves for individuals given time to adapt to SCI. Conversely, McColl and Rosenthal (50) found the opposite results. Krause and Crewe (51) reported that older persons are less likely to have an active, rewarding life after SCI than younger persons, suggesting that increased chronologic age has a negative correlation with quality of life. Krause (51), in a 20-year longitudinal study, found that although there was improvement for participants in the areas of time engaged in employment, sitting tolerance, education, and numbers of hospitalizations, self-rated adjustment decreased. Dijkers (52) found the highest levels of life satisfaction with individuals who were married, competitively employed, and had the highest levels of education. Lowest satisfaction was reported for individuals who were separated, residing in nursing homes or long-stay hospitals, retired or unemployed, and had the lowest levels of education. This study found a positive correlation of time since injury and satisfaction with life, but age had no effect. Individuals from ethnic minorities and with lower levels of education reported less life satisfaction as a result of higher levels of handicap and lower levels of social participation. Leisure satisfaction was found to be the most significant predictor of life satisfaction in another study (53), although there is no correlation between physical activity and subjective well-being (54). No correlation was found in relation to level of injury; that is, paraplegia versus tetraplegia (55).

As one begins to look critically at what variables appear to have direct impact on quality of life, it becomes very obvious that many of the social issues facing individuals after SCI influence their quality of life. Clearly adequate finances, education, employment, leisure, and family support have a critical bearing on one's satisfaction in life. Whiteneck found that persons with SCI reported, in descending order, the top five environmental barriers to their satisfaction with life as being the natural environment, transportation, need for help in the house, availability of health care, and governmental policies (56). The role of ethnicity warrants further investigation, but the impact of handicap as it relates to community reintegration is apparent.

Aging

Aging with a spinal cord injury is no longer uncommon. Many individuals live with a spinal cord injury 20, 30, 40, and 50 years post-injury. As a result, these individuals experience many of the same medical conditions and psychosocial issues that same age non-SCI individuals experience, e.g. hypertension, diabetes, congestive heart failure, chronic obstructive pulmonary disease, social isolation, and decrease in social functioning. They also experience issues related to their SCI and often times these issues are gender specific. Women with SCI have characterized their aging experience as "accelerated," and men have characterized it as "complicated." Women reported more effects of pain, fatigue, and skin problems, and more transportation problems. Men experienced more health problems, more diabetes, and more adaptive equipment changes (57). A 30-year longitudinal study by Krause (58) indicated changes in life satisfaction, general health, activities, and adjustment over three decades among individuals with SCI. He found a mixed pattern of changes over the 30 years with increases noted during the first 15-year period in sitting tolerance, educational and employment outcomes, satisfaction with employment, and adjustment. Although these changes tended to remain stable during the last 15 years, subtle changes were suggested in some areas, with clear declines noted in terms of diminished sitting tolerance, an increase in the number of physician visits, and decreased satisfaction with one's social life and sex life. Charlifue found that as a person with SCI ages there was a general decline in community integration over time in terms of physical independence, mobility, occupation, social integration, and life satisfaction. (59)

CONCLUSION

It is incumbent on rehabilitation professionals who work with individuals with SCI throughout the lifespan to systematically review and assess the status of these key social issues that are so important to quality of life. Life situations change, and we must be prepared to assist our patients with those changes. A divorce for someone with SCI can have a far more devastating impact than for someone who is able-bodied; there may be a need to look for new wheelchair-accessible housing and find a new caregiver in addition to the usual stressors associated with divorce. The death or illness of a parent, if that parent was the primary caregiver, can produce equally devastating consequences. Offering guidance and support in developing a back-up system of care and planning for the future has increased significance in working with individuals with SCI. What might be an inconvenience for an able-bodied person may constitute a genuine psychosocial emergency for someone with SCI. Failure to address and resolve these issues may lead to costly health complications as well.

References

1. Treischmann RB. Spinal Cord Injuries: *Psychological, Social, and Vocational Rehabilitation* 2nd ed. New York: Demos Publishing, 1987.
2. Moore LI. *Behavioral changes in male spinal cord injured following two types of psychosocial rehabilitation experience*. (Doctoral dissertation, Saint Louis University, 1989). Dissertation Abstracts International.
3. Kreuter M, Sullivan M, Siosteen A. Sexual adjustment and spinal cord injury focusing on partner experiences. *Paraplegia* 1994; 32:225–235.
4. Weitzenkamp DA, Gerhart KA, Charlifue SW, Whiteneck GG. Spouses of spinal core injury survivors: The added impact of caregiving. *Arch Phys Med Rehabil* 1997; 78:822–827.
5. Sheija A. Efficacy of support groups for spouses of patients with spinal cord injury and its impact on their quality of life. *Int J Rehab Research* 2005; 28(4):379–383.
6. El Ghatit AZ, Hanson RW. Outcome of marriages existing at the time of a male's spinal cord injury. *J Chronic Dis* 1975; 28:383–388.
7. DeVivo MJ, Fine PR. Spinal cord injury: Its short-term impact on marital status. *Arch Phys Med Rehabil* 1985; 66:501–504.
8. DeVivo M, Richards JS. Community reintegration and quality of life following spinal cord injury. *Int Med Soc Paraplegia* 1992; 30:108–112.
9. Crewe N, Athelstan G, Krumberger BA. Spinal cord injury: A comparison of preinjury and postinjury marriages. *Arch Phys Med Rehabil* 1979; 60:252–266.
10. Crewe N, Krause J. Prediction of long term survival among persons with spinal cord injury: An 11-year prospective study. *Rehabil Psychol* 1988; 32:205–213.
11. Kreuter M, Sullivan M, Siosteen A. Sexual adjustment after spinal cord injury comparison of partner experiences in pre- and post-injury relationships. *Paraplegia* 1994; 32:759–770.
12. Phelps J. Spinal cord injury and sexuality in married or partnered men. *Arch Sexual Behavior* 2001; 30(6):591–602.
13. Crewe NM, Krause JS. Marital status and adjustment to spinal core injury. *J Am Paraplegia Soc* 1992; 15:14–18.
14. Buck FM, Hohmann GW. Personality, behavior, values, and family relations of children of fathers with spinal cord injury. *Arch Phys Med Rehabil* 1981; 62:432–438.
15. Buck FM, Hohmann GW. Child adjustment as related to severity of paternal disability. *Arch Phys Med Rehabil* 1982; 63:249–253.
16. Alexander CJ. Mothers with spinal cord injuries: impact on marital, family, and children's adjustment. *Area Phys Med Rehabil* 2002; 83(1):24–30.
17. Brown JS, Giesy B. Marital status of persons with spinal cord injury. *Soc Sci Med* 1986; 23(3):313–322.
18. Ernst JL, Thomas LM, Hahnstadt WA, Piskule AA. The self-identified long-term care needs of persons with SCI. *SCI Psychosoc Process* 1988; 10(4):127–132.

19. *Webster's Illustrated Encyclopedic Dictionary.* Montreal: Tormont Publications, 1990.

20. Fuhrer MJ, Rintala DH, Hart KA, Clearman R, Young ME. Depressive symptomatology in persons with spinal cord injury who reside in the community. *Arch Phys Med Rehabil* 1993; 74:255–260.

21. *Spinal Cord Injury: Facts and Figures at a Glance.* Birmingham, Alabama: National Spinal Cord Injury Statistical Center, 1999.

22. Conroy L, Mckenna K. Vocational outcome following spinal cord injury. *Spinal Cord* 1999; 37:624–633.

23. El Ghatit A, Hanson R. Variables associated with obtaining and sustaining employment among spinal cord injured males: A follow-up of 760 veterans. *J Chronic Dis* 1978; 31:363–369.

24. Tomassen PCD, Post MWM, van Asbeck FWA. Return to work after spinal cord injury. *Spinal Cord* 2000; 38:51–55.

25. McAweeney MJ, Forchheimer, M, Tate DG. Identifying the unmet independent living needs of persons with spinal cord injury. *J Rehabil* 1996; Jul/Aug/Sept:29–34.

26. Elliott TR, Shewchuk RM. Social support and leisure activities following severe physical disability: Testing the mediating effects of depression. *Basic and App Soc Psych* 1995; 16(4):471–487.

27. Kerstin W., What promotes physical activity after spinal cord injury? *Disabil Rehabil* 2006; 28(8):481–488.

28. Gioia MC. Psychological impact of sports activity in spinal cord injury patients. *Scand J Med Sci Sports* 2006; 16(6):412–416.

29. Hall KM, Dijkers M, Whiteneck G, Brooks CA, Krause JS. The Craig Handicap Assessment and Reporting Technique (CHART): Metric properties and scoring. *Top Spinal Cord Inj Rehabil* 1998; 4:16–30.

30. Kerr W, Thompson M. Acceptance of disability of sudden onset in paraplegia. *Int J Parapleg* 1992; 10:94–102.

31. James M, DeVivo MJ, Richards SJ. Postinjury employment outcomes among African-American and white persons with spinal cord injury. *Rehabil Psychol* 1993; 38(3):151–164.

32. Kemp B, Karuse JS, Adkins R. Depression among African Americans, Latinos and Caucasians with spinal cord injury: An exploratory study. *Rehabil Psychol* 1999; 44(3):235–247.

33. Krause JS, Coker J, Charlifue S, Whiteneck GC. Depression and subjective well-being among 97 American Indians with spinal cord injury: A descriptive study. *Rehabil Psychol* 1999; 44(4):354–372.

34. DeGraff, AH. *Home Health Aides: How to Manage the People Who Help You.* Clifton Park, NY: Saratoga Access Publications, 1988.

35. Ulciny G, Adler A, Kennedy S, Jones M. *A Step-by-Step Guide to Training and Managing Personal Attendants. Part One: Consumer Guide.* Part Two: Agency Guide 1987.

36. *Managing Personal Assistants: A Consumer Guide.* Washington, DC: Paralyzed Veterans of America, 2000.

37. Frost FS, Brenna D, Roach MJ. Opportunities in community placement: An innovative personal care assistant training program in the inner city. *Top Spinal Cord Inj Rehabil* 1999; 4(3):94–102.

38. Dijkers M. Community integration: Conceptual issues and measurement approaches in rehabilitation research. *Top Spinal Cord Inj Rehabil* 1998; 4(10):1–15.

39. Dunn M. Social discomfort in the patient with spinal cord injury. *Arch Phys Med Rehabil* 1977; 58:257–260.

40. Song Hy. Modeling social integration in persons with spinal cord injury. *Disabil Rehabil* 2005; 27(3):131–141.

41. Means BL, Bolton B. Recommendations for expanding employability services provided by independent living programs. *J Rehabil* 1994; 4:20–25.

42. Tate DG, Forchheimer M, Maynard F, et al. Predicting depression and psychological distress in persons with spinal cord injury based on indicators of handicap. *Am J Phys Med Rehabil* 1994; 73:175–183.

43. Gerhart KA, Johnson RL, Whiteneck G. Health and psychosocial issues of individuals with incomplete and resolving spinal cord injuries. *Paraplegia* 1992; 30:282–287.

44. Edlund M, Tancredi LR. Quality of life: An ideological critique. *Perspect Biol Med* 1985; 28:591–607.

45. Hornquist JO. The concept of quality of life. *Scand J Soc Med* 1982; 10:57–61.

46. Cohen C. On quality of life: Some philosophical reflections. *Circulation* 1982; 66(Suppl 3):29–33.

47. Campbell A. Subjective measures of well-being. *American Psychologist* 1976; 31:117–124.

48. Krause JS, Crewe NM. Chronological age, time since injury, and time of measurement: Effect on adjustment after spinal cord injury. *Arch Phys Med Rehabil* 1991; 72:91–100.

49. Schulz R, Decker S. Long-term adjustment to physical disability: The role of social support, perceived control, and self-blame. *J Pers Soc Psychol* 1985; 48:1162–1172.

50. McColl MA, Rosenthal C. A model of resource needs of aging spinal cord injured men. *Paraplegia* 1994; 32:261–270.

51. Krause JS. Changes in adjustment after spinal cord injury: a 20-year longitudinal study. *Rehab Psychol* 1998; 43(1):41–55.

52. Dijkers MPJM. Correlates of life satisfaction among persons with spinal cord injury. *Arch Phys Med Rehabil* 1999; 80:867–876.

53. Coyle CP, Lesnik-Emmas S, Kinney WB. Predicting life satisfaction among adults with spinal cord injuries. *Rehab Psychol* 1994; 39(2):95–112.

54. Manns PJ, Chad KE. Determining the relation between quality of life, handicap, fitness, and physical activity for persons with spinal cord injury. *Arch Phys Med Rehabil* 1999; 80:1566–1571.

55. Fuhrer MD, Rintala DH, Hart KA, Clearman R, Young ME. Relationship of life satisfaction to impairment, disability and handicap among persons with spinal cord injury living in the community. *Arch Phys Med Rehabil* 1992; 73:552–557.

56. Whiteneck G. Environmental factors and their role in participation and life satisfaction after spinal cord injury. *Arch Phys Med Rehabil* 2004; 85(11): 1793–1803.

57. McColl, MA. Aging, gender, and spinal cord injury. *Arch Phys Med Rehabil* 2004; 85(3): 363–367.

58. Krause JS. Aging after spinal cord injury: a 30 year longitudinal study. *J Spinal Cord Med* 2006; 29(4): 371–376.

59. Charlifue S. Community integration in spinal cord injury of long duration. *Neuro Rehabilitation* 2004; 19(2): 91–101.

79 Caring for Spinal Cord Injury with Complementary and Alternative Medicine

An-Fu Hsiao

Biomedicine has been the dominant medical paradigm for much of the twentieth century. Although it has made significant contributions to improving the quality of medical care and served as a very effective paradigm for treating acute illnesses, biomedicine has not been as successful for treatment of chronic illnesses and its costs have spiraled out of control. In 2001 healthcare consumed 15% of the U.S. gross domestic product (GDP), the highest proportion of GDP in the world. In spite of these high expenditures, patients with chronic illnesses, including chronic low back pain, irritable bowel syndrome, fibromyalgia, and other functional syndromes, are not effectively treated by the current biomedical model (1–3). Furthermore, patients are dissatisfied with conventional medicine due to its adverse effects, medical errors, impersonal care, and rising healthcare costs (4–6). At the same time we are witnessing a rapid increase in the use and popularity of complementary and alternative medicine (CAM) (7, 8). The Office of Alternative Medicine Research Methodology (1995) defined CAM as "a broad domain of healing resources that encompasses all health systems, modalities, and practices, and their accompanying theories and beliefs, other than those intrinsic to the politically dominant health system of a particular society or culture in a given historical period" (9).

Consumers turn to CAM and use it concurrently with conventional medicine to treat their illnesses and promote wellness. Many patients perceive CAM to be more effective, safer, and more congruent with their health beliefs, such as holism, naturalism, and vitalism, than conventional medicine (10). A national survey in 1997 showed that 42% of individuals that year used one of 16 CAM therapies for chronic conditions such as chronic low back pain, allergies, fatigue, arthritis, headache, hypertension, depression, and others (8). Consumers spent an estimated $27 billion out-of-pocket for CAM therapy in 1997. Persons with disability, including those with spinal cord injury (SCI), are increasingly turning to CAM treatments and using them concurrently with conventional medical treatment to treat chronic conditions that are not adequately treated by conventional medicine alone. One study showed that adults with disability are twice as likely to use prayer or spiritual healing compared with able-bodied adults (11). Because there is very high prevalence of CAM use in SCI population, it is important for clinicians to have basic understanding of the efficacy and safety of common CAM modalities in order to have open discussion with their patients about their CAM use (12).

We plan to briefly review the history and evolution of CAM because it will serve as an appropriate context for understanding the conflicts between biomedical and CAM paradigms. Conventional medicine has moved within a very short period of time from hostility to CAM to incorporation of CAM (13). Conventional medicine is incorporating CAM into medical education and clinical practice. This new medical paradigm is referred to as integrative medicine. Consumer demands and political lobbying are two major forces that have contributed to the recent interest in CAM and integrative medicine (14, 15). With the knowledge that Americans spend a significant amount of out-of-pocket money for CAM care, Congress created the Office of Alternative Medicine (OAM) in the National Institutes of Health in 1993. OAM initially was "the result of political maneuver, not a scientific endeavor" (15, 16). OAM then became the National Center for Complementary and Alternative Medicine (NCCAM) to be eligible for more funding in 1995. The current budget for NCCAM is approximately $100 million. Similarly, state legislatures have responded to their constituents' increased demands for access and coverage of CAM and integrative medicine by requiring the inclusion of CAM as a part of healthcare coverage. For example, in 1993 Washington State passed a law to mandate all healthcare insurers to include CAM as a part of healthcare coverage.

Biomedicine has responded to CAM's challenge by developing integrative medicine (17, 18). By 1998, it was reported that at least a dozen major medical schools had created programs in integrative medicine, including the University of Arizona, UCLA, Columbia, Harvard, UCSF, the University of Maryland, and others (19, 20). However, each school is idiosyncratically developing its integrative medicine center (20, 21). Ninety-one out of 125 medical schools include CAM as a part of their curriculum. The curriculum of these courses varies greatly. Although medical students have responded favorably and pushed for the inclusion of integrative medicine as a part of their curriculum, the responses of faculty have varied from supportive to hostile (22).

Managed care organizations viewed the increased demand for CAM and integrative medicine as an opportunity to increase market share (23). From 1997 to 1998, managed care organizations reported growth of CAM coverage from 43% to 67% (24). Nearly one-half of members of HMOs are covered for CAM services. Surveys of HMOs suggest that the main reasons to include CAM coverage were consumer demand, state mandate, effectiveness, and cost-effectiveness of CAM (14, 24). Increased growth of CAM coverage by managed care organizations is continuing to accelerate as the consumers' demand for CAM services increases over the next decade.

Although much of the literature has focused on CAM use in the able-bodied population, little is known about CAM use in the SCI population. The purpose of this chapter is to conduct a systematic literature review on CAM modalities that are commonly use by persons with SCI using an evidenced-based approach. Although we recognize the importance of using an evidence-based approach to evaluate the effectiveness of CAM treatments, we found that there were few randomized controlled trials (RCT) of CAM modalities for persons with SCI in the medical literature. In those instances, we plan to present results of studies conducted in the able-bodied population and try to extrapolate them to the SCI population. Another goal of this chapter is to provide an overview of efficacy and safety of CAM modalities for clinicians who are interested to develop an adequate level of CAM knowledge or "CAM literacy" in order to open channels of communication with their patients who are CAM users. In this chapter, we plan to classify the strength of evidence into four levels by adopting the U.S. Preventive Services Task Force (USPSTF) classification for grading the strength of the policy recommendation, thereby allowing a consistent interpretation of conclusions across all CAM modalities. Each grade is described below and corresponds to the levels of evidence as indicated in bold letters below:

- Effective: sufficient strong and consistent evidence of positive effects (B)
- Promising: evidence is trending positive, but insufficient (C)
- Inconclusive: evidence is conflicting or difficult to interpret, insufficient (I)
- Ineffective: sufficient strong and consistent evidence of negative or no effect (D)

ACUPUNCTURE

Acupuncture increasingly is accepted as a viable, adjunctive medical treatment in the United States (8, 25, 26). Manual acupuncture and its potent alternative, electroacupuncture, have been used for centuries in the East to treat many diseases. Stimulation of acupoints, located on the skin along pathways called meridians, may improve the flow of qi or vital force, thereby restoring homeostasis and restoring health. In 1997, the NIH held a conference on acupuncture and issued a consensus statement stating that there is strong evidence to support use of acupuncture in dental pain, post-chemotherapy-related nausea and vomiting, and post-operative nausea and vomiting (27). It also stated that acupuncture is a promising treatment for a number of chronic conditions, including osteoarthritis, low back pain,

headache, addiction, stroke rehabilitation, and others. There has been substantial research done to elucidate the neurophysiologic mechanisms of acupuncture in treatment of pain (28, 29). Early animal studies showed that acupuncture caused the release of endorphins in the central nervous system and acupuncture-induced analgesia can be reversed by naloxone, an opioid receptor blocker (30, 31). More recently, imaging studies using fMRI and PET have demonstrated acupuncture enhance neuronal activities in the areas of hypothalamus, periacqueductal gray, and limbic system, which are important for modulations of cardiovascular functions, pain, and emotions (32, 33).

Patients with SCI have turned to acupuncture as an adjunctive treatment for chronic conditions that have not been well treated by conventional medicine alone, such as myofascial shoulder pain, neuropathic pain, and restoration of neurologic functions. Myofascial shoulder pain resulting from upper-limb overuse is a common medical complication associated with SCI and can lead to substantial disability and loss of independence. Because there is lack of effective treatment for shoulder pain, many SCI patients have used acupuncture as an adjunctive therapy to pain medications to decrease their pain and preserve their independence. There are two randomized controlled trials that have supported acupuncture's effectiveness for treatment of myofascial shoulder pain in SCI patients, and both of the trials were conducted by the same group of investigators (34, 35). In the more recent trial done in 2007, Dyson-Hudson et al. (35) randomized 17 patients to either acupuncture or sham acupuncture group, consisted of minimal needling of non-acupuncture points. Subjects received 10 treatments over five weeks and the shoulder pain intensity decreased significantly for both the acupuncture and sham acupuncture groups, 66% and 43% respectively. However, the magnitude of decrease in pain intensity did not differ significantly between these two groups, suggesting that sham acupuncture was just as effective as the true acupuncture. Although this study used randomization and was well designed, its main limitation is the small sample size, which may mask the difference between the acupuncture and sham acupuncture interventions.

Neuropathic pain is another common complication for persons with SCI. Current pain medications, such as narcotics and gabapentin (Neurontin), have limited effectiveness and are not well tolerated by some patients. To investigate the efficacy of acupuncture for below-level neuropathic pain, Rapson et al. (36) conducted a retrospective cohort study and found that 66% of SCI patients (24 out of 36) showed decrease in neuropathic pain intensity. This study also showed that SCI patients with bilateral, symmetric, and constant burning pain were most likely to benefit from acupuncture. However, this study design is weaker because of lack of a control group and small sample size. Many SCI patients have tried using acupuncture to improve their neurologic functions. To evaluate the efficacy of acupuncture for restoring neurologic functions in patients with acute SCI injury, Wong et al. (37) randomized 100 patients with acute SCI (ASIA A and B) to either acupuncture or control group, with both groups receiving standard rehabilitation care. The study showed that the acupuncture group, which received electroacupuncture and auricular acupuncture, showed improvement in motor nerve, sensory nerve, and functional levels at hospital discharge and one-year follow-up. Although this study had a strong design and a large sample size, it is unclear whether the improvement is clinically significant or not. In addition, the high treatment intensity, five treatments per week, and the application of acupuncture immediately after SCI injury may limit its clinical use in the United States.

In summary, acupuncture is found to be a "promising" treatment (Grade C) for treatment of myofascial shoulder pain. There is "inconclusive" evidence (Grade I) for treatment of below-level neuropathic pain and restoration of neurologic functions.

In terms of complications from acupuncture in the SCI population, acupuncture is generally very safe and well tolerated by patients. Common side effects include pain and minor bleeding at the site of needle insertion. Although some have raised the concern that acupuncture may be associated with elevated blood pressure in SCI patients at risk for developing autonomic dysreflexia, my own clinical experience with SCI patients has not supported such association. Averill et al. (38) conducted a small study (n = 15) to evaluate the risk of developing higher blood pressure and autonomic dysreflexia in SCI patients (SCI at or above T8). They found that three out of 15 subjects (20%) developed elevations of systolic blood pressure (20 mmHg or higher), "suggesting a pattern of imminent autonomic dysreflexia." In the discussion section, the authors pointed out that none of the three subjects developed symptoms of autonomic dysreflexia, and their blood pressure normalized after additional 30 minutes of monitoring. To ensure safety of SCI patients receiving acupuncture, it is important to monitor blood pressure before and after acupuncture treatment.

CHIROPRACTIC CARE AND SPINAL MANIPULATION

Chiropractors represent the third-largest healthcare profession in the United States, and there are about 60,000 chiropractors. Despite of the historical political conflicts and turf battles between chiropractors and allopathic physicians, chiropractic care is becoming a part of mainstream healthcare (13, 39). Persons with disability, including those with SCI, often have chronic neck and low back pain, and have used spinal manipulation to decrease their pain and improve quality of life. Chiropractic healing focuses on diagnosing and treating musculoskeletal disorders that affect the nervous system. Chiropractic care is based on the philosophy of vitalism—that is, the body has an innate life force that travels through the nervous system and the role of healing is to stimulate the body to heal itself. People with disabilities often use chiropractic care as an adjunctive therapy to their conventional medical care. One study showed that 23% of SCI patients with chronic pain used chiropractic care (40). Because there are no good randomized controlled studies to assess the efficacy of spinal manipulation in SCI patient population, we will present randomized controlled studies in the able-bodied population and extrapolate them to the SCI population. Overall, there is a large body of evidence to support the efficacy of spinal manipulation as an adjunctive treatment for chronic neck and low-back pain in the able-bodied population (41–43). To investigate the effectiveness of spinal manipulation for treatment of chronic neck pain, Brontfort et al. (44) randomized 191 subjects to one of three groups: (1) rehabilitation neck exercise, (2) spinal manipulation, or (3) rehabilitation neck exercise plus spinal manipulation. This study found that exercise with spinal manipulation was more effective in improving pain and health-related quality of life

compared with spinal manipulation or exercise alone at 12-month follow-up. In addition, the exercise with spinal manipulation also used the least amount of pain medications and had the highest satisfaction of care. This was a very well-conducted randomized controlled trial with adequate sample size.

To evaluate the efficacy of spinal manipulation for treatment of low-back pain, Cherkin et al. (43) randomized 321 adults with chronic low back pain to one of three groups: (1) physical therapy, (2) chiropractic manipulation, or (3) educational booklet. The chiropractic group had less severe symptoms than the educational booklet group. The physical therapy and chiropractic group were both effective in decreasing severity of low-back pain and had similar costs of care, $437 versus $429 over the 2-year period. This was rigorously conducted, evidenced by the large sample size, appropriate outcome measures, and minimal rate of attrition. This study showed that physical therapy and chiropractic manipulation had similar effects and costs in caring for chronic low back pain.

In summary, chiropractic manipulation is found to be an "effective" adjunctive treatment (Grade B) for treatment of chronic neck and low back pain in the able-bodied population. However, there is lack of clinical trials to assess the efficacy of manipulation targeting the SCI population. In addition, many patients with SCI have biomechanical changes from vertebral injury, spinal instrumentation, and/or vertebral osteoporosis, which potentially put them at higher risk for spinal manipulation compared with the able-bodied population. Although physicians often worry about the potential risk of spinal manipulation in causing spinal cord injury, chiropractic manipulation is considerably safer than pain medications in the general population. For example, one study conducted by RAND Corporation showed that 1.5 serious complications occur from every one million cervical manipulations. In contrast, 1,000 serious complications occur per million of over-the-counter painkillers. Complication rates from pain medications or chiropractic manipulation are unknown in persons with SCI. Therefore clinicians should consider such issues prior to referral to qualified chiropractors for treatment of neck and low-back pain in persons with SCI.

HERBS AND SUPPLEMENTS

There is very high prevalence of herbs and supplements used by both able-bodied and SCI populations (40). Although many current pharmaceutical medications have connections to botanical plants, herbs and supplements rely on natural substances, containing a multitude of active ingredients, whereas pharmaceutical medications often contain one active ingredient. Medicinal plants have been an important part of the healing traditions for most major civilizations. For instance, Chinese medicine healers have been using Chinese herbal medicine for over 1,000 years. Similarly, Native Americans have long used medicinal plants to cure infections and to enable them to participate in healing ceremonies. Europeans have a long tradition of using supplements as adjunctive therapies to conventional drugs. In contrast, the U.S. Congress established the Dietary Supplement Health and Education Act (DSHEA) in 1994, which classified herbs and supplements as dietary supplements. This legislation came about largely due to the lobbying efforts of herbal manufacturers and aimed to limit the role of FDA from regulating herbs and supplements

(45). The DSHEA has contributed to the lack of quality control for herbs and supplements and incentive for herbal manufacturers to conduct rigorous research to support the effectiveness of their products.

Persons with disabilities often use herbs and supplements to treat their pain, depression, and prevent urinary tract infections. Because there are no good randomized controlled studies to assess the efficacy of herbs and supplements for SCI patients, we will present randomized controlled studies in the able-bodied population and extrapolate them to the SCI population. Persons with SCI commonly take glucosamine/chondroitin to treat osteoarthritis of the hand and knee. There are many high-quality randomized controlled trials conducted in Europe to support the efficacy of glucosamine/chondroitin for treatment of osteoarthritis of knee (46, 47). NCCAM recently sponsored a large, multi-center randomized controlled trial, Glucosamine/chondroitin Arthritis Intervention Trial (GAIT). This study randomized 1,583 patients with knee osteoarthritis to one of five groups: (1) 1500 mg of glucosamine hydrochloride, (2) 1200 mg of chondroitin, (3) combination of glucosamine and chondroitin, (4) 200 mg of Celebrex, or (5) placebo. The study found that glucosamine and chondroitin alone or in combination did not reduce pain effectively (48). Interestingly, an exploratory analysis showed that the combination of glucosamine and chondroitin was more effective at reducing pain in patients with moderated to severe osteoarthritis compared with the Celebrex and placebo groups, 79%, 69%, and 54% respectively. Overall, the GAIT trial showed that the combination of glucosamine/chondroitin is ineffective for treatment of mild osteoarthritis; however, there is preliminary evidence to show that it is effective for treatment of moderate to severe osteoarthritis of the knee. Glucosamine/chondroitin is well tolerated and has few side effects. One potential side effect is the elevation of blood sugars in diabetic patients. There are currently no reported herb-drug interactions.

St. John's wort is another common herbal medication used by SCI patients for treatment of depression. The efficacy of St. John's wort for treatment of mild to moderate depression has been demonstrated in a number of randomized controlled trials and meta-analyses (49–51). St. John's wort is well-tolerated but has few adverse effects, including photosensitization, particularly in fair-skinned individuals, nausea, and vomiting. Because St. John's wort is metabolized by the liver's cytochrome P450 enzymes, there are numerous herb-drug interactions (52). Concomitant use of St. John's wort with serotonin reuptake inhibitors may cause serotonin syndrome. Additional herb-drug interactions include the following: breakthrough bleeding with those on oral contraceptives, acute rejection of organ transplant patients taking cyclosporine, and potential lower plasma levels of antiretroviral medications. Because St. John's wort causes numerous, significant herb-drug interactions, it is imperative for clinicians to ask their patients who are taking St. John's wort about their use of conventional medications as well.

Many persons with SCI often suffer from neurogenic bladder and recurrent urinary tract infections (UTIs). Thus, many have used cranberry supplements and juice to prevent recurrence of UTI. The potential mechanisms of cranberry include inhibition of bacteria from attachment to bladder lining and promotion of flushing out of bacteria with urine stream (53). A literature review by Cochrane Review identified four randomized controlled trials but concluded that the quality of the trials were poor (54). In SCI population, one pilot study supported that cranberry juice will decrease attachment of bacteria to bladder lining (55). Overall, there is preliminary evidence to support the efficacy of cranberry as a prophylactic treatment for prevention of UTI. Cranberry juice and tablets are generally well tolerated and have few side effects. In SCI persons with diabetes mellitus, they may consider taking the tablets instead of juice because of the sugar content of the juice, and very high dose of cranberry can lead to diarrhea. Theoretically, cranberry can enhance the excretion of drugs eliminated in urine or increase effect of certain antibiotics in the urinary tract.

In summary, glucosamine/chondroitin is found to be a "promising" treatment (Grade C) for treatment of osteoarthritis of knee pain. St. John's wort is also found to be a "promising" treatment (Grade C) for treatment of mild to moderate depression. Cranberry juice and supplements are found to be an "inconclusive" treatment (Grade I) for prophylactic treatment of UTIs. These three herbs and supplements are generally well tolerated and have fewer side effects compared with conventional medications. However, it is important for clinicians to be aware of the adverse herb-drug interactions of St. John's wort with serotonin reuptake inhibitors, cyclosporine, oral contraceptives, protease inhibitors, and others.

HOMEOPATHY

Homeopathy was founded by Samuel Hahnemann in the early nineteenth century. Approximately 3% of consumers have used a homeopathic remedy during the past 12 months (8). Homeopathy, however, remained one of the more controversial CAM modalities because of the lack of understanding of its underlying mechanism. Two main philosophical tenets for homeopathy are treating like with like and the most diluted solutions are most potent. For example, a homeopathic solution, 30X, is prepared by serially diluting a mother tincture with nine parts of water and vigorously shaken for a total of 30 times. Thus, a homeopathic solution may contain only few molecules of the original substance. The homeopaths believe that the diluted solutions are very potent because of the vigorous shaking between each dilution and potential transfer of energy into the solutions. However, many scientists and physicians believe that homeopathic solutions act mainly through the placebo effect and violate the western scientific principle of the dose-response curve.

Persons with SCI have used homeopathic remedies to treat anxiety, chronic pain, traumatic brain injury, and other chronic illnesses. Because there are no randomized controlled trials on SCI patients, we will present randomized controlled studies in the able-bodied population and extrapolate them to the SCI population. Bonne et al. (56) conducted a randomized controlled trial to assess the efficacy of homeopathic treatment for generalized anxiety. This study randomized 44 patients to a 10-week trial of individualized homeopathic treatment versus placebo. This rigorous study showed that homeopathic treatment was just as effective as placebo in reducing levels of anxiety.

In contrast, a randomized controlled trial showed that homeopathic treatment was more effective than placebo in improving symptoms of patients with mild traumatic brain injury (57). This study randomized 60 patients to a homeopathic treatment versus placebo group and found the homeopathic group had a greater improvement in the symptoms and functional levels for mild traumatic brain injury patients. This study also concluded that homeopathic treatment had few side effects and can be safely used with conventional medications. To assess the efficacy of homeopathic treatment on fibromyalgia, Bell et al. (58) conducted a rigorous randomized controlled trial. In this study, 62 subjects were randomized to individually tailored homeopathic treatment versus placebo. This study found that those receiving homeopathic treatment had a greater improvement in tender point count, tender point pain, quality of life, and depression symptoms.

In summary, homeopathic treatment is found to be "inconclusive" treatment (Grade I) for generalized anxiety. However, homeopathy is found to be a "promising" treatment (Grade C) for mild traumatic brain injury and fibromyalgia. Homeopathic treatments generally are very safe because of their diluted state, and there have been minimal reported cases of herb-drug interactions.

ELECTROMAGNETIC HEALING

Although early interest in magnetic and electromagnetic fields focused on their potential association with cancer, there has been increased interest in the application of magnetic and electromagnetic field for healing purposes, coinciding with the rise of the CAM movement. Ancient healers in China, Japan, and Europe have used magnetic materials for treatment of disease. In 1600 William Gilbert, the personal physician of the English Queen, used "load stones" to treat the illnesses of the English Queen and ordinary citizens. After World War II, magnetotherapy developed in Japan and later in the former Soviet Union. Magnetotherapeutic devices were registered under the Drug Regulation Act of 1961 and were commonly used by patients and clinicians, largely through the effort of Kyochi Nakawa. During the past 25 years, the most common clinical application of electromagnetic fields have been in the areas of bone unification, pain, reduction, and soft tissue edema (59).

There are preliminary experimental and clinical evidence to support the use of electromagnetic fields for restoring of nerve functions caused by SCI. In a case series of four SCI patients, the application of transcranial magnetic stimulation resulted in significant corticospinal inhibition and clinical improvement in sensory and motor functions for incomplete SCI patients (60). However, this study is limited by the small sample size and lack of adequate control group. In two experimental studies, pulsed electromagnetic fields stimulation led to improvement in functions, reduction of lesion size of SCI injury, and increased nerve growth factor levels in cats and rats. Although these two studies provided potential mechanism of how electromagnetic fields can facilitate the recovery of neurologic functions in animals with SCI injury, more studies are needed to elucidate the actual mechanism of how electromagnetic fields can influence the neuroplasticity of CNS neurons.

In the area of neuropathic pain, Weintraub et al. (61) conducted a randomized controlled trial to determine if wearing multipolar, magnetic shoe insoles can reduce neuropathic pain and improve health-related quality of life for patients with diabetic neuropathy. This was a large, multi-center trial that randomized 375 subjects to a magnetic insole group and a sham insole group. The study found that wearing magnetic shoe insoles can significantly reduce the severity of neuropathic pain and

improve quality of life in 4-month follow-up. This was a high-quality randomized controlled trial with large sample size and multiple study sites. Electromagnetic fields may have potential application in the treatment of myofascial pain in the SCI population. To assess the efficacy of electromagnetic fields for treatment of postpolio patients with myofascial pain, Valbona et al. (62) conducted a small randomized controlled trial with fifty patients. Subjects were randomized to electromagnetic or placebo group. The authors found that the application of electromagnetic fields over tender points can significantly reduce the intensity of the trigger point pain compared with subjects who received the placebo treatment.

In summary, electromagnetic healing is found to be "inconclusive" treatment (Grade I) for restoration of neurologic functions caused by SCI injury. Electromagnetic healing is found to be a "promising" treatment (Grade C) for diabetic neuropathy and myofascial pain. Although there are some preliminary experimental and clinical studies supporting the efficacy of electromagnetic healing, we need to conduct additional high-quality clinical trials to build stronger evidence to support the efficacy of electromagnetic healing for diabetic neuropathy, myofascial pain, and restoration of neurologic functions. Electromagnetic healing is generally very safe and does not adversely interact with most conventional medical treatment.

DISCUSSION

Our chapter aims to review to some of the CAM modalities commonly used by persons with SCI. We purposely focused our literature review on these five CAM modalities, including acupuncture, chiropractic, herbs and supplements, homeopathy, and electromagnetic healing, because they have a stronger body of literature to support their efficacy. We did not include other CAM modalities, such as naturopathy, prayer, therapeutic touch, and others, because they have a weaker scientific body to support their efficacy. Table 79.1 summarizes the different grade of evidence for these CAM modalities. There is a large variation of level of evidence across CAM modalities and clinical indications in the able-bodied population, whereas there are few high-quality randomized controlled trials targeting persons with SCI. For instance, chiropractic care has the strongest evidence and is found to be an "effective" (Grade B) adjunctive treatment for chronic neck and low-back pain. Acupuncture is found to be a "promising" (Grade C) adjunctive treatment for myofascial shoulder pain, but an "inconclusive" (Grade I) treatment for below-level neuropathic pain and restoration of neurologic functions. Cranberry is found to be a "promising" (Grade C) prophylactic treatment for urinary tract infection. Interestingly, electromagnetic healing is found to be a "promising" (Grade C) treatment for diabetic neuropathy and myofascial pain, but an "inconclusive" treatment for restoration of neurologic functions. Although more researchers are beginning to conduct high quality clinical trials to assess the effectiveness of CAM for treatment of chronic illnesses, we need more funding and research dedicated to assessing how CAM modalities can be effectively and safely integrated with conventional treatment in the SCI and disabled populations.

Because many persons with SCI are using CAM without discussion with their healthcare providers (10, 63), it is also important for clinicians caring for persons with SCI to query CAM use in an open-minded, nonjudgmental manner. This

Table 79.1   Use of Complementary and Alternative Medicine in SCI: Summary of the Evidence from Systematic Literature Reviews

INDICATIONS	GRADE
Acupuncture	
Myofascial shoulder pain	C (as adjunct)
Below-level neuropathic pain	I
Restoration of neurologic functions	I
Chiropractic Care	
Low back pain	B (as adjunct)
Neck pain	B (as adjunct)
Herbs and Supplements	
Glucosamine/chondrotin	C
Osteoarthritis of knee	
St. John's wort	C
Depression	
Cranberry	I
Prophylaxis of urinary tract infection	
Homeopathy	
Generalized anxiety disorder	I
Traumatic brain injury	C
Fibromyalgia	C
Electromagnetic healing	
Restoration of neurologic functions	I
Diabetic neuropathy	C
Myofascial pain	C

Grade B: *Effective: sufficient strong and consistent evidence of positive effect.*
Grade C: *Promising: evidence is trending positive, but insufficient.*
Grade I: *Inconclusive: evidence is conflicting or difficult to interpret, insufficient.*
Grade D: *Ineffective: sufficient strong and consistent evidence of negative or no effect.*

openness is vital in encouraging patients to disclose their CAM use, which may prevent adverse herb-drug interactions and detect side effects of CAM treatment. In addition, it may be important for clinicians to gain knowledge about various CAM modalities and practitioners, which will enable appropriate referral to qualified CAM practitioners and development of a coordinated care plan. To optimize the quality of care for persons with SCI it is important that we use an evidence-based approach to appropriately integrate CAM modalities with conventional care. Furthermore, we need to be open-minded and query use of CAM in order to develop a safe, integrative care plan for persons with SCI.

References

1. McWhinney I. Are we on the brink of a major transformation of clinical method. *Can Med Assoc* 1986; 135(5):873–878.
2. Aaron L, Buchwald D. A review of the evidence for overlap among unexplained clinical conditions. *Ann Intern Med* 2001; 134:868–881.
3. Sharpe M, Carson A. "Unexplained" somatic symptoms, functional syndromes, and somatization: do we need a paradigm shift? *Ann Intern Med* 2001; 134:926–930.
4. Goldstein M. *Alternative Health Care: Medicine, Miracle, or Mirage.* Philadelphia: Temple University Press; 1999.
5. Furnham A, Bhagrath R. A comparison of health beliefs and behaviours of clients of orthodox and complementary medicine. *Br j Clin Psychiatry* 1993; 32:237–246.
6. Furnham A, Forey J. The attitudes, behaviors, and beliefs of patients of conventional vs. complementary alternative medicine. *J Clin Psychiatry* 1994; 50:458–469.
7. Eisenberg D, Kessler RC, Foster C, et al. Unconventional medicine in the United States. *NEJM* 1993; 328:246–252.
8. Eisenberg D, Davis RB, Ettner SL, Appel S, Wilkey S, Rompay MV, Kessler RC. Trends in alternative medicine use in the United States, 1990–1997. *JAMA.* 1998; 280(18):1569–1575.
9. Defining and describing complementary and alternative therapies. CAM Research Methodology Conference. *Alternat Ther Health Med* 1997; 3:49–57.
10. Astin J. Why patients use alternative medicine. Results of a national study. *JAMA* 1998; 279:1548–1553.
11. Hendershot G. Mobility limitations and complementary and alternative medicine: are people with disabilities more likely to pray? *Am J Public Health* 2003; 93:1079–1080.
12. Johnston L. *Alternative Medicine and Spinal Cord Injury: Beyond the Banks of the Mainstream.* New York: Demos Medical Publishing; 2006.
13. Coulter I. Integration and paradigm clash. In: Tovey PEG, Adams J, eds. *The Mainstreaming of Complementary and Alternative Medicine: Studies in Social Context.* London and New York: Routledge Taylor & Francis Group; 2004; 103–122.
14. Pelletier K, Astin J, Haskell WL. Current trends in the integration and reimbursement of CAM by managed care organizations and insurance providers: 1998 update and cohort analysis. *AM J Health Promot* 1999; 14(2):125–133.
15. Trachtman P. NIH looks at the implausible and the inexplicable. *Smithsonian* 1994; 25:110–123.
16. Marwick C. Time for a new head, new approach at OAM. *JAMA* 1994; 272(23):1569–1575.
17. Gaudet T. Integrative medicine: the evolution of a new approach to medicine and medical education. *Integrative Med* 1998; 1:67–73.
18. Weil A. The significance of integrative medicine for the future of medical education. *Am J Med* 2000; 108:441–443.
19. Hui K, Zylowska L, Hui EK, et al. Introducing integrative East-West medicine to medical students and residents. *J Alternat Complem Med* 2002; 4:507–515.
20. Berman B. Complementary medicine and medical education. *Br Med J* 2001; 322:121–122.
21. Wetzel M, Eisenberg DM, Kaptchuk TJ. Courses involving complementary and alternative medicine at US medical schools. *JAMA.* 1998; 280:784–787.
22. Wetzel M, Kaptchuk TJ, Haramati A, Eisenberg DM. Complementary and alternative medical therapies: implications for medical education. *Ann Intern Med* 2003; 138(3):191–196.
23. Weeks J. Major trends in the integration of complementary and alternative medicine. In: Faass N, ed. *Integrating Complementary Medicine into Health Systems.* Gaithersburg, MD: Aspen Pub; 2001:4–11.
24. *Landmark Report II HMOs and Alternative Therapy.* Sacramento: Landmark Healthcare Inc; 1999.
25. Barnes P, Powell-Griner E, McFann K, Nahin RL. *Complementary and alternative medicine use among adults: United States, 2002:* Vital Health and Statistics; 2004.
26. Barnes L. The acupuncture wars: the professionalizing of American acupuncture- a view from Massachusetts. *Med Anthropol* 2003; 3:261–301.
27. *Acupuncture: NIH Consensus Statement.* Washington DC: NIH; 1997.
28. Stux G, Pomeranz B. *Basics of Acupuncture.* 4th ed. Berlin: Springer; 1998.
29. Wang S, Kain ZV, White P. Acupuncture analgesis: 1. the scientific basis. *Anesth Analg* 2008; 106:602–610.
30. Han J, Tang J. Tolerance to electroacupuncture and its cross tolerance to morphine. *Neuropharmacology* 1981; 20:593–596.
31. Han J, Tang J. Acupuncture: neuropeptide release produced by electrical stimulation of different frequencies. *Neuroscience* 2003; 26:17–22.
32. Wu M, Hsieh JC, Xiong J, Yang CF, Pan HB, Chen YC, Tsai G, Rosen BR, Kwong KK. Central nervous pathway for acupuncture stimulation: localization of processing with functional MR imaging of the brain- preliminary experience. *Radiology* 1999; 212:133–141.
33. Hui K, Liu J, Mkris N, Gollub RL, Chen AJ, Moore CI, Kennedy DN, Rosen BR, Kwong KK. Acupuncture modulates the limbic system and subcortical gray structures of the human brain: evidence from fMRI studies in normal subjects. *Human Brain Mapp* 2000; 9:13–25.

34. Dyson-Hudson TA, Shiflett SC, Kirshblum SC, Bowen JE, Druin EL. Acupuncture and Trager psychophysical integration in the treatment of wheelchair user's shoulder pain in individuals with spinal cord injury. *Arch Phys Med Rehabil* Aug 2001; 82(8):1038–1046.

35. Dyson-Hudson T, Kadar P, LaFountaine M, Emmons R, Kirshblum SC, Tulsky D, Komaroff E. Acupuncture for chronic shoulder pain in persons with spinal cord injury: a small-scale clinical trial. *Arch Phys Med Rehabil* 2007; 88:1276–1283.

36. Rapson L, Wells N, Pepper J, Majid N, Boon H. Acupuncture as a promising treatment for below-level central neuropathic pain: a retrospective study. *J Spinal Cord Med* 2003; 26:21–26.

37. Wong AM, Leong CP, Su TY, Yu SW, Tsai WC, Chen CP. Clinical trial of acupuncture for patients with spinal cord injuries. *Am J Phys Med Rehabil* Jan 2003; 82(1):21–27.

38. Averill A, Cotter AC, Nayak S, Matheis RJ, Shiflett SC. Blood pressure response to acupuncture in a population at risk for autonomic dysreflexia. *Arch Phys Med Rehabil* Nov 2000; 81(11):1494–1497.

39. Coulter I. An institutional philosophy of chiropractic. *Chiropractic J Australia* 1991; 21:136–141.

40. Nayak S, Matheis RJ, Agostinelli S, Shifleft SC. The use of complementary and alternative therapies for chronic pain following spinal cord injury: a pilot survey. *J Spinal Cord Med* Spring 2001; 24(1):54–62.

41. Van Tulder M, Koes BW, Bouter LM. Conservative treatment of acute and chronic non-specific low back pain: a systematic review of the most common interventions. *Spine* 1997; 22:2128–2156.

42. Shekelle P, Coulter I. Cervical spine manipulation: summary report of a systematic review of the literature and a multidisciplinary expert panel. *J Spinal Disorder* 1997; 10(3):223–228.

43. Cherkin DD, Barlow R, et al. A comparison of physical therapy, chiropractic manipulation, and provision of an educational booklet for the treatment of patients with low back pain. *NEJM* 1998; 339:1021–1029.

44. Bronfort G ER, Nelson B, Aker PD, Goldsmith CH, Vernon H. A randomized clinical trial of exercise and spinal manipulation for patients with chronic neck pain. *Spine* 2001; 7(788–99).

45. Seamon M, Clauson KA. Ephedra: yesterday, DSHEA, and tomorrow- a ten year perspective on the Dietary Supplement Health and Education Act of 1994. *J Herb Pharmacother* 2005; 5(3):67–86.

46. McAlindon T, LaValley MP, Gulin JP, Felson DT. Glucosamine and chondroitin for treatment of osteoarthritis: a systematic quality assessment and meta-analysis. *JAMA* 2000; 283:1469–1475.

47. Cibere J, Kopec JA, Thorne A, Singer J, Canvin J, Robinson DB, Pope J, Hong P, Grant E, Esdaile JM. Randomized, double-blind, placebo-controlled glucosamine discontinuation trial in knee osteoarthritis. *Arthritis Rheum* 2004; 51(5):738–745.

48. Clegg D, Reda DJ, Harris CL, et al. Glucosamine, chondroitin sulfate, and the two in combination for painful knee osteoarthritis. *NEJM* 2006; 354:795–808.

49. Philipp M, Kohnen R, Hiller KO. Hypericum extract versus imipramine or placebo in patients with moderate depression: randomized multi-center study of treatment for eight weeks. *Br Med J* 1999; 319:1534–1538.

50. Woelk H. Comparison of St. John's wort and imipramine for treating depression: randomized controlled trial. *Br Med J* 2000; 421:536–539.

51. Linde K, Ramirez G, Mulrow CD, Pauls A, Weidenhammer W, Melchart D. St. John's wort for depression—an overview and meta-analysis of randomized controlled trials. *Br Med J* 1996; 313:253–258.

52. Fugh-Berman A. Herb-drug interactions. *Lancet* 2000; 355:134–138.

53. Avron J, Manone M, Gurwitz JH, Glynn RJ, Choodnovsky I, Lipsitz LA. Reduction of bacteriuria and pyuria after ingestion of cranberry juice. *JAMA* 1994; 272:590.

54. Jepson R, Mihaljevic L, Craig J. *Cranberries for preventing urinary tract infections.* Oxford: Cochrane Library; 2000.

55. Reid G, Hsieh J, Potter P. Cranberry juice consumption may reduce biofilms on uroepithelial cells: pilot study in spinal cord injured patients. *Spinal Cord* 2001; 39:26–30.

56. Bonne O, Shemer Y, Gorali Y, Katz M, Shalev A. A randomized, double-blind, placebo-controlled study of classical homeopathy in generalized anxiety disorder. *J Clin Psychiatry* 2003; 64:282–287.

57. Chapman E, Weintraub RJ, Milburn MA, Pirozzi, TO, Woo E. Homeopathic treatment of mild traumatic brain injury: a randomized, double-blind, placebo-controlled clinical trial. *J Head Trauma Rehabil* 1999; 14:521–542.

58. Bell I, Lewis DA, Brooks AJ, Schwartz GE, Lewis SE, Walsh BT, Baldwin CM. Improved clinical status in fibromyalgia patients treated with individualized homeopathic remedies versus placebo. *Rheumatology* 2004; 43:577–582.

59. Markov M. Magnetic field therapy: a review. *Electromagnetic Biology and Medicine* 2007; 26:1–23.

60. Belci M, Catley M, Husain M, Frankel HL, Davey NJ. Magnetic brain stimulation can improve clinical outcome in incomplete spinal cord injured patients. *Spinal Cord* 2004; 42:417–419.

61. Weintraub M, Wolfe GI, Barohn RA, et al. Static magnetic field therapy for symptomatic diabetic neuropathy. *Arch Phys Med Rehabil* 2003; 84:736–746.

62. Vallbona C, Hazlewood, CF, Jurida G. Response to pain to static magnetic fields in postpolio patients: a double-blind pilot study. *Arch Phys Med Rehabil* 1997; 78:1200–1203.

63. Ahn AC, Ngo-Metzger Q, Legedza ATR, Massagli MP, Clarridge BR, Phillips RS. Use of Complementary and alternative medical therapies in Chinese and Vietnamese Americans: prevalence, associated factors, and the effects of patient-clinician communication. *Am J Public Health* 2006; 96(4):647–653.

80 The Financial Impact of Spinal Cord Dysfunction*

Rosemarie Filart

AVAILABLE SOURCES PROVIDE A SPECTRUM OF COSTS

Spinal cord dysfunction from traumatic or nontraumatic causes can have a far-reaching impact on the individual and the nation. An individual with a spinal cord dysfunction can experience a mild to substantial decrease in mobility, cognition, participation in activities of daily living and community integration, as well as a decline in multiple physiologic functions. In spinal cord medicine, the overall rehabilitation program includes goals to facilitate the return of functional independence, reduce morbidity and mortality, improve quality of life, and facilitate community reintegration of individuals following spinal cord dysfunction. Community reintegration in this chapter broadly refers to both the return of individuals to the workforce and avocational activities. The individual following spinal cord dysfunction is the focus of the rehabilitation management, and therefore, rehabilitation goals are tailored to the individual's progess, needs, and goals. The rehabilitation team, specialists, primary care provider, family, and friends, among others, with the individual, allocate resources to address and reach the individual's specific rehabilitation goals.

Health economics analyzes the impact of allocating healthcare resources for the individual and the nation. In a subset of health economics, costs in terms of expenditures are used to explain the financial impact of providing care. The financial impact of the allocated and utilized resources for providing care will be reviewed in this chapter and described in terms of available cost information. Cost data will be derived from the literature and databases of provider and of vendor charges and payer expenditures, noting that charges do not necessarily equate to expenditures. To this end, the aim of this chapter is to summarize the financial impact of the care of individuals with spinal cord dysfunction from available charges and expenditures data. Of a practical note, because each individual with a spinal cord dysfunction is unique, the author recommends to use actual costs

and cost estimates based on the specifics of that particular individual when calculating total cost for the individual's healthcare.

There are costs of care following spinal cord dysfunction that are necessary to recognize but are difficult to quantify and sparsely available in the literature. Because of the limited available information, these costs will not be covered in this chapter. These are the costs attributed to psychosocial stresses. Individuals following spinal cord dysfunction, caregivers, family, and friends experience psychosocial stresses due to the subsequent radical changes in life and reallocation of time to provide care and support. These stresses impact the affected individuals' function and community reintegration in varying degrees. The financial component of these stresses is referred to as intangible costs and is notably difficult to accurately quantify.

Not covered in this chapter is the financial component derived from providing research resources for spinal cord dysfunction. Complementary to the care perspective is the research perspective for the cure or repair, as well as for the care of spinal cord dysfunction, whether the spinal cord dysfunction etiology is traumatic or nontraumatic in origin. Although not covered in this chapter, it is noteworthy to recognize the critical importance of resources for basic science, clinical, translational, community-based, prevention, economics, and other types of research to develop the cure or repair of acute and chronic spinal cord dysfunction, as well as to better understand and continuously improve the care and access to care for affected individuals.

AVAILABLE FINANCIAL DATA ARE ESTIMATES

Costs of an illness are estimates and represent only a specific portion of the real costs. The real costs of an illness are difficult to fully and exactly determine. To improve the delivery and access to care, the health and medical care community, administrators, policymakers, economists, and researchers work in earnest to research and understand the financial and economic aspects of illnesses. At the same time, experts recognize that the financial and economic impact of an illness on individuals involves not only the charges and expenditures for comprehensive medical services, goods, and workforce productivity losses related to having an illness, but also

---

*Dr. Rosemarie Filart contributed to this article in her personal capacity. The views expressed are her own and do not necessarily represent the views of the National Institutes of Health or the United States Government.

more complex factors. Some of these complex factors include the welfare of individuals and intangible costs. Welfare costs can be roughly assessed from surveying individuals for their willingness to pay for goods and services and from traditional methods of estimating costs of healthcare that would not be incurred by healthy individuals. Intangible costs such as psychosocial stresses due to the radical changes in life following an illness and reallocation of time of affected individuals, family and friends are difficult to accurately quantify. Therefore, available costs are estimations that can be reasonably calculated. These cost estimates represent a portion of the overall costs of an illness to individuals and the nation (1–7).

COST PROJECTIONS ARE LIMITED

Notable limitations are observed in the available cost information. The sources of cost information describe dollar costs in several ways, such as provider and vendor charges for goods and services, payer reimbursements to providers and vendors, and out-of-pocket expenses of individuals. A limitation in solely considering provider and vendor charges is the possible overestimation of the financial impact on individuals. Payers and payer representatives negotiate and can reduce rates of payment of the provider and vendor charges. Consequently, the reduction of charges will reduce payer expenditures.

Another limitation involves solely considering surveys to collect data because surveys can underestimate or overestimate costs. The limited accuracy of survey data stem from potential survey participant recall bias and other inherent methodological limitations. In the last edition of this chapter, Monroe Berkowitz presented his research team's elegant analyses on direct and indirect costs utilizing a combination of surveys of individuals and provider and vendor charge data. These authors also noted the aforementioned potential limitations (1, 2, 7, 9). In this new chapter edition, cost studies are presented more broadly to include charge information from medical center databases and payer expenditure information, as well as Monroe Berkowitz's research and other survey analyses.

The unavailability of the reimbursement breakdown by specific services and goods is another limitation. Lastly, side-by-side comparisons are not possible with studies whose data are derived from different types of costs and different research methodologies.

TOPICS NOT COVERED IN THIS CHAPTER

In determining effective allocation and utilization of resources and healthcare strategies to improve accessible, effective and efficient healthcare, functional outcomes, quality of life, and community reintegration of individuals with spinal cord dysfunction, further research such as economics, outcomes, and comparative effectiveness research is needed. However, there is limited published research elucidating the financial impact among individuals following spinal cord dysfunction. Therefore, research such as comparative effectiveness of specific interventions and resources will not be covered in this chapter. Likewise, outcome indices such as functional independence measure (FIM) efficiencies and gain, American Spinal Injury Association (ASIA) motor efficiency scores, and length of stay efficiencies will not be described. However, length of stay (LOS), an outcome index, will be mentioned in the context of overall hospital stay costs.

There is limited financial analysis literature available regarding the pediatric spinal cord dysfunction population. Therefore, costs attributed to the care of individuals with pediatric spinal cord dysfunction will not be covered in this chapter. Also, there is limited information on health economic descriptions of costs and health economic methods that evaluate the economic costs of spinal cord dysfunction. These methods can include surveying the population to determine cost of illness (COI), willingness to pay, the quality of life years (QALY) method, the human capital approach (HCA), and the friction cost method (7, 8). There is controversy surrounding which method is the best to evaluate the costs of an illness. Numerous individual, social, and regional factors add complexity to economic evaluations. Determination of the merit or the benefits of different economic methods of evaluation is beyond the scope of this chapter. Also, medical economics pertaining to either provider practice management or medical-legal environments are beyond the scope of this chapter.

INDIVIDUAL AND SOCIAL FACTORS ARE CONSIDERED

Individual and social factors are important considerations in economic analyses. The factors can include an individual's diagnosis, severity of illness, comorbidities, impairments, and function. Factors related to an individual's clinical treatment can include insurance payment plans, pharmaceuticals, technologies (medical testing, supplies, devices, and equipment), and services (hospitals, healthcare providers, ancillary, home care, outpatient services, community reintegration, return-to-work programs, and environmental modifications). Other important individual factors include an individual's avocational and vocational goals. Societal economic factors relate to employment, community, and social networks. These factors are complex and difficult to quantify. Also, costs can relate to the regional differences in providing care, equipment, supplies, and transportation. Inevitably, costs of healthcare are also impacted by the environment relative to the payers and payment systems. This chapter will include individual and social factors considerations in determining financial impact of spinal cord dysfunction (7).

TERMINOLOGY IN THIS CHAPTER

Medical care includes the continuum of care such as emergency care services, inpatient hospital care, outpatient services, home health, subacute stay, and long-term facilities. Similarly, rehabilitation care includes acute care consultation, acute care inpatient rehabilitation, outpatient rehabilitation, home health rehabilitation services, subacute rehabilitation, and long-term care. Different methods have been used to calculate costs of selected medical services and have included primarily direct costs. Direct costs refer to costs incurred directly from the healthcare of individuals with spinal cord dysfunction. Therefore, these costs are generated from medical services such as emergency medical treatment, inpatient hospital stay, outpatient visits, medications, rehabilitation, continuing care, and informal caregiver services or goods, such as equipment and modified vehicles. Indirect costs are costs not directly related to the healthcare of individuals due to spinal cord dysfunction and have predominantly included the loss of workforce productivity and human capital. Therefore, indirect costs have been referred to also as "productivity costs." In spinal cord dysfunction literature, indirect costs have been occasionally measured. Berkowitz et al. have measured indirect costs, primarily calculating the loss of workforce productivity and human capital (1, 2, 7).

Costs are derived from individuals with traumatic causes of spinal cord dysfunction (which will be referred to also as traumatic SCI), and when data are available, of individuals with nontraumatic causes. Nontraumatic causes include such conditions as vascular myelopathy, intradural or extradural spinal cord compression, and spinal cord degeneration (ICD-9 code 336). In traumatic and nontraumatic causes of spinal cord dysfunction, the spinal cord is disturbed, causing motor and/or sensory deficits. The resulting clinical severity can be described as incomplete or complete paraplegia/tetraplegia depending on the affected spinal cord levels. In varying degrees, these neurological deficits negatively impact an individual's ability to perform activities of daily living, ambulate, and participate in vocational and avocational activities. It is important to recognize that traumatic and nontraumatic causes of spinal cord dysfunction have different mechanisms of spinal cord disruption, clinical presentations, progress, complications, and natural histories. Therefore, individuals will require tailored medical management and rehabilitation. Consequently, the overall economics, including the financial impact of an illness, can differ widely among individuals with spinal cord dysfunction. This is an important consideration when determining resource allocation (10).

REVIEW OF AVAILABLE FINANCIAL DATA

Studies provide insight into the costs for healthcare of individuals with spinal cord dysfunction using provider and vendor charges. These charges are derived from an individual's average daily inpatient hospital stay, aggregate inpatient hospital stay, and annual comprehensive medical care. From these charges, major third-party payers tabulate annual aggregate reimbursement payments on behalf of their beneficiaries. The annual aggregate comprehensive care reimbursements for all their beneficiaries with spinal cord dysfunction are described here.

This section is divided into two parts. The first part is organized in relation to the 2002 Centers of Medicare and Medicaid Services (CMS) Medicare inpatient rehabilitation facility payment policy implementation (IRF-PPS). This payment policy has been updated since the last version of this chapter. The second part provides costs reported by other payer systems including the Veteran's Administration Medical Centers (VAMC), CMS Medicaid, and the Healthcare Cost and Utilization Project (HCUP).

Payment Policy Prior to Medicare's Inpatient Rehabilitation Facilities Prospective Payment Systems

CMS Provides Influential Government-Sponsored Programs

CMS provides federal government–sponsored health insurance programs and includes Medicare and Medicaid programs. Medicare is the health insurance program for persons under 65 years of age with certain disabilities or end stage renal disease and for persons 65 years or older. Medicaid is the health insurance program that is state administered for persons and

families with certain low-income status or low resources. Along with Children's Health Insurance Program (CHIP), the Medicare and Medicaid programs accounted for slightly more than one-third of the country's total healthcare expenditures and almost three-fourths of all public spending on healthcare in 2007. The U.S. federal government estimated spending in 2008 was 16.6% and projected in 2009 to be 17.6% of the U.S. gross domestic product (GDP) on healthcare. Medicare has been one of the principal payers of U.S. health coverage for the disabled for over three decades and for the elderly for over four decades. Medicare is also the largest payer for hospital care. CMS Medicare and Medicaid program costs and policy significantly impact private insurers' payment systems and the funding of U.S. healthcare (11–14).

The Tax Equity and Fiscal Responsibility Act (TEFRA) of 1982 were enacted before the CMS's current Inpatient Rehabilitation Facilities Prospective Payment System (IRF-PPS) was implemented for the care of Medicare beneficiaries. Under TEFRA, CMS reimbursed rehabilitation facilities for the care of Medicare beneficiaries based on the average costs incurred per discharge. Chan et al. reported that the average charges per individual Medicare beneficiary with traumatic SCI admitted to a freestanding inpatient rehabilitation hospital were approximately $44,000 at the base year (in 1994 dollars) and less for the years before and after the base year. As expected, LOS correlated with the higher charges in the base years in comparison to the years prior to and after the base years (15–18).

Under TEFRA, Medicare beneficiaries' average IRF LOS declined through 2001. Short-stay transfers increased from freestanding rehabilitation units to skilled nursing facilities (SNF) and nursing homes (NH). In the years shortly before the IRF-PPS implementation from 1999–2000, there were increases in short-stay transfers from IRFs to acute care hospitals (16, 19–22).

Model Systems Spinal Cord Injury Centers Provide Costs from their National Database

The Model Systems Spinal Cord Injury Centers (MSCIC) treat 10%–15% of persons in the United States who incur a new traumatic SCI and subsequently provide persons with a continuum of comprehensive care. The National Institute on Disability and Rehabilitation Research (NIDRR) provides funding for the MSCIC. The National Spinal Cord Injury Statistical Center (NSCIC) is the Centers' current repository of their standardized national spinal cord injury database. Although this database is not population based, it provides long-term outcomes information about persons surviving an SCI who were treated at one of the MSCICs (23–25).

The NSCISC collects incremental provider and vendor charge data on persons with SCI, following admission to their facilities. The charges are the direct costs incurred toward providing healthcare for a person. Indirect costs are defined as the self-reported losses in wages and fringe benefits. Of note, the data on the actual dollars reimbursed to the providers by third-party payers and patients are not collected in the database. The NSCICS database includes charges by providers and vendors of emergency care services, acute medical-surgical care, acute rehabilitation, nursing home care, outpatient services and providers, durable equipment, environmental modifications, medications, supplies, attendant care, household assistance, vocational rehabilitation, and miscellaneous items (23–25).

MSCIC Report Average Daily Inpatient Charges for an Individual

Average daily inpatient charges were reviewed by Seel et al. Authors reported charges incurred by individuals with paraplegia, whose injuries occurred 60 days before, admitted from 1988 to 1998 into one of the MSCICs. The average acute care daily hospital charges ranged from $2,990 to $3,334, and average inpatient rehabilitation charges ranged from $1,133 to $1,313 in 2001 dollars (26).

MSCIC Report Average Hospital Stay Charges for an Individual

Total inpatient rehabilitation bills for a particular hospital stay were reviewed in the literature. Cifu et al. analyzed hospital charges for individuals who incurred a traumatic SCI and were admitted from the late 1980s to the mid-1990s into one of the MSCICs. Authors noted that the average acute care hospital charges were approximately $60,000 for an average LOS of 13 days and approximately $59,000 for an average inpatient rehabilitation stay of 57 days (27–28). Mckinley et al. analyzed charges between individuals who incurred a traumatic versus a nontraumatic spinal cord dysfunction who were admitted from 1992 to 1999 into one of the MSCICs. Authors reported a significant difference in LOS and total inpatient rehabilitation charges. Individuals following a traumatic SCI had nearly double the average LOS (41 days) and utilized greater inpatient rehabilitation services in comparison to individuals with nontraumatic spinal cord dysfunction (LOS of 22 days). Consequently, the average total inpatient rehabilitation charges were significantly different between these two groups. Authors report that the average costs of an inpatient rehabilitation stay for individuals with traumatic SCI was approximately 2.6 times greater than for individuals with nontraumatic spinal cord dysfunction ($25,000 vs. $66,000) in their analysis (29).

NSCISC Analyses Provide Average Annual Comprehensive Care Charges for an Individual

Annual comprehensive care charges are available in the literature. DeVivo et al. analyzed the charges from the NSCISC database for those incurring a traumatic SCI from 1990 to 1995, who were admitted into one of the national MSCICs. Charges included costs from hospitalizations, outpatient care, medications, equipment and supplies, environmental modifications, attendant and household assistance, vocational rehabilitation, and miscellaneous items. Table 80.1 summarizes these costs. The comprehensive charges in the first year following the onset of an SCI were greater than in subsequent years. This is due to the initial comprehensive acute medical, surgical, and rehabilitation hospital care and medical services. Investments in equipment were greater than in each of the subsequent years.

Motor vehicle crashes account for 42% of traumatic SCIs (24). DeVivo et al. estimated the first-year charges were $233,947 ± $15,554 for an individual whose injury resulted from a motor vehicle crash. The subsequent annual charges were $33,439 ± $3,601 in 1995 dollars.

Table 80.1   Average Annual Comprehensive Care Charges for Individuals with Traumatic SCI

AVERAGE ANNUAL CHARGES IN THOUSAND DOLLARS	ORIGINAL DATA IN 1992 ($000)		INFLATED BY CPI-MEDICAL CARE TO ANNUAL 2008 DOLLARS ($000)	
	FIRST YEAR	ANNUAL POST-INJURY	FIRST YEAR	ANNUAL POST-INJURY
High tetraplegia (C1–C4)	$417.1	$74.7	$798.8	$143.1
Low tetraplegia (C5–C8)	$269.3	$30.6	$515.7	$58.6
Paraplegia	$152.4	$15.5	$291.9	$29.7
Incomplete motor injury at any spinal level	$122.9	$8.6	$235.4	$16.5

AVERAGE ANNUAL CHARGES IN THOUSAND DOLLARS	ORIGINAL DATA IN 1996 DOLLARS ($000)		INFLATED BY CPI-MEDICAL CARE TO ANNUAL 2008 DOLLARS ($000)	
	FIRST YEAR	ANNUAL POST-INJURY	FIRST YEAR	ANNUAL POST-INJURY
Tetraplegia	$340.0	$9.0	$542.4	$14.4
Paraplegia	$174.0	$9.9	$277.6	$15.8
Less severe incomplete motor and sensory incurred at any spinal level	$144.3	$3.1	$230.2	$4.9

*Inflation adjusted by Consumer Price Index-Medical Care to annualized 2008 dollars.
Sources: 1992 data from DeVivo et al. (3, 4); 1996 data from Berkowitz et al. (1, 2).

Berkowitz Performed Comprehensive Analyses

Berkowitz et al. performed comprehensive analysis on the costs of traumatic SCI derived from two Rutgers University surveys combined with information from the NSCISC. They published their findings on medical and hospital costs. The analyses had 500 respondents. Hospital costs were based on hospital charges and not on payers' reimbursements.

In the first year following a traumatic SCI, the total annual medical charges for the care of an individual with tetraplegia (ASIA A, B, or C) averaged $340,000 in 1996 dollars. Converting to 2008 dollars using the inflation index (the annual consumer price index for medical care, CPI-mc), the total annual medical charges average $542,400. This sum includes charges for acute medical care, inpatient rehabilitation, emergency medical services, rehospitalization, outpatient services, medications, supplies, attendant care, and vocational rehabilitation (1–4). For the care of an individual with paraplegia (ASIA A, B, or C), the authors estimated an annual average for acute medical care, inpatient rehabilitation, and other costs in the first year following the injury to be $174,000 in 1996 dollars. Converting to 2008 dollars, the annual average is $277,600. Authors estimated an average annual charge of $144,300 in 1996 dollars for individuals with less severe incomplete SCI (ASIA D). This average annual charges are $230,200 in 2008 dollars. In 1996 the annual costs following a traumatic SCI, annual medical costs were estimated to be an average of $9,000 for an individual with tetraplegia (ASIA A–C), $9,900 for an individual with paraplegia (ASIA A–C), and $3,100 for an individual with less severe incomplete injury (ASIA D). In 2008 dollars, the estimated average annual costs are $14,400, $15,800, and $5,000, respectively. Table 80.1 includes the original 1996 data and the calculations by the annual CPI-mc to 2008 dollars.

It is clear that the comprehensive medical care, and consequently the charges, in the first year were greater than in subsequent years. This is consistent with the findings by DeVivo et al. and can be explained by the expected initial greater investment in the first year for the care of individuals following an SCI (1–4).

Analyses of Cost Projections have Limitations

There are limitations to the projections described in the DeVivo et al. and Berkowitz et al. analyses. When the costs are inflation-adjusted to 2008 dollars using the annual CPI-mc, the broad assumption is that similar hospital care, healthcare services, technology, and goods were utilized in 2008 as when the original data were collected in the 1990s. This assumption might not necessarily be accurate. Also, these analyses' hospital charges may become overestimations of the current actual costs because acute medical-surgical hospital and rehabilitation LOS are dramatically less in recent years than they were in the 1990s (1–4).

Of note, the Berkowitz et al. analyses are not able to be directly compared to the DeVivo et al. analyses because of their different age categories and severity-of-injury and costs information sources. However, these analyses provide an appreciation for the range of estimated annual costs for individuals with traumatic spinal cord dysfunction. Table 80.1 presents these analyses' range of cost estimates from provider and vendor charge data (1–4).

After the Inpatient Rehabilitation Facilities–Prospective Payment Systems Implementation

CMS Implemented New Rehabilitation Payment Systems

CMS moved from a facility-specific, cost-based TEFRA system to the IRF-PPS to track inpatient rehabilitation services. Implemented on January 2002 and monitored over the years, the IRF-PPS remains the current Medicare inpatient rehabilitation payment system for Medicare beneficiaries. The goal of the IRF-PPS is to improve access to rehabilitative care and to promote efficient use of resources. CMS revised its payment schedule based on categories called diagnosis related groups (DRG). CMS implemented the IRF-PPS nationally, except for in Maryland (a waiver State), through Indian Health Services, and at critical access hospitals. Under the new payment system, IRFs are paid based on their case mix at a predetermined rate (16, 19–22, 31, 32).

With the IRF-PPS implementation in 2002, there were observed reductions in relative resource use and continued decline in LOS. Postacute rehabilitation care and outpatient services played a more significant role. The reductions and the average costs of healthcare depended on the type and location of hospitals. Despite inflation and completing acute rehabilitation and medical care with a shorter hospital stay, the average cost per hospital stay did not increase as much as the rate of decline in LOS. A slowed acceleration of the cost per day was noted at an estimated 16.6% (16, 19–22, 31, 32).

Transfers from the IRF to acute care hospitals increased, on average. Also, transfers back to the IRF for additional care decreased in 2002, in comparison with the late 1990s. Interrupted stays are inpatient hospital stays that are interrupted by a transfer to and from acute care services. The number of interrupted stays less than 3 days decreased, and interrupted stays for 3 days or greater increased. Freestanding rehabilitation hospitals experienced a higher percentage of interrupted stays longer than 3 days than did rehabilitation units. Short-stay transfers slightly decreased from rehabilitation units to skilled nursing facilities (SNF) and nursing homes (NH). However, short-stay transfers from freestanding units to SNF and NH increased (16, 19–22, 31, 32).

The CMS Database Provides Aggregate Expenditures for Medicare Beneficiaries

Available CMS Medicare aggregate medical expenditures for beneficiaries following traumatic and nontraumatic spinal cord conditions were extracted from the 2002 beneficiaries' claims data. The claims data is derived from the CMS Medicare Services Reimbursement Database of the Chronic Condition Data Warehouse. There were an estimated 10.3 million FFS claims registered for more than 160,000 Medicare beneficiaries in 2002 with traumatic (identified as those with medical events associated with a diagnosis code 806 or 952 in the claim) and nontraumatic spinal cord dysfunction (identified as those with medical events associated with a diagnosis code 336 in the claim). For FFS reimbursements alone, CMS Medicare reported aggregate expenditures of an estimated $3.9 billion to provide comprehensive care. This estimate excludes information on premium payments to prepaid plans, and therefore represents a portion of the total 2002 payments provided

Table 80.2 Estimated Annual Aggregate Costs of the Care of Individuals Following a Spinal Cord Dysfunction Derived from Reimbursement Claims Data or Survey of Individuals (in millions of dollars)

Type	Study	2002	2004	2007
Traumatic spinal cord dysfunction	VA, 2007	$756	$907	$1,036*
	All plans, Medicaid, 2007	$696	$756*	$855*
Nontraumatic spinal cord dysfunction	All plans, Medicaid, 2007	$494	$536*	$607*

*Inflation adjusted by Consumer Price Index-Medical Care to annualized dollars for the given year. To obtain the VA 2007 data, the aggregate costs were approximately $992 million dollars in 2006 and converted to 2007 annualized dollars.

Traumatic is defined as those following a traumatic spinal cord injury associated with diagnoses coded as ICD-9 952 with or without 806. *Nontraumatic* is defined as those with a nontraumatic cause of spinal cord dysfunction associated with medical events with the principle diagnoses coded as ICD-9 code 336.

Sources: References 33, 34, 37, 38.

Table 80.3 Comparison of Average Charges before and after IRF-PPS Implementation from the Model Systems Spinal Cord Injury Centers—National Spinal Cord Injury Database (in thousands of dollars)

	Pre-IRF PPS-Cost Based		Post-IRF PPS
	1973–1981	1997–2001	2002–2006
Average LOS in days	108	50 (–58.7)	45 (–62.6)
Mean charge*	$146.9	$122.0 (–$34.9)	$107.3 (–$44.7)
Mean charge* per day	$1.4	$2,400 ($0.9)	$2.5 ($1.0)

*In 2005 dollars, adjusted by the Consumer Price Index—Medical Care.

Parentheses include the change from the 1973–1981 period. The negative sign depicts the decrease in comparison to the 1973–1981 period.

Source: Reference 30.

for Medicare beneficiaries. Table 80.2 summarizes these costs (33, 34, 37, 38).

NSCISC Provides Average Hospital Stay Charges for an Individual

From the NSCIC, DeVivo reported that the MSCIC inpatient rehabilitation average LOS decreased by 5 days and the average hospital stay costs decreased by nearly $15,000 from 1997–2001 to 2002–2006. When comparing the data from the years 1973–1981 with that of 2002–2006, the MSCIC inpatient rehabilitation average LOS decreased by 62.6 days. The average hospital stay costs decreased by $45,000, whereas the daily charges increased by $1,000. There are several feasible proposed explanations for the increased daily charges. One is that services were elevated in order to address the care needs for a shorter LOS. Two is that the utilization of updated care services and different products and technology increased costs in the later years. Overall, the decline in LOS contributed to the decrease in average total inpatient rehabilitation charges for the pre-IRS-PPS years to the post-IRS-PPS years 2002–2006 (3–6). Table 80.3 describes the charges (30).

National Costs are Estimated from Government Funded Surveys

The Medical Expenditure Panel Survey (MEPS) has been used to produce national estimates of healthcare expenditures for the United States civilian noninstitutionalized population. The Agency for Healthcare Research and Quality, National Center for Health Statistics, and Centers for Disease Control cosponsor the MEPS. The MEPS Household Component is conducted through a series of interviews to households to obtain person and household longitudinal healthcare usage information. Due to the small number of persons each year in the MEPS sample who are reported to have

received medical care for traumatic or nontraumatic spinal cord dysfunction (identified as those with medical events associated with ICD-9 codes of 952, 336, or 806), expenditure data were pooled across all currently available years of expenditure data (1996–2004) to produce estimates with at least minimum acceptable levels of statistical precision. Expenditures include payments by all payers, as well as individuals' out-of-pocket expenses (34).

From the MEPS pooled information, the estimated average annual population of survey respondents with spinal cord dysfunction over the period is about 216,000 persons per year (95% CI: 171,000 to 260,000 persons). Their estimated total annual healthcare expenditures were reportedly $1.7 billion (95% CI: $850 million to $2.6 billion) per year in 2004 dollars for comprehensive care. Expenditures from 1996–2004 were inflated to 2004 using the personal healthcare price index. From the MEPS, it is estimated that about $1 of every $10 was paid out of pocket for the care of persons with spinal cord dysfunction. These comprehensive care expenditures include payments for emergency services, inpatient care, ambulatory services, home health services, prescription medications, and other miscellaneous items and services (i.e., ambulance services, assistive and adaptive equipment, orthopedic or prosthetic items, and environmental adaptive modifications). Of note, these estimates do not include expenses incurred by persons with spinal cord dysfunction who lived in institutions or any expenses for over-the-counter drugs. Other limitations to the information extracted from the MEPS are similar to that inherent in survey methodology and retrospective data. Table 80.7 summarizes the pooled information. (34).

VETERANS ADMINISTRATION

The Veterans Administration (VA) provides a federally funded healthcare system for our veterans. The VA medical center (VAMC) system is a vital healthcare resource to veterans. It is not directly affected by the CMS payment policy. Following a stay at acute care medical facilities, eligible veterans can be transferred to a VAMC for inpatient or outpatient SCI care.

Table 80.4   VA Medical Care Costs for Veterans Following a Traumatic SCI, FY2000 (in thousand of dollars)

	NUMBER OF VETERANS	OUTPATIENT MEAN COSTS PER VETERAN	INPATIENT MEDICAL/ SURGICAL MEAN COSTS PER VETERAN	INPATIENT OTHER MEAN COSTS PER VETERAN	PHARMACY MEAN COSTS PER VETERAN	ALL PERSONS' CUMULATIVE TOTAL COSTS FOR FY2000	MEAN TOTAL COSTS PER VETERAN
Spinal cord injury	19,234	$3.5	$5.7	$15.1	$2.8	$512,120.5	$27.0
Diabetes	617,571	$2.4	$2.8	$1.2	$1.3	$4,760,600.0	$7.7
Chronic heart failure	173,006	$3.3	$7.9	$2.2	$1.5	$2,587,942.1	$14.9

Source: Reference 36.

Yu et al. reported the average per diem direct and indirect costs for VAMC care. Veterans with spinal cord dysfunction visited 24 VAMCs from fiscal year 1998 to 2000. The average costs were $859 per day (range of $410–$1,560 per day) in 2000 dollars (35, 36).

Large Variations Seen in Aggregate VA Medical Care Costs for their Beneficiary Populations

Yu et al. compiled data from the Veterans Affairs Health Care Systems Quality Enhancement Research Initiative. Authors found that 0.46% of veterans of a national VA database had incurred an SCI. Although this represents only a small portion, these veterans had high medical costs. Care for these veterans had the largest variation of the mean total costs, in comparison with the care of other conditions such as diabetes and chronic heart failure. Although medical events associated with diabetes and chronic heart failure had higher overall total medical care costs than did medical events associated with SCI, the VAMC paid less on average for each veteran's medical care to treat diabetes or chronic heart failure than to treat SCI. These costs are shown in Table 80.4. Authors reported fiscal year 2000 (FY 2000) costs in 2000 dollars. The mean total costs were estimated from inpatient services, outpatient clinics, and outpatient pharmacy data (35, 36).

Aggregate VA Medical Center Expenditures Provide Annual Estimates

The VAMC estimated the average cost per year and total costs to provide comprehensive care for veterans with traumatic and nontraumatic causes of spinal cord dysfunction. Table 80.5 summarizes the costs. In fiscal year 2006, VAMC expenditures averaged $38,239 for the care of each veteran with SCI. This tabulates to a total of over $992 million for the care of nearly 26,000 veterans with SCI. The data were extracted from the Department of Veterans Affairs report on "Maintaining Capacity to provide for the Specialized Treatment and Rehabilitative Needs of Disabled Veterans, FY 2006." Furthermore, the data were generated from the decision support system (DSS) cost accounting system using production unit costs associated with veterans. Direct, indirect, and other costs are included in the total cost calculation. The department's fiscal year runs from October 1 through September 30 of the following year. The cost data reflect healthcare utilization at 155 hospitals, 135 nursing homes, 45 domiciliaries, 881 outpatient clinics, 207 veterans' centers, and contracted care. There are twenty-three VAMC regional SCI centers, which provide primary, specialty, and SCI-specific care. The range of VAMC care visits is from one to multiple visits. From 2001 to 2006, there was a cumulative increase in the number of veterans with traumatic SCI and a subsequent increase in

Table 80.5   Veterans Administration Medical Center Annual Costs 2001–2006 for the Care of Veterans with Traumatic SCI (in millions of dollars)

	FY2001	FY2002	FY2003	FY2004	FY2005	FY2006
Estimated total costs	$692.55	$755.98	$828.95	$907.31	$967.08	$992.49
Number of veterans	24,014	24,490	24,798	25,368	25,768	25,955
Average costs per veteran	$0.028	$0.030	$0.033	$0.035	$0.037	$0.038

Source: Reference 37.

utilization of VAMC resources. Additionally, the average VAMC expenditure per year for each veteran with traumatic SCI increased by nearly $10,000 from 2001 to 2006. Healthcare for Veterans is a necessity in our society. Table 80.4 summarizes the cost estimates (36, 37).

CENTERS OF MEDICARE AND MEDICAID SERVICES: THE MEDICAID PROGRAM

CMS Estimates Aggregate Medicaid Expenditures for its Beneficiary Population

In 2009, an estimated 17% of the 51 million Medicaid beneficiaries reported being disabled (14). Available data on Medicaid's aggregate medical expenditures for individuals following traumatic and nontraumatic spinal cord conditions were extracted from the CMS reimbursement databases of 2002 estimated beneficiaries' claims data. Medicaid expenditures include comprehensive care as described by CMS Medicare and Medicaid benefits. This Medicaid cost information refers to Medicaid beneficiaries whose medical events are associated with traumatic (identified as those with medical events associated with an ICD-9 diagnosis code 952 in the claim) and nontraumatic spinal cord diagnosis (identified as those with medical events associated with an ICD-9 diagnosis code 336 in the claim). From the CMS Medicaid Analytic eXtract Reimbursement database, the aggregate 2002 expenditures for fee-for-service (FFS) and premium payments of prepaid plans were $1.2 billion in comprehensive care for approximately 44,700 Medicaid beneficiaries with traumatic or nontraumatic spinal cord dysfunction. The FFS reimbursements alone were $1.15 billion for approximately 42,500 Medicaid beneficiaries (38).

WORKER'S COMPENSATION AND EMPLOYER CONTRIBUTIONS

Worker's Compensation is a state-regulated no-fault insurance for work-related injury and illness and is financed by a state fund, employers, or private businesses. Enacted by law, this insurance provides employees with coverage of medical expenses, lost wages, rehabilitation services, and spousal death benefits (39).

Worker's Compensation Estimates Average Annual Payments for an Individual

Analyzing Worker's Compensation insurer data, Webster et al. reported the actual average annual payments of sixty-two beneficiaries who incurred work related SCIs between 1988 and 1999 in 2000 dollars. In the first year of injury, the average annual payments were $431,000–$561,000 for those with tetraplegia. To compare, those average annual payments range from $602,000 to $783,000 in 2008 dollars. Individuals with high or low tetraplegia did not have statistically significant cost differences. Annual payments were $130,000–131,000 for each of the subsequent 4 years postinjury. These annual payments range from $181,000 to $183,000 in 2008 dollars. In contrast, for beneficiaries with less severe spinal cord injury classified under ASIA D, the average annual payments were $178,000 (CI: $131,000–$225,000) in the first year and $30,000 (CI: $14,000–$55,000) for each of the

subsequent 4 years postinjury. To compare, these average annual payments become $248,000 in the first year and $42,000 in subsequent years, when converted to 2008 dollars (40).

Employer Health and Productivity Analyses Report SCI in the Top Ten for Costs

Goetzel et al. performed a health and productivity analysis of individuals who were included in a health and productivity management employer database from 1997 to 1999 and reported "traumatic spinal and spinal cord injury" as being among the top ten physical health conditions with high total expenditures. For employees with "traumatic spinal and spinal cord dysfunction," employers paid an average total health and productivity payment of $62.16 (1999 annualized dollars) per eligible employee per year, with 53% of these costs being due to sick leave or short-term disability. In comparison, authors noted that the musculoskeletal condition mechanical low back pain had higher employer healthcare payments. Employers paid $90.24 total in healthcare payments per eligible employee with mechanical low back disorders (no spinal or spinal cord injury), with 41% of these costs being due to sick leave or short-term disability (41).

MEDICAL-SURGICAL INPATIENT HOSPITAL CARE

The Healthcare Cost and Utilization Project (HCUP) is a national healthcare database funded by the Agency for Healthcare Research and Quality and reports healthcare estimates from nonfederal community hospitals regardless of payer. HCUP includes national estimates of inpatient hospital charges, excluding physician fee charges. The 2001–2005 HCUP data exclude charge information from freestanding rehabilitation hospitals, as well as outpatient, home-based, and long-term hospital care. This database generates estimates for inpatient care in nonrehabilitation community hospitals. HCUP cost estimates were generated for inpatient care of persons with nontraumatic spinal cord dysfunction (defined as those with medical events associated with a principal diagnosis code of ICD-9 336). HCUP cost estimates for persons with traumatic SCI are defined as those with medical events associated with the principal diagnosis code ICD-9 952 or 806 (42).

Cost containment of healthcare resources continues to be increasingly more visible due to the growing percentage of the cost of healthcare relative to the GDP. Consequently, inpatient hospital care in nonrehabilitation hospitals has also evolved over the years. Average inpatient LOS decreased from 2001 to 2005, whereas estimated annual aggregate inpatient hospital charges increased moderately. Further research is needed to elucidate these findings. One explanation might be that the increased costs, though moderate, are due to more costly hospital services, medications, and technology. The estimated aggregate charges varied among the type of nontraumatic spinal cord dysfunction recorded in the HCUP database and are summarized in Table 80.6 as a range. If the 2005 estimated annual aggregate inpatient hospital charges were adjusted by the annual CPI-mc to 2008 dollars, then the aggregate annual charges range from $10.7 million (SE $1.8 million) to $55.9 million (SE $8.6 million) in 2008 dollars. There was a wider range of estimated aggregate charges and LOS for persons with traumatic SCI than those reported for persons with nontraumatic spinal cord dysfunction.

Table 80.6   Average Annual Aggregate Charges and LOS for Only Acute Medical Surgical Care in Nonrehabilitation Hospitals

	2005	2008*
Nontraumatic		
Range of estimated aggregate charges (millions of dollars)	$9.5 (SE $1.6) to $49.7 (SE $7.6)	$10.7 (SE $1.8) to $55.9 (SE $8.6)
Range of estimated LOS (days)	5.1 (SE 0.3) to 9.9 (SE 1.2)	—
Traumatic		
Range of estimated aggregate charges (millions of dollars)	$3.3 (SE 1.0) to $139.4 (SE 17.8)	$3.7 (SE 1.1) to $157.0 (SE 20.0)
Range of estimated LOS (days)	5 (SE 1.3) to 19.3 (SE 2.3)	

*Inflation adjusted by Consumer Price Index-Medical Care to annualized 2008 dollars from the 2005 data.

For these HCUP estimates, *nontraumatic spinal cord dysfunction* is defined as the principal diagnosis coded as ICD-9 336. The Range of Aggregate Charge Estimates is based on the database's recorded different types of nontraumatic spinal cord dysfunction.

For these HCUP estimates, *traumatic spinal cord dysfunction* is defined as the principal diagnoses coded as ICD-9 806 or 952. The Range of Aggregate Charge Estimates is based on the database's recorded different types of traumatic spinal cord dysfunction.

Source: Reference 42.

Further research is needed to elucidate these differences in cost estimates, as well as in resource utilization and outcomes. Table 80.6 summarizes these inpatient nonrehabilitation hospital care cost estimates (42).

DURABLE MEDICAL EQUIPMENT, ASSISTIVE TECHNOLOGY, ENVIRONMENTAL MODIFICATIONS, AND MOBILITY EQUIPMENT

Definitions

Durable medical equipment (DME) is defined by the Centers of Medicare and Medicaid Services "as equipment which can withstand repeated use; is primarily and customarily used to serve a medical purpose; generally is not useful to a person in absence of an illness or injury; and is appropriate for use in the home." Assistive technology (AT) is defined broadly to include any technology that increases, maintains, or improves the "functional capabilities of individuals with disabilities," according to the Assistive Technology Act of 1998. For this chapter, environmental modifications refer to control and adapted living physical modifications that facilitate the function and independence of the individual. Mobility equipment refers to both manual and powered mobility equipment and vehicles, as well as to vehicle modifications for driving (32, 33, 38, 44, 45).

CMS Medicare Estimates Aggregate Expenditures for DME

For the fiscal year 2002, CMS Medicare medical reimbursements for DME were estimated at $12.7 million for FFS alone. These are aggregate expenditures for over 73,000 claims by Medicare beneficiaries with spinal cord dysfunction (identified as those with medical events associated with a primary or secondary diagnosis code of 336, 806, or 952 in the claim) (33).

Survey Reports Costs of AT for Working Persons

Hedrick et al. surveyed working-age civilians and veterans with chronic spinal cord dysfunction from 1998 to 2002 to assess the costs of assistive technology. Their findings confirmed that powered mobility and residential control devices were the most expensive category of assistive technologies, followed by manual mobility, exercise equipment, and residential control devices. Also, persons with tetraplegia had higher average costs for all devices compared to persons with paraplegia. The assistive technologies important in employment for both civilians and veterans were manual mobility and manual devices for environmental control and adapted living, power mobility and power control devices for environmental control and adapted living, prosthetics and orthotics, assistive computer technology, and augmentative and alternative communication devices. Persons who were self-employed had a higher cost burden than persons employed by private industry or the government (43, 44).

Home Modifications are a Large Portion of Environmental Modifications

The low-technology modifications may include DME, such as off-the-shelf access ramps, grab bars, and raised toilet seats, which are paid out of pocket or reimbursed by payers such as CMS Medicare and Medicaid, and private insurers. The high-technology modifications such as patient lifts, chair lifts or structural changes such as widening doorways or modifying bathroom facilities are provided by some payers with limited benefits. (43, 44) Berkowitz et al. estimated home modifications cost $21,000 in 1996 dollars. When adjusted by the annual CPI-mc to 2008 dollars, the costs are over $33,500 (1, 2).

NSCISC Reports that a Majority Utilize Manual Wheelchairs

The NSCISC reported that approximately 69% of individuals discharged from their inpatient rehabilitation centers utilized either a wheelchair or scooter as their primary form of mobility in 2006. Of these individuals, approximately 42% reported using primarily a manual wheelchair and 25% primarily a power wheelchair (NSCICI 2006 annual report). Manual wheelchairs can be an individual's primary or secondary mode of mobility. Hedrick et al. surveyed individuals with spinal cord dysfunction from 1998 to 2002 and noted that the average cost was $1,560 ± $1,000 for civilians and $1,080 ± $560 for veterans (44). Manual wheelchairs can range in cost from $500 to $4000 (45).

Depending on an individual's function and level of independence, power wheelchairs can also be an individual's primary or secondary mode of mobility. In an October 2007 report, the most popular reimbursable power wheelchair was paid by Medicare on the average of $4,024, whereas consumer prices ranged among Internet vendors from $1,452 to $6,149. The CMS reported that the Medicare fee schedule average amounts for all the reimbursable power mobility devices "exceeded the median Internet prices by 45% in the first quarter of 2007." CMS reimbursement schedules continue to be refined (45, 46).

Personal Vehicle Modifications Allow for Driving Accessibility and Independence

Personal vehicle modifications for driving accessibility are to be tailored to the individual's function and transportation needs. An individual may work with driver rehabilitation specialists and evaluators, vehicle modification vendors and manufacturers, and a medical rehabilitation team to identify the specifications for an accessible personal vehicle (see Chapter 62). Some payers provide limited accessible vehicle benefits. These include the Veterans Administration, worker's compensation, Medicaid waiver programs (home and community-based services), state vocational rehabilitation agencies, mobility rebate programs, and private organizations, depending on the eligibility requirements. Costs of adapting a vehicle for driving varies, depending on the type of modifications, on the manufacturer, and on available financial assistance. When this chapter was written, a new vehicle with modifications was estimated to average from $20,000 to $80,000. Costs of high-tech or low-tech modifications to a used car or to an individual's own vehicle, as well as maintenance, registration, and licenses, are other economic considerations for drivers (47–50).

State Agencies Estimate Rehabilitation Technologies Expenditures

State vocational rehabilitation agencies can provide rehabilitation technology services such as equipment, assistive technology, and vehicle modifications when no other comparable benefit is available from other payers. Rehabilitation technology expenditures in 2002 were estimated at $96 million among state vocational rehabilitation agencies (47–50).

ASSISTANCE CARE

Assistance care refers to diagnostic, therapeutic, rehabilitative, or personal assistance. Healthcare payers provide limited benefits and define assistance care differently. Depending on the type of assistance care, these services can be provided by family, friends, or paid professionals such as nurses, home health aides, or personal attendants (51).

The request for specifically personal assistance or attendant care can depend on factors such as the individual's function, neurologic impairment, health, and avocational and vocational pursuits. In a 1996 survey, Berkowitz et al. reported that an estimated 55% of their survey respondents had assistance care, which provided services from 1 hour a week to continuous care. Having paid assistance can depend on factors such as extent of unpaid assistance and healthcare payer benefits. Of individuals with assistance care, two-thirds had paid professional assistants or attendants (1, 2).

In 2002, CMS Medicare medical expenditures for home health agency (HHA) care were an estimated $27 million for FFS plans alone. This comprises over 10,000 HHA claims for Medicare beneficiaries with traumatic or nontraumatic spinal cord dysfunction (identified as those with medical events associated with a primary or secondary diagnosis code of ICD-9 336, 806, or 952 in the claim) (33).

WORKFORCE PRODUCTIVITY COSTS AND EMPLOYMENT LOSS

An important factor in the quality of life for individuals following a spinal cord dysfunction is employment status (1, 2, 44). Employment, work hours, and income decrease to varying degrees and different timeframes for individuals following a spinal cord dysfunction. With unemployment, state and federal expenses subsequently increase, and the costs shift to society. Return to the workforce improves an individual's personal satisfaction, social relationships, and community reintegration, as well as decreasing the financial impact on society. Researchers have reported that positive determinants for returning to work include such factors as accessibility in the workplace, owning a vehicle modified to drive independently, education beyond high school, assistance with activities of daily living, and age. Specific job characteristics reported to impact the return to work include computer use and the ability to work from home. Resource allocation to reduce barriers for individuals with a spinal cord dysfunction who are able to return to work is advantageous to both the individual and society (1, 2, 44, 52–59).

Berkowitz et al. calculated indirect costs (loss of workforce productivity) through the human capital economic method to describe the loss of the individual's workforce productivity. Authors estimated that indirect costs accounted for approximately 65% of the total estimated costs in the care of an individual following a traumatic SCI in 1996. The authors calculated indirect costs based on the individual's education and employment prior to incurring a traumatic SCI and at the time of their survey. Depending on the age of onset and level and severity of the injury among other factors, the indirect costs among the survey respondents were within the average range of $13,393 to $15,714 per year per individual in 1996 dollars. In comparison, if these costs were adjusted to 2008 dollars using the annual CPI-mc, the average range becomes $21,400 to $25,100 per year per individual. The costs associated with loss of workforce productivity are reduced when the individuals return to work and continue employment. Government, payer, and private industry funded programs such as vocational rehabilitation, social work programs, and employee-based transition to work assistances aid individuals in returning to the work force. These programs and related assistances facilitate community reintegration, improve quality of life, and resume a level of work force productivity (1, 2).

LIFETIME COSTS

From the onset of spinal cord dysfunction, individuals can be affected for life, especially those persons with moderate and severe conditions. The financial impact depends on numerous factors such as the extent of recovery, functional independence, age of onset, medical complications, inflation, and the cost of services and goods.

Lifetime costs for the care of individuals with spinal cord dysfunction have been estimated by several authors and have primarily focused on the care following traumatic spinal cord injuries. A range of lifetime costs provides an appreciation of the effect of different life expectancies and discount rates from two separate analyses of lifetime costs. To compute net present value, calculations modeled several discount rates including 2%, 4% and 6% to discount future benefits and costs. The outcomes are summarized in this chapter to elucidate the spectrum of estimated lifetime costs depending on the chosen discount rate.

There is a cautionary note: an assumption in these calculations is that substantial medical care and resources are needed throughout an individual's life following a spinal cord dysfunction, regardless of the extent of injury, recovery and functional outcome. Therefore, estimations of lifetime costs of care for an individual are more accurate when based on the specifics of the particular individual.

NSCIC Data Estimate Lifetime Costs for Survivors Ages 25 and 50

From the NSCISC, DeVivo et al. estimated lifetime direct costs for an individual injured at age 25 with high tetraplegia to be $1.6 million, and at age 50 with the same injury to be $0.9 million in 1992 (2% discount rate). For an individual at age 25 with paraplegia, the estimate was $0.5 million, and at age 50 with paraplegia, $0.4 million in 1992 (2% discount rate). When a 4% discount rate was used, the lifetime cost estimates were less. Lifetime costs were greater when an individual incurred an SCI at age 25 than at age 50. The assumption here was that a 25-year-old person lives with an SCI for a greater number of years than a 50-year-old, and consequently incurs more lifetime healthcare costs (3–6). When these costs are adjusted to 2008 dollars using the annual CPI-mc, estimated lifetime costs (direct costs only) for individuals with tetraplegia range from $1.5 to $3.1 million when the age of onset is 25 years old and $1.0 to $1.7 million when the age of onset is 50 years old; with paraplegia ranging from $0.8 to $1 million when the age of onset is 25 years old and $1.0 to $1.7 million when the age of onset is 50 years old; and with less severe incomplete injuries ranging from $0.6 to $1.0 million when the age of onset is 25 years old and $0.4 to $0.8 million when the age of onset is 50 years old. Table 80.7 provides a further breakdown of these dollars by discount rates of 2% and 4%.

According to DeVivo et al., the indirect costs (loss of workforce productivity with earnings and benefits) for an individual

Table 80.7   Two Analyses: Lifetime Direct Costs for Individuals with Traumatic SCI (in millions of dollars) (1–4)

Age of Onset	Original Data in 1992 Dollars (2% discount rate)		Inflated by CPI-Medical Care to Annual 2008 Dollars (2% discount rate)		Original Data in 1992 Dollars (4% discount rate)		Inflated by CPI-Medical Care to Annual 2008 Dollars (4% discount rate)	
	25 Y.O.	50 Y.O.	25 Y.O.	50 Y.O.	25 Y.O.	50 Y.O.	25 Y.O.	50 Y.O.
High tetraplegia (C1–C4)	$1.6	$0.9	$3.1	$1.7	$1.3	$0.9	$2.5	$1.7
Low tetraplegia (C5–C8)	$0.9	$0.6	$1.7	$1.2	$0.8	$0.5	$1.5	$1.0
Paraplegia (T1–S5)	$0.5	$0.4	$1.0	$0.8	$0.4	$0.3	$0.8	$0.6
Less severe incomplete motor and sensory injury incurred at any spinal level	$0.4	$0.3	$0.8	$0.6	$0.3	$0.2	$0.6	$0.4

	Original Data in 1996 Dollars (4% discount rate)	Inflated by CPI-Medical Care to Annual 2008 Dollars (4% discount rate)	Original Data in 1996 Dollars (6% discount rate)	Inflated by CPI-Medical Care to Annual 2008 Dollars (6% discount rate)
Tetraplegia (age of onset at 37 y.o.)	$0.9	$1.4	$0.8	$1.3
Paraplegia (age of onset at 31 y.o.)	$0.5	$0.8	$0.4	$0.6
Less severe incomplete motor and sensory incurred at any spinal level (age of onset at 40 y.o.)	$0.3	$0.5	$0.3	$0.5

*Inflation adjusted by Consumer Price Index-Medical Care to annualized 2008 dollars.
Sources: 1992 data from DeVivo et al. (3, 4); 1996 data from Berkowitz et al. (1, 2).

at age 25 with high tetraplegia were $1.8 million, and at age 50 with the same injury were $0.7 million in 1992 (2% discount rate). The loss of workforce productivity for an individual at age 25 with paraplegia was $1.28 million, and at age 50 was $0.5 million (2% discount rate). When the discount rate was raised to 4%, the lifetime costs were notably lower (3–6).

Survey Estimates Lifetime Costs for Survivors Injured at Ages 31 and 37

In a separate analysis, Berkowitz et al. estimated lifetime costs in 1996 dollars for different age and injury categories. For an individual with tetraplegia injured at age 37, the estimates were $0.88 million in direct costs and $0.44 million in indirect costs for a total of $1.3 million dollars in 1996 dollars (4% discount rate). Similarly, for an individual with paraplegia at age 31, the estimates were $0.5 million in direct costs and $0.5 million in indirect costs for a total cost of $1 million in 1996 dollars (4% discount rate). When the discount rate was raised to 6%, the lifetime costs were notably lower. Total lifetime costs were greater for individuals following tetraplegia than for individuals following paraplegia. In Table 80.7 the 2008 direct cost estimates were derived from 1996 data adjusted for inflation with the annual CPI-mc, and discounted at 4% and 6% (1, 2).

Factors to Consider when Reviewing these Estimates

Both of these lifetime cost estimates were derived from comprehensive 1990s analyses. In the absence of recent data, these estimates provide available information on estimated lifetime costs adjusted to the latest annualized dollars and modeled using different discount rates to estimate the present value of expected costs.

There are limitations to these lifetime cost estimations. These analyses' hospital charges may become overestimations of the current actual costs because acute hospital and rehabilitation LOS costs are dramatically lower in recent years than they were in the 1990s. Of note, these two analyses used different life tables to determine lifetime cost estimates, making the two analyses not comparable.

When reviewing these two analyses' lifetime costs originally derived from 1990s data, additional key factors may affect their relevance to recent years, such as the rise in the average age of onset of a traumatic SCI by 10 years since the 1970s and the advent of different care services and technologies. The spectrum of ages and varied causes of injury and severity of illness consequently affect the utilization of care services and goods and alter lifetime costs.

Despite the limitations, these two analyses are elegant studies that provide comprehensive estimations of lifetime costs for the care of individuals with traumatic SCI. To determine the current lifetime costs, further research is needed.

CONCLUSION

Spinal cord dysfunction from traumatic or nontraumatic causes can have far-reaching consequences for the individual and the nation. For individuals with traumatic spinal cord dysfunction alone, the incidence is reportedly 12,000 new cases per year, and the prevalence is reportedly 259,000 (range of 229,000 to 306,000) among those alive in 2008 (24). From the MEP survey pooled

data, the estimated average annual population of survey respondents with spinal cord dysfunction (traumatic and nontraumatic causes) over the 1996–2004 period is reportedly 216,000 persons per year (95% CI: 171,000 to 260,000 persons) (34).

The financial impact of spinal cord dysfunction on the individual and the nation is complex, multifaceted, and encompasses more than just the health care charges and expenditures. Therefore, it is difficult to fully and accurately quantify. Not covered in this chapter because of the limited available information, but recognized as important components of the overall financial impact, are the welfare and intangible costs such as costs attributed to the affected individual's psychosocial stresses. Because each individual with a spinal cord dysfunction is unique, the author recommends to use actual costs and compute cost estimates based on the specifics of that particular individual.

To determine the financial impact of spinal cord dysfunction, this chapter summarized the available cost information of healthcare resources for the care of individuals with spinal cord dysfunction. In summary, notable points include (1) cost studies, provider data, vendor data, and payer data estimate costs of care for persons with spinal cord dysfunction; (2) payers can affect healthcare resource utilization and financial impact; (3) there are wide variations in cost estimates depending on the parameters of the cost study and database; (4) cost differences are reported between nontraumatic and traumatic causes of SCI; (5) further research is needed to determine, assess, and provide feasible healthcare strategies; and (6) cost estimates describe a portion of the healthcare financial impact of spinal cord dysfunction on affected individuals and the nation.

Cost Studies, Provider Data, Vendor Data, and Payer Data Estimate Healthcare Costs for Persons with Spinal Cord Dysfunction

Collaborative efforts among affected individuals, healthcare providers, payers, the government, researchers, economists, and other interested groups can lead to more effective and efficient healthcare and healthcare delivery and a better understanding of the financial impact of the care for individuals with spinal cord dysfunction. From available financial data, lifetime costs (direct costs), using several discount rates, were higher among those of a younger age (25 years old) than of an older age (50 years old), with the assumption that a 25-years-old would have a longer lifespan. Also, lifetime costs for individuals with paraplegia were estimated to average at least 30% less than that for individuals with tetraplegia. As reported in several analyses, lifetime costs varied depending on factors such as the age of onset, severity and level of injury, and adjustments made by discount rates (Table 80.7). Indirect costs, defined as those associated with the loss of workforce productivity or human capital, were within the average range $21,400 to $25,100 per year per individual depending on factors such as age of onset and the level and severity of the injury. These costs are in 2008 dollars using the annual CPI-mc (1–4).

Payers Affect Healthcare Resource Utilization and Financial Impact

Payers play a tremendous role in determining the healthcare resource utilization and financial impact of the healthcare services and goods for individuals with spinal cord dysfunction.

Furthermore, CMS Medicare policies influence the overall payer environment. The costs of inpatient rehabilitation stays were impacted by the CMS Medicare IRF-PPS policy implementation in 2002. Under the IRF-PPS, there were decreases in healthcare resource allocation and utilization and continued decreases in LOS at inpatient rehabilitation facilities. Medicare reported that the average provider charges did not increase as much as LOS decreased. The LOS depended on patient and hospital factors. Medicare reported decreased average LOS to 19 days (range: 17–24) for Medicare beneficiaries with traumatic SCI and 13 days (range: 12–16) for those with nontraumatic spinal cord dysfunction. The NSCIC noted a decrease in average LOS to an average of 45 days for persons with traumatic SCI. With the IRF-PPS, there were consequential shifts in the utilization of resources of acute care hospitals, long-term facilities, and outpatient services in order to provide continued care.

In years to come, improvements toward accessible, efficient, and effective healthcare and advancements in functional outcomes, quality of life, and community reintegration of persons with spinal cord dysfunction will continue to be critical measures of success of healthcare resource utilization and investments in care services and goods (16, 19). To this end, payers, providers, and beneficiaries alike recognize the primary importance of the access to care for individuals following spinal cord dysfunction. With recent and upcoming significant changes in the national and state level payer policies and economic healthcare strategies and therefore allocation and utilization, it will be especially important to track and analyze the impact upon individuals with spinal cord dysfunction.

A Wide Range of Cost Estimates is a Notable Finding

A range of aggregate comprehensive care cost estimates are presented from available cost studies and payer databases. The VA expenditures were approximately $992 million for the care of nearly 26,000 Veterans with spinal cord dysfunction in 2006. Converting to 2008 dollars with the annual CPI-mc, the VA expenditures are approximately $1 billion. For the care of individuals with either traumatic or nontraumatic spinal cord dysfunction, CMS paid providers and vendors for aggregate comprehensive care an estimated range greatly dependent on the insurance plan. Table 80.2 summarizes these cost estimates.

For the care of individuals with traumatic SCI, the costs were greatest among those individuals with tetraplegia and least among those with less severe incomplete injuries, regardless of the level of injury (33, 34, 37, 38). Annual costs were significantly less in years subsequent to the first year following an SCI (1–4). Tables 80.1 and 80.7 summarize these cost estimates.

Consistent Cost Differences were Reported

Although there were different estimates, cost studies described consistent cost differences for the care of individuals following traumatic and nontraumatic spinal cord dysfunction regardless of the IRF-PPS implementation. Aggregate annual comprehensive care costs were greater and average LOS were longer among individuals with traumatic spinal cord dysfunction than among individuals with nontraumatic spinal cord dysfunction. Table 80.2 summarizes these aggregate costs. The aggregate costs and LOS

differences might be explained by the differences in study population, medical comorbidities, treatments, and affected individuals' rehabilitation goals (16, 19, 29, 33, 34, 37, 38).

Further Research is Needed to Assess Optimal and Feasible Healthcare Strategies

As a nation, we continue to grapple with healthcare resource allocation and utilization. Consensus has not yet been reached on optimal and feasible healthcare strategies. Technologies, healthcare and payer support will continue to evolve. Reimbursement policies, such as the CMS policies, are designed to reduce direct costs (costs directly related to spinal cord dysfunction) while improving access to care.

Berkowitz et al. proposed that the reduction of indirect costs (loss of workforce productivity or human capital) also improves the quality of life of individuals following spinal cord dysfunction. Although spinal cord dysfunction can restrict vocational pursuits, there are individuals who are able to return to work. For these individuals, several studies identified measures that significantly improve the probability of work reentry and/or continued employment. The successful implementation and utilization of these measures, as well as return to work programs, can reduce indirect costs and improve the quality of life of individuals. These measures included enhancing individuals' level of education and vocational rehabilitation, permitting work from home where ADL assistance can be provided, modifying vehicles for independent driving, and having a computer-based job and an accessible workplace.

Further research such as basic, clinical, translational, prevention, community-based, economic studies, financial analyses, and comparative effectiveness research are needed to identify optimal and feasible healthcare strategies to improve accessible, efficient, and effective medical care; functional outcomes; quality of life; and community reintegration of individuals with spinal cord dysfunction (1, 2, 7, 8, 13, 14, 43–60). Direct comparisons of the data and more detailed understandings of costs are limited because of the different data collection methodologies and limited cost breakdowns in the cost studies, provider data, vendor data, and payer data. These and other cost information limitations demonstrate the challenges in cost analysis research.

Cost Estimates Describe a Portion of the Financial Impact of Spinal Cord Dysfunction on the Nation and the Individual

The financial impact of spinal cord dysfunction on the nation and individual described in this chapter is a compilation of cost estimates of the healthcare resources provided for individuals with spinal cord dysfunction. The real total costs of care are difficult to fully and exactly quantify. This is true because the real total costs include not only the costs for healthcare services and goods in the care of an affected individual, but also components that are notably difficult to quantify such as the impact of psychosocial stresses, the reallocation of time to perform activities of daily living, changes in professional and avocational pursuits, and other intangibles affecting individuals, family and friends (1–4).

Moreover, each individual with spinal cord dysfunction is unique. Therefore, each individual experiences different degrees of decline and recovery of function and health, as well as varying levels of social support and community reintegration. Each individual has a different prognosis and medical surgical course, as well as a uniquely tailored and dynamic rehabilitation plan. Therefore, to best estimate total costs of healthcare for an individual, calculations should be based on the specifics of the particular individual.

ACKNOWLEDGMENT

Special appreciation is expressed to Douglas Hough, Ph.D., from the Carey Business School, Johns Hopkins University, for his editorial review.

References

1. Berkowitz M, O'Leary PK, Kruse DL, Harvey C. *Spinal Cord Injury: An Analysis of Medical and Social Costs.* New York: Demos Publishers, 1998.

2. Berkowitz M, Harvey C, Wilson SE, Greene CG. *The Economic Consequences of Traumatic Spinal Cord Injury.* New York: Demos Publishers, 1992.

3. DeVivo MJ, Whiteneck GG, Charles ED Jr. The economic impact of SCI. In: Stover SL, DeLisa JA, Whiteneck GG, eds. *SCI: Clinical Outcomes from the Model Systems.* Gaithersburg, MD: Aspen Publishers, 1995.

4. DeVivo MJ. Economics of Spinal Cord Injury. Spinal Cord Injury Information Center. www.spinalcord.uab.edu.

5. DeVivo MJ. Sir Ludwig Guttmann Lecture: trends in spinal cord injury rehabilitation outcomes from model systems in the United States: 1973–2006. *Spinal Cord* 2007; 45(11):713–721.

6. DeVivo MD. 2006 Annual Statistical Report. National Spinal Cord Injury Statistical Center. University of Alabama at Birmingham.

7. Tarricone R. Cost-of-illness analysis: what room in health economics? *Health Policy* 2006; 77(1):51–63.

8. Korthals-de Bos I, van Tulder M, van Dieten H, Bouter L. Economic evaluations and randomized trials in spinal disorders: principles and methods. *Spine* 2004; 29(4):442–448.

9. Berkowitz M. Costs of spinal cord injury. In: Lin V, Hammond MC, eds. *Spinal Cord Medicine: Principles and Practice.* New York: Demos Publishers, 2003.

10. Wolfbane Cybernetic Ltd. International Classification of Diseases, Revision 9, 1975. http://www.wolfbane.com/icd/icd9h.htm.

11. Centers of Medicaid and Medicare Services. CBO Testimony Statement of Donald B. Marron, Acting Director, Medicaid Spending Growth and Options for Controlling Costs before the Special Committee on Aging, United States Senate, July 13, 2006. www.cms.hhs.gov.

12. Elmendorf DW. Health care reform and the federal budget letter to the Honorable Kent Conrad and the Honorable Judd Gregg. Congressional Budget Office June 16, 2009. www.cbo.gov.

13. Foster RS, Clemens MK. Medicare financial status, budget impact, and sustainability—which concept is which? *Health Care Financing Review* 2005–2006; 27(2).

14. Klees BS, Wolfe CJ, Curtis, CA, Office of the Actuary Centers for Medicare & Medicaid Services Department of Health and Human Services. Brief summaries of Medicare & Medicaid, Title XVIII and Title XIX of The Social Security Act as of November 1, 2009. www.cms.hhs.gov.

15. Rielinger JA. Preparing for the inpatient rehabilitation PPS-prospective payment system case study, Metro Health Center for Rehabilitation, Cleveland, Ohio. *Health Finance Manage* 2001; 55(12):52–55.

16. Beeuwkes Buntin M, Carter GM, Hayden O, Hoverman C, et al. Inpatient Rehabilitation Facility Care Use Before and After Implementation of the IRF Prospective Payment System Rand Corp. Supported by the Centers for Medicare and Medicaid Services, RAND, 2006. http://www.rand.org/.

17. Chan L, Koepsell TD, Deyo RA, Esselman PC, et al. The effect of Medicare's payment system for rehabilitation hospitals on length of stay, charges, and total payments. *N Engl J Med* 1997; 337(14):978–985.

18. Chan, L. The state-of-the-science: challenges in designing postacute care payment policy. *Arch Phys Med Rehabil* 2007; 88(11):1522–1525.

19. Carter GM, Relles DA, Wynn BO, Kawata JH, et al. CMS charted RAND report reviewed the differences in pre-IRF-PPS and early IRF-PPS implementation. Interim Report on an Inpatient Rehabilitation Facility Prospective Payment System. Supported by the Centers for Medicare and Medicaid Services, RAND, July 2000. http://www.rand.org/.

20. Leavitt, MO. Report to Congress: Utilization and Beneficiary Access to Services Post-Implementation of the Inpatient Rehabilitation Facilities Prospective Payment System. Health and Human Services, August 15, 2005:1–161. http://www.cms.hhs.gov/InpatientRehabFacPPS/Downloads/IRF_Report_to_Congress08_2005.pdf

21. McCue MJ, Thompson JM. Early effects of the prospective payment system on inpatient rehabilitation hospital performance. *Arch Phys Med Rehabil* 2006; 87(2):198–202.

22. Johnson RL, Brooks CA, Whiteneck GG. Cost of traumatic spinal cord injury in a population-based registry. *Spinal Cord* 1996; 34(8):470–480.

23. UAB Spinal Cord Injury Model System, Spinal Cord Injury Information Network, funded by the National Institute on Disability and Rehabilitation Research (NIDRR), U.S. Department of Education, November 2007. http://www.spinalcord.uab.edu/show.asp?durki=21392.

24. National Spinal Cord Injury Statistical Center. Spinal Cord Injury: Facts and Figures at a Glance 2009. Birmingham, AL, June, 2009. www.nscisc.uab.edu/public_content/facts_figures_2009.aspx.

25. National Institute on Disability and Rehabilitation Research (NIDRR). Model Systems of Care, U.S. Department of Education, 2007. http://www.ed.gov/rschstat/research/pubs/res-program.html#DRRP.

26. Seel RT, Huang ME, Cifu DX, Kolakowsky-Hayner SA, McKinley WO. Age-related differences in LOS, hospitalization costs, and outcomes for an injury matched sample of adults with paraplegia. *J Spinal Cord Med* 2001; 24:241–250.

27. Cifu DX, Seel RT, Kreutzer JS, McKinley WO. A multicenter investigation of age-related differences in lengths of stay, hospitalization charges, and outcomes for a matched tetraplegia sample. *Arch Phys Med Rehabil* 1999; 80(7):733–740.

28. Cifu DX, Huang ME, Kolakowsky-Hayner SA, Seel RT. Age, outcome, and rehabilitation costs after paraplegia caused by traumatic injury of the thoracic spinal cord, conus medullaris, and cauda equina. *J Neurotrauma* 1999; 16(9):805–815.

29. McKinley WO, Seel RT, Gadi RK, Tewksbury MA. Nontraumatic vs. traumatic spinal cord injury: a rehabilitation outcome comparison. *Am J Phys Med Rehabil* 2001; 80(9):693–699; quiz 700, 716.

30. DeVivo MJ. Causes and costs of spinal cord injury in the United States. *Spinal Cord* 1997; 35(12):809–813.

31. Paddock SM, Escarce JJ, Hayden O, Buntin MB. Did the Medicare Inpatient Rehabilitation Facility Prospective Payment System Result in Changes in Relative Patient Severity and Relative Resource Use? *Med Care* 2007; 45:123–130.

32. Centers of Medicaid and Medicare Services. Medicare Advantage Payment Guide for Out of Network Payments, June 15, 2006 Update. Centers of Medicaid and Medicare Services. http://www.cms.hhs.gov/MedicareAdvtgSpecRateStats/Downloads/oon-payments.pdf

33. Clark WD, Waldron C. Personal communication regarding available (2002) Medicare reimbursements, Chronic Condition Data Warehouse, Centers for Medicare and Medicaid Services, Office of Research Development and Information, Information and Methods Group, October 2007.

34. Machlin S. Personal communication regarding statistics of the Agency for Healthcare Research and Quality Medical Expenditure Panel Survey 1996–2004, Agency for Healthcare Research and Quality, Rockville, MD, August 2007.

35. Yu W, Wagner TD, Chen S, Barnett PG. Average cost of VA rehabilitation, mental health, and long-term hospital stays. *Med Care Res Rev* 2003; 60(3):40S–53S.

36. Yu W, Cowper D, Berger M, Kuebeler M, et al. Using GIS to profile healthcare costs of VA Quality-Enhancement Research Initiative diseases. *J Med Syst* 2004; 28(3):271–285.

37. Hendricks R. Personal communication regarding the Department of Veterans Affairs Report on Maintaining Capacity to Provide for the Specialized Treatment and Rehabilitative Needs of Disabled Veterans FY2006, Veterans Administration Medical Centers Spinal Cord Injury Services Office, Seattle, WA, July 2007.

38. Clark WD, Anderson K, Personal communication regarding available (2002) Medicaid expenditures from the Medicaid Analytic eXtract reimbursement database, the Centers for Medicare and Medicaid Services, Office of Research Development and Information, Division of Research on State Programs and Special Populations, July 2007.

39. Workman's Compensation Insurance Net. Workmen's Compensation Insurance Law—Know Your Facts. November 2007. http://www.workmanscompinsurance.net/laws.html.

40. Webster B, Giunti G, Young A, Pransky G, Nesathurai S. Work-related tetraplegia: cause of injury and annual medical costs. *Spinal Cord* 2004; 42(4):240–247.

41. Goetzel et al. The health and productivity cost of burden of the "top 10" physical and mental health conditions affecting six large US employers. *J Occup Environ Med* 2003; 45:5–14.

42. Agency for Healthcare Research and Quality. HCUPnet. Healthcare Cost and Utilization Project (HCUP), 1993–2005. Rockville, Maryland. http://hcupnet.ahrq.gov/.

43. Moore T, O'Connell B. Compendium of Home Modification and Assistive Technology Policy and Practice across the States. Volume I: Final Report. Prepared by Abt Associates, Inc. October 27, 2006. Prepared for Office of Disability, Aging and Long-Term Care Policy, Office of the Assistant Secretary for Planning and Evaluation, U.S. Department of Health and Human Services, Contract #HHS-100–03–0008.

44. Hedrick B, Pape TL, Heinemann AW, Ruddell JL, Reis J. Employment issues and assistive technology use for persons with spinal cord injury. J Rehabil Res Dev 2006; 43(2):185–198.

45. The Wheelchair Site. Moxy Media. Ontario, Canada. 2007; http://www.thewheelchairsite.com/manual-wheelchairs.aspx.

46. Levinson DR. A Comparison of Medicare Program and Consumer Internet Prices for Power Wheelchairs, Department of Health and Human Services, Office of Inspector General, October 2007, oei-04-07-00160.

47. National Highway Traffic Safety Administration. Adapting Motor Vehicles for People with Disabilities. National Highway Traffic Safety Administration Brochure. http://www.nhtsa.dot.gov/cars/rules/adaptive/brochure/brochure.html.

48. New York State Education Department Office of Vocational and Educational Services for Individuals with Disabilities (VESID) 441.00P Vehicle Modifications, Adaptive and Automotive Equipment Procedure, January 2006. http://www.vesid.nysed.gov/vrpolicy/policies/pro441.htm.

49. Freiman MP, Mann WC, Johnson J, Lin S, Locklear C. Public Funding and Support of Assistive Technologies for Persons with Disabilities. AARP Public Policy Institute. 2006. http://www.aarp.org/2006_04_assist.pdf.

50. McKinley W, Tewksbury MA, Sitter P, Reed J, Floyd S. Assistive technology and computer adaptations for individuals with spinal cord injury. *NeuroRehabilitation* 2004; 19:141–146.

51. Weitzenkamp DA, Whiteneck GG, Lammertse DP. Predictors of personal care assistance for people with spinal cord injury. *Arch Phys Med Rehabil* 2002; 83:1399–1405.

52. Drainoni M-L, Houlihan B, Williams S, Vedrani M, et al. Patterns of internet use by persons with spinal cord injuries and relationship to health-related quality of life. *Arch Phys Med Rehabil* 2004; 85:1872–1879.

53. Lidal IB, Huynh TK, Biering-Sørensen F. Return to work following spinal cord injury: a review. *Disabil Rehabil* 2007; 29(17):1341–1375.

54. Putzke JD, Richards JS, Hicken BL, DeVivo MJ. Predictors of life satisfaction: a spinal cord injury cohort study. *Arch Phys Med Rehabil* 2002; 83:555–561.

55. Tasiemski T, Bergstrom E, Savic G, Gardner BP. Sports, recreation and employment following spinal cord injury—a pilot study. *Spinal Cord* 2000; 38:173–184.

56. Young AE, Murphy GC. A social psychology approach to measuring vocational rehabilitation intervention effectiveness. *J Occup Rehabil* 2002; 12:175–189.

57. Crewe NM. A 20-year longitudinal perspective on the vocational experiences of persons with spinal cord injury. *Rehabil Couns Bull* 2000; 43:122–133.

58. Dowler R, Richards JS, Putzke JD, Gordon W, Tate D. Impact of demographic and medical factors on satisfaction with life after spinal cord injury: a normative study. *J Spinal Cord Med* 2001; 24:87–91.

59. Fiedler IG, Indermuehle DL, Drobac W, Laud P. Perceived barriers to employment in individuals with spinal cord injury. *Top Spinal Cord Inj Rehabil* 2002; 7:73–82.

60. Boschen KA, Tonack M, Gargaro J. Long-term adjustment and community reintegration following spinal cord injury. *Int J Rehabil Res* 2003; 26:157–164.

81 The Prevention of Spinal Cord Injury

Philip R. Fine
Phillip Jeffrey Foster, Jr.
Andrea Underhill

Epidemiologically, spinal cord injury (SCI) is a comparatively rare phenomenon (1). This is fortunate because its catastrophic consequences typically include a spectrum of residual, lifelong disabilities. Depending on one's perspective, the significant acute care and long-term management achievements growing out of Sir Ludwig Guttman's seminal work following WWII have been either a blessing or a curse (2, 3). For example, today it is not uncommon for a substantial proportion of SCI persons to anticipate a near-normal life expectancy (1, 4). However, for many C1–C2 ventilator-dependent tetraplegics, whose average life expectancy is shorter than those SCI patients whose lesions are at a lower neurological level and, as a result are considered less severe, the demands of "normal" day-to-day living can be difficult, expensive, and in many instances devoid of meaningful quality (5). Moreover, an SCI invariably negatively affects the life experience of family members, especially caregivers, friends, and the community within which the SCI patient resides, so the scope of its impact can be overwhelming (5).

ETIOLOGIC CONTEXT

The National Spinal Cord Injury Database (NSCID) has been the epicenter of SCI data collection, reduction, and analysis for more than three decades. It manages carefully collected information derived from persons with new spinal cord injuries who are admitted to one of several world-class hospitals. Together, these hospitals and their affiliated academic research centers form a network that is the federally sponsored Model Spinal Cord Injury System (MSCIS) (6). Ongoing analyses of MSCIS data have revealed changing trends in the epidemiology of traumatic SCI. Virtually all of this information is interesting and much of it is quite useful, because epidemiologic data, if interpreted properly, can provide a template for evidence-based management decisions and even certain aspects of prevention practice.

For example, Ho and coworkers used NSCID data to describe the most common cause of SCIs between the years 2000 and 2003. As in all previous years, motor vehicle crashes were the leading cause, accounting for approximately 51% of SCI across all age groups during the 36-month study period. That figure was up slightly from approximately 49% for the period between 1973 and 1979 (7).

It is of more than casual interest that rates for falls as a cause of SCIs have increased progressively over the last three decades, climbing from 16.5% in the 1970s to 23.8% between 2000 and 2003 (7). In addition, even though falls remained the second most common cause of SCI across all age groups, it was the only etiology that showed a steady, measurable increase over the past 30-plus years. When data were stratified by age group, falls were determined to be the most common cause of SCIs in people over age 60.

Falls are becoming increasingly common as a cause of both injury and death. In fact, each year in the United States, nearly one third of older adults experience a fall (8). Given that SCI is but one consequence of falls, it is no real surprise that falls have become the second leading cause of SCIs.

It is also worth noting that the number of persons in the United States who were age 85 and older increased from approximately 1.5 million in 1970 to approximately 4.2 million by 2000, a breathtaking 280% increase. Thus, the dramatic increase in fall-related SCIs appears to be a predictable byproduct of an aging population. Consider: since 1970 the number of individuals living in the United States over age 65 increased from 20.1 million in 1970 to 35.0 million by 2000 (74%). With the number of persons age 65 and older having increased so much over that 30-year period and the rate of fall-related SCIs having also increased, it is chilling to think about what might happen over the next 10 to 15 years when a cohort of "baby boomers," the 76 million Americans born between 1946 and 1964, enter the population of persons over 65 years of age. Given the trends reflected in these data, the question should be asked: "Will this substantial increase in the number of persons age 65 and older translate to an even greater increase in fall-related SCIs over the next 10 to 15 years?" At least one prominent inquiry suggests this is likely to be the case.

In a study from Finland, Kannus and coworkers (9) documented a 131% increase in the incidence of fall-related SCIs between 1970 and 2004. This increase paralleled a substantial increase in the number of Finns age 50 and older, which ballooned approximately 66% (1.15 million to approximately 2 million) in the same 34-year period. Viewed another way, in 1970 Finns age 50 and older comprised approximately 25% of the overall Finnish population. By 2004 that proportion had increased to more than 36%. Kannus et al. concluded that the increase in the number and incidence of fall-related SCIs was a function of the increasing age of the Finnish population. Although we acknowledge this is but one study, there is well-documented evidence linking elderly persons to an increased risk of fall-related injury in general and SCIs in particular. Thus, it seems reasonable to posit that as more and more U.S. citizens enter the 65-plus years of age cohort, the number of persons at increased risk for falling in general, as well as for fall-related SCIs, will increase proportionately, or perhaps even disproportionately.

Consequently, at least for the United States, trend data suggest we may be facing a very expensive, high-stakes numbers game with more than 70 million people currently at risk for fall-related injuries and the proportion of those over age 65 increasing annually. In this regard, it seems warranted to emphasize that the baby boomer generation did not contribute to the 2.5% increase in the number of Americans 65 and older documented by the Year 2000 Census (10).

Examination of other causes of SCI shows that the rates associated with sports have been declining, from 14.4% between 1973 and 1979 to 9% between 2000 and 2003 (7). NSCID analysts determined that violence as an etiology increased from 13.3% between 1973 and 1979 to a high of 21.8% in the 1990s. Since then, violence as a leading etiology declined to 11.2% between 2000 and 2003. Comparing these figures to international SCI statistics, with the exception of acts of violence, the etiologies of SCI were similar in other countries, including Denmark, Taiwan, and Spain (7).

For the record, Ho et al. went on to posit: "Successful fall-prevention education for the elderly may mitigate the prevalence of SCI in this population" (7). We offer, without comment, the observation that Ho and coworkers qualified their assertion by suggesting that fall prevention education "may" reduce the incidence of fall-related SCIs, and they did not cite any etiology, other than falls, as possibly being amenable to primary interventions.

THE PREVENTION PARADIGM AND SCI

As in public health practice in general, the prevention paradigm for injury control consists of primary, secondary, and tertiary components. As it pertains to injury control, primary prevention focuses on the sum total of intervention efforts intended to stop the occurrence of an event having injury-producing potential. Secondary prevention encompasses the sum total of intervention efforts intended to reduce the severity of injuries. Finally, tertiary prevention encompasses the sum total of intervention efforts used to restore functional capacity after an injury has occurred.

Interventions can be active or passive. Active interventions, which require specific behavior(s) on the part of the person or populations being protected, are more difficult to implement and have lower coefficients of compliance (11). Passive interventions, which require no specific behavior(s) on the part of the person or populations being protected, are usually far more effective than active interventions (11).

Primary interventions intended to prevent SCIs from ever occurring are the most desirable among all intervention efforts. The caveat is, of course, if they really work. Proving that they work requires demonstrating that the interventions are not merely well-intended activities that fulfill society's laudable need to "do something . . . anything."

It is a given that prevention efforts can never prevent 100% of potential SCIs. Thus, secondary prevention efforts intended to reduce or thwart the development of serious medical complications assume a position of utmost significance in the SCI-prevention paradigm. Results of impressive clinically oriented secondary prevention efforts in SCI medicine are well documented elsewhere in this textbook, so we are not elaborating on them in this chapter.

For many persons with SCI, comprehensive and lifelong rehabilitation success represents the final frontier of the post-injury odyssey. In the context of the prevention paradigm, these efforts are referred to collectively as tertiary prevention. Because tertiary prevention is also addressed elsewhere in this textbook, the information and discussion that follow are confined to primary prevention, the goal of which is to stop SCI from happening in the first place.

THE STATE OF THE SCIENCE

It is not arguable that attempting to prevent SCIs from ever occurring is a praiseworthy goal. Thus, we willingly accepted the editor's invitation to update our original chapter (12). To accomplish this, we conducted an exhaustive review of the primary SCI prevention literature for the period between late 2001 and early 2007. We proceeded in this manner because preparation of the SCI Prevention chapter for the first edition included an exhaustive review of the literature prior to 2003. Surprisingly, we were struck more by what we did not find than by what we found. We discovered that precious little (pro or con) had been written about primary SCI prevention in peer-reviewed journals since the first edition of this textbook was published.

The conspicuous absence of peer-reviewed publications on primary prevention of SCI caused us to broaden our methodology and scope of inquiry. Subsequently, we communicated with several recognized SCI workers who were also members of the American Spinal Injury Association (ASIA). We also communicated with two highly regarded professionals long affiliated with ASIA in important administrative and programmatic capacities.

Almost everyone we contacted had been involved to varying degrees in primary prevention activities during ASIA's early years—1973 through the mid-1980s. Their responses to our inquiries were remarkably similar: they reported being unaware of any current primary prevention activities in which ASIA was involved or had been involved for some time; they didn't know what had become of ASIA's Prevention Committee; and they were unaware of any primary SCI prevention programs of which the efficacy had been unequivocally demonstrated on the basis of a rigorous, independent evaluation.

The substance of the recurring message from a subset of historically dedicated SCI workers who had previously championed primary prevention, coupled with the paucity of current literature on the topic, began to confirm our growing suspicion: for whatever reasons, leaders in the field of SCI medicine and research appear to have become somewhat disenchanted with primary prevention programs whose usefulness had not been or could not be proven. Our reaction is that the field is not back-sliding; rather, it is maturing.

From the most compelling comments we elicited and the limited data we were able to gather, the working experts concluded that even the best general injury prevention education programs reach far too few people to be effective at the population level. In other words, SCI prevention education programs are far too specific to be effective. We concur (G. Whiteneck, M. Dijkers, written communication, April 2007).

Despite becoming increasingly skeptical that the "Holy Grail" of primary SCI prevention existed but had simply not been discovered, we turned our attention to the Cochrane Collaboration, which for us is the court of last resort. The Cochrane Collaboration, an independent, international, not-for-profit organization, is dedicated to making up-to-date, accurate information about the effects of healthcare practices readily available worldwide. It produces and disseminates systematic reviews of healthcare interventions and promotes the search for evidence in the form of clinical trials and other studies of interventions. Founded in 1993 and named after the British epidemiologist Archie Cochrane, the organization's major product is the Cochrane Database of Systematic Reviews, published quarterly as part of *The Cochrane Library* (13).

To our amazement, at the time we conducted our analysis, we found only six reviews dealing specifically with spinal cord injury in the Cochrane Collaboration (24), and none dealt with primary prevention. Rather, the reviews identified on their Web site, at that time, included gangliosides for acute spinal cord injury (P Chinnock), pharmacological interventions for spasticity following spinal cord injury (M Tarrico), spinal fixation surgery for acute traumatic spinal cord injury (A Bagnall), spinal immobilization for trauma patients (I Kwan), spinal injuries centers (SICs) for acute traumatic spinal injury (L Jones), and steroids for acute spinal cord injury (M Bracken).

This is not meant to convey the impression that all primary preventive interventions are without merit. Some, albeit a small number, appear to do what they are designed to do. For example, a largely effective active primary intervention is use of properly designed protective helmets (14–16) and other safety equipment coupled with safety-driven rule changes in certain physically violent contact sports (e.g., prohibition of spearing tackles in American football) (17–19). In the absence of compelling evidence to the contrary, however, it is our conclusion that, for the most part, only secondary and tertiary interventions make impacts on SCIs in any meaningful or measurable way (20–26).

Primary interventions like bicycle helmets and rider-education programs actually target the prevention of head and brain injury, not spinal cord injury (27). Others that advocate more generic programs, such as "falls prevention," really do not target prevention of spinal cord injuries; rather, they target the reduction of falls in general. We cannot minimize the importance of such programs, because falls have become the second leading cause of SCIs in the United States, but we have concluded that this is more likely related to an aging population characterized by less motor vehicle crash exposure coupled with a higher likelihood of falling, a hazard known to be associated with advancing years than with any meaningful SCI-related fall-prevention program (28).

DOES ANYTHING WORK?

The short answer is "yes, probably," but the degree and extent to which most primary interventions seem to work is more likely by default than design.

Consider: Having established that motor vehicle crashes are the leading cause of SCIs and that a disproportionate number of motor vehicle crashes are caused by and/or involve drunk drivers, anti-drunk driving legislation and its associated enforcement is an example of primary prevention. In this case, the intent is to keep motor vehicle crashes caused by intoxicated drivers from ever occurring. Although it is true that state legislatures across the country have adopted tough, anti-drunk driving laws, it cannot be demonstrated, much less proven with any measure of scientific certainty, that such laws result directly in a significant reduction in motor vehicle crash mortality and morbidity statistics including catastrophic trauma, such as SCIs. Intellectual honesty demands that a variety of other factors be considered. For example, improved roadway characteristics, vehicle design that is inherently safer today than in the past, a documented reduction in per capita alcohol consumption, and the like are all factors capable of influencing a measured reduction in alcohol-related motor vehicle crash rates, and hence, morbidity and mortality statistics (29).

Another example of the difficulty associated with attempting to link cause to effect is reflected in the outcome of Congressional action, taken in 1996, abolishing what was at the time a 20-year-old federally imposed 55 mph speed limit. Despite dire predictions of enormous increases in traffic-related fatalities by many highway safety advocates, lawmakers returned the authority to set speed limits to individual states. It is interesting that early statistics suggested the dire projections did not materialize. According to the Insurance Institute for Highway Safety-Highway Loss Data Institute, however, studies reported in January 2007 that deaths on rural interstates increased 25–30% when states began increasing speed limits from 55 to 65 mph in 1987. In 1989 about two-thirds of this increase—19%, or 400 deaths—was attributed to increased speed, the rest to increased travel (30–32).

A 1999 Institute study of the effects of the 1995 repeal of the national maximum speed limit indicates this trend continues. Researchers compared the numbers of motor vehicle occupant deaths in 24 states that raised speed limits during late 1995 and 1996 with corresponding fatality counts in the six years before the speed limits were changed, as well as with fatality counts from seven states that did not change speed limits. The Institute estimated a 15% increase in fatalities on interstates and freeways (33).

Elsewhere, scientists at the Land Transport Safety Authority of New Zealand conducted a separate study to evaluate effects of increasing speed limits from 65 mph to either 70 or 75 mph. Based on deaths in states that did not change their speed limits, states that increased speed limits to 75 mph experienced 38% more deaths per million vehicle miles traveled than expected—an estimated 780 more deaths. States that increased speed limits to 70 mph experienced a 35% increase, resulting in approximately 1,100 more deaths (34).

Nonetheless, the data suggest that although speed is a factor in highway traffic fatalities, today's motor vehicle crash environment is inherently safer than it was nearly 30 years ago (29).

Returning to the etiology responsible for most SCI—motor vehicle crashes—the classic example of an effective secondary preventive intervention is the seat belt/shoulder harness restraint system. The premise is quite simple: if the seat belt/shoulder harness is used correctly, it is likely that any injury, if sustained, will be substantially less severe than without the seat belt/shoulder harness being used. Although "secondary" in character, the seat belt/shoulder harness restraint system is an active intervention requiring the vehicle occupant to make a conscious decision to use it. Secondary interventions can also be passive, meaning that the intervention requires no conscious act on the part of the person to be protected, as is the case of supplemental restraint systems or air bags.

A third example of secondary prevention can be demonstrated from the emergency medical service (EMS) perspective. Specifically, the speed and manner in which the injury site is reached by EMS personnel, coupled with the way in which an injured person is immobilized and extricated from a motor vehicle crash by first-responders, is believed to influence the eventual extent of neurologic sequelae if SCI has occurred. In such cases, the underlying assumption is always that there has been neurologic trauma to the spinal cord. Accordingly, state-of-the-art EMS protocols routinely call for use of comparatively elaborate immobilization techniques of the injured as they are removed from injury sites and transported to trauma centers.

Historically, the operative axiom has long been "better safe than sorry." In the case of possible SCI, conventional wisdom has driven the adoption of elaborate procedures intended to reduce the probability that a neurologically incomplete spinal cord lesion grows worse or even becomes the much more serious neurologically complete injury. It is of more than casual interest, however, that recently the efficacy, in fact the necessity, of elaborate spinal immobilization of most crash victims is being questioned. This somewhat controversial challenge to a long-standing EMS practice is yet another example of how conventional wisdom (read: practice) is now being questioned when conclusive supporting evidence simply does not exist (35, 36).

Preservation of life in the field, during transport as well as acute medical care in emergency and trauma centers are the remaining elements of secondary prevention. These responses encompass a spectrum of finely honed medical and surgical services provided to trauma patients for the purposes of resuscitation, stabilization, treatment, and correction of life-threatening defects or insults.

With regard to secondary prevention among persons with SCI, the emphasis shifts to the prevention of common, costly, and debilitating secondary medical conditions and complications such as pressure ulcers, respiratory infections, pneumonia and atelectasis, autonomic dysreflexia, urinary tract infections, deep vein thrombosis, pulmonary embolism, heterotopic ossification, as well as a wide range of behavioral and psychosocial pathologies.

With regard to rehabilitation, it is clear we are well beyond a point in medical achievement where rehabilitation is optional. There are two reasons for this. First, society no longer refuses to treat gravely injured people, even those with catastrophic conditions who have exceptionally poor prognoses. Second, because of significant advancements in emergency and acute care, many people now survive who in the past would have died soon after being injured.

A substantial amount of research firmly establishes the clinical benefits and economic savings associated with the early, aggressive, and highly expert application of rehabilitation practice and technology to SCI patients. In fact, most injury-related cost estimates described in the injury literature use SCI and TBI as models because their documentation is superior to cost estimates for virtually all other injuries (37).

When comparing injury prevention-education programs to other kinds of interventions (such as the secondary and tertiary interventions described in the preceding examples), it is likely, although admittedly untested at this time, that most current changes detected in the etiology, severity, and characteristics of SCI and its victims are due to (a) real, measurable differences in population demographics, and (b) continually improving secondary interventions, some of which are active, requiring adoption of a particular behavior such as using seat belts. Others are passive and require nothing behaviorally from the person being protected. These passive interventions include biomechanical design improvements of the motor vehicle/occupant interface (e.g., enhanced restraint system configurations, airbags) along with markedly better highways, intensified traffic law-enforcement programs, improved emergency response, and qualitatively improved early and acute care of injured persons on site.

Not surprisingly, there is considerable evidence that those most likely to sustain an SCI do so as a consequence of repetitive risk-taking behaviors. Experience suggests and data confirm that young males, older drivers who habitually operate vehicles while intoxicated, and persons with criminal histories of weapon use are not likely to be affected by lectures, classes, campaigns, billboards, or public service announcements extolling the virtues and benefits of "clean living" and safe behaviors even if they include "frightening scare tactics" advocated by some workers from the disciplines of criminal justice and penology.

SCIENCE, PSEUDOSCIENCE, PREVENTION PROGRAMS, AND NONSENSE

Primary prevention programs are rarely subject to rigorous, objective evaluation. Moreover, on those rare occasions when attempts have been made to critically evaluate the utility, effectiveness, and efficiency of a few rather high-profile (38) prevention activities, the results have been disappointing. Unexpectedly, some reactions to less-than-favorable findings have been embarrassing from a professional standpoint. For example, in his 2003 article published in *Policy Review*, Gorman (38) provides an exceptionally compelling account of two incidents illustrating the extent to which pseudoscientific zealots masquerading as intellectually honest scholars will go to protect their sacred cows. He describes with clarity and elegance how "academic pseudoscience (often) looks, at least superficially, like real science, in that it formulates theories and hypotheses, measures and quantifies phenomena, and conducts statistical analyses." But, as Gorman points out, "while it may display some of the accoutrements of science, it lacks its underlying substance." The short excerpt that follows is central to the focus of this chapter:

> In November 2001, a bizarre incident occurred at a conference sponsored by the Center for Substance Abuse Prevention (CSAP) in Washington, D.C. Christina Hoff Sommers of the American Enterprise Institute was invited to address an assembled audience

of CSAP staff, grantees, and consultants concerning the agency's intentions to fund "Boy Talk," a prevention program for young men designed to influence such behaviors as drug use and violence. Sommers is a critic of this type of gender-specific exercise in health education, and she suggested to the CSAP audience that the effectiveness of such programs and the commitment of dollars to them should be informed by scientific evidence regarding their effectiveness. She observed that "Girl Power!"—the program on which "Boy Talk" was based—remained unsupported by empirical evidence despite having been the recipient of federal funds for the past six years. At this point, a CSAP official informed Sommers that she should end her presentation, apparently because the "Girl Power!" program was off limits. Whether Sommers had been informed of this taboo before she began her talk is not clear, but given the association between the two programs it seems reasonable that the experiences concerning one be used to inform implementation of the other. Anyway, Sommers appears to have soldiered on with her presentation, for within minutes she was apparently instructed to "shut the f—up, bitch" by a member of the audience, causing much merriment among the assembled group of professionals.

Over the summer, I had a similar, although not as overtly censorial or hostile experience while presenting at the Tenth Annual Meeting of the Society for Prevention Research in Seattle, Washington. While nobody dropped the F-bomb on me or called me "bitch," the response to my attempt to examine the scientific base of some widely advocated prevention programs was an ad hominem attack coupled with defensive arguments justifying the violation of basic tenets of evaluation practice in prevention research (38).

It is possible, perhaps likely, that we will incur similar wrath from those who continue to promote a variety of specific primary prevention efforts despite the lack of evidence proving their value. Nonetheless, we can only conclude that primary prevention efforts in general, as well as specific activities targeting injuries such as SCI, have enormous potential for yielding little if any return on investment. Said simply, they are, in almost every well-intended instance, a waste of time and money.

A classic, and to many one of the most stunning, example of the practice we have chosen to describe as "The Emperor Has No Clothes Syndrome" is the historically sacrosanct driver-education program for public high school students. Although supporters argue that driver-education programs are responsible for lower motor vehicle–related mortality statistics, rather convincing evidence exists that driver-education programs are responsible for increasing death and injury because such programs encourage more younger drivers—drivers in the highest-risk age groups—to be on the highways (11, 39, 40, 41). Other critics suggest that given the unappreciated complexity of the driving task and the inherent limitations of driver-education programs, there is little reason such programs might work at all, because no current driver-education program can effectively perform those tasks required of it (42–46).

Another classic example of "The Emperor Has No Clothes Syndrome" is the acclaimed but useless Drug Abuse Resistance Education Program (DARE), a primary intervention that spread to schools across the United States following its inception in 1983. Suffice it to say, DARE has been shown to be as ineffective as high-school driver training. For example, a 3-year study commissioned by the National Institute of Justice in the early 1990s determined that, whereas DARE increased children's self-esteem, helped polish social skills, and improved attitudes toward police,

it did not and does not have a measurable effect on drug abuse, the fundamental purpose of the intervention program. Nonetheless, there are countless settings throughout the country where it remains active and intact because, as one former police chief stated, "I don't care if it doesn't work; it looks like I'm doing something and that's all that matters to these parents" (C. Trucks [former Homewood, Alabama, police chief], oral communication; April 1997).

The point is, that in the absence of rigorous evaluation criteria and practices, even the most promising, logical-sounding, and emotionally appealing interventions may fall far short of their intended purpose. Thus, before adopting a primary prevention program for SCI (or any other injuries), that program should be subjected to the litmus test of rigorously documented evidence of the intervention's effectiveness. Such data are often difficult to acquire, but in this era of the demand for increasing accountability, such data are not merely desirable, they are mandatory. In today's highly competitive health-promotion arena, primary prevention resources are much too scarce to squander on programs that sound good on paper and "feel good" during execution but do not work in practice.

EVALUATION

Entire textbooks have been written on the evaluation process and its meaning in health promotion. Depending on the perspective of the user or consumer of evaluative information, the reasons given for evaluating differ. Moreover, precisely where one stands relative to evaluation depends on how one regards policy and program. As different as these reasons may appear, a common thread binding them is the need to know what works . . . and what doesn't. The products of evaluation can helpfully inform each of these parties and other stakeholders. Their enlightenment can provide support for continuing and improving useful programs and for discontinuing unproductive programs and reallocating resources.

Evaluation may be defined in several ways. To some, it is a means to determine the extent to which a program has succeeded or failed. To others, evaluation serves as a management tool to improve planning and implementation or to influence policy-making. Many see it as collecting data from participants to determine their degree of satisfaction with or acceptance of the program's process and content. Still others believe it is a waste of time and money. Regardless of the viewpoint, most program evaluations should be concerned with the following five broad questions (47):

- Is the intervention reaching the target population?
- Is it being implemented in the ways specified?
- Is it effective?
- How much does it cost?
- What are its costs relative to its documented effectiveness?

One of the first steps in evaluation planning is to conduct a needs assessment and to prepare objectives. Common excuses or rationales for not conducting a comprehensive program evaluation invariably cite not enough time, not enough resources, and circumstances that simply preclude a formal evaluation. In such instances, it is our conclusion that program staffs determine, almost arbitrarily, what a program can or cannot achieve.

Determination of need usually involves some combination of the following: (1) a review of existing research on the target health problem and associated behaviors (typically, there is emphasis on the knowledge, attitudes, and skills of populations similar to the target population; environmental influences; and the role and responsibility of relevant professionals and social support resources); (2) a review of existing data sources related to the nature, frequency, and circumstances surrounding the health problems, health behaviors, and educational level(s) of the target population(s); (3) the collection of original data on the knowledge, beliefs, and attitudes of the target population: the health professionals; and (4) significant involvement regarding the health problem(s) and health behaviors of interest (48). Table 81.1 summarizes some of the more common needs

Table 81.1 Common Needs Assessment Methodologies

METHOD	ADVANTAGES	DISADVANTAGES	COSTS
Telephone surveys	Potential short response time Difficult questions answered Access to population based on phone availability	Labor intensive Questionable validity Access to specific respondents limited by availability	High
E-mail/mail surveys	Wide distribution Potential anonymity of respondents Validity of results	Lengthy process Variable, low response rate Limited number of questions viable Respondent bias Mailing list required Cost for nonrespondents	Low
Delphi Process	Pooled responses Spans distance and time High motivation and commitment of respondents Equal representation or response Consistent respondent contact and buy-in	Reduced clarification opportunities	High
Key informant technique	Expert information Time-efficient Ability to clarify questions and responses	Difficult to select valid experts Representativeness of respondents Agenda of respondent (vested interests) Need to base judgments on limited number of responses	Low
Focus groups	Convenient Creative atmosphere Targeted and focused question areas Ease of clarification	Qualitative information Limited representativeness Dependent on moderator skill Data preliminary in nature	Low
Community forum	Easy to conduct Open to advertised audience People can participate on their own terms Tends to attract interested people	Difficult to get representative mix Participants tend to be representatives of special interest groups or zealots Must be moderated effectively to keep from generating into a gripe session Data analysis can be time-consuming and difficult (validity and reliability)	Low
Nominal group process	Direct involvement of targeted groups Planned interactivity with respondents Toleration of diverse opinions Creative atmosphere	Time commitment Competing issues Participant bias Segmented planning involvement	Low
Literature review	Ease of acquisition of information Peer-reviewed information Provides foundation of information Provides historical perspective	Timeliness of data Need to make information relevant to "local" situation External validity	Low
Socioeconomic indicators	Availability of standardized data Snapshot perspective Time-efficient	Validity of data in question Interpretation of data open to question Data become dated Time-consuming to collect	Low

assessment methodologies and cites some of their inherent advantages and limitations.

In general, program staff should probably set modest expectations for their programs, although it seems to be human nature in such instances to be overly ambitious. Moreover, trying to retrospectively evaluate something that cannot be easily evaluated represents a common problem with which program staff must deal.

Program evaluators need to approach the development and revision of an evaluation plan with insights into how different parts, methods, and designs relate to one another conceptually and operationally. Adjustments in one component or method almost always affect another dimension. Attention to detail at the outset will, in general, improve the ability to revise and adapt the plan as it unfolds (49).

Four specific types of evaluations can be used to organize approaches to evaluation of primary prevention health-promotion and education programs: (1) Process Evaluation, (2) Formative Evaluation, (3) Impact Evaluation, and (4) Evaluation Research. The purposes, methods, and characteristics of each are interrelated, and the general characteristics of each evaluation type appear in Table 81.2.

Table 81.2   General Characteristics by Type of Evaluation

LEVEL	SELECTED GENERAL CHARACTERISTICS
1. Process Evaluation (quality assurance)	Applies nonexperimental designs Monitors procedures-effort-activity Examines structure and process Conducts observational analyses Performs qualitative observations Monitors effort-activity Reviews: audits data and records
2. Formative Evaluation	Assesses immediate or short-term impact Field-tests measurement and intervention methods Emphasizes internal validity Employs qualitative evaluation methods
3. Impact (program, summative)	Assesses behavioral impact Emphasizes internal validity Uses simple analyses and comparisons Applies tested interventions Employs formative and summative evaluation methods
4. Evaluation Research	Tests hypothesis on behavior change Uses multivariate analyses Improves knowledge base Grounded in theory—tests new methods Emphasizes internal and external validity Assesses behavior impact and health outcome

CAN A CASE BE MADE FOR PRIMARY PREVENTION?

In a word, the answer to the question is "Yes," but there are caveats. Prevention research has revealed two important requisites: first, successful prevention strategies must incorporate theory-based interventions and methods, and second, prevention strategies can be improved upon in virtually all instances by adopting and implementing underlying theory.

The use of theory in prevention programs can help provide a better understanding of the nature of targeted health behaviors, and theory can explain the dynamics of behavior, processes for changing behavior, and the effects of external influences on behavior. Whereas theory alone does not and cannot produce effective prevention programs, theory-based planning, implementation, and monitoring does. Theory is important in determining what to look for (research strategy), what to achieve (preventive intervention goals), and in helping explain the outcome of interventions. Finally, theory enables us to consider ideas and strategies that we might otherwise never have envisioned (50).

Many theories are associated with the social and behavioral sciences, but their practical application demands an understanding of epidemiology and physical sciences. Further, experience has demonstrated that no single theory is dominant in prevention programs. In fact, one of the major problems facing public health workers is the challenge of adapting a particular theory so that it works with a particular issue. To meet this sort of challenge, the fit must be logical and consistent with everyday observations. Also, the theoretic strategy should be similar to those used successfully in other programs, and for reproducibility and validity, the theory should be supported by rigorously derived evidence.

PREVENTION EFFORTS: DATA GATHERING AND NEEDS ASSESSMENT

The first and most critical step in the planning process is the acquisition of accurate, comprehensive data describing and characterizing the target community. To this end, several assessment strategies can be used to collect data. Each assessment strategy is categorized into one of the following areas: Assessment with Individuals, Assessment with Groups, Literature Review, and Socioeconomic Indicators. For more about these indicators, see Table 81.3.

Designing an effective intervention requires a well-choreographed balancing act. Proposed curtailment of personal liberty must be carefully scrutinized and weighed against the expected benefit to society as a whole. For example, although passive strategies (e.g., automatic seat belts) are likely to be more effective than those requiring radical behavioral changes, alienation of the public may become an unintended consequence. On the other hand, attempting to coax a target population into long-term behavior modification is also fraught with difficulty and may not be realistic, or it may run the risk of appearing to "blame the victim" or place an inordinate burden of responsibility for injury prevention on the individual. Gielen (51) examined the tension between those in the field of injury prevention who endorse circumventing the role of individual behavior through the provision of automatic or passive protection and those who support

Table 81.3   Assessment Strategies for Data Collection

I. Assessment with Individuals
  1. Single Step
     Telephone
     Mail
     Email
  2. Multi Step (Delphi)
  3. Interviews (Face to Face)
  4. Key Informant

II. Assessment with Groups
  1. Nominal Group
  2. Focus Group
  3. Community Forum
  4. Electronic Conferencing

III. Literature Review

IV. Socioeconomic Indicators

attempting to change the behavior of the individual. Ideally, the two approaches can complement one another and provide a stronger framework for effective intervention than either approach by itself. Another facet of this controversy entails designing interventions that successfully meld educational, legal, and engineering components. As one might expect, striking a balance can be challenging at best and an exercise in frustration at worst.

While pondering the merits and pitfalls of various injury-prevention programs, it may be helpful to keep in mind that optimal strategies often reflect the following principles: (a) priority and emphasis should be given to countermeasures that will most effectively reduce injury losses, regardless of their relative causal importance or position (order of occurrence) in the sequence of events; (b) a mixed strategy should usually be employed, incorporating countermeasures addressed to the pre-event, event, and post-event phases of the injury control sequence; (c) preference should be given to passive measures that protect automatically without any action on the individual's part; (d) neither mechanical failure nor human action should result in injury or property damage (the fail-safe principle); and (e) cost-effectiveness should be considered. It should be noted that effective injury control is, in essence, practical problem solving at its best. In fact, some of the most innovative interventions have arisen through the vision of individuals who recognized unmet needs or threats to personal safety and who subsequently endeavored to address those needs in the most practical manner available. And, despite that which we have described, practical experience suggests that this does not always require adopting that which researchers deem classic health-behavior theories and models (12).

Clearly, primary prevention has the potential to be the most cost-effective form of injury control, but it is also the most abstract and elusive. It is difficult to measure precisely something that does not happen in the absence of historically accurate surveillance data. Moreover, cause-effect relationships are notoriously difficult to prove, especially when attempting to ascribe change to something as complex as human behavior (12).

Measures to prevent injuries or lessen the severity of their consequences have been used since ancient times (11, 52).

Today, the rapidly expanding field of injury prevention and control has become a complex mixture of disciplines whose primary link is a common mission to reduce injury-related morbidity, mortality, and disability. Modern injury control theoreticians and practitioners come from disciplines as diverse as medicine, engineering, sociology, psychology, epidemiology, health education, health promotion, political science, and criminal justice (49).

Last but not least, the obvious lesson distilled from all of this is that the SCI that is least expensive, easiest to manage medically, psychologically, socially, and vocationally, and has the best long-term prognosis is the one that does not happen.

Current thinking as reflected by a striking reduction in the number of educationally oriented primary prevention initiatives strongly suggests that more and more workers regard people who are at the greatest risk for sustaining catastrophic injuries, including SCI, to be risk takers whose behaviors are not likely to be influenced by educational efforts. Thus, it is our recommendation that any primary intervention be subjected to rigorous evaluation. Then, if the intervention's efficacy cannot be proven or if its cost-benefit ratio is unrealistic, it should be discontinued, no matter how emotionally appealing it might appear on its surface.

References

1. National Spinal Cord Injury Statistical Center. Spinal cord injury: facts and figures at a glance. June 2006. *J Spinal Cord Med* 2007; 30:79–80.
2. Fine PR, Kuhlemeier KV, DeVivo MJ, Stover SL. Spinal cord injury: An epidemiologic perspective. *Paraplegia* 1979; 17:237–250.
3. Charles ED, Van Matre JG, Miller JM. Spinal cord injury—a cost benefit analysis of alternative treatment models. *Paraplegia* 1974; 12(3):222–231.
4. DeVivo MJ, Fine PR, Maetz HM, Wheat R. Prevalence of spinal cord injury: a re-estimation employing life-table techniques. *Arch Neurol* 1980; 37(11):707–708.
5. Bosshart HT. Social issues in spinal cord injury. In: Lin VW, ed. *Spinal Cord Medicine: Principles and Practice.* New York: Demos Medical Publishing, Inc; 2003; 941–947.
6. DeVivo MJ. Model spinal cord injury systems of care. In: Lin VW, ed. *Spinal Cord Medicine: Principles and Practice.* New York: Demos Medical Publishing, Inc; 2003; 955–957.
7. Ho CH, Wuermser LA, Priebe MM, Chiodo AE, Scelza WM and Kirshblum SC. Spinal cord injury medicine.1.Epidemiology and Classification. *Arch Phys Med Rehabil* 2007; 88(3 Suppl 1):S49–S54.
8. National Center for Injury Prevention and Control. Falls among older adults: An overview. http://www.cdc.gov/ncipc/duip/preventadultfalls.htm. Accessed April 3, 2007.
9. Kannus P, Palvanen M, Niemi S, Parkkari J. Alarming rise in the number and incidence of fall-induced cervical spine injuries among older adults. *Journal of Gerontology: Medical Sciences* 2007; 62A(2):180–183.
10. Smith DI, Spraggins RE. Gender: 2000: Census 2000 Brief. Washington, DC:US Department of Commerce; 2001.
11. National Committee for Injury Prevention and Control. Injury prevention: Meeting the challenge. *Am J Prev Med.* 1989; 5(3 Suppl):1–303.
12. Fine PR, Sykes-Horn W, Terry K. The prevention of spinal cord injury. In: Lin VW, ed. *Spinal Cord Medicine: Principles and Practice.* New York: Demos Medical Publishing, Inc; 2003; 885–928.
13. The Cochrane Collection. What is The Cochrane Collaboration? http://www.cochrane.org/docs/descrip.htm. Accessed April 3, 2007.
14. Vardy J, Clinton E, Graham A. Audit of an intervention to decrease cycle related head injuries in primary school children. *Inj Prev* 2006; 12:271–272.
15. Gittelman MA., Pomerantz WJ, Groner JI, Smith GA. Pediatric all-terrain vehicle-related injuries in Ohio from 1995 to 2001: Using the Injury Severity Score to determine whether helmets are a solution. *Pediatrics* 2006; 117: 2190–2195.

16. Kloss FR, Tuli T, Haechl O, Gassner R. Trauma injuries sustained by cyclists. *Trauma* 2006; 8:77–84.

17. Pelletier JC. Sports related concussion and spinal injuries: the need for changing spearing rules at the National Capital Amateur Football Association. *J Can Chiropr Assoc* 2006; 50(3):195–208.

18. McIntosh AS, McCrory P. Preventing head and neck injury. *Br J Sports Med* 2005; 39:314–318.

19. Heck JF, Clarket KS, Peterson TR, Torg JS, Weis, MP. National Athletic Trainers' Association position statement: head-down contact and spearing in tackle football. *J Athl Train* 2004; 39(1):101–111.

20. Sege RD, Hatmaker-Flanigan E, De Vos E, Levin-Goodman R, Spivak H. Anticipatory guidance and violence prevention: results from family and pediatrician focus groups. *Pediatrics* 2006; 117:455–463.

21. Rivara FP, Mock C. The 1,000,000 lives campaign. *Inj Prev* 2005; 11:321–323.

22. Klein KS, Thompson D, Scheidt PC, Overpeck MD, Gross LA. The HBSC international investigators. Factors associated with bicycle helmet use among young adolescents in a multinational sample. *Inj Prev* 2005; 11:288–293.

23. Hagel B, Pless IB, Goulet C. The effect of wrist guard use on upper-extremity injuries in snowboarders. *Am J Epidemiol* 2005; 162:149–156.

24. Hagel BE, Pless IB, Goulet C, Platt RW, Robitaille Y. Quality of information on risk factors reported by ski patrols. *Inj Prev* 2004; 10:275–279.

25. Sheikh A, Cook A, Ashcroft R. Making cycle helmets compulsory: ethical arguments for legislation. *J R Soc Med* 2004; 97:262–265.

26. Doll L, Binder S. Injury prevention research at the Centers for Disease Control and Prevention. *Am J Public Health* 2004; 94:522–524.

27. The Cochrane Collaboration. Cochrane Injuries Group: Spinal Cord Injury. http://www.cochrane-injuries.lshtm.ac.uk/Review%20links%20Dec06.htm#spinal. Accessed April 3, 2007.

28. Australian Government Department of Health and Ageing. National Falls Prevention for Older People Initiative. http://www.health.gov.au/internet/wcms/Publishing.nsf/Content/health-pubhlth-strateg-injury-falls-index.htm. Accessed April 4, 2007.

29. Fine PR, Tomasek AD, Horn WS, Rousculp MD. Unintentional Injury. In: Raczynski JM, DiClemente RJ, eds. *Handbook of Health Promotion and Disease Prevention*. New York: Kluwer Academic/Plenum Publishers; 1999:309–334.

30. Baum HM, Wells JK, Lund AK. The fatality consequences of the 65 mph speed limits, 1989. *J Safety Res* 1991; 22:171–177.

31. Baum HM, Lund AK, Wells JK. The mortality consequences of raising the speed limit to 65 mph on rural interstates. *Am J Public Health* 1989; 79:1392–95.

32. Baum HM, Lund AK, Wells JK. Motor vehicle crash fatalities in the second year of 65 mph speed limits. *J Safety Res* 1991; 21:1–8.

33. Farmer CM, Retting RA, Lund, AK. Changes in motor vehicle occupant fatalities after repeal of the national maximum speed limit. *Accid Anal Prev* 1999; 31:537–4.

34. Patterson TL, Frith WJ, Povey LJ, Keall MD. The effect of increasing rural interstate speed limits in the United States. *Traffic Inj Prev* 2002; 3:316–20.

35. Hauswald M, Braude D. Spinal immobilization in trauma patients: is it really necessary? *Curr Opin Crit Care* 2002; 8(6):566–570.

36. Bunn F, Kwan I, Roberts I, Wentz R. Effectiveness of pre-hospital trauma care. Report to the World Health Organization. January 2001. Available at www.cochrane-injuries.lshtm.ac.uk/Pre-HospFINALReport2.pdf. Accessed April 4, 2007.

37. Institute of Medicine, Division of Health Sciences Policy. Enabling America: assessing the role of rehabilitation science and engineering. Washington, DC: National Academy Press; 1997.

38. Gorman, D M Prevention programs and scientific nonsense. *Policy Review* Feb–Mar 2003; 117: 65–75.

39. Robertson LS. *Injuries: Causes, Control Strategies and Public Policy.* Lexington, MA: Lexington Books; 1983.

40. Robertson LS. Crash involvement of teenaged drivers when driver education is eliminated from high school. *Am J Public Health* 1980; 70:599–603.

41. Robertson LS, Zador PL. Driver education and fatal crash involvement of teenaged drivers. *Am J Public Health* 1978; 68:959–965.

42. Waller PF. Young drivers: reckless or unprepared? In: Mayhew DR, Simpson HM, Donelson AC, eds. *Young Driver Accidents: In Search of Solutions.* Traffic Injury Research Foundation of Canada;1985: 103–146.

43. Stock JR, Weaver JK, Ray HW, Brink JR, Sadof MG. *Evaluation of Safe Performance Secondary Driver Education Curriculum Demonstration Project.* Washington, DC: National Highway Traffic Safety Administration;1983.

44. Lund AK, Williams AF, Zador P. High School Driver Education: Further Evaluation of the DeKalb County Study. *Accid Anal Prev* 1986; 18:349–357.

45. Smith MF. Summary of Preliminary Results. Follow-up Evaluation: Safe Performance Curriculum Driver Education Project. Paper presented at annual conference of the American Driver and Traffic Safety Education Association; 1987.

46. Potvin LP, Champagne F, Laberge-Nadeau C. Mandatory driver training and road safety: the Quebec experience. *Am J Public Health* 1988; 78:1206–1209.

47. Rossi P, Freeman H, Wright S. *Evaluation: A systematic approach.* Beverly Hills, CA: Sage; 1979.

48. Simons-Morton B, Greene W, Gottlieb N. *Introduction to Health Education and Health Promotion.* 2nd ed. Prospect Heights, IL: Waveland Press, Inc.;1995.

49. Windsor R, Baronowski T, Clark N, Cutter G. *Evaluation of Health Promotion, Health Education, and Disease Prevention Programs.* 2nd ed. London: Mayfield Publishing Company; 1994.

50. Glanz K, Rimer B. Theory at a glance: A guide for health promotion practice. National Institutes of Health: National Cancer Institute; 1997.

51. Gielen AC. Health Education and Injury Control: Integrating approaches. *Health Educ Q* 1992; 19(2):203–218.

52. Healthy People 2000 Progress Review. Unintentional Injury. Department of Health & Human Services. United States Public Health Service; 1996.

82 Model Spinal Cord Injury Systems of Care

Michael J. DeVivo

At the beginning of World War II, the prognosis for persons with spinal cord injury (SCI) was so poor, especially for those who had neurologically complete injuries, that rehabilitation was not usually even contemplated. Incidence was reasonably low, and most persons with SCI survived no more than 1 or 2 years. However, during the war, the British were faced with the catastrophic circumstances of many air raid casualties and military personnel receiving SCIs. As a result, in 1943 British authorities, led by Sir Ludwig Guttmann, established a new spinal care unit at the Stoke Mandeville Hospital in Aylesbury and introduced the concept of comprehensive treatment and rehabilitation for people with SCI (1). Eventually, Stoke Mandeville Hospital was designated as the National Spinal Injuries Center and began admitting people with SCI from throughout the United Kingdom. Shortly thereafter, Donald Munro established the first SCI unit in the United States (US) at Boston University Hospital. The US Veterans Administration (VA) also established specialized SCI programs at six VA hospitals (1). Treatment outcomes for people with SCI improved dramatically through a combination of the enhanced knowledge and expertise that could be obtained only through treatment of sufficient numbers of similar patients, coupled with general medical advances such as the development of antibiotics and other methods of surgical and medical management of the sequelae of SCI.

By 1970 the success of the SCI programs at Stoke Mandeville Hospital and the VA led the Rehabilitation Services Administration (RSA) in the US Department of Health, Education and Welfare (HEW) to begin supporting research and demonstration projects for Model Systems for the treatment of the SCI civilian population that would be comparable to the programs at Stoke Mandeville and the VA. When HEW was split into separate departments, the SCI Model Systems demonstration projects were placed in the Department of Education, where they remain today. Currently, the SCI Model System program is housed in the National Institute on Disability and Rehabilitation Research (NIDRR) within the Office of Special Education and Rehabilitative Services.

The first SCI Model System was funded in Phoenix, Arizona, combining the resources of Good Samaritan Medical Center, Barrow Neurological Institute, St. Joseph's Hospital, the Arizona Highway Patrol, Arizona State Rehabilitation Agency, and Arizona State University into a regional system of care. In 1973 six additional SCI Model Systems were funded in Alabama, New York, Texas, Illinois, Virginia, and California (2). In 1974 new SCI Model Systems were funded in Colorado and Washington, and in 1975 another Model System in Massachusetts was funded. By 1982 seventeen SCI Model Systems were being funded by NIDRR.

In each case, initial funding was awarded through an open competition announced in the Federal Register. Once a program had achieved Model System status, additional funding each year was obtained through noncompeting continuation applications. However, beginning in 1982, all existing SCI Model Systems were required to re-compete periodically for the continued designation and funding of their programs. As a result, membership in the SCI Model System program has changed over time, with some Model Systems losing or reacquiring funding at the same time that new locations were being funded (Table 82.1). Currently, there are fourteen SCI Model Systems with annual funding for each that is between $449,417 and $489,000. The current Model System grants expire on September 30, 2011.

MISSION

Originally, the Model System program was designed and intended to demonstrate the innovative, comprehensive, and multidisciplinary methods of treatment of people with SCI and to evaluate the benefits of these treatment methods. However, after conducting an external review of the Model System program in 1999, NIDRR concluded that the value of a comprehensive integrated system of care for people with SCI had been demonstrated and was widely accepted (3–7). Therefore, NIDRR shifted the focus of the program to reduce emphasis on demonstration of Model System treatment effectiveness in favor of the establishment of centers of excellence for the conduct of high-quality individual and collaborative SCI research (8).

Table 82.1 SCI Model Systems and their Years of Participation in the Program

MODEL SYSTEM LOCATION	YEARS
Alabama, Birmingham	1973–2011
Arizona, Phoenix	1973–1985
California, Downey	1980–1981, 1983–2006
California, Northridge	1982
California, San Jose	1973–1985, 1990–2006
Colorado, Englewood	1974–2011
District of Columbia, Washington	2006–2011
Florida, Miami	1979–1981, 1984–1985, 2000–2006
Georgia, Atlanta	1982–2011
Illinois, Chicago	1973–2000, 2006–2011
Louisiana, New Orleans	1983–1985
Massachusetts, Boston	1976–1990, 1995–2011
Michigan, Ann Arbor	1985–2011
Michigan, Detroit	1982–2000
Minnesota, Minneapolis	1982
Missouri, Columbia	1979–1981, 1995–2006
New York, Mount Sinai	1990–2011
New York, NYU	1973–1990
New York, Rochester	1982–1990
New Jersey, West Orange	1990–2011
Ohio, Cleveland	1995–2000, 2006–2011
Pennsylvania, Philadelphia	1979–2011
Pennsylvania, Pittsburgh	2000–2011
Texas, Houston	1973–2011
Virginia, Fishersville	1973–1983, 1985–1990
Virginia, Richmond	1995–2006
Washington, Seattle	1974–1985, 1990–2011
Wisconsin, Milwaukee	1995–2000

MODEL SYSTEM REQUIREMENTS

Currently, there are seven basic requirements that each SCI Model System must meet to qualify for funding (9). First, each SCI Model System is still required to establish a multidisciplinary system of providing rehabilitation services specifically designed to meet the needs of individuals with SCI, including emergency medical services, acute care, vocational and other rehabilitation services, community and job placement, and long-term community follow-up and health maintenance. However, although all these required components of care must be present and coordinated into a single cohesive program at each Model System, there is considerable flexibility in the methods used to meet these requirements. As a result, no two Model Systems are set up in exactly the same way. Therefore, no unique Model System of care exists for persons with SCI, but rather a broad outline of the services that should be provided and methods to provide them efficiently (10).

The second requirement is that each SCI Model System must address the needs of people with disabilities who come from traditionally underserved populations. Although not specified in the Federal Register announcement, these underserved populations include, among others, nonwhite racial and ethnic groups, people residing in rural areas, and people with inadequate or no health insurance or financial resources. The services to be provided include both direct medical and consultative services,

opportunities to participate in research, and targeted information dissemination.

Each SCI Model System must ensure participation of individuals with disabilities in all aspects of its research. This concept requires that individuals with disabilities be involved in the conceptualization, design, planning, and conduct of research, as well as in the interpretation of results and dissemination of findings, and it ensures that projects will be perceived to have high priority and relevance to the daily lives of individuals who have SCI.

Each SCI Model System must also contribute data on at least thirty new patients it serves each year to a national SCI Model Systems database. Although the actual data to be collected have changed over time, currently these data include basic patient demographics, measures of injury severity, information on the occurrence of associated injuries, surgical procedures that occur during hospitalization, length of stay in acute care and rehabilitation, patient status at hospital discharge, functional independence, and follow-up medical, vocational, and psychosocial data gathered at the 1st, 5th, 10th, 15th, 20th, 25th, 30th, and 35th anniversary of injury (2, 11).

The national SCI Model Systems database began in Phoenix in 1975, using independent funding from RSA. Funding for that activity was terminated in 1981. In 1983 the SCI Model System in Alabama reinitiated the national database, using funding contributed by each of the other Model Systems. In 1984 NIDRR reinstituted direct federal funding of the national SCI Model Systems database through a supplemental award to the National Spinal Cord Injury Statistical Center (NSCISC), located at the Model System in Alabama, where the database remains today (12). Beginning in July 2001, funding of the NSCISC at the Model System in Alabama has occurred through a separate open competition and subsequent cooperative agreement with NIDRR. The current cooperative agreement expires on September 30, 2011, in conjunction with the expiration of current SCI Model System grants, at which time a new open competition will presumably occur (13).

Beginning in 2006, to enhance database continuity given the changes in Model Systems over time shown in Table 82.1, the NSCISC was required to implement procedures to acquire follow-up data on persons already enrolled in the database from Model Systems whose funding was discontinued (13). As a result, the NSCISC has subcontracted with several former Model Systems to continue acquiring and submitting follow-up data on their patients, thereby reducing losses to follow-up and the potential bias they might cause.

The fifth requirement of a Model System is that it must conduct one or two site-specific SCI research projects that test innovative approaches that contribute to rehabilitation interventions and evaluating outcomes in accordance with the focus areas identified in the NIDRR Long Range Plan. Focus areas include employment outcomes, maintaining health and function, technology for access and function, independent living and community integration, the refinement of measures of medical rehabilitation effectiveness, and the impact of national telecommunications and information policy on the access of people with SCI to related education, work, and other opportunities. An extensive review of the history and outcomes of SCI Model Systems research programs has been published (14).

SCI Model Systems are also required to propose at least one collaborative research module project and participate in at least one collaborative research module project with other Model Systems. Module projects are typically extensions of the NSCISC database (additional variables on a focused topic). At the beginning of the funding cycle, the SCI Model System project directors, in conjunction with NIDRR, selected the projects that would be implemented from among the proposals that had been peer-reviewed and approved by NIDRR.

Finally, the seventh requirement of a Model System is that it must coordinate with the NIDRR-funded Model Systems Knowledge Translation Center, located at the University of Washington, to provide scientific results and information for dissemination to clinical and consumer audiences using culturally appropriate methods of community outreach and education.

COLLABORATIVE RESEARCH

A few of the SCI Model Systems began participating in specific collaborative research protocols other than the national database in 1982, when the Medical Rehabilitation Research and Training Center, located at the SCI Model System in Alabama, secured funding for a study of long-term survival of patients treated at Model Systems (15, 16). By 1985 specific collaborative research protocols among the Model Systems were a required part of each application for designation and funding as a Model System (17). This continued until 2000, when applicants for Model System designation were required only to demonstrate the capacity for participating in collaborative research, but did not have to include specific protocols in their grant applications.

A separate competition for the funding of collaborative research projects was held in 2001, and three grants were awarded by NIDRR (18). These included a study of upper limb pain, a study of lifetime outcomes and needs as persons with SCI get older, and a study of pharmacological management of dyslipidemia and cardiovascular disease in persons with tetraplegia (17). Most, but not all, of the Model Systems participated in one of the three collaborative projects (three to five Model Systems per project). Separating the collaborative research proposals from the original Model System applications allowed each proposal to obtain a more thorough scientific peer review and also created the potential for larger-scale projects with bigger budgets (up to $350,000 per project per year) to be funded. It also allowed non-Model Systems to participate in the research as long as they collaborated with at least two existing SCI Model Systems.

In 2006 NIDRR again established a separate funding mechanism for SCI Model System collaborative projects with substantially increased budgets. Two projects were funded, each with a budget of approximately $5.8 million spread over 5 years. One project under the leadership of Craig Hospital is entitled "Improving Spinal Cord Injury Rehabilitation Outcomes," and the other, under the leadership of the University of Washington, is entitled "Controlled Trial of Venlafaxine XR for Depression after Spinal Cord Injury."

ORGANIZATIONAL STRUCTURE

Each SCI Model System has a project director, who is typically but not always a physician (generally a physiatrist or an orthopedic surgeon). Generally, a second doctoral-level nonphysician serves as either a co-director or as director of research. In those instances when the project director is a nonphysician, then the co-director is typically a physician. Each Model System also has one or more data collectors assigned to gather and submit information on its patients to the NSCISC, and it provides funding for other personnel involved in the specific research projects proposed in the grant application. Clinical services are generally not funded by the Model System grant, unless they are newly designed services being evaluated as part of a specific research project.

The project directors and co-directors (or directors of research) meet every 6 months with the NSCISC director and the NIDRR project officer in Washington, D.C. An Executive Committee is established at the beginning of each grant cycle, and one of the project directors is elected to chair the Executive Committee and the biannual project director meetings. During these meetings, future collaborative efforts and progress on current activities are discussed, and decisions are made concerning the scope and content of the national database.

CONCLUSION

The SCI Model Systems have an illustrious history of developing new treatment protocols and evaluating their effectiveness, conducting epidemiologic and health services research, assessing long-term psychosocial and health outcomes of persons treated at Model Systems, and advocating to government and private entities on behalf of persons with SCI (19). The Model Systems have individually and collectively produced thousands of professional and consumer-oriented training materials, presentations, and publications since the inception of the program (7). These training and dissemination activities have led to the development of other high-quality SCI treatment programs throughout the country. These programs often include all the required clinical elements of a Model System, although they may not be officially designated as Model Systems. The continued development of additional coordinated, multidisciplinary treatment programs is essential to increase access to high-quality care for all individuals with SCI.

The increased focus of the Model System program on collaborative research is an important step forward that will undoubtedly improve our capability to study the occurrence, risk factors, and effective treatments of the relatively rare sequelae of SCI. The national database created by the Model Systems is by far the largest and most productive SCI database in the world, including over 25,000 patients injured since 1973 (1). With continued funding from NIDRR, during the next 5 years efforts will be undertaken to link this database with other sources of information and databases to enhance our research capability and advance our knowledge of SCI to the next level.

R*eferences*

1. Tulsky DS. The impacts of the model SCI system: historical perspective. *J Spinal Cord Med* 2002; 25:310–315.
2. Stover SL, DeVivo MJ, Go BK. History, implementation, and current status of the national spinal cord injury database. *Arch Phys Med Rehabil* 1999; 80:1365–1371.
3. DeVivo MJ, Kartus PL, Stover SL, Fine PR. Benefits of early admission to an organised spinal cord injury care system. *Paraplegia* 1990; 28:545–555.
4. Heinemann AW, Yarkony GM, Roth EJ, Lovell L, Hamilton B, Meyer PR, Brown JT. Functional outcome following spinal cord injury: A comparison of specialized spinal cord injury center vs general hospital acute care. *Arch Neurol* 1989; 46:1098–1102.

5. Oakes DD, Wilmot CB, Hall KM, Sherck JP. Benefits of early admission to a comprehensive trauma center for patients with spinal cord injury. *Arch Phys Med Rehabil* 1990; 71:637–643.

6. Donovan WH, Carter RE, Bedbrook GM, Young JS, Griffiths ER. Incidence of medical complications in spinal cord injury: Patients in specialised, compared with non–specialised centres. *Paraplegia* 1984; 22:282–290.

7. Apple DF, Hudson LM, eds. *Spinal Cord Injury: The Model.* Proceedings of the National Consensus Conference on Catastrophic Illness and Injury, December 1989. Atlanta: Shepherd Center for Treatment of Spinal Injuries, 1990.

8. DeVivo MJ, Jackson AB, Dijkers MP, Becker BE. Current research outcomes from the model spinal cord injury care systems. *Arch Phys Med Rehabil* 1999; 80:1363–1364.

9. Federal Register. 2006; 71(38):9891–9892.

10. Kirshblum SC. Clinical activities of the model spinal cord injury system. *J Spinal Cord Med* 2002; 25:339–344.

11. DeVivo MJ, Go BK, Jackson AB. Overview of the national spinal cord injury statistical center database. *J Spinal Cord Med* 2002; 25:335–338.

12. DeVivo MJ. The history of the national spinal cord injury statistical center database, 1973–2000, with epidemiological findings from the United States and other countries. *Eur Med Phys* 2000; 36:109–114.

13. Federal Register. 2006; 71(82): 25472–25476.

14. Tate DG, Forchheimer M. Contributions from the model systems programs to spinal cord injury research. *J Spinal Cord Med* 2002; 25:316–330.

15. DeVivo MJ, Kartus PL, Stover SL, Rutt RD, Fine PR. Seven-year survival following spinal cord injury. *Arch Neurol* 1987; 44:872–875.

16. DeVivo MJ, Kartus PL, Stover SL, Rutt RD, Fine PR. Cause of death for patients with spinal cord injuries. *Arch Intern Med* 1989;149:1761–1766.

17. Richards JS. Collaborative research in the model spinal cord injury systems: process and outcomes. *J Spinal Cord Med* 2002; 25:331–334.

18. Federal Register. 2000; 65(248): 81492–81514.

19. Elliott TR, Richards JS, DeVivo MJ, Jackson AB, Stover SL. Spinal cord injury Model Systems of care: The legacy and the promise. *NeuroRehabil* 1994; 4:84–90.

83 VA Spinal Cord Injury and Disorders System of Care

Margaret C. Hammond

The United States can trace its benefits system for veterans to when the Pilgrims passed a law requiring the colony to support disabled soldiers. Veteran benefits and services were provided by various bureaus until the formal designation of the Veterans Administration in 1930. The Department of Veterans Affairs (VA) was subsequently established as a cabinet-level position in 1989. The VA provides healthcare through the Veterans Health Administration (VHA), benefits for compensation and pension through the Veterans Benefits Administration, and management of the National Cemetery System. The overall mission of the VHA includes the provision of healthcare, medical education and health professions training, backup medical care to the Department of Defense, and research. Healthcare is currently provided to enrolled veterans with service-connected as well as non–service-connected conditions.

Designated VA spinal cord injury (SCI) centers developed during World War II. The SCI system of care now includes twenty-three SCI centers and a network of providers organized in SCI support clinics and SCI primary care teams. There were approximately 26,000 veterans with spinal cord injury and disorders (SCI/D) served by the VHA in fiscal year 2008, of whom approximately 13,000 veterans received SCI specialty care. The definition of SCI/D includes patients with stable and nonprogressive neurologic deficits (etiologies include traumatic lesions, intraspinal nonmalignant neoplasms, vascular insults, degenerative changes to column with myelopathy, inflammatory disease, and demyelinating disease). Patients with demyelinating disease in active relapse or with extensive intracranial involvement receive shared services from Neurology, Rehabilitation Medicine, and SCI.

A sharing agreement with the Department of Defense allows the VA to provide for the care needs of newly SCI-injured active-duty personnel (prior to conversion to veteran status). Since the onset of Operation Enduring Freedom and Operation Iraqi Freedom, 493 active duty service members with SCI have been treated in VA SCI Centers; 159 were injured in theater.

MISSION

The VA provides a continuum of healthcare to veterans from the time of injury or onset of disorder throughout the life course, delivering integrated primary and specialty care. The mission of the SCI/D program is to support, promote, and maintain the health, independence, quality of life, and productivity of individuals with SCI/D throughout their lives. This is accomplished through the efficient delivery of rehabilitation; medical and surgical care for complications of injury or concurrent illness; patient and family education; psychologic, social, and vocational care; research; and professional training of all disciplines in the continuum of care for persons with SCI/D. Improvements to the long-term health and prevention of secondary complications are pursued through the provision of annual comprehensive preventive health evaluations. Such evaluations include components of general primary care as well as SCI-specific care. The mission is also accomplished through the provision of home structural modifications, home health services, respite care, and extended care (such as nursing home placement) for eligible veterans.

STRUCTURE

A "hub and spoke" model best describes the organizational structure. The hubs consist of the twenty-three SCI centers, which have dedicated specialized interdisciplinary care teams. All acute rehabilitation and complex specialty care is provided in the SCI center, including primary care for those veterans living within reasonable proximity to the SCI center. Each SCI center has a designated catchment area of "spoke" facilities (VA facilities without an SCI center) with whom they share responsibility for patient care. Each spoke facility has a designated and SCI support clinic or SCI primary care team (typically a physician, nurse, and social worker) who provide basic medical and limited specialty care closer to the veteran's home. Referrals are made to the SCI centers as needed. SCI support clinic personnel have attended a national training program and have completed a "mini-residency" at the SCI center to which they refer patients.

The Chief Consultant for SCI/D Services, who provides oversight for the program, is the principal advisor and reports through the Chief Officer of Patient Care Services to the Under Secretary for Health of the Veterans Health Administration on the healthcare issues of veterans with SCI/D. The SCI/D Program Office promotes excellence through participation in local, network, and national workgroups; service on national clinical practice guidelines initiatives; provision of national training programs; participation in studies on staffing and resources; fostering the hub and spoke model; promotion of the Accreditation Council on Graduate Medical Education (ACGME) accreditation of SCI Medicine residency sites and the Commission on Accreditation of Rehabilitation Facilities (CARF) accreditation; and liaison to internal and external stakeholders and advocacy groups. Educational efforts include delivery of several national training programs each year and the authorship of the continuing education package on "Medical Care for Persons with SCI," distributed to more than 16,000 physicians in the VA system. The text highlights what is unique and different about the medical care of those with SCI. Other initiatives include the development of outcome measures, the development of referral guidelines, policies on the central decision-making authority for changes in the program and on SCI extended care services, specification of the required number of beds and staff in several key clinical areas, promotion of telemedicine and teleconsultation, and development of the Spinal Cord Dysfunction Outcomes (SCIDO) application. Formerly the SCD Registry, it began as an administrative tool to track people served in the SCI program. It has evolved to include administrative and clinical applications. It links with other VA databases; thus, one can track demographics, the admission or discharge of patients, laboratory utilization, pharmacy, appointments, and clinical outcomes. SCIDO was scheduled for release in 2010.

The VHA currently provides training sites for most of the ACGME-approved training programs in SCI Medicine. In addition, the VA provides a 1–2-year advanced fellowship training in SCI Medicine for interested individuals. Finally, VHA has an extensive portfolio of SCI basic, medical rehabilitation, and health systems research.

The VA system of spinal cord injury care is unique in its ability to provide lifelong comprehensive care to veterans. Such care is delivered through a network of access involving SCI centers and non-SCI center VA facilities. Requirements regarding the SCI/D program structure, resources, and clinical care are set forth in VHA Handbooks 1176.1 and 1176.02.

84 International Perspectives on Spinal Cord Injury Care

Fin Biering-Sørensen

Internationally the possibilities for individuals contracting a traumatic or nontraumatic spinal cord injury (SCI) are very different. This is both with regard to their acute treatment, rehabilitation, resettling, and possibilities to have an active life afterwards in the society. The information available regarding treatment and rehabilitation possibilities are likewise variable for individuals in different areas of the world.

The societies are very different with regard to accessibility for wheelchair users and general possibilities for reintegration, in particular for individuals with multifaceted disabilities after an SCI; and in certain areas of the world the possibilities are very limited.

According to Reilly (1), neurotrauma, including SCI, in many countries and particularly in the younger age group kills more people than AIDS or cancer, but unlike these diseases the causes are known and preventable. The costs to communities in terms of suffering and economics are enormous. Common causes are road traffic accidents, falls, and violence. This affects particularly the developing world, where it consumes already overstretched health resources. There is general agreement on the principles of clinical management, but often there are difficulties in applying early and effective care in countries with the greatest need because of a shortage of facilities and expertise.

Consumer associations for people with SCI have grown strong in many developed countries, but here again there are less developed countries, where no one or any organization can support the individuals with SCI or talk their case to the government, politicians, local authorities etc.

The present chapter is an overview, although very incomplete, of certain fields of relevance when evaluating the possibilities for people with SCI in various parts of the world.

EPIDEMIOLOGY

Literature reviews for the years 1975–1995 (2) and 1995–2005 (3) show the overall incidences per million inhabitants per year of traumatic SCI were 13–71 (average 34.4) in the early and 10–83 (average 29.5) in the later period. The prevalence rates per million inhabitants were found to be 110–1120 (average 554) in the early and 223–755 (average 485) in the later period. Corresponding to a higher incidence in Northern America, the average prevalence rates per million inhabitants were 681 and 755, and for Europe 250 and 252 for the two periods (3). Unfortunately, data from other parts of the world are very scarce.

But according to Motivation (http://www.motivation .org.uk/_history/index.html), the World Health Organization (WHO) estimates that the average life expectancy of a paraplegic in a developing country is between 2 and 3 years. Further epidemiological information on traumatic spinal cord injuries worldwide is available in other chapters.

In a study from Victoria, Australia (4), the average age-adjusted incidence rate of nontraumatic SCI in adults was 26.3 per million per year in the period 2000–2006, and this was significantly greater than the reported incidence for traumatic SCI. The incidence of nontraumatic SCI increased with age, and men had a higher incidence than women. The most common diagnoses reported for nontraumatic SCI are degenerative disc diseases, spinal canal stenosis, tumors, vascular disease, inflammatory conditions, and spina bifida (4–6). The literature on spina bifida gives incidences from 0.9 to 36 per 10,000 births. This large variation includes a significant decline from the seventies and eighties to the nineties in certain countries; differences associated with inclusion of stillbirth and preterm terminations of the pregnancies, varying patterns of neural tube defects in different populations, and the use of folate (7). There is a growing worldwide awareness regarding individuals with nontraumatic SCI; for example in South Africa, SCI caused by HIV is a major challenge (8).

TREATMENT AND REHABILITATION

Facilities

Table 84.1 gives information on the systems for acute care, treatment, and rehabilitation for individuals with SCI and how the hospital care is paid in various countries around the world.

Table 84.1 Systems for Acute Care and Treatment and Rehabilitation for Individuals with SCI, and How Hospital Care Is Paid For in Various Countries

Country and Population (Contact Person(s))	System of Acute Care	System of Treatment and Rehabilitation	Who Pays for Hospital Care
Denmark 5.4 million (Fin Biering-Sørensen)	*Traumatic*: 2 neurosurgical departments. *Nontraumatic*: Variety of departments in particular neurosurgical and neurological.	Two centers for spinal cord lesions for those with significant deficits. Those with very mild spinal cord lesions may go to a variety of departments.	Publicly paid. Everything covered by tax payments.
United Kingdom (UK): England, Wales, Scotland & Northern Ireland 60 million (Martin R. McClelland)	*Traumatic*: Mostly by spinal orthopedic surgeons, occasionally by neurosurgeons in major trauma centers and associated with spinal injuries centers. *Nontraumatic*: By neurologists and neurosurgeons in most large hospitals.	Ten centers in UK. Some have orthopedics surgeons and carry out spinal surgery in-house; some use their spinal orthopedics colleagues or only take patients after the acute phase. Some are not inclined to take psychiatrically disturbed patients because they don't have the psychiatry back-up. Not all take ventilator-dependent patients	Medical care is free to all UK citizens through taxation. There is reciprocity for all European Union citizens.
Romania 22.3 million (Aurelian Anghelescu and Gelu Onose)	One dedicated spinal injury center in neurosurgical department *Traumatic*: Sporadically operated on another 3 Emergency Hospitals in Bucharest and 4 neurosurgical departments in the country *Nontraumatic*: Variety of neurosurgical departments in university hospitals in Bucharest and in the country.	One dedicated spinal injury post-acute rehabilitation department. Five important rehabilitation centers for post-acute and chronic patients. Two of these and 3 in Spas Balnear centers have SCI care skills for SCI with significant deficits. Sporadically, chronic patients go to district general rehabilitation wards and some other spa units.	Publicly paid. Covered by tax payments, i.e., National Health System Insurance.
Russia 141.7 million (Vladimir Baskov)	*Traumatic*: Neurosurgical or traumatologic departments at major regional clinical centers. *Nontraumatic*: Neurological or neurosurgical departments.	Neurosurgical departments of major multi-profile hospitals. Rehabilitation at health centers of neurological profile.	Publicly and insurance-company paid.
India 1 billion (H. S. Chhabra)	*Traumatic*: Various orthopedics and neurosurgical departments. One dedicated spinal injury center in New Delhi. *Nontraumatic*: Variety of departments.	Several centers in different parts of the country. One tertiary and four regional dedicated spinal injury centers in the civil set-up and two dedicated spinal injury centers in armed forces.	1. Government. 2. Insurance (1.08% of the population). 3. The company (where the patient is employed). 4. The patient.
China 1.3 billion (Jianan Li)	*Traumatic*: Mostly by spinal orthopedic surgeons, some by neurosurgeons in major general hospitals. *Nontraumatic*: By neurologists and/or neurosurgeons in major general hospitals depending on spinal cord pathology.	Spinal surgeries are conducted in all of the 946 major general hospitals (more than 800 beds) and some of the 5,156 district hospitals (200 to 800 beds) in China. The number of surgeries is more than 40,000 cases per year. However, high quality and quantity of spinal rehabilitation services are limited in a few centers, even though most major hospitals have basic rehabilitation services in the department of rehabilitation medicine.	1. Government medicare for government officers. 2. Public medicare (insurance) for general population. 3. Work injury compensation and/or insurance from government. 4. Traffic Accident Insurance Fund. 5. Employers (national and/or private). 6. Health cooperative fund in the rural areas. 7. Personal fund.

Japan 120 million (Shinsuke Katoh)	*Traumatic:* Depends on each domestic emergency system. In the metropolitan cities, mostly by spinal orthopedics surgeons, occasionally by neurosurgeons in major trauma centers or in large hospitals. In the domestic area, some especially, with central SCI, by general orthopedic surgeons. *Nontraumatic:* By orthopedic spinal surgeons, occasionally by neurosurgeons in most large hospitals.	Only some hospitals in the public organizations have systems to give total care. Most undergo the initial treatment by orthopedic spinal surgeons, occasionally by neurosurgeons in the local larger hospitals. They and referral hospitals rarely have SCI specialists on urology or rehabilitation.	Publicly paid, covered by tax payments and by patients themselves (up to 1,000 US$ per month).
Australia 21 million (Douglas Brown)	*Traumatic:* In an acute hospital containing the spinal cord center or feeding directly to the spinal rehabilitation home service. Some patients are treated in a trauma center before referral to acute spinal hospital. *Nontraumatic:* Treated in a major hospital by different medical specialties according to presentation and causation.	Six spinal cord services in Australia are either comprehensive services covering the acute, rehabilitation ongoing care or are rehabilitation services with close links to an acute hospital.	Non-compensable patients are paid from the public purse. Compensable patients are paid through the compensating body, usually workers, compensation or transport accident.
Brazil 180 million (Iulia Maria D'Andrea Greve)	*Traumatic:* In general hospitals, taken care of by neurosurgical or orthopedic doctors. One specialized SCI unit at an orthopedic department in Sao Paulo. *Nontraumatic:* Variety of departments.	15–18 rehabilitation units across the country, without automatic transfer from the general hospital of the acute phase. The patient is discharged from the general hospital, and after that, the family and the patient find themselves a rehabilitation unit.	60% Federal Health Public System (universal). 20% State Health System (university hospital), public. 15% private insurance system and most of the acute care and some rehabilitation care. 5% private only, without insurance.
Chile 17 million (Gerardo Correa)	*Traumatic (work accidents):* 3 work-related private trauma hospitals.	3 rehab departments located in work related trauma hospitals, one private rehabilitation center	4.3 millions workers affiliated to nonprofit private insurance companies. Funds provided an obligatory insurance paid by employers.
Adults 11.5 million	*Traumatic (other accidents) and Nontraumatic:* Variety of departments. There is one public hospital with many deficits in acute attention and two private clinics.	One private rehabilitation center. General rehabilitation departments in private clinics. One community center of rehabilitation (Catholic church).	80% in the private sector: health companies* and self-paid. 20% in the public sector: covered by tax payments.
Children 5.5 million	One public hospital with many deficits in acute attention, and two private clinics.	One rehabilitation center (Teletón Foundation), and one rehabilitation department in a public hospital. General rehabilitation departments in private clinics.	Teletón Foundation: financed by campaigns of people's donations. Public sector: covered by tax payments.
USA 300 million (William Donovan and Marcalee Sipski Alexander)	*Traumatic:* Patients are seen at an acute care hospital. The type of care they receive will depend on whether it is a trauma center, spinal injury center or not. Additionally, patients may be transferred to a regional center with neurosurgery or orthopedic spinal surgery, if the initial treating hospital and patient desire. A significant determinant of the treatment they receive is whether they have insurance or not. *Nontraumatic:* Various departments.	There are multiple SCI centers: 14 designated by government as model systems; 23 Veterans of America (VA) system centers. From these centers there are varying numbers of community outreach programs. Also, there are over 100 centers that are CARF accredited as SCI treatment centers and are privately funded through insurance. These centers should have a comprehensive follow-up program. Finally, patients may just be seen in a local hospital.	1. Federal government: VA** and Medicare—insurance for chronically disabled and people over 65. 2. Local government: Medicaid-insurance for the indigent. 3. Private insurance for those who have it 4. Workman's compensation for people who are injured while at work.

continued on next page

Table 84.1 (Continued)

COUNTRY AND POPULATION (CONTACT PERSON(S))	SYSTEM OF ACUTE CARE	SYSTEM OF TREATMENT AND REHABILITATION	WHO PAYS FOR HOSPITAL CARE
			5. Vocational rehabilitation—will pay in some states when patients have no funds. 6. Personal funds. 7. Charity care may be given at some local hospitals. 25–30% have no health insurance, but some are eligible for VA and Medicaid.
South Africa 46 million (Rob Campbell)	Fragmented healthcare system with no specific systems for SCI and consisting of: 1. State-run referral hospitals in larger centers with varying levels of care (level 1 trauma centers with acute SCI units to small orthopedic units in district hospitals with no specific systems of care for SCI). 2. Private hospitals with well-established trauma centers, but without specific acute SCI units. Care overseen by orthopedic and neurosurgeons.	Fragmented systems of care with great variation in quality and type of care: 1. (State) Some of the 9 provinces are well run, but with scarce resources and under-staffed general rehabilitation units (no specifically SCI units); most under the control of orthopedic units, but some independently run. 2. (State) Other provinces have no specific provision for rehabilitation as a separate activity and provided rehabilitation within general orthopedic wards. 3. (Private) About 10 general rehabilitation units in the major centers provide rehabilitation for those with insurance and those injured on duty.	1. The public health care system is almost fully covered by the state from tax, but funding is fragmented at national, provincial, and local government levels. This results in inconsistencies in staffing, resources and policies. Depending on the patients' income status, small co-payments may be required for some. 2. Medical Aids (insurance) cover care for about 20% of the population—predominantly to facilitate care in private hospitals. 3. The Department of Labour runs the Compensation Commission, which is required to pay for hospital care for all individuals injured on duty. 4. The Road Accident Fund (Department of Transport) may sometimes cover hospital care for individuals injured in motor vehicle accidents, but the existence of a "fault system" and protracted litigation in proving eligibility usually exclude treatment in the acute phase and in the rehabilitation phase.

*Each dependent worker pays for himself and his/her family 7% of his/her monthly wage to a private-for-profit health insurance company, which administers the insurance and covers partially expenses due to hospitalization and ambulatory care. Health expenses coverage in these companies is individual, with no solidarity: i.e., higher wages mean higher health expenses coverage. Patients must always pay part of the cost.

**The VA treats approximately 26,000 veterans with SCI and disorders each year. Services include acute rehabilitation and treatment for complications related to SCI (Margaret C. Hammond; see Chapter 83).

The information was collected for the purpose of this chapter and by the help of physicians working with SCI in their respective countries. This gives an idea of the variety of situations experienced in different countries around the world.

In another similar survey in twenty-one countries across Europe representing a population of 416 million, the number of hospital facilities and beds for treatment and rehabilitation were estimated. The number of hospitals/units treating acute traumatic SCI per million inhabitants ranged from 3.9 to 0.16. The number of beds available for this function was 7.7 (median) per million inhabitants. For the rehabilitation of patients with SCI there were 0.5 (median) rehabilitation facilities per million inhabitants, and the number of beds was 13.5 (median) per million inhabitants. The most decentralized system for the acute treatment of traumatic SCI was Finland with 3.92 hospitals per million inhabitants. The most centralized treatment in the acute phase was reported for England and Italy with 0.16–0.17 acute hospitals per million. This mean generally is both acute treatment and rehabilitation, which is centralized in the reporting European countries. The rather low number of beds reported in some countries may imply that some of the SCI patients will not have their rehabilitation in a designated center for this purpose (7).

Service Delivery and Outcomes in Rehabilitation for SCI

Green et al. (9) analyzed information collected between 1998 and 2006, and stored in databases in Australia, Finland, South Africa, and the United States (Table 84.2). Common data could be identified for all countries, e.g. age, FIM scores on admission and discharge, and living situation after discharge. These items can be used to measure outcomes, such as functional improvement and percentage of patients discharged home. However, there are problems of interpretation; e.g. when does the rehabilitation episode start—in Australia and the United States it starts in acute care, but in Finland and South Africa it follows acute care. This together with differences in age, tetra-/paraplegia, complete/incomplete injury, FIM scores, and the other information related to case mix in Table 84.2, shows how difficult a comparison between countries is. To exemplify, the business rules for the data collection have an effect on the outcome variables. For example, when is day one for calculation of length of stay, and when is the admission FIM scored? The services available may influence both the length of stay and the percentage of individuals who can be discharged home. Australia has designated rehabilitation units, including special SCI units, and outpatient and community services may follow. At the same time, there are various outpatient and inpatient options in the United States. In Finland, there is treatment in specialized SCI units after acute care and life-long follow-up as out- or inpatient. But the variability in outcomes is due to differences in patient case mix and services provided. If outcome measures are adjusted for the case mix, the remaining differences will largely be because of differences in services provided by the various countries. However, it is important to consider differences in business rules surrounding the collection of the data in interpreting the results.

Reimbursement and Pension

Table 84.3 gives information on systems for payment of home adaptations or rehousing, wheelchair(s), devices (e.g., catheters), medicine, and pension for individuals with SCI in the same countries around the world as in Table 84.1. Even though the data must be taken with caution, they give an insight in the very different options for individuals in various countries around the world and even within the same country. Smaller countries will general have an easier task in having uniform systems than larger countries.

Return to Work

Already in 1954, Donald Munroe was preoccupied with the possibilities of making persons with SCI capable of working and stated that persons "with full self-care ability should be able and should be expected to go to work" (10). In 2001 the International Classification of Functioning, Disability and Health (ICF) was introduced by WHO (11). This classification stresses the importance of "participation in activities," including participation in productive work. Many societies regard work as a key indicator to social integration. Because traumatic SCI often affects young adults, return to work and employment is often an important

Table 84.2 Information Collected between 1998 and 2006 from Databases in Australia,[a] Finland,[b] South Africa,[c] and the United States[d]

	AUSTRALIA	FINLAND	SOUTH AFRICA	UNITED STATES
Number of facilities	81	15	13	147
Number of episodes	3,464	1,628	396	9,847
First episodes only	Yes	No	Mixed	Mixed
Percent nontraumatic SCI	63%	49%	40%	70%
Average length of stay (days)	49	32	69	20
Average FIM change	18	6	26	20
Percentage discharged home	78	74	72	73

[a]Australasian Rehabilitation Outcomes Center.
[b]Qualisan Ltd.
[c]South African Database for Functional Medicine.
[d]eRehabData.
Source: Reference 9.

Table 84.3 Systems for Payment of Home Adaptations or Rehousing, Wheelchair(s), Devices, Medicine, and Pensions for Individuals with Spinal Cord Injury (SCI) in Various Countries

Country (Contact Person(s))	Who Pays for Home Adaptations or Rehousing	Who Pays for Wheelchair(s)	Who Pays for Devices (e.g., Catheters)	Who Pays for Medicine	Who Pays for Pension after Spinal Cord Lesion
Denmark (Fin Biering-Sørensen)	Publicly by the municipality, i.e., by tax.	Publicly by the municipality, i.e., by tax.	Publicly by the municipality, i.e., by tax.	In part publicly by the municipality, i.e., by tax; certain amount self-paid.	Basic pension by state/municipality, i.e., by tax. Several have additional private pensions or work-related pensions.
United Kingdom (UK): England, Wales, Scotland & Northern Ireland (Martin R. McClelland)	The local council is responsible for home adaptations or rehousing. This is "means tested"; i.e., it is free to those who cannot afford it. If patients own their own home, or if they have significant savings, then they have to contribute to the cost of adaptations, rehousing, or going into a nursing home.	The wheelchair is provided by the "Wheelchair Services" where the patient lives. Sometimes the Wheelchair Services will provide a wheelchair only when the patient returns to their home. Many Wheelchair Services will offer a "voucher" system; i.e., they will contribute to the cost of a privately purchased wheelchair if this one is more expensive than might be provided.	These are provided on prescription through the National Health Service. The vast majority of long-term disabled people do not have to pay the set prescription charge.	In part publicly by the municipality, i.e., by tax; certain amount self-paid.	Persons employed before their injury and unable to return to work will receive a pension from the company that employed them. The size of this pension will depend on the number of years they have worked. All patients will also receive a "disability" and a "mobility" allowance (through taxation). This is not "means tested," but people over 65 years old don't get mobility allowance. Care input (e.g., help washing/dressing) is not regarded as healthcare and is "means tested"; i.e., it depends on how much money and income the patient has.
Romania (Aurelian Anghelescu and Gelu Onose)	Ambulance (home transport) paid by National Health System Insurance (NHSI): in rare cases, private ambulance service. Home modifications: theoretically law protected, but practically, overwhelmingly self-paid by patient. In scarce cases, by charity (sponsorship). Cost of nursing home is publicly covered (exception: self-paid luxury settlement)	Publicly, by the NHSI (for the standard model of wheel chair). Electric wheelchair covered 3/4 by the patient.	Publicly during the hospitalization. For chronic cases, theoretically, publicly, by the NHSI (30 intermittent catheters and 2–3 urinary bags/month); practically, an important amount is self-paid.	Publicly, during hospitalization. After discharge publicly, by the NHSI (great majority) are 50–90% compensated/discount). For children and chronically severe disabled persons (including complete tetra/paraplegia): theoretically free of charge.	Basic pension by state and local municipality (social aid for patient's personal assistant). Disabled persons, employed before their injury, will until 65 years receive an invalidity pension from the state (function of previous period of labor); afterward they get the usual "age" pension. Possible to apply for (persons over 35 years, optionally) the private pension system and/or cumulated private pension and insurance for accidents and/or decease.
Russia (Vladimir Baskov)	Self paid.	Publicly by social insurance.	Publicly by social insurance for fixed amount, excess self-paid.	Publicly by social insurance for fixed amount, excess self-paid.	Basic pension by state with municipality, i.e., by tax.
India (H. S. Chhabra)	Self paid.	1. Government for poor patients. 2. Government for those employed in government sector. 3. Patients themselves. 4. The company where the patient is employed. 5. Insurance (1.08% of the population).	1. Government for those employed in government sector. 2. Patients themselves. 3. The company where the patient is employed.	1. Government (during hospitalization only) and for those employed in government sector. 2. Patients themselves. 3. The company where the patient is employed. 4. Insurance (during hospitalization and 1 month after discharge).	Government for those employed in government sector and if injury took place while on duty.

China (Jianan Li)	Primarily personal funds. Occasionally paid by the employers and/or work injury compensation fund.	Primarily personal funds. Occasionally paid by the employers, medical insurance, and/or work injury compensation fund.	Majority of medicine paid by the same source of insurance and/or fund unless some imported and nutritional medicine.	Government retirement fund. Some by employers. Social fund for people under the poverty line. Family support.
Japan (Shinsuke Katoh)	Publicly by the municipality, i.e. by tax.	Publicly, covered by tax payments (limited) and patients themselves.	Patients' own public health insurance covers 70%, others self-paid.	Basic pension by state/municipality, i.e. by tax.
Australia (Douglas Brown)	Non-compensable patients: home modifications paid for out of their own pocket, a charity, or the state health department. Compensable patients have home modifications paid for by the compensating body	Paid for by state health department for non-compensable patients. Compensating bodies pay for all equipment for their clients.	Public (non-compensable) patients have their medicines paid for through the Federal Government Pharmaceutical Scheme. Compensable patients have their medicines paid for by the compensating body.	Non-compensable patients receive a federal government pension. Compensable patients have income from their compensating body, usually at a level of 80–85% of their pre-employment income.
Brazil (Julia Maria D'Andrea Greve)	Self-paid.	Most self-paid, minority by government—Federal Health System.	Self-paid and Federal State Health System.	For regular employee before injury, the public system of insurance (part of the income and total of the income in work injury). For those not working at the time of injury, there is a small income (minimal national salary) that the patient has to ask for and prove the incapacity.
Chile (Gerardo Correa) *Work accidents*	Generally self-paid. In some cases there may be financial support from the municipality or the employer	Insurance company.	Insurance company.	Insurance company.
Adults *Other:*	Generally self-paid. In some cases there may be financial support from the municipality.	Private sector: health companies, some complementary health insurances, and self-paid. Public sector: covered by tax payments.	Private sector: self-paid. Public sector: mainly self-paid, in part covered by tax payments.	If salary employed, he/she pays 13% of monthly wage in order to get disability or old age retirement pension. If the patient doesn't have salary, there is a minimal pension from the municipality.
Children	Generally the patient's family (self-paid). In some cases they may have financial support from the municipality.	Public sector: covered by tax. Private sector: health companies, some complementary health insurances and patient's family.	Private sector: patient's family (self-paid). Public sector: mainly self-paid, in part covered by tax.	Depending on family income, there is an economic aid from the municipality.
USA (William Donovan & Marcalee Sipski Alexander)	Primarily personal funds. Persons going to an extended care facility may be paid by government (Medicaid, Medicare, or Veterans Administration (VA)* If the patient has worker's compensation, it is possible that modifications to the home or nursing home costs will be paid publicly.	Wheelchairs may be paid for by private insurance, Medicaid, Medicare, or VA.* Personal funds or charity often necessary to supplement these costs	May be paid by private insurance, Medicaid, Medicare, or VA.* Personal funds or charity often necessary to supplement these costs	People are eligible for federal social security disability insurance after 2 years of disability. If they are a veteran, depending on the relationship of their injury to service, they may be eligible for a pension. If they are employees with worker's compensation, they will generally get some type of payment. Some people may also have privately paid disability insurance either through their employer or through independent purchase.

continued on next page

Table 84.3 *(Continued)*

COUNTRY (CONTACT PERSON(S))	WHO PAYS FOR HOME ADAPTATIONS OR REHOUSING	WHO PAYS FOR WHEELCHAIR(S)	WHO PAYS FOR DEVICES (E.G., CATHETERS) CORD LESION	WHO PAYS FOR MEDICINE	WHO PAYS FOR PENSION AFTER SPINAL
South Africa (Rob Campbell)	No coordinated policy in place. Almost always funded by the individuals and their families. The Road Accident Fund (RAF) is liable for home alterations for individuals with proven eligibility.	Depending on the income of the individual, the cause of the SCI, and the region in which the individual lives: *State sector:* National policy provides for provision of wheel chair for all who need them—but funding and administrative problems often mean that inadequate and inappropriate chairs are provided, or no chairs are available. Some individuals have to pay for their own chairs. *Medical insurance:* Almost all medical insurers make some provision for wheelchairs and other equipment—but this is almost always insufficient to purchase adequate equipment. *Compensation Commissioner:* All individuals who are injured on duty are covered for all equipment and chairs. *RAF:* Individuals who manage to prove eligibility for funding after motor vehicle accidents are well funded for wheel chairs. *Private funding:* Many individuals, from any of the above, partially or fully fund their own chairs, given the administrative and policy framework barriers that exist.	*The public health system* provides free devices to all individuals with "disability," but logistics are unreliable, especially in smaller and rural centers. *The Compensation Commissioner* covers all devices for those injured on duty—but administrative barriers often make this difficult and unreliable. *RAF* covers those with proven eligibility. *Medical insurers* at least partly cover devices for their members.	*The public health system* provides medication to all individuals with "disability," but logistics are unreliable, especially in smaller and rural centers. *The Compensation Commissioner* covers all medication for those injured on duty—but administrative barriers often make this difficult and unreliable. *RAF* covers those with proven eligibility. *Medical insurers* at least partly cover medication for their members.	*The state (Department of Social Welfare)* provides a disability grant of around R800 per month to those who can prove that they have no other source of income greater than this. *Compensation Commissioner/Department of Labour* provides for individuals who are injured on duty a lifelong pension. *RAF* provides for individuals with proven eligibility a lump sum payment for loss of income. *Private disability insurance* holders may receive a lump sum payment or a pension from their insurer.

*The VA pays for medications, supplies, wheelchairs, and catheters. Services include home care services, attendant support for bladder and bowel care, respite and hospice care. Compensation is provided to service-connected veterans and pension for low-income disabled veterans. There is also a housing grant for home modifications (Margaret C. Hammond; see Chapter 83) goal. In addition, obtaining work has psychological, social, financial, and political implications, and employment means better self-esteem, higher life satisfaction, and sense of well being (12).

In a review it was found that 21–67% of individuals working at the time of their SCI returned to work after injury (12). The employment rate among persons with SCI ranged from 11.5% to 74%. The frequency of return to work was higher in persons injured at a younger age, with less severe injuries, higher functional independence, and the employment rate improved with time after SCI. Further, individuals who sustained their SCI during childhood or adolescence had higher adult employment rates. The most common barriers to employment were problems with transportation, health, and physical limitations, lack of work experience, education or training, physical or architectural barriers, discrimination by employers, and loss of benefits. In addition, individuals with SCI discontinued working at a younger age. Outside Europe, North America, and Australia, single studies only were found for the period 2000–2006, from Japan, Taiwan, Turkey, Saudi Arabia, and India (12). The frequencies of employment reported in these investigations were in the middle of the ranges given above, and the issues reported were similar, although the challenges are different depending on the setting.

There are special challenges related to education and employment possibilities in persons with SCI or with other disabilities living in developing countries. Taking the high national unemployment rates, poverty, and cultural differences in most of these countries into consideration, it is understandable that only little information is available on the employment conditions for persons with SCI. In 2000, the report "Disability issues, trends and recommendations for the World Bank" claimed that "Employment statistics for people with disabilities are virtually nonexistent in developing countries" (13). Levy et al. (14) described that of 136 persons with SCI in a study from Zimbabwe, only 13% were employed, and most of them spent their day doing "nothing." In the report "Implementation of the United Nations standard rules on the equalization of opportunities for persons with disabilities" from 2006, it was stated that the social stigma associated with disability still makes it common to "hide" family members with disabilities and to restrict their access to education, rehabilitation services, and job opportunities (15). In August 2006, the United Nations presented the "Convention on the rights of persons with disabilities" to promote, protect, and ensure the full and equal enjoyment of all human rights by persons with disabilities, including education and employment (16).

Because of the high unemployment rates in individuals with SCI, it is important as suggested by Bricout (17) to do research in telework, as this possibility has been well elucidated in the nondisabled population but not in the population with SCI. In addition, return to work related to Web accessibility has been little studied for spinal cord-injured patients outside the United States and is a topic to explore further. The employment conditions for persons with SCI in developing countries have been studied to little extent, and are a challenge for future research.

RESEARCH

Here are a few examples of international and other special initiatives related to research in SCI.

The International Campaign for Cures of Spinal Cord Injury Paralysis (ICCP)

(www.campaignforcure.org)

ICCP is a body of affiliated not-for-profit organizations working to fund research into cures for paralysis caused by SCI. The ICCP coalition mission is "to expedite the discovery of cures for Spinal Cord Injury Paralysis."

ICCP members represent many of the leading SCI research fundraising charities around the world. Those organizations met to determine the ways in which their collaborative efforts can hasten progress in this field. In 1998 in Charlottesville, Virginia, they signed a "Statement of Intent," and the ICCP was formed (Table 84.4).

ICCP has developed Guidelines for the conduct of clinical trials for SCI (18–21).

Spinal Cord Outcomes Partnership Endeavor (SCOPE)

SCOPE, which was initiated 2007, has the mission "To enhance the development of human study protocols (e.g. clinical trials) that will accurately validate therapeutic interventions for SCI leading to the adoption of improved best practices."

The overall goals include facilitation of communication, coordination and collaboration between basic scientists, clinical researchers, academic institutions, industry, government agencies, not-for-profit organizations, and foundations to improve functional outcomes and quality of life for people living with SCI. This involves translation of novel discoveries, identification of accurate, sensitive, and reliable outcome tools, development of clinical trial and clinical practice protocols, continual updating and integration of new knowledge, dissemination of the teaching of valid therapeutic interventions, and facilitation of training in validated best practices in order to create and distribute materials to support knowledge translation.

National Spinal Cord Injury Statistical Center (NSCISC)

(http://main.uab.edu/show.asp?durki=10766)

The University of Alabama at Birmingham's Department of Rehabilitation Medicine received grants in 1983 to establish a

---

Table 84.4 The International Campaign for Cures of Spinal Cord Injury Paralysis Membership (http://www.campaignforcure.org/)

- Christopher Reeve Foundation*
- French Institute for Spinal Cord Research (Institut Pour la Recherche sur la Moelle Épinière)
- Japan Spinal Cord Foundation
- The Miami Project to Cure Paralysis*
- Paralyzed Veterans of America*
- Rick Hansen Man in Motion Foundation*
- Spinal Cure Australia (formerly known as Australasian Spinal Research Trust*)
- Neil Sachse Foundation (formerly Spinal Treatment Australia)
- Spinal Research (International Spinal Research Trust)*
- Wings for Life

*Founding member.

national SCI data center. This was in continuation of the National Spinal Cord Injury Data Research Center that served the Model SCI Care Systems Project 1973–1981. The NSCISC supervises and directs the collection, management, and analysis of the world's largest SCI database with data from the network of the federally sponsored regional Model Spinal Cord Injury Care Systems located throughout the United States. In each of these settings, data on SCI patients are collected for acute, rehabilitation, and follow-up, and submitted to the NSCISC. Apart from maintaining the national SCI database, NSCISC conducts database-oriented research. For more information see Chapter 82.

European Multicenter Study about Spinal Cord Injury (EMSCI)

(www.emsci.org)

EMSCI was established as a multicenter project for future therapeutic interventions in human SCI and was sponsored by the International Research Institute for Paraplegia in Zurich, Switzerland.

Within the frame of this project, all patients with acute traumatic SCI will be tested and documented within a fixed time schedule (acute, 4, 12, 24, and 48 weeks) after SCI and must comply with clearly defined inclusion criteria. The examinations consist of a standard set of neurologic, neurophysiologic, and functional assessments. The collected data from each center is sent to the coordinating center in Zurich to be joined into a central database. A total of 17 SCI centers from six countries build up a close collaboration to discuss, plan, and realize prospective studies.

INTERNATIONAL SPINAL CORD INJURY STANDARDS AND DATA SETS

From the global perspective, there is an increasing need for international standards, data, and measures pertaining to SCI.

International Spinal Cord Injury Standards

The International Standards for the Neurological Classification of Spinal Cord Injury (ISNCSCI) (22) are used to document impairments of motor and sensory function after SCI. The ISNCSCI is being used to document remaining spinal cord function, but these standards do not assess the spinal cord components of autonomic function that affect a majority of organs. Therefore, autonomic standards are under development by representatives from the American Spinal Injury Association (ASIA), and the International Spinal Cord Society (ISCoS) (23). The goal of these standards is to describe the impact on various organ system functions of the SCI. The standards shall allow clinicians and researchers to describe the effects of SCI on cardiovascular, broncho pulmonary, urinary bladder, bowel, sexual, and sudomotor functions. Because of anatomic relationships, the standards will include a general anatomic diagnosis for the impact of SCI on urinary bladder, bowel, and sexual function. A secondary classification will describe a more detailed impact of injury on each of these separate organ systems. A similar though separate process is used for the autonomic control of cardiovascular and sudomotor function, including thermoregulation. The standards

will be posted on the Web sites of ISCoS (www.iscos.org.uk) and ASIA when finalized(www.asia-spinalinjury.org).

International Spinal Cord Injury Data Sets

Likewise, common International SCI Data Sets should be collected on individuals with SCI to facilitate comparisons regarding injuries, treatments, and outcomes between patients, centers, and countries. Many countries have established SCI databases. To obtain the kind of success as for the ISNCSCI, it is important that the data sets are simple and perceived relevant to the clinicians so that they will use them. In addition, it will be imperative that these data sets can be both easily retrieved and available for use for no cost and without any specific restrictions (24).

The process for establishing International SCI Data Sets started at an international meeting on SCI data collection and analysis in Vancouver, Canada, in 2002. An overall structure and terminology has been developed following the format of the International Classification of Function (ICF) (24). Figure 84.1 illustrates the general structure of the International SCI Data Sets.

The *Core Data Set* was the first one to be developed (25). The purpose of the Core Data Set is to standardize the collection and reporting of a minimal amount of information necessary to evaluate and compare results of published studies. The data included in the Core Data Set are recommended as a descriptive table in most publications, including individuals with SCI.

Basic Question

This is a question, which with an affirmative answer implies that it is possible to go on to one or more specific data set(s) with more detailed information on the particular topic. There will not be such questions for all data sets.

Basic SCI Data Set

This is the minimal number of data elements, which should be collected in daily clinical practice for a particular topic. This means that the various International Basic SCI Data Sets may be the basis for a structured record in centers worldwide caring for persons with SCI. Examples of actual and possible SCI Data Sets are seen in Figure 84.1.

Extended SCI Data Set

This is a more detailed data set that may be used as optional for a topic, but may be recommended for specific research studies within the particular area. The ICECI (International Classification of External Causes of Injury) (www.iceci.org) for SCI is being developed in cooperation between WHO and an ISCoS group based in Australia.

Module

A Module may consist of a basic question, an International Basic and Extended SCI Data Set, and other data (e.g. specific scoring-systems) that are appropriate for the particular module.

For development of further data sets, topic-specific expert working groups are created. The establishment of working groups in the various areas is done in cooperation with relevant

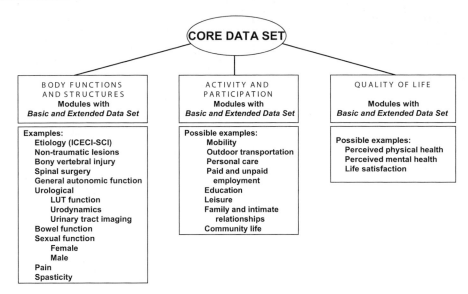

Figure 84.1 International spinal cord injury data sets.

international societies and organizations working with the respective topics and approved by ISCoS and ASIA.

For each data set, a syllabus including definitions, instructions on how to collect each data item, and coding schemes are developed.

International organizations and societies within the fields of SCI, rehabilitation, neurosurgery, orthopedic surgery, etc. are invited to appoint members to join the review process for the International SCI Data Set, and a process for approval and endorsement of the data sets by relevant (International) Organizations and Societies has been established.

As soon as a new International SCI Data Set is developed it will be disseminated at meetings, and published in international journals and through the Web sites of ISCoS (www.iscos.org.uk), and ASIA (www.asia-spinalinjury.org). For each data set, training cases will be created when relevant and made accessible through the same Web sites.

International Classification of Functioning, Disability, and Health (ICF) Core Sets

The ICF Core Sets for SCI are selections of items of the ICF that are relevant to persons with SCI. These core sets are developed in cooperation between the ICF Research Branch of the WHO Collaboration Centre of the Family of International Classifications in Germany, the Classification, Assessment, and Terminology (CAT) team, the Disability and Rehabilitation (DAR) team at WHO, ISCoS and the International Society for Physical and Rehabilitation Medicine, and partner institutions across the world (26).

ICF categories relevant for SCI have been identified in four worldwide studies with representatives from all the WHO regions: Africa, the Americas, South-Eastern Asia, Europe, Eastern Mediterranean, and Western Pacific. This was conducted during 2006–2007 by means of an empirical study, a systematic review of outcomes and measures used in SCI research, an expert survey, and focus groups and semi-structured interviews with persons with SCI.

Consensus about items to be part of a Comprehensive and Brief ICF Core Set for SCI in the early postacute and the chronic situation was reached in a final ICF Core Set Consensus Conference held in November 2007 in Nottwil, Switzerland. Subsequent field testing will be necessary to validate this first version of ICF Core Sets for SCI.

ORGANIZATIONS FOR PROFESIONALS

A variety of organizations exist worldwide. Here are a few examples of the larger ones and those that are international or have a more multidisciplinary membership. It should be remembered that many other organizations in their membership and meetings include SCI professionals and topics, including rehabilitation, neurosurgical, orthopedic surgical, and urological associations.

International Spinal Cord Society (ISCoS)

(www.iscos.org.uk)

The International Medical Society of Paraplegia was founded in 1961 with Sir Ludwig Guttmann as the President. Dr. Guttmann founded the Spinal Unit at Stoke Mandeville Hospital, Aylesbury, United Kingdom in February 1944. In 1952, he founded the International Stoke Mandeville Games, and doctors from the various countries who accompanied their teams to these games began to meet and discuss their clinical work and research. Therefore it was decided to start the society with its first official meeting in 1961. The Annual Scientific Meetings were held at Stoke Mandeville Hospital, except in Olympic years when they were held in association with the Paralympic Games. From 1979 the meetings have been held in different countries (see Table 84.5), and in addition there are Regional Meetings around the world supported by the society. The society changed its name to the International Spinal Cord Society (ISCoS) in 2001.

ISCoS serves as an international, impartial, nonpolitical, and nonprofit association with the purpose to study all problems relating to traumatic and nontraumatic SCI. This includes causes,

Table 84.5   Location of the Annual Scientific Meetings 1992–2008 of the International Medical Society of Paraplegia (since 2001, International Spinal Cord Society)

1992	Barcelona, Spain, in conjunction with the Paralympic Games
1993	Gent, Belgium
1994	Kobe, Japan
1995	New Delhi, India
1996	Atlanta, USA, in conjunction with the Paralympic Games
1997	Innsbruck, Austria—joint meeting with the Deutchsprachige Medizinische Gesellschaft für Paraplegie
1998	Iguassu, Brazil
1999	Copenhagen, Denmark—joint meeting with the Scandinavian Medical Society of Paraplegia
2000	Sydney, Australia, in conjunction with the Paralympic Games
2001	Nottwill, Switzerland
2002	Vancouver, Canada—joint meeting with American Spinal Injury Association
2003	Beijing, China
2004	Athens, Greece, in conjunction with the Paralympic Games
2005	Munich, Germany—joint meeting with the Deutchsprachige Medizinische Gesellschaft für Paraplegie
2006	Boston, USA—joint meeting with American Spinal Injury Association
2007	Reykjavik, Iceland—joint meeting with the Nordic Spinal Cord Society
2008	Durban, South Africa—joint meeting with the South African Spinal Cord Association

Table 84.6   International Spinal Cord Society (ISCoS)–Affiliated Societies, 2007

- American Paraplegia Society (APS)
- American Spinal Injury Association (ASIA)
- Asian Spinal Cord Network (ASCoN)
- Association Francophone Internationale des Groupes d'Animation de la Paraplégie (AFIGAP)
- Australian and New Zealand Spinal Cord Society (ANZSCoS)
- Chinese Association of Rehabilitation for the Disabled Society of Spinal Cord Injuries (CARDP-SOSCI)
- Deutchsprachige Medizinische Gesellschaft für Paraplegie (DMGP)
- Dutch-Flemish Society of Paraplegia (NVDG)
- Japan Medical Society of Spinal Cord Lesions (JASCoL)
- Latin American Society of Paraplegia (SLAP)
- Nordic Spinal Cord Society (NoSCoS)
- Societá Medica Italiana di Paraplegia (SoMIPar)
- Southern African Spinal Cord Association (SASCA)
- Spanish Society of Paraplegia (SEP)
- Spinal Cord Society - Indian Chapter
- Turkish Society of Spinal Cord Diseases (TrSCD)

prevention, basic and clinical research, medical and surgical management, clinical practice, education, rehabilitation, and social reintegration. Therefore, ISCoS among other things shall work in close collaboration with other national and international organizations, to encourage the most efficient use of available resources worldwide and provide a scientific exchange by collecting and disseminating information through publications, correspondence, exhibits, regional and international seminars, symposia, conferences, etc.

ISCoS shall advise, encourage, guide, and support the efforts of those responsible for the care, education, and training of medical professionals and professionals allied to medicine related to patients with SCI, and when requested, correlate these activities throughout the world. To facilitate this process, ISCoS encourages the creation of affiliated societies throughout the world. The ISCoS-affiliated societies in 2007 can be seen in Table 84.6.

Asian Spinal Cord Network (ASCoN)

(www.ascononline.org.in)

ASCoN was initiated after a conference in Bangladesh in 2001. ASCoN consists of members representing 46 organizations in 16 countries in Asia: Afghanistan, Bangladesh, Bhutan, Cambodia, India, Indonesia, Japan, Korea, Laos, Myanmar, Malaysia, Nepal, Pakistan, Sri Lanka, Thailand, and Vietnam.

The members share and learn from each other with regard to all aspects of SCI management, from initial treatment to reintegration of the patient. The information flow goes through a newsletter, exchange visits, short training courses, annual conferences, and the development of ASCoN Guiding Principles for Management of Spinal Cord Injuries.

American Spinal Injury Association (ASIA)

(www.asia-spinalinjury.org)

The early 1970s brought support for the concept of a model of care from the Rehabilitation Services Administration, which created the "model SCI systems" program. It was out of this initiative the ASIA was created in 1973.

The mission of the ASIA is to promote and establish standards of excellence for all aspects of health care of individuals with SCI from onset throughout life, to educate members, other healthcare professionals, patients, and their families, as well as the public on all aspects of SCI and its consequences in order to prevent injury, improve care, increase availability of services, and maximize the injured individual's potential for full participation in all areas of community life. In addition to fostering research, which aims at preventing SCI, improving care, reducing consequences of disability, and finding a cure for both acute and chronic SCI, it facilitates communication between members and other physicians, allied health care professionals, researchers, and consumers.

American Paraplegia Society (APS)

(www.apssci.org)

Founded in 1954, the APS is dedicated to improving the quality of medical care delivered to persons with SCI. In view of the diversity in spinal cord medicine, one of the major functions of APS is to foster the interchange of ideas in both clinical and basic science. APS is organized and functions exclusively for educational purposes. Its goals are to advance SCI patient care, promote research related to SCI, and provide a forum for the review of scientific findings.

Multidisciplinary Association of Spinal Cord Injury Professionals (MASCIP)

(www.mascip.co.uk)

MASCIP provides a professional forum to promote standards in clinical practice, foster research, and encourage the development of health and social care services for people with SCI. MASCIP exists to enable all professions and grades of staff associated with the care and welfare of people with SCI, both within and outside of SCI Centers, to articulate professional issues and concerns. MASCIP will lobby service commissioners, healthcare providers, and the Department of Health on issues of significant professional concern.

INFORMATION

Journals

Many journals bring important topics to SCI-interested professionals. There are three peer-reviewed and indexed journals specialized to SCI:

Spinal Cord (www.nature.com/sc/index.html) is the official journal of ISCoS. Formerly named Paraplegia. It provides coverage of all aspects of spinal cord injury and disease.

The Journal of Spinal Cord Medicine is the official publication of APS (www.apssci.org). Formerly named The Journal of the American Paraplegia Society, it covers basic science, translational research, clinical studies, and expert commentary.

Topics in Spinal Cord Injury Rehabilitation (www.thomasland .com) started in 1994 as a source of developments in SCI patient care; it has an interdisciplinary and practical approach.

Spinal Cord Injury Rehabilitation Evidence (SCIRE)

(www.icord.org/scire/home.php)

SCIRE synthesizes the published evidence on rehabilitation strategies and community based programs for improvement of functional outcome and quality of life for people living with SCI. It is the intention to revise SCIRE continuously as new research knowledge appears.

The Consortium for Spinal Cord Medicine Clinical Practice Guidelines

See www.pva.org "Publications," and Chapter 85 of this volume.

As part of their mission, Paralyzed Veterans of America (PVA) produces a wide range of publications. News and information relevant for wheelchair users are available on research, travel, architecture, and daily living activities.

The Consortium's clinical practice guidelines for health care professionals and companion consumer guides help people living with SCI put this information to use in their daily lives. These publications provide guidance and address questions on SCI subjects ranging from pressure ulcers, to bladder and bowel care, to expected outcomes one year out from injury. The guidelines can be downloaded free of charge to enable health care professionals and people with SCI from all over the world to benefit from these unique products. Some consumer guides are available in Spanish.

ParaDoc

(www.paradoc.org)

ParaDoc is a database created by the joint initiatives of the Education Committee of the ISCoS and the Swiss Paraplegics Foundation. ParaDoc is based in the library of the Swiss Paraplegic Centre in Nottwil, Switzerland. Its aim is to collect publications and references concerning education and training on the subject of SCI and to promote the exchange of information on an international basis, especially towards developing countries. ParaDoc as a nonprofit project needs the help of everybody interested in SCI in collecting data concerning education and training.

Spinal Cord Injury Information Network

(www.spinalcord.uab.edu)

This network, which includes various information of interest for professionals and people with SCI, is funded through the University of Alabama, Birmingham, SCI Model System.

CONSUMER ASSOCIATIONS

In many parts of the world, there are consumer associations taking action to improve the possibilities for individuals with SCI. These initiatives are political, for example to gain better treatment and rehabilitation facilities and reintegration possibilities, as well as practical with individual advices regarding how to obtain the best economic support from the society, etc.

In many countries there are no specific organizations for people with SCI, as they are organized together with other disabled people in various disability societies.

A few of the larger consumer associations are given below.

European Spinal Cord Injury Federation (ESCIF)

(www.escif.org)

ESCIF was started in Nottwil, Switzerland, in 2005 to facilitate sharing of experience and promoting expertise across Europe for people living with a SCI. The organization will communicate and distribute knowledge and expertise, and will generate ideas, research, and awareness with the ultimate aim and vision to create a high quality of life for all people with SCI.

Members of ESCIF are independent national organizations whose objective is to represent people with SCI in their country. A maximum of one organization per country can hold membership in the ESCIF. In 2007, nineteen European countries were members of ESCIF.

National Spinal Cord Injuries Association (NSCIA)

(www.spinalcord.org)

NSCIA was founded in 1948, and is dedicated to improving the quality of life for Americans living with the results of SCI and their families. NSCIA educates and empowers survivors of SCI to achieve and maintain the highest levels of independence, health, and personal fulfillment. This is fulfilled by providing a

Peer Support Network and by raising awareness about SCI through education programs and linking people with SCI to each other. The education programs are developed to address information and issues important for members, policy makers, the general public, and the media, and include injury prevention, improvements in medical, rehabilitative, and supportive services, research, and public policy formulation.

Paralyzed Veterans of America (PVA)

(www.pva.org)

PVA works to maximize the quality of life for people with SCI, including quality health care, research and education, veterans' benefits and rights, accessibility and the removal of architectural barriers, sports programs, and disability rights. PVA was founded in 1946 and has developed expertise on a wide variety of issues involving the special needs of people who have experienced SCI. Central in its mission is the evidence-based clinical practice guidelines (see above).

United Spinal Association

(www.unitedspinal.org)

United Spinal Association was founded in 1946 by paralyzed veterans to help enable people with disabilities to lead full and productive lives. The mission is to provide expertise, create access to resources, and strengthen hope. The activities include promotion of research, advocating for civil rights and independence, educating the public and enlisting its help, providing services to veteran members, providing participatory events for children and young adults, and providing guidance and motivation through a Peer Mentoring program.

CONCLUSION

The possibilities for individuals acquiring a SCI are very different depending on where and whom you are. Therefore it is an obligation for those who have the means and knowledge to educate and upgrade governments, local authorities, professionals, the public awareness, relatives, and the SCI individuals themselves as much as possible to be able to provide the best possible treatment, rehabilitation, and reintegration of everyone who contracts an SCI.

Naturally the best approach is to prevent as many of the spinal cord injuries as possible. This will primarily apply to traumatic SCI, including preventing many road traffic accidents, falls from height, and violence, work, sport, and leisure accidents. A good and systematic registration will be a first step to identify where it is best to intervene. Some nontraumatic SCI may also be preventable.

For more patients to survive and live a fruitful life, it is imperative to be aware of prevention of complications like pressure ulcers and urinary tract disorders. Treatment and rehabilitation of individuals with SCI is a complex and expensive task due to the need of a large, multispeciality, multiprofessional team approach to obtain optimal results. Therefore more developed countries have to take responsibility for the less developed countries—but also within developed countries there may be large variations, which may need to be addressed. The responsibility is to support the governments, authorities, professionals, and consumers with necessary knowledge, such as by making this freely available over the internet. In addition, it is important to investigate the most cost-effective means of prevention and evidence-based treatment of SCI. International cooperative research will be essential in the future to achieve the best solutions.

ACKNOWLEDGMENTS

Thanks to all who contributed and helped making this chapter: Marcalee Sipski Alexander (USA), Aurelian Anghelescu (Rumania), Vladimir Baskov (Russia), Marianne Bint (UK), Douglas Brown (Australia), Rob Campbell (South Africa), Susan Charlifue (USA), H.S. Chhabra (India), Gerardo Correa (Chile), William Donovan (USA), Janette Green (Australia), Julia Maria D'Andrea Greve (Brazil), Margaret C. Hammond (USA), Shinsuke Katoh (Japan), Paul Kennedy (UK), Jianan Li (China), Martin R. McClelland (UK), Gelu Onose (Rumania) and John Steeves (Canada).

References

1. Reilly P. The impact of neurotrauma on society: an international perspective. *Prog Brain Res* 161:3–9, 2007.
2. Blumer CE, Quine S. Prevalence of spinal cord injury: an international comparison. *Neuroepidemiology* 14:258–268, 1995.
3. Wyndaele M, Wyndaele J-J. Incidence, prevalence and epidemiology of spinal cord injury: what learns a worldwide literature survey? *Spinal Cord* 44:523–529, 2006.
4. New PW, Sundararajan V. Incidence of non-traumatic spinal cord injury in Victoria, Australia: a population-based study and literature review. *Spinal Cord* 2007 Dec 11; [Epub ahead of print]
5. Garcia-Reneses J, Herruzo-Cabrera R, Martinez-Moreno M. Epidemiological study of spinal cord injury in Spain 1984–1985. *Paraplegia* 28:180–90, 1991.
6. McKinley WO, Seel RT, Hardman JT. Nontraumatic spinal cord injury: Incidence, epidemiology, and functional outcome. *Arch Phys Med Rehabil* 80:619–23, 1999.
7. Biering-Sørensen F. Incidence of spinal cord lesions in Europe. In: Biering-Sørensen F, ed. Management of spinal cord lesions. State of the Art. *Clichéfa Grafisk* 2002, pp. 5–12. Can be downloaded from www.paraplegi.rh.dk.
8. Bhigjee AI. Neurological manifestations of HIV infection in Kwazulu-Natal South Africa. *J Neurovirol* 11 Suppl 1:17–21, 2005.
9. Green J, Valvanne-Tommila H, Loubser H, Fleming S, Gordon R, Paunio P, Marosszeky J. Detecting Differences in Service Delivery and Outcomes in Rehabilitation for Spinal Cord Dysfunction using Data from Australia, Finland, South Africa and the United States. 4th World Congress of the International Society of Physical and Rehabilitation Medicine, Seoul, Korea, June 10–14, 2007.
10. Munroe D. The rehabilitation of patients totally paralyzed below the waist, with special reference to making them ambulatory and capable of earning their own living. V. An end-result study of 445 cases. *New Engl J Med* 250:4–14, 1954.
11. World Health Organisation. International Classification of Functioning, Disability and Health: ICF. Geneva: WHO; 2001.
12. Lidal IB, Huynh TK, Biering-Sorensen F. Return to work following spinal cord injury: a review. *Disabil Rehabil* 15; 29(17):1341–75, 2007.
13. Metts RL. Disability issues, trends and recommendations for the World Bank. http://web.worldbank.org/WBSITE/EXTERNAL/TOPICS/EXTSOCIALPROTECTION/EXTDI 2000.
14. Levy LF, Makarawo S, Madzivire D, Bhebhe E, Verbeek N, Parry O. Problems, struggle and some success with spinal cord injury in Zimbabwe. *Spinal Cord* 36(3):213–8, 1998.
15. Inter-country meeting for the Eastern Mediterranean Region in Egypt 2006. Implementation of the United Nations standard rules on the equalization of opportunities for persons with disabilities. http://www.who.int/disabilities/publications/dar_cairo_2006_standard_rules. 2006.
16. United Nations. Convention on the rights of persons with disabilities. http://www.un.org/disabilities/convention. 2006.

17. Bricout JC. Using telework to enhance return to work outcomes for individuals with spinal cord injuries. *NeuroRehabilitation* 19(2):147–59, 2004.

18. Fawcett JW, Curt A, Steeves JD, Coleman WP, Tuszynski MH, Lammertse D, Bartlett PF, Blight AR, Dietz V, Ditunno J, Dobkin BH, Havton LA, Ellaway PH, Fehlings MG, Privat A, Grossman R, Guest JD, Kleitman N, Nakamura M, Gaviria M, Short D. Guidelines for the conduct of - clinical trials for spinal cord injury as developed by the ICCP panel: spontaneous recovery after spinal cord injury and statistical power needed for therapeutic clinical trials. *Spinal Cord* 45(3): 190–205, 2007.

19. Steeves JD, Lammertse D, Curt A, Fawcett JW, Tuszynski MH, Ditunno JF, Ellaway PH, Fehlings MG, Guest JD, Kleitman N, Bartlett PF, Blight AR, Dietz V, Dobkin BH, Grossman R, Short D, Nakamura M, Coleman WP, Gaviria M, Privat A. International Campaign for Cures of Spinal Cord Injury Paralysis. Guidelines for the conduct of clinical trials for spinal cord injury (SCI) as developed by the ICCP panel: clinical trial outcome measures. *Spinal Cord* 45(3):206–221, 2007.

20. Tuszynski MH, Steeves JD, Fawcett JW, Lammertse D, Kalichman M, Rask C, Curt A, Ditunno JF, Fehlings MG, Guest JD, Ellaway PH, Kleitman N, Bartlett PF, Blight AR, Dietz V, Dobkin BH, Grossman R, Privat A. International Campaign for Cures of Spinal Cord Injury Paralysis. Guidelines for the conduct of clinical trials for spinal cord injury as developed by the ICCP Panel: clinical trial inclusion/exclusion criteria and ethics. *Spinal Cord* 45(3):222–231, 2007.

21. Lammertse D, Tuszynski MH, Steeves JD, Curt A, Fawcett JW, Rask C, Ditunno JF, Fehlings MG, Guest JD, Ellaway PH, Kleitman N, Blight AR, Dobkin BH, Grossman R, Katoh H, Privat A, Kalichman M. International Campaign for Cures of Spinal Cord Injury Paralysis. Guidelines for the conduct of clinical trials for spinal cord injury as developed by the ICCP panel: clinical trial design. *Spinal Cord* 45(3):232–242, 2007.

22. Marino RJ, Barros T, Biering-Sorensen F, Burns SP, Donovan WH, Graves DE, Haak M, Hudson LM, Priebe MM. International standards for neurological classification of spinal cord injury. *J Spinal Cord Med* 26(suppl.1):S50-S56, 2003.

23. Krassioukov AV, Karlsson AK, Wecht JM, Wuermser LA, Mathias CJ, Marino RJ. Assessment of autonomic dysfunction following spinal cord injury: Rationale for additions to International Standards for Neurological Assessment. *J Rehabil Res Dev* 44(1):103–112, 2007.

24. Biering-Sørensen F, Charlifue S, DeVivo M, Noonan V, Post M, Stripling T, Wing P. International Spinal Cord Injury Data Sets. *Spinal Cord* 44(9):530–534, 2006.

25. DeVivo M, Biering-Sorensen F, Charlifue S, Noonan V, Post M, Stripling T, Wing P. International Spinal Cord Injury Core Data Set. *Spinal Cord* 44(9):535–540, 2006.

26. Biering-Sørensen F, Scheuringer M, Baumberger M, Charlifue SW, Post MWM, Montero F, Kostanjsek N, Stucki G. Developing core sets for persons with spinal cord injuries based on the International Classification of Functioning, Disability and Health as a way to specify functioning. *Spinal Cord* 44(9):541–546, 2006.

85 Consortium for Spinal Cord Medicine Clinical Practice Guidelines

Thomas Stripling
Caryn J. Cohen
Kim S. Nalle

Spinal cord medicine services are complicated and costly. Comprehensive care is intensive, lengthy, interdisciplinary, and frequently fragmented. Add the recent emphasis on cost reduction in both the private-sector managed care environment and the Department of Veterans Affairs, and healthcare providers are faced with the major challenge of achieving optimal clinical outcomes with ever-restricted resources. The Consortium for Spinal Cord Medicine (Consortium) Clinical Practice Guidelines was established to meet this challenge.

HISTORY

Paralyzed Veterans of America

Paralyzed Veterans of America is a nonprofit, congressionally chartered veterans' service organization that (a) advocates for its members; (b) promotes and funds spinal cord medicine, research, and education; (c) provides veterans benefits litigation; and (d) closely monitors and analyzes changes in the nation's healthcare system. In its 1995 publication, *Strategy 2000, Phase II: Meeting the Special Health Care Needs of America's Veterans,* Paralyzed Veterans recognized the benefits of promoting the development of evidence-based clinical practice guidelines (CPGs) for spinal cord medicine.

After extensive study of guideline development, applications, and uses (1–4), the Health Policy Department of Paralyzed Veterans concluded that scientific, evidence-based clinical practice guidelines (CPGs) could improve the quality of care (5–7), improve clinical outcomes (8–10), enhance program performance (6), facilitate health professional education (11), decrease medicolegal liability (12), and contain costs for all Americans with spinal cord injury (SCI) or disease (8, 13). Paralyzed Veterans decided to take a lead role by establishing the Consortium for Spinal Cord Medicine to write, publish, and disseminate CPGs in 1995.

Consortium for Spinal Cord Medicine

The Consortium comprises twenty-two health professional, payer, and consumer organizations, all having an interest to develop, publish, and disseminate evidence-based clinical practice guidelines (Table 85.1). A governing Steering Committee, consisting of one representative with experience in guideline development from each Consortium-member organization, manages and guides the development process. Steering Committee members share responsibility to (a) identify guideline topics; (b) select development panel chairs and nominate panelists; (c) establish and maintain a responsive guideline development process; (d) monitor the progress of each guideline topic panel to maintain good management; (e) develop and conduct a comprehensive publication and dissemination plan; and (f) foster a guideline evaluation/review mechanism to help measure clinical and service program outcomes.

The Consortium's mission is to enhance the quality, appropriateness, and cost-effectiveness of care delivered to people with SCI through scientifically rigorous, evidence-based practice. To achieve this goal, the following objectives were delineated by the Steering Committee:

- To develop and update professional clinical practice guidelines based on scientific evidence, expert consensus, and consumer input
- To develop and update companion consumer guides as informational tools for persons with spinal cord injury, family members, and caregivers
- To develop strategies for the dissemination of guidelines and consumer guides
- To promote the use of clinical practice guidelines as an essential component of healthcare delivery and usage
- To encourage implementation processes to promote the use of clinical practice guidelines and support outcome evaluations of the guidelines
- To promote an SCI research agenda for the domestic and international practice community that builds on existing scientific evidence

The Consortium is financed and administered primarily by Paralyzed Veterans of America. The Consortium's administration

Table 85.1   Consortium Member Organizations

Academy of Spinal Cord Injury Professionals
  • Spinal Cord Injury Nurses
  • Spinal Cord Injury Psychologists and Social Workers
  • Paraplegia Society
American Academy of Orthopaedic Surgeons
American Academy of Physical Medicine and Rehabilitation
American Association of Neurological Surgeons
American College of Emergency Physicians
American Congress of Rehabilitation Medicine
American Occupational Therapy Association
American Physical Therapy Association
American Psychological Association
American Spinal Injury Association
Association of Academic Physiatrists
Association of Rehabilitation Nurses
Christopher and Dana Reeve Foundation
Congress of Neurological Surgeons
Insurance Rehabilitation Study Group
International Spinal Cord Society
Paralyzed Veterans of America
Society of Critical Care Medicine
U.S. Department of Veterans Affairs
United Spinal Association

is under the auspices of the Research & Education Department with an immediate team of the Associate Director for Practice Guidelines and the Manager of Practice Guidelines. The Consortium has received support also from generous sponsors interested in specific topics and dissemination.

CLINICAL PRACTICE GUIDELINES

Evidence-based clinical practice guidelines can make healthcare provision more consistent, more measurable, and more cost conscious. CPGs also can forge a practical link between healthcare policy and the scientific knowledge that guides clinical practice (14, 15). Guidelines merge the current published scientific evidence and professional consensus necessary for providers to more efficiently prescribe the most appropriate treatments for specific clinical conditions. Similarly, guidelines provide consumers with the knowledge needed to participate in their care and rehabilitation to restore health and independence (6), and to facilitate a sense of self-control in care choices and options. Guidelines provide specific evidence-based information to enhance professional and patient education (11), reduce variations in practice (6, 16, 17), provide milestones for clinical management, and promote an accepted disease-specific or injury-specific standard of care (6).

When understood and used properly, guidelines can promote cost effectiveness by increasing efficiency, and in some cases, reducing the need for costly tests and services (17). For example, the guideline entitled *Prevention of Thromboembolism in Spinal Cord Injury,* 2nd edition, educates healthcare providers about the life-threatening dangers of the condition and details safe and effective interventions. This document encourages clinicians to act quickly—prescribing the most appropriate tests and procedures available—when a patient presents with symptoms

that may indicate the onset of this condition. Proceeding in this manner will likely cut costs associated with the onset of thromboembolism, thus lessening the need for more extensive and potentially lengthier services, while simultaneously improving patient outcome.

The Consortium's national success has exceeded all expectations, in large part due to the uniqueness of its structure and management. Because it is coordinated by a recognized national consumer organization with a reputation for providing effective service and advocacy for individuals with spinal cord injury and disease (SCI&D), its credibility is readily accepted in the practice community, enabling the Consortium to produce timely quality publications. Unlike other guideline development groups, the Consortium includes third-party payer organizations and consumers affected by SCI. This results in CPGs that reflect the patient's perspective and gives the consumer an increased feeling of ownership (18, 19, 20). In the course of CPG development Paralyzed Veterans provides facilitation and a neutral environment for consensus building.

During the 13 years the Consortium has been functioning, some important lessons have been learned. First, guideline development panels must represent every discipline necessary in the clinical decision-making process (21, 22). When issues arise requiring a specific area of expertise, it is important that a panelist is available to give the needed input—thus avoiding scheduling delays and additional costs. Second, an evidence-based approach to guideline development is necessary to produce credible and acceptable clinical practice guidelines (21, 22). Recommendations based solely on expert opinion do not carry the scientific weight needed for healthcare provider and consumer confidence. Biddle and Fraher (23) provide a critical review and detailed discussion of the "lessons learned" between 1996 and 1999 by the methodologic support team for the Consortium.

Definitions

Whether called practice guidelines, protocols, or parameters, guidelines have existed for decades (15). In this day of evidence-based medicine, guidelines have become widely accepted by the healthcare community as appropriate tools for physicians, nurses, therapists, and consumers in making healthcare decisions. Although not commonly understood, there are differences between clinical practice guidelines, clinical pathways, and clinical algorithms that are important to recognize (24). Clinical practice guidelines are evidence-based recommendations for healthcare providers to use when making healthcare decisions (25). Clinical pathways are institution-specific plans for organizing and sequencing the delivery of services by an interdisciplinary team (26, 27). Clinical algorithms are written instructions that organize the sequence of steps for a given treatment or condition (24). Evidence-based clinical practice guidelines can be used as the building blocks for clinical pathways and algorithms.

Recommendations that are based on current published scientific research findings and graded for scientific strength are considered "evidence-based" recommendations. To achieve an evidence-based guideline, each Consortium guideline development panel requires the support of a methodologic team of experts (7). This team conducts initial and secondary-level literature searches, evaluates the quality and strength of the scientific evidence, and grades the literature. This process often includes creating evidence tables to describe the citations, the type and quality of the reported research, and performing meta-analyses to aggregate the results of topic-specific research projects (particularly controlled clinical trials). These processes provide more conclusive information by using pooled data.

GUIDELINE DEVELOPMENT PROCESS

Basing a guideline on more than the expert opinion and consensus of healthcare providers has, in the last decade, been embraced and encouraged (20). The Agency for Healthcare Research and Quality (AHRQ) adopted a successful approach to guideline development wherein, whenever possible, scientific evidence and formal analytic methods are used as a basis for recommendations (28). Using this process, AHRQ was the primary federal agency actively producing and publishing evidence-based clinical practice guidelines in the 1980s and 1990s.

In 1997 AHRQ redirected its guideline development efforts in favor of supporting twelve new Evidence-Based Practice Centers (EPCs). The charge to each EPC was to undertake scientific analyses and evidence synthesis and create evidence reports and technology assessments on the prevention, diagnosis, treatment, and management of common diseases and clinical conditions. These evidence reports often provide a scientific foundation for organizations and specialty groups to develop CPGs and other tools to improve quality of care.

The Consortium adopted a modified version the AHRQ guideline development process, insisting that wherever possible, all guidelines are based on the most recent scientific evidence available. The Consortium's approach to the development of evidence-based guidelines is both innovative and cost efficient. The Consortium has achieved a successful and highly accepted process for guideline development based on three key elements. First, the Consortium itself is interdisciplinary, as is each of the development panels it manages. The Consortium's twenty-two member organizations and governing Steering Committee reflect the multiple needs of the spinal cord medicine community by representing all the disciplines that serve this specialized population. Accordingly, each guideline development panel is built on this same model—inclusion rather than exclusion.

The second key element in the Consortium's success is its responsiveness to the needs of its constituency. Each guideline development panel is asked to adhere to a strict publication production timeline, thereby getting the most current scientific evidence out to the field in a timely manner.

Finally, the Consortium focuses on real-life expert medical experience in those cases where the scientific literature has not yet been produced to support known clinical realities. The Consortium makes the best use of the time and expertise of the clinicians and other healthcare professionals serving as panel members, along with expert reviewers from the field, and selects topic consultants.

Twelve Steps to Success

The Consortium's process for developing clinical practice guidelines consists of twelve steps that lead to panel consensus and organizational approval. After the governing Steering Committee selects a topic, it chooses a panel chair. Qualifications for the panel chair stipulate demonstrated leadership in the topic area, a strong publication history, and experience in guideline development (11). Working with the panel chair, the Steering Committee determines which disciplines must be represented on the panel to ensure comprehensive topic development. Nominations are made and the selected individuals are extended invitations to serve as expert panelists. Working with a methodology consultant, the panel develops a detailed explication of the topic (i.e., an outline of the specific issues to be included in the guideline). The methodologist searches the international literature, grades and ranks the quality of the research studies found in the search, and prepares evidence tables and other specialized studies as warranted (13, 29, 30).

Based on their areas of expertise, panel members are assigned to write specific sections of the guideline, and a draft document is generated. The panel works together to refine the document to ensure its accuracy and completeness. Numerous critical reviews and panel discussions result in an iterative process that leads to panel consensus. Recommendations are discussed and voted on to determine the level of panel enthusiasm for each recommendation, and edits are made to resolve any discrepant opinions. Charts, graphs, and algorithms are added as necessary.

Each Consortium-member organization selects several topic-specific experts to review and comment on the draft guideline produced by the panel. These reviewers, the Steering Committee, and select outside experts and consumers review the document.

Reviewers' comments are assembled, analyzed, and collected in databases. This information is presented to the panel for deliberation. After panel discussion and agreement, the draft guideline is revised to reflect the concerns expressed by the reviewers and is sent for a legal review. Because the development and field review phases can alter a draft guideline repeatedly and sometimes in countermeasure, and the legal review can reveal significant conflicts, the Consortium requires that all working documents and draft guidelines be held in strict confidence by panelists and members. If there are no legal concerns about the draft guideline, the document is formatted and published.

CONSORTIUM SUCCESSES

To date, the Consortium has developed and published nine professional guidelines covering bladder management, respiratory management, neurogenic bowel, depression, autonomic dysreflexia, thromboembolism, preservation of upper limb, pressure ulcer management, and expected outcomes along with five companion consumer guides on autonomic dysreflexia, neurogenic bowel, depression, pressure ulcer, and expected outcomes. Several Consortium publications have been translated into Spanish. A wall poster and wallet card for autonomic dysreflexia have been produced in English and Spanish.

The Consortium encourages the development of collateral products but does not make a practice of endorsing such products. Collateral products might include training curriculum, videos, book chapters, monographs, pamphlets, etc. Although these products are certainly worthwhile, the Consortium does not want the production of such collateral products to distract from its primary mission of producing CPGs.

Consortium-member organizations including the Academy of Spinal Cord Injury Professionals, the American Academy of Physical Medicine and Rehabilitation, the Department of Veterans Affairs, and others have sanctioned the guidelines for use by their members, but the Consortium has not pursued official organizational endorsement because of the difficulties of coordinating separate administrative processes that could complicate publication of the final products. However, member organizations and others can independently endorse guideline and consumer guide with Paralyzed Veterans' approval.

Updated, second-edition guidelines for the acute management of autonomic dysreflexia (AD) and the prevention of thromboembolism (DVT) have been completed. The Consortium has a rigorous review process for maintaining the relevance and accuracy of all published products. All CPGs and consumer guides are available as free downloads at www.PVA.org.

Future Publications

The Consortium's most recent publication is a new guideline titled "Early Acute Management in Adults with Spinal Cord Injury." Its companion consumer guide will focus on frequently asked questions following SCI. A panel is currently working on the topic of sexuality and reproductive health following spinal cord injury.

Future topics for development will include

- Psychosocial adjustment following SCI
- Carbohydrate and lipid processing following SCI
- Spasticity treatment

Promoting an Evidence-Based Research Agenda

The Consortium encourages development of collaborative research on spinal cord medicine. With assistance from its professional member organizations, the Consortium generates ideas for new research to improve the published evidence that will lead to improvement in healthcare and healthcare policies.

CONCLUSION

Healthcare providers should consider clinical practice guidelines to be an excellent management tool in providing care to their patients (5). Guidelines provide scientific evidence and professional consensus to more effectively treat and manage clinical conditions. The identification of research gaps is an important derivative of the Consortium's mission (33, 34). Healthcare providers should educate themselves and their colleagues on the proper use and benefits of evidence-based clinical practice guidelines.

References

1. Eddy DM. Clinical decision making: From theory to practice. Designing a practice policy. Standards, guidelines, and options. *JAMA* 1990; 263(3077):3081–3084.

2. Eddy DM. *A Manual for Assessing Health Practices and Designing Practice Policies: The Explicit Approach.* Philadelphia: American College of Physicians, 1992.

3. Woolf SH. *AHCPR Interim Manual for Clinical Practice Guideline Development.* U.S. Dept. of Health & Human Services, Public Health Service: Agency for Health Care Policy and Research, 1991.

4. Woolf SH, DiGuiseppi CG, Atkins D, Kamerow DB. Developing evidence-based clinical practice guidelines: Lessons learned by the U.S. Preventive Services Task Force. *Annu Rev Public Health* 1996; 17:511–538.

5. Carnett WG. Clinical practice guidelines: A tool to improve care. *Qual Manag Health Care* 1999; 8(1):13–21.

6. Harris JS. Development, use, and evaluation of clinical practice guidelines. *J Occup Environ Med* 1997; 39(1):23–34.

7. Heffner JE. Does evidence-based medicine help the development of clinical practice guidelines? *Chest* 1998; 113:172S–178S.

8. Cluzeau FA, Littlejohns P. Appraising clinical practice guidelines in England and Wales: The development of a methodologic framework and its application to policy. *Jt Comm J Qual Improv* 1999; 25(10):514–521.

9. Grimshaw JM, Russell IT. Effect of clinical guidelines on medical practice: A systematic review of rigorous evaluations. *Lancet* 1993; 342(8883):1317–1322.

10. Handley MR, Stuart ME, Kirz HL. An evidence-based approach to evaluating and improving clinical practice: Implementing practice guidelines. *HMO Pract* 1994; 8(2):75–83.

11. Heffner JE. The overarching challenge. *Chest* 2000; 118:1S–3S.

12. Woolf SH, Grol R, Hutchinson A, Eccles M, et al. Clinical guidelines: Potential benefits, limitations, and harms of clinical guidelines. *BMJ* 1999; 318:527–530.

13. Connis RT, Nickinovich DG, Caplan RA, Arens JF. The development of evidence-based clinical practice guidelines. Integrating medical science and practice. *Int J Technol Assess Health Care* 2000; 16(4):1003–1012.

14. Woolf SH. Evidence-based medicine and practice guidelines: An overview. *Cancer Control* 2000; 7(4):362–367.

15. Gundersen L. The effect of clinical practice guidelines on variations in care. *Ann Intern Med* 2000; 133:317.

16. Woolf SH. Do clinical practice guidelines define good medical care? The need for good science and disclosure of uncertainty when defining 'best practices.' *Chest* 1998; 113:166S–171S.

17. Kaegi L. AMA clinical quality improvement forum ties it all together: From guidelines to measurement to analysis and back to guidelines. *Jt Comm J Qual Improv* 1999; 25(2):95–106.

18. Brouwers MC, Browman GP. Development of clinical practice guidelines: Surgical perspective. *World J Surg* 1999; 23(12):1236–1241.

19. Gunn IP. Evidence-based practice, research, peer review, and publication. *CRNA* 1998; 9(4):177–182.

20. Lohr KN, Eleazer K, Mauskopf J. Health policy issues and applications for evidence-based medicine and clinical practice guidelines. *Health Policy* 1998; 46(1):1–19.

21. Helou A, Lorenz W, Ollenschlager G, Reinauer H, Schwartz FW. Methodological standards of the evidence-based approach of clinical guidelines development in Germany. Consensus between the scientific community, self-governed bodies and practice. *Z Arztl Fortbild Qualitatssich* 2000; 94(5):330–339.

22. Shekelle PG, Woolf SH, Eccles M. Clinical guidelines: Developing guidelines. *BMJ* 1999; (318):593–596.

23. Biddle AK, Fraher EP. Developing clinical practice guidelines for spinal cord medicine. Lessons learned. *Phys Med Rehabil Clin N Am* 2000; 11(1):227–243, x–xi.

24. *Clinical Practice Guidelines: Primer.* Management Decision and Research Center; Washington, DC: VA Health Services Research and Development Service, 1998.

25. Jackson R, Feder G. Guidelines for clinical guidelines: A simple, pragmatic strategy for guideline development. *BMJ* 1998; 317:427–428.

26. Garbin BA. Introduction to clinical pathways. *JHQ* 1995; 17(6):6–9.

27. Holloway RG Jr, Ringel SP. Narrowing the evidence-practice gap: Strengthening the link between research and clinical practice. *Neurology* 1998; 50:319–321.

28. McCormick KA, Fleming B. Clinical practice guideline. The Agency for Health Care Policy and Research fosters the development of evidence-based guidelines. *Health Prog* 1992; 73(10):30–34.

29. Auston I, Cahn MA, Seldon CR. Literature search methods for the development of clinical practice guidelines. In: *Clinical Practice Guideline*

Development: Methodology Perspectives. U.S. Dept. of Health & Human Services, Public Health Service: Agency for Health Care Policy and Research 1994; 123–127.

30. Marriott R. Providing library support for the development of clinical guidelines. *Health Libraries Review* 1998; 16(2):132–134.

31. Gosfield AG. Clinical practice guidelines and the law: Applications and implications. *Health Law Handbook* 1994; 65–99.

32. Gosfield AG. Measuring performance and quality: The state of the art and legal concerns. *Health Law Handbook* 1995; 31–67.

33. Briss PA, Zaza S, Pappaioanou M, Fielding J, et al. Developing an evidence-based guide to community preventive services—methods. The Task Force on Community Preventive Services. *Am J Prev Med* 2000; 18(1 Suppl):35–43.

34. Heffner JE, Alberts WM, Irwin R, Wunderink R. Translating guidelines into clinical practice: Recommendations to the American College of Chest Physicians. *Chest* 2000; 118:70S–73S.

86 Subspecialty Certification in Spinal Cord Injury Medicine

Margaret C. Hammond

For those individuals practicing in spinal cord injury (SCI) medicine, the existence of a unique fund of knowledge and skill set, different from that acquired in basic specialty training, is easily appreciated. However, obtaining formal recognition of spinal cord injury medicine as a recognized subspecialty by the American Board of Medical Specialties required decades of effort. Multiple prominent leaders in the field engaged in this process over the years. One can trace the roots of the specialty to the 1930s, when modern methods of treating patients with SCI developed. Over the years, specialized treatment facilities developed and clinical experience and research documented the existence of a unique body of knowledge. Organizations composed of multispecialty practitioners reflected the multiple needs of such patients. The American Paraplegia Society (APS), American Spinal Injury Association, the International Medical Society of Paraplegia, and special interest groups within various specialties developed to provide a forum for those physicians whose primary commitment is to serve the person with SCI or other spinal cord disorders. Such organizations are dedicated to improving patient care, recognizing and educating providers, promoting research, and providing a forum for the exchange of ideas.

Within such organizations dedicated to SCI care, the need for subspecialty recognition was discussed over the years, and various options for recognition were considered. Constraints and critical influencing variables, such as the scope of the subspecialty, the particular organization to develop the proposal, the accrediting or certifying body, the potential of such existing oversight bodies to approve the subspecialty, and the willingness of practitioners to accept a formal designation process, changed over the years. At one point in the mid-1980s, interested parties decided to focus instead on the process of fellowship training.

In 1991 the American Paraplegia Society Board of Directors decided to explore the feasibility of obtaining certification from an American Board of Medical Specialties Member Board. The largest proportion of APS members were certified in Physical Medicine and Rehabilitation; thus the American Board of Physical Medicine and Rehabilitation (ABPM&R) was the logical Board to represent the application. The ABPM&R was willing to pursue this process, and Dr. Joel DeLisa was appointed Chair of the Subcommittee on SCI Medicine to develop the application.

The field was defined as "the subspecialty that addresses the prevention, diagnosis, treatment, and management of traumatic spinal cord injury (SCI) and nontraumatic etiologies of spinal cord dysfunction by working in an interspecialty manner. Care is provided on a lifelong basis and covers related medical, physical, psychological, and vocational disabilities and complications. This care encompasses patients of all ages" (1).

The proposal included specification of the scope of the field, documentation supporting a unique fund of knowledge, delineation of existing treatment facilities, membership of relevant organizations, and documentation of fellowship training programs. The purpose of subspecialty certification is "to enhance the quality of care available to individuals with spinal cord dysfunction through training a cadre of highly expert clinicians, teachers, and investigators." Those receiving certification must demonstrate special expertise in clinical knowledge and skill in SCI medicine, as well as improve the rehabilitation and care of individuals with SCI. They must also provide expert primary diagnostic and management services for those complex and severe clinical problems related to SCI that require interspecialty management in SCI centers. In addition, they must provide support to the principal care providers of persons with SCI who practice in non-SCI centers, by rendering follow-up care to prevent and manage complications related to SCI. They are also looked upon to improve the quality and teaching of SCI medicine in residency programs of related primary specialties. This is accomplished by stimulating the availability of subspecialists with additional knowledge and skills in SCI medicine, as well as increasing research directed toward the problems of individuals with spinal cord dysfunction, while also recognizing potential faculty members with special interests in SCI Medicine. Other duties are to improve interspecialty and interdisciplinary communication and cooperation among specialists caring for persons with SCI and to provide access to diplomates of all ABMS member Boards, particularly from specialties directly related to the care of people with SCI. These specialties include anesthesiology, emergency medicine, family practice, internal medicine, neurology, neurosurgery, orthopedic surgery, pediatrics, physical medicine and rehabilitation, plastic surgery, and urology (1).

The ABMS granted authority to the ABPM&R to issue certificates of special qualifications in SCI medicine in 1995. The certificate is awarded to candidates who meet the practice and education requirements and who successfully complete a proctored examination in the subspecialty. The practice track requirement was 3 years of practice experience, primarily in SCI medicine. Beginning in 2008, all applicants are required to complete an ACGME-accredited training program in SCI medicine.

In a separate process, the Residency Review Committee (RRC) for PM&R developed program requirements in SCI medicine. The extensive approval process required the circulation of draft requirements to the sponsoring organizations of the Accreditation Council for Graduate Medical Education (ACGME), to all other RRCs, to Program Directors, and to interested parties. After multiple revisions and the completion of the consensus building process, in 1996, the ACGME approved the program requirements for residency training in SCI medicine. Although technically referred to as *residents* by the ACGME, such trainees are often called *fellows*. The accreditation of designated training programs is considered by the RRC on behalf of the ACGME on a twice-yearly basis. At this time, there are nineteen training programs with ACGME approval.

There are 560 individuals holding certification in Spinal Cord Injury Medicine.

Reference

1. *Subspecialty Certification in SCI Medicine Booklet of Information.* Available from the American Board of Physical Medicine and Rehabilitation, 3015 Allegro Park Lane, Rochester MN 55902–4139 or www.abpmr.org.

87 The Commission on Accreditation of Rehabilitation Facilities

Sophia Chun

The history of Commission on Accreditation of Rehabilitation Facilities (CARF) dates back to the 1960s, when two organizations, the National Rehabilitation Association and the Association of Rehabilitation, began work in development of standards for sheltered workshops and for medically oriented rehabilitation centers, respectively. The two organizations' pioneering works in standards development formed the basis for the earliest CARF standards.

CARF, a private, nonprofit organization formally established in 1966, is currently the preeminent standards-setting and accrediting body promoting and advocating for the delivery of quality rehabilitation care for persons served. Its mission is to promote the quality, value, and optimal outcomes of services through a consultative accreditation process that centers on enhancing the lives of person serviced. It does this by establishing standards of quality for organizations to use as guidelines in developing and offering their programs or services to consumers. The CARF standards are developed with input from consumers, rehabilitation professionals, state and national organizations, and funders. Every year the standards are reviewed and new ones are developed to keep pace with changing conditions and current consumer needs. CARF has accredited over 17,000 locations in 10 countries, with more than 1,000 surveyors across the United States, Canada, and Europe. Specific to Spinal Cord System of Care, as of 2007, there are 81 facilities at 93 locations that are CARF accredited in Spinal Cord System of Care. Although CARF maintains its strong emphasis on rehabilitation, it has also moved beyond rehabilitation into the broader area of human services such as aging, child, and youth services.

BENEFITS OF CARF ACCREDITATION

Accreditation by CARF ensures to consumer/stakeholders, i.e. patients, insurers/funding source, referral agencies, medical and other professionals in the health field, businesses, community leaders and service organizations, that the program is reviewed by an impartial external organization and that it meets or exceeds the internationally recognized, consumer-focused standards of quality established for rehabilitation care. CARF accreditation builds confidence with the stakeholders/ consumers about the quality of services provided.

The CARF accreditation process is based on the concept of peer review, networking, and sharing ideas. One of the hallmarks of CARF is the use of a consultative rather than inspective approach to the survey process. Using a consultative approach, the surveyors interview the persons served, families, staff members, funders, and other stakeholders; observe program practices; review appropriate documentation; answer questions about important concepts in the standards; and provide suggestions to further improve the organization's operations and programs. The recommendations and suggestions provided by the CARF survey are designed to be used by the organization to continue to refine and improve its services, operations, evaluations, methods, organizational structure, and policies. In addition, the CARF staff is available by telephone or e-mail to answer questions regarding the interpretation of standards and provide consultation.

Programs seeking CARF accreditation and those that are CARF accredited receive other practical benefits, including having access to the many resources provided by CARF, including free newsletters such as "CARF Connection," which provides timely tips, resources, and updates about CARF accreditation and business practices, and the "Promising Practices," which features innovative and best practices for continuous quality improvement and removal of barriers.

In addition, providers accredited by CARF may be eligible to receive discounts on their insurance premiums in acknowledgement of their commitment to performance improvement and quality assurance. In summary, in addition to being an accrediting body, CARF can be seen as a collaborative partner in an ongoing effort to improve service delivery and care.

Recognizing the many benefits of being CARF accredited, the Veterans Affairs Healthcare System has made it mandatory to be accredited by CARF. The National Spinal Cord Injury Association also provides lists of CARF-accredited organizations to consumers.

NAVIGATING THE CARF STANDARDS MANUAL

For those not familiar with CARF, it is often thought of as equivalent or similar to Joint Commission for the Accreditation of Hospitals (JCAHO) for rehabilitation services. However, there are many standards in CARF that are specific to CARF, and it is important for hospital and program administration to understand and appreciate the different emphasis, as successful preparation or outcome in a JCAHO survey does not ensure success in CARF. One of the purposes of this chapter is to outline the CARF accreditation process, which will allow better understanding of the background behind CARF standards.

The Spinal Cord System of Care is under the CARF Medical Rehabilitation Accreditation. Although the name of the sections may change over time, the CARF standards manual for Medical Rehabilitation can be essentially divided into three sections: Section 1-Business Practice/Aspire to Excellence™, Section 2-Rehabilitation Process, and Section 3.A to 3.K, which is the Program Specific Standards. Spinal Cord System of Care (SCSC) 3.B. is one of the eleven specific programs that CARF accredits under medical rehabilitation.

The other medical rehabilitation programs that can be accredited by CARF include Comprehensive Integrated Inpatient Rehabilitation Programs, (3.C) Interdisciplinary Pain Rehabilitation Programs, (3.D) Brain Injury Programs, (3.E) Outpatient Medical Rehabilitation Programs, (3.F) Home- and Community-Based Rehabilitation Programs, (3.G) Medical Rehabilitation Case Management, (3.H) Health Enhancement Program, (3.I.) Pediatric Family-Centered Rehabilitation Programs, (3.J) Occupational Rehabilitation Programs, (3.K) Stroke Specialty Programs.

Section 1—Business Practice/Aspire to Excellence™ and Section 2—Rehabilitation Process are applicable to all programs seeking CARF accreditation. Please refer to the CARF Medical Rehabilitation Standards Manual regarding specific applicable standards within Section 2-Rehabilitation Process for various programs. For section 3, one would reference only the specific section(s) that applies to the program seeking accreditation.

SPINAL CORD SYSTEM OF CARE ACCREDITATION

CARF first developed specialty standards for spinal cord rehabilitation in 1983. The standards progressed from spinal cord injury to spinal cord system of care that must include an inpatient hospital-based rehabilitation program as well as an outpatient component. With this new addition of standards, if the Spinal Cord System of Care also provides a residential, home and community-based, or vocational component of care, they must also seek accreditation in these specific areas to assure consumers that all CARF-accredited programs for spinal cord injury are backed by standards to assess their quality delivery framework.

Section 1. Business Practice/Aspire to Excellence™

In addition to evaluating rehabilitation quality, CARF emphasizes the quality of business performance, which can be a distinctive difference from Joint Commission. The business practice section attempts to evaluate various aspects of quality of business performance, including Input from Stakeholders, Accessibility, Information Management and Performance Improvement, Rights of Persons Served, Health and Safety, Human Resources, Leadership, Legal Requirements, Financial Planning and Management, and Governance. If the program seeking CARF accreditation is part of a larger organization, some of these areas such as financial planning and management, governance, or legal requirement may involve active participation of the organization's leadership in addition to the program leadership. Although this section has undergone several significant changes in the name and the organization of the standards, there have not been changes to its basic principles of focus on evaluating business/organization performance. It is of note that many of the standards are integrated. For example, under the business practice/Aspire to Excellence™ section, CARF would evaluate if leadership takes information obtained from stakeholders and turns it into operational practice to be used for competitive advantage, business growth, innovation, solving problems, and challenges facing the program/organization.

Section 2. Rehabilitation Process

The key features of the rehabilitation process are the organization/program's responsibility to affect positive change in functional ability of persons served while protecting and promoting their rights. Persons served are treated with dignity and respect, and all personnel are aware of their rights as well as the rights of the persons served. The integrated team possesses clarity and affects reduction of redundancy in records of persons served. Predicted outcomes are achieved, and patients served are reintegrated into their community of choice.

The rehabilitation process section evaluates the program from pre-admission assessment to discharge of the persons served by the program, with emphasis on processes to ensure that there is adequate communication amongst the team members, that the records of persons contain relevant information to facilitate achievement of rehabilitation goals, and that the rights, safety, and security of persons served are protected.

Section 3B. Spinal Cord System of Care (SCSC)

Persons with spinal cord injury or dysfunction can be served in programs that are not specifically accredited in Spinal Cord System of Care, such as in Comprehensive Integrated Inpatient Rehabilitation Programs (CIIRP), however, a program seeking accreditation in Spinal Cord System of Care (SCSC) would need to meet additional standards specifically associated with caring for persons with spinal cord dysfunction that demonstrate a coordinated, case-managed, integrated service with both inpatient and outpatient component. The organization seeking SCSC accreditation must demonstrate evidence of an inpatient component that provides integrated medical and rehabilitation services that are provided 24 hours per day, 7 days per week in a licensed hospital, and an outpatient component that provides a structured, coordinated, comprehensive nonresidential program. The Spinal Cord System of Care needs to demonstrate formal links with key components of care that address the lifelong needs of the persons served. Such linkages include emergent care, acute hospitalization, other inpatient rehabilitation programs, skilled nursing care, home care, and other outpatient and medical rehabilitation programs, community-based services, residential services, vocational services, primary care, specialty consultants, and long-term care.

The organization seeking Spinal Cord System of Care accreditation is to be accountable for and serves as a resource to the persons served, their families/support systems, and continuum-of-care providers through its:

- Identification of care options and linkages with services/programs with demonstrated competencies in spinal cord dysfunction
- Achievement of predicted outcomes
- Conservation of funding to meet lifelong needs
- Provision and facilitation of medical interventions
- Facilitation of opportunities for interaction with individuals with activity limitations
- Focus on lifelong follow-up that addresses impairment, activity, participation, and quality of life
- Provision of education and training
- Identification of regulatory, legislative, and financial implications

The Spinal Cord System of Care accredited program is responsible for developing, facilitating, and ensuring demonstration of competencies that address the unique needs of the persons served. These competencies are established for the persons served, their families/support systems, and personnel.

The Spinal Cord System of Care accredited program must also encompass care that advocates for full inclusion and enhances the lives of the persons served within their families/support systems, communities, and life roles, and demonstrate how the outcomes information are shared with relevant stakeholders.

THE CARF SURVEY PROCESS

Preparation

The first step in a successful Spinal Cord System of Care CARF survey is to consult with a designated CARF Resource Specialist. The organization should proceed to order the standards manual and survey preparation guides, which are available at the CARF Web site, www.carf.org. Second, the organization should perform a self-evaluation. This would include a development of an interdisciplinary CARF work group composed of key members of the rehabilitation team, which may include physicians, nursing, social workers, a case manager, therapists, a data manager, etc. This group should set timeframes to conform to any standards that are not in conformance along with the responsible persons. Various resources are available from the CARF Web site, to aid in the self-evaluation process and preparation for the survey. Although there are no set guidelines on how the documentation is to be organized, all relevant policies and procedures, as well as written materials demonstrating conformance to the standards, should be readily available to the surveyors. Please note that to be eligible to maintain or retain accreditation, the standards must have been used for a minimum of 6 months.

Once the organization/program has decided to pursue CARF accreditation, the Intent to Survey application must be filed. The intent to survey application informs CARF about the leadership of the organization, the demographics of persons served, specific programs seeking accreditation, size and number of location of the organization, performance improvement activities, and the commitment to the accreditation process. Current information on application timetable can be found on www.carf.org Web site.

Approximately 1 month prior to the timeframe that is based on when CARF receives the intent to survey application, the organization will be notified in writing of date(s) and the name(s) of the surveyor(s). Public notification of the survey needs to be posted at least 30 days prior to the survey date to inform all the stakeholders regarding the upcoming survey as well as to give an opportunity for the stakeholders to communicate directly to the CARF survey team members. Communication between the organization to be surveyed and the surveyor will need to occur to coordinate an agenda for the survey days. A room should be set aside for the surveyors to be able to review documents and have a place to work. The organization should plan for and invite those individuals who will be attending the orientation and the exit conference.

DAY OF SURVEY

Attempt should be made by the surveyors and the organization being surveyed to follow the set agenda, which will include orientation to CARF by the surveyors, a tour, interviews of key personnel and administrative leadership, observation of team, set times for documentation review, and exit conference. The organization should plan for and invite those individuals who would attend the orientation and exit conferences. Individuals to consider inviting to the orientation and/or the exit conference include key organization management, staff members, persons served, representatives of the governance, referral sources, and/or third-party funding sources.

During the exit conference, the surveyors will share their findings, which will include the organization's strengths, exemplary conformance to standards, and areas that the organization should seek improvements.

The Standards Conformance Rating System (Scors®)

The CARF Standards Conformance Rating System, which was developed by a cross-divisional technical task force in May 1997, provides an objective, precision-driven assessment of conformance to CARF standards. The system incorporates a four point scale: (0) = Non-Conformance, (1) = Partial Conformance, (2) = Conformance, (3) = Exemplary Conformance. The ratings may be used in making an accreditation decision only after CARF has had the opportunity to analyze several years of data and is not summed up to determine the accreditation decision at this time.

Other items for consideration during the survey process include utilizing the consultative expertise of the survey team for suggestions. Please note that suggestions are suggestions and do not count toward the survey outcome. The surveyors may request a copy of the survey preparation guide and that policy and procedure manual(s) be brought to the hotel the day before the survey begins.

AFTER THE SURVEY

The survey team prepares a detailed written report that is sent to CARF. After an editing process, the report is sent to the accreditation committee of the CARF Board of Trustees and the final survey report and letter of outcome is sent approximately 8–10 weeks after the survey. The organization must submit a Quality Improvement Plan for any recommendations cited on the report within 90 days after receipt of the letter of outcome. CARF maintains contact with the organization during the tenure of accreditation. Organizations are encouraged to contact CARF as needed to help maintain conformance to the CARF standards. There are various CARF seminars and conferences that are excellent ways to receive updates and other important information about the accreditation process and the standards.

ACCREDITATION OUTCOME

There are four possible accreditation outcomes: Three-Year Accreditation, One-Year Accreditation, Provisional, and Nonaccreditation.

Three-Year Accreditation

This is the highest level of accreditation an organization may be awarded. The organization meets each of the CARF Accreditation Conditions and shows substantial fulfillment of the standards. Its services and practices are designed and implemented to benefit the people it serves. Its services, personnel, and documentation clearly indicate that present conditions represent an established pattern of total operation and that these conditions are likely to be maintained or improved in the foreseeable future.

One-Year Accreditation

The organization meets each of the CARF Accreditation Conditions. Although there are deficiencies in relation to the standards, there is evidence of the organization's capability and commitment to correct the deficiencies or make progress toward their correction. On balance, the services are benefiting those served and the organization appears to be protecting their health, welfare, and safety.

Provisional Accreditation

A Provisional Accreditation may be awarded only once, for a period of 1 year, after an organization has received a One-Year Accreditation as the result of the previous site survey. The organization must be functioning at the level of a Three-Year Accreditation at the end of the tenure of the Provisional Accreditation, or it will receive a survey outcome of Nonaccreditation.

Nonaccreditation

The organization has major deficiencies in several areas of the standards, and there are serious questions as to the rehabilitation benefits, health, welfare, or safety of its clients; the organization has failed over time to bring itself into substantial conformance to the standards; or the organization has failed to meet any one of the CARF accreditation conditions. An organization receiving a Nonaccreditation status has to wait 6 months to reapply.

*R*eference

1. CARF Medical Rehabilitation Standards Manual (July 2007–2008). CARF International 4891 East Grant Road, Tucson, AZ 85712; (888)281–6531 (Web site: www.carf.org).

88 Health Industry and Product Information

Pamela E. Wilson
Jerry Clayton

Spinal cord injury (SCI) affects all aspects of a person's life and lifestyle. In equipping an individual and his or her family to deal with these changes, information is one of the most powerful tools that can be provided. A variety of resources are available to educate both the medical professional and their patient. Although by no means complete, the information included in this chapter should serve as an introduction to information of both a scientific and practical nature that will serve as a resource to the clinician as well as the patient and family. Helpful information can be gleaned from both the print media and the Internet. Details from the medical community and experience from patients and their families come together to create a complete resource and a means to foster the quality of life for all of those involved.

SCIENTIFIC JOURNALS RELEVANT TO SCI

Journals with a Focus on Spinal Cord and Brain Injury

- *Archives of Physical Medicine and Rehabilitation* (Philadelphia, PA; W.B. Saunders Co.)
- *Journal of Neurotrauma*—The official journal of the National Neurotrauma Society. (New York; M.A. Liebert)
- *Journal of Spinal Cord Medicine*—The official journal of the American Paraplegia Society. (Jackson Heights, NY; American Paraplegia Society)
- *Spinal Cord*—The official journal of the International Medical Society of Paraplegia; formerly known as Paraplegia. (Houndmills, Basingstoke, Hampshire, U.K.: Macmillan Press)

Journals Focused on Neurology/Neuroscience Information Pertinent to SCI

- *Annals of Neurology* (Boston, MA; Little, Brown and Co.)
- *Journal of Child Neurology* (Hamilton, Ontario; Decker Periodicals)

- *Journal of Neuroscience*—The official journal of the Society for Neuroscience (Baltimore, MD; The Society for Neuroscience)
- *Journal of Neurotrauma*—The official journal of the National and International Neurotrauma Societies (New York: May Ann Liebert, Inc.)
- *Nature Neuroscience* (New York: Nature America Inc.)
- *Neurology*—The official journal of the American Academy of Neurology (Boston, MA; Little, Brown, and Co.)
- *Neuron* (Cambridge, MA; Cell Press)
- *Neuroscience* (Oxford, New York; Pergamon Press)

The reader is advised to utilize any one of several services that allow you to search the medical literature for specific topics. One of the major sites is sponsored by the U.S. government through the National Library of Medicine and is entitled MEDLINE/PubMed. This is available free to all via the internet and can be accessed at http://www.nlm.nih.gov.

GENERAL INFORMATION ON DISABILITY, LIFESTYLE, AND HEALTHCARE RESOURCES

Information on SCI can be obtained from a variety of sources both in print and via the internet. Listed below are some key resources for those interested in gaining more information pertaining to spinal cord injury.

PRINT MEDIA

Books

- Conditioning with Physical Disabilities/Kevin F. Lockette, Ann M. Keyes. Champaign, IL: Human Kinetics, 1994.
- The HealthSouth spinal cord injury handbook for patients and their families/Richard C. Senelick, Karla R. Dougherty. Birmingham, AL: Healthsouth Press, 1998.
- Sexuality after spinal cord injury: answers to your questions/by Stanley H. Ducharme and Kathleen M. Gill. Baltimore: Paul H. Brookes Pub., 1997.

Consumer Publications Focused on Disabilities and Lifestyles

Exceptional Parent
Boston, MA: Psy-Ed Corp.
http://www.eparent.com/

This magazine is for parents and professionals alike. It has general interest stories, but also has review articles on multiple topics related to disabilities. Has a yearly resource guide published on a vast array of disability resources.

Accent on Living
Bloomington, IL, Cheever Pub. Co.
http://findarticles.com/p/articles/mi_m0803

Focuses on individuals with physical disabilities and active lifestyles. General-interest articles and helpful hints.

New Mobility
Horsham, PA, No Limits Communications Inc.
http://www.newmobility.com

Geared toward the active wheelchair population with a focus on lifestyle and culture.

Paraplegia News
New York, Paralyzed Veterans of America
http://www.pvamagazines.com/pnnews/

Focuses on the wheelchair population, with an emphasis on sports, recreation, and lifestyle. Has a nice review section on SCI research updates.

Sports'n Spokes
Phoenix, AZ, N. Crase
http://www.pvamagazines.com/sns/

Mainly focused on wheelchair sports and recreational activities. Has an excellent annual review of wheelchairs and handcycles.

WE Magazine and WeMedia Sports
New York, R. Coppola
http://www.wemedia.com

Magazine and Web site geared toward multidisabilities. These include human interest stories, lifestyle, disability updates, product information, and sports. Web site is unique in following and televising multidisabled events (e.g., Paralympics).

INTERNET-BASED RESOURCES

Commercial And Organizational

Craig Hospital
http://www.craighospital.com

Craig Hospital is a center of excellence for rehabilitation medicine and research located in Denver, Colorado, and is well known for its care of spinal cord and traumatic brain-injured patients. The hospital's site provides information relevant to the SCI patient and family, with many links to resources around the world.

Cure Paralysis Now
http://www.cureparalysisnow.org/

This informational Web site reflects the efforts of an advocacy group based in Texas to promote legislation supportive of research into a cure for SCI. The site also contains a very complete list of other SCI-related organizations throughout the United States.

Paralyzed Veterans of America (PVA)
801 Eighteenth Street, NW
Washington, DC 20006–3517
E-mail: info@pva.org
http://www.pva.org

The PVA has spent a considerable amount of time and research to develop information booklets on the many aspects of SCI. A partial list of topics that may be obtained through the organization follows:

- An Introduction to Spinal Cord Injury: Understanding the Changes, 3rd edition
- Constipation and Spinal Cord Injury: A Guide to Symptoms and Treatment
- In Touch With Kids
  - Rebecca Finds a New Way (under 10 years old)
  - Follow Your Dreams (11 to 13 years old)
  - Tell It Like It Is (teens and up)
- Inform Yourself: Alcohol, Drugs, and Spinal Cord Injury
- Skin Care: Preventing Ulcers
- The Quest for Cure: Restoring Function After Spinal Cord Injury
- Yes, You Can! A Guide to Self-Care for Persons with Spinal Cord Injury Revised Edition

The Rehabilitation and Research Center (RRC)
http://www.tbi-sci.org

The Santa Clara Valley Medical Center in Santa Clara, California, is the home of the Rehabilitation and Research Center for Traumatic Brain Injury and Spinal Cord Injury. Its Web site provides information on research activities taking place at the institution, as well as elsewhere. Also, part of the site provides access and links to many resources directly related to SCI. Of particular interest is the SCI Web Ring, sponsored by the RRC. The RRC provides access to over 100 member Web sites that share an interest in SCI. Links range from commercial and organizational to personal.

Shepherd Center
http://www.shepherd.org/

The Shepherd Center in Atlanta, Georgia, is a nonprofit hospital "devoted to the medical care and rehabilitation of people with spinal cord injury and disease." The site contains general information on disabilities, resources, and research. Can link up with research base in regard to etiology, incidence, prevalence, and complications.

Spinal Cord Injury Research Links
http://www.proneuron.com/Links/index.html

This site provides links to SCI treatment centers, organizations, and support groups.

Spinal Research
http://www.spinal-research.org

Organization based in the United Kingdom focused on funding research "that will end the permanence of paralysis caused by spinal cord injury and in doing so improve the quality of life of paralyzed people." Disseminates information and supports research internationally.

Government and University

ClinicalTrials.gov
http://www.clinicaltrials.gov/

This is a Web site containing information pertinent to all clinical trials sponsored by the U.S. government. Completely searchable. An excellent way to find out what is currently being studied relevant to SCI and its sequelae.

Disabilityinfo.gov
http://www.disabilityinfo.gov

This site is a collaborative effort amongst 22 government agencies developed to provide individuals with disabilities a central resource for information related to living with a disability.

National Center for Injury Prevention and Control (NCIPC)
http://www.cdc.gov/ncipc

The Center for Disease Control (CDC) maintains the NCIPC, which has a very informative Web site. Within this site is a listing of injury-related Internet sites, some of which are specifically directed towards SCI.

National Institutes of Health
http://www.nih.gov

This is the major health-related U.S. government institute. Its focus is on health-related issues and scientific research. A part of the institute, the National Library of Medicine (http://www.nlm.nih.gov), is designed to dispense health information to the professional and to the consumer. Its consumer-related site is located at http://www.nlm.nih.gov/medlineplus.

Spinal Cord Injury Information Network, University of Alabama
http://www.spinalcord.uab.edu

This site is part of the University of Alabama's participation in the federally sponsored SCI model systems program. Site provides a large variety of up-to-date information and resources. Main section includes frequently asked questions, breaking news, and feedback. User can link into a chat room about SCI. Associated with the site is the National Spinal Cord Injury Statistical Center, which has the world's largest database on SCI.

Private

Disability Resources Page
http:// www.makoa.org

Web site hosted by Jim Lubin contains many references to sites with pertinent information. Spinal Cord Injury sites are a small portion of all that is available on this site. Information ranges from private education organizations to research institutes (private and government) and equipment manufacturers. Site has been maintained and kept current since 1994.

Spinal Cord Injury Resource Center
http://www.spinalinjury.net

Site has basic information relative to the anatomy, physiology, and complications associated with SCI. Research updates and tips on finding rehabilitation centers and recommended readings are also found.

ADAPTIVE TECHNOLOGY RESOURCES

Assistive Technology

Assistive technology is the use of assistive devices and technology to enhance the quality of life and provide access to home, work, and community. The following references provide a broad spectrum of contacts, equipment manufacturers, and general information about assistive technology and disabilities.

Abledata
http://www.abledata.com

Provides information on thousands of assistive technology products. Consumers can browse by name, manufacturer, or group.

Alliance for Technology Access
http://www.ataccess.org

National nonprofit organization that can provide information on assistive technology. Associated with 40 centers nationwide, which allow the user to try out software and hardware and other resources.

Closing the Gap
http://www.closingthegap.com

Great resource listing up-to-date products and software including descriptions, uses, and prices. A bimonthly newspaper and international conference listing are also provided.

Rehabilitation Engineering and Assistive Technology Society of North America (RESNA)
http://www.resna.org

An organization based in Arlington, Virginia, that is geared toward professionals with an interest in assistive technology and disabilities. Their stated purpose is "to improve the potential of people with disabilities to achieve their goals through the use of technology." The organization provides information about assistance programs that facilitate access to various private and governmental programs focusing on the use of technology to improve the daily lives of individuals with disabilities.

The American Occupational Therapy Association
http://www.aota.org

Web site providing a variety of information about occupational therapy, and the information located in the technology special interest section is excellent.

WHEELCHAIRS AND SEATING SYSTEMS

One of the most important decisions that an individual will make after SCI is about the purchase of a wheelchair. With technology changing rapidly, it is essential to be informed on the latest design and development. If an individual has limited resources available for purchasing a wheelchair, a phone-order distributor can be cost effective. These companies can be found in the wheelchair magazines.

Books on Wheelchairs

A Guide to Wheelchair Selection: How to Use the ANSI/ RESNA Wheelchair Standards to Buy a Wheelchair
Available from the Paralyzed Veterans of America (PVA).

This book was written to explain how ANSI/RESNA standards are helpful in prescribing and selecting the right wheelchair.

The Manual Wheelchair Training Guide by Peter Axelson and Company

PAX Press
P.O. Box 8317
Santa Cruz, CA 95060–8317

This book was written for manual wheelchair users and anyone who trains or assists this population. Has instructional text and helpful hints. Lots of illustrations.

Internet-Based Wheelchair Resources

Rehab Central
http://www.rehabcentral.com

This site's emphasis is on seating and positioning. Interactive evaluation form and recommendations provided. Provides resources for rehabilitation products and assistive devices.

Informed Consumer's Guide to Wheelchair Selection
http://www.abledata.com/abledata_docs/icg_whel.htm

Descriptive Web site on general types of wheelchair mobility. Has lots of useful information and allows the user to print out fact sheets.

The Wheelchair Manual
http://www.thewheelchairguide.com

Comprehensive Web site describing all U.S.A.-made wheelchairs plus some imported wheelchairs. Has information on manual, power, and sports wheelchairs.

Seating Systems

Seating and positioning systems are of major import when designing the optimal mobility platform for individuals with disabilities. Not only must they provide a stable and comfortable position, seating systems must also accommodate a wide variety of orthopedic anomalies. The ability of the cushion/seating system must also function to prevent skin damage under a variety of conditions. All of these considerations make prescribing seating systems an important and non-trivial task. There are many manufacturers of cushions and seating systems around the world providing excellent products.

The online community Web site entitled "WheelchairNet," based at the University of Pittsburgh and funded by the U.S. Department of Education, has done an excellent job of identifying many of the reputable manufacturers as part of their approach to providing information to the wheelchair-using community at large. These resources are an excellent place to start. http://www.wheelchairnet.org/index.html

TELEPHONE ADAPTATIONS

The use of a telephone is essential in today's culture. It provides a link to the outside world, but also is a critical safety device. The main problems encountered involve the manipulation of the telephone. Regional phone companies may provide some free services, including phone overlays and free dialing. The consumer should explore these services. Modifications can be made to phones, including large push button adapters. These can be accessed by a universal cuff or a mouthstick. Sip and puff dialing can also be installed. Headsets and speaker phones can be used. A preliminary listing of accessible telephone manufacturers can be found on the Disability Resources page maintained by Jim Lubin (see above) at http://www.makoa.org/ecu.htm.

ENVIRONMENTAL CONTROL UNITS (ECUs)

These devices are designed to interface the person to the environment. They were traditionally used by people with severe disabilities but recent trends have made them popular with the general public.

ECUs can provide a safe environment and access to home controls such as lights, television, VCRs, stereos, thermostats, doors, and kitchen equipment. The types of control are activated by household wiring, infrared, radio frequency, ultrasound, or computer. An excellent resource listing can be found on the Disability Resources Page maintained by Jim Lubin (see above) at http://www.makoa.org/ecu.htm.

HOME MODIFICATIONS

Universal design concepts are a relatively new idea. This concept uses the philosophy that homes should be built without environmental barriers. If new homes are built, the necessary modifications should include an assessment of computer and technology needs.

The Center for Universal Design at North Carolina State University
http://www.design.ncsu.edu/cud/

The Center for Universal Design (CUD) is a national information, technical assistance, and research center that evaluates, develops, and promotes accessible and universal design in housing, commercial and public facilities, outdoor environments, and products.

Another avenue for accessible housing is to explore the idea of accessible modular homes and recreational vehicles. For more information see:

Cardinal Homes
http://www.cardinalhomes.com/

A commercial builder of modular homes that incorporates accessibility features into its designs for the disabled community.

Hygienicare
http://www.hygienicare.com/

Commercial company that dedicates much of their site to information regarding accessibility. Builders of wheelchair-accessible mobile homes/recreational vehicles.

Paralyzed Veterans of America (PVA)
http://www.pva.org

A variety of information is available through the PVA Web site relevant to making modifications to older homes.

Miscellaneous Resources
Many other Web sites with a focus on accessibility can be found by searching the internet using such key words as ramps, stairglides, and elevators.

AUTOMOBILE ADAPTATIONS

The decision on what type of vehicle to purchase and what modifications it will need is a major expenditure and should be thoroughly researched. For users who load their wheelchairs, the options are extensive. Traditionally, two-door vehicles were recommended, but today any automatic vehicle is an option. The consumer who prefers to have a van and lift has fewer options available. Things to consider when evaluating a vehicle include:

- Tilt steering wheel
- Rear window defroster and windshield wipers
- Power windows
- Power seat adjustment
- Power mirrors
- Where the wheelchair will be placed (front or back seat)
- Ease of access to control panel
- Power brakes
- Power steering
- Type of wheelchair lifts
- Height of vehicle
- Ease of handcontrol installation
- Steering wheel modifications
- Tie down systems

Daimler-Chrysler, Ford, and General Motors offer a rebate program for disabled consumers purchasing a new automobile. Information can be obtained on their Web sites.

Hand controls or aftermarket modifications allow individuals without control of the lower extremities the ability to properly use the acceleration and braking mechanism of a vehicle. These can be portable or stationary. Most major cities have a number of businesses specializing in automobile adaptation. A partial list of manufacturers with links can be found at WheelchairNet (http://www.wheelchairnet.org) in their products and services section.

Consultation with experts in assistive technology and its application may facilitate helping the patient. One such professional group located in Denver, Colorado, and accessible on the internet is "Assistive Technology Partners" (http://www.uchsc.edu/atp). An excellent general text on the subject that also contains a long list of resources entitled "Assistive Technology: An interdisciplinary approach" is available from Churchill/Livingstone publishing (New York).

ORGANIZATIONS WHOSE GOAL IS TO PROVIDE SUPPORT AND EDUCATION FOR SCI INDIVIDUALS AND/OR FUND SCI-DIRECTED RESEARCH

American Paraplegia Society
7520 Astoria Blvd.
Jackson Heights, NY 11370
Phone: (718) 803–3782
Fax: (718) 803–0414
E-mail: aps@epva.org
Web address: http://www.apssci.org

American Society for Neural Transplantation and Repair (ASNTR)
Donna C. Morrison

Department of Neurosurgery MDC-78
Center for Aging and Brain Repair
University of South Florida COM
12901 Bruce B Downs Blvd
Tampa FL 33612–4799
Phone: (813) 974–3154
Fax: (813) 974–3078
Email: dmorriso@hsc.usf.edu
Web address: http://www.asntr.org

Christopher Reeve Paralysis Foundation (CRPF)
500 Morris Avenue
Springfield, NJ 07081
Phone: (800) 225–0292/ (973) 379–2960
Fax: (973) 912–9433
E-mail: Send messages from within their Web site.
Web address: http://www.crpf.org

National Neurotrauma Society
c/o Linda Garcia
PO Box 143060
Gainesville, FL 32614 USA
Phone: (352) 271–1169
Fax: (352) 271–3060
E-mail: LindaHou@aol.com
Web address: http://www.edc.gsph.pitt.edu/neurotrauma

National Spinal Cord Injury Association
8701 Georgia Avenue, Suite 500
Silver Spring, MD 20910
Phone (301) 588–6959
Fax (301) 588–9414
Help Line (800) 962–9629
E-mail: info@spinalcord.org
Web address: http://www.spinalcord.org

Paralyzed Veterans of America

Spinal Cord Research Foundation (SCRF)
801 Eighteenth Street, NW
Washington, DC 20006–3517
Phone: (202) 416–7659/ (800) 424–8200 ext. 659
TTY: (202) 416–7622
Fax: (202) 416–7641
E-mail: scrf@pva.org
Web address: http://www.pva.org/scrf

The SCRF is a branch of the PVA whose function is to support research directed at SCI. Education is also a major focus.

The Miami Project to Cure Paralysis
PO Box 016960 (R48)
Miami, FL 33101–6960
Phone: (305) 243–6001/ (800) STAND_UP
Fax: (305) 243–6017
E-mail: mpinfo@miamiproject.med.miami.edu
Web address: http://www.miamiproject.miami.edu

The Miami Project to Cure Paralysis is a Center of Excellence at the University of Miami School of Medicine focused on research toward a cure for paralysis resulting from SCI.

Index

Note: Page numbers followed by *f* indicate a figure; those followed by *t* indicate a table.